VOLUME 1

Kirklin/Barratt-Boyes

Cardiac Surgery

Morphology, Diagnostic Criteria, Natural History, Techniques, Results, and Indications

THIRD EDITION

Nicholas T. Kouchoukos, M.D.
Attending Surgeon, Division of Cardiovascular and Thoracic Surgery
Missouri Baptist Medical Center
St. Louis, Missouri
Formerly, John W. Kirklin Professor of Surgery
Division of Cardiothoracic Surgery, Department of Surgery
University of Alabama at Birmingham, School of Medicine and Medical Center
Birmingham, Alabama

Eugene H. Blackstone, M.D.
Head, Clinical Research Department of
Thoracic and Cardiovascular Surgery
Staff, Department of Biostatistics and Epidemiology
The Cleveland Clinic Foundation
Cleveland, Ohio
Professor of Surgery, University of Toronto
Toronto, Ontario, Canada
Formerly, University of Alabama at Birmingham
Cardiovascular Surgical Research Professor
Birmingham, Alabama

Donald B. Doty, M.D.
Attending Surgeon
Department of Cardiovascular Medicine and Surgery
LDS Hospital
Clinical Professor, Department of Surgery, University of Utah
Salt Lake City, Utah
Formerly, Fellow in Thoracic Surgery
University of Alabama at Birmingham
Birmingham, Alabama

Frank L. Hanley, M.D.
Professor of Surgery
Director, Pediatric Heart Center
Stanford University Medical Center
Stanford, California

Robert B. Karp, M.D.
Formerly, Professor of Surgery
Chief of Cardiac Surgery
University of Chicago
Chicago, Illinois
Formerly, Professor of Surgery
Department of Surgery
University of Alabama at Birmingham
School of Medicine and Medical Center
Birmingham, Alabama

Illustrations by **Jill A. Rhead, M.A.**
Salt Lake City, Utah

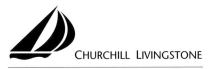

CHURCHILL LIVINGSTONE
An Imprint of Elsevier Science

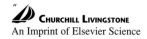

Churchill Livingstone
An Imprint of Elsevier Science

The Curtis Center
Independence Square West
Philadelphia, Pennsylvania 19106

NOTICE

Medicine is an ever-changing field. Standard safety precautions must be followed, but as new research and clinical experience broaden our knowledge, changes in treatment and drug therapy may become necessary or appropriate. Readers are advised to check the most current product information provided by the manufacturer of each drug to be administered to verify the recommended dose, the method and duration of administration, and contraindications. It is the responsibility of the licensed prescriber, relying on experience and knowledge of the patient, to determine dosages and the best treatment for each individual patient. Neither the publisher nor the authors assume any liability for any injury and/or damage to persons or property arising from this publication.

Previous editions copyrighted 1986, 1993

Library of Congress Cataloging-in-Publication Data
Kirklin/Barratt-Boyes cardiac surgery : morphology, diagnostic criteria, natural history, techniques, results, and indications / Nicholas T. Kouchoukos ... [et al.] ; illustrations by Jill A. Rhead.—3rd ed.
    p. ; cm.
    Includes bibliographical references and index.
    ISBN 0-443-07526-3
    1. Heart—Surgery.   I. Title: Cardiac surgery.   II. Kirklin, John W. (John Webster). cardiac surgery.   III. Kouchoukos, Nicholas T.
    [DNLM: 1. Cardiac Surgical Procedures—methods.   2. Cardiovascular Diseases—surgery. WG 169 K585 2003]
RD598.K547 2003
617.4'12059—dc21   2003050148

Acquisitions Editor: Richard H. Lampert
Senior Developmental Editor: Ellen Baker Geisel
Publishing Services Manager: Patricia Tannian
Senior Project Manager: Anne Altepeter
Book Design Manager: Gail Morey Hudson
Cover Design and Illustrations: Jill A. Rhead

Printed in the United States of America

Last digit is the print number: 9 8 7 6 5 4 3 2 1

Kirklin/Barratt-Boyes

Cardiac Surgery

Morphology, Diagnostic Criteria, Natural History, Techniques, Results, and Indications

THIRD EDITION

Acknowledgments

The authors gratefully acknowledge the assistance of the following individuals and organizations whose contributions made publication of this textbook possible:

St. Louis, Missouri: Suzan Murphy, R.N.; Judith F. Kunkel
The Missouri Baptist Health Care Foundation.

Cleveland, Ohio: Tess Knerik; Janet Blackstone, M.S.; Luci Mitchin
The Cleveland Clinic Foundation

Salt Lake City, Utah: Barbara H. Hafen, Jill A. Rhead, M.A.

Stanford, California: Daria P. Graham, Sam Suleman, Norman Silverman, M.D.

Chicago, Illinois: Maria Siambekos; Kathy Prazuch; Peter Koenig, M.D.;
Roberto Lange, M.D.

Elsevier Science
St. Louis, Missouri: Ellen Baker Geisel, Anne Altepeter, Kristen Mandava

Preface to Third Edition

The decision to prepare the third edition of *Cardiac Surgery* was made with considerable trepidation by the five new authors. Updating and expanding the content of the highly successful second edition, which was written almost entirely by John Kirklin and Sir Brian Barratt-Boyes, provided us with a formidable and stimulating challenge. What is lost in this new edition is the intense personal involvement of these two pioneers of cardiac surgery, for whom portions of each chapter's "Historical Note" were at one time their future, then their present, and now their past.

Except for Frank Hanley, all of us received our cardiothoracic surgical education at the University of Alabama Medical Center under the tutelage of John Kirklin, and we were fortunate to serve as faculty members in the Department of Surgery at the University of Alabama at Birmingham School of Medicine during the period that he served as Chair of the Department and Director of the Division of Cardiothoracic Surgery. We have all, including Dr. Hanley, been profoundly influenced by his teachings, intellect, and vision, and by his commitment to improving the quality of cardiac surgery by rigorous clinical and laboratory investigations, superb clinical care, and disciplined training of young surgeons. Although our interactions with Sir Brian Barratt-Boyes have been less frequent and less intense, he exemplifies these same attributes, and he has been an inspiration to us as well. The systematic approach to cardiac surgery that these two pioneering surgeons developed and promulgated has been a major fixture in our professional careers. The decision to author the third edition was, in large part, influenced by our desire to perpetuate their philosophic approach to cardiac surgery. Thus, the general format of the first and second editions has been maintained.

All chapters present in the second edition have been substantially revised. Each chapter was rewritten with input from at least two of the five authors. All five authors participated in revising Chapters 1, 2, 3, 5, and 7. Chapter 4 (Anesthesia for Cardiovascular Surgery) was revised by Dr. J.G. Reves, our former colleague at the University of Alabama at Birmingham, who is now Vice President for Medical Affairs at the Medical College of South Carolina, and his former colleagues from Duke University, Dr. Hilary P. Grocott and Dr. Frank Stem. The content, and in some instances the title, of several of the chapters relating to treatment of congenital heart disease and thoracic aortic disease have been altered to reflect current knowledge and practice. New chapters have been added on managing endocarditis, diseases of pulmonary arteries, and diseases of systemic veins. Echocardiographic, computed tomographic, and magnetic resonance images have been added to many of the chapters. They reflect important advances in the diagnosis of congenital and acquired diseases of the heart and great vessels.

In his foreword to the first edition, the late Dr. Dwight McGoon wrote:

Whether a text is more valuable if each of its various chapters is written by a highly selected authority on the subject, or more valuable if written entirely by one or a handful of authors, with consequent advantages of consistency of style and integration of presentation is debatable. . . . The question is especially irrelevant with respect to this book since, though it has only two authors, each chapter reflects their combined outstanding authority on that subject. Thus this text retains the advantages of both approaches. One wonders if this phenomenon can ever again be possible.

We recognized the potential dangers of five authors writing separate portions of this edition: (1) loss of uniformity in style, expression, and nomenclature; (2) redundancy; (3) loss of precision and organization of material within each chapter; and (4) failure to cross-reference other chapters that amplify general concepts and management of patients (Chapters 1 to 6) or chapters written by different authors. In part, this challenge was met by at least dual authorship of each chapter and by a number of author meetings. In part it was also met by a process of universal review. Specifically, Dr. Blackstone was designated as the final arbiter because he had worked intensely with Dr. Kirklin in the production of both the first and second editions. After review of each edited chapter by the primary author, copy-edited material was forwarded to Cleveland, where Dr. Blackstone and his editorial assistant, Tess Knerik, edited, revised, reorganized, questioned, and adjudicated the entire content of each chapter. Subsequently, they reviewed all page proofs after they were returned by the primary author. Our hope was that this intensive process not only would answer Dr. McGoon's implied question—"One wonders if this phenomenon can ever again be possible in terms of achieving precision?"—but also would improve the book's accuracy and comprehensiveness.

As in the previous two editions, Part I discusses basic concepts of cardiac surgery: anatomy, support techniques, myocardial management, anesthesia, postoperative care, and methodology for generating new knowledge from previous experience. These core chapters are applicable to the broad audience of medical professionals who care for patients with cardiac disease. The remaining chapters (Parts II to VI) discuss specific acquired and congenital diseases of the heart and great vessels. This edition has retained, in these later sections, presentation of "Indications for Operation" at the end of each chapter, because the indications are the derivatives of comparisons of various outcomes (results) of alternative forms of treatment, including no treatment (natural history). All illustrations of surgical procedures from the second edition have been redrawn, and many new illustrations have been added. We are deeply indebted to the artist, Jill Rhead, M.A. She worked closely with Dr. Doty, who reviewed all of these illustrations for accuracy and consistency. The drawings of surgical procedures are, with few exceptions, oriented as the operative field is seen from the position of the surgeon. In the case of open cardiac operations, this is from the patient's right side.

The abbreviation *UAB* has been retained, and is used to identify data and illustrations from the University of Alabama at Birmingham; similarly, *GLH* identifies those from Green Lane Hospital in Auckland, New Zealand. The bibliographic references are again designated using the first letter of the surname of the first author and a number (such as L4), rather than simply a number. This convention is simple and convenient, and allows the reader to easily locate a given author's publication among the alphabetically arranged references. New references for the third edition within each alphabetic subheading either replaced references from the second edition or were added at the end of the list. The abbreviation *CL* is used throughout to denote 70% confidence limits around the point estimate. The reasons for presenting 70% rather than 95% or 50% confidence limits are presented in Chapter 6.

The second edition looked toward cardiac surgery and health care in general becoming more regulated, making the evidence-based approach to indications for operative intervention even more important. The third edition is written at a time of great change for the specialty of cardiac surgery. Percutaneous catheter–based interventions are being used increasingly to treat patients with coronary atherosclerotic heart disease, hypertrophic obstructive cardiomyopathy, diseases of the thoracic aorta, and congenital cardiac lesions such as patent ductus arteriosus, coarctation of the aorta, atrial septal defect, and pulmonary stenosis. Implantable cardioverter–defibrillator devices have largely replaced operative procedures for ventricular arrhythmias. This edition is written under the assumption that these advances must not only be acknowledged but also embraced. Improvement of current surgical procedures and development of new techniques to treat those conditions not yet amenable to percutaneous intervention are essential if cardiac surgery is to thrive in the future.

It is our hope that this book will be of value to cardiac surgeons who care for patients with congenital and acquired heart disease and with disorders of the major vessels in the chest, as well as to cardiologists and interventional cardiologists who treat children and adults with these conditions, anesthesiologists, intensivists, pulmonologists, imaging experts, trainees in all of these specialties, cardiovascular nurses, and others.

Nicholas T. Kouchoukos, M.D.
Eugene H. Blackstone, M.D.
Donald B. Doty, M.D.
Frank L. Hanley, M.D.
Robert B. Karp, M.D.

Contents

I General Considerations

1 Anatomy, Dimensions, and Terminology

This chapter describes normal cardiac and great artery anatomy and dimensions, as well as the terminology usually employed.

CARDIAC CHAMBERS AND MAJOR VESSELS

Accurate diagnosis of congenital heart defects depends in part on identification of cardiac chambers and major vessels by their morphology, regardless of their spatial positions (Fig. 1-1).

Right Atrium

The right atrium (Fig. 1-2) is the chamber of the heart that normally receives systemic venous drainage from the inferior and superior venae cavae. It also normally receives the major portion of coronary venous drainage from the coronary sinus. Morphologic characteristics important for identification of the right atrium are the presence of the limbus of the fossa ovalis, which surrounds the valve of the fossa ovalis (septum primum) superiorly, anteriorly, and posteriorly; a wide-based, blunt-ended, right-sided atrial

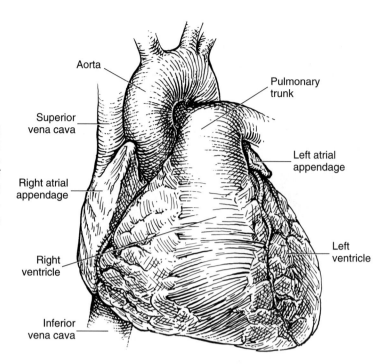

Figure 1-1 Surface anatomy of the heart. The left atrial appendage is long and narrow, whereas the right atrial appendage is short and blunt. The aorta originates posterior and to the right of the pulmonary artery at the base of the heart, but is anterior and to the right by the pericardial reflection. The right ventricle occupies most of the anterior aspect of the heart, with the left ventricle forming the apex and posterior aspects.

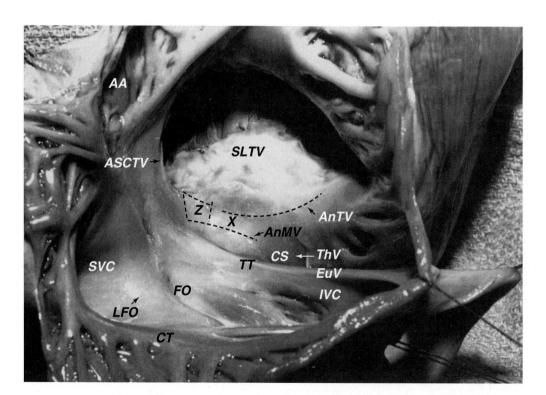

Figure 1-2 Interior of the normal right atrium, viewed from the right side at operation.

Key: *AA,* Atrial appendage; *AnMV,* position of mitral valve anulus on the other side of the septum, indicated by the dotted line; *AnTV,* anulus of tricuspid valve, indicated by the dotted line; *ASCTV,* anteroseptal commissure of tricuspid valve; *CS,* orifice of coronary sinus; *CT,* crista terminalis (the inside of the sulcus terminalis); *EuV,* eustachian valve; *FO,* fossa ovalis, sometimes called the septum primum; *IVC,* orifice of inferior vena cava; *LFO,* limbus of fossa ovalis (this is C-shaped and extends anteriorly and posteriorly to enclose the fossa ovalis); *SLTV,* septal leaflet of tricuspid valve; *SVC,* orifice of superior vena cava; *ThV,* thebesian valve; *TT,* tendon of Todaro; *X,* muscular portion of atrioventricular septum; *Z,* membranous portion of atrioventricular septum.

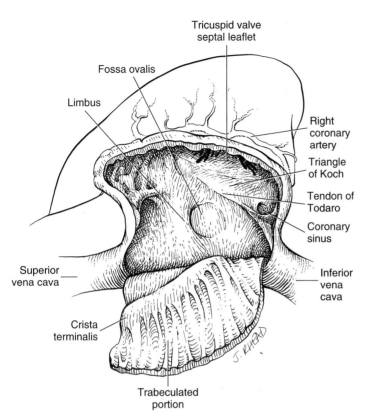

Tricuspid valve
septal leaflet

Fossa ovalis

Limbus

Right
coronary
artery

Triangle
of Koch

Tendon of
Todaro

Coronary
sinus

Superior
vena cava

Inferior
vena
cava

Crista
terminalis

Trabeculated
portion

Figure 1-3 Interior of the right atrium, oriented as at operation. The right atrium receives the superior and inferior venae cavae. The trabeculated portion is separated from the smooth portion by the crista terminalis. The fossa ovalis is located in the center of the atrial septum, surrounded on its superior, anterior, and posterior aspects by the limbus. The coronary sinus is positioned inferiorly. The coronary sinus, along with the tendon of Todaro and the anulus of the septal leaflet of the tricuspid valve, form the boundaries of the triangle of Koch. The atrioventricular node and proximal portions of the bundle of His, portions of the specialized conduction system, lie within the triangle of Koch. The right coronary artery lies in the atrioventricular groove, the anatomic point of separation of the right atrium and right ventricle.

appendage; the eustachian valve at the orifice of the inferior vena cava and the thebesian valve at the orifice of the coronary sinus; and the crista terminalis, which separates the trabeculated from the nontrabeculated portion of the atrium (Fig. 1-3).

The normal structures are sometimes expressed in an excessive or unusual manner. These are not themselves functionally important abnormalities, but they are usually associated with important cardiac malformations. Thus, the eustachian and thebesian valves may be sufficiently prominent so as to appear to divide the right atrium into two parts, a not infrequent finding in tricuspid atresia.[T7] The right atrial appendage may be juxtaposed leftward, and the left atrial appendage is less frequently juxtaposed rightward. Juxtaposition of the atrial appendages is usually associated with important cardiac malformations.[A14]

Clinically, the definitive morphologic features of the right atrium may be difficult to recognize.[B1] Occasionally, the atrial septum is seen well enough in angiographic profile to delineate the limbus of the fossa ovalis, and sometimes the right atrial appendage is outlined sufficiently to differentiate its shape from that of the left atrial appendage. The fact that the hepatic portion of the inferior vena cava usually drains into the right atrium often makes it possible to determine the location of the right atrium by passage of a catheter from the inferior vena cava to the heart.

The atria are not in normal position in some patients; in these cases, the wide-based, blunt-ended right atrial appendage is the most secure indicator that an atrium is morphologically a right atrium. Other indicators of the morphology of the atria, and of atrial situs, include venous drainage and the situs indicated by the pulmonary artery and bronchial anatomy.[P1,S1,V1,V2]

Left Atrium

The left atrium (Fig. 1-4) is the cardiac chamber that normally receives pulmonary venous drainage from the four pulmonary veins. The septal surface of the left atrium is characterized by the flap valve of the fossa ovalis (septum primum), in contrast to the limbus of the fossa ovalis present on the right atrioseptal surface. The left atrial appendage is long and narrow, in contrast to the bluntness of the right atrial appendage, and is the best indicator that the atrium is morphologically a left atrium. There is no crista terminalis at the base of the left atrial appendage, the only trabeculated structure in the left atrium.

In general, at cardiac catheterization, the location of the left atrium is determined by exclusion after identifying the position of the right atrium as described above. With normal pulmonary venous connection, the left atrium may be well opacified after a right ventricular or pulmonary artery injection.

Right Ventricle

The right ventricle has a large sinus portion that surrounds and supports a tricuspid atrioventricular (AV) valve and includes the apex and a smaller *infundibulum,* or outlet portion, which supports a semilunar valve. The inlet and outlet valves of the right ventricle are thus widely sepa-

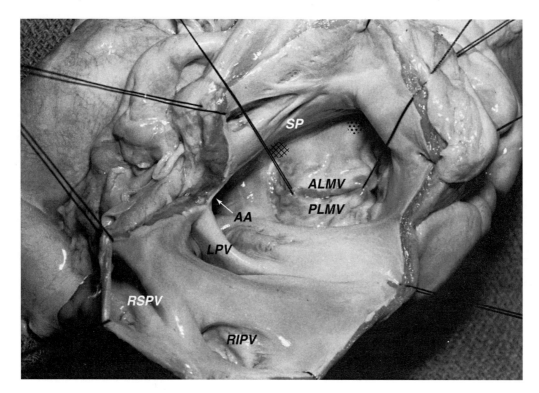

Figure 1-4   Interior of the normal left atrium, viewed from the right side at operation, as, for example, during mitral valve operations. The stippled area indicates the position of the right trigone, which contains the bundle of His. Crosshatching marks the left trigone, the area of greatest risk to the aortic valve during mitral valve replacement.

Key: *AA,* Base of atrial appendage; *ALMV,* anterior leaflet of mitral valve; *LPV,* orifices of left pulmonary veins; *PLMV,* posterior leaflet of mitral valve; *RIPV,* orifice of right inferior pulmonary vein; *RSPV,* orifice of right superior pulmonary vein; *SP,* septum primum.

rated. The entire sinus portion of the right ventricle and most of the infundibulum (both free wall and septum) are coarsely trabeculated.

The septal surface of the right ventricle is divided into an inlet portion, a trabecular portion (sometimes called the apical trabecular portion), and an outlet portion[A7,S12] (Fig. 1-5). Alternatively, the septal surface of the right ventricle may be divided into *posterior* (basal), *middle, apical* (anterior), and *infundibular* (conal) portions (Fig. 1-6). The inlet portion of the ventricular septum surrounds and supports the tricuspid valve.[1] The trabecular portion is that portion with the coarse trabecular pattern typical of the right ventricle (see Fig. 1-6). The outlet portion of the right ventricular aspect of the ventricular septum is smooth but complex and has three components. The largest is the conal (infundibular) septum, which separates the pulmonary from the aortic and tricuspid valves. Only part of the conal septum is interventricular (see Fig. 1-5), and in some

malformations, such as double outlet right ventricle, none of it may be. Thus, it must be emphasized that the most distal cephalad portion of the infundibular septum is not, strictly speaking, part of the ventricular septum, because in the normal heart, the pulmonary valve arises from the apex of a cone of muscle and does not have a septal attachment.[A7,B7] A second part of the outlet portion of the septum is the anterior (superior) extension, or division, of the septal band (or trabecula septomarginalis). A third small, very anterior portion is a narrow extension superior to the trabecular septum.

Laterally to the right, the infundibular (conal) septum imperceptibly merges with the free right ventricular wall immediately beyond its attachment to the membranous septum; at that point, it can be called the *parietal extension* (band) of the infundibular septum (Fig. 1-7).[S14] The parietal band lies anterior to the right aortic sinus (see Fig. 1-7), partially overlying that portion of the free wall of the right ventricle termed the *ventriculoinfundibular fold.* Many surgeons call the infundibular septum and the parietal band the *crista superventricularis.* Medially and to the left, the conal (infundibular) septum merges with the trabecular portion of the septum between the limbs of the particularly prominent, smooth, Y-shaped muscle bundle called the *septal band,* or *trabecula septomarginalis* (TSM)[A1,T1] (Fig. 1-8). The septal band extends apically to become continu-

---

[1] The phrase *inlet septum* is in some ways undesirable because the term has developmental implications,[A5] and the large inlet septum on the right ventricular side is not duplicated on the left side. The use of the term *trabecular* to describe a portion of the sinus septum is also undesirable in some ways, because part of the infundibular septum is also trabeculated (see Fig. 1-5).

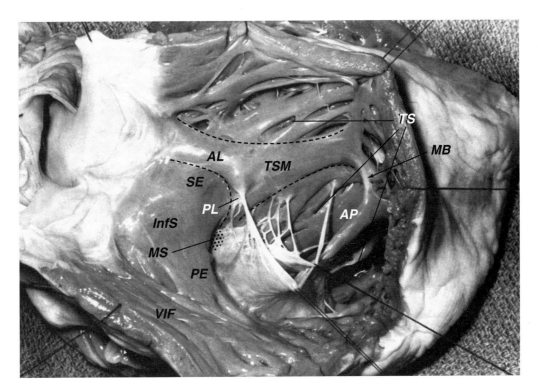

Figure 1-5   Interior of the normal right ventricle, particularly the trabecular and outlet portions, oriented as at operation. The conal or infundibular septum separates the pulmonary from the tricuspid valve, and only its rightward portion and inferior part of its central portion form part of the interventricular septum (see also Fig. 1-6). The entire outlet portion of the septum of the infundibulum is composed of the septal extension of the infundibular septum, the anterior limb of the septal band (trabecula septomarginalis, TSM), and, in front of that, a heavily trabeculated portion of septum.

Key: *AL,* Anterior (superior) limb of TSM; *AP,* anterior papillary muscle; *InfS,* infundibular (conal) septum; *MB,* moderator band; *MS,* position of membranous septum; *PE,* parietal extension of infundibular septum (parietal band); *PL,* posterior limb of TSM, giving origin to the medial papillary muscle; *SE,* septal extension of infundibular septum; *TS,* trabeculated portion of septum, part of which lies in the infundibulum and the remainder in the sinus portion of the ventricle; *TSM,* trabecula septomarginalis (septal band); *VIF,* ventriculoinfundibular fold.

ous with the *moderator band,* a prominent trabeculation running from the septum to the free wall.

The junction between the outlet and sinus (trabecular) portions of the right ventricle is clearly demarcated only along the lower margin of the outlet portion of the septum. The incomplete muscular ridge formed by the outlet septum (here, specifically, the infundibular or conal septum) and the parietal band, together with the septal and moderator bands, forms a natural line of division between the posteroinferior sinus portion and the anterosuperior outlet portion of the ventricle.[V3] It is in this area that ventricular septal defects most commonly occur; the morphology of the area gives the name "junctional," or "conoventricular," to these defects.

The papillary muscle arrangement supporting the three leaflets of the tricuspid valve is different from that of the mitral valve in the left ventricle. In the case of the tricuspid valve, in addition to a single large anterior papillary muscle attached to the anterior free wall that fuses with the moderator band, there are multiple smaller posterior papillary muscles attached partly to the posterior (inferior) free wall and partly to the septum, and a group of small septal papillary muscles. The lowermost of these small septal muscles attaches posterior to the trabecula septomarginalis (septal band) (see Fig. 1-5) and the uppermost, called the medial (conal) papillary muscle (muscle of Lancisi, or muscle of Luschka), to the posterior limb of the septal band (Fig. 1-9).

Left Ventricle

The left ventricle consists of a larger *sinus* portion, which supports a bicuspid (mitral) atrioventricular (AV) valve and includes the apex, and a much smaller *outlet* (outflow) portion beneath a semilunar valve. The inlet and outlet valves of the left ventricle lie juxtaposed within its base, and inflow and outflow portions are separated by the anterior mitral leaflet (Fig. 1-10).

The entire free wall of the left ventricle and apical half to two thirds of the septum are trabeculated (Fig. 1-11; see also Fig. 1-10), but the trabeculations are characteristically fine compared with those in the right ventricle.[B1] The septal surface of the left ventricle may be considered to have a *sinus* portion, most of which is trabeculated, and a smooth *outlet* (outflow) portion (see Fig. 1-11). The part of the

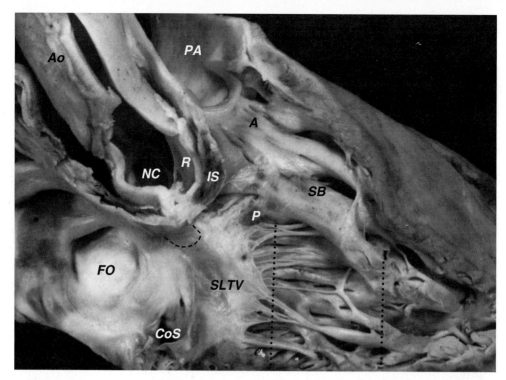

Figure 1-6 Right ventricular side of the septum after the right atrium, right ventricle, and pulmonary artery have been exposed by removing their anterior walls and the rightward portion of aorta and parietal band (or parietal extension of the infundibular septum). The entire right ventricular septum is displayed, together with the relationship of the infundibular septum to the aortic root. In this heart, the infundibular septum is less prominent than in some. The dashed line defines the atrioventricular portion of the membranous septum. The dotted lines define the arbitrary division of the sinus septum into posterior (beneath septal tricuspid leaflet), middle, and apical portions. The specimen corresponds to a right anterior oblique projection in cineangiography.

Key: *A,* Left anterior division septal band; *Ao,* aorta; *CoS,* coronary sinus; *FO,* fossa ovalis; *IS,* cut end of infundibular septum; *NC,* noncoronary aortic sinus; *P,* right posterior division of septal band; *PA,* pulmonary artery; *R,* right coronary aortic sinus; *SB,* septal band (trabecula septomarginalis); *SLTV,* septal tricuspid leaflet.

Figure 1-7 Demonstration of the interrelationships between the right ventricular aspect of the ventricular septum and other structures in a longitudinal coronal section through the heart.

Key: *AA,* Ascending aorta; *LC,* left coronary cusp; *LPC,* left pulmonary cusp; *MPM,* medial papillary muscle; *NC,* noncoronary cusp; *RC,* right coronary cusp; *TSM,* trabecula septomarginalis (septal band); *TV,* tricuspid valve.

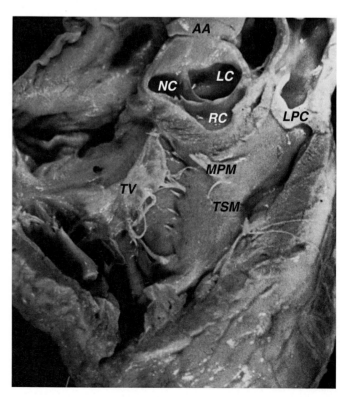

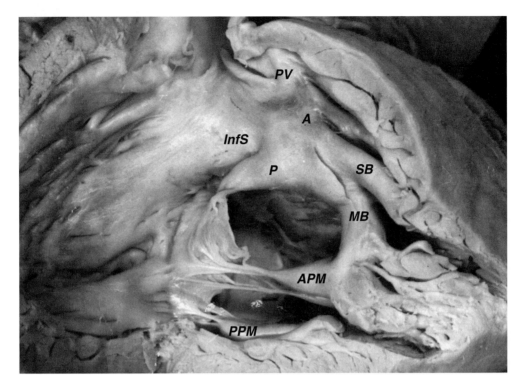

Figure 1-8   Interior of the right ventricle after it has been opened close to the anterior septal margin and along its acute margin inferiorly, and the anterior wall hinged to the right. The specimen is oriented anatomically, with the aorta and pulmonary artery at the top. The pulmonary artery also has been opened. The attachments of the septal band are clearly demonstrated.

Key: *A*, Left anterior division of septal band; *APM*, anterior papillary muscle; *InfS*, infundibular (conal) septum; *MB*, moderator band; *P*, right posterior division of septal band giving origin to the medial papillary muscle; *PPM*, posterior papillary muscle; *PV*, pulmonary valve; *SB*, septal band (trabecula septomarginalis).

sinus portion of the septum immediately beneath the mitral valve may be termed the *inlet septum,* and the rest of the sinus portion the *trabecular septum* (Fig. 1-12). The outlet (outflow) portion lies in front and to the right of the anterior mitral leaflet, corresponding to the inlet portion on the right ventricular side of the septum, and includes the atrioventricular septum (Fig. 1-13). In contrast to the right ventricular side, where the septal tricuspid leaflet is the only valvar attachment to the septum, on the left ventricular side the rightward half of the anterior mitral valve leaflet attaches to the septum posteriorly, and the right and part of the noncoronary aortic cusps attach to it anteriorly (see Fig. 1-12). The leftward half of the anterior mitral leaflet is in fibrous continuity with the aortic valve in an area termed the *aortic–mitral anulus* (Fig. 1-14; see also Figs. 1-12 and 1-13). The anteriorly placed right ventricular infundibular (conal) septum lies opposite the aortic valve (Fig. 1-15). It may occasionally be displaced into the left ventricular outflow beneath the aortic valve; occasionally, muscle may also extend between the aortic and mitral valves, forming a true infundibulum to the left ventricle (see Fig. 1-10). The papillary muscles are called *anterolateral* (or simply *anterior*) and *posteromedial (posterior).* No papillary muscles attach to the left side of the ventricular septum.

Myoarchitecture of the Ventricles

The adult ventricular mass is made up of a three-dimensional network of myocardial cells.[S30] This network is highly structured and arranged in layers in which the myocardial cells have a preferred orientation. In all hearts, the ventricular wall is arranged in three different layers: superficial (subepicardial), middle, and deep (subendocardial). The superficial and deep layers are present in both right and left ventricles, whereas the middle layer is only present in the left ventricle. The superficial and deep layers are anchored at the ventricular orifices to fibrous structures of the central fibrous skeleton of the heart. This suggests that myocardial contraction plays an active role in cardiac valve function. The middle layer, unique to the left ventricle, shows a circumferential pattern. No planes of fibrous septation are present between the three layers. Instead, the distinction between one layer and the next is made by a change in direction of the muscle fibers. This is particularly evident in the ventricular septum, where the superficial layer of the right ventricle invaginates at the interventricular sulcus to form a thin muscular layer that forms the right side of the ventricular septum, covering the circumferentially arranged muscle fibers of the middle layer of the left ventricle. There are age-related changes in the direction of

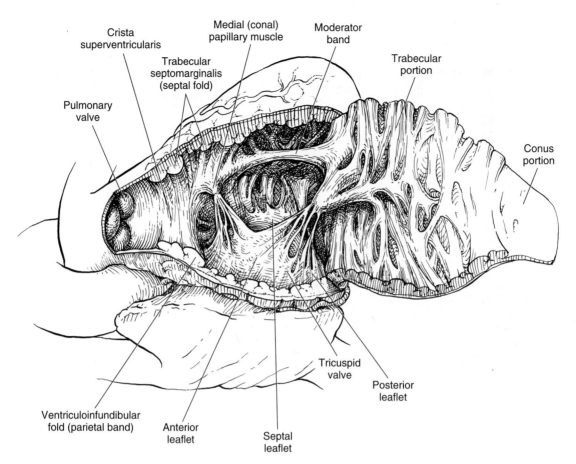

Figure 1-9   Interior of the right ventricle, oriented as at operation. The right ventricle is divided into three portions: inlet, containing the tricuspid valve and surrounding ventricular septum; sinus, or coarse trabecular portion; and outlet, or conus portion, containing the infundibular septum and pulmonary valve. The right lateral extension of the infundibular septum merges with the right ventricle as the ventriculoinfundibular fold (parietal band). Medially and to the left, the infundibular septum merges with the right ventricle to form the Y-shaped muscle bundle called the *trabecular septomarginalis* (septal band). The septal band extends to the apex as the moderator band. An important landmark is the medial (conal) papillary muscle of the tricuspid valve.

Figure 1-10   Interior of the left ventricle after anterior ventricular and aortic walls have been excised, leaving the obtuse margin, posterior free wall, and septum intact. The specimen is oriented anatomically. The posterior (mural) leaflet of the mitral valve lies against the posterior free wall, whereas the anterior mitral leaflet hinges in part from the fibrous subaortic curtain and in part from the septum and separates the outflow portion of the ventricle from the remaining sinus portion. The arrow indicates left ventricular outflow. Papillary muscles and chordae tendineae support the mitral valve.

Key: *APM*, Anterior papillary muscle; *ALMV*, anterior leaflet of mitral valve; *P*, posterior free wall; *PLMV*, posterior leaflet of mitral valve; *PPM*, posterior papillary muscle; *S*, septal surface.

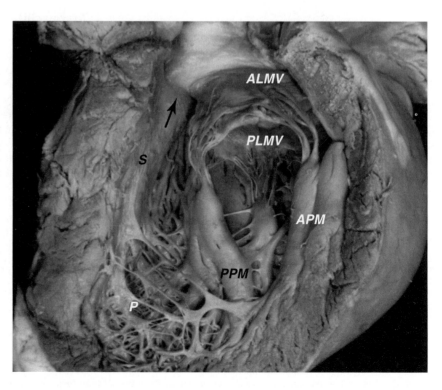

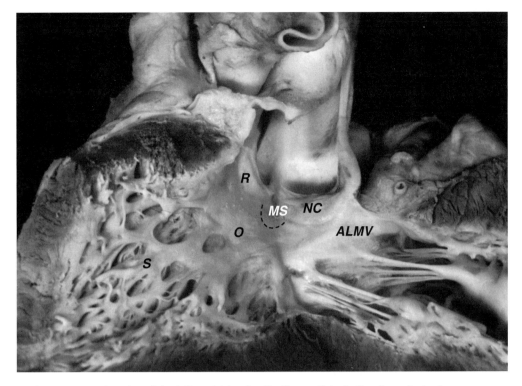

Figure 1-11 Interior of the left ventricle after the free wall, including the mitral valve apparatus, has been displaced to the observer's right and away from the septal surface by a fish-mouth incision into the left ventricle and aorta to demonstrate the sinus and outlet portions of the septum.

Key: *ALMV*, Anterior leaflet of mitral valve; *MS*, membranous septum; *NC*, noncoronary aortic cusp; *O*, outlet septum; *R*, right coronary aortic leaflet; *S*, sinus septum.

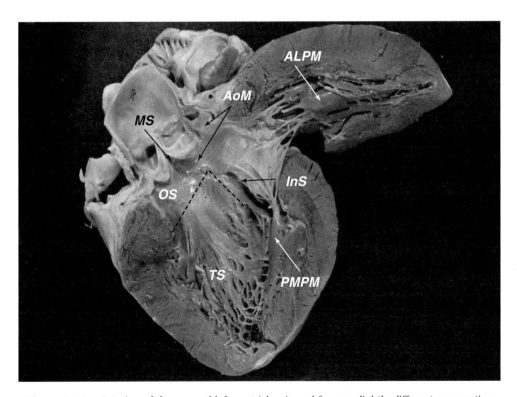

Figure 1-12 Interior of the normal left ventricle, viewed from a slightly different perspective than that of Fig. 1-11 to demonstrate inlet, outlet, trabecular, and membranous portions of the septum.

Key: *ALPM*, Anterolateral papillary muscle; *AoM*, aortic-mitral anulus (continuity); *InS*, inlet septum; *MS*, membranous septum; *OS*, outlet septum; *PMPM*, posteromedial papillary muscle; *TS*, trabecular septum.

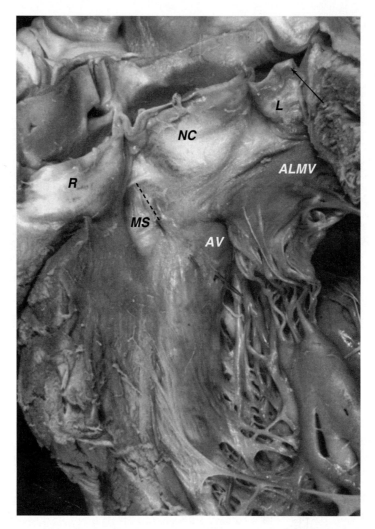

Figure 1-13   Ventricular septum from its left ventricular side, displaying the relationship between the outflow portion and the aortic and mitral valves. Pins protrude along the line of attachment of the tricuspid septal leaflet to the right ventricular side of the septum. Septal tissue inferior to this and the dashed line correspond to the right ventricular inflow, and septal tissue superior to it corresponds to the atrioventricular septum. The arrow indicates a nodulus Aranti. (In this specimen, also shown in Fig. 1-11, the right coronary artery ostium is located eccentrically near the R–NC commissure.)

Key: *ALMV,* Anterior leaflet of mitral valve; *AV,* atrioventricular septum (muscular portion); *L,* left aortic cusp; *MS,* membranous septum, with the atrioventricular portion superior to the dashed line and the interventricular portion inferior to it; *NC,* noncoronary aortic cusp; *R,* right aortic cusp.

the muscle fibers in the superficial layer. With advancing fetal and infant age, muscle fiber arrangement progresses from a horizontal to an oblique orientation.[S21] This change is especially evident in the right ventricle and probably reflects the changing pressure gradient between right and left ventricles.

The anatomy of the muscular subpulmonary infundibulum was studied by Merrick and colleagues.[M8] They point out that there is a free-standing sleeve of myocardium supporting the pulmonary valve that is separate from the underlying anatomic ventricular septum. This may be identified by changing directions of myocardial muscle fibers,

referred to by surgeons as "layers" of the septum. This anatomic feature makes possible the safe separation of the pulmonary trunk from the right ventricular outflow tract for use as a valve substitute (autograft).

Great Arteries

The *aorta* is the great artery arising from the base of the heart that normally gives rise to the systemic and coronary arteries. The identity of the aorta is established by recognizing it as the vessel of origin of the brachiocephalic arteries, which never arise from the pulmonary artery. It is not so

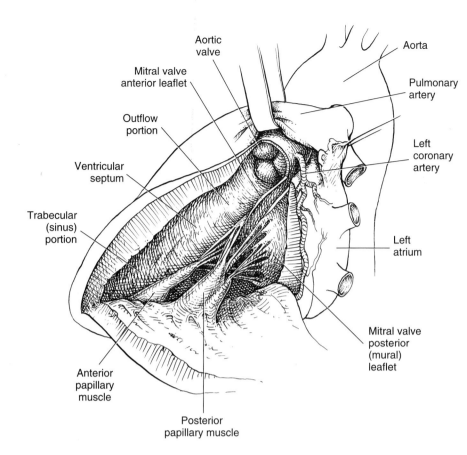

Figure 1-14   Interior of left ventricle, lateral view. The trabecular and outflow portions of the ventricular septum are demonstrated. The inflow portion is beneath and behind the mitral valve. The anterior leaflet of the mitral valve is in fibrous continuity with the aortic valve. The passageway below the aortic valve, bounded by the outflow portion of the ventricular septum and the anterior leaflet of the mitral valve, is called the *left ventricular outflow tract*. The mitral valve is supported by two papillary muscles, anterior and posterior, arising from the free wall of the left ventricle.

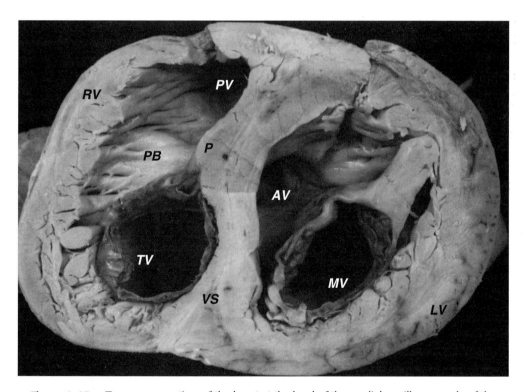

Figure 1-15   Transverse section of the heart at the level of the medial papillary muscle of the tricuspid valve, showing the curvature of the septum that results in the right ventricular infundibulum lying superior and anterior to the aortic valve. Curvature of papillary muscles of the mitral valve is also shown. (Specimen is from a 9-month-old patient with a patent ductus arteriosus and pulmonary hypertension.)

Key: *AV,* Aortic valve; *LV,* left ventricle; *MV,* mitral valve; *P,* posterior division of the septal band and medial papillary muscle; *PB,* parietal band (parietal extension of infundibular septum); *PV,* pulmonary valve; *RV,* right ventricle; *TV,* tricuspid valve; *VS,* ventricular septum.

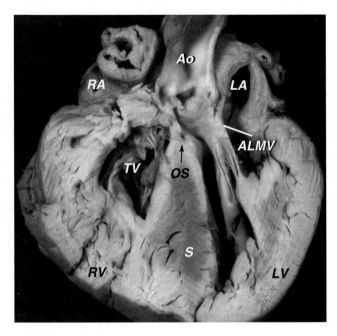

Figure 1-16   Oblique section of a heart from which the superior portion of both ventricles has been removed, including the entire right ventricular infundibulum and pulmonary artery and front half of the aorta. The sharp rightward angulation of the outflow portion of the left ventricular septum is well seen, as is the manner in which the anterior leaflet of the mitral valve contributes one boundary to the left ventricular outflow.

Key: *ALMV,* Anterior leaflet of mitral valve; *Ao,* aorta; *LA,* left atrium; *LV,* left ventricle; *OS,* left ventricular outflow septum; *RA,* right atrium; *RV,* right ventricle; *S,* septum; *TV,* tricuspid valve.

definitively the vessel of origin of the coronary arteries, as occasionally one, or rarely both, coronary arteries may arise from the pulmonary artery.[O1]

The *pulmonary trunk* (main pulmonary artery) is the great artery that normally gives rise to the pulmonary arterial system. As noted above, the main pulmonary trunk characteristically has no brachiocephalic vessels arising from it. At angiography, the differentiation between pulmonary trunk and aorta may require careful study, as the brachiocephalic vessels may opacify with the pulmonary trunk by filling through a patent ductus arteriosus. The pulmonary valve is normally anterior, and the aortic valve posterior and to the right in individuals with visceral and atrial situs solitus.

ATRIAL SEPTUM

See "Right Atrium" and "Left Atrium."

VENTRICULAR SEPTUM

The right and left ventricular septal surfaces are asymmetric, related mainly to the presence of an infundibulum in the right ventricle only. In addition, the higher pressure in the left ventricle makes the sinus septal surface concave on the left side and convex on the right (see Fig. 1-15), a feature that is accentuated during ventricular systole. The axes of the right and left ventricular outflow tracts differ. That of the right ventricle is almost vertically oriented, whereas that of the left ventricle angles sharply to the right (Fig. 1-16), a feature profiled cineangiographically in the left anterior oblique (LAO) view and in the parasternal long axis view by two-dimensional echocardiography.[B1,B2]

Muscular Septum

See "Right Ventricle" and "Left Ventricle."

Membranous Septum

The membranous septum (pars membranacea) is the fibrous part of the cardiac septum separating the left ventricular outflow tract from, in part, the right ventricle and, in part, the right atrium. The line of division between these components is determined by the attachment of the tricuspid valve anulus to the septum (see Fig. 1-12). On the right ventricular side of this attachment is the *interventricular component,* whereas on the right atrial side it forms the membranous portion of the atrioventricular septum.

Atrioventricular Septum

The atrioventricular septum is the portion of the cardiac septum that lies between the right atrium and the left ventricle. It consists of a superior membranous portion and an inferior muscular portion. The atrioventricular septum is apparent because the septal attachment of the tricuspid valve is more apical than the septal attachment of the anterior leaflet of the mitral valve (Fig. 1-17). Viewed from the left ventricular side, the muscular component forms part of the outlet septum (see Fig. 1-13). The AV node lies in the atrial septum adjacent to the junction between the membranous and muscular portions of the atrioventricular septum, and the bundle of His passes toward the right trigone between these two components (Fig. 1-18).

CONDUCTION SYSTEM

The following description is based on studies of hearts without congenital defects.[B6] Abnormalities of the conduction system are associated with certain congenital cardiac malformations and are determined primarily by the alignment between atrial and ventricular septal structures and the pattern of ventricular architecture[A8,A10] (see Chapters 41 and 42).

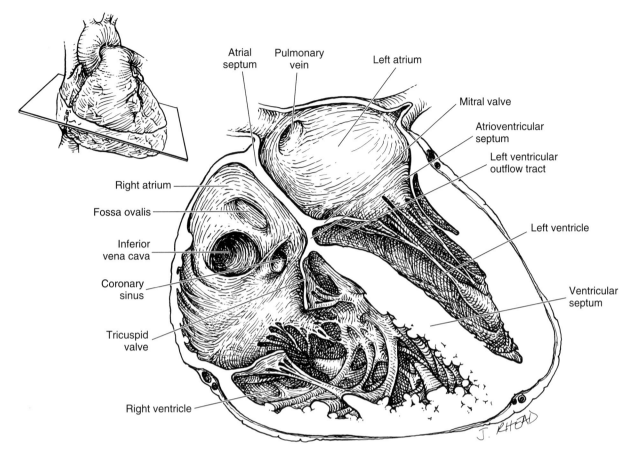

Atrial septum

Pulmonary vein

Left atrium

Mitral valve

Atrioventricular septum

Left ventricular outflow tract

Right atrium

Fossa ovalis

Inferior vena cava

Coronary sinus

Tricuspid valve

Right ventricle

Left ventricle

Ventricular septum

Figure 1-17 Cardiac septation. The atrioventricular septum lies between the left ventricle and right atrium. The septal attachment of the tricuspid valve is more toward the apex of the heart than is the attachment of the mitral valve. The left ventricular outflow tract is angulated to the right.

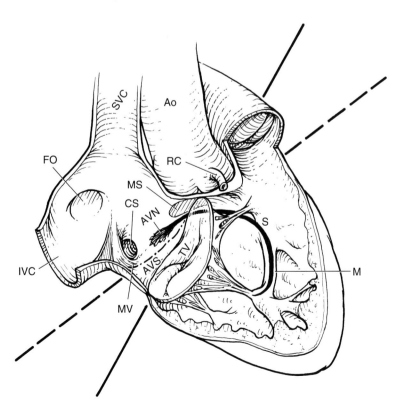

Figure 1-18 Diagram of the right heart, aortic root, and conduction tissue, at approximately 65° right anterior oblique projection. The plane of the mitral valve attachment *(dashed line)* corresponds to the atrial edge of the muscular atrioventricular septum and the inferior edge of the membranous septum, but differs from the plane of the tricuspid valve *(solid line)*. The muscular portion of the atrioventricular septum is frequently smaller than depicted. (Modified from McAlpine.[M4])

Key: *Ao,* Ascending aorta; *AVN,* atrioventricular node extending into the bundle of His and the right bundle branch; *AVS,* muscular atrioventricular septum; *CS,* coronary sinus; *FO,* fossa ovalis; *IVC,* inferior vena cava; *M,* moderator band; *MS,* membranous septum, crossed by the attachment of the tricuspid valve; *MV,* mitral valve anulus; *RC,* right coronary artery; *S,* portion of septal band (trabecula septomarginalis); *SVC,* superior vena cava; *TV,* tricuspid valve.

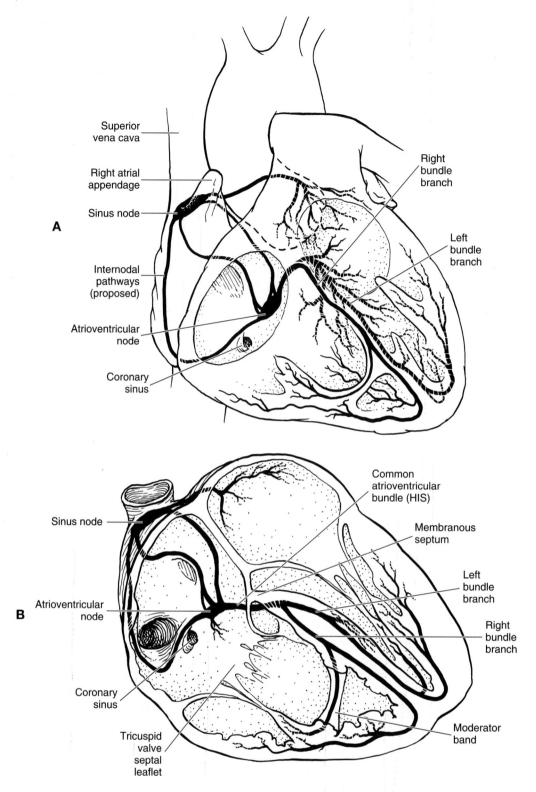

Figure 1-19 Cardiac conduction system. **A,** The sinus node is located on the anterolateral aspect of the junction between the superior vena cava and right atrial appendage. Internodal pathways are not well defined anatomically and are presented here as proposed pathways. The atrioventricular node lies in the triangle of Koch. The right and left bundle branches spread out on the subendocardial surfaces of the right and left aspects of the ventricular septum. **B,** This section of the heart, taken more posterior than that shown in (**A**), demonstrates the location of the atrioventricular node in the triangle of Koch, bounded by the coronary sinus, anulus of the tricuspid valve septal leaflet, and tendon of Todaro. The common atrioventricular bundle (bundle of His) continues from the atrioventricular node to penetrate the central fibrous body and reach the posteroinferior margin of the membranous septum. The left bundle branch spreads over the left ventricular aspect of the ventricular septum. The right bundle branch continues on the right ventricular surface of the ventricular septum into the moderator band.

Sinus Node

The sinus node is located along the anterolateral aspect of the junction between the superior vena cava and the right atrial appendage[H1,J1,L6,T2] (Fig. 1-19). In rare cases, it extends medially across the crest of the caval–atrial junction. The node is superficial, lying just beneath the epicardial surface in the sulcus terminalis, and is approximately $15 \times 5 \times 1.5$ mm.[J1] It is pierced by the relatively large sinus node artery. (For details of the blood supply, see "Coronary Arteries.")

Internodal Pathways

The spread of activation between sinus node and AV node occurs preferentially through the muscle bundles delimited by the orifices of the right atrium (see Fig. 1-19).[S2,S3] Considerable histologic and electrophysiologic investigation has been carried out to determine whether pathways of specialized conduction tissue exist within these broad muscle bundles and connect the sinoatrial (SA) and AV nodes. Investigators have not found discrete internodal tracts composed of homogeneous cells or fibers, although some have identified Purkinje-like cells in the major muscle bundles of adult hearts.[J2,J3,L1,T3] Controversy continues as to whether these pale cells seen in the atrial myocardium are Purkinje-type cells and whether they form the preferential conduction pathways.

Atrioventricular Node

The AV node lies directly on the right atrial side of the central fibrous body (right trigone) in the muscular portion of the atrioventricular septum, just anterosuperior to the ostium of the coronary sinus.[J4,T2] At times, its posterior margin has been found to lie directly against the coronary sinus ostium.[J4] It has a flattened oblong shape, with an average dimension in adults of $1 \times 3 \times 6$ mm. Its left surface lies against the mitral anulus. Viewed from the right atrium, the AV node can be localized within a triangle, described by Koch (Fig. 1-20), formed by the tricuspid anulus, the tendon of Todaro (the continuation of the eustachian valve that runs to the central fibrous body), and the coronary sinus ostium. The opening of the coronary sinus is usually a good landmark for the nodal triangle.[S25] In hearts with abnormal orifice of the coronary sinus, however, the nodal triangle is variable in relation to the coronary sinus. Examples of variability are when the coronary sinus opens to the left of the ventricular septum, when there is malalignment between atrial and ventricular septal structures, and when the atrial septum is absent.

Bundle of His and Bundle Branches

The common AV bundle (bundle of His) is a direct continuation of the AV node. The bundle passes through the rightward part of the right trigone of the central fibrous body to reach the posteroinferior margin of the membranous ventricular septum. This area is just inferior to the commissure between the tricuspid valve's septal and anterior leaflets (see Fig. 1-19, B). Its diameter in the region of the central fibrous body is about 1 mm.[J4] The bundle courses along the posteroinferior border of the membranous

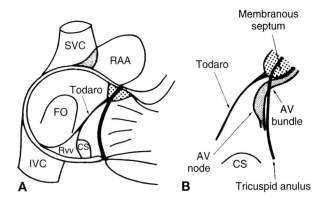

Figure 1-20 Anatomic and surgical aspects of the conduction system. **A,** Diagram of the triangle of Koch within the right atrium. The triangle is defined by the tendon of Todaro, orifice of the coronary sinus, and tricuspid anulus. **B,** Diagram showing the relationship of the atrioventricular node and atrioventricular bundle (bundle of His) to the triangle of Koch. The atrioventricular node lies within the triangle, and the atrioventricular bundle is located at the apex of the triangle. (From Anderson and colleagues.[A3])

Key: AV, Atrioventricular; CS, coronary sinus; FO, fossa ovalis; IVC, inferior vena cava; RAA, right atrial appendage; Rvv, right venous valve; SVC, superior vena cava.

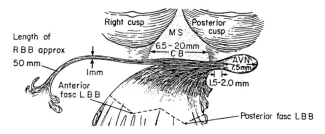

Figure 1-21 Diagram of the atrioventricular conduction system and its relationship to the membranous septum and aortic valve, viewed from the left ventricular side. The atrioventricular node is in the atrioventricular septum on the right atrial side of the right trigone, which is beneath the nadir of the posterior (noncoronary) cusp of the aortic valve. The common atrioventricular bundle courses along the posteroinferior margin of the membranous septum, giving off fibers that form the left bundle branch. This region lies beneath the commissure of right and noncoronary (posterior) aortic cusps. The right bundle branch originates from the common atrioventricular bundle in the region of the anteroinferior border of the membranous septum. (From Titus.[T2])

Key: approx, Approximately; AVN, atrioventricular node; CB, branching portion of common atrioventricular bundle; fasc, fascicle; LBB, left bundle branch; MS, membranous septum; RBB, right bundle branch.

septum and crest of the muscular ventricular septum, giving off fibers that form the left bundle branch. This branching occurs beneath the commissure between the right and noncoronary cusps in close proximity to the aortic valve, over a distance of 6.5 to 20 mm, after which the remaining fibers form the right bundle branch (Fig. 1-21). The bundle of His lies on the left side of the ventricular septal crest in about 75% to 80% of human hearts and on the right side of the crest in the remainder.[M1] In the latter situation, the His bundle connects to the left bundle by a relatively narrow stem.[M2]

The left bundle branch fans out over the left ventricular septal surface, gradually forming two or three main radiations.[D1,S4,T2] It is not uncommon for the anterior and posterior subdivisions to be accompanied by a central, third radiation that originates from the His bundle or from both of the former subdivisions. The anterior radiation travels toward the base of the anterolateral papillary muscle of the left ventricle. The wider posterior subdivision courses toward the base of the posteromedial papillary muscle. Multiple peripheral anastomoses occur among the subdivisions of the left bundle branch system as it distributes to the left ventricle.[D1]

The right bundle branch originates from the bundle of His in the region of the anteroinferior margin of the membranous septum and courses along the right ventricular septal surface, passing just below the medial papillary muscle and along the inferior margin of the septal band and the moderator band to the base of the anterior papillary muscle.[L1] The fibers then fan out to supply the walls of the right ventricle. Proximally, the right bundle averages about 1 mm in diameter.[T2] It is usually subendocardial in its proximal portion, intramyocardial in its middle portion, and again subendocardial near the base of the anterior papillary muscle.[T2] Ventricular septal defects associated with mal-

alignment of portions of the ventricular septum affect these relationships to some extent.[T4]

CARDIAC VALVES

The interrelationships among the heart valves in normally formed hearts are remarkably uniform.[M3] The aortic valve occupies a central position, wedged between the mitral and tricuspid valves, whereas the pulmonary valve is situated anterior, superior, and slightly to the left of the aortic valve (Fig. 1-22). The anuli of the mitral and tricuspid valves merge with each other and with the membranous septum to form the fibrous skeleton of the heart.[G1] The core of the skeleton is the central fibrous body, with its two extensions, the right and left fibrous trigones. The right fibrous trigone forms a dense junction between the mitral and tricuspid anuli, the left ventricular–aortic junction below the non-coronary cusp, and the membranous septum. The trigone is pierced by the bundle of His. The left fibrous trigone, situated more anteriorly and to the left, lies between the left ventricular–aortic junction and the mitral anulus. The tendon of the infundibulum is a fibrous band joining the more superiorly placed pulmonary valve to the central cardiac skeleton. The tendon of Todaro also joins the central fibrous body (see "Atrioventricular Node").

By virtue of similarities in morphology and function, the heart valves naturally fall into two groups: AV (mitral and

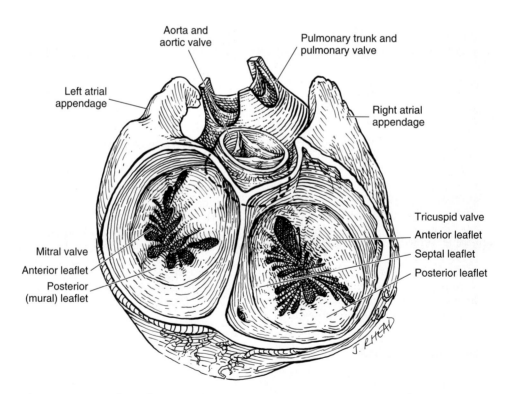

Figure 1-22   Cardiac valves viewed from superior aspect. The interrelationships of the heart valves are shown, with the aorta and semilunar aortic valve wedged between the mitral and tricuspid valves. The pulmonary trunk and semilunar pulmonary valve are anterior and slightly to the left of the aortic valve. The left atrioventricular valve, or mitral valve, has two leaflets: anterior, or septal, and posterior, or mural. The tricuspid valve has three leaflets: anterior, septal, and posterior. The blunt and broad-based right atrial appendage is contrasted to the long and narrow left atrial appendage, providing identification of the anatomic structures.

tricuspid) valves and semilunar (aortic and pulmonary) valves.

Mitral Valve

The AV valve of the left ventricle, the mitral valve, is bicuspid, with an anterior (aortic, or septal) leaflet and a posterior (mural, or ventricular) leaflet (Fig. 1-23). Tissue that could be called *commissural leaflets* is usually present at the commissures between these two leaflets. The combined area of the two mitral leaflets is twice that of the mitral orifice, resulting in a large area of coaptation.[P2,S5] When this large area of coaptation is lost because of malalignment of the leaflets, undue stress is placed on the chordae tendineae, and they may rupture. Although there has been some controversy as to the definition of commissural areas, particularly in regard to clefts in the posterior leaflet, Silver and colleagues describe chordae tendineae that define the limits of the septal (anterior) and posterior leaflets.[L2,R1] Rusted and colleagues found the depth of commissures in the normal mitral valve averaged 0.7 to 0.8 cm and never exceeded 1.3 cm in the 50 hearts they studied.[R2]

The larger *septal* (anterior, or aortic) *leaflet* is roughly triangular in shape, with the base of the triangle inserting on about one third of the anulus. The septal leaflet has a relatively smooth, free margin with few or no indentations. A distinct ridge separates the region of closure (rough zone)

from the remaining leaflet (clear zone).[R1] The clear zone is devoid of direct chordal insertions. The septal leaflet is in fibrous continuity with the aortic valve through the aortic–mitral anulus and forms a boundary of the left ventricular outflow tract.[W1] This region of continuity occupies about one fourth of the mitral anulus and corresponds to the region beneath half the left coronary cusp and half the noncoronary cusp of the aortic valve. The limits of this attachment are demarcated by the right and left fibrous trigones (Fig. 1-24). The commissure between the left and noncoronary sinuses of the aortic valve is located directly over the middle of the anterior leaflet of the mitral valve (Fig. 1-25; see also Fig. 1-24). These points do not correspond to the commissures of the mitral valve (see Fig. 1-4). The AV node and bundle of His are at risk of surgical damage adjacent to the right trigone.

The smaller *posterior leaflet* inserts into about two thirds of the anulus and typically has a scalloped appearance. Ranganathan and colleagues found the posterior leaflet to be divided into three segments in 46 of the 50 normal mitral valves they studied.[R1] The posterior leaflet has rough and clear zones corresponding to those of the anterior leaflet, as well as a basal zone close to the anulus, which receives chordae directly from left ventricular trabeculae.[L2,R1]

The mitral valve leaflets may be described using a segmental classification. The valve leaflets are segmented into six sections, A1 to A3 for the septal and P1 to P3 for

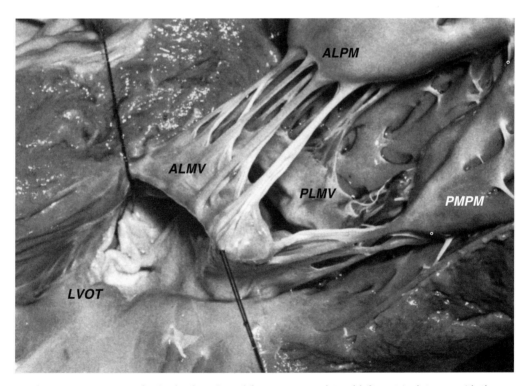

Figure 1-23   Normal mitral valve, viewed from an anterolateral left ventriculotomy, with the anterolateral left ventricular wall held forward and to the observer's right.

Key: *ALMV,* Anterior leaflet of mitral valve; *ALPM,* anterolateral papillary muscle; *LVOT,* left ventricular outflow tract; *PLMV,* posterior leaflet; *PMPM,* posteromedial papillary muscle.

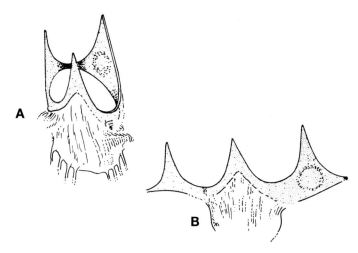

Figure 1-24 Diagram of the crownlike area of attachment of the aortic valve. **A,** View from the direction of the mitral valve. This area is in continuity with the membranous septum and anterior (septal) leaflet of the mitral valve. The subaortic curtain is the aortic-mitral anulus. The posterior commissure of the aortic valve is directly over the midpoint of the anterior leaflet of the mitral valve. **B,** The aortic wall flattened out, illustrating the U-shaped attachment of the aortic valve. (From Zimmerman.[Z1])

the posterior. Sections A1 and P1 represent the anterolateral sections, A2 and P2 the middle sections, and A3 and P3 the posteromedial sections (see Fig. 1-25, *C*). This segmental classification has been useful in describing morphology observed at operation,[K7] multiplane two-dimensional transesophageal echocardiography,[F3] and three-dimensional echocardiography.[C4]

The majority of *chordae tendineae* to the mitral valve originate from the two large papillary muscles of the left ventricle, the anterolateral and the posteromedial. Each leaflet receives chordae from both papillary muscles, and the majority insert on the free leaflet edge.[R2] The papillary muscles are often thought of as a fingerlike structure protruding into the left ventricular cavity from the ventricular wall. Perhaps this is because these muscles are frequently visualized in two dimensions by angiography or echocardiography. Actually, the papillary muscles have a somewhat crescent shape that conforms to the curvature of the free wall of the left ventricle. This is reasonable, because the papillary muscles and chordae tendineae are derived embryologically by undermining of the left ventricular myocardium.

One hundred normal human hearts were examined at autopsy by Victor and Nayak.[V16] The papillary muscles and arrangement of the chordae were evaluated and categorized. The anterolateral papillary muscle is attached by chordae tendineae to the left half of the anterior and posterior leaflets (as viewed by a surgeon through the usual right side approach to the mitral valve), whereas the posteromedial papillary muscle is attached by chordae tendineae to the right side half of both anterior and posterior leaflets. The papillary muscles are considered an anterolateral "group" and a posteromedial "group" because there was often more than a single papillary muscle

"belly." There were patterns of mostly single or two muscle bellies, but occasionally three, four, or even five bellies were observed. When there are three muscle bellies, the papillary muscle supporting the chordae to the commissure arises separately from the ventricular wall. Commissural chordae are shorter than the others and usually originate from the highest tip of the papillary muscle.

Variations of the chordal attachments were also described. There were usually 4 to 12 chordae originating from each papillary muscle group (range 2 to 22). Chordal branching resulted in a number of chordae inserting to the mitral valve leaflet, ranging from 12 to 80. Acar and colleagues proposed a clinical morphologic classification of the papillary muscles.[A15] A single, undivided papillary muscle is referred to as type I. Type II refers to papillary muscles cleaved in a sagittal plane into two heads that separately support the anterior and posterior leaflets of the mitral valve. Type III papillary muscles are cleaved in a coronal plane, forming an individual head that supports the commissural chordae. Type IV refers to papillary muscles divided into multiple heads, with a separate papillary muscle originating as a separate muscular band close to the mitral anulus, which supports short chordae to the commissure. Tandler defined three orders of chordae.[T1] Those of the first order insert on the free margin of the leaflet; those of the second order insert a few to several millimeters back from the free edge, and those of the third order insert at the base of the leaflet (applicable only to the posterior leaflet). Lam and colleagues reclassified chordae into rough zone (including strut chordae), cleft, basal, and commissural chordae.[L2] These investigators suggest that this classification provides a clear definition of mitral valve leaflets and should be useful in studying mitral valve function.

The mitral valve is designed to allow the largest possible orifice during the diastolic phase of ventricular filling so that there will not be the slightest obstruction at low pressures in the left atrium and left ventricle. The mitral valve opens as the anterior leaflet swings anteriorly away from the posterior leaflet. The orifice dimensions are enhanced by flexion of the anterior leaflet (see Fig. 1-25). During systole, the mitral valve closes under the full load of left ventricular contraction. The anterior leaflet straightens and extends toward the posterior leaflet. The posterior leaflet functions like a shelf to stop the movement of the anterior leaflet as the leaflets appose.

Tricuspid Valve

The AV valve of the right ventricle, or tricuspid valve, has three leaflets: anterior, posterior, and septal (Fig. 1-26). Its orifice is roughly triangular and is larger than the mitral orifice. The anulus is relatively indistinct, especially in the septal region. The leaflets and chordae tendineae are thinner than those of the mitral valve.[B3,G2]

The *anterior leaflet* (actually anterosuperior in position) is the largest of the three leaflets and may have notches creating subdivisions. Silver and colleagues found a notch close to the anteroseptal commissure in 47 of the 50 anterior leaflets they examined.[S6] This notch was occasionally as deep as a commissure, but could be differentiated from a true commissure by the type of chordal attachments.

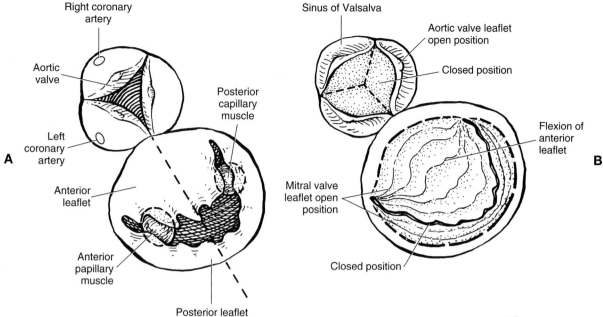

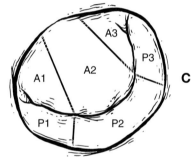

Figure 1-25   Anatomic relationships of the mitral and aortic valves. **A,** The commissure between the left and noncoronary sinuses of the aortic valve is located directly above the midpoint of the anterior leaflet of the mitral valve. The dashed line represents the midpoint of both the anterior and posterior leaflets of the mitral valve, separating the chordal attachments to the anterior and posterior papillary muscles. **B,** The three-leaflet, semilunar aortic valve opens widely during systole, without touching the aortic wall, owing to the sinuses of Valsalva. During diastole, the mitral valve opens not only as the anterior leaflet swings away from the posterior leaflet but also as it flexes, to create the widest possible orifice. This is illustrated as a series of flexion lines. **C,** Segmental classification used to describe morphology of the mitral valve at surgery and two-dimensional and three-dimensional echocardiography.

The chordae attaching to the anterior leaflet arise from the anterior and medial papillary muscles.

The *posterior leaflet* (actually inferior in position) is usually the smallest and commonly is scalloped. Its chordae originate from the posterior and anterior papillary muscles.

The *septal leaflet* is usually slightly larger than the posterior leaflet. Its chordae arise from the posterior and septal papillary muscles. Most of this leaflet attaches to the membranous and muscular portions of the ventricular septum, although part may attach to the posterior wall of the right ventricle. The transition between the attachments to posterior wall and septum is associated with a fold in the leaflet.[S6]

Of major surgical importance is the proximity of the conduction system to the septal leaflet and its anteroseptal commissure. The membranous septum usually lies beneath the septal leaflet inferior to the anteroseptal commissure, but the attachments at the septal and anterior leaflets are variable, so that parts of either may attach to the membranous septum. The bundle of His penetrates the right trigone beneath the interventricular component of the membranous septum (usually about 5 mm inferior to the commissure) and runs along the crest of the muscular septum ("Conduc-

tion System"). That portion of the septal leaflet between the membranous septum and the commissure extends around the tricuspid anulus, away from the septum, to the right ventricular free wall (see Fig. 1-2). This portion of the tricuspid valve may form a flap over some ventricular septal defects (VSDs).[S7]

Aortic Valve

The aortic valve is normally tricuspid and is composed of delicate cusps and sinuses of Valsalva. These components form three cuplike structures that constitute the entire valve mechanism; the valve is in fibrous continuity with the anterior leaflet of the mitral valve and the membranous septum (see Fig. 1-25).

The free edge of each cusp is of tougher consistency than the remainder of the cusp. At the midpoint of each free edge is a fibrous *nodulus Aranti*. On either side of each nodulus is an extremely thin, crescent-shaped portion of the cusp termed the *lunula* (see Fig. 1-13). The lunulae are occasionally fenestrated near the commissures. These regions form the area of coaptation during valve closure.

The aortic sinuses (sinuses of Valsalva) are dilated

pockets of the aortic root that form the outer component of the three cuplike closing structures of the aortic valve (see Fig. 1-25). The coronary arteries arise from two of the aortic sinuses. The walls of the sinuses are considerably thinner than the wall of the aorta proper,[Z1] an important consideration in the design of proximal aortotomies.

The crown-shaped anulus, fibrous trigones, aortic cusps, aortic sinuses, and sinotubular junction share a dynamic coordinated action to provide unidirectional transmission of large volumes of blood pumped intermittently through the channel while maintaining laminar flow, minimal resistance, optimal coronary artery flow, and least damage to blood elements during widely variable and frequently changing conditions.[Y1]

The origins of the coronary arteries are the basis of a nomenclature for the sinuses and cusps. The ostia of the right and left coronary arteries identify the right and left sinuses and cusps. The sinus and cusp without an associated coronary artery are termed *noncoronary.* Several other nomenclatures for the cusps and sinuses have been described (see "Morphology" in Chapter 38).[B3,G2,K1]

Pulmonary Valve

The structure of the pulmonary valve is similar to that of the aortic valve.[G2] The pulmonary valve normally has three cusps, with a nodule at the midpoint of each free edge and lunulae and thin, crescent-shaped coaptive surfaces on both sides of the nodules. The pocket behind each cusp is the sinus. Major differences from the aortic valve are

(1) the lighter construction of the pulmonary valve cusps,[G1,G2] (2) the normal absence of coronary artery origins, and (3) the normal lack of fibrous continuity with the anterior tricuspid valve leaflet. The pulmonary valve cusps are supported entirely by freestanding musculature, having no direct relationship with the ventricular septum.[M8] The pulmonary valve is lifted away from the ventricular septum by the subpulmonary infundibulum. The first septal branch of the left anterior descending artery pierces the ventricular septum below the shortest part of the subpulmonary infundibulum. The artery is protected by the subpulmonary infundibulum.

The pulmonary valve cusps have been described by several terminologies,[B3,G2,K1] but are usually named by their relationships to the aortic valve. They are thus termed *right, left,* and *anterior* (nonseptal). Kerr and Goss found that a commissure of the pulmonary valve was adjacent to a commissure of the aortic valve in 199 of the 200 specimens they studied.[K1] These investigators suggested that the cusps of each arterial valve should be termed *right adjacent, left adjacent,* and *opposite* (or, as suggested by Anderson, right facing, left facing, and nonfacing) in relationship to the adjacent commissure of each valve.

CORONARY ARTERIES

From an anatomic point of view, the coronary artery system divides naturally into two distributions, left and right. From the standpoint of the surgeon, the coronary artery system is divided into four parts: the left main coronary artery, the

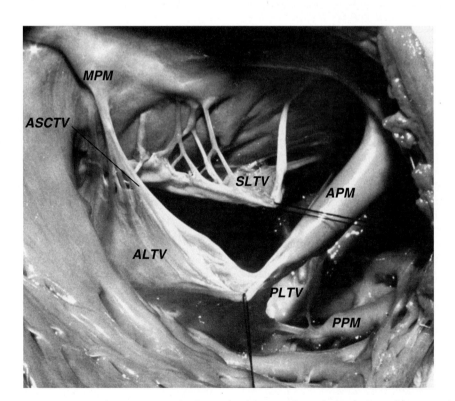

Figure 1-26   Normal open tricuspid valve, viewed from in front through the right ventricular cavity.

Key: *ALTV,* Anterior leaflet; *APM,* anterior papillary muscle; *ASCTV,* anteroseptal commissure; *MPM,* medial papillary muscle; *PLTV,* posterior leaflet; *PPM,* posterior papillary muscle; *SLTV,* septal leaflet.

left anterior descending coronary artery and its branches, the left circumflex coronary artery and its branches, and the right coronary artery and its branches. The branches of each of the last three vessels must also be familiar to the surgeon.

The major coronary arteries form a circle and a loop about the heart[D2,S8] (Fig. 1-27). The circle is formed by the right coronary and left circumflex arteries as they traverse the atrioventricular sulci. The loop between the ventricles and at right angles to the circle is formed by the left anterior descending coronary artery and the posterior descending coronary artery as they encircle the septum. The

blood supply to the back of the left ventricle streams down as a series of parallel obtuse marginal arteries coming from the posterior half of the circle, formed on the left by the left circumflex artery and on the right (in hearts with a dominant right coronary circulation) by the extension of the right coronary artery across the crux cordis, the area along the posterior aspect of the atrioventricular groove where the atrial and ventricular septa meet, termed the *right posterolateral segment*. This latter segment supplies inferior surface (marginal) branches to the inferior (diaphragmatic) surface of the left ventricle. Although the right coronary artery may not supply a large portion of the posterior left ventricular wall, it nevertheless serves the left side of the heart to a greater extent than it does the right side in terms of the number and volume of vessel segments involved.[Z2] A right dominant artery does not necessarily supply branches to the inferior surface of the left ventricle, however, because it may terminate only as the posterior descending artery. The blood supply to the anterior portion of the left ventricle comes from the diagonal branches of this portion of the loop, the left anterior descending coronary artery. That to the lateral part of the anterior portion comes from the first branches of both the left anterior descending and circumflex arteries. The ventricular septum receives its blood supply from the loop that encircles it, formed by the left anterior descending coronary artery in front and the posterior descending artery behind.

Variability in the origin of the posterior descending artery is expressed by the term *dominance*. A right dominant coronary circulation is one in which the posterior descending coronary artery is a terminal branch of the right coronary artery. A left dominant circulation, which occurs in about 10% to 15% of hearts, is one in which the posterior descending coronary artery is a branch, usually the last one, of the left circumflex coronary artery. Left dominance occurs more frequently in males than in females. This distinction as to whether the right or left coronary artery supplies the posterior descending artery is important in

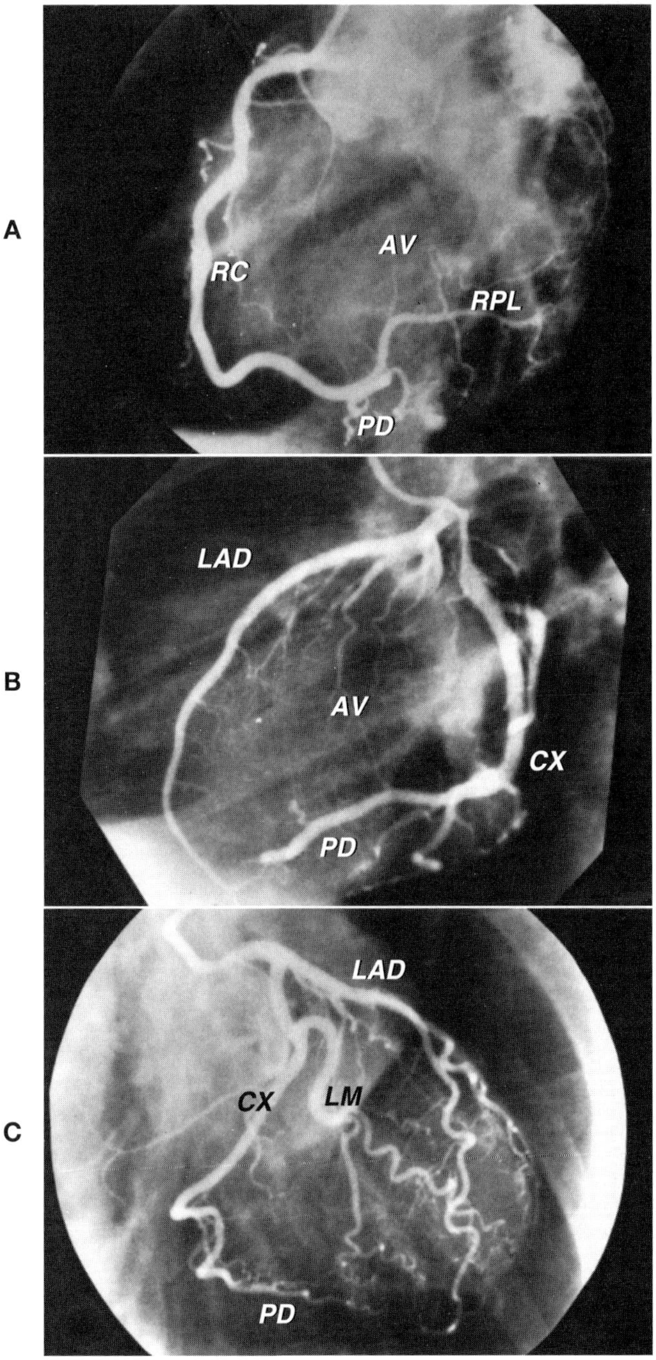

Figure 1-27 Coronary angiograms, demonstrating the circle-loop concept of coronary artery anatomy. The circle is formed by right coronary and left circumflex arteries and is displayed in the left anterior oblique (LAO) projection. The loop is formed by left anterior descending and posterior descending arteries and is demonstrated in the right anterior oblique (RAO) projection. **A,** Right coronary injection in the LAO projection. The circulation is right dominant. The right coronary artery, which forms the right component of the circle, is visualized. **B,** Left coronary injection in the LAO projection. Note that this is a left dominant circulation. The left circumflex artery, which forms the left component of the circle, is visualized. **C,** Left coronary injection in RAO projection. The left dominant circulation allows demonstration of both components of the loop: left anterior descending and posterior descending arteries.

Key: *AV,* Atrioventricular node artery; *CX,* left circumflex artery; *LAD,* left anterior descending artery; *LM,* left marginal artery; *PD,* posterior descending artery; *RC,* right coronary artery; *RPL,* right posterolateral artery.

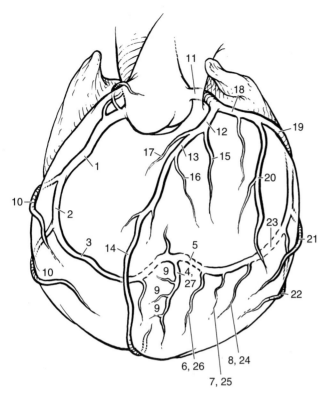

Figure 1-28 Diagram of the anatomic segments of the coronary arteries for use in locating lesions in individual patients. *(1, 2, 3)* Proximal, mid-, and distal portions of right coronary artery. *(4, 27)* Posterior descending coronary artery, which, as the dotted segments proximal to it indicate, may arise from the right *(4)* or left *(27)* system. *(5)* Right posterolateral segment, an extension of the right coronary artery in association with right dominant systems. *(6, 7, 8)* From it come several inferior surface (marginal) branches, called *right posterolateral arteries*, to the back of the left ventricle. Left dominant systems have a comparable left posterolateral segment leading to the posterior descending artery. *(9)* Inferior septal branches of the posterior descending artery. *(10)* Acute marginal branches of right coronary artery. *(11)* Left main coronary artery. *(12, 13, 14)* Proximal, mid-, and distal portions of the left anterior descending coronary artery. *(15, 16)* First and second diagonal branches. The first diagonal may originate near the bifurcation of the left main coronary artery, and was formerly called *ramus intermedius*. Additional diagonal branches may be present. *(17)* First septal branch of the left anterior descending artery. *(18, 19)* Proximal and distal portions of the left circumflex coronary artery. *(20, 21, 22)* First, second, and third obtuse marginal branches of the circumflex artery, the first usually being a large vessel. *(23)* Extension of the circumflex artery, called the *left AV artery*, present only in patients with a left dominant system. In such patients, this vessel gives off further inferior surface ("marginal") branches to the back of the left ventricle, called *left posterolateral arteries (24, 25, 26)*, before terminating in the left posterior descending coronary artery *(27)*. (Modified from the National Heart, Lung, and Blood Institute Coronary Artery Surgery Study [CASS].[C1])

evaluating patients with coronary artery disease and in the planning of coronary artery bypass grafting.

The following is a general description of coronary artery anatomy in normal hearts.[B4,F1,G3,J5,M4,S8,V4] As with the conduction system, some congenital cardiac malformations are associated with abnormalities of the coronary arteries. The nomenclature is based on the United States National Heart, Lung, and Blood Institute's *Proposal and Manual of Operations for Collaborative Studies in Coronary Artery Surgery*[N1] (Fig. 1-28) and the American Heart Association's coronary artery disease reporting system.[A2] Both systems include rules for defining the various segments of the major coronary arteries. Figure 1-29 is also supplied to provide a more dimensional representation of the coronary arteries on the surface of the heart and should be studied along with the brief descriptions that follow.

Left Main Coronary Artery

The left main coronary artery extends from the ostium in the left sinus of Valsalva to its bifurcation into the left anterior descending and left circumflex branches. Its usual length is 10 to 20 mm, with a range of 0 to 40 mm. It normally courses between the pulmonary trunk and the left atrial appendage to reach the left atrioventricular groove. Occasionally, additional vessels originate from the left main coronary artery and course parallel to the diagonal branches of the left anterior descending branch.[J5] Such an additional artery (formerly called a *ramus intermedius*) is termed the *first diagonal branch* of the left anterior descending artery. Rarely (in 1% of persons), the left main coronary artery is absent, the left anterior descending and left circumflex coronary arteries originating directly from the aorta via separate ostia.

Left Anterior Descending Coronary Artery

Beginning as a continuation of the left main coronary artery, the left anterior descending coronary artery courses along the anterior interventricular sulcus to the apex of the heart. Part of it may be buried in muscle. In most cases, this artery extends around the apex into the posterior interventricular sulcus, supplying the apical portion of both right and left ventricles.[J5] This vessel supplies branches to the right ventricular free wall (usually small), to the septum, and to the left ventricular free wall. One or more branches to the right ventricle connect with infundibular branches from the proximal right coronary artery. This important route for collateral flow is the *loop of Vieussens*. The *septal arteries* arise almost perpendicularly from the left anterior descending coronary artery, a characteristic that is sometimes helpful in the angiographic identification of the anterior descending artery. A variable number of *diagonal arteries* course obliquely between the anterior descending and left circumflex arteries and supply the left ventricular free wall anteriorly and laterally.

Variations in the left anterior descending artery are infrequent, although in about 4% of hearts, it exists as two parallel vessels of about equal size. It may terminate before the apex or extend as far as the posterior atrioventricular groove.

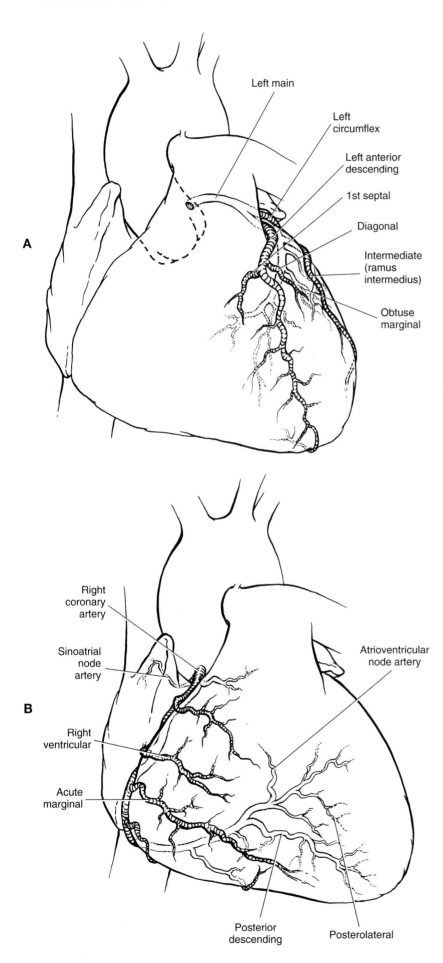

Figure 1-29   Coronary arteries. **A,** Left coronary artery. The left main coronary artery originates from the aorta and divides to form the *left anterior descending* and *left circumflex coronary arteries.* Branches of the left anterior descending artery on the surface of the heart are termed *diagonal arteries,* whereas those coursing into the ventricular septum are called *septal arteries.* Branches of the left circumflex artery on the posterior wall of the surface of the left ventricle are termed *obtuse marginal arteries.* A large artery originating near the left main coronary bifurcation and supplying the obtuse margin between the diagonal branches of the left anterior descending and circumflex marginal branches was formerly called an *intermediate branch* or *ramus intermedius.* **B,** Right coronary artery, right dominant pattern. The right coronary artery originates from the aorta and courses in the atrioventricular groove. Branches of the right coronary artery supplying blood to the right ventricle are called *right ventricular branches,* except for the nearly constant and often large branch at the acute margin of the heart, termed the *acute marginal artery.* The right coronary artery divides at the crux of the heart into the right posterior descending branch, which courses over the posterior aspect of the ventricular septum, and the right posterolateral segment artery, which continues in the atrioventricular groove, providing branches to the posterior wall of the left ventricle. Arterial branches to the specialized conduction system frequently arise from the right coronary artery. The sinoatrial node branch originates from the proximal portion of the right coronary artery. The atrioventricular node branch originates from the U-bend in the posterior lateral segment of the right coronary artery.

Left Circumflex Coronary Artery

The left circumflex coronary artery originates from the left main coronary artery at about a 90° angle, with its initial few centimeters lying medial to the base of the left atrial appendage. The sinus node artery occasionally originates from the first few millimeters of the left circumflex artery. Rarely, the circumflex artery terminates before the obtuse margin. A large branch originating from the proximal left circumflex artery and coursing around the left atrium near the atrioventricular groove is termed the *atrial circumflex artery*. The ventricular branches of the circumflex artery, the *obtuse marginal arteries,* supply the obtuse margin of the heart and may be embedded in the muscle. Often, their position can then be identified at operation by the altered (reddish or light tan) color of the overlying thin muscle layer compared with that of the remainder of the ventricular wall. Those branches supplying the inferior surface of the left ventricle in a heart with a left dominant system (or in one with a codominant system in which the right coronary artery gives rise only to a posterior descending artery) are termed *left posterolateral (mar-ginal) arteries.* In hearts with a left dominant system, the left circumflex coronary artery gives rise to the *posterior descending artery* at or usually before the crux. Variations in the origin and length of the left circumflex artery, and in the number and size of its marginal branches, are common.

Right Coronary Artery

The right coronary artery usually is a single large artery, and it courses down the right atrioventricular groove. Branches supplying the anterior right ventricular free wall

exit from the atrioventricular sulcus in a looping fashion because of the depth of the right coronary artery in the sulcus. In this same area, the anterior right atrial artery arises, and this branch often gives origin to the sinus node artery. More distally, a lateral right atrial artery usually arises[B9] (this artery is frequently severed when an oblique right atriotomy is made). In the region of the acute margin of the heart, a relatively constant long branch of the right coronary artery arises, the *acute marginal artery,* which courses most of the way to the apex of the heart. The right coronary artery in most hearts crosses the crux, where it takes a characteristic deep U-turn, giving off the *atrioventricular node artery* at the apex of the turn. The right coronary artery then terminates by bifurcating into the *right posterior descending coronary artery* and the *right postero-lateral segment artery.* The *posterior descending coronary artery* descends in the posterior interventricular sulcus for a variable distance, giving rise to septal, right ventricular, and left ventricular branches. Variations in its anatomy are numerous, and it frequently arises before the crux. The right posterolateral segment of the right coronary artery gives origin to marginal branches to the inferior surface of the left ventricle in most hearts with a right dominant system.

Variations in the right coronary artery are common. It may have a dual origin from the right sinus of Valsalva. In about 10% of hearts, it bifurcates within a few millimeters of the aortic ostium, forming two diverging trunks of equal size. In half the cases, the artery supplying the infundibulum of the right ventricle arises separately from the aortic sinus and is then termed the *conus artery.*[J5,S9] The *sinoatrial node (sinus node) artery* originates from the second or third centimeter of the right coronary artery

Figure 1-30   Blood supply of the ventricular septum. Most of the septum is supplied by the left anterior descending coronary artery via large septal arteries. Septal arteries from the posterior descending artery are relatively small. In this right dominant circulation, note the origin of the atrioven-tricular node artery from the characteristic U-turn of the right coronary artery. (Modified from James and Burch.[J6])

Key: *AV,* Atrioventricular.

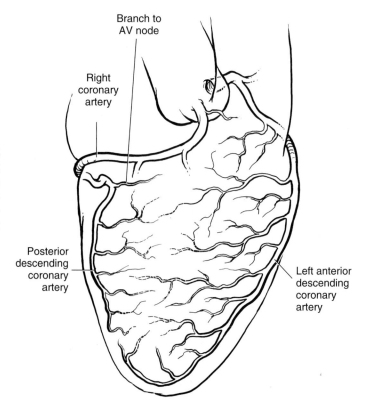

in many hearts (see "Coronary Arterial Supply to Specialized Areas of the Heart").[J5] The acute marginal artery crosses the diaphragmatic surface of the right ventricle in 10% to 20% of hearts and reaches the anterior aspect of the diaphragmatic portion of the ventricular septum, to which it gives branches.[A11]

Coronary Arterial Supply to Specialized Areas of the Heart

The predominant blood supply to the ventricular septum is from the left anterior descending coronary artery via four to six large septal arteries 70 to 80 mm in length.[J6,J7] In contrast, the septal arteries from the posterior descending coronary artery (except for the AV node artery) are rarely more than 15 mm in length (Fig. 1-30). They supply only a small zone of the ventricular septum near the posterior interventricular sulcus and in the region of the AV node. The septal arteries from the posterior descending artery may, however, serve as an important source of collateral circulation. Until their final terminations, the septal arteries from both anterior and posterior descending arteries course along the right ventricular side of the septum, where pressure is lower than on the left side.[J6] In the 10% of hearts with a left dominant circulation, the entire blood supply is from the left coronary artery.

The sinus node artery is a single artery in 89% and double in 11% of hearts.[S22] Its origin is from the right coronary artery in 55% to 65% of cases and from the left circumflex or left main coronary artery in the remainder. When it arises from the right coronary artery, it courses posteriorly and superiorly over the anterior wall of the right atrium beneath the right atrial appendage to the base of the superior vena cava (Fig. 1-31). The sinus node artery may penetrate the interatrial septum in its course to the superior vena cava. It then encircles the cava clockwise or counterclockwise, or bifurcates and encircles it in both directions. If the sinus node artery arises from the left circumflex artery, it courses over the left atrial wall, variably penetrates the interatrial septum, and ascends to the base of the superior vena cava, encircling that vessel as when it originates from the right coronary artery.

The AV node artery arises from the characteristic U-turn of the right coronary artery as it crosses the crux of the heart. The AV node is usually supplied by the dominant coronary artery. The AV node artery courses superiorly and anteriorly and terminates with a distinctive angulation.[S8] An important accessory blood supply to the AV node is *Kugel's artery,* which originates from the proximal segment of either the right coronary artery or the left circumflex artery and courses through the interatrial septum to the crux of the heart to anastomose with the AV node artery. In the

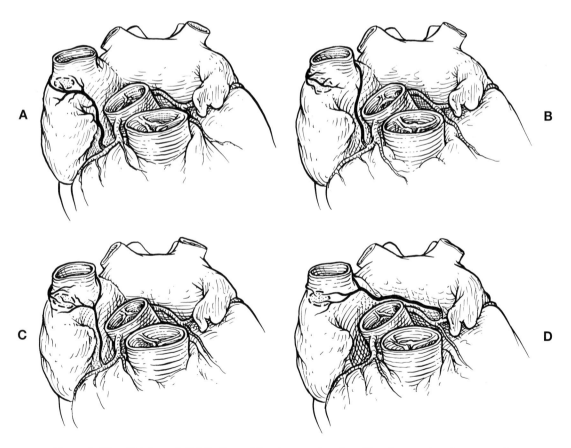

Figure 1-31   Origin and distribution of the sinus node artery. The sinus node artery may arise from the right coronary artery and encircle the base of the superior vena cava in (**A**) a clockwise direction or (**B**) a counterclockwise direction, or it may (**C**) bifurcate and encircle it in both directions. It may also arise from (**D**) the left circumflex artery and encircle the base of the superior vena cava as in **A**, **B**, or **C**. (Modified from Lewis and colleagues.[L7])

atrial septum, Kugel's artery anastomoses with branches of the sinus node artery.[J5] Kugel's artery is the source of the blood supply to the AV node in 40% of normal hearts.[A16] The right superior descending artery supplied the AV node in 70% of hearts studied by Abuin and Nieponice.[A16] This atrial vessel has its origin within the first centimeter of the right coronary artery, giving branches to the ventriculoinfundibular fold of the right ventricle, penetrating the right atrium, and continuing along the anterior border of the fossa ovalis. The artery goes through the central fibrous body and supplies the bundle of His and the area within the triangle of Koch, including the AV node. Kugel's artery and the right superior descending artery are placed at risk of injury in operations requiring dissection around the right coronary artery (aortic root replacement, Ross procedure) and in the atrioventricular groove (extended transseptal approaches to the mitral valve).[A17]

The bundle of His and the proximal few millimeters of the main bundle branches are supplied by the AV node artery. The remainder of the bundle branches and the Purkinje arborization within the septum are supplied by septal arteries originating from the left anterior descending artery.

The anterolateral papillary muscle of the right ventricle, located near the junction of apical septum and free wall, is supplied by branches from the left anterior descending artery. The anterolateral papillary muscle of the left ventricle is supplied primarily by one or more branches from the left anterior descending coronary artery, but it may also be supplied by circumflex marginal branches. The arterial supply of the posteromedial papillary muscle of the left ventricle is from terminal branches of the right or circumflex arteries, depending on the distribution of these arteries to the inferior surface of the left ventricle.

DIMENSIONS OF NORMAL CARDIAC AND GREAT ARTERY PATHWAYS

Cardiac and great artery pathways with normal dimensions accommodate blood flow at rest and during exercise and stress with little or no pressure drop across the pathway. In some patients being considered for cardiac surgery, however, dimensions are so small as to preclude a satisfactory outcome; therefore, prediction of outcome based on dimensions of a pathway becomes important. A major problem in predicting outcome in a patient simply from the subjective evaluation of the size of a structure is that this evaluation may be grossly inaccurate because of unconscious comparison of the size of the structure in question with that of a neighboring unusually large structure. Prediction of outcome simply from subjective evaluation is also affected by the preformed bias of the observer, as well as by inexperience. Therefore, measurements and their relationship to outcome are required for reproducible, accurate predictions, and decisions must be made regarding the methods for expressing the dimensions.

Dimensions of the Pathway

The measured dimension is usually expressed as diameter of the pathway. Occasionally, a circular shape is assumed and the dimension is transformed to cross-sectional area. Under some circumstances, cross-sectional area can be measured directly. In other circumstances, an elliptical shape is assumed, and major and minor axes are measured and area calculated with an equation that applies to ellipses.

Use of observed (measured) dimensions generally requires their being related to normal dimensions, which vary with body size and age. Normal dimensions may also vary according to imaging modality, image projection (e.g., anteroposterior versus lateral), phase of the cardiac cycle, method of fixation in the case of specimens, and other factors. These must be specifically controlled in making the measurements.

Dimensions have been measured in autopsy specimens,[C4,C5,R3,U1] by cineangiography (in which dimensions must be corrected for magnification), by echocardiography (M-mode, two-dimensional, three-dimensional[C3,N4,S23,S24]), and in a few instances by magnetic resonance imaging (MRI). However, normal values are not available in each of these modalities; therefore, dimensions need to be related to normal values that are available, even if from another modality. Echocardiography has evolved as the most commonly used modality for measuring these dimensions. Pathway dimensions have been determined by echocardiography at nearly all ages of life, from fetal to age 90. Hornberger and colleagues[H6] established dimensions by high-resolution two-dimensional echocardiography for the fetal aortic arch in 92 fetuses age 16 to 38 weeks gestation to facilitate diagnosis of left heart and aortic abnormalities, particularly coarctation. Skelton and colleagues[S27] followed changes in cardiac dimensions of preterm infants during the first month of life, suggesting that there are differences from term infants, with the preterm babies showing mild left ventricular dysfunction. Pathway dimensions for hearts from birth to about 20 years have been determined by M-mode[K8] and two-dimensional[S26] echocardiography. Daubeney and colleagues'[D4] prospective study aimed at developing equations relating cardiac dimensions to body area over the range of 0.1 to 2.0 m^2 is particularly useful (see Appendix 1D). A number of studies in adults use two-dimensional echocardiography (transthoracic or transesophageal) with pathway dimensions measured directly or derived from Doppler ultrasound measurements and the continuity equation. The age range is often wide, but there are populations studied at mean age 23,[D5] 28,[S28] 33,[D6] 45,[C6] and 53 years.[S29] Swinne and colleagues[S29] call attention to age-associated changes in left ventricular outflow tract geometry observed in normal subjects, mostly after age 70. These changes consist of a more acute septoaortic angle or septal bulge that is not associated with left ventricular outflow tract obstruction. These may represent degenerative changes associated with aging.

Normalization of Pathway Dimensions

Pathway dimensions may be used without any normalization to body size or age. Thus, some cardiologists who work exclusively with adult patients express aortic size simply in centimeters. This method is not recommended, not only for the obvious reason that it is unacceptable when the population being considered consists of patients who range from very young to very old, but also because it takes no account of differences between adults of differing size.

Normalization may be based on age, height, weight, or body surface area. Normalization to body size generally is termed *indexing*. Normalization may also be to another structure, such as the size of the descending aorta at the diaphragm. Normalization to another body structure generally is termed a *ratio*. The preference is for normalization to body surface area of the patient, very simply obtained by dividing the value of the dimension by the body surface area. This allows the dimension (or other variable) to be expressed "per square meter body surface area." This preference presumes a strictly linear relation between the dimension and body surface area, which may be inaccurate.

Indexed cross-sectional area and diameter, in normal individuals, of mitral and tricuspid valves, left ventricular–aortic junction (aortic valve "anulus"), right ventricular infundibulum, and right ventricular–pulmonary trunk junction (pulmonary valve "anulus") are summarized in Table 1-1 according to the modality in which the dimension was measured; those for the pulmonary trunk, right and left pulmonary arteries, and descending thoracic aorta at the diaphragm are summarized in Table 1-2. Values for the diameter of the upper descending thoracic aorta on both sides of the ductus arteriosus are also available.[V14] These tables are not intended as a source of normalized dimensions in patients, but rather as a reference and guide to the appendices to this chapter, which contain specific regression equations and nomograms for calculating mean normal values and their standard deviations for use in patients.

Standardization of Dimensions

Values of dimensions are made useful by standardizing them to body size. They are expressed as deviation from their mean normal value for body size in terms of number of standard deviations from the mean. Standardization takes into account the fact that values in normal individuals of the same size vary. The mathematical framework for standardization of dimensions is the normal distribution domain, because of its mathematical flexibility and tractability. This framework may require transformation of the dimension scale of the variable under consideration to comply with assumptions of the normal distribution.

A less desirable alternative is standardization according to percentiles (the 50th percentile is the median). This method is commonly used in relating body weight or height to age. Although percentiles are easily expressed, the method has the major disadvantage that the relationships cannot be reduced to equations. This increases the difficulty of relating dimensional data to outcome.

Once in the normal distribution domain, any given value for a dimension can be expressed in terms of the number of standard deviations of the given value from the mean value of that dimension in normal individuals. This is the *Z* value, or *Z* score (Fig. 1-32). The transformation to a dimensionless *Z* value is as follows:

$$Z = \frac{\text{Observed dimension}^{(1)} - \text{Mean normal dimension}^{(2)}}{\text{Standard deviation around mean normal dimension}^{(3)}}$$

■ **TABLE 1-1   Summary of Indexed Dimensions of Cardiac Pathways in Normal Individuals** [a]

Structure, Modality, and Source	Cross-Sectional Area (mm² · m⁻² BSA)	Diameter (mm · m⁻² BSA)
Mitral Valve		
Autopsy		
Rowlatt et al.[R3]	343	26
Westaby et al.[W2]	425	17
Angiography		
None		
Two-dimensional echocardiography		
King et al.[K4]	602	34
Riggs et al.[R4]	471	30
Pollick et al.[P3]	420	
Ormiston et al.[O2]	380	
Tricuspid Valve		
Autopsy		
Rowlatt et al.[R3]	507	32
Westaby et al.[W2]	576	20
Angiography		
Bull et al. (not normals)[B10]	1065	46
Alboliras et al.[A12]	547	33
Two-dimensional echocardiography		
King et al.[K4]	611	35
Tei et al.[T5]	610	
LV–Aortic Junction (Aortic "Anulus")		
Autopsy		
Rowlatt et al. (children)[R3]	156	18
Westaby et al. (adults; age 58)[W2]	239	13
Krovetz (children)[K5]	180	
Krovetz (adults; age 50)[K5]	310	
Angiography		
Sievers et al. (children)[S13]	291	24
Two-dimensional echocardiography		
Pollick et al. (children)[P3]	180	
Habbal and Somerville (≤1.5 m² BSA)[H2]	212	20
Habbal and Somerville (>1.5 m² BSA)[H2]	249	13
Hanséus (from diameter)[H3]	236	22
Hanséus (from area)[H3]	236	22
RV Infundibulum		
Angiography		
Sievers et al. (systole)[S13]	138	17
Sievers et al. (diastole)[S13]	311	25
Infundibular RV–Pulmonary Trunk Junction (Pulmonary "Anulus")		
Autopsy		
Rowlatt et al.[R3]	194	20
Westaby et al. (adults)[W2]	260	13
Angiography		
Bini M, Naftel DC, Blackstone EH (unpublished observations; 1984)	279	24
Sievers et al.[S13]	280	24
Two-dimensional echocardiography		
Hanséus et al. (short axis)[H3]	281	24

Key: *BSA*, Body surface area; *LV*, left ventricle; *RV*, right ventricle.

[a] Normalization is in terms of body surface area.

where (1) is the observed dimension or its appropriate transformation in scale in the patient, who is of a known size (body surface area), and (2) and (3) refer to corresponding values in normal individuals of the same body surface area as the patient, obtained from regression analysis and equations.

■ **TABLE 1-2 Summary of Indexed Dimensions of Aortic and Pulmonary Arterial Pathways in Normal Individuals**[a]

Structure, Modality, and Source	Cross-Sectional Area (mm² · m⁻² BSA)	Diameter (mm · m⁻² BSA)
Pulmonary Trunk		
Autopsy		
None		
Angiography		
Bini M, Naftel DC, Blackstone EH (unpublished observations; 1984)	346	32
Sievers et al.[S13]	347	26
Two-dimensional echocardiography		
Snider et al.[S15]	217	21
Right Pulmonary Artery		
Autopsy		
None		
Angiography		
Bini M, Naftel DC, Blackstone EH (unpublished observations; 1984) (origin, midportion, prebranching)	174, 137, 180	21, 18, 22
Sievers et al. (prebranching)[S13]	186	19
Two-dimensional echocardiography		
Snider et al. (mid-RPA, short axis)[S15]	82	13
Snider et al. (mid-RPA, long axis)[S15]	110	15
Left Pulmonary Artery		
Autopsy		
None		
Angiography		
Bini M, Naftel DC, Blackstone EH (unpublished observations; 1984) (origin, prebranching)	134, 136	19, 19
Sievers et al. (prebranching)[S13]	161	17
Two-dimensional echocardiography		
None		
Right Pulmonary Artery Plus Left Pulmonary Artery		
Autopsy		
None		
Angiography		
Bini M, Naftel DC, Blackstone EH (unpublished observations; 1984)	320	41
Nakata et al.[N2]	330	
Sievers et al.[S13]	347	36
Descending Thoracic Aorta at Diaphragm		
Autopsy		
None		
Angiography		
Sievers et al. (children, systole)[S13]	153	17
Bini M, Naftel DC, Blackstone EH (unpublished observations; 1984) (children, systole)	129	19
Arvidsson (normals and abnormals)[A13]	120	15
Two-dimensional echocardiography		
Hanséus et al.[H3]	97	14

Key: *BSA*, Body surface area; *RPA*, right pulmonary artery.

[a] Normalization is in terms of body surface area.

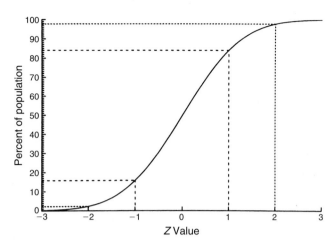

Figure 1-32 Depiction of relationship of the *Z* value of a patient's dimension to the percentage of a population of normal individuals with that specific dimension or a smaller one. The exact percentage, on vertical axis, related by dashed lines to the patient *Z* value, is the percentile of normal individuals with the corresponding *Z* value. A patient with a specific *Z* value has the dimension of the corresponding percentile of the normal population.

Appendix 1B includes dimensions, obtained at autopsy, of various cardiac and pulmonary artery pathways in normal individuals. In Appendix 1C the dimensions were obtained at in vivo cineangiography, and in Appendix 1D at in vivo two-dimensional echocardiography. Appendix 1E compares pathway dimensions in normal individuals from different measurement modalities. Additional reliable information is contained in other sources, for example, Roman and colleagues.[R5]

Dimensions of the Pulmonary Arteries

Indexing and standardizing the dimensions of the pulmonary arteries present special problems because of the multiplicity of methods that have been used. These dimensions in patients are usually measured on cineangiograms. They have been important in considering treatment for patients with tetralogy of Fallot and pulmonary stenosis, tetralogy of Fallot with pulmonary atresia, and conditions for which the Fontan operation is performed.

Among the different methods for expressing dimensions of the pulmonary arteries are the McGoon ratio,[B11,P4] the sum of the diameters of the prebranching portions of the right and left pulmonary arteries, pulmonary artery area index (PAAI),[S18] cross-sectional area index (Nakata index),[N2] and *Z* value. The *Z* value is the preferred method. It should be applied to more distal portions of the pulmonary arteries as well.

To facilitate transformation of already published dimensions of the pulmonary arteries in patients with congenital heart disease to a different normalization, relationships between the values obtained by these various methods are shown in Appendix 1F.

Relating Dimensions to Outcome

The goal is an equation expressing the continuously variable relationship between normalized dimensions of the patient and some outcome event (e.g., death, freedom from reoperation, postrepair P$_{RV/LV}$, cardiac index). Obtaining the equation may require detailed studies and complex analyses, but once obtained, the equation is made easy to use by expressing it in a nomogram. This process is the basis of many of the depictions in the subsequent chapters.

As is already evident from Appendixes 1B, 1C, and 1D, the normalization used in relating dimensions to outcome can be to measurements made at autopsy, at cineangiography, at two-dimensional echocardiography, at MRI, or other imaging method. Although in theory it may seem proper to normalize measurements made on cineangiography, for example, using normalizing equations based on cineangiographic measurements, this is in fact unnecessary. All that is important is that the same method of normalizing the patient's dimensions be used in predicting outcome as was used in the previous studies that determined the relationship between the dimensions and outcome. Thus, for example, in normalizing measurements of the dimensions of the tricuspid valve made at cineangiography, one might like to use equations based on cineangiographic measurements. Unfortunately, an insufficient number of measurements is made at cineangiography in normal individuals to generate equations for indexing or standardizing tricuspid measurements by this modality. Equations for standardization of tricuspid measurements using measurements obtained by two-dimensional echocardiography are available, as are measurements made at autopsy (Rowlatt and colleagues[R3]). Based on these practical considerations, normalization to autopsy or echocardiographic measurements may be used for standardizing tricuspid dimensions to a Z value, even though these measurements are made by cineangiography. Thus, the nomogram shown in Appendix Fig. 1B-2 or that in Appendix Fig. 1D-3 or the actual equation described in Appendix 1D may be used.

However, once a disparate standardization of a dimension is related to outcome, the user of that relationship must make that identical standardization.

This is analogous to the use of a ruler. Rulers may be subdivided into inches or centimeters. However, once a scale is chosen, it must be used consistently.

DIMENSIONS OF NORMAL VENTRICLES

Normal ventricular volumes, masses, and dimensions, assuming normal myocardial contractility and loading conditions, can accommodate normal blood flow at rest and during exercise. Sometimes the dimensions of the left or right ventricle are smaller or larger than those of the other, leading to problems in simply *judging* the normality of the size and its relationship to outcome, for the same reasons as in the case of pathway dimensions.

Accurate and precise ventricular diameters,[P5] volumes, and masses are difficult to obtain because ventricles may have unusual shapes. Nevertheless, a number of useful studies have been done that use M-mode and two-

dimensional directed M-mode echocardiography to determine left ventricular volume and mass and to relate these dimensions to body size over the life course of humans.[D7,G6,G7,H7] Particularly interesting is de Simone and colleagues'[D8] study of left ventricular mass in overweight children and adults. They found that height is the best means of normalizing left ventricular mass. Vasan and colleagues[V15] provide "cut" limits for range of normal values (90th and 95th percentiles) for ventricular mass and thickness and atrial and ventricular dimensions derived from nearly 5000 subjects in the Framingham Heart Study. Bull and colleagues[B10] proposed making surgical decisions based on the size (in terms of Z values) of the AV valve guarding the entrance to the ventricle, rather than on the size of the ventricle itself.

The Z value method (standardization) can be used to describe patients' ventricular volumes and masses, although this general body of knowledge is not yet well developed, in part because of methodologic problems. The Z value method can also be used for diameters. Table 1-3 gives the mean values for normal individuals of various body sizes, as an approximation and for guidance rather than for use in calculating patient-specific Z values. Appendix Fig. 1G-1 presents the information in a form from which patient-specific Z values can be calculated.

TERMINOLOGY AND CLASSIFICATION OF HEART DISEASE

Understanding the morphology of heart disease is fundamental to its surgical treatment. Morphology could be described fully using any one of a number of systems of terminology and classification. However, appropriate and accurate terminology and classification are important because they greatly facilitate understanding and teaching of cardiac morphology, diagnosis, and surgical treatment. Also, they determine the method of categorization of cases, a procedure that is essential to the study of groups of patients.

The system of terminology and classification used here evolved over many years, to a considerable extent in response to clinical, and particularly surgical, needs. It was based originally on the teaching of Edwards and his pupil, Becu. It has been profoundly influenced and modified on numerous occasions by the work of Van Praagh; has benefited through the years from the work of Van Mierop and of Lev and his colleague Bharati; and by the concepts of Anderson.[A18]

Following the ideas of Lev, terminology based on the somewhat shifting sands of embryology has been avoided as much as possible. Any terms that have embryologic implications are used only because they have become conventional. This is not to deny the importance of the science of embryology but, rather, to emphasize the importance of precise description of morphology.

Complete description of a cardiac anomaly includes the anatomic variables listed in Box 1-1.[B1,B12,K2,K3,S10,V6]

Nomenclature and classification schemes are essential for accurate data reporting and establishment of databases. The Society of Thoracic Surgeons Congenital Heart Sur-

■ **TABLE 1-3** Summary of Indexed Dimensions of Ventricular Volumes, Wall Thicknesses, and Masses in Normal Individuals[a]

Structure	Dimension · m^{-2} BSA
Left Ventricle	
Volume (mL)	
Angiography	
End-diastolic	
Graham et al.[G4]	67
Lange et al.[L9]	58
Nakazawa et al.[N3]	66
Thilenius and Arcilla[T6]	61
End-systolic	
Lange et al.[L9]	16
Thilenius et al.[T6]	16
Wall thickness (mm)	
Autopsy	
Rowlatt et al.[R3]	13
Two-dimensional echocardiography	
Henry et al. (diastolic)[H4]	9.9
Henry et al. (systolic)[H4]	15
Septum (mm)	
Two-dimensional echocardiography	
Henry et al. (diastolic)[H4]	10
Henry et al. (systolic)[H4]	13
Mass (g)	
Angiography	
Graham et al.[G4]	88
Two-dimensional echocardiography	
Henry et al.[H4]	95
Right Ventricle	
Volume (mL)	
Angiography	
End-diastolic	
Graham et al.[G4]	58
Lange et al.[L9]	68
Nakazawa et al.[N3]	67
Thilenius and Arcilla[T6]	74
End-systolic	
Graham et al.[G4]	37
Lange et al.[L9]	25
Thilenius and Arcilla[T6]	29
Wall thickness (mm)	
Autopsy	
Rowlatt et al. (conal)[R3]	5.3
Rowlatt et al. (inlet)[R3]	5.6
Heart Weight (g)	
Autopsy	
Kitzman et al. (adult females)[K6]	186
Kitzman et al. (adult males)[K6]	187
Rowlatt et al. (children)[R3]	112
Scholz et al. (female infants and children)[S16]	110
Scholz et al. (male infants and children)[S16]	114

Key: *BSA,* Body surface area.

[a] Normalization is in terms of body surface area.

gery Nomenclature and Database Project was organized to standardize nomenclature and reporting strategies and to establish an international database.[M7] The framework of this effort will serve as a guideline for future efforts at classification of cardiac morphology.

BOX 1-1 Anatomic Variables in the Complete Description of a Cardiac Anomaly

Situs of the thoracic viscera and atria
Situs of the ventricles
Completeness of the ventricles
Dominance of the ventricles
    Balanced ventricles
    Right ventricular (left hypoplasia)
    Left ventricular (right hypoplasia)
Cardiac connections
    Atrioventricular
    Ventriculoarterial
Cardiac and arterial positions
    Heart
    Atria
    Ventricles
    Great arteries
Defects or malformations
Conventional diagnosis (when available)

Situs of the Thoracic Viscera and Atria

The possible situs of the thoracic viscera and atria are (1) situs solitus, or usual situs, (2) situs inversus, and (3) situs ambiguus. *Situs solitus* means that the right–left relationships of the asymmetric viscera and the atria are usual. That is, the right (eparterial) and left (hyparterial) main stem bronchi are normally positioned, the right atrium is to the right of the left atrium, and the left atrium is to the left. *Situs inversus* indicates that the right–left relationships are the opposite of usual. In chemical language, these are isomers. With rare exceptions, atrial and thoracic visceral situs are the same (concordant). *Situs ambiguus* is the absence of lateralization in the thoracic organs and atrial chambers[V1,V2]; in the latter case, this condition is termed *atrial isomerism* (see Chapter 44). It is usually, but not invariably, associated with the lack of abdominal lateralization, that is, asplenia or polysplenia.

In *asplenia* and *polysplenia,* the usually asymmetric structures tend to be symmetric. In both, in contrast to normal, the length of the right and left main stem bronchi is the same, as is the relation of each bronchus to its pulmonary artery and the configuration of the artery.[L3,P1,V2] People with *asplenia* tend to have bilateral right-sidedness and right atrial isomerism, a condition identified[S10,S11] by finding the right-type configuration of main stem bronchus and its pulmonary artery on both left and right sides (the bronchus is relatively short and posterior and superior to the pulmonary artery, which bifurcates into an upper and lower trunk).[B5,L3,S11] Patients with *polysplenia* tend to have bilateral left-sidedness[M5] and left atrial isomerism, with the left-type configuration of the main stem bronchus and its pulmonary artery on both sides (the bronchus is anterior and inferior to the pulmonary artery, which gives off individual branches, rather than a discrete trunk, to the upper lobe). A determination of situs can sometimes be made by study of the plain chest radiograph.[S1] When there is situs ambiguus, a common atrium is often present, and only the morphology of the atrial appendages indicates whether there is right or left atrial isomerism (see Chapter 44). Complex forms of congenital heart disease tend to occur in patients with atrial isomerism,[L4,L5,M5,S11] although, in rare cases, the heart is normal.

Situs of the Ventricles

In situs solitus, ventricles are said to have normal (usual, concordant) situs when the morphologically right ventricle is anterior and to the right of the morphologically left ventricle, which is posterior and to the left. Van Praagh's term *D-loop*[V6,V9,V10] may be used to describe this ventricular situs, or isomer, as may his term *right-handedness,*[V7,V13] also used by Anderson.[A9] *D-loop* indicates that the *sinus portion* of the morphologically right ventricle is to the right vis-à-vis that of the left. In hearts with D-loop (as described by Van Praagh[V7]), direction of blood flow in the right ventricle is from right to left through the right-sided tricuspid valve and inflow (sinus) portion to the usually left-sided outflow portion (infundibulum). D-loop, or right-handedness, can also be defined as existing when the palmar surface of the right hand can be placed on the septal surface of the right ventricle such that the thumb is in the inlet (tricuspid valve), the wrist is in the apical trabecular component, and the fingers are in the outlet (pulmonary valve).

In situs solitus, ventricles are said to be *inverted* when the morphologically right ventricle is more or less posterior and to the left of the morphologically left ventricle. Van Praagh's term *L-loop* applies here, as does the term *left-handedness.* In L-loop, the sinus (inlet) portion of the morphologically right ventricle is to the left vis-à-vis that of left ventricle; that is, internal organization is opposite of that in D-loop, and direction of blood flow is from the left-sided tricuspid valve to the right-sided infundibulum. L-loop, or left-handedness, can also be defined as existing when the palmar surface of the left hand can be placed on the septal surface of the right ventricle such that the thumb is in the inlet, the wrist is in the apical trabecular component, and the fingers are in the outlet. L.M. Bargeron (UAB; personal communication) suggested that, looking through the right ventricle's AV valve toward its apex, in D-loop the septal structures are to the left and in L-loop they are to the right.

In atrial situs inversus, L-loop is the normal (usual, concordant) situs, and D-loop is the inverted situs. The definitions of loop, or handedness, are independent of atrial or visceral situs and are thus the same as just described. Because there are two possible ventricular situses (D-loop and L-loop) in both atrial situs solitus and atrial situs inversus, there are four basic hearts, an idea expressed many years ago by Stanger, Edwards, and colleagues[S12] (see Appendix 1A).

When thoracic and atrial situs are ambiguus, only ventricular situs can be described, and its relationship to thoracic and atrial situs is "ambiguus."

Completeness of the Ventricles

Both the right and left ventricle may be considered to have inlet, sinus, and outlet portions when complete. Either ventricle may be incomplete (or rudimentary). For example, the inlet portion of the right ventricle is absent in hearts with tricuspid atresia.

Dominance of the Ventricles

Normally, the size (area on biplane cineangiogram) of the two ventricles is similar and can be said to be *balanced.* In many kinds of cardiac conditions, one ventricle is larger, or dominant, and the smaller one and can be severely hypoplastic. The dominance may be mild, moderate, or severe. Generally, a ventricle is said to be dominant only when the other ventricle is too small to maintain adequate pulmonary or systemic blood flow.

Cardiac Connections

Information about cardiac connections is fundamental in describing any malformed heart and requires elucidation at both atrioventricular and ventriculoarterial levels. The *atrioventricular connection* may be *concordant* (right atrium[2] connects to right ventricle; left atrium connects to left ventricle), *discordant* (right atrium connects to left ventricle; left atrium connects to right ventricle), *univentricular* (atria connect to only one ventricle; see Chapter 42 for more details of this subset), or *ambiguus* (situs ambiguus of atria). When an AV valve is straddling, it is considered to be connected to the ventricle into which more than 50% of the valve orifice faces. As Bharati and colleagues have pointed out, it is pertinent to distinguish between straddling of the *valve anulus* across the septum and of the *chordal attachments* into an inappropriate ventricle.[B8] Milo and colleagues suggested that the term *overriding* be used when referring to the anulus, and *straddling* when referring to chordal attachments.[M6]

The *ventriculoarterial connection* may be concordant (left ventricle connects wholly or nearly so to aorta; right ventricle to pulmonary artery) or discordant (right ventricle connects to aorta; left ventricle to pulmonary artery, commonly called transposition of the great artery[V8]). As with atrioventricular connections, when a semilunar valve is overriding a ventricular septal defect, it is considered to be connected to the ventricle from which more than 50% of the valve area arises. The connection may also be *double outlet* (the great arteries arise wholly or for the most part from one ventricle).

The ventriculoarterial connection may be considered *single outlet* when there is a common arterial trunk (truncus arteriosus communis) or only a single artery, usually the aorta, connected to a ventricle. In the latter case, there is usually pulmonary atresia, and categorization as single-outlet ventriculoarterial connection, although morphologically precise, considerably complicates the presentation of information in many types of congenital heart disease. Alternatively, the ventriculoarterial connections can be termed concordant, discordant, or double outlet by identifying the connection, although atretic, of the pulmonary artery to a ventricle. Even when there is a ventriculopulmonary artery discontinuity, this is often possible. For example, when the morphology is typical for tetralogy of Fallot, except that there is only a single ventricular outlet because

---

[2] The adjectives *left* and *right* used to modify atrium or ventricle mean "morphologically right" or "morphologically left." The position of the chamber is referred to as "right-sided" or "left-sided."

of pulmonary atresia, the condition is called tetralogy of Fallot with pulmonary atresia (see Chapter 24).

Cardiac and Arterial Positions

Normally, the cardiac apex points to the left, a situation called *levocardia.* The term *dextrocardia* applies when the cardiac apex points to the right, and *mesocardia* when it is in the midline. There is merit to using the term *dextroversion* to denote dextrocardia with situs solitus of the viscera and atria, and *levoversion* to denote levocardia with situs inversus. Dextroversion and levoversion alter the geometry and position of all cardiac chambers. Thus, the position of the heart is important surgically, but it is not a basic abnormality, as is D- or L-loop. The left atrium is generally to the left and the right atrium to the right in situs solitus, and vice versa in situs inversus.

Position of the ventricles is determined primarily, but not exclusively, by the ventricular situs (loop or handedness). The morphologically right ventricle is usually anterior and to the right in D-loop, and the left ventricle posterior and to the left. Generally, with L-loop (inverted ventricles), the morphologically left ventricle is anterior and to the right, and the morphologically right ventricle posterior and to the left. However, the ventricles may be side by side or directly anteroposterior to each other, with either ventricle in either position. Ventricles may also be in a superoinferior (over and under) position; this occurs most commonly with L-loop, but can occur with D-loop.[V7] This, and probably other positional anomalies, are most clearly seen by echocardiographic and angiographic study and may be entirely overlooked by autopsy studies. Positional interrelations are not basic pathologic entities, but rotational anomalies producing variations of the four basic hearts.

The possible positions of the origins of the great arteries are nearly infinite around the 360° of a circle, but may be simplified as (1) normal, with aorta to the right (in visceroatrial situs solitus) or left (in inversus) and somewhat posterior to the pulmonary artery; (2) aorta anterior to the pulmonary artery, either directly or somewhat to the right (D-malposition[V8]); (3) aorta to the left of the pulmonary artery (L-malposition); and (4) aorta posterior to the pulmonary artery.

Normally, the great arteries tend to cross rather than to run parallel. In contrast, when the great arteries are malposed, their first portions are usually parallel.[D3]

As indicated, these are all positional arterial abnormalities and are not basic parts of a malformation. However, certain probabilities exist. For example, the inflow portion of the right ventricle is usually on the side of the aortic origin.

Atrioventricular Flow Pathways

In normal hearts, atrioventricular flow pathways are more or less parallel. In cases of crisscross atrioventricular flow pathways, they cross over each other. The term *crisscross hearts* was introduced by Ando and colleagues[A6] and by Anderson and colleagues[A4] in 1974, but the condition had been described earlier by Lev and Rowlatt in 1961.[L8]

The phrase *crisscross* has led to confusion and controversy. One point of view is that in some abnormal hearts, the pathways cross when viewed on cineangiography. Another point of view is that this is an illusion.[V11] In any event, *crisscross* has no implications with regard to internal ventricular architecture or atrioventricular connections. The crisscross of the flow pathways is produced by positional abnormalities of the ventricles (often a superior–inferior position). Hypoplasia of the inflow or sinus of the right ventricle often contributes to crisscross. In most cases of crisscross, there is ventriculoarterial discordance and either discordant ventriculoarterial connections or double outlet right ventricle.

Defects and Abnormalities

Defects involving cardiac septa, chambers, and valves occur as more or less isolated anomalies, but are more common when connection and rotational anomalies exist. Such defects must be described separately for each heart, along with segmental situs, connections, and positions of the heart. Possible defects include atrial septal defect, ventricular septal defect, atrioventricular canal, anomalous systemic and pulmonary venous connections, congenital valvar and subvalvar lesions, straddling AV valves, and abnormalities of septal morphology, including conal infundibular development.

Conventional Diagnoses

As a summarizing convenience, certain old and widely used phrases that are in themselves not anatomically specific, but are well understood by surgeons, continue to be useful. In each instance, morphology denoted by a given phrase must be defined, in part because others may use the same phrase (e.g., *transposition of the great arteries*) differently. Such phrases include *AV canal* (see Chapter 20), *tetralogy of Fallot* (see Chapter 24), *Taussig-Bing heart* (see Chapter 39), *complete transposition of the great arteries* (see Chapter 39), *double outlet ventricle* (see Chapters 39 and 40), *corrected transposition of the great arteries* (see Chapter 41), *isolated ventricular inversion* (see Chapter 41), and *anatomically corrected malposition of the great arteries* (see Chapter 43). In the interest of readability, the text does not use quotation marks for these phrases, because, once defined, they are used primarily for convenience.

Symbolic Convention of Van Praagh

Van Praagh's symbolic convention for the heart, for example, S,D,D heart, is widely used and is a convenient and concise way of expressing certain anatomic features and relations.[V5] The first symbol refers to situs (isomerism) of thoracic viscera and atria (S for solitus, I for inversus). The second symbol indicates situs (isomerism) of the ventricles in terms of D-loop and L-loop (see "Situs of the Ventricles"). When taken with the first symbol, it is of fundamental significance in designating which of the four basic hearts, or isomeric combinations, is present. The third symbol refers to position of the aortic origin (D for right-sided, L for left-sided).

APPENDIXES

APPENDIX 1A

Illustrative Models of Congenital Heart Disease

Van Praagh's symbolic representation may be combined with those of atrioventricular and ventricular arterial connections as shown in the figures. In Van Praagh's convention, the first letter (S or I) refers to atrial position (solitus or inversus), the second letter (D or L) to ventricular loop, and the third letter to position of the origin of the aorta (recognized by its two coronary ostia) in relation to origin of the pulmonary trunk.[V12] Arrangement of boxes and abbreviations is identical in all similar models presented.

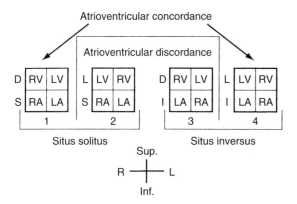

Figure 1A-1   Model of atrioventricular connections of the four basic hearts, excluding situs ambiguus.

Key: *D,* D ventricular loop; *I,* situs inversus; *Inf.,* inferior; *L,* L ventricular loop; *LA,* left atrium; *LV,* left ventricle; *RA,* right atrium; *RV,* right ventricle; *S,* situs; *Sup.,* superior.

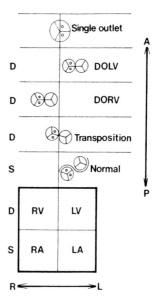

Figure 1A-3   Model of varieties of ventriculoarterial connection. Aortic origin in transposition of the great arteries and the double outlet ventricles (DORV, DOLV) is indicated by *D* when it lies to the right of the pulmonary artery origin and *L* when it lies to the left. When aortic origin is anterior, it is almost always superior to the pulmonary trunk; when side by side, both origins are usually at the same level. Vertical line above the box represents position of the ventricular septum.

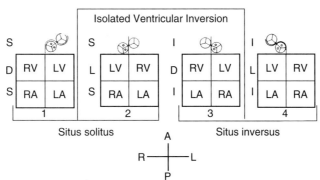

Figure 1A-2   Model of four so-called normal hearts, that is, hearts with atrioventricular and ventriculoarterial concordant connections. Vertical line above the box represents position of the ventricular septum. Note that in situs inversus, the aortic origin lies to the left of the pulmonary trunk origin.

APPENDIX 1B

Normal Pathway Dimensions from Autopsy Specimens

Rowlatt and colleagues provided extensive information about the dimensions (measured as circumference) of cardiac valves in formalin-fixed autopsy specimens from apparently normal children.[R3] Because it is the diameter that is usually measured by echocardiography, angiography, and in the operating room, circumferences have been transformed to diameter, assuming that valve orifices are perfectly circular and using the equation

$$\text{Diameter} = \frac{\text{Circumference}}{\pi}$$

These dimensions can also be expressed in terms of cross-sectional area, using for the transformation the equation

$$\text{Area} = \pi \left[\frac{\text{Diameter}}{2} \right]^2$$

Krovetz[K5] and Westaby and colleagues[W2] also made measurements in autopsy specimens from adults that are compatible with those of Rowlatt and colleagues.[R3] These investigators added the information that as adults age, the size of the aortic orifice gradually enlarges. Eckner and colleagues measured pressure-fixed autopsy specimens and found dimensions similar to but slightly larger than those of Rowlatt and colleagues.[E1]

Scholz and colleagues also present extensive information on cardiac dimensions obtained in autopsy specimens.[S16] Their findings and equations are generally similar to those of Rowlatt and colleagues, except that they find the valve dimensions are best normalized to the age and gender of the individual (rather than to body surface area). These investigators believe that the predicted values from their regression equations are applicable to either fresh or fixed specimens, and that they compare well with systolic anular dimensions obtained by imaging techniques in living subjects.

Most of the information in this book relating dimensions in patients to those obtained at autopsy uses equations derived from the work of Rowlatt and colleagues[R3] to compute the mean normal value and standard deviation, based on the patient's body surface area. Dimensions were expressed as circumference and body surface area as cm^2 by Rowlatt and colleagues. For use in this text, these have been transformed into diameter (assuming that the cross-section was a perfect circle) and m^2. Diameters of cardiac valves for normal individuals are summarized in Table 1B-1.

Capps and colleagues[C5] analyzed 6801 fresh autopsied hearts for valve cryopreservation over the range of 0.18 to 3.55 m^2 body surface area. Mean indexed aortic valve area ($n = 4636$) was 2.02 ± 0.52 $cm^2 \cdot m^{-2}$. Mean diameters of each valve within ranges of body surface area are given in Table 1B-2. Regression equations useful for predicting mean normal aortic and pulmonary valve diameters are given for males, females, and overall in Table 1B-3. This analysis ignores increase in valve size due to aging, which, though normal, may be considered a degenerative process.

■ **TABLE 1B-1   Diameters (mm) of Normal Cardiac Valves** [a]

BSA (m²)	Mitral		Tricuspid		Aortic		Pulmonary	
	Mean	±SD	Mean	±SD	Mean	±SD	Mean	±SD
0.25	11.4	9.8-13.0	13.4	11.8-15.0	7.2	6.2-8.2	8.4	7.3-9.6
0.30	12.5	10.9-14.2	14.9	13.3-16.5	8.1	7.1-9.1	9.3	8.2-10.5
0.35	13.5	11.9-15.2	16.2	14.5-17.8	8.8	7.8-9.8	10.1	8.9-11.2
0.40	14.4	12.7-16.0	17.3	15.6-18.9	9.5	8.5-10.5	10.7	9.6-11.9
0.45	15.1	13.5-16.7	18.2	16.6-19.9	10.1	9.1-11.1	11.3	10.2-12.5
0.50	15.8	14.1-17.4	19.1	17.5-20.7	10.6	9.6-11.6	11.9	10.7-13.0
0.60	16.9	15.3-18.6	20.6	19.0-22.2	11.4	10.4-12.5	12.8	11.6-13.9
0.70	17.9	16.3-19.5	21.9	20.3-23.5	12.2	11.2-13.2	13.5	12.4-14.7
0.80	18.7	17.1-20.4	23.0	21.4-24.6	12.8	11.8-13.8	14.2	13.0-15.3
0.90	19.5	17.8-21.1	24.0	22.3-25.6	13.4	12.4-14.4	14.8	13.6-15.9
1.00	20.1	18.5-21.8	24.8	23.2-26.5	13.9	12.9-14.9	15.3	14.1-16.4
1.20	21.3	19.7-22.9	26.3	24.7-28.0	14.8	13.8-15.8	16.2	15.0-17.4
1.40	22.3	20.6-23.9	27.6	26.0-29.2	15.6	14.6-16.6	17.0	15.8-18.1
1.60	23.1	21.5-24.8	28.7	27.1-30.3	16.2	15.2-17.2	17.6	16.5-18.8
1.80	23.9	22.2-25.5	29.7	28.1-31.3	16.8	15.8-17.8	18.2	17.1-19.4
2.00	24.5	22.9-26.2	30.6	28.9-32.3	17.3	16.3-18.3	18.7	17.6-19.9

Key: *BSA,* Body surface area; *SD,* standard deviation.

[a] Values are based on measurements made in hearts obtained at autopsy from apparently normal children (the oldest was 15 years of age).[R3] The relationship of these measurements to those obtained in other modalities is shown in Appendix Figures 1E-1 to 1E-4.

■ **TABLE 1B-2   Left Ventricular–Aortic Junction (Aortic Valve) and Right Ventricular–Pulmonic Junction (Pulmonary Valve) Diameters in Males and Females According to Body Surface Area (BSA) Range**

BSA Range (m²)	Males Aortic Valve n	Males Aortic Valve Diameter (mm)	Males Pulmonary Valve n	Males Pulmonary Valve Diameter (mm)	Females Aortic Valve n	Females Aortic Valve Diameter (mm)	Females Pulmonary Valve n	Females Pulmonary Valve Diameter (mm)
0.21–0.30	19	8.8 ± 1.0	39	10.4 ± 2.3	20	9.1 ± 0.8	30	10.0 ± 1.1
0.31–0.40	34	10.0 ± 1.6	38	11.7 ± 2.0	30	9.9 ± 0.8	36	11.2 ± 1.2
0.41–0.50	57	11.2 ± 0.9	58	13.3 ± 1.6	32	11.4 ± 1.4	31	13.2 ± 2.2
0.51–0.60	64	12.3 ± 1.2	68	14.5 ± 1.3	50	11.9 ± 1.2	54	13.9 ± 1.6
0.61–0.70	70	13.5 ± 1.3	73	16.0 ± 1.8	35	12.5 ± 1.3	36	15.0 ± 1.8
0.71–0.80	57	14.1 ± 1.1	64	16.6 ± 1.5	31	13.9 ± 1.5	36	16.4 ± 1.8
0.81–0.90	37	14.6 ± 1.5	39	17.6 ± 2.0	30	14.3 ± 1.3	30	17.5 ± 1.9
0.91–1.00	48	15.6 ± 1.3	61	18.7 ± 1.9	32	15.4 ± 1.4	35	18.1 ± 2.0
1.01–1.10	42	16.3 ± 1.5	51	19.5 ± 1.8	30	15.6 ± 1.4	36	18.9 ± 2.0
1.11–1.20	42	17.2 ± 1.9	45	20.4 ± 1.9	21	16.8 ± 1.8	22	19.6 ± 1.6
1.21–1.30	25	17.1 ± 1.6	39	20.6 ± 1.8	23	17.8 ± 2.1	27	20.7 ± 1.9
1.31–1.40	38	18.7 ± 1.7	55	21.6 ± 2.1	47	18.5 ± 2.2	71	21.6 ± 2.3
1.41–1.50	39	19.1 ± 2.3	44	22.3 ± 2.5	122	19.6 ± 2.0	150	22.4 ± 2.1
1.51–1.60	52	20.7 ± 2.4	69	23.5 ± 2.3	175	19.9 ± 1.9	218	22.8 ± 2.1
1.61–1.70	125	20.8 ± 2.1	135	23.7 ± 2.4	267	20.5 ± 1.8	317	23.5 ± 2.0
1.71–1.80	223	21.5 ± 2.0	230	24.5 ± 2.4	218	21.0 ± 1.6	285	24.1 ± 2.0
1.81–1.90	350	22.3 ± 2.1	417	25.2 ± 2.2	148	21.3 ± 1.6	167	24.1 ± 1.9
1.91–2.00	466	22.6 ± 1.7	518	25.7 ± 2.1	109	21.5 ± 1.4	122	24.6 ± 2.0
2.01–2.10	453	23.0 ± 1.8	525	26.2 ± 2.1	77	21.6 ± 1.4	75	24.8 ± 2.0
2.11–2.20	266	23.6 ± 1.9	309	26.8 ± 2.0	46	21.9 ± 1.5	68	25.0 ± 1.8
2.21–2.30	172	23.8 ± 1.8	210	26.8 ± 2.0	31	21.8 ± 1.5	39	25.5 ± 1.9
2.31–2.40	115	24.1 ± 1.9	134	27.3 ± 1.9	25	22.0 ± 1.5	34	25.0 ± 3.1
2.41–2.50	85	24.4 ± 1.9	133	27.5 ± 1.7	11	22.5 ± 1.6	14	26.0 ± 2.3
2.51–2.60	43	24.8 ± 1.8	45	27.8 ± 1.8	8	22.6 ± 1.2	7	26.0 ± 1.5
2.61–2.70	33	25.2 ± 2.3	47	28.1 ± 1.9	8	22.3 ± 1.0	8	26.1 ± 2.1
2.71–2.80	8	24.3 ± 2.4	15	27.5 ± 2.5	8	22.0 ± 1.7	8	26.1 ± 2.3
2.81–2.90	8	25.8 ± 1.8	21	28.2 ± 1.3	3	22.3 ± 1.5	5	26.2 ± 2.3

(Data modified from CryoLife, Inc., 1999.)

Key: BSA (m²) = 0.024265 • weight (kg)$^{0.5378}$ • height (cm)$^{0.3964}$ (from Haycock and colleagues[H5]).

■ **TABLE 1B-3   Regression Coefficients of Valve Anulus Diameter (mm) on BSA (m²)[a]**

Structure	n	Intercept (b₀)	Slope (b₁)	SD
Male				
AVD	2993	2.785 ± 0.0025	0.4777 ± 0.0037	0.08927
PVD	3508	2.936 ± 0.0022	0.4455 ± 0.0032	0.08835
Female				
AVD	1643	2.769 ± 0.0029	0.4517 ± 0.0050	0.09293
PVD	1972	2.913 ± 0.0028	0.4425 ± 0.0047	0.09563
Overall				
AVD	4636	2.778 ± 0.0019	0.4727 ± 0.0030	0.09167
PVD	5480	2.926 ± 0.0018	0.4483 ± 0.0027	0.09179

(Modified from Capps and colleagues.[C5])

Key: *AVD*, Aortic valve anulus diameter; *BSA*, body surface area; *PVD*, pulmonary valve anulus diameter; *SD*, standard deviation.

[a] General form of equation: predicted diameter = exp(intercept + slope • Ln[BSA]), where exp is the base of the natural logarithms (Ln).

APPENDIX 1C

Normal Pathway Dimensions from Cineangiography

Bini and colleagues measured the cardiac and great artery dimensions, at peak systole and in diastole, on cineangiograms made in both anteroposterior and lateral projections in 42 normal children (Bini M, Naftel DC, Blackstone EM: unpublished study; 1984). Median age of the children was 12 months, range 2 days to 16 years. Twenty-five percent were 2 months of age or younger, and 25% were 67 months of age or older. Twenty-four were males and 18 were females. Consideration of adoption was usually the indication for study. Structures measured included midportion of the right ventricular infundibulum and junction of the right ventricle and pulmonary artery ("anulus");

distal end of the pulmonary trunk; origin, midportion, and immediately prebranching portion of the right pulmonary artery; origin and immediately prebranching portion of the left pulmonary artery; and aorta immediately downstream to the aortic valve, immediately before the takeoff of the innominate artery, and immediately above the diaphragm. By dividing the measured internal diameter of the cardiac catheter in the same frame by the known internal diameter of the catheter, a correction factor was calculated and used to correct the measured value for magnification.

To account for increased scatter of dimension data as body surface area increased, logarithmic transformations were made of both dimension and body size. Individual regression equations (derived only when the number of observations was greater than 10) were developed for each location, and individually for systole and diastole in the anteroposterior and lateral projections. Mean normal diameter and standard deviation according to body surface area were derived from these equations. A similar analysis of cineangiographic measurements was made earlier by Sievers and colleagues.[S13] Both groups, working without knowledge of the other, found logarithmic transformation to express the relations best. Information for the equations is presented in Tables 1C-1 and 1C-2. The equations may be used to calculate the mean normal dimensions and standard deviations of the right ventricular outflow tract and pulmonary arteries for a specific body surface area, for use in determining the Z value of the dimension of a structure in a patient.

Dimensions of a part of the left ventricular tract and aorta were also determined by Bini and by Sievers and their colleagues[S13] (Bini M, Naftel DC, Blackstone EH: unpublished study; 1984) (see Tables 1C-1 and 1C-2). Clarkson and Brandt made measurements of the aorta in cineangiograms of normal infants and young children,[C2] similar to those of Bini and colleagues.

Most of the information is this book relating patient dimensions to Z values based on cineangiographic measurements uses regression equations derived from the measurements made by Bini and colleagues, which are similar to those made by Sievers and colleagues[S13] (see Tables 1C-1 and 1C-2). Unfortunately, they did not measure the tricuspid valve. These equations are used to calculate normal mean

■ **TABLE 1C–1   Coefficients of the Linear Regression Equation Relating Diameter in the Anteroposterior Projection to Body Surface Area in Normal Subjects[a]**

Structure	Systole					Diastole					Average[b]				
	n	Scale Factor (Intercept)	Exponent (Slope)	SD (Logarithmic Domain)	r	n	Scale Factor (Intercept)	Exponent (Slope)	SD (Logarithmic Domain)	r	n	Scale Factor (Intercept)	Exponent (Slope)	SD (Logarithmic Domain)	r
RV infundibulum	—	—	—	—	—	—	—	—	—	—	—	—	—	—	—
Pulmonary trunk															
Right ventricular–PA junction	29	2.897	0.6033	0.1406	0.94	26	2.929	0.5460	0.1260	0.94	26	2.909	0.5647	0.1200	0.94
Midportion	—	—	—	—	—	—	—	—	—	—	—	—	—	—	—
Right pulmonary artery															
Origin	34	2.787	0.6768	0.1519	0.94	34	2.672	0.6557	0.1478	0.94	34	2.732	0.6664	0.1452	0.95
Midportion	32	2.671	0.6886	0.1636	0.94	32	2.562	0.6591	0.1587	0.94	32	2.619	0.6751	0.1550	0.94
Prebranching	34	2.784	0.6340	0.1422	0.94	34	2.684	0.5924	0.1743	0.91	34	2.737	0.6149	0.1498	0.93
Left pulmonary artery															
Origin	17	2.692	0.7079	0.1470	0.95	17	2.592	0.6803	0.1428	0.95	7	2.645	0.6947	0.1329	0.96
Prebranching	27	2.694	0.7075	0.1650	0.94	26	2.605	0.6652	0.1908	0.94	26	2.651	0.6860	0.1692	0.93
RPA + LPA diameters	27	3.450	0.6727	0.1318	0.96	26	3.340	0.6171	0.1504	0.96	26	3.400	0.6484	0.1421	0.94
Aorta															
Left ventricular–aortic junction	—	—	—	—	—	—	—	—	—	—	—	—	—	—	—
Commissural level	31	2.960	0.5057	0.1488	0.91	31	2.872	0.5137	0.1596	0.90	31	2.918	0.5095	0.1513	0.91
Preinnominate	28	2.899	0.5183	0.1173	0.94	28	2.803	0.5232	0.1265	0.93	28	2.852	0.5208	0.1178	0.94
Descending thoracic at diaphragm	35	2.506	0.4694	0.1530	0.89	35	2.447	0.4814	0.1701	0.87	35	2.478	0.4755	0.1580	0.88

(From Bini M, Naftel DC, Blackstone EH: Unpublished study; 1984.)

Key: *LPA*, Left pulmonary artery; *r*, correlation coefficient; *PA*, pulmonary artery; *RV*, right ventricular; *RPA*, right pulmonary artery; *SD*, standard deviation.

[a]Normal structure size (diameter or cross-sectional area) is calculated as Ln[size(diameter or cross-sectional area)] = scale factor + exponent • Ln(BSA), where body surface area (BSA) is expressed as square meters. Size can then be obtained by exponential transformation (e taken to the power of the logarithm). If diameter is used, coefficients are as shown in the table. If cross-sectional area is used, a circular lumen is assumed and the coefficients modified by multiplying the scale factor by 2 and subtracting 0.2415645 from the value obtained [Ln(π) − 2Ln(2)], by multiplying the exponent by 2, and by multiplying the standard deviation by 2. In all instances $P < .0001$.

The Z value (number of standard deviations a structure is above or below normal size) is calculated from the observed size as the logarithm of the observed size minus the calculated logarithm of normal size, divided by the standard deviation. Because the analysis uses the logarithmic transformation, Z obtained using diameters is identical to one using cross-sectional area.

All logarithms are natural logarithms.

[b](Systolic + diastolic diameters)/2.

■ **TABLE 1C–2   Coefficients of the Linear Regression Equation Relating Diameter in the Lateral Projection to Body Surface Area in Normal Subjects[a]**

| | Systole | | | | | Diastole | | | | | Average[b] | | | | |
Structure	n	Scale Factor (Intercept)	Exponent (Slope)	SD (Logarithmic Domain)	r	n	Scale Factor (Intercept)	Exponent (Slope)	SD (Logarithmic Domain)	r	n	Scale Factor (Intercept)	Exponent (Slope)	SD (Logarithmic Domain)	r
RV infundibulum	23	2.549	0.4080	0.1337	0.89	23	2.929	0.3450	0.1153	0.89	23	2.7600	0.3720	0.1080	0.91
Pulmonary trunk															
Right ventricular–PA junction	29	2.863	0.4664	0.1326	0.92	29	2.898	0.4602	0.1120	0.94	29	2.883	0.4642	0.1115	0.94
Midportion	22	3.127	0.6292	0.1327	0.95	25	2.965	0.5725	0.1350	0.94	22	3.052	0.6037	0.1254	0.95
Right pulmonary artery															
Origin	—	—	—	—	—	—	—	—	—	—	—	—	—	—	—
Midportion															
Prebranching															
Left pulmonary artery															
Origin	—	—	—	—	—	—	—	—	—	—	—	—	—	—	—
Prebranching	19	2.639	0.7213	0.1922	0.90	19	2.500	0.7146	0.2447	0.85	19	2.573	0.7178	0.2101	0.88
RPA + LPA diameters	—	—	—	—	—	—	—	—	—	—	—	—	—	—	—
Aorta															
Left ventricular–aortic junction	24	2.929	0.4220	0.1249	0.90	24	2.833	0.4440	0.1406	0.89	24	2.879	0.4320	0.1302	0.90
Commissural level	29	2.985	0.5310	0.1896	0.87	29	2.896	0.5174	0.1987	0.85	29	2.942	0.5247	0.1910	0.86
Preinnominate	27	2.864	0.5098	0.1609	0.87	27	2.811	0.5209	0.1625	0.87	27	2.838	0.5151	0.1591	0.88
Descending thoracic at diaphragm	27	2.462	0.4576	0.1817	0.82	27	2.389	0.4546	0.1751	0.83	27	2.427	0.4564	0.1755	0.83

(From Bini M, Naftel DC, Blackstone EH: Unpublished study; 1984, except for the values for the RV infundibulum, which are from Sievers and colleagues.[513])

[a,b] Key and footnotes a and b are identical to those for Table 1C-1.

values and standard deviations according to the patient's body surface area; then the equation given in the earlier section entitled "Standardization of Dimensions" is used to calculate the Z value. These equations and nomograms are for diameter. Some prefer to express the dimensions of the pulmonary arteries as cross-sectional area. Because of the logarithmic transformation used in the Bini and Sievers analyses, the Z value for cross-sectional area is the same as that for diameter.

APPENDIX 1D

Normal Pathway Dimensions from Two–Dimensional Echocardiography

Dimensions obtained by two-dimensional echocardiography are sometimes measured and expressed as length of anulus (without a commitment as to the shape of the orifice), sometimes as the shortest axis (anteroposterior) and the longest axis (lateral), and sometimes as cross-sectional area measured directly on the two-dimensional echocardiographic image, without an assumption as to shape. Sometimes both the smallest and largest dimensions in a cardiac cycle are measured and expressed.

King and colleagues provided two-dimensional echocardiographic measurements of the largest diameter of the mitral and tricuspid valves in apparently normal children.[K4] These can be used for determining the normal mean values and standard deviations necessary for calculating the Z values in individual patients. Tei and colleagues provided similar measurements of the tricuspid valve.[T5] Their mean value for area was 6.1 ± 0.9 cm$^2 \cdot$ m^{-2} at the moment when the valve was largest, and 4.1 ± 0.6 cm$^2 \cdot$ m^{-2} when it was smallest; anular circumference was 7.8 ± 0.7 cm$^2 \cdot$ m^{-2} and 5.2 ± 0.5 cm$^2 \cdot$ m^{-2}, respectively. These values correspond well with the data presented by King and colleagues. Riggs and colleagues[R4] presented information on mitral valve area and diameters in normal children and derived a regression equation normalizing these to body surface area. These values are similar to those of King and colleagues[K4] with regard to the anteroposterior dimensions, but are smaller in the lateral dimensions. Pollick and colleagues reported dimensions in normal children that were similar to those obtained by Riggs.[P3]

Daubeney and colleagues[D4] have provided a comprehensive cata-log of cardiac structural dimensions by two-dimensional echocardiography in normal infants and children. Definition of each dimension and the two-dimensional echocardiographic view in which it was measured are given in Table 1D-1. For the most part, a regression equation was developed using body surface area in the logarithmic transformation domain. The regression equation is

$$\text{Ln[Mean normal diameter (mm)]} = \text{Intercept} + \text{Slope} \cdot \text{Ln(BSA)}$$

where mean normal diameter is specific for body surface area (BSA), BSA is expressed in square meters, and Ln is the natural logarithm. The values for the intercept and the slope, as well as for the standard deviations (root mean square error), are presented in Table 1D-2. Values are the largest ones during the cardiac cycle, nearly always at end-diastole. The Z value equation (see "Standardization of Dimensions") can then be used to calculate the Z value. More simply, a nomogram (Fig. 1D-1) may be used.

Dimensions of mitral and tricuspid valves were measured using two-dimensional echocardiography by King and colleagues.[K4] Based on these data, regression equations were developed for mean normal diameter (logarithmic transformation) and body surface area (logarithmic transformation) as shown in Table 1D-3. A digital nomogram is presented in Table 1D-4.

Dimensions of the left ventricular–aortic junction (aortic "anulus") in normal children were measured using two-dimensional echocardiography by Habbal and Somerville.[H2] Their regression equation relating mean normal value to body surface area is

$$\text{Mean normal value} = 17.20[1 - \exp(-2.486 \cdot \text{BSA})] + 0.4663 \cdot \text{BSA}^{4.622}$$

where Ln is the natural logarithm, and exp is e, the base of the natural logarithms. The standard deviation is 0.09717. The standard deviation was obtained in the log-log domain to stabilize the variability. Therefore, as in the case of the analysis of cineangiographic data by Bini and colleagues and the analysis of two-dimensional echocardiography by Daubeney and colleagues,[D4] the Z value for cross-sectional area in a given patient is the same as for diameter, because of the logarithmic transformations used.

Snider and colleagues measured, in children, cross-sectional dimensions of the right pulmonary artery and pulmonary trunk[S15] using two-dimensional echocardiography. The regression equation is

$$\text{Mean normal diameter (mm)} = \text{Intercept} + \text{Slope} \cdot \sqrt{\text{BSA}}$$

where BSA is expressed in square meters. Values for the intercept and slope are given in Table 1D-5. Insufficient numeric data are presented to permit derivation of the standard deviation for the mean normal diameter; therefore, Z values cannot be derived from this analysis.

■ TABLE 1D-1   Cardiac Dimensions Measured, Echocardiographic Views Used, and Definitions of Each Measurement

Cardiac Dimension	Echocardiographic View	Definition
Tricuspid valve	Apical four chamber	Distance between "hinge points" of leaflets at level of anulus
RV–pulmonic junction	Parasternal short axis	Distance between "hinge points" of attachment of the valve
Pulmonary trunk	Parasternal short axis	Diameter of pulmonary trunk half-way between RV–pulmonic junction and bifurcation
Right pulmonary artery	Parasternal short axis	Diameter immediately beyond bifurcation
Left pulmonary artery	Parasternal short axis	Diameter immediately beyond bifurcation
Mitral valve (anteroposterior)	Parasternal long axis	Distance between "hinge points" of leaflets at level of anulus
Mitral valve (lateral)	Apical four chamber	Distance between "hinge points" of leaflets at level of anulus
LV–aortic junction	Parasternal long axis	Distance between "hinge points" of attachment of the valve
Sinuses of Valsalva	Parasternal long axis	Maximum anteroposterior diameter of aortic root at level of sinuses of Valsalva
Sinotubular junction	Parasternal long axis	Maximum anteroposterior diameter of aortic root at level of sinotubular junction

Key: *LV*, Left ventricular; *RV*, right ventricular.

■ TABLE 1D-2   Regression Equations Relating Cardiac Dimension and Body Surface Area[a]

Structure	n	Intercept	Slope	SD	r
Tricuspid valve	120	1.084	0.4945	0.08121	0.97
RV–pulmonic junction	105	0.6367	0.5028	0.1143	0.95
Pulmonary trunk	80	0.6067	0.4941	0.1430	0.93
Right pulmonary artery	81	0.1396	0.5495	0.1294	0.95
Left pulmonary artery	112	0.2024	0.6039	0.1446	0.94
Mitral valve (anteroposterior)	124	0.9445	0.5022	0.09403	0.96
Mitral valve (lateral)	124	0.9651	0.4658	0.09167	0.96
Aortic valve	122	0.5183	0.5347	0.06726	0.98
Sinuses of Valsalva	122	0.7224	0.5082	0.07284	0.98
Sinotubular junction	85	0.5417	0.5490	0.08656	0.98

(From Daubeney and colleagues.[D4])

Key: *LV*, Left ventricular; *r*, correlation coefficient; *RV*, right ventricular; *SD*, standard deviation (root mean square error).

[a] The form of the equation is Ln[mean normal value of structure] = intercept + slope·Ln[BSA], where *Ln* is the natural logarithm and *BSA* is body surface area (m^2). The structures are expressed in cm or cm^2. Z can be calculated as Z = [Ln(measured structure) − Ln(mean normal value)]/SD.

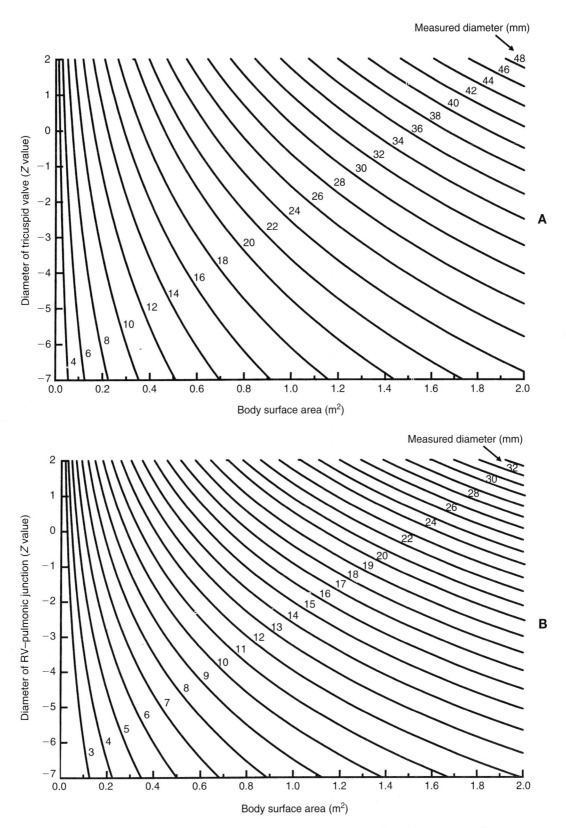

Figure 1D-1   Nomograms expressing measured diameter of the indicated structure (isobars) in an individual of a given body surface area (horizontal axis) as a Z value (vertical axis). Mean normal values and standard deviations used in equations to calculate Z values were obtained from Daubeney and colleagues[D4] (see Table 1D-2). **A**, Tricuspid valve. **B**, Right ventricular–pulmonic junction (pulmonary valve).   *Continued*

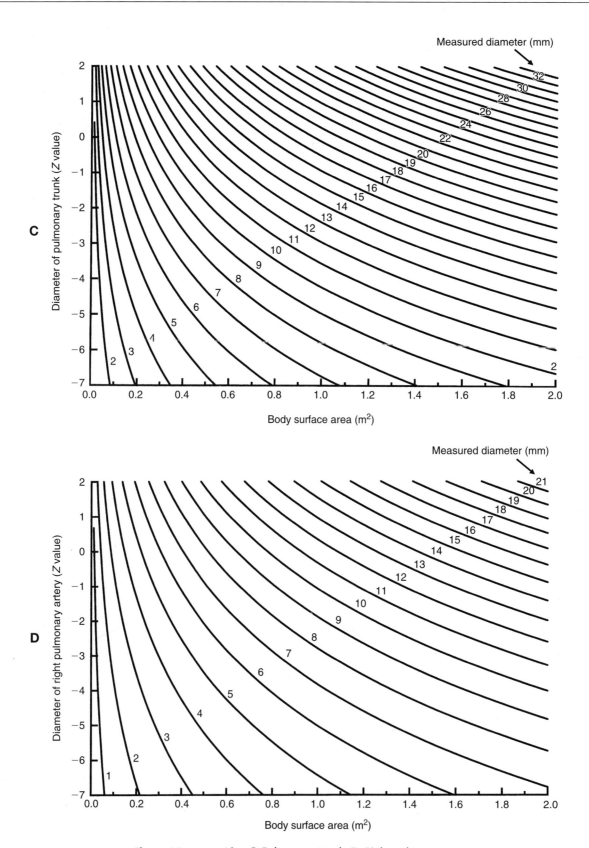

Figure 1D-1—cont'd **C,** Pulmonary trunk. **D,** Right pulmonary artery.

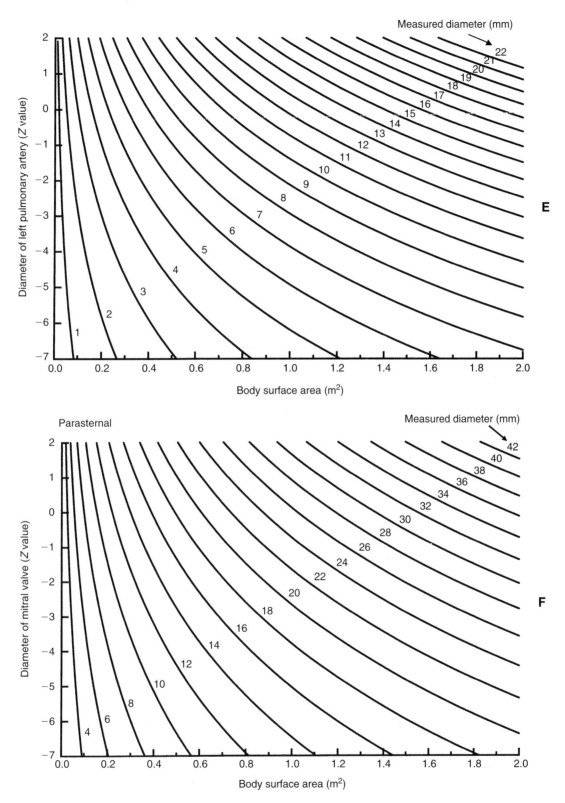

Figure 1D-1–cont'd   **E,** Left pulmonary artery. **F,** Mitral valve (anteroposterior, parasternal long axis view).

Continued

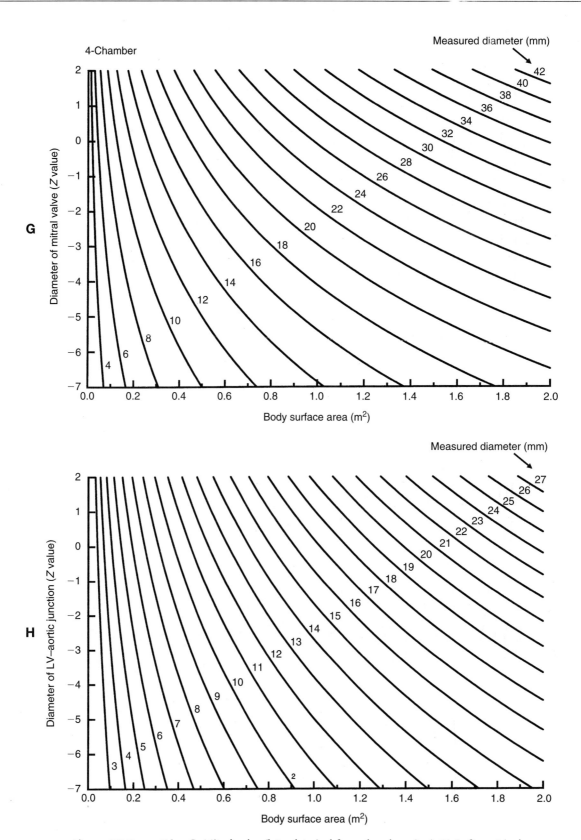

Figure 1D-1—cont'd **G,** Mitral valve (lateral, apical four-chamber view). **H,** Left ventricular–aortic junction (aortic valve).

Key: *LV,* Left ventricular.

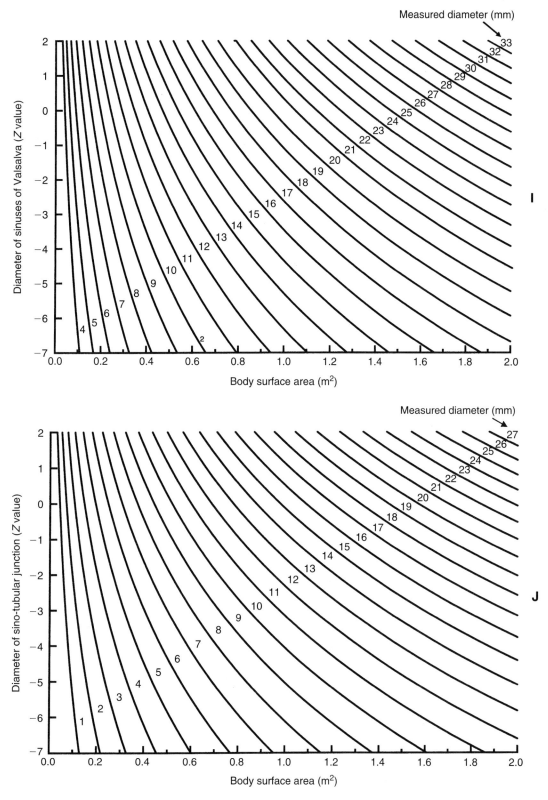

Figure 1D-1—cont'd   I, Sinuses of Valsalva. **J**, Sinotubular junction.

■ **TABLE 1D-3**   **Values for the Intercept, Slope, and Standard Deviation Describing Normal Echocardiographic Diameters**

Structure and Axis	Intercept	Slope	SD
Mitral valve			
Anteroposterior [a]	23.9	8.56	1.8
Lateral [b]	32.3	12.47	3.2
Tricuspid valve	34.4	12.29	3.4

(Based on data from King and colleagues.[K4])

Key: *SD,* Standard deviation.

[a] Measured in parasternal long-axis projection.

[b] Measured in four-chamber view.

■ **TABLE 1D-4**   **Diameters of Mitral and Tricuspid Valves in Normal Children, Using Echocardiography to Measure Dimension of the Valve**

	Mitral Valve				Tricuspid Valve Major Axis (Lat)	
	Minor Axis (A-P)		Major Axis (Lat)			
BSA	Mean (mm)	±SD	Mean (mm)	±SD	Mean (mm)	±SD
0.25	12.0	10.2-13.8	15.0	11.8-18.2	15.4	12.0-18.8
0.30	13.6	11.8-15.4	17.3	14.1-20.5	17.6	14.2-21.0
0.35	14.9	13.1-16.7	19.2	16.0-22.4	19.5	16.1-22.9
0.40	16.1	14.3-17.9	20.9	17.7-24.1	21.1	17.7-24.5
0.45	17.1	15.3-18.9	22.3	19.1-25.5	22.6	19.2-26.0
0.50	18.0	16.2-19.8	23.7	20.5-26.9	23.9	20.5-27.3
0.60	19.5	17.7-21.3	25.9	22.7-29.1	26.1	22.7-29.5
0.70	20.8	19.0-22.6	27.9	24.7-31.1	28.0	24.6-31.4
0.80	22.0	20.2-23.8	29.5	26.3-32.7	29.7	26.3-33.1
0.90	23.0	21.2-24.8	31.0	27.8-34.2	31.1	27.7-34.5
1.00	23.9	22.1-25.7	32.3	29.1-35.5	32.4	29.0-35.8
1.20	25.5	23.7-27.3	34.6	31.4-37.8	34.6	31.2-38.0
1.40	26.8	25.0-28.6	36.5	33.3-39.7	36.5	33.1-39.9
1.60	27.9	26.1-29.7	38.2	35.0-41.4	38.2	34.8-41.6
1.80	28.9	27.1-30.7	39.6	36.4-42.8	39.6	36.2-43.0
2.00	29.8	28.0-31.6	40.9	37.7-44.1	40.9	37.5-44.3

(Based on data from King and colleagues.[K1])

Key: *A-P,* Anteroposterior; *BSA,* body surface area; *Lat,* lateral; *SD,* standard deviation.

■ **TABLE 1D-5**   **Coefficients for Use in the Normal Pulmonary Arterial Dimension Equation**

Structure and View (in Diastole)	Intercept	Slope
Right pulmonary artery		
Suprasternal long axis	−0.0149	11.84
Parasternal short axis	1.50	8.31
Suprasternal short axis	−0.0372	11.60
Pulmonary trunk		
Parasternal short axis	0.946	15.44

(Based on data from Snider and colleagues.[S15])

APPENDIX 1E

Comparison of Pathway Dimensions from Different Measurement Modalities

Comparisons between Cineangiographic Dimensions and Those Obtained at Autopsy

The relationship of measurements obtained by imaging techniques to those obtained from autopsy specimens is arguable, but as was expressed earlier, this is not critical in studies relating dimensions to outcome when the Z value is used. Differences relating to measurement modalities are nonetheless interesting.

Dimensions obtained from autopsy data are probably the most complete and reliable dimensions available. Even among postmortem direct measurements of dimensions, however, differences exist. As stated earlier, Scholz and colleagues found that dimensions are similar in both fresh and fixed specimens (except that when pressure fixation is used, the tricuspid valve and right heart dimensions are somewhat larger) and that dimensions in autopsy specimens from normal children are similar to those obtained by imaging techniques.[S16] However, Alboliras and colleagues obtained data indicating that autopsy measurements should be multiplied by 1.04 to be comparable to cineangiographic measurements.[A12] Bull and colleagues derived a multiplication factor of 1.4 for this purpose.[B10]

A comparison of the carefully performed cineangiographic measurements of Sievers and colleagues[S13] with those of Rowlatt and colleagues[R3] indicates that the normal dimensions for the left ventricular–aortic junction were about 40% larger cineangiographically than at autopsy (Fig. 1E-1). A similar comparison of the dimensions of the right ventricular–pulmonary artery junction indicated that in subjects of less than about 1 m^2 body surface area, cineangiographic measurements were about 17% larger, and that in larger subjects, cineangiographic measurements were 33% larger (Fig. 1E-2).

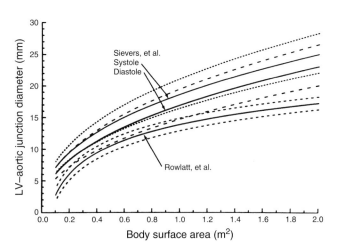

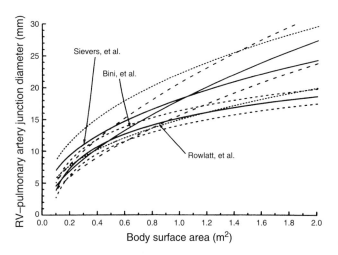

Figure 1E-1   Relation between diameter of the left ventricular–aortic junction (aortic "anulus") and body surface area, according to whether the measurements were made in fixed autopsy specimens (Rowlatt and colleagues[R3]) or by cineangiography (Sievers and colleagues[S13]). Solid lines represent continuous point estimates of the relations, and dashed lines enclose 70% confidence interval.

Figure 1E-2   Relation between diameter of the right ventricular–pulmonary artery junction (pulmonary "anulus") and body surface area, according to whether measurements were made on fixed autopsy specimens (Rowlatt and colleagues[R3]) or by cineangiography (Sievers and colleagues[S13] and Bini M, Naftel DC, Blackstone EH: Unpublished study; 1984). Meanings of the depictions are as described for Fig. 1E-1.

Sepehri and colleagues found that in diseased states in children, dimensions of the left ventricular–aortic junction obtained at autopsy were similar to those obtained from cineangiography, whereas those of the mitral valve obtained by cineangiography were approximately 16% larger than those obtained at autopsy.[S17] These same investigators, using a perfusion fixation technique, found the tricuspid valve to be about 50% larger by cineangiography and the pulmonary valve about 14% larger, thereby confirming the statements of Scholz and colleagues.[S16]

Comparisons between Two-Dimensional Echocardiographic Dimensions and Those Obtained at Autopsy

An informal comparison between the echocardiographic measurements of the mitral valve by King and colleagues[K4] and those obtained at autopsy by Rowlatt and colleagues[R3] suggests that in subjects who have less than about 0.5 m² body surface area, the echocardiographic dimensions are about 33% larger (Fig. 1E-3). A similar comparison between the echocardiographic dimensions ob-

tained by Riggs and colleagues[R4] and those obtained in autopsy specimens by Rowlatt and colleagues[R3] indicates that the dimensions were similar in small subjects, but the echocardiographically determined dimensions were about 20% larger in patients with body surface areas greater than 1 m².

Other Comparisons

Formal comparisons of dimensions of cardiac structures in normal subjects obtained by angiography and echocardiography are missing. However, N.C. Nanda (personal communication; 1989) believes that in diseased states, echocardiographic dimensions are slightly larger than angiographic ones, probably because different bordering structures are used to define the dimension in these two different imaging techniques.

It is particularly difficult to compare dimensions derived from all three modalities. However, a comparison made for the tricuspid valve suggests that there is considerable difference in dimensions obtained using different measurement modalities (Fig. 1E-4).

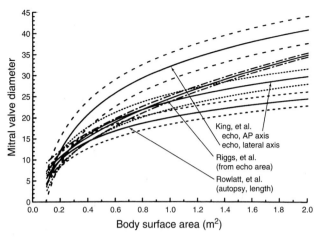

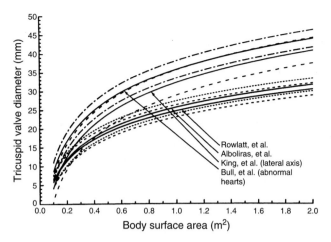

Figure 1E-3   Relation between diameter of the mitral valve orifice and body surface area, according to whether the measurements were made in fixed autopsy specimens (Rowlatt and colleagues[R3]) measuring circumference or by echocardiography (King and colleagues[K4] measuring major and minor axes; Riggs and colleagues[R4] measuring area directly). Meanings of the depictions are as described for Fig. 1E-1.

Key: *AP*, Anterior–posterior.

Figure 1E-4   Relation between diameter of the tricuspid valve and body surface area, according to whether the measurements were made in fixed autopsy specimens (Rowlatt and colleagues[R3]), by cineangiography (Alboliras and colleagues,[A12] Bull and colleagues[B10]), or by echocardiography (King and colleagues[K4]). Meanings of the depictions are as described for Fig. 1E-1.

APPENDIX 1F

Comparison of Methods for Normalizing the Dimensions of Pulmonary Arteries

Four data sets were used to derive the interrelationships among three methods of expressing the dimensions of the right and left pulmonary arteries: (1) 35 normal children among the 42 studied by Bini and colleagues (see Appendix 1C), (2) 168 patients who had undergone repair of tetralogy of Fallot with pulmonary stenosis, whose cineangiograms were made before any surgical procedure,[S20] (3) 215 patients with tetralogy of Fallot and pulmonary atresia,[S19] and (4) 106 patients who had undergone the Fontan operation.[F2]

The comparisons are expressed in Figs. 1F-1, 1F-2, and 1F-3.

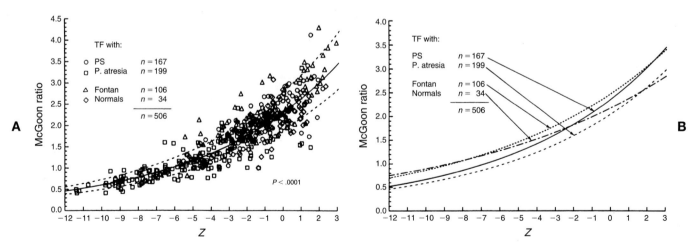

Figure 1F-1   Relation between the McGoon ratio and the *Z* value for summed diameters of the right and left pulmonary arteries just before the takeoff of their first branch. **A,** Analysis of all patients as a single group. Symbols represent an individual patient's values, the solid line represents the continuous point estimate of the relation, and dashed lines enclose 70% confidence interval. The regression equation is

$$\text{McGoon ratio} = 2.355 \cdot \exp(0.1356 \cdot Z)$$

where exp is *e*, the base of the natural logarithms. **B,** Individual analysis of each of the four groups. No confidence limits are displayed.

Key: *P,* Pulmonary; *PS,* pulmonary stenosis; *TF,* tetralogy of Fallot.

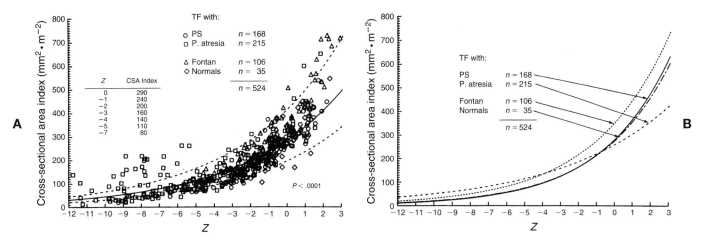

Figure 1F-2   Relation between cross-sectional area index (mm^2 · m^{-2}), the so-called Nakata index, and Z value for summed diameters of the right and left pulmonary arteries just before takeoff of their first branch. **A,** Analysis of all patients as a single group. Meanings of the depictions are as described for Fig. 1F-1. The regression equation is

$$\text{CSA index} = 288.6 \cdot \exp(0.1856 \cdot Z)$$

where exp is *e*, the base of the natural logarithms. **B,** Individual analysis of each of the four groups. No confidence limits are displayed.

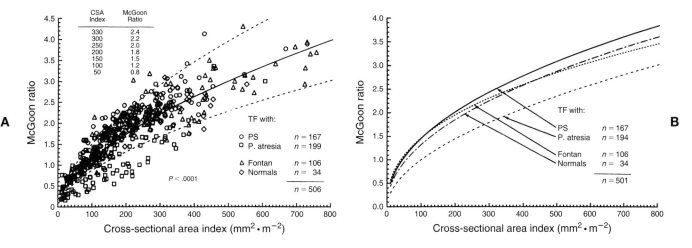

Figure 1F-3   Relation between the McGoon ratio and cross-sectional area index (mm^2 · m^{-2}). **A,** Analysis of all patients as a single group. Meanings of the depictions are as described for Fig. 1F-1. The regression equation is

$$\text{McGoon ratio} = 0.07332 \cdot \text{CSA Index}^{0.5992}$$

B, Individual analysis of each of the four groups. No confidence limits are displayed.

Key: *CSA,* Cross-sectional area; *P,* pulmonary; *PS,* pulmonary stenosis; *TF,* tetralogy of Fallot.

APPENDIX 1G

Normal Ventricular Volume, Masses, and Dimensions from Different Measurement Modalities

Right and left ventricular dimensions and area, left ventricular wall thickness and mass, and septal thickness were measured by echocardiography (Table 1G-1).[D4] Regression equations are presented in Table 1G-2. The information is presented in pairs of figures (Fig. 1G-1).

In addition to the measurements of Daubeney and colleagues,[D4] the relation between right ventricular end-diastolic volume (RVEDV) and body surface area (BSA) was presented by Graham and colleagues,[G5] Thilenius and Arcilla,[T6] Nakazawa and colleagues,[N3] and Lange and colleagues.[L9] Graham's equation and its use for Z values is

$$\text{Ln (mean normal RVEDV, mL)} = 4.162 + 1.340 \text{ Ln (BSA, m}^2)$$

and

$$Z = \frac{\text{Ln (observed RVEDV)} - \text{Ln (mean normal RVEDV)}}{0.2710}$$

where 0.2710 is the standard deviation and Ln is the natural logarithm.

The relation between right ventricular end-systolic volume (RVESV) and BSA was presented by Graham and colleagues,[G5] Thilenius and Arcilla,[T6] and Lange and colleagues.[L9] Graham's equation and its use for Z values is

$$\text{Ln (mean normal RVESV, mL)} = 3.692 + 1.284 \text{ Ln (BSA, m}^2)$$

and

$$Z = \frac{\text{Ln (observed RVESV)} - \text{Ln (normal RVESV)}}{0.3211}$$

The mean normal value for right ventricular infundibular wall thickness from Rowlatt and colleagues[R3] is 2.962 ± 0.779 mm and

$$Z = \frac{\text{Observed wall thickness} - 2.962}{0.779}$$

The mean normal value for right ventricular wall thickness in the area of the tricuspid valve is 3.117 ± 1.55 mm and

$$Z = \frac{\text{Observed wall thickness} - 3.117}{1.155}$$

The relation between heart weight and BSA was studied by Kitzman and colleagues,[K6] Scholz and colleagues,[S16] and Rowlatt and colleagues[R3] (Table 1G-3; see p. 61). The regression equation in all cases is

$$\text{Ln (mean normal heart weight, g)} = \text{Intercept} + \text{Slope} \cdot \text{Ln (BSA, m}^2)$$

The values are for intercept and slope. The Z value equation for heart weight is

$$Z = \frac{\text{Ln (observed weight)} - \text{Ln (normal weight)}}{\text{SD}}$$

where SD is standard deviation.

■ TABLE 1G-1 Cardiac Dimensions Measured, Echocardiographic Views Used, and Definitions of Each Measurement

Cardiac Dimension	Echocardiographic View	Definition
RV inflow	Apical four chamber	Ventricular length from midpoint of plane of tricuspid valve anulus to apex of RV
RV outflow	Subcostal parasagittal	Perpendicular from RV free wall to midpoint of RV pulmonic junction
RV area	Apical four chamber	Maximal area bordered by RV endocardium (excludes area of papillary muscles)
LV inflow	Apical four chamber	Ventricular length from midpoint of plane of mitral valve anulus to apex of LV
LV end-diastolic dimension	M-mode, parasternal long axis	M-mode measurement of a line of inquiry of the two-dimensional echocardiogram at the level of the tips of the mitral leaflet at onset of QRS
LV end-systolic dimension	M-mode, parasternal long axis	M-mode measurement of a line of inquiry of the two-dimensional echocardiogram at the level of the tips of the mitral leaflet, narrowest dimension
LV area	Apical four chamber	Maximal area bordered by LV endocardium (excludes area of papillary muscles)
Interventricular septum	M-mode, parasternal long axis	M-mode measurement of a line of inquiry of the two-dimensional echocardiogram at the level of the tips of the mitral leaflet at onset of QRS
LV posterior wall	M-mode, parasternal long axis	M-mode measurement of a line of inquiry of the two-dimensional echocardiogram at the level of the tips of the mitral leaflet at onset of QRS
LV mass[a]	M-mode, parasternal long axis	M-mode measurement of a line of inquiry of the two-dimensional echocardiogram at the level of the tips of the mitral leaflet at onset of QRS

(Modified from Daubeney and colleagues.[D4])

Key: *LV*, Left ventricular; *RV*, right ventricular.

[a] Derived from LV end-diastolic dimension (LVEDd), diastolic LV posterior wall thickness (PW), and diastolic septal thickness (S) as: LV mass (g) = 1.04 $[(\text{LVEDd} + \text{PW} + \text{S})^3 - \text{LVEDd}^3] - 13.6$.[D9]

■ TABLE 1G-2 Regression Equations Relating Cardiac Dimension and Body Surface Area[a]

Structure	n	Intercept	Slope	SD	r
RV inflow	119	1.823	0.4962	0.1086	0.95
RV outflow	101	1.943	0.6185	0.1009	0.97
RV area	116	2.795	0.9566	0.1753	0.97
LV inflow	121	1.893	0.4936	0.09847	0.96
LV end-diastolic dimension	110	0.08230	1.392	0.08230	0.97
LV end-systolic dimension	110	0.1205	0.9209	0.4661	0.93
LV area	120	3.141	1.020	0.1806	0.97
Interventricular system[b]	86	0.1978	0.003832	0.1257	0.73
LV posterior wall[c]	102	0.3131	0.007282	0.1067	0.74
LV mass	103	4.211	1.288	0.4209	0.89

(Modified from Daubeney and colleagues.[D4])

[a] Key and footnote *a* are identical to those for Table 1D-2.

[b] The form of this equation is mean normal value of structure = intercept + slope·height (cm).

[c] The form of this equation is mean normal value of structure = intercept + slope·weight (kg).

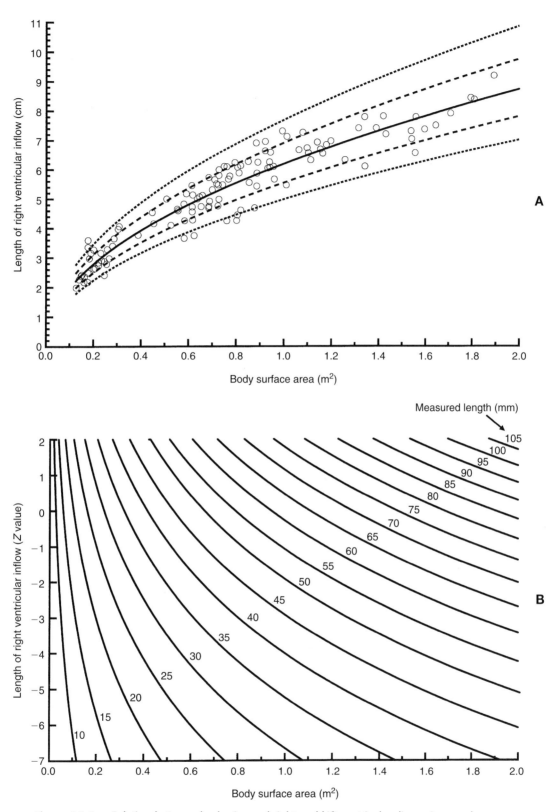

Figure 1G-1   Relation between body size and right and left ventricular dimensions and area, and left ventricular wall thickness and mass. The expression of body size, height, weight, or body surface area that best correlated with the cardiac measurement is used. Presentation of the figures is in pairs, with the raw data points in the first panel, on which is superimposed the line of regression and confidence limits equivalent to 1 and 2 standard deviations, and Z value and body size in the second panel as in Fig. 1D-1. **A,** Right ventricular inflow length and body surface area. **B,** Right ventricular inflow length, relating measured value and body surface area to Z value.   *Continued*

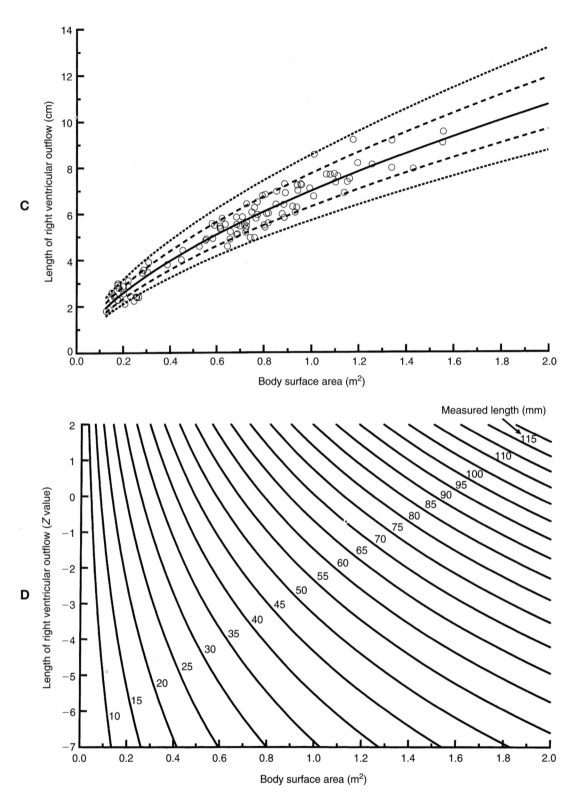

Figure 1G-1—cont'd   C, Right ventricular outflow length and body surface area. **D,** Right ventricular outflow length, relating measured value and body surface area to Z value.

Continued

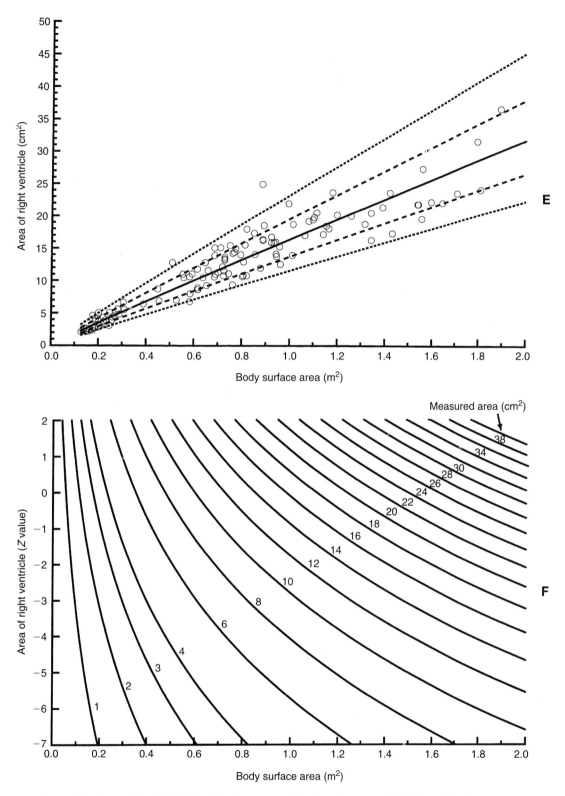

Figure 1G-1—cont'd   E, Right ventricular area and body surface area. **F,** Right ventricular area, relating measured value and body surface area to *Z* value.   *Continued*

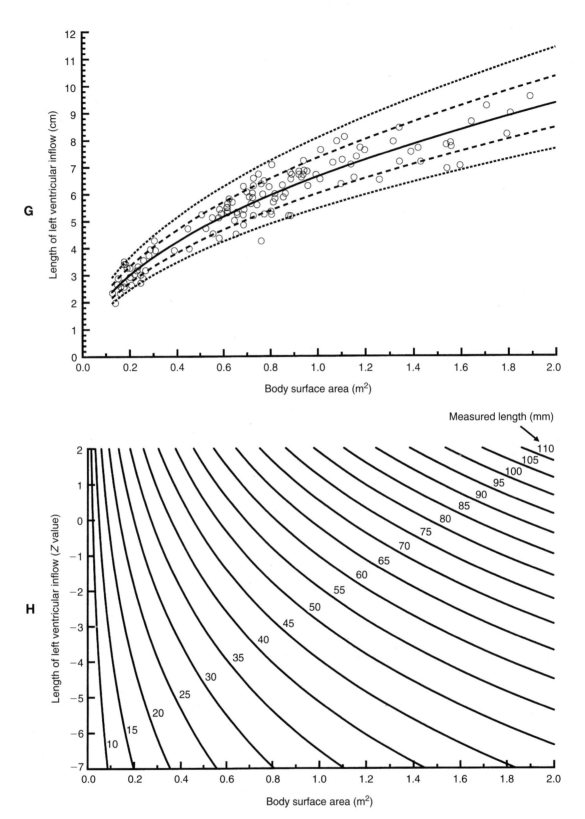

Figure 1G-1—cont'd   G, Left ventricular inflow length and body surface area. **H**, Left ventricular inflow length, relating measured value and body surface area to *Z* value.   *Continued*

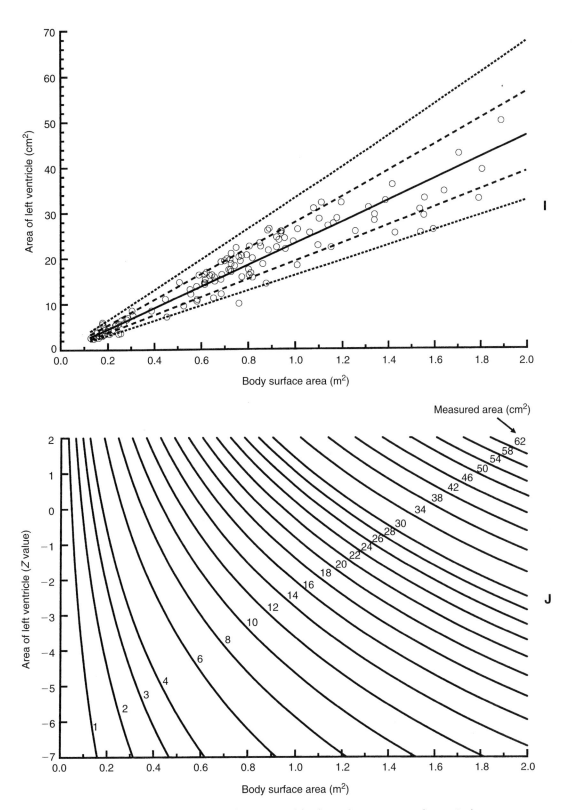

Figure 1G-1—cont'd   I. Left ventricular area and body surface area. **J,** Left ventricular area, relating measured value and body surface area to *Z* value.   *Continued*

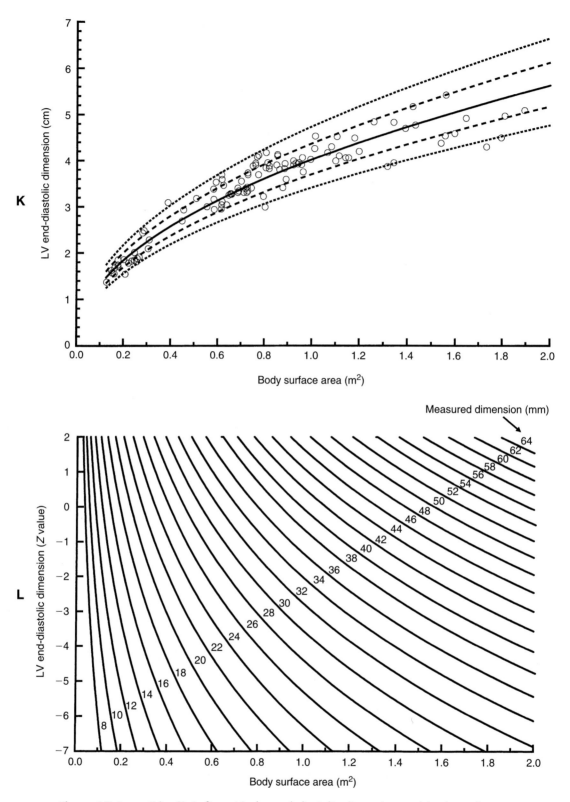

Figure 1G-1—cont'd **K**, Left ventricular end-diastolic dimension and body surface area. **L**, Left ventricular end-diastolic dimension, relating measured value and body surface area to Z value.

Key: *LV*, Left ventricular.

Continued

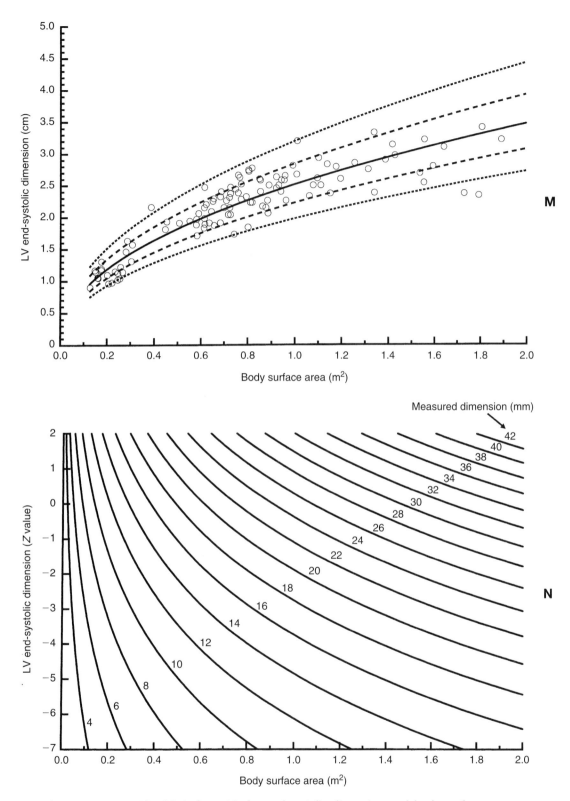

Figure 1G-1—cont'd M, Left ventricular end-systolic dimension and body surface area. **N**, Left ventricular end-systolic dimension, relating measured value and body surface area to Z value.

Key: *LV*, Left ventricular.   *Continued*

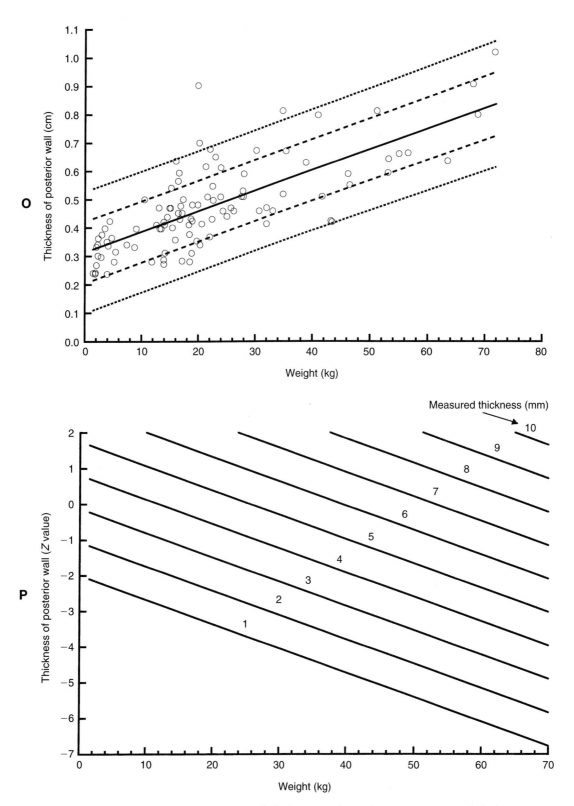

Figure 1G-1–cont'd   O, Posterior wall thickness and weight. **P,** Posterior wall thickness, relating measured value and weight to Z value.   *Continued*

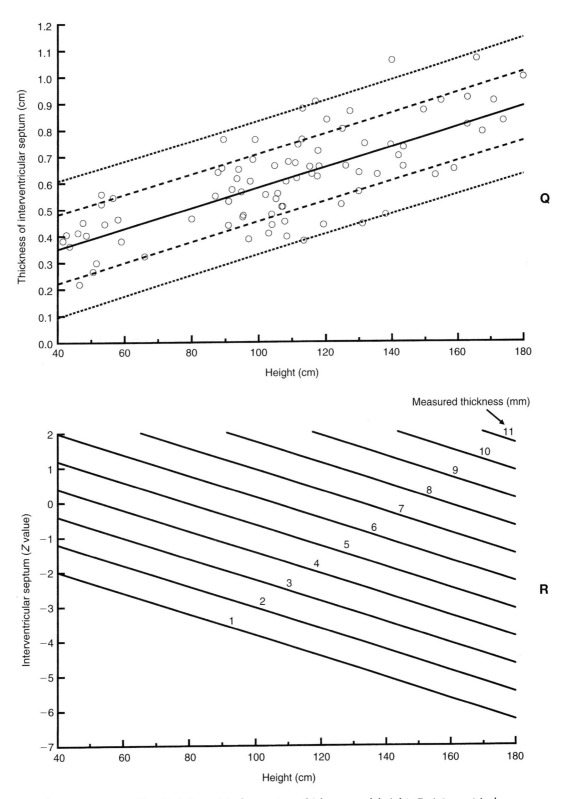

Figure 1G-1—cont'd   Q, Interventricular septum thickness and height. **R,** Interventricular septum thickness, relating measured value and height to Z value.

Key: *LV,* Left ventricular.   *Continued*

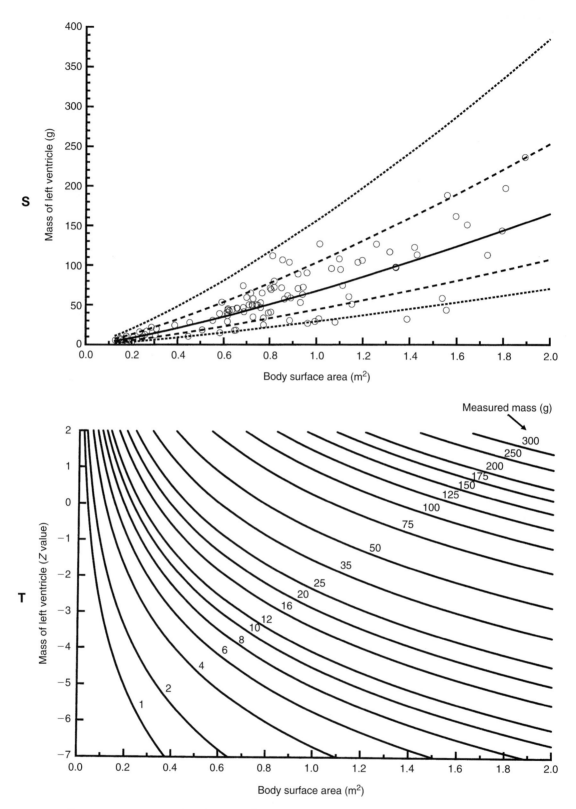

Figure 1G-1–cont'd **S**, Left ventricular mass and body surface area. **T**, Left ventricular mass, relating measured value and body surface area to *Z* value.

■ **TABLE 1G–3   Regression Coefficients for Use in Estimating Mean Normal Heart Weight from Body Surface Area**

Source	Intercept	Slope	SD
Kitzman et al. (adults)[K6]			
Females	5.162	0.8167	0.237
Males	5.204	0.9471	0.144
Scholz et al. (children)[S16]			
Females	4.748	1.127	0.202
Males	4.806	1.210	0.197
Rowlatt et al. (children)[R3]	4.785	1.201	0.1844

Key: *SD,* Standard deviation.

REFERENCES

A

1. Anderson RH, Becker AE, Van Mierop LH. What should we call the "crista"? Br Heart J 1977;39:856.
2. Ad Hoc Committee for Grading of Coronary Artery Disease, Council on Cardiovascular Surgery, American Heart Association. American Heart Association committee report: a reporting system on patients evaluated for coronary artery disease. Circulation 1975;51:5.
3. Anderson RH, Becker AE, Wenink AC. The development of the conducting tissues. In Roberts NK, Gelband H, eds. Cardiac arrhythmias in the neonate, infant, and child. East Norwalk, Conn: Appleton & Lange, 1977, p. 1.
4. Anderson RH, Shinebourne EA, Gerlis LN. Criss-cross atrioventricular relationships producing paradoxical atrioventricular concordance or discordance: their significance to nomenclature of congenital heart disease. Circulation 1974;50:176.
5. Anderson RH. Embryology of the ventricular septum. In Anderson RH, Shinebourne EA, eds. Pediatric cardiology 1977. Edinburgh: Churchill Livingstone, 1978, p. 103.
6. Ando M, Takao A, Cho E. Criss-cross heart by abnormal rotation of ventricular loop: diagnostic considerations for complex cardiac anomaly. Proc Pediatr Circ Soc 1974;4.
7. Anderson RH, Becker AE. Cardiac anatomy. Edinburgh: London: Churchill Livingstone, 1980.
8. Anderson RH, Ho SY, Becker AE. The surgical anatomy of the conduction tissues. Thorax 1983;38:408.
9. Anderson RH. Criss-cross hearts revisited: a question of definition. Pediatr Cardiol 1982;3:305.
10. Anderson RH, Ho SY, Becker AE. The clinical anatomy of the cardiac conduction system. In Rowlands DJ, ed. Recent advances in cardiology. Edinburgh: Churchill Livingstone, 1984.
11. Adams J, Treasure T. Variable anatomy of the right coronary artery supply to the left ventricle. Thorax 1985;40:618.
12. Alboliras ET, Julsrud PR, Danielson GK, Puga FJ, Schaff HV, McGoon DC, et al. Definitive operation for pulmonary atresia with intact ventricular septum. J Thorac Cardiovasc Surg 1987;93:454.
13. Arvidsson H. Angiocardiographic measurements in congenital heart disease in infancy and childhood. I. The size of the ascending and descending aorta. Acta Radiol [Diagn] (Stockh) 1963;1:981.
14. Anjos RT, Ho SY, Anderson RH. Surgical implications of juxtaposition of the atrial appendages: a review of forty-nine autopsied hearts. J Thorac Cardiovasc Surg 1990;99:897.
15. Acar C, Tolan M, Berrebi A, Gaer J, Rouezo R, Marchix T, et al. Homograft replacement of the mitral valve: graft selection, technique of implantation, and results in forty-three patients. J Thorac Cardiovasc Surg 1996;111:367.
16. Abuin G, Nieponice A. New findings on the origin of the blood supply to the atrioventricular node: clinical and surgical significance. Tex Heart Inst J 1998;25:113.
17. Abuin G, Nieponice A, Martinez S, Fernando C. The role of atrial vessels in aortic root and mitral valve operations. Ann Thorac Surg 2000;70:1234.
18. Anderson RH, Ho SY. Sequential segmental analysis: description and categorization for the millennium. Cardiol Young 1997;7:98.

B

1. Brandt PW, Calder AL. Cardiac connections: the segmental approach to radiologic diagnosis in congenital heart disease, Curr Probl Diagn Radiol 1977;7:1.
2. Bargeron LM Jr, Elliott LP, Soto B, Bream PR, Curry G. Axial cineangiography in congenital heart disease. I. Concept, technical and anatomic considerations. Circulation 1977;56:1075.
3. Barry A, Patten BM. The structure of the adult heart. In Gould SE, ed. Pathology of the heart and blood vessels, 5th ed. Springfield, Ill.: Charles C. Thomas, 1968, p. 91.
4. Baltaxe HA, Amplatz K, Levin DC. Coronary angiography. Springfield, Ill.: Charles C. Thomas, 1973.
5. Brandt HM, Liebow AA. Right pulmonary isomerism associated with venous, splenic, and other abnormalities. Lab Invest 1958;7:469.
6. Bharati S, Lev M, Kirklin JW. Cardiac surgery and the conduction system, 2nd ed. Mount Kisco, N.Y.: Futura, 1992.
7. Bartelings MM, Gittenberger-de Groot AC. The outflow tract of the heart—embryologic and morphologic correlations. Int J Cardiol 1989;22:289.
8. Bharati S, McAllister HA Jr, Lev M. Straddling and displaced atrioventricular orifice valves. Circulation 1979;60:673.
9. Busquet J, Fontan F, Anderson RH, Ho SY, Davies MJ. The surgical significance of the atrial branches of the coronary arteries. Int J Cardiol 1984;6:223.
10. Bull C, de Leval MR, Mercanti C, Macartney FJ, Anderson RH. Pulmonary atresia and intact ventricular septum: a revised classification. Circulation 1982;66:266.
11. Blackstone EH, Kirklin JW, Bertranou EG, Labrosse CJ, Soto B, Bargeron LM Jr. Preoperative prediction from cineangiograms of postrepair right ventricular pressure in tetralogy of Fallot. J Thorac Cardiovasc Surg 1979;78:542.
12. Becker AE, Anderson RH. Cardiac pathology. An integrated text and colour atlas. London: Churchill Livingstone, 1983.

C

1. Principal investigators of CASS and their associates. The National Heart, Lung, and Blood Institute Coronary Artery Surgery Study (CASS). Circulation 1981;63:1.
2. Clarkson PM, Brandt PW. Aortic diameters in infants and young children: normative angiographic data. Pediatr Cardiol 1985;6:3.
3. Chatel D, Martin-Bouyer Y, Acar C, Bouchoucha H, Sableyrolles JL, Jebara V, et al. Three-dimensional modeling of the anatomy of the heart and great vessels. Surg Radiol Anat 1993;15:341.
4. Chauvel C, Bogino E, Clerc P, Fernandez G, Vernhet JC, Becat A, et al. Usefulness of three-dimensional echocardiography for the evaluation of mitral valve prolapse: an intraoperative study. J Heart Valve Dis 2000;9:341.

5. Capps SB, Elkins RC, Fronk DM. Body surface area as a predictor of aortic and pulmonary valve diameter. J Thorac Cardiovasc Surg 2000;119:975.
6. Cohen GI, White M, Sochowski RA, Klein AL, Bridge PD, Stewart WJ, et al. Reference values for normal adult transesophageal echocardiographic measurements. J Am Soc Echocardiogr 1995;8:221.

D
1. Demoulin JC, Kulbertus HE. Histopathological examination of concept of left hemiblock. Br Heart J 1972;34:807.
2. Daves ML. Cardiac roentgenology: the loop and circle approach. Radiology 1970;95:157.
3. De la Cruz MV, Berrazueta JR, Arteaga M, Attie F, Soni J. Rules for diagnosis of arterioventricular discordances and spatial identification of ventricles: crossed great arteries and transposition of the great arteries. Br Heart J 1976;38:341.
4. Daubeney PE, Blackstone EH, Weintraub RG, Slavid Z, Scanlon J, Webber SA. Relationship of the dimension of cardiac structures to body size: an echocardiographic study in normal infants and children. Cardiol Young 1999;9:402.
5. Drexler M, Erbel R, Muller U, Wittlich N, Mohr-Kahaly S, Meyer J. Measurement of intracardiac dimensions and structures in normal young adult subjects by transesophageal echocardiography. Am J Cardiol 1990;65:1491.
6. Davidson WR Jr, Pasquale MJ, Fanelli C. A Doppler echocardiographic examination of the normal aortic valve and left ventricular outflow tract. Am J Cardiol 1991;67:547.
7. Daniels SR, Kimball TR, Morrison JA, Khoury P, Meyer RA. Indexing left ventricular mass to account for differences in body size in children and adolescents without cardiovascular disease. Am J Cardiol 1995;76:699.
8. de Simone G, Daniels SR, Devereux RB, Meyer RA, Roman MJ, de Divitiis O, et al. Left ventricular mass and body size in normotensive children and adults: assessment of allometric relations and impact of overweight. J Am Coll Cardiol 1992;20:1251.
9. Devereux RB, Reichek N. Echocardiographic determination of left ventricular mass in man. Anatomic validation of the method. Circulation 1977;55:613.

E
1. Eckner FA, Brown BW, Davidson DL, Glagov S. Dimensions of normal human hearts after standard fixation by controlled pressure coronary perfusion. Arch Pathol 1969;88:497.

F
1. Fulton WF. The coronary arteries. Springfield, Ill: Charles C. Thomas, 1965.
2. Fontan F, Fernandez G, Costa F, Naftel DC, Tritto F, Blackstone EH, et al. The size of the pulmonary arteries and the results of the Fontan operation. J Thorac Cardiovasc Surg 1989;98:711.
3. Foster GP, Isselbacher EM, Rose GA, Torchiana DF, Akins CW, Picard MH. Accurate localization of mitral regurgitation defects using multiplane transesophageal echocardiography. Ann Thorac Surg 1998;65:1025.

G
1. Gray H. Anatomy of the human body. Goss CM, ed. Philadelphia: Lea & Febiger, 1973, p. 543.
2. Gross L, Kugel MA. Topographic anatomy and histology of the valves in the human heart. Am J Pathol 1931;7:445.
3. Gensini GG. Coronary arteriography. Mount Kisco, N.Y.: Futura, 1975.
4. Graham TP Jr, Jarmakani JM, Canent RV Jr, Morrow MN. Left heart volume estimation in infancy and childhood: reevaluation of methodology and normal values. Circulation 1971;43:895.
5. Graham TP Jr, Jarmakani JM, Atwood GF, Canent RV Jr. Right ventricular volume determinations in children: normal values and observations with volume or pressure overload. Circulation 1973;47:144.

6. Gutgesell HP, Rembold CM. Growth of the human heart relative to body surface area. Am J Cardiol 1990;65:662.
7. Gruppo Ligure Della Societa Italiana De Ecografia Cardiovascolare. Developments of allometric equations to establish normal limits for M-mode echocardiographic measurements in the Italian population. G Ital Cardiol 1996;26:503.

H
1. Hudson RE. The human pacemaker and its pathology. Br Heart J 1960;22:153.
2. Habbal ME, Somerville J. Size of the normal aortic root in normal subjects and in those with left ventricular outflow obstruction. Am J Cardiol 1989;63:322.
3. Hanseus K, Bjorkhem G, Lundstrom NR. Dimensions of cardiac chambers and great vessels by cross-sectional echocardiography in infants and children. Pediatr Cardiol 1988;9:7.
4. Henry WL, Ware J, Gardin JM, Hepner SI, McKay J, Weiner M. Echocardiographic measurements in normal subjects: growth-related changes that occur between infancy and early adulthood. Circulation 1978;57:278.
5. Haycock GB, Schwartz GJ, Wisotsky DH. Geometric method for measuring body surface area: a height–weight formula validated in infants, children, and adults. J Pediatr 1978;93:62.
6. Hornberger LK, Weintraub RG, Pesonen E, Murillo-Olivas A, Simpson IA, Sahn C, et al. Echocardiographic study of the morphology and growth of the aortic arch in the human fetus: observations related to the prenatal diagnosis of coarctation. Circulation 1992;86:741.
7. Huwez FU, Houston AB, Watson J, McLaughlin S, Macfarlane PW. Age and body surface area related normal upper and lower limits of M mode echocardiographic measurements and left ventricular volume and mass from infancy to early adulthood. Br Heart J 1994;72:276.

J
1. James TN. Anatomy of the human sinus node. Anat Rec 1961;141:109.
2. James TN. The connecting pathways between the sinus node and the AV node and between the right and left atrium in the human heart. Am Heart J 1963;66:498.
3. Janse MJ, Anderson RH. Specialized internodal atrial pathways: fact or fiction? Eur J Cardiol 1974;2:117.
4. James TN. Morphology of the human atrioventricular node, with remarks pertinent to its electrophysiology. Am Heart J 1961;62:756.
5. James TN. Anatomy of the coronary arteries. New York: Hoeber, 1961.
6. James TN, Burch GE. The blood supply of the human interventricular septum. Circulation 1958;17:391.
7. James TN. Anatomy of the coronary arteries in health and disease. Circulation 1965;32:1020.

K
1. Kerr A Jr, Goss CM. Retention of embryonic relationship of aortic and pulmonary valve cusps and a suggested nomenclature. Anat Rec 1956;125:777.
2. Kirklin JW. Introduction. In Kirklin JW, ed. Advances in cardiovascular surgery. Orlando, Fla: Grune & Stratton, 1973, p. 3.
3. Kirklin JW, Pacifico AD, Bargeron LM Jr, Soto B. Cardiac repair in anatomically corrected malposition of the great arteries. Circulation 1973;48:153.
4. King DH, Smith EO, Huhta JC, Gutgesell HP. Mitral and tricuspid valve anular diameter in normal children determined by two-dimensional echocardiography. Am J Cardiol 1985;55:787.
5. Krovetz LJ. Age-related changes in size of the aortic valve anulus in man. Am Heart J 1975;90:569.
6. Kitzman DW, Scholz DG, Hagen PT, Ilstrup DM, Edwards WD. Age-related changes in normal human hearts during the first 10 decades of life. II. A quantitative anatomic study of 765 specimens from subjects 20 to 99 years old. Mayo Clin Proc 1988;63:137.
7. Kumar N, Kumar M, Duran CM. A revised terminology for recording surgical findings of the mitral valve. J Heart Valve Dis 1995;4:70.

8. Kampmann C, Wiethoff CM, Wenzel A, Stolz G, Betancor M, Wipperman CF, et al. Normal values of M mode echocardiographic measurements of more than 2000 healthy infants and children in central Europe. Heart 2000;83:667.

L

1. Lev M, Bharati S. Anatomy of the conduction system in normal and congenitally abnormal hearts. In Roberts NK, Gelband H, eds. Cardiac arrhythmias in the neonate, infant, and child. East Norwalk, Conn: Appleton & Lange, 1977, p. 29.
2. Lam JH, Ranganathan N, Wigle ED, Silver MD. Morphology of the human mitral valve. I. Chordae tendineae: a new classification. Circulation 1970;41:449.
3. Landing BH, Lawrence TK, Payne VC, Wells TR. Bronchial anatomy in syndromes with abnormal visceral situs, abnormal spleen, and congenital heart disease. Am J Cardiol 1971;128:456.
4. Lev M, Liberthson RR, Golden JG, Eckner FA, Arcilla RA. The pathologic anatomy of mesocardia. Am J Cardiol 1971;28:428.
5. Liberthson RR, Hastreiter AR, Sinha SN, Bharati S, Novak GM, Lev M. Levocardia with visceral heterotaxy–isolated levocardia: pathologic anatomy and its clinical implications. Am Heart J 1973;85:40.
6. Lev M. The conduction system. In Gould SE, ed. Pathology of the heart and blood vessels, 3rd ed. Springfield, Ill: Charles C. Thomas, 1968, p. 183.
7. Lewis AB, Lindesmith GG, Takahashi M, Stanton RE, Tucker BL, Stiles QR, et al. Cardiac rhythm following the Mustard procedure for transposition of the great vessels. J Thorac Cardiovasc Surg 1977;73:919.
8. Lev M, Rowlatt UF. The pathological anatomy of mixed levocardia: a review of 13 cases of atrial or ventricular inversion with or without corrected transposition. Am J Cardiol 1961;9:216.
9. Lange PE, Onnasch DG, Schaupp GH, Zill C, Heintzen PH. Size and function of the human left and right ventricles during growth: normative angiographic data. Pediatr Cardiol 1982;3:205.

M

1. Massing GK, Liebman J, James TN. Cardiac conduction pathways in the infant and child. In Engle MA, ed. Pediatric cardiology. Philadelphia: FA Davis, 1974, p. 27.
2. Massing GK, James TN. Anatomical configuration of the His bundle and proximal bundle branches in the human heart. Circulation 1976;53:609.
3. Merkin RJ. Position and orientation of the heart valves. Am J Anat 1969;125:375.
4. McAlpine WA. Heart and coronary arteries. Berlin: Springer-Verlag, 1975.
5. Moller JH, Nakib A, Anderson RC, Edwards JE. Congenital cardiac disease associated with polysplenia: a developmental complex of bilateral "left-sideness." Circulation 1967;36:789.
6. Milo S, Ho SY, Macartney FJ, Wilkinson JL, Becker AE, Wenink AC, et al. Straddling and over-riding atrio-ventricular valves: morphology and classification. Am J Cardiol 1979;44:1122.
7. Mavroudis C, Jacobs JP. The Society of Thoracic Surgeons Congenital Heart Surgery Nomenclature and Database Project. Ann Thorac Surg 2000;69:S372.
8. Merrick AF, Yacoub MH, Ho SY, Anderson RH. Anatomy of the muscular subpulmonary infundibulum with regard to the Ross procedure. Ann Thorac Surg 2000;69:556.

N

1. National Heart, Lung, and Blood Institute. Proposal and Manual of Operations for Collaborative Studies in Coronary Artery Surgery. Contract No. I-HV-32973. Washington, DC: National Heart, Lung, and Blood Institute, 1975.

2. Nakata S, Ihai Y, Takanashi Y, Kurosawa H, Tezuka M, Nakazaw M, et al. A new method for the quantitative standardization of cross-sectional area of the pulmonary arteries in congenital heart diseases with decreased pulmonary blood flow. J Thorac Cardiovasc Surg 1984;88:610.
3. Nakazawa M, Marks RA, Isabel-Jones J, Jarmakani JM. Right and left ventricular volume characteristics in children with pulmonary stenosis and intact ventricular septum. Circulation 1976;53:884.
4. Nelson TR, Pretorius DH, Sklansky M, Hagen-Ansert S. Three-dimensional echocardiographic evaluation of fetal heart anatomy and function: acquisition, analysis, and display. J Ultrasound Med 1996; 15:1.

O

1. Ogden JA. Congenital anomalies of the coronary arteries. Am J Cardiol 1970;25:474.
2. Ormiston JA, Shah PM, Tei C, Wong M. Size and motion of the mitral valve anulus in man. I. A two-dimensional echocardiographic method and findings in normal subjects. Circulation 1981;64:113.

P

1. Partridge JB, Scott O, Deverall PB, Macartney FJ. Visualization and measurement of the main bronchi by tomography as an objective indicator of thoracic situs in congenital heart disease. Circulation 1975;51:188.
2. Perloff JK, Roberts WC. The mitral apparatus: functional anatomy of mitral regurgitation. Circulation 1972;46:227.
3. Pollick C, Pittman M, Filly K, Fitzgerald PJ, Popp RL. Mitral and aortic valve orifice area in normal subjects and in patients with congestive cardiomyopathy: determination by two dimensional echocardiography. Am J Cardiol 1982;49:1191.
4. Piehler JM, Danielson GK, McGoon DC, Wallace RB, Fulton RE, Mair DD. Management of pulmonary atresia with ventricular septal defect and hypoplastic pulmonary arteries by right ventricular outflow obstruction. J Thorac Cardiovasc Surg 1980;80:552.
5. Pearlman JD, Triulzi MO, King ME, Newell J, Weyman AE. Limits of normal left ventricular dimensions in growth and development: analysis of dimensions and variance in the two-dimensional echocardiograms of 268 normal healthy subjects. J Am Coll Cardiol 1988;12:1432.

R

1. Ranganathan N, Lam JH, Wigle ED, Silver MD. Morphology of the human mitral valve. II. The valve leaflets. Circulation 1970;41:459.
2. Rusted IE, Scheifley CH, Edwards JE. Studies of the mitral valve. I. Anatomic features of the normal mitral valve and associated structures. Circulation 1952;6:825.
3. Rowlatt JF, Rimoldi JH, Lev M. The quantitative anatomy of the normal child's heart. Pediatr Clin North Am 1963;10:499.
4. Riggs TW, Lapin GD, Paul MH, Muster AJ, Berry TE. Measurement of mitral valve orifice area in infants and children by two-dimensional echocardiography. J Am Coll Cardiol 1983;1:873.
5. Roman MJ, Devereux RB, Kramer-Fox R, Loughlin J. Two-dimensional echocardiographic aortic root dimensions in normal children and adults. Am J Cardiol 1989;64:507.

S

1. Soto B, Pacifico AD, Souza AS Jr, Bargeron LM Jr, Ermocilla R, Tonkin IL. Identification of thoracic isomerism from the plain chest roentgenogram. Am J Roentgenol 1978;131:995.
2. Spach MS, King TD, Barr RC, Boaz DE, Morrow MN, Herman-Giddens S. Electrical potential distribution surrounding the atria during depolarization and repolarization in the dog. Circ Res 1969;24:857.

3. Spach MS, Lieberman M, Scott JC, Barr RC, Johnson EA, Kootsey JM. Excitation sequences of the atrial septum and AV node in isolated hearts of the dog and rabbit. Circ Res 1971;29:156.

4. Spach MS, Huang S, Armstrong SI, Canent RV Jr. Demonstration of peripheral conduction system in human hearts. Circulation 1963; 28:333.

5. Silverman ME, Hurst JW. The mitral complex. Am Heart J 1968; 76:399.

6. Silver MD, Lam JH, Ranganathan N, Wigle ED. Morphology of the human tricuspid valve. Circulation 1971;43:333.

7. Sherman FE. Ventricular septal defect. In Sherman FE, ed. An atlas of congenital heart disease. Philadelphia: Lea & Febiger, 1963, p. 170.

8. Soto B, Russell RO Jr, Moraski RE. Radiographic anatomy of the coronary arteries: an atlas. Mount Kisco, N.Y.: Futura, 1976.

9. Schlesinger MJ, Zoll PM, Wessler S. The conus artery: a third coronary artery. Am Heart J 1949;38:823.

10. Shinebourne EA, Macartney FJ, Anderson RH. Sequential chamber localization: logical approach to diagnosis in congenital heart disease. Br Heart J 1976;38:327.

11. Stanger P, Rudolph AM, Edwards JE. Cardiac malpositions. Circulation 1977;56:159.

12. Stanger P, Benassi RC, Korns ME, Jue KL, Edwards JE. Diagrammatic portrayal of variations in cardiac structure, reference to transposition, dextrocardia and the concept of four normal hearts. Circulation 1968;37:IV1.

13. Sievers HH, Onnasch DG, Lange PE, Bernhard A, Heintzen PH. Dimensions of the great arteries, semilunar valve roots, and right ventricular outflow tract during growth: normative angiocardiographic data. Pediatr Cardiol 1983;4:189.

14. Soto B, Ceballos R, Kirklin JW. Ventricular septal defects: a surgical viewpoint. J Am Coll Cardiol 1989;14:1291.

15. Snider AR, Enderlein MA, Teitel DF, Juster RP. Two-dimensional echocardiography determination of aortic and pulmonary artery sizes from infancy to adulthood in normal subjects. Am J Cardiol 1984;53:218.

16. Scholz DG, Kitzman DW, Hagen PT, Ilstrup DM, Edwards WD. Age-related changes in normal human hearts during the first 10 decades of life. I. A quantitative anatomic study of 200 specimens from subjects from birth to 19 years old. Mayo Clin Proc 1988;63:126.

17. Sepehri B, Fisher EA, Eckner FA, Hastreiter AR. Correlation of angiographic and autopsy right ventricular dimensions in infants and children. Circulation 1980;62:416.

18. Shimazaki Y, Kawashima Y, Hirose H, Nakano S, Matsuda H, Kitamura S, et al. Operative results in patients with pseudotruncus arteriosus. Ann Thorac Surg 1983;35:294.

19. Shimazaki Y, Maehara T, Blackstone EH, Kirklin JW, Bargeron LM Jr. The structure of the pulmonary circulation in tetralogy of Fallot with pulmonary atresia. J Thorac Cardiovasc Surg 1988;95:1048.

20. Shimazaki Y, Blackstone EH, Kirklin JW, Jonas RA, Mandell V, Colvin EV. The dimensions of the right ventricular outflow tract and pulmonary arteries in tetralogy of Fallot and pulmonary stenosis. J Thorac Cardiovasc Surg 1992;106:692.

21. Sanchez-Quintana D, Garcia-Martinez V, Climent V, Hurle JM. Morphological changes in the normal pattern of ventricular myoarchitecture in the developing human heart. Anat Rec 1995;243:483.

22. Sow ML, Ndoye JM, Lo EA. The artery of the sinuatrial node: anatomic considerations based on 45 injection-dissections of the heart. Surg Radiol Anat 1996;18:103.

23. Salustri A, Roelandt JR. Ultrasonic three-dimensional reconstruction of the heart. Ultrasound Med Biol 1995;21:281.

24. Sapin PM, Gopal AS, Clarke GB, Smith MD, King DL. Three-dimensional echocardiography compared to two-dimensional echocardiography for measurement of left ventricular mass anatomic validation in an open chest canine model. Am J Hypertens 1996;9:467.

25. Seo JW, Zuberbuhler JR, Ho SY, Anderson RH. Surgical significance of morphological variations in the atrial septum in atrioventricular septal defect for determination of the site of penetration of the atrioventricular conduction axis. J Cardiac Surg 1992;7:324.

26. Sheil ML, Jenkins O, Sholler GF. Echocardiographic assessment of aortic root dimensions in normal children based on measurement of a new ratio of aortic size independent of growth. Am J Cardiol 1995;75:711.

27. Skelton R, Gill AB, Parsons JM. Reference ranges for cardiac dimensions and blood flow velocity in preterm infants. Heart 1998;80:281.

28. Singh B, Mohan JC. Doppler echocardiographic determination of aortic and pulmonary valve orifice areas in normal adult subjects. Int J Cardiol 1992;37:73.

29. Swinne CJ, Shapiro EP, Jamart J, Fleg JL. Age-associated changes in left ventricular outflow tract geometry in normal subjects. Am J Cardiol 1996;78:1070.

30. Sanchez-Quintana D, Garcia-Martinez V, Hurle JM. Myocardial fibre architecture in the human heart. Acta Anat 1990;138:352.

T

1. Tandler J. Anatomie des Herzens: Handbuch des Anatomie des Menshen, vol. 3, part 1. Jena: Gustav Fischer, 1913, p. 84.

2. Titus JL. Normal anatomy of the human cardiac conduction system. Mayo Clin Proc 1973;48:24.

3. Truex RC. The sinoatrial node and its connections with the atrial tissues. In Wellens HJ, Lie KI, Janse MJ, eds. The conduction system of the heart. Philadelphia: Lea & Febiger, 1976, p. 209.

4. Tamiya T, Yamashiro T, Matsumoto T, Ogoshi S, Seguchi H. A histological study of surgical landmarks for the specialized atrioventricular conduction system, with particular reference to the papillary muscle. Ann Thorac Surg 1985;40:599.

5. Tei C, Pilgrim JP, Shah PM, Ormiston JA, Wong M. The tricuspid valve anulus: study of size and motion in normal subjects and in patients with tricuspid regurgitation. Circulation 1982;66:665.

6. Thilenius OG, Arcilla RA. Angiographic right and left ventricular volume determination in normal infants and children. Pediatr Res 1984;8:67.

7. Trento A, Zuberbuhler JR, Anderson RH, Park SC, Siewers RD. Divided right atrium (prominence of the eustachian and thebesian valves). J Thorac Cardiovasc Surg 1988;96:457.

U

1. Ursell PC, Byrne JM, Fears TR, Strobino BA, Gersony WM. Growth of the great vessels in the normal human fetus and in the fetus with cardiac defects. Circulation 1991;84:2028.

V

1. Van Mierop LH, Wiglesworth FW. Isomerism of the cardiac atria in the asplenia syndrome. Lab Invest 1962;11:1303.

2. Van Mierop LH, Eisen S, Schiebler GL. The radiographic appearance of the tracheobronchial tree as an indicator of visceral situs. Am J Cardiol 1970;26:432.

3. Van Mierop LH. Anatomy and embryology of the right ventricle. In Edwards JE, Ley M, Abell MR, eds. The heart. Baltimore: Williams & Wilkins, 1974.

4. Vlodaver Z, Amplatz K, Burchell HB, Edwards JE. Coronary heart disease: clinical angiographic and pathologic profiles. New York: Springer-Verlag, 1976.

5. Van Praagh R. The segmental approach to diagnosis in congenital heart disease: birth defects. Original Article Series 1972;8:4.

6. Van Praagh R, Ongley PA, Swan HJ. Anatomic types of single or common ventricle in man. Am J Cardiol 1964;13:367.

7. Van Praagh S, LaCorte M, Fellows KE, Bossina K, Busch HJ, Keck EW, et al. Superior–inferior ventricles: anatomic and angiocardiographic findings in 10 post-mortem cases. In Van Praagh R, Takao A, eds. Etiology and morphogenesis of congenital heart disease. Mount Kisco, N.Y.: Futura, 1980, p. 317.

8. Van Praagh R, Van Praagh S. Isolated ventricular inversion: a consideration of the morphogenesis, definition and diagnosis of non-transposed and transposed great arteries. Am J Cardiol 1966;17:395.

9. Van Praagh R, Van Praagh S, Vlad P, Keith JD. Anatomic types of congenital dextrocardia: diagnostic and embryologic implications. Am J Cardiol 1964;13:510.

10. Van Praagh R, Plett JA, Van Praagh S. Single ventricle: pathology, embryology, terminology, and classification. Herz 1979;4:113.

11. Van Praagh R, Weinberg PM, Van Praagh S. Malposition of the heart. In Moss AJ, Adams FH, Emmanouilides GC, eds. Heart disease in infants, children and adolescents. Baltimore: Williams & Wilkins, 1977, p. 395.

12. Van Praagh R. Terminology of congenital heart disease: glossary and commentary. Circulation 1977;56:139.

13. Van Praagh R, David I, Gordon D, Wright B, Van Praagh S. Ventricular diagnosis and designation. In Godman MJ, ed. Pediatric cardiology, vol. 4. London: Churchill Livingstone, 1981, p. 153.

14. Van Meurs-van Woezik H, Debets T, Klein HW. Internal diameters of the ventriculo-arterial junctions and great arteries of normal infants and children: a database for evaluation of congenital cardiac malformations. Int J Cardiol 1989;23:303.

15. Vasan RS, Larson MG, Levy D, Evans JC, Benjamin EJ. Distribution and categorization of echocardiographic measurements in relation to reference limits: the Framingham Heart Study: formulation of a height- and sex-specific classification and its prospective validation. Circulation 1997;96:1863.

16. Victor S, Nayak VM. Variations in the papillary muscles of the normal mitral valve and their surgical relevance. J Card Surg 1995;10:597.

W

1. Walmsley R, Watson H. The outflow tract of the left ventricle. Br Heart J 1966;28:435.

2. Westaby S, Karp RB, Blackstone EH, Bishop SP. Adult human valve dimensions and their surgical significance. Am J Cardiol 1984;53:552.

Y

1. Yacoub MH, Kilner PJ, Birks EJ, Misfeld M. The aortic outflow and root: a tale of dynamism and crosstalk. Ann Thorac Surg 1999;68:S37.

Z

1. Zimmerman J. The functional and surgical anatomy of the aortic valve. Isr J Med Sci 1969;5:862.

2. Zamir M. Tree structure and branching characteristics of the right coronary artery in a right-dominant human heart. Cardiovasc Anat 1996;12:593.

2

Hypothermia, Circulatory Arrest, and Cardiopulmonary Bypass

Hypothermic Circulatory Arrest

HISTORICAL NOTE

In 1950, Bigelow and colleagues, in their publications on experimental hypothermia produced by surface cooling, introduced the concept that whole body hypothermia might be useful in cardiac surgery.[B1,B2] They subsequently reported cooling dogs to 20°C by surface cooling, with recovery after 15 minutes of circulatory arrest.[B4] In 1951, Boerema and colleagues reported experimental studies indicating that when animals were cooled by a femoral–femoral shunt through a cooling coil, up to 15 minutes of circulatory arrest (produced by inflow stasis) were tolerated without apparent ill effect.[B3] In 1953, Lewis and Taufic reported successful repair of an atrial septal defect in a 5-year-old girl using surface cooling, and, in the same year, Swan and colleagues reported successful results in a series of patients treated using the same technique.[L1,S1] In 1958, Sealy and colleagues reported successful clinical cases in which hypothermia was combined with cardiopulmonary bypass (CPB).[S2] In 1959, Drew and colleagues reported experimental studies in which CPB (using the subject's own lungs as the oxygenator) was used to cool and rewarm the subject, and operations were done during circulatory arrest at 15° C.[D1] In 1960, Guiot and colleagues and Weiss and colleagues reported use of hypothermia and circulatory arrest for cardiac surgery in human subjects.[G1,W1] In 1961, Kirklin and colleagues of the Mayo Clinic reported the results of operation with hypothermic circulatory arrest in 52 patients, using Drew's technique in 23 and a pump-oxygenator in 29.[K1] In 1963, Horiuchi and colleagues from Tohoku University reported using surface cooling to 25°C and circulatory arrest during repair of ventricular septal defect in 18 infants younger than 1 year of age, with 16 survivors.[H1] Dillard and colleagues modified this technique to permit surface cooling to hypothermic temperatures of 17° to 20°C, and extension of the duration of circulatory arrest to 60 minutes.[D2] In 1967, they reported successful repair of total anomalous pulmonary venous connection in four infants by this method of surface cooling and rewarming.[D2] Similar experiences with this and other congenital malformations were reported by Hikasa and colleagues and Wakusawa and colleagues.[H2,W2] In 1970, Barratt-Boyes and colleagues in New Zealand reported the repair of a variety of malformations during hypothermic circulatory arrest in 34 infants weighing less than 10 kg using surface cooling to 22° to 27°C, followed by a brief period of CPB to reduce the temperature further, as well as rewarming with CPB.[B5] In 1973, Hamilton and colleagues reported operations with hypothermic circulatory arrest in 18 infants using only CPB for cooling (core cooling).[H3] These experiences and subsequent modifications in technique opened the way for safer intracardiac surgery in neonates and infants.

Use of hypothermic circulatory arrest in combination with CPB in adults was first reported by Barnard and Schrire in 1963.[B44] Two patients with aneurysms of the ascending aorta and aortic arch underwent replacement of the involved aortic segments using hypothermia to an esophageal temperature of approximately 10°C and short intervals of circulatory arrest. One survived. In 1964, Borst and colleagues reported successful repair of an arteriovenous fistula involving the aortic arch using a period of hypothermic circulatory arrest.[B45] In 1969, Lillehei and colleagues reported use of partial CPB, hypothermia, and circulatory arrest for management of ruptured mycotic aneurysms, ruptured left ventricles, and other complicated cardiac pathology.[L8] The first series of patients with aneurysms of the aortic arch that were successfully resected during an interval of hypothermic circulatory arrest was reported by Griepp and colleagues in 1975.[G21]

HYPOTHESES

A basic hypothesis underlying use of circulatory arrest for cardiac and aortic surgery is that there is a safe duration of this state, the length of which is inversely related to the temperature of the organism during the arrest period. A safe period of circulatory arrest is characterized by absence of detectable functional or structural organ derangements in the early or late postoperative period. Structural derangements without apparent functional correlates are of concern, particularly in the central nervous system, because of an implied loss of neurologic reserve that may be important to the individual in later life.

Temperature of the organism is not easily defined or described. In normal humans, temperature gradients between areas of the body at rest are small, so that a single representation of inner body temperature is generally acceptable.[B6] When hypothermia is produced by surface cooling, internal temperature gradients are relatively small, although the skin and muscles become cooler than the inner organs, and rectal temperature is substantially lower than nasopharyngeal temperature.[C1] During cooling by hypothermic perfusion with CPB (core cooling), the relationship of rectal to nasopharyngeal temperature is reversed, and regional differences in temperature are considerable, although they can be lessened by prolonging the period of cooling.[C1] Thus, when the latter technique is used wholly or in part to induce hypothermia, the specific site of temperature measurement, as well as the limitations in interpretation of the measurements themselves, must be noted.

Another hypothesis is that hypothermia, without itself producing damage, reduces metabolic activity to the extent that the available energy stores in the various organs maintain cell viability throughout the ischemic period of circulatory arrest, and thus allow normal structure and function to return after reperfusion is accomplished. The magnitude of reduction of oxygen consumption is hypothesized to be directly related to safe duration of circulatory arrest.

OXYGEN CONSUMPTION DURING HYPOTHERMIA

Oxygen consumption is considered a measure of metabolic activity. Therefore, the magnitude of its decrease by hypothermia (in the anesthetized subject in whom shivering is prevented) is an index of the degree of reduction of metabolic activity. Use of oxygen consumption as such a marker is reasonable, because for all practical purposes, tissue and cellular stores of oxygen do not exist. Thus, the body is dependent on circulation to bring oxygen to tissues in amounts determined by oxygen consumption.

Relationship between Oxygen Consumption and Body Temperature

Energy requirements of the body, reflected in part by oxygen consumption ($\dot{V}_{O_2}$), are reduced during hypothermia, reflecting dependence of the rate of biochemical reactions on temperature.[F1] Quantitative interrelations have been expressed mathematically in various ways (Box 2-1). Some have used a *linear model*. Others, including Harris and colleagues, have used a *model based on the Arrhenius equation,* which states that the logarithm of the rate of a chemical reaction is inversely proportional to the reciprocal of the absolute temperature.[H4] The nomogram describing this relationship is S-shaped (similar to the oxygen dissociation curve) such that at high temperatures, the reaction rate ceases increasing with temperature (reaches an asymptote).

At physiologic temperatures, biochemical systems operate only on the upswing of the curve. Thus, particularly when the range of temperatures is relatively small, this relationship finds *numerical expression in the van't Hoff law,* which relates the logarithm of a chemical reaction rate directly to temperature. Conveniently, according to this equation, the reaction rate increases by two to three times for an increase in temperature of 10°C. Chemists use the symbol Q_{10} for this multiple.

Because oxygen uptake is the expression of all oxidative reactions, both direct and indirect, the logarithm of $\dot{V}_{O_2}$ might be expected to be directly proportional to temperature. In general, this appears to be so. Whether the observed decline in $\dot{V}_{O_2}$ during clinical hypothermia can be accounted for entirely on this physicochemical basis is doubtful, however (see "Oxygen Consumption during Hypothermia in Tissue Slices and Isolated Organs" later in this section).

Total Body Oxygen Consumption after Surface Cooling

When hypothermia is induced by cooling the surface of anesthetized humans or experimental animals, cooling is rather uniform throughout the body, and temperatures of internal organs and regions differ by less than 2°C.[C1] Therefore, values for whole body oxygen consumption at various body temperatures are probably useful, and the relative magnitude of reduction can be assumed to be similar throughout the body.

Good data in this area are available from the animal experiments of Bigelow and colleagues, Ross, and Penrod.[B2,P1,R1] Data for surface cooling in humans are sparse, although Harris estimated Q_{10} to lie between 1.9 and 4.2 in 10 surface-cooled infants.[H5] The experimental

---

BOX 2-1   Kinetics of Oxygen Consumption

The relationship of oxygen consumption to perfusion flow rate and temperature is not linear; that is, a unit increase in flow or temperature does not increment oxygen consumption a constant amount. A number of formal mathematical models (see Box 6-7 in Chapter 6) have been proposed that relate, in particular, metabolic activity and temperature based on fundamental thermodynamics. These models provide a good starting point for examining oxygen consumption data for other empiric relations, such as with blood flow.

Arrhenius Equation

The Arrhenius equation relates reaction rate k to temperature T, the universal gas constant R, activation energy E_a, and a constant related to molecular collision as:

$$k = Ae^{-\frac{E_a}{RT}}$$

where e is the base of the natural logarithms. If logarithms are taken of both sides of this equation, one obtains the following:

$$Ln[k] = Ln[A] - \frac{E_a}{RT}$$

Constants A, R, and E_a are coalesced (a, b) to obtain a log-inverse equation:

$$Ln[k] = a - \frac{b}{T}$$

Therefore, one can examine the correlation of the logarithm of oxygen consumption and inverse temperature to see if the data are consistent with this relation.

van't Hoff Law (Q_{10})

Another relation is expressed in the van't Hoff law, which is generally formulated in terms of change in metabolic rate (k) per 10°C change in temperature (Q_{10}):

$$Q_{10} = \left(\frac{k_1}{k_2}\right)^{\frac{10}{T_1 - T_2}}$$

If $T_1 - T_2$ is 10°, then Q_{10} is simply the ratio of k_1 to k_2 (the metabolic rates at each temperature). This relation can be derived from the parameter b in the Arrhenius equation.

Hyperbolic Equation

Metabolic rate (reflected in oxygen consumption, $\dot{V}_{O_2}$) and blood flow rate ($\dot{Q}$) should be independent until blood flow becomes limiting. This suggests a hyperbolic relation between the two variables:

$$\frac{1}{\dot{V}_{O_2}} = \frac{1}{c} + \frac{d}{\dot{Q}}$$

where c is the asymptotic (limit of $\dot{V}_{O_2}$) value of $\dot{V}_{O_2}$ as $\dot{Q}$ becomes large (metabolic rate independent of flow).

Empiric Relations

Actual data may be better characterized by (1) a linear relation (rare), (2) a log–linear (exponential) relation, (3) a log–log relation, (4) an inverse–log relation, or a more complex relation. Many of these models can be fitted to data using linear regression (see Box 6-7 in Chapter 6) by logarithmic or inverse transformations of scale. Others require iterative nonlinear optimization methods to obtain parametric estimates (see Box 6-14 in Chapter 6).

---

data were reanalyzed using (1) a linear equation, (2) the Arrhenius equation, and (3) the van't Hoff law. The van't Hoff law best fits this combined set of data (Fig. 2-1) and is considered the most appropriate model for this purpose.[B2,P1,R1] This model also best fits the relation between temperature and cerebral oxygen consumption during CPB in humans.[C28]

Kent and Peirce studied $\dot{V}_{O_2}$ in experimental animals during hypothermia produced by combined surface and core cooling.[K2] Their data are similar to those obtained from surface cooling alone.

Oxygen Consumption during Hypothermia in Tissue Slices and Isolated Organs

Data from the studies described could lead to an underestimation of true oxygen demand, because only areas in which perfusion of the microcirculation continues can participate in oxygen consumption (tissue and cellular stores of oxygen being trivial). In theory at least, a considerable part of the reduction in oxygen consumption from surface cooling could be from shutting down of the microcirculation of portions of the body or from arteriovenous shunting. New technologies, particularly magnetic resonance imaging (MRI), may resolve some of these questions.[N1,S29]

Studies of tissue slices at various temperatures show that oxygen consumption is in fact reduced by hypothermia.[F2-F4] These studies and those of isolated organs suggest that Q_{10}, although differing from tissue to tissue, is on average about 2 (for references and a table of Q_{10} values, see Harris and colleagues[H6]). Measurement of human whole body $\dot{V}_{O_2}$ before and after heating, rather than cooling, indicates a Q_{10} in this same range (about 1.9) (see "Hypothermia" under Brain Protection in Section 3 of Chapter 4).[S3] Vasodilatation caused by heating presumably ensures access of oxygen to the tissues, and this Q_{10} probably represents true tissue oxygen requirement. A Q_{10} greater than 1.9 associated with cooling may therefore indicate that oxygen delivery has been compromised by inadequate flow rate. Fuhrman and colleagues have spent many years investigating this possibility. They showed that, in general, there was a close agreement between resting $\dot{V}_{O_2}$ at 37°C and tissue slice respiration.[F4,M1] However, rats cooled by immersion to 18°C exhibited a 33% lower $\dot{V}_{O_2}$ than would be expected from studies of tissue slice respiration at this temperature.[F3] The discrepancy was not accounted for either by inhomogeneities in whole body temperature or by known changes in Q_{10} exhibited by some tissues (in part related to altered function at reduced temperatures). The precise mechanism remains unknown. It could be due to arteriovenous shunting or to shutting down of perfusion to some areas of the body. Microvascular physiologists have referred to the latter as a decrease in *effective capillary density*. This may result not only from reduced cardiac output and vasoconstriction but also from changes in blood viscosity, geometry, and compliance of red blood cells, plasma "skimming," and clumping of formed blood elements.

Some studies of tissue slices and isolated, perfused organs show a relative reduction of oxygen consumption at any degree of hypothermia that is *greater* than in those of the body as a whole (Table 2-1). This may be related to known species differences in tissue respiration, to suboptimal

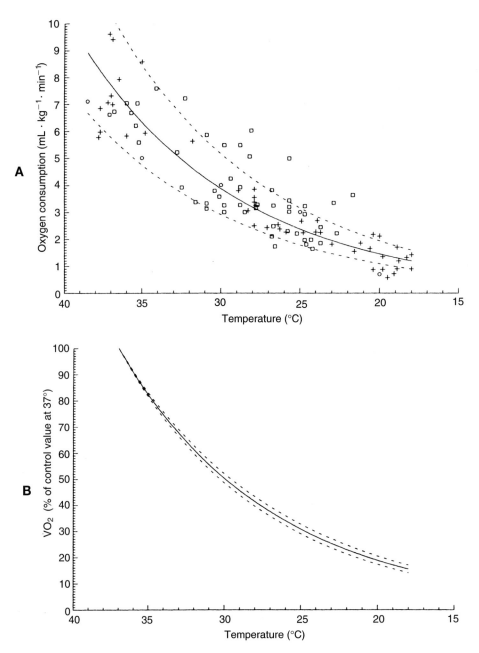

Figure 2-1   Temperature and oxygen consumption. (Note reversal of temperature scale from normothermia to hypothermia.) **A,** Figure contains two depictions. One is a group of symbols representing data points relating measured whole body oxygen consumption ($\dot{V}o_2$) to body temperature in dogs made hypothermic by surface cooling. (Crosses are data points from Ross[R1]; circles from Bigelow and colleagues[B2]; squares from Penrod.[P1]) From these, a regression equation, the second depiction, was derived, showing the van't Hoff relation between $\dot{V}o_2$ and temperature (Appendix Equation 2A-1). Solid line (representing the point estimates) and dashed lines (enclosing 70% confidence intervals) are nomograms of the equation. Slope indicates a Q_{10} of 2.7. **B,** Nomogram of the same equation, with oxygen consumption expressed as percentage of control value at 37°C.

conditions for tissue respiration in the studies with tissue slices, or to increased oxygen consumption during whole body perfusion caused, for example, by catecholamine release.[M1]

A striking fact from both whole body and tissue and organ studies is that oxygen consumption is not reduced to near zero at temperatures close to 0°C.[H19,M28,R10] Metabolic activity is therefore continuing and the time limits of safe circulatory arrest must be finite. Furthermore, this continuing metabolic activity causes a tendency for organs and systems to rewarm during the arrest period. Donald and Kerr showed in dog brains cooled to 1° to 2°C that an increase in temperature occurred during a 30-minute period of circulatory arrest and that this was in part related to the gradient between brain and room temperature and in part to continuing metabolic activity in the brain.[D3]

■ **TABLE 2-1   Oxygen Consumption ($\dot{V}o_2$)** [a]

Organ	Tissue Slices (Rats) [b]			Isolated *In Situ* Organs (Dogs) [c] (Cooling Coil Shunt)			Isolated *In Situ* Organs (Dogs) [d] (Surface Cooling)		
	37°C	25°C	% $\dot{V}o_2$ Reduction	37°C	25°C	% $\dot{V}o_2$ Reduction	37°C	25°C	% $\dot{V}o_2$ Reduction
Brain	1.98 ± 0.31	0.73 ± 0.139	63	5.16 ± 0.90	3.54 ± 0.90	31	4.31 ± 0.64	1.46 ± 0.30	66
Kidney	3.87^{e}	1.63^{e}	58	5.58 ± 1.98	0.96 ± 0.36	83	–	–	–
Muscle	0.76	0.36	53	0.90 ± 0.30	0.30 ± 0.12	67	–	–	–

[a] Expressed as mL · h^{-1} · g^{-1} wet weight $\pm$ SD. Data have been rearranged and recalculated to allow for comparisons.
[b] Data from Fuhrman.[F2]
[c] Data from Holobut and colleagues.[H19]
[d] Data from Rosomoff and Holaday.[R10]
[e] Kidney cortex.

OTHER PHENOMENA DURING HYPOTHERMIA AND CIRCULATORY ARREST

No-Reflow Phenomenon

It is only a hypothesis that a numerical relationship exists between oxygen consumption and safe circulatory arrest time at any given temperature. In fact, existence of a necessary and close relationship between the two over a wide range of temperatures would be surprising in view of other phenomena that occur during circulatory arrest. One of these is regional vascular occlusion in the brain and probably in all organs and tissues, leading to the no-reflow phenomenon.[A2] This is an obstructive lesion of the microcirculation that prevents local reperfusion and leads to additional damage after the general circulation of blood has been reestablished. The no-reflow phenomenon could theoretically damage the brain after hypothermic circulatory arrest. However, Norwood and colleagues have shown experimentally that this phenomenon develops as a result of severe hypoxia or anoxia, not because of circulatory arrest per se.[N8] They have also shown that hypothermia to 20°C prevents the no-reflow phenomenon with 90 minutes of anoxia, produced by continuing perfusion at an arterial PaO_2 of about 10 mmHg. Thus, this phenomenon may represent, at least in part, hypoxic endothelial cell injury, with alteration in the expression of the endothelial relaxing and constricting factors.[K16] In experimental studies, hypoxia, followed by reoxygenation, results in an almost twofold increase in the release by endothelial cells of endothelin-1, the most powerful vasoconstrictor yet identified.[G25] Other experimental studies have shown that this response can be blunted when the ischemia is induced under hypothermic conditions.[Z4] Thus, hypothermia may provide protection against hypoxic endothelial cell injury. Hypoxia may also promote a procoagulant response in endothelial cells that can result in intravascular microthrombosis.[G26,S31] Edema, as well as neutrophil and platelet plugging, may also contribute to the impaired perfusion that occurs following ischemia, despite what appears to be adequate restoration of blood flow.[B46,R26]

Changes in Plasma Volume

Chen and colleagues demonstrated progressive hemoconcentration and decrease in plasma volume during surface cooling of infants to 25°C, an observation supporting their own and previous experimental studies.[C14,D15] This may represent sequestration of plasma in portions of the vascular bed and leakage of plasma into the interstitial fluid compartment.

DAMAGING EFFECTS OF CIRCULATORY ARREST DURING HYPOTHERMIA

It is generally agreed that the brain has the shortest safe circulatory arrest time of any organ or region of the body, although occasionally the kidney seems to be damaged by a period of circulatory arrest when the brain is not. Although other organs and regions can be severely damaged by long periods of circulatory arrest, their safe arrest times are generally longer than that of the brain.

Brain Function and Structure: Risk Factors for Damage

The possibly damaging effects of circulatory arrest on the brain (see Chapter 4), as well as the risk factors related to it in patients undergoing cardiac operations during hypothermic circulatory arrest, are incompletely understood. Furthermore, the conduct of cooling and rewarming by CPB and the damaging effects of CPB itself likely contribute to or interact with the injury produced by circulatory arrest per se.

Duration of total arrest of cerebral blood flow is clearly a determinant of the amount of brain damage, but the safe duration of circulatory arrest to the brain (the duration within which irreversible structural or functional damage does not occur) is affected by a few known risk factors and no doubt by other risk factors that are as yet poorly understood. Furthermore, in patients undergoing cardiac surgery, brain damage that occurs in the setting of hypothermic circulatory arrest is rarely diffuse. In adults, it is usually manifested by specific intellectual or motor deficits, whereas in neonates, infants, and small children it is more likely to be manifested by seizures or choreoathetoid movements. This may be related to the phenomenon of *selective neuronal vulnerability,* that is, a heightened sensitivity of specific neuron groups to ischemic injury. This sensitivity has been correlated with the concentration of specific membrane receptors whose density in specific areas varies with age.[G17,R19] Concentration of these receptors is transiently high in the basal ganglia in the neonatal period, which may relate to the appearance of choreoathetosis as a result of ischemic injury in the very young.

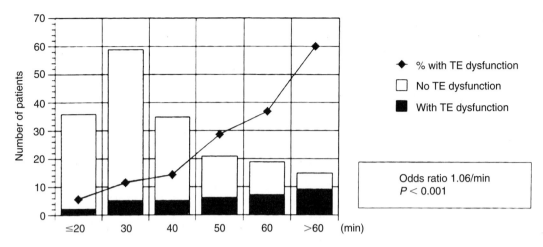

Figure 2-2   Prevalence of temporary (TE) neurologic dysfunction as a function of duration of circulatory arrest time. (From Ergin and colleagues.[E12])

Risk factors for irreversible structural and functional brain damage from circulatory arrest, in addition to duration of the arrest, include mean and regional brain temperature during circulatory arrest, rate of cooling and rewarming, cerebral blood flow and distribution during cooling, arterial blood pressure during cooling and reperfusion, electrical activity before arrest, biochemical milieu and catecholamine levels during cooling and circulatory arrest, absence of pharmacologic interventions before and after the cessation of cerebral blood flow, and total management of reperfusion.

Temperature and Duration

Most clinical studies of the relationship of temperature to safety of a given circulatory arrest time are flawed by lack of information about the temperature of the brain itself and by the variety of sites of measurement of temperature (tympanic membrane, nasopharynx, rectum, midesophagus, bladder, extremity skin) used to estimate safety.[B36] There is little consistent correlation between some of these sites, although temperature of the tympanic membrane and nasopharynx most closely resembles the mean temperature of the brain.[C25,G1,W1] For this reason, these sites should be used whenever possible.

Animal experiments and clinical experiences indicate that when the brain is cooled to 15° to 20°C, *circulatory arrest of 30 minutes or less* is tolerated without development of evident structural or functional damage.[F6-F8,K3,R21,T15,W3] During such a period, adenosine triphosphate (ATP) concentrations decline to 35% of initial values, but return rapidly to normal during reperfusion.[K3] Evidence that *circulatory arrest of 45 minutes* at these temperatures is unsafe is less secure.[R21,S5,T15]

Considerable information supports the inference that *circulatory arrest of 60 minutes or more* at temperatures of 15° to 18°C is associated with irreversible structural or functional damage, although it may be tolerated without evident damage by some subjects under some circumstances. In experimental studies by Folkerth and colleagues and Fisk and colleagues, histologic evidence of anoxic brain damage was found in all animals subjected to hypothermic circulatory arrest for 45 to 60 minutes, although some animals survived without evident func-

tional abnormality.[F6-F8] Half (2 of 4) of the animals studied by Kramer and colleagues showed no recovery of ATP when subjected to 60 minutes of hypothermic circulatory arrest.[K3]

Other clinical studies have found fewer problems associated with 60 minutes or more of hypothermic circulatory arrest. Particularly striking is the experience of Coselli and colleagues, who found no clinical evidence of brain damage attributed to hypothermic circulatory arrest (mean nasopharyngeal temperature 16.9°C, range 10.1° to 24.1°C) in 56 patients with arrest times ranging from 14 to 109 minutes (median 36 minutes).[C25] Comprehensive neuropsychometric studies were not undertaken. Hemiparesis or hemiplegia attributed to cerebral edema developed in 3 of 51 surviving patients (6%; CL 3%-11%).

Temporary neurologic dysfunction (postoperative confusion, agitation, delirium, obtundation, or transient parkinsonism without localizing signs) can occur in up to 20% of survivors of operations on the thoracic aorta in which hypothermic circulatory arrest is used.[E12] Incremental risk factors associated with development of this complication are duration of hypothermic circulatory arrest and increasing age of the patient.[E12] Prevalence of temporary neurologic dysfunction increases substantially among patients in whom the duration of circulatory arrest exceeds 60 minutes (Fig. 2-2). Although postoperative delirium is not permanent, it can be an important complication. Among a group of patients undergoing pulmonary thromboendarterectomy, circulatory arrest times of greater than 50 minutes were a powerful risk factor for its occurrence.[W21]

Some evidence supports the concept that continuous perfusion of the brain for 60 or more minutes at low temperature also produces neurologic sequelae in a few patients (see "Evidence of Gross Neurologic Damage").[M11] However, cold (10° to 15°C) continuous perfusion of brains already at 15°C resulted in no intellectual or other deficit in trained rhesus monkeys.[W3]

Characteristics of the Cooling Process

Uneven cooling of the brain is probably a risk factor for brain damage, although evidence is largely indirect.[B36] Almond and colleagues conducted experiments in dogs undergoing hypothermic circulatory arrest for 30 minutes.[A3] Results

■ **TABLE 2-2   Major Neurologic Events after Hypothermic Circulatory Arrest**

Method	No. of Patients	Circulatory Arrest (min)	Major Neurologic Events[a]		
			No.	%	CL
Surface cooling to 28°C, then core cooling	80	42.5 ± 13.6	0	0	0-2
Core cooling only	138	42.8 ± 15.4	8	6	4-9
TOTAL	218[b]				
P				.03	

(Data from Stewart and colleagues.[S5])

Key: *CL*, 70% confidence limits.

[a] Excludes seizures followed by uneventful convalescence.
[b] Repair of ventricular septal defect (VSD), tetralogy of Fallot, transposition of the great arteries, and atrioventricular septal defects. Mean temperature ± standard deviation during arrest for both groups was 19.7 ± 1.76°C.

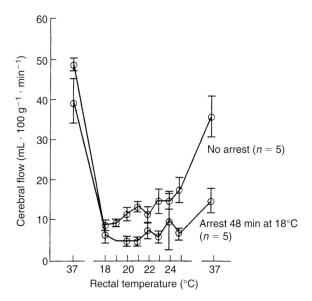

Figure 2-3   Cerebral blood flow ($mL \cdot 100\ g^{-1} \cdot min^{-1}$) in gerbils after induction of and recovery from hypothermia by surface cooling. Along the horizontal axis is rectal temperature. Break between 37°C and 18°C represents 48 minutes of circulatory arrest (total bilateral carotid artery occlusion) at 18°C (arrest group) or continuing hypothermic perfusion (no arrest group). Note that cerebral blood flow was lower during rewarming in those animals that had total cessation of cerebral blood flow for 48 minutes. (From Kirklin.[K15])

were interpreted to indicate structural and functional brain damage when cooling by CPB was done with the perfusate 20°C colder than the patient. These investigators believed that this did not occur when the blood was only 4° to 6°C cooler than the patient. However, the damage might have been related to the short period of cooling required with the very cold blood, producing uneven brain cooling, as suggested by the work of Zingg and Kantor.[Z1] The longer period of cooling required with the blood only 4° to 6°C colder than the subject probably produced more uniform cooling. In their patients, Stewart and colleagues noted a considerably higher prevalence of major neurologic events after circulatory arrest when core cooling by CPB alone was used, compared with surface cooling first to 28°C, followed by core cooling (Table 2-2).[S5] A reasonable presumption is that the more rapid core cooling resulted in uneven cooling of the brain. In another study in neonates and infants, rapid core cooling was associated with more evidence of neurologic deficits after hypothermic circulatory arrest than more prolonged core cooling.[B41] Again, a reasonable presumption is that prolonged core cooling results in more uniform cooling of the brain.

Cerebral Blood Flow during Cooling and Rewarming

The relationship of cerebral blood flow during cooling, before establishing hypothermic circulatory arrest, to safety of the arrest period has received little investigation. However, related to this is the suggestion in the earlier literature that reduced arterial blood pressure during CPB without circulatory arrest contributes to postoperative neurologic dysfunction, presumably because the hypotension resulted in reduced cerebral blood flow.[B32,J4,S20,S21] This possibility now appears less certain (see "Cerebral Blood Flow" under Distribution of Blood Flow in Section 2).

More recently, when cerebral blood flow was measured during operations involving hypothermic circulatory arrest in children, Greeley and colleagues observed that patients with increased oxygen extraction before circulatory arrest may be particularly vulnerable to cerebral injury.[G13] In a subsequent study, they demonstrated that during cooling, a parallel reduction in cerebral oxygen consumption and cerebral blood flow occurred.[G19] However, in three of four patients who were subsequently found to have sustained

neurologic injury, oxygen extraction before the period of circulatory arrest was increased, suggesting that cerebral blood flow during this period was inadequate to sustain metabolic requirements. Other studies in children have confirmed the observation that cerebral blood flow generally decreases with temperature during cooling, and that coupling with cerebral metabolism is maintained even at low temperatures when ventilation is managed according to the alpha-stat strategy.[G6,H35,V8]

Information is available about the magnitude and effect of cerebral blood flow during rewarming. An experimental study found that cerebral blood flow was reduced during rewarming after circulatory arrest (Fig. 2-3). This phenomenon occurs in humans during cardiac surgery, with or without circulatory arrest, and may affect outcome.[G6] In infants, cerebral blood flow is reduced during rewarming immediately after hypothermic circulatory arrest and after achieving normothermia.[G6] Based on measurements of jugular venous oxygen saturation, oxygen delivery appears to be adequate during this period of reduced flow.[V9] In a study of 255 adult patients undergoing elective coronary artery bypass grafting with or without associated cardiac valve replacement, Croughwell and colleagues observed a decline in postoperative cognitive function in 38%.[C34] The severity of decline was related to greater arteriovenous oxygen content difference between radial artery and jugular venous blood ($CavO_2$) during rewarming. This increase in oxygen extraction was associated with a low jugular venous oxygen saturation and low cerebral blood flow.

Biochemical Milieu

Only incomplete information is available in this area as well; it is uncertain whether some variables are actual risk

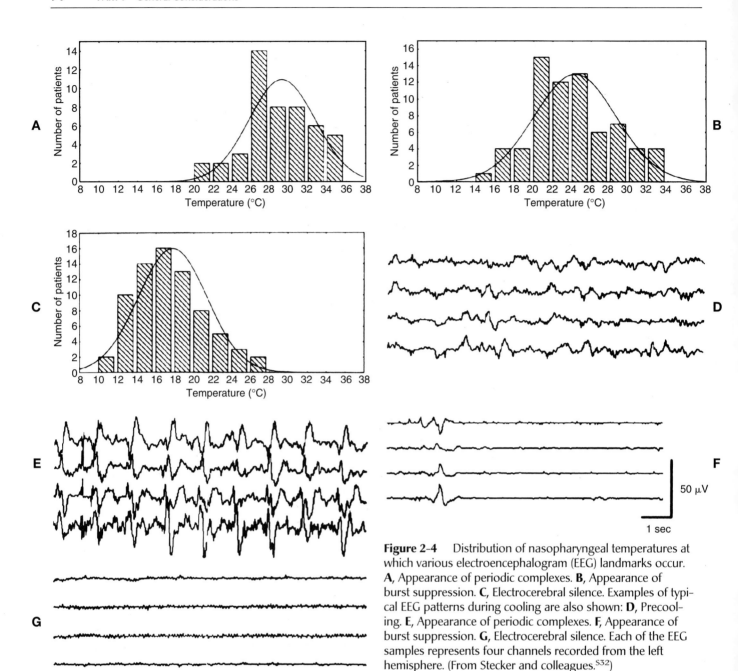

Figure 2-4   Distribution of nasopharyngeal temperatures at which various electroencephalogram (EEG) landmarks occur. **A,** Appearance of periodic complexes. **B,** Appearance of burst suppression. **C,** Electrocerebral silence. Examples of typical EEG patterns during cooling are also shown: **D,** Precooling. **E,** Appearance of periodic complexes. **F,** Appearance of burst suppression. **G,** Electrocerebral silence. Each of the EEG samples represents four channels recorded from the left hemisphere. (From Stecker and colleagues.[S32])

factors or surrogates for the real risk factor. Thus, arterial blood pH and Pco_2 during cooling may have important direct effects on brain tissue at the beginning of the period of circulatory arrest, and thereby on outcome, but they also influence cerebral blood flow, and perhaps its distribution, during cooling (see "Controlled Variables" in Section 2). Any effect they may have on neurologic outcome, which is uncertain, could be through either mechanism.

Brunberg and colleagues and Anderson and colleagues suggested that increased tissue glucose, such as is usually present at the beginning of the arrest period, may lead to excessive glycolysis and acidosis during the arrest period, possibly resulting in tissue damage from lactic acid accumulation.[A20, B7] It is this possibility that makes it imprudent to use glucose solutions for priming the pump-oxygenator and for intravenous infusion when a period of circulatory arrest is contemplated.[D21]

Based on the work of Choi and of Olney and colleagues, evidence has accumulated indicating that the neuroexcitatory amino acids—particularly glutamate, the major transmitter mediating synaptic excitation in the mammalian central nervous system—have potent neurotoxic activity during conditions of depleted cellular energy such as hypoxia or ischemia, when the synaptic reuptake of these amino acids, a highly energy-dependent process, is compromised.[C35,O8] Resulting overaccumulation of glutamate leads to excessive excitation of the glutamate receptors, leading to an increase in intracellular calcium and eventual neuronal cell injury and death. This process has been observed in experimental animals after 2 hours of circulatory arrest.[R22] Neuronal necrosis is selective and corresponds closely to the distribution of excitatory amino acid receptors.[R23] The hippocampus, cerebellum, and basal ganglia, which have high concentrations of glutamate re-

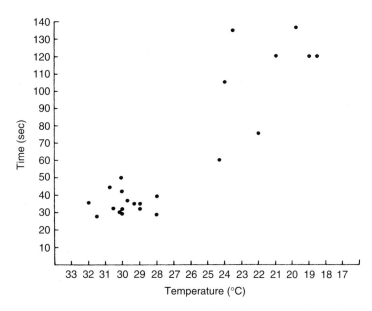

Figure 2-5   Relationship of interval (seconds) from beginning of circulatory arrest to appearance of electroencephalographic quiescence, and nasopharyngeal temperature at time of circulatory arrest. (Note reversal of temperature scale.) (Redrawn from Harden and colleagues.[H7])

ceptors, are characteristically most vulnerable to this injury, implying excitation as an underlying mechanism.[R22,R23]

Other experimental studies by Fessatidis and colleagues have demonstrated, using histopathologic techniques, that the cerebellum is the most vulnerable area of the brain to prolonged periods (more than 70 minutes) of hypothermic (15°C) circulatory arrest.[F22,F23]

Electroencephalogram before Arrest

Electroencephalographic criteria for safe circulatory arrest are conflicting. In a study by Coselli and colleagues, the longest recorded durations of safe circulatory arrest in adults were in situations in which a full formal electroencephalogram (EEG) had recorded *electrocerebral silence* (no electrical activity of cerebral origin at maximal gain, 2 $\mu V \cdot mm^{-1}$) for 3 minutes before the arrest.[C25] In this study, mean nasopharyngeal temperature at this point was 16.9°C (range 10.1° to 23.1°C).

In a subsequent study by Stecker and colleagues of 109 adult patients undergoing hypothermic circulatory arrest, electrocerebral silence was achieved at a mean nasopharyngeal temperature of 17.8°C (range 12.5°C to 27.2°C).[S32] This required cooling, using a standardized protocol, for a mean of 27.5 minutes (range 12 to 50 minutes). Distributions of times to cool to various EEG events are shown in Fig. 2-4. The time to cool to electrocerebral silence was prolonged by high hemoglobin concentration, low arterial partial pressure of carbon dioxide, and slow cooling rates. Only 60% of patients demonstrated electrocerebral silence by either a nasopharyngeal temperature of 18°C or a cooling time of 30 minutes. Although cooling to an end point such as electrocerebral silence provides a more reproducible effect of hypothermia on the nervous system than cooling to a specific temperature (such as 12.5°C,

which was sufficient to produce electrocerebral silence in all patients in this study), the optimal temperature for circulatory arrest could not be determined.[S32]

Others have found that in infants and children cooled to a nasopharyngeal temperature of 18.5°C, the EEG was characterized by continuous phasic activity.[C3,H7,S4,W4] During cooling, however, there was a gradual disappearance of fast components and an increase in slow components. Occasionally, repetitive, rapid discharges occurred. Such reports indicate that when circulatory arrest is established, electrocerebral silence develops after an interval that is inversely related to nasopharyngeal temperature at the beginning of the arrest period[H7,K3] (Fig. 2-5). However, Reilly and colleagues reported persistent electroencephalographic activity during circulatory arrest, perhaps reflecting activity in the white matter and cerebellum.[R2] This is of interest because of the occasional postoperative occurrence of choreoathetoid movements in humans and high-stepping gaits in experimental animals. These abnormalities may be due in part to uneven brain cooling secondary to regional differences in flow during cooling.

Also, when CPB is resumed after circulatory arrest in infants, electroencephalographic activity is absent initially and then gradually returns as rewarming proceeds.[C3] In general, after 20 to 30 minutes of rewarming, the EEG has returned approximately to its control condition.[C3] This latent period, between resumption of whole body perfusion for rewarming and time of return of reasonably normal EEG activity, is believed by Weiss and colleagues to be related to the important metabolic (oxygen) debt that develops during the arrest period.[W4] This in turn is influenced by brain temperature during arrest and by duration of the arrest. Weiss and colleagues observed that when circulatory arrest lasted less than 40 minutes, electroencephalographic activity always reappeared within less than 20 minutes, whereas longer periods of circulatory arrest were followed by longer and more varied latent periods.[W4]

In adults, Stecker and colleagues observed that lower nasopharyngeal temperatures at the time of circulatory arrest resulted in a slower return to continuous activity.[S33] Prolonged time to recovery of continuous EEG activity and higher temperature at which the EEG first became continuous were associated with increased risk of neurologic injury. Patients who sustained postoperative neurologic injury also had a longer period of circulatory arrest (52 ± 21 min) than patients who did not (37 ± 12 min) ($P = .006$).

Age of the Patient

Although it has been stated that very young patients suffer less brain damage from hypothermic circulatory arrest than do older patients, there is little factual support for this concept. Relative to the general population, cognitive, language, and motor performances are significantly reduced at 4 years in infants younger than 3 months in whom circulatory arrest has been employed.[B47] In adults in whom circulatory arrest is used, increasing age is an important predictor of both stroke and temporary neurologic dysfunction.[E1,E12] Temporary neurologic dysfunction is a marker for long-term functional neurologic deficit.[E13]

Effects of Brain Damage
Evidence of Gross Neurologic Damage

Choreoathetosis has occurred early postoperatively in infants and children undergoing hypothermic circulatory arrest.[B7,B8,C4,S5] When it occurs, choreoathetosis usually develops 2 to 6 days postoperatively. As time passes, the movements usually lessen in severity. If mild, they disappear completely, but if severe, they or hypotonia may persist. Brunberg and colleagues found no correlation between circulatory arrest time or depth of cooling (between $16°$ and $20°C$) and development of choreoathetosis.[B7] These reports suggest that this specific complication occurs in 1% to 12% of patients and that its residual effects are permanent in some. When choreoathetosis occurs, it is often in the setting of prolonged circulatory arrest.[S5]

However, choreoathetosis has been observed in infants and children subjected to deep hypothermic CPB without circulatory arrest.[D22] There are suggestions that this complication can result from perfusion of the brain with very cold blood for a prolonged period at relatively high flows.[B39,B40,D22,E11] This is the basis for the recommendation that arterial temperature not be reduced to less than $15°C$.

The cause of choreoathetosis is unclear. Deep hypothermia per se may cause neurologic injury. Egerton and colleagues reported that continuous hypothermic perfusion at $10°$ to $12°C$ produced moderate or severe brain damage, including choreoathetosis, in 10 of 16 patients (63%; CL 46%-77%).[E11] Air or particulate embolization to the brain may be a contributing factor. When circulatory arrest is used, choreoathetosis may be related to uneven brain cooling, leading to the continued metabolic activity in the white matter and cerebellum observed by Reilly and colleagues,[R2] and perhaps uneven brain reperfusion related to vascular changes implicated in the no-reflow phenomenon.[C5,G2,H8,H9,O1] The

latter finding lends support to the rationale for using hemodilution during cooling, because absence of red cells in the perfusion used just before circulatory arrest to the brain eliminates the no-reflow phenomenon.[A2] Use of the alpha-stat strategy of acid–base balance has also been implicated as a causative factor.[J9]

Seizures have occurred in the early postoperative period in 5% to 10% of patients undergoing hypothermic circulatory arrest.[B7,B9,B10,C4,V5] Because seizures are usually transient and followed by uneventful convalescence, they have not been considered major neurologic events. However, in an analysis from the Boston Circulatory Arrest Study involving 171 children with D-transposition of the great arteries, transient postoperative clinical and EEG seizures were associated with worse neurodevelopmental outcomes at ages 1 and 2.5 years, as well as neurologic and MRI-detected abnormalities at 1 year of age.[R24]

The comments made concerning possible causes of choreoathetosis are also applicable to seizures. However, it is well known that infants are highly susceptible to seizures from disturbances of thermoregulation and fluid balance, as well as from metabolic disorders, especially those related to glucose and calcium, and many of these factors may be operative in these patients.

More severe and gross evidence of brain damage has uncommonly occurred after hypothermic circulatory arrest in infants and children, including *coma* either dating from surgery or developing some hours later, followed by *lasting impairment* or *death*. In a study by Stewart and colleagues, three (1.4%; CL 0.6%-2.7%) such instances occurred among 218 young patients undergoing repair of the common types of congenital heart disease with hypothermic circulatory arrest.[S5] Five other patients developed choreoathetosis. All these events occurred in the group of patients in whom core cooling alone was used. None occurred in patients in whom the duration of circulatory arrest was less than 45 minutes, and the probability of developing major neurologic events increased as circulatory arrest time increased beyond this (Fig. 2-6).

Focal neurologic damage resulting in serious neurologic impairment (stroke) occurs in adult patients following hypothermic circulatory arrest. Ergin and colleagues demonstrated that this form of injury is related to older age ($P < .0001$) particularly beyond 60 years, presence of clot or atheroma in the aortic arch ($P < .0001$), as well as longer duration of hypothermic circulatory arrest ($P < .0001$).[E12]

Postoperative Intellectual Capacity

The effect of hypothermic circulatory arrest on late postoperative intellectual capacity and behavior in infants and children has been difficult to study. Problems in testing small infants preoperatively so that each may serve as his or her own control contribute to the difficulty. Associated congenital developmental disorders, possible adverse effects before operation of severe congenital heart disease, and effects of other perioperative events complicate interpretation of the data. In general, late postoperative studies suggest that when circulatory arrest is less than 60 minutes at nasopharyngeal temperatures of about $20°C$, intellectual capacity and development are not adversely affected.[H10] When arrest is longer than 60 minutes, intellectual development may be adversely affected.

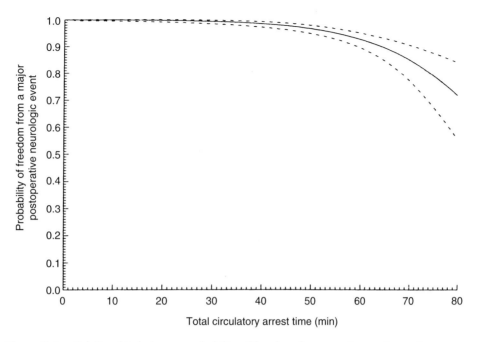

Figure 2-6   Relationship between probability of freedom from a major postoperative neurologic event and hypothermic circulatory arrest time in 219 infants under 3 months of age (eight events) undergoing open intracardiac operations. (See Appendix 2A, Equation 2A-5.) (Data from Stewart and colleagues.[S5])

■ **TABLE 2-3   Results of Intelligence Testing Some Years after Surgery Performed in Infancy Using Hypothermic Circulatory Arrest**

		IQ <80			
		"Explained" by:			
Investigators	No. of Patients Tested	Preoperative Events	Postoperative Events	Unexplained	Total (%)
Stevenson et al.[S7]	36	3	0	1	4 (11)
Dickinson and Sambrooks[D4]	38	3	1	3	7 (18)
Clarkson et al.[C4]	72	6	1	5	12 (16)
TOTAL	146	12 (8%; CL 6%–11%)	2 (14%; CL 0.5%–3.2%)	9 (6.2%; CL 4.1%–9.0%)	23 (16%; CL 13%–19%)

Key: *CL,* 70% confidence limits; *IQ,* intelligence quotient.

Results of psychomotor testing in 146 children undergoing cardiac surgery during hypothermic circulatory arrest early in the experience with this technique, obtained by combining the three largest reported series, are summarized in Table 2-3.[C4,D4,S7] Late postoperatively, 23 of the 146 (16%; CL 13%-19%) had an intelligence quotient (IQ) of 80 or less, more than one standard deviation below the test mean. In approximately half these patients, preoperative events were considered likely to account for the low scores. In the remainder, an occasional child suffered an adverse perioperative event, but the low scores were unexplained in nine (6.2%; CL 4.1%-9.0%) patients.

Wells and colleagues obtained data on intellectual and psychological development in children that caused them to question the idea that 60 minutes of circulatory arrest at 18°C is safe.[W16] They found that the verbal ($P = .06$), quantitative ($P = .07$), and general cognitive ($P = .003$) IQ scores of patients with an arrest time of 50 minutes or more were lower late postoperatively than those of patients with an arrest time of less than 50 minutes.

The first randomized clinical trial comparing prevalence of brain injury after corrective heart surgery in infants with D-transposition of the great arteries using deep hypothermia, predominantly with circulatory arrest or low-flow CPB, was conducted at Boston Children's Hospital.[N10] This study demonstrated that infants in whom circulatory arrest was used had a higher prevalence of neurologic abnormalities and poorer mental function at 1 year of age, and poorer expressive language and motor development at 2.5 years of age. Follow-up studies of the same cohort at 4 years of age showed that use of circulatory arrest is associated with worse motor coordination and planning but not with lower IQ or worse overall neurologic status.[B47] However, neither IQ nor overall neurologic status was correlated with duration of circulatory arrest. In the cohort as a whole, cognitive, language, and motor performance were reduced relative to the general population.[B47]

In summary, data for infants and children are somewhat conflicting. There is general agreement that arrest times of longer than 60 minutes at 18° to 20°C may be associated

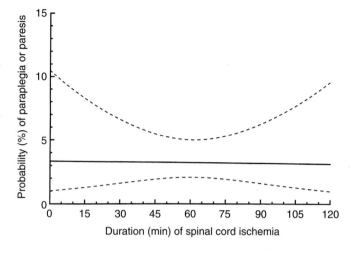

Figure 2-7   Risk of paraplegia or paresis according to duration of spinal cord ischemia. Dashed lines represent 70% confidence limits. *P* value for relationship is .98. (From Kouchoukos and colleagues.[K17])

with impairment of intellectual function and development, and some of the data suggest that arrest periods of longer than 45 minutes may not be entirely safe.

Spinal Cord Function

The spinal cord is less susceptible to ischemic injury than the brain, as evidenced by absence of sensory or motor deficits of the trunk or the upper and lower extremities of infants, children, and adults who have been subjected to intervals of hypothermic circulatory arrest of up to 60 minutes. Hypothermia also provides important protection of the spinal cord during ischemic intervals produced by aortic clamping. In a clinical study of hypothermic CPB and circulatory arrest (mean interval of arrest 38 minutes, range 8 to 62 minutes) for operations on the descending thoracic and thoracoabdominal aorta in 161 patients, prevalence of paraplegia or paresis (a severe injury resulting from spinal cord ischemia) remained constant and less than 3.5% for ischemic (but hypothermic) intervals of up to 138 minutes[K17] (Fig. 2-7).

Renal Function and Structure
Experimental Studies

At normothermia, at least in rats, 20 minutes of circulatory arrest to the kidney produces no histochemical evidence of cell death, whereas 30 minutes produces extensive cell death in the distal portion of the proximal convoluted tubules, with scattered areas of cell death being seen at 25 minutes.[V2] Vogt and Farber identified progressive accumulation of lactic acid during ischemia as a causative factor, and rapid decrease of ATP to 20% of control values as an indicator of impending renal death.[V2]

Hypothermia prolongs the safe circulatory arrest time for the dog kidney. Ninety minutes of circulatory arrest after surface cooling to 18° to 20°C produces no late morphologic changes in the kidney.[R3] However, precise relationships among temperature, duration of circulatory arrest, and morphologic and functional renal damage are not clear. Gowing and Dexter suggest that minimal morphologic changes evolve in the kidney after 60 minutes of circulatory arrest at 21°C.[G3] It is apparent, however, that at any temperature, the safe circulatory arrest time for the kidney is longer than it is for the brain and shorter than it is

for the liver. In addition, a scattered loss of cells through cell death probably results in no detectable loss of renal function, whereas this may not be true in the brain.

As with other organs, the question of damaging effects of hypothermia per se is not fully resolved. Ward found fewer morphologic and functional derangements of the kidney after 90 minutes of circulatory arrest at 15°C than at either lower or higher temperatures.[W6] This suggests that temperatures less than 15°C may damage the kidney.

Studies in Humans

Important oliguria beginning about 12 hours postoperatively occasionally complicates recovery of infants operated on with hypothermic circulatory arrest for less than 60 minutes. Venugopal and colleagues reported four deaths (3%; CL 2%-6%) from renal failure among 130 patients operated on with surface-induced hypothermic circulatory arrest.[V5] Among patients who died, renal failure was the mode of death in 14%.

The primary cause of the renal failure appears to be low cardiac output after operation. However, in at least some cases, severe oliguria develops when the hemodynamic state of the patient appears to be adequate. In view of the finding in experimental studies that morphologic and functional damage to the kidney does not occur after 60 minutes of circulatory arrest at temperatures of 18° to 20°C (Fig. 2-8), damaging effects from CPB must be implicated. In part, this may be the result of low cardiac output preceding and following the interval of circulatory arrest. In part, it may be due to damage to the kidneys by free hemoglobin and by circulating toxins that appear during CPB (see Section 2). Free hemoglobin has been found in the renal tubules of some of these patients at autopsy.

In 161 adult patients undergoing resection of the distal aortic arch and descending thoracic and thoracoabdominal aorta in whom hypothermic circulatory arrest was used (mean nasopharyngeal temperature, 14.5°C; mean interval, 38 minutes; longest interval, 62 minutes), prevalence of postoperative renal failure requiring dialysis among 157 operative survivors was 2.5% (4 patients).[K17] Among the subgroup of 18 operative survivors who had evidence of renal dysfunction preoperatively (serum creatinine level >1.5 mg · dL^{-1}), none developed renal failure that required dialysis.

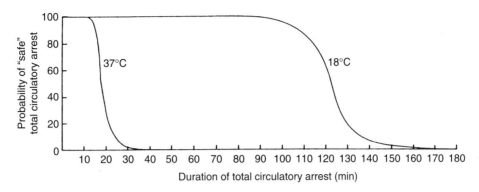

Figure 2-8 Freehand nomogram for the kidney of the relation between probability of safe total circulatory arrest and duration of circulatory arrest at two temperatures. The normothermic relationship is based on the work of Vogt and Farber[V2] and the hypothermic one on data presented in the text.

Liver Function

Studies in dogs suggest that complete hepatic circulatory arrest for 45 minutes or more at 37°C is followed by serious functional derangements.[A4,B19] The normothermic liver of humans resumes normal function after its complete isolation from the circulation for 35 to 40 minutes.[H11] With hypothermia (20° to 22°C), 60 minutes of circulatory arrest does not produce structural or functional abnormalities in the liver.[R3]

SAFE DURATION OF CIRCULATORY ARREST

The preceding information does not allow formulation of a table or an equation relating safe duration of circulatory arrest to various temperatures based on rigorously derived rules. Knowledge of biologic systems in general indicates that if adequate information were available, relationships should be expressed as probability of no functional or structural damage (that is, probability of safe circulatory arrest) at a given temperature, rather than as an absolute value.

In addition to the data already presented, a few other comments are indicated. Early experience at the Mayo Clinic suggested that 45 minutes was the maximum safe duration even when nasopharyngeal temperature was reduced to 20°C.[K1]

Fig. 2-9, *A* shows three curves relating probability of safe circulatory arrest to arrest time at nasopharyngeal temperatures of 37°, 28°, and 18°C. These estimates are based on available information, but because of lack of data they have not been rigorously derived. To emphasize that each curve would have a degree of uncertainty even if considerable data were available, the 70% confidence limits around the continuous point estimate for 18°C are shown in Fig. 2-9, *B*. The preceding pages indicate that histologic changes in the central nervous system, without functional abnormalities, are the most sensitive indicators of lack of complete safety of the arrest period used. The portrayal at 18°C of essentially complete safety of 30 minutes of circulatory arrest is consistent with all available information. The portrayal of essentially complete safety of arrest of 45 minutes for at least 70% of subjects is also consistent with the facts, and the damage produced within this period

is likely to be structural and without permanent functional sequelae. Most patients will have some structural evidence of damage from 60 minutes of arrest, but only about 10% to 20% will have evident functional damage, and in many of them the manifestations will be transient.

Other support systems, such as continuous CPB at normothermia or with moderate or deep hypothermia, with or without low perfusion flow rates, have their own potential for damaging one or more organ systems. Furthermore, the heart disease being treated has the potential for producing damage. An inaccurate repair can produce damage, and such inaccuracies are more likely to result when surgical exposure is poor. The surgical team must therefore weigh the relative risks of these and other factors in deciding in an individual patient whether circulatory arrest should be used and, if it is to be used, its duration and temperature during the arrest period (see Section 3 for additional details).

SECTION 2

Whole Body Perfusion during Cardiopulmonary Bypass

CPB for cardiac surgery is conceptually simple, and equipment is available to accomplish it with relative ease. Most or all of the patient's systemic blood, which normally returns to the right atrium, is diverted into a device in which oxygen is supplied to the blood and carbon dioxide is removed. The newly arterialized blood is pumped from the device into the aorta. Among the complexities of CPB are that blood does not naturally (1) circulate through nonendothelially lined channels, (2) contain gaseous and particulate emboli, and (3) experience nonphysiologic shear stresses. Also, the body is unaccustomed to absence of any appreciable pulmonary blood flow and to presence of only minimally pulsatile aortic pressure. In addition to CPB, the patient undergoing cardiac surgery experiences all of the stress responses characteristic of major surgical procedures and trauma.

What is truly remarkable is that most human subjects survive operation and CPB, and they convalesce in a

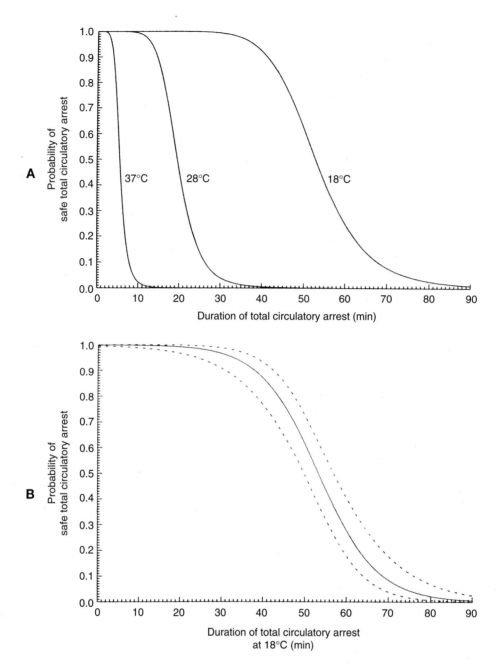

Figure 2-9 Probability of safe (absence of structural or functional damage) circulatory arrest according to duration. **A,** Estimate at nasopharyngeal temperatures of 37°, 28°, and 18°C. **B,** Estimate at 18°C with dashed lines representing 70% confidence limits. Number of experiments in the literature concerning 40 minutes of circulatory arrest at 18°C nasopharyngeal temperature is estimated at 20 as a basis for calculating these confidence limits. Note that at 30 minutes safe arrest is highly likely and that at 45 minutes it is probable. Other data suggest that at 45 minutes, damage will probably be only structural and without evident functional sequelae.

reasonably normal manner. However, almost every patient retains, for a time, a few demonstrable stigmata from the procedure; some have major morbidity, and a few die of their response to CPB. Prevalence of these unfavorable outcomes in a group of patients is in part determined by identifiable risk factors, but determinants of their occurrence and severity in an individual patient have not been completely defined.

When essentially all systemic venous blood returns to the pump-oxygenator instead of to the heart, the situation is termed *total cardiopulmonary bypass*. When some systemic venous blood returns to the right atrium and right ventricle and is pumped into the lungs, from which it passes back into the left atrium and is pumped by the left ventricle into the aorta, the situation is termed *partial cardiopulmonary bypass*. Partial CPB has long been known to be better tolerated than complete CPB. Reasons for this have not been clearly defined, but continuation of at least some pulmonary blood flow is a likely explanation. The remainder of this section is concerned with total CPB.

HISTORICAL NOTE

The historical aspects of CPB for cardiac surgery are not easily described, because it is almost impossible to determine who first conceived the idea of diverting the circulation of a patient to an oxygenator outside the body and pumping it back to the arterial system to allow surgery to be performed on or within the heart. References to extracorporeal gas exchange in blood go back to the last part of the nineteenth century. For example, Frey and Gruber worked with an "oxygenator" in 1885.[F9] Subsequently, scores of laboratory studies with oxygenators and pumps were reported. However, serious consideration of pump-oxygenators for cardiac surgery had to await development of modern anesthesia, modern surgical methods, and, particularly, scientific developments such as discovery and use of heparin and manufacture of biocompatible plastic materials. Without doubt, John Gibbon, with his pioneering experimental work at Massachusetts General Hospital in Boston in the late 1930s, was a major contributor to development of CPB and its advancement to the stage of successful clinical application.[G4] Gibbon's work was interrupted by World War II, but when he came to Jefferson Medical College in Philadelphia after military service, he resumed work with CPB, its pathophysiology, and the equipment required for it. Most of the medical and surgical world took little note of his work and, in fact, considered it unlikely to lead to any useful purpose. However, Gibbon persevered. In 1953, he performed the first successful operation in which the patient was totally supported by CPB when he repaired an atrial septal defect in a young woman using a pump-oxygenator.[G5] Unfortunately, his subsequent four patients died of a variety of problems, and he became discouraged with the method (Gibbon JH Jr: personal communication; 1955).

Meanwhile, a few others began to work with pump-oxygenators for CPB during the late 1940s. Among them were Clarence Dennis and his colleagues at the University of Minnesota. His laboratory studies led him to make what may have been the first attempt to use a pump-oxygenator for clinical cardiac surgery in 1951.[D5] Dennis and Richard Varco operated on a patient thought to have an atrial septal defect. These surgeons believed they had done a satisfactory repair, but the patient died. Autopsy showed that the lesion was in fact a partial atrioventricular septal defect and misinterpretation of the anatomy was a major factor in the patient's death. In Stockholm, Viking Bjork and Åke Senning also worked during the late 1940s and early 1950s with CPB.[B12,S9] In related efforts, Clarence Crafoord was an early user of this method for removal of an atrial myxoma.[C6]

After Dennis' unsuccessful effort, C. Walton Lillehei and his colleagues at the University of Minnesota began working in the laboratory with controlled cross-circulation, using another intact subject as the "oxygenator."[C7] Their experimental studies led them to adopt the now discarded "azygos flow principle," which presumed that only low perfusion flow rates were needed.[A5] In April 1954, they began a spectacular series of operations for congenital heart disease using "controlled cross-circulation" with the mother or father as the oxygenator.[W7] Although this particular technique was soon abandoned, the work of Lillehei and colleagues brought into being the modern era of open intracardiac surgery.

Experimental work at the Mayo Clinic with pump-oxygenators began in the early 1950s under the direction of John Kirklin.[D6,J1] This led to the first use of CPB with a pump-oxygenator at the Mayo Clinic on March 22, 1955, when a ventricular septal defect was successfully repaired, and subsequently to the world's first published series of intracardiac operations performed with use of CPB and a pump-oxygenator.[K4] These procedures were performed using the Mayo-Gibbon pump-oxygenator, which was designed and constructed in the engineering shops of the Mayo Clinic.[K5,K9,K15,K18] Use of a pump-oxygenator for CPB during cardiac surgery expanded rapidly, and today the method is used many times a day in hospitals in almost every country in the world.

UNIQUENESS OF CARDIOPULMONARY BYPASS

The patient whose arterial blood flow is temporarily provided by means of a pump-oxygenator is in an abnormal state that affects most, if not all, physiologic processes. Throughout evolution, blood has passed only through channels lined with endothelial cells, but during CPB, it is passed across nonendothelial foreign surfaces. As a result and perhaps because of other factors, virtually all humoral and cellular components of the inflammatory response are acutely activated, and probably some of the more slowly reactive specific immune responses are activated as well, at least initially.[K9] The general stress response, seen after surgery and trauma, also occurs to a major degree.

During total CPB, a number of physiologic variables are under direct external control, in contrast to the situation in intact humans. These include total systemic blood flow ("cardiac" output); input pressure waveform; systemic venous pressure; pulmonary venous pressure; hematocrit and chemical composition of the initial perfusate; arterial oxygen, carbon dioxide, and nitrogen levels; and temperature of the perfusate and patient.

Another group of variables is determined in part by the externally controlled variables but in large part by the patient. These include systemic vascular resistance, total body oxygen consumption, mixed venous oxygen levels, lactic acidemia and pH, regional and organ blood flow, and organ function.

A third group of largely uncontrolled variables includes, to a greater or lesser degree, all components of the process of inflammation, incited in large part by the organism recognizing the foreign surfaces across which blood passes as "nonself."

These features make the patient who has undergone CPB a unique organism, at least for a few days. Recognition of this, as well as a detailed knowledge of the post-CPB state, is necessary for delivery of optimal postoperative care (see Chapter 5).

CONTROLLED VARIABLES

Arterial Output to the Patient

Arterial output (outflow) from the pump-oxygenator to the subject is achieved by generation of a large pressure gradient by a pump. The most commonly used type of arterial pump is the *roller pump* (originally used by

DeBakey for blood transfusion[D8]). It generates a relatively nonpulsatile flow and is simple, reliable, and relatively inexpensive. In clinical use, roller pumps are generally set to be nearly occlusive.[1] When they are occlusive, trauma to the formed elements in blood is increased; when they are too nonocclusive, they are unable to maintain the same rate of flow against the wide range of resistances (pressure differentials of 30 to 300 mmHg) offered by arterial cannulae and the patient's systemic vascular resistance. The tubing passing through the roller pump head is most often Tygon (a special nontoxic surgical grade of polyvinyl), but during hypothermia, Tygon tubing decreases in elasticity and filling volume; thus, stroke volume of the pump is slightly decreased. Silicone rubber tubing does not have this disadvantage and may be used in the roller pump head when hypothermia is required. Volume output of the roller pump is more certain to be that predicted when output resistance is high than when a high negative pressure is generated on the input side. When generated negative pressure on the input side exceeds about 200 mmHg, volume output of the roller pump becomes less predictable.

The controlled vortex (centrifugal) pump is also commonly used for cardiac surgery and for closed-chest support of patients in whom both arterial and venous cannulation are accomplished centrally or peripherally (termed cardiopulmonary support, CPS). Flow generated by a controlled vortex pump varies with changes in resistance to flow into and out of the pump. When pressure in the output line reaches about 500 mmHg, both outflow from and inflow into the pump become zero. When pressure in the inflow line decreases to about −500 mmHg, both inflow and outflow become zero. Therefore, in contrast to the roller pump, revolutions per minute (rpm) of the controlled vortex pump cannot be used to estimate flow. Instead, a flowmeter must be placed on the arterial (output) or venous (input) line. However, if the arterial line becomes completely occluded, either intentionally or by accident, flow immediately ceases, but pressure in the arterial line will rise no higher than 500 mmHg, and it is unlikely that the tubing will rupture or a junction will give way. Blood trauma is similar in controlled vortex and roller pumps. Although air can be entrapped within the controlled vortex pump, it, like the roller pump, can transmit air bubbles from the venous to the arterial lines.

Venous Input from the Patient

The venous input (inflow) into the pump-oxygenator from the patient is achieved by a negative pressure gradient from patient to machine. The negative pressure required to move blood from the patient to the pump-oxygenator is considerably less than the pressure required to move blood from the pump-oxygenator to the patient, because of the different characteristics of the venous and arterial systems

of the patient and to some extent of the venous and arterial cannulae.

Sufficient negative pressure for venous input into the pump-oxygenator can be generated by

- Creating a controlled vacuum within a venous reservoir
- Using a siphon system in which gravity creates the negative pressure
- Using a pump to create the negative pressure within the venous line from the patient

Vacuum-Assisted Venous Return

The ideal method for creating negative pressure for venous input into the pump-oxygenator is by controlled vacuum in a small reservoir. The patient and machine can be at the same level, the negative pressure does not rise above the controlled level if the cannula becomes occluded, and the amount of negative pressure can be varied as needed. Most importantly, the two pressures (that is, output pressure to the patient and input pressure from the patient) are uncoupled and can be varied independently.

Use of a hard-shelled reservoir in currently available oxygenators and a vacuum regulator connected to wall suction that is set at −40 to −60 cm H_2O has allowed vacuum-assisted venous return (VAVR) to become widely accepted.[F20,T23] VAVR permits use of smaller venous cannulae, smaller reservoirs, considerably shorter tubing, and low priming volume. It is of considerable value for cardiac operations performed in infants and through small incisions in children and adults (see Special Situations and Controversies in Section 3).[O7,T23] In a study by Banbury and colleagues at The Cleveland Clinic Foundation, VAVR was found to reduce priming volume from 2.0 ± 0.4 L to 1.4 ± 0.4 L ($P < .0001$), to increase hematocrit both on bypass and immediately postbypass ($P < .0001$), and to reduce use of blood products both intraoperatively and postoperatively from 39% of patients to 19% ($P = .002$).[B54]

Siphon (Gravity) Drainage

A common method of generating the negative pressure gradient is through siphonage. Disadvantages of this approach include an imposed difference in the levels of patient and pump-oxygenator, the relatively narrow range of negative pressures that can be generated in the operating room by its use, and its interruption by large boluses of air in the venous line. Most importantly, the need for a reservoir increases the filling (priming) volume of the pump-oxygenator. It is, however, simple, reliable, effective, and inexpensive.

Venous Pumping

The controlled vortex pump permits direct pumping from the patient's venous system and is more convenient than a roller pump. The potentially large pressure gradient between the tip of the venous cannula and the right atrium or venae cavae must be controlled in some way, to prevent "fluttering" of the walls of the right atrium or venae cavae around the end of the venous cannulae. One way of accomplishing this is to use small venous cannulae to impose a considerable resistance between the pump and the tip of the cannula, rather than between the tip of the

---

[1] In the laboratory, this is defined as a fall of 1 inch per minute of a column of water in tubing held vertically above the roller pump. Clinically, when the pump-oxygenator is fully primed, the system is pressurized to 300 mmHg measured by an onboard manometer. The roller heads are adjusted to allow a slight pressure drop over 1 minute.

cannula and the patient's venous system. This is fortuitously advantageous in percutaneous peripheral cannulation, because an 18- or 20-French venous cannula of some length can be easily passed into the venous system of a normal-sized adult and provides adequate venous drainage. It also facilitates minimally invasive cardiac surgery. By contrast, 28- to 32-French catheters are required when gravity drainage is used.

Gas Exchange

The device for gas exchange, the oxygenator, is a highly important component of pump-oxygenators. Not only does it regulate tension of gases in the arterial blood emerging from the pump-oxygenator, but it is also the largest area of foreign surface with which the blood comes into contact, and therefore probably the component of the pump-oxygenator in which the most blood damage occurs. This contact occurs in the boundary layer of the blood, which is made very large in the oxygenator to facilitate gas exchange. Only a small proportion of the formed and unformed elements of the blood comes into contact with the surfaces of the tubing and pumps.

Gas exchange occurs directly across the blood–gas interface in bubble oxygenators, in rotating disk and cylinder oxygenators, and in stationary vertical screen oxygenators. It occurs across a multitude of tiny pores in so-called membrane oxygenators of the hollow-fiber, microporous polypropylene, and other types, in which there are still blood–gas interfaces. However, damage to the blood is less in these types of "membrane oxygenators" than in bubble oxygenators.[V15] Only in the true silicone rubber membrane oxygenator, of the type devised by Kolobow and colleagues, is there no blood–gas interface.[K14] This allows CPB to be used for more than 24 hours with reasonable safety.

Because of their efficiency, hollow-fiber and true membrane oxygenators do not depend on minute ventilation (gas flow) to the oxygenator for CO_2 regulation under most circumstances. Rather, the ventilating gas flow rate and composition are regulated independently. This allows precise regulation of arterial Po_2 and Pco_2.

Arterial Oxygen Levels

With present-day oxygenators, maintaining PaO_2 at about 250 mmHg is easily accomplished. Higher PaO_2 is unnecessary and theoretically subjects patients to the risk of oxygen toxicity and bubble formation. PaO_2 lower than about 85 mmHg results in a declining arterial oxygen content (according to the oxygen dissociation curve of blood) and a corresponding reduction of tissue and mixed venous oxygen levels. Shepard demonstrated that when arterial oxygen saturation fell below 65% in dogs undergoing normothermic CPB, total body oxygen consumption ($\dot{V}o_2$) fell, indicating hypoxic cell damage.[S10]

PaO_2 is related to temperature of the patient, which is related to $\dot{V}o_2$ (see Fig. 2-1), blood flow rate ($\dot{Q}$), performance of the oxygenator, and, in a complex fashion, to ventilating gas flow rate and composition (see "Gas Exchange" earlier in this section). Reducing the patient's body temperature reduces $\dot{V}o_2$ and increases $P\bar{v}o_2$, resulting in increased PaO_2. During rewarming by perfusion from the

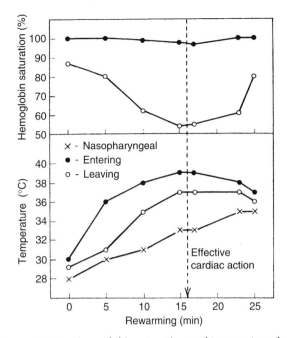

Figure 2-10   Hemoglobin saturation and temperature during rewarming. Note sharp decrease in mixed venous oxygen saturation, shown by open circles in the upper panel, as rewarming proceeds. "Entering" temperatures are those in the arterial tubing and "leaving" temperatures those in the venous return tubing. (From Theye and Kirklin.[T1])

pump-oxygenator, the increasing $\dot{V}o_2$ and the metabolic debt that has accumulated result in relatively low mixed venous oxygen levels[T1-T3] (Fig. 2-10). This period, then, places maximal demands on the oxygen transfer capacity of the oxygenator.[L2,T2,T3]

Arterial Carbon Dioxide Pressure

Arterial carbon dioxide pressure ($PaCO_2$) is controllable during CPB by varying the ratio between gas flow rate into the oxygenator ($\dot{V}$, or ventilation $\cdot$ min^{-1}) and blood flow rate through the oxygenator ($\dot{Q}$).[H13] This is facilitated by use of microporous or true membrane oxygenators, because gas flow rate is not the force driving blood through the oxygenator, as is the case in bubble oxygenators, and arterial oxygen levels are well maintained over a wide range of gas flow rates. Inline Pco_2 and pH meters facilitate control of $PaCO_2$ and pH.

Some clinical perfusions for cardiac surgery are performed at normothermia (approximately 37°C) and others at various levels of hypothermia: mild (30° to 35°C), moderate (25° to 30°C), or deep (<25°C). Therefore, it is necessary to consider the strategy for control line $PaCO_2$ and, indirectly, pH. The "alpha-stat" strategy is based on (1) using the pH *measured at 37°C and uncorrected* for the temperature of the patient's blood, and (2) maintaining this level at 7.4. That is, the ventilation of the oxygenator is maintained at the level appropriate for a body temperature of 37°C, no matter how deep the hypothermia. This "hyperventilation" during hypothermia results in a decrease in $PaCO_2$ and an increase in pH when the values for these are corrected for the temperature of the patient's blood. Swan and Reeves, Rahn and colleagues have all emphasized that at low temperatures, neutrality exists at a higher pH than at normothermia, because of the change of the dissociation constant of water with temperature.[R5-R7,S11] The alpha-stat strategy results in optimal function of a number of important enzyme systems, including lactate dehydrogenase, phosphofructokinase, and sodium-potassium ATPase.[Y1]

In contrast, the "pH-stat" strategy strives for the same values of pH and $PaCO_2$, *corrected to the temperature of the patient's blood,* during hypothermia as at normothermia. This represents a state of respiratory acidosis and hypercarbia. Cerebral blood flow usually increases under these circumstances. This may be considered advantageous in some situations, but so-called luxury perfusion may expose the brain to larger numbers of microemboli than would otherwise be the case, and therefore could be disadvantageous.[H29,J8]

At a cellular enzyme level, the alpha-stat strategy may be preferable, but which is preferable in clinical cardiac surgery in neonates, children, and adults is the subject of current investigation.[J9] The alpha-stat strategy results in a lower $PaCO_2$, which may adversely affect cerebral blood flow.[V3] This may be of particular importance for patients with cyanotic congenital heart disease, such as tetralogy of Fallot with pulmonary atresia, for whom low $PaCO_2$ may result in pulmonary vasodilatation in addition to cerebral vasoconstriction.[M22] Thus, there can be a steal of blood from the cerebral to the pulmonary vascular bed.[K19,W25] The pH-stat technique may depress cardiac function.[B29] However, at least in dogs, regional distribution of blood flow during normothermic and hypothermic full-flow CPB is similar with the alpha-stat and pH-stat strategies.[B28]

Heparin Levels

Before CPB is established, the patient is anticoagulated by intravenous or intracardiac injection of heparin, usually in a dose of 300 to 400 U · kg^{-1} body weight (sometimes expressed as 3 to 4 mg · kg^{-1}). (The details of dosage of heparin and protamine, and of the activated clotting time, are given later in "Heparinization and Later Protamine Administration" under Preparation for Cardiopulmonary Bypass in Section 3). Heparin, one of a heterogeneous group of biologic products called glycosaminoglycans, has an approximate molecular weight of 3000 to 100,000. A purified form derived from porcine intestinal mucosa may be used, but more often the form derived from bovine lung is employed. Experimental and limited prospective clinical studies suggest that lung heparin may be preferable for CPB, because bovine lung heparin has a more reliable protamine neutralization response.[S6] Heparin binds to and activates antithrombin III, which is responsible for virtually all the anticoagulant activity of heparin.

Heparin concentrations in plasma can now be measured directly; the usual values during CPB are 3.5 to 4.0 U · mL^{-1}. Usually these measurements correlate well with the activated clotting time (ACT).[W9] One exception is the situation of antithrombin III deficiency, a state of heparin resistance.[B52,B53] Two or three times the usual dose of heparin may be required to produce satisfactory anticoagulation, that is, an ACT of 480 seconds. If only the heparin level is measured, initiation of CPB might produce thrombosis in the pump-oxygenator system and introduce thrombus into the patient. The most common cause of antithrombin III deficiency is previous exposure to heparin in a dose-dependent fashion.[E14,S34] Treatment is based on replenishing antithrombin III, either with fresh frozen plasma or with antithrombin III concentrate.

Although heparin used in the manner described has been clinically satisfactory, activation of the clotting cascade during CPB is not completely neutralized. At least factor XII, factor XI, and prekallikrein are activated, and high-molecular-weight kininogen is cleared.[C20] Thus, markers of fibrin formation can be detected in most patients during and early after CPB, and fibrin emboli can occur.[D10] In most patients, this subclinical coagulation does not cause the concentrations of the soluble coagulation factors to become sufficiently low during or early after CPB to cause bleeding.[H22]

Increasing the dose of heparin does not prevent subclinical coagulation during CPB.[G16] By contrast, maintaining ACT at 300 to 350 seconds, rather than 450 seconds, results in no more subclinical plasma coagulation than does the traditional method, requires less heparin, and may be associated with less bleeding after operation.[C26,G16]

The use of aprotinin has affected the concepts of heparinization for CPB for intracardiac surgery, because this agent may prolong both the clotting time and the ACT, depending on the method of measurement (see "Fibrinolytic Cascade" under Response Variables later in this section).[H40,N12,W27] An optimal recommendation when aprotinin is used is to administer the usual initial dose of heparin and add additional heparin to maintain the ACT above 700 seconds, if the activating agent is celite (diatomaceous earth). Kaolin is a more dependable activating agent, giving ACTs in the presence of aprotinin similar to those without aprotinin in vitro and during CPB.[F28,W28] Therefore, a preferable method when aprotinin is used during CPB is to use kaolin as the activating agent and maintain the usual ACT at 480 seconds. Alternatively, the heparin concentration is measured at intervals and is kept above 3 mg · kg^{-1}.

Perfusate

Diluent

The diluent (which is used to prime the pump-oxygenator system, wholly or in part, and for any erythrocyte-free additions during CPB) is a balanced electrolyte solution, with a near-normal pH and an ion content resembling that of plasma. There is some evidence for the concept that in both adults and very young patients, it is disadvantageous to include either glucose or lactate in the priming solution[M17,M18] (see "Biochemical Milieu" under Damaging Effects of Circulatory Arrest during Hypothermia in Section 1). However, priming solutions containing glucose and lactate are used in some centers.[M3]

In pump-oxygenator systems without a venous reservoir or using vacuum-assisted venous return, mixing of blood and prime may be partially or wholly avoided, with residual prime discarded.

Hemoglobin Concentration

At some institutions, in adult patients and even in very young patients, no effort is made to control the hemoglobin concentration or hematocrit during CPB. Instead, the pump-oxygenator is routinely filled initially with a balanced salt solution.

In intact humans at 37°C, the normal hematocrit of 0.40 to 0.50 is optimal rheologically and for oxygen transport (assuming a normal red blood cell hemoglobin concentration).[C8] This provides sufficient oxygen delivery to maintain normal mitochondrial Po_2 levels of about 0.05 to 1.0 mmHg and average intracellular Po_2 levels of about 5 mmHg, these being reflected in normal oxygen levels ($P\bar{v}O_2$) of about 40 ($S\bar{v}O_2$ of about 75%) in mixed venous blood. When the hematocrit is abnormally high, oxygen content is high, but the increased viscosity tends to decrease blood flow. The rate of oxygen transport varies directly with hematocrit (because oxygen content varies directly with hematocrit, assuming normal red blood cell hemoglobin concentrations and adequate oxygenation) and inversely with the viscosity of blood (which is also determined primarily by hematocrit). Hypothermia increases the viscosity of blood; therefore, at low temperatures, a lower hematocrit is more appropriate than at 37°C.

A lower-than-normal hematocrit appears desirable during hypothermic CPB because the perfusate has a lower apparent viscosity and low shear rates, and provides better perfusion of the microcirculation. Thus, a hematocrit of about 0.20 may be optimal during moderately and deeply hypothermic CPB, although a low hematocrit could predispose the patient to neurologic dysfunction, particularly when it exists during a period of low CPB flow and particularly in elderly individuals. During rewarming, a higher hematocrit may be desirable because of the increased oxygen demands, and the higher apparent viscosity of a higher hematocrit is appropriate during normothermia. This may be achieved by ultrafiltration (see "Components" under Pump-Oxygenator in Section 3) at this time, or by adding packed red blood cells if the blood volume is too low to allow this.

The need for and amount of additional blood or packed red blood cells to achieve a desired hemoglobin concentration during CPB can be determined before the start of CPB (Box 2-2). If the calculated hematocrit is in the desired range, a blood-free priming solution is used. If the calculated Hct is lower than desired, an appropriate amount of blood (or packed red blood cells) is added.

Banked blood preferably less than 48 hours old is used, but older blood is accepted for adults when necessary. Banked blood is rendered calcium-free by the anticoagulant solution (citrate-phosphate-dextrose, or CPD) and is acidotic, so additions of heparin, calcium, and buffer may be required before placing it in the pump-oxygenator, before or during CPB. However, in at least a few institutions, no calcium is added before placing the blood in the pump-oxygenator, and none is added thereafter until the patient's nasopharyngeal temperature reaches about 28°C during the rewarming process. Then the ionized calcium level is measured, and an appropriate amount of calcium is added. (The normal level is about 1.2 mmol · L^{-1}, with total calcium being about 2.5 mmol · L^{-1} or 10 mg · dL^{-1}.) This practice results in extremely low levels of ionized calcium when CPB is first established. Unduly high levels of ionized calcium could be more deleterious (see Chapter 3). A reasonable practice would be to add initially 3 mL of

---

BOX 2-2   Algorithm for Calculating Patient–Machine Hematocrit

The need for and amount of additional packed red blood cells to achieve a desired hemoglobin concentration early after commencing bypass is determined by the patient's blood volume (VpB) and hemoglobin concentration prior to CPB (expressed as hematocrit, HCTp), and the volume of pump-oxygenator prime (VmB) and its hemoglobin concentration (expressed as hematocrit, HCTm). Patient blood volume is estimated as

$$VpB = 1000f \cdot wt,$$

where f is the proportion of body weight attributable to blood volume; $f = 0.08$ for infants and children up to 12 years of age, $f = 0.065$ for older patients, and wt is weight in kg. More complex regression equations are available for more accurate estimates.[N13]

Patient (VpRBC) and machine (VmRBC) red cell volumes are

$$VpRBC = VpB \cdot HCTp$$
$$VmRBC = VmB \cdot HCTm.$$

Then, mixed patient-machine hematocrit (HCTpm) is

$$HCTpm = (VpRBC + VmRBC)/(VpB + VmB).$$

If no blood is in the prime,

$$HCTpm = VpRBC/(VpB + VmB).$$

These calculations may be included in a computer-prepared printout for the perfusionist, available before the patient comes to the operating room.

---

calcium chloride (10%) rather than 5 mL for each unit of banked blood used, and then add no more until the ionized calcium is measured.

Albumin Concentration

Concentration of albumin in the mixed patient–machine blood volume, as well as of hemoglobin, is affected by the amount of hemodilution. Theoretically, according to the Starling law of transcapillary fluid exchange (see "Pulmonary Venous Pressure" later in this section), a reduction of albumin and thus of the colloidal osmotic pressure of the plasma accentuates movement of fluid out of the vascular space into the interstitial space. That this occurs is indicated by the work of Cohn and colleagues, who showed that the extracellular fluid volume increases more rapidly when hemodilution is used than when it is not.[C9]

However, during CPB, microvascular permeability to macromolecules is increased[S18]; some of the administered albumin leaks into the interstitial fluid and has an unfavorable effect on the relationships expressed in the Starling law. Homologous albumin may provoke an allergic response, which increases microvascular permeability and causes leakage of albumin into the interstitial fluid.

These complex interrelations probably explain the failure of a randomized trial to find a favorable effect from adding homologous albumin to the prime in adults.[M16] Whether albumin concentration should be maintained at normal levels in some special situations remains arguable.

Other colloidal solutions (dextran 40, dextran 70, hydroxyethyl starch) can also be added to the priming solution to attenuate the loss of fluid from the intravascular space.

However, none of them has been conclusively shown to have a beneficial effect.

Other Additives

Practices vary regarding the addition of substances and drugs to the perfusate (by administering them into the priming volume of the pump-oxygenator or patient before CPB, or into the patient or pump-oxygenator during CPB) other than basic balanced salt solution and blood and its required additives.

Use of an *osmotic diuretic* may be advisable. Mannitol (about 0.5 g $\cdot$ kg^{-1}), a pure osmotic diuretic, can be included as part of the prime. Mannitol also has the advantage of being an effective agent against the oxygen-free radicals that are generated during CPB.[E8,M15] Glucose (added to the prime of the pump-oxygenator in sufficient quantity to obtain a glucose concentration of about 350 mg $\cdot$ dL^{-1} in the prime) also produces a diuresis. However, its use in the priming volume and its administration during and early after CPB, employing more than moderate hypothermia, may be unwise in view of the strong suggestion that hyperglycemia during cooling and early after hypothermic circulatory arrest increases the probability of brain damage.[A20,E7,S19]

Administration of a potent diuretic during CPB is generally useful. Incorporation of furosemide in the pump prime is practiced by many groups. It may be more advantageous to give it as a bolus in a dose of 1 to 2 mg $\cdot$ kg^{-1} at the start of rewarming, either after an interval of circulatory arrest or moderately or deeply hypothermic CPB.

The short-acting *adrenergic α-receptor blocking agent* phentolamine is capable of antagonizing the vasoconstriction produced by catecholamines and has been shown to produce more uniform body cooling and rewarming and improved tissue perfusion when given during CPB.[B30] A bolus of 0.2 mg $\cdot$ kg^{-1} is administered just after the start of CPB and the initiation of cooling. When circulatory arrest is used, an additional dose of 0.2 mg $\cdot$ kg^{-1} is administered with the resumption of CPB for rewarming.

Alternatively, the long-acting adrenergic α-receptor blocking agent phenoxybenzamine can be used in infants and children and produces total α-blockade for 8 to 10 hours. It is given in a dose of 1 mg $\cdot$ kg^{-1} about 15 minutes before commencing CPB and at the beginning of rewarming after the period of circulatory arrest.[L7] A continuous infusion of nitroprusside during cooling and again during rewarming is preferred to either of these by some groups. Nitroprusside reduces arterial blood pressure (by about 25 mmHg), yet maintains cerebral blood flow during moderately hypothermic CPB.[R8]

Opinions differ about the advisability of routinely administering (or adding to the perfusate) *corticosteroids* and the appropriate agent to use. Available evidence suggests that corticosteroids improve tissue perfusion and lessen the increase in extracellular water that usually accompanies CPB.[N6] Although some studies have reported improved clinical status when steroids are given in the manner described, this matter remains controversial.[J2] Methylprednisolone in a single dose of 30 mg $\cdot$ kg^{-1} or dexamethasone in a single dose of 1 mg $\cdot$ kg^{-1} given at the onset of CPB and not repeated may be advantageous. These agents do not appear to reduce complement activation, but there is evidence to support the hypothesis that they do attenuate complement-mediated leukocyte activation, particularly that associated with reperfusion of the heart and lungs in the latter part of CPB.[H36,H37,J2,K10,T18]

The powerful *antifibrinolytic agent* aprotinin is a biologic product that acts as a serine proteinase inhibitor. It may have a favorable effect on some of the platelet membrane–specific receptors, specifically GPIb. Aprotinin has been shown in several randomized studies to reduce bleeding after CPB by about 50% without demonstrable adverse effect in the patients studied.[B14,B48,F11,F17,R17,V13,V14,W20] A small initial dose (500 kallikrein inactivator units [KIU], or 0.05 mL) is administered intravenously just after the induction of anesthesia to test for sensitivity of the patient to the drug, but sensitivity is rarely seen unless the drug has been previously given.[D18] The pump-oxygenator prime (in adults) is arranged to contain 1 x 10^6 KIU, or 100 mL of the drug, in a concentration of 10,000 units $\cdot$ mL^{-1} in a normal saline solution, although some protocols arrange for the prime to include 2 x 10^6 KIU (200 mL). Before CPB is established, a continuous infusion of aprotinin is begun. During the first 20 to 30 minutes, 2 x 10^6 KIU (200 mL) is administered; thereafter, 0.5 x 10^6 KIU $\cdot$ h^{-1} (50 mL $\cdot$ h^{-1}) is given. This is continued throughout CPB or until 6 hours have elapsed, whichever comes first. No further doses are administered. Aprotinin affects the results of the celite-based ACT test. Special practices regarding heparin administration are indicated when aprotinin is used (see "Heparin Levels" earlier in this section).

Epsilon-aminocaproic acid and tranexamic acid are two other antifibrinolytic agents that can be administered before, during, and after CPB to reduce bleeding and the need for allogeneic blood transfusions.[C30,L9,M26,M27,N9] Epsilon-aminocaproic acid is administered using an empirical dose of 10 g before the skin incision, 10 g during the procedure, and 10 g in the early postoperative period.[V10] Alternatively, it can be given at a dose of 150 mg $\cdot$ kg^{-1} at the time of the skin incision, with an additional 30 mg $\cdot$ kg^{-1} for 4 hours upon initiation of CPB.[B49] Tranexamic acid is given at a dose of 1 g before the skin incision, 500 mg in the pump prime, and 400 mg $\cdot$ h^{-1} during the procedure.[C30]

Changes during Cardiopulmonary Bypass

During CPB for cardiac surgery, blood loss in the operative field, gradual increase in interstitial fluid, and urinary output combine to steadily deplete the patient–machine blood volume. Usual practice is for the perfusionist to add increments of a balanced electrolyte solution to maintain the volume at a safe level; in adults, sometimes up to 2000 mL is added. Unless special precautions are taken, such as avoiding return of irrigating fluids to the pump-oxygenator by cardiotomy pump suckers and using ultrafiltration during the final stages of CPB, severe hemodilution results and persists into the postbypass period.

In neonates and infants, ultrafiltration immediately after CPB (before removal of the cannulae) is often advisable using the modified ultrafiltration (MUF) technique introduced by Elliot.[E15] Its efficacy has been confirmed by others.[D24,T25] In children and adults, ultrafiltration may be performed during the latter part of CPB if the hematocrit is below about 0.25 and there is excess volume in the pump-oxygenator. If not, it may be performed after discontinuing CPB, slowly circulating blood through the patient before any cannulae are removed. A third option, and one

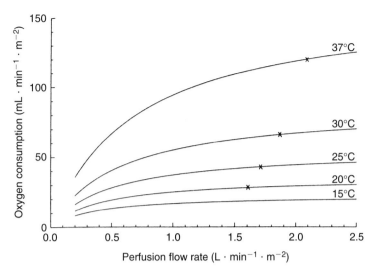

Figure 2-11   Nomogram of equation expressing relationship of oxygen consumption ($\dot{V}o_2$) to perfusion flow rate ($\dot{Q}$) and temperature (T). Small Xs have been added to represent perfusion flow rates used clinically at these temperatures (see Appendix 2A, Equation 2A-3).

that is frequently used, is ultrafiltration of the volume remaining in the pump-oxygenator after CPB is discontinued and the venous cannulae have been removed. Hemoconcentrated pump-oxygenator volume is then infused slowly into the patient before the arterial cannula is removed (see "Pump-Oxygenator" under Completing the Operation in Section 3).

Total Systemic Blood Flow

Although total CPB has generally been considered to require separate caval cannulation and occlusive tapes around each cannula, a single large, properly designed, and properly positioned venous cannula can direct all venous return to the pump-oxygenator and provide total CPB.

During total CPB, systemic blood flow (perfusion flow rate) is controlled by the perfusionist. It can be set at an arbitrary level or may be kept equal to the venous return from the patient. A rational approach is to set it at an arbitrary level.

In clinical practice, when body temperature is at 28°C or greater, a flow of 2.5 L · min^{-1} · m^{-2} is usually chosen for infants and children younger than about 4 years of age and a flow of 2.2 L · min^{-1} · m^{-2} for older patients. For adults with a body surface area of 2.0 m^2 or more, a flow of 1.8 to 2.0 L · min^{-1} · m^{-2} may be chosen, to avoid the disadvantage of high flow through the oxygenator. When moderate hypothermia is chosen, the CPB flow can safely be reduced to about 1.7 L · min^{-1} · m^{-2} for prolonged periods (Fig. 2-11). When cardiac operations are performed with body temperature reduced to 18° to 20°C in neonates, infants, or adults, CPB flows of 1 L · min^{-1} · m^{-2} are adequate for prolonged periods, at least as judged by persistence of the somatosensory evoked response (SSER) under these circumstances.[W19] Flows as low as 0.5 L · min^{-1} · m^{-2} (20 to 30 mL · min^{-1} · kg^{-1}) have been shown to be adequate at these temperatures to maintain cerebral oxygen consumption and ATP levels for at least 30 to 60 minutes (see Chapter 4).[F5,M19,R15,S28]

When flow rates are lower than optimal for more than a

BOX 2-3   Mixed Venous Oxygen Levels

Mixed venous oxygen saturation ($S\bar{v}o_2$), mixed venous oxygen pressure ($P\bar{v}o_2$), and mixed venous oxygen content ($C\bar{v}o_2$) may all be used to express mixed venous oxygen levels. The equation is

$$C\bar{v}o_2 = 1.38 \cdot S\bar{v}o_2 \cdot [Hb] + P\bar{v}o_2 \cdot 0.003$$

where $C\bar{v}o_2$ is in mL · dL^{-1}, [Hg] is hemoglobin concentration in g · dL^{-1}, $S\bar{v}o_2$ is a decimal fraction, and $P\bar{v}o_2$ is in mmHg.

short time, $\dot{V}o_2$ is considerably subnormal (less than 85% of the asymptote of the temperature-specific curve in Fig. 2-11 is considered subnormal), primarily as a result of perfusion of less than the total capillary bed. Also, the areas of the capillary bed that are open are underperfused, resulting in lactic acidemia and metabolic acidosis.

$P\bar{v}o_2$ and saturation ($S\bar{v}o_2$) have been widely used as indices of adequate perfusion flow rate (see Box 2-3; for references, see Harris and colleagues[H12]), the assumption being that these values reflect average cellular Po_2. If flow rate is high and the entire microcirculation perfused, this is true. However, it has been shown that during CPB, with perfusion rates within the conventional range, $S\bar{v}o_2$ is inversely related to $\dot{V}o_2$.[H12] This might have been predicted from the Fick equation:

$$\dot{V}o_2 = \dot{Q}(Cao_2 - C\bar{v}o_2)$$

$$(2\text{-}1)$$

where Cao_2 is arterial oxygen content, $C\bar{v}o_2$ is mixed venous oxygen content, and $\dot{Q}$ is flow rate.

If $\dot{V}o_2$ and Cao_2 are fixed, $C\bar{v}o_2$ increases with $\dot{Q}$. If, instead, $\dot{Q}$ and Cao_2 are fixed, $C\bar{v}o_2$ increases as $\dot{V}o_2$ decreases, and $\dot{V}o_2$ may decrease, despite a perfectly "adequate" $\dot{Q}$, if the capillary bed is not evenly perfused. In this case the distance between perfused capillaries and many tissue cells increases, and these cells do not obtain their oxygen requirement. In effect, this amounts to a shunt of arterial blood into the venous system. This effective shunt may at times amount to half the total flow. Rudy and colleagues, using microspheres in normothermic rhesus monkeys during CPB, found that shunting was only 1.4% of total flow rate.[R4]

A high $P\bar{v}O_2$ or $S\bar{v}O_2$ does not, therefore, mean that cellular oxygenation is satisfactory, whatever the $\dot{Q}$. A $\dot{V}O_2$ at or near the whole body requirement does. The $\dot{V}O_2$ is not difficult to calculate during CPB; the problem is, rather, to decide what the oxygen requirement is in a given case.[H4,H12] Moreover, if $\dot{V}O_2$ is less than the usual levels at conventional $\dot{Q}$, increasing $\dot{Q}$ probably will not increase $\dot{V}O_2$ (see Fig. 2-11). The fault is not in $\dot{Q}$ but in the capillary bed or at the cellular level.

As might be expected, high flow rate is achieved at the expense of some loss of safety and convenience in other variables. Blood trauma in the oxygenator is probably greater when high blood flows pass through it. With a bubble oxygenator, risks of gaseous emboli are also greater. Pressure gradients across the arterial cannula are greater at high flows. This increases cavitation, blood trauma, and the risk of bubbles forming as blood emerges from the cannula.

Arterial Pressure Waveform

CPB is usually conducted in such a manner that the arterial pressure pulse is very narrow and essentially nonpulsatile, but, if desired, a pulsatile arterial input can be achieved in several ways. One is by using left ventricular ejection. With no tapes around the caval cannulae, arterial flow to the patient may be temporarily increased over venous return, or venous return may be temporarily reduced by partially occluding the venous tubing. Atrial pressures and thus ventricular filling pressures are increased, left ventricular ejection augments systemic blood flow, and a somewhat pulsatile arterial blood flow results. In other words, pulsation is achieved by partial CPB. This mechanism is used during cooling and rewarming whenever cardiac action is sufficiently vigorous to prevent overdistention of the heart during the process. The procedure of partial CPB produces not only some arterial pressure pulsations, but some pulmonary blood flow as well, with its favorable effect.

A pulsatile waveform can also be produced by using intraaortic balloon pumping during bypass.[P2] A third method is to use a pulsatile arterial pump.

The effects on the organism of using a system that results in a pulsatile rather than nonpulsatile arterial waveform during CPB have been questioned since the beginning of clinical CPB. An already complex problem is still further complicated by an almost universal failure to describe the energy of the pulsatile flow in a proper manner, such as by *energy equivalent pressure.*[S16]

Intuitively, pulsatile flow seems advantageous over nonpulsatile flow. Several physiologic studies lend strong support to this idea, demonstrating that with nonpulsatile flow, vascular resistance increases, red blood cells aggregate, renal function is impaired, renin is released, and cellular hypoxia leads to metabolic acidosis.[G8,G9,M7,W11] However, it is not clearly established that pulsatile flow during CPB results in fewer functional derangements than does nonpulsatile flow. A number of studies have concluded that pulsatile perfusion is beneficial, but not all of them

present convincing evidence, and several have found little or no benefit.[A13,B18,D12,H18,J3,M8,N3,N4,S14,S15,T8-T12,W12,W13] Extensive reviews of this subject have been presented.[H28,M9]

A randomized clinical study by Singh and colleagues investigated pulsatile versus nonpulsatile flow during moderately hypothermic (25° to 30°C) CPB.[S14] No statistically significant differences between the two techniques were found in whole body oxygen consumption, blood lactate concentration, systemic vascular resistance, urine flow, or thermal gradients. Thus, no evidence was found that pulsatile flow improved the perfusion of the microcirculation during clinical CPB. It is possible that pulsatile flow would result in fewer functional derangements at lower flows than were used in this study.[D12,N7,O3,S10] Bixler and colleagues found that nonpulsatile perfusion at a mean pressure of 50 mmHg of a hypertrophied fibrillating dog's heart resulted in subendocardial ischemia, whereas pulsatile flow did not.[B18] When the mean perfusion pressure was 80 mmHg, neither pulsatile nor nonpulsatile flow resulted in subendocardial ischemia.

It is also possible, but not proven, that pulsatile flow has an advantage over nonpulsatile flow in infants. Williams and colleagues drew this conclusion from a clinical study in which they found more rapid cooling and rewarming and greater urine flow with pulsatile flow.[W14] Results of this study are difficult to interpret, however. Finally, pulsatile flow could prove beneficial in high-risk patients who come to operation desperately ill with end-stage disease (low cardiac output, acidosis, or renal failure).[H38]

Currently, there is insufficient evidence to conclude that pulsatile flow from the pump-oxygenator importantly reduces the ill effects of the relatively short periods of CPB required for cardiac surgery in the great majority of patients.

Systemic Venous Pressure

During CPB, systemic venous pressure is determined by the methods used,[K5] because

$$P\bar{v} = f \frac{\dot{Q}, \text{viscosity}}{\text{Cannula size, venous tubing size, venous negative pressure}}$$

$$(2\text{-}2)$$

where $P\bar{v}$ is mean systemic venous pressure, $\dot{Q}$ is systemic blood flow rate, and f means "a function of." The cross-sectional area and length of the single or multiple venous cannulae, and to a lesser extent (because it usually has a large diameter) those of the venous tubing, are fixed factors determining venous pressure during total CPB. For this reason, the largest venous cannulae compatible with the clinical situation are commonly used, mindful of the need for the cannulae to lie loosely, not snugly, in the caval veins. When smaller cannulae are used, the other variables in Equation 2-2 can be manipulated. For example, systemic blood flow can be reduced or suction applied to the venous return to ensure an acceptable venous pressure (see "Vacuum-Assisted Venous Return" earlier in this section).

There is no apparent physiologic advantage in having a central venous pressure greater than zero during total CPB. Increasing the venous pressure requires more intravascular volume and often additional priming volume. Venous pressure should therefore be kept close to zero, and certainly not more than 10 mmHg, to minimize increases in extracellular fluid.

Pulmonary Venous Pressure

Ideally, pulmonary venous pressure should be at zero during total CPB, and certainly not more than 10 mmHg. Undue elevations are dangerous because they produce increased extravascular lung water and eventually gross pulmonary edema, according to the Starling law of transcapillary fluid exchange.[3]

$$P_c - P_t = \pi_c - \pi_t$$

$$(2\text{-}3)$$

where P_c is effective blood pressure within the capillary, P_t is tissue turgor pressure (interstitial fluid pressure), π_c is osmotic pressure of the plasma (colloid) inside the capillary, and π_t is osmotic pressure of the extracellular fluid (tissue colloid osmotic pressure).

Increase in extracellular lung water is related to the duration of elevation of pulmonary venous or pulmonary capillary pressure, other things being equal. Not only can pulmonary edema result, but a combination of the damaging effects of CPB and increased pulmonary venous pressure can lead to pulmonary hemorrhage. Maintaining a very low pulmonary venous pressure will not always eliminate these complications.

Maintenance of a low pulmonary venous pressure can be ensured by monitoring left atrial pressure in patients undergoing CPB (see Section 3). In most clinical settings, there is little tendency for pulmonary venous pressure to increase. If it does, the pulmonary venous system can be decompressed by suction on either a catheter (or an opening) in the pulmonary trunk, because no valves are present in pulmonary veins, or a catheter inside the left atrium or left ventricle.

Temperature

Since the introduction by Brown and colleagues of an efficient heat exchanger for extracorporeal circulation, temperature of the perfusate, and secondarily of the patient, has been controlled by the perfusionist.[B13] In decisions regarding temperature of the patient during CPB, several facts must be considered. Flexibility of CPB is achieved when it is combined with hypothermia. Hypothermia of even moderate degree appears to blunt some of the damaging effects of CPB.[M20,T19] It allows use of lower pump flow rates with less blood trauma, and achieves better myocardial protection and protection of other organs than does normothermic CPB.[C36] Systemic hypothermia also provides a margin of safety for organ protection if equipment failure occurs. The patient's body temperature is the most important determinant of the length of the safe circulatory arrest time (see Section 1).

Moderate hypothermia is used in many patients, and we consider at least mild hypothermia (31° to 34°C) to be advisable in essentially all cases. A nasopharyngeal temperature of 14° to 20°C is chosen when circulatory arrest is required.

During core cooling, blood entering the patient's aorta can be kept 10° to 14°C below the nasopharyngeal temperature to minimize the tendency for gas to come out of solution when the cold blood is warmed by the patient. This is a conservative recommendation, in that some groups use the coldest perfusate temperature that can be obtained (4° to 5°C) once CPB is initiated.

Because blood is damaged by temperatures greater than 42°C and the boundary layer of blood next to the wall surface of the heat exchanger probably reaches the temperature of that surface, and thus of the water on the other side of the wall, water temperature should not exceed 42°C during rewarming. Blood temperature should not exceed 39.5°C during rewarming. Solubility of gas in blood is decreased when blood is warmed, but this is not a problem when the heat exchanger is upstream (proximal) to the oxygenator. When it is downstream (distal) to the oxygenator, it is a potential problem during rewarming, and a bubble trap may be interposed in the arterial tubing downstream to both. In general, maintenance of a temperature gradient from the heat exchanger to the blood of not more than 10° to 12°C will prevent bubble formation.

RESPONSE VARIABLES

Alberts and colleagues state in their textbook: "There is a paradox in the growth of scientific knowledge. As information accumulates in ever more intimidating quantities, disconnected facts and impenetrable mysteries give way to rational explanations, and simplicity emerges from chaos. The essential principles of a subject gradually come into focus."[A17] The patient response to CPB using current techniques and equipment is still largely described by "disconnected facts and impenetrable mysteries," but considerable effort has been made to begin both to develop simplicity and to reduce chaos. Continued interest in this response has stimulated the search for more cohesive knowledge and for ways of minimizing unfavorable outcomes of cardiac surgery using CPB and whole body perfusion from a pump-oxygenator.

Unfavorable aspects of the response of the patient to CPB and use of a pump-oxygenator were evident during the early days of open cardiac surgery, but tended to be overlooked in the excitement generated by this new technology. Subsequently, surgeons observed that (1) diffuse bleeding was more common than after other types of surgery; (2) some patients, particularly small ones, became edematous during the procedure; (3) occasionally severe and truly malignant hyperthermia occurred with no demonstrable infection; (4) pulmonary dysfunction was sometimes unexpectedly prominent; and (5) the heart often did not perform as well as anticipated after its repair. Yet they also noted that many patients appeared to be free of these developments, and most survived. Since then, more information has been gathered, but not as much as is desirable.

Whole Body (Nonspecific) Inflammatory Response to Use of a Pump-Oxygenator

Diversion of blood through nonendothelialized channels to, through, and from pumps and the oxygenator appears to stimulate the organism to recognize the extracorporeal system as "nonself." Thus, potential is present for the specific (immune) and nonspecific (inflammatory) response systems to be activated. Specific immune responses of an immunologically naive (unprepared) patient are slow to develop and are not in evidence during the first few days after CPB. In any event, they are generally not strong. Nonspecific inflammatory responses appear rapidly, and in a few patients they dominate the early minutes, hours, and days after use of a pump-oxygenator. We initially called this response the *whole body inflammatory response,* which we hypothesized unified the many diffuse responses to exposure of blood to abnormal events.[B57] It is now often called the *systemic inflammatory response syndrome* (SIRS) because processes other than CPB can stimulate it.

Humoral Response

Initial response is probably a humoral response and is initiated by the contact of plasma with the foreign surfaces of the tubing and pump-oxygenator, and with air. Gas exchange requires a large surface area; it is therefore in the oxygenator that the greatest stimulus to this response occurs. Humoral response appears to begin with the "activation" of specialized plasma proteins, developed and conditioned through centuries of life to recognize and repel transcutaneous invaders. Whereas previously this invasion has generally been a relatively small, localized, and often extravascular process, in the patient exposed to a pump-oxygenator it is a massive intravascular process. Even though the patient is heparinized, parts of the coagulation cascade respond virtually immediately to the activating capability of the foreign surface, as do the complement, kallikrein, fibrinolytic, and other cascades. Activation of Hageman factor (factor XII) may be the initial event in the activation of these cascades, although platelets appear to be independently activated at about the same time. Thus, nearly all the split products resulting from these multiple activations can be found in the patient's blood during and, for a time, after bypass. Mechanisms for their disappearance have not been elucidated, but presumably they are to some extent metabolized, taken up by specific cell-surface receptors, dissipated into extravascular fluids, including peritoneal and pleural fluids, and excreted in the urine.

Products of activation of these cascades have powerful physiologic effects, both directly and by activation of other systems and cells. The *complement* cascade, once activated, results in the production of powerful *anaphylatoxins* (C3a and C5a) that increase vascular permeability, cause smooth muscle contraction, mediate leukocyte chemotaxis, and facilitate neutrophil aggregation and enzyme release.[G7,H16] Complement activation occurs through either the classic or the alternative pathway.

Contact activation of Hageman factor also immediately initiates the *kallikrein–bradykinin* cascade, resulting in the production of bradykinin. Plasma kallikrein circulates in the blood as a precursor, *prekallikrein,* 75% of which is bound to the high-molecular-weight kininogen (HMWK) in the plasma. Bradykinin, formed largely from HMWK, increases vascular permeability, dilates arterioles, initiates smooth muscle contraction, and elicits pain. Kallikrein also activates Hageman factor and plasminogen to form plasmin, again demonstrating the complex interactions and feedback loops between the various reactions of blood to nonself.

Once activated, the contact activation system overcomes its normal regulating system, and all the responses are amplified. Because plasma kallikrein leads to the conversion of plasminogen to plasmin, whose basic function in the circulation is to digest fibrin clots and thrombi, the fibrinolytic cascade is activated by this and other humoral and cellular mechanisms.

Cellular Response

Blood cells and endothelial cells participate in the nonspecific inflammatory response to the use of a pump-oxygenator. Lymphocytes (both antibody-forming B cells and T cells) are part of the specific immune system and, as indicated earlier, participate little in the response to CPB in the usual immunologically naive patient. Eosinophilic granulocytes also seem to have limited participation. Basophilic granulocytes (mast cells) may well participate, but the extent to which they do so is not clear, and the same is true of the natural killer (NK) cells within the leukocyte family. Monocytes, once activated, participate in the cellular response.

Neutrophilic granulocytes (polymorphonuclear leukocytes) play a major role in the response to CPB. Neutrophils are activated by complement and by other soluble inflammatory mediators. When activated, neutrophils migrate directionally toward areas of higher complement concentration (usually in the tissues, but during CPB probably in blood); they change their shape, become more adhesive, and secrete cytotoxic substances, including oxygen-derived free radicals. Of importance—and possibly a clue as to why most patients recover uneventfully from cardiac operations in which CPB is used despite the strong humoral and cellular response—is the fact that complement can also desensitize neutrophils, thereby reducing their ability to participate in the inflammatory response.[D20] Neutrophils are also activated by other humoral agents participating in the cascades in the blood, including kallikrein, as well as by other inflammatory mediators (cytokines) generated by cells, including tumor necrosis factor (TNF) and platelet activating factor (PAF). These molecules also have been shown to increase in amounts both during and early after CPB.

Platelets are strongly affected by CPB using a pump-oxygenator, but in a complex manner that has been well summarized by Edmunds and colleagues.[E5,E9] As in the case of neutrophils, platelets must be aroused from their normally passive state (activated); this occurs within 1 minute of the start of CPB. The precise initial trigger is uncertain, but possibilities include direct surface contact, abnormal shear stresses, mechanical lysis, exposure to adenosine diphosphate, and unidentified chemical agonists. The mechanism for activation of platelets is exposure on the surface of the platelet of numerous specific membrane receptors. Exposure of the fibrinogen glycoprotein receptors (GPIIb-IIIa complex), and subsequent binding of fibrinogen to them, are essential for adherence of platelets to the foreign surfaces of the pump-oxygenator and for their aggregation. Many other specific receptor sites are expressed and exposed by activated platelets. Control, feedback, and amplification mechanisms regulate platelets as well as the humoral systems, all of which are involved in the response to CPB.

Endothelial cells do not pass through the pump-oxygenator, but their complex activities are affected while the patient is connected to it. Triggering mechanisms are not clearly defined, but they probably include abnormal pressures and shear stresses, localized ischemia, and increased concentrations of normal and abnormal substances and cells in the blood. As a result, endothelial surface receptors are exposed, substances are elaborated and extruded, and spaces between the endothelial cells and their membranes are enlarged.[B17,S8,V11]

Endothelial and other cells, particularly those in the locally ischemic areas that surely exist during CPB, express phospholipid molecules derived from arachidonic acid (eicosanoids). These are important mediators of inflammation and include the prostaglandins, thromboxanes, leukotrienes, and lipoxins. Other cells in areas of acute inflammation that may be present during CPB can produce soluble factors called cytokines that normally act on other cells to regulate their function, but after CPB, they can induce elevation of body temperature, among other things.

Metabolic Response

Magnitude of the acute elevation of catecholamine levels in the blood that develops during CPB (see "Catecholamine Response" later in this section) is a measure of severity of the stress reaction induced by most cardiac surgery using CPB. Thus, in addition to the responses induced by CPB, cardiac operations and CPB induce the important perturbations associated with other major operations and trauma. Characteristics of this "metabolic response to stress" have been intensively studied by a number of investigators and clinicians. Among the first was Cuthbertson in 1930,[C27] and among the most prominent, Francis D. Moore.[M21] The essence of this process has been well summarized by Wilmore[W22]:

> The human body responds to these stresses with dramatic resilience. For example, following injury, clotting mechanisms are immediately activated to reduce blood loss; body fluids shift from the extravascular compartment to restore blood volume; blood flow is redistributed to ensure perfusion of vital organs; and respiratory and renal functions compensate to maintain acid-base neutrality and body fluid tonicity. Following these acute adaptations, other changes occur; these responses are more gradual and prolonged but are apparently necessary for recovery of the injured organism. A variety of immunologic alterations are initiated; leukocytes are mobilized, macrophages and specialized T cells are produced, and "acute phase" plasma proteins are synthesized by the liver. Inflammatory cells invade the injured area, set up a perimeter defense, and engulf the dead and dying cells and other wound contaminants. These initial steps are followed rapidly by ingrowth of blood vessels, appearance of fibroblasts that build collagen scaffolding, and a host of other local changes that aid wound repair.
>
> Local changes that occur at the injury site are accompanied by systemic alterations in body physiology and metabolism. Cardiac output is elevated, minute ventilation is increased, and the patient becomes febrile. Lipolysis and skeletal muscle proteolysis are accelerated, providing an ongoing fuel supply and an immediate source of amino acids that are utilized for wound healing and synthesis of "acute phase" proteins and new glucose. The glucose provides essential energy for the brain and other vital organs and for healing of the wound.

Phenomena associated with CPB not only produce their own damage but also interfere with the "metabolic response to stress," a process that is necessary for recovery. Uneventful recovery of most patients after cardiac surgery means that a vast array of control and counteractive phe-

nomena of both humoral and cellular types is in place, many of which await discovery and exploitation.

Details of the Whole Body Inflammatory Response
Neutrophil Activation

During CPB, an initial mild leukopenia develops, which soon returns to baseline values.[K7] Similar changes occur without an oxygenator in the system and are in part the result of transient movement of leukocytes out of the vascular system.[K8] By the end of CPB, leukocytosis is present, consisting primarily of mature segmented forms of neutrophils (coming primarily from the bone marrow, most of which are activated).[Q1,R16] Leukocyte count often increases to a peak of 12,000 to 24,000 cells · mL^{-3} at 24 to 28 hours postoperatively. Both T and B lymphocytes are decreased early after CPB, and T-cell function is decreased.[R16]

Pulmonary sequestration of neutrophils occurs during CPB.[C10] An inflammatory response follows their disruption and release of proteolytic and vasoactive substances and powerful lysosomal enzymes, contributing to the increased vascular permeability associated with CPB (see "Complement Activation" later in this section).[A14,S18] Also, activation of neutrophils during CPB by the C3a and C5a complement fragments liberates oxygen-derived free radicals; this contributes to the damaging effects of CPB.[E8,T7] Neutrophil elastase, a connective tissue protease and product of neutrophil activation that appears in plasma, is considerably increased by CPB, and the peak concentration correlates positively and closely with the duration of CPB.[H27]

Such proteases break down elastin, collagen, and fibronectin, destroying extracellular structures, and contribute to the capillary leak that leads to postoperative extracellular volume overload and electrolyte imbalance.[F24]

Neutrophils in healthy persons are distinct cells. By inference, these cells are resting and unready for the numerous deleterious effects they exert during and early after CPB. However, when stimulated, neutrophils transiently aggregate and cluster with each other and to other cell types, such as vascular endothelial cells.[P4,R9] The process of aggregation and clustering is rapid, is mediated by cell adhesion molecules (CAMs), and is a critical step in development of inflammatory and immune responses. In myocardial infarction, anti-CAM antibodies of specific types, which can be produced by monoclonal techniques and can attenuate or prevent neutrophil aggregation and clustering, have been shown to considerably reduce the extent of cell death produced by ischemia and reperfusion.[S23]

Gillinov and colleagues used the anti-inflammatory agent NPC15669 to inhibit neutrophil adhesion in a CPB model and found a marked decrease in pulmonary injury.[G18]

Nifedipine, infused during CPB in doses of about 6 μg · kg^{-1} · h^{-1}, appears to inhibit neutrophil activation.[R16] Hypothermia has been shown to delay, though not prevent, the expression of neutrophil adherence molecules.[J10,L5] Further investigations along these lines may lead to attenuation of the damaging effects of CPB.

Platelet Response

In vitro test circuits show that the platelet count (corrected for dilution) decreases within 2 minutes of the beginning of extracorporeal circulation to about 80% of the pre-CPB level. By 8 minutes, the count has decreased to about 70% of the pre-CPB level and then stays close to that level during the rest of CPB and the period therafter.[Z2] Decrease in platelet count during clinical CPB tends to be greater than this because of hemodilution.[H25] Cardiotomy sucker systems substantially reduce platelet count.[E2] Interestingly, membrane oxygenators tend to reduce more than bubble oxygenators.[C13,E4] As a result of these and other factors, the number of platelets in circulating blood after CPB is decreased to about 60% of the prebypass value and does not correlate with the duration of CPB.[A6,F10,H15,H22,K6]

Sequestration of platelets in the liver and other organs during CPB in humans is slight and therefore not a factor in reducing the platelet count.[H24] Something more fundamental than mere loss of platelets by adhesion to foreign surfaces is involved, because the platelet count continues to be low in some patients for as long as 72 hours postoperatively. One factor may be the reduced survival time of platelets after CPB.[H24] Shear stresses likely do not reduce either the number or the function of platelets.[A7,S12,T6]

More complex and probably more important than the change in numbers are qualitative changes that occur in the platelets of patients undergoing CPB. Normally, platelets adhere only to cut ends of blood vessels and to subendothelial surfaces (presumably because subendothelial collagen causes them to adhere). Once CPB begins, platelets start almost immediately to adhere to foreign (nonendothelial) surfaces.[B16,D7] Once this process begins, platelets also begin to clump (aggregate), primarily on the foreign surfaces to which they have already adhered.[D11] There is some evidence that the initial aggregation is in very small clumps that are capable of deaggregating. If the stimulus is strong, however, these primary aggregates are transformed into larger aggregates. It is believed that only then do platelets begin to release the contents of their granules and to be irreversibly activated.[A8,Z2] Aggregates break off on occasion and become particulate emboli. Either platelets aggregate and disaggregate for many days after CPB or the aggregates formed during CPB persist in the circulation, because platelet aggregates can be seen passing through the retinal vessels of patients for days after cardiac surgery with CPB.

As blood circulates normally through endothelially lined tubes, platelets are generally inactive or dormant. The stimulus to platelet adherence and aggregation on the surfaces of the pump-oxygenator system, whatever it may be, also activates the platelets, a process that changes their form and internal architecture. This activation causes platelets to expose or assemble specific membrane receptors on their surfaces, for example, membrane glycoproteins IIb and IIIa (which bind fibrinogen) and GPIb (which binds von Willebrand factor), with a resultant cascade of further platelet adherence to the foreign surfaces and aggregation.[G14] The activation process simultaneously affects platelet granules, which are concentrations of selectively sequestered intraplatelet substances. These substances include (1) serotonin, ATP, adenosine diphosphate, pyrophosphate, and calcium, in the "dense bodies"; (2) α_1-antitrypsin, β-thromboglobulin, platelet factor 4, and platelet-derived growth factor; and (3) lysosomes. When activated, prostaglandin synthesis (arachidonic acid cascade) and

other reactions take place in the surface membrane of the platelet as well as within the cell and lead to external secretion of the highly reactive components of the platelet granules. The entire process may well contribute to a number of the damaging effects of CPB.

As is usual in the humoral and cellular cascades, the same processes that lead to platelet activation lead virtually simultaneously to processes that inhibit it. This proceeds because platelets, like most cells in humans, contain adenylate cyclase, which converts ATP to cyclic adenosine monophosphate (cyclic AMP); this conversion is greatly stimulated by the products of the arachidonic acid cascade. The arachidonic cascade is known to be accelerated by CPB. Cyclic AMP, in sufficient amounts, leads to inhibition of platelet adhesion, aggregation, change of shape, and secretion. This is part of the normal autoregulatory process, but it may be abnormally amplified during CPB.

Although platelet adherence to the foreign surfaces of the pump-oxygenator is the initial feature of the platelet response to CPB, and is surely accompanied by other major and complex responses, there remains a degree of uncertainty about subsequent events. There are even doubts as to whether platelet depletion and dysfunction are the primary causes of the bleeding tendency that is usually present after cardiac surgery. In any event, a short time after the tumultuous first few minutes of CPB, about 60% of circulating platelets have a normal smooth discoid form, as do about 80% 8 minutes after the start of CPB and at the end of CPB.[Z2] The implication is that either these platelets have never been activated (because they have just been released into the bloodstream or because foreign surfaces of the pump-oxygenator, passivated by absorption and denaturation of fibrinogen and albumin, no longer activate platelets[A7,P11,S13]), or they have been reversibly activated and returned to an inactive state. The latter is supported by the work of Zilla and colleagues, but is contested by Edmunds.[E5,Z2] Sufficient irreversible activation occurs that partially degranulated platelets, platelets with damaged membranes, and platelet fragments can be recovered both during and at the end of CPB, along with a large number of normal-appearing platelets.[E5,W18] Thus, by the end of CPB, platelet aggregability is reduced by 60% and bleeding time is prolonged, abnormalities that may persist more than 24 hours.[Z3]

Most of the events during CPB that profoundly depress platelet function appear to take place initially in the platelet membranes. During CPB, there appears to be a loss or inactivation of the functionally important glycoprotein-specific surface receptor sites.[M5,W17,W18] It is possible that abnormal shear stresses are partly responsible.[Z3] The GPIb receptor (to which plasma von Willebrand factor must bind for platelet adhesion) is markedly reduced shortly after the onset of CPB and remains low throughout bypass (Fig. 2-12). The GPIIb and IIIa receptors (which bind fibrinogen in a process that leads to platelet aggregation in the presence of extracellular calcium) are markedly reduced by the end of CPB.[M5,W18] Other changes in the platelet membranes may occur. Zilla has postulated, as have others, that the key to preventing loss of platelet function during CPB, and therefore to preventing the sometimes strong bleeding tendency associated with cardiac surgery, is

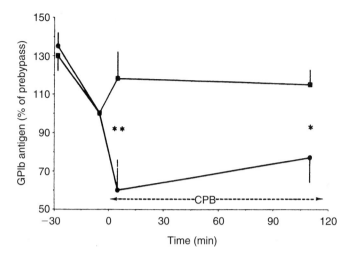

Figure 2-12   GPIb antigen on platelet membrane from patients on cardiopulmonary bypass (CPB), untreated (placebo) (closed circles), and aprotinin (closed squares). At 5 minutes of CPB and at end of CPB, differences unlikely to be due to chance were observed. Results are given as mean ± standard error. (From van Oeveren and colleagues.[V14])

to avert loss of action of the platelet membrane–specific receptor glycoproteins.[Z3]

Whatever the mechanisms and despite the high probability that development of platelet abnormalities is inherent in CPB as it is currently used, these alterations can be favorably influenced. The true membrane oxygenator, made from silicone rubber, appears to cause less platelet (and erythrocyte) damage than occurs with bubble oxygenators.[B27] Aprotinin may further lessen the development of platelet abnormalities (see Fig. 2-12 and "Other Additives" earlier in this section).

Complement Activation

Complement is a group of circulating glycoproteins that function as a part of the body's response to various kinds of injury, such as traumatic, immunologic, or foreign body insults.[J5] The complement system can be activated upon contact of blood with nonbiologic surfaces, perhaps by way of Hageman factor, but other substances, such as thrombin and plasmin, can also activate it.

Complement activation during CPB was reported by Hairston, Parker, and Hammerschmidt and their colleagues.[H17,H21,P5] Complement consumption during CPB was demonstrated by Chiu and Samson.[C19] Chenoweth and colleagues identified C3a, a complement breakdown product, in blood shortly after commencing CPB for cardiac surgery, and found that its continuing production was directly related to body temperature and perfusion flow rate.[C10] The result is that more than 50% of patients have serum C3a levels above 1000 $ng \cdot mL^{-1}$ at the end of operation with CPB (Fig. 2-13). Complement activation has also been demonstrated to occur during hemodialysis from exposure of blood to the dialysis membrane.[A11,C11,C12] Complement activation in this setting is through the alternative pathway, with depletion of C3 but not C1.[C11,C12] During CPB, activation is also through the alternative pathway.[C13,K11] Further complement activation by the clas-

sic pathway occurs after administration of protamine at the end of CPB[K11]; this may add to the whole body inflammatory response in some patients.[N5]

Magnitude of complement activation is affected by several factors, which probably interact with still other factors in complex ways.[V4,V7] The nature of the foreign surface has some effect; nylon is apparently a particularly potent complement activator.[C10] True membrane oxygenators are weaker activators of complement than are bubble oxygenators.[C22] Duration of CPB has a weak positive effect on the final level of C3a, but administration of protamine has a considerably stronger effect.[C22,C23,K11] Pretreatment of the patient with methylprednisolone or other steroids may decrease the amount of complement activation.[C22]

Adverse effects of complement activation relate to depletion of a component (complement) necessary for normal immune response and to adverse effects of the intravascular production of anaphylatoxins (C5a and C3a). Hairston and colleagues showed a decreased ability of postbypass serum to inhibit the growth of certain bacteria and related this in part to complement depletion.[H17] Adverse effects of anaphylatoxins probably account for the degree of complement activation as a risk factor for morbidity after clinical CPB (Table 2-4, Fig. 2-14).

Pulmonary sequestration of polymorphonuclear leukocytes and neutropenia have been shown to develop during hemodialysis and to be temporally related to complement activation.[C11] Similar observations have been made during CPB (see "Neutrophil Activation" earlier in this section).[C10,W10] That these changes are functionally significant is evident from the increased alveolar–arterial oxygen difference that develops during hemodialysis and after CPB, and from the pulmonary edema observed after CPB.[C12] Activation of complement has been shown to be directly involved in production of pulmonary edema.[E6] These findings suggest that neutrophil-mediated pulmonary endothelial injury (see "Cellular Response" earlier in this section) and increased lung vascular permeability, perhaps also mediated by reactive oxygen metabolites, may contribute to the adverse effects of CPB on pulmonary function.[P10] Similar sequestrations may take place in other organs.

That important complement activation is dependent on a large proportion of blood in the boundary layer (such as in an oxygenator or hemodialysis coil) is evident from the demonstration in sheep that a simple veno-venous shunt produces no adverse effects on white blood cells, platelets, or pulmonary artery pressure. Addition of an oxygenator to the circuit results in a decrease in circulating white blood cells and in platelets (presumably from pulmonary sequestration) and in a marked increase in pulmonary artery pressure. Fountain and colleagues showed that infusion of complement-activated plasma produces the same result.[F12]

Kallikrein Activation

Another humoral amplification system involves kallikrein and bradykinin. Several studies have shown important amounts of bradykinin to be present during CPB.[E3,F13,P7] Hypothermia itself apparently results in production of bradykinin. Apparently, immaturity, such as is present in young infants, results in less effective elimination of bradykinin.[F13] Exclusion of the pulmonary circulation probably

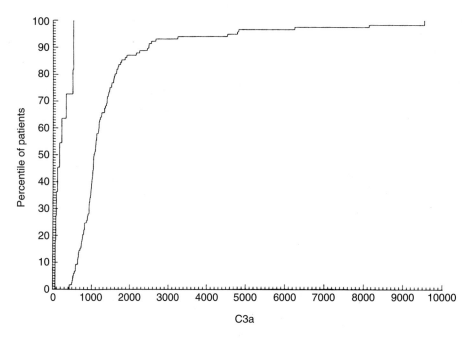

Figure 2-13 C3a levels at end of cardiopulmonary bypass, expressed in a cumulative percentile plot. Steep vertical line on the left represents closed cases, 100% of which had near-normal or normal levels. Curve on the right represents open cases, virtually all of which had increased levels. Fifty percent of patients had levels greater than 1000 ng·mL^{-1}, and 25% had levels greater than 1600 ng·mL^{-1}. (From Kirklin and colleagues.[K10])

■ **TABLE 2-4 Incremental Risk Factors for Morbidity after Cardiopulmonary Bypass**

Incremental Risk Factor	Logistic Coefficient ± SD	P
Higher C3a levels (ng·mL^{-1}) 3 hours after CPB	.0006 ± 0.00033	.07
Longer elapsed time of CPB (min)	.017 ± 0.0048	.0004
Younger age at operation [a]	−.71 ± .131	<.0001
Intercept	2.0 ± 60	

(Based on data from Kirklin and colleagues.[K10])

Key: *CPB,* Cardiopulmonary bypass; *SD,* standard deviation.

[a] Natural logarithmic transformation.

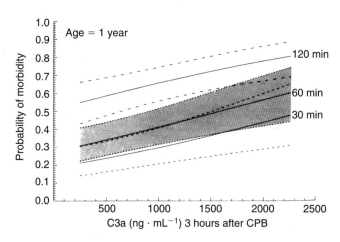

Figure 2-14 Nomogram of probability of morbidity after cardiopulmonary bypass (CPB), according to level of C3a. Relationships are shown for three different CPB times in a patient 1 year of age. (From Kirklin and colleagues.[K10])

also reduces the ability of the organism to cope with circulating bradykinin, because the lungs are the main site of bradykinin elimination. Bradykinin, a small peptide, is a powerful vasodilator, and this effect is probably important in the overall response of the organism to CPB.

Nagaoka and Katori demonstrated a reduction in peripheral resistance and in fluid requirement during CPB accompanied by the administration of aprotinin.[N2] This agent is known to neutralize the kallikrein–bradykinin system.

Coagulation Cascade

Coagulation, the formation of fibrin clots, is largely inhibited by heparin during CPB (see "Heparin Levels" under Controlled Variables earlier in this section), but the coagulation cascade is in part activated. Related or unrelated to this, coagulation is often defective for a period of time *after* CPB.

Normally, in the presence of damaged endothelium or an exposed subendothelium, platelets and soluble components of the coagulation cascade are activated. Through the *contact phase,* the *intrinsic phase,* and the *extrinsic phase* of activation, prothrombin is converted to thrombin, which acts on fibrinogen to produce fibrin monomers that polymerize spontaneously to form a fibrin clot. Were CPB to be started in a nonheparinized patient, the contact phase and intrinsic phase would be rapidly activated, and within a very short time the pump-oxygenator would be filled with clot.

Because of the incomplete blockade of the coagulation cascade by heparin, small amounts of fibrin form even during routine CPB.[D10] Many of the soluble coagulation factors are mildly reduced by the end of CPB.[H22] Most authorities believe that these changes are insufficient by themselves to be responsible for the bleeding tendency following CPB.

Fibrinolytic Cascade

The fibrinolytic cascade, another humoral amplification system, is probably activated to some degree in all operations in which CPB is used. Important hyperfibrinolysis was shown to be present in 159 (20%) of 774 patients undergoing coronary artery bypass grafting.[L4]

Naturally occurring inactive plasminogen (normally incorporated within thrombi) is transformed into the active fibrinolytic agent plasmin under certain circumstances, and measurable blood plasmin levels have been demonstrated in patients shortly after initiation of CPB.[B15] Because conversion of plasminogen to plasmin is facilitated by kallikrein, which also results from activation of Hageman factor, the fibrinolytic cascade may be initiated during CPB by activation of factor XII. However, extrinsic plasminogen activator expressed by endothelial cells has been shown to be the major stimulant for conversion of plasminogen to plasmin, and thus for the fibrinolytic cascade.[S25] A reasonable explanation for this behavior of endothelial cells during CPB is the abnormally high levels of such substances as catecholamines, bradykinins, and other molecules generated.[S25]

Because plasmin also serves as an activator of complement, prekallikrein, and possibly Hageman factor, the intravascular activation of plasminogen into plasmin (which in intact humans is usually a localized phenomenon) may continue to stimulate cascades of all the humoral amplification systems. Breakdown products of fibrinogen (produced to some extent by the coagulation cascade during CPB), when acted upon by plasmin, have been shown experimentally to lead to important pulmonary dysfunction. This is another example of the powerful effects of the intravascular occurrence of events that are usually localized and extravascular in intact humans.

For a time, it was conventional wisdom that excessive bleeding after CPB was primarily the result of platelet depletion and dysfunction.[H22] Currently, several lines of information strongly suggest that activation of the fibrinolytic cascade also contributes importantly to postoperative bleeding after cardiac surgery in which CPB has been used.[B14,H20,V1,W9] One of these is the favorable effect of aprotinin on bleeding, with most reports indicating a 50% reduction in bleeding after CPB when this drug is administered.[B14,B38,E10,H32,H33] However, its action is probably not limited to the antifibrinolytic effect of inhibition of plasmin. Plasmin itself appears to cause platelet aggregation, and its inhibition by aprotinin could therefore favorably affect platelets as well as fibrinolysis.[E10]

Arachidonic Acid Cascade

The completely cellular arachidonic acid cascade is activated by a disturbance of the cell membrane, which in turn activates phospholipase A_2. This releases arachidonic acid from the phospholipid fraction of the cell, but the arachidonic acid can also come from intracellular lipid pools. The cascade proceeds through the prostaglandin–endoperoxide (cyclooxygenase) pathway. Stationary, migrating, and intravascular cells are susceptible to the arachidonic acid cascade and liberate the active products, which exhibit a very short half-life.

The lung, bypassed during CPB, is a major site of the synthesis, release, and degradation of the eicosanoids (products of the arachidonic acid cascade), although not necessarily the cellular source of those compounds. Prostacyclin and prostaglandin E_2 (PGE_2) production appears to be sharply increased shortly after CPB is begun, but later when the CPB becomes partial and some blood again passes through the lung, the levels decrease.[F16] By contrast, thromboxane B_2 production (thromboxane B_2 is a stable metabolite of thromboxane A_2) becomes apparent and reaches peak levels when total CPB becomes partial bypass as the lungs again are perfused.[F16] Many researchers believe that most of the thromboxane A_2 comes from platelets, even though release occurs to a great extent in the lungs. Platelet activating factor (PAF), another product of the cascade, appears to be an important mediator of inflammation.[D19]

Leukotriene B_4, a product of the arachidonic cascade that promotes plasma leakage and leukocyte adhesion, is also increased during and for a time after CPB.[J2]

Details and overall effects of activation of the arachidonic acid cascade during CPB are not completely understood. However, there is at least evidence that the magnitude of the release of both of these eicosanoids during CPB is greatest in the very young.[G15] The activation releases agents that are somewhat counteracting, including the vasoconstricting agent thromboxane A_2, a PAF, and the vasodilating and platelet-inhibiting factors prostacyclin and PGE_2.

Cytokines

Cytokines are soluble factors elaborated by cells of the immune system, such as T-cell lymphocytes, that normally act on other cells to regulate their function. During CPB, cytokines such as the interleukins elaborate other mediators of the inflammatory process, such as tumor necrosis factor (TNF), leukocyte adhesion molecules, and PAF, which in turn continue the process.

Interleukin-1 is an intracellular derivative of stimulated mononuclear phagocytes and a mediator of fever, of changes in endothelial cell function and permeability, and of decreased vascular resistance.[D17] Its concentration in monocytes is increased during CPB and again 24 hours later.[H26] A positive correlation has been found between intracellular interleukin-1 activity and the temperature of the patient 24 hours after CPB.[H26] The interrelation between complement activation (which activates monocytes), prostaglandins (which also mediate interleukin-1 production), and interleukin-1 illustrates the complexity of the whole body inflammatory response to CPB and the problems inherent in efforts to prevent its damaging effects.

Interleukin-6 and interleukin-8 levels rapidly increase after initiation of CPB.[D13] Degree of cytokine response appears to correlate with the duration of CPB and aortic clamping.[H39]

Other Mediators of Inflammation

TNF is released by activated monocytes (and macrophages) and is increased in many patients in the later stages of

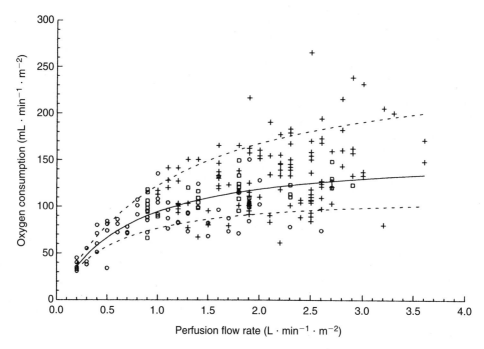

Figure 2-15   Relationship of total body oxygen consumption ($\dot{V}_{O_2}$) to perfusion flow rate ($\dot{Q}$) at normothermia during nonpulsatile cardiopulmonary bypass. Figure contains two depictions. One is a scattergram of data from animal experiments ($n = 213$) performed at about 37°C by Cheng and colleagues[C2] ($n = 33$), Paneth and colleagues[P8] ($n = 60$), and Starr[S27] ($n = 120$). Note that scatter of data increases as flow increases. Second depiction is solid and dashed lines (presented as in Fig. 2-1), which is a solution of the hyperbolic equation (Appendix Equation 2A-2) derived from these data. The hyperbolic equation is chosen because the correlation coefficient, r, was .69, whereas it was .39, .54, and .52 for the linear equation,[S27] log-log equation,[H4] and Arrhenius equation,[P8] respectively.

CPB and during subsequent hours.[J2] It is known to increase endothelial cell permeability and open interendothelial cell spaces, thereby promoting development of interstitial edema.[B33,B34]

Endotoxin, a powerful stimulant of complement and endothelial activation, is also a potent agonist of release of TNF from macrophages and is elevated in some patients after CPB.[B46,B51,F25,F26,H39,K20] Endotoxin release may be the result of translocation of bacteria from the gut as the result of splanchnic ischemia and possibly impaired function of Kupffer cells in the liver.[T24]

Protein Denaturation

Proteins are denatured by a blood–gas interface such as in a bubble or stationary vertical film oxygenator, but are denatured considerably less in microporous and true membrane oxygenators.[L3] Denaturation of albumin has a nonspecific effect, but denaturation of immunoglobulins yields degradation products that activate the complement cascade.[T16]

Oxygen Consumption
Total Body Oxygen Consumption

Theoretically, total body oxygen consumption during CPB at normothermia (37°C) should be that of an intact human under anesthesia, if all parts of the microcirculation are perfused. Yet, in two studies in humans, $\dot{V}_{O_2}$ during normothermic CPB at flows of 1.8 to 2.4 $L \cdot min^{-1} \cdot m^{-2}$ was highly variable. Values of 74 to 162 $mL \cdot min^{-1} \cdot m^{-2}$ were found in one study[M2]; in the other study, which consisted of 12 patients, mean ± standard deviation of $\dot{V}_{O_2}$ was 131 ± 20 $L \cdot min^{-1} \cdot m^{-2}$.[L2]

A combined analysis of experimental studies in animals during normothermic CPB[C2,P8,S27] indicates a best-fit hyperbolic relationship between the perfusion flow rate and $\dot{V}_{O_2}$ (Fig. 2-15). Flow rate in these studies was expressed in $L \cdot min^{-1} \cdot m^{-2}$. (These units were not used in the excellent study of Andersen and Senning, nor could the data be recalculated in these terms, hence their exclusion.[A1]) The following linear regression equation was derived from the data:

$$\dot{V}_{O_2} = 0.4437 \cdot (\dot{Q} - 62.7) + 71.6$$

(2-4)

where $\dot{V}_{O_2}$ is oxygen consumption, expressed as a percentage of measured control value before bypass, and $\dot{Q}$ is flow from the pump-oxygenator, expressed as $mL \cdot kg^{-1} \cdot min^{-1}$ (correlation coefficient = 0.83). Andersen and Senning noted, however, that flow and oxygen consumption must meet at zero and that the control value for $\dot{V}_{O_2}$ was usually reached at high flows (100 to 125 $mL \cdot kg^{-1} \cdot min^{-1}$).[A1] Visual observation of their scattergram suggests that the hyperbolic model derived from the combined analysis fits their data and ideas well.

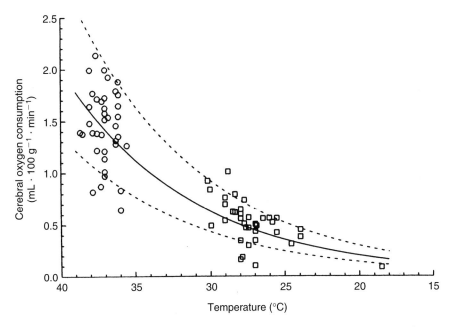

Figure 2-16   Relation between body temperature (nasopharyngeal) and cerebral oxygen consumption ($CMRO_2$) during full flow ($2\ L \cdot min^{-1} \cdot m^{-2}$) cardiopulmonary bypass, which is presumed to be applicable to all ages. The equation (van't Hoff) is

$$CMRO_2 = 0.021e^{0.1147 \cdot T}$$
$$r = .85, P < .001$$

where e is the base of the natural logarithms and T is temperature in °C. (Based on data from Croughwell and colleagues.[C28])

Temperature of the patient is also related to $\dot{V}_{O_2}$ during CPB, as it is in intact, anesthetized, nonshivering subjects. Harris and colleagues were first to express mathematically the interrelation between perfusion flow rate, temperature, and $\dot{V}_{O_2}$, but their data covered a narrow range of temperature.[H4] Complete data of the type desired are not available. Using the experimental data at 37°C just described and the relation of $\dot{V}_{O_2}$ to flow at 20°C measured during CPB in humans, a multivariable equation and nomogram have been developed (see Fig. 2-11) portraying the relations of $\dot{V}_{O_2}$ to flow at various temperatures.[F5]

Pulsatility of the arterial input does not affect $\dot{V}_{O_2}$, at least during flow rates greater than about 1.4 $L \cdot min^{-1} \cdot m^{-2}$, nor does the strategy (pH-stat versus alpha-stat) of managing the acid–base balance.[A15] Other factors that may affect $\dot{V}_{O_2}$ include amount of developed pericapillary edema and amount and type of catecholamine release.

Cerebral Oxygen Consumption

Cerebral oxygen consumption is important during CPB (see "Brain Protection" in Chapter 4), particularly hypothermic CPB at low flow, because cerebral $\dot{V}_{O_2}$ that is reduced below the usual ("normal") value at a given temperature implies incomplete or uneven cerebral perfusion (*decreased effective capillary density*). An equation has been developed from the data of Croughwell and colleagues that appears to be the best expression available of the normal relation, during CPB at full flow ($2.0\ L\ min^{-1} \cdot m^{-2}$), between cerebral $\dot{V}_{O_2}$ and temperature during CPB. It is presumably applicable to all ages [C28] (Fig. 2-16). Assuming that cerebral oxygen consumption at 37°C before CPB is

the same as that at 37°C during CPB is inappropriate, because whole body $\dot{V}_{O_2}$ on CPB is a little less than off CPB. This may be from presumed uneven perfusion on CPB.

Cerebral oxygen consumption does not appear to change with the variations in cerebral blood flow that occur during clinical CPB.[F14,S24] This is consistent with findings in experimental studies. For example, Fox and colleagues found that in monkeys on CPB at 20°C, cerebral oxygen consumption was the same at CPB flow rates of 0.5 and 1.6 $L \cdot min^{-1} \cdot m^{-2}$, even though cerebral blood flow at 0.5 was 50% of that at 1.6.[F5]

Mixed Venous Oxygen Levels

Although mixed venous oxygen levels are related to the controlled variables of perfusion flow rate, the hemoglobin concentration of the perfusate, and the arterial oxygen tension as expressed by the Fick equation (see Equation 2-1), they are also related to the patient's response in terms of $\dot{V}_{O_2}$ and thus to some partially controllable variables that affect $\dot{V}_{O_2}$, such as pH and 2,3-diphosphoglyceric acid levels in the red blood cells.[S17]

When most of the microcirculation is known to be perfused, mixed venous oxygen levels reflect the mean value for tissue oxygen levels. Thus, the assumption can be made that when mixed venous oxygen levels during CPB are relatively normal ($P\bar{v}O_2$, 30 to 40 mmHg; $S\bar{v}O_2$, 60% to 70%) and total body oxygen consumption is relatively normal, tissue oxygen levels are relatively normal, and the whole body perfusion is meeting the patient's metabolic demands (see "Total Systemic Blood Flow" under Controlled Variables earlier in this section).

Metabolic Acid–Base Status

Metabolic acidosis tends to develop during CPB, even when "adequate" flow rates are used.[A15] This is probably related to the uneven distribution of flow during CPB, with the consequent development of underperfused areas that release lactic acid.[C16] Resultant metabolic acidosis is usually not severe, and the concentration of lactic acid rarely exceeds $5 \text{ mmol} \cdot \text{L}^{-1}$.[H6]

Hemolysis

Hemolysis of red blood cells during CPB has long been recognized. During the early years of open heart surgery, plasma hemoglobin levels during and after operation were monitored as an index of damage caused by the pump-oxygenator. However, serum hemoglobin levels during clinical CPB do not accurately reflect the amount of hemolysis, because hemoglobin either bound to haptoglobins or free when haptoglobin binding sites are saturated is continuously removed from the circulating blood by the reticuloendothelial system and kidneys.[D11] When the plasma-free hemoglobin level exceeds about $40 \text{ mg} \cdot \text{dL}^{-1}$, hemoglobin casts may form in renal tubules. There is little likelihood of renal shutdown from this effect unless the plasma hemoglobin level exceeds $100 \text{ mg} \cdot \text{dL}^{-1}$.

Han and colleagues found plasma-free hemoglobin levels to be $8.3 \pm 1.3 \text{ mg} \cdot \text{dL}^{-1}$ before CPB, $33 \pm 3.6 \text{ mg} \cdot \text{dL}^{-1}$ 10 minutes after the start of CPB, and $91 \pm 8.4 \text{ mg} \cdot \text{dL}^{-1}$ after CPB.[H15] The plasma-free hemoglobin level may be still higher several hours after CPB. Classically, this has been explained as continuing destruction of erythrocytes damaged, but not destroyed, during CPB.

Red blood cell mass often declines still further during the first 3 or 4 postoperative days. Although in the past this has been attributed to the shortened half-life of damaged erythrocytes, the entire matter of hemolysis during and after CPB may be considerably more complex than this finding suggests. C5b-9, a product of complement activation, is deposited on the surface of erythrocytes during CPB. This may play a major role in hemolysis associated with CPB.[S22]

Systemic Vascular Resistance and Arterial Blood Pressure

At the onset of normothermic or moderately hypothermic CPB, systemic vascular resistance usually decreases abruptly. It then gradually increases toward normal throughout the period of CPB and may become higher than normal.[C17,M10] Considerable variation exists from patient to patient in systemic vascular resistance and thus in systemic arterial blood pressure during perfusion. In patients with coronary artery disease, a high systemic vascular resistance tends to develop during CPB.[W8]

Precise mechanisms underlying these variations in systemic vascular resistance during clinical CPB have not been identified, except in one situation. When, after a protracted period of global myocardial ischemia, cardiac reperfusion is commenced, systemic arterial pressure and resistance decrease within about 30 to 45 seconds.[D16] This interval coincides with the time it takes the cardiac reperfusate to appear in the coronary sinus, return to the pump-oxygenator via the venous cannula, pass through that machine, and be returned to the patient. Contents of the coronary sinus blood first appearing after an appreciable period of global myocardial ischemia likely contain vasodilating substances that develop in the heart during the ischemic period. Some studies have suggested that this blood contains a large number of leukocytes that have been sequestered in the heart during global myocardial ischemia.[B55,B56,S35]

In general, it is unnecessary and unwise to manipulate systemic vascular resistance pharmacologically during CPB. However, some evidence indicates that cerebral blood flow is lower than desirable when mean arterial blood pressure during normothermic or moderately hypothermic CPB goes below about 40 mmHg. Therefore, when blood pressure is lower than 40 mmHg for more than a few minutes during rewarming, the rational pharmacologic approach is to increase systemic vascular resistance (see Chapter 4), hence arterial blood pressure. Increasing the perfusion flow rate above usual values during rewarming is ineffective in increasing arterial pressure. When systemic vascular resistance becomes so high during this phase of CPB that mean arterial blood pressure increases to more than 100 mmHg, it is prudent to pharmacologically reduce it to less than that level (see Chapter 4).

Distribution of Blood Flow

Distribution of blood flow during CPB cannot be assumed to be similar to that when the circulation is intact. Distribution (and thus regional and organ blood flow) during CPB has the potential to vary according to age of the patient, amount of hemodilution, perfusion flow rate, arterial pulse contour, any pharmacologic manipulation, temperatures of the perfusate and patient, and arterial P_{CO_2}, pH, and P_{O_2}. The effect of some of these on distribution of blood flow is unclear. There may well be species differences, making data based on human subjects the most useful in the clinical setting.[R4]

Cerebral Blood Flow

Under conditions that often pertain in adults undergoing cardiac operations (nonpulsatile perfusion; flow $1.6 \text{ L} \cdot \text{min}^{-1} \cdot \text{m}^{-2}$; temperature $\pm 25°C$), cerebral blood flow (measured by radioactive xenon clearance) is about $25 \text{ mL} \cdot \text{min}^{-1} \cdot 100 \text{ g brain tissue}^{-1}$, with some variability depending on $PaCO_2$.[G11] During CPB in monkeys, a similar value has been found (using microspheres), representing about 6% of total systemic blood flow.[F14]

In humans, cerebral blood flow during CPB is no less in elderly patients than in other adult patients, and it appears to be proportionally similar in neonates and infants to that in adults.[B31,G12,G13] Thus, *age* appears to have little effect on the proportion of total flow represented by cerebral blood flow under usual circumstances of CPB.

During normothermic and moderately hypothermic CPB in adults and elderly patients, cerebral blood flow is not importantly altered with variations of *mean arterial blood pressure.*[B31,G12] This is similar to the situation in normal awake adult humans, in whom cerebral blood flow does not vary significantly with variations of arterial blood pressure (mean) from about 60 to 150 mmHg. When arterial blood pressure during CPB falls below about 40 mmHg, cerebral blood flow may decline appreciably, with a concomitant decrease in cerebral oxygen consumption.[F18,T17] A reasonable inference is that in adults on CPB, arterial blood pressure need not be manipulated pharmacologically unless it is less than 40 mmHg.

By contrast, during deep hypothermic CPB, at least in neonates, infants, and children, cerebral blood flow is dependent on arterial blood pressure.[G12,G13,G19] Corresponding variations in cerebral oxygen consumption have not been established with certainty. In view of this, arterial blood pressure should probably be kept above about 25 mmHg in this setting, at least in young patients.

The effect of decreased *CPB flow rate* on cerebral blood flow in humans is incompletely understood, in part because of the interaction between CPB flow rate and arterial blood pressure (see Chapter 4).[F18] However, during moderately hypothermic CPB at the usual flow rates, there appears to be a direct correlation between CPB flow and cerebral blood flow, despite the poor or absent correlation between arterial blood pressure and cerebral blood flow.[S24]

Cerebral blood flow during CPB is affected by *arterial carbon dioxide pressure* ($PaCO_2$). Hypercarbia increases cerebral blood flow, whereas hypocarbia decreases it.[G11,M14,P6] In children undergoing hypothermic CPB, the flow increases $1.2 \; mL \cdot min^{-1} \cdot 100 \; g$ brain tissue^{-1} for every 1-mmHg increase in $PaCO_2$ (measured at 37°C) between 33 and 50 mmHg.[K12] Infants have a slightly blunted response. Data gathered by Kern and colleagues are compatible with the hypothesis that, under usual conditions of hypothermic CPB, the metabolic needs of the brain are met with a $PaCO_2$ value of 33 mmHg.[K12]

Although "autoregulation of cerebral blood flow" has been described during normothermic and moderately hypothermic CPB, it may well be that it is the remainder of the body, not the brain, that accomplishes autoregulation. This was suggested by the experimental studies of Fox and colleagues.[F14]

Cerebral blood flow during CPB may at times be excessive in relation to cerebral oxygen consumption. For example, Croughwell and colleagues found that during CPB and reduction of the patient's body temperature from 37°C to 28°C, cerebral blood flow decreased less than cerebral oxygen consumption. This was referred to as a situation of "luxuriant cerebral blood flow," accompanied by a narrowing of the cerebral arteriovenous oxygen difference.[C28] Similar "luxury perfusion" can result from hypercarbia, and it has been argued that this increases the risk of cerebral damage by microemboli.[H30,H31] This is an argument against use of pH-stat strategy for control of $PaCO_2$ during CPB.

Cutaneous Blood Flow

Clinical information strongly suggests that blood flow to the skin is severely reduced during nonpulsatile CPB in humans. The small "bald spot" that develops on the back of the head after CPB in some patients is probably the result of the pressure produced by the weight of the head on an area of poorly perfused skin in contact with even a well-padded pillow during operation. Ease with which burns are produced by the cautery pad may also be the result of poor blood flow to the skin during CPB.

Venous Tone

Veins constrict during CPB, increasing venous tone. It remains high for some hours afterward.[G10,R12] The mechanism has not been determined with certainty, but high levels of circulating catecholamines probably play an important role.

Catecholamine Response

Response of circulating epinephrine (released primarily from the adrenal medulla) and norepinephrine (which overflows into the bloodstream from generalized sympathetic nervous system discharge) has been studied by many groups, with somewhat conflicting results.[H5,H14,P3,T4,T5] However, it is now clear that CPB is associated with a massive catecholamine release, greater than that from nearly any other form of stress. With the onset of CPB in adult patients with coronary artery disease, plasma epinephrine levels increase; they begin to decline after bypass[W8] (Fig. 2-17, *A*). Persisting elevation 1 hour after operation occurs only in patients with postoperative hypertension.

Plasma norepinephrine levels do not increase in adult patients who remain normotensive postoperatively, but in those with postoperative hypertension it increases at the start of operation and reaches a peak at the start of CPB (Fig. 2-17, *B*). It remains elevated at 1 hour postoperatively in this group. These patients show arterial blood pressure responses typical for patients undergoing CPB, with a striking decrease at the onset of CPB from reduced systemic arteriolar resistance (Fig. 2-17, *C*).

Mean arterial blood pressure 1 hour after operation correlates positively with both plasma epinephrine and norepinephrine levels. Neonates, infants, and young children also demonstrate marked increase in catecholamine concentration during CPB.[A9,A10,R14,W8]

Sympathetic–adrenal system discharge during, and in some patients after, operation is presumably related to use of CPB. The increased catecholamine response, particularly of norepinephrine, is partly attributable to the fact that during CPB, blood does not pass through the lungs, where norepinephrine is largely inactivated.[R14]

Adrenal Cortical Hormones

Clinical studies nearly uniformly demonstrate large increases in cortisol and adrenocorticotropic hormones with initiation of CPB.[A10,T11,T14] After CPB, patients exhibit markedly elevated levels of cortisol (free and total) for more than 24 hours.[U2] It is not clearly established whether the elevated corticosteroid concentrations during CPB are deleterious or beneficial.

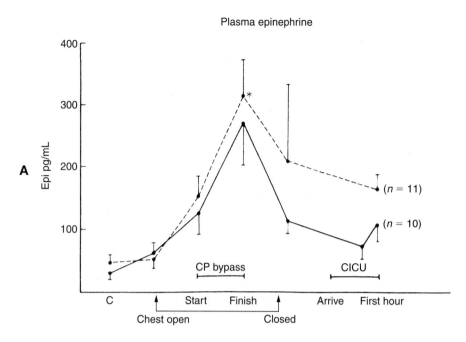

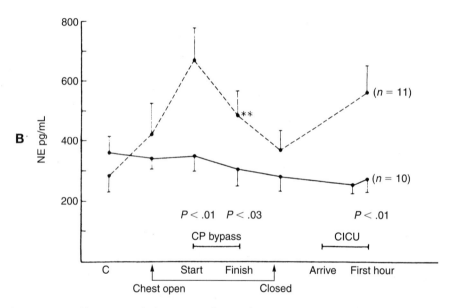

Figure 2-17   Plasma catecholamines and arterial pressures (mean ± SE) in patients undergoing cardiopulmonary bypass (CPB) for coronary artery bypass grafting at various stages of operation and early postoperative period. Solid lines represent patients who were normotensive early postoperatively, and dashed lines those who were hypertensive. **A,** Epinephrine (Epi). **B,** Norepinephrine (NE).

Key: *CICU,* Cardiac intensive care unit; *CP,* cardiopulmonary.   *Continued*

Vasopressin

Vasopressin, or antidiuretic hormone (ADH), is secreted by the pituitary gland and is a potent regulator of renal water excretion. Cardiac operations employing CPB are associated with large increases in ADH concentration that exceed those during other major surgical procedures; they can persist into the early postoperative period.[K21,V12,W5]

Body Composition

After CPB, extracellular fluid volume is increased.[B22,C18] The increase is in the interstitial fluid compartment, as shown by increased interstitial fluid pressure during CPB.[C18,R13] Plasma volume tends to be decreased.[C18] The magnitude of increase in extracellular fluid volume is directly related to duration of CPB (Fig. 2-18) and is greater

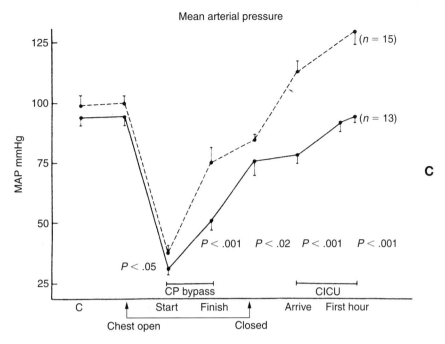

Figure 2-17, cont'd. **C,** Mean arterial blood pressure *(MAP)*. (From Wallach and colleagues.[W8])

Key: *CICU,* Cardiac intensive care unit; *CP,* cardiopulmonary.

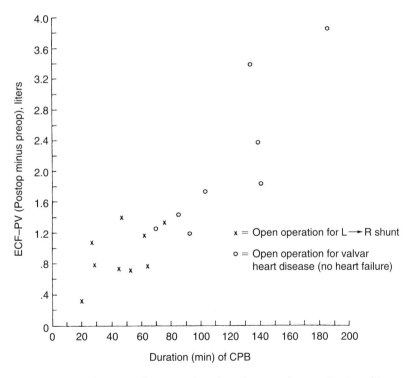

Figure 2-18 Relation between duration of cardiopulmonary bypass *(CPB)* and increment in ECF-PV soon after operation (patients with heart failure are not included). (From Cleland and colleagues.[C18])

Key: *ECF,* Extracellular fluid; *PV,* plasma volume.

when hemodilution is used.[C9] The large thoracic duct lymph flow occurring during CPB is related to this tendency of the interstitial fluid volume to increase.[B21] Also, exchangeable sodium is increased after CPB, while total exchangeable potassium is decreased.[P9] Amount and concentration of intracellular potassium are decreased.[P9]

These acute changes are probably, at least in part, the result of some of the damaging effects of CPB, including increases in capillary permeability, which probably facilitate the changes in body composition.[B57,C37,D25,M29,T26,T27] Neurohumoral alterations resulting from a period of relatively nonpulsatile flow may also be contributing factors.

Thermal Balance

Heat is lost during CPB. A study of six adult patients cooled to 30°C during bypass lasting 130 minutes showed a mean net loss of 1000 kJ of heat (1 kilocalorie = 4.2 kJ) by the end of the hypothermic interval.[D9] Loss to the heat exchanger and pump circuit was 840 kJ, and evaporative and convective loss was 380 kJ; the patient's metabolism supplied 220 kJ. During rewarming to a nasopharyngeal temperature of 37°C, the pump-oxygenator returned 670 kJ to the patient. Loss of heat during the period of anesthesia preceding bypass was not accounted for. Patients therefore left the operating room with a deficit of at least 330 kJ, equivalent to more than 1.5 hours of basal energy production. This deficit has to be restored during the early postoperative period, and the extra metabolism necessary to do this places a strain on the circulation that at times may be substantial. When deeper hypothermia is used, the problem is magnified, because muscle rewarms slowly and heat loss during operation is greater. It is necessary to bear in mind that the temperature of the muscles and body fat remains considerably lower than that of the nasopharynx after a short period of rewarming.

After CPB, a hypermetabolic state exists for at least 6 hours, sometimes longer. Oxygen consumption and carbon dioxide production are increased during this period, and body temperature may rise precipitously.[C24,T21] The possible relationship between intracellular levels of interleukin-1 and hyperpyrexia is discussed earlier in this section under "Cytokines."

AGENTS OF DAMAGE

Foreign Surfaces

Recognition by the cells that the surfaces in the pump-oxygenator system are foreign is a fundamental inciting agent for the damaging effects of CPB, as just described.[E16,E17] All elements of blood, formed and soluble, are affected. These phenomena were perhaps first reported by Lee and colleagues in 1972 and termed protein denaturation.[L3] In the subsequent 30 years, further effects on the complement cascade, white cell, and platelet elements and humoral and endothelial systems have been described. Selectins, kallikreins, kinins, leukotrienes, TNF, proteases, cytokines, and others are activated, liberated, or suppressed during CPB, presumably by exposure to foreign or nonbiologic surfaces or the blood–gas interface.

Because it is only in the boundary layer of flowing blood that the foreign surface is encountered, opportunity for damage is directly related to the proportion of the blood that is flowing there. Thus, it is in the oxygenator, where this proportion is deliberately made as large as possible to promote efficient gas exchange, that the opportunity for surface interactions and damage is greatest. This includes bubble oxygenators, because gases themselves are recognized as foreign surfaces when in direct contact with blood. It is next greatest in the heat exchanger, next in filters, and least in tubing and reservoirs.

Some artificial surfaces are more interactive with blood than others; nylon may be a particular offender.[C10] Surfaces may be "passified" to some extent in the initial few minutes of CPB by the deposition on them of denatured albumin, platelets, and other substances, but in oxygenators this is disadvantageous to gas exchange.[G28] Experimentally, some of the surfaces of certain parts of pump-oxygenator systems have been "seeded" with endothelial cells, but this has not yet been made practicable.

Shear Stresses

Shear stresses are generated by blood pumps, suction systems, abrupt acceleration and deceleration of blood, and cavitation around the end of the arterial cannula. They are an important abnormal event during CPB for the leukocyte. This is in part because leukocytes are the largest formed blood element and are normally exposed to nonendothelialized surfaces, and because they are capable of exiting from the vascular space by diapedesis and by migrating via chemotactic gradients. They are also capable of phagocytosis and, because of their proteolytic and enzymatic components, of digesting almost any biological material. Martin demonstrated that shear stresses not only increase leukocyte disruption but also increase degranulation and adherence, and decrease aggregation, chemotactic migration, and phagocytosis in nondisrupted leukocytes.[M4]

Erythrocytes are damaged during CPB primarily by shear stresses. The amount of hemolysis and liberated free hemoglobin increases linearly as shear increases.[S12] In CPB systems, hemolysis is much less without the oxygenator in the system, and bubble oxygenators have been shown to produce more hemolysis than membrane oxygenators.[A12,C13,M5] Interaction of the damaging effects is again demonstrated by the fact that the critical shear stress for erythrocytes is lowered by presence of an unphysiologic surface. Intracardiac sucker systems are particularly damaging to erythrocytes, not only because of high shear stresses and deceleration injury but also because negative pressures are more damaging to erythrocytes than positive ones.

Incorporation of Foreign Substances

In intact humans, foreign substances rarely enter the arterial bloodstream, although when they do, the well-recognized pathologic state of arterial thromboembolism may develop. During CPB for cardiac surgery, air bubbles, particulate matter from the pump-oxygenator, platelet aggregates and fragments, fibrin aggregates, denatured protein particles, atheroma, and chylomicrons may be contained in the arterial blood and may be distributed throughout the patient's arterial system.[B11,B24,C15,D14,R11]

Microembolization is greatest during the first 5 to 10 minutes of CPB.[C15] Perhaps related to this, the total amount of microembolization is not correlated with the duration of CPB.[B11] The amount does seem to be decreased by a small-pore filter in the arterial tubing of the pump-oxygenator, but this is arguable.[B11] Microembolization is greater when bubble oxygenators, rather than membrane oxygenators, are used.[B25,B42] Embolized particles, whatever they may be, usually cause only transient obstructions to flow; thus, after 5 to 10 days, there is usually little evidence of their presence.[B26] Nevertheless, there is some correlation between depressed neuropsychometric test scores postoperatively and number of microemboli.[B11,F21]

There are many potential sources of microemboli. In some instances, pump-oxygenator surfaces have fine deposits of debris[R11]; this has led some to advocate preliminary filtration of blood that has passed through the system, before CPB is established. Gas bubbles are commonly found in the arterial input to the patient; these must have multiple sources, although they have been shown to be more prevalent when bubble oxygenators are used. There is some suggestion, from the work of Clark and colleagues and Donald and Fellows, that large gradients between the water bath and the blood in the heat exchanger (that is, rapid cooling and rewarming) are accompanied by a showering of gaseous microemboli.[C15,D14] Adhesion and aggregation of platelets during CPB (see "Platelet Response" earlier in this section) and formation of fibrin despite heparinization (see "Humoral Response" earlier in this section) contribute importantly to microembolization.[B11] Intracardiac sucker systems incorporate gaseous macroemboli and microemboli, fibrin, platelet aggregates, and debris into the blood, some of which cannot be removed before the blood is returned to the patient.

Gradual improvements in the techniques and equipment for CPB have decreased the prevalence of foreign substances and cellular debris entering the patient's arterial system during cardiac surgery.[A16,B11] This problem remains important and the subject of research, because it probably contributes to neuropsychiatric abnormalities after CPB and to cardiac, pulmonary, and other subsystem dysfunction.[B11]

Heparin

Heparin is administered before and during CPB to prevent coagulation of blood (see "Heparin Levels" under Controlled Variables earlier in this section, and see "Heparinization and Later Protamine Administration" under Preparation for Cardiopulmonary Bypass in Section 3). It is an agent of damage, in part because it is an imperfect anticoagulant that permits formation of microthrombi in the pump-oxygenator that can embolize to the patient. In rare instances, heparin produces an adverse effect, such as severe thrombocytopenia.

Efforts continue to be made to avoid heparinizing patients in the usual manner, primarily by making surfaces of the pump-oxygenator biocompatible. The most common method involves bonding heparin to these surfaces.[V4]

Contraindications to use of unfractionated heparin in-

clude heparin-induced thrombocytopenia (HIT), heparin allergy, or protamine allergy. Currently, alternative agents are undergoing laboratory and clinical investigation. These include low-molecular-weight heparin and heparinoids, ancrod (a defibrinogenating agent derived from pit viper venom), hirudin (a coagulation inhibitor derived from the salivary glands of the medicinal leech), and coagulation factor inhibitors such as factor IXia, an inhibitor of factor IXa, and argatroban, an inhibitor of factor IIa.[F27]

Protamine

Protamine is generally necessary after terminating CPB to reverse the effect of heparin. In addition, however, it is an agent with damaging effects because it activates the complement cascade through the classic pathway, and occasionally provokes temporary (5 to 15 minutes) severe bronchospasm, elevation of pulmonary vascular resistance, and hypotension.[K11,L6] Whether prevalence of these untoward reactions is reduced by slow administration of the drug or by infusing into the left atrium or aorta rather than the right atrium is arguable.

PREVENTION OF UNDESIRABLE RESPONSES

True prevention of the fundamentally disadvantageous and undesirable responses to CPB has eluded the cardiovascular surgical community despite intensive efforts. Developments in molecular biology may provide techniques that may some day accomplish this. To date, only palliative measures are available, some of which are described in "Other Additives" under Controlled Variables.

SAFE DURATION OF TOTAL CARDIOPULMONARY BYPASS

Partial CPB is better tolerated than total CPB, and its safe duration is measured in days if a true membrane oxygenator is used (see "Cardiopulmonary Support and Extracorporeal Membrane Oxygenation" in Section 1 of Chapter 5). Safe duration of *total* CPB is much shorter and is measured in hours, although not fully defined. The safety of CPB is known to be adversely affected by certain incremental risk factors.

Duration of CPB is clearly a risk factor for morbidity (Fig. 2-19) and mortality after cardiac surgery. However, the relationship between duration of total CPB and morbidity and mortality is affected by other risk factors as well. Type of oxygenator is probably one such risk factor; in general, true membrane oxygenators are the safest, followed by microporous oxygenators. Bubble oxygenators are generally the least safe. In contrast to moderate or deep hypothermia, normothermia throughout most of the period of total CPB is arguably a risk factor that affects the relationship between duration of CPB and unfavorable outcomes (see "General Comments and Strategy" in Section 3). Absence of hemodilution is probably a risk factor. Very low venous oxygen levels, although no doubt interrelated with some of the previously mentioned risk factors, appear to increase the risk of unfavorable events after CPB.

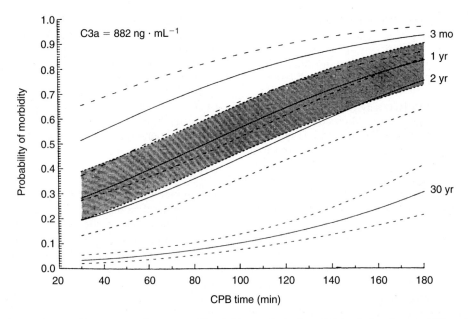

Figure 2-19   Nomogram from a multivariable analysis (see Table 2-4) of probability of morbidity (cardiac, pulmonary, renal, and coagulation dysfunction) after cardiopulmonary bypass *(CPB)* according to its duration. Relationships are shown for four age groups at a C3a level of 882 ng · mL^{-1} (median value in the study). Dashed lines enclose 70% confidence intervals. (From Kirklin and colleagues.[K10])

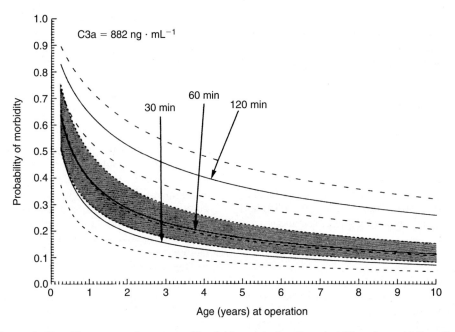

Figure 2-20   Nomogram from a multivariable analysis of probability of morbidity after cardiopulmonary bypass (CPB) according to age at operation at three different CPB times. Dashed lines enclose 70% confidence intervals. (From Kirklin and colleagues.[K10])

It is arguable that age of the patient is a risk factor for unfavorable outcome events after CPB, but the impression is that very young age (Fig. 2-20) and very old age have an unfavorable effect on the relation between duration of CPB and prevalence of unfavorable outcomes. Immature patients may have a greater tendency to develop increased capillary permeability than older patients, although this has not been well documented. Strength of the patient's humoral and cellular responses to CPB also affects this relationship, with greater complement activation appearing to have an unfavorable effect (see Table 2-4).

Thus, the relationship between safety and duration of total CPB depends on a number of factors that have mitigated against a complete understanding of it. Safe duration is surely measured in hours, not in minutes or days, and is surely closer in general to 3 hours than 1 hour.

Clinical Methodology of Cardiopulmonary Bypass

GENERAL COMMENTS AND STRATEGY

CPB should be used as a flexible clinical tool, recognizing its physiologic limitations, risks, and damaging effects. CPB is combined with at least some degree of hypothermia in many situations for the reasons given in the previous sections. An important advantage of hypothermia is that it allows safe periods of very low perfusion flow rate (about $0.5 \, \text{L} \cdot \text{min}^{-1} \cdot \text{m}^{-2}$) or circulatory arrest, when needed. However, the possible advantages of normothermic CPB continue to be explored. These include lower systemic vascular resistance and higher cardiac output in the early postoperative period and less blood loss.[T22] However, decreased oxygen saturation (<50%) in the cerebral venous blood has also been observed, particularly during the early period of CPB.[C29]

Size of the arterial and venous cannulae is determined primarily by perfusion flow rate and type of venous return. However, total perfusion flow rate, even at normothermia, is not an absolute quantity, but encompasses a range of acceptable values. Thus, if the surgical situation compels use of smaller cannulae, perfusion flow rate can be set at a smaller value or assisted venous return (vacuum, centrifugal pump) can be used.[B54,F20,O7,T23] Two venous cannulae may be used as a routine or only for congenital heart disease operations, including those in small infants, and operations in the right atrium, such as tricuspid valve surgery. A single two-stage venous cannula, having additional holes that come to lie in the right atrium while the tip is in the inferior vena cava (IVC), may be used for coronary artery bypass grafting; for operations on the aortic valve, mitral valve, and ascending aorta; for some operations for congenital heart disease; and for combinations of these procedures. Such a cannula has been shown experimentally to decompress the right heart efficiently.[B23] On occasion, a single venous cannula may also be used with conventional CPB and without aortic clamping for simple operations such as replacement of a valved extracardiac conduit.

Method of cannulation, use of left atrial and left ventricular vents, monitoring catheters, and indeed all aspects of clinical CPB should be flexible within certain limits. The combined knowledge and experience of the surgeon, anesthesiologist, and perfusionist should allow adaptation to the surgical situation while ensuring the greatest possible safety for the patient.

POSITIONING MONITORING DEVICES

Monitoring devices used for various cardiac operations in infants, children, and adults and specific positioning are discussed in Chapter 4.

POSITIONING PATIENT

The surgeon should collaborate with the anesthesiologist to position the patient correctly for operation, because an improperly positioned patient can make the operation more difficult. For a median sternotomy, both arms may be placed at the side to permit optimal access for the surgical team and to avoid traction on the brachial plexus during operation. Alternatively, a carefully positioned arm board can be used for the left arm (and for venous and arterial catheters).

Particularly in infants, a pad is placed under the back to project the chest forward and extend the neck. The patient's trunk must not be rotated, and the arms at the side must be secured and protected to prevent compression of the ulnar nerve at the elbow. A cautery pad is placed under the buttocks or the back. Pads for external defibrillation may also be placed on the anterolateral left chest and the back. A draping framework is placed over the head of the patient and extended to either side to screen the patient's head and the anesthesiologist from the sterile field. A urethral catheter containing a thermistor is inserted into the bladder. A thermistor probe is positioned in the nasopharynx.

PREPARING SURGICAL FIELD

The skin of the anterior thorax and abdomen is prepared with an antiseptic solution after mechanically cleansing it. In most patients, both groins should be prepared as well and draped into the surgical field so that the femoral vessels can be cannulated if necessary. Both legs are surgically prepared in their entirety for individuals undergoing coronary artery bypass grafting.

Appropriate sterile drapes are applied. Draping must shield the surgical field from the anesthesiologist, while at the same time allowing him or her an unobstructed view into the field.

Finally, the surgical field is covered by an impervious adhesive plastic sheet, in part to prevent the side drapes from falling away from the skin. It also prevents the drapes in the vicinity of the wound from becoming wet and thus losing their sterility.

Pump tubing is passed from the operating table to the perfusionist, who completes the CPB circuit. Tubing for infusion of cardioplegia, pericardial irrigation, suction, and venting is also positioned.

INCISION
Primary Median Sternotomy

A straight vertical midline skin incision is generally made in patients undergoing CPB through a median sternotomy. This incision commences several centimeters below the suprasternal notch and extends to the tip of the xiphoid.

An exception may be made in prepubertal girls in whom a bilateral submammary skin incision is made that follows the fourth intercostal space. A flap of skin and subcutaneous tissue is raised superiorly and inferiorly to expose the full length of the sternum for a vertical sternotomy. However, this incision may cause underdevelopment of the breasts in girls of this age and should be used judiciously. When used in female patients of all ages, this incision may cause hypesthesia or anesthesia of the anterior chest wall.

The exact midline over the sternum is scored with the cautery. A retractor elevates the upper angle of the vertical skin incision, placing the underlying tissues on tension. The soft tissue is separated from the superior surface of the manubrium, and a right-angled clamp is passed over the denuded manubrium into the space behind, hugging the bone. The clamp is spread to create a space for the tip of the sternal saw. The suprasternal ligament is cut with the cautery.

The blade of an electric or air-driven saw is held snugly against the posterior surface of the manubrium with the cutting edge against the superior manubrial surface. After activating the saw, the surgeon cuts the manubrium and sternum, staying precisely in the midline. The tip of the saw is kept elevated so the toe of the saw hugs the back of the sternum. During sawing, the anesthesiologist should cease ventilating the patient and exert no pressure on the lungs so that the soft tissue and pleura will fall away from the sternum. Drifting away from the midline with the saw must be avoided, because the sternum will not spread evenly and its later closure will be more difficult.

Alternatively, the sternum can be divided from the bottom up. The xiphoid process is mobilized or excised, and the tip of the blade is introduced beneath it. In neonates and infants, the xiphoid process may be excised, the costal margin on either side elevated by sharp retractors, and sharp, well-aligned scissors used to cut the sternum in the midline, from below upward.

When the incision is properly made, the pleural spaces are infrequently entered. A thin layer of bone wax is spread over the bone marrow, primarily where the bleeding is active. When the sternum is fragile, as in older patients, it is better to avoid wax altogether. Bleeding points in the cut edge of the anterior and posterior sternal periosteum are cauterized, but excessive cauterization should be avoided. A retractor is inserted and opened just enough to permit dissection. After a few minutes, it is opened further. It should be opened no more than is necessary for the procedure, because excessive retraction, particularly of the upper half of the sternum, may cause rib fractures, injury to the brachial plexus, and damage to the stellate ganglion.

Dissection continues by incising the fascia that envelops the thymus gland. The right and left lobes of the thymus are separated up to the level of the innominate vein. In infants and children, and occasionally in adults, the thymus may be subtotally resected, leaving only the cervical portion cephalad to the innominate vein, to avoid expanding hematomas that may cause postoperative bleeding.

The pericardium is then opened longitudinally in the midline from the diaphragm below to the innominate vein above. Where this incision meets the diaphragm, care must be taken not to incise the parietal peritoneum. If entry is made into the peritoneal cavity, the opening is sutured to avoid sequestration of blood and fluid in it. The pericardium is cut at right angles to the longitudinal incision at its diaphragmatic end, further on the left than on the right, after pushing back the pleura to avoid entering the pleural spaces. Pericardial stay sutures are then placed.

Alternative Primary Incisions

Incisions other than a full median sternotomy are being used with increasing frequency. These incisions and the techniques of cannulation required for their use are de-

scribed at the end of this section in "Special Situations and Controversies."

The remainder of the general discussion on the clinical methods of CPB focuses on the median sternotomy approach to the pericardial cavity and its contents.

Secondary Median Sternotomy

The surgeon must estimate preoperatively the chances that catastrophic hemorrhage will develop from sternotomy. This affects the decision regarding whether to cannulate peripheral vessels and establish CPB before sternotomy. It is helpful to study the chest radiograph and any available cineangiograms. However, cross-sectional imaging by computed tomography (CT) or MRI provides the most useful information. When one of the great arteries, right ventricle, or a right ventricle–to–pulmonary artery conduit is in close proximity to the back of the sternum, peripheral cannulation, establishment of CPB, and induction of moderate hypothermia before sternotomy are prudent precautions.

When a previous sternotomy has been performed, an oscillating saw is used as a routine. Properly used with a light touch by the operator, this saw allows the sternum to be split without damage to underlying structures. Once the sternum is divided, a sharp handheld retractor is inserted to elevate the lower left sternal fragment. Dissection is commenced just beneath the xiphisternum, dividing the tissues *just* behind the sternum. Working from below upward, the surgeon frees the left sternal edge in this manner to the level of the suprasternal notch. The same maneuver is repeated on the right side. Returning to the left sternal edge, the surgeon fully elevates it with two retractors and carries the dissection leftward, keeping fairly close to the sternum until the divided edge of the pericardium is identified (when the pericardium has not been sutured at the first operation, it retracts well away from the midline). The left edge of the pericardium is separated from the underlying ventricle with scissors. This plane is usually easily developed inferiorly above the diaphragm. This limited left-sided dissection is carried superiorly also, over the pulmonary trunk, avoiding damage to the tip of the left atrial appendage and left phrenic nerve. If the left internal thoracic artery was used as a bypass graft during the previous operation, it must be identified and protected.

The rib spreader is then inserted and opened. The right-sided structures usually must also be completely dissected. The plane of dissection for this is also most easily developed inferiorly above the diaphragm. It is often best accomplished partly from below and partly from above at the anterior and right lateral margins of the aorta.

It is very important during dissection of the aorta to remain outside the adventitial layer. The outer edge of the superior vena cava (SVC) is then dissected. The inferior and superior dissections can frequently be easily connected by blunt dissection with the finger posteriorly, just in front of the right pulmonary veins and left atrium. Finally, the lateral right atrium is carefully freed, leaving a piece of pericardium attached to the atrium if it is too densely adherent. This is often at the site of previously placed purse-string sutures. To permit later clamping, the aorta requires further dissection, particularly posteriorly in front of the right pulmonary artery and on the left lateral margin.

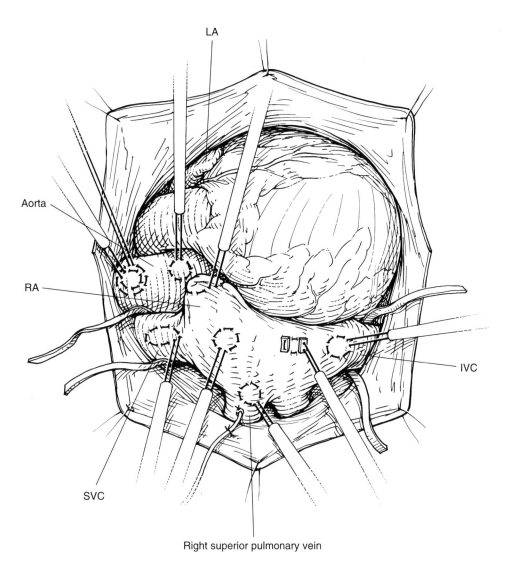

Figure 2-21   Schematic representation showing positions of sites for cannulae and catheters. As indicated in the text, not all are used in each patient.

Key: *IVC,* Inferior vena cava; *LA,* left atrium; *RA,* right atrium; *SVC,* superior vena cava.

Further dissection should be avoided unless it is necessary for proper exposure. Operations in which more extensive dissection may be necessary include redo coronary artery bypass grafting and repairs inside the right ventricle (see later chapters). When further mobilization is necessary, it is usually deferred until CPB has been established. The heart can then be emptied and dissection performed more precisely, with no hemodynamic disturbances. However, perfusion at this stage should be normothermic to prevent ventricular fibrillation and overdistention of the heart. If the heart cannot be completely mobilized, the left pleural space may be entered and opened widely, because this allows cardiac defibrillation and the usual de-airing maneuvers at the end of operation.

PREPARATION FOR CARDIOPULMONARY BYPASS

Once the pericardial stay sutures are inserted, size and any abnormalities of the cardiac chambers are noted, anomalies of systemic venous return (especially a persistent left SVC)

or pulmonary venous return are sought, and the heart is palpated for evidence of mitral, tricuspid, or aortic valve disease. A left atrial monitoring catheter may be inserted at this time or later, just before discontinuation of CPB. For this, a No. 3-0 silk purse-string stitch is placed on the right superior pulmonary vein just posterior to the right atrium (Fig. 2-21). A fine polyvinyl catheter is threaded into a 16-gauge Tuohy needle, the needle is inserted into the left atrium through the purse string, the catheter is advanced about 2 cm, the needle is withdrawn, and the purse string is tied. A No. 5-0 silk stitch is placed in the adjacent pericardium and tied snugly around the catheter, very near the purse string. The other end of the catheter is brought through the skin and attached to a pressure gauge.

Siting and Purse-String Sutures for Aortic Cannulation

The site for cannulation of the aorta should be within the pericardial reflection whenever possible, because the aorta where the pericardium is fused onto the anterior surface is tougher and better for cannulation than is that part outside (beyond and downstream to) the reflection. In this location, the cannulation site is proximal (upstream) to the origin of the innominate artery. The site should be a little to the left side of the anterior aortic surface (to the right side in patients with right aortic arch) as an added precaution against the cannula tip entering the innominate artery. At times in infants, in children with a previously constructed Waterston anastomosis or with truncus arteriosus, in adults with short ascending aortas or ascending aortic aneurysms, and in those about to undergo primary or redo coronary artery bypass grafting, the pericardial reflection over the cephalad end of the ascending aorta can be dissected off the aorta, the aorta retracted inferiorly, and the purse-string sutures placed on the anterior aortic wall at the level of, or if necessary distal (downstream) to, the orifice of the innominate artery on the aortic arch. In such situations, care is taken to position the aortic clamp proximal (upstream) to the orifice of the innominate artery.

Two purse-string sutures of No. 2-0 or 3-0 polyester or polypropylene are placed. They should catch only the adventitia and must not penetrate into the lumen. Tourniquets are placed on these sutures. When the aorta is scarred from a previous operation, a single pledgeted No. 3-0 polypropylene box stitch may be used at the cannulation site. A purse-string stitch is also placed for the cardioplegic needle or venting cannula (see Fig. 2-21).

The aorta of older patients, particularly those with coronary artery disease, may be atherosclerotic, and manipulation, cannulation, and clamping it may result in dislodgement and embolization of atheroma. It is prudent to perform epiaortic ultrasonographic scanning of the aorta in such patients to detect severe atherosclerosis and to position cannulae and clamps in areas where the atherosclerotic disease is minimal or absent (see Chapter 53).

Siting and Purse-String Sutures for Venous Cannulation

Purse-string sutures for venous cannulation can be placed before or after heparinization and aortic cannulation.

Number and sites of these purse strings depend on the perfusion technique to be used. When a single venous cannula is used, only a right atrial appendage purse-string suture is needed.

When two venous cannulae are used, the SVC and IVC may be cannulated directly. This approach is an old one, but has been refined by availability of smaller cannulae. With this method, venous drainage and exposure within the atria and ventricles are excellent, even in small infants. An oval-shaped purse string is placed on the presenting surface of the SVC (see Fig. 2-21), and a tape is placed around the SVC. For this, an incision is made in the pericardial reflection over the right pulmonary artery on the medial side of the SVC and again lateral to the SVC. These incisions allow a right-angled clamp to be passed easily around the SVC to grasp the tape and pull it through. The tape is placed in a rubber or plastic tourniquet. Alternatively, the SVC can be cannulated through a purse string in the right atrial appendage. To pass a tape around the IVC, the pericardial reflection posterior to the IVC and just inferior to the right inferior pulmonary vein is incised. This

maneuver clearly delineates the inferior border of the right inferior pulmonary vein and left atrium. It establishes a free communication between the two pericardial spaces, which permits better circulation of the external cooling fluid, and provides a space for the IVC tape to be placed. Alternatively, the IVC can be mobilized by first passing the fingers to the right of and behind the cava, and breaking down the pericardial reflection posteriorly by blunt dissection. The hand is then removed and a right-angled clamp is substituted. The tip of this instrument is exposed by retracting the lateral right atrial wall superiorly and to the left. Usually, the clamp slides around the IVC without further dissection. Occasionally, tissue must be divided with scissors working lateral to the right atrium and below the inferior pulmonary vein. Then the surgeon, with tissue forceps or a sponge, retracts the right atrium superiorly and to the left to expose the presenting surface of the IVC, which may require limited dissection from the diaphragm. A purse-string stitch is placed at the junction of the right atrium and IVC, or on the IVC itself, in a transverse oval shape (see Fig. 2-21).

Heparinization and Later Protamine Administration

Measurement of activated clotting time (ACT) and calculation of a heparin dose-response curve allows heparin and protamine doses to be individualized for each patient.[B15] First, a baseline, or control, ACT is established after sternotomy. Heparin (300 to 400 $U \cdot kg^{-1}$ or 3 to 4 $mg \cdot kg^{-1}$) is then given. After 3 to 5 minutes, the ACT is again determined. Additional heparin is given, as needed, to achieve an ACT of greater than 400 seconds. Cannulation is then performed. Heparin (3 $U \cdot mL^{-1}$) is added to the priming volume of the pump-oxygenator (for example, 5000 U for a 1600-mL clear solution). After CPB is established, the ACT is determined every 30 minutes, and additional heparin is given to maintain the ACT at greater than 400 seconds during normothermic CPB, and at greater than 480 seconds during hypothermic CPB (less than 30°C). The ACT should be measured more frequently if it does not respond appropriately to additional doses of heparin. (See cautions about the interference of aprotinin and other factors with interpretation of ACT, particularly when measured with celite, in "Other Additives" in Section 2.)

Protamine sulfate is given at the end of CPB, after removal of all cannulae. This biologic product, obtained from the sperm of fish, is a simple protein of low molecular weight. It is a heparin antagonist, forming with heparin a heparin–protamine complex. Protamine has a rapid onset of action. However, the heparin–protamine complex may be partially metabolized or may react with fibrinolysin, thus freeing heparin and causing the so-called *heparin rebound*.

Several methods are available to calculate the dosage of protamine to be administered at the end of CPB.[M25] These methods and their advantages and disadvantages are listed in Table 2-5. A widely used method involves administering 1.0 to 1.5 mg of protamine for each 100 units (or each milligram) of heparin. One milligram of protamine neutralizes approximately 85 units of heparin. Extra protamine is

■ **TABLE 2-5 Comparison of Methods for Calculating Protamine Dosage**

Method	Advantages	Disadvantages
Fixed dose (1.0-1.5 mg heparin · kg⁻¹)	Simple Not reliant on ACT	Inadequate or excessive protamine Potential for increased coagulation times with standard doses
ACT/heparin dose-response curves	Rapid, easy to use in OR More accurate protamine administration Decreased blood product requirements	No correlation between ACT and heparin levels Relies on ACT Dependence on plasma volume
Heparin levels	Less protamine given Not reliant on ACT	Requires peripheral laboratory Time consuming Assumes point on static curve
Protamine titration	Less protamine required than fixed dose Decreased postoperative bleeding No rebound effect seen with small protamine doses	Variability between heparin and protamine preparations Dependence on blood volume estimate Several steps for potential error Assumes point on static curve

(Modified from Moorman and colleagues.[M25])

Key: *ACT*, Activated clotting time; *OR*, operating room.

given to prevent heparin rebound associated with heparin release from tissue stores or from heparin–protamine aggregates, and to compensate for the probable shorter biologic half-life of protamine.[M25]

Arterial Cannulation

After heparin has been administered, the adventitia within the purse string is incised. With the aorta stabilized by a gauze sponge under the surgeon's left index finger, a digitally controlled stab wound of sufficient length is made within the purse string. The aortic cannula can then be slipped into the aorta easily and usually bloodlessly. Care is taken to adjust the cannula so that 5 to 10 mm projects into the aorta, and the obliquely angled open end is positioned so that it faces distally into the aortic arch.

The tourniquet on the purse-string suture is secured, and the cannula is tied to it. The arterial cannula is connected to the arterial tubing from the pump-oxygenator and carefully de-aired. All clamps are then removed from this tubing (unless the arterial pump is of the controlled vortex type). This technique may be used in adults, children, and infants.

Alternatively, in infants and small children, a fine side-biting clamp (Cooley or Castaneda) is used. All layers of the aorta, including the adventitia, are thicker in these small patients, and an excluding clamp will not damage the intima. The excluded portion of aorta is opened longitudinally with a knife. The purse-string stitch is then positioned, and the cannula tip is inserted in the opening while releasing the clamp. With this technique, the arterial cannula can have a long tip beyond the collar and is positioned so that this tip lies in the transverse portion of the aortic arch, safely beyond the origin of the innominate artery. Alternatively, the arterial cannula may have a very short tip beyond its collar, and the cannula will be perpendicular to the aorta after its insertion.

Venous Cannulation

When a single venous cannula is to be used, a suitable clamp is placed across the right atrial appendage, the appendage is opened, hemostats or forceps are placed on both edges, and the cannula is inserted into the right atrium.

A single two-stage venous cannula of variable diameter may be used in adults undergoing coronary artery bypass grafting, aortic valve replacement, or in some cases of mitral valve replacement. When properly positioned, the tip will be in the IVC and the side holes will be in the mid-right atrium.

When two venous cannulae and caval taping are to be used, a clamp is placed across the right atrial appendage, the appendage is opened, and one and then the other venous cannula is inserted through this opening. One is guided into the SVC and one into the IVC. Alternatively, direct caval cannulation can be used. The right atrium adjacent to the IVC is retracted by the surgeon with tissue forceps or a sponge, a stab wound is made in the center of the IVC purse string, and the cannula is inserted. A stab wound is made in the center of the purse string on the SVC, and this venous cannula is inserted. CPB is then established.

Direct caval cannulation can be difficult in neonates and small infants when the heart is large. In these small patients, exposure of the IVC can lead to severe hypotension.

After the cannulae are inserted, each tip must lie directly parallel to the walls of the vena cava, with the tip of the SVC cannula pointing upward and that of the IVC downward. Otherwise, venous obstruction will result. Precision in positioning the tips of the cannulae can be obtained by attaching the cannulae to the Y connector on the venous line in exactly the right orientation before their insertion. When exposure of the IVC is particularly difficult, the SVC may be cannulated first, partial CPB established, and the IVC then exposed for placing the tape and purse-string suture and for inserting the cannula.

Two venous cannulae inserted directly into the cavae as described are well suited for operations in children, infants, and neonates down to a body weight of about 2.5 kg. When the cannulae are placed as described, venous drainage is excellent; this can be verified by routine measurement of SVC pressure through an indwelling small catheter previously introduced into the internal jugular vein. An advantage of direct caval cannulation, in cases in which the major portion of the operation is performed during hypothermic circulatory arrest, is that the heart may be opened and the exposure arranged during the latter part of cooling and before the arrest period. The cardiac chambers can be closed during rewarming. A disadvantage is that, when the heart is closed, the inferior caval cannula must be repositioned into the right atrium to prevent its distention by blood returning from the coronary sinus, SVC, or both.

COMMENCING CARDIOPULMONARY BYPASS AND LEFT HEART VENTING

On command from the surgeon, the perfusionist commences CPB. The surgeon removes the arterial and venous line clamps (if present). The perfusion flow is gradually increased to about 2.2 L · min^{-1} · m^{-2}, and after the proper flow has been obtained, perfusion cooling (if indicated) is begun.

In neonates and infants undergoing deep hypothermia, the priming volume of the pump may be maintained at a temperature of 18° to 22°C, 30°C, or 37°C. If a cold prime is used, myocardial function is immediately affected after establishing CPB. Heart rate slows and contraction is impaired. The contribution to total blood flow by the heart rapidly diminishes. Therefore, the arterial pump must reach full flow rapidly to maintain adequate systemic perfusion. The heart should be carefully observed during this period for ventricular distention, especially in infants and neonates with low ventricular compliance and a heart less tolerant of excessive preload. If distention occurs, pump flow must be reduced and the venous cannulae repositioned. If cardiac contractility is maintained during initiation of CPB, it is preferable to maintain ventilation until full flow is achieved.

For operations in adults and older children, the venting catheter is inserted from the right side directly into the left atrium through a purse-string stitch positioned at the junction of the right superior pulmonary vein and the left atrium (see Fig. 2-21). The stitch should pick up atrial wall and the adventitia of the pulmonary vein, and should not be large enough to compromise the pulmonary vein orifice when tied down. In most cases a long, angled catheter is used, and it is advanced through the mitral valve into the left ventricle. This must be done precisely, in view of the possibility that air can be introduced into the heart and embolize to the brain unless the aorta has been clamped. Therefore, venous pressure is increased by reducing venous drainage to increase the volume of blood in the heart. A small incision is made within the purse string, and the venting catheter is introduced. After the venting catheter has been advanced into the left atrium, the left hand is placed behind the heart to palpate the tip of the vent and guide it toward the mitral valve and into the left ventricle. The same precautions with respect to air are necessary as the vent is withdrawn at the end of the operation.

For operations in the right atrium or right ventricle in which increased pulmonary venous return is anticipated, venting of the left heart can be performed as described in the previous paragraph. Alternatively, when two venous cannulae are used for operations in the right ventricle or right atrium, the caval tapes are secured after cooling has been initiated and the right atrium opened through a small oblique atriotomy. If a patent foramen ovale or atrial septal defect is present, a sump catheter is placed partially across this and into the left atrium. If neither is present, a stab wound is made in the fossa ovalis directly beneath the superior limbus. If this landmark is not used and the stab wound is imprecisely made, the vent may come to lie outside the heart rather than in the left atrium. Because the sump catheter lies only partially across the septal hole, it removes both left and right atrial blood. The right atrium remains open during the repair.

If the right superior or inferior pulmonary vein is not accessible for venting, the pulmonary trunk and the apex of the left ventricle are alternative sites. If the pulmonary trunk is used, a catheter or sump is inserted through a purse string in it immediately above the pulmonary valve. Drainage and decompression of the left heart may be suboptimal with this technique. If the left ventricle is to be vented directly, a pledgeted mattress suture of No. 2-0 or 3-0 polyester or polypropylene is placed near, but not at, the apex of the heart on the anterolateral wall, and a catheter or sump is introduced after the ventricle has been incised with a stab blade.

For operations in which the heart is not opened, such as coronary artery bypass grafting, the left heart can be vented through the ascending aorta proximal to the aortic clamp, using a needle vent that can be connected either to the venous line (gravity drainage) or directly to the reservoir of the pump-oxygenator using a roller pump.

CARDIOPULMONARY BYPASS DURING OPERATION AND REWARMING

When the desired perfusion flow rate is achieved, perfusate temperature is reduced, the aorta is clamped, and cardioplegic solution is infused (see Chapter 3). Cooling by the perfusate is continued until the nasopharyngeal temperature reaches the desired level, and then the perfusate temperature is stabilized at that level. A broad range of temperatures can be used. In most cases, the nasopharyngeal temperature should be lowered to at least 32°C. When the temperature is lowered to less than this level, perfusion flow rate can be safely reduced. For example, if 25°C is chosen, then the flow can be safely reduced to 1.6 L · min^{-1} · m^{-2}. Brief periods of lower flow may be used.

After completing most or all of the repair, rewarming is begun. It is usually at this point that preparation for myocardial reperfusion is commenced. The precise moment for commencing rewarming depends on the strategy used for myocardial management (see Chapter 3). For rewarming, the water in the heat exchanger is raised to 42°C; the arterial blood temperature should not exceed 39°C. It is advantageous, but not essential, to have the nasopharyngeal temperature at 37°C for about 10 minutes before CPB is discontinued, lest there be an excessive downward drift of temperature in the postbypass period.

DE-AIRING THE HEART

After completing the repair and as the cardiac chambers are closed or as coronary artery bypass grafting is being completed, the heart must be freed of as much air as possible before it begins to eject into the systemic circulation. Special maneuvers are necessary to avoid air embolism, as has clearly been demonstrated by intraoperative echocardiography.[M12,O4,V6] The exact steps and sequences and the time of de-airing may vary, but the principles are well established: (1) the heart is filled with fluid (blood or electrolyte solution) before closing to minimize air entrapment; (2) the heart must be reperfused and beating; (3) residual air is aspirated from the heart before allowing it to eject; (4) the lungs are intermittently ventilated to express air from the pulmonary veins; and (5) continuous suction is applied on a needle vent or catheter in the ascending aorta as the heart commences ejecting blood to retrieve any air that may have remained in the heart or pulmonary veins (alternatively, a freely bleeding stab wound may be used).[H23] The exact technique used will depend in part on the method used for myocardial management (see Chapter 3).

One technique can be illustrated with the procedure for aortic valve replacement:

1. As the suture line for aortic closure is being completed, suction on the left atrial vent is discontinued, and flow is reduced to allow the heart to fill with blood. If blood is not freely escaping from the most anterior portion of the aortotomy before completing this suture line, fluid (saline or Ringer's lactate) is injected into the opened aorta with a syringe. The suture line is completed. A needle vent connected to tubing from the pump-oxygenator is inserted into the ascending aorta. The anesthesiologist should *gently* inflate the lungs to remove air from the pulmonary veins into the left atrium. Vigorous inflation is not advisable, because when the lungs collapse, air can be drawn into the left ventricle through the still opened aorta.

2. With a large-bore needle connected to a 20-mL syringe or to a catheter from the pump-oxygenator, the left atrium is aspirated through its dome beneath the aorta. Air is almost invariably obtained. Aspiration is combined with gentle ventilation on two or three occasions until no further air appears. The left atrial appendage is inverted to evacuate air.

3. The heart is gently pulled forward and to the right, and needle aspiration of the left ventricular cavity is performed through the front of the left ventricular apex. This is a simple and effective way of removing the pocket of air that is almost always present at this site. The maneuver can be repeated several times.

4. The operating table is tilted with the patient's head down.

5. Perfusion flow rate is temporarily reduced as the aortic clamp is slowly released. Blood and air are gently aspirated from the needle vent in the ascending aorta. Left ventricular overdistention must be prevented.

6. The left atrial vent is removed while the lungs are gently inflated and the central venous pressure is slowly increased to evacuate any residual air. The purse-string suture is secured. The heart is electrically defibrillated if not already beating. The left ventricle is shaken with the left hand several times.

7. Central venous pressure is *slowly* raised by the perfusionist. The heart begins to eject. Air may then appear in the aortic vent suction line. When the central venous pressure has been elevated to 10 mmHg and the heart has ejected for several minutes, CPB flow is slowly reduced. The ventricle is again shaken and CPB is discontinued.

8. The table is leveled. Suction on the aortic needle is reduced and then discontinued, the needle is removed, and the stitch is tied. These maneuvers should not be hurried. The longer the aortic needle vent is in use, the better, and it should not be removed until the heart has been ejecting well for some time.

Transesophageal two-dimensional echocardiography (TEE) is commonly used to monitor removal of air from the heart before CPB is discontinued. There is little doubt that TEE enables the operating team to identify the presence of even small amounts of intracardiac and intraaortic air.[F15,S26] Because small amounts of intracardiac air have a low probability of causing any detectable damage, adherence to a strict protocol for removal of air, such as the one described above, will suffice for most patients.[R18,T20] The clinical benefit conferred by TEE during operations in which standard de-airing procedures are used has not been conclusively demonstrated. However, TEE may be of particular value during operations employing small incisions, or during operations in which the left-sided cardiac chambers are not fully mobilized, add some of the usual maneuvers for removal of air, such as aspiration and manipulation of the left ventricle, cannot be used.

Flooding the operative field with carbon dioxide has been used for displacing air from the cardiac chambers. Its use was first reported by Nichols and colleagues in 1988.[N11] It is currently used in a few cardiac surgical practices. The theoretical value of this technique is that carbon dioxide will displace air from the operative field because it is a heavier gas and because carbon dioxide emboli, if they occur, are better tolerated than air emboli.[K13] It may have a role in operations performed through small incisions or during reoperative procedures. However, the potential for inducing profound systemic hypercarbia and acidosis exists.[B20,O2] Thus, frequent monitoring of arterial blood gases and electrolytes is necessary when the technique is used.

COMPLETING CARDIOPULMONARY BYPASS

As rewarming is being completed, two temporary pacing wire electrodes are positioned on the lateral wall of the right atrium.[W15] The bared end of the shielded wire electrode is secured to the atrium with No. 5-0 sutures or with small clips. In most patients, one or two pacing wire electrodes are similarly sutured to the right ventricular myocardium on the anterior or inferior surface.

When the patient has been rewarmed to a nasopharyngeal temperature of 37°C, perfusion flow rate is gradually decreased until the right and left atrial and aortic pressures are adequate, and CPB is then discontinued. The venous cannulae are removed and the purse-string sutures are tied. Protamine is administered slowly (see "Heparinization and Later Protamine Administration" earlier in this section).

Positioning the Chest Tubes

There is considerable surgeon-to-surgeon difference in the location and number of chest tubes that are placed before closure of the median sternotomy incision. In general, the tubes are placed after CPB is discontinued and protamine has been administered, to avoid unnecessary bleeding. If the pleural spaces have not been entered, then one or two tubes are placed. A single tube can be positioned in the anterior mediastinum and brought out through a stab wound in the midline just below the sternotomy incision. Alternatively, two tubes, one in the anterior mediastinum as described and one (an angled tube) in the inferior–posterior portion of the pericardial cavity, are brought out through stab wounds in the epigastric region on both sides of the midline. If the left pleural space has been entered, as often occurs when the left internal thoracic artery is dissected from the parasternal area, a tube is positioned with the tip well posterior and inferior in the pleural space to ensure maximum removal of fluid. This tube can be brought out through the epigastrium in the midline below the sternotomy incision or through a stab wound on the lateral chest wall.

COMPLETING THE OPERATION

After CPB is discontinued, aside from ensuring adequate hemodynamics, the surgeon's primary task is to obtain hemostasis. This should be accomplished in a systematic fashion. All cardiac and aortic suture lines and purse strings are inspected. Fine (No. 4-0 or 5-0) single or pledgeted polypropylene sutures can be placed in the adventitia or epicardium to control bleeding from suture lines.

Generally, electrocautery suffices to control bleeding from the mediastinal tissues and around the sternum. Troublesome bleeding from the sternum itself can be managed by tying heavy, encircling, absorbable sutures around it. The wound should be closed only after hemostasis is secure.

The pericardium is generally left open after operations with CPB through a median sternotomy. A few stitches may, however, be placed at the upper end to partially cover a particularly prominent aorta or an aortic graft. Reoperations have not posed a problem with this technique. Advantages of leaving the pericardium open are (1) good drainage into the pericardium (and then out through the drainage tubes) of blood from the mediastinal and substernal tissues, thus preventing hematomas from developing in that area; and (2) reduction (but not elimination) of the tendency of retained blood to produce a positive intrapericardial pressure, thus lowering ventricular transmural pressure (tamponade).

Secure closure of the sternum is critically important. Stainless steel wire sutures are used, with the most cephalad one or two placed through the manubrium, the next three or four through the sternum or around the sternum close to the bone, and the most inferior one or two through the sternum. Different sizes of stainless steel sutures are available to match the patient's size. The wires are twisted, not tied, to bring the sternum together; in adults, these are further twisted with an instrument to ensure that the sternal fragments are securely approximated. If the sternal edges are thin or fragmented, wire sutures can be passed vertically in the parasternal position in front of and behind the costal cartilages on one or both sides. These vertical sutures can then be incorporated into the closure by the transverse wire sutures.[R25] Absorbable sutures are used for closing the muscles over the sternum and the linea alba. The skin is closed with a subcuticular absorbable suture or with metal staples.

Some patients have a suboptimal hemodynamic state as preparations are made to close the chest.[J6] In most of them, the sternum should probably not be closed, because this frequently further depresses cardiac function. Rather, the sternum, subcutaneous tissue, and skin are left unsutured. An impervious sheet of silicone rubber is cut to fit into the cutaneous defect and is sutured to the skin edges with a running monofilament suture. An occlusive but not constrictive dressing is applied to the anterior chest wall. This maneuver is lifesaving in some patients.[B43,F19,G20,J6,J7,M23,M24,O5,O6,R20,U1] Usually a secondary closure can be performed 2 to 7 days later.

PUMP-OXYGENATOR

The available apparatus for CPB changes continually, but some general points are important.

Components

A *venous reservoir* is currently used and is positioned to provide adequate siphonage by gravity, if gravity drainage is used.[P8] Alternatively, the venous reservoir may be a hard-shell device used for vacuum-assisted venous return. Such a reservoir allows escape of any air returning with the venous blood and provides storage of excess volume. This reservoir is generally incorporated within the housing of the oxygenator. Although useful, venous reservoirs substantially increase priming volume of the pump-oxygenator system.

The *oxygenator* is probably the most varied and yet most important part of the system, while at the same time it is probably the most damaging part of the extracorporeal apparatus. Microporous and true membrane oxygenators have advantages over bubble oxygenators and are currently indicated for cardiac surgery (see "Gas Exchange" under Controlled Variables in Section 2).

An efficient *heat exchanger* is necessary. This may be integral within the oxygenator or freestanding. Integrated heat exchangers have generally been less efficient than freestanding ones, but they reduce priming volume.

The *arterial pump* is most commonly a roller pump. It should be adjusted before each perfusion so as to be slightly nonocclusive, and should be calibrated at frequent intervals so that the flow rate can be accurately established. A centrifugal pump may also be used.

The *arterial line pressure* in the pump-oxygenator must be continuously monitored. When this pressure exceeds 250 to 300 mmHg, risk of disruption of the arterial line and of cavitation in the region of the arterial cannula increases. A proper arterial line pressure is ensured by a properly positioned cannula of adequate size.

The advantages, disadvantages, and need for a low-porosity *filter* in the *arterial line* remain somewhat controversial.[S29] A randomized study by Walker and colleagues (Walker DR, Blackstone EH, Kirklin JW, Karp RB, Kouchoukos NT, Pacifico AD, et al: unpublished data; 1976) showed good neuropsychiatric function (determined by specialized testing) in patients after coronary artery bypass grafting, whether or not a low-porosity arterial filter was present in the circuit. A similar study in patients undergoing open cardiotomy provided the same result.[A16] However, studies using transcranial Doppler ultrasound have shown that gaseous microemboli, more prevalent with bubble than with membrane or hollow fiber oxygenators, can be considerably reduced by 40-μm filters in the arterial line of the pump-oxygenator.[B37,P12,P13] Currently, routine use of a low-porosity filter of this type in the arterial line appears to be beneficial.

The exact filter to be used and its compatibility with the other components of the pump-oxygenator must be determined within each institution performing cardiac surgery.

A *device for ultrafiltration* is incorporated into the circuit of the pump-oxygenator, usually between the cardiotomy reservoir and the arterial line. During CPB, if there is excess volume in the pump-oxygenator, the device is activated for removal of serum water by ultrafiltration (see "Perfusate" under Controlled Variables in Section 2).

The CPB circuit generally should contain at least two *cardiotomy suction* ports for return of blood from the opened heart. This blood may contain particulate matter and boluses of air and must be passed through a low-porosity filter and defoamed in a separate chamber open to air before it is returned to the circuit. During the perfusion, blood should be promptly aspirated from the pericardium with these suckers. Blood left too long in the pericardium before being aspirated can promote thrombolysis. Ideally, these lines should be activated by a continuously and rapidly variable high-capacity vacuum system. Because this has so far proved to be impractical, roller pumps are used. With this system, when the open end of the line is blocked, the suction rapidly increases; this may damage either the tissue or the blood. Thus, constant monitoring of the roller pumps is necessary.

Priming Volume

Each component of the pump-oxygenator adds to the priming volume, which explains why many cardiac surgical groups are unwilling to add unessential components to their system. However, pump-oxygenator systems can be so oversimplified to reduce priming volume that safety may be compromised. Even with the most stringent efforts, the typical pump-oxygenator system currently in use has a priming volume considerably larger than is ideal.

Future Developments

Pump-oxygenator systems have not changed in their fundamental design since 1955. A few innovative modifications have been developed, but few have been adopted.[T13] Development of an integrated oxygenator–heat exchanger–pump-filter system, probably based on a controlled vortex pump and an efficient membrane oxygenator, will constitute a major advance in overall simplicity and reduction of priming volume. Collection of venous return into a vacuum-controlled small reservoir or by a special system incorporating direct pumping from the venous cannulae will complete development of a new generation of pump-oxygenators, which will be compact, require a very small priming volume, and be located at the level of the operating table near the head of the patient. Since the second edition of this book, one such device incorporating many of these features has been introduced for clinical testing.

SPECIAL SITUATIONS AND CONTROVERSIES

One Versus Two Venous Cannulae

Use of a single two-stage venous cannula is optimal for many cardiac operations (coronary artery bypass grafting, aortic valve replacement, and in many instances mitral valve replacement) in adult patients and is widely practiced. The technique is likewise optimal in neonates, infants, and children when the entire repair (including closure of the cardiac chambers) is performed during hypothermic circulatory arrest.

A single venous cannula may also be used in operations in which part of the repair is done during circulatory arrest, but a portion is left to be performed during CPB. Although convenient, the method has some disadvantages. Unless assisted venous return is used, an air lock may occur in the venous line during operations within the right ventricle or pulmonary trunk, with the air entering the right atrium through the tricuspid valve. When this happens, venous return to the pump-oxygenator stops abruptly and blood floods the right side of the heart. The perfusionist must not reduce the perfusion flow rate, but instead the intracardiac sucker is positioned outside the heart to keep blood from overflowing from the pericardial well, while the air lock is moved down the venous line and expelled into the venous reservoir. Principles for use of the single venous cannula in this setting are the same as those already described, including the need for the tip of the cannula to be in the IVC, while its side holes remain in the right atrium.

Cardiopulmonary Bypass Established by Peripheral Cannulation

Closed-chest cannulation of the femoral artery and vein for CPB was practiced at the Mayo Clinic during the 1960s for establishing hypothermic circulatory arrest in patients undergoing intracranial operations.[M13] It has since been used with increasing frequency to establish CPB before opening the sternum in reoperations in which there is a high probability of entering a cardiac chamber or a major artery during sternotomy. In these situations, a vertical or oblique incision in the groin crease is made over the femoral vessels. After identifying the inguinal ligament and working just inferior to it, the common femoral artery and vein are dissected, and a tape is placed around each. After the patient has been heparinized, a clamp is placed on the distal common femoral artery, any branches are occluded with ligature loops or small clamps, a clamp is placed proximally, and a transverse incision is made between the clamps. The arterial cannula is inserted into the vessel and, as the proximal clamp is removed, is gently advanced. The tape is snugged down around the cannula using a tourniquet, and the cannula is connected to the arterial line of the pump-oxygenator with the usual precautions to eliminate air. A large (No. 28 to 32 French) long cannula is similarly inserted into the common femoral vein. This cannula must be advanced over the sacral promontory and into the IVC.[W23] When the right femoral vein is used, this is usually easily accomplished. If the left femoral vein is used, it is often necessary to first insert a guide wire, positioning the tip in the right atrium or the adjacent IVC, then a small bore catheter which is passed over the wire, and then the venous cannula, which is inserted over the smaller catheter. After securing the tape and removing the smaller catheter and the guide wire, the cannula is connected to the venous line of the pump-oxygenator.

Femoral artery cannulation may result in peripheral embolization, local thrombosis, or aortic dissection. Additionally, in the presence of an existing acute or chronic aortic dissection, retrograde flow from femoral cannulation may result in central malperfusion. An alternative is use of either axillary artery. Advantages include absence of malperfusion, establishment of brain blood flow during otherwise whole body circulatory arrest, and presumably lack of retrograde particulate embolization. The axillary artery is exposed below and parallel to the lateral two thirds of the clavicle. The pectoralis major muscle is divided in the direction of its fibers and the clavipectoral fascia incised, exposing the pectoralis minor muscle, which may be divided or retracted laterally. Using sharp dissection, the artery is dissected from surrounding tissue, taking care not to injure the brachial plexus. Proximal and distal control of the axillary artery is obtained. After administration of heparin, the artery is cannulated, preferably through a short length of 8- or 10-mm polyester tubing anastamosed end-to-side to the artery.[G27,S36]

Currently, indications for peripheral cannulation have been expanded to include operations performed through small midline or lateral chest incisions (see "Alternative Primary Incisions" earlier in this section), resuscitation of preoperative and postoperative cardiac surgical patients, and support of high-risk patients during percutaneous catheter interventions.

Both arterial and venous cannulation can be accomplished by percutaneous techniques. The pump-oxygenator should be used in conjunction with a controlled vortex pump or vacuum assisted venous return, which permits use of smaller (No. 22 or 24 French) venous cannulae.

Blood Conservation

Since the earliest days of clinical use of CPB, there has been concern about the relatively large amounts of allogeneic blood that often must be administered during and early after operations. This concern has been magnified by the prevalence of cardiac operations requiring CPB and the possibility of acquiring deadly diseases such as hepatitis and human immunodeficiency virus. Methods of testing the suitability of donor blood have improved greatly in recent years, and currently in well-regulated institutional settings, risk of acquiring such diseases from transfused blood is small (see Chapter 5).

A major reason for the near-routine use of non-blood solutions for the initial priming of the pump-oxygenator is the desire to minimize use of allogeneic blood. Removal of 500 to 800 mL of blood from adult patients with hematocrits greater than 33% to 35% after induction of anesthesia is safe and is commonly performed. The blood is collected in bags containing CPD anticoagulant, as used by blood banks, and is left unrefrigerated in the operating room. (Refrigeration even for a short time renders platelets less effective.) This blood is not used during CPB, but rather is administered for its hemostatic as well as blood volume

effects after protamine is given and major bleeding has been controlled. Donation of blood by the patient several weeks before the operation, as well as by relatives and friends, is widely practiced. This blood has the disadvantages associated with stored blood.

The pump-oxygenator should incorporate one of the compact ultrafiltration devices currently available (see "Pump-Oxygenator" earlier in this section). This provides the capability of concentrating the blood left in the machine after CPB, including plasma proteins (in contrast to cell-saver systems), and preparing it for prompt administration to the patient.

Blood aspirated from the surgical field by a standard high-power sucker during and after the cardiac operation can be processed through a cell-saver system.[M6] These systems separate, wash, and to some extent concentrate the erythrocytes, which are then transfused to the patient. Anticoagulation is provided by heparin that is added to the apparatus. The components of plasma are lost.

Postoperatively for about 12 hours, shed blood from the mediastinal and pleural tubes can be collected in the reservoir and returned intravenously to the patient.[C21] This blood has been defibrinated in the patient before its collection and has the disadvantage of having essentially no clotting factors.

Most of the bleeding after cardiac surgery results from coagulation disturbances associated with CPB, related primarily to platelet dysfunction and activation of the fibrinolytic cascade (see Chapter 5 and "Response Variables" in Section 2).

Prophylactic administration of antifibrinolytic drugs (epsilon-aminocaproic acid, tranexamic acid, and aprotinin) decreases the frequency of reoperations for bleeding and the need for allogeneic blood transfusions in patients after operations employing CPB.[L9] Comparative studies have demonstrated equivalent effectiveness of these three agents.[C30,L9,M26,M27,N9,W24] Aprotinin is substantially more expensive than the other two drugs, however.[B50,C30]

Left Superior Vena Cava

A left superior vena cava (LSVC) presents no problems in operations in which a single venous cannula is used. When other techniques for venous cannulation are used, several options exist. A simple method is to use cannulae in the superior and inferior venae cavae and to pick up the LSVC flow by the sump sucker that is positioned partially across the atrial septum (see "Commencing Cardiopulmonary Bypass and Left Heart Venting" earlier in this section) or in the coronary sinus ostium.

Alternatively, the LSVC may be taped so that the cava can be occluded completely for short periods when exposure in the right atrium is suboptimal. As another alternative, a pressure-monitoring needle may be inserted into the LSVC, or the pressure in the left jugular vein may be monitored. As a test, the LSVC is clamped below the needle (downstream). If the monitored pressure does not increase, it may be assumed that the vein can be safely occluded during CPB. If the pressure increases substantially, an additional (third) cannula is inserted into the LSVC either via the right atrium and coronary sinus ostium or directly via a purse string where the vein enters the pericardium lateral to the left atrial appendage. The latter is most easily done after CPB has been established but before the right atrium is opened. When three cannulae are in use, two Y-connectors are required to connect the venous return to the single venous pump line.

Left Atrial Pressure Monitoring

Knowledge of left atrial pressure both intraoperatively and postoperatively is important. The most direct way of measuring this pressure is to insert a fine polyvinyl catheter into the left atrium. There is danger of accidental introduction of air into the left atrial line and of cerebral embolization from a tiny thrombus on its tip, but these complications are rare. The only major complication has been occasional bleeding when the catheter is removed. This can be significant enough in small infants to require immediate blood replacement and, rarely, reoperation. Even in neonates and small infants, bleeding after removal has not been encountered when removal is delayed until at least 48 hours postoperatively.

A less satisfactory but more commonly used alternative is to introduce a catheter into the pulmonary artery for intraoperative and postoperative monitoring (as discussed earlier). Unless pulmonary vascular disease is present, the pulmonary artery diastolic pressure approximates mean left atrial pressure. Many groups routinely insert a Swan-Ganz catheter after induction of anesthesia, rather than using a left atrial catheter as described (see "Operative Monitoring" in Section 2 of Chapter 4).

Alternative Primary Incisions
Minimal Sternotomy and Thoracotomy

Currently, a number of smaller incisions are being used for procedures on the cardiac valves, the ascending aorta and aortic arch, and the coronary arteries in adults, and for correction of congenital cardiac defects in children and in adults.[A18,C31,C32,D23,G22-G24,L10,L11] The various incisions that have been used are shown in Fig. 2-22. They can be classified into three general types: a partial midline sternotomy (upper, lower, or middle), a parasternal incision with resection of one or more costal cartilages, and a more lateral approach through an intercostal space, with or without resection of a segment of costal cartilage or rib, and with or without partial or total transection of the sternum. The commonly used minimal incisions for coronary artery bypass grafting and for valve replacement or repair are described in Chapters 7, 11, 12, and 13.

Putative advantages of these "mini" or "minimal access" incisions, when compared with the full sternotomy, include reduced blood loss, less pain and therefore a lowered requirement for analgesic agents, a more rapid convalescence with a reduced hospital stay, a reduced prevalence of infection, a better cosmetic result, and lower overall costs. In a number of observational studies that have compared minimal incisions with a full sternotomy, these advantages have not been consistently observed.[A19,C33,G23,H34,L11,L12,S30,W26] In many instances, duration of CPB and total time of operation are prolonged with the minimal incisions. The resulting increase in operating room costs often offsets the reduced costs achieved by a shorter hospital stay.

It appears likely that the trend to use smaller incisions will continue as new instruments and cannulae are developed that facilitate performing procedures on the heart and great vessels through smaller openings. However, until clear advantages of minimal incisions are demonstrated, full sternotomy should continue to be used. Cardiac surgeons must be competent and experienced in use of the full sternotomy before attempting procedures through small incisions. Furthermore, they must recognize that the potential or real advantages of small incisions may be outweighed by the disadvantages that can result from limited exposure.

Right Anterolateral Thoracotomy

A right anterolateral thoracotomy through the fourth or fifth intercostal space may be used for cosmetic reasons in young women with developing breasts, for mitral and tricuspid valve operations, and for repair of atrial septal defects. It may also be used in patients who require reoperation only on the tricuspid valve and for reoperations on the mitral valve after one or more previous procedures. This approach provides excellent access to the left and right atria, although the field may be relatively restricted and cannulation of the ascending aorta may be difficult. When the aorta is inaccessible or when coronary artery bypass grafts have been anastomosed to the ascending aorta during a previous operation, the common femoral or axillary artery is used (see "Cardiopulmonary Bypass Established by Peripheral Cannulation" earlier in this section).

A double-lumen endotracheal tube is used to permit collapse of the right lung and enhanced exposure. The patient is positioned with the right side elevated 30 to 40 degrees. The right arm is flexed at the elbow and kept at the patient's side. The left arm lies at the side. Groin areas are draped into the operative field. The skin incision follows the intercostal space to be entered and extends laterally to the anterior axillary line. The intercostal muscle is divided and a retractor placed. The pleural cavity is entered and the intercostal muscles are further divided laterally beneath the skin incision if exposure is not optimal. The collapsed lung is gently retracted posteriorly and the pericardium is incised vertically 1 to 2 cm anterior and parallel to the phrenic nerve. If cannulation of both venae cavae is required, the cannulae are inserted through purse-string sutures in the SVC and in the right atrial wall adjacent to the IVC. Alternatively, a long cannula can be positioned in the IVC after insertion in the common femoral vein, or a two-stage long cannula can be inserted in the femoral vein and the openings positioned in the SVC and IVC. The aorta is cannulated on its right anterolateral aspect. For primary operations, the remainder of the procedure is similar to a median sternotomy approach.

For reoperations on the mitral valve, particularly after a previous coronary artery bypass grafting procedure, cannulation and clamping of the ascending aorta may not be possible. In this situation, myocardial management is accomplished by hypothermic fibrillation. Temperature of the perfusate is lowered until the heart fibrillates or until the nasopharyngeal temperature reaches 18° to 22°C. At that temperature, an external fibrillator is applied to the myocardium to induce ventricular fibrillation. The heart must be

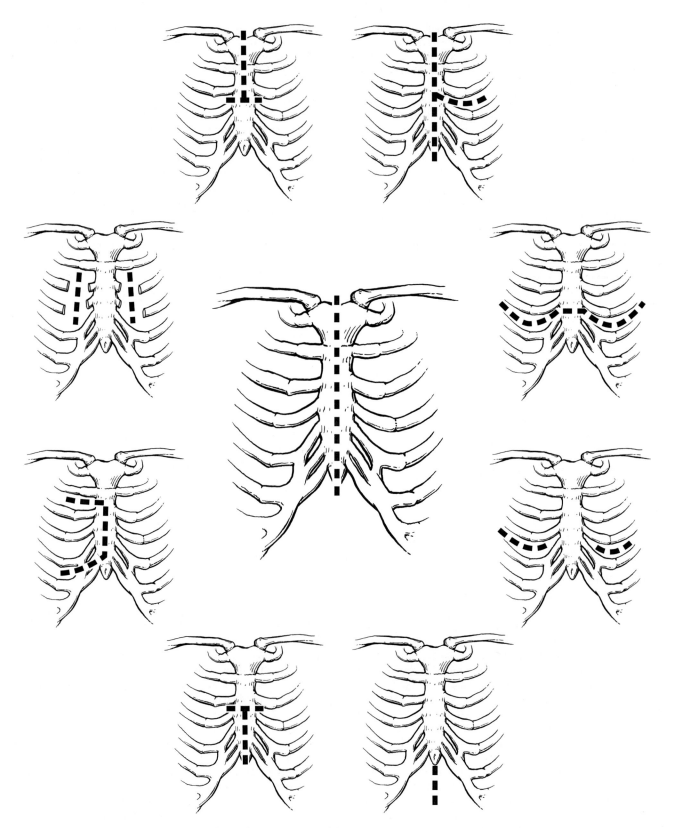

Figure 2-22 Currently used sternotomy and thoracotomy incisions *(dashed lines)* for cardiac operations.

maintained hypothermic and in a fibrillating state to avoid ejection of air into the ascending aorta. Rewarming is not initiated until the left atrium has been closed. A soft rubber catheter attached to a cardiotomy suction line is positioned in the left ventricle through the mitral valve or a prosthesis, and is brought out through the atriotomy incision. Continuous suction is applied to this catheter during rewarming to evacuate air from the left ventricle. The catheter is removed just before CPB is discontinued and the left atrial suture line is secured.

SECTION 4
Clinical Methodology of Hypothermic Circulatory Arrest

GENERAL COMMENTS AND STRATEGY

Although opinions differ regarding the appropriate use of hypothermic circulatory arrest, there is no doubt that it is essential to some operative procedures. For many other procedures it may be chosen, knowing that other options exist and that there is no certainty that one method is superior to another. Time limits and safeguards of the arrest period are discussed in Section 1.

TECHNIQUE IN ADULTS

The technique for establishing hypothermic circulatory arrest in adult patients is described in detail in Chapter 53 under "Replacement of the Aortic Arch" and "Replacement of the Thoracoabdominal Aorta."

TECHNIQUE IN NEONATES, INFANTS, AND CHILDREN
Preparation for Cardiopulmonary Bypass

Preparation of the patient is the same as described for CPB in general (see Section 3). Historically, surface cooling was employed as an adjunct to core cooling. Now, most institutions use a cooling blanket and packing of ice around the head. These maneuvers, plus a cool operating room, usually reduce the body temperature of the patient to 30° to 32°C by the time CPB is initiated. The ice bags remain in place around the head until perfusion rewarming is begun after the period of circulatory arrest.

Cannulation

The aortic cannula is inserted into the ascending aorta in the usual manner. In some cases, particularly in small infants, it is inserted near or into the innominate artery. It is critically important to remember that although the purse string around the aortic cannula may be hemostatic, it does not protect against the passage of air. This is important, because when CPB is temporarily discontinued to establish circulatory arrest, the arterial pump may be sufficiently nonocclusive that suction initiated by gravity develops in the arterial system. With the aorta at essentially zero pressure, such suction draws air into the aorta and the cannula from the site of cannula insertion. The purse-string suture cannot be made snug enough to prevent this. Therefore, just before CPB is discontinued, the perfusionist clamps the arterial tubing and then discontinues CPB, making this suction-driven air entry impossible because the arterial system has been "pressurized." Just as CPB is recommenced, the perfusionist removes the clamp. These precautions are unnecessary if a clamp is placed on the aorta *distal* to the aortic cannula. The aortic cannula can then be used for delivery of cardioplegic solution.

Commonly, a single venous cannula is used (see "Siting and Purse-String Sutures for Venous Cannulation" and "One Versus Two Venous Cannulae" in Section 3). Two venous cannulae and caval tapes may be used even if the patient weighs less than 3 kg. This allows maximal flexibility. The caval tapes are often left loose and then tightened during cooling and periods of low flow. Some procedures can be performed at low flow rate with a single venous cannula.

Cardiopulmonary Bypass for Cooling

After CPB is established, cooling is begun as described in Section 3. Relatively high CPB flows, 2.2 to 2.5 $L \cdot min^{-1} \cdot m^{-2}$, are used. The nasopharyngeal temperature in neonates and small infants can sometimes decrease to 18°C within 10 minutes. However, rapid cooling has been demonstrated to be suboptimal for circulatory arrest (see "Characteristics of the Cooling Process" in Section 1), probably because it is not homogeneous. Therefore, the cooling period should last at least 20 minutes and may at times approach 30 minutes.

The target temperature and its most appropriate site of measurement remain controversial (see "Brain Function and Structure: Risk Factors for Damage" in Section 1). A nasopharyngeal temperature of 16° to 18°C is a reasonable criterion to establish circulatory arrest.

Management of gas exchange during cooling is also controversial (see "Arterial Carbon Dioxide Pressure" in Section 2). In any event, arterial P_{CO_2}, and thus arterial pH, the important variables, are quite controllable with membrane oxygenators and on-line measurement of arterial pH and P_{CO_2}. The most commonly used method (alpha-stat) is the maintenance during cooling of arterial pH, measured at 37°C and *not* corrected to the patient's blood temperature, at the prebypass level by varying $PaCO_2$. Usually some reduction of ventilation of the membrane oxygenator is required, with a consequent elevation of $PaCO_2$ measured at 37°C.

During cooling, dilatation of the heart must be avoided. It may be necessary to manipulate the position of the venous cannulae to ensure adequate drainage. A single infusion of cardioplegic solution will usually suffice if circulatory arrest does not exceed 30 minutes.

Circulatory Arrest

Time constraints of safe circulatory arrest are discussed in Section 1. There is no secure evidence that interposing a short period of CPB increases safe duration of circulatory arrest, presumably because cerebral blood flow is low early after resumption of CPB and presumably inhomogeneously distributed under that condition[S28] (see Fig. 2-3). However, when time constraints are anticipated, intermittent perfusion to interrupt hypothermic circulatory arrest may be useful.[L13]

Cardiac Operation

The right atrial cannula is often removed from the heart. The heart is opened where appropriate, and repair is performed. The right atrium is usually opened to close any atrial communication, including a patent foramen ovale.

When the intracardiac repair is completed, the cardiotomy is closed.

Rewarming

Precise details of the rewarming with CPB and the time of its initiation, myocardial management, cardiac de-airing, and removal of the aortic clamp are highly interrelated and primarily dependent on the method of myocardial management. Each surgical group should determine these protocols for itself, using the principles described in this chapter and in Chapter 3.

APPENDIX

APPENDIX 2A

Equations

The equation derived from the data in Figure 2-1 is

$$\log_{10} \dot{V}_{O_2} = -0.69 \pm 0.061 + 0.043 \pm 0.0021 \cdot \text{temperature}$$

(2A-1)

where P for intercept and slope <.0001, SD of regression = 0.12, and r^2 = .80.

Correlation (r^2) of the data in Fig. 2-15 to a linear model[S27] was .39; to a log-log model[H4] .54; to the Arrhenius[P8] equation (log $\dot{V}_{O_2}$ proportional to flow^{-1}) .52; and to a hyperbolic model .69. The equation for Fig. 2-15 is

$$1/\dot{V}_{O_2} = 0.0062 \pm 0.00024 + 0.0044 \pm 0.00020/\text{flow}$$

(2A-2)

where $\dot{V}_{O_2}$ is oxygen consumption (mL · min^{-1} · m^{-2}) at 37°C; flow is perfusion flow rate (L · min^{-1} · m^{-2}) during CPB; P for intercept and slope <.0001; SD of regression = 0.0024; and r^2 = .69.

The equation represented by the nomogram in Fig. 2-11 is

$$1/\dot{V}_{O_2} = 0.168 \cdot 10^{-0.0387 \cdot T} + 0.0378 \cdot \dot{Q}^{-1} \cdot 10^{-0.0253 \cdot T}$$

(2A-3)

where T is temperature in °C.

This was derived as follows. The relationship between $\dot{V}_{O_2}$ and $\dot{Q}$ at 37°C was established from published animal experimental data (Fig. 2-15 and Equation 2A-2). Fox and colleagues established these relationships at 20°C in humans during CPB.[F5] The equation is

$$1/\dot{V}_{O_2} = 0.0284 + 0.0118 \cdot \dot{Q}^{-1}$$

(2A-4)

In mating these for the curves at intermediate temperatures, the first coefficient in Equation 2A-3 (relating to maximum oxygen consumption at limitless flow) followed Q_{10}, which happened to be 2.4. The second coefficient (relating flow slope change to temperature) followed a Q_{10} of 1.8. Both the experimental data at 37°C and the data of Fox and colleagues at 20°C are described by Equation 2A-3.

The logistic equation for Figure 2-6 is

$$Z = -7.3 \pm 1.56 + 0.08 \pm 0.026 \cdot \text{TCA}$$

(2A-5)

where TCA is circulatory arrest time (minutes), P for intercept <.0001, and P for TCA = .002. Also, among the 211 patients without such events, TCA time was 42 ± 14.0 (SD) minutes, compared with 59 ± 10.2 for the eight patients with such events (P = .0008).

REFERENCES

A

1. Andersen MN, Senning A. Studies in oxygen consumption during extracorporeal circulation with a pump-oxygenator. Ann Surg 1958;148:59.

2. Ames A 3rd, Wright RL, Kowada M, Thurston JM, Majno G. Cerebral ischemia. II. The no-reflow phenomenon. Am J Pathol 1968;52:437.

3. Almond CH, Jones JC, Snyder HM, Grant SM, Meyer BW. Cooling gradients and brain damage with deep hypothermia. J Thorac Cardiovasc Surg 1964;48:890.

4. Alivisatos CN, Filippakis M. Quelques données expérimentales sur l'arrêt provisoire de la circulation afférente du foie. J Chir (Paris) 1971;101:191.

5. Andreasen AT, Watson F. Experimental cardiovascular surgery. Br J Surg 1952;39:548.

6. Addonizio VP Jr, Strauss JF 3rd, Colman RW, Edmunds LH Jr. Effects of prostaglandin E$_1$ on platelet loss during in vivo and in vitro extracorporeal circulation with a bubble oxygenator. J Thorac Cardiovasc Surg 1979;77:119.

7. Addonizio VP Jr, Macarak EJ, Nicolaou KC, Edmunds LH Jr, Colman RW. Effects of prostacyclin and albumin on platelet loss during in vitro simulation of extracorporeal circulation. J Am Soc Hematol 1979;53:1033.

8. Addonizio VP Jr, Smith JB, Strauss JF 3rd, Colman RW, Edmunds LH Jr. Thromboxane synthesis and platelet secretion during cardiopulmonary bypass with bubble oxygenator. J Thorac Cardiovasc Surg 1980;79:91.

9. Anand KJ, Hansen DD, Hickey PR. Hormonal-metabolic stress responses in neonates undergoing cardiac surgery. Anesthesiology 1990;73:661.

10. Anand KJ, Hickey PR. Halothane-morphine compared with high-dose sufentanil for anesthesia and postoperative analgesia in neonatal cardiac surgery. N Engl J Med 1992;326:1.

11. Aljama P, Bird PA, Ward MK, Feest TG, Walker W, Tanboga H, et al. Haemodialysis-induced leucopenia and activation of complement: effects of different membranes. Proc Eur Dial Transplant Assoc 1978;15:144.

12. Alon L, Turina M, Gattiker R. Membrane and bubble oxygenator: a clinical comparison in patients undergoing aortocoronary bypass procedures. Herz 1979;4:56.

13. Azariades M, Wood AJ, Awang Y, Lennox SC. A qualitative analysis of pulsatile perfusion: effects on cortisol response to cardiopulmonary bypass surgery. Thorac Cardiovasc Surg 1986;34:163.

14. Addonizio VP Jr, Strauss JF 3rd, Chang LF, Fisher CA, Colman RW, Edmunds LH Jr. Release of lysosomal hydrolases during simulated extracorporeal circulation. J Thorac Cardiovasc Surg 1982;84:28.

15. Alston RP, Singh M, McLaren AD. Systemic oxygen uptake during hypothermic cardiopulmonary bypass. Effects of flow rate, flow character, and arterial pH. J Thorac Cardiovasc Surg 1989;98:757.

16. Aris A, Solanes H, Camara ML, Junque C, Escartin A, Caralps JM. Arterial line filtration during cardiopulmonary bypass. Neurologic, neuropsychologic, and hematologic studies. J Thorac Cardiovasc Surg 1986;91:526.

17. Alberts B, Johnson A, Lewis J, Raff M, Roberts K, Walter P. Molecular biology of the cell, 4th ed. New York: Garland, 2002.

18. Aklog L, Adams DH, Couper GS, Gobezie R, Sears S, Cohn LH. Techniques and results of direct-access minimally invasive mitral valve surgery: a paradigm for the future. J Thorac Cardiovasc Surg 1998;116:705.

19. Asher CR, DiMengo JM, Arheart KL, Weber MM, Grimm RA, Blackstone EH, et al. Atrial fibrillation early postoperatively following minimally invasive cardiac valvular surgery. Am J Cardiol 1999;84:744.

20. Anderson RV, Siegman MG, Balaban RS, Ceckler TL, Swain JA. Hyperglycemia increases cerebral intracellular acidosis during circulatory arrest. Ann Thorac Surg 1992;54:1126.

B

1. Bigelow WG, Lindsay WK, Greenwood WF. Hypothermia: its possible role in cardiac surgery. Ann Surg 1950;132:849.

2. Bigelow WG, Lindsay WK, Harrison RC, Gordon RA, Greenwood WF. Oxygen transport and utilization in dogs at low body temperatures. Am J Physiol 1950;160:125.

3. Boerema I, Wildschut A, Schmidt WJ, Broekhuysen L. Experimental researches into hypothermia as an aid in the surgery of the heart. Arch Chir Neerl 1951;3:25.

4. Bigelow WG, Callaghan JC, Hopps JA. General hypothermia for experimental intracardiac surgery. Ann Surg 1950;132:531.

5. Barratt-Boyes BG, Simpson MM, Neutze JM. Intracardiac surgery in neonates and infants using deep hypothermia. Circulation 1970;61,62:III73.

6. Burton AC. Human calorimetry. II. The average temperature of the tissues of the body. J Nutr 1935;9:261.

7. Brunberg JA, Reilly EL, Doty DB. Central nervous system consequences in infants of cardiac surgery using deep hypothermia and circulatory arrest. Circulation 1974;50:II60.

8. Bergouignan M, Fontan F, Trarieux M, Julien J. Syndromes choréiformes de l'enfant au décours d'interventions cardiochirurgicales sous hypothermie profonde. Rev Neurol (Paris) 1961;105:48.

9. Barratt-Boyes BG, Neutze JM, Clarkson P, Shardey GC, Brandt PW. Repair of ventricular septal defect in the first two years of life using profound hypothermia-circulatory arrest techniques. Ann Surg 1976;184:376.

10. Belsey RH, Keen G, Skinner DB. Profound hypothermia in cardiac surgery. J Thorac Cardiovasc Surg 1968;56:497.

11. Blauth CI, Arnold JV, Schulenberg WE, McCartney AC, Taylor KM. Cerebral microembolism during cardiopulmonary bypass. Retinal microvascular studies in vivo with fluorescein angiography. J Thorac Cardiovasc Surg 1988;95:668.

12. Bjork VO. Brain perfusions in dogs with artificially oxygenated blood. Acta Chir Scand 1948;96:137.

13. Brown IW Jr, Smith WW, Emmons WO. An efficient blood heat exchanger for use with extracorporeal circulation. Surgery 1958;44:372.

14. Bidstrup BP, Royston D, Sapsford RN, Taylor KM. Reduction in blood loss and blood use after cardiopulmonary bypass with high dose aprotinin (Trasylol). J Thorac Cardiovasc Surg 1989;97:364.

15. Backmann F, McKenna R, Cole ER, Najafi H. The hemostatic mechanism after open-heart surgery. I. Studies on plasma coagulation factors and fibrinolysis in 512 patients after extracorporeal circulation. J Thorac Cardiovasc Surg 1975;70:76.

16. Baier RE, Dutton RC. Initial events in interactions of blood with a foreign surface. J Biomed Mater Res 1969;3:191.

17. Boyle EM Jr, Pohlman TH, Johnson MC, Verrier ED. Endothelial cell injury in cardiovascular surgery: the systemic inflammatory response. Ann Thorac Surg 1997;63:277.

18. Bixler TJ, Magee PG, Flaherty JT, Gardner TJ, Gott VL. Beneficial effects of pulsatile perfusion in the hypertrophied ventricle during ventricular fibrillation. Circulation 1979;60:1.

19. Bernhard WF, McMurray JD, Curtis GW. Feasibility of partial hepatic resection under hypothermia. N Engl J Med 1955;253:159.

20. Burbank A, Ferguson TB, Burford TH. Carbon dioxide flooding of the chest in open-heart surgery. A potential hazard. J Thorac Cardiovasc Surg 1965;50:691.

21. Baue AE, Nusbaum M, Anstadt G, Blakemore WS. The pattern of lymphatic flow during extracorporeal circulation. J Thorac Cardiovasc Surg 1965;50:648.

22. Breckenridge IM, Digerness SB, Kirklin JW. Validity of concept of increased extracellular fluid after open heart surgery. Surg Forum 1969;20:169.

23. Bennett EV Jr, Fewel JF, Ybarra J, Grover FL, Trinkle JK. Comparison of flow differences among venous cannulas. Ann Thorac Surg 1983;36:59.

24. Brennan RW, Patterson RH Jr, Kessler J. Cerebral blood flow and metabolism during cardiopulmonary bypass: evidence of microembolic encephalopathy. Neurology 1971;21:665.

25. Blauth C, Smith P, Newman S, Arnold J, Siddons F, Harrison MJ, et al. Retinal microembolism and neurophysiological deficit following clinical cardiopulmonary bypass: comparison of a membrane and a bubble oxygenator. Eur J Cardiothorac Surg 1989;3:135.

26. Blauth C, Arnold J, Kohner EM, Taylor KM. Retinal microembolism during cardiopulmonary bypass demonstrated by fluorescein angiography. Lancet 1986;2:837.

27. Boonstra PW, Vermeulen FE, Leusink JA, de Nooy EH, van Zalk A, Soons JB, et al. Hematological advantage of a membrane oxygenator over a bubble oxygenator in long perfusions. Ann Thorac Surg 1986;41:297.

28. Bove EL, West HL, Paskanik AM. Hypothermic cardiopulmonary bypass: a comparison between alpha and pH stat regulation in the dog. J Surg Res 1987;42:66.

29. Becker H, Vinten-Johansen J, Buckberg GD, Robertson JM, Leaf JD, Lazar HL, et al. Myocardial damage caused by keeping pH 7.40 during systemic deep hypothermia. J Thorac Cardiovasc Surg 1981;82:810.

30. Bridges KG, Reichard GA Jr, MacVaugh H 3rd, Kues JR, Cevallos WH, Lechman MJ, et al. Effect of phentolamine in controlling temperature and acidosis associated with cardiopulmonary bypass. Crit Care Med 1985;13:72.

31. Brusino FG, Reves JG, Smith LR, Prough DS, Stump DA, McIntyre RW. The effect of age on cerebral blood flow during hypothermic cardiopulmonary bypass. J Thorac Cardiovac Surg 1989;97:541.

32. Branthwaite MA. Cerebral blood flow and metabolism during open heart surgery. Thorax 1974;29:633.

33. Beutler B, Cerami A. Cachectin. More than a tumor necrosis factor. N Engl J Med 1987;316:379.

34. Brett J, Gerlach H, Nawroth P, Steinberg S, Godman G, Stern D. Tumor necrosis factor/cachectin increases permeability of endothelial cell monolayers by a mechanism involving regulatory G proteins. J Exp Med 1989;169:1977.

35. Ballinger WF II, Vollenweider H, Templeton JY 3rd, Pierucci L Jr. Acidosis of hypothermia. Ann Surg 1961;154:517.

36. Busto R, Dietrich WD, Globus MY, Valdes I, Scheinberg P, Ginsberg MD. Small differences in intraischemic brain temperature critically determine the extent of ischemic neuronal injury. J Cereb Blood Flow Metab 1987;7:729.

37. Berman L, Marin F. Micropore filtration during cardiopulmonary bypass. In Taylor KM, ed. Cardiopulmonary bypass. London: Chapman and Hall, 1986, p. 361.

38. Blauhut B, Brucke P, Nacek S, Doran JE, Spath P, Lungsgaard-Hansen P. Effects of high-dose aprotinin on blood loss, platelet function, fibrinolysis complement and renal function after cardiopulmonary bypass. J Thorac Cardiovasc Surg 1991;101:958.

39. Barratt-Boyes BG. Choreoathetosis as a complication of cardiopulmonary bypass. Ann Thorac Surg 1990;50:693.

40. Bjork VO, Hultquist G. Brain damage in children after deep hypothermia for open heart surgery. Thorax 1960;15:284.

41. Bellinger DC, Wernovsky G, Rappaport LA, Mayer JE, Castaneda AL, Farrell DM, et al. Cognitive development of children following early repair of transposition of the great arteries using deep hypothermic circulatory arrest. Pediatrics 1991;87:701.

42. Blauth CI, Smith PL, Arnold JV, Jagoe JR, Wootton R, Taylor KM, et al. Influence of oxygenator type on the prevalence and extent of microembolic retinal ischemia during cardiopulmonary bypass. Assessment of digital image analysis. J Thorac Cardiovasc Surg 1990;99:61.

43. Bex JP, de Riberolles C, Lecompte Y, Marchand M, Menu P, Fiemeyer A, et al. Compression cardiaque lors de la fermeture du sternum après correction de cardiopathies congénitales complexes. Ann Chir 1980;34:198.

44. Barnard CN, Schrire V. The surgical treatment of acquired aneurysm of the thoracic aorta. Thorax 1963;18:101.

45. Borst HG, Schaudig A, Rudolph W. Arteriovenous fistula of the aortic arch: repair during deep hypothermia and circulatory arrest. J Thorac Cardiovasc Surg 1964;48:443.

46. Boyle EM Jr, Pohlman TH, Cornejo CJ, Verrier ED. Endothelial cell injury in cardiovascular surgery: ischemia-reperfusion. Ann Thorac Surg 1996;62:1868.

47. Bellinger DC, Wypij D, Kuban KC, Rappaport LA, Hickey PR, Wernovsky G, et al. Developmental and neurological status of children at 4 years of age after heart surgery with hypothermic circulatory arrest or low-flow cardiopulmonary bypass. Circulation 1999;100:526.

48. Bidstrup BP, Harrison J, Royston D, Taylor KM, Treasure T. Aprotinin therapy in cardiac operations: a report on use in 41 cardiac centers in the United Kingdom. Ann Thorac Surg 1993;55:971.

49. Bennett-Guerrero E, Sorohan JG, Canada AT, Ayuso L, Newman MF, Reves JG, et al. Epsilon-aminocaproic acid plasma levels during cardiopulmonary bypass. Anesth Analg 1997;85:248.

50. Bennett-Guerrero E, Sorohan JG, Gurevich ML, Kazanjian PE, Levy RR, Barbera AV, et al. Cost-benefit and efficacy of aprotinin compared with epsilon-aminocaproic acid in patients having repeated cardiac operations: a randomized, blinded clinical trial. Anesthesiology 1997;87:1373.

51. Butler J, Rocker GM, Westaby S. Inflammatory response to cardiopulmonary bypass. Ann Thorac Surg 1993;55:552.

52. Baron JM. Hypercoagulable states: clinical and laboratory diagnosis. Clin Comment 1988;4:1988.

53. Bidstrup BP. Monitoring of systemic anticoagulation during cardiopulmonary bypass. Ann Thor Surg 1996;61:781.

54. Banbury MK, White JA, Blackstone EH, Cosgrove DM 3rd. Vacuum-assisted venous return reduces blood usage. J Thorac Cardiovasc Surg (in press).

55. Bhujle R, Li J, Shastri P, Gaffke JN, Clift JE, Ye YW, et al. Influence of cardiopulmonary bypass on platelet and neutrophil accumulations in internal organs. ASAIO J 1997;43:M739.

56. Brix-Christensen V, Tonnesen E, Hjortdal VE, Chew M, Flo C, Marqversen J, et al. Neutrophils and platelets accumulate in the heart, lungs, and kidneys after cardiopulmonary bypass in neonatal pigs. Crit Care Med 2002;30:670.

57. Blackstone EH, Kirklin JW, Stewart RW, Chenoweth DE. Damaging effects of cardiopulmonary bypass. In Wu KK, Rossi EC, eds. Prostaglandins in clinical medicine. Chicago: Year Book Medical Publishers, 1982;355.

C

1. Civalero LA, Moreno JR, Senning A. Temperature conditions and oxygen consumption during deep hypothermia. Acta Chir Scand 1962;123:179.

2. Cheng HC, Kusunoki T, Bosher LH Jr, McElvein RB, Blake DA. A study of oxygen consumption during extracorporeal circulation. Trans Am Soc Artif Intern Organs 1959;5:273.

3. Cohen ME, Olszowka JS, Subramanian S. Electroencephalographic and neurological correlates of deep hypothermia and circulatory arrest in infants. Ann Thorac Surg 1977;23:238.

4. Clarkson PM, MacArthur BA, Barratt-Boyes BG, Whitlock RM, Neutze JM. Developmental progress following cardiac surgery in infancy using profound hypothermia and circulatory arrest. Circulation 1980;62:855.

5. Chiang J, Kowada MD, Ames A 3rd, Wright RL, Majno G. Cerebral ischemia. III. Vascular changes. Am J Pathol 1968;52:455.

6. Crafoord C, Norberg B, Senning A. Clinical studies in extracorporeal circulation with a heart-lung machine. Acta Chir Scand 1957;112:220.

7. Cohen M, Lillehei CW. A quantitative study of the "azygos factor" during vena caval occlusion in the dog. Surg Gynecol Obstet 1954;98:225.

8. Chien S. Present state of blood rheology. In Messmer K, Schmid-Schonbein H, eds. Hemodilution: theoretical basis and clinical application. Basel: Karger, 1972, p. 1.

9. Cohn LH, Angell WW, Shumway NE. Body fluid shifts after cardiopulmonary bypass. I. Effects of congestive heart failure and hemodilution. J Thorac Cardiovasc Surg 1971;62:423.

10. Chenoweth DE, Cooper SW, Hugli TE, Stewart RW, Blackstone EH, Kirklin JW. Complement activation during cardiopulmonary bypass: evidence for generation of C3a and C5a anaphylatoxins. N Engl J Med 1981;304:497.

11. Craddock PR, Fehr J, Dalmasso AP, Brigham KL, Jacob HS. Pulmonary vascular leukostasis resulting from complement activation by dialyzer cellophane membranes. J Clin Invest 1977;59:879.

12. Craddock PR, Fehr J, Brigham KL, Kronenberg RS, Jacob HS. Complement and leukocyte-mediated pulmonary dysfunction in hemodialysis. N Engl J Med 1977;296:769.

13. Clark RE, Beauchamp RA, Magrath RA, Brooks JD, Ferguson TB, Weldon CS. Comparison of bubble and membrane oxygenators in short and long perfusions. J Thorac Cardiovasc Surg 1979;78:655.

14. Chen RY, Wicks AE, Chien S. Hemoconcentration induced by surface hypothermia in infants. J Thorac Cardiovasc Surg 1980;80:236.

15. Clark RE, Dietz DR, Miller JG. Continuous detection of microemboli during cardiopulmonary bypass in animals and man. Circulation 1976;54:III74.

16. Clowes GH Jr, Neville WE, Sabga G, Shibota Y. The relationship of oxygen consumption, perfusion rate, and temperature to the acidosis associated with cardiopulmonary circulatory bypass. Surgery 1958;44:220.

17. Cordell AR, Spencer MP, Meredith JH. Studies of peripheral vascular resistance associated with total cardiopulmonary bypass. I. Peripheral resistance under conditions of normothermia and normotension. J Thorac Cardiovasc Surg 1960;40:421.

18. Cleland J, Pluth JR, Tauxe WN, Kirklin JW. Blood volume and body fluid compartment changes soon after closed and open intracardiac surgery. J Thorac Cardiovasc Surg 1966;52:698.

19. Chiu RC, Samson R. Complement (C3, C4) consumption in cardiopulmonary bypass, cardioplegia, and protamine administration. Ann Thorac Surg 1984;37:229.
20. Colman RW. Surfaces in mediated defense reactions: the plasma contact activation system. J Clin Invest 1984;73:1249.
21. Cosgrove DM, Amiot DM, Meserko JJ. An improved technique for autotransfusion of shed mediastinal blood. Ann Thorac Surg 1985;40:519.
22. Cavarocchi NC, Pluth JR, Schaff HV, Orszulak TA, Homburger HA, Solis E, et al. Complement activation during cardiopulmonary bypass. Comparison of bubble and membrane oxygenators. J Thorac Cardiovasc Surg 1986;91:252.
23. Cavarocchi NC, Schaff HV, Orszulak TA, Homburger HA, Schnell WA, Pluth JR. Evidence for complement activation by protamine-heparin interaction after cardiopulmonary bypass. Surgery 1985;98:525.
24. Chiara O, Giomarelli PP, Biagioli B, Rosi R, Gattinoni L. Hypermetabolic response after hypothermic cardiopulmonary bypass. Crit Care Med 1987;15:995.
25. Coselli JS, Crawford ES, Beall AC Jr, Mizrahi EM, Hess KR, Patel VM. Determination of brain temperatures for safe circulatory arrest during cardiovascular operation. Ann Thorac Surg 1988;45:638.
26. Cardoso PF, Yamazaki F, Keshavjee S, Schaefers HF, Hsieh CM, Wang LS, et al. A reevaluation of heparin requirements for cardiopulmonary bypass. J Thorac Cardiovasc Surg 1991;101:153.
27. Cuthbertson DP. The disturbance of metabolism produced by bone and non-bony injury, with notes on certain abnormal conditions of bone. Biochem J 1930;24:1244.
28. Croughwell N, Smith LR, Quill T, Newman M, Greeley W, Kern F, et al. The effect of temperature on cerebral metabolism and blood flow in adults during cardiopulmonary bypass. J Thorac Cardiovasc Surg 1992;103:549.
29. Cook DJ, Oliver WC Jr, Orszulak TA, Daly RC. A prospective, randomized comparison of cerebral venous oxygen saturation during normothermic and hypothermic cardiopulmonary bypass. J Thorac Cardiovasc Surg 1994;107:1020.
30. Casati V, Guzzon D, Oppizzi M, Bellotti F, Franco A, Gerli C, et al. Tranexamic acid compared with high-dose aprotinin in primary elective heart operations: effects on perioperative bleeding and allogeneic transfusions. J Thorac Cardiovasc Surg 2000;120:520.
31. Cosgrove DM 3rd, Sabik JF, Navia JL. Minimally invasive valve operations. Ann Thorac Surg 1998;65:1535.
32. Chitwood WR Jr, Wixon CL, Elbeery JR, Moran JF, Chapman WH, Lust RM. Video-assisted minimally invasive mitral valve surgery. J Thorac Cardiovasc Surg 1997;114:773.
33. Chaney MA, Durazo-Arvizu RA, Fluder EM, Sawicki KJ, Nikolov MP, Blakeman BP, et al. Port-access minimally invasive cardiac surgery increases surgical complexity, increases operating room time, and facilitates early postoperative hospital discharge. Anesthesiology 2000;92:1637.
34. Croughwell ND, Newman MF, Blumenthal JA, White WD, Lewis JB, Frasco PE, et al. Jugular bulb saturation and cognitive dysfunction after cardiopulmonary bypass. Ann Thorac Surg 1994;58:1702.
35. Choi DW. Glutamate neurotoxicity and diseases of the nervous system. Neuron 1988;1:623.
36. Cameron DE, Gardner TJ. Principles of clinical hypothermia. Cardiac surgery: state of the art reviews. 1988;2:13.
37. Cremer J, Martin M, Redl H, Bahrami S, Abraham C, Graeter T, et al. Systemic inflammatory response syndrome after cardiac operations. Ann Thorac Surg 1996;61:1714.

D

1. Drew CE, Keen G, Benazon DB. Profound hypothermia. Lancet 1959;1:745.
2. Dillard DH, Mohri H, Hessel EA II, Anderson HN, Nelson RJ, Crawford EW, et al. Correction of total anomalous pulmonary venous drainage in infancy utilizing deep hypothermia with total circulatory arrest. Circulation 1967;35:I105.

3. Donald DE, Kerr FW. The response of dogs to perfusion and arrest of circulation at near zero cerebral temperatures. J Surg Res 1964;63:243.
4. Dickinson DF, Sambrooks JE. Intellectual performance in children after circulatory arrest with profound hypothermia in infancy. Arch Dis Child 1979;54:1.
5. Dennis C, Spreng DS Jr, Nelson GE, Karlson KE, Nelson RM, Thomas JV, et al. Development of a pump-oxygenator to replace the heart and lungs: an apparatus applicable to human patients and application to one case. Ann Surg 1951;134:709.
6. Donald DE, Harshbarger HG, Hetzel PS, Patrick RT, Wood EH, Kirklin JW. Experiences with a heart-lung bypass (Gibbon type) in the experimental laboratory: preliminary report. Mayo Clin Proc 1955;30:113.
7. Dutton RC, Edmunds LH Jr. Measurement of emboli in extracorporeal perfusion systems. J Thorac Cardiovasc Surg 1973;65:523.
8. DeBakey MD. Simple continuous flow blood transfusion instrument. New Orleans Med Surg J 1934;87:386.
9. Davis FM, Parimelazhagan KN, Harris EA. Thermal balance during cardiopulmonary bypass with moderate hypothermia in man. Br J Anaesth 1977;49:1127.
10. Davies GC, Sobel M, Salzman EW. Elevated plasma fibrinopeptide A and thromboxane B_2 levels during cardiopulmonary bypass. Circulation 1980;61:808.
11. Dutton RC, Edmunds LH Jr, Hutchinson JC, Roe BB. Platelet aggregate emboli produced in patients during cardiopulmonary bypass with membrane and bubble oxygenators and blood filters. J Thorac Cardiovasc Surg 1974;67:258.
12. Dunn J, Kirsh MM, Harness J, Carroll M, Straker J, Sloan H. Hemodynamic, metabolic, and hematologic effects of pulsatile cardiopulmonary bypass. J Thorac Cardiovasc Surg 1974;68:138.
13. Dybdahl B, Wahba A, Lien E, Flow TH, Waage A, Qureshi N, et al. Inflammatory response after open heart surgery. Circulation 2002;105:685.
14. Donald DE, Fellows JL. Relation of temperature, gas tension and hydrostatic pressure to the formation of gas bubbles in extracorporeally oxygenated blood. Surg Forum 1960;10:589.
15. D'Amato HE, Hegnauer AH. Blood volume in the hypothermic dog. Am J Physiol 1953;173:100.
16. Digerness SB, Kirklin JW, Naftel DC, Blackstone EH, Kirklin JK, Samuelson PN. Coronary and systemic vascular resistance during reperfusion after global myocardial ischemia. Ann Thorac Surg 1988;46:447.
17. Durum SK, Schmidt JA, Oppenheim JJ. Interleukin 1: an immunological perspective. Annu Rev Immunol 1985;3:263.
18. Dietrich W, Spath P, Zuhlsdorf M, Dalichau H, Kirchhoff PG, Kuppe H, et al. Anaphylactic reactions to aprotinin reexposure in cardiac surgery: relation to antiaprotinin immunoglobulin G and E antibodies. Anesthesiology 2001;95:64.
19. Dillon PK, Duran WN. Effect of platelet-activating factor on microvascular permselectivity: dose-response relations and pathways of action in the hamster cheek pouch microcirculation. Circ Res 1988;62:732.
20. Dreyer WJ, Smith CW, Entman ML. Neutrophil activation during cardiopulmonary bypass (invited letter). J Thorac Cardiovac Surg 1991;102:318.
21. D'Alecy LG, Lundy EF, Barton KJ, Zelenock GB. Dextrose containing intravenous fluid impairs outcome and increases death after eight minutes of cardiac arrest and resuscitation in dogs. Surgery 1986;100:505.
22. DeLeon S, Ilbawi M, Arcilla R, Cutilletta A, Egel R, Wong A, et al. Choreoathetosis after deep hypothermia without circulatory arrest. Ann Thorac Surg 1990;50:714.
23. Doty DB, DiRusso GB, Doty JR. Full-spectrum cardiac surgery through a minimal incision: mini-sternotomy (lower half) technique. Ann Thorac Surg 1998;65:573.
24. Daggett CW, Lodge AJ, Scarborough JE, Chai PJ, Jaggers J, Ungerleider RM. Modified ultrafiltration versus conventional ultrafiltration: a randomized prospective study in neonatal piglets. J Thorac Cardiovasc Surg 1998;115:336.

25. Davies MG, Hagen PO. Systemic inflammatory response syndrome. Br J Surg 1997;84:920.

E

1. Ergin MA, Griepp EB, Lansman SL, Galla JD, Levy M, Griepp RB. Hypothermic circulatory arrest and other methods of cerebral protection during operations on the thoracic aorta. J Card Surg 1994;9:525.

2. Edmunds LH Jr, Saxena NC, Hillyer P, Wilson TJ. Relationship between platelet count and cardiotomy suction return. Ann Thorac Surg 1978;25:306.

3. Ellison N, Behar M, MacVaugh H 3rd, Marshall BE. Bradykinin, plasma protein fraction and hypotension. Ann Thorac Surg 1980; 29:15.

4. Edmunds LH Jr, Ellison N, Colman RW, Niewiarowski S, Rao AK, Addonizio VP Jr, et al. Platelet function during cardiac operation: comparison of membrane and bubble oxygenators. J Thorac Cardiovasc Surg 1982;83:805.

5. Edmunds LH Jr. Blood platelets and bypass. J Thorac Cardiovasc Surg 1989;97:470.

6. Egan TM, Saunders NR, Luk SC, Cooper JD. Complement-mediated pulmonary edema in sheep. J Surg Res 1988;45:204.

7. Ekroth R, Thompson RJ, Lincoln C, Scallan M, Rossi R, Tsang V. Elective deep hypothermia with total circulatory arrest: changes in plasma creatine kinase BB, blood glucose, and clinical variables. J Thorac Cardiovasc Surg 1989;97:30.

8. England MD, Cavarocchi NC, O'Brien JF, Solis E, Pluth JR, Orszulak TA, et al. Influence of antioxidants (mannitol and allopurinol) on oxygen free radical generation during and after cardiopulmonary bypass. Circulation 1986;74:III134.

9. Edmunds LH, Addonizio VP. Extracorporeal circulation. In Colman RW, Hirsh J, Marder VJ, Salzman EW, eds. Hemostasis and thrombosis, 2nd ed. Philadelphia: JB Lippincott, 1987, p. 901.

10. Edmunds LH Jr, Niewiarowski S, Colman RW. Aprotinin J Thorac Cardiovasc Surg 1991;101:1103 (invited letter).

11. Egerton N, Egerton WS, Kay JH. Neurologic changes following profound hypothermia. Ann Surg 1963;157:366.

12. Ergin MA, Galla JD, Lansman L, Quintana C, Bodian C, Griepp RB. Hypothermic circulatory arrest in operations on the thoracic aorta. Determinants of operative mortality and neurologic outcome. J Thorac Cardiovasc Surg 1994;107:788.

13. Ergin MA, Uysal S, Reich DL, Apaydin A, Lansman SL, McCullough JN, et al. Temporary neurological dysfunction after deep hypothermic circulatory arrest: a clinical marker of long-term functional deficit. Ann Thorac Surg 1999;67:1887.

14. Esposito RA, Culliford AT, Colvin SB, Thomas SJ, Lackner H, Spencer FC. Heparin resistance during cardiopulmonary bypass. The role of heparin pretreatment. J Thorac Cardiovasc Surg 1983;85:346.

15. Elliot MJ. Ultrafiltration and modified ultrafiltration in pediatric open heart operations. Ann Thorac Surg 1993;56:1518.

16. Edmunds LH Jr. Inflammatory response to cardiopulmonary bypass. Ann Thorac Surg 1998;66:S12.

17. Edmunds LH Jr. Blood-surface interactions during cardiopulmonary bypass. J Card Surg 1993;8:404.

F

1. Fuhrman GJ, Fuhrman FA. Oxygen consumption of animals and tissues as a function of temperature. J Gen Physiol 1959;42:715.

2. Fuhrman FA. Oxygen consumption of mammalian tissues at reduced temperatures. In Dripps RD, ed. The physiology of induced hypothermia. Washington, DC: National Academy of Sciences, National Research Council, 1956, p. 50.

3. Field J II, Belding HS, Martin AW. An analysis of the relation between basal metabolism and summated tissue respiration in the rat. I. The post-pubertal albino rat. J Cell Comp Physiol 1939;14:143.

4. Fuhrman FA, Fuhrman GJ, Farr DA, Fail JH. Relationship between tissue respiration and total metabolic rate in hypo- and normothermic rats. Am J Physiol 1961;201:231.

5. Fox LS, Blackstone EH, Kirklin JW, Stewart RW, Samuelson PN. Relationship of whole body oxygen consumption to perfusion flow rate during hypothermic cardiopulmonary bypass. J Thorac Cardiovasc Surg 1982;83:239.

6. Folkerth TL, Angell WW, Fosburg RG, Oury JH. Effect of deep hypothermia, limited cardiopulmonary bypass, and total arrest on growing puppies. In Roy PE, Rona G, eds. Recent advances in studies on cardiac structure and metabolism, Vol 10. Baltimore: University Park, 1975, p. 411.

7. Fisk GC, Wright JS, Turner BB, Baker WC, Hicks RG, Lethlean AK, et al. Cerebral effects of circulatory arrest at 20°C in the infant pig. Anaesth Intens Care 1974;2:33.

8. Fisk GC, Wright JS, Hicks RG, Anderson RM, Turner BB, Baker WC, et al. The influence of duration of circulatory arrest at 20°C on cerebral changes. Anaesth Intens Care 1976;4:126.

9. Frey MV, Gruber M. Untersuchungen über den Stoffwechsel isolierter Organe: Ein Respirations-Apparat für isolierte Organe. Arch F Physiol 1885;9:519.

10. Friedenberg WR, Myers WO, Plotka ED, Beathard JN, Kummer DJ, Gatlin PF, et al. Platelet dysfunction associated with cardiopulmonary bypass. Ann Thorac Surg 1978;25:298.

11. Fritz H, Wunderer G. Biochemistry and applications of aprotinin, the kallikrein inhibitor from bovine organs. Arzneimittelforschung 1983;33:479.

12. Fountain SW, Martin BA, Musclow CE, Cooper JD. Pulmonary leukostasis and its relationship to pulmonary dysfunction in sheep and rabbits. Circ Res 1980;46:175.

13. Friedli B, Kent G, Olley PM. Inactivation of bradykinin in the pulmonary vascular bed of newborn and fetal lambs. Circ Res 1973;33:421.

14. Fox LS, Blackstone EH, Kirklin JW, Bishop SP, Bergdahl LA, Bradley EL. Relationship of brain blood flow and oxygen consumption to perfusion flow rate during profoundly hypothermic cardiopulmonary bypass. J Thorac Cardiovasc Surg 1984;87:658.

15. Furuya H, Suzuki T, Okumura F, Kishi Y, Uefuji T. Detection of air embolism by transesophageal echocardiography. Anesthesiology 1983;58:124.

16. Faymonville ME, Deby-Dupont G, Larbuisson R, Deby C, Bodson L, Limet R, et al. Prostaglandin E₂, prostacyclin, and thromboxane changes during nonpulsatile cardiopulmonary bypass in humans. J Thorac Cardiovac Surg 1986;91:858.

17. Fraedrich G, Weber C, Bernard C, Hettwer A, Schlosser V. Reduction of blood transfusion requirement in open heart surgery by administration of high doses of aprotinin—preliminary results. Thorac Cardiovasc Surg 1989;37:89.

18. Feddersen K, Aren C, Nilsson NJ, Radegran K. Cerebral blood flow and metabolism during cardiopulmonary bypass with special reference to effects of hypotension induced by prostacyclin. Ann Thorac Surg 1986;41:395.

19. Fanning WJ, Vasko JS, Kilman JW. Delayed sternal closure after cardiac surgery. Ann Thorac Surg 1987;44:169.

20. Fried DW, Zombolas TL, Weiss SJ. Single pump mechanically aspirated venous drainage (SPMAVD) for cardiac reoperation. Perfusion 1995;10:327.

21. Fearn SJ, Pole R, Wesnes K, Faragher EB, Hooper TI, McCollum CN. Cerebral injury during cardiopulmonary bypass: emboli impair memory. J Thorac Cardiovasc Surg 2001;121:1150.

22. Fessatidis IT, Thomas VL, Shore DF, Hunt RH, Weller RO, Goodland F, et al. Assessment of neurological injury due to circulatory arrest during profound hypothermia. An experimental study in vertebrates. Eur J Cardiothorac Surg 1993;7:465.

23. Fessatidis IT, Thomas VL, Shore DF, Sedgwick ME, Hunt RH, Weller RO. Brain damage after profoundly hypothermic circulatory arrest: correlations between neurophysiologic and neuropathologic findings. An experimental study in vertebrates. J Thorac Cardiovasc Surg 1993;106:32.

24. Faymonville ME, Pincemail J, Duchateau J, Paulus JM, Adam A, Deby-Dupont G, et al. Myeloperoxidase and elastase as markers of leukocyte activation during cardiopulmonary bypass in humans. J Thorac Cardiovasc Surg 1991;102:309.

25. Finn A, Naik S, Klein N, Levinsky RJ, Strobel S, Elliott M. Interleukin-8 release and neutrophil degranulation after pediatric cardiopulmonary bypass. J Thorac Cardiovasc Surg 1993;105:234.

26. Frering B, Philip I, Dehoux M, Rolland C, Langlois JM, Desmonts JM. Circulating cytokines in patients undergoing normothermic cardiopulmonary bypass. J Thorac Cardiovasc Surg 1994;108:636.

27. Frederiksen JW. Cardiopulmonary bypass in humans: bypassing unfractionated heparin. Ann Thorac Surg 2000;70:1434.

28. Feindt P, Seyfert UT, Volkmer I, Straub U, Gams E. Celite and kaolin produce differing activated clotting times during cardiopulmonary bypass under aprotinin therapy. Thorac Cardiovasc Surg 1994;42:218.

G

1. Guiot G, Rougerie J, Arfel G, Dubost C, Blondeau P. Le "grand froid" en neurochirurgie: possibilités et perspectives d'avenir. Neurochirurgie 1960;6:332.

2. Ginsberg MD, Myers RE. The topography of impaired microvascular perfusion in the primate brain following total circulatory arrest. Neurology 1972;22:998.

3. Gowing NF, Dexter D. The effects of temporary renal ischemia in normal and hypothermic rats. J Pathol 1956;72:519.

4. Gibbon JH Jr. The maintenance of life during experimental occlusion of the pulmonary artery followed by survival. Surg Gynecol Obstet 1939;69:602.

5. Gibbon JH Jr. Application of a mechanical heart and lung apparatus to cardiac surgery. Minn Med 1954;37:171.

6. Griepp EB, Griepp RB. Cerebral consequences of hypothermic circulatory arrest in adults. J Card Surg 1992;7:134.

7. Goldstein IM, Brai M, Osler AG, Weissmann G. Lysosomal enzyme release from human leukocytes: mediation by the alternate pathway of complement activation. J Immunol 1973;111:33.

8. Giron F, Birtwell WC, Soroff HS, Deterling RA Jr. Hemodynamic effects of pulsatile and nonpulsatile flow. Arch Surg 1966;93:802.

9. German JC, Chalmers GS, Hirai J, Mukherjee ND, Wakabayashi A, Connolly JE. Comparison of nonpulsatile and pulsatile extracorporeal circulation on renal tissue perfusion. Chest 1972;61:65.

10. Gall WE, Clarke WR, Doty DB. Vasomotor dynamics associated with cardiac operations. I. Venous tone and the effects of vasodilators. J Thorac Cardiovasc Surg 1982;83:724.

11. Govier AV, Reves JG, McKay RD, Karp RB, Zorn GL, Morawetz RB, et al. Factors and their influence on regional cerebral blood flow during nonpulsatile cardiopulmonary bypass. Ann Thorac Surg 1984;38:592.

12. Greeley WJ, Ungerleider RM, Kern FH, Brusino FG, Smith LR, Reves JG. Effects of cardiopulmonary bypass on cerebral blood flow in neonates, infants, and children. Circulation 1989;80:I209.

13. Greeley WJ, Ungerleider RM, Smith LR, Reves JG. The effects of deep hypothermic cardiopulmonary bypass and total circulatory arrest on cerebral blood flow in infants and children. J Thorac Cardiovasc Surg 1989;97:737.

14. Gluszko P, Rucinski B, Musial J, Wenger RK, Schmaier AH, Colman RW, et al. Fibrinogen receptors in platelet adhesion to surfaces of extracorporeal circuit. Am J Physiol 1987;252:H615.

15. Greeley WJ, Bushman GA, Kong DL, Oldham HN, Peterson MB. Effects of cardiopulmonary bypass on eicosanoid metabolism during pediatric cardiovascular surgery. J Thorac Cardiovasc Surg 1988; 95:842.

16. Gravlee GP, Haddon WS, Rothberger HK, Mills SA, Rogers AT, Bean VE, et al. Heparin dosing and monitoring for cardiopulmonary bypass. J Thorac Cardiovasc Surg 1990;99:518.

17. Greenamyre T, Penney JB, Young AB, Hudson C, Silverstein FS, Johnston MV. Evidence for transient perinatal glutamatergic innervation of globus pallidus. J Neurosci 1987;7:1022.

18. Gillinov AM, Redmond JM, Zehr KJ, Wilson IC, Curtis WE, Bator JM, et al. Inhibition of neutrophil adhesion during cardiopulmonary bypass. Ann Thorac Surg 1994;57:126.

19. Greeley WJ, Kern FH, Ungerleider RM, Boyd JL 3rd, Quill T, Smith LR, et al. The effect of hypothermic cardiopulmonary bypass and total circulatory arrest on cerebral metabolism in neonates, infants, and children. J Thorac Cardiovasc Surg 1991;101:783.

20. Gielchinsky I, Parsonnet V, Krishnan B, Silidker M, Abel RM. Delayed sternal closure following open-heart operation. Ann Thorac Surg 1981;32:273.

21. Griepp RB, Stinson EB, Hollingsworth JF, Buehler D. Prosthetic replacement of the aortic arch. J Thorac Cardiovasc Surg 1975; 70:1051.

22. Gundry SR, Shattuck OH, Razzouk AJ, del Rio MJ, Sardari FF, Bailey LL. Facile minimally invasive cardiac surgery via ministernotomy. Ann Thorac Surg 1998;65:1100.

23. Grossi EA, Zakow PK, Ribakove G, Kallenbach K, Ursomanno P, Gradek CE, et al. Comparison of post-operative pain, stress response, and quality of life in port access vs. standard sternotomy coronary bypass patients. Eur J Cardiothorac Surg 1999;16:S39.

24. Gillinov AM, Banbury MK, Cosgrove DM. Hemisternotomy approach for aortic and mitral valve surgery. J Card Surg 2000;15:15.

25. Gertler JP, Ocasio VH. Endothelin production by hypoxic human endothelium. J Vasc Surg 1993;18:178.

26. Gertler JP, Weibe DA, Ocasio VH, Abbott WM. Hypoxia induces procoagulant activity in cultured human venous endothelium. J Vasc Surg 1991;13:428.

27. Gillinov AM, Sabik JF, Lytle BW, Cosgrove DM. Axillary artery cannulation. J Thorac Cardiovasc Surg 1999;118:1153.

28. Gorman JH 3rd, Edmunds LH Jr. Blood anesthesia for cardiopulmonary bypass. J Card Surg 1995;10:270.

H

1. Horiuchi T, Koyamada K, Matano I, Mohri H, Komatsu T, Honda T, et al. Radical operation for ventricular septal defect in infancy. J Thorac Cardiovasc Surg 1963;46:180.

2. Hikasa Y, Shirotani H, Mori C, Kamiya T, Asawa Y. Open heart surgery in infants with the aid of hypothermic anesthesia. Arch Jpn Chir 1967;36:495.

3. Hamilton DI, Shackleton J, Rees GJ, Abbott T. Experience with deep hypothermia in infancy using core cooling. In Barratt-Boyes BG, Neutze JM, Harris EA, eds. Heart disease in infancy. Baltimore: Williams & Wilkins, 1973, p. 52.

4. Harris EA, Seelye ER, Squire AW. Oxygen consumption during cardiopulmonary bypass with moderate hypothermia in man. Br J Anaesth 1971;43:1113.

5. Harris EA. Metabolic aspects of profound hypothermia. In Barratt-Boyes BG, Neutze JM, Harris EA, eds. Heart disease in infancy. Baltimore: Williams & Wilkins, 1973, p. 65.

6. Harris EA, Seelye ER, Barratt-Boyes BG. Respiratory and metabolic acid-base changes during cardiopulmonary bypass in man. Br J Anesth 1970;42:912.

7. Harden A, Pampiglione G, Waterston DJ. Circulatory arrest during hypothermia in cardiac surgery: an EEG study in children. Br Med J 1966;2:1105.

8. Hallenbeck JM, Bradley ME. Experimental model for systematic study of impaired microvascular reperfusion. Stroke 1977;8:238.

9. Hallenbeck JM. Prevention of postischemic impairment of microvascular perfusion. Neurology 1977;27:3.

10. Haka-Ikse K, Blackwood MJ, Steward DJ. Psychomotor development of infants and children after profound hypothermia during surgery for congenital heart disease. Dev Med Child Neurol 1978;20:62.

11. Huguet C, Nordlinger B, Bloch P, Conard J. Tolerance of the human liver to prolonged normothermic ischemia. Arch Surg 1978;113:1448.

12. Harris EA, Seelye ER, Barratt-Boyes BG. On the availability of oxygen to the body during cardiopulmonary bypass in man. Br J Anesth 1974;46:425.

13. Hallowell P, Austen G, Laver MB. Influence of oxygen flow rate on arterial oxygenation and acid-base balance during cardiopulmonary bypass with use of a disc oxygenator. Circulation 1967;35:119.

14. Hine IP, Wood WG, Mainwaring-Burton RW, Butler MJ, Irving MH, Booker B. The adrenergic response to surgery involving cardiopulmonary bypass, as measured by plasma and urinary catecholamine concentrations. Br J Anaesth 1976;48:355.

15. Han P, Turpie AG, Butt R, LeBlanc P, Genton E, Bunstensen S. The use of β-thromboglobulin release to assess platelet damage during cardiopulmonary bypass. Presented at the Combined Meeting of the Royal Australasian College of Surgeons and Royal Australasian College of Physicians, Sydney, Australia, February 24-29, 1980.

16. Hugli TE. Chemical aspects of the serum anaphylatoxins. Contemp Top Mol Immunol 1978;7:181.

17. Hairston P, Manos JP, Graber CD, Lee WH Jr. Depression of immunologic surveillance by pump-oxygenation perfusion. J Surg Res 1969;9:587.

18. Habal SM, Weiss MB, Spotnitz HM, Parodi EN, Wolff M, Cannon PJ, et al. Effects of pulsatile and nonpulsatile coronary perfusion on performance of the canine left ventricle. J Thorac Cardiovasc Surg 1976;72:742.

19. Holobut W, Modrzejewski E, Stazka W. Irrigation sanguine et consommation d'oxygène de divers organes en tempèrature normale et en hypothermie. J Physiol (Paris) 1969;61:507.

20. Holloway DS, Summaria L, Sandesara J, Vagher JP, Alexander JC, Caprini JA. Decreased platelet number and function and increased fibrinolysis contribute to postoperative bleeding in cardiopulmonary bypass patients. Thromb Haemost 1988;59:62.

21. Hammerschmidt DE, Stroncek DF, Bowers TK, Lammi-Keefe CJ, Kurth DM, Ozalins A, et al. Complement activation and neutropenia occurring during cardiopulmonary bypass. J Thorac Cardiovasc Surg 1981;81:370.

22. Harker LA, Malpass TW, Branson HE, Hessel EA II, Slichter SJ. Mechanism of abnormal bleeding in patients undergoing cardiopulmonary bypass: acquired transient platelet dysfunction associated with selective alpha-granule release. Blood 1980;56:824.

23. Harlan BJ, Kyger ER 3rd, Reul GJ Jr, Cooley DA. Needle suction of the aorta for left heart decompression during aortic cross-clamping. Ann Thorac Surg 1977;23:259.

24. Hope AF, Heyns AD, Lotter MG, van Reenen OR, de Kock F, Badenhorst PN, et al. Kinetics and sites of sequestration of indium 111-labeled human platelets during cardiopulmonary bypass. J Thorac Cardiovasc Surg 1981;81:880.

25. Hennessy VL Jr, Hicks RE, Niewiarowski S, Edmunds LH Jr, Colman RW. Function of human platelets during extracorporeal circulation. Am J Physiol 1977;232:H622.

26. Haeffner-Cavaillon N, Roussellier N, Ponzio O, Carreno MP, Laude M, Carpentier A, et al. Induction of interleukin-1 production in patients undergoing cardiopulmonary bypass. J Thorac Cardiovasc Surg 1989;98:1100.

27. Hind CR, Griffin JF, Pack S, Latchman YE, Drake HF, Jones HM, et al. Effect of cardiopulmonary bypass on circulating concentrations of leucocyte elastase and free radical activity. Cardiovasc Res 1988;22:37.

28. Hickey PR, Buckley MJ, Philbin DM. Pulsatile and nonpulsatile cardiopulmonary bypass: review of a counterproductive controversy. Ann Thorac Surg 1983;36:720.

29. Henriksen L. Brain luxury perfusion during cardiopulmonary bypass in humans. A study of the cerebral blood flow response to changes in CO_2, O_2, and blood pressure. J Cereb Blood Flow Metab 1986;6:366.

30. Henriksen L, Hjelms E. Cerebral blood flow during cardiopulmonary bypass in man: effect of arterial filtration. Thorax 1986;41:386.

31. Henriksen L. Evidence suggestive of diffuse brain damage following cardiac operations. Lancet 1984;1:816.

32. Harder MP, Eijsman L, Roozendaal KJ, van Oeveren W, Wildevuur CR. Aprotinin reduces intraoperative and postoperative blood loss in membrane oxygenator cardiopulmonary bypass. Ann Thorac Surg 1991;51:936.

33. Havel M, Teufelsbauer H, Knobl P, Dalmatiner R, Jaksch P, Zwolfer W, et al. Effect of intraoperative aprotinin administration on postoperative bleeding in patients undergoing cardiopulmonary bypass. J Thorac Cardiovasc Surg 1991;101:968.

34. Hamano K, Kawamura T, Gohra H, Katoh T, Fujimura Y, Zempo N, et al. Stress caused by minimally invasive cardiac surgery versus conventional cardiac surgery: incidence of systemic inflammatory response syndrome. World J Surg 2001;25:117.

35. Hillier SC, Burrows FA, Bissonnette B, Taylor RH. Cerebral hemodynamics in neonates and infants undergoing cardiopulmonary bypass and profound hypothermic circulatory arrest: assessment by transcranial Doppler sonography. Anesth Analg 1991;72:723.

36. Hill GE, Alonso A, Spurzem JR, Stammers AH, Robbins RA. Aprotinin and methylprednisolone equally blunt cardiopulmonary bypass-induced inflammation in humans. J Thorac Cardiovasc Surg 1995;110:1658.

37. Hall RI, Smith MS, Rocker G. The systemic inflammatory response to cardiopulmonary bypass: pathophysiological, therapeutic, and pharmacological considerations. Anesth Analg 1997;85:766.

38. Hornick P, Taylor K. Pulsatile and nonpulsatile perfusion: the continuing controversy. J Cardiothorac Vasc Anesth 1997;11:310.

39. Hennein HA, Ebba H, Rodriguez JL, Merrick SH, Keith FM, Bronstein MH, et al. Relationship of the proinflammatory cytokines to myocardial ischemia and dysfunction after uncomplicated coronary revascularization. J Thorac Cardiovasc Surg 1994;108:626.

40. Hunt BJ, Segal H, Yacoub M. Aprotinin and heparin monitoring during cardiopulmonary bypass. Circulation 1992;86:II410.

J

1. Jones RE, Donald DE, Swan HJ, Harshbarger HG, Kirklin JW, Wood EH. Apparatus of the Gibbon type for mechanical bypass of the heart and lungs: Preliminary report. Mayo Clin Proc 1955;30:105.

2. Jansen NJ, van Oeveren W, van den Broek L, Oudemans-van Straaten HM, Stoutenbeek CP, Joen MC, et al. Inhibition by dexamethasone of the reperfusion phenomena in cardiopulmonary bypass. J Thorac Cardiovasc Surg 1991;102:515.

3. Jacobs LA, Klopp EH, Seamone W, Topaz SR, Gott VL. Improved organ function during cardiac bypass with a roller pump modified to deliver pulsatile flow. J Thorac Cardiovasc Surg 1969;58:703.

4. Javid H, Tufo HM, Najafi H, Dye WS, Hunter JA, Julian OC. Neurological abnormalities following open-heart surgery. J Thorac Cardiovasc Surg 1969;58:502.

5. Jacob HS, Craddock PR, Hammerschmidt DE, Moldow CF. Complement-induced granulocyte aggregation: an unsuspected mechanism of disease. N Engl J Med 1980;302:789.

6. Jogi P, Werner O. Hemodynamic effects of sternum closure after open-heart surgery in infants and children. Scand J Thorac Cardiovasc Surg 1985;19:217.

7. Josa M, Khuri SF, Braunwald NS, VanCisin MF, Spencer MP, Evans DA, et al. Delayed sternal closure. An improved method of dealing with complications after cardiopulmonary bypass. J Thorac Cardiovasc Surg 1986;91:598.

8. Johnsson P, Messeter K, Ryding E, Kugelberg J, Stahl E. Cerebral vasoreactivity to carbon dioxide during cardiopulmonary perfusion at normothermia and hypothermia. Ann Thorac Surg 1989;48:769.

9. Jonas, RA. Optimal pH strategy for hypothermic circulatory arrest. J Thorac Cardiovasc Surg 2001;121:204.

10. Johnson M, Haddix T, Pohlman T, Verrier ED. Hypothermia reversibly inhibits endothelial cell expression of E-selectin and tissue factor. J Card Surg 1995;10:428.

K

1. Kirklin JW, Dawson B, Devloo RA, Theye RA. Open intracardiac operations: use of circulatory arrest during hypothermia induced by blood cooling. Ann Surg 1961;154:769.

2. Kent B, Peirce EC II. Oxygen consumption during cardiopulmonary bypass in the uniformly cooled dog. J Appl Physiol 1974;37:917.

3. Kramer RS, Sanders AP, Lesage AM, Woodhall B, Sealy WC. The effect of profound hypothermia on preservation of cerebral ATP content during circulatory arrest. J Thorac Cardiovasc Surg 1968;56:699.

4. Kirklin JW, DuShane JW, Patrick RT, Donald DE, Hetzel PS, Harshbarger HG, et al. Intracardiac surgery with the aid of a mechanical pump-oxygenator system (Gibbon type): report of eight cases. Mayo Clin Proc 1955;30:201.

5. Kirklin JW, Theye RA. Whole-body perfusion from a pump oxygenator for open intracardiac surgery. In Gibbon JH Jr, ed. Surgery of the chest. Philadelphia: W.B. Saunders, 1962, p. 694.

6. Kalter RD, Saul CM, Wetstein L, Soriano C, Reiss RF. Cardiopulmonary bypass: associated hemostatic abnormalities. J Thorac Cardiovasc Surg 1979;77:427.

7. Kusserow BK, Larrow R, Nichols J. Perfusion- and surface-induced injury in leukocytes. Fed Proc 1971;30:1516.

8. Kusserow BK, Machanic B, Collins FM Jr, Clapp JF 3rd. Changes observed in blood corpuscles after prolonged perfusions with two types of blood pumps. Trans Am Soc Artif Intern Organs 1965;11:122.

9. Kirklin JW. A letter to Helen. J Thorac Cardiovasc Surg 1979;78:643.

10. Kirklin JK, Westaby S, Blackstone EH, Kirklin JW, Chenoweth DE, Pacifico AD. Complement and the damaging effects of cardiopulmonary bypass. J Thorac Cardiovasc Surg 1983;86:845.

11. Kirklin JK, Chenoweth DE, Naftel DC, Blackstone EH, Kirklin JW, Bitran DD, et al. Effects of protamine administration after cardiopulmonary bypass on complement, blood elements, and the hemodynamic state. Ann Thorac Surg 1986;41:193.

12. Kern FH, Ungerleider RM, Quill TJ, Baldwin B, White WD, Greeley WJ, et al. Cerebral blood flow response to changes in arterial carbon dioxide tension during hypothermic cardiopulmonary bypass in children. J Thorac Cardiovasc Surg 1991;101:618.

13. Kunkler A, King H. Comparison of air, oxygen and carbon dioxide embolization. Ann Surg 1959;149:95.

14. Kolobow T, Zapol WM, Sigman RL, Pierce J. Partial cardiopulmonary bypass lasting up to seven days in alert lambs with membrane lung blood oxygenation. J Thorac Cardiovasc Surg 1970;60:781.

15. Kirklin JW. The movement of cardiac surgery toward the very young. In Crupi G, Parenzan L, Anderson RH, eds. Perspectives in pediatric cardiology. Vol 2. Pediatric cardiac surgery, part 1. Mount Kisco, N.Y.: Futura, 1989, p. 3.

16. Kourembanas S, Marsden PA, McQuillan LP, Faller DV. Hypoxia induces endothelin gene expression and secretion in cultured human endothelium. J Clin Invest 1991;88:1054.

17. Kouchoukos NT, Masetti P, Rokkas CK, Murphy SF, Blackstone EH. Safety and efficacy of hypothermic cardiopulmonary bypass and circulatory arrest for operations on the descending thoracic and thoracoabdominal aorta. Ann Thorac Surg 2001;72:699.

18. Kirklin JW. Open-heart surgery at the Mayo Clinic. The 25th anniversary. Mayo Clin Proc 1980;55:339.

19. Kirshbom PM, Skaryak LR, DiBernardo LR, Kern FH, Greeley WJ, Gaynor JW, et al. pH-stat cooling improves cerebral metabolic recovery after circulatory arrest in a piglet model of aortopulmonary collaterals. J Thorac Cardiovasc Surg 1996;111:147.

20. Kalfin RE, Engelman RM, Rousou JA, Flack JE 3rd, Deaton DW, Kreutzer DL, et al. Induction of interleukin-8 expression during cardiopulmonary bypass. Circulation 1993;88:II401.

21. Kaul TK, Swaminathan R, Chatrath RR, Watson DA. Vasoactive pressure hormones during and after cardiopulmonary bypass. Int J Artif Organs 1990;13:293.

L

1. Lewis FJ, Taufic M. Closure of atrial septal defects with the aid of hypothermia: experimental accomplishments and the report of one successful case. Surgery 1953;33:52.

2. Levin MB, Theye RA, Fowler WS, Kirklin JW. Performance of the stationary vertical-screen oxygenator (Mayo-Gibbon). J Thorac Cardiovasc Surg 1960;39:417.

3. Lee WH Jr, Krumhaar D, Fonkalsrud EW, Schjeide OA, Maloney JV Jr. Denaturation of plasma proteins as a cause of morbidity and death after intracardiac operations. Surgery 1961;50:29.

4. Lambert CJ, Marengo-Rowe AJ, Leveson JE, Green RH, Thiele JP, Geisler GF, et al. The treatment of postperfusion bleeding using epsilon-aminocaproic acid, cryoprecipitate, fresh-frozen plasma, and protamine sulfate. Ann Thorac Surg 1979;28:440.

5. Le Deist F, Menasche P, Kucharski C, Bel A, Piwnica A, Bloch G. Hypothermia during cardiopulmonary bypass delays but does not prevent neutrophil-endothelial cell adhesion. A clinical study. Circulation 1995;92:II354.

6. Lowenstein E, Johnston WE, Lappas DG, D'Ambra MN, Schneider RC, Daggett WM, et al. Catastrophic pulmonary vasoconstriction associated with protamine reversal of heparin. Anesthesiology 1983;59:470.

7. Li DM, Mullaly R, Ewer P, Bell B, Eyres RL, Brawn WJ, et al. Effects of vasodilators on rates of change of nasopharyngeal temperature and systemic vascular resistance during cardiopulmonary bypass in anaesthetized dogs. Aust N Z J Surg 1988;58:327.

8. Lillehei CW, Todd DB Jr, Levy MJ, Ellis RJ. Partial cardiopulmonary bypass, hypothermia, and total circulatory arrest: a lifesaving technique for ruptured mycotic aortic aneurysms, ruptured left ventricle, and other complicated cardiac pathology. J Thorac Cardiovasc Surg 1969;58:530.

9. Levi M, Cromheecke ME, de Jonge E, Prins MH, de Mol BJ, Briet E, et al. Pharmacological strategies to decrease excessive blood loss in cardiac surgery: a meta-analysis of clinically relevant endpoints. Lancet 1999;354:1940.

10. Loulmet DF, Carpentier A, Cho PW, Berrebi A, d'Attellis N, Austin CB, et al. Less invasive techniques for mitral valve surgery. J Thorac Cardiovasc Surg 1998;115:772.

11. Laussen PC, Bichell DP, McGowan FX, Zurakowski D, DeMaso DR, del Nido PJ. Postoperative recovery in children after minimum versus full-length sternotomy. Ann Thorac Surg 2000;69:591.

12. Liu J, Sidiropoulos A, Konertz W. Minimally invasive aortic valve replacement (AVR) compared to standard AVR. Eur J Cardiothorac Surg 1999;16:S80.

13. Langley SM, Chai PJ, Miller SE, Mault JR, Jaggers JJ, Tsui SS, et al. Intermittent perfusion protects the brain during deep hypothermic circulatory arrest. Ann Thorac Surg 1999;68:4.

M

1. Martin AW, Fuhrman FA. The relationship between summated tissue respiration and metabolic rate in the mouse and dog. Physiol Zool 1955;28:18.

2. Moffitt EA, Kirklin JW, Theye RA. Physiologic studies during whole body perfusion in tetralogy of Fallot. J Thorac Cardiovasc Surg 1962;44:180.

3. Metz S, Keats AS. Benefits of a glucose-containing priming solution for cardiopulmonary bypass. Anesth Analg 1991;72:428.

4. Martin RR. Alterations in leukocyte structure and function due to mechanical trauma. In Hwang NH, Gross DR, Patel DJ, eds. Quantitative cardiovascular studies: clinical and research applications of engineering principles. Baltimore: University Park, 1979, p. 419.

5. Musial J, Niewiarowski S, Hershock D, Morinelli TA, Colman RW, Edmunds LH Jr. Loss of fibrinogen receptors from the platelet surface during simulated extracorporeal circulation. J Lab Clin Med 1985;105:514.

6. Mayer ED, Welsch M, Tanzeem A, Saggau W, Spath J, Hummels R, et al. Reduction of postoperative donor blood requirement by use of the cell separator. Scand J Thorac Cardiovasc Surg 1985;19:165.

7. Many M, Soroff HS, Birtwell WC, Giron F, Wise H, Deterling RA Jr. The physiologic role of pulsatile and nonpulsatile flow. II. Effects of renal function. Arch Surg 1967;95:762.

8. Maddoux G, Pappas G, Jenkins M, Battock D, Trow R, Smith SC Jr, et al. Effect of pulsatile and nonpulsatile flow during cardiopulmonary bypass on left ventricular ejection fraction early after aortocoronary bypass surgery. Am J Cardiol 1976;37:1000.

9. Mavroudis C. To pulse or not to pulse. Ann Thorac Surg 1978;25:259.

10. McGoon DC, Moffitt EA, Theye RA, Kirklin JW. Physiologic studies during high flow, normothermic, whole body perfusion. J Thorac Cardiovasc Surg 1960;39:275.

11. Molina JE, Einzig S, Mastri AR, Bianco RW, Marks JA, Rasmussen TM, et al. Brain damage in profound hypothermia: perfusion versus circulatory arrest. J Thorac Cardiovasc Surg 1984;87:596.

12. Mills NL, Ochsner JL. Massive air embolism during cardiopulmonary bypass. J Thorac Cardiovasc Surg 1980;80:708.

13. Michenfelder JD, Kirklin JW, Uihlein A, Svien HJ, MacCarty CS. Clinical experience with a closed-chest method of producing profound hypothermia and total circulatory arrest in neurosurgery. Ann Surg 1964;159:125.

14. Murkin JM, Farrar JK, Tweed WA, McKenzie KN, Cuirauden G. Cerebral autoregulation and flow/metabolic coupling during cardiopulmonary bypass: the influence of $PaCO_2$. Anesth Analg 1987;66:825.

15. Magovern GJ Jr, Bolling SF, Casale AS, Bulkley BH, Gardner TJ. The mechanisms of mannitol in reducing ischemic injury: Hyperosmolarity or hydroxyl scavenger? Circulation 1984;70:I91.

16. Marelli D, Paul A, Samson R, Edgell D, Angood P, Chiu R. Does the addition of albumin to the prime solution in cardiopulmonary bypass affect clinical outcome? J Thorac Cardiovasc Surg 1989;98:751.

17. McKnight CK, Elliott MJ, Pearson DT, Holden MP, Alberti KG. The effects of four different crystalloid bypass pump-priming fluids upon the metabolic response to cardiac operation. J Thorac Cardiovasc Surg 1985;90:97.

18. Milne EM, Elliott MJ, Pearson DT, Holden MP, Orskov H, Alberti KG. The effect on intermediary metabolism of open-heart surgery with deep hypothermia and circulatory arrest in infants of less than 10 kilograms body weight. A preliminary study. Perfusion 1986;1:29.

19. Miyamoto K, Kawashima Y, Matsuda H, Okuda A, Maeda S, Hirose H. Optimal perfusion flow rate for the brain during deep hypothermic cardiopulmonary bypass at 20°C. J Thorac Cardiovasc Surg 1986;92:1065.

20. Moore FD Jr, Warner KG, Assousa S, Valeri CR, Khuri SF. The effects of complement activation during cardiopulmonary bypass. Ann Surg 1988;208:95.

21. Moore FD. Metabolic care of the surgical patient. Philadelphia: W.B. Saunders, 1959.

22. Mavroudis C, Brown GL, Katzmark SL, Howe WR, Gray LA Jr. Blood flow distribution in infant pigs subjected to surface cooling, deep hypothermia, and circulatory arrest. J Thorac Cardiovasc Surg 1984;87:665.

23. Martinez MJ, Albus RA, Barry MJ, Bowen TE. Treatment of cardiac compression after cardiopulmonary bypass. Am J Surg 1984;147:400.

24. Murphy DA. Delayed closure of the median sternotomy incision. Ann Thorac Surg 1985;40:76.

25. Moorman RM, Zapol WM, Lowenstein E. Neutralization of heparin anticoagulation. In Gravelee GP, Davis RF, Utley JR, eds. Cardiopulmonary bypass: principles and practice. Baltimore: Williams & Wilkins, 1993, p. 384.

26. Maineri P, Covaia G, Realini M, Caccia G, Ucussich E, Luraschi M, et al. Postoperative bleeding after coronary revascularization. Comparison between tranexamic acid and epsilon-aminocaproic acid. Minerva Cardioangiol 2000;48:155.

27. Munoz JJ, Birkmeyer NJ, Birkmeyer JD, O'Connor GT, Dacey LJ. Is epsilon-aminocaproic acid as effective as aprotinin in reducing bleeding with cardiac surgery?: a meta-analysis. Circulation 1999;99:81.

28. McCullough JN, Zhang N, Reich DL, Juvonen TS, Klein JJ, Spielvogel D, et al. Cerebral metabolic suppression during hypothermic circulatory arrest in humans. Ann Thorac Surg 1999;67:1895.

29. Markewitz A, Lante W, Franke A, Marohl K, Kuhlmann WD, Weinhold C. Alterations of cell-mediated immunity following cardiac operations: clinical implications and open questions. Shock 2001;16:10.

N

1. Norwood WI, Norwood CR, Ingwall JS, Castaneda AR, Fossel ET. Hypothermic circulatory arrest: 31-phosphorus nuclear magnetic resonance of isolated perfused neonatal rat brain. J Thorac Cardiovasc Surg 1979;78:823.

2. Nagaoka H, Katori M. Inhibition of kinin formation by a kallikrein inhibitor during extracorporeal circulation in open-heart surgery. Circulation 1975;52:325.

3. Nakayama K, Tamiya T, Yamamoto K, Izumi T, Akimoto S, Hashizume S, et al. High-amplitude pulsatile pump in extracorporeal circulation with particular reference to hemodynamics. Surgery 1963;54:798.

4. Nieminen MT, Philbin DM, Rosow CE, Lowenstein E, Triantafillou A, Levine FH, et al. Temperature gradients and rewarming time during hypothermic cardiopulmonary bypass with and without pulsatile flow. Ann Thorac Surg 1983;35:488.

5. Nordstrom L, Fletcher R, Pavek K. Shock of anaphylactoid type induced by protamine: a continuous cardiorespiratory record. Acta Anaesth Scand 1978;22:195.

6. Niazi Z, Flodin P, Joyce L, Smith J, Mauer H, Lillehei RC. Effects of glucocorticosteroids in patients undergoing coronary artery bypass surgery. Chest 1979;76:262.

7. Nakamura K, Koga Y, Sekiya R, Onizuka T, Ishii K, Chiyotanda S, et al. The effects of pulsatile and non-pulsatile cardiopulmonary bypass on renal blood flow and function. Jpn J Surg 1989;19:334.

8. Norwood WI, Norwood CR, Castaneda AR. Cerebral anoxia: effect of deep hypothermia and pH. Surgery 1979;86:203.

9. Nuttall GA, Oliver WC, Ereth MH, Santrach PJ, Bryant SC, Orszulak TA, et al. Comparison of blood-conservation strategies in cardiac surgery patients at high risk for bleeding. Anesthesiology 2000;92:674.

10. Newburger JW, Jonas RA, Wernovsky G, Wypij D, Hickey PR, Kuban KC, et al. A comparison of the perioperative neurologic effects of hypothermic circulatory arrest versus low-flow cardiopulmonary bypass in infant heart surgery. N Engl J Med 1993;329:1057.

11. Nichols HT, Morse DP, Hirose T. Coronary and other air embolism occurring during open heart surgery. Prevention by the use of gaseous carbon dioxide. Surgery 1988;43:236.

12. Najman DM, Walenga JM, Fareed J, Pifarre R. Effects of aprotinin on anticoagulant monitoring: implications in cardiovascular surgery. Ann Thorac Surg 1993;55:662.

13. Nadler SB, Hidalgo JU, Bloch T. Prediction of blood volume in normal human adults. Surgery 1961;51:224.

O

1. Olsson Y, Hossmann KA. The effect of intravascular saline perfusion on the sequelae of transient cerebral ischemia. Acta Neuropathol (Berl) 1971;17:68.

2. O'Connor BR, Kussman BD, Park KW. Severe hypercarbia during cardiopulmonary bypass: a complication of CO_2 flooding of the surgical field. Anesth Analg 1998;86:264.

3. Ogata T, Ida Y, Nonoyama A, Takeda J. Sasaki H. A comparative study on the effectiveness of pulsatile and non-pulsatile blood flow in extracorporeal circulation. Nippon Geka Hokan 1960;29:59.

4. Oka Y, Inoue T, Hong Y, Sisto DA, Strom JA, Frater RW. Retained intracardiac air. J Thorac Cardiovasc Surg 1986;91:329.

5. Odim JN, Tchervenkov CI, Dobell AR. Delayed sternal closure: a lifesaving maneuver after early operation for complex congenital heart disease in the neonate. J Thorac Cardiovasc Surg 1989;98:413.

6. Ott DA, Cooley DA, Norman JC, Sandiford FM. Delayed sternal closure: a useful technique to prevent tamponade or compression of the heart. Cardiovasc Dis (Bull Texas Heart Inst) 1978;5:15.

7. Ojito JW, Hannan RL, Miyaji K, White JA, McConaghey TW, Jacobs JP, et al. Assisted venous drainage cardiopulmonary bypass in congenital heart surgery. Ann Thorac Surg 2001;71:1267.

8. Olney JW, Ho OL, Rhee V, DeGubareff T. Neurotoxic effects of glutamate. N Engl J Med 1973;289:1374.

P

1. Penrod KE. Oxygen consumption and cooling rates in immersion hypothermia in the dog. Am J Physiol 1949;157:436.
2. Pappas G, Winter SD, Kopriva CJ, Steele PP. Improvement of myocardial and other vital organ functions and metabolism with a simple method of pulsatile flow (IABP) during clinical cardiopulmonary bypass. Surgery 1975;77:34.
3. Philbin DM, Levine FH, Emerson CW, Buckley MJ, Coggins CH, Moss J, et al. The renin-catecholamine vasopressin response to cardiopulmonary bypass with pulsatile flow (abstract). Circulation 1979;59,60:II34.
4. Patarroyo M, Makgoba MW. Leucocyte adhesion to cells in immune and inflammatory responses. Lancet 1989;2:1139.
5. Parker DJ, Cantrell JW, Karp RB, Stroud RM, Digerness SB. Changes in serum complement and immunoglobulins following cardiopulmonary bypass. Surgery 1972;71:824.
6. Prough DS, Stump DA, Roy RC, Gravlee GP, Williams T, Mills SA, et al. Response of cerebral blood flow to changes in carbon dioxide tension during hypothermic cardiopulmonary bypass. Anesthesiology 1986;64:576.
7. Pang LM, Stalcup SA, Lipset JS, Hayes CJ, Bowman FO Jr, Mellins RB. Increased circulating bradykinin during hypothermia and cardiopulmonary bypass in children. Circulation 1979;60:1503.
8. Paneth M, Sellers R, Gott VL, Weirich WL, Allen P, Read RC, et al. Physiologic studies upon prolonged cardiopulmonary bypass with the pump-oxygenator with particular reference to (1) acid-base balance, (2) siphon canal drainage. J Thorac Surg 1947;34:570.
9. Pacifico AD, Digerness S, Kirklin JW. Acute alterations of body composition after open intracardiac operations. Circulation 1970;41:331.
10. Perkowski SZ, Havill AM, Flynn JT, Gee MH. Role of intrapulmonary release of eicosanoids and superoxide anion as mediators of pulmonary dysfunction and endothelial injury in sheep with intermittent complement activation. Circ Res 1983;53:574.
11. Packham MA, Evans G, Glynn MF, Mustard JF. The effect of plasma proteins on the interaction of platelets with glass surfaces. J Lab Clin Med 1969;73:686.
12. Padayachee TS, Parsons S, Theobold R, Gosling RG, Deverall PB. The effect of arterial filtration on reduction of gaseous microemboli in the middle cerebral artery during cardiopulmonary bypass. Ann Thorac Surg 1988;45:647.
13. Padayachee TS, Parsons S, Theobold R, Linley J, Gosling RG, Deverall PB. The detection of microemboli in the middle cerebral artery during cardiopulmonary bypass: a transcranial Doppler ultrasound investigation using membrane and bubble oxygenators. Ann Thorac Surg 1987;44:298.

Q

1. Quiroga MM, Miyagishima R, Haendschen LC, Glovsky M, Martin BA, Hogg JC. The effect of body temperature on leukocyte kinetics during cardiopulmonary bypass. J Thorac Cardiovasc Surg 1985;90:91.

R

1. Ross DN. Hypothermia. II. Physiological observations during hypothermia. Guys Hosp Rep 1954;103:116.
2. Reilly EL, Brunberg JA, Doty DB. The effect of deep hypothermia and total circulatory arrest on the electroencephalogram in children. Electroencephalogr Clin Neurophysiol 1974;36:661.
3. Rittenhouse EA, Mohri H, Reichenbach DD, Merendino KA. Morphological alterations in vital organs after prolonged cardiac arrest at low body temperature. Ann Thorac Surg 1972;13:564.
4. Rudy LW Jr, Heymann MA, Edmunds LH Jr. Distribution of systemic blood flow during cardiopulmonary bypass. J Appl Physiol 1973;34:194.
5. Reeves RB. Temperature-induced changes in blood acid-base status: pH and P_{CO_2} in a binary buffer. J Appl Physiol 1976;40:752.
6. Reeves RB. Temperature-induced changes in blood acid-base status: donnan rCl and red cell volume. J Appl Physiol 1976;40:762.

7. Rahn H, Reeves RB, Howell BJ. Hydrogen ion regulation, temperature and evolution. Am Rev Respir Dis 1975;112:165.
8. Rogers AT, Prough DS, Stump DA, Gravlee GP, Angert KC, Roy RC, et al. Cerebral blood flow does not change following sodium nitroprusside infusion during hypothermic cardiopulmonary bypass. Anesth Analg 1989;68:122.
9. Ryhanen P, Herva E, Hollmen A, Nuutinen L, Pihlajaniemi R, Saarela E. Changes in peripheral blood leukocyte counts, lymphocyte subpopulations, and in vitro transformation after heart valve replacement. J Thorac Cardiovasc Surg 1979;77:259.
10. Rosomoff HL, Holaday DA. Cerebral blood flow and cerebral oxygen consumption during hypothermia. Am J Physiol 1954;179:85.
11. Reed CC, Romagnoli A, Taylor DE, Clark DK. Particulate matter in bubble oxygenators. J Thorac Cardiovasc Surg 1974;68:971.
12. Reid DJ, Digerness SB, Kirklin JW. Changes in whole body venous tone and distribution of blood after open intracardiac surgery. Am J Cardiol 1968;22:621.
13. Rosenkranz ER, Utley JR, Menninger FJ 3rd, Dembitsky WP, Hargens AR, Peters RM. Interstitial fluid pressure changes during cardiopulmonary bypass. Ann Thorac Surg 1980;30:536.
14. Reves JG, Karp RB, Buttner EE, Tosone S, Smith LR, Samuelson PN, et al. Neuronal and adrenomedullary catecholamine release in response to cardiopulmonary bypass in man. Circulation 1982;66:49.
15. Rebeyka IM, Coles JG, Wilson GJ, Watanabe T, Taylor MJ, Adler SF, et al. The effect of low-flow cardiopulmonary bypass on cerebral function: an experimental and clinical study. Ann Thorac Surg 1987;43:391.
16. Riegel W, Spillner G, Schlosser V, Horl WH. Plasma levels of main granulocyte components during cardiopulmonary bypass. J Thorac Cardiovasc Surg 1988;95:1014.
17. Royston D, Bidstrup BP, Taylor KM, Sapsford RN. Effect of aprotinin on need for blood transfusion after repeat open-heart surgery. Lancet 1987;2:1289.
18. Rodigas PC, Meyer FJ, Haasler GB, Dubroff JM, Spotnitz HM. Intraoperative 2-dimensional echocardiography: ejection of microbubbles from the left ventricle after cardiac surgery. Am J Cardiol 1982;50:1130.
19. Rothman SM, Olney JW. Glutamate and the pathophysiology of hypoxic-ischemic brain damage. Ann Neurol 1986;19:105.
20. Riahi M, Tomatis LA, Schlosser RJ, Bertolozzi E, Johnston DW. Cardiac compression due to closure of the median sternotomy in open heart surgery. Chest 1975;67:113.
21. Reich DL, Uysal S, Sliwinski M, Ergin MA, Kahn RA, Konstadt SN, et al. Neuropsychologic outcome after deep hypothermic circulatory arrest in adults. J Thorac Cardiovasc Surg 1999;117:156.
22. Redmond JM, Gillinov AM, Zehr KJ, Blue ME, Troncoso JC, Reitz BA, et al. Glutamate excitotoxicity: a mechanism of neurologic injury associated with hypothermic circulatory arrest. J Thorac Cardiovasc Surg 1994;107:776.
23. Redmond JM, Gillinov AM, Blue ME, Zehr KJ, Troncoso JC, Cameron DE, et al. The monosialoganglioside, GM1, reduces neurologic injury associated with hypothermic circulatory arrest. Surgery 1993;114:324.
24. Rappaport LA, Wypij D, Bellinger DC, Helmers SL, Holmes GL, Barnes PD, et al. Relation of seizures after cardiac surgery in early infancy to neurodevelopmental outcome. Boston Circulatory Arrest Group. Circulation 1998;97:773.
25. Robicsek F, Daugherty HK, Cook JW. The prevention and treatment of sternum separation following open-heart surgery. J Thorac Cardiovasc Surg 1977;73:267.
26. Rezkalla SH, Kloner RA. No-reflow phenomenon. Circulation 2002;105:656.

S

1. Swan H, Zeavin I, Blount SG Jr, Virtue RW. Surgery by direct vision in the open heart during hypothermia. JAMA 1953;153:1081.

2. Sealy WC, Brown IW Jr, Young WG Jr. A report on the use of both extracorporeal circulation and hypothermia for open heart surgery. Ann Surg 1958;147:603.

3. Shapiro H, Stoner EK. Body temperature and oxygen uptake in man. Ann Phys Med 1966;8:250.

4. Setiey A, Challamel MJ, Champsaur G, Samuel D, Courjon J. Effects of profound hypothermia with circulatory arrest on the intra-operative electroencephalogram of the infant. Rev Electroencephalogr Neurophysiol Clin 1975;5:103.

5. Stewart RW, Blackstone EH, Kirklin JW. Neurological dysfunction after cardiac surgery. In Parenzan L, Crupi G, Graham G, eds. Congenital heart disease in the first three months of life. Medical and surgical aspects. Bologna, Italy: Patron Editore, 1981, p. 431.

6. Shore-Lesserson L, Gravlee GP. Anticoagulation for cardiopulmonary bypass. In Gravlee GP, Davis RF, Kurusz M, Utley JR, eds. Cardiopulmonary bypass. Philadelphia: Lippincott Williams & Wilkins, 2000, p. 436.

7. Stevenson JG, Stone EF, Dillard DH, Morgan BC. Intellectual development of children subjected to prolonged circulatory arrest during hypothermic open heart surgery in infancy. Circulation 1974;50:II54.

8. Sellke FW, Boyle EM Jr, Verrier ED. Endothelial cell injury in cardiovascular surgery: the pathophysiology of vasomotor dysfunction. Ann Thorac Surg 1996;62:1222.

9. Senning A. Ventricular fibrillation during extracorporeal circulation: used as a method to prevent air-embolisms and to facilitate intracardiac operations. Acta Chir Scand 1952;171:1.

10. Shepard RB. Whole body oxygen consumption during hypoxic hypoxemia and cardiopulmonary bypass circulation. In Proceedings of the Tenth International Symposium on Space Technology and Science, Tokyo, 1973, p. 1307.

11. Swan H. Thermoregulation and bioenergetics: patterns for vertebrate survival. New York: Elsevier, 1974, p. 183.

12. Solen KA, Whiffen JD, Lightfoot EN. The effect of shear, specific surface, and air interface on the development of blood emboli and hemolysis. J Biomed Mater Res 1978;12:381.

13. Salzman EW, Merrill EW, Binder A, Wolf CF, Ashford TP, Austen WG. Protein-platelet interaction on heparinized surfaces. J Biomed Mater Res 1969;3:69.

14. Singh RK, Barratt-Boyes BG, Harris EA. Does pulsatile flow improve perfusion during hypothermic cardiopulmonary bypass? J Thorac Cardiovasc Surg 1980;79:827.

15. Sink JD, Chitwood WR Jr, Hill RC, Wechsler AS. Comparison of nonpulsatile and pulsatile extracorporeal circulation on renal cortical blood flow. Ann Thorac Surg 1980;29:57.

16. Shepard RB, Simpson DC, Sharp JF. Energy equivalent pressure. Arch Surg 1966;93:730.

17. Swan H, Sanchez M, Tyndall M, Koch C. Quality control of perfusion: monitoring venous blood oxygen to prevent hypoxic acidosis. J Thorac Cardiovasc Surg 1990;99:868.

18. Smith EE, Naftel DC, Blackstone EH, Kirklin JW. Microvascular permeability after cardiopulmonary bypass. An experimental study. J Thorac Cardiovasc Surg 1987;94:225.

19. Siemkowicz E, Gjedde A. Post-ischemic coma in the rat: effect of different pre-ischemic blood glucose levels on cerebral metabolic recovery after ischemia. Acta Physiol Scand 1980;110:225.

20. Stockard JJ, Bickford RG, Schauble JF. Pressure-dependent cerebral ischemia during cardiopulmonary bypass. Neurology 1973;23:521.

21. Stockard JJ, Bickford RG, Myers RR, Aung MH, Dilley RB, Schauble JF. Hypotension-induced changes in cerebral function during cardiac surgery. Stroke 1974;5:730.

22. Salama A, Hugo F, Heinrich D, Hoge R, Muller R, Kiefel V, et al. Deposition of terminal C5b-9 complement complexes on erythrocytes and leukocytes during cardiopulmonary bypass. N Engl J Med 1988;318:408.

23. Simpson PJ, Todd RF 3rd, Fantone JC, Mickelson JK, Griffin JD, Lucchesi BR. Reduction of experimental canine myocardial reperfusion injury by a monoclonal antibody (anti-Mo1, anti-CD11b) that inhibits leukocyte adhesion. J Clin Invest 1988;81:624.

24. Soma Y, Hirotani T, Yozu R, Onoguchi K, Misumi T, Kawada K, et al. A clinical study of cerebral circulation during extracorporeal circulation. J Thorac Cardiovasc Surg 1989;97:187.

25. Stibbe J, Kluft C, Brommer EJ, Gomes M, de Jong DS, Nauta J. Enhanced fibrinolytic activity during cardiopulmonary bypass in open-heart surgery in man is caused by extrinsic (tissue-type) plasminogen activator. Eur J Clin Invest 1984;14:375.

26. Spotnitz HM. Two-dimensional ultrasound and cardiac operations. J Thorac Cardiovasc Surg 1982;83:43.

27. Starr A. Oxygen consumption during cardiopulmonary bypass. J Thorac Cardiovasc Surg 1959;38:46.

28. Swain JA, McDonald TJ Jr, Griffith PK, Balaban RS, Clark RE, Ceckler T. Low-flow hypothermic cardiopulmonary bypass protects the brain. J Thorac Cardiovasc Surg 1991;102:76.

29. Sellman M, Hindmarsh T, Ivert T, Semb BK. Magnetic resonance imaging of the brain before and after open heart operations. Ann Thorac Surg 1992;53:807.

30. Szwerc MF, Benckart DH, Wiechmann RJ, Savage EB, Szydlowski GW, Magovern GJ Jr, et al. Partial versus full sternotomy for aortic valve replacement. Ann Thorac Surg 1999;68:2209.

31. Spiess BD. Ischemia—a coagulation problem? J Cardiovasc Pharmacol 1996;27:S38.

32. Stecker MM, Cheung AT, Pochettino A, Kent GP, Patterson T, Weiss SJ, et al. Deep hypothermic circulatory arrest: I. Effects of cooling on electroencephalogram and evoked potentials. Ann Thorac Surg 2001;71:14.

33. Stecker MM, Cheung AT, Pochettino A, Kent GP, Patterson T, Weiss SJ, et al. Deep hypothermic circulatory arrest: II. Changes in electroencephalogram and evoked potentials during rewarming. Ann Thorac Surg 2001;71:22.

34. Staples MH, Dunton RF, Karlson KJ, Leonardi HK, Berger RL. Heparin resistance after preoperative heparin therapy or intraaortic balloon pumping. Ann Thorac Surg 1994;57:1211.

35. Semb AG, Forsdahl K, Vaage J. Granulocyte and eicosanoid gradients across the coronary circulation during myocardial reperfusion in cardiac surgery. Eur J Cardiothorac Surg. 1990;4:543.

36. Sabik JF, Lytle BW, McCarthy PM, Cosgrove DM. Axillary artery: an alternative site of arterial cannulation for patients with extensive aortic and peripheral vascular disease. J Thorac Cardiovasc Surg 1995;109:885.

T

1. Theye RA, Kirklin JW. Vertical film oxygenator performance at 30°C and oxygen levels during rewarming. Surgery 1963;54:569.

2. Theye RA, Kirklin JW, Fowler WS. Performance and film volume of sheet and screen vertical-film oxygenators. J Thorac Cardiovasc Surg 1962;43:481.

3. Theye RA, Donald DE, Jones RE. The effect of geometry and filming surface on the priming volume of the vertical-film oxygenator. J Thorac Surg 1962;43:473.

4. Turley K, Roizen M, Vlahakes GJ, Graham B, Ebert PA. Catecholamine response to deep hypothermia and total circulatory arrest in the infant lamb. Circulation 1980;62:I175.

5. Tan CK, Glisson SN, El-Etr AA, Ramakrishnaiah KB. Levels of circulating norepinephrine and epinephrine before, during, and after cardiopulmonary bypass in man. J Thorac Cardiovasc Surg 1976;71:928.

6. Tamari Y, Aledort L, Puszkin E, Degnan TJ, Wagner N, Kaplitt MJ, et al. Functional changes in platelets during extracorporeal circulation. Ann Thorac Surg 1975;19:639.

7. Ts'ao C, Lin CY, Glagov S, Replogle RL. Disseminated leukocyte injury during open-heart surgery. Arch Pathol 1973;95:357.

8. Taylor KM, Bain WH, Maxted KJ, Hutton MM, McNab WY, Caves PK. Comparative studies of pulsatile and nonpulsatile flow during cardiopulmonary bypass. I. Pulsatile system employed and its hematologic effects. J Thorac Cardiovasc Surg 1978;75:569.

9. Trinkle JK, Helton NE, Wood RE, Bryant LR. Metabolic comparison of a new pulsatile pump and a roller pump for cardiopulmonary bypass. J Thorac Cardiovasc Surg 1969;58:562.

10. Trinkle JK, Helton NE, Bryant LR, Griffen WO. Pulsatile cardiopulmonary bypass: clinical evaluation. Surgery 1970;68:1074.

11. Taylor KM, Wright GS, Reid JM, Bain WH, Caves PK, Walker MS, et al. Comparative studies of pulsatile and nonpulsatile flow during cardiopulmonary bypass. II. The effects on adrenal secretion of cortisol. J Thorac Cardiovasc Surg 1978;75:574.

12. Taylor KM, Wright GS, Bain WH, Caves PK, Beastall GS. Comparative studies of pulsatile and nonpulsatile flow during cardiopulmonary bypass. III. Response of anterior pituitary gland to thyrotropin-releasing hormone. J Thorac Cardiovasc Surg 1978;75:579.

13. Turina M, Housman LB, Intaglietta M, Schauble J, Braunwald NS. An automatic cardiopulmonary bypass unit for use in infants. J Thorac Cardiovasc Surg 1972;63:263.

14. Taylor KM, Jones JV, Walker MS, Rao S, Bain WH. The cortisol response during heart-lung bypass. Circulation 1976;54:20.

15. Treasure T, Naftel DC, Conger KA, Garcia JH, Kirklin JW, Blackstone EH. The effect of hypothermic circulatory arrest time on cerebral function, morphology, and biochemistry. J Thorac Cardiovasc Surg 1983;86:761.

16. Tamiya T, Maeo Y, Okada T, Ogoshi S, Fujimoto S, Yasui H. Significance of the concentrated red cells and albumin priming method with particular reference to anaphylatoxin generation. J Thorac Cardiovasc Surg 1992;103:78.

17. Tanaka J, Shiki K, Asou T, Yasui H, Tokunaga K. Cerebral autoregulation during deep hypothermic nonpulsatile cardiopulmonary bypass with selective cerebral perfusion in dogs. J Thorac Cardiovasc Surg 1988;95:124.

18. Tennenberg SD, Bailey WW, Cotta LA, Brodt JK, Solomkin JS. The effects of methylprednisolone on complement-mediated neutrophil activation during cardiopulmonary bypass. Surgery 1986;100:134.

19. Taggart DP, Fraser WD, Borland WW, Shenkin A, Wheatley DJ. Hypothermia and the stress response to cardiopulmonary bypass. Eur J Cardiothorac Surg 1989;3:359.

20. Topol EJ, Humphrey LS, Borkon AM, Baumgartner WA, Dorsey DL, Reitz BA, et al. Value of intraoperative left ventricular microbubbles detected by transesophageal two-dimensional echocardiography in predicting neurologic outcome after cardiac operations. Am J Cardiol 1985;56:773.

21. Tulla H, Takala J, Alhava E, Huttunen H, Kari A. Hypermetabolism after coronary artery bypass. J Thorac Cardiovasc Surg 1991;101:598.

22. Tonz M, Mihaljevic T, von Segesser LK, Schmid ER, Joller-Jemelka HI, Pei P, et al. Normothermia versus hypothermia during cardiopulmonary bypass: a randomized, controlled trial. Ann Thorac Surg 1995;59:137.

23. Toomasian JM, McCarthy JP. Total extrathoracic cardiopulmonary support with kinetic assisted venous drainage: experience in 50 patients. Perfusion 1998;13:137.

24. Taggart DP, Sundaram S, McCartney C, Bowman A, McIntyre H, Courtney JM, et al. Endotoxemia, complement, and white blood cell activation in surgery: a randomized trial of laxatives and pulsatile perfusion. Ann Thorac Surg 1994;57:376.

25. Thompson LD, McElhinney DB, Findlay P, Miller-Hance W, Chen MJ, Minami M, et al. A prospective randomized study comparing volume-standardized modified and conventional ultrafiltration in pediatric cardiac surgery. J Thorac Cardiovasc Surg. 2001;122:220.

26. Taylor KM. Honored Guest's Address. A practical affair. J Thorac Cardiovascular Surg 1999;118:394.

27. Taylor KM. SIRS—the systemic inflammatory response syndrome after cardiac operations. Ann Thorac Surg 1996;61:1607.

U

1. Ugorji CC, Turner SA, McGee MG, Fuhrman TM, Cooley DA, Norman JC. Transascending aortic intraaortic balloon insertion with delayed sternal closure: A retrospective analysis. Cardiovasc Dis (Bull Texas Heart Inst) 1980;7:307.

2. Uozumi T, Manabe H, Kawashima Y, Hamanaka Y, Monden Y. Plasma cortisol, corticosterone and non-protein-bound cortisol in extra-corporeal circulation. Acta Endocrinol (Copenh) 1972;69:517.

V

1. Vander Salm TJ, Ansell JE, Okike ON, Marsicano TH, Lew R, Stephenson WP, et al. The role of epsilon-aminocaproic acid in reducing bleeding after cardiac operation: a double-blind randomized study. J Thorac Cardiovasc Surg 1988;95:538.

2. Vogt MT, Farber E. On the molecular pathology of ischemic renal cell death. Reversible and irreversible cellular and mitochondrial metabolic alterations. Am J Pathol 1968;53:1.

3. Venn GE, Sherry K, Klinger L, Newman S, Treasure T, Harrison M, et al. Cerebral blood flow during cardiopulmonary bypass. Eur J Cardiothorac Surg 1988;2:360.

4. Videm V, Mollnes TE, Garred P, Svennevig JL. Biocompatibility of extracorporeal circulation. In vitro comparison of heparin-coated and uncoated oxygenator circuits. J Thorac Cardiovasc Surg 1991;101:654.

5. Venugopal P, Olszowka J, Wagner H, Vlad P, Lambert E, Subramanian S. Early correction of congenital heart disease with surface-induced deep hypothermia and circulatory arrest. J Thorac Cardiovasc Surg 1973;66:375.

6. van der Linden J, Casimir-Ahn H. When do cerebral emboli appear during open heart operations? A transcranial Doppler study. Ann Thorac Surg 1991;51:237.

7. Videm V, Svennevig JL, Fosse E, Semb G, Osterud A, Mollnes TE. Reduced complement activation with heparin-coated oxygenator and tubings in coronary bypass operations. J Thorac Cardiovasc Surg 1992;103:806.

8. van der Linden J, Wesslen O, Eckroth R, Tyden H, von Ahn H. Transcranial Doppler-estimated versus thermodilution-estimated cerebral blood flow during cardiac operations. Influence of temperature and arterial carbon dioxide tension. J Thorac Cardiovasc Surg 1991;102:95.

9. van der Linden J, Priddy R, Eckroth R, Lincoln C, Pugsley W, Scallan M, et al. Cerebral perfusion and metabolism during profound hypothermia in children. A study of middle cerebral artery ultrasonic variables and cerebral extraction of oxygen. J Thorac Cardiovasc Surg 1991;102:103.

10. Vander Salm TJ, Kaur S, Lancey RA, Okike ON, Pezzella AT, Stahl RF, et al. Reduction of bleeding after heart operations through the prophylactic use of epsilon-aminocaproic acid. J Thorac Cardiovasc Surg 1996;112:1098.

11. Verrier ED, Boyle EM Jr. Endothelial cell injury in cardiovascular surgery. Ann Thorac Surg 1996;62:915.

12. Viinamaki O, Nuutinen L, Hanhela R, Karinen J, Pekkarinen A, Hirvonen J. Plasma vasopressin levels during and after cardiopulmonary bypass in man. Med Biol 1986;64:289.

13. van Oeveren W, Jansen NJ, Bidstrup BP, Royston D, Westaby S, Neuhof H, et al. Effects of aprotinin on hemostatic mechanisms during cardiopulmonary bypass. Ann Thorac Surg 1987;44:640.

14. van Oeveren W, Eijsman L, Roozendaal KJ, Wildevuur CR. Platelet preservation by aprotinin during cardiopulmonary bypass. Lancet 1988;1:644.

15. van Oeveren W, Kazatchkine MD, Descamps-Latscha B, Maillet F, Fischer E, Carpentier A, et al. Deleterious effects of cardiopulmonary bypass. A prospective study of bubble versus membrane oxygenation. J Thorac Cardiovasc Surg 1985;89:888.

W

1. Weiss M, Piwnica A, Lenfant C, Sprovieri L, Laurent D, Blondeau P, et al. Deep hypothermia with total circulatory arrest. Trans Am Soc Artif Intern Organs 1960;6:227.

2. Wakusawa R, Shibata S, Saito H, Chiba T, Hosoi N, Sasaki T, et al. Clinical experience in 525 cases of open-heart surgery under simple profound hypothermia. Jpn J Anesth 1968;18:240.

3. Wolin LR, Massopust LC Jr, White RJ. Behavioral effects of autocerebral perfusion, hypothermia and arrest of cerebral blood flow in the rhesus monkey. Exp Neurol 1973;39:336.

4. Weiss M, Weiss J, Cotton J, Nicolas F, Binet JP. A study of the electroencephalogram during surgery with deep hypothermia and circulatory arrest in infants. J Thorac Cardiovasc Surg 1975;70:316.

5. Wu W, Zbuzek VK, Bellevue C. Vasopressin release during cardiac operation. J Thorac Cardiovasc Surg 1980;79:83.

6. Ward JP. Determination of the optimum temperature for regional renal hypothermia during temporary renal ischaemia. Br J Urol 1975;47:17.

7. Warden HE, Cohen M, Read RC, Lillehei CW. Controlled cross circulation for open intracardiac surgery. J Thorac Surg 1954;28:331.

8. Wallach R, Karp RB, Reves JG, Oparil S, Smith LR, James TN. Pathogenesis of paroxysmal hypertension developing during and after coronary artery bypass surgery: a study of hemodynamic and humoral factors. Am J Cardiol 1980;46:559.

9. Wolk LA, Wilson RF, Burdick M, Selik N, Brown J, Starricco A, et al. Changes in antithrombin, antiplasmin, and plasminogen during and after cardiopulmonary bypass. Am Surg 1985;51:309.

10. Wilson JW. Pulmonary morphologic changes due to extracorporeal circulation: a model for "the shock lung" at cellular level in humans. In Forscher BK, Lillehei RC, Stubbs SS, eds. Shock in low- and high-flow states: proceedings of a symposium at Brook Lodge, Augusta, Michigan. Amsterdam: Excerpta Medica, 1972, p. 160.

11. Wilkens H, Regelson W, Hoffmeister FS. The physiologic importance of pulsatile blood flow. N Engl J Med 1962;267:443.

12. Wesolowski SA, Sauvage LR, Pinc RD. Extracorporeal circulation: the role of the pulse in maintenance of the systemic circulation during heart-lung bypass. Surgery 1955;37:663.

13. Wright G, Sanderson JM. Brain damage and mortality in dogs following pulsatile and non-pulsatile blood flows in extracorporeal circulation. Thorax 1972;27:738.

14. Williams GD, Seifen AB, Lawson NW, Norton JB, Readinger RI, Dungan TW, et al. Pulsatile perfusion versus conventional high-flow nonpulsatile perfusion for rapid core cooling and rewarming of infants for circulatory arrest in cardiac operation. J Thorac Cardiovasc Surg 1979;78:667.

15. Waldo AL, MacLean WA. Diagnosis and treatment of cardiac arrhythmias following open heart surgery: emphasis on the use of atrial and ventricular epicardial wire electrodes. Mount Kisco, N.Y.: Futura, 1980.

16. Wells FC, Coghill S, Caplan HL, Lincoln C. Duration of circulatory arrest does influence the psychological development of children after cardiac operation in early life. J Thorac Cardiovasc Surg 1983;86:823.

17. Wachtogel YT, Musial J, Jenkin B, Niewiarowski S, Edmunds LH Jr, Colman RW. Loss of platelet alpha 2-adrenergic receptors during simulated extracorporeal circulation: prevention with prostaglandin E1. J Lab Clin Med 1985;105:601.

18. Wenger RK, Lukasiewicz H, Mikuta BS, Niewiarowski S, Edmunds LH Jr. Loss of platelet fibrinogen receptors during clinical cardiopulmonary bypass. J Thorac Cardiovasc Surg 1989;97:235.

19. Wilson GJ, Rebeyka IM, Coles JG, Desrosiers AJ, Dasmahapatra HK, Adler S, et al. Loss of the somatosensory evoked response as an indicator of reversible cerebral ischemia during hypothermic, low-flow cardiopulmonary bypass. Ann Thorac Surg 1988;45:206.

20. Wildevuur CR, Eijsman L, Roozendaal KJ, Harder MP, Chang M, van Oeveren W. Platelet preservation during cardiopulmonary bypass with aprotinin. Eur J Cardiothorac Surg 1989;3:533.

21. Wragg RE, Dimsdale JE, Moser KM, Daily PO, Dembitsky WP, Archibald C. Operative predictors of delirium after pulmonary thromboendarterectomy. J Thorac Cardiovasc Surg 1988;96:524.

22. Wilmore DW. Homeostasis: bodily changes in trauma and surgery. In Sabiston DC, ed. Textbook of surgery, 13th ed. Philadelphia: W.B. Saunders, 1986, p. 23.

23. Wenger RK, Bavaria JE, Ratcliffe MB, Bogen D, Edmunds LH Jr. Flow dynamics of peripheral venous catheters during extracorporeal membrane oxygenation with a centrifugal pump. J Thorac Cardiovasc Surg 1988;96:478.

24. Wong BI, McLean RF, Fremes SE, Deemar KA, Harrington EM, Christakis GT, et al. Aprotinin and tranexamic acid for high transfusion risk cardiac surgery. Ann Thorac Surg 2000;69:808.

25. Wong PC, Barlow CF, Hickey PR, Jonas RA, Castaneda AR, Farrell DM, et al. Factors associated with choreoathetosis after cardiopulmonary bypass in children with congenital heart disease. Circulation 1992;86:II118.

26. Walther T, Falk V, Metz S, Diegeler A, Battelini R, Autschbach R, Mohr FW. Pain and quality of life after minimally invasive versus conventional cardiac surgery. Ann Thorac Surg 1999;67:1643.

27. Wang JS, Lin CY, Hung WT, Thisted RA, Karp RB. In vitro effects of aprotinin on activated clotting time measured with different activators. J Thorac Cardiovasc Surg 1992;104:1135.

28. Wang JS, Lin CY, Hung WT, Karp RB. Monitoring of heparin-induced anticoagulation with kaolin-activated clotting time in cardiac surgical patients treated with aprotinin. Anesthesiology 1992;77:1080.

Y

1. Yancey PH, Somero GN. Temperature dependence of intracellular pH: Its role in the conservation of pyruvate apparent Km values of vertebrate lactate dehydrogenases. J Comp Physiol 1978;125:129.

Z

1. Zingg W, Kantor S. Observations on the temperatures in the brain during extracorporeal differential hypothermia. Surg Forum 1960; 11:192.

2. Zilla P, Fasol R, Groscurth P, Klepetko W, Reichenspurner H, Wolner E. Blood platelets in cardiopulmonary bypass operations. Recovery occurs after initial simulation, rather than continual activation. J Thorac Cardiovasc Surg 1989;97:379.

3. Zilla P. Reply to: Blood platelets and bypass. J Thorac Cardiovasc Surg 1989;98:797.

4. Zhang JX, Wolf MB. Effect of cold on ischemia-reperfusion-induced microvascular permeability increase in cat skeletal muscle. Cryobiology 1994;31:94.

Myocardial Management during Cardiac Surgery with Cardiopulmonary Bypass

To whatever extent possible, injury to the myocardium must be avoided during operations utilizing cardiopulmonary bypass (CPB). During these operations, alterations of myocardial blood flow and oxygen demand are often imposed that, unmodified, might injure cellular energetics and morphology. We have chosen to call the following general discussion one of *management* rather than *protection* of the myocardium. Most efforts at management will result in protection of function. However, some techniques at times result in injury; at other times perhaps one or another technique may improve myocardial function. Almost all the techniques of myocardial management introduced in the past are in use today by one or more surgical groups, and at this time there is little secure evidence that one method is superior to another, or that the same method is optimal under all circumstances.[F14] This chapter is written, nonetheless, with the bias that few if any methods currently available perfectly protect the heart from the damaging effects of an appreciable period of global myocardial ischemia, but that such a method may evolve with additional knowledge. Emphasis is given to methods that are currently satisfactory.

HISTORICAL NOTE

In the early years of cardiac surgery, little mention was made of the possibility that fatal or nonfatal low cardiac output in the early postoperative period was related to damaging effects of the cardiac operation itself. Indeed, in two reviews of complications of open heart operations published in 1965[W1] and 1966,[R1] early postoperative low cardiac output was discussed extensively, but no mention was made of myocardial necrosis as a complication of the surgery or as a cause of low cardiac output, nor of temporary depression of myocardial function (stunning) as a result of the operation itself. Then, in 1967, Taber, Morales, and Fine described scattered small areas of myocardial necrosis, estimated to involve about 30% of the left ventricular myocardium, in a group of patients dying early after cardiac operations, and implicated this as the etiology of the patients' low cardiac output.[T1] Najafi and colleagues showed in 1969 that acute diffuse subendocardial myocardial infarction was found frequently in patients who died early after valve replacement; these investigators suggested that this was related to methods of intraoperative management of the myocardium.[H1,N1] They discussed the possibility that disturbances of the myocardial oxygen supply–demand ratios might be implicated, and that proper perfusion of the subendocardial layer of the myocardium was a particular problem during CPB.

When coronary artery bypass grafting began during the early 1970s, cardiologists and cardiac surgeons soon noted that a disturbingly high proportion of surgical patients developed a transmural myocardial infarction perioperatively (immediately before, during, or within 24 hours of operation).[A1,B1] Although first widely publicized in connection with coronary artery bypass grafting, the development of transmural myocardial infarction was soon shown to be a complication of cardiac surgery in general. In 1973, in a consecutive series of patients with normal coronary arteries who had undergone various open cardiac operations, Hultgren and colleagues documented a 7% occurrence of acute transmural myocardial infarction.[H2] These investigators recognized that "there is clearly an urgent need to further improve the protection of the heart during [cardiac] surgery." Various autopsy studies have confirmed that acute transmural myocardial infarction, as well as scattered myocardial necrosis and confluent subendocardial necrosis, can occur after cardiac surgery despite the presence of normal coronary arteries.[R2] The rarely occurring extreme manifestation of ischemic damage, "stone heart,"[C1] was recognized at about that time and has been confirmed to be essentially a massive myocardial infarction developing during reperfusion.[K1,L1]

Development of knowledge in this area was facilitated by improved methods of identifying myocardial necrosis during life and, to some degree at least, quantifying its extent. Electrocardiographic criteria for diagnosing transmural myocardial infarction and ischemic changes were clarified[R3] and applied to postoperative patients. Appearance of cardiac-specific enzymes in plasma was shown to correlate well with other evidence of myocardial necrosis,[D1,O1,R4] and their concentrations shown to correlate directly with the amount of muscle that had become necrotic, as judged by other criteria.[G1,K2,K9] Recently, isoforms of troponin I and T have been demonstrated to be sensitive and somewhat specific serum markers of myocardial injury following CPB.[C17,M27,T10] Koh and colleagues have shown that serum levels of troponin were related to duration of ischemic time during cardioplegia, and elevated serum levels were associated with the occurrence of delayed post-clamp recovery of ventricular function.[K17] Radionuclide imaging was also used to identify the presence and extent of perioperative myocardial infarctions.[R5,R6]

With these methods, a number of clinical studies have supported the finding of autopsy studies that myocardial necrosis is an important and frequent complication of conventional cardiac surgery. In 1974, the frequency of myocardial necrosis in patients convalescing well was demonstrated in a study of isolated aortic valve replacement.[S1] Although hospital mortality was low (2%), 15% of the patients developed electrocardiographic evidence of transmural myocardial infarction, and 70% developed isoenzymatic evidence of myocardial necrosis. In 1974, it was shown that even after the short and simple operation for repair of an uncomplicated atrial septal defect, 12 (92%) of 13 adult patients and all 6 children developed isoenzymatic evidence of myocardial necrosis. Myocardial necrosis was demonstrated by enzymatic methods in children undergoing surgery for a number of different congenital cardiac defects.[N2]

In 1975, data were collected that indicated that early postoperative cardiac output was inversely proportional to the extent of myocardial necrosis (Fig. 3-1) and, thus, that the amount of myocardial necrosis was a determinant of the early postoperative condition of the patient and of the probability of survival[R7] (Fig. 3-2). Subsequently, it became clear that *myocardial stunning* also occurs after cardiac surgery, as well as after regional myocardial ischemia from coronary artery disease.[B24] This also results in a period of low cardiac output of variable duration, albeit without myocardial necrosis in some patients.

It is difficult to identify the individual who first thought about special methods of myocardial management to protect the heart itself from damage during operations. Probably the first special method was retrograde coronary perfusion for surgery on the aortic valve, reported by Lillehei and colleagues in 1956,[L18] and subsequently by Gott and colleagues.[G10] "Elective cardiac arrest" was advocated by Melrose in 1955,[M9] and its use at that time by Cleland in London was for intracardiac exposure, not myocardial management. The first deliberate attempts to protect the myocardium other than by simply perfusing it may have been made by Hufnagel and colleagues in 1961, who introduced profound cardiac cooling using ice slush,[H8] and Shumway and Griepp and colleagues, who used ice cold saline for the same purpose.[G2,S17,S18] Pharmacologic intervention, designed to provide myocardial protection against

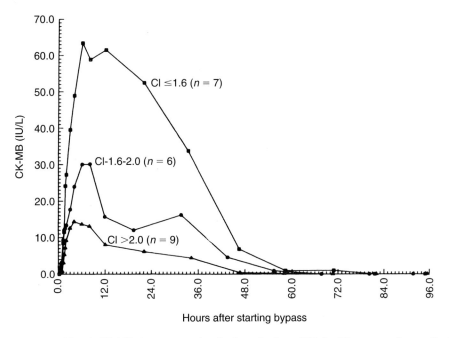

Figure 3-1   Blood CK-MB isoenzyme level after starting CPB in 22 consecutive patients undergoing isolated mitral valve replacement. Operations were performed in 1975 with simple cold ischemic arrest. Geometric mean values are portrayed. Patients are grouped according to range of cardiac index 4 to 6 hours postoperatively. Note high levels of CK-MB in patients with low cardiac index (≤1.6) and low levels in patients with higher cardiac index (>2.0). The overall correlation of CK-MB (duration, peak, and integrated area) and cardiac index was $r = -0.4, P = .04$.

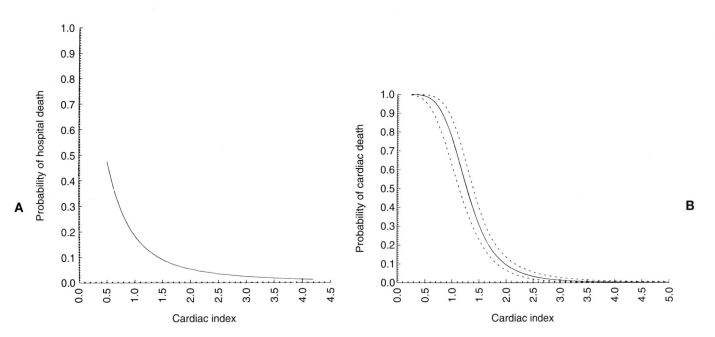

Figure 3-2   **A,** Relationship between early postoperative cardiac index and probability of hospital death in patients undergoing mitral valve surgery ($P < .05$), cold ischemic arrest, or intermittent ischemic arrest. **B,** Probability of acute cardiac death, from early postoperative low cardiac output, according to level of cardiac index in 139 infants and children undergoing open intracardiac repair. Dashed lines encompass 70% confidence limits. (**A** from Appelbaum and colleagues[A3]; **B** from Parr and colleagues[P11]; see publications for data, equation, and statistics.)

the damaging effect of ischemia, began during the 1970s, before the surgical induction of global myocardial ischemia and as more knowledge of the pathophysiology of myocardial ischemia evolved.[N8] In the late 1970s, Clark and colleagues accumulated evidence of the favorable effect of nifedipine, a calcium channel-blocking agent.[C9-C11]

The concept of reducing global myocardial ischemic damage by inducing immediate cessation of electromechanical activity, cardioplegia, was discussed generally by cardiac surgeons during the late 1950s, during which time cold Melrose solution was used for this purpose at the Mayo Clinic. Lack of any apparent advantage led to abandonment of the method. The concept remained largely unused in the United States for many years thereafter, but in Europe, Hoelscher,[H7,H19] Spieckerman and colleagues,[B25] Bretschneider and colleagues,[B7,B15,B26] and Kirsch[K14] continued investigations of induced cardioplegia. Sondergaard reported clinical use of Bretschneider's solution in 1967,[S22] and in 1972 Kirsch and Rodewald and colleagues reported use of Kirsch cardioplegic solution in clinical cardiac surgery.[K5] Working with the latter group, Bleese and colleagues reported a hospital mortality in 1979 of 11.5% among 26 patients undergoing complex operations with cold procaine–magnesium cardioplegia and global myocardial ischemic times greater than 150 minutes.[B23] At about the same time, Hearse and Braimbridge and their colleagues in London were exploring the induction of reversible cardiac arrest[H9] and its clinical application; their work has continued until the present. Gay and Ebert studied and advocated potassium-induced cardioplegia in 1973,[G3] as did Roe and colleagues in 1977.[R11] Randomized trials soon confirmed the advantages of cold cardioplegia.[C6] Buckberg identified blood as the optimal cardioplegic vehicle in 1979.[B9] In the past several years, Wechsler, Damiano, and others began experiments using concepts of membrane hyperpolarization (nearer the resting state) via ATP-sensitive K^+ channels rather than hyperkalemic cell membrane depolarization.[C18,L19] Aprikalim and pinacidil are examples of K^+ channel openers.[M21]

In 1960, Danforth, Naegle, and Bing showed the rapidity with which myocardial energy supply is replenished after ischemia when electromechanical quiescence is continued for a few minutes into the reperfusion period.[D3] This key observation remained unused until Buckberg and colleagues in 1978, probably independently, identified this phenomenon and showed experimentally that improved outcome could be obtained through the use of an initially hyperkalemic reperfusate.[F1] Subsequently, these investigators modified the reperfusate.[F6] For acutely energy-deficient hearts, they introduced warm induction of cardioplegia with an enriched, modified, hyperkalemic blood perfusate.[R20] Control of perfusion pressure during reperfusion and continuance of controlled reperfusion until full recovery were additional contributions to cardioplegic and reperfusion techniques.[D4]

The mode of delivery of the cardioplegic vehicle is the latest contribution to cardioplegic management. Buckberg[D9] in North America and Menasche[M13] in Europe have documented the efficacy and safety of retrograde and combined antegrade–retrograde infusion in valvar and coronary surgery. Metabolic demands of the heart are reduced by approximately 85% by sustained potassium arrest, even at normothermia. Therefore, using the delivery concepts of Buckberg and Menasche, Lichtenstein[L20] and Salerno[S24] reasoned that warm continuously delivered blood cardioplegia containing minimal amounts of potassium would provide adequate oxygen, substrate, and buffer to the arrested, nonworking heart. The aorta is clamped and the heart is maintained quiet and flaccid, but perfused.

NEED FOR SPECIAL MEASURES OF MYOCARDIAL MANAGEMENT

Conditions during Cardiopulmonary Bypass

The heart of intact humans is perfused by blood, ejected from the left ventricle, that leaves the aorta via the right and left coronary arteries. Blood is continuously modified by the organism so as to be correct in its composition and free of damaging materials, such as gaseous or particulate microemboli. The amount and distribution of myocardial blood flow (hence myocardial oxygen supply) are continuously regulated, primarily in response to myocardial oxygen demand. This flow is determined by the coronary perfusing pressure (aortic pressure), tension in the various layers of the myocardium (related in part to ventricular wall thickness and size), and coronary vascular resistance. An appropriate coronary vascular resistance depends on proper function of the coronary endothelial cells and underlying smooth muscle. The ratio between the flow to the inner one fourth of the myocardium (the subendocardial layer) and that to the outer one fourth (the subepicardial layer) in normal hearts with intact circulation is maintained at 1 or a little larger. Although blood flow to the subepicardial layer occurs during both systole and diastole, blood flow to the subendocardial layer of the left ventricle occurs essentially only during diastole, because intramyocardial tension during systole closes the branches of the coronary arteries that pass perpendicularly through the myocardium to arborize in the subendocardium. The well-known vulnerability to ischemia of the left ventricular subendocardial layer in shock, ventricular hypertrophy, and coronary artery disease, as well as during cardiac surgery, is dependent in part on this relationship, but in part on other factors as well, including a higher rate of oxygen consumption in the subendocardial layer.[B32]

During CPB, the heart is deprived of most of these protective regulatory factors. During total CPB, blood enters the arterial system through a cannula in the ascending aorta or at a more distal point. It then passes retrogradely into the most proximal part of the aorta and is distributed through the right and left coronary ostia into the coronary arteries. Arterial pulse pressure is narrow (essentially nonpulsatile), and mean arterial blood pressure is variable. The heart is usually more or less empty and thus smaller than usual, thereby increasing intramyocardial tension and transmural and subendocardial vascular resistance, and decreasing flow to the subendocardial layer.[A2,S2] The effect is particularly powerful in the small heart and hypothermic heart.[S2] Ventricular fibrillation increases intramyocardial tension still more. Coronary vascular resistance during CPB is also affected by circulating vasoactive agents (see "Details of the Whole Body Inflammatory Response" in Section 2 of Chapter 2). The perfusate is diluted blood of variable composition with highly abnormal physiochemical properties. The blood may contain microemboli of several kinds, and leukocytes and platelets with altered mechanical and humoral functions.

Thus, there is little reason to assume that the empty perfused human heart on CPB, even when beating, is managed optimally. Furthermore, clinical experience refutes that view.

Vulnerability of the Diseased Heart

In most patients undergoing cardiac surgery, coronary blood supply or the myocardium, or both, is not normal, and is therefore particularly susceptible to ischemic and reperfusion damage.

Hypertrophied ventricles have long been known to be particularly susceptible to ischemic and reperfusion damage.[S10] This vulnerability is a result of several factors. Transmural gradients of energy substrate utilization are markedly elevated, increasing the vulnerability of the subendocardium to ischemic damage.[B32] Xanthine oxidase levels are markedly elevated, increasing the opportunity for elaboration of oxygen-derived free radicals. Superoxide dismutase levels are markedly decreased, reducing the natural defenses against oxygen-derived free radicals.[B39] Also, wall characteristics of the hypertrophied ventricle make reperfusion of the subendocardium even more difficult than under normal circumstances.

The heart of the patient with chronic heart failure is chronically depleted in energy charge and is particularly susceptible to additional acute depletion and damage during ischemia and reperfusion. (*Energy charge* describes the energy-producing capacity of the particular combination of adenine nucleotides present in mitochondria and cytoplasm of myocytes of a particular heart. Normally, it is 0.85. It would be 1.0 if the nucleotides were present only as ATP, but 0.0 if they were present only as adenosine monophosphate.[A15,A16]) The hearts of experimental animals made cyanotic have been shown to be considerably more susceptible to ischemic and reperfusion damage than are normal hearts.[J13] This may pertain also to severely ill, cyanotic patients. It is well known that the heart of a patient coming to the operating room in a hemodynamically unstable state or in cardiogenic shock is highly sensitive to the damaging effects of global myocardial ischemia.

Surgical Requirements

Cardiac operations can be performed with the heart perfused and either beating, in ventricular fibrillation, or in diastolic arrest. However, the probability of a precise and complete surgical procedure without air embolization is greatest when the heart is bloodless and mechanically quiescent. These optimal conditions are provided by global myocardial ischemia, but they necessitate appropriate myocardial management to limit the damage that would otherwise result from the period of global myocardial ischemia. The changes associated with myocardial ischemia and those changes associated with reperfusion are not often discussed as separate events. Much of the literature does not allow interpretation of one or the other as a separate event. In contrast, the surgeon, by his or her manipulations, has a unique opportunity to control and influence each separately.

Therefore, the following discussion must, for strategic purposes, attempt to distinguish the role of ischemia from that of reperfusion.

DAMAGE FROM GLOBAL MYOCARDIAL ISCHEMIA

Damage from a period of ischemia may result in a variable, and sometimes prolonged, period (many days) of both systolic and diastolic dysfunction without muscle necrosis.[E2,H10] This condition is now termed *myocardial stunning*.[B24,B27] A period of ischemia may also result in irreversible damage *(myocardial necrosis)*. Some investigators have obtained information indicating that this can develop after as little as 20 minutes of normothermic ischemia (in the subendocardium).[J1,J2] Others have obtained evidence that at least 6 hours of normothermic myocardial ischemia is compatible with myocardial cell survival throughout the myocardium.[B28] Ischemic damage involves myocardial cells (myocytes), vascular endothelium, and specialized conduction cells (which, with many cardioplegic techniques, may be the last to recover).

Overall reviews of the damage from myocardial ischemia, and of the potentially damaging effect of reperfusion, are available.[H15,N9] Nayler and Elz stress the extreme heterogeneity among cells (and by implication among hearts) in the rate of progression of ischemic damage, as well as in the rapidity of the chain of events of ischemia (i.e., the switch from aerobic to anaerobic glycolysis occurs within seconds of onset of ischemia). They also emphasize the key role of calcium in reperfusion injury.[N9] The stiffness of cardiac muscle resulting from uncontrolled reperfusion after a period of ischemia is caused by the massive influx of calcium into mitochondria and cytoplasm of myocytes, as well as by edema and capillary disruption.[B40]

Although the phrase *global myocardial ischemia* is appropriately used to describe the situation during cardiac surgery when the aorta is clamped, some blood flow, originating in mediastinal arteries, continues from noncoronary collaterals.[B11] Generally, noncoronary collateral flow is less than 3% of total coronary flow. However, in patients with cyanotic congenital heart disease, advanced ischemic heart disease, extensive pericarditis, and other conditions, coronary collateral flow may be sufficient to initiate electromechanical activity in the heart rendered quiescent by cardioplegia, but insufficient to prevent continuing and important ischemia.

Myocardial Cell Stunning

Surgeons have long known that patients may have severely depressed cardiac function after cardiac surgery, without evidence of myocardial necrosis, and that the duration of the depressed function may last minutes or days. Some instances of delayed recovery of cardiac function after cardiac surgery may be related to initially incomplete reperfusion of the microvasculature of the heart. However, *myocardial stunning* probably underlies at least some instances of prolonged postoperative low cardiac output. In general, *stunning* occurs after a state of acutely diminished myocardial blood flow followed by adequate reperfusion. After establishment of "normal" blood flow, there remains for a time diminished contractility, that is, perfusion–contractility mismatch.[1]

Myocardial stunning, which can follow even brief periods of myocardial ischemia, is characterized by systolic and diastolic dysfunction in the absence of myocardial necrosis.[B27,E2,H10,P8] Myocardial stunning has been attributed to reduced oxygen consumption, which might protect against myocardial necrosis. This hypothesis is denied by the fact that stunned myocardium has a high, not low, oxygen consumption.[B29] Some have suggested that stunning may be a consequence of abnormal energy transduction or utilization secondary to depletion of high-energy phosphates. Stunned myocardium, however, responds to inotropic stimulation, indicating the presence of adequate adenosine triphosphate (ATP) to produce active contraction.[E7] Myocardial stunning is, then, a form of myocardial cell damage caused by ischemia and reperfusion.[B33] Stunning, like myocardial necrosis, tends to begin in the subendocardial layers and progress outward; recovery during reperfusion proceeds in the reverse direction.[B31]

Current information makes it unlikely that stunning is the result of prolonged postischemic depletion of myocardial cell energy charge.[B24] It does not appear to be the result of a continuing postischemic impairment of coronary blood flow or coronary reserve.[J5] It may be caused in part by the release of oxygen-derived free radicals, presumably by activated neutrophils and probably occurring to a major degree during the first few minutes of reperfusion.[B30,B33] Experimentally, introduction of superoxide dismutase and catalase (free radical scavengers) before an ischemic period results in nearly full restoration of contractile indices upon reperfusion, compared with prolonged depression in controls.[P3] Stunning may be caused in part by an ischemia-induced increase in influx of calcium into the myocardial cells.[M14,P9,P10] This possibility has led to the hypothesis that cardiac stunning is related to a defect in calcium-mediated excitation–contraction coupling that results from the excess calcium.[B24] This hypothesis must be reconciled with evidence that, after short periods of ischemia, excess intracellular calcium that rapidly accumulates with the onset of reperfusion soon leaves the cells.[M14]

Techniques of myocardial management designed to minimize myocardial necrosis are probably effective against myocardial stunning as well. Thus, for optimal results, these techniques should be used even when the period of global myocardial ischemia is less than that anticipated to result in myocardial cell death.

---

[1]*Myocardial Hibernation*

If stunning is characterized as a perfusion–contraction mismatch, hibernation is a perfusion–contraction match; in the latter, both are low.[R27] Generally, hibernation is a chronic, potentially reversible state of segmental (less often, global) contractile dysfunction. Theoretically, dobutamine echocardiography, thallium scintigraphy, and positron emission tomography can distinguish hibernating from nonviable myocardium. However, the difference between stunned and hibernating segments may be vague. Marban[M23] suggests that a decrease in Ca^{2+} transients at a cellular level is responsible for the contractile dysfunction in hibernation, whereas a decrease in myofilament Ca^{2+} responsiveness accounts for the excitation-contraction decoupling seen in stunning.

Myocardial Cell Necrosis

Myocardial necrosis after cardiac surgery is the end stage of a complex process initiated by the onset of global myocardial ischemia, maintained by continuing ischemia, and aggravated by reperfusion. The final link in the chain of events, reperfusion, can be favorably modified so as to prevent necrosis, unless the duration of myocardial ischemia is excessive; "excessive" in this context has not yet been defined.[B14]

Immediately after the onset of ischemia, contractile force declines rapidly, as does myocardial pH.[C14,G6] Oxidative metabolism, electron transport, and ATP production by oxidative phosphorylation (which take place in mitochondria) decline rapidly. Some ATP is still produced by relatively inefficient anaerobic glycolysis. Fatty acid utilization is rapidly reduced, while fatty acid acyl-CoA derivatives accumulate because of continuing uptake of fatty acids by myocardial cells. Intracellular acidosis develops because of accumulation of lactate and protons in the myocardial cytoplasm, suppressing anaerobic glycolysis. These developments contribute to damage to the cell membrane and to loss of control of cell size, with consequent cell swelling, intracellular accumulation of calcium, and other disturbances of membrane ion transport.[L7] This entire process acutely diminishes myocardial energy charge and glycogen reserves, while adenosine, inosine, and other nucleotides that are the results of ATP catabolism and the building blocks for ATP repletion leave the cell. Ultrastructural changes during this early phase are limited to loss of glycogen granules and some intracellular and organelle swelling.

As the duration of ischemia lengthens, intracellular metabolic deterioration continues, still more fatty acids accumulate within the myocytes, and diastolic arrest occurs. Loss of control of sarcolemmal membrane permeability, which begins within 15 minutes of onset of ischemia,[H18] continues, and nonspecific membrane permeability increases. Adenosine, lactate, and other small molecules leak still more rapidly out of the cell, as do cytoplasmic proteins and enzymes; these appear in the cardiac interstitium and in the lymph.[L7] As macromolecules within myocardial cells are converted to smaller, more osmotically active molecules by ischemic metabolic conversion, cell swelling proceeds more rapidly.[T8] Cellular metabolism and ATP production nearly cease, and glycogen stores are depleted.[M1] As glycolysis and mitochondrial function are totally lost, cellular autolysis begins, and cell contents leak more extensively into the interstitial space and cardiac lymph.

In many laboratory preparations, as the depletion of ATP continues and finally reaches critical levels, myocardial *contracture* begins to occur.[G5] The classic belief has been that once contracture is completed, functional recovery is suddenly more difficult, and the time to this end point has been an important criterion in many studies in isolated rat heart preparations.[A13] However, the time to contracture (1) is highly species dependent, (2) is unknown but probably quite long in humans, and (3) in the rat heart, at least, has a greatly different implication in crystalloid versus blood-perfused preparations.[W2] The appearance of contracture does indicate that the content of ATP has been depleted to a critically low level. Contracture first develops in the subendocardium, be-

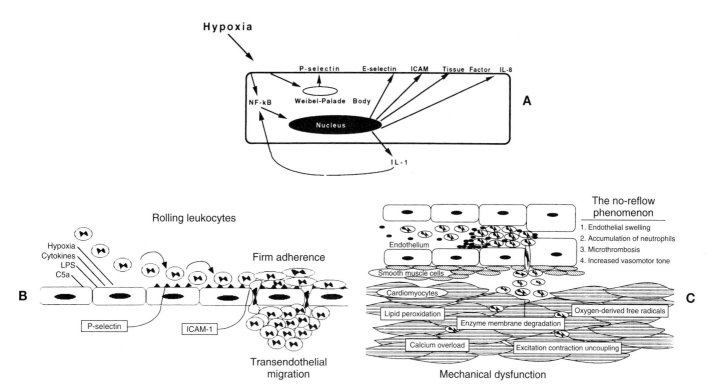

Figure 3-3   **A,** Hypoxic endothelial cell activation. Hypoxia stimulates Weibel-Palade bodies to release P-selectin and activates NF-κB. NF-κB is translocated to the nucleus, where it promotes transcription of E-selectin, intracellular adhesion molecule (ICAM), tissue factor, interleukin-8 (IL-8), and interleukin-1 (IL-1). Interleukin-1 feeds back to promote more endothelial cell activation through activation of NF-κB. **B,** Neutrophil adhesion is a multistep process that involves contact between neutrophils and members of the selectin family of adhesion molecules (P-selectin, E-selectin) expressed on the activated endothelium. These low-affinity bonds result in rolling and slowing of leukocytes. As this occurs, neutrophils become activated, and a firm bond forms between integrins on the leukocyte surface (that is, CD 11/18) and adhesion molecules on the endothelium (that is, intracellular adhesion molecule-1, vascular cell adhesion molecule, platelet-endothelial cell adhesion molecule). *LPS,* Lipopolysaccharide. **C,** The no-reflow phenomenon. Hypoxia results in activation of the endothelial cell layer, which promotes leukocyte adhesion and degranulation, endothelial swelling, platelet activation, microthrombosis, and increased vasomotor tone. This contributes to impaired microcirculatory flow, despite what appears to be adequate perfusion through the large epicardial arteries. Adherent neutrophils infiltrate the underlying myocardium and promote lipid peroxidation, enzymatic degradation of membranes, calcium overload, and excitation-contraction uncoupling. Collectively, these events result in impaired myocardial function. (From Boyle and colleagues.[B43])

cause of its higher metabolic rate and consequent more rapid depletion of ATP.[A9,B32,J4,L9,V1] Contracture develops more rapidly in hypertrophied than in normal hearts,[B32] and is delayed in its onset by hypothermia.

Where the process becomes truly irreversible along this course of events, and cell death becomes inevitable, is not known with certainty.

Endothelial Cell Damage

As in the case of myocytes, distinguishing between ischemic endothelial cell damage and reperfusion damage is difficult. Endothelial cell swelling develops during ischemia[S7] and becomes more prominent during reperfusion, and secretion of endothelial relaxing factor, as well as of endothelin, the constricting factor, is affected. Boyle and Verrier have reviewed the role of the endothelium in events associated with ischemia and reperfusion[B43] (Fig. 3-3). There is endothelial cell activation following hypoxia, anoxia, or ischemia. Activated endothelial cells express proinflammatory properties, including induction of leukocyte adhesion molecules. These result in neutrophil accumulation at the arterial wall and release of oxygen-derived free radicals. Intracellular adhesion molecules (ICAM) are upregulated (see Fig. 3-3). Endothelial cell selectins (E and P) are also involved in the hypoxic inflammatory response, and theoretically, may ultimately contribute to small-vessel occlusion (no-reflow) occasionally seen after myocardial ischemia. Impaired microcirculatory flow, membrane degradation, and enzyme dysfunction result then in poor mechanical function (see Fig 3-3). After prolonged ischemia, endothelial cell damage is marked and apparent during reperfusion with unmodified blood and without control of pressure, with sufficient endothelial cell damage that necrosis occurs and large intraluminal projections develop, some of which are cast off into the lumen.[K8] Thus, myocardial endothelial cells probably also participate, along with other endothelial cells in the body, in the "whole body inflammatory response" to cardiopulmonary bypass (see "Details of the Whole Body Inflammatory Response" in Section 2 of Chapter 2).

These ischemic changes in the coronary vascular endothelium play an important role in changes in coronary vascular resistance that have been observed in humans during reperfusion after global myocardial ischemia,[D4] and in the "no-reflow" phenomenon seen after prolonged ischemia, particularly in the inner half of the myocardium.[K8] In children, cytokines such as IL-8 are liberated during CPB[F15] and may contribute to neutrophil adhesion and migration. Burns and colleagues[B44] and Kilbridge and colleagues[K18] report endothelial expression of P-selectin, E-selectin, and ICAM in myocardial biopsies taken during cardioplegic ischemic arrest in infants undergoing complex repairs. However, the degree to which endothelial activation and related subsequent events contribute to impaired microcirculatory flow and myocardial dysfunction during cardiac surgery is unknown.

Specialized Conduction Cell Damage

The specialized conduction cells become nonfunctional early in the course of global myocardial ischemia in humans; it may be speculated that their recovery takes longer than does recovery of myocytes. Some support for this is that, 5 or so minutes after initially hyperkalemic reperfusion, the ventricular myocardium in some patients responds well and strongly to direct ventricular pacing, although it is quiescent with atrial pacing or without pacing. Then, after 5 or so more minutes, sinus rhythm may appear. Also, when blood cardioplegia and uncontrolled normokalemic reperfusion are used, about 50% of patients have atrioventricular (AV) conduction disturbances when CPB is discontinued.[B35] This appears to be a form of specialized conduction cell stunning rather than necrosis, because these disappear by the time of hospital discharge in most of the patients in whom it had developed. Even third-degree AV block persisting as long as 2 months has been observed to give way to sinus rhythm.[B35] The validation of this speculation remains to be obtained, however. These changes might also be ascribed to variation of the specialized conduction fibers' sensitivity to chemical components of the cardioplegia infusate.[O5]

DAMAGE FROM REPERFUSION

The morphologic changes following normal blood reperfusion of ischemic myocardium have been authoritatively presented by Jennings and Reimer.[J14] They stress the complexity of the process, including cell swelling, contraction band necrosis, calcium loading of mitochondria, accelerated washout of creatine kinase early in reperfusion, and the particular vulnerability of the subendocardium. It is clear that there can be no reperfusion damage in the absence of prior ischemia. What is not clear is whether there can be reperfusion damage in the absence of ischemic *damage*.[R28] Clearly, limitation of the duration of ischemia

and modification of the conditions during ischemia are fundamental to limiting reperfusion injury.

The following discussion assumes some degree of spontaneous ischemia (coronary obstructive disease) or induced ischemia (low blood flow or aortic clamping); it pertains to uncontrolled reperfusion, which is reperfusion by unmodified blood without control of pressure or flow.

Myocardial Cell Damage

The response of myocardial cells to uncontrolled reperfusion depends in large part on the time-related point along the pathway to cell death that has been reached during the ischemic period. Yet the critical point at which the "explosive cellular response" to uncontrolled reperfusion can be expected is not known with certainty. In the past, it has been defined, in the isolated rat heart, as the point at which contracture appears (a definition that is of little help in humans undergoing cardiac surgery because the time to contracture, if it occurs, is unknown but probably quite long). Also, when the rat heart is blood perfused (rather than crystalloid perfused), reperfusion after contracture results in good return of function.[W2]

When uncontrolled reperfusion is initiated after global myocardial ischemia in cardiac surgery, the response may be only myocardial stunning. A more severe response consists of reperfusion arrhythmias, particularly ventricular tachycardia and ventricular fibrillation. The more prolonged and the larger the area of myocardial ischemia, the more frequent, severe, and intractable the arrhythmias.[B19] A still more severe response is the hard and fibrillating heart, sometimes termed the *stone heart*.[C1,H3,K1,L1] The *stone heart phenomenon* may involve only some regions of the heart, typically the basilar portion of the left ventricle and the subendocardium. This phenomenon indicates that the heart has undergone severe damage and may be considered to have approached the critical point of "no return." It has not necessarily reached this point, because the stone heart is, at least under some circumstances, capable of recovery. The histologic features of these advanced forms of reperfusion damage include disruption of the regular myofibrillar pattern and evident contraction bands.[M2]

Clearly, the strong influx of calcium into myocytes, and particularly its accumulation in mitochondria, are obvious and fundamental features of reperfusion injury.[I1,N7,O4,S3,S9] However, many other types of events are ongoing, most well under way within 1 or 2 minutes of uncontrolled reperfusion.

Chemotactic factors of cardiac subcellular origin, activated endothelial cells, activated complement fragments, such as C5a, and cytokines are generated locally in ischemic myocardium.[D7,M19,R9] This process activates circulating neutrophils, which accumulate and play an important role in initiating and sustaining reperfusion injury.[B16,C8,E3,M16] Neutrophils plug myocardial capillaries as reperfusion continues because of their large size and their active adherence to ischemically damaged endothelial cells.[E4] Leukocytes, and in particular neutrophils, release large amounts of oxygen-derived free radicals in these circumstances.[F3,H17,M17] Activated neutrophils also release arachidonic acid metabolites[M18] that cause endothelial injury, vasoconstriction, and platelet aggregation. During reperfusion, certain leukotrienes are also released from platelets and endothelial cells.[I4,R21]

Oxygen-derived free radicals generated during reperfusion represent one of the fundamental processes that produce damage.[A14,P6] Oxygen-derived free radicals are characterized by the presence of unpaired electrons and include superoxide (O_2), hydrogen peroxide (H_2O_2), and the hydroxyl radical (OH). Normally, myocardial cells are constantly exposed to superoxide anions in very small amounts, produced in (1) mitochondria (where 95% of oxygen consumption occurs) during electron transport, (2) cell cytoplasm during prostaglandin synthesis and metabolism and oxidation of tissue catecholamines, (3) vascular endothelium by xanthine oxidase–catalyzed reactions, and (4) extracellular fluids by activated neutrophils. Normally, these very small amounts of oxygen-derived free radicals are well controlled. Superoxide dismutase, which is normally present in myocytes, catalyzes the transformation of superoxide anions to hydrogen peroxide and water; metabolism of hydrogen peroxide to water and oxygen is accomplished by either catalase or glutathione peroxidase, or both.[A14]

The very onset of uncontrolled reperfusion can produce large amounts of oxygen-derived free radicals because of profound alterations imposed on this exquisite system by ischemia. Ischemia progressively decreases the cellular levels of the scavenger superoxide dismutase and also increases metabolic end products of ATP catabolism, such as hypoxanthine and xanthine. These catabolites may participate in producing oxygen-derived free radicals by supplying free radical substrates to endothelial xanthine oxidase.[A5] Also, during ischemia, normally present xanthine dehydrogenase is converted to xanthine oxidase. Superoxide anions are generated at the start of uncontrolled reperfusion. Xanthine oxidase is the catalyst for reoxygenation and metabolism of the considerable amounts of hypoxanthine and xanthine generated during ischemia. A chain reaction results, leading to the generation of other free radicals and of a direct attack by them on unsaturated fatty acids within cell membranes. As part of this chain reaction, iron plays a key role in converting relatively innocuous superoxide radicals into highly damaging hydroxyl radicals.[B21] Peroxidation of membrane lipids has been shown to result in increased membrane permeability, decreased calcium transport into the sarcoplasmic reticulum, and altered mitochondrial function,[A14] setting the stage for myocardial stunning or necrosis.

Endothelial Cell Damage

Reperfusion damage to the heart involves more than the myocytes. For example, myocytes surrounding a necrotic area of myocardium may be perfectly viable and functioning 1 hour after the start of reperfusion, only to become necrotic over the subsequent few hours.[A6] This has been shown to be due to delayed closure of coronary arterioles and capillaries and to the resulting no-reflow phenomenon. The endothelial cells of large coronary arteries appear to be little affected by the damaging effects of ischemia and reperfusion.[Q1] The coronary microvasculature is profoundly affected, however, and the resultant endothelial dysfunction appears to develop rapidly with the onset of

reperfusion.[Q1,T9] This damage appears to be minimal after ischemia itself, but is incited almost exclusively by reperfusion.[Q1] In addition to changes in endothelial cell function (see below), the endothelial cell swells, activated neutrophils and platelets aggregate and adhere to the endothelium, and microvascular obstruction can develop.[A6,N3,V4]

This rapidly induced reperfusion injury to the endothelial cells severely impairs normal endothelium-dependent relaxations to neutrophils and platelets as well as to thrombin, acetylcholine, and bradykinin.[K16,M21,P12,V5] These alterations could play some role in the observed progressive increase in coronary vascular resistance during reperfusion. In addition, with damage to endothelial cells, smooth muscle beneath the cells is exposed, allowing additional mediators to induce direct smooth muscle contraction.

In addition to these phenomena, coronary vessels are compressed by myocardial areas with high wall tension and hemorrhage and by myocardial cell swelling. This all may lead to inhomogeneous distribution of the uncontrolled, unmodified blood reperfusate or actual "no-flow," further aggravating reperfusion injury in the clinical setting. These unfavorable events are particularly damaging after prolonged (more than 24 hours) cardiac preservation,[S19] as may eventually be required for cardiac transplantation.

Specialized Conduction Cell Damage

Little specific information is available about reperfusion injury to the specialized conduction cells.

ADVANTAGEOUS CONDITIONS DURING ISCHEMIA

Advantageous conditions during ischemia delay the time required for the ischemic myocardium to reach the hypothetical *critical point* in the course of ischemic injury. This is classically considered the point at which uncontrolled, unmodified blood reperfusion produces explosive cell damage and accelerated myocardial necrosis, rather than recovery. For this discussion, it is this critical point that must be delayed. The common denominator may be delay in severe reduction of the energy charge of the myocardium.

Circumstances that decrease the rate of ATP utilization (or its surrogate, myocardial oxygen consumption) lengthen the *safe ischemic interval*. These circumstances include immediate cessation of electromechanical activity and hypothermia.[F4] The interrelationships are such that a great advantage is obtained by reducing myocardial temperature from 37° to 27°C, a lesser advantage by reducing temperature from 27° to 17°C, and a still smaller advantage by reducing temperature further (Fig. 3-4).[H9] However, for longer periods of arrest (6 hours), Rosenfeldt found an increase in protection with stepwise cooling from 20° to 4°C.[R29] In a different experimental preparation, Balderman and colleagues[B47] found less satisfactory ventricular performance after 120 minutes of ischemia at temperatures of 6° and 10°C compared with 14° and 18°C.

Preoperative enhancement of cardiac substrates seems advantageous, but has been little used in cardiac surgery to date. Myocardial glycogen content can be increased by an intravenous infusion of a glucose–insulin–potassium solution during the 12 hours preceding operation.[L8,O3] This

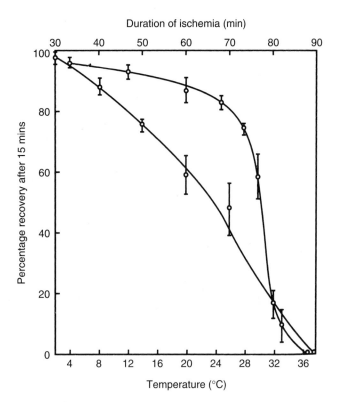

Figure 3-4   Relation between duration of global myocardial ischemia and percentage recovery of left ventricular systolic function and between temperature of the heart during ischemic arrest and percentage recovery. Note the linear relation between duration of ischemia and percentage recovery (indicated by circles, with standard error represented by vertical bars). Note the curvilinear relation between temperature and recovery, such that most of the advantage was obtained by temperature reduction to about 22°C. (From Hearse and colleagues.[H9])

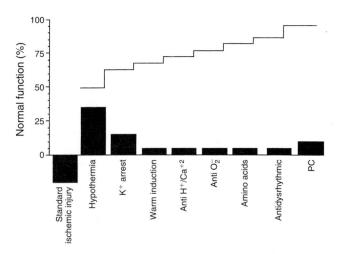

Figure 3-5   Conceptual incremental beneficial effects of the various components of current myocardial management. The top staircase line represents the amount of protection, expressed as percent normal ventricular function, that is added cumulatively by each component. The bottom solid bars represent the individual protection of each component. *PC,* Preconditioning. (From Cleveland and colleagues.[C19])

can be combined with continuous retrograde coronary sinus infusion of a similar solution during the ischemic period.[L15,L16]

Acute substrate enhancement before cold cardioplegia and ischemia by initial infusion of warm, hyperkalemic, modified and substrate-enriched blood has been shown to benefit hearts that have become energy depleted before the cardiac operation.[R18,R20,R22] The continuation of the pressure-controlled, warm, enriched blood infusion, for a few minutes after the onset of asystole, takes advantage of increased coronary flow and better distribution brought about by cardiac asystole.[S11]

Preischemic administration of drugs such as lidoflazine has been shown to be advantageous,[D2,F9,F10] although the mechanism of their favorable effect remains arguable (see "Drug-Mediated Myocardial Protection" later in this chapter).

Preischemic pharmacologic myocardial conditioning may surface as an additional tactic to limit damage during an induced ischemic interval and as an adjunct to surgical myocardial management. Ischemia-induced cardiac preconditioning has been shown to reduce infarct size in dogs[M24] and swine.[S27] Several reports suggest that in humans, prodromal angina may limit infarct size.[K19,O6] Adenosine activation and α_1-adrenergic stimulation are two pathways

suggested as mediators of preconditioning.[B45,L21] Protein kinase C has been identified as at least one of the factors that when activated by adenosine or phenylephrine results in protection by myocardial conditioning in laboratory animals[M25,T11] (Fig. 3-5). Experimentally in sheep, preconditioning has been produced by CPB alone and the response suppressed by α_1-adrenergic blockade or adenosine receptor blocker.[B46]

ADVANTAGEOUS CONDITIONS DURING REPERFUSION

Advantageous conditions during reperfusion (1) minimize the persistence of myocardial stunning into the post-CPB period, (2) provide for optimal recovery of function of reversibly damaged myocardium, and (3) resuscitate myocytes that would otherwise have undergone necrosis.

Buckberg and colleagues evolved the methods and demonstrated the advantages of controlling reperfusion.[F1,F6] These ideas now constitute a clinically useful body of knowledge. In essence, the advantageous conditions consist of the following:

1. Maintaining electromechanical quiescence during the first 3 to 5 minutes of reperfusion, to permit more rapid repletion of myocardial energy charge, minimize regional heterogeneity of reperfusion flow, minimize myocardial energy expenditure until recovery has been established, and minimize intracellular accumulation of calcium
2. Combating accumulated myocardial acidosis by controlling pH of the initial reperfusate and providing a large buffering capacity, to permit more prompt morphologic, biochemical, and functional recovery
3. Minimizing damage from oxygen-derived free radicals
4. Reducing ionized calcium in the initial reperfusate to help minimize intracellular accumulation of calcium

5. Increasing availability of substrate for repletion of myocardial energy charge
6. Maintaining a low perfusion pressure (about 30 mmHg) during the first 60 to 120 seconds of reperfusion, to minimize endothelial cell damage and swelling, during which time reactive hyperemia, usually present, allows this low pressure to be maintained with adequate volume and distribution of flow
7. Maintaining a flow sufficient to encourage near-uniform myocardial distribution of the reperfusate
8. Continuing control of the reperfusion pressure and flow until myocyte, endothelial cell, and specialized conduction cell recovery is essentially complete.

Specific comments about the individual items follow, and the details of establishing these advantageous conditions during clinical cardiac surgery are described in "Cold Cardioplegia, Controlled Aortic Root Perfusion, and (When Needed) Warm Cardioplegic Induction" later in this chapter. New information continues to accumulate, and current practices must be changed whenever sufficient information becomes available to indicate the possibility of improving results by modifying methods.

Blood

Blood as the reperfusion vehicle has been shown to be superior to crystalloid solutions.[B9,C13,D8,E5,E6,F5,F8,K10,N12,R17,S13,S14,T7] The advantage is due in part to the red blood cell component, although it may not relate to the oxygen transport capacity of the red blood cells.[I3] Among other things, red blood cells contain abundant oxygen-derived free radical scavengers, which have been shown to be important.[J14] The minimal effective level of the hematocrit in the reperfusate is 0.15 to 0.20.[I3] The buffering capacity of blood proteins, especially their histidine and imidazole groups, is also advantageous.

Leukocyte Depletion

There is little doubt that activated leukocytes play an important role in reperfusion damage. Depletion of leukocytes from the blood reperfusate (by filtration) has been shown to reduce reperfusion injury considerably.[C15] This is, however, impractical for clinical cardiac surgery and may not in fact be necessary.

Substrate

Addition of the amino acids L-glutamate and aspartate to solutions used to reperfuse the heart after an ischemic insult has been shown by Rosenkranz and by Buckberg and colleagues to be beneficial to metabolic and functional recovery.[L11,L12,R18,R19] Their early work has been confirmed by Choong and Gavin[C12] and others.[G9]

The addition of adenosine during reperfusion was theorized to improve postischemic function; there is now experimental support for its efficacy.[B12] The delay in repletion of ATP after ischemic injury may well be related to lack of availability of adenosine, an important component of the process of rebuilding ATP stores,[A5,R25,S21,V3] because it presumably converted to inosine and, as such, is washed out of cells during reperfusion.[R4]

Hydrogen Ion Concentration

The initial reperfusate should contain adequate buffering capacity to combat the intracellular acidosis developed during the ischemic period (see "Blood" in the previous discussion). Various buffering agents have been used, but hydroxymethyl aminomethane (Tris) and histidine have particularly favorable characteristics.[B15,H12,N5,R12,T6]

Calcium

During reperfusion, perfusate calcium content should be low to minimize the influx of calcium into potentially damaged myocytes. However, calcium should not be totally absent from either cardioplegic or reperfusion solutions, to avoid the calcium paradox.[H11,Y2,Z1,Z2]

Potassium

Hyperkalemic reperfusion permits rapid repletion of ATP[D3] and improved functional recovery, even in the face of ischemic contracture and myocardial accumulation of calcium.[D5] It also promotes better myocardial blood flow.[D6] Therefore, if controlled reperfusion is elected, the initial reperfusate should contain sufficient potassium to maintain electromechanical quiescence for at least 2 to 3 minutes, and preferably 5 to 10 minutes. The sufficient concentration is about 12 mmol $\cdot$ L^{-1}.

The advantages of hyperkalemic reperfusion in clinical cardiac surgery have been confirmed in a randomized trial by Teoh and colleagues,[T2] although these advantages may be difficult to demonstrate in low-risk patients undergoing uncomplicated coronary artery bypass grafting[F14,R15] (Fig. 3-6).

Pressure

After a period of myocardial ischemia, coronary vascular endothelial cells are in a state in which they are easily damaged by high reperfusion pressure[O2,S20] (Shangyi J, Hongxi S, Gongshong L: unpublished data; 1987), but that state appears to be rapidly reversed by gentle reperfusion. Therefore, in clinical cardiac surgery, it is prudent to keep reperfusion pressure at about 30 mmHg for the first 60 to 120 seconds of reperfusion. Because of reactive hyperemia present at that time,[D5] the reperfusion flow rate may, nonetheless, be large.

Some experimental studies have suggested that reperfusion pressure should be no higher than 50 mmHg, lest excessive myocardial edema develop; others have suggested that it may be as high as 100 mmHg. These differences may be the result of species differences. In any event, in a canine model, improved myocardial function and no more myocardial edema resulted from 1 hour of hyperkalemic reperfusion at 80 mmHg (with electromechanical quiescence) than from normokalemic reperfusion and rapid resumption of cardiac activity.[A11] The importance of maintaining a sufficient coronary perfusion pressure at this stage has been well documented in the diastolically arrested canine heart exhibiting maximal coronary vasodilation. In that model, endocardial flow falls steeply when coronary perfusion pressure is reduced from 70 mmHg to 40 mmHg.[A10] Reduction of perfusion pressure to 20 mmHg

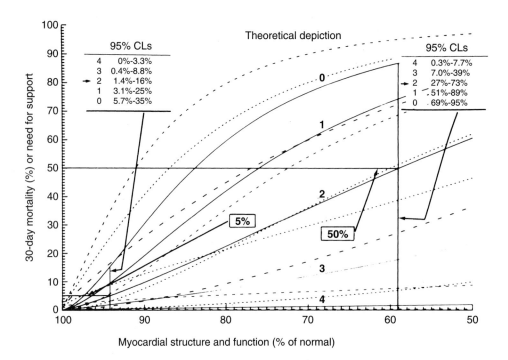

Figure 3-6   Theoretical depiction of preoperative energy charge and state of hypertrophy of the heart (represented as percent normal myocardial structure and function) along the horizontal axis, and percent survival of the patient without important catecholamine or mechanical support along the vertical axis. Isobars represent variable degrees of myocardial management; zero represents no special management and implies the normothermic beating heart or the normothermic briefly arrested heart; 4 represents the most complete myocardial management possible, including (when necessary) warm induction of cardioplegia (see "Cold Cardioplegia, Controlled Aortic Root Reperfusion, and [When Needed] Warm Cardioplegic Induction" later in this chapter). Note that in low-risk patients, there is only a small difference in outcome according to the type of myocardial management, whereas in patients with loss of cardiac reserves, outcome differences are large and easily discernible. Thus, in a low-risk patient (myocardial status 95% of normal), 95% confidence intervals of percent survival without support all overlap, except those for management 4, and percent survival is only a little lower with management 4. In contrast, when myocardial status is 63% of normal, the confidence limits (CLs) largely do not overlap, and differences are relatively easily discerned.

leads to substantially increased heterogeneity of flow (Fig. 3-7). Clinical experience at UAB demonstrated the efficacy and safety, after the first 60 to 120 seconds, of maintaining reperfusion pressure between 50 and 75 mmHg, or at the preoperative diastolic arterial blood pressure of the patient, whichever was lower.[D4,F16]

Flow and Resistance

At the beginning of reperfusion, coronary resistance is very low, primarily as a result of reactive hyperemia, with additive effects from the cold temperature of the myocardium and the action of vasoactive substances, such as adenosine and lactic acid, that accumulate during the ischemic period. Thus, coronary blood flow is very high initially, even with low reperfusion pressure, but begins to fall within a few minutes of the beginning of reperfusion.

Subsequently, reperfusion flow is usually about 150 mL · min^{-1} in adults (about 100 mL · min^{-1} · m^{-2} body surface area). This is about 40 mL · min^{-1} · 100 g^{-1} of heart muscle,[D4] approximately half the value for normal hearts, but it appears to be adequate in the nonworking empty

heart being reperfused under these conditions. In similar experimental models of normal hearts, flow after the initial hyperemia is higher and near control level.[R13]

Temperature

In practice, the temperature of the reperfusate is initially about 35°C, because of the characteristics of the heat exchange mechanism in the reperfusion circuit. After 2 to 3 minutes, the temperature rises to 37°C. There may be advantages to this gradual return to normothermia. Normothermia is advantageous to the normal function of enzyme systems.

Suppression of Formation of Oxygen-Derived Free Radicals and Enhancement of Free Radical Scavengers

Allopurinol, a xanthine oxidase inhibitor, given just before reperfusion, protects the previously ischemic isolated rat heart from reperfusion injury, presumably by slowing the conversion of hypoxanthine and xanthine to superoxide

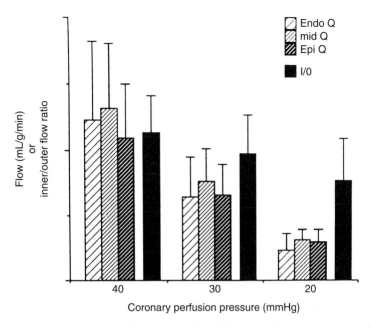

Figure 3-7   Information obtained from an isolated blood-perfused canine model, with the heart diastolically arrested and with maximal coronary vasodilatation. Variation in coronary perfusion pressure is along the horizontal axis, coronary flow rate (or inner/outer flow ratio) is along the vertical axis, and the columns represent endomyocardial, midmyocardial, and epimyocardial flow rates, and the inner/outer flow ratio. Note that as coronary perfusion pressure was reduced, perfusion of the subendocardium progressively declined out of proportion to the decline in the other layers. Accordingly, the inner/outer ratio fell. Also, heterogeneity of flow increased with decreasing perfusion pressure (increased height of vertical bars). (From Aldea and colleagues.[A10])

ions.[B17] Deferoxamine, given just before reperfusion, is also protective in experimental models, presumably by chelating iron and slowing the formation of the highly damaging hydroxyl radicals from superoxide radicals.[B2,B17] The free radical scavengers superoxide dismutase and catalase protect against reperfusion injury when given before ischemia in experimental studies.[G7,J11,P3,S15] Their use during early reperfusion has also been shown to be advantageous in experimental models.[J10] However, the use of blood as the reperfusate, with its naturally occurring free radical scavengers, appears to obviate the need for these agents in clinical cardiac surgery.[J3]

Duration

Recovery is not complete at the end of the hyperkalemic phase of controlled reperfusion. This may be because, at this time (1) cellular recovery from ischemia is incomplete, and (2) inhomogeneity of myocardial perfusion probably persists. Controlled normokalemic reperfusion with adequate aortic root pressure should be continued until the heart is beating forcefully and is in sinus rhythm. This stage is usually reached 10 to 20 minutes after the beginning of reperfusion. In an experimental study, this length of time has been shown to be required for return of normal coronary vascular resistance, myocardial oxygen consumption, myocardial lactate levels, and ventricular function.[R13]

Although ATP levels have not yet returned to normal,[R13] at this stage the heart itself is able to generate an adequate

coronary perfusion pressure. Controlled aortic root reperfusion can therefore be discontinued by removing the aortic clamp, with proper precautions (see "Cold Cardioplegia, Controlled Aortic Root Reperfusion, and [When Needed] Warm Cardioplegic Induction" later in this chapter).

Reperfusion as described above, with the aorta clamped, has been called "hot shot."[T2] In practice, "controlled" reperfusion (with the aorta clamped) may not be necessary. Reperfusion by pump flow supported by pharmacologic manipulation may be entirely adequate.

METHODS OF MYOCARDIAL MANAGEMENT DURING CARDIAC SURGERY

The objective of any type of myocardial management during CPB should be limitation of injury during ischemia by some combination of myocardial hypothermia, electromechanical arrest, washout, O_2 and other substrate enhancement, oncotic manipulation, and buffering.

No single method of myocardial management is unequivocally the best. Many different methods are in use by surgeons obtaining good results. Surgeons necessarily make a decision as to the method to be used each time they perform a cardiac operation, often based on "preferences" rather than on rigorous comparisons between methods. A number of factors influence the surgeon's "preference":

1. The surgeon's specific surgical techniques or operative sequencing that influence duration of aortic clamping

2. The strength of the surgeon's desire to have a quiet, bloodless heart
3. The strength of the conviction that cardiac surgery without myocardial necrosis or residual stunning is desirable and possible despite the added complexity to achieve these goals
4. The institutional environment
5. Costs

Continuous Normokalemic Coronary Perfusion

Empty Beating Heart

The earliest intracardiac operations were performed on normothermic, perfused, empty beating heart.[B3] Experimental studies had been interpreted as showing "normal left ventricular function" after 30 minutes to 3 hours of CPB with the heart perfused, empty, and beating.[E1,N4]

Current information indicates that the method is not ideal. Water tends to accumulate in the myocardium during CPB; as a result, ventricular distensibility in dog models is decreased by nearly 50% after 3 hours of CPB with the heart perfused, empty, and beating. The distribution of coronary blood in the normothermic, beating, empty (and thus small) heart is abnormal.[A21] The change in myocardial compressive forces and left ventricular wall geometry with the empty beating heart have been shown to impede intracoronary collateral flow supplying potentially ischemic areas of myocardium.[M3] The occurrence of transmural myocardial infarction has been shown to be 15% when individual coronary artery perfusion was used for aortic valve replacement, with isoenzymatic evidence of myocardial necrosis in 70% of patients, proportions as high as in patients randomly assigned to cold ischemic arrest.[S1]

Despite these considerations, the method can serve well for various procedures, and under certain circumstances may be combined with other methods of myocardial management.[S24]

Mild or moderate whole body, and thus cardiac, hypothermia are often combined with this method. McGoon and colleagues[M7] reported a series of 100 consecutive cases of isolated aortic valve replacement using this method, with no hospital deaths, evidence that, properly used, the method can provide good results.[M8]

Perfusion of Individual Coronary Arteries

Individual coronary artery cannulation is necessary when perfusion of the empty beating heart is used for surgery on the aortic valve.[L2,M4] After CPB is established, the aorta is clamped (stopping the flow of blood into the aortic root and ostia of the right and left coronary arteries), and an incision is made into the first part of the ascending aorta. Small individual cannulae are placed into the ostia of the right and left coronary arteries, and, by way of a separate pump, blood is infused into both. The cannulae tips are at least 3 to 4 mm long.

This technique works well in most patients, but it is not ideal. The tip of the cannula may extend beyond the bifurcation of the left main coronary artery, so that only the left anterior descending or circumflex artery is perfused. In about 1% of patients, these two arteries arise separately from the aortic sinus, making proper individual cannulation

even more difficult. The prevalence of left dominant systems in patients with aortic stenosis secondary to congenital bicuspid valves is higher than normal; in left dominant systems, the left main coronary artery is shorter than normal,[H4,K3,M5] again making individual coronary perfusion more difficult. In about 50% of patients, the conus artery supplying the infundibulum of the right ventricle arises separately from the aortic sinus and is not perfused by a cannula inserted into the right coronary ostium. Also, mechanical injury to the coronary ostia can occur whenever techniques of direct coronary ostial cannulation are used; this results in intraoperative myocardial infarction and late coronary ostial stenosis.[C4,H5,L3,M6,R8,S4,Y1]

The method in practice is not without periods of global myocardial ischemia. One occurs between aortic clamping and initiation of right and left coronary artery perfusion. This interval varies, depending on the sequences elected by the surgeon, but can seldom be reduced below 2 to 3 minutes. If exposure for the operation is hampered by leakage of blood around the cannulae, coronary perfusion may have to be discontinued for short periods during the procedure.

When this method is used, the flow rate is of obvious importance, and information obtained for patients in whom the flow was delivered separately and directly into the right and left coronary arteries during aortic valve replacement provides useful information in this regard.[B5,H20] This information indicates that total coronary blood flow of about 200 to 250 mL · min^{-1} (approximately 120 to 150 mL · min^{-1} · m^{-2}) is optimal, at least at 30°C. This flow is comfortably below the 300-mL · min^{-1} level, which under some circumstances produces histologic evidence of myocardial damage.[I1] Yet it is sufficient to prevent undesirable vasoconstriction, which leaves part of the microcirculation without flow, or at least underperfused.

When this method is used, the heart should be kept beating; therefore, the perfusate should be warmer than 30°C. Spanos and colleagues[S5] showed that when ventricular fibrillation persisted throughout the period of coronary perfusion, risk of perioperative infarction and death was higher than if the heart were beating. This would be expected from knowledge of subendocardial blood flow during ventricular fibrillation.[B4,H6]

Hypothermic Fibrillating Heart

In continuous coronary perfusion with ventricular fibrillation, fibrillation can be maintained by an electrical current, which is necessary when the perfusion is at 37°C, or it may be spontaneously or electrically induced and maintained by moderately hypothermic (25° to 30°C) coronary perfusion. The latter condition is desirable. The coronary perfusion can be through the intact aortic root (as in coronary artery bypass grafting) or by individual coronary perfusion cannulae during aortic valve replacement.

A number of theoretical objections to the method can be raised. For example, perfusion of the subendocardium is impaired during CPB and ventricular fibrillation, particularly in hearts with ventricular hypertrophy. However, good clinical results have been obtained using either normothermic CPB and electrically maintained ventricular fibrillation or moderate hypothermia and ventricular fibrillation sustained only by hypothermia, or profound cardiac hypothermia and ventricular fibrillation. Akins has reported excellent results from coronary artery bypass grafting using the latter method.[A8,A12] Time constraints must apply to this method, as to most others, but they have not been defined.

The surgical conditions that exist with this method are better than with the beating heart, but most surgeons find them less satisfactory than with a cardioplegic technique.

Moderately Hypothermic Intermittent Global Myocardial Ischemia

Use of intermittent cardiac ischemia with moderate cardiac hypothermia requires conducting CPB with the perfusate temperature at 25° to 30°C. The surgeon works on or in the heart intermittently for periods of 10 to 15 minutes, during which time the ascending aorta is clamped (to stop coronary perfusion) or individual perfusion into the coronary ostia is interrupted. Between these periods, the aortic clamp is released (or individual coronary perfusion resumed) for 3 to 5 minutes. When the technique is used optimally, the heart is made to beat (not fibrillate) during this interval. This was the method most commonly used during the 1960s and early 1970s and is used by some surgeons today.

The clinical results can be good, as was demonstrated by McGoon and by Bonchek and colleagues.[A19,B42,M8] McGoon's analysis of one group of patients—those receiving valved extracardiac conduits—indicated no relationship between the proportion of nonsurvivors in the experience and cumulative aortic clamp time. However, because 35% of the 468 patients in the group had low cardiac output postoperatively[M8] (in which subset the mortality was 52%), the method must have been producing myocardial damage. However, Reduto and colleagues found no difference in left ventricular performance early after coronary artery bypass grafting, regardless of whether this or cold cardioplegic myocardial protection was used.[R16]

The method does not provide optimal exposure for operations inside the heart, but does provide reasonable working conditions for the coronary artery bypass grafting. Unless the heart is electrically fibrillated just before the aortic clamping, it continues to beat during much of the ischemic period, making precise repair difficult. Each time coronary perfusion is recommenced, coronary (and perhaps systemic) air embolization may occur, despite precautions against it. A considerable amount of blood comes into the heart during periods of coronary perfusion, stressing the intracardiac sucker systems and thereby increasing blood damage and interfering with the smooth and efficient flow of the operation. Moreover, each time the coronary arteries are perfused in this uncontrolled manner, a reperfusion injury may occur.

Profoundly Hypothermic Global Myocardial Ischemia

The heart may be profoundly cooled by the perfusate and/or by filling the pericardium with very cold saline solution, after which the aorta is aortic-clamped. The cardiac operation is done during a single period of aortic clamping.[B6,C5,G2,H8,K4,P1,S6] In clinical practice, myocardial temperature is generally about 22°C with these methods[C6]; most surgeons believe that this allows 45 to 60 minutes of safe global myocardial ischemia.

This technique provides better operating conditions than do those discussed earlier, and good results have been obtained with it. Despite this important consideration, a randomized study of patients undergoing aortic valve replacement showed that this technique results in as much myocardial necrosis as does continuous individual coronary perfusion.[S1]

Profoundly hypothermic cardiac ischemia without cardioplegia may be preferred for infant cardiac surgery in which hypothermic circulatory arrest is used. Part of the rationale for this preference is that no perfusate passes through the heart to rewarm or inadequately reperfuse it during circulatory arrest, as may happen when CPB is continued.

Drug-Mediated Myocardial Protection

Both β-adrenergic receptor-blocking and calcium channel-blocking drugs, in conjunction with one of the other methods, have been used as part of the myocardial management by some groups.[C9,C10,M12] The calcium channel-blocking agents, verapamil and diltiazem, have seemed particularly advantageous, because of their prevention of calcium influx into cells and coronary vasodilatory effects.[B20,L14] However, these drugs are potent negative ionotropes and produce prolonged electromechanical quiescence, at least when used clinically in cardioplegic solutions.[B38,C7]

Particularly good results have been obtained by giving lidoflazine intravenously just before CPB and using moderately hypothermic intermittent cardiac ischemia.[F9,F10,K11] Lidoflazine is believed to be a nucleotide transport inhibitor, which results in increased myocardial accumulation of endogenous adenosine during ischemia, increased lactate extraction during reperfusion, and improved postischemic function.[C16] The basic action of lidoflazine is complex and appears to be different from that of β-blocking and calcium channel-blocking drugs.

Certain drugs have been shown in experimental studies to reduce reperfusion damage related to oxygen-derived free radicals (see "Advantageous Conditions during Reperfusion" earlier in this chapter). However, when using blood cardioplegia and pressure-controlled, initially hyperkalemic blood reperfusion, incorporation of free radical scavengers has not been demonstrated to provide additional protection.

Cold Cardioplegia (Multidose)

A number of techniques for cold cardioplegia provide good results. An encyclopedic review of all the available methods recommended by clinical and experimental studies would serve little purpose, particularly because it has been provided in two texts.[H15,R24]

Cardioplegic Solution

There are both asanguinous solutions and those that are mixed with blood (at a 2:1 or 4:1 blood:solution ratio), and extracellular solutions and intracellular solutions as distin-

■ TABLE 3-1   Asanguinous Cardioplegic Solutions (as Prepared Commercially)

Components	Plegisol — St. Thomas II	CAPS [a] — Buckberg	Bretschneider	ViaSpan — UW	Units
K^+	16	60	10	125	mEq/L or mmol/L
Na^+	110	[b]	15	30	mEq/L or mmol/L
Cl^-	128	[b]	50	41.5	mEq/L or mmol/L
Ca^{2+}	2.4/1.2	–	–	–	mEq/L / mmol/L
Mg^{2+}	32/16	–	8/4	5/2.5	mEq/L / mmol/L
$PO_4{}^{2-}$	–	–	–	50/25	mEq/L / mmol/L
Histidine	–	–	198	–	mmol/L
Tryptophan	–	–	2	–	mmol/L
Ketoglutarate	–	–	1	–	mmol/L
Glucose	–	4	–	–	g/L
Mannitol	–	–	30	–	mmol/L
THAM (0.3 mol)	–	200	–	–	mL
CPD	–	50	–	–	mL
Raffinose	–	–	–	30	mmol/L
K-Lactobionate	–	–	–	100	mmol/L
Allopurinol	–	–	–	1	mmol/L
Adenosine	–	–	–	3	mmol/L
Hydroxyethyl starch	–	–	–	50	g/L
Glutathione	–	–	–	5	mmol/L
pH	7.8	7.65	7.1	7.4	
Osmolarity	280	~350	310	320	mOsm/L
Additives [c]					
$NaHCO_3{}^-$	10	–	25	–	mEq/L or mmol/L
0.46 mol aspartate glutamate [d]	–	–	250	–	mL
Insulin	–	–	–	40	units/L
Dexamethasone	–	–	–	16	mmol/L

[a] This formulation is intended for dilution by 2 or 4 parts blood (perfusate) to solution.

[b] Concentration is diluent dependent.

[c] Added to the commercially prepared solutions.

[d] For warm induction and reperfusion strategies only.

BOX 3-1   Elements to Limit Ischemic Damage during Induced Myocardial Ischemia

Electromechanical arrest
  Depolarization: (K^+) (Ca^{2+} channel blockers)
  Hyperpolarization: (Na^+-K^+ channel openers)
Hypothermia
  Perfusate
  External cooling
  Cold infusate
Substrate enhancement
  Oxygenation of crystalloid or blood
  Glucose-insulin
  Glutamate-aspartate
Buffering
  HCO_3
  THAM
  Histidine
  Imidazole buffers
  Blood
Washout of metabolites
  Repeated infusion
Control of Ca^{2+} flux
  CPD blood
  Low [Ca^{2+}]
Antioxidants
  Mannitol
  Allopurinol
Uniform delivery, antegrade, and retrograde

---

guished by their potassium concentrations (Table 3-1). Some believe that the components of the solution, particularly K^+ concentrations, should be altered according to solution temperature, timing of infusion (initial, maintenance, and terminal), and presumed energy state of the myocardium. In general, K^+ concentration is lowered for maintenance, and substrates are added for energy-depleted hearts. Delivery can be intermittent (multidose) or continuous; in the latter case the K^+ concentration is lower than for intermittent delivery (Box 3-1).

Hyperkalemic cold sanguineous cardioplegia is advantageous[B50] and is preferred, although asanguineous cardioplegia may work equally well. The Buckberg formulation (cold oxygenated hyperkalemic blood–crystalloid mixture, with lowered free calcium concentration, added glucose, and added buffering capacity) may be preferable to simple hyperkalemic blood (see Table 3-1). The latter, however, is less costly because it involves only transferring blood perfusate from the CPB oxygenator to a separate reservoir–heat exchanger–pump system, adding sufficient potassium chloride to make it cardioplegic (potassium concentration about 22 mmol · L^{-1}).

Technique of Antegrade Infusion

After CPB is established with the perfusate at 32°C (under which conditions ventricular fibrillation should not develop), an aortic root catheter is inserted through a previously placed purse-string stitch, attached to the cardioplegia line, and de-aired. Optionally, the pressure line of the cannula may be attached to a strain gauge for continuous measurement of aortic root pressure. The aorta is clamped as soon as the aortic root catheter is in place, and in any event before the heart has been cooled sufficiently by the whole body perfusion that it becomes arrhythmic or develops ventricular fibrillation.

Cold cardioplegic infusion is begun promptly at a flow of 150 mL · min^{-1} · m^{-2} (based on the data for continuous direct coronary perfusion described earlier in this chapter) for 3 minutes in adults; the average adult is given a dose of about 750 mL. In infants and children with a body surface area of less than 1 m^2, the infusion is given at the same flow rate (150 mL · min^{-1} · m^{-2} body surface area), but for only 2 minutes. Occasionally the monitored aortic root pressure is less than 30 mmHg, in which case the flow rate, but not the total dose, is increased. However, low aortic root perfusion pressure may be due to aortic regurgitation, hidden by the action of a left ventricular vent; the surgeon must be certain that this is not the situation. In patients with severe ischemic heart disease, the aortic root pressure sometimes rises above 75 mmHg, but the flow should not be reduced.

External cooling of the heart may be established while the cardioplegic infusion is being administered. An isolating pad can be placed between the heart and the left side of the pericardium containing the phrenic nerve. A thin layer of ice slush (or ice-cold saline) is placed over the anterior surface of the heart. Later, whenever the heart will be in a stable position for a time, a thin layer of ice slush can be placed on the surface. The slush is never placed in the pericardial space itself, because left phrenic nerve damage may result. As the slush melts, the fluid is aspirated with the high-vacuum sucker. If it is surgically inconvenient, the slush is omitted.

Neither the left nor the right ventricle is allowed to become distended at any time. A left ventricular vent (introduced through a right pulmonary vein) is used for some operations, suction through an aortic root catheter for others, and simple needle aspiration of the ventricle across the ventricular septum for others.

Cardioplegic solution is reinfused about every 25 minutes.[L6,N6] The initial flow rate is used, and the surgeon must be certain that the aortic valve has closed as the infusion begins. If it has not, a few pinches of the proximal aorta usually accomplish valve closure. Reinfusion is given for 30 to 60 seconds. After the first infusion, the potassium concentration of any subsequently infused cardioplegic solution is reduced to about 10 mmol · L^{-1}.

Should serum potassium levels reach 7 to 8 mEq · L^{-1} (a rare occurrence), a bolus injection of 400 mg · kg^{-1} of glucose (as 50% glucose) and 0.2 unit · kg^{-1} of soluble insulin may be given after the beginning of myocardial reperfusion. Because the levels of both whole body intracellular potassium[P4] and circulating insulin[C3] are abnormally low at this point, these maneuvers are physiologically reasonable.

Technique of Retrograde Infusion

Retrograde infusion of cardioplegic solutions directly into the coronary sinus was suggested by Lillehei and colleagues in 1956.[L18] Many have found this technique as effective as antegrade infusion,[A20] although the right ventricle, particularly its midportion, and the right atrium are less well perfused. When instead retrograde infusion is administered through the right atrium and right ventricle, this problem may be avoided.[F13,G11,M10,M13,P2,R23,S8] Retrograde coronary sinus infusion is particularly advantageous in the presence of acutely developing high-grade coronary artery stenoses or obstructions.[G8]

The surgeon should arrange to deliver either antegrade or retrograde cardioplegia, or both. Either before or after CPB has been established, a purse-string stitch is placed in the right atrial wall, and a small stab wound is made in the middle, through which the retrograde infusion catheter is introduced and under digital control manipulated into the coronary sinus.[B13] The catheter is attached to one arm of the cardioplegia infusion line and de-aired. The pressure measuring arm of the catheter is connected to a manometer. Coronary sinus pressure must not be allowed to rise above 50 mmHg during coronary sinus infusion.

Indications for combined antegrade–retrograde or totally retrograde infusion vary among surgeons,[B8] in part because no clear advantage of retrograde over antegrade infusion of cardioplegic solutions has been identified in patients undergoing elective operations.[F2] However, for aortic valve replacement and during mitral valve operations, reinfusions of cardioplegic solution are often more conveniently given by the retrograde method. The same may be true for many operations performed through the right atrium for congenital heart disease.

A conscious decision to utilize both the antegrade and retrograde routes of cardioplegia routinely, delivered in either an alternating sequential fashion or simultaneously, has evolved in the practice of some institutions.[B48] This method allows rapid electromechanical quiescence, protects against uneven cardioplegic distribution, and may maximize the duration of ischemia while avoiding cardioplegia overdose. The combined approach has also been successful in pediatric patients.[D10]

Thus, we believe retrograde cardioplegia is better viewed as synergistic and complementary to antegrade cardioplegia rather than as the sole method of myocardial management.[B48]

Severe obstructive manifestations of coronary artery disease are perhaps the best example for the superiority of retrograde cardioplegia. These include left main lesions and acute coronary syndromes.

Various procedures on the aortic valve and the ascending aorta demanding long clamp times are safely accomplished using coronary ostial infusion supplemented by retrograde infusion. These include acute aortic dissections and the Ross procedure.

Retrograde cardioplegic myocardial protection has some disadvantages. It clearly has various degrees of maldistribution to the right ventricle.[A22,A23,W3] There is the odd occasion when a left superior vena cava is encountered and is unrecognized. Infrequently, the retrograde cannula cannot be placed or is dislodged. There may be less satisfactory protection in hearts with severe left ventricular hypertrophy. Application may be difficult in children and sometimes impossible in neonates. Coronary sinus rupture is a well-known complication. (It can be dealt with before separation from CPB by closure of the rupture with fine suture or oversewing the sinus at the site of rupture). Finally, retrograde cardioplegia demands more cannulae, and in some situations seems to clutter the field in greater measure than its benefit.

Results of Cold Cardioplegia

Despite several randomized trials and numerous observational studies, the quantitative advantage of the cold cardioplegic technique over other methods of myocardial management in low-risk patients is not unequivocally defined. This alone suggests that it may be small in routine operations performed with reasonable dispatch. The technique facilitates the cardiac operation, and it is the technique most widely used today.

Even with cold cardioplegia, the "safe" duration of the global myocardial ischemic time is not unlimited. Furthermore, it varies according to preoperative ventricular hypertrophy, ventricular function, and energy charge of the myocardium. In general, it is probably about 100 minutes with this particular technique and without controlled reperfusion.

Antegrade cardioplegia has proved safe and effective over many years and in many clinical settings. It is easily accomplished and requires little special equipment. However, myocardial protection in some situations is admittedly imperfect using classic antegrade cardioplegia, and thus outcomes may be improved with retrograde cardioplegia delivery.

Retrograde delivery may be superior or synergistic in redo coronary artery bypass grafting, particularly in the presence of narrowed or obstructed saphenous vein grafts or with an open left internal thoracic artery to an obstructed left anterior descending coronary artery. When coronary artery bypass grafting is planned in the presence of mild aortic regurgitation (valve not replaced), retrograde cardioplegia is optimal for induction and maintenance. This is also true for other procedures with mild aortic regurgitation in which the aorta need not be opened for direct infusion.

Single-Dose Cold Cardioplegia in Neonates and Infants

An opinion has been expressed elsewhere in this chapter that (1) no compelling evidence exists that a different method of myocardial management is required in neonates and infants than in older patients, even though some of the characteristics of the heart in these small patients are different from those in older patients, and (2) the optimal method of myocardial management in general remains arguable.

A method that has given excellent results in neonates and infants is single-dose, oxygenated St. Thomas solution (see Table 3-1). Using a simple pressure bag, it is infused into the aortic root proximal to the aortic clamp. The dose is 20 mL · kg^{-1}. The dose is not repeated.

An exception is the first stage of the hypoplastic left heart operation (Norwood operation). The ascending aorta is thin and small in this situation. Simple cold ischemic arrest may be used, primarily because this avoids insertion of a needle into the delicate ascending aorta.

Continuous Cardioplegic Coronary Perfusion
Cold Perfusion

Continuous antegrade cold blood cardioplegia has been used as an alternative to single-dose and multidose intermittent cold cardioplegia. Khuri and colleagues have reported data from measurement of myocardial pH indicating that, at least in hypertrophied hearts, the myocardial milieu is more normal, although not completely normal, with this method than

with intermittent cold cardioplegia.[K9] A similar inference was drawn by Bomfim and colleagues from their clinical studies of the method.[B10] Anecdotal clinical experiences suggest that retrograde continuous cold cardioplegic perfusion through the coronary sinus also provides an excellent method of myocardial management during cardiac surgery. Some have used this method after giving an initial antegrade dose of cold cardioplegia. Under experimental conditions, cold retrograde blood cardioplegia after initial antegrade cold blood cardioplegia was found to maintain optimal myocardial pH.[J12]

Warm Perfusion

Continuous warm blood cardioplegia, administered by antegrade infusion or by retrograde coronary sinus infusion after an initial antegrade dose, has also been used for coronary artery bypass grafting and other cardiac operations.[L4,S24,S25] Some groups have found recovery of ventricular function better with the use of warm continuous blood cardioplegia than with intermittent cold cardioplegia.[Y5] Others have found similar efficacy between warm and cold.[M26] Although continuous warm blood cardioplegia provides good protection of the myocardium, it is surgically inconvenient for certain operations.

Cold Cardioplegia, Controlled Aortic Root Reperfusion, and (When Needed) Warm Cardioplegic Induction

In the belief that control of all aspects of the reperfusion may be even more important than details of cold cardioplegia, and that acutely ill patients coming to the operating room require a special form of myocardial management, the technique described in this section may be used. During reperfusion the heart is separated from the ongoing events in the remainder of the body for a brief time. The technique is surgically convenient, prolongs the operation only mildly, is essentially devoid of ventricular fibrillation, minimizes myocardial stunning and myocardial necrosis, and appears to result in better postoperative cardiac performance than methods previously used (Fig. 3-8).[F14] Yet the proof of its advantages has remained as difficult to obtain as for other techniques, which probably accounts for the fact that it is not, as yet, widely used in its entirety.

Some may wish to use simpler methods for routine operations and to restrict the use of this method for more complex, high-risk operations. The problems with such a plan are the usual operational disadvantages of a surgical method that is used infrequently rather than routinely (see "Human Error" in Chapter 6), and the fact that even routine operations have a small mortality and occasionally considerable morbidity, which may be nearly eliminated by more perfect myocardial management.

Circuitry

A small separate system on the pump-oxygenator, with its own miniaturized heat exchanger^2 and two pumps, manages aortic root (and/or retrograde) infusions. It enables the solution of choice to be infused at controlled temperature

---

^{2} Bentley (surface, stainless steel; priming volume, 120 mL; efficiency 0.8) or Shiley (surface, anodized aluminum; priming volume, 150 mL; efficiency 0.6).

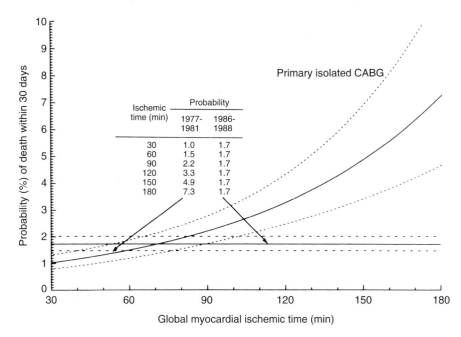

Figure 3-8   Relation between global myocardial ischemic time (minutes) and probability of death within 30 days of operation. The two depictions are nomograms of multivariable equations describing the UAB experience with isolated primary coronary artery bypass grafting from 1977 to 1981 ($n = 3872$) and from 1986 to 1988 ($n = 2351$). Cold cardioplegia was used in both eras, but in the later era, controlled aortic root reperfusion was used in patients with longer global myocardial ischemic times. Solid lines depict the continuous estimate of probability, and dashed lines enclose 70% confidence intervals around the estimate. (From Kirklin and colleagues.[K6])

and pressure. Although the circuitry seems complex, from the surgeon's standpoint its use is simple and extremely flexible. Perfusionists have demonstrated their ability to manage it both effectively and efficiently.

Technique for Elective Surgery

After the operation is completed, using cardioplegic myocardial management and with the aortic clamp still in place, controlled aortic root reperfusion is begun, initially using warm, hyperkalemic, modified, and enriched blood cardioplegia. The aortic root pressure is kept at 30 mmHg for the first 60 to 120 seconds of the reperfusion, for the reasons discussed earlier. The flow is then increased until the aortic root pressure is 50 to 75 mmHg in adults (or to the normal systemic arterial diastolic pressure in infants and children whose body surface area is less than 1 m²). A total of 500 mL of the modified blood reperfusate is administered. For patients with a body surface area of less than 1.5 m², the reperfusate volume = 500 × BSA ÷ 1.5. Once that has been infused, the perfusionist continues the controlled aortic root reperfusion by arranging the circuit so that aortic root perfusion continues with normothermic, normokalemic, unmodified blood.

During the controlled aortic root reperfusion, the surgeon must concentrate on avoiding ventricular distention, the adverse effects of which have been fully documented.[A18,B41]

The heart remains flaccid and electromechanically quiescent for 2 to 10 minutes after the onset of the controlled aortic root reperfusion. During this time, the coronary resistance may rise, requiring the perfusionist to reduce the flow rate to maintain a constant aortic root pressure. Should that occur, boluses of 5 mL of nitroglycerin[3] may be administered into the line by the surgeon, although the value of this is uncertain.

When the period of quiescence passes and cardiac action

begins, the initial rhythm frequently is AV dissociation. Very rarely, it is ventricular fibrillation.[F14] The controlled aortic root perfusion continues. Small-volume pulmonary ventilation is begun, because the right ventricle pumps some blood through the lungs. Even the vented left ventricle will eject some blood into the isolated aortic root. The perfusionist must be alert to the need to reduce the aortic root perfusion flow rate to keep the aortic root pressure from becoming excessively high (greater than 120 mmHg). At times, the perfusionist may need to place suction on the aortic root pressure catheter to prevent this problem.

Controlled aortic root perfusion is continued until sinus rhythm has returned and ventricular contractions are strong. The interval between the beginning of the controlled aortic root reperfusion and the reaching of these end points is usually 10 to 25 minutes. When the end points cannot be reached, myocardial management was in some way imperfect, and the patient almost certainly will require pharmacologic or mechanical support after CPB.

When the end points are reached, the perfusionist places strong suction (rather than perfusion) on the aortic root catheter and partly occludes the venous line so that some blood passes into the right ventricle and through the lungs; the anesthesiologist intermittently inflates the lung to assist in moving any air that is present out of the pulmonary veins and left atrium into the left ventricle, which ejects it into the aortic root. The suction on the aortic root catheter evacuates any mobilized boluses of air, as the surgeon ballots the left atrium and pulmonary veins. These procedures are repeated several times. Although strong suction continues on the aortic root catheter, the aortic clamp is released. As the clamp is released, the patient's blood volume is rapidly augmented to bring the left atrial or pulmonary artery wedge pressure to 6 to 10 mmHg, so that the heart's ejection will continue to maintain a good systemic arterial pressure and a good coronary perfusion pressure. Thereafter, the usual detailed de-airing procedure is followed (see "De-Airing the Heart" in Section 3 of Chapter 2). CPB is then discontinued; usually

---

[3] One milligram of nitroglycerin in 5 mL of a balanced salt solution.

nothing remains but to establish hemostasis and close the chest.

Technique for Energy-Depleted Hearts

Patients who come to operation in acute cardiac failure with hemodynamic instability or are severely cyanotic have energy-depleted hearts. Specific efforts to improve the energy charge of the heart before submitting it to the period of global myocardial ischemia probably result in better cardiac structure and function postoperatively.[R10,R22] Survival should thereby be enhanced.

After making the median sternotomy, CPB at 35°C is established as expeditiously as possible. The aortic root catheter is inserted. The aorta is clamped, and warm hyperkalemic, modified and enriched blood infusion is begun. The infusion is given at the usual flow rate for the induction of cardioplegia and continued for 5 minutes. The perfusionist then makes the cardioplegic solution as cold as possible, while the aortic root infusion of the same cardioplegic solution continues for another 3 minutes.

Subsequent cold infusions are given every 20 to 30 minutes as usual, except with a potassium concentration of about 10 mmol · L^{-1}. After completion of the cardiac procedure, the warm reperfusion is performed in the standard manner. (See "Special Situations and Controversies" in this chapter for details on myocardial management when an acute coronary occlusion immediately precedes the operation.)

ANCILLARY MEASURES FOR PREVENTING MYOCARDIAL DAMAGE

Important myocardial necrosis can develop between induction of anesthesia and start of CPB in as many as 30% to 40% of patients undergoing coronary artery bypass grafting when anesthetic and supportive management is suboptimal (Roe CR: unpublished data; 1976). Lell and colleagues have shown that this proportion can fall to almost 3% under optimum circumstances.[L5] No doubt patients other than those undergoing coronary artery bypass grafting are also at risk of developing myocardial damage during this period, particularly those with marked ventricular hypertrophy or reduced myocardial energy charge. Proper intraoperative management before and after CPB avoids increased myocardial oxygen demand (which can be caused by arterial hypertension, tachycardia, and increased endogenous catecholamine secretion from anxiety and excitement). It avoids high ventricular end-diastolic pressures and the concomitant detrimental effect on perfusion of the subendocardium.[H13] Good management maintains an optimal myocardial oxygen supply by maintaining adequate arterial oxygen levels and arterial blood pressure and adjusts ventricular preload and afterload to achieve a reasonable compromise between adequacy of cardiac output and avoidance of deleterious effects (see Chapter 4 for details).

Important perioperative myocardial necrosis can develop because of events occurring after CPB, either before or after the patient leaves the operating room. These may be events that produce imbalances between myocardial oxygen demand and supply. The use of catecholamines for treatment of low cardiac output early after CPB can result in myocardial necrosis.[H14,M11,P5]

SPECIAL SITUATIONS AND CONTROVERSIES

Species and Model Differences

Possible species and model differences pose a major problem in generating inferences regarding myocardial management during cardiac surgery in human subjects. For example, extensive myocardial edema is frequently observed after ischemia and reperfusion in experimental studies of many different types in many different animal models.[R14] Yet in clinical experience it has been rarely evident, except for instances of prolonged and severe damage and of some operations in young patients. In support of this, a careful study in humans using two-dimensional echocardiography failed to disclose any increase in left ventricular mass (a reasonably sensitive indicator of increased myocardial water) after uncomplicated cardiac operations in which cardioplegia was used. By contrast, the same study in a dog model showed a marked sudden increase in left ventricular mass.[S12]

Inferences from studies in isolated supported heart models, usually rat heart, are generally transferred to human cardiac surgery with some difficulty. This difficulty is considerably increased when the isolated heart models are perfused with a crystalloid solution, because such models behave differently from blood-perfused models.[W2]

Inferences from studies of immature hearts in animal models are transferred with difficulty to cardiac surgery in neonates and infants, because the relationship of age-defined cardiac immaturity in one species to that in another is uncertain.

These considerations emphasize that confirmation must continually be sought of the applicability to humans of inferences derived from animal models.

Neonates and Infants

Certain cardiac events begin at birth and change the characteristics of the neonatal heart into those of a mature heart. The time frame of many of these events is not known. As a result, the rather noncompliant neonatal heart[L13,R26] gradually becomes more compliant and proceeds from having little functional reserve[T3,T4] to having that of the mature heart. Coronary reserve may be greater in immature hearts.[T5]

In general, the normal neonatal and infant heart is believed to be more resistant to ischemic and reperfusion damage than is the normal adult heart, even when both are protected by hypothermia during the ischemic period.[B18,G4] This greater resistance is not necessarily present in hearts of cyanotic neonates and children or those in acute or chronic heart failure.

Ischemic Damage

The cell membrane (sarcolemma) of myocytes from immature hearts is generally believed to be more resistant to the calcium paradox and other forms of calcium damage than that of myocytes from mature hearts.[C2] Related to this is the finding that the sarcolemma of immature hearts binds calcium more effectively than that of mature hearts.[B34] All this points to greater stability of the sarcolemma of immature hearts and tighter glycocalyceal junction, and consequently to greater resistance to the intracellular influx of calcium during and after ischemia.[F12,N11] (However, some data suggest *less* membrane stability and less resistance to calcium influx in the *newborn,* in contrast to the *neonatal,* heart.[P7]) By contrast, immature hearts do not have as good a capacity to sequester (immobilize) intracellular calcium as do mature hearts,[S23] making them more vulnerable to damage once calcium has entered the cells.[F12]

The adult myocardium normally relies primarily on fatty acids to produce energy for myocardial contraction and cell survival. This is also true in the neonatal heart; in contrast to the adult heart, the neonatal heart has relatively large glycogen stores, and thus a relatively large capacity for anaerobic glycolysis. This feature begins to disappear shortly after birth[H16] and has disappeared completely by about 2 months of age. ATP utilization appears to be slower in immature hearts, because of lower contractile energy requirements.[A4] These mechanisms, and perhaps others, probably provide to both neonatal and immature but otherwise normal infant hearts a higher tolerance to ischemia than that possessed by adult hearts.[B36,B37,F11,G4,J7,N10,S6,Y3]

Larger stores of amino acids in neonatal hearts also contribute to their increased capacity for anaerobic metabolism, including ATP production, and this persists throughout infancy. This anaerobic ATP production appears to be for the transamination and substrate level phosphorylation of glutamate and pyruvate.[J6] This may be expected to result in better maintenance of cellular integrity during ischemia and thereby better functional recovery after ischemia than experienced by adult hearts. These considerations also help explain the demonstrated value of amino acid supplementation for improving tolerance of the immature heart to ischemia and hypoxia.[J8,M15] However, some have found the immature myocardium (less than about 18 months old) to be deficient in cytosolic 5'-nucleotidase and thereby less able than mature myocardium to convert cyclic AMP and inosine back to ATP.[L10]

Reperfusion Damage

Complement activation and leukocyte infiltration play as important a role in reperfusion injury in immature hearts as they do in mature hearts.[B16] Other than this, little is known about possible differences in susceptibility of immature hearts to reperfusion (as compared with ischemic) injury, compared with mature hearts.

Abnormal Immature Hearts

These characteristics of normal neonatal and infant myocardium may or may not be characteristic of abnormal neonatal or infant hearts. Neonates and infants who come to cardiac surgery are unlikely to have normal myocardium, because they are usually either cyanotic or in heart failure, or both. Julia and colleagues have shown that immature hearts in acute cardiac failure or recently subjected to hypoxia develop profound functional depression after periods of ischemia well tolerated by normal immature hearts.[J13] Thus, neonates and infants who come to open heart surgery probably have hearts that are *not* unusually resistant to the damaging effects of global myocardial ischemia. Cyanosis, both acute and chronic, accelerates the damaging effect of global myocardial ischemia and lessens

postischemic recovery, probably as a result of its effect on myocardial metabolism.[F7,L17,V2]

Buckberg[B49] has demonstrated experimentally that cyanotic neonates and infants may suffer myocardial injury simply by exposure to reoxygenation during CPB, particularly the initial stages of CPB. This hypoxemic/reoxygenation injury may be avoidable by beginning CPB at the ambient oxygen tension of the hypoxemic subject. Reoxygenation injury is linked to oxidant damage and a lack of antioxidant reserve capacity in cyanotic immature myocardium. Reoxygenation is associated with elevation of conjugated dienes, generation of hydroxyl radicals causing lipid peroxidation, and release of nitric oxide. Buckberg's studies further suggest that adding desferrioxamine and antioxidants (*N*-[2-mereoptoproprionyl]-glycine, catalase, and coenzyme Q_{10}) to the CPB prime might limit in vivo oxidant damage and improve myocardial functional reserve. The importance of these observations made in animal preparations has yet to be clarified in human neonatal myocardial management.

Methods of Myocardial Management

The effectiveness of cold cardioplegia in the immature heart is arguable. A paper by Bull and colleagues is often cited in the introduction to experimental papers on the subject, in support of the idea that cold cardioplegia as used in adults is not effective in young patients.[B22] However, these investigators found the "safe" ischemic time to be 65 minutes when intermittent aortic clamping was used and 85 minutes when cold cardioplegia was used.[B22] Another early experience found cold crystalloid cardioplegia advantageous in neonates and infants,[K13] as did Schachner and colleagues in a small randomized trial.[S16]

From experimental models, many different and sometimes conflicting inferences have been derived. In one experimental study, cold cardioplegia was found to reduce ischemic injury in immature hearts.[A7] Multidose administration of cardioplegic solutions was shown to be disadvantageous in immature hearts.[K15] Various crystalloid solutions have been found experimentally to be superior to others for use in immature hearts. Other experimental studies have shown that including glutamate and aspartate in the warm induction of cardioplegia and in the reperfusate provides additional benefit.[F7,J9,K12]

One point of view, compatible with all available evidence but not with the opinions of some, is that the basic methodology for myocardial management in neonates, infants, and children should be similar to that in adults. Little concerted effort has been made to overcome the technical difficulty of accomplishing this in very small hearts. For example, in many operations in neonates, the procedure is done largely through the right atrium; retrograde infusion of the sanguineous cardioplegic solution into the coronary sinus should be particularly convenient. In fact, the feasibility, safety, and efficiency of retrograde coronary sinus infusion of the cardioplegic solution have already been demonstrated in the arterial switch operation.[Y4]

When using the technique of cold cardioplegia, controlled aortic root reperfusion, and (when needed) warm cardioplegic induction, all catheters, cannulae, doses, flow rates, and pressures should be scaled appropriately to small patients, as has been described.

Aortic Valve Surgery

Unless the aortic valve is completely competent, which is uncommon, the induction of cold cardioplegia for aortic valve repair or replacement is best accomplished by direct infusion of the solution into the coronary ostia, preceded by retrograde induction via the coronary sinus. The apparently complex sequence about to be described is unnecessary for cardioplegia with the capability for retrograde delivery, but is needed until retrograde *reperfusion* is established as a useful modality.

The circuit is modified at the operating table in such cases by placing a Y connector in the antegrade cardioplegia tubing, one distal arm of which connects to the aortic root infusion catheter and the other to a second Y, to each arm of which an O-ring direct coronary perfusion cannula is connected. A clamp is placed just beyond the first Y, on the tubing leading to the second Y and the direct coronary perfusion cannulae. After CPB has been established and the aortic root catheter has been inserted, properly connected, de-aired, and the line leading to it clamped and the line to the second Y unclamped, the aorta is clamped, and the aortic root is opened transversely but not completely. One of the O-ring cannulae is inserted into the left coronary ostia and about three fifths of the initial cardioplegic infusion given. A second O-ring cannula is similarly placed in the right coronary ostium and the remaining two fifths of the cardioplegic infusion given. Ideally, and when easily accomplished, both infusions are given simultaneously. A No. 5-0 or 6-0 polypropylene suture is placed around each of the cannulae, brought out of the adjacent aortic wall, and secured with a "snugger." Subsequent cardioplegic infusions may be given in this manner or retrogradely via the coronary sinus (see "Technique of Retrograde Infusion" earlier in this chapter).

A major reason for preferring this arrangement for the induction and maintenance of cardioplegia lies in the reperfusion phase. All devices for aortic valve replacement, except the allograft, autograft, and stentless xenograft valve inserted free hand or as an aortic root replacement, leak a variable but usually considerable amount of blood from the aortic root back through the sewing ring, at least, into the left ventricle. The left ventricular vent can keep the ventricle decompressed, but maintenance of desired aortic root pressure frequently becomes impossible during reperfusion via the aortic root. Therefore, the usually warm and initially hyperkalemic modified blood reperfusion after aortic valve surgery is infused through the direct coronary perfusion cannulae. Many surgeons use simultaneous retrograde coronary sinus infusion as an adjunct to this reperfusion phase, beginning with substrate-enhanced hyperkalemic blood, then switching to normothermic normokalemic blood. While this is proceeding, closure of the aortotomy begins. The left ventricular vent keeps the operative field dry even after cardiac action begins. The last few sutures of the aortotomy closure are placed but left loose.

When the heart is beating well and the criteria previously described for ceasing the controlled aortic root reperfusion are met, suction on the left ventricular vent is reduced to a low level or stopped. If necessary, the venous tubing is occluded briefly to drive a little blood through the lungs and back into the left ventricle. Blood ejected by the left ventricle now essentially fills the aortic root and escapes through the loose part of the suture line. An assistant clamps the tubing leading to the Y connector with its direct coronary perfusion cannulae and unclamps the line to the aortic root catheter, the perfusionist places mild suction on the aortic root catheter, and the surgeon removes the "snuggers" on the sutures around the coronary cannulae; the sutures and then the cannulae are removed, and the aortotomy sutures are snugged and tied. Because the heart is beating well, aortic root pressure (being monitored by the aortic root cannula as usual) may tend to rise, but the perfusionist controls this by increasing suction on the aortic root pressure monitoring catheter as needed. The aortic clamp is still in place, so systemic air embolization is not possible.

By mildly occluding the venous line, the perfusionist causes the left ventricle to receive sufficient blood so that its ejection maintains an aortic root pressure of about 100 mmHg systolic. Suction continues on the aortic root catheter, minimal or no suction is on the left ventricular vent, and usual de-airing procedures are accomplished (see Chapter 2). The aortic clamp is then removed, and the entire de-airing procedure is repeated. The remainder of the operation proceeds in the usual manner.

When aortic regurgitation is mild in patients requiring aortic valve replacement or other operations, the initial cardioplegic infusion may be administered antegradely in the usual way through the unopened aortic root or retrogradely via the previously placed coronary sinus cannula. If the aortic root infusion maintains an adequate pressure in the aortic root, and thus confirms that runoff is minimal, the left atrial vent line is clamped, the infusion continued, and the left ventricle gently massaged manually during the infusion period. This prevents left ventricular distention and assists in perfusing the coronary arteries. If runoff is excessive, an aortotomy is made and the cold cardioplegic infusion is given directly into the coronary ostia (see "Perfusion of Individual Coronary Arteries" earlier in this chapter).

Coexisting Mild Aortic Regurgitation

Some cardiac operations are complicated by the presence of aortic regurgitation, too mild to justify aortic valve replacement (or repair), but sufficient to complicate myocardial management. If an appropriate aortic root pressure can be maintained during induction of cold cardioplegia and reperfusion, then standard aortic root infusions are used.

If the regurgitation is such that an appropriate aortic root pressure *cannot* be achieved during the administration of the cold cardioplegic solution, or during reperfusion, cold cardioplegic solution is administered retrogradely through the coronary sinus. In the reperfusion phase, the heart can be carried through the initially warm hyperkalemic reperfusion and then the normokalemic reperfusion until cardiac action fully resumes, using exclusively retrograde perfusion through the coronary sinus.

Acute Occlusion of the Left Anterior Descending Coronary Artery

Patients brought to the operating room shortly after acute occlusion of the left anterior descending coronary artery (LAD) are usually hemodynamically unstable or in cardiogenic shock. Because of both the acute occlusion and the hemodynamic state, these patients present a special problem. The principles set down and tested by Allen and Buckberg and colleagues form the basis for the management program described here.[A17] These principles include (1) the initial controlled administration of warm cardioplegic solution (see "Cold Cardioplegia, Controlled Aortic Root Reperfusion, and [When Needed] Warm Cardioplegic Induction" earlier in this chapter), administered antegradely for 2½ minutes and retrogradely (through the coronary sinus) for 2½ minutes; (2) use of at least a vein graft to the LAD (or another coronary vessel if it is responsible for the acute infarction); and (3) prolonged (20 minutes) controlled reperfusion with hyperkalemic modified blood of the LAD (or another coronary artery if it was the culprit responsible for the area of acute ischemia).

The general plan of the operation is as described under "Technique of Operation" in Chapter 7. Initial warm cardioplegia (administered as just described) followed by usual cold cardioplegia produces cardiac quiescence. During the grafting procedure, it is supplemented in the usual manner by additional intermittent infusions of the cold cardioplegic solutions. Antegrade and retrograde routes of infusion are used alternately, or as dictated by ease of delivery, or by number of grafts in place.

Large Noncoronary Collateral Flow

Occasionally, in patients with long-standing severe coronary artery disease, noncoronary collateral blood flow may be large and, under the usual circumstances of the coronary operation, can actually restart cardiac electromechanical activity by washing out the cardioplegic solution, despite cardiac venting and multidose cardioplegia. Clinical experience indicates that under these circumstances, the risk of important myocardial damage is increased. Therefore, at the first sign of this development, the whole body perfusate temperature is made as cold as possible until the patient's temperature reaches 20°C; the perfusate temperature is then set at 20°C and CPB flow reduced to about $1 \, L \cdot min^{-1} \cdot m^{-2}$. Another dose of cold cardioplegia is then administered.

Active Rheumatic Pericarditis Necessitating Multiple Valve Surgery

Patients with active rheumatic pericarditis necessitating multiple valve surgery present special problems because of their extensive and vascular pericardial adhesions. If divided, these adhesions cause excessive bleeding and contribute an excessive collateral coronary flow. Such patients are critically ill, usually with aortic and mitral regurgitation. If cold cardioplegia is used, low-flow hypothermic perfusion and repeated cardioplegic infusions are necessary.

Reoperative Surgery

Reoperative coronary artery bypass grafting also may present special issues for myocardial management. In general, cardioplegic myocardial protection should be established early in the procedure—usually before mobilization of the cardiac mass. Antegrade and retrograde infusions are complementary; it is thus imperative that the retrograde catheter be placed accurately in the coronary sinus. This can be accomplished by minimal sharp dissection over the acute margin of the right ventricle followed by posterior freeing using finger dissection. In most cases a patent internal thoracic artery graft should be identified by careful dissection, partially mobilized, and occluded during the cardioplegic period. Occasionally, it can be left open and CPB conducted at low flow and 20°C.

Whether patent vein grafts should remain in situ is controversial; however, for induction of cardioplegia, aortic root antegrade infusion along with retrograde infusion with saphenous veins grafts left in place seems the surest way to obtain close to optimal delivery of the cardioplegic solution.

Because of adhesions the myocardium tends to rewarm more quickly than usual. More frequent cardioplegia infusion and/or low systemic perfusion temperature are appropriate.

REFERENCES

A

1. Assad-Morell JL, Wallace RB, Elveback LR, Gau GT, Connolly DC, Barnhorst DA, et al. Serum enzyme data in diagnosis of myocardial infarction during or early after aorta-coronary saphenous vein bypass graft operations. J Thorac Cardiovasc Surg 1975;69:851.

2. Archie JP Jr. Determinants of regional intramyocardial pressure. J Surg Res 1973;14:338.

3. Appelbaum A, Kouchoukos NT, Blackstone EH, Kirklin JW. Early risks of open heart surgery for mitral valve disease. Am J Cardiol 1976;37:201.

4. Abd-Elfattah A, Murphy C, Salter D, Goldstein J, Morris J, Wechsler A. Biochemical basis for tolerance of the newborn heart to ischemic injury: development differences in adenine nucleotide degradation between ischemic immature and adult canine myocardium. A possible role of sarcolemmal 5′ nucleotidase. Presented at the International Symposium on Myocardial Protection, Boston, May 9-11, 1985.

5. Abd-Elfattah AS, Jessen ME, Lekven J, Doherty NE III, Brunsting LA, Wechsler AS. Myocardial reperfusion injury. Role of myocardial hypoxanthine and xanthine in free radical-mediated reperfusion injury. Circulation 1988;78:III224.

6. Ambrosio G, Weisman HF, Mannisi JA, Becker LC. Progressive impairment of regional myocardial perfusion after initial restoration of postischemic blood flow. Circulation 1989;80:1846.

7. Avkiran M, Hearse DJ. Protection of the myocardium during global ischemia. Is crystalloid cardioplegia effective in the immature myocardium? J Thorac Cardiovasc Surg 1989;97:220.

8. Akins CW. Noncardioplegic myocardial preservation for coronary revascularization. J Thorac Cardiovasc Surg 1984;88:174.

9. Anderson PG, Bishop SP, Digerness SB. Transmural progression of morphologic changes during ischemic contracture and reperfusion in the normal and hypertrophied rat heart. Am J Pathol 1987; 129:152.

10. Aldea GS, Austin RE Jr, Flynn AE, Coggins DL, Husseini W, Hoffman JI. Heterogeneous delivery of cardioplegic solution in the absence of coronary artery disease. J Thorac Cardiovasc Surg 1990;99:345.

11. Addetia AM, O'Reilly BF, Walsh GW, Reid P. Prolonged asystole during intraoperative myocardial reperfusion. An experimental study. Ann Thorac Surg 1988;45:482.

12. Akins CW, Carroll DL. Event-free survival following nonemergency myocardial revascularization during hypothermic fibrillatory arrest. Ann Thorac Surg 1987;43:628.

13. Allen DG, Orchard CH. Myocardial contractile function during ischemia and hypoxia. Circ Res 1987;60:153.

14. Ambrosio G, Weisfeldt ML, Jacobus WE, Flaherty JT. Evidence for a reversible oxygen radical-mediated component of reperfusion injury: reduction by recombinant human superoxide dismutase administered at the time of reflow. Circulation 1987;75:282.

15. Acar C, Partington MT, Buckberg G. Studies of controlled reperfusion after ischemia. XVIII. Reperfusion conditions. Attenuation of the regional ischemic effect by temporary total vented bypass before controlled reperfusion. J Thorac Cardiovasc Surg 1990;100:737.

16. Atkinson DE. The control of citrate synthesis and breakdown. In Lowenstein JM, ed. Citric acid cycle, control and compartmentation. New York: Marcel Dekker, 1967, p. 137.

17. Allen BS, Buckberg GD, Schwaiger M, Yeatman L, Tillisch J, Kawata N, et al. Studies of controlled reperfusion after ischemia. Early recovery of regional wall motion in patients following surgical revascularization after eight hours of acute coronary occlusion. J Thorac Cardiovasc Surg 1986;92:636.

18. Allen BS, Okamoto F, Buckberg GD, Bugyi H, Leaf J. Studies of controlled reperfusion after ischemia. XIII. Reperfusion conditions: critical importance of total ventricular decompression during regional reperfusion. J Thorac Cardiovasc Surg 1986;92:605.

19. Antunes MJ, Bernardo JE, Oliveira JM, Fernandes LE, Andrade CM. Coronary artery bypass surgery with intermittent aortic cross-clamping. Eur J Cardiothorac Surg 1992;6:189.

20. Arom KV, Emery RW. Coronary sinus cardioplegia. Clinical trial with only retrograde approach. Ann Thorac Surg 1992;53:965.

21. Archie JP Jr. Intramyocardial pressure. Effect of preload on transmural distribution of systolic coronary blood flow. Am J Cardiol 1975;35:904.

22. Allen BS, Winkelmann JW, Hanafy H, Hartz RS, Bolling KS, Ham J, et al. Retrograde cardioplegia does not adequately perfuse the right ventricle. J Thorac Cardiovasc Surg 1995;109:1116.

23. Aronson S, Jacobsohn E, Savage R, Albertucci M. The influence of collateral flow on the antegrade and retrograde distribution of cardioplegia in patients with an occluded right coronary artery. Anesthesiology 1998;89:1099.

B

1. Brewer DL, Bilbro RH, Bartel AG. Myocardial infarction as a complication of coronary bypass surgery. Circulation 1973;47:58.

2. Bernard M, Menasche P, Pietri S, Grousset C, Piwnica A, Cozzone PJ. Cardioplegic arrest superimposed on evolving myocardial ischemia. Improved recovery after inhibition of hydroxyl radical generation by peroxidase or deferoxamine. A ^{31}P nuclear resonance study. Circulation 1988;78:III164.

3. Buckberg GD, Olinger GN, Mulder DG, Maloney JV Jr. Depressed postoperative cardiac performance: prevention by adequate myocardial protection during cardiopulmonary bypass. J Thorac Cardiovasc Surg 1975;70:974.

4. Buckberg GD, Brazier JR, Nelson RL, Goldstein SM, McConnell DH, Cooper N. Studies of the effects of hypothermia on regional myocardial blood flow and metabolism during cardiopulmonary bypass. I. The adequately perfused beating, fibrillating, and arrested heart. J Thorac Cardiovasc Surg 1977;73:87.

5. Barratt-Boyes BG, Harris EA, Kenyon AM, Lindop CA, Seelye ER. Coronary perfusion and myocardial metabolism during open-heart surgery in man. J Thorac Cardiovasc Surg 1976;72:133.

6. Brody WR, Reitz BA. Topical hypothermic protection of the myocardium. Ann Thorac Surg 1975;20:66.

7. Bretschneider HJ, Hubner G, Knoll D, Lohr B, Nordbeck H, Spieckermann PG. Myocardial resistance and tolerance to ischemia. Physiological and biochemical basis. J Cardiovasc Surg 1975;16:241.

8. Bhayana JN, Kalmbach T, Booth FV, Mentzer RM Jr, Schimert G. Combined antegrade/retrograde cardioplegia for myocardial protection. A clinical trial. J Thorac Cardiovasc Surg 1989;98:956.

9. Buckberg GD. A proposed "solution" to the cardioplegic controversy. J Thorac Cardiovasc Surg 1979;77:803.

10. Bomfim V, Kaijser L, Bendz R, Sylven C, Morillo F, Olin C. Myocardial protection during aortic valve replacement. Cardiac metabolism and enzyme release following continuous blood cardioplegia. Scand J Thorac Cardiovasc Surg 1981;15:141.

11. Brazier J, Hottenrott C, Buckberg G. Noncoronary collateral myocardial blood flow. Ann Thorac Surg 1975;19:426.

12. Bolling SF, Bies LE, Bove EL, Gallagher KP. Augmenting intracellular adenosine improves myocardial recovery. J Thorac Cardiovasc Surg 1990;99:469.

13. Buckberg GD. Antegrade/retrograde blood cardioplegia to ensure cardioplegic distribution: operative techniques and objectives. J Card Surg 1989;4:216.

14. Braunwald E. Myocardial reperfusion, limitation of infarct size, reduction of left ventricular dysfunction, and improved survival. Should the paradigm be expanded? Circulation 1989;79:441.

15. Bretschneider HJ. Myocardial protection. Thorac Cardiovasc Surg 1980;28:295.

16. Breda MA, Drinkwater DC, Laks H, Bhuta S, Corno AF, Davtyan HG, et al. Prevention of reperfusion injury in the neonatal heart with leukocyte-depleted blood. J Thorac Cardiovasc Surg 1989;97:654.

17. Bodenhamer RM, DeBoer LW, Geffin GA, O'Keefe DD, Fallon JT, Aretz TH, et al. Enhanced myocardial protection during ischemic arrest. Oxygenation of a crystalloid cardioplegic solution. J Thorac Cardiovasc Surg 1983;85:769.

18. Bove EL, Gallagher KP, Drake DH, Lynch MJ, Fox M, Forder J, et al. The effect of hypothermic ischemia on recovery of left ventricular function and preload reserve in the neonatal heart. J Thorac Cardiovasc Surg 1988;95:814.

19. Bolli R, Patel B. Factors that determine the occurrence of reperfusion arrhythmias. Am Heart J 1988;115:20.

20. Balderman SC, Chan AK, Gage AA. Verapamil cardioplegia. Improved myocardial preservation during global ischemia. J Thorac Cardiovasc Surg 1984;88:57.

21. Badylak SF, Simmons A, Turek J, Babbs CF. Protection from reperfusion injury in the isolated rat heart by postischaemic deferoxamine and oxypurinol administration. Cardiovasc Res 1987;21:500.

22. Bull C, Cooper J, Stark J. Cardioplegic protection of the child's heart. J Thorac Cardiovasc Surg 1984;88:287.

23. Bleese N, Doring V, Kalmar P, Krebber HJ, Pokar H, Rodewald G. Clinical application of cardioplegia in aortic cross-clamping periods longer than 150 minutes. J Thorac Cardiovasc Surg 1979;27:390.

24. Braunwald E. The stunned myocardium. Newer insights into mechanisms and clinical implications (letter to the editor). J Thorac Cardiovasc Surg 1990;100:310.

25. Bonhoeffer K, Standfuss K, Spieckerman PG. Der sauerstoffrerbrauch des hunderherzens nach karioplegie durch extrazellularen natriumentzug und novocain applikation. Pfluegers Arch Ges Physiol 1964;281:19.

26. Bretschneider HJ. Uberlebenszeit und wiederbelebungszeit des herzens bei normo-und hypothermie. Verh Dtsch Ges Kreislaufforsch 1964;30:11.

27. Braunwald E, Kloner RA. The stunned myocardium: prolonged, postischemic ventricular dysfunction. Circulation 1982;66:1146.

28. Beyersdorf F, Allen BS, Buckberg GD, Acar C, Okamoto F, Sjostrand F, et al. Studies on prolonged acute regional ischemia. I. Evidence for preserved cellular viability after 6 hours of coronary occlusion. J Thorac Cardiovasc Surg 1989;98:112.

29. Bavaria JE, Furukawa S, Kreiner G, Ratcliffe MB, Streicher J, Bogen DK, et al. Myocardial oxygen utilization after reversible global ischemia. J Thorac Cardiovasc Surg 1990;100:210.

30. Bolli R, Patel BS, Jeroudi MO, Lai EK, McCay PB. Demonstration of free radical generation in "stunned" myocardium of intact dogs with the use of the spin trap α-phenyl N-tert-butyl nitrone. J Clin Invest 1988;82:476.

31. Bolli R, Patel BS, Hartley CJ, Thornby JI, Jeroudi MO, Roberts R. Nonuniform transmural recovery of contractile function in stunned myocardium. Am J Physiol 1989;257:H375.

32. Bladergroen MR, Takei H, Christopher TD, Cummings RG, Blanchard SM, Lowe JE. Accelerated transmural gradients of energy compound metabolism resulting from left ventricular hypertrophy. J Thorac Cardiovasc Surg 1990;100:506.

33. Bolli R, Jeroudi MO, Patel BS, Aruoma OI, Halliwell B, Lai EK, et al. Marked reduction of free radical generation and contractile dysfunction by antioxidant therapy begun at the time of reperfusion. Evidence that myocardial "stunning" is a manifestation of reperfusion injury. Circ Res 1989;65:607.

34. Boucek RJ Jr, Shelton ME, Artman M, Landon E. Myocellular calcium regulation by the sarcolemmal membrane in the adult and immature rabbit heart. Basic Res Cardiol 1985;80:316.

35. Baerman JM, Kirsh MM, de Buitleir M, Hyatt L, Juni JE, Pitt B, et al. Natural history and determinants of conduction defects following coronary artery bypass surgery. Ann Thorac Surg 1987; 44:150.

36. Baker JE, Boerboom LE, Olinger GN. Age-related changes in the ability of hypothermia and cardioplegia to protect ischemic rabbit myocardium. J Thorac Cardiovasc Surg 1988;96:717.

37. Bove EL, Stammers AH. Recovery of left ventricular function after hypothermic global ischemia. Age-related differences in the isolated working rabbit heart. J Thorac Cardiovasc Surg 1986;91:115.

38. Barner HB, Swartz MT, Devine JE, Williams GA, Janosik D. Diltiazem as an adjunct to cold blood potassium cardioplegia. A clinical assessment of dose and prospective randomization. Ann Thorac Surg 1987;43:191.

39. Batist G, Mersereau W, Malashenko BA, Chiu RC. Response to ischemia-reperfusion injury in hypertrophic heart. Role of free-radical metabolic pathways. Circulation 1989;80:III10.

40. Beyersdorf F, Okamoto F, Buckberg GD, Sjostrand F, Allen BS, Acar C, et al. Studies on prolonged acute regional ischemia. II. Implications of progression from dyskinesia to akinesia in the ischemic segment. J Thorac Cardiovasc Surg 1989;98:224.

41. Buckberg GD. The importance of venting the left ventricle (editorial). Ann Thorac Surg 1975;20:488.

42. Bonchek LI, Burlingame MW, Vazales BE, Lundy EF, Gassmann CJ. Applicability of noncardioplegic coronary bypass to high-risk patients. Selection of patients, technique, and clinical experience in 3000 patients. J Thorac Cardiovasc Surg 1992;103:230.

43. Boyle EM Jr, Pohlman TH, Cornejo CJ, Verrier ED. Ischemia-reperfusion injury. Ann Thorac Surg 1996;62:S24.

44. Burns SA, DeGuzman BJ, Newburger JW, Mayer JE Jr, Neufeld EJ, Briscoe DM. P-selectin expression in myocardium of children undergoing cardiopulmonary bypass. J Thorac Cardiovasc Surg 1995; 110:924.

45. Banerjee A, Locke-Winter C, Rogers KB, Mitchell MB, Brew EC, Cairns CB, et al. Preconditioning against myocardial dysfunction after ischemia and reperfusion by an α₁-adrenergic mechanism. Circ Res 1993;73:656.

46. Burns PG, Krunkenkamp IB, Caldarone CA, Gaudette GR, Bukhari EA, Levitsky S. Does cardiopulmonary bypass alone elicit myoprotective preconditioning? Circulation 1995;92:II447.

47. Balderman SC, Binette JP, Chan AW, Gage AA. The optimal temperature for preservation of the myocardium during global ischemia. Ann Thorac Surg 1983;35:605.

48. Buckberg GD, Beyersdorf F, Allen BS, Robertson JM. Integrated myocardial management: background and initial application. J Card Surg 1995;10:68.

49. Buckberg G. Studies of hypoxemic/reoxygenation injury. J Thorac Cardiovasc Surg 1995;110:1163.

50. Buckberg GD. Oxygenated cardioplegia: blood is a many splendored thing. Ann Thorac Surg 1990;50:175.

C

1. Cooley DA, Reul GJ, Wukasch DC. Ischemic contracture of the heart: "stone heart." Am J Cardiol 1972;29:575.

2. Chizzonite RA, Zak R. Calcium-induced cell death. Susceptibility of cardiac myocytes is age-dependent. Science 1981;213:1508.

3. Chiu RC, McArdle HA. Levels of plasma cyclic AMP and insulin in cardiac surgery. J Thorac Cardiovasc Surg 1978;75:286.

4. Chawla SK, Najafi H, Javid H, Serry C. Coronary obstruction secondary to direct cannulation. Ann Thorac Surg 1977;23:135.

5. Cohn LH, Collins JJ Jr. Local cardiac hypothermia for myocardial protection. Ann Thorac Surg 1974;17:135.

6. Conti VR, Bertranou EG, Blackstone EH, Kirklin JW, Digerness SB. Cold cardioplegia versus hypothermia for myocardial protection. Randomized clinical study. J Thorac Cardiovasc Surg 1978;76:577.

7. Christakis GT, Fremes SE, Weisel RD, Tittley JG, Mickle DA, Ivanov J, et al. Diltiazem cardioplegia. A balance of risk and benefit. J Thorac Cardiovasc Surg 1986;91:647.

8. Chatelain P, Latour JG, Tran D, de Lorgeril M, Dupras G, Bourassa M. Neutrophil accumulation in experimental myocardial infarcts: relation with extent of injury and effect of reperfusion. Circulation 1987;75:1083.

9. Clark RE, Ferguson TB, West PN, Shuchleib RC, Henry PD. Pharmacological preservation of the ischemic heart. Ann Thorac Surg 1977;24:307.

10. Clark RE, Christlieb IY, Spratt JA, Henry PD, Fischer AE, Williamson JR, et al. Myocardial preservation with nifedipine. A comparative study at normothermia. Ann Thorac Surg 1981;31:3.

11. Clark RE, Christlieb IY, Ferguson TB, Weldon CS, Marbarger JP, Biello DR, et al. The first American clinical trial of nifedipine in cardioplegia. A report of the first 12 month experience. J Thorac Cardiovasc Surg 1981;82:848.

12. Choong YS, Gavin JB. L-Aspartate improves the functional recovery of explanted hearts stored in St. Thomas' Hospital cardioplegic solution at 4°C. J Thorac Cardiovasc Surg 1990;99:510.

13. Catinella FP, Cunningham JN Jr, Spencer FC. Myocardial protection during prolonged aortic cross-clamping. Comparison of blood and crystalloid cardioplegia. J Thorac Cardiovasc Surg 1984;88:411.

14. Cobbe SM, Poole-Wilson PA. The time of onset and severity of acidosis in myocardial ischaemia. J Mol Cell Cardiol 1980;12:745.

15. Chiba Y, Muraoka R, Ihaya A, Morioka K, Sasaki M, Uesaka T. Leukocyte depletion and prevention of reperfusion injury during cardiopulmonary bypass: a clinical study. J Thorac Cardiovasc Surg 1993;1:350.

16. Chang-Chun C, Masuda M, Szabo Z, Szerafin T, Szecsi J, Van Belle H, et al. Nucleoside transport inhibition mediates lidoflazine-induced cardioprotection during intermittent aortic crossclamping. J Thorac Cardiovasc Surg 1992;104:1602.

17. Caputo M, Dihmis W, Birdi I, Reeves B, Suleiman MS, Angelini GD, et al. Cardiac troponin T and troponin I release during coronary artery surgery using cold crystalloid and cold blood cardioplegia. Eur J Cardiothoracic Surg 1997;12:254.

18. Cohen NM, Wise RM, Wechsler AS, Damiano RJ Jr. Elective cardiac arrest with a hyperpolarizing adenosine triphosphate-sensitive potassium channel opener. A novel form of myocardial protection? J Thorac Cardiovasc Surg 1993;106:317.

19. Cleveland JC Jr, Meldrum DR, Rowland RT, Banerjee A, Harken AH. Optimal myocardial preservation: cooling, cardioplegia, and conditioning. Ann Thorac Surg 1996;61:760.

D

1. Dixon SH Jr, Limbird LE, Roe CR, Wagner GS, Oldham NH Jr, Sabiston DC Jr. Recognition of postoperative acute myocardial infarction. Application of isoenzyme techniques. Circulation 1973; 48:III137.

2. Ver Donck L, Van Reempts J, Vandeplassche G, Borgers M. A new method to study activated oxygen species induced damage in cardiomyocytes and protection by Ca²⁺–antagonists. J Mol Cell Cardiol 1988;20:811.

3. Danforth WH, Naegle S, Bing RJ. Effect of ischemia and reoxygenation on glycotic reactions and adenosine-triphosphate in heart muscle. Circ Res 1960;8:965.

4. Digerness SB, Kirklin JW, Naftel DC, Blackstone EH, Kirklin JK, Samuelson PN. Coronary and systemic vascular resistance during reperfusion after global myocardial ischemia. Ann Thorac Surg 1988;46:447.

5. Digerness SB, Tracy WG, Andrews NF, Bowdoin B, Kirklin JW. Reversal of myocardial ischemic contracture and the relationship to functional recovery and tissue calcium. Circulation 1983;68:II34.

6. Domalik-Wawrzynski LJ, Powell WJ Jr, Guerrero L, Palacios I. Effect of changes in ventricular relaxation on early diastolic coronary blood flow in canine hearts. Circ Res 1987;61:747.

7. Dreyer WJ, Smith CW, Michael LH, Rossen RD, Hughes BJ, Entman ML, et al. Canine neutrophil activation by cardiac lymph obtained during reperfusion of ischemic myocardium. Circ Res 1989;65:1751.

8. Daggett WM Jr, Randolph JD, Jacobs M, O'Keefe DD, Geffin GA, Swinski LA, et al. The superiority of cold oxygenated dilute blood cardioplegia. Ann Thorac Surg 1987;43:397.

9. Drinkwater DC, Laks H, Buckberg GD. A new simplified method of optimizing cardioplegic delivery without right heart isolation. Antegrade/retrograde blood cardioplegia. J Thorac Cardiovasc Surg 1990;100:56.

10. Drinkwater DC Jr, Cushen CK, Laks H, Buckberg GD. The use of combined antegrade-retrograde infusion of blood cardioplegic solution in pediatric patients undergoing heart operations. J Thorac Cardiovasc Surg 1992;104:1349.

E

1. Ebert PA, Greenfield LJ, Austen WG, Morrow AG. Experimental comparison of methods for protecting the heart during aortic occlusion. Ann Surg 1962;155:25.

2. Ellis SG, Henschke CI, Sandor T, Wynne J, Braunwald E, Kloner RA. Time course of functional and biochemical recovery of myocardium salvaged by reperfusion. J Am Coll Cardiol 1983;1:1047.

3. Engler RL, Dahlgren MD, Peterson MA, Dobbs A, Schmid-Schonbein GW. Accumulation of polymorphonuclear leukocytes during 3-hour experimental myocardial ischemia. Am J Physiol 1986;251:H93.

4. Engler R. Consequences of activation and adenosine-mediated inhibition of granulocytes during myocardial ischemia. Fed Proc 1987; 46:2407.

5. Engelman RM, Rousou JH, Lemeshow S, Dobbs WA. The metabolic consequences of blood and crystalloid cardioplegia. Circulation 1981; 64:II67.

6. Engleman RM, Rousou JH, Dobbs W, Pels MA, Longo F. The superiority of blood cardioplegia in myocardial preservation. Circulation 1980;62:162.

7. Ellis SG, Wynne J, Braunwald E, Henschke CI, Sandor T, Kloner RA. Response of reperfusion-salvaged, stunned myocardium to inotropic stimulation. Am J Heart 1984;107:13.

F

1. Follette DM, Fey KH, Steed DL, Foglia RP, Buckberg GD. Reducing reperfusion injury with hypocalcemic, hyperkalemic, alkalotic blood during reoxygenation. Surg Forum 1978;29:284.

2. Fiore AC, Naunheim KS, Kaiser GC, Willman VL, McBride LR, Pennington DG, et al. Coronary sinus versus aortic root perfusion with blood cardioplegia in elective myocardial revascularization. Ann Thorac Surg 1989;47:684.

3. Ferrara N, Bonaduce D, Abete P, Leosco D, Longobardi G, Canonico V, et al. Role of increased cholinergic activity in reperfusion induced ventricular arrhythmias. Cardiovasc Res 1987;21:279.

4. Freedman BM, Pasque MK, Pellom GL, Deaton DW, Frame JR, Wechsler AS. Effects of delay in administration of potassium cardioplegia to the isolated rat heart. Ann Thorac Surg 1984;37:309.

5. Feindel CM, Tait GA, Wilson GJ, Klement P, MacGregor DC. Multidose blood versus crystalloid cardioplegia. Comparison by quantitative assessment of irreversible myocardial injury. J Thorac Cardiovasc Surg 1984;87:585.

6. Follette DM, Fey K, Buckberg GD, Helly JJ Jr, Steed DL, Foglia RP, et al. Reducing postischemic damage by temporary modification of reperfusate calcium, potassium, pH, and osmolarity. J Thorac Cardiovasc Surg 1981;82:221.

7. Fujiwara T, Kurtts T, Anderson W, Heinle J, Mayer JE Jr. Myocardial protection in cyanotic neonatal lambs. J Thorac Cardiovasc Surg 1988;96:700.

8. Fremes SE, Christakis GT, Weisel RD, Mickle DA, Madonik MM, Ivanov J, et al. A clinical trial of blood and crystalloid cardioplegia. J Thorac Cardiovasc Surg 1984;88:726.

9. Flameng W, Xhonneux R, Borgers M. Myocardial protection in open heart surgery. In Wauquier A, Borgers M, Amery WK, eds. Protection of tissues against hypoxia. Amsterdam: Elsevier, 1982.

10. Flameng W, Borgers M, Van der Vusse GJ, Demeyere R, Vandermeersch E, Thone F, et al. Cardioprotective effects of lidoflazine in extensive aorto-coronary bypass grafting. J Thorac Cardiovasc Surg 1983;85:758.

11. Fischer JH, Isselhard W. Metabolic patterns in several tissues of newborn rabbits during ischemia. Biol Neonate 1975;27:235.

12. Frank JS, Rich TL. Ca depletion and repletion in rat heart: age-dependent changes in the sarcolemma. Am J Physiol 1983;245:H343.

13. Fabiani JN, Deloche A, Swanson J, Carpentier A. Retrograde cardioplegia through the right atrium. Ann Thorac Surg 1986;41:101.

14. Fontan F, Madonna F, Naftel DC, Kirklin JW, Blackstone EH, Digerness S. Modifying myocardial management in cardiac surgery: a randomized trial. Eur J Cardiothorac Surg 1992;6:127.

15. Finn A, Naik S, Klein N, Levinsky RJ, Strobel S, Elliott M. Interleukin-8 release and neutrophil degranulation after pediatric cardiopulmonary bypass. J Thorac Cardiovasc Surg 1993;105:234.

16. Fontan F, Madonna F, Naftel DC, Kirklin JW, Blackstone EH, Digerness S. The effect of reperfusion pressure on early outcomes after coronary artery bypass grafting. A randomized trial. J Thorac Cardiovasc Surg 1994;107:265.

G

1. Gray RJ, Shell WE, Conklin C, Ganz W, Shah PK, Miyamoto AT, et al. Quantification of myocardial injury during coronary artery bypass graft. Circulation 1978;58:II38.

2. Griepp RB, Stinson EB, Shumway NE. Profound local hypothermia for myocardial protection during open-heart surgery. J Thorac Cardiovasc Surg 1973;66:731.

3. Gay WA Jr, Ebert PA. Functional, metabolic, and morphologic effects of potassium-induced cardioplegia. Surgery 1973;74:284.

4. Grice WN, Konishi T, Apstein CS. Resistance of neonatal myocardium to injury during normothermic and hypothermic ischemia arrest and reperfusion. Circulation 1987;76:V150.

5. Gott VL, Dutton RC, Young WP. Myocardial rigor mortis as an indicator of cardiac metabolic function. Surg Forum 1962;13:172.

6. Garlick PB, Radda GK, Seeley PJ. Studies of acidosis in the ischaemic heart by phosphorus nuclear magnetic resonance. Biochem J 1979;184:547.

7. Gardner TJ, Stewart JR, Casale AS, Downey JM, Chambers DE. Reduction of myocardial ischemic injury with oxygen-derived free radical scavengers. Surgery 1983;94:423.

8. Gundry SR, Kirsh MM. A comparison of retrograde cardioplegia versus antegrade cardioplegia in the presence of coronary artery obstruction. Ann Thorac Surg 1984;38:124.

9. Gharagozloo F, Melendez FJ, Hein RA, Laurence RG, Shemin RJ, DiSesa VJ, et al. The effect of amino acid L-glutamate on the extended preservation ex vivo of the heart for transplantation. Circulation 1987;76:V65.

10. Gott VL, Gonzalez JL, Zuhdi MN. Retrograde perfusion of the coronary sinus for direct-vision aortic surgery. Surg Gynecol Obstet 1957;104:319.

11. Guiraudon GM, Campbell CS, McLellan DG, Kostuk WJ, Purves PD, MacDonald JL, et al. Retrograde coronary sinus versus aortic root perfusion with cold cardioplegia: randomized study of levels of cardiac enzymes in 40 patients. Circulation 1986;74:III105.

H

1. Henson DE, Najafi H, Callaghan R, Coogan P, Julian OC, Eisenstein R. Myocardial lesions following open heart surgery. Arch Pathol 1969;88:423.
2. Hultgren HN, Miyagawa M, Buch W, Angell WW. Ischemic myocardial injury during cardiopulmonary bypass surgery. Am Heart J 1973; 85:167.
3. Hearse DJ, Garlick PB, Humphrey SM. Ischemic contracture of the myocardium: mechanisms and prevention. Am J Cardiol 1977;39:986.
4. Hutchins GM, Nazarian IH, Bulkley BH. Association of left dominant coronary arterial system with congenital bicuspid aortic valve. Am J Cardiol 1978;42:57.
5. Hazan E, Rioux C, Dequirot A, Mathey J. Postperfusion stenosis of the common left coronary artery. J Thorac Cardiovasc Surg 1975;69:703.
6. Hottenrott C, Maloney JV Jr, Buckberg G. Studies of the effects of ventricular fibrillation on the adequacy of regional myocardial flow. I. Electrical vs. spontaneous fibrillation. J Thorac Cardiovasc Surg 1974;68:615.
7. Hoelscher B. Studies by electron microscopy on the effects of magnesium chloride-procainamide or potassium citrate on the myocardium in induced cardiac arrest. J Cardiovasc Surg (Torino) 1967;8:163.
8. Hufnagel CA, Conrad PW, Schanno J, Pifarre R. Profound cardiac hypothermia. Ann Surg 1961;153:790.
9. Hearse DJ, Stewart DA, Braimbridge MV. Cellular protection during myocardial ischemia: the development and characterization of a procedure for the induction of reversible ischemic arrest. Circulation 1976;54:193.
10. Heyndrickx GR, Millard RW, McRitchie RJ, Maroko PR, Vatner SF. Regional myocardial function and electrophysiological alterations after brief coronary artery occlusion in conscious dogs. J Clin Invest 1975;56:978.
11. Holland CE Jr, Olson RE. Prevention by hypothermia of paradoxical calcium necrosis in cardiac muscle. J Mol Cell Cardiol 1975;7:917.
12. Holmdahl MH, Nahas GG. Volume of distribution of C^{14}-labeled tris (hydroxymethyl) aminomethane. Am J Physiol 1962;202:1011.
13. Hoffman JI. Determinants and prediction of transmural myocardial perfusion. Circulation 1978;58:381.
14. Haft JI, Kranz PD, Albert FJ, Fani K. Intravascular platelet aggregation in the heart induced by norepinephrine. Microscopic studies. Circulation 1972;46:698.
15. Hearse DJ, Braimbridge MV, Jynge P. Ischemia and reperfusion: the progression and prevention of tissue injury. In Protection of the ischaemic myocardium: cardioplegia. New York: Raven Press, 1981, p. 21.
16. Hoerter J. Changes in the sensitivity to hypoxia and glucose deprivation in the isolated perfused rabbit heart during perinatal development. Pflugers Arch 1976;363:1.
17. Hammond B, Hess ML. The oxygen free radical system: potential mediator of myocardial injury. J Am Coll Cardiol 1985;6:215.
18. Harper IS, Lochner A. Sarcolemmal integrity during ischaemia and reperfusion of the isolated rat heart. Basic Res Cardiol 1989;84:208.
19. Hoelscher B, Just OH, Merker HJ. Studies by electron microscope on various forms of induced cardiac arrest in dog and rabbit. Surgery 1961;49:492.
20. Harris EA, Parimelazhagan KN, Seelye ER, Barratt-Boyes BG. Optimization of coronary perfusion rate during cardiac surgery in man. J Thorac Cardiovasc Surg 1979;77:662.

I

1. Isom OW, Kutin ND, Falk EA, Spencer FC. Patterns of myocardial metabolism during cardiopulmonary bypass and coronary perfusion. J Thorac Cardiovasc Surg 1973;66:705.

2. Iverson LI, Young JN, Ennix CL Jr, Ecker RR, Moretti RL, Lee J, et al. Myocardial protection: a comparison of cold blood and cold crystalloid cardioplegia. J Thorac Cardiovasc Surg 1984;87:509.
3. Illes RW, Silverman NA, Krukenkamp IB, Yusen RD, Chausow DD, Levitsky S. The efficacy of blood cardioplegia is not due to oxygen delivery. J Thorac Cardiovasc Surg 1989;98:1051.
4. Ito BR, Roth DM, Engler RL. Thromboxane A_2 and peptidoleukotrienes contribute to the myocardial ischemia and contractile dysfunction in response to intracoronary infusion of complement C5a in pigs. Circ Res 1990;66:596.

J

1. Jennings RB, Sommers HM, Smyth GA, Flack HA, Linn H. Myocardial necrosis induced by temporary occlusion of a coronary artery in the dog. AMA Arch Pathol 1960;70:68.
2. Jennings RB, Sommers HM, Herdson PB, Kaltenbach JP. Ischemic injury of myocardium. Ann N Y Acad Sci 1969;156:61.
3. Julia PL, Partington MT, Buckberg GD. Superiority of blood cardioplegia over crystalloid cardioplegia in limiting reperfusion damage: importance of endogenous oxygen free-radical scavengers in red blood cells. Surg Forum 1988;39:221.
4. Jones RN, Attarian DE, Currie WD, Olsen CO, Hill RC, Sink JD, et al. Metabolic deterioration during global ischemia as a function of time in the intact normal dog heart. J Thorac Cardiovasc Surg 1981;81:264.
5. Jeremy RW, Stahl L, Gillinov M, Litt M, Aversano TR, Becker LC. Preservation of coronary flow reserve in stunned myocardium. Am J Physiol 1989;256:H1303.
6. Julia PL, Kofsky ER, Buckberg GD, Young HH, Bugyi HI. Studies of myocardial protection in the immature heart. I. Enhanced tolerance of immature versus adult myocardium to global ischemia with reference to metabolic differences. J Thorac Cardiovasc Surg 1990;100:879.
7. Jarmakani JM, Nagatomo T, Nakazawa M, Langer GA. Effect of hypoxia on myocardial high-energy phosphates in the neonatal mammalian heart. Am J Physiol 1978;235:H475.
8. Julia P, Young HH, Buckberg GD, Kofsky ER, Bugyi HI. Studies of myocardial protection in the immature heart. II. Evidence for importance of amino acid metabolism in tolerance to ischemia. J Thorac Cardiovasc Surg 1990;100:888.
9. Julia P, Young HH, Buckberg GD, Kofsky ER, Bugyi HI. Studies of myocardial protection in the immature heart. IV. Improved tolerance of immature myocardium to hypoxia and ischemia by intravenous metabolic support. J Thorac Cardiovasc Surg 1991;101:23.
10. Jolly SR, Kane WJ, Bailie GD, Abrams GD, Lucchesi BR. Canine myocardial reperfusion injury. Its reduction by the combined administration of superoxide dismutase and catalase. Circ Res 1984;54:277.
11. Johnson DL, Lahorra JA, Gott VL, Gardner TJ. Reducing intraoperative myocardial acidosis by continuous cardioplegic perfusion via the coronary sinus. J Surg Res 1988;44:625.
12. Jurmann MJ, Schaefers HJ, Dammenhayn L, Haverich A. Oxygen-derived free radical scavengers for amelioration of reperfusion damage in heart transplantation. J Thorac Cardiovasc Surg 1988;95:368.
13. Julia P, Kofsky ER, Buckberg GD, Young HH, Bugyi HI. Studies of myocardial protection in the immature heart. III. Models of ischemic and hypoxic/ischemic injury in the immature puppy heart. J Thorac Cardiovasc Surg 1991;101:14.
14. Jennings RB, Reimer KA. Factors involved in salvaging ischemic myocardium: effect of reperfusion of arterial blood. Circulation 1983;68:I25.

K

1. Katz AM, Tada M. The "stone heart" and other challenges to the biochemist. Am J Cardiol 1977;39:1073.
2. Kirklin JW. Nature of the problem, in Cardioplegia Workshop. An International Exchange of Ideas, June 23, 1979. Deerfield, Ill: Travenol Laboratories, 1979, p. 1.
3. Kronzon I, Deutsch P, Glassman E. Length of the left main coronary artery: its relation to the pattern of coronary arterial distribution. Am J Cardiol 1974;34:787.

4. Koster JK Jr, Cohn LH, Collins JJ Jr, Sanders JH, Muller JE, Young E. Continuous hypothermic arrest versus intermittent ischemia for myocardial protection during coronary revascularization. Ann Thorac Surg 1977;24:330.

5. Kirsch U, Rodewald G, Kalmar P. Induced ischemic arrest. Clinical experience with cardioplegia in open-heart surgery. J Thorac Cardiovasc Surg 1972;63:121.

6. Kirklin JW. The science of cardiac surgery. Eur J Cardiothorac Surg 1990;4:63.

7. Kirklin JW, Conti VR, Blackstone EH. Prevention of myocardial damage during cardiac operations. N Engl J Med 1979;301:135.

8. Kloner RA, Ganote CE, Jennings RB. The "no-reflow" phenomenon after temporary coronary occlusion in the dog. J Clin Invest 1974;54:1496.

9. Khuri SF, Warner KG, Josa M, Butler M, Hayes A, Hanson R, et al. The superiority of continuous cold blood cardioplegia in the metabolic protection of the hypertrophied human heart. J Thorac Cardiovasc Surg 1988;95:442.

10. Krukenkamp IB, Silverman NA, Levitsky S. The effect of cardioplegia oxygenation on the correlation between the linearized Frank–Starling relationship and myocardial energetics in the ejecting postischemic heart. Circulation 1987;76:V122.

11. Kates RA, Dorsey LM, Kaplan JA, Hatcher CR Jr, Guyton RA. Pretreatment with lidoflazine, a calcium-channel blocker. Useful adjunct to heterogenous cold potassium cardioplegia. J Thorac Cardiovasc Surg 1983;85:278.

12. Kofsky E, Julia P, Buckberg GD, Young H, Tixier D. Studies of myocardial protection in the immature heart. V. Safety of prolonged aortic clamping with hypocalcemic glutamate/aspartate blood cardioplegia. J Thorac Cardiovasc Surg 1991;101:33.

13. Kirklin JK, Blackstone EH, Kirklin JW, McKay R, Pacifico AD, Bargeron LM Jr. Intracardiac surgery in infants under age 3 months: incremental risk factors for hospital mortality. Am J Cardiol 1981;48:500.

14. Kirsch U. Untersuchungen zum eintritt der totenstarre an ischaemischen meer-schweinchenherzen in normothermie. Der einfluss von procain, kalium, und magnesium. Arzneimforsch 1970;20:1071.

15. Kempsford RD, Hearse DJ. Protection of the immature heart. Temperature-dependent beneficial or detrimental effects of multidose crystalloid cardioplegia in the neonatal rabbit heart. J Thorac Cardiovasc Surg 1990;99:269.

16. Ku DD. Coronary vascular reactivity after acute myocardial ischemia. Science 1982;218:576.

17. Koh TW, Hooper J, Kemp M, Ferdinand FD, Gibson DG, Pepper JR. Intraoperative release of troponin T in coronary venous and arterial blood and its relation to recovery of left ventricular function and oxidative metabolism following coronary artery surgery. Heart 1998;80:341.

18. Kilbridge PM, Mayer JE, Newburger JW, Hickey PR, Walsh AZ, Neufeld EJ. Induction of intercellular adhesion molecule-1 and E-selectin mRNA in heart and skeletal muscle of pediatric patients undergoing cardiopulmonary bypass. J Thorac Cardiovasc Surg 1994;107:1183.

19. Kloner RA, Shook T, Przylenk K, Davis VG, Junio L, Matthews RV, et al. Previous angina alters in-hospital outcome in TIMI 4. A clinical correlate to preconditioning? Circulation 1995;91:37.

L

1. Lie JT, Sun SC. Ultrastructure of ischemic contracture of the left ventricle ("stone heart"). Mayo Clin Proc 1976;51:785.

2. Littlefield JB, Lowicki EM, Muller WH Jr. Experimental left coronary artery perfusion through an aortotomy during cardiopulmonary bypass. J Thorac Cardiovasc Surg 1960;40:685.

3. Lesage CH Jr, Vogel JH, Blount SG Jr. Iatrogenic coronary occlusive disease in patients with prosthetic heart valves. Am J Cardiol 1970;26:123.

4. Lichtenstein SV, Ashe KA, el Dalati H, Cusimano RJ, Panos A, Slutsky AS. Warm heart surgery. J Thorac Cardiovasc Surg 1991;101:269.

5. Lell WA, Walker DR, Blackstone EH, Kouchoukos NT, Allarde R, Roe CR. Evaluation of myocardial damage in patients undergoing coronary-artery bypass procedures with halothane–N$_2$O anesthesia and adjuvants. Anesth Analg 1977;56:556.

6. Lucas SK, Elmer EB, Flaherty JT, Prodromos CC, Bulkley BH, Gott BL, et al. Effect of multiple-dose potassium cardioplegia on myocardial ischemia, return of ventricular function, and ultrastructural preservation. J Thorac Cardiovasc Surg 1980;80:102.

7. Leaf A. Maintenance of concentration gradients and regulation of cell volume. Ann N Y Acad Sci 1959;72:396.

8. Lolley DM, Ray JF III, Myers WO, Sautter RD, Tewksbury DA. Importance of preoperative myocardial glycogen levels in human cardiac preservation. Preliminary report. J Thorac Cardiovasc Surg 1979;78:678.

9. Lowe JE, Cummings RG, Adams DH, Hull-Ryde EA. Evidence that ischemic cell death begins in the subendocardium independent of variations in collateral flow or wall tension. Circulation 1983;68:190.

10. Lofland GK, Abd-Elfattah AS, Wyse R, de Leval M, Stark J, Wechsler AS. Myocardial adenine nucleotide metabolism in pediatric patients during hypothermic cardioplegic arrest and normothermic ischemia. Ann Thorac Surg 1989;47:663.

11. Lazar HL, Buckberg GD, Manganaro AJ, Becker H, Maloney JV Jr. Reversal of ischemic damage with amino acid substrate enhancement during reperfusion. Surgery 1980;88:702.

12. Lazar HL, Buckberg GD, Manganaro AJ, Becker H. Myocardial energy replenishment and reversal of ischemic damage by substrate enhancement of secondary blood cardioplegia with amino acids during reperfusion. J Thorac Cardiovasc Surg 1980;80:350.

13. Lee JC, Downing SE. Left ventricular distensibility in newborn piglets, adult swine, young kittens, and adult cats. Am J Physiol 1974;226:1484.

14. Lange R, Ingwall J, Hale SL, Alker KJ, Braunwald E, Kloner RA. Preservation of high-energy phosphates by verapamil in reperfused myocardium. Circulation 1984;70:734.

15. Lolley DM, Hewitt RL, Drapanas T. Retroperfusion of the heart with a solution of glucose, insulin, and potassium during anoxic arrest. J Thorac Cardiovasc Surg 1974;67:364.

16. Lolley DM, Hewitt RL. Myocardial distribution of asanguineous solutions retroperfused under low pressure through the coronary sinus. J Cardiovasc Surg (Torino) 1980;21:287.

17. Lupinetti FM, Wareing TH, Huddleston CB, Collins JC, Boucek RJ Jr, Bender HW Jr, et al. Pathophysiology of chronic cyanosis in a canine model. Functional and metabolic response to global ischemia. J Thorac Cardiovasc Surg 1985;90:291.

18. Lillehei CW, DeWall RA, Gott VL, Varco RL. The direct vision correction of calcific aortic stenosis by means of a pump oxygenator and retrograde coronary sinus perfusion. Dis Chest 1956;30:123.

19. Lawton JS, Sepic JD, Allen CT, Hsia PW, Damiano RJ Jr. Myocardial protection with potassium-channel openers is as effective as St. Thomas' solution in the rabbit heart. Ann Thorac Surg 1996;62:31.

20. Lichtenstein SV, Ashe KA, el Dalati H, Cusimano RJ, Panos A, Slutsky AS. Warm heart surgery. J Thorac Cardiovasc Surg 1991;101:269.

21. Liu GS, Thornton J, Van Winkle DM, Stanley AW, Olsson RA, Downey JM. Protection against infarction afforded by preconditioning is mediated by A$_1$-adenosine receptors in rabbit heart. Circulation 1991;84:350.

M

1. Moulder PV, Blackstone EH, Eckner FA, Lev M. Pressure-derivative loop for left ventricular resuscitation. Arch Surg 1968;96:323.

2. Martin AM Jr, Hackel DB. An electron microscopic study of the progression of myocardial lesions in the dog after hemorrhage shock. Lab Invest 1966;15:243.

3. Miyamoto AT, Robinson L, Matloff JM, Norman JR. Perioperative infarction: effects of cardiopulmonary bypass on collateral circulation in an acute canine model. Circulation 1978;58:I147.

4. Muller WH Jr, Warren WD, Dammann JF Jr, Beckwith JR, Wood JE Jr. Surgical relief of aortic insufficiency by direct operation on the aortic valve. Circulation 1960;21:587.

5. Murphy ES, Rosch J, Rahimtoola SH. Frequency and significance of coronary arterial dominance in isolated aortic stenosis. Am J Cardiol 1977;39:505.

6. Midell AI, DeBoer A, Bermudez G. Postperfusion coronary ostial stenosis: incidence and significance. J Thorac Cardiovasc Surg 1976;72:80.

7. McGoon DC, Pestana C, Moffitt EA. Decreased risk of aortic valve surgery. Arch Surg 1965;91:779.

8. McGoon DC. Alternatives to cardioplegia, in Cardioplegia Workshop. An International Exchange of Ideas, June 23, 1979, Deerfield, Ill: Travenol Laboratories, 1979, p. 23.

9. Melrose DG, Dreyer B, Bentall HH, Baker JBE. Elective cardiac arrest. Preliminary communication. Lancet 1955;2:21.

10. Menasche P, Kucharski K, Mundler O, Veyssie L, Subayi JB, Pimpec F, et al. Adequate preservation of right ventricular function after coronary sinus cardioplegia. A clinical study. Circulation 1989; 80:III19.

11. Mueller HS, Evans R, Ayres SM. Effect of dopamine on hemodynamics and myocardial metabolism in shock following acute myocardial infarction in man. Circulation 1978;57:361.

12. Magovern GJ, Dixon CM, Burkholder JA. Improved myocardial protection with nifedipine and potassium-based cardioplegia. J Thorac Cardiovasc Surg 1981;82:239.

13. Menasche P, Kural S, Fauchet M, Commin P, Bercot M, Touchot B, et al. Retrograde coronary sinus perfusion: a safe alternative for ensuring cardioplegic delivery in aortic valve surgery. Ann Thorac Surg 1982;34:647.

14. Marban E, Koretsune Y, Corretti M, Chacko VP, Kusuoka H. Calcium and its role in myocardial cell injury during ischemia and reperfusion. Circulation 1989;80:IV17.

15. Matsuoka S, Jarmakani JM, Young HH, Uemura S, Nakanishi T. The effect of glutamate on hypoxic newborn rabbit heart. J Mol Cell Cardiol 1986;18:897.

16. Mullane KM, Kraemer R, Smith B. Myeloperoxidase activity as a quantitative assessment of neutrophil infiltration into ischemic myocardium. J Pharmacol Methods 1985;14:157.

17. McCord JM. Superoxide radical: a likely link between reperfusion injury and inflammation. Adv Free Radical Biol Med 1986;2:325.

18. Mehta JL, Nichols WW, Mehta P. Neutrophils as potential participants in acute myocardial ischemia: relevance to reperfusion. J Am Coll Cardiol 1988;11:1309.

19. Martin SE, Chenoweth DE, Engler RL, Roth DM, Longhurst JC. C5a decreases regional coronary blood flow and myocardial function in pigs: implications for a granulocyte mechanism. Circ Res 1988;63:483.

20. Mehta JL, Nichols WW, Donnelly WH, Lawson DL, Saldeen TG. Impaired canine coronary vasodilator response to acetylcholine and bradykinin after occlusion-reperfusion. Circ Res 1989;64:43.

21. Maskal SL, Cohen NM, Hsia PW, Wechsler AS, Damiano RJ Jr. Hyperpolarized cardiac arrest with potassium-channel opener, aprikalim. J Thorac Cardiovasc Surg 1995;110:1083.

22. Menashe P, Piwnica A. Cardioplegia by way of the coronary sinus for valvular and coronary surgery. J Am Coll Cardiol 1991;18:628.

23. Marban E. Myocardial stunning and hibernation. The physiology behind the colloquialisms. Circulation 1991;83:681.

24. Murry CE, Jennings RB, Reimer KA. Preconditioning with ischemia: a delay of lethal cell injury in ischemic myocardium. Circulation 1986;74:1124.

25. Mitchell MB, Meng X, Ao L, Brown JM, Harken AH, Banerjee A. Preconditioning of isolated rat heart is mediated by protein kinase C. Circ Res 1995;76:73.

26. Martin TD, Craver JM, Gott JP, Weintraub WS, Ramsay J, Mora CT, et al. Prospective, randomized trial of retrograde warm blood cardioplegia: myocardial benefit and neurologic threat. Ann Thorac Surg 1994;57:298.

27. Mair P, Mair J, Seibt I, Wieser C, Furtwaengler W, Waldenberger F, et al. Cardiac troponin T: a new marker of myocardial tissue damage in bypass surgery. J Cardiothorac Vasc Anesth 1993;7:674.

N

1. Najafi H, Henson D, Dye WS, Javid H, Hunter JA, Callaghan R, et al. Left ventricular hemorrhagic necrosis. Ann Thorac Surg 1969;7:550.

2. Neutze JM, Drakeley MJ, Barratt-Boyes BG, Hubbert K. Serum enzymes after cardiac surgery using cardiopulmonary bypass. Am Heart J 1974;88:425.

3. Nishida M, Kuzuya T, Hoshida S, Kim Y, Kitabatake A, Kamada T, et al. Polymorphonuclear leukocytes induced vasoconstriction in isolated canine coronary arteries. Circ Res 1990;66:253.

4. Nelson RL, Goldstein SM, McConnell DH, Maloney JV Jr, Buckberg GD. Studies of the effects of hypothermia on regional myocardial blood flow and metabolism during cardiopulmonary bypass. V. Profound topical hypothermia during ischemia in arrested hearts. J Thorac Cardiovasc Surg 1977;73:201.

5. Nahas GG. The pharmacology of tris (hydroxymethyl) aminomethane (THAM). Pharmacol Rev 1962;14:447.

6. Nelson RL, Fey KH, Follette DM, Livesay JJ, DeLand EC, Maloney JV Jr, Buckberg GD. Intermittent infusion of cardioplegic solution during aortic cross-clamping. Surg Forum 1976;27:241.

7. Nayler WB, Poole-Wilson PA, Williams A. Hypoxia and calcium. J Mol Cell Cardiol 1979;11:683.

8. Nayler WG, Ferrari R, Williams A. Protective effect of pretreatment with verapamil, nifedipine and propranolol on mitochondrial function in the ischemic and reperfused myocardium. Am J Cardiol 1980;46:242.

9. Nayler WG, Elz JS. Reperfusion injury: laboratory artifact or clinical dilemma? Circulation 1986;74:215.

10. Nishioka K, Nakanishi T, Jarmakani JM. Effect of ischemia on calcium exchange in the rabbit myocardium. Am J Physiol 1984;247:H177.

11. Nakanishi T, Young HH, Shimizu T, Nishioka K, Jarmakani JM. The relationship between myocardial enzyme release and Ca^{2+} uptake during hypoxia and reoxygenation in the newborn and adult heart. J Mol Cell Cardiol 1984;16:519.

12. Novick RJ, Stefaniszyn HJ, Michel RP, Burdon FD, Salerno TA. Protection of the hypertrophied pig myocardium. A comparison of crystalloid, blood, and Fluosol-DA cardioplegia during prolonged aortic clamping. J Thorac Cardiovasc Surg 1985;89:547.

O

1. Oldham HN Jr, Roe CR, Young WG Jr, Dixon SH Jr. Intraoperative detection of myocardial damage during coronary artery surgery by plasma creatine phosphokinase isoenzyme analysis. Surgery 1973;74:917.

2. Okamoto F, Allen BS, Buckberg GD, Bugyi H, Leaf J. Studies of controlled reperfusion after ischemia. XIV. Reperfusion conditions: importance of ensuring gentle versus sudden reperfusion during relief of coronary occlusion. J Thorac Cardiovasc Surg 1986;92:613.

3. Oldfield GS, Commerford PJ, Opie LH. Effects of preoperative glucose-insulin-potassium on myocardial glycogen levels and on complications of mitral valve replacement. J Thorac Cardiovasc Surg 1986;91:874.

4. Opie LH. Proposed role of calcium in reperfusion injury. Int J Cardiol 1989;23:159.

5. O'Riordain DS, al Delamie TY, Aherne T. Low potassium cardioplegia: its effect on the incidence of complete heart block following cardiac surgery. Ir J Med Sci 1989;158:257.

6. Ottani F, Galvani M, Ferrini D, Sorbello F, Limonetti P, Pantoli D, et al. Prodromal angina limits infarct size. A role for ischemic preconditioning. Circulation 1995;91:291.

P

1. Pupello DF, Blank RH, Bessone LN, Connar RG, Carlton LM Jr. Local deep hypothermia for combined valvular and coronary heart disease. Ann Thorac Surg 1976;21:508.

2. Partington MT, Acar C, Buckberg GD, Julia P, Kofsky ER, Bugyi HI. Studies of retrograde cardioplegia. I. Capillary blood flow distribution to myocardium supplied by open and occluded arteries. J Thorac Cardiovasc Surg 1989;97:605.

3. Przyklenk K, Kloner RA. Superoxide dismutase plus catalase improve contractile function in the canine model of the "stunned myocardium." Circ Res 1986;58:148.

4. Pacifico AD, Digerness S, Kirklin JW. Acute alterations of body composition after open intracardiac operations. Circulation 1970;41:331.

5. Piscatelli RL, Fox LM. Myocardial injury from epinephrine overdosage. Am J Cardiol 1968;21:735.

6. Pryor WA. The role of free radical reactions in biological system. In Pryor WA, ed. Free radicals in biology. New York: Academic Press, 1976, p. 1.

7. Pridjian AK, Levitsky S, Krukenkamp I, Silverman NA, Feinberg H. Developmental changes in reperfusion injury. A comparison of intracellular cation accumulation in the newborn, neonatal, and adult heart. J Thorac Cardiovasc Surg 1987;93:428.

8. Patel B, Kloner RA, Przyklenk K, Braunwald E. Postischemic myocardial "stunning": a clinically relevant phenomenon. Ann Intern Med 1988;108:626.

9. Przyklenk K, Kloner RA. Effect of verapamil on postischemic "stunned" myocardium: importance of the timing of treatment. J Am Coll Cardiol 1988;11:614.

10. Przyklenk K, Ghafari GB, Eitzman DT, Kloner RA. Nifedipine administered after reperfusion ablates systolic contractile dysfunction of postischemic "stunned" myocardium. J Am Coll Cardiol 1989;13:1176.

11. Parr GV, Blackstone EH, Kirklin JW. Cardiac performance and mortality early after intracardiac surgery in infants and young children. Circulation 1975;51:867.

12. Pearson PJ, Schaff HV, Vanhoutte PM. Acute impairment of endothelium-dependent relaxations to aggregating platelets following reperfusion injury in canine coronary arteries. Circ Res 1990;67:385.

Q

1. Quillen JE, Sellke FW, Brooks LA, Harrison DG. Ischemia-reperfusion impairs endothelium-dependent relaxation of coronary microvessels but does not affect large arteries. Circulation 1990;82:586.

R

1. Rosky LP, Rodman T. Medical aspects of open-heart surgery. N Engl J Med 1966;274:833.

2. Roberts WC, Bulkley BH, Morrow AG. Pathologic anatomy of cardiac valve replacement: a study of 224 necropsy patients. Prog Cardiovasc Dis 1973;15:539.

3. Rose GA, Blackburn H. Cardiovascular survey methods. Geneva: World Health Organization, 1968, p. 137.

4. Roe CR, Wagner GS, Young WG Jr, Curtis SE, Cobb FR, Irvin RG. Relation of creatine kinase isoenzyme MB to postoperative electrocardiographic diagnosis in patients undergoing coronary-artery bypass surgery. Clin Chem 1979;25:93.

5. Righetti A, Crawford MH, O'Rourke RA, Hardarson T, Schelbert H, Daily PO, et al. Detection of perioperative myocardial damage after coronary artery by-pass graft surgery. Circulation 1977;55:173.

6. Righetti A, O'Rourke RA, Schelbert H, Henning H, Hardarson T, Daily PO, et al. Usefulness of preoperative and postoperative Tc-99m (Sn)-pyrophosphate scans in patients with ischemic and valvular heart disease. Am J Cardiol 1977;39:43.

7. Richardson JV, Kouchoukos NT, Wright JO 3rd, Karp RB. Combined aortic valve replacement and myocardial revascularization: results in 220 patients. Circulation 1979;59:75.

8. Reed GE, Spencer FC, Boyd AD, Engelman RM, Glassman E. Late complications of intraoperative coronary artery perfusion. Circulation 1973;47,48:III80.

9. Rossen RD, Michael LH, Kagiyama A, Savage HE, Hanson G, Reisberg MA, et al. Mechanism of complement activation after coronary artery occlusion: evidence that myocardial ischemia in dogs causes release of constituents of myocardial subcellular origin that complex with human C1q in vivo. Circ Res 1988;62:572.

10. Rosenkranz ER, Okamoto F, Buckberg GD, Robertson JM, Vinten-Johansen J, Bugyi HI. Safety of prolonged aortic clamping with blood cardioplegia. III. Aspartate enrichment of glutamate-blood cardioplegia in energy-depleted hearts after ischemic and reperfusion injury. J Thorac Cardiovasc Surg 1986;91:428.

11. Roe BB, Hutchinson JC, Fishman NH, Ullyot DJ, Smith DL. Myocardial protection with cold, ischemic, potassium-induced cardioplegia. J Thorac Cardiovasc Surg 1977;73:366.

12. Robin ED, Wilson RJ, Bromberg PA. Intracellular acid-base relations and intracellular buffers. Ann N Y Acad Sci 1961;92:539.

13. Rosenfeldt FL, Rabinov M, Newman M. Coronary blood flow and myocardial metabolism during reperfusion after hypothermic cardioplegia in the dog. Eur J Cardiothorac Surg 1987;1:91.

14. Rosenblum HM, Haasler GB, Spotnitz WD, Lazar HL, Spotnitz HM. Effects of simulated clinical cardiopulmonary bypass and cardioplegia on mass of the canine left ventricle. Ann Thorac Surg 1985;39:139.

15. Roberts AJ, Woodhall DD, Knauf DG, Alexander JA. Coronary artery bypass graft surgery: clinical comparison of cold blood potassium cardioplegia, warm cardioplegic induction, and secondary cardioplegia. Ann Thorac Surg 1985;40:483.

16. Reduto LA, Lawrie GM, Reid JW, Whissenand HH, Noon GP, Kanon D, et al. Sequential postoperative assessment of left ventricular performance with gated cardiac blood pool imaging following aortocoronary bypass surgery. Am Heart J 1981;101:59.

17. Roberts AJ, Moran JM, Sanders JH, Spies SM, Lichtenthal PR, Kaplan KJ, et al. Clinical evaluation of the relative effectiveness of multidose crystalloid and cold blood potassium cardioplegia in coronary artery bypass graft surgery: a nonrandomized matched-pair analysis. Ann Thorac Surg 1982;33:421.

18. Rosenkranz ER, Buckberg GD, Laks H, Mulder DG. Warm induction of cardioplegia with glutamate-enriched blood in coronary patients with cardiogenic shock who are dependent on inotropic drugs and intra-aortic balloon support. J Thorac Cardiovasc Surg 1983;86:507.

19. Rosenkranz ER, Okamoto F, Buckberg GD, Vinten-Johansen J, Edwards H, Bugyi H. Advantages of glutamate-enriched cold blood cardioplegia in energy-depleted hearts. Circulation 1982;66:II151.

20. Rosenkranz ER, Vinten-Johansen J, Buckberg GD, Okamoto F, Edwards H, Bugyi H. Benefits of normothermic induction of blood cardioplegia in energy-depleted hearts, with maintenance of arrest by multidose cold blood cardioplegic infusions. J Thorac Cardiovasc Surg 1982;84:667.

21. Rossen RD, Swain JL, Michael LH, Weakley S, Giannini E, Entman ML. Selective accumulation of the first component of complement and leukocytes in ischemic canine heart muscle. A possible initiator of an extra myocardial mechanism of ischemic injury. Circ Res 1985;57:119.

22. Rosenkranz ER, Okamoto F, Buckberg GD, Vinten-Johansen J, Robertson JM, Bugyi H. Safety of prolonged aortic clamping with blood cardioplegia. II. Glutamate enrichment in energy-depleted hearts. J Thorac Cardiovasc Surg 1984;88:402.

23. Rhodes GR, Syracuse DC, McIntosh CL. Evaluation of regional myocardial nutrient perfusion following selective retrograde arterialization of the coronary vein. Ann Thorac Surg 1978;25:329.

24. Roberts AJ. Myocardial protection in cardiac surgery. New York: Marcel Dekker, 1987.

25. Reimer KA, Hill ML, Jennings RB. Prolonged depletion of ATP and of the adenine nucleotide pool due to delayed resynthesis of adenine nucleotides following reversible myocardial ischemic injury in dogs. J Mol Cell Cardiol 1981;13:229.

26. Romero T, Covell J, Friedman WF. A comparison of pressure-volume relations of the fetal, newborn, and adult heart. Am J Physiol 1972;222:1285.

27. Redwood SR, Ferrari R, Marber MS. Myocardial hibernation and stunning: from physiological principles to clinical practice. Heart 1998;80:218.

28. Robicsek F, Schaper J. Reperfusion injury: fact or myth? J Card Surg 1997;12:133.

29. Rosenfeldt FL. The relationship between myocardial temperature and recovery after experimental cardioplegic arrest. J Thorac Cardiovasc Surg 1982;84:656.

S

1. Sapsford RN, Blackstone EH, Kirklin JW, Karp RB, Kouchoukos NT, Pacifico AD, et al. Coronary perfusion versus cold ischemic arrest during aortic valve surgery. A randomized study. Circulation 1974;49:1190.

2. Steed D, Follette D, Foglia R, Buckberg G. Unavoidable subendocardial underperfusion during bypass, especially in infants (abstract). Circulation 1977;56:III248.

3. Shen AC, Jennings RB. Myocardial calcium and magnesium in acute ischemic injury. Am J Pathol 1972;67:417.

4. Sharratt GP, Rees P, Conway N. Myocardial infarction complicating aortic valve replacement. J Thorac Cardiovasc Surg 1976;71:869.

5. Spanos PK, Brown AL Jr, McGoon DC. The significance of intraoperative ventricular fibrillation during aortic valve replacement. J Thorac Cardiovasc Surg 1977;73:605.

6. Schraut W, Lamberti JJ, Kampman K, Anagnostopoulos C, Replogle R, Glagov S. Does local cardiac hypothermia during cardiopulmonary bypass protect the myocardium from long-term morphological and functional injury? Ann Thorac Surg 1977;24:315.

7. Schaper J, Schwarz F, Kittstein H, Kreisel E, Winkler B, Hehrlein FW. Ultrastructural evaluation of the effects of global ischemia and reperfusion on human myocardium. Thorac Cardiovasc Surg 1980;28:337.

8. Stirling MC, McClanahan TB, Schott RJ, Lynch MJ, Bolling SF, Kirsh MM, et al. Distribution of cardioplegic solution infused antegradely and retrogradely in normal canine hearts. J Thorac Cardiovasc Surg 1989;98:1066.

9. Shen AC, Jennings RB. Kinetics of calcium accumulation in acute myocardial ischemic injury. Am J Pathol 1972;67:441.

10. Schaper J, Scheld HH, Schmidt U, Hehrlein F. Ultrastructural study comparing the efficacy of five different methods of intraoperative myocardial protection in the human heart. J Thorac Cardiovasc Surg 1986;92:47.

11. Sabiston DC JR, Gregg DE. Effect of cardiac contraction on coronary blood flow. Circulation 1957;15:14.

12. Spotnitz WD, Clark MB, Rosenblum HM, Lazar HL, Haasler GB, Collins RH, et al. Effect of cardiopulmonary bypass and global ischemia on human and canine left ventricular mass: evidence for interspecies differences. Surgery 1984;96:230.

13. Singh AK, Farrugia R, Teplitz C, Karlson E. Electrolyte versus blood cardioplegia: randomized clinical and myocardial ultrastructural study. Ann Thorac Surg 1982;33:218.

14. Shapira N, Kirsh M, Jochim K, Behrendt DM. Comparison of the effect of blood cardioplegia to crystalloid cardioplegia on myocardial contractility in man. J Thorac Cardiovasc Surg 1980;80:647.

15. Shlafer M, Kane PF, Kirsh MM. Superoxide dismutase plus catalase enhances the efficacy of hypothermic cardioplegia to protect the globally ischemic, reperfused heart. J Thorac Cardiovasc Surg 1982;83:830.

16. Schachner A, Vladutiu A, Montes M, Koreyni-Both A, Levinsky L, Levy M, et al. Myocardial protection in infant open heart surgery. Scand J Thor Cardiovasc Surg 1983;17:101.

17. Shumway NE, Lower RR. Topical cardiac hypothermia for extended periods of anoxic arrest. Surg Forum 1960;10:563.

18. Shumway NE, Lower RR, Stofer RC. Selective hypothermia of the heart in anoxic cardiac arrest. Surg Gynec Obstet 1959;109:750.

19. Susilo AW, van der Laarse A, Scheltema H, van Ark E, Los GJ, van Rijk GL, et al. Progressive coronary vasoconstriction during 25 hours of myocardial preservation in vitro impairs functional capacity following preservation. Eur J Cardiothorac Surg 1989;3:544.

20. Sawatari K, Kadoba K, Bergner KA, Daitch JA, Mayer JE Jr. Influence of initial reperfusion pressure after hypothermic cardioplegic ischemia on endothelial modulation of coronary tone in neonatal lambs. Impaired coronary vasodilator response to acetylcholine. J Thorac Cardiovasc Surg 1991;101:777.

21. Swain JL, Sabina RL, McHale PA, Greenfield JC Jr, Holmes EW. Prolonged myocardial nucleotide depletion after brief ischemia in the open-chest dog. Am J Physiol 1982;242:H818.

22. Sondergaard T, Senn A. Klinische Erfahrungen in der Kardioplegie nach Bretschneider. Langenbecks. Arch Chir 1967;319:661.

23. Seguchi M, Harding JA, Jarmakani JM. Developmental change in the function of sarcoplasmic reticulum. J Mol Cell Cardiol 1986;18:189.

24. Salerno TA, Houck JP, Barrozo CA, Panos A, Christakis GT, Abel JG, et al. Retrograde continuous warm blood cardioplegia: a new concept in myocardial protection. Ann Thorac Surg 1991;51:245.

25. Salerno TA. Myocardial temperature management during aortic clamping for cardiac surgery—protection, preoccupation, and perspective (invited letter). J Thorac Cardiovasc Surg 1992;103:1019.

26. Schott RJ, Rohmann S, Braun ER, Schaper W. Ischemic preconditioning reduces infarct size in swine myocardium. Circ Res 1990;66:1133.

T

1. Taber RF, Morales AR, Fine G. Myocardial necrosis and the postoperative low-cardiac-output syndrome. Ann Thorac Surg 1967;4:12.

2. Teoh KH, Christakis GT, Weisel RD, Fremes SE, Mickle DA, Romaschin AD, et al. Accelerated myocardial metabolic recovery with terminal warm blood cardioplegia. J Thorac Cardiovasc Surg 1986;91:888.

3. Teitel DF, Sidi D, Chin T, Brett C, Heymann MA, Rudolph AM. Developmental changes in myocardial contractile reserve in the lamb. Pediatr Res 1985;19:948.

4. Thornburg KL, Morton MJ. Filling and arterial pressures as determinants of left ventricular stroke volume in fetal lambs. Am J Physiol 1986;251:H961.

5. Toma BS, Wangler RD, DeWitt DF, Sparks HV Jr. Effect of development on coronary vasodilator reserved in the isolated guinea pig heart. Circ Res 1985;57:538.

6. Tait GA, Booker PD, Wilson GJ, Coles JG, Steward DJ, MacGregor DC. Effect of multidose cardioplegia and cardioplegic solution buffering on myocardial tissue acidosis. J Thorac Cardiovasc Surg 1982;83:824.

7. Takamoto S, Levine FH, LaRaia PJ, Adzick NS, Fallon JT, Austen WG, et al. Comparison of single-dose and multiple-dose crystalloid and blood potassium cardioplegia during prolonged hypothermic aortic occlusion. J Thorac Cardiovasc Surg 1980;79:19.

8. Tranum-Jensen J, Janse MJ, Fiolet WT, Krieger WJ, D'Alnoncourt CN, Durrer D. Tissue osmolality, cell swelling, and reperfusion in acute regional myocardial ischemia in the isolated porcine heart. Circ Res 1981;49:364.

9. Tsao PS, Aoki N, Lefer DJ, Johnson G III, Lefer AM. Time course of endothelial dysfunction and myocardial injury during myocardial ischemia and reperfusion in the cat. Circulation 1990;82:1402.

10. Taggart DP, Hadjinikolas L, Hooper J, Albert J, Kemp M, Hue D, et al. Effects of age and ischemic times on biochemical evidence of myocardial injury after pediatric cardiac operations. J Thorac Cardiovasc Surg 1997;113:728.

11. Tsuchida A, Liu Y, Liu GS, Cohen MV, Downey JM. Alpha1-adrenergic agonists precondition rabbit ischemic myocardium independent of adenosine by direct activation of protein kinase C. Circ Res 1994;75:576.

V

1. Van Trigt P, Jones RN, Olsen CO, Peyton RB, Currie WD, Pellon GL, et al. Sonomicrometric determination of ischemic contracture of the left ventricle. J Thorac Cardiovasc Surg 1982;83:298.

2. Visner MS, Arentzen CE, Ring WS, Anderson RW. Left ventricular dynamic geometry and diastolic mechanics in a model of chronic cyanosis and right ventricular pressure overload. J Thorac Cardiovasc Surg 1981;81:347.

3. Vary TC, Angelakos ET, Schaffer SW. Relationship between adenine nucleotide metabolism and irreversible ischemic tissue damage in isolated perfused rat heart. Circ Res 1979;45:218.

4. Vane JR, Anggard EE, Botting RM. Regulatory functions of the vascular endothelium. N Engl J Med 1990;323:27.

5. Van Benthuysen KM, McMurty IF, Harwitz LD. Reperfusion after acute coronary occlusion in dogs impairs endothelium-dependent relaxation to acetylcholine and augments contractile reactivity in vitro. J Clin Invest 1987;79:265.

W

1. Williams JF Jr, Morrow AG, Braunwald E. The incidence and management of "medical" complications following cardiac operations. Circulation 1965;32:608.

2. Walters HL III, Digerness SB, Naftel DC, Waggoner JR III, Blackstone EH, Kirklin JW. The response to ischemia in blood perfused vs. crystalloid perfused isolated rat heart preparations. J Mol Cell Cardiol 1992;24:1063.

3. Winkelmann J, Aronson S, Young CJ, Fernandez A, Lee BK. Retrograde-delivered cardioplegia is not distributed equally to the right ventricular free wall and septum. J Cardiothorac Vasc Anesth 1995;9:135.

Y

1. Yates JD, Kirsh MM, Sodeman TM, Walton JA Jr, Brymer JF. Coronary ostial stenosis, a complication of aortic valve replacement. Circulation 1974;49:530.

2. Yates JC, Dhalla NS. Structural and functional changes associated with failure and recovery of hearts after perfusion with Ca^{2+}-free medium. J Mol Cell Cardiol 1975;7:91.

3. Young HH, Shimizu T, Nishioka K, Nakanishi T, Jarmakani JM. Effect of hypoxia and reoxygenation on mitochondrial function in neonatal myocardium. Am J Physiol 1983;245:H998.

4. Yonenaga K, Yasui H, Kado H, Nakamura Y, Shiokawa Y, Yamamoto T, et al. Myocardial protection by retrograde cardioplegia in arterial switch operation. Ann Thorac Surg 1990;50:238.

5. Yau TM, Ikonomidis JS, Weisel RD, Mickle DA, Ivanov J, Mohabeer MK, et al. Ventricular function after normothermic versus hypothermic cardioplegia. J Thorac Cardiovasc Surg 1993;105:833.

Z

1. Zimmerman AN, Daems W, Hulsmann WC, Snijder J, Wisse E, Durrer D. Morphological changes of heart muscle caused by successive perfusion with calcium-free and calcium-containing solutions (calcium paradox). Cardiovasc Res 1967;1:201.

2. Zimmerman AN, Hulsmann WC. Paradoxical influence of calcium ions on the permeability of the cell membranes of the isolated rat heart. Nature 1966;211:646.

Anesthesia for Cardiovascular Surgery

The practice of anesthesiology has undergone major changes over the past two decades. Nowhere has this change been more apparent than in the field of cardiac surgery. Where once the anesthesiologist's sole responsibility was to ensure hypnosis, amnesia, analgesia, and paralysis during surgery (traditional concepts of anesthesia), the contemporary anesthesiologist is an integral member of the surgical team who evaluates the patient in the preoperative setting, provides comprehensive intraoperative care and monitoring, and may provide postoperative intensive care.

It was once widely believed that there was an "ideal" cardiac anesthetic[L1]; it has now become clear that no such ideal exists, but rather an optimal balance of hemodynamics, anesthetic goals, and surgical necessity.[M1,R1]

Anesthetic management of patients undergoing cardiovascular surgery follows the same principles that govern anesthesia for other surgical procedures. During the preoperative visit the anesthesiologist collates the information provided by the history, physical examination, and laboratory results and decides on the best form of anesthetic

■ TABLE 4-1 Cardiac Grid: Desired Objectives during Induction and Maintenance of Anesthesia

Cardiac Lesion	Objective				
	Heart Rate	Rhythm	Contractility	Preload	Afterload
Coronary artery disease	–	Sinus	+	+	+
Tamponade	++	Sinus	++	++	++
Aortic stenosis	+	Sinus	++	++	++
Aortic regurgitation	++	Sinus	+	+	– –
Mitral stenosis	–	Sinus	+	+	+
Mitral regurgitation	++	Sinus	+	–	– –
Hypertrophic obstructive cardiomyopathy	–	Sinus	–	++	++
Coarctation of the aorta	0	Sinus	+	+	P_{AO} –, P_{PA} +
Aortopulmonary shunt	0	Sinus	0	+	–
Fontan physiology	–	Sinus	+	+	–
Tetralogy of Fallot	+	Sinus	0	+	–

Key: +, Increase; –, decrease; P_{AO}, systemic (aorta) pressure; P_{PA}, pulmonary artery pressure.

management. Successful outcome depends on carrying out these plans in an orderly sequence. Coordination and communication between the anesthesiologist and the surgeon are essential so that even the most difficult problems, both in the operating room and during the postoperative period, can be handled in a calm, efficient manner by an experienced team working together daily.

SECTION 1
Anesthetic Management

TYPICAL PROTOCOLS FOR ANESTHESIA AND SUPPORTIVE CARE FOR CARDIOVASCULAR OPERATIONS

Anesthetic management of the cardiac surgical patient begins in the preoperative setting, where the patient undergoes evaluation by the anesthetic team. Anesthetic evaluation has several goals:

■ To gain a thorough understanding of the proposed procedure in order to deal with its potential anesthetic implications
■ To identify potential risks associated with the procedure relative to the patient's overall condition
■ To review and understand diagnostic studies in order to select the most appropriate anesthetic
■ To assess the underlying pathophysiology of the disease process, because each cardiac condition presents unique features and objectives that must be considered when planning induction and maintenance of anesthesia

The desired physiologic objectives relating to various cardiac conditions can be conceptualized in tabular form by placing each into a grid (Table 4-1).

Apart from the condition requiring surgical intervention, assessment of ventricular function is essential. *Left ventricular ejection fraction* (LVEF) can be determined at cardiac catheterization or by other diagnostic modalities such as echocardiography or nuclear imaging. LVEF provides the anesthesiologist with information about cardiac reserve and tolerance to potential hemodynamic challenges during anesthetic induction, endotracheal intubation, and impending surgical manipulations. Preoperative assessment of ventricular function should be supplemented by intraoperative

transesophageal echocardiography (TEE)[D1] because function may be different at operation. For example, sympathetic neural stimulation and catecholamine release during induction and intubation elevate peripheral resistance, resulting in apparent decreased ventricular function as assessed by LVEF. Conversely, many anesthetics lower heart rate, resulting in increased LVEF.

Although each patient presents individual problems that affect anesthetic management and supportive care, typical protocols can be used.

PATIENTS UNDERGOING CORONARY ARTERY BYPASS GRAFTING WITH CARDIOPULMONARY BYPASS
Procedures

Coronary artery bypass grafting (CABG) employing cardiopulmonary bypass (CPB) may be performed using a median sternotomy, smaller incisions, or port-access surgery (see Chapter 2). Anesthetic management is essentially the same for all.

At the preoperative visit, current medications are reviewed. Resting, angina-free heart rate and blood pressure are recorded. Presence of exercise-induced angina, pulmonary venous hypertension, or heart failure is noted. Calm discussion by the anesthesiologist of premedication, anesthetic management, and other aspects of the operation is important to alleviate anxiety and prevent excessive catecholamine release.

Premedication given 1 hour before anesthetic induction usually consists of diazepam (10 to 15 mg) and methadone (10 mg) administered orally, but a number of benzodiazepine/opiate combinations can be used. Interventions before induction include placement of a blood pressure cuff, electrocardiogram (ECG) leads, and a single peripheral intravenous (IV) infusion catheter. Usually a peripheral arterial cannula is inserted using local anesthesia to avoid painful maneuvers that may precipitate myocardial ischemia. Often, central access is established via the internal jugular vein with a catheter after further local anesthesia has been administered. A pulmonary artery catheter or central venous catheter may be inserted at this time. After induction with midazolam (or thiopental) and fentanyl, muscle relaxation is achieved with pancuronium or vecuronium, and ventilation is controlled for at least 4 minutes with oxygen. Pancuronium may transiently increase blood pressure and heart rate, but fre-

■ **TABLE 4–2   Hemodynamic Effects of Anesthetic Drugs**

Drug	Hemodynamic Effect					
	CI	BP	SVR	P$_{LVED}$	HR	Contractility
d-Tubocurarine	↓	↓	↓	↓	↑	↔
Diazepam	↓	↓	↓	↔	↔	↔
Dimethyl tubocurarine	↑	↔↑	↔↓	↔↓	↑	↔
Droperidol	↔↑	↓	↓	↓	↑	↔
Enflurane	↓	↓	↓	↔↓	↔↓	↓
Fentanyl	↔	↓	↓	↔	↔	↔
Halothane	↓	↓	↔↓	↔↑	↔↑↓	↓
Innovar	↔↑	↓	↓	↓	↔	↔
Isoflurane	↔	↓	↓	↔	↑	↓
Ketamine	↑	↑	↑	↑	↑	↑
Methoxyflurane	↓	↓	↓	↔	↔	↓
Midazolam	↔	↔	↔↓	↓	↑	↔↓
Morphine	↔↑	↔↓	↓	↔↑	↓	↔
Nitrous oxide	↓	↔↓	↔↑	↑	↔↓	↓
Pancuronium	↑	↑	↔	↓	↑	?
Succinylcholine	↓	↔↓	↓	↓	↑↓	?
Thiopental	↔↓	↔	↑	↔	↑	↓
Vecuronium	↔	↔	↔	↔	↔	↔

Key: ↓, Decrease; ↑, increase; ↔, no change; ?, insufficient data; *CI*, cardiac index; *BP*, blood pressure; *SVR*, systemic vascular resistance; *P$_{LVED}$*, left ventricular end-diastolic pressure; *HR*, heart rate.

quently does not in patients who have received beta-adrenergic receptor antagonists. Maintenance of anesthesia is achieved with continuous infusion of midazolam and fentanyl with or without isoflurane.[T1]

Before and after orotracheal intubation, all or some of the following interventions may be necessary to control the determinants of myocardial oxygen supply and demand:

- Administration of fluid (crystalloid, colloid) to ensure adequate circulating blood volume, cardiac output, and coronary perfusion
- Administration of volatile anesthetics (e.g., isoflurane), in part to control myocardial contractility, but also for supplemental anesthesia
- Administration of additional other anesthetic agents (e.g., diazepam, midazolam, fentanyl, droperidol) to assist in control of blood pressure and heart rate (Table 4-2)
- Administration of vasodilators (e.g., sodium nitroprusside, nitroglycerin) to optimize ventricular wall tension (afterload) (Table 4-3)
- Administration of vasoconstrictors (e.g., phenylephrine) to increase aortic pressure and improve coronary blood flow (Table 4-4)
- Administration of agents (e.g., dopamine) to increase myocardial contractility (Table 4-5)

During anesthetic induction, reduced plasma volume,[C1] present in many patients with ischemic heart disease, may result in hypotension. It is usually responsive to volume administration.

During operation, agents are administered to provide a depth of anesthesia that is compatible with the changing levels of operative stimulation.[R2] If hypertension or tachycardia persists, additional vasodilators, beta-adrenergic antagonists, or both are administered. Vasoconstrictors and inotropic drugs are sometimes necessary to correct hypotension that is unresponsive to volume administration or results from excessive cardiac manipulation.

As CPB is discontinued, the four variables affecting cardiac output (performance)—preload, afterload, heart rate, and contractility—are adjusted according to principles outlined in Chapter 2. The adjustments utilize central venous pressure and left atrial pressure (P$_{LA}$) (directly or as reflected by pulmonary capillary wedge pressure [P$_{PCW}$] or pulmonary artery diastolic pressure), arterial blood pressure, ECG, and TEE.

In the closing stages of operation, anesthetics and muscle relaxants are managed so that their effects will persist only into the first 1 or 2 hours of convalescence in the intensive care unit, with a view toward tracheal extubation a few hours later.

Effectiveness of these simple methods of anesthetic management in minimizing perioperative myocardial necrosis is well established.[L1,M2,R2]

Rationale

Management of patients during myocardial revascularization procedures is directed toward preventing myocardial damage from atherosclerotic heart disease, inadequacies of anesthesia, or surgical techniques. Thus, anesthetic management is designed to provide an optimum myocardial oxygen supply–demand ratio.[P1,R3-R5] Although this is important in every cardiac surgical patient, it is critically important for preventing myocardial ischemia or stunning in patients with coronary artery disease.

Myocardial oxygen demand is directly related to heart rate, myocardial contractility, wall tension (afterload),[B1,S1] *and myocardial temperature* (see Chapter 3). Tachycardia increases myocardial ischemia.[S2] Catecholamine release (or administration) increases contractility and thus myocardial oxygen demand. Systemic arterial hypertension increases intraventricular pressure, increasing left ventricular volume and thus wall tension and oxygen demand, as described by the Laplace relationship.

Myocardial oxygen supply is directly related to arterial oxygen content and coronary blood flow. In turn, arterial oxygen content is dependent on hemoglobin concentration, oxygen partial pressure, and variables affecting oxyhemoglobin dissociation, and coronary blood flow is dependent on aortic diastolic pressure for the left ventricular

■ **TABLE 4-3** Comparison of Pharmacologic Properties of Vasodilators

Generic	Trade Name	Action	Prominent Vasodilatation	Onset (min)	Duration	Adult Dosage IV
Sodium nitroprusside	Nipride	Direct	Arteriovenous	1/2	2-4 min	0.2-8.0 $\mu g \cdot kg^{-1} \cdot min^{-1}$ infusion
Nitroglycerin	Nitrostat	Direct	Venous	1-2	10 min	0.8 mg; 5 $\mu g \cdot kg^{-1} \cdot min^{-1}$ infusion
Diazoxide	Hyperstat	Direct	Arterial	1-2	4-12 h	3-5 $mg \cdot kg^{-1}$ bolus
Trimethaphan	Arfonad	Ganglionic blockade	Arteriovenous	1-2	4-8 min	10-50 $\mu g \cdot kg^{-1} \cdot min^{-1}$ infusion
Hydralazine	Apresoline	Direct	Arterial	10-20	3-4 h	5.0-7.5 mg bolus
Labetalol	Trandate	α_1- and β-adrenergic blockade	Arteriovenous	2-3	2-4 h	0.25-1.0 $mg \cdot kg^{-1}$ bolus 0.02-2.5 $mg \cdot min^{-1}$ infusion
Phentolamine	Regitine	α_1-and β-adrenergic blockade	Arteriovenous	1-2	20 min	20 $\mu g \cdot kg^{-1} \cdot min^{-1}$ infusion
Prazosin	Minipress	α_1-adrenergic blockade	Arteriovenous	30-60	2-3 h	2-20 mg b.i.d. orally
Enalapril	Vasotec	ACE inhibitor	Arterial	15	6-7 h	1.25-5.0 mg bolus
Nifedipine	Procardia	Calcium antagonist	Arterial	5-15	2-4 h	10-20 mg sublingual
Nicardipine	Cardene	Calcium antagonist	Arteriovenous	5-10	2-4 h	4-12 $mg \cdot min^{-1}$ infusion
Isradipine	Dynacirc	Calcium antagonist	Arteriovenous	5-10	5-6 h	0.007-0.15 $mg \cdot kg^{-1}$ bolus 8-40 $\mu g \cdot min^{-1}$ infusion

(From Braunwald[B18] and Reves and colleagues.[R13])

Key: *NA*, Not available in a parenteral formulation; *ACE*, angiotensin–converting enzyme.

■ **TABLE 4-4** Adrenergic Receptor Stimulation and Dosages of Vasoconstrictors

Vasoconstrictor		Activity					
		Vascular		Cardiac			
Generic	Trade Name	α_1	β_2	β_1	Onset	Duration	Initial Adult Dosage
Methoxamine	Vasoxyl	++++	0	0	++	++	0.5-2.0 mg bolus
Phenylephrine	Neo-Synephrine	++++	0	0	++	+++	0.1-0.5 mg bolus
Norepinephrine	Levophed	++++	+	++	++++	+	0.05-2.0 $\mu g \cdot kg^{-1} \cdot min^{-1}$ [a]
Ephedrine	None	+++	0	++	++	++++	2.5-5.0 mg bolus
Vasopressin	Pitressin	0	0	0	++	++	0.04-0.12 $U \cdot min$

Key: Number of + signs denotes increasing activity; α, alpha-adrenergic; β, beta-adrenergic.

[a] See Appendix 5C in Chapter 5.

■ **TABLE 4-5** Agents to Improve Cardiac Performance

Agent		Activity				
		Vascular		Cardiac	Phosphodiesterase	
Generic	Trade Name	α_1	β_1	β_2	Inhibition	Initial Adult Dose
Dopamine	Inotropin	++	++	+	0	2-10 $\mu g \cdot kg^{-1} \cdot min^{-1}$
Dobutamine	Dobutrex	+	+++	+	0	2-10 $\mu g \cdot kg^{-1} \cdot min^{-1}$
Amrinone	Inocor	0	0	0	+	0.05-2.0 $mg \cdot kg^{-1}$ bolus, then 5-10 $\mu g \cdot kg^{-1} \cdot min^{-1}$ infusion
Milrinone	Primacor	0	0	0	+	50 $\mu g \cdot kg^{-1}$ bolus, then 0.5 $\mu g \cdot kg^{-1} \cdot min^{-1}$ infusion
Isoproterenol	Isuprel	0	++++	++++	0	0.05-0.2 $\mu g \cdot kg^{-1} \cdot min^{-1}$ [a]
Epinephrine	Adrenalin	+++	++	+	0	0.05-0.2 $\mu g \cdot kg^{-1} \cdot min^{-1}$ [a]

Key: Number of + signs denotes increasing time; α, alpha-adrenergic; β, beta-adrenergic.

[a] See Appendix 5C in Chapter 5.

subendocardial layer and aortic systolic and diastolic pressure for outer myocardial layers. Coronary blood flow is also inversely related to coronary vascular resistance; a decrease in vascular resistance of the normal myocardium secondary to increased metabolic demands or selective vasodilatation, in the face of a relatively fixed cardiac output, may result in decreased perfusion of areas supplied by stenotic coronary arteries. This is pertinent to the use of inotropic and vasodilator agents in patients with ischemic heart disease. By increasing the metabolic demands of normal tissue, inotropic agents may shunt blood away from jeopardized myocardium, causing ischemia. By lowering perfusion pressure or by selectively dilating vessels supplying normal myocardium, vasodilators may result in an intercoronary steal syndrome.[C2] Coronary collateral flow will supply some oxygen to the ischemic area, but this is not predictable. A blood hemoglobin level of about 10 to 12 $g \cdot dL^{-1}$, normal systemic blood pressure, and P_{PCW} of 8 to 14 mmHg are optimal for myocardial oxygen delivery. A higher P_{PCW} reflects increased left ventricular cavity pressure during diastole, which can result in a reduction of the left ventricular myocardial perfusion gradient (approximated by arterial pressure minus P_{LA}).

Effects of various anesthetic agents on the determinants of myocardial oxygen supply and demand are discussed in detail in Section 4. It is important to remember that all interventions entail risks. Use of potent and potentially harmful pharmacologic agents must therefore be selective. Transient alterations in hemodynamic variables may be better tolerated than the complications resulting from aggressive polypharmacy. Unfortunately, lack of a single reliable index of myocardial ischemia necessitates use of

■ **TABLE 4-6   Comparison of Beating and Arrested Heart Techniques for Coronary Artery Bypass Grafting**

Technique	Advantages	Disadvantages
Beating heart off CPB	Avoids CPB May afford small incisions	Field movement Target limitation No intracardiac procedures
Arrested heart on CPB	Security of CPB Motionless field Intracardiac procedures possible	Damaging effects of CPB

(From Fontana.[F4])

Key: *CPB,* Cardiopulmonary bypass.

■ **TABLE 4-7   Distinctive Features of Off-Pump Coronary Artery Bypass (OPCAB)** [a]

Feature	Implications
Potential for extreme hemodynamic instability and dysrhythmias	Monitoring choices: TEE, PA catheter, CVP, ECG, continuous CO Understand management options: ischemic preconditioning, coronary shunt, conversion to CPB, circulatory support systems (right heart, left heart), inotropic agents Need for standby CPB
Requirement for "quiet" surgical field	Mechanical stabilizers used; pharmacologically induced bradycardia Avoid vagolytic anesthetic drugs One-lung ventilation occasionally required or requested
Poor access to epicardium (MIDCAB)	Defibrillation and pacing capabilities, if desired, must be provided by means that do not require direct epicardial contact if surgery is performed via thoracotomy.
CPB not used	Reduced doses of heparin; reversal with protamine optional
Hypothermia possible	Active warming measures encouraged
Options for incision	Several options available for pain management, depending on incision site
Cost containment	"Fast track" or "appropriately timed extubation" especially important
Anesthetic choices and postoperative pain management	Should meet "fast-track" goals

Key: *TEE,* Transesophageal echocardiography; *PA,* pulmonary artery; *CVP,* central venous pressure; *ECG,* electrocardiogram; *CO,* cardiac output; *CPB,* cardiopulmonary bypass; *MIDCAB,* minimally invasive direct coronary artery bypass.

[a] Compared with "standard" coronary artery bypass grafting with CPB.[S3]

multiple variables to assess the need for intervention. For example, ST-segment depression in the absence of hemodynamic changes may represent a nonspecific finding that does not require treatment. On the other hand, ischemia associated with hemodynamic changes may be present without detectable ST-segment changes. TEE is a sensitive and specific indicator of wall motion abnormalities resulting from myocardial ischemia.[D1] Rarely, however, the only manifestation of ischemia may be a rise in pulmonary artery diastolic pressure, P_{PCW}, or P_{LA}.

PATIENTS UNDERGOING CORONARY ARTERY BYPASS GRAFTING WITHOUT CARDIOPULMONARY BYPASS

Procedures

Myocardial revascularization of the beating heart without use of CPB is an alternative technique, called *off-pump coronary artery bypass* (OPCAB). Preoperative assessment, fundamental anesthesia management, monitoring, and goals of management are identical to those for operations that entail CPB. Table 4-6 provides a comparison of beating and arrested cardiac operations.

Myocardial revascularization without CPB has certain distinctive features (Table 4-7) that make anesthetic management challenging. A double lumen endotracheal tube or other means to isolate a lung may be required to facilitate harvest of the corresponding internal thoracic artery. Heparin is usually administered in doses of 100 to 200 U · kg^{-1}, and activated clotting time is kept between 250 and 300 seconds (see Chapter 2). Drugs, alone or in combination, are used to produce a lower heart rate and less vigorous contraction of the myocardium; these include esmolol, metoprolol, diltiazem, verapamil, adenosine, neostigmine, and edrophonium. These agents are used in addition to maneuvers employed by the surgeon to stabilize the coronary artery and remove blood from the site of the anastomosis. Because the heart is physically distorted and often lifted from its normal position, hypotension is common. Hypotension is treated by placing the patient in the head-down position and administering vasopressors such as phenylephrine or norepinephrine. This positioning also facilitates surgical exposure of the lateral and inferior walls of the left ventricle. It is important that the anesthesiologist assist the surgeon during this part of the procedure in ways not required when the patient is on CPB, including manual ventilation with low tidal volumes and continued monitoring for myocardial ischemia. Because the standard ECG is often uninterpretable in the distorted heart, assessment of

ischemia requires integrating information provided by TEE. However, elevation and distortion of the heart may preclude optimal TEE imaging.

Occlusion of the coronary artery for 3 to 5 minutes may be performed before starting the coronary artery anastomosis. Although this may produce ischemic preconditioning, it more likely provides a preview of hemodynamic decompensation that may occur during arterial anastomosis. While the surgeon performs the anastomosis, the anesthesiologist treats any arrhythmias or hemodynamic disturbances. With reperfusion of the distal myocardium, arrhythmias can occur, but they are usually self-limiting.

Techniques are generally used intraoperatively to permit early extubation either at the conclusion of operation or within 1 to 2 hours postoperatively. Treatment of pain is similar for patients with median sternotomy incisions and lateral thoracotomy.

Rationale

Goals and rationale of managing patients undergoing CABG without CPB are the same as for those with CPB.[S3] A major difference between on-pump and off-pump techniques is that the heart can be more or less protected from ischemia with cardioplegic agents during operations with CPB. In this regard, inhalation techniques that reduce myocardial contractility and heart rate are important adjuncts to IV anesthetics that have little effect on contractility but reduce heart rate. These techniques are useful for reducing myocardial oxygen consumption. Maintaining adequate coronary perfusion pressure often requires use of vasopressors and is best achieved with a pure alpha-adrenergic agonist drug rather than one with beta-adrenergic activity that increases myocardial oxygen consumption.

SURGERY FOR VALVAR HEART DISEASE

Procedures

Anesthetic management for patients undergoing valvar procedures depends on individual valve pathology.

During the preoperative visit, patient history and physical examination are used to gain an understanding of the functional derangements produced by the valvar disease. Detailed review of the preoperative transthoracic and transesophageal echocardiograms, as well as cardiac catheterization data, is essential to plan appropriate anesthetic management. Evidence of heart failure, particularly with ongoing pulmonary edema, is particularly important because effects of lung injury frequently induced by CPB can be exacerbated by preexisting pulmonary edema. Cardiac dysrhythmias, most prominently atrial fibrillation, are common in these patients. A review of the patient's medications often reveals conditions for which he or she is receiving prophylaxis or treatment (e.g., atrial fibrillation, heart failure, thromboembolism).

Because intraoperative TEE generally is routinely performed, a history of esophageal conditions that might preclude use of TEE is important. Examples include previous esophageal surgery, esophageal strictures with ongoing dysphagia, esophageal bleeding caused by varices, and esophageal diverticulum.

Preoperative management of patients with valvar heart disease is similar to that for patients with coronary artery disease. Premedication consists of a combination of diazepam (10 to 15 mg) and methadone (10 mg). After placement of monitoring devices, a peripheral arterial cannula is inserted. Central venous access is desirable, and catheters can be inserted with the patient awake (before induction of anesthesia) or after general anesthetics are given. A pulmonary artery catheter or later a left atrial catheter is routinely used during these procedures.

Although no single anesthetic technique can be applied to all patients, specific hemodynamic objectives for each cardiac valvar lesion dictate how an anesthetic should be administered (see Table 4-1). To meet these objectives, administration of adjunctive therapies, including volume administration, vasoconstrictors, vasodilators, and beta-receptor blockers, is frequently required.

Increasing use of smaller surgical incisions has broadened the anesthesiologist's role. He or she is required not only to administer anesthetic agents and perform TEE but also to insert percutaneous cannulae for access approaches (e.g., Heartport), coronary sinus perfusion, pulmonary artery venting, and venous drainage.

After intubation, TEE is used to confirm the diagnosis, determine the status of other valves, and assess the severity of valvar dysfunction. Altered loading conditions induced by anesthesia can alter the apparent severity of valvar dysfunction; for example, in patients undergoing operations for mitral regurgitation, reduced preload and afterload accompanying anesthesia often lessen the severity of the regurgitation. It is thus important to assess the severity of valvar dysfunction under conditions similar to those the patient experiences daily. This may require administration of vasopressors or volume to elevate the blood pressure to a level encountered preoperatively, or at times to even higher levels. TEE also permits assessment of overall myocardial performance. Once the valve has been repaired or replaced, TEE is used to assess adequacy of the procedure (see Section 2, "Operative Monitoring").[S4]

Rationale

The most common abnormalities for which patients present for valvar surgery involve the mitral and aortic valves.

Mitral Regurgitation

The important pathophysiologic manifestation of mitral regurgitation is volume overload of the left ventricle that is generally well tolerated because of increased compliance of the left atrium, until onset of heart failure with severe pulmonary venous hypertension. Anesthetic considerations include improving hemodynamic performance with judicious vasodilatation to decrease the backward regurgitant flow and increase the forward ejection from the left ventricle.[S22] Decreasing the systemic arterial pressure lower than that consistent with coronary perfusion must be avoided. Maintenance of a normal or slightly increased heart rate also aids in minimizing the regurgitant flow.

The situation is more complex in ischemic mitral regurgitation. Segmental wall dysfunction, combined with left ventricular dilatation, leads to ventricular remodeling that results in increased sphericity. Anesthetic and hemodynamic management are the same as for nonischemic mitral regurgitation except that left ventricular function must be supported at times and coronary flow maintained.

Mitral Stenosis

Mitral stenosis is usually associated with slow deterioration of cardiac function, frequently accelerated by atrial fibrillation. Pulmonary vascular resistance may increase, resulting finally in right-sided heart failure with or without tricuspid regurgitation. Major hemodynamic problems are decreased left ventricular filling and reduced cardiac output. To achieve adequate left ventricular filling, high left atrial pressure and volume are required. Anesthetic considerations include maintenance of this volume and filling pressure, as well as a heart rate slow enough to permit adequate left ventricular diastolic filling time. It may be necessary to slow a rapid ventricular rate.

Aortic Stenosis

Patients with aortic stenosis frequently have a long asymptomatic period and thus present for surgery with marked left ventricular hypertrophy with or without heart failure. They may also have concomitant coronary artery disease (see Chapter 12). Anesthetic management is influenced by the presence of the thick, noncompliant left ventricle with outflow obstruction. Thus, the ventricle requires a high filling pressure. Heart rate must be kept near normal, fast enough to maintain cardiac output but not so fast that myocardial oxygen consumption becomes excessive. Mild vasodilatation may be helpful in increasing cardiac output (especially in patients with left ventricular dysfunction), but care must be taken to maintain arterial pressures consistent with adequate coronary artery perfusion, especially in the presence of coronary artery disease.[C18,G17]

Aortic Regurgitation

Patients with aortic regurgitation may be acutely or chronically ill. Those with acute disease resulting from infective endocarditis, aortic dissection, or dehiscence of a previously inserted aortic prosthetic valve frequently have more marked heart failure, related in part to the normal size of the left ventricle. The chronic form of aortic regurgitation caused by rheumatic heart disease or aortic root dilatation is usually better tolerated because of the larger ventricular volume; however, when heart failure is present in patients with aortic regurgitation, compensation has reached its limit. Specific considerations for anesthetic management include minimizing regurgitant (backward) flow and maximizing forward flow. Regurgitant flow into the ventricle is decreased by shortening diastole, by increasing heart rate, or at least by avoiding bradycardia. A high systolic pressure suggests the need for vasodilatation,[S22] but excessive vasodilatation may lower coronary artery perfusion pressure below safe levels.

Patients may present with a mixed lesion (stenosis and regurgitation) of a single valve, with multiple valve lesions, or with concomitant coronary artery disease. Although these factors may complicate the anesthetic plan, they can be controlled through judicious use of anesthetic and adjuvant agents.

INFANTS AND CHILDREN UNDERGOING CARDIOPULMONARY BYPASS (OPEN PROCEDURES)

Substantial improvements have been made in anesthetic management of children with congenital heart disease. This is particularly true for management of neonates and patients undergoing staged repair of single-ventricle malformations. The anesthesiologist must possess a comprehensive understanding of each congenital malformation and its altered physiology, as well as a broad knowledge of pediatric medicine and pediatric cardiology.

In the acutely ill child who requires ventilatory and inotropic support preoperatively, anesthetic management must be carefully constructed to optimize cardiac output, and in those with shunt-dependent physiology, to balance systemic and pulmonary blood flow. Increasingly, children outside the newborn period arrive for cardiac operations on the same day as admission. Thus, the anesthesiologist must have access to the history and all cardiac diagnostic information before meeting with the child and family. In many centers a formalized conference occurs regularly to review historical, radiographic, echocardiographic, and cardiac catheterization data. Associated problems, such as reactive airway disease, airway anomalies, renal dysfunction, and congenital syndromes, are discussed. Presence of shunts, patches, and conduits affects selection of anesthetic and surgical approaches. Previous aortopulmonary shunts or subclavian flap repair for coarctation of the aorta may reduce blood flow to the left or right arm and result in reduced blood pressure in that extremity.

Laboratory Evaluation

Laboratory evaluation should include analysis of hemoglobin, hematocrit, pulse oximetry, and serum electrolytes in patients receiving diuretics or those with renal insufficiency. An elevated hematocrit in a normovolemic child reflects the magnitude and chronicity of cyanosis. Hematocrit levels above 60% may predispose the patient to capillary sludging and stroke. Because of liberalized feeding guidelines that allow administration of clear liquids up to 3 hours before induction, admission for preoperative intravenous hydration is no longer required in many of these patients. However, it is important to achieve adequate hydration in cyanotic infants.

Premedication

Premedication is used to achieve adequate sedation and maintain respiratory and hemodynamic stability. In children with complex congenital heart disease, premedication is directed toward decreasing oxygen consumption, improving oxygen saturation, and promoting satisfactory anesthetic induction. Oral administration is effective and widely accepted. Most centers use $0.5 \ mg \cdot kg^{-1}$ of midazolam orally 10 to 20 minutes before anesthetic induction, up to a maximum dose of 15 mg. Dosage is adjusted based on age and clinical condition. Dosages of $0.7 \ mg \cdot kg^{-1}$ may be used in hemodynamically stable younger children, with lower doses of $0.3 \ mg \cdot kg^{-1}$ in children with reduced myocardial reserve. Generally, children under the age of 6 months do not require premedication.

Physiologic Monitoring

Physiologic monitoring includes routine noninvasive monitoring as well as an arterial catheter, central venous catheter, and temperature probes. In term newborns and young children, a 22-gauge radial arterial catheter is preferred. In small babies or premature infants, a 24-gauge catheter is used. Posterior tibial and dorsalis pedis arterial catheters should be avoided because of their tendency to function poorly after CPB. Femoral artery catheters may be used, but because of future need for cardiac catheterizations, they are not preferred. Use of an umbilical artery catheter for up to 7 days is appropriate for newborns.

Many centers employ percutaneous central venous catheters as a standard monitoring tool. Others rely on directly placed transthoracic catheters to obtain information for separation from CPB. In patients who require inotropic agents or parenteral nutrition for long intervals postoperatively, placement of a percutaneous indwelling central (PIC) venous catheter should be strongly considered. Percutaneous venous catheters tend to be larger and may have an increased risk for vascular thrombosis around them.

Alternatively, transthoracic catheters may be placed before or after repair of the malformation. However, these fail to provide central access for administration of medication late postoperatively and do not allow central venous pressure monitoring in the prebypass period or effective monitoring of superior vena cava (SVC) pressure during CPB. Similarly, in the absence of a jugular venous catheter, ineffective venous drainage from the head, induced by malfunction of the SVC cannula, is not readily identified during CPB. Although not universally employed, direct measurement of left atrial, right atrial, and pulmonary artery pressures via small indwelling catheters provides more accurate assessment of central pressures than other methods used to guide treatment in the postbypass period.

Temperature

Thermistor probes are placed for measurement of rectal temperature and either nasopharyngeal or tympanic membrane temperature. Nasopharyngeal and tympanic membrane temperatures provide a reasonable estimate of brain temperature. Large gradients between the rectal and nasopharyngeal or tympanic membrane temperature may reflect inadequate total-body cooling and may predispose the patient to unanticipated warming during periods of circulatory arrest or low-flow CPB.

Intraoperative Echocardiography

Intraoperative echocardiography is important for evaluating function and anatomy during the operative procedure. In the postinduction period, TEE provides an opportunity to assess the anatomy and revise the operative plan if necessary.[M3] It permits assessment of systolic and diastolic function, identification of valvar dysfunction, and estimation of pulmonary artery pressure. These observations may lead to modifying the anesthetic plan. After CPB, previously unidentified malformations and residual defects can be identified and corrected in the same operative setting, which may reduce morbidity and mortality.[U1]

Anesthetic Agents

A wide variety of anesthetic drugs have been successfully and safely used, including inhalation agents such as sevoflurane or halothane and intravenous agents such as propofol, fentanyl, midazolam, thiopental, or ketamine (intravenous or intramuscular). [L2,W1] For critically ill neonates, opioid drugs with or without benzodiazepine are generally preferred. Fentanyl is most often used, titrated in 5- to 10-μg · kg^{-1} increments with or without midazolam (0.1 mg · kg^{-1} per increment) until the patient is no longer responsive. A nondepolarizing muscle relaxant is then administered. Alternatively, combined infusions of opioids and benzodiazapines may be used,[K2] generally pancuronium, 0.1 to 0.2 mg · kg^{-1}. Pancuronium causes a mild vagal blockade and an increase in heart rate. This effect, which is undesirable in adults with coronary artery disease, is appropriate in infants and children, who have a greater dependence on heart rate for augmenting cardiac output. Additionally, use of an opioid tends to reduce heart rate, and pancuronium will prevent this reduction.

Ventilation

In infants and children who are not critically ill, controlled induction with sevoflurane and air or oxygen is used after establishing noninvasive monitoring. Sevoflurane has become the preferred agent for induction based on its more rapid onset of action and better hemodynamic profile compared with halothane.

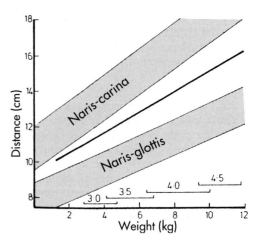

Figure 4-1 Relationship of naris–trachea distance and tracheal tube size (in millimeters of internal diameter) to body weight in infants with congenital cardiac lesions. (From Neutze and colleagues.[N8])

Key: *Heavy line,* naris to midtrachea; *shaded areas,* 75% confidence intervals for naris to carina and naris to glottis.

An orotracheal or nasotracheal tube of proper diameter and length is introduced and fixed in position (Fig. 4-1).[N8]

High fractional concentration of inspired oxygen (FIo$_2$) is avoided in children with shunt physiology or a nonrestrictive ventricular septal defect. Oxygen is a potent pulmonary vasodilator, and use of high concentrations can reduce systemic cardiac output (Q̇s) by diverting more of the cardiac output through the shunt into the pulmonary circulation. Similarly, a low partial pressure of arterial carbon dioxide (PaCO$_2$) can reduce pulmonary vascular resistance (PVR), increase pulmonary blood flow, and reduce blood flow to the systemic circulation. Increased PaCO$_2$ increases PVR and thus also may be hazardous in patients with intracardiac or extracardiac shunts. Therefore, induction with reduced FIo$_2$ and a normal or slightly elevated PaCO$_2$ is helpful in balancing blood flow between the systemic and pulmonary circulations. This is particularly important because all inhaled and most intravenous anesthetics decrease overall cardiac contractility and total cardiac output.

Maintenance of Anesthesia

A combination of an opioid, usually fentanyl, and an inhalation anesthetic, usually isoflurane, is used for maintenance of anesthesia. In general, children with limited cardiac reserve are maintained primarily on an opioid anesthetic, with low concentrations of inhalation agent as a supplement when tolerated. In patients in whom early extubation is planned, anesthesia in the postbypass period is maintained with an inhalation anesthetic, and use of fentanyl is limited. Historically, use of high-dose opioids has been advocated to blunt the stress response in neonates and infants.[H1,H2] More recently, lower doses of opioids have proved to be equally effective, with less release of inflammatory mediators and a lesser degree of endothelial injury.[G2] Alternatively, caudal anesthesia with opioids can be used for patients undergoing operations that require short duration of CPB or no CPB. A single dose of preservative-free morphine (0.5 to 1 mg · kg^{-1}) is administered after induction of anesthesia; it provides excellent pain control during the procedure and in the early postoperative period. Maintenance of anesthesia is accomplished with inhalation isoflurane and supplemental midazolam. This technique facilitates early extubation and provides excellent pain control for up to 12 hours postoperatively.

INFANTS AND CHILDREN UNDERGOING DEEP HYPOTHERMIA WITH OR WITHOUT CIRCULATORY ARREST

In neonates and infants who require complex operative repairs, hypothermic low-flow CPB or hypothermic circulatory arrest may be used. During the prebypass period, the patient's temperature should be maintained above 30° to 32°C to minimize the effects of hypothermia on cardiac output and prevent dysrhythmias. Using CPB, the patient is cooled to between 15° and 20°C nasopharyngeal and tympanic membrane temperature. The goal is to achieve optimal and uniform cooling through a combination of core cooling using CPB and surface cooling using a cooling blanket beneath the patient. Room temperature is lowered after arterial and venous catheter placement. When circulatory arrest is planned, ice packs are placed around the child's head after initiating CPB.

Cardiopulmonary Bypass

With initiation of CPB, cooling is started. In neonates and infants undergoing deep hypothermia, the pump prime may be maintained at a temperature of 18° to 22°C (cold), 30°C (moderate), or 37°C (warm). If a cold prime is used, myocardial function is immediately affected after establishing CPB. Heart rate slows and contraction is impaired. The contribution to total blood flow by the heart rapidly diminishes. Therefore, the arterial pump must reach full flow rapidly to maintain adequate systemic perfusion.

Duration of cooling before reducing flow to low levels or initiating circulatory arrest is generally 20 to 25 minutes. Cooling should proceed at a controlled rate so that temperature does not fall more than 1°C per minute (see Chapter 2). A reduced rate of head or rectal cooling may indicate suboptimal tissue perfusion or a malpositioned probe. If pump flow is inadequate, vasodilators (e.g., phentolamine, phenoxybenzamine, nitroglycerin) can be used. Inhalation anesthetics are used to maintain anesthesia. During cooling and before circulatory arrest, arterial blood gases and hematocrit are measured and necessary adjustments made.

In children the appropriate arterial blood gas management strategy during deep hypothermia is controversial. Some studies have suggested a role for "pH-stat" technique during operations involving deep hypothermia.[D2] The pH-stat method may provide better cerebral blood flow during the cooling and rewarming periods, particularly in patients with aortopulmonary collaterals.[K3] Studies in noncyanotic animals suggest that pH stat may not be beneficial and that

crossover strategies using the pH-stat method followed by "alpha-stat" technique may be preferable.[S5] Data are unclear, but suggest that pH stat may have a role in select patients and that crossover strategies may be another option (see Chapter 2).[B2]

Separation from Cardiopulmonary Bypass

The patient is rewarmed to 35.5° to 36°C, the heart is filled and allowed to eject, arterial blood gases are obtained to ensure adequate acid–base balance, and calcium level is corrected to normal values in neonates and infants. Pacing wires are applied to the heart and tested, and the heart rate is maintained at an age-appropriate level using atrial or atrioventricular sequential pacing, if needed. In most patients, low-dose dopamine (5 µg · kg^{-1} · min^{-1}) is begun prior to weaning from CPB.

If high doses of inotropic agents are required despite adequate preload and ventilatory support, presence of a residual anatomic defect or poor adaptation to new loading conditions resulting from the operative repair may be contributing factors. TEE is helpful for determining the cause of the low output state.

Rationale for Specific Therapies
Right Ventricular Dysfunction (Pulmonary Ventricle)

Primary right ventricular dysfunction may occur after intracardiac surgery in neonates, infants, and children. Diagnosis of right ventricular dysfunction is suggested by high right-sided filling pressures, liver engorgement, hypotension, tachycardia, and reduced cardiac output and systemic venous desaturation (low mixed-venous saturation).

Treatment of right ventricular dysfunction is directed toward improving oxygen delivery by increasing preload, augmenting contractility directly or indirectly, enhancing coronary perfusion, and reducing afterload.

The right ventricle is generally less responsive to inotropic support than the left ventricle and therefore may require higher doses of inotropic agents. Epinephrine enhances right ventricular contractility.[M4] In addition, it may lower pulmonary vascular resistance and improve systemic arterial pressure, which may augment right ventricular coronary blood flow. Coronary perfusion pressure is often reduced with right ventricular dysfunction.[V1,V2] Maintenance of a normal to slightly elevated systolic arterial pressure will maximize coronary perfusion and augment right ventricular contractility.

Mechanical ventilation should be adjusted to optimize preload and decrease afterload. The right ventricle is extremely sensitive to alterations in intrathoracic pressure. Although slight hyperventilation may be beneficial to decrease pulmonary vascular resistance, positive-pressure ventilation, positive end-expiratory pressure, and other ventilatory strategies that increase mean airway pressure will increase afterload and reduce preload.

If these measures are unsuccessful, *extracorporeal membrane oxygenation* (ECMO) should be implemented (see Chapter 5). EMCO unloads the right ventricle and favorably shifts the oxygen supply–demand ratio, often allowing the injured myocardium to recover.

Left Ventricular Dysfunction (Systemic Ventricle)

After separation from CPB, the contractile state of the systemic ventricle may be depressed. Contributing factors include preoperative condition of the myocardium (myocardial hypertrophy, elevated end-diastolic pressure, systolic dysfunction), response of the myocardium to the new loading conditions imposed by the operative repair, effects of deep hypothermia on myocardial compliance, suboptimal myocardial management, and residual anatomic problems.[B3-B8,G3,G4,J1]

Systemic ventricular dysfunction is managed by optimizing preload, afterload, and heart rate (see Chapter 5). Tachycardia (greater than 180 to 190 beats · min^{-1}) may impair ventricular function in newborns and infants and should be treated with beta-adrenergic blocking agents and, if necessary, vasopressors. When heart rate is less than 120 to 130 beats · min^{-1} atrial or atrioventricular sequential, pacing is appropriate.

If inotropic support is necessary, it is usually initiated with dopamine (5 to 10 mg · kg^{-1} · min^{-1}) (see Table 4-4). Infusion of calcium intravenously is an important step to augment ventricular contractility in pediatric patients. Epinephrine is also a potent inotropic agent and is particularly useful in patients with important systemic ventricular dysfunction.

Clinical studies of the effects of milrinone in pediatric patients have shown considerable benefit, especially in those whose myocardium is afterload sensitive, such as patients who have had an arterial switch operation.[B9,C3] Pharmacokinetic studies suggest that milrinone at a loading dose of 50 μg · kg^{-1} followed by an infusion of 0.5 to 1.0 μg · kg^{-1} · min^{-1} is optimal.

Management of Hypoplastic Left Heart Physiology

In the preinduction period, ductal patency must be maintained with prostaglandins to ensure systemic cardiac output. Management depends on optimizing systemic oxygen delivery (by increasing cardiac output) and restricting pulmonary blood flow.

In patients with hypoplastic left heart physiology, pulmonary vascular resistance decreases within hours of delivery, thereby redistributing blood flow away from the systemic circulation. Excessive pulmonary blood flow can be reduced by mild hypoventilation, lowering FIo$_2$ to 0.21, and adding carbon dioxide (CO_2) to the ventilatory circuit. During administration of CO_2, the patient must be sedated or given a muscle relaxant to eliminate increased respiratory effort. Supplemental CO_2 not only reduces pulmonary blood flow, but also allows administration of supplemental oxygen. When transporting patients with hypoplastic left heart physiology to the operating room, monitoring of hemodynamic state and arterial oxygen saturation (SaO$_2$) is essential.

Before discontinuing CPB, ionized calcium levels and hematocrit must be optimized to ensure adequate oxygen-carrying capacity. Myocardial function is supported by judicious use of inotropes. Tidal volume is increased to account for a reduction in lung compliance, and minute ventilation is adjusted to maintain a PaCO$_2$ of 30 to 35 mmHg. After separation from CPB, FIo$_2$ is adjusted to maintain SaO$_2$ between 70% and 80%.

Modified ultrafiltration has been shown to improve myocardial function, decrease lung water, and remove inflammatory mediators in patients with hypoplastic left heart physiology as well as other complex malformations (see Chapter 2).

Excessive pulmonary blood flow is less common in the immediate postbypass period. After modified ultrafiltration and before chest closure, the anesthesiologist should estimate (Q̇p/Q̇s) and attempt to adjust FIo$_2$ and minute ventilation accordingly.

Closure of the chest can markedly reduce lung compliance and worsen hemodynamics. Leaving the chest open may improve pulmonary blood flow and heart filling by reducing mean airway pressure.

Rationale for Management of Fontan, Hemifontan, and Bidirectional Glenn Procedures

Patients undergoing a bidirectional Glenn or hemifontan procedure usually have had either a pulmonary trunk band or a systemic pulmonary artery shunt in the neonatal period. Cardiac performance may be impaired by either a small noncompliant ventricle or a large dilated ventricle, the latter resulting from excessive aortopulmonary shunt flow. Inotropic support may therefore be necessary in the prebypass period as well as postoperatively.

After the bidirectional Glenn or hemifontan procedure, cardiac output is generally well maintained because inferior vena cava flow mixes with pulmonary venous blood in the physiologic left atrium. Low systemic arterial saturation and reduced pulmonary blood flow, however, are problems in the postoperative period. A marked discrepancy between end-tidal carbon dioxide (PetCO$_2$) and PaCO$_2$ is an early sign of reduced pulmonary blood flow. If pulmonary blood flow is reduced with no residual cardiac abnormalities, cardiac output should be optimized and interventions to lower pulmonary vascular resistance employed.

INFANTS AND CHILDREN NOT UNDERGOING CARDIOPULMONARY BYPASS (CLOSED PROCEDURES)

The most common procedures that do not involve CPB are *palliative* (systemic-pulmonary artery shunting and pulmonary trunk banding) or *corrective* (ligation of patent ductus arteriosus or repair of coarctation of the aorta).

Palliative Procedures

Palliative procedures are performed under general anesthesia, with monitoring of systemic arterial pressure. Measurement of arterial pressure, SaO$_2$, and PetCO$_2$ are necessary to assess adequacy of the palliative procedure. Important reduction in PetCO$_2$ after pulmonary trunk banding indicates that pulmonary blood flow may be excessively reduced. This is followed by a precipitous drop in SaO$_2$. If the banding procedure is optimal, systemic arterial blood pressure should increase by approximately 10 to 15 mmHg. The gradient between PetCO$_2$ and PaCO$_2$ should be about 6 to 10 mmHg. Arterial saturation should be no lower than 75% to 80%, and pulmonary arterial pressure should decrease to about 50% of systemic pressure.

Closure of Patent Ductus Arteriosus

Anesthetic considerations for closure of patent ductus arterisosus (PDA) depend on the size of the ductus and clinical condition and age of the patient. Babies with a large PDA and low pulmonary vascular resistance generally present with excessive pulmonary blood flow and heart failure. Neonates and premature infants also may have left ventricular dysfunction from coronary ischemia due to substantial diastolic runoff to the pulmonary circuit. Thus, patients range from the relatively healthy young child to the sick ventilatory-dependent premature infant on inotropic agents. Healthy children can tolerate a variety of anesthetic techniques, culminating in extubation in the operating room and use of epidural/caudal analgesia. Symptomatic neonates and premature infants require a carefully controlled anesthetic and fluid management plan.

Most infants who fail medical management consisting of indomethacin, diuretics, and fluid restriction require admission to a neonatal intensive care unit. A common finding is sepsis, so it is important to ascertain a history of medical treatment and verify negative blood cultures before surgical intervention. Most premature neonates with ductal patency are operated on in the neonatal intensive care unit, thereby avoiding transport hazards, such as hypothermia, multiple transfers to and from infant incubators, inadvertent extubation, and venous access disruption.

In the neonatal intensive care unit the patient is positioned on a warmer, and access to the patient must be shared among the anesthesiologist, surgeon, surgical assistant, and scrub nurse. Careful positioning of an IV catheter and rapid access to a manual resuscitator or equivalent should be established before the baby is draped. Anesthesia is induced with fentanyl (usually in 5-µg aliquots) to maintain appropriate arterial pressure and perfusion. Muscle relaxation is obtained with pancuronium to prevent reduction in heart rate and preserve cardiac output. The patient is temporarily ventilated on 100% oxygen and is weaned once both lungs are allowed to expand after ductal closure. Manual ventilation is often necessary during retraction of the lung in small neonates or in those with preexisting increased oxygen requirements.

Complications include ligation of a pulmonary artery or the aorta. If SaO_2 remains low and $PetCO_2$ decreases, this alerts the anesthesiologist to possible pulmonary artery ligation. Evaluation of pulses in the lower extremities before and after repair also helps ensure that the aorta is patent.

In older children, PDAs are often closed in the interventional cardiac catheterization laboratory. Large PDAs or those with a short segment, however, often require intervention in the operating room under combined general and regional anesthesia.

Coarctation of the Aorta

Coarctation of the aorta is a common cardiac defect and in infants often is associated with anomalies of the mitral valve and left ventricular outflow tract, and with malformation of the great arteries. As with PDA, neonatal repairs are performed in critically ill patients. Coarctation in the newborn is typically associated with left ventricular dysfunction, and these patients may be receiving prostaglan-

dins to ensure ductal patency. Usually they are also receiving mechanical ventilation and inotropic agents. A central intravenous catheter, arterial catheter, and peripheral intravenous catheter are normally placed for operation. Optimal placement of an arterial pressure catheter is in the right radial artery so that pressure can be monitored during clamping of the aorta. If right-sided arterial access is not achieved, a blood pressure cuff is placed on the right arm and the arterial catheter in the left arm or lower extremity. Anesthesia is administered with a combination of fentanyl and an inhalation agent. During aortic clamping, proximal systemic arterial pressure is allowed to rise by 20% to 25% over baseline to optimize perfusion to the spinal cord. Intravascular volume loading with 10 to 20 mL · kg^{-1} of crystalloid is given just before removal of the aortic clamp. The anesthetic concentration is decreased, and additional fluid is administered until arterial pressure rises. In inotrope-dependent neonates, 1 mL · kg^{-1} of bicarbonate is administered before clamp release.

Avoidance of hyperthermia along with mild cooling is appropriate for patients undergoing aortic coarctation repair. Intraoperative hyperthermia has been associated with risk of spinal cord ischemia and paraplegia.[C17] A target temperature of approximately 35°C is appropriate.

In older subjects, postrepair rebound hypertension caused by heightened baroreceptor reactivity often occurs and requires therapy. After aortic clamp release, systemic hypertension is most effectively lowered by institution of beta-adrenergic blockade using esmolol or combined alpha and beta blockade with labetalol. Sodium nitroprusside may be a necessary adjunct to control refractory hypertension; however, it increases calculated wall stress in the absence of beta-adrenergic blockade by accelerating dP/dt. An effective alternative to nitroprusside is the calcium channel blocker nicardipine.

PATIENTS UNDERGOING OPERATIONS ON ASCENDING AORTA, AORTIC ARCH, AND DESCENDING THORACIC AORTA

Patients presenting for procedures on the thoracic aorta (ascending, arch, and descending) may be in extremis, thus limiting the degree of preoperative anesthetic assessment. In elective cases a standard preoperative interview and examination can be performed. The anesthesiologist must clearly understand the details of the proposed operation. For example, surgery on the descending thoracic aorta requires lateral decubitus positioning as well as temporary deflation of the left lung.

Because of the possibility of major hemorrhage, insertion of large-bore IV catheters is essential. Intraarterial catheters and other monitoring devices can usually be placed before induction. A pulmonary artery catheter is placed. The site for arterial access depends on the location of the aortic disease as well as the surgical approach. Generally, a right radial arterial catheter is used to avoid inaccurate readings from the left radial artery, which can occur when the subclavian artery is diseased or requires clamping during the aortic procedure. Monitoring of arterial pressure at a distal site (femoral or dorsalis pedis artery) is useful when left heart bypass will be used to ensure adequate perfusion pressure distal to the occluded aortic segment. This additional arterial access can be obtained after anesthetic induction.

Use of beta-adrenergic drugs (e.g., esmolol, labetalol) and a vasodilator (e.g., nitroprusside) may be necessary to limit the extent of the aortic dissection or rupture (if present) by reducing wall tension and decreasing shear forces exerted on the aorta. This should be done before induction of anesthesia to compensate for rapid changes that may occur during induction. Induction is generally accomplished with a combination of narcotics, benzodiazepines, other hypnotics, and muscle relaxants. If the procedure is emergent, requiring rapid endotracheal intubation in a patient who is at risk for aspiration, a rapid-acting hypnotic (e.g., etomidate) and a paralytic agent (e.g., succinylcholine) are administered. In the elective setting a slower induction can be performed using vecuronium or pancuronium.

If the ascending aorta or aortic arch will be replaced through a median sternotomy, a single-lumen endotracheal tube is appropriate. If the descending aorta will be repaired or replaced through a median sternotomy or a left thoracotomy, one-lung ventilation will be required. A double-lumen or single-lumen endotracheal tube with an endobronchial blocker can be used. Fiberoptic bronchoscopy is necessary to confirm proper placement of the double-lumen endotracheal tube or endobronchial blocker.

TEE is helpful in assessing location and extent of an aortic dissection or other aortic disease. Often the site of an intimal disruption can be identified. A disruption in the aortic arch that extends into the descending aorta may influence the surgical approach. When aortic disease involves the ascending aorta, evaluation of the aortic valve is important. Proximal extension of a dissection toward the aortic anulus results in aortic regurgitation. In addition, obstruction of the right coronary artery can occur and can often be identified both by location of the intimal flap and presence of an inferior regional wall motion abnormality. After repair, TEE is of value in assessing the adequacy of the repair as well as providing information about myocardial function.

If the operative repair involves the descending thoracic or thoracoabdominal aorta, the spinal cord is at risk for ischemic injury. Techniques for protection of the spinal cord during surgery are discussed in Chapter 53 and Box 4-1. The prevalence of paraplegia after operations on the thoracic and thoracoabdominal aorta is variable.[M5]

Measurement of temperature is particularly important during operations on the thoracic aorta. For operations on the descending aorta, mild hypothermia (30° to 32°C) may provide protection of the spinal cord. For operations on the aortic arch, hypothermic circulatory arrest is often necessary (see Chapters 2, 52, and 53).

PATIENTS UNDERGOING PERICARDECTOMY FOR CONSTRICTIVE PERICARDITIS AND PERICARDIAL TAMPONADE

Decreased cardiac output resulting from acute cardiac tamponade or a chronic constrictive process may require surgical intervention. Cardiac output is reduced because of inadequate diastolic filling of the ventricles. Intrapericardial pressure greater than intraventricular pressure results in

---

BOX 4-1   Techniques for Spinal Cord Protection during Thoracic Aorta Surgery

Surgical Technique
Minimizing aortic clamp time
Minimizing vascular interruption (avoiding ligation of intercostal arteries, use of staged aortic clamping)
Reimplanting intercostal arteries

"Neuroanesthesia" Adjuncts
Moderate hyperventilation (PaCO₂ 30-32 mmHg)
Mannitol (1 g · kg⁻¹ intravenously)

Distal Perfusion Techniques
Vascular shunts (Gott shunt)
Left atrial–femoral artery bypass
Femoral–femoral bypass

Optimization of Hemodynamics/Spinal Cord Hydrodynamics
Lower CVP (phlebotomy)
Lower CSF pressure (CSF drainage)

Hypothermia
Epidural/spinal cord cooling
Systemic hypothermia (mild to moderate or deep)

Pharmacologic
(theoretic)

Key: *PaCO₂,* Partial pressure of arterial carbon dioxide; *CVP,* central venous pressure; *CSF,* cerebrospinal fluid.

---

inadequate ventricular filling, decreased ventricular end-diastolic transmural pressure, and reduced cardiac output.[M6,R6,S6] Increased heart rate and elevated venous pressure are compensatory mechanisms that offset the increase in intrapericardial pressure.

Regardless of the cause of cardiac tamponade, principles of anesthetic management are the same (see Table 4-1). A satisfactory regimen includes induction with ketamine (1 mg · kg⁻¹) and pancuronium (0.1 mg · kg⁻¹) and subsequent administration of nitrous oxide and isoflurane. Alternatively, etomidate (0.2 to 0.6 mg · kg⁻¹) can be used for induction. Positive-pressure ventilation in the presence of cardiac tamponade may depress cardiac output, and maintenance of spontaneous breathing until the chest is opened may be advisable.[M6,S7]

Except in the case of constrictive pericarditis, cardiac performance immediately improves after incision of the pericardium.[V3] In patients with uremic pericardial effusion and evidence of tamponade, drugs that are primarily metabolized and excreted by the kidney should be avoided. Fluid must be administered cautiously, and serum potassium must be measured.[K4,P2]

PATIENTS UNDERGOING CARDIAC TRANSPLANTATION

Management objectives must take into account the cause of heart failure, commonly associated arrhythmias, likelihood of previous heart surgery, and medications, including anticoagulants, that the patient may be taking, as well as the urgency of operation.

Because of the relatively urgent time frame for heart transplantation, the anesthesiologist often has limited opportunity to assess and interact with the patient preoperatively. Ideally, an anesthesiology preoperative consultation will have been performed at the time a patient is placed on the transplant waiting list, but this is not always possible. Some management objectives differ from those for other types of heart surgery (see Chapter 49).

Understanding the cause of heart failure leading to transplantation is an important aspect of preoperative assessment. Considerations are different for the patient with end-stage ischemic heart disease than for one with dilated cardiomyopathy. A patient with ischemic cardiomyopathy is prone to additional myocardial ischemia resulting from anxiety induced by the forthcoming operation. The possibility of ischemia needs to be monitored (through close verbal patient contact and with multilead ECG) and anxiety and its consequences aggressively treated (e.g., intravenous nitroglycerin).

Ventricular arrhythmias are common in these patients, and many receive long-term antiarrhythmic therapy. Often, automatic defibrillators have been implanted and require special consideration. Unlike other types of pacemakers, the defibrillator must be turned off before operation because the electrocautery artifact will be interpreted as a malignant arrhythmia, triggering a countershock from the device that may itself precipitate an arrhythmia. Many patients with severe left ventricular dysfunction or atrial fibrillation are receiving anticoagulation and require replacement of coagulation factors at a later stage in the operation.

The patient with ischemic cardiomyopathy may have had previous coronary artery bypass grafting (CABG), with risks of bleeding from adhesions and disruption of the heart or major vessels at sternotomy. Large-bore IV access is essential to prepare for major blood loss, but venous access can be limited because of the chronicity of illness. Indwelling central venous access catheters for induction and maintenance of anesthesia are desirable, and the preferred site is the left jugular vein, because the right side will be used subsequently as access for myocardial biopsy.

Patients may have eaten shortly before arrival in the operating room. Administration of an oral nonparticulate antacid and IV H_2 receptor blocker (e.g., ranitidine 50 mg) and gastric motility agent (e.g., metoclopramide 10 mg) can be useful to prevent aspiration of gastric contents. Anxiolytic sedatives (e.g., IV midazolam 0.015 to 0.03 mg $\cdot$ kg^{-1} in divided doses) are administered during preinduction placement of IV and arterial catheters. This may prevent psychological stress–induced ischemia. Central venous access may have to be instituted after induction because heart failure–related dyspnea may make supine positioning of the patient difficult. Immunosuppressive therapy is generally initiated in the preinduction period. The immunocompromised state induced in these patients necessitates strict asepsis during catheter placement.

Anesthesia induction proceeds in much the same manner as for the patient undergoing CABG. Because of the critical nature of their disease, these patients have little if any hemodynamic reserve. In general, higher doses of narcotics (e.g., fentanyl) and benzodiazepines (e.g., midazolam) are used to induce and maintain anesthesia. These negate the need for any other anesthetics that may have adverse hemodynamic effects while ensuring an adequate level of anesthesia.

Administration of the antifibrinolytic and antiinflammatory agent aprotinin is useful because these patients often have long duration of CPB and are prone to excessive bleeding. Aprotinin is typically administered after a test dose using an IV bolus (2×10^6 KIU, with 2×10^6 KIU into the CPB pump prime) and subsequent IV infusion (0.5×10^6 KIU $\cdot$ h^{-1}), preferably just before incision and continuing until the end of operation. Plans for treating a coagulopathy need to be formulated before the end of CPB, including the potential need for several different blood products.

Weaning from CPB after heart transplant warrants special consideration of both left and right ventricular function. The normal (nonhypertrophied) donor right ventricle faces elevated afterload imposed by pulmonary hypertensive changes and thus has a greater potential for dysfunction than after other cardiac operations. This requires liberal use of inotropic support. Although epinephrine and isoproterenol are useful, a phosphodiesterase inhibitor such as milrinone (50 μg $\cdot$ kg^{-1} as IV bolus, followed by IV infusion of 0.5 μg $\cdot$ kg^{-1} $\cdot$ min^{-1}) is typically added as a second-line agent. If right ventricular dysfunction persists, inhaled nitric oxide is added to provide further afterload reduction. Often, these agents are maintained well into the postoperative period. Typically, extubation also is delayed, necessitating continued sedation.

SECTION 2
Operative Monitoring

Comprehensive perioperative care of the cardiac patient requires the ability to detect organ dysfunction through various monitoring systems, thereby allowing modification of the patient's care as necessary. Choice of monitors is based on both patient and surgical factors.

Overall age-adjusted hospital mortality for cardiac surgery has trended down over the past two decades. Refinement in both surgical technique and anesthetic ability has allowed patients who otherwise would have been denied surgery because of their high risk to proceed successfully through operation to recovery. Part of the reason for this success has been the ability to identify problems that might occur during operation by means of better monitoring techniques. However, as a result of a sicker and an older cohort presenting for surgery, certain organ morbidities have increased. Notably, both number and proportion of neurologic-related deaths from cardiac surgery have increased.[A1,E3,G5,T2]

Except for cardioplegia and its utility to improve myocardial management, no greater advance has come in organ monitoring and protection than that directed toward the brain. New methods to measure brain function have improved the understanding of the neurologic morbidity that may accompany cardiac surgery.[N1] At Duke University, a comprehensive neurologic monitoring system has been applied to patients considered at increased risk for neurologic injury (Fig. 4-2). This system selectively includes transcranial Doppler (TCD) color flow imaging, near-infrared spectroscopy (NIRS), multichannel electroencephalography (EEG), and jugular bulb oxygen saturation (SjvO$_2$) monitoring, in addition to routine use of TEE to help provide information regarding stroke risk by assessing atheromatous involvement of the aorta.

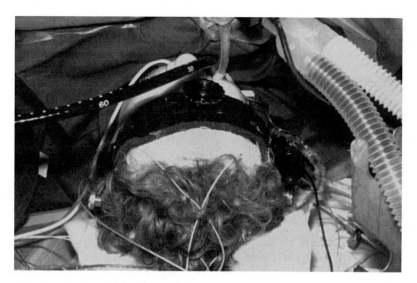

Figure 4-2   Comprehensive neurologic monitoring system consisting of a jugular bulb oxygen saturation catheter, transcranial Doppler, near-infrared spectroscopy, multichannel electroencephalography, and transesophageal echocardiography. At Duke University, this system has been used on patients deemed at increased risk for neurologic injury. Various combinations of monitors are used selectively on other patients.

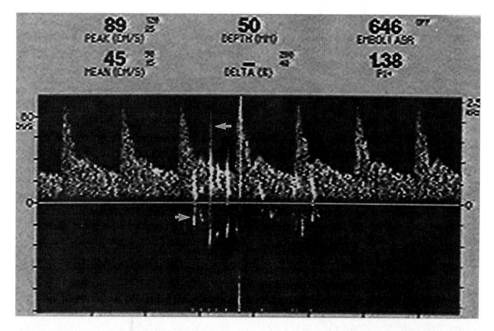

Figure 4-3   Transcranial Doppler (TCD) signals in a patient undergoing coronary artery bypass grafting. TCD provides information on blood flow velocity (an indirect measure of cerebral blood flow) as well as microembolic phenomena. Arrows depict high-intensity signals that represent cerebral microemboli (either gaseous or particulate).

Neurocognitive dysfunction after cardiac operations is related to microembolic load.[P3] TCD imaging has been used during cardiac surgery to detect microemboli (Fig. 4-3). The image shows multiple high-intensity signals representing microemboli, both gaseous and particulate, passing through the middle cerebral artery (MCA). The drawback to TCD is the inability to differentiate between the two types of microemboli. TCD using blood flow velocity signals can also estimate relative changes in cerebral blood flow during CPB,[V4,W2] although there is con-

siderable debate as to its accuracy[N2] and therefore its applicability.

Hemodynamic monitoring includes electrocardiography (to determine heart rate, rhythm, and morphology) and measurement of arterial, central venous (or P_{RA}), pulmonary artery, and left atrial pressures. Continuous automated ECG monitoring systems allow detection of ST-segment changes.[J2,P4] In a multicenter study, ECG predicted myocardial infarction in patients undergoing CABG based on the occurrence of ST-segment changes in the first 8 to

BOX 4-2 Indications and Complications of Pulmonary Artery Catheterization

Indications
1. Monitoring of pulmonary artery pressure
2. Measurement of pulmonary artery wedge pressure to estimate left atrial pressure, left ventricular end–diastolic pressure, and left ventricular preload
3. Pulmonary artery and pulmonary artery wedge pressure waveform analysis (e.g., giant regurgitant *c* and *v* waves in mitral regurgitation)
4. Measurement or continuous monitoring of cardiac output
5. Measurement or continuous monitoring of mixed venous hemoglobin saturation

Complications
Catheter Placement
1. Arrhythmias, including supraventricular tachyarrhythmias, atrial fibrillation, ventricular extrasystoles, ventricular tachycardia, ventricular fibrillation, right bundle branch block, and complete heart block
2. Misplaced catheter tip
3. Air embolism

Catheter Residence (Late Complications)
1. Mechanical problems, including catheter entrapment, coiling, knotting, and tip migration
2. Introducer sheath problems
3. Balloon rupture
4. Thrombosis, pulmonary embolism
5. Thrombocytopenia
6. Pulmonary infarction
7. Infection, including endocarditis
8. Other structural damage to the endocardium, tricuspid valve, pulmonic valve, or pulmonary artery, resulting in pulmonary artery rupture or pseudoaneurysm

Misinterpretation or Misuse of Catheter-Derived Data

(Modified from Mark and colleagues.[M16])

16 hours after aortic clamp removal.[J3] ECG is also useful during CPB to detect persistent electrical activity under aortic clamping, prompting additional cardioplegia administration.

After its introduction in the 1970s for management of critically ill patients, pulmonary artery (PA) catheterization became widely used in cardiac surgery. Undoubtedly, use of the PA catheter improved understanding of perioperative cardiac physiology. Along with this knowledge, however, it also became apparent that the information gained from the PA catheter might be offset by potential complications, although these occur infrequently.[C19] A selective rather than universal approach to PA catheter use is therefore suggested. Box 4-2 lists the indications and complications of PA catheterization.

Cardiac output can be measured directly by PA catheter thermodilution[G16,M17] or indirectly by a number of different methods, including mixed venous oxygen saturation,[D4] by either intermittent sampling of PA blood or continuous oximetry.[C20] During cardiac surgery, Doppler examination of aortic blood flow velocity,[G13,H6] arterial pulse wave contour analysis,[A3,K1] and capnography using the modified Fick principle[F5,Z2] have also been used to estimate cardiac output.[S21]

As noted earlier, one of the most important advancements in monitoring during cardiac surgery is TEE. It has proven effective for both diagnosing morphologic entities and elucidating normal and abnormal physiology, and is cost effective (Figs. 4-4 to 4-6). Since the advent of intraoperative TEE, cardiac anesthesiologists not only monitor heart function but also participate in diagnosing heart disease and assist in surgical techniques[E1,H3,P10] (Box 4-3). TEE allows a real-time estimate of ejection fraction, myo-

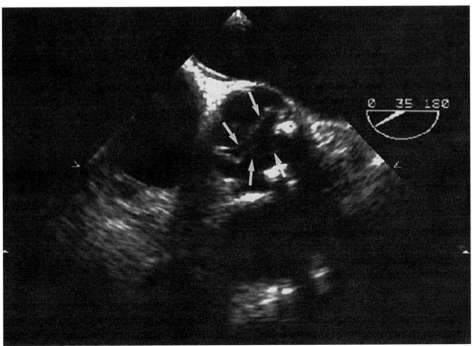

Figure 4-4 Transesophageal echocardiographic image of aortic stenosis as seen by the arrows outlining the stenotic orifice. In addition to the stenosis, this valve is congenitally bicuspid.

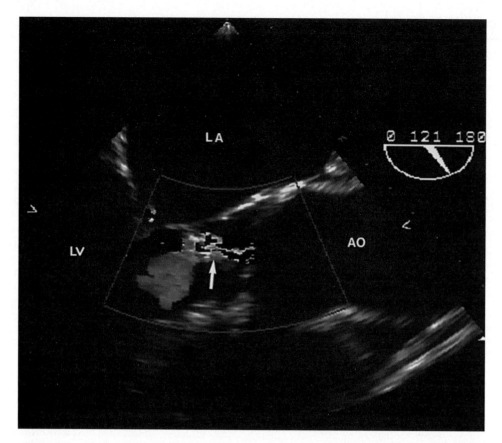

Figure 4-5   Transesophageal echocardiographic image of aortic regurgitation demonstrating a long-axis view of the left ventricular *(LV)* outflow tract, left atrium *(LA)*, aortic valve, and ascending aorta *(AO)*. The regurgitant jet *(arrow)* can be seen using color flow Doppler imaging.

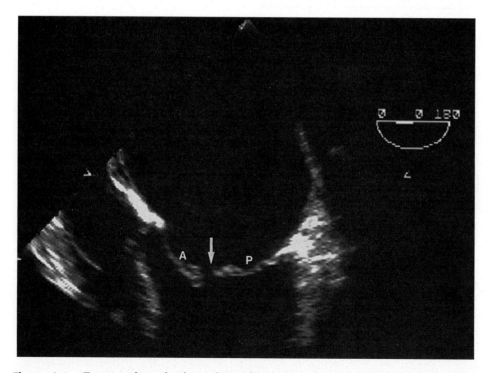

Figure 4-6   Transesophageal echocardiographic image of mitral stenosis. Stenotic mitral orifice *(arrow)* is a result of rheumatic degeneration of both the anterior *(A)* and posterior *(P)* leaflets. The anterior leaflet is shaped in a "hockey stick" pattern, a characteristic sign of rheumatic mitral degeneration.

BOX 4-3 Perioperative Transesophageal Echocardiography (TEE) Practice Guidelines

Category I Indications
Supported by the strongest evidence or expert opinion; TEE is frequently useful in improving clinical outcomes in these settings and is often indicated, depending on individual circumstances (e.g., patient risk, practice setting).

- Intraoperative evaluation of acute, persistent, and life-threatening hemodynamic disturbances in which ventricular function and its determinants are uncertain and have not responded to treatment
- Intraoperative use in valve repair
- Intraoperative use in congenital heart surgery for most lesions requiring cardiopulmonary bypass
- Intraoperative use in repair of hypertrophic obstructive cardiomyopathy
- Intraoperative use for endocarditis when preoperative testing was inadequate or extension of infection to perivalvular tissue is suspected
- Preoperative use in unstable patients with suspected thoracic aortic aneurysms, dissection, or disruption who need to be evaluated quickly
- Intraoperative assessment of aortic valve function in repair of aortic dissections with possible aortic valve involvement
- Intraoperative evaluation of pericardial window procedures
- Use in intensive care unit for unstable patients with unexplained hemodynamic disturbances, suspected valve disease, or thromboembolic problems (if other tests or monitoring techniques have not confirmed the diagnosis or patients are too unstable to undergo other tests)

Category II Indications
Supported by weaker evidence and expert consensus; TEE may be useful in improving clinical outcomes in these settings, depending on individual circumstances, but appropriate indications are less certain.

- Perioperative use in patients with increased risk of myocardial ischemia or infarction
- Perioperative use in patients with increased risk of hemodynamic disturbances
- Intraoperative assessment of valve replacement
- Intraoperative assessment of repair of cardiac aneurysms

- Intraoperative evaluation of removal of cardiac tumors
- Intraoperative detection of foreign bodies
- Intraoperative detection of air emboli during cardiotomy, heart transplant operations, and upright neurosurgical procedures
- Intraoperative use during intracardiac thrombectomy
- Intraoperative use during pulmonary embolectomy
- Intraoperative use for suspected cardiac trauma
- Preoperative assessment of patients with suspected acute thoracic aortic dissections, aneurysms, or disruption
- Intraoperative use during repair of thoracic aortic dissections without suspected aortic valve involvement
- Intraoperative detection of aortic atheromatous disease or other sources of aortic emboli
- Intraoperative evaluation of pericardiectomy and pericardial effusion or evaluation of pericardial surgery
- Intraoperative evaluation of anastomotic sites during heart and/or lung transplantation
- Monitoring of placement and function of assist devices

Category III Indications
Little current scientific or expert support; TEE is infrequently useful in improving clinical outcomes in these settings, and appropriate indications are uncertain.

- Intraoperative evaluation of myocardial perfusion, coronary artery anatomy, or graft patency
- Intraoperative use during repair of cardiomyopathies other than hypertrophic obstructive cardiomyopathy
- Intraoperative use for uncomplicated endocarditis during noncardiac surgery
- Intraoperative monitoring for emboli during orthopedic procedures
- Intraoperative assessment of repair of thoracic aortic injuries
- Intraoperative use for uncomplicated pericarditis
- Intraoperative evaluation of pleuropulmonary diseases
- Monitoring placement of intraaortic balloon pumps, automatic implantable cardiac defibrillators, or pulmonary artery catheters
- Intraoperative monitoring of cardioplegia administration

(From American Society of Anesthesiologists.[P10])

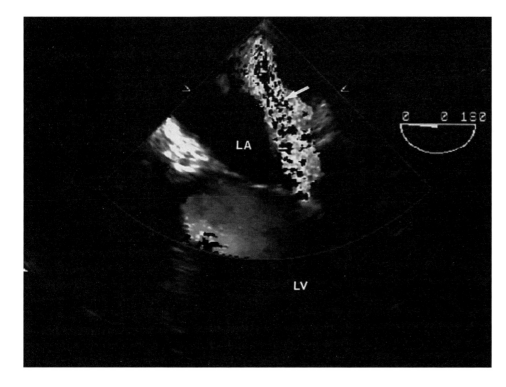

Figure 4-7 Transesophageal echocardiographic image of mitral regurgitation. Regurgitant flow *(arrow)* from the left ventricle *(LV)* is seen within the left atrium *(LA)*.

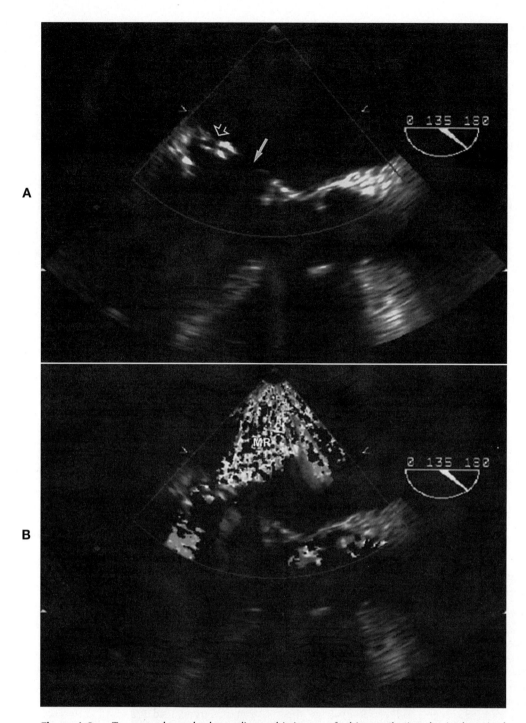

Figure 4-8   Transesophageal echocardiographic image of a bioprosthetic valve in the mitral position. **A**, Defect *(open arrow)* in the lateral anular structure of the bioprosthesis *(solid arrow)* can be seen. **B**, Color flow Doppler image of the lateral aspect of the anulus demonstrates periprosthetic leakage with resulting mitral regurgitation.

cardial ischemia (as segmental wall dysfunction), and valve function[B10,S8] (Fig. 4-7). During valve surgery, TEE can be used to assess the type and severity of lesion as well as the valve function after repair or replacement. Figure 4-8 illustrates periprosthetic leakage after placement of a bioprosthetic valve. TEE aided in determining the cause and location of the mitral regurgitation. TEE can be used to guide fluid therapy, vasopressor and inotropic support, and antiischemic therapy,[B10] particularly during high-risk CABG.[S9] TEE also supplements epiaortic scanning for defining atheromatous disease in the aorta and its associated risk of stroke.[H4,S10]

SECTION 3
Cardiopulmonary Bypass and the Brain

While undergoing CPB, the patient deviates from normal physiology in a number of important ways. As noted in Chapter 2, circulation is nonpulsatile, perfusion flow is generally lower than normal, body temperature is often decreased, hemodilution is intentionally created, and the lungs are excluded from the circulation. The blood is pumped through conduits with biologically foreign surfaces, resulting in rheologic abnormalities and protein denaturation, among many other damaging effects (see Chapter 2).

BRAIN PROTECTION

Hypothermia

Both hypothermia and general anesthesia protect the potentially ischemic brain. Various levels of hypothermia are maintained during CPB to protect organ morphology and function when the potential exists for ischemia, which may result from nonpulsatile and lower-than-normal flows. The brain is the organ of greatest concern and requires optimal protection during CPB (see Chapter 2). Cerebral metabolic rate for oxygen ($CMRo_2$) has been shown to be directly related to brain temperature (Fig. 4-9).[C4] A convenient way to express the effect of temperature on $CMRo_2$ is to calculate the change of metabolism during cooling or warming for a temperature change of 10°C (the Q_{10}). During CPB the brain Q_{10} is 2.8 for adults (Fig. 4-10)[C4] and is slightly higher in infants (see Section 2 of Chapter 2).[G6]

It has been postulated[M7] and experimentally confirmed in animals[S11] and humans[W3] that temperature and general anesthesia affect brain oxidative metabolism differently. Cerebral metabolism supports cellular function (electrical activity of neuronal transmission of impulses) and cellular integrity (maintenance of cellular homeostasis). The functional component of cerebral metabolism accounts for 60% of metabolism, and cellular integrity accounts for the remainder.[M7] General anesthetics affect primarily the functional component, whereas temperature affects both function and integrity. In clinical practice, there will always be a combined effect of general anesthesia and hypothermia, but as shown in dogs, *temperature* provides the most important cerebral protection from anoxia.[M7]

Although suppression of cerebral metabolism is the dominant protective effect of low temperature, other temperature-dependent mechanisms exist. Hypothermia attenuates the release of excitotoxic amino acids (aspartate and glutamate),[B11] reduces calcium influx, hastens the recovery of protein synthesis,[W4] diminishes membrane-bound protein kinase C activity,[B12] and increases the time to onset of ischemic depolarization.[N3] In addition, salutary effects of hypothermia on mediators of the inflammatory response include reduced formation of reactive oxygen species[G7] and suppressed nitric oxide synthase activity.[K5] Each activity, unfettered, can injure the brain.

A number of studies have examined the effect of temperature during CPB on neurologic and cognitive function after cardiac surgery[B13,B14,E1,E2,G8,G9,K6,M8-M10,P5,S12]

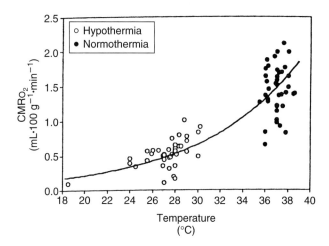

Figure 4-9 Cerebral metabolic rate for oxygen ($CMRo_2$) is expressed in relation to temperature based on the van't Hoff equation $Ln(CMRo_2) = a + b*T$, where *Ln* is the natural logarithmic function, *a* is the intercept, *b* is the slope, and *T* is temperature in °C. (From Croughwell and colleagues.[C4])

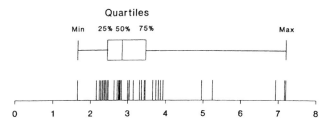

Figure 4-10 Box-and-whisker plot illustrates the quartile measurements of Q_{10} for the brain (cerebral oxygen consumption change for a temperature change of 10°C). Each line represents a calculated Q_{10} from an individual patient. Fifty percent of the data lies between 2.4 (lower quartile) and 3.4 (higher quartile); this data range is represented by the large rectangle. The median Q_{10} on nonpulsatile cardiopulmonary bypass is 2.8. (From Croughwell and colleagues.[C4])

(Table 4-8). Several major trials have also examined the effects of normothermic or hypothermic CPB on cerebral outcome after cardiac surgery. The Warm Heart Investigators trial examined normothermic (33° to 37°C, n = 860) versus moderately hypothermic (25° to 30°C, n = 872) coronary bypass surgery and found no difference in either 30-day mortality or prevalence of stroke.[R5] This is in contrast to a study by Martin and colleagues of 1001 patients in which the normothermic CPB group had a higher occurrence of stroke (normothermic 3.1%, moderately hypothermic 1.0%, P <.02).[M9] Results of the neurocognitive outcomes in these two studies coincided, however. In subgroup analyses from the Martin (n = 138) and Warm Heart Investigators trials (n = 201), no differences were demonstrated in neurocognitive outcome.[M8,M10] In the study of Grigore and colleagues of 300 patients undergoing normothermic (36°C) versus moderately hypothermic (28°C) CPB, there again was no effect of temperature on neurocognitive outcome.[G9]

Methodologic differences among the three studies partly explain the divergent results. Of particular importance was

■ **TABLE 4-8   Effect of Temperature on Neurologic and Neurocognitive Dysfunction in Patients Undergoing Coronary Artery Bypass Grafting**

Study	Year Published	Type	n	Neurologic Dysfunction	Neurocognitive Dysfunction	Temperature (°C)
Grigore et al.[G9]	2001	Randomized	300	No relationship to temperature	No relationship to temperature	28, 36
Engelman et al.[E1]	1999	Randomized	291	No relationship to temperature	Not investigated	20, 32, 37
Plourde et al.[P5]	1997	Randomized	62	No relationship to temperature	No relationship to temperature	28, 35
Mora et al.[M8]	1996	Randomized	138	Higher in 35°C group	No relationship to temperature	28, 35
Engelman et al.[E2]	1996	Randomized	130	Trend toward a higher prevalence in 20°C group	Not investigated	20, 32, 37
Singh et al.[S12]	1995	Clinical study	2585	No relationship to temperature	Not investigated	25-30, 37
Martin et al.[M9]	1994	Randomized	1001	Higher in 35°C group	Not investigated	28, 35
Warm Heart Investigators[R5]	1994	Randomized	1732	No relationship to temperature	Not investigated	25-30, 33-37
McLean et al.[M10]	1994	Randomized	201	No relationship to temperature	No relationship to temperature	28, 34

how "normothermia" was both defined and maintained. In the Warm Heart Investigators trial (where neither stroke nor neurocognitive dysfunctional differences were demonstrated), the normothermic group was actually mildly hypothermic, with temperature allowed to "drift" during CPB (at times reaching as low as 33°C). In the Martin study (where prevalence of stroke differed but neurocognitive outcome did not), a bladder temperature of 35°C or greater was maintained by actively warming the arterial inflow blood to 37°C. This active warming has been shown to cause cerebral hyperthermia.[C5,G10] The fact that Martin and colleagues did not measure nasopharyngeal temperature (which is higher than bladder temperature) likely resulted in their warm group being slightly hyperthermic. Grigore and colleagues' normothermic group (where no difference in neurocognition was demonstrated) was maintained at 35.5° to 36.5°C, in effect representing an intermediate temperature group between the other two trials. Most studies (see Table 4-8) show little effect of temperature within the ranges quoted. However, the data may be interpreted as consistent with the recommendation that in adults, a perfusion temperature of 32° to 34°C with hemodilution is acceptable. (For a discussion of deep hypothermia and the effect of core cooling, see "Temperature and Duration" under Hypothermia and Circulatory Arrest in Chapter 2).

Hemoglobin Concentration

If perfusion flow rate remains constant, as it usually does during CPB in the brain because of autoregulation, and if PaO_2 remains constant, as it usually does during CPB, the major determinant of oxygen delivery is hemoglobin concentration (see Chapter 2).

In the earliest days of CPB, the perfusate was adjusted to provide a normal hemoglobin concentration, and hemodilution was not allowed. With the advent of hypothermia, however, intentional hemodilution became standard practice. In humans at 37°C the normal hematocrit of 40% is rheologically optimal for maximal oxygen transport.[C6] This provides sufficient oxygen delivery to maintain normal mitochondrial oxygen partial pressure levels of about 0.05 to 1.0 mmHg and average intracellular Po_2 levels of about 5 mmHg, as reflected in normal venous oxygen levels of about 40 mmHg and venous oxygen saturation of about 75%. Hypothermia increases apparent blood viscosity within the normal hematocrit range. When hematocrit is abnormally high or when temperature is abnormally low, the resulting increased viscosity decreases microcirculatory blood flow. Although oxygen transport varies directly with hematocrit, it varies inversely with the apparent blood viscosity. Thus, during moderate hypothermic CPB, hematocrit levels of 20% to 25% are desirable for optimal oxygen transport, although severe reduction of hematocrit may predispose the patient to neurologic dysfunction.[C6]

In animals subjected to MCA occlusion, resultant infarct size was increased by reducing hematocrit levels.[L5,R7] In humans during hypothermic CPB, the level of hemodilution at which the risk of neurologic damage outweighs the rheologic benefit is unknown. During the past two decades, because of concerns about the safety of the blood supply, intentional hemodilution to hematocrits less than 18% evolved and was reported to be acceptable.[C7,C8,J4,L3,L4,O1,P6,S13,Z1] This practice is being questioned now,[F1] especially in high-risk and elderly patients who possess less powerful compensatory mechanisms. The safe lower limit of hematocrit during CPB is unknown in humans, although in a recent canine CPB study the "critical hematocrit value" for the brain during normothermic CPB was 14%. This low hematocrit value was compensated for by increased cerebral blood flow, but below a hematocrit of 14% brain oxygenation and oxygen utilization decreased.[C9] In the same model, hypothermia (28°C) reduced the "critical hematocrit" to 11%.[C10] Hemoglobin concentration at the start of CPB can be predicted from the estimated blood volume and red cell volume of the patient, and priming volume and red cell volume of the heart-lung machine (see "Diluent" under Whole Body Perfusion during Cardiopulmonary Bypass in Chapter 2).

Perfusion Pressure

Perfusion pressure during CPB is the product of perfusion flow rate, usually 1.6 to 2.4 $L \cdot min^{-1} \cdot m^{-2}$, and systemic vascular resistance (see "Systemic Vascular Resistance and Arterial Blood Pressure" under Whole Body Perfusion during Cardiopulmonary Bypass in Chapter 2). The brain has a pressure–flow relationship that is described by autoregulatory curves. With autoregulation intact, as it is during CPB (during alpha-stat strategy of arterial blood gas management), cerebral blood flow is relatively constant over a wide range of perfusion pressures.[A2,S14] During CPB the relationship of cerebral blood flow to perfusion pressure is 1.8 $mL \cdot min^{-1} \cdot 100 \ g^{-1}$ for every 10-mmHg change in

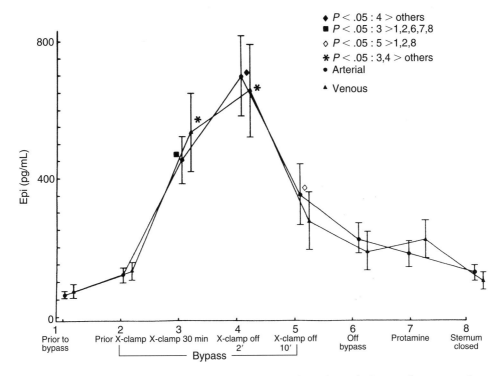

Figure 4-11 Plasma epinephrine concentration at various times during cardiac surgery ($n = 28$; vertical bars represent ±1 standard error). Note the significantly elevated level at the end of aortic clamping. (From Reves and colleagues.[R12])

perfusion pressure.[N4] The relationship is more pronounced in normothermic patients than hypothermic patients. Evidence indicates that insulin-dependent diabetic patients do not have normal autoregulation during CPB,[C11] and cerebral blood flow is more pressure dependent. Cerebral blood flow is also perfusion pressure dependent in patients with elevated $PaCO_2$ or during pH-stat strategy of arterial blood gas management (see "Arterial Carbon Dioxide Pressure" under Whole Body Perfusion during Cardiopulmonary Bypass in Chapter 2).

Over the past 35 years a number of studies on the effect of perfusion pressure on clinical outcomes have reported persistently conflicting results.[G11,N5,S15,S16,T3] A higher perfusate pressure might be helpful in patients with known arterial obstructions, such as those with carotid artery stenosis of greater than 90% or severe renal artery stenosis, although supportive evidence is limited. Diabetic patients and older patients may also benefit from a higher perfusion pressure. Otherwise, the bulk of the evidence suggests that maintaining a perfusion pressure of 30 to 50 mmHg or greater is satisfactory for most cardiac surgical patients.[G18]

BLOOD GAS MANAGEMENT

Arterial blood gas pressures are monitored during CPB to measure adequacy of oxygenation and CO_2 exchange. Cooling blood causes a right shift in CO_2 dissociation (increased solubility) and thus a trend toward alkalemia. Therefore, it is important to decide whether the arterial blood gas pressures are temperature corrected (pH stat) or

not (alpha stat), as described in "Arterial Carbon Dioxide Pressure" under Whole Body Perfusion during Cardiopulmonary Bypass in Chapter 2. Generally, CPB monitoring and management are done without temperature correction. With alpha-stat management, blood is taken from a hypothermic patient (32°C) and measured at 37°C. The resulting partial pressures are uncorrected for the patient's temperature, and thus during CPB the patient is alkalotic. CO_2 is not added to the gas mixture flowing into the oxygenator. With pH-stat management and blood gases measured at 37°C, the partial pressures are corrected for the patient's temperature using published nomograms, and CO_2 is added to the gas mixture to correct the respiratory alkalosis and low $PaCO_2$. The differences between these two methods of management and measurement relate to the temperature-dependent solubility of CO_2 in blood caused by temperature.

pH-stat management tends to obliterate the pressure autoregulation of cerebral blood flow. In adults, alpha-stat management is used, preserving pressure autoregulation.[B15,M8,M11,N6,P7,S14]

ANESTHETIC DRUG MANAGEMENT

CPB influences anesthetic drug management.[R8] On initiation of CPB, a brief but dramatic drop can occur in blood levels of anesthetic drugs because of the dilution effect of CPB prime. This is rapidly corrected by equilibration of the perfusate with the vast reservoir of drugs in the tissues. Using EEG information (Bispectral Index [BIS]), there is a decrease of 1.12 BIS units for each degree centigrade

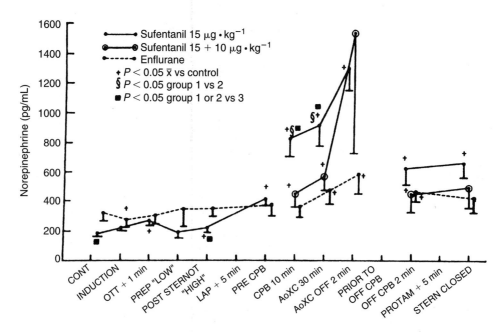

Figure 4-12   Plasma norepinephrine concentration at various times during cardiac surgery (vertical bars represent 1 standard error). (From Samuelson and colleagues.[S17])

Key: *CONT,* Control/baseline; *OTT + 1 min,* 1 minute after orotracheal intubation; *PREP "LOW,"* lowest systolic blood pressure during prepping; *POST STERNOT "HIGH,"* highest systolic blood pressure after sternotomy; *LAP + 5 min,* 5 minutes after left atrial catheter placement; *PRE CPB,* preceding cardiopulmonary bypass; *CPB 10 min,* 10 minutes into cardiopulmonary bypass; *AoXC 30 min,* 30 minutes after aortic clamp placed; *AoXC OFF 2 min,* 2 minutes after aortic clamp removed; *PRIOR TO OFF CPB,* immediately before coming off cardiopulmonary bypass; *OFF CPB 2 min,* 2 minutes after coming off cardiopulmonary bypass; *PROTAM + 5 min,* 5 minutes after protamine administration; *STERN CLOSED,* at sternal closure.

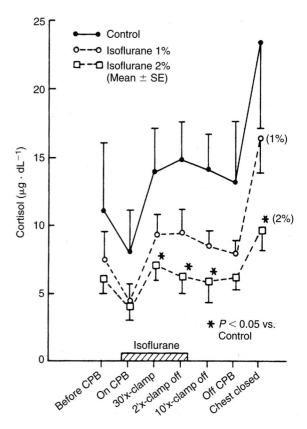

Figure 4-13   Plasma cortisol levels (μg/dL) measured at different times during coronary artery bypass grafting (vertical bars represent 1 standard error). (From Flezzani and colleagues.[F3])

Key: *CPB,* Cardiopulmonary bypass; *x-clamp,* aortic cross-clamp.

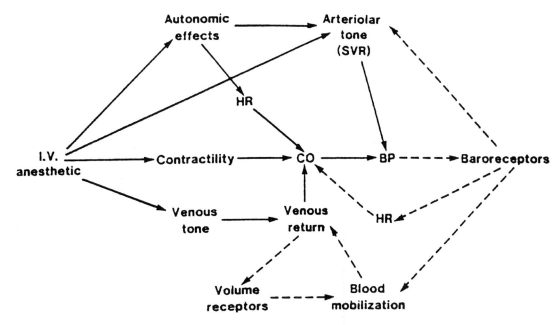

Figure 4-14   Hemodynamic effects and compensatory changes occurring with administration of most intravenous anesthetics. Individual variations from this overall generalization are addressed within the text.

Key: *BP*, systemic blood pressure; *CO*, cardiac output; *HR*, heart rate; *I.V.*, intravenous; *SVR*, systemic vascular resistance.

decrease in body temperature.[M14] This decrease, coupled with a general reduction in drug biotransformation with hypothermia,[F2] means that during CPB there is less requirement for anesthetic agents with hypothermia than normothermia.

Just as CPB influences anesthetic drug management, so do anesthetic agents alter CPB response. CPB (and aortic clamping) elicits numerous hormonal responses, including an increase in epinephrine and norepinephrine levels (Figs. 4-11 and 4-12). Also, both stress and adrenergic responses to CPB can be modulated by various anesthetic agents. Perioperative cortisol increases are blunted by administration of volatile anesthetics during CPB (Fig. 4-13).[F3] Additionally, anesthetics effectively decrease the norepinephrine response to CPB (Fig. 4-14).[S17] The degree to which depth of anesthesia affects these responses is not clear. How modulation of these stress responses influences patient outcome is also uncertain.

SECTION 4
Anesthetic Techniques and Pharmacology

Anesthetic techniques can be divided into four categories. The first is *general anesthesia,* which is accomplished with a wide variety of intravenous and inhalation drugs. Most general anesthetics are given with a *hypnotic* (usually a barbiturate or benzodiazepine), an *analgesic* (an opioid and/or inhalation drug), and a *muscle relaxant* (neuromuscular blocking agents). A second form of anesthesia is *neuroaxial blockade,* which is accomplished by placing a local anesthetic in either the subarachnoid or epidural space. A third technique is a *regional nerve block* with a local anesthetic, which by itself is rarely used in cardiac surgery. A final anesthetic technique involves *sedation* of the patient and local anesthetic infiltration at the surgical site, referred to as *monitored anesthesia care* (MAC). Except possibly for a pericardiocentesis for cardiac tamponade or pacemaker insertion, MAC is not used during cardiac surgery.

Loss of consciousness as seen in normal sleep[K7,S18] results in diminished heart rate, cardiac output, and blood pressure. Most drugs used for general anesthesia have hemodynamic effects, which, along with loss of consciousness, cause an overall hypotensive effect. Neuroaxial blockade with local anesthetics produces hypotension as a result of dermatomal level–dependent sympathetic nervous system blockade. This results in vasodilatation with reductions in both preload and afterload, thereby producing hypotension. The effects of neuroaxial blockade on cardiac sympathetic activity, as well as myocardial blood flow and metabolism, have been studied during CABG.[K8,S19]

Epidural anesthesia combined with general anesthesia lowers the prevalence of operative hypertension, but is associated with an increased prevalence of hypotension and may result in hypertension when it dissipates postoperatively.[G12] Thoracic epidural anesthesia for CABG has been adopted by many surgical programs for effective postoperative analgesia. Epidural anesthesia outside the setting of cardiac surgery requiring CPB has proven safe and effective for treatment of thoracic dermatomal pain, with a very low occurrence of neurologic complications (0.07%).[C12,G1] There are concerns, however, regarding epidural or spinal hematoma formation in patients who will be anticoagulated for CPB.[V5]

	IV	Inhalation	Neuroaxial	Peripheral
Cardiac output	0 to −	−	− to 0	0
Systemic vascular resistance	− to 0	−	− −	0
Contractility	0	−	0	0
Heart rate	0	−	0	0
Stroke volume	0	−	0	0

(From Rao and colleagues.[R14])

Key: *IV,* Intravenous administration; *0,* no change; *−,* decrease.

GENERAL ANESTHETIC CARDIOVASCULAR PHARMACOLOGY

Major cardiovascular effects of inhalation, intravenous, and sedative anesthetics are summarized in Table 4-9.[D3,R9,R10] To avoid problems with overgeneralization, details for certain anesthetic techniques and common drugs are discussed here.

Thiopental is the oldest and most extensively used IV anesthetic agent. Its rapid, highly predictable hypnotic effect and overall safety profile are responsible for its continued popularity since its introduction by Lundy and Waters in 1934.[L6] The principal hemodynamic change produced by thiopental is a decrease in myocardial contractility. Increases in heart rate result in a compensatory attempt to preserve cardiac output. Mean arterial pressure (P_{ART}) is maintained or slightly reduced. When thiopental is given in the setting of known or occult hypovolemia (which can include poorly controlled hypertensive patients or patients undergoing aggressive diuresis for heart failure), there can be a profound reduction in cardiac output and blood pressure.[P8] Fig. 4-14 provides a generalized view of the hemodynamic consequences of IV anesthetics.

IV *midazolam* is the most common benzodiazepine used in cardiac anesthetic practice today. This water-soluble agent is unique among benzodiazepines and characterized by rapid onset, short duration of action, and relatively rapid plasma clearance.[R11] Midazolam is often used in cardiac surgery as a hypnotic and amnestic drug. The hemodynamic effects in CABG patients are relatively minor after IV administration (0.2 mg · kg^{-1}). Changes of potential importance include a slight decrease in P_{ART} (20%) and a small increase in heart rate, with maintenance of cardiac index. Filling pressures are usually unchanged or slightly decreased in patients who have normal ventricular function, but can be importantly decreased in patients with an elevated P_{PCW}.

Interactions between midazolam and other drugs are generally mild and predictable. An exception is the interaction with fentanyl; important hypotension may occur, similar to that with diazepam and fentanyl.[T1] However, midazolam in reduced doses (0.05 to 0.1 mg · kg^{-1}) is routinely combined with fentanyl for induction and maintenance of general anesthesia during cardiac surgery without adverse hemodynamic sequelae.[N7,T1]

Ketamine produces rapid hypnosis and profound analgesia, and respiratory and cardiovascular functions are depressed less than with most other induction agents. Although itself a direct myocardial depressant, ketamine's unique sympathomimetic feature, causing endogenous catecholamine release, results in a compensatory stimulation of the cardiovascular system. The most prominent hemodynamic changes are increases in heart rate, cardiac index, systemic vascular resistance, and systemic and pulmonary artery pressures. Disturbing psychomimetic effects (vivid dreams, hallucinations, emergence phenomena), as well as undesirable increases in myocardial oxygen consumption, have limited the routine use of ketamine. Small doses of concomitantly administered midazolam, however, can prevent most of these undesirable side effects.

Etomidate, an imidazole derivative, is an IV anesthetic often used for anesthetic induction in the setting of hemodynamic compromise. After administration, almost no changes in heart rate, blood pressure, or filling pressures occur in healthy patients; this stable profile is similar even for those with important ischemic heart disease. In aortic and mitral valve disease, however, there may be up to a 20% reduction in blood pressure.[C13]

Propofol, an alkylphenol, is a new IV hypnotic.[K9] After IV induction with 1.5 to 2.0 mg · kg^{-1} and a maintenance infusion of 50 to 100 kg · min^{-1}, P_{ART} decreases by 15% to 40%. Its effect on heart rate is variable. Most studies have demonstrated reductions in systemic vascular resistance (9% to 30%), cardiac index, stroke volume, and left ventricular stroke work index. Usually, propofol alone or in combination with other anesthetics causes decreases in arterial pressure and cardiac index secondary to both increased vasodilatation and decreased myocardial contractility.

DRUGS FOR ANESTHETIC MAINTENANCE

The goal of anesthetic maintenance is to ameliorate surgical stress and to reduce stresses associated with CPB. Importantly, patients should be sufficiently anesthetized so they do not recall events that occurred during the operation. To achieve optimal anesthetic depth, therapeutic anesthetic drug levels must be maintained, generally with continuous infusions of the IV drugs and with in-line vaporizers (during CPB a vaporizer is placed in the fresh-gas circuit of the oxygenator). The BIS monitor facilitates assessment of the level of consciousness.[G14]

Maintenance of anesthesia is accomplished with continued administration of IV or inhalation anesthetics, or both. Contemporary inhalation anesthesics comprise only six drugs: the volatile liquids *halothane, enflurane, isoflurane, sevoflurane,* and *desflurane* and the inert gas *nitrous oxide* (N_2O). Unlike IV anesthetic drugs, the cardiovascular effects of the inhalational agents are more similar to one another than different. Except for N_2O, all exert a direct, dose-dependent negative inotropism and produce vasodilatation.[B16,M12,P9] As with the IV agents, their hemodynamic effect depends on several factors, including the individual drug, overall cardiovascular status of the patient, and any concurrent pharmacologic therapy.

There are small differences in the degree of myocardial depression produced by the individual drugs, as well as differences in the mechanisms by which contractility is depressed. In healthy patients, halothane and enflurane reduce cardiac output more than isoflurane. Depressant effects of the volatile anesthetics on myocardial contractility in diseased states such as ischemic heart disease are additive[M13] and depend on age, premedication, and adjuvant drugs. Inhalation anesthetics can be used to "smooth" anesthetic maintenance and to reduce the need for larger doses of IV drugs. Inhalation agents are removed from the body relatively rapidly, making them useful for early extubation protocols.

Opioids have long been used to provide analgesia during general anesthesia for cardiac surgery as well as to reduce pain postoperatively. The drugs typically used are morphine, fentanyl, sufentanil, alfentanil, and remifentanil. *Morphine* differs from the others because it causes more hemodynamic perturbations. Because of its inherent release of histamine, morphine causes vasodilatation-induced hypotension. The other synthetic opioids are devoid of this action, and their administration is generally marked by maintenance of systemic vascular resistance. All opioids tend to be vagomimetic, with a resultant decrease in heart rate. In general, opioids exert little effect on cardiac output, stroke volume, cardiac filling, or baroreflex function. Their interaction with benzodiazepines, however, can cause vasodilatation and hypotension. Intrathecal opioids have been used for postoperative analgesia, but their role in the setting of cardiac surgery has not yet been clearly defined.

EMERGENCE FROM ANESTHESIA

The choice of both induction and maintenance agents must also take into account issues related to duration of effect and timing of emergence from anesthesia. In the past the issue of emergence was relegated to the intensive care unit because patients were generally deeply anesthetized with combinations of high doses of narcotics and benzodiazepines. Current anesthetic techniques focus on managing emergence from anesthesia so that intubation time is minimized. Anesthetic planning must take into account the procedure performed and the individual patient's characteristics in order to determine when emergence from anesthesia would be most appropriate. For example, a 40-year-old, otherwise healthy male who undergoes single-vessel CABG without CPB should emerge from anesthesia more rapidly than an 80-year-old patient with poor left ventricular function who undergoes difficult reoperative CABG with prolonged CPB.

Anesthetic levels are decreased toward the end of the operation such that any residual in the circulation will serve to bridge the gap between operating room and intensive care unit. There are as many different techniques for this as there are individual anesthesiologists, but a common technique is to discontinue the inhaled anesthetic and start a continuous infusion of propofol or midazolam to allow sufficient sedation for the first few hours in the intensive care unit. These infusions can be titrated downward as time to emergence and extubation nears. Additional analgesia may be needed during this time, for which small doses of morphine or another narcotic are commonly used.

Pressure for cost containment from national and managed health care systems has stimulated efforts to decrease the time that cardiac surgery patients spend in the operating room, intensive care unit, and hospital. Changes have emerged in surgical techniques and procedures (e.g., minimally invasive surgery) and in anesthetic management that reflect these efforts. Terminology such as "facilitated extu-

TABLE 4-10 Neuromuscular Blocking Agents

Drug	Type	Dosage (mg · kg⁻¹)ᵃ	Duration of Actionᵇ
Succinylcholine	Depolarizing	1.0-1.5	Ultrashort
Mivacurium	Nondepolarizing	0.2-0.25	Short
Atracurium	Nondepolarizing	0.5-0.6	Intermediate
cis-Atracurium	Nondepolarizing	0.05-0.1	Intermediate
Vecuronium	Nondepolarizing	0.1-0.15	Intermediate
Rocuronium	Nondepolarizing	0.6-1.0	Intermediate
Pancuronium	Nondepolarizing	0.1-0.12	Long
d-Tubocurarine	Nondepolarizing	0.5-0.6	Long
Metocurine	Nondepolarizing	0.3-0.4	Long
Doxacurium	Nondepolarizing	0.05-0.08	Long

ᵃ Dose required for intubation (generally two to three times that required for maintenance of neuromuscular blockade).

ᵇ Duration of action depends on multiple variables, including total dose administered, concomitantly administered volatile anesthetics, temperature, serum electrolytes, and integrity of metabolic mechanisms. In general, *ultrashort* refers to duration of less than 10 minutes; *short* less than 30 minutes; *intermediate* less than 60 minutes; and *long* greater than 60 minutes.

bation," "early extubation," and "fast tracking" are used interchangeably to describe the strategy whereby patients are extubated, transferred out of the intensive care unit, and discharged from the hospital much earlier than previously thought advisable or achievable. A more logical term is *appropriately timed extubation,* which takes into account many variables that determine timing of extubation.[G15,H5] Although there has been considerable debate, early extubation has been shown to be safe, to reduce costs, and to allow better resource utilization.[C14,C16]

NEUROMUSCULAR BLOCKING AGENTS

Neuromuscular blocking agents, or muscle relaxants, are administered to facilitate endotracheal intubation, provide patient immobility, and facilitate mechanical ventilatory support. Because neuromuscular blocking agents do not produce analgesia, sedation, or amnesia, they cannot substitute for other supportive care in the potentially conscious patient. Therefore, muscle paralysis should not be performed without the assurance of adequate sedation or general anesthesia.

Muscle-relaxing drugs are classified according to their mechanism of action. The two main categories are depolarizing and nondepolarizing (Table 4-10). *Depolarizing* neuromuscular blocking agents, of which succinylcholine is the prototype, mimic the action of acetylcholine, a neuromuscular junction transmitter producing sustained membrane permeability changes that, until the drug dissipates, prevent further depolarization at the postsynaptic membrane. Onset of muscle paralysis is usually rapid (60 to 90 seconds) after IV administration. *Nondepolarizing* blockers are competitive antagonists for acetylcholine binding, thus preventing depolarization at the neuromuscular junction. Because of the relative excess of receptors, greater than 70% must be blocked before there is clinically significant muscle weakness. Therefore, the onset of paralysis using nondepolarizing agents compared with depolarizing agents is much slower, requiring several minutes for the full paralyzing effect. Onset is also somewhat dose dependent and can be hastened with higher doses of the nondepolarizing agent.

Many factors can alter muscle relaxant distribution, metabolism, and elimination, leading to wide variability in dosing requirements. Renal disease, hepatic disease, protein binding, age, temperature, and concomitant drug administration alter their pharmacodynamics. Major differences among nondepolarizing neuromuscular blocking agents include duration of blockade (intermediate versus long acting), mechanisms of metabolism and clearance, and autonomic side effects. The most widely used drug, *pancuronium,* provides an excellent long-acting state of muscle relaxation, but may increase heart rate, particularly if administered rapidly or in large doses. *Atracurium* has two unique mechanisms of metabolism: Hoffman degradation (which occurs at a predictable in vivo rate such that clearance of the drug is unaltered even in the presence of severe hepatic or renal disease) and ester hydrolysis.[S20] *Vecuronium* has the lowest autonomic side effect profile and produces little hemodynamic alteration. Newer intermediate-acting nondepolarizing neuromuscular blocking agents include *cis-atracurium* and *rocuronium.* In general, cis-atracurium can be considered similar to atracurium and rocuronium similar to vecuronium in terms of onset, duration, and side effects.

Depolarizing relaxants cannot be pharmacologically reversed, but depend on plasma cholinesterase (pseudocholinesterase) to provide enzymatic degradation with cessation of blocking effects. Patients with a prolonged effect due to pseudocholinesterase deficiency may improve with IV enzyme administration through a plasma transfusion. However, sedation and ventilatory support until the drug is metabolized are generally sufficient and advisable.

Nondepolarizing relaxants can be reversed once the patient has partially recovered neuromuscular function, as evidenced by at least some movement (twitch) present on a neuromuscular blocking agent monitor. Anticholinesterase drugs (e.g., edrophonium, neostigmine, physostigmine, pyridostigmine) inhibit the acetylcholinesterase enzyme and permit accumulation of the acetylcholine at the postsynaptic junction. Acetylcholine competitively displaces residual nondepolarizing muscle relaxants. Problems in routine reversal of nondepolarizing drugs can complicate the clinical situation. Anticholinesterases increase ganglionic neural transmission (often precipitating bradycardia), necessitating concomitant administration of an anticholinergic drug such as atropine or glycopyrrolate. Duration of action of the competitive reversal agent may be shorter than duration of the muscle relaxant, which may lead to unexpected postreversal weakness and potential muscle paralysis. With proper administration and monitoring, however, nondepolarizing relaxants and reversal agents can provide periods of optimal surgical relaxation.

LOCAL ANESTHETICS

In the cardiac surgical patient, local anesthetics are used for intercostal blocks, insertion of IV and intraarterial catheters, removal of sternal wires, and other minor procedures. In addition, the patient is exposed to local anesthetics in the catheterization laboratory. Epidural instillation of local anesthetics has been suggested for pain relief after median sternotomy and thoracotomy.[B17] Their specific membrane-altering properties (sodium channel blockade) explain the use of many drugs with local anesthetic properties for treatment of cardiac dysrhythmias.

In a manner analogous to the neuromuscular blocking agents, local anesthetics interfere with neural transmission to produce their effects, although by different mechanisms. Local anesthetics act within the nerve membrane, where they inhibit transmission of nerve action potentials by reducing membrane permeability to sodium and displacing ionized calcium. Thus, the threshold potential for depolarization is not reached, and an action potential is not conducted. Duration of action of a local anesthetic is proportional to the time it is in direct contact with the nerve fiber and depends on its protein-binding characteristics. Subsequent recovery of conduction occurs spontaneously. Onset of action is related to the lipophilicity and ionic state of the local anesthetic. Potency is generally a function of lipophilicity.

Most local anesthetics, except for cocaine, produce peripheral vasodilatation by direct relaxation of vascular smooth muscle. *Epinephrine* is often added to local anesthetic solutions to produce local vasoconstriction, reduce systemic drug absorption, and thus maintain a high drug concentration at the injection site.

There are important differences in the pathways of drug metabolism for the two classes of local anesthetics (esters and amides) as well as differences in their potential for producing allergic reactions and other side effects. Ester local anesthetics are metabolized by plasma cholinesterase with *p*-aminobenzoic acid (PABA) as a metabolite. PABA makes esters more likely to produce allergic reactions than amide local anesthetics, which are metabolized in the liver to multiple metabolites, none of which is particularly allergenic. However, preservative agents (e.g., methylparaben) may be added to ester or amide local anesthetics, which may cause allergic reactions. True allergy to local anesthetics is extremely rare. Patients presenting with a history of local anesthetic allergy should be questioned as to the nature of the allergy. Allergy can be misdiagnosed, often being confused with the effects of the epinephrine added to local anesthetic solutions to prolong duration.

Toxicity associated with local anesthetics arises from a relative or absolute overdose of the drug from unrecognized intravascular injection, or from excessive intravascular absorption. Toxicity can produce both central nervous system (CNS) and cardiovascular effects.[C15] Fortunately, toxicity of local anesthetics is progressive, with CNS toxicity occurring well before the more serious cardiac toxicity. CNS toxicity is manifested by lightheadedness, tinnitus, and circumoral numbness, often followed by generalized seizures. With further increases in plasma local anesthetic concentration, signs of cardiovascular toxicity occur in the cardiac conduction system, myocardium, and vascular smooth muscle. Cardiac electrical effects include increases in the ratio of the effective refractory period to the action potential duration, with prolonged PR and QRS intervals, atrioventricular nodal dysrhythmias, and ultimately sinus bradycardia and arrest. Effects on cardiac muscle are predominantly negatively inotropic and directly related to local anesthetic potency.

Dosages should be adjusted based on site of injection, use of vasoconstrictors, comorbid disease, and volume of drug necessary (Table 4-11).

Treatment of local anesthetic toxicity involves securing an airway and establishing ventilation. Seizures may be treated with benzodiazepines or barbiturates. Cardiovascular toxicity can be treated with catecholamines, atropine, and bretylium as necessary. A newer local anesthetic, *ropivacaine* (an isomer of bupivacaine), appears to have a more favorable side effect profile with considerably less cardiotoxicity.

■ **TABLE 4-11   Doses and Toxic Levels of Local Anesthetics**

Drug	Dosage ($mg \cdot kg^{-1}$)	Toxic Blood Levels ($\mu g \cdot mL^{-1}$)
Esters		
Procaine	10-12	20
Chloroprocaine	7-10	20
Tetracaine	2	1.5-4.0
Amides		
Lidocaine	5-7	5-10
Mepivacaine	5-7	5-10
Bupivacaine	2-4	1.5-4.0
Prilocaine	6-8	5-10
Etidocaine	3-5	1.5-4.0

REFERENCES

A

1. Arrowsmith JE, Grocott HP, Newman MF. Neurologic risk assessment, monitoring and outcome in cardiac surgery. J Cardiothorac Vasc Anesth 1999;13:736.
2. Arrowsmith J, Grocott HP, Reves JG, Newman MF. Central nervous system complications of cardiac surgery. Br J Anaesth 2000;84:378.
3. Alderman EL, Branzi A, Sanders W, Brown BW, Harrison DC. Evaluation of pulse contour method of determining stroke volume in man. Circulation 1972;46:546.

B

1. Braunwald E. Thirteenth Bowditch lecture. The determinants of myocardial oxygen consumption. Physiologist 1969;12:65.
2. Bellinger DC, Wypij D, du Plessis AJ, Rappaport LA, Riviello J, Jonas RA, et al. Developmental and neurologic effects of alpha-stat versus pH-stat strategies for deep hypothermic cardiopulmonary bypass in infants. J Thorac Cardiovasc Surg 2001;121:374.
3. Berner M, Oberhansli I, Rouge JC, Jaccard C, Friedli B. Chronotropic and inotropic supports are both required to increase cardiac output early after corrective operations for tetralogy of Fallot. J Thorac Cardiovasc Surg 1989;97:297.
4. Baylen B, Meyer RA, Korfhagen J, Benzing G III, Bubb ME, Kaplan S. Left ventricular performance in the critically ill premature infant with patent ductus arteriosus and pulmonary disease. Circulation 1977;55:182.
5. Berner M, Jaccard C, Oberhansli I, Rouge JC, Friedli B. Hemodynamic effects of amrinone in children after cardiac surgery. Intens Care Med 1990;16:85.
6. Berner M, Rouge JC, Friedli B. The hemodynamic effect of phentolamine and dobutamine after open-heart operations in children: influence of the underlying heart defect. Ann Thorac Surg 1983;35:643.
7. Borow KM, Keane JF, Castaneda AR, Freed MD. Systemic ventricular function in patients with tetralogy of Fallot, ventricular septal defect and transposition of the great arteries repaired during infancy. Circulation 1981;64:878.
8. Borow KM, Green LH, Castaneda AR, Keane JF. Left ventricular function after repair of tetralogy of Fallot and its relationship to age at surgery. Circulation 1980;61:1150.
9. Bailey JM, Miller BE, Lu W, Tasone SR, Kanter KR, Tam VK. The pharmacokinetics of milrinone in pediatric patients after cardiac surgery. Anesthesiology 1999;90:1012.
10. Bergquist BD, Leung JM, Bellows WH. Transesophageal echocardiography in myocardial revascularization: I. Accuracy of intraoperative real-time interpretation. Anesth Analg 1996;82:1132.
11. Busto R, Globus MY, Dietrich WD, Martinez E, Valdes I, Ginsberg MD. Effect of mild hypothermia on ischemia-induced release of neurotransmitters and free fatty acids in rat brain. Stroke 1989;20:904.
12. Busto R, Globus MY, Neary JT, Ginsberg MD. Regional alterations of protein kinase C activity following transient cerebral ischemia: effects of intraischemic brain temperature modulation. J Neurochem 1994; 63:1095.
13. Berntman L, Welsh FA, Harp JR. Cerebral protective effect of low-grade hypothermia. Anesthesiology 1981;55:495.
14. Busto R, Dietrich WD, Globus MY, Valdes I, Scheinberg P, Ginsberg MD. Small differences in intra-ischemic brain temperature critically determine the extent of ischemic neuronal injury. J Cereb Blood Flow Metab 1987;7:729.
15. Bashein G, Townes BD, Nessly ML, Bledsoe SW, Hornbein TF, Davis KB, et al. A randomized study of carbon dioxide management during hypothermic cardiopulmonary bypass. Anesthesiology 1990;72:7.
16. Brown BR Jr, Crout JR. A comparative study of the effects of five general anesthetics on myocardial contractility. I. Isometric conditions. Anesthesiology 1971;34:236.
17. Bromage PR, Camporesi E, Chestnut D. Epidural narcotics for postoperative analgesia. Anesth Analg 1980;59:473.
18. Braunwald E. Vasodilator therapy: a physiologic approach to the treatment of heart failure. N Engl J Med 1977;297:331.

C

1. Cohn L, Klovekorn P, Moore FD, Collins JJ Jr. Intrinsic plasma volume deficits in patients with coronary artery disease. Effects of myocardial revascularization. Arch Surg 1974;108:57.
2. Chiariello M, Gold M, Gold HK, Leinbach RC, Davis MA, Maroko PR. Comparison between the effects of nitroprusside and nitroglycerin on ischemic injury during acute myocardial infarction. Circulation 1976;54:766.
3. Chang AC, Atz AM, Wernovsky G, Burke RP, Wessel DL. Milrinone: systemic and pulmonary hemodynamic effects in neonates after cardiac surgery. Crit Care Med 1995;23:1907.
4. Croughwell N, Smith LR, Quill T, Newman M, Greeley W, Kern F, et al. The effect of temperature on cerebral metabolism and blood flow in adults during cardiopulmonary bypass. J Thorac Cardiovasc Surg 1992;103:549.
5. Cook DJ, Orszulak TA, Daly RC, Buda DA. Cerebral hyperthermia during cardiopulmonary bypass in adults. J Thorac Cardiovasc Surg 1996;111:268.

6. Chien S. Present state of blood rheology. In Messmer K, Schmid-Schoenbein H, eds. Hemodilution: theoretical basis and clinical applications. Basel: Karger, 1972.

7. Cohn LH, Fosberg AM, Anderson WP, Collins JJ Jr. The effects of phlebotomy, hemodilution and autologous transfusion on systemic oxygenation and whole blood utilization in open heart surgery. Chest 1975;68:283.

8. Cosgrove DM, Loop FD, Lytle BW, Gill CC, Golding LR, Taylor PC, et al. Determinants of blood utilization during myocardial revascularization. Ann Thorac Surg 1985;40:380.

9. Cook DJ, Orszulak TA, Daly RC, MacVeigh I. Minimum hematocrit for normothermic cardiopulmonary bypass in dogs. Circulation 1997;96:II200.

10. Cook DJ, Oliver WC Jr, Orszulak TA, Daly RC, Bryce RD. Cardiopulmonary bypass temperature, hematocrit, and cerebral oxygen delivery in humans. Ann Thorac Surg 1995;60:1671.

11. Croughwell N, Lyth M, Quill JJ, Newman M, Greeley WJ, Smith LR, et al. Diabetic patients have abnormal cerebral autoregulation during cardiopulmonary bypass. Circulation 1990;82:IV407.

12. Chaney MA. Intrathecal and epidural anesthesia and analgesia for cardiac surgery. Anesth Analg 1997;84:1211.

13. Colvin MP, Saege TM, Newland PE, Weaver EJ, Waters AF, Brookes JM, et al. Cardiorespiratory changes following induction of anaesthesia with etomidate in patients with cardiac disease. Br J Anaesth 1979;51:551.

14. Cheng DC. Pro: early extubation after cardiac surgery decreases intensive care unit stay and cost. J Cardiothorac Vasc Anesth 1995;9:460.

15. Covino BG, Wildsmith JA. Clinical pharmacology of local anaesthetic agents. In Cousins MJ, Bridenbaugh PO, eds. Neural blockade in clinical anaesthesia and management of pain, 3rd ed. Philadelphia: Lippincott, 1998, p. 97.

16. Chamorro C, de Latorre FJ, Montero A, Sanchez-Izquierdo JA, Jareno A, Moreno JA, et al. Comparative study of propofol versus midazolam in the sedation of critically ill patients: results of a prospective, randomized, multicenter trial. Crit Care Med 1996;24:932.

17. Crawford FA Jr, Sade RM. Spinal cord injury associated with hyperthermia during aortic coarctation repair. J Thorac Cardiovasc Surg 1984;87:616.

18. Cohn JN, Franciosa JA. Vasodilator therapy of cardiac failure. N Engl J Med 1977;297:27.

19. Connors AF Jr, Speroff T, Dawson NV, Thomas C, Harrell FE Jr, Wagner D, et al. The effectiveness of right heart catheterization in the initial care of critically ill patients. JAMA 1996;276:889.

20. Carey JS, Hughes RK. Cardiac output: clinical monitoring and management. Ann Thorac Surg 1969;7:150.

D

1. de Bruijn NP, Clements FM. Transesophageal echocardiography. Boston: Martinus Nijhoff, 1987.

2. du Plessis AJ, Jonas RA, Wypij D, Hickey PR, Riviello J, Wessel DL, et al. Perioperative effects of alpha-stat versus pH-stat strategies for deep hypothermic cardiopulmonary bypass in infants. J Thorac Cardiovasc Surg 1997;114:991.

3. Dentz ME, Grichnik KP, Sibert KS, Reves JG. Anesthesia and postoperative analgesia. In Sabiston DC, ed. Textbook of surgery: the biological basis of modern surgical practice, 15th ed. Philadelphia: WB Saunders, 1997, p. 186.

4. Divertie MB, McMichan JC. Continuous monitoring of mixed venous oxygen saturation. Chest 1984;85:423.

E

1. Engelman RM, Pleet AB, Rousou JA, Flack JE III, Deaton DW, Pekow PS, et al. Influence of cardiopulmonary bypass perfusion temperature on neurologic and hematologic function after coronary artery bypass grafting. Ann Thorac Surg 1999;67:1547.

2. Engleman RM, Pleet AB, Rousou JA, Flack JE III, Deaton DW, Gregory CA, et al. What is the best perfusion temperature for coronary revascularization? J Thorac Cardiovasc Surg 1996;112:1622.

3. Estafanous FG, Loop FD, Higgins TL, Tekyi-Mensah S, Lytle BW, Cosgrove DM 3rd, et al. Increased risk and decreased morbidity of coronary artery bypass grafting between 1986 and 1994. Ann Thorac Surg 1998;65:383.

F

1. Fang WC, Helm RE, Kreiger KH, Rosengart TK, DuBois WJ, Sason C, et al. Impact of minimum hematocrit during cardiopulmonary bypass on mortality in patients undergoing coronary artery surgery. Circulation 1997;96:II194.

2. Flezzani P, Alvis MJ, Jacobs JR, Schilling MM, Bai S, Reves JG. Sufentanil disposition during cardiopulmonary bypass. Can J Anaesth 1987;34:566.

3. Flezzani P, Croughwell ND, McIntyre RW, Reves JG. Isoflurane decreases the cortisol response to cardiopulmonary bypass. Anesth Analg 1986;65:1117.

4. Fontana GP. Minimally invasive cardiac surgery. Chest Surg Clin North Am 1998;8:871.

5. Franciosa JA. Evaluation of CO_2 rebreathing cardiac output method in seriously ill patients. Circulation 1977;55:449.

G

1. Greenspun HG, Adourian UA, Fonger JD, Fan JS. Minimally invasive direct coronary artery bypass (MIDCAB): surgical techniques and anesthetic considerations. J Cardiothorac Vasc Anesth 1996;10:507.

2. Gruber EM, Laussen PC, Casta A, Zimmerman AA, Zurakauski D, Red R, et al. Stress response in infants undergoing cardiac surgery: a randomized study of fentanyl bolus, fentanyl infusion and fentanyl-midazolam infusion. Anesth Analg 2001;92:822.

3. Girardin E, Berner M, Rouge JC, Rivest RW, Friedli B, Paunier L. Effect of low dose dopamine on hemodynamic and renal function in children. Pediatr Res 1989;26:200.

4. Graham TP Jr. Ventricular performance in congenital heart disease. Circulation 1991;84:2259.

5. Gardner TJ, Homeffer PJ, Manolio TA, Pearson TA, Gott VL, Baumgartner WA, et al. Stroke following coronary bypass grafting: a ten year study. Ann Thorac Surg 1985;40:574.

6. Greeley WJ, Kern FH, Ungerleider RM, Boyd JL III, Quill T, Smith LR, et al. The effect of hypothermic cardiopulmonary bypass and total circulatory arrest on cerebral metabolism in neonates, infants, and children. J Thorac Cardiovasc Surg 1991;101:783.

7. Globus MY, Busto R, Lin B, Schnippering H, Ginsberg MD. Detection of free radical activity during transient global ischemia and recirculation: effects of intraischemic brain temperature modulation. J Neurochem 1995;65:1250.

8. Globus MY, Busto R, Dietrich WD, Martinez E, Valdes I, Ginsberg MD. Intra-ischemic extracellular release of dopamine and glutamate is associated with striatal vulnerability to ischemia. Neurosci Lett 1988;91:36.

9. Grigore AM, Mathew J, Grocott HP, Reves JG, Blumenthal JA, White WD, et al. A prospective randomized trial of normothermic versus hypothermic cardiopulmonary bypass on cognitive function after coronary artery bypass graft surgery. Anesthesiology 2001;95:1110.

10. Grocott HP, Newman MF, Croughwell ND, White WD, Lawry E, Reves JG. Continuous jugular venous versus nasopharyngeal temperature monitoring during hypothermic cardiopulmonary bypass for cardiac surgery. J Clin Anesth 1997;9:312.

11. Gold J, Charlson ME, Williams-Russo P, Szatrowski TP, Peterson JC, Pirraglia PA, et al. Improvement of outcomes after coronary artery bypass. A randomized trial comparing intraoperative high versus low mean arterial pressure. J Thorac Cardiovasc Surg 1995;110:1302.

12. Garnett RL, MacIntyre A, Lindsay P, Barber GG, Cole CW, et al. Perioperative ischaemia in aortic surgery: combined epidural/general anaesthesia and epidural analgesia vs general anaesthesia and i.v. analgesia. Can J Anaesth 1996;43:769.

13. Gabe IT, Gault JH, Ross J, Mason DT, Mills CJ, Schillingford JP, et al. Measurement of instantaneous blood flow velocity and pressure in conscious man with a catheter-tip velocity probe. Circulation 1969;40:603.

14. Glass PS, Bloom M, Kearse L, Rosow C, Sebel P, Manberg P. Bispectral analysis measures sedation and memory effects of propofol, midazolam, isoflurane and alfentanil in healthy volunteers. Anesthesiology 1996;86:836.

15. Gayes JM, Emery RW. The MIDCAB experience: a current look at evolving surgical and anesthetic approaches. J Cardiothorac Vasc Anesth 1997;11:625.

16. Ganz W, Donoso R, Marcus HS, Forrester JS, Swan HJ. A new technique for measurement of cardiac output by thermodilution in man. Am J Cardiol 1971;27:392.

17. Grose R, Nivatpumin T, Katz S, Yinintsoi T, Scheuer J. Mechanism of nitroglycerin effect in valvular aortic stenosis. Am J Cardiol 1979;44:1371.

18. Govier AV, Reves JG, McKay RD, Karp RB, Zorn GL, Morawetz RB, et al. Factors and their influence on regional cerebral blood flow during nonpulsatile cardiopulmonary bypass. Ann Thorac Surg 1984;38:592.

H

1. Hickey PR, Hansen DD, Wessel DL, Lang P, Jonas RA, Elixson EM. Blunting of stress responses in the pulmonary circulation of infants by fentanyl. Anesth Analg 1985;64:1137.

2. Hickey PR, Hansen DD, Wessel DL, Lang P, Jonas RA. Pulmonary and systemic hemodynamic responses to fentanyl in infants. Anesth Analg 1985;64:483.

3. Hodgins L, Kisslo JA, Mark JB. Perioperative transesophageal echocardiography: the anesthesiologist as cardiac diagnostician. Anesth Analg 1995;80:4.

4. Hartmann G, Yao FS, Bruefach M III, Barbut D, Peterson JC, Purchell MH, et al. Severity of aortic atheromatous disease diagnosed by transesophageal echocardiography predicts stroke and other outcomes associated with coronary artery surgery: a prospective study. Anesth Analg 1996;83:701.

5. Higgins TL. Safety issues regarding early extubation after coronary artery bypass surgery. J Cardiothorac Vasc Anesth 1995;24:24.

6. Huntsman LL, Stewart DK, Barnes SR, Franklin SB, Colocousis JS, Hessel EA. Noninvasive Doppler determination of cardiac output in man: clinical validation. Circulation 1983;67:593.

J

1. Jaccard C, Berner M, Rouge JC, Oberhansli I, Friedli B. Hemodynamic effect of isoprenaline and dobutamine immediately after correction of tetralogy of Fallot. Relative importance of inotropic and chronotropic action in supporting cardiac output. J Thorac Cardiovasc Surg 1984;87:862.

2. Jopling MW. Pro: automated electrocardiogram ST-segment monitoring should be used in the monitoring of cardiac surgical patients. J Cardiothorac Vasc Anesth 1996;10:678.

3. Jain U, Laflamme CJ, Aggarwal A, Ramsay JG, Comunale ME, Ghashal S, et al. Electrocardiographic and hemodynamic changes and their association with myocardial infarction during coronary artery bypass surgery. Anesthesiology 1997;86:576.

4. Jones J, Rawitscher RE, McLean TR, Beall AC Jr, Thornby JI. Benefit from combining blood conservation measures in cardiac operations. Ann Thorac Surg 1991;51:541.

K

1. Kouchoukos NT, Sheppard LC, McDonald DA. Estimation of stroke volume in the dog by a pulse contour method. Circulation 1970;26:611.

2. Kern FH, Ungerleider RM, Jacobs JR, Boyd JL III, Reves JG, Goodman D, et al. Computerized continuous infusion of intravenous anesthetic drugs during pediatric cardiac surgery. Anesth Analg 1991;72:487.

3. Kirshbom PM, Skaryak LA, DiBernardo LR, Kern FH, Greeley WJ, Gaynor JW, et al. Effects of aortopulmonary collaterals on cerebral cooling and cerebral metabolic recovery after circulatory arrest. Circulation 1995;92:II490.

4. Konchigeri HN, Levitsky S. Anesthetic considerations for pericardectomy in uremic pericardial effusion. Anesth Analg 1976;55:378.

5. Kader A, Frazzini VI, Baker CJ, Solomon RA, Trifilette RR. Effect of mild hypothermia on nitric oxide synthesis during focal cerebral ischemia. Neurosurgery 1994;35:272.

6. Keykhah MM, Welsh FA, Hagerdal M, Harp JR. Reduction of the cerebral protective effect of hypothermia by oligemic hypotension during hypoxia in the rat. Stroke 1982;13:171.

7. Khatri IM, Freis ED. Hemodynamic changes during sleep. J Appl Physiol 1967;22:867.

8. Kirno K, Friberg P, Grzegorczyk A, Milocco I, Ricksten SE, Lundin S. Thoracic epidural anesthesia during coronary artery bypass surgery: effects on cardiac sympathetic activity, myocardial blood flow and metabolism, and central hemodynamics. Anesth Analg 1994;79:1075.

9. Kay B, Rolly G. I.C.I. 35868, a new intravenous induction agent. Acta Anaesthesiol Belg 1977;28:303.

L

1. Lell WA, Walker DR, Blackstone EH, Kouchoukos NT, Allarde R, Roe CR. Evaluation of myocardial damage in patients undergoing coronary-artery bypass procedures with halothane-N_2O anesthesia and adjuvants. Anesth Analg 1977;56:556.

2. Laishley RS, Burrows FA, Lerman J, Roy WL. Effect of anesthetic induction regimens on oxygen saturation in cyanotic congenital heart disease. Anesthesiology 1986;65:673.

3. Lilleaasen P. Moderate and extreme haemodilution in open heart surgery. Blood requirements, bleeding and platelet counts. Scand J Cardiovasc Surg 1977;11:97.

4. Lowenstein E. Blood conservation in open heart surgery. Cleve Clin Q 1981;48:112.

5. Lee SH, Heros RC, Mullan JC, Korosue K. Optimum degree of hemodilution for brain protection in a canine model of focal cerebral ischemia. J Neurosurg 1994;80:469.

6. Lundy JS. From this point in time: some memories of my part in the history of anesthesia. J Am Assoc Nurse Anesth 1966;24:95.

M

1. Mora CT, Dudek C, Torjman MC, White PF. The effects of anesthetic technique on the hemodynamic response and recovery profile in coronary revascularization patients. Anesth Analg 1995;81:900.

2. McDaniel HG, Reves JG, Kouchoukos NT, Smith LR, Rogers WJ, Samuelson PN, et al. Detection of myocardial injury after coronary artery bypass grafting using a hypothermic, cardioplegic technique. Ann Thorac Surg 1982;33:139.

3. Muhiudeen Russell IA, Miller-Hance WC, Silverman NH. Intraoperative transesophageal echocardiography for pediatric patients with congenital heart disease. Anesth Analg 1998;87:1058.

4. McGovern JJ, Cheifetz IM, Craig DM, Bengur AR, Quick G, Ungerleider RM, et al. Right ventricular injury in young swine: effects of catecholamines on right ventricular function and pulmonary vascular mechanics. Pediatr Res 2000;48:763.

5. Mauney MC, Blackbourne LH, Langenburg SE, Buchanan SA, Kron IL, Tribble CG. Prevention of spinal cord injury after repair of the thoracic or thoracoabdominal aorta. Ann Thorac Surg 1995;59:245.

6. Moller CT, Schoonbee CG, Rosendorff C. Haemodynamics of cardiac tamponade during various modes of ventilation. Br J Anaesth 1979;51:409.

7. Michenfelder JD, Theye RA. The effects of anesthesia and hypothermia on canine cerebral ATP and lactate during anoxia produced by decapitation. Anesthesiology 1970;33:430.

8. Mora C, Henson MB, Weintraub WS, Murkin JM, Martin TD, Craver JM, et al. The effect of temperature management during cardiopulmonary bypass on neurologic and neuropsychologic outcomes in patients undergoing coronary revascularization. J Thorac Cardiovasc Surg 1996;112:514.

9. Martin TD, Craver JM, Gott JP, Weintraub WS, Ramsay J, Mora CT, et al. Prospective, randomized trial of retrograde warm blood cardioplegia: myocardial benefit and neurologic threat. Ann Thorac Surg 1994;57:298.

10. McLean RF, Wong BI, Naylor CD, Snow WG, Harrington EM, Gawel M, et al. Cardiopulmonary bypass, temperature, and central nervous system dysfunction. Circulation 1994;90:II250.

11. Murkin JM, Farrar JK, Tweed WA, McKenzie FN, Guiraudon G. Cerebral autoregulation and flow/metabolism coupling during cardiopulmonary bypass: the influence of $PaCO_2$. Anesth Analg 1987;66:825.

12. Merin RG. Are the myocardial functional and metabolic effects of isoflurane really different from those of halothane and enflurane? Anesthesiology 1981;55:398.

13. Mallow JE, White RD, Cucchiara RF, Tarhan S. Hemodynamic effects of isoflurane and halothane in patients with coronary artery disease. Anesth Analg 1976;55:135.

14. Mathews JP, Weatherwax KJ, East CJ, White WD, Reves JG. Bispectral analysis during cardiopulmonary bypass: the effect of hypothermia on the hypnotic state. J Clin Anesth 2001;13:301.

15. Moulton MJ, Creswell LL, Mackey ME, Cox JL, Rosenbloom M. Obesity is not a risk factor for significant adverse outcomes after cardiac surgery (discussion by Reves JG, Howell S). Circulation 1996;94:II87.

16. Mark JB, Slaughter TF, Reves JG. Cardiovascular monitoring. In Miller RD, Miller ED Jr, Reves JG, Ross A, eds. Anesthesia, 5th ed. Philadelphia: Churchill Livingstone, p. 1117.

17. Mathur M, Harris EA, Yarrow S, Barratt-Boyes BG. Measurement of cardiac output by thermodilution in infants and children after open heart operations. J Thorac Cardiovasc Surg 1976;72:221.

N

1. Newman MF, Murkin JM, Roach G, Croughwell ND, White WD, Clements FM, et al. Cerebral physiologic effects of burst suppression doses of propofol during nonpulsatile cardiopulmonary bypass. CNS subgroup of McSPI. Anesth Analg 1995;81:452.

2. Nuttall GA, Cook DJ, Fulgham JR, Oliver WC Jr, Proper JA. The relationship between cerebral blood flow and transcranial Doppler blood flow during hypothermic cardiopulmonary bypass in adults. Anesth Analg 1996;82:1146.

3. Nakashima K, Todd MM, Warner DS. The relation between cerebral metabolic rate and ischemic depolarization. A comparison of the effects of hypothermia, pentobarbital, and isoflurane. Anesthesiology 1995;82:1199.

4. Newman MF, Croughwell ND, White WL, Lowry E, Baldwin BI, Clements FM, et al. Effect of perfusion pressure on cerebral blood flow during normothermic cardiopulmonary bypass. Circulation 1996;94:II353.

5. Nussmeier NA, Arlund A, Slogoff S. Neuropsychiatric complications after cardiopulmonary bypass: cerebral protection by a barbiturate. Anesthesiology 1986;64:165.

6. Newman MF, Croughwell ND, Blumenthal JA, White WD, Lewis JB, Smith LR, et al. Effects of aging on cerebral autoregulation during cardiopulmonary bypass: association with postoperative cognitive dysfunction. Circulation 1994;90:II243.

7. Newman M, Reves JG. Pro: midazolam is the sedative of choice to supplement narcotic anesthesia. J Cardiothorac Vasc Anesth 1993;7:615.

8. Neutze JM, Moller CT, Harris EA, Horsburgh MP, Wilson MD, eds. Intensive care of the heart and lungs. 3rd ed. Oxford: Blackwell Scientific, 1982, p. 281.

O

1. Ochsner JL, Mills NL, Leonard GL, Lawson N. Fresh autologous blood transfusion with extracorporeal circulation. Ann Surg 1973;177:811.

P

1. Phillips PA, Marty AT, Miyamoto AM, Brewer LA III. A clinical method for detecting subendocardial ischemia after cardiopulmonary bypass. J Thorac Cardiovasc Surg 1975;69:30.

2. Posner MA, Reves JG, Lell WA. Aortic valve replacement in a hemodialysis-dependent patient: anesthetic considerations—a case report. Anesth Analg 1975;54:24.

3. Pugsley W, Klinger L, Paschalis C, Treasure T, Harrison M, Newman S. The impact of microemboli during cardiopulmonary bypass on neuropsychological functioning. Stroke 1994;25:1393.

4. Proctor LT, Kingsley CP. Con: ST-segment analysis—who needs it? J Cardiothorac Vasc Anesth 1996;10:681.

5. Plourde G, Leduc AS, Monn JE, DeVarennes B, Latter D, Symes J, et al. Temperature during cardiopulmonary bypass for coronary artery operations does not influence postoperative cognitive function: a prospective, randomized trial. J Thorac Cardiovasc Surg 1997;114:123.

6. Paone G, Silverman NA. The paradox of on-bypass transfusion thresholds in blood conservation. Circulation 1997;96:II205.

7. Prough DS, Stump DA, Troost BT. $PaCO_2$ management during cardiopulmonary bypass: intriguing physiologic rationale, convincing clinical data, evolving hypothesis? Anesthesiology 1990;72:3.

8. Pedersen T, Engbaek J, Klausen NO, Sorensen B, Weiberg-Jorgensen F. Effects of low-dose ketamine and thiopentone on cardiac performance and myocardial oxygen balance in high-risk patients. Acta Anaesthesiol Scand 1982;26:235.

9. Price ML, Price HL. Effect of general anesthetics on contractile response of rabbit aorta strips. Anesthesiology 1962;23:16.

10. Practice guidelines for perioperative transesophageal echocardiography. A report by the American Society of Anesthesiologists and the Society of Cardiovascular Anesthesiologists Task Force on Transesophageal Echocardiography. Anesthesiology 1996;84:986.

R

1. Reves JG, Sladen RN, Newman MF. Cardiac anesthetic: is it unique? Anesth Analg 1995;81:895.

2. Reves JG, Samuelson PN, Lell WA, McDaniel HG, Kouchoukos NT, Rogers WJ, et al. Myocardial damage in coronary artery bypass surgical patients anaesthetized with two anaesthetic techniques: a random comparison of halothane and enflurane. Can Anaesth Soc J 1980;27:238.

3. Reves JG, Samuelson PN, Lell WA, Allarde RR, Younes HM, Oget S. Anesthesia for coronary artery surgery: an evolution in anesthetic management. Ala J Med Sci 1977;14:394.

4. Reves JG, Samuelson PN, Younes HM, Lell WA. Anesthetic considerations for coronary artery surgery. Anesthesiol Rev 1977;4:19.

5. Randomised trial of normothermic versus hypothermic coronary bypass surgery. The Warm Heart Investigators. Lancet 1994;343:559.

6. Reddy PS, Curtiss EI, O'Toole JD, Shaver JA. Cardiac tamponade: hemodynamic observation in man. Circulation 1978;58:265.

7. Reasoner DK, Ryu KH, Hindman BJ, Cutkomp J, Smith T. Marked hemodilution increases neurologic injury after focal cerebral ischemia in rabbits. Anesth Analg 1996;82:61.

8. Reves J. Anesthesia during cardiopulmonary bypass: does it matter? In Tinker JH, ed. Cardiopulmonary bypass: current concepts and controversies. New York: WB Saunders, 1989, p. 69.

9. Reves JG, Gelman S. Cardiovascular effects of intravenous anesthetic drugs. In Covino BG, Rehder K, Strichartz G, eds. Effects of anesthesia. Baltimore: Williams & Wilkins, 1985, p. 179.

10. Reves JG, Greeley WJ, Grichnik K, Leslie JB, Leone B. Anesthesia and supportive care for cardiothoracic surgery. In Sabiston DC Jr, Spencer FC, eds. Surgery of the chest. 6th ed. Philadelphia: WB Saunders, 1995, p. 117.

11. Reves JG, Fragen RJ, Vinik HR, Greenblatt DJ. Midazolam: pharmacology and uses. Anesthesiology 1985;62:310.

12. Reves JG, Karp RB, Buttner EE, Tosone S, Smith LR, Samuelson PN, et al. Neuronal and adrenomedullary catecholamine release in response to cardiopulmonary bypass in man. Circulation 1982;66:49.

13. Reves JG, Sheppard LC, Wallach R, Lell WA. Therapeutic uses of sodium nitroprusside and an automated method of administration. Int Anesthesiol Clin 1978;16:51.

14. Rao S, Sherbaniuk RW, Prasad K, Lee SJ, Sproule BJ. Cardiopulmonary effects of diazepam. Clin Pharmacol Ther 1973;14:182.

S

1. Sonnenblick EH, Ross J Jr, Braunwald E. Oxygen consumption of the heart: newer concepts of its multifactorial determination. Am J Cardiol 1968;22:328.

2. Slogoff S, Keats AS. Does perioperative myocardial ischemia lead to postoperative myocardial infarction? Anesthesiology 1985;62:107.

3. Schell R, Gundry S, Grichnik K. Anesthesia for minimally invasive cardiac surgery. In Estafanous FG, Barash PG, Reves JG, eds. Cardiac anesthesia: principles and clinical practice, 2nd ed. Philadelphia: Lippincott Williams & Wilkins, 2001.

4. Sheikh KH, de Bruijn NP, Rankin JS, Clements FM, Stanley T, Wolfe WG, et al. The utility of transesophageal echocardiography and Doppler color flow imaging in patients undergoing cardiac valve surgery. J Am Coll Cardiol 1990;15:363.

5. Skaryak LA, Chai PJ, Kern FH, Greeley WJ, Ungerleider RM. Blood gas management and degree of cooling: effects on cerebral metabolism before and after circulatory arrest. J Thorac Cardiovasc Surg 1995;110:1649.

6. Shabetai R, Fowler NO, Guntheroth WG. The hemodynamics of cardiac tamponade and constrictive pericarditis. Am J Cardiol 1970;26:480.

7. Stefaniszyn HJ, Novick RJ, Salerno TA. Toward a better understanding of the hemodynamic effects of protamine and heparin interaction. J Thorac Cardiovasc Surg 1984;87:678.

8. Svensson LG, Hess KR, D'Agostino RS, Entrup MH, Hreib K, Kimmel WH, et al. Reduction of neurologic injury after high-risk thoracoabdominal aortic operation. Ann Thorac Surg 1998;66:132.

9. Savage RM, Lytle BW, Aronson S, Navia JL, Licina M, Stewart WJ, et al. Intraoperative echocardiography is indicated in high-risk coronary artery bypass grafting. Ann Thorac Surg 1997;64:368.

10. Sylivris S, Calafiore P, Matalanis G, Rosalion A, Yuen HP, Buxton BF, et al. The intraoperative assessment of ascending aortic atheroma: epiaortic imaging is superior to both transesophageal echocardiography and direct palpation. J Cardiothorac Vasc Anesth 1997;11:704.

11. Steen PA, Newberg L, Milde JH, Michenfelder JD. Hypothermia and barbiturates: individual and combined effects on canine cerebral oxygen consumption. Anesthesiology 1983;58:527.

12. Singh AK, Bert AA, Feng WC, Rotenberg FA. Stroke during coronary artery bypass grafting using hypothermic versus normothermic perfusion. Ann Thorac Surg 1995;59:84.

13. Szecsi J, Batonyi E, Liptay P, Orosi P, Medgyessy I, Petterffy A. Early clinical experience with a simple method for autotransfusion in cardiac surgery. Scand J Cardiovasc Surg 1989;23:51.

14. Schell RM, Kern FH, Greeley WJ, Schulman SR, Frasco PE, Croughwell ND, et al. Cerebral blood flow and metabolism during cardiopulmonary bypass. Anesth Analg 1993;76:849.

15. Savageau JA, Stanton BA, Jenkins CD, Klein MD. Neuropsychological dysfunction following elective cardiac operation. Early assessment. J Thorac Cardiovasc Surg 1982;84:585.

16. Slogoff S, Reul GJ, Keats AS, Curry GR, Crum ME, Elmquist BA, et al. Role of perfusion pressure and flow in major organ dysfunction after cardiopulmonary bypass. Ann Thorac Surg 1990;50:911.

17. Samuelson PN, Reves JG, Kirklin JK, Bradley E Jr, Wilson KD, Adams M. Comparison of sufentanil and enflurane-nitrous oxide anesthesia for myocardial revascularization. Anesth Analg 1986;65:217.

18. Stocker F, Herschkowitz N, Bossi E, Stoller M, Cross TA, Aue WP, et al. Cerebral metabolic studies in situ by 31P-nuclear magnet resonance after hypothermic circulatory arrest. Pediatr Res 1986;20:867.

19. Stenseth R, Berg EM, Bjella L, Christensen O, Levang OW, Gisvold SE. Effects of thoracic epidural analgesia on coronary hemodynamics and myocardial metabolism in coronary artery bypass surgery. J Cardiothorac Vasc Anesth 1995;9:503.

20. Stenlake JB, Waigh RD, Urwin J, Dewar GH, Coker GG. Atracurium: conception and inception. Br J Anaesth 1983;5:3S.

21. Schinman MM, Evans GT, Brown MA, Rapaport E. Simplified direct Fick techniques for measurement of cardiac output in seriously ill patients. Am Heart J 1972;83:61.

22. Stone JG, Hoar PF, Calabro JR, DePetrillo MA, Bendixen HH. Afterload reduction and preload augmentation improve the anesthetic management of patients with cardiac failure and valvular regurgitation. Anesth Analg 1980;59:737.

T

1. Theil D, Stanley TE, White WD, Goodman DK, Glass PS, Bai SA, et al. Midazolam and fentanyl continuous infusion anesthesia for cardiac surgery: a comparison of computer-assisted versus manual infusion systems. J Cardiothorac Vasc Anesth 1993;7:300.

2. Tuman KJ, McCarthy RJ, Najafi H, Ivankovich AD. Differential effects of advanced age on neurologic and cardiac risks of coronary artery operations. J Thorac Cardiovasc Surg 1992;104:1510.

3. Treasure T, Smith PL, Newman S, Schneidau A, Joseph P, Ell P, et al. Impairment of cerebral function following cardiac and other major surgery. Eur J Cardiothorac Surg 1989;3:216.

U

1. Ungerleider RM, Greeley WJ, Kanter RJ, Kisslo JA. The learning curve for intraoperative echocardiography during congenital heart surgery. Ann Thorac Surg 1992;54:691.

V

1. Vlahakes GJ, Turley K, Hoffman JI. The pathophysiology of failure in acute right ventricular hypertension: hemodynamic and biochemical correlations. Circulation 1981;63:87.

2. Vlahakes GJ, Turley K, Hoffman JI. Mechanism of failure in acute right ventricular hypertension. Surg Forum 1979;30:214.

3. Viola AR. The influence of pericardectomy on the hemodynamics of chronic constrictive pericarditis. Circulation 1973;48:1038.

4. van der Linden J, Wesslen O, Ekroth R, Tyden H, von Ahn H. Transcranial Doppler-estimated versus thermodilution-estimated cerebral blood flow during cardiac operations. J Thorac Cardiovasc Surg 1991;102:95.

5. Vandermeulen EP, Van Aken H, Vermylen J. Anticoagulants and spinal-epidural anesthesia. Anesth Analg 1994;79:1165.

W

1. William GD, Jones TK, Hanson KA, Morray JP. The hemodynamic effects of propofol in children with congenital heart disease. Anesth Analg 1999;89:1411.

2. Weyland A, Stephan H, Kazmaier S, Weyland W, Schorn B, Grune F, et al. Flow velocity measurements as an index of cerebral blood flow: validity of transcranial Doppler sonographic monitoring during cardiac surgery. Anesthesiology 1994;81:1401.

3. Woodcock TE, Murkin JM, Farrar JK, Tweed WA, Guiraudon GM, McKenzie FN. Pharmacologic EEG suppression during cardiopulmonary bypass: cerebral hemodynamic and metabolic effects of thiopental or isoflurane during hypothermia and normothermia. Anesthesiology 1987;67:218.
4. Widmann R, Miyazawa T, Hossmann KA. Protective effect of hypothermia on hippocampal injury after 30 minutes of forebrain ischemia in rats is mediated by postischemic recovery of protein synthesis. J Neurochem 1993;61:200.

Z

1. Zubiate P, Kay JH, Mendez AM, Krohn BG, Hochman R, Dunne EF. Coronary artery surgery. A new technique with the use of little blood, if any. J Thorac Cardiovasc Surg 1974;68:263.
2. Zeidifard E, Silverman M, Godfrey S. Reproducibility of indirect (CO_2) Fick method for calculation of cardiac output. J Appl Physiol 1972;33:141.

5 Postoperative Care

The primary determinants of success of a cardiac operation are events in the operating room. However, some patients who are seriously ill when they leave the operating room can survive and have a good long-term result when postoperative care is appropriate and intensive. Conversely, ill-advised or overly energetic interventions early after operation can put a patient at risk who would otherwise convalesce normally.

Normal convalescence is not normal physiology. For instance, care early after open intracardiac operations is complicated by the whole body inflammatory response to cardiopulmonary bypass (CPB). However, the major issue relating to abnormalities of postoperative convalescence currently is the degree of preoperative morbidity in terms of both circulatory derangements and comorbid subsystem abnormalities. Conceptual and management errors are made, and unnecessary tests and interventions are used, because of failure to realize that a patient undergoing CPB is, for a time afterward, in a special biologic situation to which the knowledge and rules applicable to other humans may or may not apply.

Fortunately, despite these problems and because of knowledge that has been generated, postoperative care can and should be simple for many patients undergoing cardiac operations. These are the patients experiencing an *uncomplicated,* or *normal, convalescence,* devoid of any findings or events that increase the probability of hospital death or complications or a suboptimal late result. Generally, these patients have adequate function of all subsystems, as determined by standard criteria. As long as this pattern of normal convalescence continues, testing and intervention can be safely minimized. In these situations, expeditious discharge from the intensive care unit can be accomplished and a short subsequent hospital stay anticipated. Alertness to deviations from the pattern of an uncomplicated convalescence is mandatory, because deviations are an indication for closer observation and possibly more intensive testing and treatment. Therefore, analysis of early convalescence can place the patient into one of three categories: optimal, suboptimal but in control, and critically ill. Each category carries therapeutic implications.

- Optimal: Routine care; no change or important modification is currently necessary or foreseeable.
- Suboptimal but in control: Careful consideration is given to a change in therapy and a new modality is likely, such as additional catecholamine support for low cardiac output or lidocaine drip for frequent premature ventricular contractions.
- Critically ill: A modification, change, or new intervention is necessary and urgent, such as treatment of oliguria or metabolic acidosis, or return to the operating room for bleeding.

Both the "suboptimal" and "critically ill" categories define abnormal convalescence.

The patient convalescing normally and without complications after cardiac surgery usually appears at a glance to be doing well. Although there is always pain, varying in intensity from patient to patient, there is no restlessness, agitation, or anxiety. Eyes and skin look normal, and the pulse is full but may be rapid. Breathing is neither labored nor excessively rapid. The patient is oriented and lucid and, whether a neonate, infant, or adult, exhibits generally appropriate behavior. Few tests and interventions are required.

When convalescence is abnormal, the observations and interventions need to be intensive and at times complex. It is particularly in these situations that care must be well organized and should follow specific patient management protocols. Such protocols allow all members of the intensive care team to be clear about the details of management.

Use of protocols is facilitated by considering the patient to be a complex, integrated system composed of a number of separate but interrelated subsystems (i.e., cardiovascular, pulmonary, renal, nervous, gastrointestinal). Care of such a patient can be accomplished effectively using a "subsystems analysis" approach.[K3] This analysis begins in the operating room as CPB is discontinued (see Chapters 2 and 4) and continues into the early and late postoperative period. This is not to say that care can be carried out in an automatic fashion. Optimal postoperative care requires overall direction by a knowledgeable and experienced physician using, when indicated, specialized methods of securing information and the skills of personnel in a dedicated cardiovascular intensive care unit.

Management of patients after cardiac surgery has become in some institutions a specialty of its own. The literature on the subject is enormous. Numerous institutions around the world, with large experiences in the surgery of both congenital and acquired heart disease, have developed their own protocols and specific systems of management. These include "fast track" protocols and critical pathways that integrate the goals of all caregivers and other interested parties. Within the context of these developments, this chapter discusses general principles, along with enough specific details to be helpful to those desiring to change or develop their own protocols.

Subsystems during Early Convalescence after Cardiac Surgery

CARDIOVASCULAR SUBSYSTEM
Cardiac Reserve

Cardiac reserve is the capacity to increase (or at least maintain) cardiac output as a response to a variety of stressful sudden developments, including increased total body oxygen consumption, increased ventricular afterload, or decreased ventricular preload. Providing that capacity are all the cardiac and extracardiac mechanisms for maintaining and increasing the force of ventricular contraction and cardiac output. Most of these reside in myocardial contractility and coronary blood flow.[1] In patients convalescing from cardiac surgery, adequacy of cardiac performance alone is insufficient for a high probability of normal convalescence and survival. There must, in addition, be adequacy of cardiac reserve.

Inadequacy of cardiac reserve may become apparent only during periods of increased oxygen consumption (from struggling or hyperthermia), suddenly increased ventricular afterload (from paroxysmal pulmonary arterial hypertension in a neonate), or acute reduction in ventricular preload (from sudden blood loss). Such inadequacies of cardiac reserve probably explain "sudden death" occurring early after cardiac surgery.

Cardiac reserve is highly dependent on the preoperative condition of the patient. When, because of disease, reserves are being nearly fully utilized to maintain adequate cardiac performance in nonstressful situations, that which remains may be insufficient to meet successfully the stresses of the intraoperative and postoperative period. Reserves probably cannot be increased before the operation, unless they are acutely impaired by a reduced myocardial energy charge.[A7] Energy charge may be increased by the cardioplegic technique used in the operating room (see "Cold Cardioplegia, Controlled Aortic Root Reperfusion, and [When Needed] Warm Cardioplegic Induction" under Methods of Myocardial Management during Cardiac Surgery in Chapter 3).

Limited cardiac reserves are specifically compensated for by many features of early postoperative care.

Adequacy

Although infrequently conceptualized and not specifically measurable, adequacy of blood flow (cardiac output) in meeting the needs of the patient during recovery from cardiac surgery is the central issue with respect to the cardiovascular subsystem. Arteries and veins are infrequently the primary limiting factors. Therefore, emphasis is on adequacy of performance of the heart itself in providing adequate blood flow to the body.

Cardiac Index

Cardiac index (cardiac output expressed as $L \cdot min^{-1} \cdot m^{-2}$) is one measure of adequacy of the cardiovascular subsys-

---

[1] The familiar exercise stress test is a test for cardiac reserve.

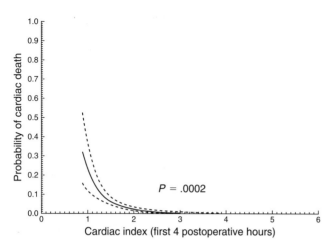

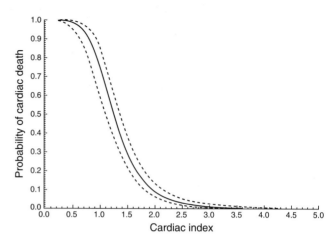

Figure 5-1   Relationship of cardiac index in the early hours after mitral valve replacement to the probability of cardiac death (UAB, 1975 to 1979). The solid line is the point estimate, and dashed lines are the 70% confidence limits. (From Conti VR, Wideman F, Blackstone EH, Kirklin JW. Unpublished study; 1979.)

Figure 5-2   Relationship of early postoperative cardiac index (average of all early postoperative values) to the probability of cardiac death in infants and small children. This graph suggests that convalescence cannot be considered normal in infants and small children unless cardiac index is about 2.0 to 2.2 $L \cdot min^{-1} \cdot m^{-2}$, somewhat higher than the value for adults. (From Parr and colleagues.[P4])

tem, as evidenced by the oft-demonstrated relation between cardiac index and survival (described by Dietzman and colleagues in 1969[D1]). In adults, a cardiac index of at least 2.0 $L \cdot min^{-1} \cdot m^{-2}$ during the first few hours in the intensive care unit and one of at least 2.4 on the morning after operation are required for normal convalescence (Fig. 5-1). This is at the lower end of the range of normal, which is 2.2 to 4.4.[B4] Infants and small children appear, in general, to require a somewhat higher cardiac index for normal convalescence (Fig. 5-2). Also, in young patients, cardiac index tends to be lower about 4 hours after operation than it was soon after discontinuing CPB, and then begins to rise after 9 to 12 hours.[B20,M4]

Cardiac indices below these values are usually inadequate for maintaining a normal convalescence; this can be formalized in the inverse relation between cardiac index early postoperatively and the probability of hospital death. This relation can be refined by considering not only cardiac output but also mixed venous oxygen levels, with lower levels worsening prognosis at any given value of cardiac output.[2]

Arterial Blood Pressure

Arterial blood pressure is an insensitive method of estimating the adequacy of cardiac output early postoperatively, primarily because systemic vascular resistance is usually elevated.[E5] This may be related to increased levels of circulating catecholamines,[W9] plasma renin,[R1] angiotensin II,

or other mechanisms. This high resistance may result in a normal or high arterial blood pressure even when cardiac output is low.

Some patients tend early postoperatively to have a low systemic arterial resistance and arterial blood pressure, even when cardiac performance is good. This may occur more frequently in children with cyanotic heart disease, adults with diabetes, and patients with sepsis or drug interactions (especially preoperative use of ACE inhibitors).[C31,M35]

Arterial hypotension is an indication for thoughtful evaluation. Children cannot be considered to be convalescing normally when mean arterial blood pressure is lower than about 10% below normal for the patient's age (Table 5-1). For adults, particularly the elderly, arterial blood pressure may mandate maintenance at or above commonly accepted normal values, to ensure adequate perfusion of various organs, such as the brain, viscera, and kidneys.

Pedal Pulses

Simple observation of pedal pulses is a commonly used, useful, but not infallible method of estimating the adequacy of cardiac output in children and young adults. Normal (grade 4) pedal pulses early postoperatively are highly, but not perfectly, correlated with adequate cardiac output and a high probability of survival (Table 5-2).[K4] In older adults, estimation of the adequacy of perfusion by amplitude of pedal pulses is often confounded by the presence of peripheral arterial occlusive disease.

Skin Temperature

Skin temperature in the foot is another indirect but reasonably reliable estimator of adequacy of cardiac output. A study of cardiac surgery in infants under 3 months of age indicated that pedal pulses and skin temperature predicted the probability of hospital death from cardiac causes and thus were reasonably good estimators of the adequacy of

---

[2] Although dye dilution or thermodilution is the standard for measuring cardiac output, caution is required in interpreting measurement values. In small subjects, confidence intervals around the measurement may be large; low core temperature may diminish accuracy; and tricuspid regurgitation, absence of an adequate mixing chamber, lack of steady state, and intracardiac shunts (as originally articulated by Stewart and Hamilton[H29,S42]) invalidate the measurement.

■ **TABLE 5-1   Normal Values for Blood Pressure According to Age**

Age ≤ years <		Systolic Pressure/ Diastolic Pressure (mmHg)	Mean[a] (mmHg)	10% > Mean Normal Value (mmHg)	10% < Mean Normal Value (mmHg)
	0.5	80/46	57	63	51[b]
0.5	1.0	89/60	70	77	63
1.0	2.0	99/64	76	84	68
2.0	4.0	100/65	77	85	69
4.0	12.0	105/65	78	86	70
12.0	15.0	118/68	85	94	74
15.0		120/70	87	96	78

(Data from Nadas and Fyler.[N2])

[a] Mean arterial blood pressure has been calculated as the diastolic pressure plus one third of the pulse pressure.

[b] 40 mmHg in infants <1 month of age.

■ **TABLE 5-2   Relation of Foot Pulse Amplitude and Foot Temperature (estimated by nursing staff) to Hospital Death from Acute Cardiac Failure in Infants under 3 Months Undergoing Cardiac Operation**

Clinical Observations	n	Hospital Deaths from Acute Cardiac Failure			
		No.	%	70% CL	
Pulses					
Absent	11	6	55	35–73	
1+	12	2	17	6–35	18/47 (38%)
2+	24	10	42	30–54	CL 30%–47%
3+	25	2	8	3–18	3/68 (4%)
4+	43	1	2	0.3–8	CL 2%–9%
TOTAL	115	21	18	14–23	
P (logistic) = .0001					
Skin Temperature					
Cold	29	15	52	41–63	
Tepid	19	4	21	11–35	
Warm	66	2	3	1–7	
TOTAL	114	21	18	15–25	
P (logistic) < .0001					

(From Kirklin and colleagues.[K33])

CL, Confidence limits.

cardiac output.[K4] As with assessment of pedal pulse amplitude, in older adults skin temperature offers guidance but not solid evidence for adequacy of perfusion (see Table 5-2).

Whole Body Oxygen Consumption

Whole body oxygen consumption is infrequently calculated, but knowledge of it is useful; in some circumstances, it is a better basis for prognostic and therapeutic inferences than cardiac output or mixed venous oxygen levels. Whole body oxygen consumption ($\dot{V}O_2$) can be calculated by a rearranged Fick equation,[3] which states:

$$\dot{V}O_2 \, (mL \cdot min^{-1} \cdot m^{-2}) = \dot{Q} \cdot (CaO_2 - C\bar{v}O_2) \tag{5-1}$$

The normal value for $\dot{V}O_2$ at 37°C is 155 mL $\cdot$ min^{-1} $\cdot$ m^{-2}. The value for whole body oxygen consumption in the

---

[3] The Fick equation states

$$\dot{Q} = \frac{\dot{V}O_2}{CaO_2 - C\bar{v}O_2} \, (L \cdot min^{-1}) \tag{5-2}$$

where $\dot{Q}$ is cardiac output in L $\cdot$ min^{-1}, $\dot{V}O_2$ is oxygen consumption in mL $\cdot$ min^{-1}, CaO_2 is arterial O_2 content in mL $\cdot$ L^{-1}, and $C\bar{v}O_2$ is mixed venous O_2 content in mL $\cdot$ L^{-1}.

The oxygen content of blood consists of combined plus dissolved oxygen:

$$Co_2 = \frac{1.38 \cdot Hb \cdot So_2}{100} + 0.03 \cdot Po_2 \, (mL \cdot L^{-1}) \tag{5-3}$$

where Hb is hemoglobin concentration in g $\cdot$ L^{-1}, So_2 is O_2 saturation as a percentage of capacity, Po_2 is O_2 tension in mmHg, 1.38 is effective O_2 capacity of 1 g of hemoglobin in mL $\cdot$ g^{-1}, and 0.03 is solubility of O_2 in blood at 37°C in mL $\cdot$ L^{-1} $\cdot$ mmHg^{-1}.

Rearranging equation 5-2 and substituting for CaO_2 from equation 5-3,

$$C\bar{v}O_2 = \frac{1.38 \cdot Hb \cdot SaO_2}{100} + 0.03 \cdot PaO_2 - \frac{\dot{V}O_2}{\dot{Q}} \tag{5-4}$$

where SaO_2 is arterial O_2 content in mL $\cdot$ L^{-1}, and PaO_2 is arterial O_2 tension in mmHg.

For a given $\dot{V}O_2$, equation 5-4 indicates that to increase $C\bar{v}O_2$, there must be an increase in SaO_2, PaO_2, Hb, or $\dot{Q}$. $C\bar{v}O_2$ varies directly with $P\bar{v}O_2$, and $P\bar{v}O_2$ varies directly with cellular Po_2 unless there is shunting in the peripheral circulation. Thus, to maximize tissue oxygen supply, there must be an increase of one or more of the following: PaO_2 (and thus SaO_2), Hb, or $\dot{Q}$.

patient recovering from cardiac surgery must be interpreted in light of his or her body temperature; residual hypothermia is the most common explanation for the somewhat low whole body oxygen consumption usually present within the first few hours after open heart surgery. This reduced $\dot{V}O_2$ is in part a result of a reduced capillary density (reduced area of capillary flow) and increased heterogeneity of capillary flow through the muscle mass and other tissues of the body in the early hours after CPB.[B19] Normally convalescing patients operated on with hypothermic CPB generally require 4 to 8 hours for this to disappear and for their peripheral perfusion to return to normal.[K21]

When $\dot{V}O_2$ is appreciably reduced below the normal level for the existing body temperature, a hazardous condition exists; indeed, one useful definition of shock is "a condition characterized by an acute reduction in $\dot{V}O_2$." Abnormally low $\dot{V}O_2$ may result from reduction or extreme heterogeneity of capillary flow (of which "no reflow" is an extreme example) in one or more organs of the body (sometimes termed a reduction in capillary density), lengthening of the diffusion path between capillaries and cells, or intracellular metabolic derangement. One or all of these may exist in patients early after cardiac surgery. When important reduction in $\dot{V}O_2$, considering the temperature, persists for more than a few hours, the probability of death increases.

Mixed Venous Oxygen Level

Mixed venous oxygen level, generally expressed as oxygen tension ($P\bar{v}O_2$) or as saturation ($S\bar{v}O_2$), is a useful index of circulatory adequacy, because it reflects to some extent mean tissue oxygen levels.[K1] When $P\bar{v}O_2$ is less than 30 mmHg, cardiac output is likely to be inadequate; when it is below about 23 mmHg, the inadequacy is apt to be severe (Fig. 5-3). However, normal or near-normal venous oxygen levels are not reassuring as to the adequacy of cardiac output, unless it is known that oxygen

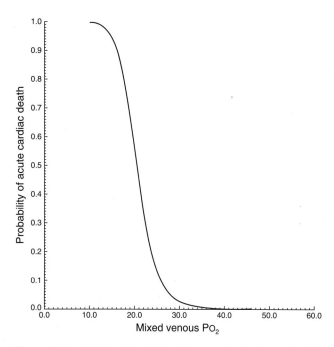

Figure 5-3   Relationship of mixed venous P_{O_2} to the probability of acute cardiac death in infants and young children. Convalescence cannot be considered normal if the value is less than about 28 mmHg. (From Parr and colleagues.[P4])

consumption is approximately normal for the existing body temperature.

In a nonsurgical but critically ill intensive care unit population, Jain and colleagues[J9] found a weak relationship between $S\bar{v}O_2$ and cardiac index. There was considerable variability among all patients in various conditions. However, when normalized for $\dot{V}O_2$ and hemoglobin concentration, the correlation coefficient improved (Fig. 5-4). Using indwelling fiberoptic reflectance oximetry,[I4] other investigators have found no or only a very weak relationship between $S\bar{v}O_2$ or $P\bar{v}O_2$ and measured cardiac index.[M32] Following CPB, changes in $S\bar{v}O_2$ may be useful in detecting low cardiac output, one of many causes of decreased oxygen delivery. Identifying decreases may be of particular value in patients coming to surgery with high severity of illness index.[V5] Online continuous oximetry is useful in critically ill patients because it reflects unanticipated events or occasionally the usefulness (or nonusefulness) of therapeutic maneuvers.[S33] These aspects of postoperative care illustrate the need for uniformity in monitoring techniques and highlight the conflict between overreliance on devices and the ability to form accurate estimates (in this case, of cardiac performance) based on previous correlations.[S33] However, many surgeons rely on continuous $S\bar{v}O_2$ monitoring to detect deviations from normal convalescence early postoperatively. Catheters that allow measurement of both $S\bar{v}O_2$ and cardiac output are optimal.

Urine Flow and Serum Potassium

Urine flow and serum potassium levels are useful indirect guides to the adequacy of cardiac output. Early postoperative oliguria suggests inadequate cardiac output and thus is often an indication for treatment of the cardiovascular subsystem. Hyperkalemia rising over a 4-hour period (with

sampling every 2 hours) to a level of about 5 mEq $\cdot$ L^{-1} is a sensitive indicator of a low or falling cardiac output in neonates and infants, hence an indication for intensifying treatment. Hyperkalemia is usually accompanied by a fall in pedal skin temperature and a rise in esophageal temperature, but it often precedes the appearance of a base deficit or of arterial hypotension.

Metabolic Acidosis

A frequently used but somewhat nonspecific and insensitive indicator of the adequacy of cardiac output is the acid-base status of blood. Metabolic acidosis during and after cardiac surgery is almost always a result of lactic acidemia. Lactate production is a byproduct of anaerobic metabolism, which most often occurs under conditions in which cardiac output and oxygen consumption are suboptimal. Occasionally, excess lactate may occur with high measured cardiac output under conditions of high metabolic rate, diabetes, sepsis, or intestinal ischemia.

Concentration of lactic acid in blood may be measured directly. Normally, little or none is present, normal values in plasma being 0.7 to 2.1 mEq $\cdot$ L^{-1}. A concentration of about 5 mEq $\cdot$ L^{-1} correlates, in general, with moderate metabolic acidosis, and one of 10 mEq $\cdot$ L^{-1} correlates with severe metabolic acidosis and usually markedly reduced cardiac output. Moderate elevation of lactic acid concentration is a common finding early after cardiac surgery, but in the normally convalescing patient, lactic acid gradually declines to normal values within 12 to 24 hours.

When arterial pH is less than about 7.4, acidosis is present, but may be the result of retention of carbon dioxide; this is reflected in an arterial $PaCO_2$ greater than 40 mmHg. Alternatively, acidosis may be "metabolic" and due primarily to accumulation of lactic acid. Quantification of metabolic acidosis is expressed by a derived value obtained from an equation after measuring arterial pH and $PaCO_2$.[S15] Either the buffer base deficit or the standard bicarbonate is calculated.[A5,A8] Most commercially available equipment calculates the buffer base deficit or excess (which takes account of the buffering capacity of blood as well as that of bicarbonate) after measuring PaO_2, $PaCO_2$, and pH of whole blood. The normal buffer base is about 48 mEq $\cdot$ L^{-1}, and the normal base excess or deficit is 0.

Cardiac Output and Its Determinants

The cardiac index in normally convalescing adults is often 2.5 to 3.5 L $\cdot$ min^{-1} $\cdot$ m^{-2} after cardiac surgery performed with modern methods of myocardial management. It is generally higher 4 to 6 hours after operation than it is in the operating room and still higher the next day (Table 5-3), although exceptions occur. Even in patients who convalesce well, some variability in cardiac output occurs. Risk factors for low cardiac output seem primarily to affect cardiac output in the operating room (Table 5-4), which in turn is strongly correlated with cardiac output 4 to 6 hours later and the next day.[F8]

Cardiac output after operations using CPB is usually correlated with age of the patient (older patients have lower outputs), morphologic lesion (for example, see Table 5-4), functional state of the patient just before operation (the higher the New York Heart Association [NYHA] class, the

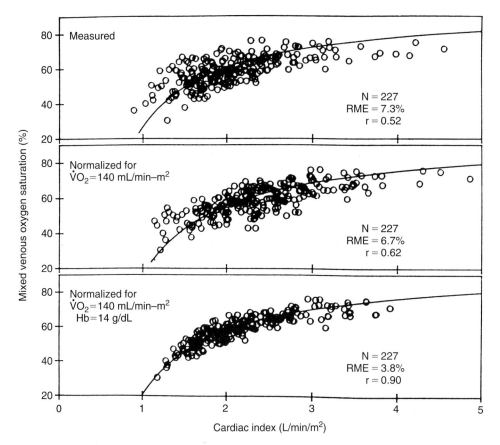

Figure 5-4   Relationship between mixed venous oxygen saturation and cardiac index in 30 patients with advanced heart failure. *Top panel,* solid line represents best fit of the Fick equation to all measured data points (N). *Center panel,* measured cardiac index normalized by calculated oxygen consumption ($\dot{V}o_2c$). *Bottom panel,* measured cardiac index normalized for hemoglobin (Hb) and $\dot{V}o_2c$. A nonlinear relationship was observed between mixed venous oxygen saturation and cardiac index (correlation coefficient = 0.52). On normalizing for differences in hemoglobin and oxygen consumption, the correlation coefficient became 0.90. Thus, the relationship between mixed venous oxygen saturation and cardiac index in a group of patients depends on the homogeneity of their hemoglobin and oxygen consumption. Furthermore, the ability of mixed venous oxygen saturation to serve as a therapeutic indicator in any given patient depends on the baseline saturation and cardiac index. (From Jain and colleagues.[J9])

■ **TABLE 5-3   Cardiac Index (L · min^{-1} · m^{-2}) after Cardiac Surgery in Adult Patients Who Convalesce Normally, According to the Interval after Operation and the Global Myocardial Ischemic Time** [a,b]

Global Myocardial Ischemic Time	Interval after Operation					
	30 min [c]		4-6 h		20-24 h	
≤ min <	n	Mean ± SD	n	Mean ± SD	n	Mean ± SD
35	46	2.81 ± 0.632	46	2.88 ± 0.689	46	3.03 ± 0.621
35 55	87	2.75 ± 0.662	86	2.91 ± 0.711	84	2.95 ± 0.655
55	25	2.56 ± 0.520	24	2.40 ± 0.325	22	2.68 ± 0.391
TOTAL	158	2.74 ± 0.632	156	2.82 ± 0.679	152	2.93 ± 0.609
P		.07		.03		.23

(Data from Fontan and colleagues.[F8])

[a] Coronary artery bypass grafting and valve replacement using antegrade cardioplegic myocardial management.

[b] Database is 160 patients undergoing operation at the University of Bordeaux, France, in 1991.

[c] In the operating room after cardiopulmonary bypass.

■ **TABLE 5-4 Correlates of Cardiac Index (L · min⁻¹ · m⁻²) in the Operating Room 30 Minutes after Completion of Cardiopulmonary Bypass**[a]

Correlates of Cardiac Index	Regression Coefficient ± SD [b]	P
Patient		
Age (years)	−0.008494 ± 0.0045	.06
NYHA class (I-V) [c]	−0.1989 ± 0.114	.08
Mitral stenosis (no [0], yes [1])	−0.5213 ± 0.24	.03
Aortic regurgitation (0,1)	0.6612 ± 0.33	.04
Procedural		
Nonenriched initial reperfusate (0,1)	−0.5339 ± 0.115	.0001
Nonhyperkalemic initial reperfusate (0,1)	−0.4633 ± 0.143	.002
CPB time (minutes)	−0.005523 ± 0.00163	.009
Concomitant variable [d]		
Heart rate (beats · min⁻¹)	0.004637 ± 0.0026	.08
Intercept (valve replacement)	3.978	
Intercept (CABG)	3.531	

(Data from Fontan and colleagues.[F8])

Key: *CABG,* Coronary artery bypass grafting; *CPB,* cardiopulmonary bypass; *NYHA,* New York Heart Association; *SD,* standard deviation.

[a] The database is as in Table 5-3. Note the different intercepts for patients undergoing coronary artery bypass grafting and those undergoing valve replacement. Left and right atrial pressures were low (±6-10) and similar in all patients.

[b] A positive sign indicates a positive correlation; a negative sign indicates a negative correlation.

[c] Active only in patients undergoing valve replacement.

[d] Variables existent at the time of measurement.

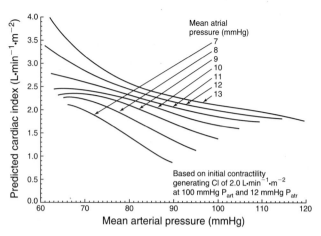

Figure 5-5 Relationship among mean arterial blood pressure, mean atrial pressure, and cardiac output after cardiac surgical procedures in infants. The nomogram depicts specific solutions of the multivariable regression equation developed by Appelbaum and colleagues.[A6] All patients in the study were in good clinical condition. Mean arterial pressure is depicted as a continuous variable along the horizontal axis, and mean atrial pressure (the higher of the two) is represented by isobars. Note that, in general, the lower the arterial pressure the higher the cardiac index, and the higher the atrial pressure the higher the cardiac index. (Data from Appelbaum and colleagues.[A6])

Key: *CI,* Cardiac index; P_{art}, mean arterial blood pressure; P_{atr}, mean atrial pressure.

lower the output), duration of CPB, and duration of global myocardial ischemia (see Table 5-4). During the early postoperative period, a heart rate within usual ranges correlates directly with cardiac output, and arterial blood pressure within usual ranges correlates inversely with it.[A6] Within the usual ranges, the higher the atrial pressures, the higher the cardiac output[A6] (Fig. 5-5).

Determinants of cardiac output are preload, afterload, myocardial contractility, and heart rate. Most normally convalescing patients require no special measures to adjust these fundamental determinants; patients with impaired or inadequate cardiac performance require at least adjustment of preload and afterload, and at times adjustment of heart rate and/or pharmacologic or interventional augmentation of contractility. In many patients who have undergone cardiac surgery, it is specifically either the left or the right ventricle that limits cardiac output, less commonly both (see "Relative Performance of Left and Right Ventricles" later in this section).

Ventricular Preload

Ventricular preload, which is correlated directly with the force of contraction, is equated with sarcomere length at end-diastole, and thus with change in ventricular volume between end-systole and end-diastole. This volume change is determined by transmural pressure during diastole, compliance and thickness of the ventricular wall, and curvature of the wall (La Place effect). Transmural geometric arrangement of fibers also plays a role, but changes little during the postoperative period.

Transmural pressure is determined by intraventricular pressure and intrapericardial pressure. Intraventricular pressure at end-diastole (which is a determinant of the force of contraction) is related to phasic changes in atrial pressure, and these are affected by blood volume and systemic

venous capacitance. The latter is decreased early after CPB.[R5] Because transmural pressure is affected by intrapericardial pressure, it is affected by closure of the pericardium and sternum, both of which increase intrapericardial pressure and decrease transmural pressure. Daughters and colleagues have demonstrated clearly that pericardial closure in the setting of cardiac surgery, both itself and independent of sternal closure, increases intrapericardial pressure, decreases transmural pressure, and unfavorably affects cardiac performance.[D3] Changes in myocardial compliance during and after cardiac operations are due primarily to changes in myocardial water content.

After cardiac surgery in patients with normal atrioventricular (AV) valves, most acute changes in preload are equated with acute changes in mean left (in the case of the left ventricle) or right (in the case of the right ventricle) atrial pressure. This is because in this setting, and when the atria are functioning normally as reservoirs,[P5] ventricular end-diastolic pressure is similar to the mean pressure in the corresponding atrium. Therefore, mean atrial pressure is measured in cardiac surgical patients to deduce ventricular end-diastolic pressure. Right atrial pressure is usually measured using a fine polyvinyl catheter introduced through the right atrial appendage or internal jugular vein. Left atrial pressure is measured through a fine catheter introduced through the right superior pulmonary vein (or the left atrial appendage in neonates and young infants). In the absence of pulmonary vascular disease and important pulmonary congestion or edema, pulmonary artery diastolic pressure is a reasonable approximation of left atrial pressure. In most adult patients following CPB, pulmonary capillary wedge

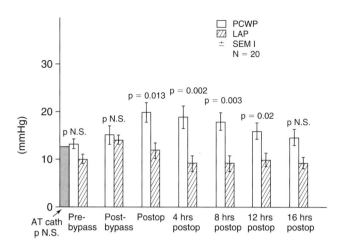

Figure 5-6   Pulmonary capillary wedge pressure (PCWP) compared with left atrial pressure (LAP) expressed as mean ± standard error (SEM). In 20 consecutive patients, PCWP exceeded LAP in the early postbypass period and was most significantly increased at 4, 8, and 12 hours after operation. These data suggest the LAP more accurately reflects left ventricular filling and is more accurate than PCWP to monitor hemodynamics postoperatively. (From Mammana and colleagues.[M33])

pressure exceeds left atrial pressure, and this discrepancy increases through the twelfth postoperative hour. It is thought that this difference is due to accumulation of interstitial lung water[M33] (Fig. 5-6).

Ventricular Afterload

In the intact ventricle, afterload is defined as systolic wall stress. This is the analogue of the load that resists shortening in the isolated papillary muscle. Other things being equal, increased afterload results in decreased stroke volume. In the intact ventricle, afterload is related to (1) ventricular transmural pressure during systole; (2) ventricular wall curvature, as determined by ventricular volume (the La Place effect); (3) ventricular wall thickness; and (4) shape of the ventricle.

Ventricular wall determinants of afterload change little during and early after operations. Instead, acute changes in afterloads of the left and right ventricles are usually produced by changes in intraventricular pressures during systole. These changes are equated with changes in proximal aortic and pulmonary arterial systolic pressures. Usually, during and early after operation, proximal pulmonary arterial pressures are monitored directly, but proximal aortic pressures are not. They must be inferred from measured radial (or femoral) artery pressures. Because of the many determinants of the magnitude of systolic amplification, systolic blood pressure at the radial artery is usually higher than in the ascending aorta. In most instances, systolic pressure variability between the aorta and peripheral arteries is not clinically important, but an awareness of it is advantageous in some situations. Mean pressures are similar in the two areas.

A tendency toward arterial hypertension is present in most adult patients early postoperatively, related to increased systemic arteriolar resistance.[G6] The precise explanation for the resulting hypertension is under continuing investigation.

This complication (1) increases ventricular afterload and thereby decreases stroke volume, (2) increases aortic wall tension and thereby encourages tearing of aortic purse-string sutures and suture lines, and (3) increases left ventricular metabolic demands that exacerbate any latent myocardial ischemia.[F5] An appropriate criterion for treatment to lower arterial blood pressure in this setting is a mean arterial blood pressure 10% above the normal value. Mean arterial blood pressure, and not systolic pressure, is monitored for this purpose, because of the interrelations between peripheral and central arterial pressures discussed earlier. However, the subject's preoperative blood pressure must be taken into account, and, to avoid cerebral complications, markedly hypertensive patients must not be rendered hypotensive. In the intensive care unit, sodium nitroprusside is generally used for this purpose (see Appendix 5A), but nitroglycerin may be preferred when myocardial ischemia is present, because it decreases coronary resistance. Negative intrathoracic pressure also increases left ventricular load-resisting shortening by increasing left ventricular transmural pressure. Positive pressure ventilation negates this effect, but labored spontaneous ventilation may augment afterload, and this may decrease cardiac output.[P17,R21]

Myocardial Contractility

When a change in stroke volume cannot be explained by a change in end-diastolic fiber length (preload) or load-resisting shortening (afterload), it is considered to result from a change in the contractile state. Contractility in a given ventricle can be acutely depressed or increased. When an attempt is made to compare ventricular contractility, from patient to patient and from time to time in the same patient, problems arise. A papillary muscle that is twice as thick as others might appear to have twice the contractility when studied in the usual way. In the ventricle, and at least theoretically in papillary muscle, data interpreted in terms of contractility must be normalized according to muscle thickness and length.

In vivo assessment of myocardial contractility and the resultant quantification of ventricular pump function are desirable goals postoperatively. The simplest representation of the capacity of the heart as a pump is a determination of any of several modifications of the Frank–Starling mechanism. For instance, the measured change in cardiac output (or stroke volume) with aliquot infusions of blood or blood substitute serves as a surrogate for assessment of contractile function. Clearly this is not reflective of intrinsic contractile properties of the myocardium, because the pressure–volume relationship is affected not only by preload but also by load-resisting shortening, myocardial compliance, and intact vagal and sympathetic reflex activity. Changes in the instantaneous ventricular pressure (or aortic pressure) over time, dp/dt, may reflect myocardial contractility, but this quantity is exquisitely sensitive to afterload and preload and cannot be assumed to be an index of contractility that can be transferred from one patient to another or within the same patient over a period of time.

The relationship between ventricular pressure and volume (pressure–volume loop) is currently the nearest approximation to an in vivo assessment of contractility. Additionally, the area within the loop represents stroke work. The end-systolic pressure and the pressure at end-

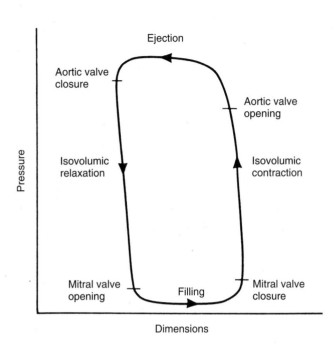

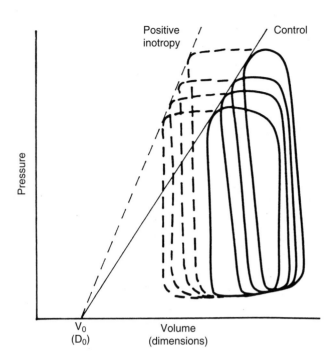

Figure 5-7 Diagrammatic representation of a pressure–dimension relationship of the left ventricle on which events of the cardiac cycle have been indicated. (From Foex and Leone.[F15])

Figure 5-8 When resistance to ejection is altered, pressure–dimension loops, at end-systole, extend to a straight line termed the *end-systolic pressure-dimension line.* The slope of this line is an index of contractility. An increase in inotropy causes an increase in the slope of the line. It can also be seen that an increase in inotropy causes a widening of the loop as ejection shortening is increased. Extrapolation of the end-systolic pressure-dimension line to zero pressure defines V_0 (or D_0), the dimension the ventricle would attain if intracavitary pressure became zero. (From Foex and Leone.[F15])

diastole of several different loops allow an expression of contractility and stiffness, respectively. The loops are composed of four segments: isovolumic contraction, ejection, isovolumic relaxation, and filling (Fig. 5-7). When ventricular volume or resistance is altered, a group of points at end-systole fall along a line, the slope of which Suga and colleagues called Emax.[S36-38] Emax is an index of contractility (Fig. 5-8). Changes of the slope in a steeper direction reflect increased inotropy. A shift in the rightward direction represents negative inotropy. The introduction of catheters and online echocardiographic border detection allow description of pressure volume loops and calculation of Emax in some intensive care unit settings. With the use of catheters to measure left ventricular pressure and transesophageal echocardiography for instantaneous border detection, pressure-volume loops and Emax (contractility at zero volume) can be interpreted online in the intensive care unit.

It is paradoxical that the least clearly and directly defined determinant of the force of cardiac contraction is the one most discussed and treated. Its specific treatment is by the administration of inotropic drugs, usually catecholamines (see "Treatment of Low Cardiac Output" later in this section).

Relative Performance of Left and Right Ventricles

During and early after cardiac operations, one of the two ventricles is usually the factor limiting cardiac performance, not both. It is usually advantageous to consider and treat patients with this concept clearly in mind. The clue of greatest importance in this regard, when the AV valves are normal, is the relation between the left and

right atrial pressures, because they represent the closest approximation available to ventricular end-diastolic pressure and, by implication, sarcomere length.[B9] When the cardiac valves are normal, the ventricle with the highest corresponding atrial pressure is the one limiting cardiac performance. Echocardiography can often provide supportive information.[S34]

Heart Rate

Sinus rhythm is optimal postoperatively, and with this rhythm a wide range of heart rates at various ages is compatible with survival (Table 5-5). The normal compensatory response to increased O_2 demand is increased heart rate. Often in the elderly and also in patients with diseased myocardium, this response is absent. It is prudent to manipulate heart rate in otherwise normally convalescing patients with slow sinus (or junctional) rhythm to improve cardiac output. For this, atrial pacing via two temporary atrial leads placed at operation is used. In these situations, atrial pacing is also helpful to suppress premature beats (both atrial and ventricular) and may limit the onset of an established arrhythmia.

■ **TABLE 5-5   Ranges of Heart Rate during Sinus Rhythm in Normally Convalescing Patients**

Age		Heart Rate
≤ years <		(beats · min⁻¹)
	1/12	120-190
1/12	6/12	110-180
6/12	12/12	100-170
1	3	90-160
3	6	80-150
6	15	80-140
15		70-130

(From Kirklin and colleagues.[K2])

Cardiac Rhythm

Disturbances of cardiac rhythm may also contribute to low cardiac output. Junctional (AV nodal) rhythm reduces cardiac output by 10% to 15%. Junctional rhythm is less efficient than sinus rhythm because the atrial contribution to ventricular filling is absent in the former. Because junctional rhythm is usually transient and its effects are easily overcome by atrial pacing (unless the rate is rapid),[H7] its presence does not connote an added immediate risk.

Prevalence and Risk Factors Associated with Atrial Fibrillation

New atrial fibrillation develops in 25% to 50% of adult patients undergoing open intracardiac operations.[L3] This arrhythmia uncommonly results in major morbidity or death, but it can complicate convalescence considerably. It is most likely to develop in patients in whom chronic atrial fibrillation has been present before operation and who have left the operating room in sinus rhythm.[D12]

The largest group of patients in whom atrial fibrillation has not been present preoperatively are those undergoing coronary artery bypass grafting (CABG). In this group, discontinuance postoperatively of a β-adrenergic receptor blocking agent that has been taken regularly before operation increases the risk of developing atrial fibrillation during the postoperative period; this complication can be expected in about 40% of such situations.[M19] Older age at operation is also a risk factor for developing atrial fibrillation postoperatively; this arrhythmia develops in about 4% of patients under 40 years of age undergoing CABG, compared with 30% of those aged 70 or older.[L3] Chronic obstructive pulmonary disease and chronic renal disease also appear to increase its prevalence.[L3] Other pre- and intraoperative variables do not appear to be correlated with development of atrial fibrillation after cardiac operation.[L3]

Prevention of Atrial Fibrillation

Although the matter has been argued at length, the prevalence of new atrial fibrillation after cardiac surgery can, in fact, be reduced by prophylaxis with a β-adrenergic receptor blocking agent.[M19,R15,S21] For this purpose, propranolol may be given in doses of 10 to 20 mg three or four times a day, beginning the morning after operation. Alternatively, atenolol (Tenormin) may be given in doses of 25 mg three times each day, which is often better tolerated than propranolol.

New atrial fibrillation after cardiac surgery increases morbidity, length of stay, and cost.[A11,N13] Morbidity includes hemodynamic compromise and, occasionally, embolic events. New postoperative atrial fibrillation is statistically correlated with advanced age, but is also seen across a wide spectrum of adult cardiac operations. The peak incidence is 2 to 3 days postoperatively, but it may occur earlier or following discharge. Postoperative atrial fibrillation is usually transient; most patients return to sinus rhythm with treatment within 2 to 3 days. Patients with preoperative atrial fibrillation are unlikely to return to sinus rhythm, especially if atrial fibrillation has been present for more than 6 months. Aggressive treatment is indicated (see "Treatment of Atrial Fibrillation" later in this section).

Premature Ventricular Contractions

Unifocal, isolated premature ventricular contractions occurring outside the T waves fewer than six times per minute are not known to increase the risk of cardiac death and are compatible with normal convalescence. Other arrhythmias indicate an abnormal convalescence and may require special management (see later section on Cardiac Arrhythmias). Rarely, atrial fibrillation or isolated premature ventricular beats occurring early (within 2 to 4 hours) after operation in the presence of hypothermia or low potassium level leads to profound ventricular instability, including ventricular fibrillation.

Causes of Acute Dysfunction (Low Cardiac Output) after Cardiac Surgery

Inadequate Operation

The surgeon's responsibility for obtaining an adequate operation demands that he or she continue to search for evidence of this postoperatively, particularly when the patient has low cardiac output. Using the methods described in this and other chapters, a search is made for residual intra- or extracardiac shunting, pathway obstructions, valvar regurgitation, graft or conduit dysfunction, or cardiac compression. If the operation is found to be inadequate in any of these regards, prompt reoperation is usually indicated.

Myocardial Dysfunction

Myocardial dysfunction was once thought to explain low cardiac output after cardiac surgery, when atrial pressures were elevated above the usual postoperative values in the absence of any other explanation. The availability of two-dimensional echocardiography in the operating room and intensive care unit, particularly TEE, makes possible the direct demonstration of ventricular wall motion, as well as an assessment of end-diastolic and end-systolic volumes. These studies can lead more directly to the inference that low cardiac output is due to myocardial necrosis or stunning, or impaired cardiac reserve in the face of increased stress. This inference can be supported by the finding of increased CK-MB isoenzyme or troponin in the serum.

Reduced Preload

Hypovolemia. The most common cause of reduced preload is overlooked hypovolemia. This may be a relative intravascular loss secondary to vasodilatation, bleeding into undrained cavities (pleural spaces, retroperitoneum, or free peritoneal space), or uncharted chest tube drainage. The most obvious cause of hypovolemia, of course, is bleeding associated with cardiotomy or CPB reflected by excessive chest tube output. Low cardiac output or low arterial blood pressure associated with low filling pressures (left or right atrial pressure, central venous pressure, or pulmonary capillary wedge pressure) is the sine qua non of hypovolemia. Echocardiography showing vigorous wall motion and small chamber size is simply confirmatory.

Occasionally there is a sympathetic response that supports blood pressure, but often this is blunted early after anesthesia. There may be reflex tachycardia, but ultimately cardiac output suffers.

Infrequently, excessive diuresis leads to relative hypovolemia and lowering of cardiac output. In this instance the picture may be complicated by hypokalemia leading to arrhythmias.

Diastolic dysfunction. In the presence of left ventricular hypertrophy, fibrosis, or myocardial edema, filling pressures do not reflect ventricular volume. In this situation, ventricular compliance is diminished. The root problem is inadequate resting (diastolic) sarcomere length. In these situations, echocardiography is especially useful. The picture is characterized by a small ventricular chamber in the presence of high filling pressure, tachycardia, small stroke volume, low arterial blood pressure, and low cardiac output. Appropriate interventions should be aimed at decreasing heart rate, initiating beta blockade, and subsequent volume infusion. Some inotropic agents may be detrimental in this situation.

Acute Cardiac Tamponade. Acute pericardial tamponade (with its resultant acute decrease in ventricular preload in the face of elevated atrial pressures) must always be considered when low cardiac output is present in the early postoperative period. Undrained intrapericardial bleeding may cause acute cardiac tamponade. It may also occur as a result of marked myocardial edema and chamber dilatation inside the closed chest, because the pericardium can be constricting under these circumstances even when it has not been resutured. Acute dilatation of the right ventricle during an acute pulmonary hypertensive crisis may result in acute atypical tamponade in neonates and infants.[K15] It is these phenomena that explain the advantage of leaving the sternum open and covering the mediastinum with an impermeable sheet sutured to the skin edges in critically ill patients, or of opening it in the intensive care unit when this form of cardiac tamponade is limiting cardiac output.[K15,L12,M21-M23,O3]

After an early period of adequate and stable cardiac output, cardiac tamponade is a likely cause of rapid deterioration that cannot be easily explained otherwise. It is usually associated with rapidly rising right and left atrial pressures that often, but not always, equalize. Often, drainage from chest tubes is initially brisk and then ceases, and serial chest radiographs show progressive widening of the cardiac and superior mediastinal shadows. Arterial pressure falls, and a paradoxical pulse may be replaced by a narrow pulse pressure. Characteristically,

arterial pressure shows a minimal response to a bolus injection of an inotrope. TEE examination is indicated as soon as cardiac tamponade from retained intrapericardial blood is suspected, and is often diagnostic.

Increased Ventricular Afterload

Increased right ventricular (RV) afterload may appear quickly as a result of a sudden rise in pulmonary artery pressure and vascular resistance. Consequently, during an episode of paroxysmal pulmonary hypertension (often provoked by intratracheal suctioning), cardiac output may fall rapidly and apparently "sudden" death may occur, particularly in neonates and infants. These outcomes are probably not purely the result of increased RV afterload, because they reflect impaired RV reserve as well.

Increased left ventricular (LV) afterload may result from a sudden elevation of systemic arterial pressure, such as may occur during suctioning, restlessness, or hypoxia. These result in a sudden increase in LV afterload that, combined with impaired LV reserves, can result in low cardiac output early postoperatively. Sustained increase in systemic arterial pressure and LV afterload is present early after cardiac operations in at least half the adult patients operated on for acquired heart disease.[E13,F5,W9]

Often, disturbances of afterload (afterload mismatch) and preload (preload reserve)[R22,R23] are neither independent nor isolated events. Increased RV afterload leads to decreased LV preload. Similarly, but not as important, increased LV afterload leads to decreased RV preload. A common situation in which a corrective operation leads to increased LV afterload is restoration of mitral valve competence or closure of a ventricular septal defect (VSD). In a physics analogy, mitral regurgitation or left to right flow through a VSD represents a pair of resistors in a parallel circuit in which $R_T = 1/r_1 + 1/r_2$, where r_1 and r_2 represent resistances in the two outflow streams and R_T is total resistance. Closure of one outflow (r) increases downstream resistance to ventricular shortening; by inference, wall tension and myocardial oxygen consumption ($M\dot{V}O_2$) increase.

Arrhythmia

Bradyarrhythmias, caused by damage to the AV node or His bundle, by hypoxemia, or by drugs, can result in low cardiac output. Tachyarrhythmias in the form of atrial fibrillation or flutter or paroxysmal atrial tachycardia may result in hypotension. The incidence of tachyarrhythmias increases during infusion of catecholamines.

Risk Factors for Low Cardiac Output

A number of circumstances increase the probability of low cardiac output after cardiac surgery. These have been determined for the most part by numerous multivariable analyses of outcomes after surgery for specific conditions (see Chapters 7 through 55).

Patient-Specific

Chronic impairment of ventricular preload, afterload, and/or contractility by any mechanism (ventricular hypertrophy, stiffness, chronic heart failure) increases the risk of low cardiac output after the cardiac surgical procedure. These are for the most part immutable risk factors for low cardiac output, because they do not change quickly after the operation. However, when a patient who had been alive and ambulatory preoperatively has inadequate cardiac output postoperatively, the assumption must be that intraoperative damage has been superimposed on the chronic state. On the other hand, certain surgical procedures, such as ablation of the regurgitant volume of aortic regurgitation (see Table 5-4), or closure of a defect with a large left-to-right shunt, have an immediately favorable impact on cardiac output. Thus, the cardiac surgical procedure itself often increases cardiac output; it is myocardial damage during the procedure that decreases it.

Acute reduction in ventricular contractility preoperatively can sometimes be ameliorated by intraoperative maneuvers. For the most part, these maneuvers are directed toward increasing an acutely reduced energy charge (see "Cold Cardioplegia, Controlled Aortic Root Reperfusion, and [When Needed] Warm Cardioplegic Induction" under Methods of Myocardial Management during Cardiac Surgery in Chapter 3).

Procedural

The most important intraoperative risk factor for low cardiac output early postoperatively, other than an incomplete operation, is a discrepancy between the duration of any global myocardial ischemia and the efficacy of the measures used for myocardial management (see complete discussion in Chapter 3). This is often reflected in the finding of long global myocardial ischemic time as a risk factor for low cardiac output and for death after operation. Coronary air embolization during CPB is said to adversely affect cardiac performance after the operation, but most air entering the coronary arteries while the heart is not supporting the circulation passes quickly into the coronary sinus and may have little deleterious effect.

The extensiveness of the "whole body inflammatory response" to CPB affects the heart as well and relates to the probability of low cardiac output after operation. This is one aspect of the association of duration of CPB with death after operation; another is that long CPB duration is sometimes the result, rather than the cause, of poor cardiac performance.

Low cardiac output can be the result of (1) an incomplete or inadequate operation; (2) acute myocardial ischemia, with or without necrosis, from impaired coronary blood flow resulting from failure of some part of a CABG operation; (3) incomplete relief of ventricular inflow or outflow obstruction; (4) important residual or created AV valve or semilunar valve regurgitation that may increase the stroke volume requirements of the ventricle; and (5) residual VSD and large left-to-right shunt that may similarly increase LV stroke volume requirements.

One of the reasons for placing temporary fine polyvinyl catheters in the left atrium, right atrium, pulmonary trunk via the right ventricle, and uncommonly the left ventricle, and for placing of temporary epicardial atrial and ventricular wires, is that they can be helpful in intraoperative and early postoperative efforts to identify an inadequate or incomplete operation as the cause of low cardiac output. TEE with color flow Doppler imaging is also important in identifying an incomplete or inadequate operation. The possibility of residual left-to-right shunting contributing to low cardiac output must always be considered after repair of congenital heart disease. With the materials now used as patches for repair of VSDs, an appreciable left-to-right shunt ($\dot{Q}p/\dot{Q}s$ greater than 1.5) early postoperatively must be assumed to represent an incomplete repair or an overlooked defect. The shunt can be quantified by double indicator dilution, a method rarely used in the current era. Sampling is from both the pulmonary artery and systemic artery, preferably simultaneously with one injection. It can also be accomplished by two separate injections and sampling from the pulmonary artery during one and the radial artery during the other.[W8] Alternatively, the left-to-right shunt may be estimated in terms of the pulmonary to systemic flow ratio by simultaneously removing samples from the radial artery, right atrium, and pulmonary artery and solving the simplified shunt equation:

$$\dot{Q}p/\dot{Q}s = \frac{SaO_2 - SvO_2}{SaO_2 - S\bar{v}O_2}$$

where SaO_2 is the percent oxygen saturation of arterial blood, SvO_2 that of blood withdrawn from the right atrium, and $S\bar{v}O_2$ that of blood withdrawn from the pulmonary artery.

TEE with color flow Doppler imaging now can sometimes settle the issue simply, although without the desirable quantification. Savage and colleagues examined the usefulness of intraoperative TEE in 82 selected high-risk CABG operations.[S34] Intraoperative TEE led to at least one major surgical management alteration in 27 (33%) patients. Using either intraoperative epicardial echocardiography or TEE, Ungerleider and colleagues found 44 indications for intraoperative revision in 1000 consecutive congenital heart repairs (4.4%).[U1] Thirty-nine of these (89%) were successful. In a number of these patients, echocardiography provided the impetus for revision when the surgeon otherwise believed the repair was adequate.

Course of Low Cardiac Output

The heart is in an especially vulnerable position early postoperatively, because its poor function adversely affects coronary blood flow; this, in turn, further worsens cardiac function. This explains the observation that low cardiac output early after cardiac operations rarely resolves spontaneously. Aggressive treatment is indicated.

With treatment, most patients with low cardiac output early postoperatively recover, and unless it was produced by a large area of myocardial necrosis, most patients have no demonstrable ill effects from it late postoperatively.

Treatment of Low Cardiac Output

Experience indicates that it is worthwhile to treat patients with low or inadequate cardiac output early after cardiac surgery intensively, because cardiac performance often improves after 1 or 2 days, followed by good recovery.

Many causes of low cardiac output are reversible. Investigating whether cardiac tamponade or compression is the cause is one of the first steps (see "Acute Cardiac Tamponade" earlier in this section). If tamponade is present and is caused by retained blood in the pericardium, emergency reoperation is indicated. If there is acute cardiac dilatation, such as may occur in a pulmonary hypertensive crisis,[D8,K17] the sternum and pericardium should be rapidly opened (if they were closed). In patients at an increased risk of low cardiac output, this complication can be prevented by leaving the sternum open at operation and closing it postoperatively.[F7,J6,L12] The pericardium should rarely be closed after cardiac operations, because this has a restrictive effect on the heart early postoperatively.[D3]

When cardiac constriction is believed not to be present, treatment is directed at increasing cardiac output by manipulating preload, afterload, contractile state, and heart rate and improving tissue oxygen levels. When these measures fail, use of devices to support the circulation must be considered. All such devices have their own risks and imponderables and, except for the intraaortic balloon pump, they are usually not used unless it seems likely that the patient will not survive without them. The decision to use such devices is always made with concern for the possibility that the patient may be left seriously disabled, even though surviving, and with knowledge of the costs of such interventions.[B29,K29]

Noninvasive Methods

When cardiac output is low, *preload* is manipulated by increasing blood volume with an appropriate fluid until the higher of the two atrial pressures is about 15 mmHg (see Appendix 5B). If the wall thickness of the LV is unusually great or its contractility or compliance is decreased, it may be helpful to raise mean left atrial pressure to 20 mmHg. However, the tendency to pulmonary edema is increased when left atrial pressure is elevated to this level. When the RV is the limiting factor in cardiac performance, right atrial pressure usually can be raised advantageously only to about 18 mmHg. Above this, a descending limb on the Starling curve usually becomes apparent, and cardiac output falls. Also, the tendency to whole body fluid retention, pleural effusion, and ascites is increased by high right atrial pressure.

When LV performance is the limiting factor, and systemic arterial blood pressure is more than 10% above normal (see Table 5-1), vasodilating agents should be used to reduce LV *afterload* to between normal and 10% above normal. Nitroprusside is generally the drug of choice, because it is a potent arterial and, to a lesser extent, venous dilator, with a short half-life (see Appendix 5A). The drug appears to be as safe in very young patients as it is in adults.[K22] Calcium-channel antagonists, such as nifedipine and diltiazem, lead to similar arteriolar vasodilatation and may improve coronary perfusion in this setting.[M18] However, their longer half-life and depressive effect on ventricular contractility make nitroprusside the preferred drug.

Rarely, in patients with severe, long-standing mitral valve disease or congenital heart disease with pulmonary vascular obstructive changes, RV dysfunction associated with elevated pulmonary artery pressure may limit cardiac performance. Reduction of RV afterload with vasodilating agents is occasionally dramatic in its increase of RV, and thus cardiac, stroke volume. Nitroprusside (0.5 to 3 $\mu g \cdot kg^{-1} \cdot min^{-1}$), nitroglycerin (0.5 to 3 $\mu g \cdot kg^{-1} \cdot min^{-1}$), or phentolamine (1.5 to 2 $\mu g \cdot kg^{-1} \cdot min^{-1}$) may be effective in this setting.[K2] In infants, maintaining near-anesthesia for 24 to 48 hours with fentanyl or another intravenously administered agent may minimize paroxysms of pulmonary artery hypertension and the consequent increased RV afterload (see "Pulmonary Hypertensive Crises" later in this section).[L4]

Alternatively, management of neonates and infants may be based on the use of the long-acting α-receptor blocking agent phenoxybenzamine (Dibenzyline) (see Appendix 5A). It is administered first at the commencement of CPB (see "Other Additives" under Perfusate in Section 2 of Chapter 2). An additional dose is usually given about 12 hours after returning to the intensive care unit.

Heart rate is adjusted to optimal levels when necessary by atrial pacing, by ventricular pacing when atrial fibrillation is present, or by AV sequential pacing when AV dissociation is present. When there are tachyarrhythmias, pharmacologic means of control may be used (see below).

If these relatively simple measures do not quickly bring cardiac performance to an adequate level, inotropic agents are begun (see Appendix 5C for details), although their disadvantages are recognized. There is no ideal inotropic agent, nor are there specific indications for specific agents. In their review, Doyle and colleagues[D16] classified inotropic drugs based on their effect on intracellular cAMP. cAMP-independent drugs include calcium, digoxin, and α-adrenergic agonists. cAMP-dependent agents include epinephrine (and levarterenol), dobutamine, and isoproterenol. These are β-adrenergic agonists that, coupled with dopaminergic drugs (dopamine), have variable effects on peripheral resistance. Phosphodiesterase inhibitors (amrinone, milrinone, enoximone) may enhance contractility while producing myocardial relaxation (lusitropism) and relaxation of vascular smooth muscle. They are not susceptible to receptor downregulation.

Initially, *dopamine* may be infused at 2.5 $\mu g \cdot kg^{-1} \cdot min^{-1}$. This dose can be increased to 15 or 20 $\mu g \cdot kg^{-1} \cdot min^{-1}$ if needed, but if a favorable response is not obtained at 10 $\mu g \cdot kg^{-1} \cdot min^{-1}$, it is not likely to be obtained at higher doses. Dopamine has the advantage of augmenting renal blood flow in addition to increasing cardiac contractility.[H3] Dopamine increases ventricular automaticity (hence the probability of ventricular arrhythmias) but to a lesser extent than does isoproterenol. At low doses (2 to 4 $\mu g \cdot kg^{-1} \cdot min^{-1}$), systemic peripheral vascular resistance is decreased or unchanged by dopamine, whereas higher doses (greater than 6 $\mu g \cdot kg^{-1} \cdot min^{-1}$) increase peripheral resistance.[G3] Tachycardia may limit the rate at which dopamine can be administered. When dopamine is not effective, *dobutamine* is gradually added in similar doses. Dobutamine, although more expensive than dopamine, appears to augment myocardial blood flow more[F6]; in general, its effectiveness is similar to that of dopamine.[D11] *Isoproterenol* may be preferred initially and is probably superior in the presence of predominantly right ventricular dysfunction and de-creased or normal heart rate because of its favorable effect on pulmonary vascular resistance.

Occasionally, hypotension exists in the presence of normal and adequate cardiac output. Under that special circumstance, *norepinephrine* administered through a cen-tral venous catheter is rational treatment. The administra-tion of a very low dose ($0.01~\mu g \cdot kg^{-1} \cdot min^{-1}$) is often sufficient under these circumstances. Under more dire circumstances, larger doses can be used.

Epinephrine is the catecholamine of choice of some, but its powerful vasoconstricting effects make it less desirable than dopamine or dobutamine. When an insufficient re-sponse is obtained from other drugs, or excessive tachy-cardia develops, epinephrine is added or substituted. The drug is initially infused at a dose of 0.01 to 0.05 $\mu g \cdot kg^{-1} \cdot min^{-1}$, which may be increased as needed.

Amrinone is also useful in patients with low cardiac output after cardiac surgery, because it combines a periph-eral vasodilatory action with its inotropic effect.[G16] This drug is different in structure and mode of action from catecholamines and also from digitalis, and it is not a β-adrenergic receptor agonist; it is a direct relaxant of vascular smooth muscle. Administration is usually initiated with a loading dose of 3 $\mu g \cdot kg^{-1}$ and is continued at an infusion rate of 5 to 20 $\mu g \cdot kg^{-1} \cdot min^{-1}$. It should be administered in a balanced salt solution, not in dextrose. The drug is effective in neonates and infants as well as adults, but in small patients, particular care is necessary to maintain an adequate blood volume because of the va-sodilatory effect of the drug.[L13] The indications for this drug versus catecholamines remain arguable. However, it appears to cause less tachycardia and fewer atrial arrhyth-mias than do catecholamines.[R16]

Additionally, 10% calcium chloride is administered in a dose of 0.1 $mmol \cdot kg^{-1}$, with supplemental doses if the ionized serum calcium level is below 1.2 $mmol \cdot L^{-1}$.

Once the acute problems have subsided, some patients in sinus rhythm appear to require chronic augmentation of ven-tricular contractile function. Use of *digitalis* in this setting has long been argued, but there is evidence that it does increase contractility.[C21] Digitalization appears to be useful, particularly in children (see ''Atrial Arrhythmias'' under Cardiac Arrhythmias later in this section), but it is not recom-mended in neonates, because digitalis may impair diastolic function.[K19]

Intraaortic Balloon Pump

The concept of intraaortic balloon pumping (IABP) to produce diastolic augmentation of coronary and systemic blood flow was elucidated by Moulopoulos, Topaz, and Kolff in 1962.[M7] The procedure was first performed clini-cally by Kantrowitz and colleagues in 1968.[K9] IABP uses the principle of diastolic counterpulsation, which augments diastolic coronary perfusion pressure, reduces systolic af-terload, favorably affects the myocardial oxygen supply–demand ratio, and augments cardiac output.

IABP is used in adult patients with inadequate cardiac performance not responsive to optimized preload, afterload, and heart rate or to moderate doses (up to 10 $\mu g \cdot kg^{-1} \cdot min^{-1}$) of dopamine or equivalent doses of dobutamine or epinephrine (see Appendix 5C). Whenever possible, the decision to insert an intraaortic balloon is made in the operating room, rather than postoperatively. It is used in preference to catecholamines postoperatively for patients with severe LV dysfunction, with or without evidence of myocardial necrosis, and for patients with evidence of myocardial necrosis and inadequate cardiac output or se-vere ventricular arrhythmias. This technique has clearly led to survival of some patients who would otherwise have died.[D9,D10,G17,P6] Survival is less than 50% if renal failure develops postoperatively.[D9] IABP has been effective not only in patients with ischemic heart disease but also in those with valvar and congenital heart disease.[D9]

Preoperative prophylactic insertion of the IABP is some-times advisable. In addition to its use in myocardial infarc-tion with low cardiac output or shock, preoperative inser-tion is often helpful in unstable angina, left main disease with ongoing ischemia, and ischemia leading to ventricular arrhythmias. In the era of more complex arterial revascular-ization, IABP support is helpful intraoperatively for pre-bypass support of patients with low ejection fractions. For patients with acute mitral regurgitation or ventricular septal rupture, insertion upon diagnosis is often lifesaving. Per-haps the most frequent indication for preoperative IABP insertion utilizing the ease and reproducibility of the cathe-terization suite is poor perfusion from either low cardiac output or peripheral arterial disease. It follows that the best survival following IABP occurs when the device is in place preoperatively.[D17]

Insertion by arterial puncture is generally used, despite its somewhat higher prevalence of vascular complica-tions,[G11] because of the technical ease of balloon insertion and removal. When the patient is still on CPB or the femoral pulse cannot be palpated because of hypotension, an incision only in the skin is made over the femoral artery. Through this incision, the femoral artery can nearly always be palpated and the arterial puncture technique used.

Important aortoiliac occlusive disease and abdominal aortic aneurysm greatly increase the risk of vascular com-plications or failure of insertion when the femoral route is used.[G7] In their presence, the balloon can be inserted into the ascending aorta through a purse-string suture. This is usually performed before discontinuing CPB. A pledgeted mattress suture of No. 2-0 or 3-0 polypropylene is placed in the midportion of the ascending aorta. A tie is placed on the shaft of the intraaortic balloon to indicate the point that should be level with the aortic wall when the balloon is in proper position within the descending aorta. An aortic stab wound is made and controlled digitally, and the balloon is introduced through the wound and passed into the descend-ing aorta. Proper position is verified by appearance of the characteristic IABP aortic pressure pulse when pumping is begun. The balloon shaft is usually brought out through the lower end of the sternotomy incision. When pumping is no longer needed, the patient is returned to the operating room, the median sternotomy reopened, and another pledgeted mattress suture placed outside the original one. As the balloon is removed, the stab wound is controlled digitally, and the pledgeted mattress suture is made snug and tied. In severe atheromatous aortic wall disease, use of other assist devices is probably indicated.

IABP is begun in a 1 : 1 ratio with ventricular diastole, as judged by electrocardiographic and arterial pressure pulse signals. Often the patient's hemodynamic state improves promptly; consideration is then given to weaning the patient from IABP as early as 6 to 12 hours after insertion. If catecholamines have also been required, they are reduced as rapidly as possible to 5 $\mu g \cdot kg^{-1} \cdot min^{-1}$ of dopamine or less, or the equivalent doses of dobutamine or epinephrine (see Appendix 5C). Once the hemodynamic state is improved, the IABP ratio is progressively reduced to 1:8 (or 1:3 with some systems). In most postoperative patients, the final reduction can be reached within 12 to 48 hours. The balloon can then be removed, using a closed method. Although objections have been raised to use of this method,[C10] most of the problems have occurred when the balloon inadvertently was inserted through the superficial, rather than the common, femoral artery. After removing the balloon percutaneously, firm pressure is applied to the groin and held for ½ hour. If the circulation to the leg becomes impaired, or if a hematoma becomes apparent, prompt exploration in the operating room is indicated.

Circulation in the leg distal to the site of balloon insertion is observed systematically. If signs of ischemia appear, generally the balloon is removed. Complications that importantly complicate convalescence occur in about 3% of patients.[K10]

Temporary Ventricular Assistance

Ventricular assist devices, probably first used in a planned fashion by Cooley and colleagues in 1969,[C14] are now used (1) for support after cardiac operations, (2) as a bridge to transplantation, and (3) as a bridge to recovery. Without ventricular assist devices, nearly all patients assisted would likely have died; however, uncertainty about this makes interpretation of outcomes and indications for assist devices difficult. It also hampers efforts to determine the direct risks of these devices. The following discussion relates to use of various temporary ventricular assist devices for cardiopulmonary failure after cardiac operations. (A discussion of use of these devices for other indications can be found in Chapter 49.)

Temporary ventricular assist devices. Low cardiac output accompanying reduced ventricular function following cardiac operations occasionally prohibits separating the patient from CPB. A thorough investigation for correctable causes of low cardiac output should be made and may include ensuring aortocoronary bypass graft patency and adequacy of flow using Doppler ultrasound flow velocity or electromagnetic flow probes, and evaluating accuracy of repairs and segmental ventricular wall motion using intraoperative TEE. Preload and afterload should be optimized, appropriate pharmacologic agents administered, and IABP instituted. When these measures are not sufficient, temporary ventricular assistance should be considered.

Use of a temporary ventricular assist device often follows a prolonged operation and a long period on CPB. Insertion of an implantable ventricular assist device or cardiac transplantation under these circumstances is not advised. Temporary support of the failing circulation allows postponing further major operative intervention until the patient's condition improves. The temporary assist system is used as a "bridge to bridge" to cardiac transplantation (see Chapter 49).

Temporary ventricular assist is set up as right or left heart bypass, or as a combined biventricular bypass circuit. Cannulae for left and right heart bypasses are introduced through the midline sternotomy utilized during the cardiac operation. (Using cannulae previously placed makes the transition from CPB to right and left heart bypass a more controlled process.) With those cannulae in place, an additional thin-walled, metal-tip, right-angle cannula (No. 28 French) is introduced into the left atrium via the right superior pulmonary vein or via the roof of the left atrium through a purse-string stitch with a short tourniquet. The purse-string stitch may be felt-reinforced if tissues are thin or friable, because bleeding around the perfusion cannulae is frequently troublesome and may require re-exploration. An arterial cannula (No. 24 French wire thin wall) is placed in the pulmonary trunk.

Left heart bypass is established by connecting the left atrial cannula to the aortic cannula via a centrifugal pump. This ventricular bypass circuit provides continuous blood flow.

Right heart bypass is established by connecting the right atrial cannula to the pulmonary trunk cannula via a centrifugal pump. Pump flow is increased gradually to 4.0 to 5.0 $L \cdot min^{-1}$ for adult patients as CPB flow is reduced and discontinued. The cannulae are brought through the fascia, muscle, and skin into the left and right upper quadrants of the abdomen at the time of insertion or connection to the extracorporeal circuit. Polytetrafluoroethylene (Teflon) felt strips are placed tightly around the cannulae in the subcutaneous tissues to seal the exit tract. In some cases the cannulae are simply brought through the wound. The midline incision may be closed primarily in some cases. More often, cardiac compression results from wound closure. The skin may then be closed, leaving the sternal edges apart; alternatively, an Esmark bandage (silicone membrane) is attached to the skin edges with staples to seal the mediastinum. The edges of the membrane are sealed with iodine ointment to eliminate ingress of air and to present a barrier to bacteria. Bulky dressings are applied and sealed to the skin with a large iodine-impregnated plastic adhesive.

Heparin-coated tubing and centrifugal pumps are desirable to reduce trauma to blood elements by providing a more blood-compatible extracorporeal circuit. Roller pumps can also be used, but seldom are, because of the perception that more blood elements are injured. A new centrifugal pump (A-Med Systems, Inc., West Sacramento, California) is miniaturized so that it can be positioned close to the patient's body (paracorporeal). Short tubing reduces foreign blood contact surface and heat loss in the extracorporeal circuit.

An alternative, pulsatile extracorporeal blood pump system is also available (ABIOMED, Inc., Danvers, Massachusetts). The pump consists of a compliant inflow chamber to which blood is drained by gravity, separated from a rigid pumping chamber by a polyurethane inflow valve. The pumping chamber is fitted with an outflow polyurethane valve. A sac within the pumping chamber is expanded pneumatically to propel the blood. The components of the system are arranged vertically and placed at the bedside. A console provides pneumatic power, senses filling of the pumping device, and synchronizes pumping, so that little attention to the system is required. Anticoagulation with heparin is necessary, and the patient must remain immobile, as with other temporary systems. It may be used in left, right, or biventricular assist configuration. Although the system provides the possible advantages of pulsatile flow and less operator attention, it costs substantially more than centrifugal pump systems.

Bypass support of a single failing ventricle is used when possible. It is frequently possible to bypass a failing RV using an extracorporeal ventricular assist system combined with IABP to support the LV. Bypass support of the failing LV seems more complicated. In theory, the LV can be sustained by left atrial to aortic bypass, while the unassisted RV continues to provide adequate pulmonary flow. Experience has shown, however, that RV function also declines. Biventricular support is usually advisable even when there is apparent isolated LV failure.

Management. Each of these devices has specific methods and equipment for insertion and late management. In general, anticoagulation with heparin followed by warfarin is required for all devices with mechanical valves, and low-dose anticoagulation with heparin, warfarin, or aspirin is used for those with biologic valves. However, management details vary among institutions.

Bleeding from the primary operative site is controlled by reversal of heparin with protamine. Platelet infusion, transfusion of fresh frozen plasma (FFP) or other blood products, and pharmacologic agents to promote normalization of the blood clotting subsystem are administered as indicated. A heparin-bonded extracorporeal circuit is adequate to prevent clotting in the short term. When bleeding from the operative site has ceased or slowed, heparin therapy is restarted. Usually this occurs within 12 hours after completing the operation. Activated clotting time (ACT) is used to monitor the heparin effect. The desired ACT is approximately 160 seconds (assuming a control level of 100 to 120 seconds).

Postoperative care of patients on left, right, or biventricular bypass is labor intensive. Continuous bedside care, often by more than one nurse, is required, as is ready availability of a cardiopulmonary perfusionist or other personnel capable of managing the extracorporeal assist system. Bleeding is frequently a nuisance or even a major complication, requiring frequent monitoring of blood clotting by ACT. Smooth operation of the system requires frequent infusion of blood products to maintain adequate atrial pressures. Body temperature is monitored continuously, and measures are taken to heat or cool the blood in the extracorporeal circuit or the patient's body with a heating/cooling blanket. The system may be fitted with ports for hemofiltration to remove excess extracellular fluid if there is marked edema. Occasionally, hemodialysis is necessary. Ventilatory assist is required.

Separating the patient from temporary ventricular assistance requires judgment and patience. There is a tendency to remove systems too early to avoid complications directly related to prolonged extracorporeal circulation. It is advisable to wait a day or so longer than to rush the process of separation. Ability of the heart to support the circulation is tested by reducing flow into the extracorporeal circuit, thereby raising atrial pressures and allowing flow through the supported ventricle. There is a limit to which flow in an

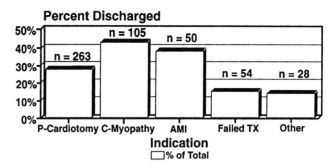

Figure 5-9   Survival to discharge from the ABIOMED worldwide experience. Demonstrated is percent discharged for each patient category. (From Jett.[J10])

Key: *AMI,* Acute myocardial infarction; *C-Myopathy,* cardiomyopathy; *P-Cardiotomy,* postcardiotomy; *TX,* transplantation.

extracorporeal circuit can be reduced without introducing danger of clotting. Flow of less than $1 \text{ L} \cdot \text{min}^{-1}$ should be avoided. Heparin levels should be maintained and duration of testing short. Cardiac function is monitored by TEE and continuous measurement of arterial and pulmonary artery pressures, atrial pressures, cardiac output, and venous oxygen saturation. If the heart cannot sustain adequate cardiac output under conditions of low-flow bypass, the separation process is abandoned, full flow is resumed, and plans are made for later attempts at separation or conversion to an implantable device. Simply removing the temporary device in anticipation that the heart will sustain adequate function is usually unsuccessful.

Results. Results are judged either by recovery and long-term survival after removal of the device or by success in maintaining the patient until cardiac transplantation is accomplished. Clearly, some patients not only survive but also have an excellent long-term functional result.[F9,G9,K18,M11,P9,P11-P16,P20,R9,R10,S20,S31] Of some importance in this regard is the finding that myocardial cellular atrophy is not a complication of prolonged ventricular assistance.[J7] These experiences document that to some extent, patients with ventricular assist devices are at risk of thromboembolism, hemorrhage, and infection.

The report of the combined registry for clinical use of mechanical ventricular assist devices summarizes experience with 965 patients.[P8] For about half of those patients, successful weaning from the device was accomplished, and about half of those weaned were discharged from the hospital alive. Two-year survival among patients discharged from the hospital was 82%, with most being in NYHA functional class I or II. A higher proportion of patients receiving LV assist devices had satisfactory outcomes than was the case in those receiving biventricular assist devices. The probability of survival was similar in patients receiving nonpulsatile, centrifugal pump devices and those receiving pulsatile pneumatic devices. Survival to discharge for the multi-institutional experience is summarized in Fig. 5-9. Individual institutions have recorded discharge rates of up to 60%, and this seems to be related to greater experience with the device and earlier establishment of support.[J10]

Indications. It is impossible to do more than tentatively suggest the indications for application of a ventricular assist device to a patient during or early after cardiac surgery. This is because of the complex scientific, surgical, ethical, moral, political, philosophical, and financial considerations necessarily involved.

There is general agreement that a low cardiac output (cardiac index less than about $1.5 \text{ L} \cdot \text{min}^{-1} \cdot \text{m}^{-2}$) and elevated ventricular diastolic pressure (reflected in high left or right atrial pressure) after continuing CPB an hour beyond the usual time of discontinuance, with IABP support and administration of catecholamines in moderate doses, indicate a low probability of survival.[H28] Trial separation from CPB has failed (usually reflected in a progressive drop of systemic arterial blood pressure, elevation of atrial pressures, reduction of venous oxygen saturation, and metabolic acidosis). Under these conditions, in institutions prepared for it and, if necessary, cardiac transplantation (even if this means transportation to another institution), temporary ventricular assistance is usually indicated. Patients with continuing low cardiac output in the intensive care unit, despite IABP and catecholamine support, also should be considered for temporary ventricular assistance. Use of temporary ventricular assistance is appropriate for patients of any age whose myocardial problem is expected to resolve within a few days, and for patients younger than 65 to 70 years of age whose myocardial problem is not expected to resolve but who are acceptable candidates for cardiac transplantation. In the latter group, the temporary device is used for support while it is determined whether there is good function of major organ systems and the patient is neurologically intact.

Further experience with ventricular assist devices may lead to discarding current criteria in favor of more liberal usage; in part, this is because LV assistance is more effective in preserving myocardial structure and function than is IABP, at least in experimental studies.[M6] In general, the younger the patient, the better the prognosis from the now repaired cardiac disease, and the fewer the other subsystem diseases and failures, the stronger the indication for temporary ventricular assistance.

Cardiopulmonary Support and Extracorporeal Membrane Oxygenation

Right and left heart bypass (biventricular assist) works only if pulmonary function is adequate to support gas exchange. In situations of severe compromise of the respiratory system, support of that system is also required. Portable CPB systems (cardiopulmonary support [CPS]) include both a centrifugal blood pump and a membrane oxygenator, with heparin-coated tubing. These systems are usually referred to as *extracorporeal membrane oxygenation* (ECMO). Successful use has been reported, particularly in infants and children,[K16,P19] and there is little doubt that in some patients, it is an effective means of biventricular support. (It may be used occasionally in venovenous configuration to support respiration in the face of severe postoperative arterial desaturation from impaired pulmonary function.[B21,M5]) This methodology has also been used in patients undergoing myocardial infarction or sustaining a catastrophic event in the cardiac catheterization laboratory, and as a support technique during angioplasty.[M24,P21]

Only two cannulae need to be inserted, one in the right atrium and the other in a systemic artery. These cannulae are

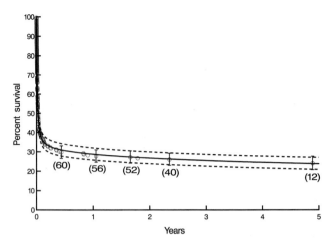

Figure 5-10 Survival after commencing extracorporeal membrane oxygenation in 202 adult patients. Each symbol represents a death positioned at the time of death on the horizontal axis and by the Kaplan–Meier estimator on the vertical axis. Vertical bars represent asymmetric 68% confidence limits. Numbers in parentheses are the number of patients remaining at risk. The solid line enclosed within dashed 68% confidence limits is the parametric estimate. (From Smedira and colleagues.[S31])

present during surgery and may simply be attached to the system. Oxygenation is achieved in a closed system, without an air-to-blood interface. Alternatively, separate venous and arterial cannulae may be inserted through the femoral artery and femoral or jugular vein by percutaneous technique (see "Cardiopulmonary Bypass Established by Peripheral Cannulation" under Special Situations and Controversies in Section 3 of Chapter 2). This places the cannulae in a position for ready control of hemorrhage. Centrally placed cannulae are removed so the wound may be closed. Percutaneous placement of cannulae and use of the CPS system can be employed for emergent support of the failing circulation at the bedside. The CPS system does not ordinarily provide decompression of the LV. LV unloading depends on total diversion of blood from the right atrium to the extracorporeal circuit and the ability of the LV to empty pulmonary venous return to the aorta. A beating heart and absence of aortic valve regurgitation are necessary.

Management. Heparin anticoagulation is required to prevent clotting or excess fibrin formation in the oxygenator membrane. The ACT is maintained at approximately 160 seconds by continuous infusion of heparin.

Results. In the pediatric population, overall survival after using ECMO for support after a cardiac operation is 30% to 40%. It may be more effective in situations complicated by pulmonary hypertension or in the presence of a two-ventricle repair compared with repairs in which there is a cavopulmonary connection or aortopulmonary shunt.[K32,L17,M34] However, Smedira and colleagues reported 30-day survival of 38% in 202 adults supported by ECMO with intent to wean or bridge to transplant (Figs. 5-10, 5-11).[S31,S39] Patients who survived 30 days had a 63% 5-year survival. Risk factors for death included older age, reoperation, subsystem failure while on ECMO, and occurrence of a neurologic event while on ECMO.

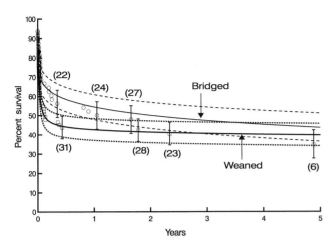

Figure 5-11   Survival after discontinuing extracorporeal membrane oxygenation (ECMO) (time zero) in 202 adult patients stratified according to the outcome of ECMO: bridged or weaned. Format of depiction is as in Figure 5-10. (From Smedira and colleagues.[S31])

In adults, ECMO seems more cumbersome than temporary LV or biventricular assistance, and hospital survival may be lower than in children.[M17]

Indications. The imponderables, and therefore the uncertainties as to the indications for this type of support after cardiac surgery, are similar to those for temporary ventricular assist devices; in addition, the need for nearly full heparinization and the presence of an oxygenator in the circuit are disadvantages of ECMO.

Cardiac Arrhythmias

Postoperative morbidity and mortality can result from cardiac arrhythmias, which may occur either when the cardiac subsystem has been otherwise functioning normally or as a complication of low cardiac output. Atrial and ventricular pacing wires, routinely placed at operation (see Chapter 2) and left for 5 to 10 days postoperatively, are of utmost importance in diagnosing and treating postoperative arrhythmias.[F1,W3-W5]

Ventricular Electrical Instability

Ventricular electrical instability includes premature ventricular contractions (PVCs), ventricular tachycardia, and ventricular fibrillation. Controversy exists concerning the proportion of postoperative patients with PVCs and some types of ventricular tachycardia who are at risk of developing ventricular fibrillation. Despite this, it is prudent to assume that such arrhythmias early postoperatively place the patient at an increased risk of sudden death. Therefore, to detect such arrhythmias, the electrocardiogram (ECG) is monitored continuously for at least the first 48 hours after operation.

The management of ventricular electrical instability occurring in cardiac surgery patients after postoperative day 1 or 2 has been importantly affected by the results of the Cardiac Arrhythmia Suppression Trial (CAST).[C15,E10,E11] This trial has shown that drugs used for the suppression of ventricular electrical instability can themselves be lethal, and that they are often ineffective. Application of these

findings to the postoperative patient and implications for treatment are not well understood. For example, CAST patients for the most part had persisting ischemia; most postoperative patients (coronary disease or not) are probably well revascularized. However, in the postoperative period many antiarrhythmic agents are proarrhythmic; therefore, treatment of ventricular arrhythmias other than ventricular tachycardia is probably not necessary.

In patients with an ejection fraction under 40% or those with postoperative ventricular tachycardia, early electrophysiologic study is indicated. Paradoxically, patients in whom such studies demonstrate acute suppression of PVCs or ventricular tachycardia with the administration of drugs have a good prognosis without drug treatment; such patients probably should be discharged from the hospital on no drug therapy. By contrast, patients whose ventricular arrhythmias cannot be suppressed with drugs have a relatively poor prognosis, and consideration should be given to implanting an Implantable Cardioverter–Defibrillator (ICD) (see "Ventricular Tachycardia/Ventricular Fibrillation in Ischemic Heart Disease" in Section 7 of Chapter 45).

When during the first day or two of convalescence, ventricular electrical instability develops in the form of PVCs occurring more than six times per minute or ventricular tachycardia persisting more than 1 minute, treatment is prudent even if cardiac performance is good (see Appendix 5D). Often, PVCs or bursts of ventricular tachycardia can be suppressed by atrial or ventricular pacing using temporary electrodes, without need for drug therapy. When the hemodynamic state is impaired by ventricular tachycardia, immediate direct current cardioversion (100 J initially in adults and, if ineffective, 200 J) is indicated. When these measures are ineffective, the advice of an experienced electrophysiologically oriented cardiologist is indicated.

Atrial Arrhythmias

The most common atrial arrhythmia after cardiac operations is atrial fibrillation. The most difficult to manage is atrial flutter. Paroxysmal atrial tachycardia is uncommon and, when persistent, requires specialized care.

Treatment of atrial fibrillation. When atrial fibrillation develops postoperatively, several protocols are appropriate for rate control. Classically, digoxin was nearly always used (for details, see Appendix 5E). When approximately two thirds of the estimated digitalizing dose has been given and has not accomplished control of the ventricular rate, oral administration of propranolol should be started unless the patient has poor ventricular function or pulmonary disease; if the situation is urgent, propranolol may be given intravenously in doses of 0.5 mg every 2 minutes, to a total intravenous dose of 4 mg in adults. Alternatively, treatment with verapamil may be initiated in doses of 40 mg orally 2 to 3 times daily. This drug may be infused intravenously in a dose of $0.075 \text{ mg} \cdot \text{kg}^{-1}$ to a maximum dose of 5 mg, but its action is very short when given in this manner, and oral administration must be started promptly.

Alternatively, in patients in whom atrial fibrillation or flutter is importantly embarrassing the circulation, amiodarone may be given intravenously.[M25,M26] A bolus dose of $5 \text{ mg} \cdot \text{kg}^{-1}$ in saline is given over a 20-minute period, followed by a continuous infusion of 0.25 to $0.5 \text{ mg} \cdot \text{min}^{-1}$

for 4 to 8 hours. This regimen has been shown to be effective slightly less often than quinidine, but it has fewer side effects.[K23,M25] Oral, long-term therapy with amiodarone may then be started.[C30,D18,K25,S35]

Using bipolar temporary atrial wires placed at operation (one each on the right atrium and left atrium), low-energy cardioversion techniques have been developed that result in an 80% conversion early postoperatively; anesthesia is not necessary.[L18]

Atrial flutter. Atrial flutter can be a difficult arrhythmia when it occurs postoperatively. Although not always successful, the best treatment is rapid atrial pacing via the two atrial epicardial wires placed at operation (see Appendix 5F). When the flutter ceases, digoxin is begun and usually continued for about 6 weeks.

Paroxysmal atrial tachycardia. Important episodes of paroxysmal atrial tachycardia or paroxysmal atrial contractions occurring after cardiac operations may also be treated by rapid atrial pacing; if these arrhythmias persist, however, the diagnostic and therapeutic advice of an electrophysiologically expert cardiologist is needed. The specific treatment depends on the precise nature of the supraventricular tachycardia. In general, administration of catecholamines should be reduced as much as possible; if additional support is necessary, amrinone is considered (see "Noninvasive Methods" under Treatment of Low Cardiac Output earlier in this section). Beta-adrenergic receptor blocking agents such as propranolol are useful (see earlier discussion). Multifocal atrial tachycardias are often best treated by verapamil given intravenously.

Junctional ectopic tachycardia (JET) may be a particularly difficult problem in children. It is associated with operations to close VSDs, perioperative transient AV block, or young age. In 70 of 71 patients with postoperative JET, Walsh and colleagues obtained control of the arrhythmia and hemodynamic stability using a combination of sedation, hypothermia to 34°C, and procainamide.[W17] Amiodarone may also be effective.[R17]

PULMONARY SUBSYSTEM

Adequacy

During Intubation

The adequacy of pulmonary function early postoperatively, while the patient is still intubated and receiving controlled ventilation, is judged by the response of arterial oxygen pressure (PaO_2) and arterial carbon dioxide pressure ($PaCO_2$) to the minute volume of ventilation and ventilating gas mixture being used. The response of the *arterial oxygen levels* can be expressed as the alveolar–arterial oxygen difference, $P(A - a)O_2$, which in intact humans is normally only a few mmHg. Nearly all patients early after cardiac operations have abnormally large alveolar–arterial oxygen differences, resulting from intrapulmonary right to left shunting of 3% to 15%.[E3,G10,H9] This assumes that no right to left intracardiac shunting is present. The response of the *carbon dioxide levels* can be expressed as the minute volume of ventilation required to maintain $PaCO_2$ at 30 to 45 mmHg. Usually this is about 15 to 20 mL · kg^{-1} in both adults and children.

When anesthesia and heavy sedation are no longer present and the ventilator is in a mode of intermittent mandatory ventilation, the patient's ventilatory rate is a useful guide to the ease with which the respiratory center's needs are met, and thus to the adequacy of pulmonary function. A patient-triggered respiratory rate, in an adult, of 8 to 12 breaths/min, with the usual tidal volume, inspiratory gases, and end-expiratory pressure, indicates adequacy of lung function.

Positive end-expiratory pressure (PEEP) may be used as a routine or on indication, with a setting of 5 to 8 cm H_2O for adults and children over 12 years of age, and 4 cm H_2O for younger patients. Unless the hemodynamic state is suboptimal, PEEP does not alter it, even in infants.[L19] PEEP is used because of studies that suggest it is associated with larger lung volumes, fewer perfused but nonventilated alveoli during ventilation, and smaller $P(A - a)O_2$ after extubation.[A4] PEEP is contraindicated in patients with chronic obstructive lung disease (to avoid air trapping and rupturing a bulla, with consequent pneumothorax) and in infants and children who have undergone a Fontan operation or cavopulmonary anastomosis (to avoid still further elevation of jugular venous pressure).

Continuous positive airway pressure (CPAP)[G4,S41] may be used in infants once their cardiovascular state is stable, obviating the need for IPPB and IMV. Should IPPB be required initially, the infant is transferred to IMV and sometimes to CPAP for several hours before extubation.

Extubation

Traditionally, continued intubation after cardiac operations has been recommended to maintain more precise control of cardiopulmonary physiology. However, early extubation may decrease intensive care unit and hospital stay. Therefore, a protocol beginning with anesthesia induction may be designed to expedite awakening and spontaneous breathing.

Once the patient has been extubated, $PaCO_2$ and PaO_2 levels, as well as the visually estimated work of breathing, are useful indices of pulmonary function. A $PaCO_2$ of less than 45 mmHg in adults, of less than 50 mmHg in young children, and of less than 55 mmHg in small infants indicates an adequate minute volume of ventilation. Values higher than these indicate inadequate alveolar ventilation. PaO_2 is often mildly depressed at this time and usually remains so for the first few days after cardiac surgery done with CPB (Fig. 5-12). This results from the somewhat widened alveolar–arterial oxygen difference. These measurements are valuable, but when a patient is comfortable and breathing easily and slowly, and the chest radiograph is essentially normal, it is highly probable that pulmonary function is adequate and convalescence will be satisfactory.

Causes of Dysfunction

After cardiac surgery with CPB, the lungs are more likely to have dysfunction, albeit mild and transient, than any organ other than the heart itself. This dysfunction has multiple causes. In part, it is caused by the absence of pulmonary blood flow during total CPB and by its near absence during partial CPB. Among other things, this results in very low sheer stresses in the pulmonary capillaries; this appears to accentuate neutrophil activation, because neutrophils appear to be exquisitely sensitive to sheer stress. Leukocytes are also activated by the general damaging effects of CPB and incite an inflammatory response in the pulmonary vasculature.[C12] During total CPB and lung

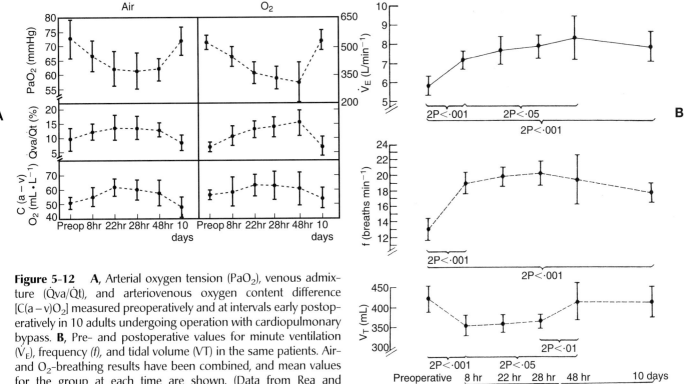

Figure 5-12   **A,** Arterial oxygen tension (PaO₂), venous admixture (Q̇va/Q̇t), and arteriovenous oxygen content difference [C(a − v)O₂] measured preoperatively and at intervals early postoperatively in 10 adults undergoing operation with cardiopulmonary bypass. **B,** Pre- and postoperative values for minute ventilation (V̇ₑ), frequency (f), and tidal volume (VT) in the same patients. Air- and O₂-breathing results have been combined, and mean values for the group at each time are shown. (Data from Rea and colleagues.[R2])

ischemia, plasma thromboxane B₂ increases, and this may contribute to a pulmonary vascular inflammatory response.[F13] Cytokines IL-6 and IL-8 increase with CPB and may also contribute to membrane damage and neutrophil activation in the lung.[B25,F14] The alveolar–capillary barrier becomes more permeable than normal[B16] and, after cardiac surgery using CPB, macromolecules enter the pulmonary interstitium, and ultimately the alveoli, promoting development of pulmonary edema. During the early hours after CPB, radioactive albumin injected intravenously can be detected in considerable quantity in fluid aspirated from the tracheobronchial tree (Digerness SB, Kirklin JW: personal communication; 1972). In 1962, Gardner and colleagues[G18] described alterations in lung surface extracts after CPB bypass. More recently, McGowan and colleagues[M27] linked postoperative disturbances of lung function and increases of alveolar polymorphonuclear leukocytes to important reduction of pulmonary surfactant activity. In addition, multiple and not yet totally defined factors encourage development of large areas of atelectasis, either segmental or occasionally lobar; in particular, the left lower lobe has a strong tendency to atelectasis, even in patients who are otherwise convalescing normally.[T9]

In some patients, direct trauma to the lungs occurs and contributes to pulmonary dysfunction. Should secretions be retained during or early after the operation, these also contribute to dysfunction. Left (and occasionally, right) phrenic nerve injury may occur after carefully performed cardiac operations, increasing the tendency to pulmonary dysfunction early postoperatively.[R8,S10] However, left lower lobe atelectasis is considerably more common than left phrenic nerve paralysis; Markand and colleagues found the left phrenic nerve to be paralyzed in only 11% of patients experiencing left lower lobe atelectasis early after

open heart operations.[M20] In most patients, the left phrenic nerve recovers from its paralysis within 6 months.[L9] Mechanical obstruction of the lower trachea or the bronchi can produce pulmonary dysfunction, which may go unrecognized unless care is taken to identify and treat it.[C16] Localized or more extensive pulmonary edema may develop in the presence of low or normal left atrial pressure, no doubt related to changes in pulmonary venular and capillary permeability, the causes of which are only partially understood; this phenomenon seems to be more marked in elderly patients.[G12,M8] Less commonly, frank pulmonary hemorrhage, developing as CPB is discontinued or early thereafter, can cause serious bronchial obstruction and contribute in a major way to pulmonary dysfunction.[S16] This is probably a more severe result of the same factors that lead to pulmonary edema in patients with normal or low left atrial pressures.

Risk Factors for Acute Dysfunction
Patient-Specific

Patient-specific risk factors for pulmonary dysfunction after cardiac surgery have long been recognized, but formal identification and quantification are rare.

In a formal observational study, *young age* at operation was identified as a risk factor, particularly when the patient was less than about 2 years old (Fig. 5-13). Similar observations were made by Lell and colleagues.[L2] Increased risk with young age is associated with the increased tendency of the very young to develop whole body edema after CPB. In the experience of most institutions, and in a study by Gallagher and colleagues, *older age,* particularly over 60 years, has also been associated with an increased prevalence of pulmonary dysfunction after cardiac sur-

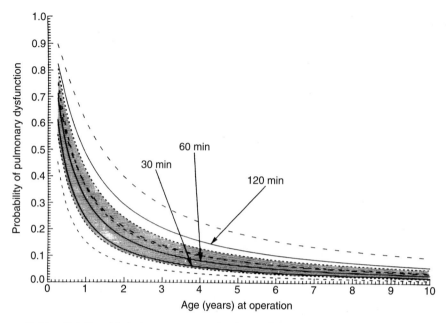

Figure 5-13 Relationship between age at operation and duration of cardiopulmonary bypass (represented by solid isobars and their dashed 70% confidence limits) to the probability of pulmonary dysfunction after cardiac surgery. The nomogram depicts specific solutions of a multivariable equation; the value entered for C3a was 882 ng · mL^{-1} (see original publication for details). (From Kirklin and colleagues.[K7])

gery.[G12] *Chronic obstructive lung disease* is an important risk factor for pulmonary dysfunction postoperatively and increases the overall risk of operation because it predisposes patients to increased work of breathing and air trapping.[R3] Preoperative *pulmonary arterial hypertension,* even when associated with low pulmonary arteriolar resistance, predisposes infants to pulmonary dysfunction and also to paroxysms of pulmonary arteriolar constriction and pulmonary hypertension early postoperatively (see "Pulmonary Hypertensive Crises" later in this section). Congenital morphometric pulmonary abnormalities, such as the *alveolar hypoplasia* that is frequently present in patients with congenital heart disease and *Down syndrome,* increase the prevalence of postoperative pulmonary dysfunction.[Y1] Some drugs given during the period before operation increase the prevalence of pulmonary complications postoperatively; *amiodarone,* used for the control of cardiac arrhythmias, is a particularly serious offender that has caused rapidly fatal pulmonary dysfunction after cardiac surgery.[D5,K12,M16]

Procedural

The *type of oxygenator* used is probably related to the amount of pulmonary dysfunction generated by the operation, with oxygenators other than membrane type being risk factors for pulmonary damage.[H8] *Proper filters* in the arterial tubing may reduce pulmonary dysfunction postoperatively.[M3] *Longer duration* of CPB is a risk factor. This is probably related, in part, to the direct correlation between the duration of CPB and the increase in the patient's extracellular water[C1,C4,P1] (Fig. 5-14). The *amount of C3a* generated by complement activation during CPB is a risk

factor for pulmonary dysfunction; this may relate to a greater amount of neutrophil activation with higher levels of C3a.[K7] The use of *external cardiac cooling,* particularly by ice slush rather than cold saline, increases the prevalence of left phrenic nerve paralysis, hence the tendency to postoperative pulmonary dysfunction.[B17,S25]

Postoperative

Postoperative events can increase the probability of pulmonary dysfunction. Elevated *left atrial pressure,* with consequent elevation of pulmonary capillary and venular pressures, aggravates the tendency toward increased lung water and pulmonary dysfunction. The longer the patient is on a ventilator, the greater are the chances of continuing pulmonary dysfunction. *Paralysis of the phrenic nerve,* and the consequent elevation of the left hemidiaphragm, predispose patients to continuing pulmonary dysfunction, particularly small patients.[R8,S10]

Course of Dysfunction after Cardiac Surgery

Mild pulmonary dysfunction in normally convalescing patients slowly improves without specific therapy except for ambulation and breathing exercises; however, residues of dysfunction may still be present 10 days after operation.[R2]

Occasionally, in the patient who appears to be convalescing normally and is out of the intensive care unit for 3 to 6 days, orthopnea and paroxysmal nocturnal dyspnea may develop insidiously. This is particularly likely to occur in patients who have marked left ventricular hypertrophy or poor left ventricular function preoperatively, and it may occur even though their left atrial pressure was

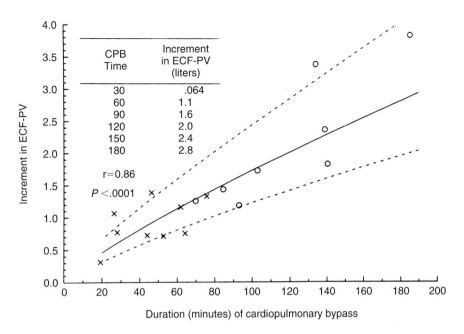

Figure 5-14 Relationship between duration of cardiopulmonary bypass and increase in interstitial fluid (ECF-PV) 4 to 6 hours after operation. x's represent patients undergoing closure of left-to-right shunts; circles represent patients operated on for valvar heart disease. Patients with heart failure were not included. The regression equation is

$$\text{Ln (ECF} - \text{PV)} = -3.248 + 0.8248 \cdot \text{Ln (CPB time)}$$

$$r = .86; \ P < .0001.$$

(Data from Cleland and colleagues.[C4])

Key: *CPB,* Cardiopulmonary bypass; *ECF,* extracellular fluid; *Ln,* natural logarithm; *PV,* plasma volume.

less than 15 mmHg when last monitored in the intensive care unit. The chest radiograph may have been normal or may have shown evidence of a mild increase in interstitial fluid. The response to diuresis in such a patient is dramatic and, as a rule, terminates the problem. The hypothesis is that fluid that has accumulated in the interstitial spaces throughout the body during and early after CPB returns to the vascular space 24 to 72 hours after operation; blood volume is thereby increased at a time when the renal response is subnormal, and diuresis and control of blood volume do not follow.[C1,P1] In this setting, left ventricular end-diastolic, left atrial, and pulmonary venous pressures rise and symptoms develop. Weight gain and other gross evidence of fluid retention may be absent.

Occasionally, patients who have convalesced without difficulty begin to cough up thick tracheobronchial secretions 48 to 72 hours after operation. Often, seemingly paradoxically, whatever dyspnea and tachypnea may have been present begins to lessen with these events. Presumably, at this time, protein-rich fluid that has been in the alveoli and interstitium of the lung since CPB (or soon thereafter) begins to be moved by ciliary action out of the terminal bronchioles and into the larger airways, from which it can be cleared by coughing.

Lung volumes are usually reversibly decreased early after cardiac surgery, particularly vital capacity and total lung volume.[A9,E12] This is probably the result of the summed effects of multiple small areas of atelectasis, occasionally left lower lobe collapse, occult pulmonary edema and pleural fluid, and reduced inspiratory efforts.[E12] These usually revert to normal within 3 to 6 months.

Management and Treatment

The goal of treatment of the pulmonary subsystem is the earliest possible return of the patient to extubated spontaneous breathing and ambulation. In an era characterized by the ability to treat intensively both large and small patients after cardiac surgery, the distinctly beneficial effects of early extubation are often forgotten. These include a decline in intrapleural pressure and an increase in left ventricular end-diastolic diameter (or volume), improved ventricular systolic function (because of increased preload associated with shifting of some of the blood volume toward the chest), and improved cardiac output.[G13]

General Measures

Patients who are convalescing normally are extubated either in the operating room or during the early hours after operation. In most intensive care units, it is advisable to extubate patients in the daytime rather than at night; this consideration is a reasonable cause of delay of extubation for a few hours. Otherwise, when pulmonary function is good, extubation should be delayed only under special circumstances, including the presence of cardiac assist devices and the possibility of early reoperation. In general, criteria for extubation include stable and satisfactory cardiac performance, lack of important cardiac arrhythmia, and appropriate awakening with satisfactory neurologic status. There should be no anticipation of return to the operating room (for example, for bleeding) and satisfactory mechanics and ventilatory lung function, as assessed by arterial blood gas analysis and a clinical estimate of inspiratory force and volume.

Treatment of patients with pulmonary dysfunction who are still intubated during the early hours after operation is in large part an intensification of the usual management, as effective specific therapy is not available. Fractional inspired oxygen (FIo_2) is appropriately adjusted upward if $P(A - a)O_2$ is large. Minute volume of respiration (not only measured, but judged visually by excursion of the chest wall) and respiratory rate are adjusted to maintain $PaCO_2$ at about 30 to 35 mmHg. The airway is kept clear by appropriate tracheal suctioning (see "Pulmonary Hypertensive Crises" later in this section for special precautions in neonates and infants). When hemoconcentration develops from leakage of plasma from the intravascular space into the interstitial space of the lungs, and at times into all other organs and the pleural and peritoneal spaces, administration of concentrated serum albumin is helpful in counteracting this trend (see Appendix 5G). Diuretics are useful, because they reduce extracellular fluid volume and, in turn, extravascular lung water. During all of this, efforts continue to reduce the ventilatory support and work toward extubation of the patient (see Appendix 5H).

Prolonged Intubation

A prolonged period of endotracheal intubation is necessary when:
- Criteria for extubation are not met
- Neurologic complications are present
- Severe dysfunction of the cardiac subsystem is present, or
- Persistent chest drainage or a residual cardiac defect make early return to the operating room likely

Prolonged intubation (beyond about 48 hours) entails problems necessitating fastidious care of the patient. A pneumothorax occasionally develops from positive-pressure breathing, usually requiring urgent aspiration and underwater drainage. Bronchospasm may become a particular problem, probably as a reflex response to proteinaceous tracheobronchial fluid often present under these circumstances. Administration of nebulized isoetharine (Bronchosol) every hour can be helpful. In extreme cases, aminophylline is given as a continuous intravenous infusion in 10% dextrose in a dose of $0.15 \ mg \cdot kg^{-1} \cdot min^{-1}$. An initial loading dose of about $4 \ mg \cdot kg^{-1}$ is given over 20 minutes. Neonates, infants, and young children who require intubation and ventilation for more than about 14 days often have phrenic nerve paralysis; in these patients, plication of the hemidiaphragm often permits prompt extubation.[V6,W14] Plication usually does not interfere with recovery of phrenic nerve and diaphragmatic function.[S9]

In those unusual circumstances when intubation in older children and adults is necessary for more than about 10 days, consideration is given to tracheostomy. Both patient comfort and effectiveness of ventilation are thereby usually increased. This procedure has disadvantages, but is sometimes helpful in weaning the patient from the ventilator. Tracheostomy is rarely performed in neonates, infants, and young children, because it is difficult to manage in this age group. Moreover, nasotracheal intubation has few complications in infants, even over a period of months, provided the endotracheal tube is of the proper diameter and length (see Chapter 4, Fig. 4-1).

Reintubation

When the patient meets all criteria for extubation, reintubation is usually not necessary. However, reintubation is indicated when:
- $PaCO_2$ rises above 50 mmHg over 4 hours
- Signs of falling cardiac output are noted
- The patient shows signs of exhaustion from breathing spontaneously
- Excessive pulmonary secretions, with ineffective coughing (the latter two are frequently combined), are evidenced

When the situation is borderline, proper management requires careful observation by senior members of the team. Reintubation should be performed by a competent professional.

Pulmonary Hypertensive Crises

Description. Pulmonary hypertensive crisis is a phrase used to describe a serious syndrome of hyperacute rise in pulmonary arterial pressure, usually accompanied by bronchospasm, often followed within seconds, or accompanied by, profound reduction in cardiac output and fall in arterial oxygen saturation; these sequelae may be irreversible. The syndrome occurs most commonly, but not exclusively, among neonates and infants who are intubated after an operation for repair of a congenital cardiac defect associated with pulmonary arterial hypertension. The pulmonary artery pressure is usually essentially normal after repair, until an episode of pulmonary hypertensive crisis. The crisis may appear spontaneously, but usually occurs during or shortly after suctioning of the endotracheal tube. Multiple crises may occur in a single patient. The prevalence of pulmonary hypertensive crises is greatest about 18 hours after operation, but they can occur before or after that time.[H17] During an acute hypertensive crisis, atypical cardiac tamponade can result from acute right ventricular dilatation.[D7,K15]

Incremental risk factors. This syndrome has been recognized for many years, but its precise cause at the time it occurs is unknown.[D4,J2,W13] Congenital cardiac defects accompanied by large pulmonary blood flow and relatively low pulmonary vascular resistance are strong *patient risk factors* for the development of the syndrome. Chief among them are truncus arteriosus and atrioventricular septal defect. The histology of the pulmonary arteries and arterioles is normal or mildly abnormal, with all changes considered to be clearly reversible.[H17] The syndrome is not seen in patients with fixed pulmonary hypertension or severe pulmonary vascular disease. *Procedural risk factors* have not been clearly identified, although absence of pulmonary blood flow during CPB, accumulation of neutrophils in the lung, and damage to pulmonary endothelial cells are known to occur and provide a favorable setting for development of pulmonary hypertensive crises. Release of arachidonic metabolites from some cells in the lung (probably pulmonary endothelial cells),[V3] failure of pulmonary endothelial cells to inactivate bradykinin,[S23] and release by injured pulmonary endothelial cells of the vasoconstrictive platelet-activating factor[R13] are probably all encouraged by events during CPB, perhaps particularly if these cells were preconditioned before operation by a high pulmonary blood flow. *Postoperative risk factors* nearly certainly include acute hypoxia, which is known to produce acute hypoxic vasoconstriction, probably using some of the mechanisms just described.[C19,S24] Catecholamine administration appears to predispose patients to these crises.

Prevention. Because pulmonary hypertensive crises may be fatal despite intense therapy, their prevention is critical. An important preventive measure in neonates and infants is maintenance of paralysis and sedation (with pancuronium, or a similar agent, and fentanyl) for at least the first 20 to 24 postoperative hours, and for at least another 24 hours or longer if the patient remains intubated (see Section 4, "General Care of Neonates and Infants," later in this chapter). Fentanyl has been shown to be a safe agent in neonates and adults, with little adverse effect on cardiac function or systemic and pulmonary circulations[H14]; pancuronium (in doses of at least $0.015 \text{ mg} \cdot \text{kg}^{-1}$) is given along with fentanyl to prevent rigidity. Fentanyl (in a dose of $25 \text{ μg} \cdot \text{kg}^{-1}$), along with pancuronium, should be given before suctioning the endotracheal tube in any neonate or infant who is not already well paralyzed and sedated, because it appears to minimize the possibility of a pulmonary hypertensive crisis. In addition to sedation, aggressive treatment of acidosis, including hyperventilation to $\text{Pco}_2 = 30$ to 34 mmHg, will also decrease the prevalence and severity of pulmonary hypertensive crises. When the monitored pulmonary artery pressure becomes paroxysmally elevated early postoperatively, efforts are made to control and reduce it. A high concentration of oxygen is maintained in the inspired air, because this is as useful an agent as exists for reducing pulmonary vascular resistance. Direct infusion of nitroprusside into the pulmonary artery has also been useful. Many agents have been advanced as being optimal on the grounds that they selectively reduce pulmonary vascular resistance, but few do so, and no clearly superior one among those has been identified.[B15,J2,P18,R14]

There are encouraging results from the use of inhaled nitric oxide to reduce pulmonary artery pressure in cardiac transplant recipients,[K25] patients on left ventricular assist devices,[A12] and generally in infants and children prone to pulmonary hypertensive crises.[B24] Journis and colleagues[J8] found that 15 of 17 children having critical pulmonary hypertension following operation for congenital heart disease responded to inhaled nitric oxide (20 ppm) after failure of conventional medical treatment (Table 5-6). Pulmonary arterial pressure decreased without a change in systemic arterial pressure but with concomitant increase of SaO_2 and SvO_2. Other investigators have also shown an increase in cardiac index and improvement of indices of right ventricular function after nitric oxide treatment.[S26] Intrapulmonary shunt fraction may decrease as well.[B23] The response in postoperative patients with valvar heart disease may be less satisfactory.[F12]

■ **TABLE 5-6** **Effects of Inhaled Nitric Oxide on Hemodynamics after Operations for Congenital Heart Defects**

	T_0 (before NO)	T_1 (20 min after NO)	*P*
HR (beats · min⁻¹)	153 ± 22	145 ± 21	.0083
Systolic P_{PA} (mmHg)	60 ± 14	40 ± 11	.0003
Mean P_{PA} (mmHg)	42 ± 14	27 ± 8	.0008
Diastolic P_{PA} (mmHg)	31 ± 14	18 ± 10	.0003
Systolic P_{AO} (mmHg)	68 ± 12	69 ± 7	.18
Mean P_{AO} (mmHg)	55 ± 11	56 ± 6	.4
Diastolic P_{AO} (mmHg)	44 ± 10	46 ± 6	.12
P_{LA} (mmHg)	7.2 ± 1.9	6.8 ± 1.5	.3
P_{CV} (mmHg)	6.6 ± 2.5	5.2 ± 1.8	.04
$S\bar{v}O_2$ (%)	50 ± 13	67 ± 12	.003
SaO_2 (%)	87 ± 8	96 ± 3	.0007

(From Journois and colleagues.[J8])

Key: *HR,* Heart rate; *NO,* nitric oxide; *P$_{AO}$,* systemic arterial pressure; *P$_{CV}$,* central venous pressure; *P$_{LA}$,* left atrial pressure; *P$_{PA}$,* pulmonary arterial pressure; *SaO$_2$,* arterial oxygen saturation; *S$\bar{v}$O$_2$,* mixed venous blood oxygen saturation.

Nitric oxide inhaled at 20 ppm reduces pulmonary artery pressure and improves $S\bar{v}O_2$, while having no effect on systemic artery pressure when given to a group of patients following operations for defects associated with pulmonary hypertension.

RENAL SUBSYSTEM

Adequacy

As a guide to the continuing evaluation of the renal subsystem, a urinary catheter is inserted preoperatively in the operating room and left for a minimum of 48 hours to monitor hourly urine flow. In some cases, consideration should be given to use of a trocar-introduced suprapubic catheter in adults, rather than a urethral catheter, because this type of catheter is more comfortable, easier to manage, and associated with less urinary tract infection.[12] Serum potassium concentration is measured every 4 hours during the first 24 postoperative hours and, if the patient is still in the intensive care unit, every 8 hours for at least the next 48 hours. Serum creatinine and blood urea nitrogen (BUN) levels are measured each morning for at least the first 48 hours.

Convalescence early after cardiac surgery can, arbitrarily, be considered adequate with regard to urine flow when urine volume is greater than $500 \text{ mL} \cdot 24 \text{ h}^{-1} \cdot \text{m}^{-2}$, or $167 \text{ mL} \cdot 8 \text{ h}^{-1} \cdot \text{m}^{-2}$, or $20 \text{ mL} \cdot 1 \text{ h}^{-1} \cdot \text{m}^{-2}$. Some prefer to use the criterion of 0.5 to $1 \text{ mL} \cdot \text{h}^{-1} \cdot \text{kg}^{-1}$ in the case of infants and small children; Srinivasan and colleagues (Srinivasan V, Levinsky L, Choh JH, Baliah T, Subramanian S: personal communication; 1981) and the Great Ormond Street Children's Hospital use $0.5 \text{ mL} \cdot \text{h}^{-1} \cdot \text{kg}^{-1}$ as their lower limit of acceptable urine flow in infants and children.

In most postoperative patients, CPB induces a diuresis early after operation. Factors responsible for this are hemodilution with a clear fluid prime (lactated Ringer's solution, D5W + ½ NS, or Plasmalyte A), and often glucose and mannitol additions to increase tubular oncotic load. Low cardiac output therefore can exist early postoperatively even in the presence of nominally adequate urine flow. The renal function is inadequate when solute excretion is insufficient to keep the serum potassium level below $5 \text{ mEq} \cdot \text{L}^{-1}$, the BUN level below $40 \text{ mg} \cdot \text{dL}^{-1}$, and the creatinine level below $1.0 \text{ mg} \cdot \text{dL}^{-1}$ (Srinivasan V, Levinsky L, Choh JH, Baliah T,

Subramanian S: personal communication; 1981). Convalescence cannot be considered normal when the urine is pink but without red blood cells early postoperatively, because this indicates a free plasma hemoglobin greater than 40 mg $\cdot$ dL^{-1} and an inordinate and potentially dangerous amount of hemolysis.

Acute renal failure requiring dialysis is rare in adults.[M28] However, postoperative renal dysfunction (doubling or greater of serum creatinine) occurs in approximately 1% of adult patients if preoperative renal function is normal. If any degree of renal dysfunction is present preoperatively, it occurs in 16% to 20% of patients, about one fifth of whom will need dialysis. Acute renal failure occurred in 61 of 2262 children (2.7%) undergoing open intracardiac operation.[P22] Acute renal failure (in patients without preexisting renal disease) after cardiac surgery is nearly always associated with low cardiac output, but rarely may occur when the other criteria of cardiac subsystem performance are satisfactory[B5,H1] (Srinivasan and colleagues: personal communication; 1981).

Causes of Acute Dysfunction after Cardiac Surgery

There are no usual intraoperative events during well-conducted cardiac operations that are damaging to renal function and can be considered causes of acute renal failure.

Risk Factors for Acute Dysfunction
Patient-Specific

Preoperative impairment of renal function that is intractable to therapy considerably increases the risk of acute renal failure early postoperatively.[A3,H1] Therefore, preoperative evaluation includes assessment of renal function. *Chronic heart failure* (preoperative NYHA class IV) considerably increases the risk of acute renal failure after operation. *Cyanotic heart disease* increases the risk of renal failure after cardiac surgery in older patients.[T1] A renal lesion is known to exist preoperatively in many such patients. This does not appear to be the case in young patients; in a study of 176 patients with tetralogy of Fallot undergoing repair, no deaths in acute renal failure were observed.[K8]

Young age is a risk factor for acute renal failure. When cardiac output is importantly reduced after cardiac surgery in neonates and infants, a prevalence of acute renal failure as high as 8% to 10% has been reported[C5,H13,R6] (Srinivasan and colleagues: personal communication; 1981). One reason for this apparently increased prevalence may be that immature kidneys have less ability to concentrate urine in the face of reduced renal blood flow. Compared with older patients, infants may develop more tissue hypoxia during and early after CPB, with a resulting increase in production of potassium, BUN, and other substances, some of which may be nephrotoxic. Uric acid levels, for example, were shown by Hencz and colleagues to rise to nephrotoxic levels (10 mg $\cdot$ dL^{-1}) in some patients within 24 hours of operation, and the levels were significantly ($P = .001$) higher in patients under 3 years of age than in older children.[H2] At the other end of the spectrum, *older age* (over 70 years) is a risk factor for the development of acute renal failure.[L14]

Procedural

A *long period of CPB* increases the risk of acute renal failure.[R6] This has been clearly demonstrated by a prospective study[K7] and is probably in part related to the damaging effects of CPB. There is an additional risk imposed by a longer duration of hypothermic circulatory arrest, particularly in infants and children.[P22] However, a CPB flow of 1.6 L $\cdot$ min^{-1} (at body temperatures of 28°C or higher) with a mean arterial blood pressure of at least 30 mmHg seems to minimize the occurrence of acute renal failure when postoperative cardiac output is good.[H1]

Several studies suggest that using a CPB prime of *whole blood* (rather than hemodilution) increases the risk of acute renal failure,[G2,W6] as does *high plasma hemoglobin level* (greater than 40 mg $\cdot$ dL^{-1}) during and early after CPB.

Postoperative

Acute reduction in cardiac output early after operation is the most common and most important risk factor for the development of acute renal failure. Yet the prevalence of acute renal failure varies among patients with low cardiac output, in part because of the role played by other risk factors. Picca and colleagues[P22] found a 79% mortality in children developing acute renal failure. High central venous pressure, low systemic blood pressure, and high dosage of dopamine or epinephrine, each associated with low cardiac output, were significant risk factors.[P22]

Aminoglycosides (for example, gentamicin) and some other *antibiotics* increase the risk of acute renal dysfunction early after operation.

Course of Dysfunction

Acute renal failure is rarely evident immediately after operation, but becomes evident 12 to 18 hours later. Its first manifestation, particularly in infants and children, is usually oliguria of increasing severity that is resistant to measures to increase cardiac output, to dopamine, and to furosemide. The oliguria is soon accompanied by a rapid rise in serum potassium concentration (probably because of acute release of potassium from hemolyzing red blood cells and from other intracellular stores of potassium) and a slower rise in BUN and creatinine. Although this form of acute renal failure is rarely the primary mode of death, it is a major contributor unless prompt and effective interventions are made. In patients who survive, and particularly in young patients, renal function usually begins to improve as cardiac output rises, and important residual renal dysfunction rarely remains.

By contrast, a less lethal form of renal dysfunction, usually occurring in adults, becomes apparent on the third or fourth postoperative day. It manifests itself by a progressive rise in BUN and creatinine levels, which usually peak at 80 to 120 mg $\cdot$ dL^{-1} and 5 to 8 mg $\cdot$ dL^{-1}, respectively, about 7 to 10 days postoperatively. Oliguria is often absent, and hyperkalemia greater than 5 mEq $\cdot$ L^{-1} usually does not develop. Spontaneous resolution occurs in about 75% of patients.[C17]

Acute renal failure (as opposed to dysfunction) after cardiac operations, treated or otherwise, is associated with subsequent hospital death in about 50% of patients.[L6] The probability of death in patients with acute renal failure severe enough to require dialysis is increased by the coexistence of cardiac subsystem dysfunction and pulmonary subsystem dysfunction. Development of infection after the beginning of dialysis is also an important risk factor for death.

Management and Treatment

One important aspect of managing the renal subsystem is a reasonable program of fluid administration (see "Fluid, Electrolyte, and Caloric Intake" in Section 2 of this chapter) early after open cardiac operations; its purpose, in part, is avoidance of the fluid overload that can easily develop with even mild impairment of renal function. There is no evidence that larger amounts of fluids reduce the prevalence of acute renal failure in this setting. The maintenance of good function in other subsystems, particularly cardiac, is a second important aspect of managing the renal subsystem after cardiac surgery.

When oliguria occurs early postoperatively, cardiac preload and afterload are optimized, and administration of dopamine at 2.5 $\mu g \cdot kg^{-1} \cdot min^{-1}$ is begun (see Appendix 5I). The direct diuretic effect of low-dose dopamine and its subsequent prevention of oliguric renal failure are controversial.[C25] At best, dopamine may increase cardiac output and/or blood pressure, resulting in greater urine volume, but its therapeutic effect on the glomerular filtration rate (GFR), creatinine clearance, and serum creatinine is doubtful,[D13,H26] particularly in high-risk patients.[D14] If these measures do not quickly suffice, furosemide (usually given as Lasix, 1 $mg \cdot kg^{-1}$ or up to 40 mg in adults) is administered intravenously. If a good response is obtained, this dosage is repeated every 6 to 12 hours for 3 days. If a response is not obtained within 30 to 60 minutes, the dose is doubled and then quadrupled, and then 8 $mg \cdot kg^{-1}$ is given. This therapy is based on the reasonable hypothesis that maintenance of urine production, even though dilute, is advantageous to renal function. When serum potassium rises above 5.5 $mEq \cdot L^{-1}$, a glucose insulin solution is given intravenously, and K-exalate enemas are used[W12] (see Appendix 5J). These are temporary palliative measures, to be used until dialysis can be initiated.

Alternatively, when urine flow does not respond to the first few doses of the furosemide schedule, infusion of a "renal cocktail" may be effective. This consists of a mixture of 400 mg of furosemide in 100 mL of 20% mannitol (both amounts are halved for small patients); it is administered continuously at a furosemide rate of 1 $mg \cdot kg^{-1} \cdot h^{-1}$. During infusion of the renal cocktail, the serum osmolarity of the patient is measured every 2 to 4 hours; if it exceeds 310 $mOsm \cdot L^{-1}$, the infusion is immediately discontinued. Otherwise, it is administered for 4 hours, discontinued for 4 hours, then administered for another 4 hours, and so forth. If a large urine flow develops, the "cocktail" is usually discontinued after 24 hours, or after 3000 mL of urine (in an adult) has been excreted. If a large urine flow does not develop within about 2 hours of beginning this infusion, it is stopped. Occasionally, in the absence of a diuretic response to furosemide, intravenous ethacrynic acid (100 mg for the adult) may be effective.

Unless oliguria and hyperkalemia respond to treatment within a few hours, especially in neonates and infants, a considerable probability of death exists.[A3,C17,H1,M28,R6] Therefore, peritoneal dialysis or continuous arteriovenous hemodialysis[P24] is initiated on an emergency basis; the urgency is in part due to the frequent coexistence of an increased extracellular fluid volume ("fluid overload") dating back to the time of CPB. More optimally, preventive measures are applied earlier, including (1) ultrafiltration during the closing phases of CPB (see "Components" under Pump-Oxygenator in Section 3 of Chapter 2)[M13,N7]; (2) limitation of fluid administration during the early hours after operation; and (3) routine placement, in neonates and infants, of a small silicone peritoneal dialysis catheter through the lower end of the incision used for the median sternotomy. The advantages of this last technique have been developed and emphasized by Mee.[M12] His protocol includes using the catheter simply as a drain initially; occasionally the tube drains large amounts of peritoneal fluid with a protein content similar to that of plasma. Should oliguria develop that is unresponsive to furosemide, or should the serum potassium rise above 5 $mEq \cdot L^{-1}$, rapid-cycle, low-volume peritoneal dialysis is recommended. The dialysates, alternatively isotonic and hypertonic, are used in volumes of 10 $mL \cdot kg^{-1}$. The potassium content is dependent on the serum potassium concentration. Particularly in neonates, infants, and children, dialysis by this or other techniques usually improves cardiac performance and decreases ventilatory requirements.[M12,Z1] Complications of such protocols are rare; the most frequent error in their use is delay in beginning the intervention.[B10,H13,N3,R6,W18]

In older children and in adults, who more commonly develop nonoliguric renal failure,[S27] conventional hemodialysis may be appropriate when indicated. However, continuous pumped or unpumped arteriovenous or venovenous hemofiltration is the technique preferred in this setting, with the unpumped technique having advantages in patients who are hemodynamically unstable.[B26,L5,M9]

NEUROPSYCHOLOGICAL SUBSYSTEM

Neuropsychological symptoms and signs after cardiac surgery are difficult to categorize, arguable as to etiology, and often overlooked. The literature concerning them is voluminous, but substantive information has emerged only relatively recently and in small amounts. Inferences from the available information are arguable.

The neuropsychological sequelae of hypothermic circulatory arrest are described separately in "Brain Function and Structure: Risk Factors for Damage" and "Effects of Brain Damage" under Damaging Effects of Circulatory Arrest during Hypothermia in Section 1 of Chapter 2. (For a discussion of the emergency treatment of seizures, one sequel of hypothermic circulatory arrest, see Appendix 5K.)

Generalized (Diffuse) Neuropsychological Function

Intelligence, problem-solving, concentration, learning, memory, error-free performance, and dexterity are components of the general neuropsychological subsystem, and all or some of these have been included in the term *cognitive functions.* It is believed that changes in these cognitive functions reflect genuine disturbances in the brain and are testable, usually by psychometric study.

Adequacy

Concentration, memory, learning, and speed of visuomotor responses have been reported to be adequate early postoperatively in less than half of patients who undergo cardiac surgery with CPB.[N5,S14,S17] However, in many patients this inadequacy (or decrease in function) is only mild (and presumably transient); in about 20% of patients it is moderate in severity, and in 5% it is severe.[S17] By contrast, after peripheral vascular surgery, mild inadequacy is present in 30% of patients, and moderate or severe disturbances in none.[S17] These findings, however, have been disputed, and the early prevalences remain uncertain.[H18,H19,M10,R7,S8] By 8 weeks after operation, at least 60% of patients have adequate (normal) cognitive functions. Six months to 5 years after operation, more than 80% of patients have adequate (normal) function of this subsystem,[S18] although Newman and colleagues observed an increase in cognitive decline between 6 months and 5 years.[N14]

These estimates from objective testing have seemed incompatible with the general experience of many physicians and surgeons with patients after open cardiac operations. The general experience is that patients are not commonly disabled by neuropsychological problems, unless they have experienced an overt stroke.[O4,T4] In no instance among a carefully studied group of 165 patients was neuropsychological dysfunction sufficient to prevent return to work.[S14]

Causes of Dysfunction

Presumably, organic changes in the brain cause disturbances of the general neuropsychological subsystem. Embolization and hypoperfusion, with resultant ischemia, have most generally been considered etiologic to these organic changes. In adults randomized to either pH-stat or alpha-stat acid-base management during CPB, cerebral blood flow was greater using the pH-stat strategy. However, patients with higher cerebral blood flow suffered greater postoperative neurophysiological impairment, inferring that hyperemia as well as hypoperfusion may be factors in postoperative cerebral dysfunction.[P23] Speculatively, the causes of both general neuropsychological subsystem dysfunction and localized subsystem dysfunction (such as strokes) are the same except in degree and/or distribution.

The emotions and moods of patients appear to be causally related to cognitive function. For example, patients who sense cognitive deterioration after CPB usually are not found to have it by objective testing; instead, they are found to have more depression postoperatively than preoperatively.[N8] Also, preoperative depression and a lower socioeconomic status appear to appreciably increase the risk of deterioration of cognitive function postoperatively.[F10] In a study of patients randomized to either coronary angioplasty or surgical revascularization, cognitive function was similar in each group after 5 years of follow-up, suggesting no lasting detrimental effect of CPB,[H21] a finding contrary to that of Newman and colleagues.[N14]

Risk Factors for Acute Dysfunction

Knowledge in this area remains incomplete, in part because of difficulty in defining and measuring the end points of acute dysfunction, as well as the variables that are possible risk factors for development of dysfunction. *Older age* at operation is a mild risk factor for diffuse neuropsychological dysfunction postoperatively.[H12] Mild or moderate carotid artery stenosis is not a risk factor.[H12] *Longer duration of CPB* has been found to be a risk factor for general neuropsychological disturbances after the cardiac operation,[N5,N6,S8,S19] as has a *greater amount of microembolization,* both particulate and gaseous.[B12,P10] Normothermic CPB (used in combination with warm myocardial management) was noted by one group to have a comparatively higher incidence of central neurologic system events than standard hypothermic perfusion.[C26] However, other studies have not corroborated these findings.[R18] Engelman and colleagues[E14] performed a randomized study to evaluate the effect of perfusion temperature on prevalence of postoperative neurologic dysfunction. Two hundred ninety-one patients were divided among perfusion temperatures of 20°, 32°, and 37°C. In the group as a whole there was a 36% prevalence of neurologic dysfunction at 1 month postoperatively but no difference in cognitive function, elemental skills, or neurologic functional capacity among the groups. Aside from that for pH-stat regulation, no other correlation has been found between total cerebral blood flow during CPB and prevalence of general neuropsychological dysfunction after operation.[V1,V2] *Oxygenators other than the membrane type* and *absence of 40 µm arterial blood filtration* somewhat increase the risk of this type of dysfunction.[B18]

Course of Dysfunction

As indicated earlier, the prevalence of general neuropsychological dysfunction declines considerably as time passes after the operation.

Management and Treatment

Management and treatment involve prevention and intelligent counseling and reassurance. The former consists of further improvements in CPB and techniques of cardiac operations. The latter is highly important in determining the final overall result of the operation, because perceived continuing dysfunction can limit the quality of life.

Mood State
Adequacy

An adequate mood state after a cardiac operation is one without unusual anxiety, depression, or euphoria, and without delirium. The prevalence of an inadequate mood state has received little study, for reasons similar to those in the case of the general neuropsychological subsystem. In one study of 759 patients undergoing CABG, 7% showed transient confusion without delirium, and in no case did delirium develop thereafter.[C20]

Causes and Risk Factors for Acute Dysfunction

Preoperative emotional characteristics of the patient play a major role in the postoperative mood state. In a study performed during the early era of open cardiac operations,

Burgess and colleagues found all patients to have acute preoperative anxiety in varying degrees; a few were frankly depressed.[B11] The absence of daily access to an empathetic individual, not part of the surgical team, preoperatively and postoperatively was an important risk factor for increased anxiety and depression postoperatively. These mood states were particularly apparent in the intensive care unit and during the first few days thereafter.

Course of Dysfunction

Most patients have some degree of anxiety during the first few postoperative days, and severe delirium occurs in 2% to 10%; 10% to 20% of patients have hallucinations and frightening dreams late postoperatively; and 10% to 20% of patients may continue to have episodic alterations in mood state after hospital discharge. In some patients, this seems to be related to difficulty in adjusting to the situational demands of life with improved cardiac function.[B11]

Management and Treatment

Daily access to an empathetic individual not identified with the surgical team, and attention to the patient as a sensitive and threatened human being by physicians, are the most important methods of prevention. When the mood state becomes severely abnormal, psychiatric assistance is required.

Localized Neuropsychological Function

Adequacy

Most patients recover from open cardiac operations without gross localized neuropsychological subsystem dysfunction, such as hemipareses or hemiplegias, and in them the subsystem performs adequately throughout convalescence. Subtle defects occur more frequently. Visual field defects are sometimes perceived by the patient and confirmed by testing, and then usually regress or disappear.[S8] Difficulty in focusing, such as is required for reading, is sometimes experienced in the early postoperative period, but it usually disappears within 2 weeks. Disturbances of memory are nearly always transient, but may be noticeable to the patient. Because of the known phenomenon of accentuation and prolongation of the patient's perception of the abnormality by fixation on it, patients and their families are provided supportive care and reassurance. Special diagnostic procedures are rarely indicated because there is essentially no effective specific therapy (see "Management" later in this section).

Gross neurologic defects, usually hemipareses or hemiplegias, are less common than neuropsychological and mood abnormalities, but they are generally more serious. The prevalence of these abnormalities after open cardiac operations is about 0.5% in relatively young patients, gradually rising with increasing age to around 5% in patients over about 65, and 8% in those over about 75.[C13,G8] In a study of 2108 patients undergoing isolated CABG, adverse cerebral outcomes occurred in 129 (6.1%). Approximately half of these were major deficits; the remainder had deterioration of intellectual function or seizures.[R19] In a related multicenter study of 271 patients undergoing CABG combined with an intracardiac procedure, adverse cerebral outcomes occurred in 43 (16%).[W19]

Causes and Risk Factors for Acute Dysfunction

These defects probably represent more severe forms of the same kinds of damage (that is, greater quantities or more sensitive locations) that cause neuropsychological and mood disturbances. Thus, they are probably the result of emboli (e.g., platelet aggregates, clusters of microbubbles, aggregates of fibrin accumulations from pump-oxygenators or tubing surfaces, boluses of air, or atherosclerotic debris or plaques dislodged from the ascending aorta) and other facets of the damaging effects of CPB. When investigated using computed tomography (CT) scans in patients with evidence of stroke after cardiac operations, the defects are typically multiple and posteriorly located in the brain. These findings are most consistent with particulate atheromatous embolization.[B28]

Older age is a risk factor for stroke after cardiac operations such as CABG, but this may be only because of the increased prevalence of atherosclerosis.[B27,W20] *Severe atherosclerosis of the ascending aorta* clearly increases the risk of perioperative stroke, as does known preexisting cerebral vascular disease.[G8] *Duration of CPB* and *low cardiac output after operation* also appear to be risk factors.[G8,K24] Cardiac microbubbles identified by intraoperative TEE have not been a risk factor for diffuse or localized neuropsychological dysfunction; furthermore, such microbubbles can rarely be eradicated by what might appear to be effective surgical maneuvers.[T8]

Management

Precise recommendations for the complete prevention of localized neurologic dysfunction remain elusive. However, certain precautions may reduce the frequency of major neurologic events, such as maintaining adequate perfusion pressure, minimizing duration of circulatory arrest, and using blood filters and appropriate de-airing procedures (see Chapter 2). In adults, Blauth and colleagues[B27] and Wareing and colleagues[W20] have stressed the importance of ascending aortic atheromatous disease as etiologic in postoperative stroke. Perioperative detection of severe atheromatous disease of the ascending aorta is facilitated by ultrasonographic interrogation by the surgeon.[D15] Management may consist of (1) modification of the techniques of aortic cannulation or aortic clamping, (2) aortic endarterectomy or resection, (3) grafting of the ascending aorta, and (4) use of an intra-aortic filter at the time of aortic clamp removal.[H27,K26,V4]

The only general therapeutic intervention that seems to be of value is use of hyperbaric oxygenation. This has been demonstrated only in patients with massive air embolization, but, even in this setting, evaluation is difficult because spontaneous recovery frequently occurs. The interval from the embolic event (which nearly always occurs in the operating room and usually during or at the end of CPB) to hyperbaric therapy plays a major role in outcome; beyond 12 to 24 hours this therapy probably is not useful.[A10,L10,L11] Because these patients, as well as many others without these localized neurologic disorders, are intubated and heavily sedated during this period, localized neuropsychological disturbances are rarely discovered within 24 hours of operation.[K29] Intense diagnostic efforts, such as lumbar puncture and CT scanning, are generally not indicated in the absence of any therapeutic implication. In addition, CT scanning may fail to be diagnostic.[A10]

Moazami and colleagues have reported the safety and efficacy of intraarterial thrombolysis in a group of 13 patients suffering strokes after cardiac operations.[M36] A "stroke" team is organized to evaluate all patients with an acute neurologic deficit recognized within 6 hours of operation. Patients with a clinically important stroke (National Institutes of Health [NIH] stroke scale >10) or isolated disabling symptoms are considered for study. They undergo emergent contrast cranial CT; evidence of hemorrhage or major early signs of infarction preclude thrombolytic therapy. Otherwise, 4-vessel arterial angiography is performed using the transfemoral approach. Digital subtraction angiography permits the site of occlusions to be located and collateral circulation evaluated. Patients with middle cerebral, internal carotid, or basilar artery occlusions are considered for thrombolysis. A No. 2.3 French microcatheter is steered to the occlusion by fluoroscopy and is embedded within or through the center of the thrombosis. Thrombolysis is attempted at 5- to 10-minute intervals for up to 2 hours. Additional mechanical manipulation of the clot is also used. Among the 13 patients studied, NIH stroke scale improved importantly in 5 (38%, CL 23% to 57%) and did not worsen appreciably in the 8 who did not improve.

The prognosis is variable, as is the case with strokes in general. In some patients the signs and symptoms gradually disappear, whereas in others there is only partial or no recovery from the neurologic defect. At times, the defects are so massive as to be fatal.

GASTROINTESTINAL SUBSYSTEM

Adequacy

Abnormalities of function of the gastrointestinal tract, including the liver and pancreas, are not clinically detectable when convalescence after cardiac surgery is normal, and oral intake is usually allowed on the morning after operation. Patients who remain intubated are exceptions; in these cases, fluid intake through a nasogastric tube is begun 12 to 24 hours after operation, gradually progressing to a nutritious one. Evidence of abdominal distention, absence of peristalsis, and hyperperistalsis is sought twice daily. If one of these develops, the gastrointestinal system is not adequate and alimentation is discontinued, investigations are begun, and intravenously administered hyperalimentation is considered.

Patients with a history of peptic ulcer disease should be given 300 mg of cimetidine (or some other histamine H_2-receptor antagonist) every 6 hours, by mouth or intravenously, during the postoperative hospitalization, beginning 6 to 12 hours after operation. Such a program is worthy of consideration as a routine.

Types of Acute Dysfunction

Acute dysfunction of the gastrointestinal subsystem is uncommon after open cardiac operations, occurring in only about 1% of patients.[L7,O5] However, important dysfunction of the gastrointestinal subsystem is followed by death during the period of hospitalization in more than 50% of those patients. Emergency operations are required for some.

Gastrointestinal Bleeding

Gastrointestinal bleeding after open cardiac operations is usually from the upper part of the gastrointestinal tract.[K11] The pathology is usually hemorrhagic gastritis or duodenitis.[K11,R11] Occasionally, a previously existing duodenal ulcer is the site of bleeding, and rarely, massive bleeding originates in the colon.[W2]

Acute Cholecystitis

Acute cholecystitis, when it develops after open cardiac surgery, may be noncalculus, but it produces the same clinical syndrome of severe pain, leukocytosis, and right upper quadrant tenderness as when it develops in other patients.[L7] Perhaps because of delay in diagnosis that has been present, mortality among patients who have developed this complication is about 75%.[L7]

Acute Pancreatitis

Some evidence of acute pancreatitis is present in about 25% of patients after open cardiac surgery and is manifested by hyperamylasemia.[R12] In most cases the increased levels of serum amylase gradually decline, with few if any clinical sequelae. Occasionally (in less than 5% of patients with elevated amylase), severe pancreatitis develops, with pancreatic abscess or hemorrhagic pancreatitis.[C18] Indiscriminate administration of large doses of calcium chloride contributes to the development of pancreatic cellular injury after cardiac surgery.[C18]

Hepatic Necrosis

Convalescence may be complicated by jaundice, with about 20% of patients having a serum bilirubin concentration of at least 3 mg · dL after cardiac surgery.[C9] Jaundice is moderate or severe (bilirubin concentration greater than 6 mg · dL) in only about 5% of patients. Severity of preoperative right atrial hypertension, hypoxia during operation, early postoperative hypotension, and amount of blood transfused perioperatively all increase the probability of postoperative jaundice.[C9,M14] Halothane, if used, and duration of CPB may be risk factors.[C9]

Provided that postoperative cardiac output is good, hepatic dysfunction can be expected to improve gradually and disappear, but when cardiac output is low, prognosis is poor. Frank hepatic necrosis may develop when cardiac output is acutely and severely reduced. The only useful treatment is that directed at improving cardiac performance and supplying adequate parenteral nutritional support.

Intestinal Necrosis

Intestinal necrosis develops uncommonly but insidiously after cardiac operations. Inevitable perforation in the area of necrosis may be overlooked for a number of days because of the multiplicity of problems associated with the causative low cardiac output.

Esophagitis

Esophagitis, when it occurs after a cardiac operation, is manifested by dysphagia, which is uncommon. Esophagitis may be related to an intrapericardial accumulation of blood or to pericarditis. When oral candidiasis is present, *Candida* esophagitis is nearly certainly the cause of dysphagia[G5] and can be diagnosed by means of esophagoscopy or radiologic study of the barium-filled esophagus.[O1] When candidal esophagitis appears, antibiotic therapy is stopped unless it is essential. Every 2 to 6 hours, 500,000 to 1 million units of nystatin are given orally, preferably in methylcellulose, to increase viscosity.[G5] Treatment is continued for 1 to 3 weeks.

Watery Diarrhea

As a complication of cardiac surgery, watery diarrhea may accompany or follow abdominal distention or appear de novo toward the end of the first week. Should it become frequent and explosive, with passage of mucus and blood, it has ominous implications. Any oral antibiotics should be discontinued when diarrhea develops. The diarrhea may be caused by ischemia of the bowel secondary to a long period of low cardiac output, and this ischemia may lead to small or large bowel infarction,[A2] or it may be a form of ulcerative colitis and proctitis. Diagnosis can be made by sigmoidoscopy and colonoscopy. If the bowel ischemia and ulceration progress, laparotomy and bowel resection are required, but even with such treatment, prognosis is poor.

Abdominal Distention

Occasionally, gas in the gastrointestinal tract produces abdominal distention within 24 to 48 hours of operation. Bowel sounds can be heard initially. Although not part of normal convalescence, this complication is usually benign and subsides after another day or so in response to fasting, use of glycerine suppositories, and application of heat to the abdomen. A rectal examination should be performed to exclude fecal impaction as a possible cause of the distention. If the distention does not promptly subside, other causes must be considered. The distention could be due to oral administration of procainamide or cephalosporins, and these drugs may need to be administered by another route. Mediastinitis and an infected median sternotomy incision may be causative and should be investigated. Abdominal distention may be the first sign of postoperative acute pancreatitis. When combined with marked weakness and fever, particularly in a patient on sodium warfarin (Coumadin), postoperative adrenal insufficiency must be excluded by appropriate tests as a possible cause.

Causes of Acute Dysfunction

Nearly all acute intraabdominal dysfunctions (inadequacies of the gastrointestinal subsystem) result from localized or generalized severe hypoperfusion of either the gastrointestinal tract or the liver, or both.[B13,K11,L7,M14,R11,W2] However, in neonates and infants, improper position of the inferior vena cava cannula during CPB and thrombosis or infection in umbilical arterial or venous catheters may cause intraabdominal problems early postoperatively.

Risk Factors for Acute Dysfunction

Preoperative *peptic ulcer disease* predisposes patients to upper gastrointestinal bleeding after cardiac operations. Other chronic diseases of the intestinal tract also seem to increase the risk of gastrointestinal complications. *Acute necrotizing enteritis,* occurring in neonates severely aci-

dotic before operation, is a risk factor for gastrointestinal dysfunction early postoperatively. *Advanced age* increases the risk of acute dysfunction of the gastrointestinal subsystem after cardiac operations, as does valvar heart disease and congenital heart disease in adults.[L7]

Long duration of CPB as a risk factor is arguable, but most believe it to be one. *Low cardiac output* requiring prolonged catecholamine support and IABP increases the risk of serious intraabdominal complications.[L7] Increased prevalence of these complications is also associated with *infection* during the postoperative period, preoperative chronic *renal failure,* and postoperative acute renal dysfunction.[O5]

Management and Treatment

Encouragement of normal convalescence is the best protection against gastrointestinal dysfunction. Routine administration of cimetidine or some other histamine H_2-receptor antagonist should be considered for any patient at increased risk of gastrointestinal complications.

Once complications appear, their precise nature is determined on an emergency basis, usually by fiberoptic endoscopic examination and with the collaboration of a gastrointestinal specialist. In the absence of massive hemorrhage or gastrointestinal perforation, or both, intense medical treatment rather than surgical intervention is advisable. In the presence of symptoms, however, the possibility of intestinal necrosis must always be entertained, even when symptoms and signs are mild.[A2]

ENDOCRINE SUBSYSTEM

Few abnormalities of the endocrine subsystem have been described as postoperative complications of cardiac surgery. An exception is acute adrenal insufficiency, found by Alford and colleagues in 5, or 0.1%, of 4364 patients.[A1] Its cause is probably hemorrhagic infarction of the adrenal gland.[A1] This can be precipitated by CPB, and the tendency toward it is aggravated by postoperative anticoagulant therapy. Symptoms generally appear between the fourth and tenth postoperative days and consist of abdominal and flank pain, abdominal distention, altered mental status, fever, and occasionally, shock. When this diagnosis is suspected, a low serum cortisol level is virtually diagnostic. The diagnosis is also highly likely if the serum cortisol level remains low 60 minutes after administration of 25 units of intravenous or intramuscular adrenocorticotropic hormone (ACTH). Later, confirmatory evidence of acute adrenal insufficiency should be obtained.[A1] Prompt treatment with intravenous cortisol and saline solutions results in rapid clearing of symptoms. Lifetime oral treatment is indicated subsequently.

Neither hypo- nor hyperthyroidism has been identified as a complication after cardiac surgery with the aid of CPB. However, an important reduction of plasma-free triiodothyronine (T_3), (although not of thyroxine [T_4]), occurs early after cardiac operations. T_3 remains low for at least 24 hours, and this has led to the suggestion that administration of T_3 to the patient at that time is associated with an increase in myocardial function and energy stores.[N11] Chronic excessive catecholamine stimulation may depress isometric force development in myocardial muscle, and Timek and colleagues[T10] found that exogenous T_3 may improve myocardial fiber shortening amplitude by accelerating Ca^{2+} transients in an in vivo preparation of catecholamine stimulation. There is some clinical evidence that exogenous T_3 (0.6 to 0.8 $\mu g \cdot Kg^{-1}$) may improve cardiac output immediately after CABG in patients with depressed ejection fraction[K31] and also in brain-dead organ donors.[S30] However, results have varied. When T_3 was given to patients expected to have an uneventful course, little change in outcome was noted.[S31] When T_3 was given to adult patients undergoing CABG in a randomized study, improvement in cardiac output and a decreased prevalence of myocardial ischemia compared with controls were noted by Mullis-Jansen and colleagues.[M31] An increase in cardiac output was also apparent after CABG in patients with depressed LV function.[K31]

HEMATOLOGIC SUBSYSTEM

Adequacy

The function of the hematologic subsystem is assessed in terms of volume of postoperative bleeding, adequacy of clotting, volume restoration, and resistance to infection (see Immune Subsystem later in this section).

Causes of Acute Dysfunction

Excessive blood loss after CPB may result from a variety of causes, either singly or in combination. A surgical (mechanical) cause must always be suspected. Reoperative procedures, complex procedures, and operations on the aorta are those most frequently associated with a mechanical etiology for bleeding. Often, if there is excessive bleeding, it is obvious within the first hour after transfer from the operating room. It is persistent but may vary in volume over successive hours, depending on hemodynamic status, coagulation status, and patient position and wakefulness. Surgical bleeding occasionally also presents as a delayed increase in chest drainage following an apparently normal early postoperative course, and this usually demands emergency reexploration. Likely causes include suture line leak, chamber rupture, or (in the case of CABG) graft disruption or mechanical erosion. Occasionally, in a patient with a low hourly blood loss persisting over 12 or more hours, a surgical cause is found at reexploration.

The occurrence of reexploration for bleeding varies between 0.5% and 5.0%,[L15] depending on institutional criteria and case mix. Moulton and colleagues[M30] identified increased patient age, preoperative renal insufficiency, operation other than CABG, and prolonged bypass time as independent risk factors for reexploration. In their series, the prevalence of reexploration was 4.2% (253/6015), and reexploration was a strong risk factor associated with increased operative mortality and morbidity, including sepsis, renal failure, respiratory failure, and atrial arrhythmias. Others report little or no increased mortality and morbidity associated with reoperation for bleeding.[H23,K27]

The prevalence of bleeding attributable to nonmechanical (nonsurgical) causes is difficult to estimate, because in many instances reexploration results in cessation of bleeding even though no single site or only a minor site of bleeding can be identified.

Disturbances of coagulation may arise from a myriad of causes. It has long been recognized that the damaging effects of CPB and the magnitude of the resulting inflammatory response are related to postoperative blood loss, presumably via cytokine activation, platelet activation and aggregation, and kallikrein stimulation of neutrophils.[K7,K28,K30] Platelet abnormalities, both quantitative and qualitative, universally occur during and after CPB. Some consider platelet dysfunction the most common and most important defect of hemostasis in the postoperative period.[C27,C28,H24,S28] The qualitative abnormalities include degranulation and membrane fragmentation attributable in part to changes in GPIb and GPIIb/IIIa receptor activity.

During CPB, coagulation factors are depleted by *dilution, activation, and consumption*. These effects center on activation of thrombin, plasmin, and fibrinogen. Antithrombin (AT III) normally inhibits thrombin and factors IV and V. Heparin leads to anticoagulation basically by enhancing the thrombin-inhibiting ability of AT III by a factor of 2000.[H25,O6] Heparin also diminishes activation of factors IX and X and cofactors V and VIII. Residual heparin may lead to excessive bleeding by its effect on thrombin. This has also been characterized as rebound heparin effect.

The rationale for use of heparin-bonded circuits is based partially on the potential to reduce contact activation inherent in the CPB apparatus.[A13,A14,G19] Contact activation is due to vibration, blood–gas interfaces, and pericardial aspiration; simple exposure of blood to tubing may lead to important fibrinolysis, diffuse intravascular coagulation, and various consumption coagulopathies.

Hypothermia that can impair thromboxane synthesis and suppress platelet aggregation may lead to coagulation defects.[D19,R20] Thus, adequate rewarming on CPB is essential. Platelet transfusion, although controversial, may be beneficial.[C29] Further prevention of coagulation difficulties involves limitation or reversal of hemodilution, efforts to avoid contact activation of platelets and blood proteins, adequate rewarming, and use of pharmacologic agents, all discussed in Chapter 2.

Treatment of Acute Dysfunction

A moderate thrombocytopenia to levels of 100,000 mL^{-1} is to be expected following CPB. A level of 70,000 mL^{-1} may meet a threshold for transfusion if there is excessive bleeding. Under ordinary circumstances, platelet counts as just noted are decreased by dilution, destruction, and aggregation. Platelet function is diminished by changes in platelet membrane receptor activity, which includes downregulation of GPIb and GPIIb/IIIa receptors. Heparin-induced thrombocytopenia (HIT) can occur in the late postoperative phase following CPB. Its prevalence is said to be 5.5% for bovine lung heparin and 1.1% for heparin derived from porcine mucosa.[W21] The syndrome is likely to occur in individuals who have repeated exposure to heparin or in those with chronic or prolonged exposure. The diagnosis must be suspected early in the course of the syndrome, because the only treatment is total heparin withdrawal. As the syndrome progresses, there may be simple thrombocytopenia, but some patients will develop disseminated intravascular coagulation and thrombosis, leading to stroke, limb ischemia, renal failure, or death. The diagnosis of HIT is made in the presence of a platelet count under 70,000. In vitro tests for platelet function reflect serotonin release during aggregation and presence of antiplatelet serum IgG, which activates complement.

Reexposure to CPB in patients having a history of HIT poses a problem. Often, the antiplatelet reaction will resolve over 4 to 12 weeks. However, if reoperation is indicated, alternatives to heparin must be considered. These include ancrod (viper venom); hirudin, which inhibits thrombin; and low molecular weight heparin. There is no experience large enough at present to choose among these agents or to suggest that any is better than reexposure to heparin.

Heparin resistance may be encountered at operation. It may result from a congenital defect in the coagulation cascade, but usually is the result of chronic heparin therapy. The diagnosis is made by an ACT less than 480 seconds after administration of a minimum of three times the calculated dose of heparin. It is treated by administration of FFP or, more appropriately, antithrombin III concentrate.

Treatment of Bleeding

Treatment of bleeding involves four interventions: pharmacologic agents, infusion of blood-derived factors, transfusion of blood products, and reexploration.

Strategies to prevent excessive bleeding, or in some cases to treat it, begin with reversal of hypothermia. The importance of remaining on CPB to achieve a core temperature (measured at the tympanic membrane or in the nasopharynx) of 37°C has been stressed elsewhere (Chapter 2). In the intensive care unit, the use of warming blankets or, in infants, overhead heaters supplements this process.

Control of arterial blood pressure using nitroglycerin, nitroprusside, or diazoxide may be helpful. The use of positive end-expiratory pressure (PEEP) has been advocated, but its effect on the magnitude of blood loss is controversial. Residual heparin effect or heparin rebound can be diagnosed by a prolonged ACT. Additional protamine can be administered, usually 50 to 75 mg in adults and 5 to 10 mg in children. (There is a remote possibility of a protamine reaction in this setting, which may vary from mild hypotension to anaphylaxis. See Section 2, "Whole Body Perfusion during Cardiopulmonary Bypass," in Chapter 2.)

Use of antifibrinolytic agents in the intensive care unit is controversial. Tranexamic acid, epsilon-aminocaproic acid (EACA), and aprotinin are each more effective when given during CPB than after (see Chapter 2). Transfusion therapies include cryoprecipitate, FFP, platelets, and whole blood or packed red blood cells (RBC). Each institution may establish different thresholds for transfusion. As an example, whole blood or packed RBCs could be given for hemoglobin under 7.0 g · 100 mL^{-1}, hematocrit under 20%, or S$\bar{v}$O$_2$ under 65%. This threshold might be raised to hemoglobin under 10.0 g · 100 mL^{-1} in severely ill or elderly patients or in those with unstable hemodynamics, because they are unlikely to increase cardiac output in response to acute anemia.

Transfusion of platelets should be considered for patients with a platelet count under 70,000 and excessive bleeding. Similarly, FFP should be administered for an INR (International Normalized Ratio) greater than 1.5 to 1.7 in patients with excessive bleeding and a history of warfarin treatment. Specific treatment with cryoprecipitate, FFP, or other components is indicated in the presence of a consumption coagulopathy as reflected by a fibrinogen level less than 200 mg · 100 mL^{-1}, a positive D-dimer assay, or the presence of fibrin degradation products.

There are strong reasons to limit or avoid transfusion of blood products in stable patients. The public, patients, and physicians have become reasonably aware of the possibility, although small, of disease transmission from transfusion. The current estimated likelihood of contamination with the human immunodeficiency virus (HIV) is 1 in 440,000 to 640,000 screened units of blood. Hepatitis B is estimated to be present in 1 per 63,000 units, and hepatitis C in 1 per 103,000 units.[L16,S29] With the routine use of polymerase chain reaction (PCR) testing or nucleic acid testing (NAT), the risk of contamination by HIV and hepatitis B will be even less. The possibility of bacterial contamination is probably slightly greater than the figures just mentioned. Hemolytic reactions occur infrequently and are not generally due to human error, but rather to a delayed reaction from previously undetectable antibody that is activated following a series of transfusions. Finally, the estimated cost for the patient of 1 unit of packed RBCs is U.S. $250 to $280, and efforts at cost control suggest prudence in transfusion will help to lower overall hospital costs.

IMMUNE SUBSYSTEM

Some have suggested that the immune subsystem is mildly depressed for several weeks after CPB. In general, however, specific immunologic responses (in contrast to general responses such as those expressed in the whole body inflammatory response) in nonsensitized patients are weak ones. Interleukin levels are increased after CPB,[M29] and some[H22] believe this to be responsible for the hyperthermia frequently present early after operation (see "Body Temperature" under Special Considerations after Cardiac Surgery in Section 2 of this chapter). In adult patients, the number of helper/inducer T-lymphocyte subsets (CD4+) is decreased after CPB and suppressor/cytotoxic T cells (CD8+) are elevated. This possible overall depression of the immune response can be modulated by pretreatment with indomethacin and thymopentin.[M29] Ultrafiltration, glucosteroids, or lymphocyte depletion may even further complicate the immune response by their salutary effects on the whole body inflammatory response.

SECTION 2
Special Considerations after Cardiac Surgery

FLUID, ELECTROLYTE, AND CALORIC INTAKE
Children and Adults

Because of the increase in extracellular fluid and total exchangeable sodium and the decrease in exchangeable potassium that develop during CPB, postoperative fluid administration early after cardiac operations should be precise. Based on pioneering work by Sturtz and colleagues,[S2] a standardized approach to fluid administration has been developed that meets the requirements. For approximately 48 hours after operation in children and adults, no sodium is administered, and minimal amounts of water (as 5% glucose in water) are given intravenously (see Appendix 5L). Larger amounts of water are disadvantageous because they result in higher urine volumes and an increased potassium loss if renal function is good, and fluid overload if renal function is impaired. A modest amount of potassium ($10 \text{ mEq} \cdot m^{-2} \cdot 24 \text{ h}^{-1}$) is given on the day of operation because large amounts generally are not needed in normally convalescing patients, despite the decrease in total exchangeable potassium; larger amounts simply escape in the urine.[B3] During the first three postoperative days, hypokalemia is not treated unless it becomes severe (serum potassium level less than $3.0 \text{ mEq} \cdot L^{-1}$). Exceptions to this are patients receiving digitalis preparations, in whom serum potassium is kept at $4.0 \text{ mEq} \cdot L^{-1}$ or more. In the presence of ventricular ectopic beats, the level is increased to 4.5 to $5.0 \text{ mEq} \cdot L^{-1}$.

Liquids are taken orally a few hours after extubation, and intravenous administration can then cease by the second postoperative day. Ability of the kidneys to excrete sodium may be impaired for some days after operation even in normally convalescing patients,[P2] so a diet low in sodium is needed until the patient's weight (measured daily) falls below preoperative level.

When extubation is delayed beyond the second postoperative day, an adequate caloric intake must be ensured. Once bowel sounds are present, caloric needs can be met through nasogastric tube feedings using an appropriate high-calorie formula. Rarely, intravenous hyperalimentation is required.

Neonates and Infants

In neonates and infants, more exacting management is required. Care is taken to avoid fluid overload from the solution used to keep the pressure-recording catheters patent. Because the infant's energy requirements are relatively large, 10% glucose is more appropriate than 5%. Small amounts of sodium are administered from the beginning, because of the requirements of infants; a special protocol that includes $250 \text{ mL} \cdot m^{-2} \cdot 24 \text{ h}^{-1}$ of a balanced salt solution is used (see Appendix 5L).

In infants, oral feeding is not begun until 8 hours after extubation. Small feedings of glucose water are then given every 4 hours; if well tolerated, an appropriate formula low in sodium is started after two or three feedings. Mothers who are breast-feeding may resume nursing their infant once he or she is strong enough. The infant must be picked up and held for the feedings, and burped thereafter. If the infant is too weak to suck, gavage feedings of the mother's milk are given through a nasogastric tube.

Gavage feedings are begun in any infant who has been intubated longer than 2 days. The fluid is placed in an open syringe or burette attached to the tube and allowed to run in slowly by gravity (see Appendix 5M). If gavage feeding is necessary for more than a few days, the baby's caloric and other metabolic needs must be calculated and a determined effort made to meet them. If this does not become possible within 48 to 72 hours, intravenous hyperalimentation is begun.

During the first 48 postoperative hours, *hypoglycemia* may develop, particularly in neonates and infants less than 3 months old. Therefore, blood glucose is routinely measured twice daily in these patients, and as a precaution against hypoglycemia, 10% dextrose in water is used in maintenance fluids (see Appendix 5L). When hypoglycemia (blood glucose level less than $80 \text{ mg} \cdot dL^{-1}$) occurs, 50 $\text{mg} \cdot \text{kg}^{-1}$ of glucose is given ($1 \text{ mL} \cdot \text{kg}^{-1}$ of 50% dextrose mixed with an equal amount of 5% glucose in water and administered intravenously over a 15-minute period). Blood glucose levels are measured 30 minutes later and at 4-hour intervals for 24 hours.

Special Problems

As indicated earlier, some *metabolic acidosis* (base deficit of $2 \text{ mEq} \cdot L^{-1}$ or greater) may be present during the early hours after cardiac surgery even when the patient is convalescing normally. It is left untreated if arterial pH is equal to or greater than 7.4 and $PaCO_2$ is equal to or greater than 30 mmHg. When $PaCO_2$ is less than 30 mmHg, the base deficit is treated before adjusting $PaCO_2$ appropriately upward. When pH is less than 7.4, the base deficit is treated (see Appendix 5N). However, if convalescence is otherwise normal, treatment is delayed for 4 to 8 hours in adults and for 2 to 4 hours in infants, by which time the base deficit may have cleared spontaneously. In infants particularly, it is best to avoid an additional sodium load whenever possible.

A mild *metabolic alkalosis* may be present 24 hours after operation in normally convalescing patients, probably related in part to the citrate load contained in the anticoagulant solution of the banked blood. Metabolic alkalosis is self-correcting under these circumstances and is not treated. When large amounts of homologous blood containing sodium citrate have been transfused, important metabolic alkalosis can occur. Metabolism of the citrate leaves bicarbonate as the only anion available to balance the sodium ions. This situation may be exacerbated after 2 to 4 days by the migration of hydrogen ions from the cells, because hydrogen ions are replaced by potassium ions, and serum potassium falls, sometimes precipitously, in association with potassium loss in the urine. Relatively large amounts of potassium chloride must be given under such circumstances (up to 200 mEq in 24 hours), but the dose should be titrated against 4-hourly serum potassium measurements. The alkalosis is associated with a fall in serum chloride and a compensatory rise in $PaCO_2$. Provided renal function is adequate, the situation will correct itself. If it continues to worsen, hydrochloric acid is given intravenously (see Appendix 5O).

BODY TEMPERATURE

The most frequently misunderstood phenomena after cardiac surgery are abnormalities in body temperature. Most normally convalescing patients are febrile for at least 4 to 5 days after operation, and in some the hyperthermia persists 2 weeks or longer[B1,D2,L1,W1] (Fig. 5-15). During this period, those unfamiliar with cardiac surgical patients frequently order numerous blood, sputum, and urine cultures; white blood cell (WBC) counts; and other special studies without any indication other than fever. The expense of

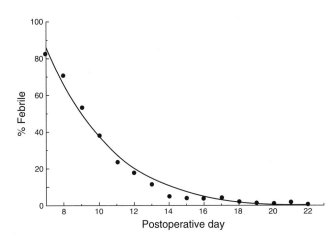

Figure 5-15   The proportion of patients febrile (temperature greater than 37.8°C) after the sixth postoperative day, starting with the group febrile on the sixth day. Note the continuation of fever in some patients to nearly 3 weeks after operation. (From Livelli and colleagues.[L1])

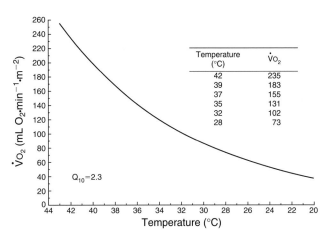

Figure 5-16   Relationship between resting whole body oxygen consumption ($\dot{V}O_2$) and body temperature. The nomogram depicts the Van't Hoff equation, in which the Q_{10} was considered to be 2.3. Confidence intervals are not placed around the point estimates, because of uncertainties as to the actual Q_{10} in this setting (see "Oxygen Consumption during Hypothermia" in Section 1 of Chapter 2 for a more complete discussion of this relation). Note the marked increase in $\dot{V}O_2$ with hyperthermia.

performing such studies is rarely justified, because the probability is low that the fever is anything other than a usual manifestation of the damaging effects of CPB.[W15] A number of hypotheses have been advanced as to the etiology of the fever, including the possibility that elevated levels of interleukin are responsible.

When the patient continues to be febrile at the time of hospital discharge, blood cultures are drawn, but discharge is allowed. Blood cultures in this setting are nearly always negative, but the patient and responsible physicians are warned that hyperthermia may continue or episodically disappear and appear. Fever may occasionally be accompanied by chills.[C13] Further blood cultures are prudent during these subsequent episodes, but the probability is high that infection is not present and that the fever will gradually disappear spontaneously.

By contrast, severe and increasing hyperthermia during the first 6 to 36 hours after operation is a potentially lethal complication. The hyperthermia does not result from infection, but its precise etiology is not known; it may relate in part to the hypermetabolic state that characterizes the early period after cardiac surgery with CPB.[C23,T5] Hyperthermia is often associated with low cardiac output and lowered blood flow through the skin, which impairs heat loss. Some simple measures may be initiated (see Appendix 5P), but in the face of a severe tendency toward hyperpyrexia, these measures may be ineffective in stopping the rise in body temperature. The condition is then an important emergency, and peritoneal dialysis is initiated, with the dialysate at room temperature or colder. The adequacy of cardiac output is maintained at as high a level as possible, because of the powerful effect of hyperthermia in increasing whole body oxygen consumption (Fig. 5-16).

Severe hyperthermia in this setting appears to have little relation to the syndrome of so-called malignant hyperthermia[N10]; the specific treatment for that syndrome has not been shown to be effective in patients with severe hyperpyrexia associated with CPB.

BLEEDING

In an era characterized by a high level of professional and public concern about infection (particularly with HIV and hepatitis), bleeding (and thus the need for transfusion) after cardiac surgery is a major concern. This influences not only management in the operating room but also early postoperative care. Special measures are important during and after cardiac surgery because of the effects of CPB on the factors that normally maintain hemostasis[L8] (see "Blood Conservation" under Special Situations and Controversies in Section 3 of Chapter 2). Use of the procedures described in Chapter 2 and appropriate care in the intensive care unit allow many patients to receive no homologous blood, lowering costs and decreasing morbidity.[B14,G15,M15,T7]

Chest drainage tubes must have been properly placed in the operating room for them to function well early postoperatively and keep the pericardial and pleural spaces free of blood (see "Positioning Chest Tubes" under Completing Cardiopulmonary Bypass in Section 3 of Chapter 2). During transport to the intensive care unit, chest tubes are connected to an underwater seal. Once the patient is in the unit, the tubes drain into an initially empty container in which a negative pressure of 10 to 15 mmHg is continuously maintained. Routine "stripping" of the chest tubes by nursing personnel is unnecessary and potentially dangerous, and the technique should be used only for clearing clots. Provisions are made for continuous precise measurement of the drainage from the chest tubes; this can be incorporated into an automated care system (see Section 5, Automated Care in the Intensive Care Unit). Reinfusion of the shed blood is useful in most circumstances (this again can be incorporated into the automated care system), but its lack of fibrinogen and high levels of fibrin degradation products must be recognized[G14,H15,S22,T6] (see Appendix 5Q and "Blood

■ **TABLE 5-7**   **Chest Drainage Criteria for Reoperation**

	Chest Drainage Indicating Reoperation				
Preoperative Weight (kg)	Hourly Amount (mL · h⁻¹)			Total Amount (ml)	
	No. of Successive Hours[a]			Hour No.[b]	
	1	2	3	4	5
5	70	60	50	120	130
6	70	60	50	130	155
7	70	60	50	150	180
8	90	70	50	175	200
9	90	80	60	195	230
10	100	90	65	220	260
12	130	100	80	260	300
14	150	120	90	300	360
16	170	140	100	350	400
18	195	150	120	390	460
20	200	175	130	450	520
25	270	220	160	540	650
30	325	260	195	650	770
35	380	300	230	760	900
40	430	350	260	800	1035
45	500	400	300	975	1150
50	500	400	300	1000	1200

[a] Reoperation is advisable if the patient has bled the amount indicated in any 1 hour (column 1), the lesser amount in column 2 during each of any 2 successive hours, or the still smaller amount (column 3) in each of any 3 successive hours.

[b] Reoperation is advisable if, by the end of the fourth or fifth postoperative hour, the patient has bled in total the amount indicated.

Conservation" Special Situations and Controversies in Section 3 of Chapter 2).

When chest drainage is excessive, prompt reoperation for bleeding is indicated. Use of specific, quantitative guidelines for reoperation (Table 5-7) results in relatively early reoperation for bleeding, and reoperation usually stops the excessive bleeding, even when no specific bleeding points are found. The advantages of this protocol include prevention of pericardial tamponade, minimization of the administration of homologous blood, and easier management of all subsystems. Nonetheless, cardiac surgeons must consider reoperations to be disadvantageous and devote their skill, time, and patience during the final stages of the operation to preventing it. These can reduce the occurrence of reoperations to nearly 0%.[N12]

When excessive bleeding continues after a reoperation at which no specific bleeding point is identified, prompt hematologic consultation and specific treatment are indicated. It is easy to regress into the indiscriminate, costly, and sometimes hazardous use of FFP and platelet concentrates, and additional doses of protamine. Optimally, specific management protocols are activated by this occurrence and include (1) repeated measurements of ACT and administration of additional protamine only when indicated (see "Heparinization and Later Protamine Administration" under Preparation for Cardiopulmonary Bypass in Section 3 of Chapter 2); (2) consideration and possibly measurement of excessive fibrinolysis, and use of either ε-aminocaproic acid or aprotinin, although these are best used prophylactically (see "Blood Conservation" under Special Situations and Controversies in Section 3 of Chapter 2); and (3) consideration of possible platelet dysfunction and/or depletion, and administration of platelet concentrates.[L8,W11]

CARDIAC TAMPONADE

Weitzman and colleagues found by echocardiographic study that 103 of 122 consecutive patients (84%; CL 80% to 88%) had pericardial effusions during recovery from cardiac surgery[W10]; a similar prevalence was found by Ikaheimo and colleagues.[13] *Large* pericardial effusions 4 to 10 days postoperatively develop in 30% of patients and are more common in patients in whom early postoperative bleeding was excessive[S12] or in cardiac transplant patients. Effusions reach their maximum size in most patients on about the tenth postoperative day, generally regressing spontaneously after that time.[13] Most pericardial effusions are asymptomatic and require no treatment.

Cardiac tamponade develops in only about 1% of patients with pericardial fluid.[13,W10] It occasionally develops in the intensive care unit, and prompt reoperation is required (see "Acute Cardiac Tamponade" under Causes of Acute Dysfunction [Low Cardiac Output] after Cardiac Surgery in Section 1).

Delayed cardiac tamponade may develop several days to several weeks after the patient leaves the operating room. Although delayed tamponade is uncommon, it is more common among patients being treated with anticoagulants. It also may have a higher prevalence when small incisions are utilized. If unrecognized, delayed tamponade can cause serious morbidity and mortality.[E2,H4,H5,M1] Clinical signs and symptoms may be subtle, but one or more of the following are usually present: progressive and unexplained weakness and lethargy; progressive dyspnea on exertion or orthopnea; unexplained hepatomegaly, ascites, or peripheral edema; elevated jugular venous pressure; pulsus paradoxus; widening of the cardiac silhouette on chest radiography; and unexplained prerenal azotemia.[K2] A chest radiograph (which should be taken routinely the day before hospital discharge or the seventh postoperative day, whichever comes first) usually shows enlargement of the cardiac silhouette before symptoms appear. Cardiac tamponade may, however, not become apparent until as late as 4 months after operation.[O2]

Treatment consists of pericardial decompression, by either pericardiocentesis or surgical drainage. Drainage is generally effected under local anesthesia through a 2-cm reopening of the incision just below the xiphoid process and aspiration of the fluid with an ordinary surgical sucker.[H6] A chest tube generally is not required.

INFECTION
Prevalence

Fortunately, important wound complications are uncommon after cardiac surgery. These complications are usually in the form of mediastinitis and sternal dehiscence. In a prospective study by Breyer and colleagues, prevalence was 0.8%,[B8] but it has been reported to be 1.5% by Culliford and colleagues and as high as 8% when bilateral internal mammary artery to coronary artery bypass grafting is performed.[C11] Reported mortality after this complication varies widely, from 6% to 70%.[C22] With early effective treatment, it is 5% to 10%.[D6]

Although edema and some hematoma formation are common in a leg from which a saphenous vein has been removed, infection occurs infrequently (1% to 2% of cases).[W16]

Risk Factors

Imperfect aseptic technique in the operating room is the basic cause of infected median sternotomy wounds. An undrained retrosternal hematoma is an incremental risk factor.[C11] This is one reason for leaving the pericardium open as a routine after cardiac operations; retrosternal bleeding falls into the pericardial space and is aspirated by the pericardial drainage tubes. Prolonged operative time is also a risk factor for development of mediastinal infections.[E9,W16] Inaccurate and insecure sternal closure increases the incidence of important sternal infections.[S11] Reoperation for bleeding is not a risk factor.

Obesity is clearly a risk factor for infection in the median sternotomy wound.[W16] The combination of diabetes, obesity, and harvesting of both internal mammary arteries has increased the prevalence of wound infections.[K13] Chronic obstructive lung disease predisposes to sternal dehiscence and infection. Male gender is a risk factor, probably related to the common practice of shaving the patient the day before operation when hair is present.

Prolonged mechanical ventilation after operation also increases the risk of infection in the median sternotomy.[N9] Corticosteroids greatly increase the risk of sternal wound infection. These drugs must therefore be discontinued completely or reduced to the lowest possible dose for several weeks (ideally, six or more) before operation. For similar reasons, in patients for whom renal transplant surgery is a planned part of management, the cardiac operation should be performed first, so that corticosteroids are not used postoperatively.

Prevention

A precise aseptic technique by the surgical, anesthetic, and perfusionist team is an essential part of the prophylaxis against infection in open cardiac operations. The many people involved and the length and complexity of the operations make bacterial contamination more likely than in shorter and simpler procedures. It has been shown clearly that control of the surgical and intensive care unit environment and awareness of the problem among personnel importantly reduce the prevalence of infection.[F11] Preoperative shaving should be done immediately before the operation, if at all.[F3]

Infection inside or around the heart, particularly when prostheses have been used, is a major threat to the patient's life. Therefore, prophylactic antibiotic therapy is recommended for cardiac operations.[F2,M2] Adequate blood levels of antibiotics should be present during operation and while any intravascular or endotracheal device is in place.[B6] Administration is therefore commenced at induction of anesthesia, an additional dose is given before CPB, and a dose is given immediately after CPB. An appropriate intermittent dosage schedule is continued through the second postoperative day or 24 hours after removal of the last intravascular or endotracheal device.[B6] The drug and dosage vary according to the prevalence of organisms and their susceptibility.

For many reasons, including to minimize the risk of infection, all intravascular and endotracheal devices should be removed as early postoperatively as possible. Infection is also minimized by simplifying postoperative care, early transfer out of the intensive care unit, early ambulation and oral alimentation, and early hospital discharge.

Treatment

Occasionally a small, localized, subcutaneous collection of serum or necrotic fat may suggest a wound infection when in fact none is present. These minor complications occur in about 2% of patients.[B8] Such collections should be left alone until it becomes clear that a wound infection is present. Even when a small amount of frank pus drains from the wound, mediastinitis should not be assumed to be present unless the sternum has become unstable, a retrosternal collection of fluid is demonstrated by CT, or drainage can be shown to be coming through the sternum from the retrosternal area. Even sternal dehiscence is not unequivocally diagnostic of infection; occasionally the dehiscence is sterile.

Unusual fever and malaise, sternal tenderness, and persistent, severe central chest pain not relieved by usual analgesics suggest the possibility of an important sternotomy infection despite the absence of obvious inflammatory changes in the skin. Under these circumstances the wound is examined twice daily for evidence of sternal instability or drainage coming through the sternum, and repeated blood and wound cultures are taken. Antibiotics are generally not begun until infection is confirmed, and they should be specific for the organisms involved.

Diagnosis of an infected wound should be made before there is extensive breakdown of the wound skin edges. CT scans may be helpful and should be obtained when diagnosis is uncertain, but it must be remembered that at least edema and some hemorrhage in the anterior mediastinum are usually present in normally convalescing patients and are visible on CT. However, the diagnosis through CT scanning of retrosternal fluid with air pockets or sternal disruption is usually indicative of mediastinitis.[K5]

As soon as the diagnosis of an infected median sternotomy incision is made, the patient is returned to the operating room and anesthetized, and a formal operation is undertaken.[S13] The entire median sternotomy incision is reopened, and all the sternal wires, other suture material, and necrotic tissue are removed. Usually, the infection is most marked immediately in front of and behind the sternum, and minimal around the heart itself. In this situation, although a few small fragments of sternum may be removed, extensive debridement of the sternum is not performed. The wound is thoroughly irrigated first with warm saline solution and then with dilute Betadine (povidone–iodine) solution. Two small (No. 16 French) chest tubes are left anteriorly for the postoperative continuous infusion of dilute povidone–iodine or antibiotic solution, and two larger tubes (No. 20 or 24 French) are left posteriorly for aspiration of fluid. Generally, the sternum is closed by rewiring, and the tissues anterior to it, including the skin, are closed en bloc by vertical mattress sutures.

The wound is irrigated continuously with 1 to 2 $mL \cdot kg^{-1} \cdot h^{-1}$ of dilute (0.5%) povidone–iodine or antibiotic solution through the anterior tubes, and suction is continuously applied to the dependent tubes.[T2] Full-strength povidone–iodine must be avoided because it injures tissue.[K6] When an antibiotic solution is used for irrigation, the level of the agent in the solution should be the same as the level in blood during maximal parenteral treatment. An input–output chart must be maintained. If the balance becomes positive, infusion is stopped until the fluid is recovered. Irrigations are not effective after 3 to 4 days, because by then the tubes have become sequestered from the retrosternal space. They are therefore removed at that time.

If the infection is extensive, more rapid recovery occurs when the wound is closed with musculocutaneous flaps[J3,J5,P7] or, when needed, omental transfer,[H20,S3] after debridement. Generally, it is prudent to perform this with the plastic surgeon, Rarely, the infection is so extensive that the wound is left open 3 to 5 days, with a bulky dressing and drainage tubes, and then the closure accomplished.[J4] These techniques are useful in infants and children as well as adults.[S6] With these protocols, most patients survive this potentially lethal complication and experience good long-term functional results.[B7,K14]

CHYLOTHORAX

Effused chyle may be present in the thoracic cavity after repair of coarctation of the aorta; after placement of Blalock–Taussig or, less frequently, polytetrafluoroethylene (PTFE) interposition shunts; or, rarely, after repair of patent ductus arteriosus.[C8,H10] In such instances, chylothorax probably results from cutting large tributaries of the thoracic duct or, less frequently, from injury to the thoracic duct itself. More complex and difficult to manage are the chylothoraces (and, on occasion, the pericardial accumulations of chyle with tamponade) that follow operations through a median sternotomy, such as the venous switch procedures for transposition of the great arteries, superior vena cava–right pulmonary artery anastomoses, and the Fontan procedure. The chylothorax probably results from the combination of inevitable transection of small lymph channels (probably in the thymus gland) and elevation of superior vena caval pressure that follows these procedures.

Chylothorax may develop immediately after operation, in which case it may not be recognized initially, because the fluid may appear to be serous. In most such cases, chylous drainage subsides spontaneously, and continuation of effective tube drainage is all that is necessary. However, chylothorax may not develop for a week or more. In that case, needle aspirations repeated every 3 to 4 days usually constitute adequate treatment. Late-appearing chylothoraces after closed operations are particularly likely to subside without operation, and the aspirations can be continued on an outpatient basis.

In early-appearing and persistently massive chylothorax, such as may occur after open cardiac operations, the outlook with conservative treatment is less favorable. Malnutrition resistant to therapy rapidly develops. When the chylothorax is a complication of the Fontan operation, its management is part of the overall management of the patient (see Chapter 27).

When chylothorax has developed as a complication of an operation performed through a lateral thoracotomy, surgical intervention is indicated if such drainage persists for more than about 7 days. The hemithorax in which the chyle is accumulating is entered through a posterolateral thoracotomy incision. The chylous leakage is sometimes easily seen and is oversewn. Unfortunately, the source is often not found, and watertight oversewing is not always possible. Under such circumstances, the thoracic duct can be sought behind the esophagus; if identified, it is doubly ligated, and this usually solves the problem. Even if these procedures are apparently successful, and certainly if they cannot be accomplished, the pleural space is scarified, and three properly placed intrapleural tubes are left for at least 96 hours, to ensure that the lung remains expanded and becomes adherent to the chest wall. Fibrin glue placed on the parietal pleura may enhance adherence.[S7] A good result is usually obtained from a combination of these maneuvers.

Rarely, after cardiac operations other than the Fontan operation, chyle accumulates in the pericardial space, with or without chylothorax. This problem was first reported after operations with CPB by Thomas and McGoon[T3] and has subsequently been reported by others. It has been reported after the Waterston anastomosis,[H11,J1] in which, of course, the pericardium is opened. It has also been reported after a Blalock–Taussig shunt in which the pericardium was not opened.[F4] This is a difficult problem, and initial management consists of wide and prompt operative drainage of the pericardium into the pleural spaces by making large pericardial windows and then draining both pleural spaces with chest tubes. Following this, the measures just described are used.

Careful attention to the nutrition of the patient is important during the period of chylous drainage, but special diets designed to minimize the drainage are usually not helpful. Fortunately, chylothoraces have never been reported to become infected.

POSTPERFUSION AND POSTCARDIOTOMY SYNDROMES

Postperfusion syndromes are complex and not yet fully understood. Whether they are totally attributable to the body's response to the damaging effects of CPB (see Chapter 2, Section 2) or have multiple etiologies is not certain.

A cytomegalic postperfusion syndrome has been described that consists of an infection with cytomegalic virus transmitted in homologous blood.[W7] The larger the volume of blood used, the greater the chance of infection.[C7] This infection produces a moderate pyrexia, beginning at about the end of the first week, associated with a "flulike illness," with the patient complaining of weakness, malaise, muscle pains, and sweating. The differential white blood count shows lymphocytosis and atypical mononuclear cells. The disease can be confirmed by demonstrating a rise in complement-fixing special antibody, and the virus can be isolated from the urine, although this is technically difficult. The Paul-Bunnell test is negative, excluding infectious mononucleosis (which can present an identical clinical picture) as a possible diagnosis. Although fever and symptoms usually persist for about 2 weeks, the disease is self-limiting, and no treatment is required. Depression is a common sequel.

The postcommissurotomy syndrome was described by Soloff and colleagues in 1953, when it was noted to follow closed mitral valve surgery.[S40] Although they interpreted the syndrome as reactivation of rheumatic fever, subsequently it became clear that this syndrome was not related to rheumatic fever and could occur after any operation that involved opening the pericardium, hence the name *post-pericardiotomy syndrome*,[11] also called the *postcardiotomy syndrome.* When Ito and colleagues coined the term *post-pericardiotomy syndrome,* they suggested that the syndrome was due to an immunologic reaction to damaged autologous tissue in the pericardial cavity.[11] Subsequent work at the same institution[E6-E8] has confirmed an "auto-immune theory" of etiology. Apparently, heart-reactive antibodies appear in significant titers in most patients undergoing cardiac surgery, but the titer is much higher in patients who develop this syndrome.[E6,E7]

Whether there are single or multiple etiologies, it is a fact that in many patients, symptoms appear a few weeks to a few months after cardiac operations. Nishimura and colleagues found the median postoperative time of onset to be 4 weeks.[N4] The most striking symptom is chest pain, both a central ache from pericarditis and severe pain from pleuritis. There may be no associated fever, but pericardial and pleural friction rubs are usually present and, often, pericardial and pleural effusions. These are usually minor but may be major, and delayed pericardial tamponade can occur. There are no specific changes in the formed blood elements. Although the disease is self-limiting, its duration is highly variable, with a median of 22 days and a range of 2 to 100 days in the study by Nishimura and colleagues.[N4] Recurrences are not uncommon, appearing in 21% of patients in the Mayo Clinic series.[N4] In some of these patients, recurrence was as long as 30 months after a previous episode. The syndrome usually recurs should reoperation be required.

The pain and effusions are often relieved by bed rest and aspirin or nonsteroidal antiinflammatory drugs. Although these symptoms are quickly resolved by prednisone, steroids should be avoided whenever possible because of their side effects. However, when symptoms persist, and once the diagnosis is secure and infection has been excluded, prednisone may be given initially in high dosage (40 mg · day^{-1}), gradually reduced, and completely discontinued within 4 to 8 weeks. Subsequent courses may be necessary.

SECTION 3
General Care of Children and Adults

The general management of older children and adults after cardiac surgery, in the absence of specific complications, is relatively simple. This section describes general aspects of care, leaving many of the details and documentation to the preceding discussions of the subsystems.

Patients leave the operating room with an arterial catheter in place and, optimally, pressure-monitoring catheters in the left and right atria and in the pulmonary trunk introduced by way of the right ventricle. One or more routes of access to large central veins are in place. The risks associated with these devices are extremely low, but care is necessary in placing them, caring for them, and removing them. Proper placement of devices (see "Completing Operation" and "Left Atrial Pressure Monitoring" in Section 3

of Chapter 2) is key to the prevention of bleeding intraoperatively or at the time of their removal. Infection is a potential risk, but only 1.5% of such catheters have positive cultures when removed postoperatively.[D8] Use of antibiotic or antiseptic gels around the site of emergence of such catheters is nonetheless a prudent precaution. Sterile technique in their management is essential.[D8]

Patients routinely come to the intensive care unit intubated and still anesthetized and with a nasogastric tube in place. They are attached to a ventilator (usually a volume-controlled one), as described in "Management and Treatment" under Pulmonary Subsystem in Section 1. Fluids to be administered until 7 AM of postoperative day 1 (the day after operation) are calculated ("calculated fluids"), and these are begun as described in "Fluid, Electrolyte, and Caloric Intake" in Section 2. The urinary catheter, placed in the operating room (usually a typical Foley catheter, although at times a suprapubic catheter), is connected to a drainage system that permits hourly urine flow to be measured conveniently. The chest tubes are attached to a container in which there is a negative pressure of about 15 mmHg. Arrangements are made for measuring the chest drainage at 5-minute intervals.

Many adult patients who are convalescing normally have systemic hypertension, at least in the early period after operation. Even when cardiac performance is good, prudence dictates controlling this hypertensive tendency. This is usually done with continuous infusion of nitroprusside (see Appendix 5A). If the hypertensive state continues, an oral hypertensive agent is usually started at the time of transfer out of the intensive care unit. The dosage should be decreased, at least temporarily, at the time of hospital discharge, as symptomatic arterial hypotension may otherwise develop. Finally, patients with impaired ventricular function and reasonable renal function may benefit from the addition of afterload reducing agents such as ACE inhibitors and Ca^{2+} channel blocking agents. This may ultimately positively affect ventricular remodeling and benefit cardiac performance.

Generally the chest tube drainage is reinfused into the patient by an automated system. The system may be "instructed" as to the level of left (or right) atrial pressure above which automatic reinfusion of shed blood is not to be performed (see Appendix 5B). When this limit is not violated, the system automatically reinfuses the chest tube drainage at a prescribed rate. The automatic chest tube drainage reinfusion is stopped 6 to 12 hours after the patient comes to the intensive care unit, at the direction of the surgeon or another responsible individual. At times the infusion of the shed blood appears to perpetuate a bleeding tendency; in this circumstance the reinfusion is promptly discontinued.

When chest tube drainage is sufficiently small that reoperation will clearly not be indicated, and when all subsystems give evidence of functioning well, consideration is given to extubation of the patient. If this cannot be safely accomplished by early evening, sedation is administered, and no attempt is made to determine whether the patient can be extubated until early the next morning. However, sedation is minimized after about 2 AM, and at about 5 AM (or at another early, convenient time) the protocol that may lead to extubation is again activated. Generally, patients can be extubated either on the day of operation or the following morning. In concert with the anesthesiologist, many operations in adults and children utilizing CPB can be conducted using short-acting drugs that allow extubation within 1 to 4 hours following transfer to the intensive care unit. It is thought that this shortens stay in the unit and decreases overall cost.

The nasogastric tube is removed just before extubation, and after extubation the head of the bed is elevated to about 30°. Deep breathing exercises and spontaneous coughing are encouraged, and chest vibration is carried out on a regular basis. Sips of water are allowed, as well as other clear liquids, but no effort is made to attain a prescribed fluid intake by mouth, the intravenous route being relied on for another 24 hours. In children the urinary catheter may be removed, but in many of them and in adults it can remain in place another day.

Chest tubes are usually removed early on the morning of the first postoperative day, as appreciable chest drainage has usually ceased by about midnight of the day of operation. When chest tubes are in the pleural space, the lower posterior tubes are removed first, and those in the upper and anterior parts of the thorax a few minutes to a few hours thereafter. This sequence allows for evacuation of air, which may have been introduced with removal of the posterior tubes. Often it is most appropriate to remove the chest tubes before extubating the patient, but this is not necessary. The intracardiac monitoring devices generally may be removed on the morning after operation in older children and adults. It is advantageous but not necessary that they be removed before removing the chest tubes. In neonates and young infants, monitoring devices should be removed before the chest tubes, and this is usually not on the first day postoperatively.

After extubating the patient and removing the intracardiac catheters and chest tubes, a final portable chest radiograph is obtained. If this is satisfactory, the arterial catheter is removed and the patient transferred either to the pediatric cardiac surgical unit or the adult cardiac surgical unit for continuation of convalescence. If the urinary catheter is still in place on the morning of postoperative day 2, it is removed; when a suprapubic catheter is used, the patient's ability to void can be tested before removing the catheter. When normal convalescence to this point is confirmed, all intravenous catheters are removed. Patients are urged to ambulate and to begin to care for themselves as much as possible.

When progress continues to be satisfactory, the patient is generally discharged from the hospital on the fifth, sixth, or seventh postoperative day; however, some institutions manage some adult patients in a highly satisfactory fashion by discharging them on the third or fourth postoperative day.[K17] Early hospital discharge implies daily follow-up in an outpatient facility or by a responsible physician for at least 2 to 3 more days.[K17] A final chest radiograph and electrocardiogram are obtained in the outpatient facility. The appropriateness of all medications and postoperative advice is ascertained at that time, and the patient is carefully instructed as to these matters. All information is conveyed to the patient's general physician or cardiologist or pediatric cardiologist, who then assumes responsibility for the patient.

At discharge, children may still be somewhat withdrawn and ill at ease, even with parents. Every effort is made to help the parents understand the normality of this situation, and they are advised of ways in which the child's return to an entirely normal relation with them can be expedited.

A program of daily exercise should be started as soon as the patient leaves the hospital and should emphasize regular walking for progressively longer periods. Patients who were active and gainfully employed before operation are urged to return to full activity (and employment in the case of adults) as soon as possible and, except under unusual circumstances, no later than 2 to 3 months after the procedure.

SECTION 4
General Care of Neonates and Infants

Neonates and infants, and some small young children, present problems of postoperative care that differ in some ways from those of adults. The principles of subsystem and overall care remain the same, but the internal milieu of even normal neonates and infants is different in some respects from that of adults. The cardiac operation has generally been more urgently indicated, and therefore these young patients often have more preoperative derangement and require more extensive operations. The cardiac reserve of neonates and infants is often less than that of adults after cardiac surgery because of the nature and seriousness of their preoperative cardiac condition. Their small airways are more apt to be suddenly obstructed by secretions. They are subject to special problems, such as episodes of pulmonary arterial hypertensive crises. Serum potassium level rises much more rapidly during oliguria in small patients than it does in older children and adults. These considerations do not necessarily indicate that very young age per se is a risk factor for death after cardiac surgery; they do indicate that special attention must be given to them. As in Section 3, we provide the general aspects of postoperative care of neonates and infants here, with details presented in the discussions of the various subsystems.

If the endotracheal tube has not been inserted through the nose initially, a nasotracheal tube may be substituted for the orotracheal tube before the patient leaves the operating room. A urinary catheter, intracardiac recording devices, epicardial myocardial wires, and intravenous access to large central veins are in place when the patient leaves the operating room, just as in adults. Intravenous access in the caval or internal jugular veins is generally avoided in patients having cavopulmonary connections, because of the risk of thrombosis. In the intensive care unit, the patient is placed on a ventilator specifically designed for small patients. Often, 2.5 to 5 $\mu g \cdot kg^{-1} \cdot min^{-1}$ of dopamine is infused, even in patients convalescing normally, and this is generally continued until the morning of postoperative day 1.

Because measuring devices and infusion of medications require some fluid, and because it is desirable to limit the total fluid intake in neonates and infants just as it is in adults, all continuously infused medications are mixed in sufficient concentration that the infusion rate does not exceed 2 to 3 $mL \cdot h^{-1}$, the minimal rate at which reasonably accurate infusions can be given. No "calculated fluids" are planned for the day of operation, and this can be reconsidered early on the morning of postoperative day 1. Calculations are made as to the amount of fluid administered not only by the intravenous route but also in flushing the pressure measuring devices, and at 7 AM of postoperative day 1 consideration is given to beginning the administration of "calculated fluids" or of continuing without them (see Appendix 5L).

Once the patient is settled on the ventilator, the status of his anesthetic and sedating medication is assessed. The goal, in general, is to keep the patient paralyzed and sedated at least until the morning of postoperative day 1. For paralysis, appropriate doses of pancuronium (or a comparable agent) are administered intravenously. This is insufficient to overcome many possibly deleterious reflexes. Therefore, fentanyl is also given as a continuous infusion of about 10 $\mu g \cdot kg^{-1} \cdot h^{-1}$, and at times at the increased dose of 15 to 25 $\mu g \cdot kg^{-1} \cdot h^{-1}$, not only for sedation but also for control of sympathetic activity.[H16,H17] Particularly when the nasotracheal tube is suctioned, the patient must be under the influence of fentanyl.[H14] Ventilation is arranged to keep arterial $PaCO_2$ at about 30 mmHg, arterial PaO_2 above 120 mmHg, and, if possible, pH at 7.45 or higher. This minimizes the tendency for pulmonary vascular resistance to rise paroxysmally (see "Pulmonary Hypertensive Crises" under Pulmonary Subsystem in Section 1).

We recommend irrigating the endotracheal tube with saline and suctioning every 2 hours, although some who do not use fentanyl favor no suctioning of the endotracheal tube. Whatever the policy, it must be recognized that this is a potentially hazardous procedure, and it should be undertaken only by skilled nurses with adequate backup should an emergency develop during or within a few minutes after suctioning.

Early on the morning of postoperative day 1, consideration is given to extubating the patient. If all subsystems appear to be functioning satisfactorily, the protocol leading to extubation is begun. A dose of dexamethasone of 0.3 $mg \cdot kg^{-1}$ is administered about 1 hour before extubation, for its presumed effect in minimizing laryngeal edema, and then 0.1 $mg \cdot kg^{-1}$ is given 2 hours later and a second dose 2 hours thereafter. Then, if the patient is awake and active, extubation is accomplished. After extubation the baby is maintained in a humidified, oxygen-enriched environment for at least another 24 hours in the intensive care unit, although care is taken to avoid excessively high PaO_2.

If all subsystems are not functioning well on the morning after operation, there should be no hesitancy to continue control of ventilation as well as paralysis and sedation for another 24 hours. However, about 70% of normally convalescing neonates and small infants can be extubated the morning after operation and the remainder usually on the morning of postoperative day 2.

Following extubation and the passage of a few hours, oral feedings can be started. For the feedings, the patient is held at least in a semi-upright position, observing the usual precautions necessary in feeding small babies (see Appendix 5M). Neonates and young infants have little nutritional reserve. When oral intake is not possible on postoperative day 1 or 2, nasogastric tube feeding is begun. If this is not promptly effective, intravenous hyperalimentation is begun (see "Fluid, Electrolyte, and Caloric Intake" in Section 2).

Intracardiac catheters should *not* be removed before postoperative day 2, to avoid bleeding after their removal. It is prudent but not mandatory to leave all chest tubes in place until after intracardiac devices have been removed.

When convalescence is not normal for any reason, management is altered appropriately, generally as described in the earlier parts of this chapter.

A special situation is presented early postoperatively by neonates and young infants when the operation leaves pulmonary blood flow coming solely from a surgically created systemic–pulmonary artery shunt (see "Special Features of Postoperative Care" in Chapter 35). In these intubated patients, magnitude of pulmonary blood flow is largely determined by the relation of the systemic to pulmonary vascular resistance.[C24,R4] When pulmonary resistance is low, pulmonary blood flow tends to be excessive and systemic blood flow small; should pulmonary vascular resistance gradually or suddenly rise, pulmonary blood flow declines, sometimes rapidly, and hypoxia develops. In this setting, pulmonary vascular resistance is largely determined by the arterial $PaCO_2$ and arterial pH. Because metabolic acidosis is always undesirable, and at least a moderately high fractional concentration of oxygen in the inspired air is desirable, manipulation of $PaCO_2$ is the best method for manipulating pulmonary vascular resistance. When pulmonary blood flow appears to be too high and systemic blood flow too low, arterial $PaCO_2$ is deliberately elevated modestly (to 40 to 45 mmHg) to increase pulmonary vascular resistance, decrease pulmonary blood flow, and increase systemic blood flow. When pulmonary blood flow seems too low and hypoxia too prominent, pulmonary arteriolar resistance is lowered by lowering the arterial $PaCO_2$ appropriately, usually to 25 to 35 mmHg.

Alterations in arterial $PaCO_2$ are conveniently accomplished by altering the tidal volume and respiratory rate. The adjustments required are usually sufficiently small that they produce no change in other important variables. Alternatively, ventilatory variables are set so that arterial $PaCO_2$ is 25 to 30 mmHg; if, with this, pulmonary blood flow seems excessive and/or systemic blood flow too low, the $PaCO_2$ is increased by simply increasing the fractional concentration of carbon dioxide in the inspired air.

SECTION 5
Automated Care in the Intensive Care Unit

Because most treatment decisions in the intensive care unit are based on use of numerical data and an orderly set of rules and logic,[K3] automation can be used for making, displaying, and storing observations and for intervening in some situations via a closed-loop computer system. These concepts were described in 1968,[S1] but the bedside hardware and computers have been continuously modified. Computers can be cost effective, prevent rules-based errors (see "Human Error" in Chapter 6), serve as "cognitive prostheses" to simplify presentation of complex multidimensional data, and provide strategic decision support to the surgical faculty, house staff, and nurses. Although there are studies and opinions to the contrary,[E4] these reflect a difference in orientation and goals and, thus, a different method of using automated care.

The intensive care unit computer may do the following:

1. Using the patient's age, height, weight, and hemoglobin level, the computer calculates and prints out surgeon-specific preoperative orders, directions for assembly and priming the pump-oxygenator, and postoperative orders.

2. At designated intervals (for example, every 2 minutes), the computer can automatically measure, numerically display, and record systemic and pulmonary artery systolic, diastolic, and mean blood pressures; right and left atrial pressures; heart rate; chest tube drainage; urine flow; and temperature. Plots of these data can be displayed on command.

3. The computer, continually sensing drainage from the chest, automatically reinfuses all the shed blood and uses the desired atrial pressure limit to interrupt infusions when the limit is exceeded (see Appendix 5B).

4. Using computer logic and the rules described under "Bleeding" in Section 2, messages can be displayed suggesting reoperation.

5. Arterial blood gas and hemoglobin levels are stored and displayed. The base excess or deficit is calculated.

When metabolic acidosis is present, the recommended dose of bicarbonate is calculated using the rules and logic in Appendix 5N.

6. The appropriate concentration and drip rate of infusion of any inotropic agent can be calculated and displayed using the rules and logic in Appendix 5C.

7. The computer regulates the infusion of nitroprusside by a closed-loop system, having been programmed with the desired mean arterial blood pressure and other relevant information, using the rules and logic in Appendix 5A.[S1,S4,S5] Studies indicate that this method of continuously maintaining a desired blood pressure is more effective than manual methods in avoiding sudden under- or overdosage.

8. The type and amount of fluid to be given intravenously after surgery is calculated according to the rules and logic in Appendix 5J, and can be printed out.

9. The computer can generate surgeon-specific antibiotic orders, including dosages, accounting for the presence of drug allergies.

10. On request, the computer displays all recent data in a tabular or plotted form for review, with the time interval between measurements (e.g., 5 minutes, 15 minutes, 30 minutes, or 1 hour) being selected by the reviewer.

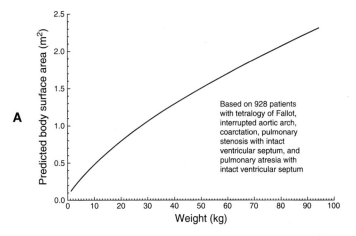

A

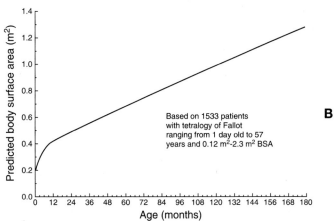

B

Figure 5-17   Nomograms of the relation between age or weight and predicted body surface area, for use in studies in which height or weight and height are not known. **A,** Relationship between weight and predicted body surface area. This is a nomogram of a nonlinear regression equation:

$$BSA(m^2) = exp[-2.3779 + 0.7389 \cdot weight(kg)^{.9728}]$$

where exp is *e*, the base of the natural logarithms.

The data are from 928 patients with tetralogy of Fallot, interrupted aortic arch, coarctation, pulmonary stenosis with intact ventricular septum, and pulmonary atresia with intact ventricular septum, in whom both weight and height were known and body surface area was calculated by the standard Boyd equation.[B22] Patients' ages ranged from a few hours to 57 years. **B,** Relationship between age and predicted body surface area:

$$BSA(m^2) = exp[-4.504 + 27.82 \cdot f(age)^3 - 45.51 \cdot f(age)^4 + 26.39 \cdot f(age)^5 - 5.238 \cdot f(age)^6]$$

where exp is *e*, the base of the natural logarithms (Ln), and f(age) = Ln(Ln[age(months) − 9]). The data are from 1533 patients with tetralogy of Fallot ranging from 1 day to 57 years of age and body surface areas ranging from 0.12 m^2 to 2.3 m^2.

SECTION 6

Body Surface Area

Because cardiac output has traditionally been normalized according to body surface area (as cardiac index), other variables related to cardiac surgical patients are optimally normalized in the same way. The computation of body surface area by the classic Boyd formula (a more general statement of the original DuBois formula) requires knowledge of height and weight, and height is not always available in clinical studies.[B22] A nomogram (see Fig. 5-17, A) can be used to estimate body surface area from weight.

In some situations, not even weight is available. In these circumstances, a nomogram (see Fig. 5-17, B) can be used to estimate body surface area based on age alone.

APPENDIXES

APPENDIX 5A

Protocol for Reducing Arterial Blood Pressure and Afterload

Sodium nitroprusside is administered intravenously (IV) continuously or intermittently as required. It acts directly on arterial and, to a lesser extent, venous smooth muscle, and thus decreases systemic and pulmonary vascular resistance and systemic venous tone. Its onset and end of action are immediate. The dose is 1 to 10 $\mu g \cdot kg^{-1} \cdot min^{-1}$ (doses larger than this are *not* used), regulated in most cases to maintain a mean arterial blood pressure 10% above the normal value for the patient's age. In patients with thick left ventricular walls or coronary artery disease, concern about coronary perfusion pressure makes a mean arterial blood pressure 20% above normal desirable (or 150 mmHg in adults). Fifty or 100 μg of sodium nitroprusside are dissolved in 150 mL of 5% glucose in water. The drug may be administered with a servo-pump using a closed-loop system[S1] under computer control[S4,S5] or with a slow-infusion pump. When nitroprusside is being administered, methods should be available for measuring blood thiocyanate levels, because values of >10 $g \cdot dL^{-1}$ are potentially toxic.[C6,P3] Toxicity is manifested by signs of intracellular suppression of oxygen consumption (elevation of mixed venous oxygen levels, narrowing of arterial–venous oxygen difference, and metabolic acidosis) and by anorexia, muscular spasms, disorientation, and convulsions. The toxicity is due largely to the formation of cyanide, the major metabolic product of sodium nitroprusside.[P3,C2] Toxicity is treated by IV infusion over 15 minutes of 150 $\mu g \cdot kg^{-1}$ of a 25% solution of sodium thiosulfate (10 $\mu g \cdot kg^{-1} \cdot min^{-1}$).

Nitroglycerin decreases venous tone but also decreases coronary resistance.[B2,C3,G1] It is therefore particularly useful when myocardial ischemia is present.[E1] Infusion rates of 0.5 to 3.0 $\mu g \cdot kg^{-1} \cdot min^{-1}$ are recommended.[K2] Nitroglycerin is absorbed into polyvinyl tubing used for IV infusion, and the concentration reaching the patient is less than planned until the tubing becomes saturated. Nitroglycerin is not as effective as nitroprusside in lowering arterial pressure.

A single-dose, longer-acting drug, *diazoxide,* is available although seldom used. The dose is 3 to 5 $\mu g \cdot kg^{-1}$. *Phentolamine* (Regitine) is another vasodilator used on occasion. It has an α-adrenergic receptor blocking effect, produces direct smooth muscle relaxation, and reduces pulmonary vascular resistance.[N1] Its recommended infusion rates are 1.5 to 2 $\mu g \cdot kg^{-1} \cdot min^{-1}$.[K2]

Phenoxybenzamine (Dibenzyline) is a noncompetitive blocker of α-receptors with a prolonged (12- to 24-hour) effect and a delayed (30- to 60-minute) onset. It acts on both arterial and venous vessels and has no important side effects. It is administered IV in a dose of 1 $mg \cdot kg^{-1}$, with the solution diluted in 20 to 50 mL of normal saline solution and infused slowly over about 15 minutes. The disadvantage of phenoxybenzamine is that its α-blocking effect is complete for at least 12 hours; thus, the drug is not used until the need for prolonged afterload reduction has been established by the patient's response to a sodium nitroprusside infusion over about 12 hours. Rather than continue infusing sodium nitroprusside at a relatively high rate, phenoxybenzamine may be substituted, and the dose repeated in 12 to 15 hours, when it is clear that its effect is wearing off. The *phosphodiesterase inhibitors* milrinone and amrinone may also produce a salutary vasodilatory effect.

APPENDIX 5B

Protocol for Optimizing Preload Using Atrial Pressure "Limit"

One of the determinants of cardiac output is resting sarcomere length, or filling volume, or preload. In most situations this is reflected by left atrial pressure (P_{LA}). To optimize postoperative cardiac performance, atrial pressure may be manipulated, often by infusion of blood or blood substitute. Elevation of P_{LA}, or volume infusion per se, has disadvantages; thus, the target P_{LA} must have an upper limit.

An avoidable or readily correctable cause of low or suboptimal cardiac output is relative or absolute hypovolemia. To treat or avoid inadequate preload, the concept of an atrial pressure limit is applicable. In practice, one must:

a. Judge or measure cardiac output
b. Decide on the most appropriate P_{LA} (or right atrial pressure, P_{RA})
c. Set an upper P_{LA} (or P_{RA}) limit
d. Design parameters to *guarantee* attainment of the desired goals, particularly adequate filling volume
e. Limit risk of overinfusion

In the operating room and intensive care unit, d) and e) are accomplished as follows:

1. A P_{LA} limit is selected to attain adequate cardiac output. (This limit is modified from case to case, and from time to time in any one case as necessary.)
2. Blood or a blood substitute is selected and infused to attain the desired P_{LA} limit. Of great importance is the fact that infusion is terminated by other parameters or limits. One of these is P_{LA}; others are either dependent variables or obligatory variables.

Dependent variables are

1. Accomplishment and persistence of a chosen cardiac output measured by thermodilution
2. Persistence of adequate cardiac output estimated by pulses, skin temperature, mentation, or urine flow
3. Achievement and maintenance of a predetermined level of systolic arterial blood pressure

Obligatory variables are

1. Maximum hourly infusion as a multiple of hourly chest drainage (e.g., 1×, 2×, or 3× measured chest drainage).
2. Increment for total infusion, based on body surface area (e.g., 250, 500, or 750 mL $\cdot m^{-2}$).

The physician's order with respect to P_{LA} therefore must have two parts:

1. The P_{LA} limit
2. The parameter by which the infusion to attain that limit is blocked. For example:

a. P_{LA} = 12 mmHg, arterial blood pressure (P_{AO}) ≤ 120 systolic
b. P_{LA} = 8 mmHg, infuse 250 mL $\cdot m^{-2}$
c. P_{LA} = 10 mmHg, infuse to limit of 2× chest drainage
d. P_{LA} = 18 mmHg, infuse for measured cardiac index (CI), ≥ 2.5 L $\cdot mm^{-1} \cdot m^{-2}$
e. P_{RA} = 16 mmHg, infuse to P_{AO} 100 systolic (e.g., following tetralogy repair).

APPENDIX 5C

Protocol for Infusion of Inotropic Agents

The rate of infusion is calculated and recorded in micrograms per kilogram body weight per minute ($\mu g \cdot kg^{-1} \cdot min^{-1}$). Using a microdrip apparatus, the number of drops per minute equals the number of milliliters per hour. The formula for milliliters per hour (drops per minute) as a function of infusion rate ($\mu g \cdot kg^{-1} \cdot min^{-1}$), body weight (kg), and concentration of catecholamine is

$$mL \cdot h^{-1} \text{ (or drops per minute)} = \frac{\text{Infusion rate } (\mu g \cdot kg^{-1} \cdot min^{-1}) \cdot \text{weight (kg)} \cdot 60}{\text{Concentration } (\mu g \cdot mL^{-1})}$$

The drug is diluted in 5% glucose and water, except in infants weighing less than 13 kg, for whom it is diluted in 10% glucose in water. A dilution is chosen that results in a drip rate of $3 \ mL \cdot h^{-1}$ or greater (drip rates lower than this cannot be managed with precision, and the line may clot), but lower than 20 to $30 \ mL \cdot h^{-1}$ in adults and lower than $10 \ mL \cdot h^{-1}$ in infants (to avoid excess fluid administration).

First, the rate of drug infusion is selected, and then the drip rate. The concentration of drug needed in the solution may be found by solving the equation above or with a nomogram (Fig. 5C-1) and boxes (Boxes 5C-1 and 5C-2).

For each drug, a "standard" rate of infusion based on past experience has been determined. Infusion rates are altered according to the hemodynamic state and response of the individual patient to the infusion. "Standard" rates of infusion should, however, be exceeded only under special circumstances.

The "standard" rates of infusion are

Dopamine	$10.0 \ \mu g \cdot kg^{-1} \cdot min^{-1}$
Dobutamine	$10.0 \ \mu g \cdot kg^{-1} \cdot min^{-1}$
Isoproterenol	$0.05 \ \mu g \cdot kg^{-1} \cdot min^{-1}$
Epinephrine	$0.1 \ \mu g \cdot kg^{-1} \cdot min^{-1}$
Norepinephrine	$0.1 \ \mu g \cdot kg^{-1} \cdot min^{-1}$

(The rate of administration of amrinone is described in "Treatment of Low Cardiac Output" under Cardiovascular Subsystem in Section 1.)

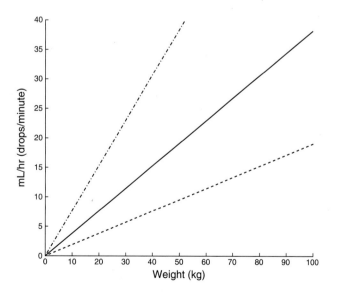

Figure 5C-1 Nomogram of drip rate (drops per minute) related to patient body weight for three different dose schedules ($\mu g \cdot kg^{-1} \cdot min^{-1}$) of inotropic agents. The desired drip rate is selected and the concentration of the drug and its dose schedule determined from Boxes 5C-1 or 5C-2.

BOX 5C-1 Representative Data for Dopamine and Dobutamine ^{a}

Adults and Children Weighing >13 kg:
1. Concentration 400 mg (10 mL) in 250 mL of 5% dextrose in water (5% glucose)
   a. - - - - - - - $5 \ \mu g \cdot kg^{-1} \cdot min^{-1}$
   b. —————— $10 \ \mu g \cdot kg^{-1} \cdot min^{-1}$ ("standard")
   c. - · - · - · - $20 \ \mu g \cdot kg^{-1} \cdot min^{-1}$
2. Concentration 800 mg (20 mL) in 250 mL of 5% dextrose in water (5% glucose)
   a. - - - - - - - $10 \ \mu g \cdot kg^{-1} \cdot min^{-1}$ ("standard")
   b. —————— $20 \ \mu g \cdot kg^{-1} \cdot min^{-1}$
   c. - · - · - · - $40 \ \mu g \cdot kg^{-1} \cdot min^{-1}$
3. Concentration 1600 mg (40 mL) in 250 mL of 5% dextrose in water (5% glucose)
   a. - - - - - - - $20 \ \mu g \cdot kg^{-1} \cdot min^{-1}$
   b. —————— $40 \ \mu g \cdot kg^{-1} \cdot min^{-1}$
   c. - · - · - · - not usually used

Infants and Small Children Weighing <13 kg:
1. Concentration 200 mg (5 mL) in 250 mL of 5% dextrose in water (10% glucose)
   a. - - - - - - - not usually used
   b. —————— $5 \ \mu g \cdot kg^{-1} \cdot min^{-1}$
   c. - · - · - · - $10 \ \mu g \cdot kg^{-1} \cdot min^{-1}$ ("standard")
2. Concentration 400 mg (10 mL) in 250 mL of 5% dextrose in water (10% glucose)
   See 1 under "Adults and children weighing >13 kg."

^{a} The dashed, solid, and dash-dot lines refer to the drip rate–body weight lines in Fig. 5C-1.

BOX 5C-2 Representative Data for Epinephrine and Norepinephrine ^{a}

Adults and Children Weighing >13 kg:
1. Concentration 4 mg in 250 mL (5% glucose)
   a. - - - - - - - $0.05 \ \mu g \cdot kg^{-1} \cdot min^{-1}$
   b. —————— $0.1 \ \mu g \cdot kg^{-1} \cdot min^{-1}$ ("standard")
   c. - · - · - · - $0.2 \ \mu g \cdot kg^{-1} \cdot min^{-1}$
2. Concentration 8 mg in 250 mL (5% glucose)
   a. - - - - - - - $0.1 \ \mu g \cdot kg^{-1} \cdot min^{-1}$ ("standard")
   b. —————— $0.2 \ \mu g \cdot kg^{-1} \cdot min^{-1}$
   c. - · - · - · - $0.4 \ \mu g \cdot kg^{-1} \cdot min^{-1}$

Infants and Small Children Weighing <13 kg:
1. Concentration 2 mg in 250 mL (10% glucose)
   a. - - - - - - - $0.025 \ \mu g \cdot kg^{-1} \cdot min^{-1}$ (not usually used)
   b. —————— $0.05 \ \mu g \cdot kg^{-1} \cdot min^{-1}$
   c. - · - · - · - $0.1 \ \mu g \cdot kg^{-1} \cdot min^{-1}$ ("standard")
2. Concentration 4 mg in 250 mL (10% glucose)
   See 1 under "Adults and children weighing >13 kg."

^{a} The dashed, solid, and dash-dot lines refer to the drip rate–body weight lines in Fig. 5C-1.

APPENDIX 5D

Protocol for Managing Some Aspects of Ventricular Electrical Instability

Early Interventions for Ventricular Electrical Instability
1. Give lidocaine as an IV bolus injection (the dose is $1 \ mg \cdot kg^{-1}$ for adults and children, although in adults the usual dose is 50 mg) if the arrhythmia is premature ventricular contraction (PVC) or ventricular tachycardia (VT) with a good hemodynamic state. If there is VT and reduction of cardiac output, use *immediate DC cardioversion* (100 and then 200 J).

2. Draw a blood sample for determination of serum K^+; when the result is available, treat hypokalemia (K^+ concentration <4.0 mEq $\cdot$ L^{-1}) if present:
   a. Administer 5 mEq K^+ as an IV bolus
   b. Administer 20 mEq K^+ in 50 mL of 5% glucose over 1 hour; then obtain repeat serum K^+ level measurement and repeat treatment until serum level is satisfactory (at least 3.5 mEq $\cdot$ L^{-1} and preferably 4.0 mEq $\cdot$ L^{-1})
   c. Double the IV maintenance K^+ dose
   d. Recheck serum K^+ level. If it is <4.0 mEq $\cdot$ L^{-1}, order oral K^+ supplement as 20% KCl, 10 mL twice a day in orange juice (60 mEq approximate daily dose).
3. If the ventricular rate is less than 80 to 90 beats/min, initiate pacing. If basic rhythm is sinus or atrioventricular (AV) junctional, use atrial pacing. When cardiac rhythm is other than sinus or AV junctional, or atrial pacing fails to result in 1:1 AV conduction, use ventricular pacing (with the ventricular wire electrode attached to negative pole of pacer). In the presence of second- or third-degree AV block, consider AV sequential pacing.

Interventions after Control of the Urgent Situation

1. If the arrhythmia recurs promptly or is not controlled by these simple measures, begin continuous IV lidocaine infusion in a dose of 20 to 50 μg $\cdot$ kg^{-1} $\cdot$ min^{-1}, or 0.02 to 0.05 mg $\cdot$ kg^{-1} $\cdot$ min^{-1}. To calculate the number of drops per minute of a solution of 2 g of lidocaine in 250 mL of solution

$$\text{Drops per minute} = \frac{\text{Dose} \cdot \text{weight (kg)} \cdot 60}{4}$$

The lidocaine level should be measured at 12 hours to prevent toxicity.
2. Additional measures to control ventricular arrhythmias:
   a. Procainamide 15 mg $\cdot$ kg^{-1} IV over 30 minutes (usually 600 mg IV can be given rapidly)
      i. Maintenance dose 500 mg IV q6h
      ii. Observe for hypotension and torsade de pointes
   b. Bretylium (a quaternary ammonium compound) 5 to 10 mg $\cdot$ kg^{-1} IV over 1 minute
      i. Maintenance dose 5 to 10 mg $\cdot$ kg^{-1} every 6 to 8 hours
   c. Amiodarone; initial loading dose 150 mg IV over 10 minutes
      i. Maintenance dose 0.5 mg $\cdot$ min^{-1} to approximately 1000 mg $\cdot$ 24 h^{-1}

APPENDIX 5E

Protocol for Acute Digitalization

Estimated Digitalizing Dose

An estimated digitalizing dose of digoxin provides a convenient guideline for the cardiac surgeon. The estimated dose of digoxin, when no digitalis has been given in the past 10 days, may be considered to be 0.9 mg $\cdot$ m^{-2} intravenously and 1.6 mg $\cdot$ m^{-2} orally. The digitalizing dose in infants may be considered 50 μg $\cdot$ kg^{-1} intravenously, and the maintenance dose 10 to 15 μg $\cdot$ kg^{-1} $\cdot$ day^{-1}.

Atrial Fibrillation

When the ventricular rate is at least 110 beats $\cdot$ min^{-1} and no contraindication to digitalis exists, *small doses of digoxin* are given by the following schedule until the ventricular rate is 90 to 110 beats $\cdot$ min^{-1}:
1. When the rate is between 110 and 120 beats $\cdot$ min^{-1}, give a dose of 0.15 mg intravenously (IV) for adults and 10% of the estimated digitalizing dose for children.
2. When the rate is 120 to 140 beats $\cdot$ min^{-1}, give an initial dose of 0.2 mg IV for adults and 15% of the estimated digitalizing dose for children.
3. When the rate exceeds 140 beats $\cdot$ min^{-1}, give an initial dose of 0.25 mg IV for adults and 20% of the estimated digitalizing dose for children.
4. Usually, several subsequent doses 2 to 3 hours apart are required, and the dose must be reassessed at each interval based on the ventricular rate.
5. When the ventricular rate is controlled, begin oral maintenance doses of digoxin 6 to 12 hours after the last IV dose (the usual oral

maintenance dose is 0.25 mg $\cdot$ day^{-1} for adults; for children, see section on sinus rhythm below).
When the ventricular rate is not controlled by the time the estimated digitalizing dose has been administered (which can occur in patients in atrial flutter-fibrillation or in those receiving catecholamines), further digoxin should be given only with caution to guard against the occurrence of digitalis toxicity before rate control is achieved. Additional measures (see "Atrial Arrhythmias" under Cardiac Arrhythmias in Section 1) are useful.

Sinus Rhythm

The digoxin dose cannot be titrated by heart rate, as in atrial fibrillation. Therefore, when digitalization is indicated, one third of the *estimated digitalizing dose of digoxin* is given, usually IV, and this dose is generally repeated 3 hours later. Six hours later, a maintenance schedule is begun, usually with one twelfth of the estimated digitalizing dose given twice daily. The serum digoxin level is measured daily for 2 days. The appropriate level is 1.5 to 2.0 μg $\cdot$ mL^{-1}.

Alternative Protocols for Acute Management of Postoperative Atrial Fibrillation

■ Digoxin (see Appendix 5D) has classically been recommended, but it may be slow to act (3 to 8 hours) and relatively ineffective at decreasing heart rate in postoperative patients with increased sympathetic activity. In the elderly or in the presence of compromised renal function, the therapeutic window is narrow and toxicity may occur.
■ In hemodynamically stable adult patients, intravenous verapamil, diltiazem, esmolol, propanolol, or amiodarone are effective alternative therapies:
   Verapamil: 5-10 mg IV as bolus; may repeat after 10-15 minutes
      Adverse effect: Infrequently hypotension, later increase of heart rate
   Diltiazem: 20 mg IV over 2 minutes, may repeat × 1
      Adverse effect: Infrequently hypotension
   Esmolol: 0.5 mg $\cdot$ kg^{-1} $\cdot$ min^{-1} IV infusion
      Adverse effect: hypotension, bronchospasm
   Propranolol: 0.05 mg $\cdot$ kg^{-1} or 5-mg bolus IV
      Adverse effect: Hypotension
   Amiodarone: 150 mg IV over 10 minutes
      Adverse effect: Rarely hypotension
■ Unstable hemodynamics
   DC cardioversion
   Amiodarone
■ Recurrent atrial fibrillation
   Procainamide 500-1000 mg p.o., 6-8 hours
   Sotalol: Initially 80 mg BID
■ Anticoagulation
   The prevalence of stroke attributable to postoperative atrial fibrillation is unknown. It seems justifiable to initiate anticoagulation if atrial fibrillation persists longer than 48 hours or is recurrent. In these instances, warfarin is recommended. If elective cardioversion is planned, intravenous heparin is recommended and is prescribed in therapeutic doses.

APPENDIX 5F

Protocol for Rapid Atrial Pacing via Atrial Wires

Rapid Atrial Pacing

The technique of rapid atrial pacing is applied to *atrial flutter*, defined as a general atrial rate of 250 to 350 beats $\cdot$ min^{-1}, with a constant beat-to-beat cycle length that *can be interrupted* by rapid atrial pacing. This is rarely possible in *atrial flutter-fibrillation*, a more rapid type of atrial flutter, with a rate >350 beats $\cdot$ min^{-1}, and is not possible in atrial fibrillation.

The electrocardiographic (ECG) limb leads are placed on the patient for monitoring, and the two atrial wires are connected to the rapid atrial pacer. Because the atrial pacing threshold is usually high during atrial flutter, output is set at 10 to 20 mA. Bipolar atrial pacing is used because the stimulus artifact then rarely distorts the ECG tracing, and the atrial complex in the ECG is clearly seen so that atrial capture can be verified.

A relatively slow pacing rate is used first, because occasionally, immediate one-to-one conduction occurs with rapid ventricular tachycardia, which is to be avoided. After this, there are several possible maneuvers for control of atrial flutter and its rapid ventricular response, as described by Waldo and MacLean.[W5]

Ramp technique

Atrial pacing is begun at a rate 10 beats · min^{-1} faster than the atrial flutter rate. The rate of atrial pacing is then gradually increased. When the typical negative atrial complex in lead II changes to a positive atrial complex, indicating capture by pacing, atrial pacing is either abruptly stopped or gradually slowed until the ventricular rate is considered satisfactory.

Constant rate technique

Pacing is initiated at a rate 10 beats · min^{-1} faster than the spontaneous atrial flutter rate. After pacing at this rate for about 30 seconds, pacing is either abruptly stopped or the pacing rate quickly slowed until the ventricular rate is considered satisfactory. If these maneuvers are unsuccessful in interrupting the atrial flutter, they are repeated, with the initial atrial pacing rate increased in increments of 10 beats · min^{-1}.

Continuous Rapid Atrial Pacing

When atrial flutter is interrupted by the procedures just described but recurs with unacceptable frequency, continuous atrial pacing at 400 to 600 beats · min^{-1} is used. This results in continuing atrial fibrillation with variable AV block. The ventricular rate can then be controlled by digoxin.

When premature atrial beats are continuous or recurrent despite pharmacologic treatment, continuous atrial pacing at about 200 to 230 beats · min^{-1} usually results in their suppression and a 2:1 AV conduction ratio with an acceptable ventricular rate.

APPENDIX 5G

Protocol for Control of Hemoconcentration

In children, occasionally, excessive capillary leakage may occur associated with elevation of hemoglobin levels, excessive temperature elevation, and a transient high cardiac output state, ultimately leading to metabolic acidosis.[S32]

If the hemoglobin level is ≥16 g · 100 mL^{-1} and there is evidence of plasma leakage from the intravascular space:
1. Give 20 mL · m^{-2} of 25% serum albumin in a syringe *slowly* (over 5 minutes) if left atrial pressure (P$_{LA}$) is <15 mmHg. If P$_{LA}$ is >15 mmHg, consider administering furosemide (Lasix) and then albumin.
2. Repeat hemoglobin measurement in 1 hour.
3. If hemoglobin measurement in step 2 is ≥16 g · 100 mL^{-1}, repeat steps 1 and 2.

APPENDIX 5H

Protocol for an Intubated Patient

1. The ventilator is used with its air heating and humidifying devices and the valves for intermittent mandatory ventilation and positive end-expiratory pressure (PEEP) functioning.
2. The patient has a well-positioned and well-secured orotracheal tube in place or, in infants and young children (for greater security and comfort) and adults in whom postoperative ventilation for more than 24 hours is likely, a well-positioned and well-secured nasotracheal tube in place (see Chapter 4).
3. Initially, the fractional concentration of oxygen (FIo$_2$) is set at 0.6, tidal volume (TV) at 12 to 20 mL · kg^{-1}, and intermittent mandatory ventilation (IMV) at 12 to 14 breaths · min^{-1} in adults, 20 to 25 breaths · min^{-1} in older children, 30 breaths/min in young children, and 30 to 40 breaths · min^{-1} in infants. End-inspiratory pressure should normally be <40 cm H$_2$O. In all situations, *visual, palpatory, and auscultatory observation* of the patient's chest must be used to confirm that TV is adequate for good air movement in and out of the lungs. These observations

must be made whenever the patient becomes restless or agitated or there is any other reason to suspect inadequate gas exchange. Except in patients with chronic obstructive lung disease and those in whom the Glenn or Fontan operation has been done, PEEP of 5 to 10 cm H$_2$O (4 cm H$_2$O in patients ≤4 years old) may be used.
4. When the patient is admitted to the ICU, baseline blood gas analysis is obtained and the ventilatory parameters are adjusted accordingly. Continuous monitoring of oxygen saturation by use of a digital infrared sensor is advisable in most patients. In adults, additional arterial blood gas analyses are not done routinely thereafter, unless there is a change in the clinical status of the patient. In neonates and children, more frequent arterial blood gas analyses are usually necessary.
5. A supine portable chest radiograph is obtained upon arrival in the intensive care unit and reviewed by a physician for placement of the tip of the endotracheal tube; the presence of pneumothorax, atelectasis, vascular congestion, or gastric distention; and the size of the mediastinal silhouette. The chest radiograph is routinely repeated the first postoperative morning.
6. Turning of the patient and sterile suctioning of the airway are performed each hour to clear retained secretions and minimize atelectasis. Suctioning is performed after hand bagging with 100% oxygen, hyperventilation for several breaths, and instillation of 1 to 5 mL of sterile saline solution down the endotracheal tube (see Section 4, "General Care of Neonates and Infants," for discussion of suctioning of the endotracheal tube in these patients). Suctioning is followed again by hand bagging with 100% oxygen. *The length of the endotracheal tube must be known,* so that the suctioning catheter can be passed with certainty beyond the tube into the trachea.
7. In patients without severe preoperative pulmonary dysfunction, criteria for extubation include the following:
   a. Patient awake and alert, indicating recovery from anesthesia and ability to protect his or her airway
   b. Satisfactory hemodynamic state
   c. Absence of important drainage from chest tubes
   d. Arterial Po$_2$ ≥ 70 mmHg or SaO$_2$ > 90% to 92% (in the absence of intracardiac right-to-left shunting) on intermittent mandatory ventilation (IMV) of 6 breaths · min^{-1} and FIo$_2$ of 0.40
   e. Spontaneous respiratory rate <25 breaths · min^{-1} in adults, <40 breaths · min^{-1} in young children, and <50 breaths · min^{-1} in infants
   f. Absence of increased work of breathing (use of accessory respiratory muscles)
   g. Normal PaCO$_2$ and pH (PaCO$_2$ may be somewhat elevated with a normal pH, if metabolic alkalosis is present)

APPENDIX 5I

Protocol for Oliguria

Indication

A urine output in the early postoperative period of <0.5 to 1.0 mL · kg^{-1} · h^{-1} in infants and children and <0.5 mL · kg^{-1} · h^{-1} (30 to 35 mL · h^{-1}) in adults.

Rationale

To reverse the nearly universal occurrence of fluid retention following CPB.

Treatment

1. Exclude low cardiac output as the cause of the oliguria.
2. Insert a urinary catheter if not already in place.
3. Administer a diuretic.
   a. Furosemide (Lasix): 1 mg · kg^{-1} for infants and children and 20 to 40 mg for adults administered intravenously (IV) as a bolus. Usually, no greater diuretic response is elicited with higher doses. However, doses of up to 180 to 240 mg may be necessary in patients with chronic heart failure, cirrhosis, and the nephrotic syndrome.
      i. The expected result is at least a doubling of the urine output over 2 to 3 hours.

ii. If the diuresis is inadequate, other diuretics may be used in adults.
b. Ethacrynic acid (Edecrin): 50 to 100 mg IV in 50 mL of solute over 30 minutes. (Ototoxicity occurs in 2% to 3% of patients.)
c. Bumetanide (Bumex): 0.5 to 2.0 mg IV over 1 to 2 minutes.
d. Torsemide (Demadex): 10 to 20 mg IV as a bolus.
e. A continuous infusion of the diuretics just mentioned may be safer and more effective in some patients. This is usually given after a bolus, if the diuretic effect is not sustained. Furosemide is given at an initial infusion rate of 20 mg $\cdot$ h^{-1}, increasing to 40 mg $\cdot$ h^{-1} if necessary. The equivalent dose of bumetanide is 1 mg $\cdot$ h^{-1}, increasing to 2 mg $\cdot$ h^{-1}, and for torsemide 10 mg $\cdot$ h^{-1}, increasing to 20 mg $\cdot$ h^{-1}.

APPENDIX 5J

Protocol (Interim Measures) for a Serum K$^+$ Level >5.5 mEq $\cdot$ L^{-1} from Acute Renal Failure

1. Give glucose and insulin solution intravenously (IV). For adults, mix 20 units of regular insulin in 50 mL of 50% dextrose and give IV over 10 minutes. For children and infants, mix 0.5 mL of regular insulin per kilogram of body weight in 2 mL of 25% dextrose per kilogram and give IV over 10 minutes.
2. Administer a sodium polystyrene sulfonate (Kayexalate) enema. For adults, mix 50 g in 200 mL of sorbitol or 20% dextrose, and give as a retention enema; hold for 30 minutes, then remove; repeat hourly as necessary. For children and infants, give 1 g $\cdot$ kg^{-1} and 10 to 50 mL of sorbitol as a retention enema (total volume of sorbitol may be increased up to about 150 mL for children up to about 10 years of age).
3. Give 1 mEq $\cdot$ kg^{-1} sodium bicarbonate IV for infants and children. For adults, give 1 ampule (44 mEq) IV.
4. If potassium levels exceed 6.5 mEq $\cdot$ L^{-1} and the patient is not receiving digoxin, give 10 mg $\cdot$ kg^{-1} of calcium chloride for infants and small children and about 200 mg $\cdot$ kg^{-1} for adults IV, to decrease the cardiovascular effects of hyperkalemia.
5. If these measures do not result in a potassium level <5.5 mEq $\cdot$ L^{-1}, then nephrology consultation should be obtained.

APPENDIX 5K

Protocol for Seizures in Infants and Children

General Comments

Generalized or focal seizures are an infrequent but potentially serious occurrence following cardiac surgery in infants and children. In such cases a number of etiologies are possible (e.g., metabolic; infectious; cerebral edema, embolism, or hemorrhage; decreased cerebral perfusion), but in most patients no specific causative factor is identified. The protocols that follow outline the initial evaluation to identify possible correctable causes and describe an initial treatment regimen; in most cases a consultation is obtained with a neurologist who is knowledgeable about cardiac surgical patients.

The following generalizations are useful:
1. In infants and small children, whether the seizure is generalized or focal is not helpful diagnostically.
2. Respiratory arrest, discoordinate respiratory activity, or sudden inability to adequately mechanically ventilate can be an indication of seizural activity in infants. Additional evidence of seizures is usually present on detailed evaluation.
3. After initial control of seizures, anticonvulsant therapy should be continued through the recovery period. Decisions regarding long-term therapy are made by the neurologist or pediatric cardiologist before hospital discharge.
4. Most children having a seizure in the early postoperative period will not have a chronic seizure disorder.
5. Choreiform movements are more serious symptoms than are seizures and are more apt to persist.

6. Because of its potential to cause cardiorespiratory depression and its short duration of action, diazepam (Valium) is best avoided as an anticonvulsant unless the patient is being artificially ventilated.

Initial Evaluation and Treatment

1. At the onset of a seizure, arterial blood gases and pH; serum glucose, calcium, and electrolytes; cardiac index; and body temperature are determined.
2. Interventions are made in an attempt to correct:
   a. pH < 7.25 or > 7.50; $PaCO_2$ < 25 mmHg; PaO_2 < 80 mmHg; and base deficit >10 to 15 mEq $\cdot$ L^{-1}. (In some patients, prompt control of seizures will correct low values.)
   b. Serum glucose level <40 mg $\cdot$ dL^{-1} in infants and <60 mg $\cdot$ dL^{-1} in older children (see "Fluid, Electrolyte, and Caloric Intake" in Section 2)
   c. Serum calcium level <7 mg $\cdot$ dL^{-1} in infants and <8 mg $\cdot$ dL^{-1} in older children
   d. Serum sodium level <125 mEq $\cdot$ L^{-1}. Usual management in this situation is restriction of salt and water intake
   e. Cardiac index <2.0 L $\cdot$ min^{-1} $\cdot$ m^{-2}
   f. Body temperature >38.6°C (>101.5°F)

Initial Anticonvulsant Therapy

When seizures are first noted, steps are taken to terminate them or, if they are no longer present, to prevent their recurrence while the chemical and other variables are being determined.
1. Give
   a. 0.1 to 0.2 mg $\cdot$ kg^{-1} of diazepam IV and
   b. 15 mg $\cdot$ kg^{-1} of phenobarbital IV over 5 to 10 minutes as a loading dose.
2. If seizures are not controlled by these measures, additional doses of diazepam (if the patient is being ventilated) may be used. (The full effect of the loading dose of phenobarbital may not be apparent for several hours, but if problems continue at this stage, consider giving a further 5 mg $\cdot$ kg^{-1}.)
3. If there has been spontaneous termination of seizure activity and prevention of recurrence is desired, omit step 1a and proceed to step 1b.
4. Continuing major seizures will rarely be a problem. If they are, a loading dose of phenytoin (Dilantin) (20 mg $\cdot$ kg^{-1} orally) is given, followed by maintenance with 3 to 4 mg $\cdot$ kg^{-1} $\cdot$ day^{-1} given orally.
5. An alternative, especially when seizures interfere with effective ventilatory support, is paralysis with pancuronium.

Maintenance Anticonvulsive Therapy

The administration of phenobarbital (2.5 mg $\cdot$ kg^{-1} $\cdot$ 12 h^{-1}) can be instituted 12 to 24 hours after giving the initial loading dose.

APPENDIX 5L

Protocol for Intravenous Fluids

In adults and children (>2 years of age or >13 kg in weight):
1. Day of operation:
   a. 500 mL of 5% glucose in water $\cdot$ m^{-2} $\cdot$ 24 h^{-1}
   b. 10 mEq of K$^+$ $\cdot$ m^{-2} $\cdot$ 24 h^{-1}
2. First and second postoperative days:
   a. 750 mL of 5% glucose in water $\cdot$ m^{-2} $\cdot$ 24 h^{-1}
   b. 20 mEq of K$^+$ $\cdot$ m^{-2} $\cdot$ 24 h^{-1}
3. Third postoperative day:
   a. 750 mL of 5% glucose in water $\cdot$ m^{-2} $\cdot$ 24 h^{-1}
   b. 350 mL of 5% glucose in saline solution $\cdot$ m^{-2} $\cdot$ 24 h^{-1} } or 1100 mL of 5% glucose in one-quarter–strength saline solution $\cdot$ m^{-2} $\cdot$ 24 h^{-1}
   c. 10 mEq of K$^+$ $\cdot$ m^{-2} $\cdot$ 24 h^{-1}
4. If oral intake has not been established on the third postoperative day, consider gavage feeding or intravenous (IV) hyperalimentation.

In infants and small children (<2 years old or <13 kg in weight):
1. Day of operation:
   a. Calculate patient's saline requirement.
      i. 250 mL $\cdot$ m^{-2} $\cdot$ 24 h^{-1} are required.

ii. If this is 75 mL or less for the individual patient, use only balanced salt solution for flushing[4] the arterial catheter; if it is 75 to 150 mL, use balanced salt solution for flushing the arterial and left atrial catheters; if it is >150 mL, flush the arterial, left atrial, and right atrial (and, if present, pulmonary artery) catheters with balanced salt solution.

iii. Give no additional sodium-coating fluids if step ii supplies the patient's needs. Otherwise, subtract the amount in step ii from the requirement and give the difference.

b. Calculate the patient's water requirement.
    i. $500 \ mL \cdot m^{-2} \cdot 24 \ h^{-1}$ of 10% glucose in water are required.
    ii. Subtract $72 \ mL \cdot$ the number of intracardiac recording catheters being flushed with 10% glucose in water from the amount in step i, and order that amount.

c. Give no potassium in the fluids.

2. Days thereafter:
  a. Calculate patient's saline requirement.
      i. $250 \ mL \cdot m^{-2} \cdot 24 \ h^{-1}$ are required.
      ii. Proceed as in 1a.
  b. Calculate patient's water requirement.
      i. $750 \ mL \cdot m^{-2} \cdot 24 \ h^{-1}$ of 10% glucose are required.
      ii. Subtract 72 mL the number of intracardiac catheters being flushed with 10% glucose in water from the amount in step (1), and order that amount.
  c. Give no potassium in the IV fluids.

3. If oral intake has not been established on the third postoperative day, consider gavage feeding or IV hyperalimentation.

Note that when medications such as lidocaine, catecholamines, and sodium nitroprusside are administered, the amount of fluid thereby infused must be determined and subtracted from the daily fluid requirement.

APPENDIX 5M

Protocol for Infant Feeding

Infants can rapidly develop a profoundly catabolic state after major surgery. Caloric intake should be raised to adequate levels as soon as possible after operation.

When respiratory assistance via an endotracheal tube continues into the third postoperative day, gavage feeding is begun unless specific contraindications exist. In extubated infants, weakness and underdevelopment may prevent proper feeding and result in aspiration, making intermittent gavage feeding necessary. The steps are as follows:

1. As a precaution, prepare the endotracheal suction catheter for immediate use.

2. Check to be certain that the nasogastric tube is in the stomach; if intermittent gavage is to be used, a feeding catheter is inserted for each feeding and then removed.
  a. Aspirate the tube. If stomach contents are not obtained or if large quantities of air with a little mucus are obtained, the tube is probably in the trachea.
  b. While listening over the stomach with a stethoscope, inject a little air and listen for the typical noise.
  c. Persistent coughing suggests that the tube is in the trachea.
  d. Absence of a normal cry suggests the tube is in the trachea (steps a, b, and d apply to patients without an endotracheal tube).

3. If these checks indicate that the tube is in the stomach and if aspiration does not reveal >10 to 15 mL of fluid in the stomach, then initial feedings can be begun. These feedings are injected slowly over 2 to 3 minutes or allowed to enter by gravity, preferably with the infant sitting upright. Otherwise, the infant is placed on his or her right side, with the head inclined to at least a 15° angle.

---

[4]An automatic, very slow (3 mL $\cdot$ h^{-1} or 72 mL $\cdot$ 24 h^{-1}), continuous infusion system for all devices attached to pressure transducers is used. The solution flushing the arterial needle must be a heparinized, balanced salt solution, to prevent arterial spasm and pain. When salt restriction is important, as in infants, a glucose solution can be used for flushing the other pressure lines.

4. The gavage feeding is given *every 3 hours* on the following schedule:
  a. Give sterile water, 10 to 15 mL $\cdot$ 1.
  b. If well tolerated, give 10% dextrose in water, 30 mL $\cdot$ 1.
  c. If well tolerated and if the residual is less than 5 mL, give Lanolac or SMA-20, 30 mL $\cdot$ 8, and, if well tolerated, full-strength Lanolac or SMA-20 in increasing amounts.

5. If needed:
  a. Consider giving SMA-27 (27 calories per ounce) if diarrhea is not present.
  b. Consider continuous drip infusion to avoid a bolus effect (residual fluid in the stomach is aspirated and measured every 2 hours).

APPENDIX 5N

Protocol for Metabolic Acidosis

Indication

Metabolic acidosis exists if the base deficit is >2 mEq $\cdot$ L^{-1} and pH is <7.35 or PaCO$_2$ is <30 mmHg.

Rationale

Treatment is directed only at the extracellular fluid, and a conservative dose of NaHCO$_3$ is given, because more can easily be administered if needed.

$$\text{Extracellular fluid volume} = 30\% \text{ body weight (kg)}$$

$$\text{Base deficit (mEq} \cdot \text{L}^{-1}) \cdot 0.3 \cdot \text{body weight (kg)}$$
$$= \text{total extracellular base deficit}$$

Treatment

1. Administer NaHCO$_3$ so that the amount of Na$^+$ (mEq) equals half the total extracellular base deficit.
2. Remeasure the base deficit in 30 to 60 minutes and repeat treatment if indicated.

Note that in acute reduction of cardiac output or cardiac arrest, much larger doses of NaHCO$_3$ are indicated (44 mEq for adults, 1 mEq $\cdot$ kg^{-1} for infants and children).

APPENDIX 5O

Protocol for Severe Metabolic Alkalosis

Indication

Severe metabolic alkalosis exists if blood pH is >7.60 or base excess >5.0 mEq $\cdot$ L^{-1}. Some surgeons use total base excess >50 mEq.

$$\text{Total base excess (mEq)} =$$
$$\text{Base excess (mEq} \cdot \text{L}^{-1}) \cdot 0.3 \ (\text{L} \cdot \text{kg}^{-1}) \cdot \text{body weight (kg)}$$

Rationale

Cardiac surgical patients who develop severe metabolic alkalosis are usually slow to convalesce and resume normal alimentation and are frequently on moderate or large diuretic programs. This complication may be more common in infants. The condition is associated with a volume-contracted state (dehydration), with potassium and chloride depletion, and, in its more severe form, with hypercapnia. The major complications of severe alkalemia include a leftward shift of the oxyhemoglobin dissociation curve, with attendant tissue hypoxia, peripheral and central chemoreceptor depression, hypoventilation, and hypoxemia; refractory cardiac arrhythmias; excessive myocardial contractility, with attendant increase in oxygen consumption; tetany; and altered calcium metabolism. Mild forms of metabolic alkalosis may be corrected with volume expansion and replacement of potassium and chloride. Severe alkalemia (pH ≥7.60) mandates aggressive therapy. The administration of hydrochloric acid corrects metabolic alkalosis directly without dependence on renal or hepatic metabolic function. Complications of hemolysis and tissue necrosis are not a problem if central venous administration of dilute hydrochloric acid is used. However, because of the respiratory depression (CO$_2$ retention and hypoxia) caused by metabolic alkalosis, the too rapid administration of hydrochloric acid may produce inappropriate hyperventilation and hypocapnia with an intracellular–extracellular hydrogen dysequilibrium. With the concomitant correction of saline and potassium chloride deficits, intravenous (IV) infusion of hydrochloric acid is a safe and desirable therapy for severe metabolic alkalosis.

Treatment

1. Use an internal jugular or right atrial catheter for infusion.
2. Prepare 0.15N hydrochloric acid in sterile water (12.5 mL concentrated hydrochloric acid [36% to 38%] diluted to a volume of 1000 mL with sterile water). One liter of 0.15N HCl contains 150 mEq of H$^+$ and 150 mEq of Cl$^-$.
3. Determine the amount of hydrochloric acid required for correction of the metabolic alkalosis. Calculate the chloride deficit and the total base excess by the formulae:

Cl$^-$ deficit = 0.3 · body weight (kg) · Cl$^-$ concentration (mEq · L^{-1})

Total base excess (mEq) =
$$0.3 \cdot \text{body weight (kg)} \cdot \text{base excess (mEq} \cdot \text{L}^{-1})$$

4. Administer the chloride deficit as 0.15N HCl over 16 to 24 hours. The maximum infusion rate should be about 0.2 mEq H$^+$ · kg^{-1} · h^{-1}. The infusion continues until the base excess is within an acceptable range, that is, <5 mEq · L^{-1}. As a check, the total base excess should be reduced to between 0 and about 1 mEq · kg^{-1}. (Infusion tubing should be changed every 12 hours and the acid infused from a glass container, because the effect of hydrochloric acid on plastic is uncertain.)
5. Correct the patient's volume deficit based on current and previous body weight by volume expansion with saline solution. Administer the maintenance daily IV fluids and sodium and potassium requirements and replace any prior deficits. Correct potassium deficit and maintain potassium level greater than 3.5 mEq · L^{-1}.
6. Monitor arterial blood gases and electrolytes every 4 to 6 hours and blood urea nitrogen and creatinine levels once or twice daily.

APPENDIX 5P

Protocol for Hyperthermia

Indication

Hyperthermia exists if rectal temperature is ≥38.3°C (≥101°F).

Rationale

Hyperthermia increases metabolic demands and, thus, myocardial oxygen consumption. Severe hyperthermia (central temperatures ≥41.1°C [≥106°F]) may permanently and severely damage the brain.

Treatment

1. If rectal temperature is ≥38.3°C (≥101°F), give acetaminophen as a rectal suppository every 4 hours. The dose in infants and children is 10 mg · kg^{-1} (rounded to the nearest 30 mg), and in adults, 650 to 1300 mg.

2. Consider using a cooling blanket or cold syringing and a fan or ice bags applied to the body.
3. If rectal temperature is ≥39.4°C (≥103°F):
   a. Insert esophageal temperature probe for continuous monitoring of central temperature and intensify efforts to improve cardiac output. Check for possible transfusion reaction.
   b. If esophageal temperature is ≥39.4°C (≥103°F):
      i. Make preparations for peritoneal dialysis with room temperature or cooled dialysate, to be initiated if simpler measures do not *promptly* control hyperthermia.
      ii. Give acetaminophen as in step 1.
      iii. Give dexamethasone, 0.25 mg · kg^{-1} IV, then 0.1 mg · kg^{-1} IV every 6 hours.
4. Give sodium nitroprusside, 1 µg · kg^{-1} · min^{-1}, to increase peripheral heat loss if arterial pressure remains acceptable with this drug; if inotropic agents are necessary, give preference to amrinone and isoproterenol.
5. Abolish muscular heat production, particularly when an infant is restless, by paralyzing with pancuronium (0.1 mg · kg^{-1}).
6. Continue efforts to improve cardiac output.

APPENDIX 5Q

Protocol for Autotransfusion

1. Several commercial chest drainage systems that accommodate autotransfusion are available. The two general types are (1) those that transfuse shed blood directly from the drainage system and (2) those that contain a drainage receptacle (a collapsible bag) that is manually transferred as an independent infusion setup.
2. A filter is optional.
3. Often there is a threshold for autoinfusion (that is, drainage >100 mL in adults).
4. A time limit for duration of autotransfusion is set for 4 to 6 hours.
5. Reinfusion of shed blood is governed by:
   a. Amount of drainage
   b. Atrial pressure limits
6. With either system the total volume of chest drainage must be noted. This is a simple arithmetic sum of volume currently occupying the chest drainage reservoir plus the amount of chest drainage autotransfused. This total is noted hourly.
7. Contraindications to autotransfusion include:
   a. Infectious endocarditis or other infection
   b. Exogenous chemicals in the mediastinum
      i. Betadine
      ii. Topical antibiotics
      iii. Hemostatic agents
      iv. Biologic glue
   c. Hematologic abnormalities, for example, sickling, diffuse intravascular coagulation, hemolysis

REFERENCES

A

1. Alford WC Jr, Meador CK, Mihalevich J, Burrus GR, Glassford DM Jr, Stoney WS, et al. Acute adrenal insufficiency following cardiac surgical procedures. J Thorac Cardiovasc Surg 1979;78:489.
2. Aldrete JS, Han SY, Laws HL, Kirklin JW. Intestinal infarction complicating low cardiac output states. Surg Gynecol Obstet 1977;144:371.
3. Abel RM, Buckley MJ, Austen WG, Barratt GO, Beck CH Jr, Fisher JE. Etiology, incidence, and prognosis of renal failure following cardiac operations. J Thorac Cardiovasc Surg 1976;71:323.
4. Ashbaugh DG, Petty TL. Positive end-expiratory pressure. J Thorac Cardiovasc Surg 1979;65:165.
5. Astrup P, Anderson OS, Jorgenson K, Engel K. The acid-base metabolism: a new approach. Lancet 1960;1:1035.
6. Appelbaum A, Blackstone EH, Kouchoukos NT, Kirklin JW. Afterload reduction and cardiac output in infants early after intracardiac surgery. Am J Cardiol 1977;39:445.

7. Atkinson DE. The energy charge of the adenylate pool as a regulatory parameter. Interaction with feedback modifiers. Biochemistry 1968;7:4030.
8. Anderson OS. Blood acid-base alignment nomogram. Scand J Clin Lab Invest 1963;15:211.
9. Ali J, Weisel RD, Layug AB, Kripke BJ, Hechtman HB. Consequences of postoperative alterations in respiratory mechanics. Am J Surg 1974;128:376.
10. Armon C, Deschamps C, Adkinson C, Fealey RD, Orszulak TA. Hyperbaric treatment of cerebral air embolism sustained during an open-heart surgical procedure. Mayo Clin Proc 1991;66:565.
11. Almassi G, Schowalter T, Nicolosi A, Aggarwal A, Moritz T, Henderson W, et al. Atrial fibrillation after cardiac surgery: a major event? Ann Surg 1997;226:501.

12. Arganziano M, Chondin B, Moazani M, Rose E, Smith C, Levin H, et al. Randomized double-blind trial of inhaled nitric oxide in LVAD recipients with pulmonary hypertension. Ann Thorac Surg 1998;65:340.

13. Aldea GS, Doursounian M, O'Gara P, Treanor P, Shapira OM, Lazar HL, et al. Heparin-bonded circuits with a reduced anticoagulation protocol in a primary CABG: a prospective randomized study. Ann Thorac Surg 1996;62:410.

14. Aldea GS, O'Gara P, Shapira OM, Treanor P, Osman A, Patalis E, et al. Effect of anticoagulation protocol on outcome in patients undergoing CABG with heparin-bonded cardiopulmonary bypass circuits. Ann Thorac Surg 1998;65:425.

B

1. Bell DM, Goldmann DA, Hopkins CC, Karchmer AW, Moellering RC Jr. Unreliability of fever and leukocytosis in the diagnosis of infection after cardiac valve surgery. J Thorac Cardiovasc Surg 1978;75:87.

2. Becker LC, Fortuin NJ, Pitt B. Effect of ischemia and antianginal drugs on the distribution of radioactive microspheres in the canine left ventricle. Circ Res 1971;28:263.

3. Breckenridge IM, Deverall PB, Kirklin JW, Digerness SB. Potassium intake and balance after open intracardiac operations. J Thorac Cardiovasc Surg 1972;63:305.

4. Barratt-Boyes BG, Wood EH. Cardiac output and related measurements and pressure values in the right heart and associated vessels. J Lab Clin Med 1958;51:72.

5. Bourgeois BF, Donath A, Paunier L, Rouge JC. Effects of cardiac surgery on renal functions in children. J Thorac Cardiovasc Surg 1979;77:283.

6. Burke JF. The effective period of preventive antibiotic action in experimental incisions and dermal lesions. Surgery 1961;50:161.

7. Bryant LR, Spencer FC, Trinkle JK. Treatment of median sternotomy infection by mediastinal irrigation with an antibiotic solution. Ann Surg 1969;169:915.

8. Breyer RH, Mills SA, Hudspeth AS, Johnston FR, Cordell AR. A prospective study of sternal wound complications. Ann Thorac Surg 1984;37:412.

9. Berglund E. Ventricular function: VI. Balance of left and right ventricular output: relation between left and right atrial pressures. Am J Physiol 1954;178:381.

10. Book K, Ohqvist G, Bjork VO, Lundberg S, Settergran G. Peritoneal dialysis in infants and children after open heart surgery. Scand J Thorac Cardiovasc Surg 1982;16:299.

11. Burgess GN, Kirklin JW, Steinhilber RM. Some psychiatric aspects of intracardiac surgery. Mayo Clin Proc 1967;42:1.

12. Blauth C, Smith P, Newman S, Arnold J, Siddons F, Harrison MJ, et al. Retinal microembolization and neuropsychological deficit following clinical cardiopulmonary bypass: comparison of a membrane and a bubble oxygenator. A preliminary communication. Eur J Cardiothorac Surg 1989;3:135.

13. Bailey RW, Bulkley GB, Hamilton SR, Morris JB, Haglund UH, Meilahn JE. The fundamental hemodynamic mechanism underlying gastric "stress ulceration" in cardiogenic shock. Ann Surg 1987;205:597.

14. Breyer RH, Engelman RM, Rousou JA, Lemeshow S. Blood conservation for myocardial revascularization. Is it cost effective? J Thorac Cardiovasc Surg 1987;93:512.

15. Bush A, Busst CM, Shinebourne EA. The use of oxygen and prostacyclin as pulmonary vasodilators in congenital heart disease. Int J Cardiol 1985;9:267.

16. Barrowcliffe MP, Jones GJ. Solute permeability of the alveolar capillary barrier. Thorax 1987;42:1.

17. Benjamin JJ, Cascade PN, Rubenfire M, Wajszczuk W, Kerin NZ. Left lower lobe atelectasis and consolidation following cardiac surgery: the effect of topical cooling on the phrenic nerve. Radiology 1982;142:11.

18. Blauth C, Griffin S, Harrison M, Klinger L, Newman S, Pugsley W, et al. Neuropsychologic alterations after cardiac operation (letter). J Thorac Cardiovasc Surg 1989;98:454.

19. Beerthuizen GI, Goris RJ, Bredee JJ, Mashhour YA, Kimmich HP, van der Kley AJ, et al. Muscle oxygen tension, hemodynamics, and oxygen transport after extracorporeal circulation. Crit Care Med 1981;16:748.

20. Burrows FA, Williams WG, Teoh KH, Wood AE, Burns J, Edmonds J, et al. Myocardial performance after repair of congenital cardiac defects in infants and children. J Thorac Cardiovasc Surg 1988;96:548.

21. Bartlett RH, Gazaaniga B, Huxtable RF, Schippers HC, O'Connor MJ, Jefferies MR. Extracorporeal circulation (ECMO) in neonatal respiratory failure. J Thorac Cardiovasc Surg 1977;74:807.

22. Boyd E. Growth of the surface area of the human body. Minneapolis: University of Minnesota Press, 1935, p. 132.

23. Bender K, Alexander J, Enon J, Skiming J. Effects of inhaled nitric oxide in patients with hypoxemia and pulmonary hypertension after cardiac surgery. Am J Crit Care 1997;6:127.

24. Beghetti M, Habre W, Friedli B, Berner M. Continuous low dose inhaled nitric oxide for treatment of severe pulmonary hypertension after cardiac surgery in pediatric patients. Br Heart J 1995;73:65.

25. Butler J, Chong GL, Baigrie RJ, Pillai R, Westaby S, Rocker GM. Cytokine responses to cardiopulmonary bypass with membrane and bubble oxygenation. Ann Thorac Surg 1992;53:833.

26. Baudouin SV, Wiggins J, Keogh BF, Morgan CJ, Evans TW. Continuous veno-venous haemofiltration following cardio-pulmonary bypass. Indications and outcome in 35 patients. Intensive Care Med 1993;19:290.

27. Blauth CI, Cosgrove DM, Webb BW, Ratliff NB, Boylan M, Piedmonte MR, et al. Atheroembolism for the ascending aorta: an emerging problem in cardiac surgery. J Thorac Cardiovasc Surg 1992;103:1104.

28. Barbut D, Grassineau D, Lis E, Heier L, Hartman GS, Isom OW. Posterior distribution of infants in strokes related to cardiac operations. Ann Thorac Surg 1998;65:1656.

29. Bashour CA, Yared JP, Ryan TA, Rady MY, Mascha E, Leventhal MJ, et al. Long-term survival and functional capacity in cardiac surgery patients after prolonged intensive care. Crit Care Med 2000;28:3847.

C

1. Cohn LH, Angell WW, Shumway NE. Body fluid shifts after cardiopulmonary bypass. I. Effects of congestive heart failure and hemodilution. J Thorac Cardiovasc Surg 1971;62:423.

2. Cottrell JE, Casthely P, Brodie JD, Patel K, Klein A, Trundorf H. Prevention of nitroprusside-induced cyanide toxicity with hydroxocobalamin. N Engl J Med 1978;298:809.

3. Chiariello M, Gold HK, Leinbach RC, Davis MA, Maroko PR. Comparison between the effects of nitroprusside and nitroglycerin on ischemic injury during acute myocardial infarction. Circulation 1976;54:766.

4. Cleland J, Pluth JR, Tauxe WN, Kirklin JW. Blood volume and body fluid compartment changes soon after closed and open intracardiac surgery. J Thorac Cardiovasc Surg 1966;52:698.

5. Chesney RW, Kaplan BS, Freedom RM, Haller JA, Drummond KN. Acute renal failure: an important complication of cardiac surgery in infants. J Pediatr 1975;87:381.

6. Cole P. The safe use of sodium nitroprusside. Anaesthesia 1978;33:473.

7. Caul EO, Mott MG, Clark SK, Perham TG, Wilson RS. Cytomegalovirus infections after open heart surgery. A prospective study. Lancet 1971;1:777.

8. Cevese PG, Vecchioni R, D'Amico DF, Cordiano C, Biàsiato R, Favia G, et al. Postoperative chylothorax. J Thorac Cardiovasc Surg 1975;69:966.

9. Chu C, Chang C, Liaw Y, Hsieh M. Jaundice after open heart surgery: a prospective study. Thorax 1984;39:52.

10. Cutler BS, Okike O, Salm TJ. Surgical versus percutaneous removal of the intra-aortic balloon. J Thorac Cardiovasc Surg 1983;86:907.

11. Culliford AT, Cunningham JN Jr, Zeff RH, Isom OW, Teiko P, Spencer FC. Sternal and costochondral infections following open-heart surgery. A review of 2,594 cases. J Thorac Cardiovasc Surg 1976;72:714.

12. Chenoweth DE, Cooper SW, Hugli TE, Stewart RW, Blackstone EH, Kirklin JW. Complement activation during cardiopulmonary bypass: evidence for generation of C3a and C5a anaphylatoxins. N Engl J Med 1981;304:497.

13. Cosgrove DM, Loop FD, Lytle BW, Baillot R, Gill CC, Golding LA, et al. Primary myocardial revascularization: trends in surgical mortality. J Thorac Cardiovasc Surg 1984;88:673.

14. Cooley DA, Liotta D, Hallman GL, Bloodwell RD, Leachman RD, Milam JD. Orthotopic cardiac prosthesis for two-staged cardiac replacement. Am J Cardiol 1969;24:723.

15. Cardiac Arrhythmia Suppression Trial (CAST) Investigators. Preliminary report: effect of encainide and flecainide on mortality in a randomized trial of arrhythmia suppression after myocardial infarction. N Engl J Med 1989;321:406.

16. Corno A, Giamberti A, Giannico S, Marino B, Rossi E, Marcelletti C, et al. Airway obstructions associated with congenital heart disease in infancy. J Thorac Cardiovasc Surg 1990;99:1091.

17. Corwin HL, Sprague SM, DeLaria GA, Norusis MJ. Acute renal failure associated with cardiac operations: a case-control study. J Thorac Cardiovasc Surg 1989;98:1107.

18. Castillo CF-D, Harringer W, Warshaw AL, Vlahakes GJ, Koski G, Zaslavsky AM, et al. Risk factors for pancreatic cellular injury after cardiopulmonary bypass. N Engl J Med 1991;325:382.

19. Cutaia MV, Rounds S. Hypoxic pulmonary vasoconstriction: physiology and pathophysiology. J Intensive Care Med 1989;4:186.

20. Calabrese JR, Skwerer RG, Gulledge AD, Gill CG, Mullen JD, Rodgers DA, et al. Incidence of postoperative delirium following myocardial revascularization: a prospective study. Cleve Clin J Med 1987;54:29.

21. Cook LS, Johnson RG, Elkins RC. Cardiovascular time course after digoxin administration in left ventricular dysfunction after coronary artery bypass grafting. Am J Cardiol 1987;59:74.

22. Cheung EH, Craver JM, Jones EL, Murphy DA, Hatcher CR Jr, Guyton RA. Mediastinitis after cardiac valve operations: impact upon survival. J Thorac Cardiovasc Surg 1985;90:517.

23. Chiara O, Giomarelli PP, Biagioli B, Rosi R, Gattinoni L. Hypermetabolic response after hypothermic cardiopulmonary bypass. Crit Care Med 1987;15:995.

24. Chang AC, Farrell PE Jr, Murdison KA, Baffa JM, Barber G, Norwood WI, et al. Hypoplastic left heart syndrome: hemodynamic and angiographic assessment after initial reconstructive surgery and relevance to modified Fontan procedure. J Am Coll Cardiol 1991;17:1143.

25. Cottee DB, Saul WP. Is renal dose dopamine protective or therapeutic? No. Crit Care Clin 1996;12:687.

26. Craver JM, Bufkin BL, Weintraub WS, Guyton RA. Neurologic events after coronary bypass grafting: further observations with warm cardioplegia (see comments). Ann Thorac Surg 1995;59:1429.

27. Czer LS. Mediastinal bleeding after cardiac surgery: etiologies, diagnostic considerations, and blood conservation methods. J Cardiothorac Anesth 1989;3:760.

28. Crittenden MD, Khuri SF. The effect of cardiopulmonary bypass on platelet function and platelet kinetics. In Attar S, ed. Hemostasis in cardiac surgery. Armonk, N.Y.: Futura Publishing, 1999, p. 3.

29. Consensus conference. Platelet transfusion therapy. JAMA 1987;257:1777.

30. Chen S, Sager P, Stevenson W, Nadamance K, Middlekauf H, Singh B. Long-term efficacy of amiodarone for the maintenance of normal sinus rhythm in patients with refractory atrial fibrillation or flutter. Am J Cardiol 1995;76:47.

31. Carrel T, Englberger L, Mohacsi P, Neidhart P, Schmidli J. Low systemic vascular resistance after cardiopulmonary bypass: incidence, etiology, and clinical importance. J Card Surg 2000;15:347.

D

1. Dietzman RH, Ersek RA, Lillehei CW, Castaneda AR, Lillehei RC. Low output syndrome: recognition and treatment. J Thorac Cardiovasc Surg 1969;57:138.

2. deVillota ED, Barat G, Astorqui F, Damaso D, Avello F. Pyrexia following open heart surgery. The role of bacterial infection. Anaesthesia 1974;29:529.

3. Daughters GT, Frist WH, Alderman EL, Derby GC, Ingels NB Jr, Miller DC. Effects of the pericardium on left ventricular diastolic filling and systolic performance early after cardiac surgery. J Thorac Cardiovasc Surg 1992;104:1084.

4. Damen J, Hitchcock JF. Reactive pulmonary hypertension after a switch operation: successful treatment with glyceryl trinitrate. Br Heart J 1985;53:223.

5. Dunn M, Glassroth J. Pulmonary complications of amiodarone toxicity. Prog Cardiovasc Dis 1989;31:447.

6. Demmy TL, Park SB, Liebler GA, Burkholder JA, Maher TD, Benckart DH, et al. Recent experience with major sternal wound complications. Ann Thorac Surg 1990;49:458.

7. Del Nido PJ, Williams WG, Villamater J, Benson LN, Coles JG, Bohn D, et al. Changes in pericardial surface pressure during pulmonary hypertensive crises after cardiac surgery. Circulation 1987;76:III93.

8. Damen J, Verhoef J, Bolton DT, Middleton NG, van der Tweel I, de Jonge K, et al. Microbiologic risk of invasive hemodynamic monitoring in patients undergoing open-heart operations. Crit Care Med 1985;13:548.

9. Downing TP, Miller DC, Stofer R, Shumway NE. Use of the intra-aortic balloon pump after valve replacement: predictive indices, correlative parameters, and patient survival. J Thorac Cardiovasc Surg 1986;94:210.

10. Downing TP, Miller DC, Stinson EB, Burton NA, Oyer PE, Reitz BA, et al. Therapeutic efficacy of intra-aortic balloon pump counterpulsation: analysis with concurrent "control" subjects. Circulation 1981;64:II108.

11. DiSesa VJ, Gold JP, Shemin RJ, Collins JJ Jr, Cohn LH. Comparison of dopamine and dobutamine in patients requiring postoperative circulatory support. Clin Cardiol 1986;9:253.

12. Douglas PS, Hirshfeld JW, Edmunds LH Jr. Clinical correlates of atrial tachyarrhythmias after valve replacement for aortic stenosis. Circulation 1985;72:II159.

13. Davis RF, Lappas DG, Kirklin JK, Buckley MJ, Lowenstein E. Acute oliguria after cardiopulmonary bypass: renal functional improvement with low-dose dopamine infusion. Crit Care Med 1982;10:852.

14. Denton M, Chertoro G, Brady H. Renal dose dopamine for the treatment of acute renal failure: scientific rationale, experimental studies and clinical trials. Kidney Int 1996;49:4.

15. Davila-Roman VG, Barzilai B, Wareing TH, Murphy SF, Kouchoukos NT. Intraoperative ultrasonographic evaluation of the ascending aorta in 100 consecutive patients undergoing cardiac surgery. Circulation 1991;84:III47.

16. Doyle AR, Dhir AK, Moors AH, Latimer RD. Treatment of perioperative low cardiac output syndrome. Ann Thorac Surg 1995;59:3.

17. Downing TP, Miller DC, Stofer R, Shumway NE. Use of intra-aortic balloon pump after valve replacement: predictive indices, correlative parameters, and patient survival. J Thorac Cardiovasc Surg 1986;92:210.

18. Deedwania P, Singh B, Ellenbogen K, Fisher S, Fletcher R, Singh S. Spontaneous conversion and maintenance of sinus rhythm by amiodarone in patients with heart failure and atrial fibrillation. Circulation 1998;98:2574.

19. Despotis GJ, Filos KS, Zoys TN, Hogue CW Jr, Spitznagel E, Lappas DG. Factors associated with excessive postoperative blood loss and hemostatic transfusion requirements: a multivariate analysis in cardiac surgical patients. Anesth Analg 1996;82:13.

E

1. Epstein SE, Kent DM, Goldstein RE, Borer JS, Redwood ER. Reduction of ischemic injury by nitroglycerin during acute myocardial infarction. N Engl J Med 1974;292:29.
2. Engelman RM, Spencer FC, Reed GE, Tice DA. Cardiac tamponade following open-heart surgery. Circulation 1970;41:II165.
3. Eltringham WK, Schroder R, Jenny M, Matloff JM, Zollinger RM Jr. Pulmonary arteriovenous admixture in cardiac surgical patients. Circulation 1968;37:II207.
4. Edmunds LH, MacVaugh H III, Stevens J, Wechsler AB, Worthington GM. Evaluation of computer-aided monitoring of patients after heart surgery. J Thorac Cardiovasc Surg 1977;74:890.
5. Estafanous FG, Tarazi RC. Systemic arterial hypertension associated with cardiac surgery. Am J Cardiol 1980;46:685.
6. Engle MA, McCabe JC, Ebert PA, Zabriskie J. The postpericardiotomy syndrome and antiheart antibodies. Circulation 1974;49:401.
7. Engle MA, Zabriskie JB, Senterfit LB, Gay WA Jr, O'Loughlin JE, Ehlers KH. Viral illness and the postpericardiotomy syndrome: a prospective study in children. Circulation 1980;62:1151.
8. Engle MA, Gay WA Jr, McCabe J, Longo E, Johnson D, Senterfit LB, et al. Postpericardiotomy syndrome in adults: incidence, autoimmunity and virology. Circulation 1981;64:II58.
9. Engelman RM, Williams CD, Gouge TH, Chase RM Jr, Falk EA, Boyd AD, et al. Mediastinitis following open-heart surgery: review of two years' experience. Arch Surg 1973;107:772.
10. Echt DS, Liebson PR, Mitchell LB, Peters RW, Obias-Manno D, Barker AH, et al. Mortality and morbidity in patients receiving encainide, flecainide or placebo. The Cardiac Arrhythmia Suppression Trial. N Engl J Med 1991;324:781.
11. Epstein AE, Bigger JT, Wyse DG, Romhilt DW, Reynolds-Haertle RA, Hallstrom AP, et al. Events in the cardiac arrhythmia suppression trial (CAST): mortality in the entire population enrolled. J Am Coll Cardiol 1991;18:14.
12. Estenne M, Yernault JC, De Smet JM, De Troyer A. Phrenic and diaphragm function after coronary artery bypass grafting. Thorax 1985;40:293.
13. Estafanous FG, Tarazi RC, Viljoen JF, el-Tawil MY. Systemic hypertension following myocardial revascularization. Am Heart J 1973;85:732.
14. Engelman R, Pleet A, Rouseau J, Flack J, Deaton D, Pekow P, et al. Influence of cardiopulmonary bypass perfusion temperature on neurologic and hematologic function after coronary artery bypass grafting. Ann Thorac Surg 1999;67:1547.

F

1. Friesen WG, Woodson RD, Ames AW, Herr RH, Starr A, Kassebaum DG. A hemodynamic comparison of atrial and ventricular pacing in postoperative cardiac surgical patients. J Thorac Cardiovasc Surg 1968;55:271.
2. Firor WB. Infection following open-heart surgery, with special reference to the role of prophylactic antibiotics. J Thorac Cardiovasc Surg 1967;53:371.
3. Fairclough J, Evans PD, Elliot TS, Newcombe RG. Skin shaving: a cause for concern. J R Coll Surg Edinb 1987;32:76.
4. Feteih W, Syamasundar R, Whisennand HH, Mardini MK, Lawrie GM. Chylopericardium: new complication of Blalock-Taussig anastomosis. J Thorac Cardiovasc Surg 1983;85:791.
5. Fremes SE, Weisel RD, Baird RJ, Mickleborough LL, Burns RJ, Teasdale SJ, et al. Effects of postoperative hypertension and its treatment. J Thorac Cardiovasc Surg 1983;86:47.
6. Fowler MB, Alderman EL, Oesterle SN, Derby G, Daughters GT, Stinson EB, et al. Dobutamine and dopamine after cardiac surgery: greater augmentation of myocardial blood flow with dobutamine. Circulation 1984;70:I103.
7. Fanning WJ, Vasko JS, Kilman JW. Delayed sternal closure after cardiac surgery. Ann Thorac Surg 1987;44:169.
8. Fontan F, Madonna F, Naftel DC, Kirklin JW, Blackstone EH, Digerness S. Modifying myocardial management in cardiac surgery: a randomized trial. Eur J Cardiothorac Surg 1992;6:127.

9. Farrar DJ, Hill DJ, Gray LA, Pennington DG, McBride LR, Pierce WS, et al. Heterotopic prosthetic ventricles as a bridge to cardiac transplantation. N Engl J Med 1988;318:333.
10. Folks DG, Freeman AM, Sokol RS, Govier AV, Reves JG, Baker DM. Cognitive dysfunction after coronary artery bypass surgery: a case-controlled study. South Med J 1988;81:202.
11. Ferrazzi P, Allen R, Crupi G, Reyes I, Parenzan L, Maisonnet M. Reduction of infection after cardiac surgery: a clinical trial. Ann Thorac Surg 1986;42:321.
12. Fullerton D, Jaggers J, Wollmering M, Piedalre F, Grover F, McIntyre R. Variable response to inhaled nitric oxide after cardiac surgery. Ann Thorac Surg 1997;63:1251.
13. Friedman M, Selke FW, Wang SY, Weintraub RM, Johnson RG. Parameters of pulmonary injury after total or partial cardiopulmonary bypass. Circulation 1994;90:II262.
14. Finn A, Naik S, Klein N, Levinsky R, Strobel S, Elliot M. Interleukin 8 release and neutrophil degranulation after pediatric cardiopulmonary bypass. J Thorac Cardiovasc Surg 1993;105:234.
15. Foex P, Leone BJ. Pressure–volume loops: a dynamic approach to the assessment of ventricular function. J Cardiothorac Vasc Anesth 1994;8:84.

G

1. Goldstein RE, Stinson EB, Scherer JL, Seningen RP, Grehl TM, Epstein SE. Intraoperative coronary collateral function in patients with coronary occlusive disease: nitroglycerin responsiveness and angiographic correlations. Circulation 1974;49:298.
2. German JC, Chalmers GS, Hirai J, Nrisingha MD, Wakabayashi A, Connolly JE. Comparison of nonpulsatile and pulsatile extracorporeal circulation on renal tissue perfusion. Chest 1972;61:65.
3. Goldberg LI. Dopamine: clinical use of an endogenous catecholamine. N Engl J Med 1974;291:707.
4. Gregory GA, Kitterman JA, Phibbs RH, Tooley WH, Hamilton WK. Treatment of the idiopathic respiratory-distress syndrome with continuous positive airway pressure. N Engl J Med 1971;284:1333.
5. Gundry SR, Borkon AM, McIntosh CL, Morrow AG. Candida esophagitis following cardiac operation and short-term antibiotic prophylaxis. J Thorac Cardiovasc Surg 1980;80:661.
6. Gall WE, Clarke WR, Doty DB. Vasomotor dynamics associated with cardiac operations. I. Venous tone and the effects of vasodilators. J Thorac Cardiovasc Surg 1982;83:724.
7. Gottlieb SO, Brinker JA, Borkon AM, Kallman CH, Potter A, Gott VL, et al. Identification of patients at high risk for complications of intraaortic balloon counterpulsation: a multivariate risk factor analysis. Am J Cardiol 1984;53:1135.
8. Gardner TJ, Horneffer PJ, Manolio TA, Pearson TA, Gott VL, Baumgartner WA, et al. Stroke following coronary artery bypass grafting: a ten-year study. Ann Thorac Surg 1985;40:547.
9. Golding LA, Crouch RD, Stewart RW, Novoa R, Lytle BW, McCarthy PM, et al. Postcardiotomy centrifugal mechanical ventricular support. Ann Thorac Surg 1992;54:1059.
10. Gillespie DJ, Didier EP, Rehder K. Ventilation-perfusion distribution after aortic valve replacement. Crit Care Med 1990;18:136.
11. Goldberg MJ, Ruabenfire M, Kantrowitz A, Goodman G, Freed PS, Hallen L, et al. Intraaortic balloon pump insertion: a randomized study comparing percutaneous and surgical techniques. J Am Coll Cardiol 1987;9:515.
12. Gallagher JD, Moore RA, Kerns D, Jose AB, Botros SB, Clark DL. Effects of advanced age on extravascular lung water accumulation during coronary artery bypass surgery. Crit Care Med 1985;13:68.
13. Gall SA Jr, Olsen CO, Reves JG, McIntyre RW, Tyson GS Jr, Davis JW, et al. Beneficial effects of endotracheal extubation on ventricular performance. J Thorac Cardiovasc Surg 1988;95:819.
14. Griffith LD, Billman GF, Daily PO, Lane TA. Apparent coagulopathy caused by infusion of shed mediastinal blood and its prevention by washing of the infusate. Ann Thorac Surg 1989;47:400.

15. Giordano GF, Goldman DS, Mammana RB, Marco JD, Nestor JD, Raczkowski AR, et al. Intraoperative autotransfusion in cardiac operations: effect on intraoperative and postoperative transfusion requirements. J Thorac Cardiovasc Surg 1988;96:382.

16. Goenen M, Pedemonte O, Baele P, Col J. Amrinone in the management of low cardiac output after open heart surgery. Am J Cardiol 1985;56:33B.

17. Golding LA, Loop FD, Petes M, Cosgrove DM, Taylor PC, Phillips OF. Late survival following use of intra-aortic balloon pumping in revascularization surgery. Ann Thorac Surg 1980;30:48.

18. Gardner R, Finley T, Tooley W. The effect of cardiopulmonary bypass on surface activity of lung extracts. Bull Soc Int Surg 1962;21:542.

19. Gu YJ, van Oerveren W, van der Kamp HJ, Akkerman C, Boonstra CW, Wildervuur CR, et al. Heparin-coating of extracorporeal circuits reduces thrombin formation in patients undergoing cardiopulmonary bypass. Perfusion 1991;6:221.

H

1. Hilberman M, Myers BD, Carrie BJ, Derby G, Jamison RL, Stinson EB. Acute renal failure following cardiac surgery. J Thorac Cardiovasc Surg 1979;77:880.

2. Hencz P, Deverall PB, Crew AD, Steel AE, Mearns AJ. Hyperuricemia of infants and children: a complication of open heart surgery. J Pediatr 1979;94:774.

3. Hollenberg NK, Adams DF, Mendell P, Abrams HL, Merrell JP. Renal vascular responses to dopamine: hemodynamic and angiographic observations in normal man. Clin Sci 1973;45:733.

4. Hockberg MS, Merrill WH, Gruber H, McIntosh CL, Henry WL, Morrow AG. Delayed cardiac tamponade associated with prophylactic anticoagulants. J Thorac Cardiovasc Surg 1978;75:777.

5. Hill JD, Johnson DC, Miller GE Jr, Kerth WJ, Gerbode F. Latent mediastinal tamponade after open heart surgery. Arch Surg 1969;99:808.

6. Hardesty RL, Thompson M, Lerberg DB, Siewers RD, O'Toole JD, Salerni R, et al. Delayed postoperative cardiac tamponade: diagnosis and management. Ann Thorac Surg 1978;26:155.

7. Harris PD, Malm JR, Bowman FO Jr, Hoffman BF, Kaiser GA, Singer DH. Epicardial pacing to control arrhythmias following cardiac surgery. Circulation 1968;37:II178.

8. Hill DG, de Lanerolle P, Kosek JC, Agiular MJ, Hill JD. The pulmonary pathophysiology of membrane and bubble oxygenators. Trans Am Soc Artif Intern Organs 1975;11:165.

9. Hedley-Whyte J, Corning H, Laver MB, Austen WG, Bendixen HH. Pulmonary ventilation-perfusion relations after heart valve replacement or repair in man. J Clin Invest 1965;44:406.

10. Higgins GB, Mulder DG. Chylothorax after surgery for congenital heart disease. J Thorac Cardiovasc Surg 1971;61:411.

11. Hawker RE, Cartmill TB, Celermajer JM, Bowdler JD. Chylous pericardial effusion complicating aorta–right pulmonary artery anastomosis. J Thorac Cardiovasc Surg 1972;63:491.

12. Harrison MJ, Schneidau A, Ho R, Smith PL, Newman S, Treasure T. Cerebrovascular disease and functional outcome after coronary artery bypass surgery. Stroke 1989;20:235.

13. Hanson J, Loftness S, Clarke D, Campbell D. Peritoneal dialysis following open heart surgery in children. Pediatr Cardiol 1989;10:125.

14. Hickey PR, Hansen DD, Wessel DL, Lang P, Jonas RA. Pulmonary and systemic hemodynamic responses to fentanyl in infants. Anesth Analg 1985;64:483.

15. Hartz RS, Smith JA, Green D. Autotransfusion after cardiac operation: assessment of hemostatic factors. J Thorac Cardiovasc Surg 1988;96:178.

16. Hickey PR, Hansen DD, Wessel DL, Lang P, Jonas RA, Elixson EM. Blunting of stress responses in the pulmonary circulation of infants by fentanyl. Anesth Analg 1985;64:1137.

17. Hopkins RA, Bull C, Summer E, Haworth SG, de Leval MR, Stark J. Pulmonary hypertensive crises following surgery for congenital heart defects in children. Eur J Cardiothorac Surg 1991;5:628.

18. Hammeke TA, Hastings JE. Neuropsychologic alterations after cardiac operation. J Thorac Cardiovasc Surg 1988;96:326.

19. Hammeke TA, Hastings JE. Reply to the Editor. (Re: Letter to the Editor. Blauth C, Griffin S, Harrison M, Klinger L, Newman S, Pugsley W, et al. Neuropsychologic alterations after cardiac operation. J Thorac Cardiovasc Surg 1989;98:454.) J Thorac Cardiovasc Surg 1989;98:455.

20. Herrera HR, Ginsburg ME. The pectoralis major myocutaneous flap and omental transposition for closure of infected median sternotomy wounds. Plast Reconstr Surg 1982;70:465.

21. Hlatky MA, Bacon C, Boothroyd D, Mahanna E, Reves JG, Newman MF, et al. Cognitive function 5 years after randomization to coronary angioplasty or coronary bypass graft surgery. Circulation 1997;II11.

22. Haeffner-Cavaillon N, Roussellier N, Ponzio O, Carreno MP, Laude M, Carpentier A, et al. Induction of interleukin-1 production in patients undergoing cardiopulmonary bypass. J Thorac Cardiovasc Surg 1989;98:1100.

23. Hill J, Rodvien R, Mielke C. Bleeding and hemorrhagic complications. In Litwak R, Jurado R, eds. Care of cardiac surgical patient. Norwalk, Conn: Appleton-Century-Crofts, 1982, p. 380.

24. Harker L. Bleeding after cardiopulmonary bypass (editorial). N Engl J Med 986;314:1446.

25. Hasnain JU. Anticoagulation for cardiopulmonary bypass. In Attar S, ed. Hemostasis in cardiac surgery. Armonk, N.Y.: Futura Publishing, 1999, p. 3.

26. Hilberman M, Maseda J, Stinson EB, Derby GC, Spencer RJ, Miller DC, et al. The diuretic properties of dopamine in patients after open-heart operation. Anesthesiology 1984;61:489.

27. Harringer W. Capture of particulate emboli during cardiac procedures in which aortic cross-clamp is used. International Council of Emboli Management Study Group. Ann Thorac Surg 2000;70:1119.

28. Hausmann H, Potapov EV, Koster A, Siniawski H, Kukucka M, Loebe M, et al. Predictors of survival 1 hour after implantation of an intra-aortic balloon pump in cardiac surgery. J Card Surg 2001;16:72.

29. Hamilton WF, Moore JW, Kinsman JM, Spurling RG. Studies on the circulation. IV. Further analysis of the injection method, and of changes in hemodynamics under physiological and pathological conditions. Am J Physiol 1932;99:534.

I

1. Ito T, Engle MA, Goldberg HP. Postpericardiotomy syndrome following surgery for non-rheumatic heart disease. Circulation 1958;17:549.

2. Ichsan J, Hunt DR. Suprapubic catheters: a comparison of suprapubic versus urethral catheters in the treatment of acute urinary retention. Aust N Z J Surg 1987;57:33.

3. Ikaheimo MJ, Huikuri HV, Airaksinen J, Korhonen UR, Linnaluoto MK, Tarkka MR, et al. Pericardial effusion after cardiac surgery: incidence, relation to the type of surgery, antithrombotic therapy, and early coronary bypass graft patency. Am Heart J 1988;116:97.

4. Inomata S, Nisikawa T, Taguchi M. Continuous monitoring of mixed venous oxygen saturation for detecting alterations in cardiac output after discontinuation of cardiopulmonary bypass. Br J Anaesthesia 1994;72:11.

J

1. Jacob T, de Leval M, Stark J, Waterston DJ. Chylopericardium as a complication of aorto-pulmonary shunt. Arch Surg 1974;108:870.

2. Jones OD, Shore DF, Rigby ML, Leijala M, Scallan J, Shinebourne EA, et al. The use of tolazoline hydrochloride as a pulmonary vasodilator in potentially fatal episodes of pulmonary vasoconstriction after cardiac surgery in children. Circulation 1981;64:II134.

3. Jurkiewicz MJ, Bostwick J III, Hester TR, Bishop JB, Craver J. Infected median sternotomy wounds: successful treatment by muscle flaps. Ann Surg 1980;191:738.

4. Johnson JA, Gall WE, Gundersen AE, Cogbill TH. Delayed primary closure after sternal wound infection. Ann Thorac Surg 1989;47:270.

5. Jeevanadam V, Smith CR, Rose EA, Malm JR, Hugo NE. Single-stage management of sternal wound infections. J Thorac Cardiovasc Surg 1990;99:256.

6. Josa M, Khuri SF, Barunwalk NS, VanCisin MF, Spencer MP, Evans DA, et al. Delayed sternal closure: an improved method of dealing with complications after cardiopulmonary bypass. J Thorac Cardiovasc Surg 1986;91:598.

7. Jacquet L, Zerbe T, Stein KL, Kormos RL, Griffith BP. Evolution of human cardiac myocyte dimension during prolonged mechanical support. J Thorac Cardiovasc Surg 1991;101:256.

8. Journois D, Pouard P, Mauriat P, Malhere T, Vouhe P, Safran D. Inhaled nitric oxide as a therapy for pulmonary hypertension after operations for congenital heart defects. J Thorac Cardiovasc Surg 1994;107:1129.

9. Jain A, Shroff SG, Janicki JS, Reddy HK, Weber KT. Relationship between mixed venous oxygen saturation and cardiac index. Nonlinearity and normalization for oxygen uptake and hemoglobin. Chest 1991;99:1403.

10. Jett GK. ABIOMED BVS 5000: experience and potential advantages. Ann Thorac Surg 1996;61:301.

K

1. Kirklin JW, Archie JP Jr. The cardiovascular subsystem in surgical patients. Surg Gynecol Obstet 1974;139:17.

2. Kirklin JK, Daggett WM Jr, Lappas DG. Postoperative care following cardiac surgery. In Johnson RA, Haber E, Austen WG, eds. The practice of cardiology, Boston: Little, Brown, 1980, p. 1110.

3. Kirklin JW, Systems analysis in surgical patients with particular attention to the cardiac and pulmonary subsystems. Macewen Memorial Lecture. Glasgow: University of Glasgow Press, 1970.

4. Kirklin JK, Blackstone EH, Kirklin JW, McKay R, Pacifico AD, Bargeron LM Jr. Intracardiac surgery in infants under age 3 months: predictors of postoperative in-hospital cardiac death. Am J Cardiol 1981;48:507.

5. Kay HR, Goodman LR, Teplick SK, Mundth ED. Use of computed tomography to assess mediastinal complications after median sternotomy. Ann Thorac Surg 1983;36:706.

6. Kratz JM, Metcalf JS, Sade RM. Pericardial injury by antibacterial irrigants. J Thorac Cardiovasc Surg 1983;85:785.

7. Kirklin JK, Westaby S, Blackstone EH, Kirklin JW, Chenoweth DE, Pacifico AD. Complement and the damaging effects of cardiopulmonary bypass. J Thorac Cardiovasc Surg 1983;86:845.

8. Kirklin JW, Blackstone EH, Jonas RA, Shimazaki Y, Kirklin JK, Mayer JE, et al. Morphologic and surgical determinants of outcome events after repair of tetralogy of Fallot and pulmonary stenosis: a two-institution study. J Thorac Cardiovasc Surg 1992;103:706.

9. Kantrowitz A, Tjonneland S, Freed PS, Phillips SJ, Butner AN, Sherman JL Jr. Initial clinical experience with intraaortic balloon pumping in cardiogenic shock. JAMA 1968;203:113.

10. Kantrowitz A, Wasfie T, Freed PS, Rubenfire M, Wajsczuk W, Schork MA. Intraaortic balloon pumping 1967 through 1982: analysis of complications in 733 patients. Am J Cardiol 1986;57:976.

11. Krasna MJ, Flancbaum L, Trooskin SZ, Fitzpatrick JC, Scholz PM, Scott GE, et al. Gastrointestinal complications after cardiac surgery. Surgery 1988;104:773.

12. Kennedy JI, Myers JL, Plumb VJ, Fulmer JD. Amiodarone pulmonary toxicity: clinical, radiologic, and pathologic correlations. Arch Intern Med 1987;147:50.

13. Kouchoukos NT, Wareing TH, Murphy SF, Pelate C, Marshall WG. Risks of bilateral internal mammary artery bypass grafting. Ann Thorac Surg 1990;49:210.

14. Kohman LJ, Auchincloss JH, Gilbert R, Beshara M. Functional results of muscle flap closure for sternal infection. Ann Thorac Surg 1991;52:102.

15. Kay PH, Brass T, Lincoln C. The pathophysiology of atypical tamponade in infants undergoing cardiac surgery. Eur J Cardiothorac Surg 1989;3:255.

16. Kanter KR, Pennington DG, Weber TR, Zambie MA, Braun P, Martychenko V. Extracorporeal membrane oxygenation for postoperative cardiac support in children. J Thorac Cardiovasc Surg 1987;93:27.

17. Krohn BG, Kay JH, Mendez MA, Zubiate P, Kay GL. Rapid sustained recovery after cardiac operations. J Thorac Cardiovasc Surg 1990;100:194.

18. Karl TR, Sano S, Horton S, Mee RB. Centrifugal pump left heart assist in pediatric cardiac operations: indications, technique, and results. J Thorac Cardiovasc Surg 1991;102:624.

19. Konishi T, Apstein CS. Deleterious effects of digitalis on newborn rabbit myocardium after simulated cardiac surgery. J Thorac Cardiovasc Surg 1991;101:337.

20. Kanter KR, Ruzevich SA, Pennington DG, McBride LR, Swartz MT, Willman VL. Follow-up of survivors of mechanical circulatory support. J Thorac Cardiovasc Surg 1988;96:72.

21. Kuttila K, Ninikoski J. Peripheral perfusion after cardiac surgery. Crit Care Med 1989;17:217.

22. Kunathai S, Sholler GF, Celermajer JM, O'Halloran M, Cartmill TB, Nunn GR. Nitroprusside in children after cardiopulmonary bypass: a study of thiocyanate toxicity. Pediatr Cardiol 1989;10:121.

23. Kay GN. Invited letter to the editor: amiodarone and quinidine for postoperative atrial arrhythmias. J Thorac Cardiovasc Surg 1990; 99:942.

24. Katz ES, Tunick PA, Rusinek H, Ribakove G, Spencer FC, Kronzon I. Protruding aortic atheromas predict stroke in elderly patients undergoing cardiopulmonary bypass: experience with intraoperative transesophageal echocardiography. J Am Coll Cardiol 1992;20:70.

25. Kieler-Jensen N, Lundin S, Rickstein SE. Vasodilation therapy after heart transplantation: effects of inhaled nitric oxide and intravenous prostacyclin, prostaglandin E$_1$ and sodium nitroprusside. J Heart Lung Transplant 1995;14:436.

26. Kouchoukos NT, Wareing TH, Daily BB, Murphy SF. Management of the severely atherosclerotic aorta during cardiac operations. J Card Surg 1994;9:490.

27. Kaiser GC, Naunheim KS, Fiore AC, Harris HH, McBride LR, Pennington DG, et al. Reoperation in the intensive care unit. Ann Thorac Surg 1990;49:903.

28. Kirklin JK. The postperfusion syndrome: inflammation and the damaging effects of cardiopulmonary bypass. In Tinker JH, ed. Cardiopulmonary bypass: current concepts and controversies. Philadelphia: WB Saunders, 1989, p. 131.

29. Karp RB, Replogle R. Long-term survival and functional capacity in cardiac surgery patients after prolonged intensive care. Crit Care Med 2000;28:3983.

30. Khuri SF, Wolfe JA, Josa M, Axford TC, Szymanski I, Assousa S, et al. Hematologic changes during and after cardiopulmonary bypass and their relationship to the bleeding time and nonsurgical blood loss. J Thorac Cardiovasc Surg 1992;104:94.

31. Klemperer JD, Klein I, Gomez M, Helm RE, Ojamaa K, Thomas SJ, et al. Thyroid hormone treatment after coronary-artery bypass surgery. N Engl J Med 1995;333:1522.

32. Kulik TJ, Moler FW, Palmisano JM, Custer JR, Mosca RS, Bove EL, et al. Outcome-associated factors in pediatric patients treated with extracorporeal membrane oxygenator after cardiac surgery. Circulation 1996;94:II63.

33. Kirklin JK, Blackstone EH, Kirklin JW, Stewart RW, Pacifico AD, Bargeron LM Jr, et al. Management of cardiac subsystem after cardiac surgery. In Parenzan L, Crupi G, Graham G, eds. Congenital heart disease in the first 3 months of life: medical and surgical aspects. Bologna: Casa Editrice, 1981, p. 39.

34. Korfer R, El-Banayosy A, Arusoglu L, Minami K, Breymann T, Selfert D, et al. Temporary pulsatile ventricular assist devices and biventricular assist devices. Ann Thorac Surg 1999;68:679.

L

1. Livelli FD Jr, Johnson RA, McEnany MT, Sherman E, Newell J, Block PC, et al. Unexplained in-hospital fever following cardiac surgery. Circulation 1978;57:968.

2. Lell WL, Samuelson P, Reves JG, Strong SD. Duration of intubation and ICU stay after open heart surgery. South Med J 1979;72:773.

3. Leitch JW, Thomson D, Baird DK, Harris PJ. The importance of age as a predictor of atrial fibrillation and flutter after coronary artery bypass grafting. J Thorac Cardiovasc Surg 1990;100:338.

4. Lynn AM, Opheim KE, Tyler DC. Morphine infusion after pediatric cardiac surgery. Crit Care Med 1984;12:863.

5. Lamer C, Valleaux T, Plaisance P, Kucharski K, Payen D, Menasche P, et al. Continuous arteriovenous hemodialysis for acute renal failure after cardiac operations (letter to the editor). J Thorac Cardiovasc Surg 1990;99:175.

6. Lange HW, Aeppli DM, Brown DC. Survival of patients with acute renal failure requiring dialysis after open heart surgery: early prognostic indicators. Am Heart J 1987;113:1138.

7. Leitman IM, Paull DE, Barie PS, Isom OW, Shires GT. Intra-abdominal complications of cardiopulmonary bypass operations. Surg Gynecol Obstet 1987;165:251.

8. Lambert GJ, Geisler GF. Routine administration of platelet concentrates (letter to the editor). Ann Thorac Surg 1985;39:293.

9. Large SR, Heywood L, Flower CD, Cory-Pearce R, Wallwork J, English TA. Incidence and aetiology of a raised hemidiaphragm after cardiopulmonary bypass. Thorax 1985;40:444.

10. Lar LW, Lai LC, Ren LW. Massive arterial air embolism during cardiac operation: successful treatment in a hyperbaric chamber under 3 ATA (letter to the editor). J Thorac Cardiovasc Surg 1990;100:928.

11. Leitch DR, Greenbaum LJ Jr, Hallenbeck JM. Cerebral arterial air embolism. I. Is there benefit in beginning HBO treatment at 6 bar? II. Effect of pressure and time on cortical evoked potential recovery. III. Cerebral blood flow after decompression from various pressure treatments. IV. Failure to recover with treatment, and secondary deterioration. Undersea Biomed Res 1984;11:221, 237, 249, 265.

12. Lincoln C, Gibson D, Kay P, Shore D. Delayed sternal closure in neonate (letter to the editor). J Thorac Cardiovasc Surg 1990;100:928.

13. Lang P, Wessel DL, Wernovsky G, Jonas RA, Mayer JE Jr, Castaneda A. Hemodynamic effects of amrinone in infants after cardiac surgery. In Crupi G, Parenzan L, Anderson RH, eds. Perspectives in pediatric cardiology. Vol 2. Pediatric cardiac surgery. Part 2. Mount Kisco, N.Y.: Futura, 1989, p. 292.

14. Leurs PB, Mulder AW, Fiers HA, Hoorntje SJ. Acute renal failure after cardiovascular surgery. Current concepts in pathophysiology, prevention and treatment. Eur Heart J 1989;10:H38.

15. Lang SJ. Reoperative strategies for the bleeding cardiovascular patient. In Krieger KH, Isom OW, eds. Blood conservation in cardiac surgery. New York: Springer-Verlag, 1998, p. 537.

16. Lackritz EM, Satten GA, Aberle-Grasse J, Dodd RY, Raimondi VP, Janssen RS, et al. Estimated risk of transmission of the human immunodeficiency virus by screened blood in the United States. N Engl J Med 1995;333:1721.

17. Luciani GB, Chang AC, Starnes VA. Surgical repair of the great arteries in neonates with persistent pulmonary hypertension. Ann Thorac Surg 1996;61:800.

18. Leibold A, Wahba A, Birnhaum DE. Low energy cardioversion with epicardial wire electrodes: new treatment of atrial fibrillation after open-heart surgery. Circulation 1998;98:883.

19. Levett JM, Culpepper WS, Lin CY, Arcilla RA, Replogle RL. Cardiovascular responses to PEEP and CPAP following repair of complicated congenital heart defects. Ann Thorac Surg 1983;36:411.

M

1. Merrill W, Donahoo JS, Brawley RK, Taylor D. Late cardiac tamponade: a potentially lethal complication of open-heart surgery. J Thorac Cardiovasc Surg 1976;72:919.

2. Myerowitz PD, Caswell K, Lindsay WG, Nicoloff DM. Antibiotic prophylaxis for open-heart surgery. J Thorac Cardiovasc Surg 1977;73:625.

3. McLennan JR, Young WE, Sykes MK. Respiratory changes after open-heart surgery. Thorax 1965;20:545.

4. Mathur M, Harris EA, Yarrow S, Barratt-Boyes BG. Measurement of cardiac output by thermodilution in infants and children after open heart operations. J Thorac Cardiovasc Surg 1976;72:221.

5. Moront MG, Katz NM, Keszler M, Visner MS, Hoy GR, O'Connell JJ, et al. Extracorporeal membrane oxygenation for neonatal respiratory failure: a report of 50 cases. J Thorac Cardiovasc Surg 1989;97:706.

6. Mickleborough LL, Rebeyka I, Wilson GJ, Gray G, Desrosiers A. Comparison of left ventricular assist and intra-aortic balloon counterpulsation during early reperfusion after ischemic arrest of the heart. J Thorac Cardiovasc Surg 1987;93:597.

7. Moulopoulos SD, Topaz S, Kolff WJ. Diastolic balloon pumping (with carbon dioxide) in the aorta: a mechanical assistance to the failing circulation. Am Heart J 1962;63:669.

8. Maggart M, Stewart S. The mechanisms and management of noncardiogenic pulmonary edema following cardiopulmonary bypass. Ann Thorac Surg 1987;43:231.

9. Morgan JM, Morgan C, Evans TW. Clinical experience of pumped arteriovenous haemofiltration in the management of patients in oliguric renal failure following cardiothoracic surgery. Int J Cardiol 1988;21:259.

10. Mills SA, Prough DS. Neuropsychiatric complications following cardiac surgery. Semin Thorac Cardiovasc Surg 1991;3:39.

11. Magovern GJ, Park SB, Maher TD. Use of a centrifugal pump without anticoagulants for postoperative left ventricular assist. World J Surg 1985;9:25.

12. Mee RB. Dialysis after cardiopulmonary bypass in neonates and infants (invited letter to the editor). J Thorac Cardiovasc Surg 1992;103:1021.

13. Magilligan DJ. Indications for ultrafiltration in the cardiac surgical patient. J Thorac Cardiovasc Surg 1985;89:183.

14. Matsuda H, Covino E, Hirose H, Nakano S, Kishimoto H, Miyamoto Y, et al. Acute liver dysfunction after modified Fontan operation for complex cardiac lesions. J Thorac Cardiovasc Surg 1988;96:219.

15. McCarthy PM, Popovsky MA, Schaff HV, Orszulak TA, Williamson KR, Taswell HF, et al. Effect of blood conservation efforts in cardiac operations at the Mayo Clinic. Mayo Clin Proc 1988;63:225.

16. Martin WJ, Rosenow EC. Amiodarone pulmonary toxicity. Recognition and pathogenesis. (Part I). Chest 1988;93:1067.

17. Muehrcke DD, McCarthy PM, Stewart RW, Foster RC, Ogella DA, Borsh JA, et al. Extracorporeal membrane oxygenation for postcardiotomy cardiogenic shock. Ann Thorac Surg 1996;61:684.

18. Mullen JC, Miller DR, Weisel RD, Birnbaum PL, Teoh KH, Madonik M, et al. Postoperative hypertension: a comparison of diltiazem, nifedipine, and nitroprusside. J Thorac Cardiovasc Surg 1988;96:122.

19. Matangi MF, Neutze JM, Graham KJ, Hill DG, Kerr AR, Barratt-Boyes BG. Arrhythmia prophylaxis after aorta-coronary bypass: the effect of minidose propranolol. J Thorac Cardiovasc Surg 1985;89:439.

20. Markand ON, Moorthy SS, Mahomed Y, King RD, Brown JW. Postoperative phrenic nerve palsy in patients with open-heart surgery. Ann Thorac Surg 1985;39:68.

21. Murphy DA. Delayed closure of the median sternotomy incision. Ann Thorac Surg 1985;40:76.

22. Milgater E, Uretzky G, Shimon DV, Silberman S, Appelbaum A, Borman JB. Delayed sternal closure following cardiac operations. J Cardiovasc Surg 1986;27:328.

23. Moggio R, Agarwal N, Pooley RW, Somberg ED, Praeger PI, Sarabu MR, et al. Delayed sternal closure as a safe adjunct to support biventricular failure after open heart surgery. Tex Heart Inst J 1986;13:155.

24. Mooney MR, Arom KV, Joyce LD, Mooney JF, Goldenberg IF, et al. Emergency cardiopulmonary bypass support in patients with cardiac arrest. J Thorac Cardiovasc Surg 1991;101:450.

25. McAlister HF, Luke RA, Whitlock RM, Smith WM. Intravenous amiodarone bolus versus oral quinidine for atrial flutter and fibrillation after cardiac operations. J Thorac Cardiovasc Surg 1990;99:911.

26. McAlister HF, Luke RA, Whitlock RM, Smith WM. Amiodarone and quinidine for postoperative atrial arrhythmias (letter to the editor). J Thorac Cardiovasc Surg 1990;100:630.

27. McGowan F, Ikegonui N, Del Nido P, Motoyama E, Kurland G, Davis P, et al. Cardiopulmonary bypass significantly reduces surfactant activity in children. J Thorac Cardiovasc Surg 1993;106:968.

28. Mangos GJ, Brown MA, Chan WY, Horton D, Trew P, Whitworth JA. Acute renal failure following cardiac surgery: incidence, outcomes and risk factors. Aust N Z J Med 1995;25:278.

29. Markewitz A, Faist E, Lang S, Endres S, Fuchs D, Reichart B, et al. Successful restoration of cell-mediated immune response after cardiopulmonary bypass by immunomodulation. J Cardiovasc Surg 1993;105:15.

30. Moulton MJ, Creswell LL, Mackey ME, Cox JL, Rosenbloom M. Reexploration for bleeding is a risk factor for adverse outcomes after cardiac operations. J Thorac Cardiovasc Surg 1996;111:1037.

31. Mullis-Jansen S, Argenziano M, Corwin S, Homma S, Weinberg A, Williams M, et al. A randomized double-blind study of triiodothyronine on cardiac function and morbidity after coronary bypass surgery. J Thorac Cardiovasc Surg 1999;117:1128.

32. Mahutte CK, Jaffe MB, Sasse SA, Chen PA, Berry RB, Sassoon CS. Relationship of thermodilution cardiac output to metabolic measurements and mixed venous oxygen saturation. Chest 1993;104:1236.

33. Mammana RB, Hiro S, Levitsky S, Thomas PA, Plachetka J. Inaccuracy of pulmonary capillary wedge pressure when compared to left atrial pressure in the early postsurgical period. J Thorac Cardiovasc Surg 1982;84:420.

34. Meliones JN, Custer JR, Snedecor S, Moler FW, O'Rourke PP, Delius RE. Extracorporeal life support for cardiac assist in pediatric patients: review of ELSO registry data. Circulation 1991;84:III168.

35. Mekontso-Dessap A, Houel R, Soustelle C, Kirsch M, Thebert D, Loisance DY. Risk factors for post-cardiopulmonary bypass vasoplegia in patients with preserved left ventricular function. Ann Thorac Surg 2001;71:1428.

36. Moazami N, Smedira NG, McCarthy PM, Katzan I, Sila CA, Lytle BW, et al. Safety and efficacy of intraarterial thrombolysis for perioperative stroke after cardiac operation. Ann Thorac Surg 2001;72:1933.

N

1. Nickerson M. Drugs inhibiting adrenergic nerves and structures innervated by them. In Goodman LS, Gilman A, eds. The pharmacological basis of therapeutics, 4th ed. New York: Macmillan, 1970, p. 559.

2. Nadas AS, Fyler DC. Pediatric cardiology. Philadelphia: WB Saunders, 1972.

3. Norman JC, McDonald HP, Sloan H. The early and aggressive treatment of acute renal failure following cardiopulmonary bypass with continuous peritoneal dialysis. Surgery 1964;56:240.

4. Nishimura RA, Fuster V, Burgert SL, Puga FJ. Clinical features and long-term natural history of the postpericardiotomy syndrome. Int J Cardiol 1983;4:443.

5. Newman S. The incidence and nature of neuropsychological morbidity following cardiac surgery. Perfusion 1989;4:93.

6. Newman S, Smith P, Treasure T, Joseph P, Ell P, Harrison M. Acute neuropsychological consequences of coronary artery bypass surgery. Curr Psych Res Rev 1987;6:115.

7. Naik SK, Knight A, Elliott M. A prospective randomized study of a modified technique of ultrafiltration during paediatric open-heart surgery. Circulation 1991;84:III422.

8. Newman S, Klinger L, Venn G, Smith P, Harrison M, Treasure T. Subjective reports of cognition in relation to assessed cognitive performance following coronary artery bypass surgery. J Psychosomat Res 1989;33:227.

9. Newman LS, Szezukowski LC, Bain RP, Perlino CA. Suppurative mediastinitis after open heart surgery: a case control study of risk factors. Chest 1988;94:546.

10. Nelson TE, Flewellen EH. The malignant hyperthermia syndrome. N Engl J Med 1983;309:416.

11. Novitzky D, Cooper DK, Swanepoel A. Inotropic effect of triiodothyronine (T3) in low cardiac output following cardioplegic arrest and cardiopulmonary bypass: an initial experience in patients undergoing open heart surgery. Eur J Cardiothorac Surg 1989;3:140.

12. Najafi H. Reoperation for excessive bleeding after cardiac operations (invited letter to the editor). J Thorac Cardiovasc Surg 1992;103:814.

13. Nickerson N, Murphy S, Davila-Roman V, Schectman K, Kouchoukos N. Obstacles to early discharge after cardiac surgery. Am J Manag Care 1999;5:29.

14. Newman MF, Kirchner JL, Phillips-Bute B, Gaver V, Grocott H, Jones RH, et al. Longitudinal assessment of neurocognitive function after coronary-artery bypass surgery. N Engl J Med 2001;344:395.

O

1. Orringer MB, Sloan H. Monilial esophagitis: an increasingly frequent cause of esophageal stenosis. Ann Thorac Surg 1978;26:364.

2. Ofori-Kraykye SK, Tyberg TI, Geha AS, Hammond GL, Cohen LS, Langou RA. Late cardiac tamponade after open heart surgery: incidence, role of anticoagulants in its pathogenesis and its relationship to the postpericardiotomy syndrome. Circulation 1981;63:1323.

3. Odim JN, Tchervenkov CI, Dobell AR. Delayed sternal closure: a lifesaving maneuver after early operation for complex congenital heart disease in the neonate. J Thorac Cardiovasc Surg 1989;98:413.

4. O'Brien DJ, Bauer RM, Yarandi H, Knauf DG, Bramblett P, Alexander JA. Patient memory before and after cardiac operations. J Thorac Cardiovasc Surg 1992;104:1116.

5. Ott MJ, Buchman TG, Baumgartner WA. Postoperative abdominal complications in cardiopulmonary bypass patients: a case-controlled study. Ann Thorac Surg 1995;59:1210.

6. Ofosu FA. Antithrombotic mechanisms of heparin and related compounds. In Lane DA, Lindahl U, eds. Heparin. Boca Raton, Fla: CRC Press, 1989, p. 433.

P

1. Pacifico AD, Digerness S, Kirklin JW. Acute alterations of body composition after open intracardiac operations. Circulation 1970;41:331.

2. Pacifico AD, Digerness S, Kirklin JW. Sodium-excreting ability before and after intracardiac surgery. Circulation 1970;41:II142.

3. Palmer RF, Lasseter KC. Drug therapy: sodium nitroprusside. N Engl J Med 1975;292:294.

4. Parr GV, Blackstone EH, Kirklin JW. Cardiac performance and mortality early after intracardiac surgery in infants and young children. Circulation 1975;51:867.

5. Parr GV, Blackstone EH, Kirklin JW, Pacifico AD, Lauridsen P. Cardiac performance early after interatrial transposition of venous return in infants and small children. Circulation 1974;50:II163.

6. Pennington DG, Swartz M, Codd JE, Merjavy JP, Kaiser GC. Intraaortic balloon pumping in cardiac surgical patients: a nine year experience. Ann Thorac Surg 1983;36:125.

7. Pairolero PC, Arnold PG. Management of recalcitrant median sternotomy wounds. J Thorac Cardiovasc Surg 1984;88:357.

8. Pae WE Jr, Miller CA, Matthews Y, Pierce WS. Ventricular assist devices for postcardiotomy cardiogenic shock: a combined registry experience. J Thorac Cardiovasc Surg 1992;104:541.

9. Pennington DG, Kanter KR, McBride LR, Kaiser GC, Barner HB, Miller LW, et al. Seven years' experience with the Pierce-Donachy ventricular assist device. J Thorac Cardiovasc Surg 1988;96:901.

10. Pugsley W, Klinger L, Pascalis C, Newman S, Harrison M, Treasure T. Do microemboli contribute to bypass related cerebral impairment? J Cardiovasc Surg 1988;29:81.

11. Pennington DG, Merjavy JP, Swartz MT, Codd JE, Barner HB, Lagunoff D, et al. The importance of biventricular failure in patients with postoperative cardiogenic shock. Ann Thorac Surg 1985;39:16.

12. Pae WE, Pierce WS, Pennock JL, Campbell DB, Waldhausen JA. Long-term results of ventricular assist pumping in postcardiotomy cardiogenic shock. J Thorac Cardiovasc Surg 1987;93:434.

13. Pennock JL, Pierce WS, Wisman CB, Bull AP, Waldhausen JA. Survival and complications following ventricular assist pumping for cardiogenic shock. Ann Surg 1983;198:469.

14. Pennington DG, Samuels LD, Williams G, Palmer D, Swartz MT, Codd JE, et al. Experience with the Pierce-Donachy ventricular assist device in postcardiotomy patients with cardiogenic shock. World J Surg 1985;9:37.

15. Pennington DG, Bernhard WJ, Golding LR, Berger RL, Khuri SF, Watson JT. Long-term follow-up of postcardiotomy patients with profound cardiogenic shock treated with ventricular assist device. Circulation 1985;72:216.

16. Pierce WS, Donachy JH, Landis DL, Brighton JA, Rosenberg G, Migliore JJ, et al. Prolonged mechanical support of the left ventricle. Circulation 1978;58:I33.

17. Pinsky MR, Summer WR, Wise RA, Permutt S, Bromberger-Barnea B. Augmentation of cardiac function by elevation of intrathoracic pressure. J Appl Physiol 1983;54:950.

18. Powers K, Fyfe DA, Taylor AB, Halushka PV, Crawford FA Jr. Treatment of pulmonary vasospasm with prazosin after atrial septal defect closure in a child (letter to the editor). J Thorac Cardiovasc Surg 1989;97:802.

19. Pennington DG, Swartz MT, Ruzevich SA, Braun PR, Klinedinst WJ, Kanter KR. Circulatory support in children. In Crupi G, Parenzan L, Anderson RH, eds. Perspectives in pediatric cardiology. Vol 2. Pediatric cardiac surgery. Part 2. Mount Kisco, N.Y.: Futura, 1989, p. 296.

20. Pennington DG, McBride LR, Swartz MT, Kanter KR, Kaiser GC, Barner HB, et al. Use of the Pierce-Donachy ventricular assist device in patients with cardiogenic shock after cardiac operation. Ann Thorac Surg 1989;47:130.

21. Phillips SJ, Zeff RH, Kongtahworn C, Skinner JR, Toon RS, Grignon A, et al. Percutaneous cardiopulmonary bypass: application and indication for use. Ann Thorac Surg 1989;47:121.

22. Picca S, Principato F, Mazera E, Corona R, Ferrigno L, Marcelletti C, et al. Risks of acute renal failure after cardiopulmonary bypass surgery in children: a retrospective 10-year case-control study. Nephrol Dial Transplant 1995;10:630.

23. Patel RL, Turtle MR, Chambers DJ, James DN, Newman S, Venn GE. Alpha-stat acid-base regulation during cardiopulmonary bypass improves neurophysiologic outcome in patients undergoing coronary artery bypass grafting. J Thorac Cardiovasc Surg 1996;111:1267.

24. Paret G, Cohen AJ, Bohn DJ, Edwards H, Taylor R, Geary D, et al. Continuous arteriovenous hemofiltration after cardiac operations in infants and children. J Thorac Cardiovasc Surg 1992;104:1225.

R

1. Roberts AJ, Niarchos AP, Subramanian VA, Abel RM, Herman SD, Sealey JE, et al. Systemic hypertension associated with coronary artery bypass surgery. J Thorac Cardiovasc Surg 1977;74:846.

2. Rea HH, Harris EA, Seelye ER, Whitlock RM, Withy SJ. The effects of cardiopulmonary bypass upon pulmonary gas exchange. J Thorac Cardiovasc Surg 1978;75:104.

3. Ratliff NB, Young WG Jr, Hackel DB, Mikat E, Wilson JW. Pulmonary injury secondary to extracorporeal circulation: an ultrastructure study. J Thorac Cardiovasc Surg 1973;65:425.

4. Rychik J, Murdison KA, Chin AJ, Norwood WI. Surgical management of severe aortic outflow obstruction in lesions other than the hypoplastic left heart syndrome: use of a pulmonary artery to aorta anastomosis. J Am Coll Cardiol 1991;18:809.

5. Reid DJ, Digerness SB, Kirklin JW. Changes in whole body venous tone and distribution of blood after open intracardiac surgery. Am J Cardiol 1968;22:621.

6. Rigden SP, Barratt TM, Dillon MJ, de Leval M, Stark J. Acute renal failure complicating cardiopulmonary bypass surgery. Arch Dis Child 1982;57:425.

7. Rodewald G, Meffert HJ, Emskotter T, Gotze P, Lachenmayer L, Lamparter U, et al. Head and heart: neurological and psychological reactions to open heart surgery. Thorac Cardiovasc Surg 1988;36:254.

8. Russell RI, Mulvey D, Laroche C, Shinebourne EA, Green M. Bedside assessment of phrenic nerve function in infants and children. J Thorac Cardiovasc Surg 1991;101:143.

9. Rose DM, Colvin SB, Culliford AT, Cunningham JN, Adams PX, Glassman E, et al. Long-term survival with partial left heart bypass following perioperative myocardial infarction and shock. J Thorac Cardiovsc Surg 1982;83:483.

10. Rose DM, Laschinger J, Grossi E, Kreger KH, Cunningham JN, Spencer FC. Experimental and clinical results with a simplified left heart assist device for treatment of profound left ventricular dysfunction. World J Surg 1985;9:11.

11. Rosemurgy AS, McAllister E, Karl RC. The acute surgical abdomen after cardiac surgery involving extracorporeal circulation. Ann Surg 1988;207:323.

12. Rattner DW, Gu ZY, Vlahakes GJ, Warshaw AL. Hyperamylasemia after cardiac surgery: incidence, significance, and management. Am Surg 1989;209:279.

13. Ryan US, Ryan JW. Relevance of endothelial surface structure to the activity of vasoactive substances. Chest 1985;88:203S.

14. Rubis LJ, Stephenson LW, Johnston MR, Nagaraj S, Edmunds LH Jr. Comparison of effects of prostaglandin E1 and nitroprusside on pulmonary vascular resistance in children after open-heart surgery. Ann Thorac Surg 1981;32:563.

15. Rubin DA, Nieminski KE, Reed GE, Herman MV. Predictors, prevention, and long-term prognosis of atrial fibrillation after coronary artery bypass graft operations. J Thorac Cardiovasc Surg 1987;94:331.

16. Royster RL, Whiteley JW, Butterworth JF IV. Amrinone therapy during emergence from cardiopulmonary bypass (letter to the editor). J Thorac Cardiovasc Surg 1991;101:942.

17. Raja P, Hawker R, Chaikitpinyo A, Cooper SG, Lau KC, Nunn GR, et al. Amiodarone management of junctional ectopic tachycardia after cardiac injury in children. Br Heart J 1994;72:261.

18. Regragui I, Birdi I, Izzat MB, Black AM, Lopatatzidis A, Day CJ, et al. The effects of cardiopulmonary bypass temperature on neurophysiologic outcome after coronary artery operations: a prospective randomized trial. J Thorac Cardiovasc Surg 1997;114:146.

19. Roach GW, Kanchuger M, Mangano CM, Newman M, Nussmeier N, Wolman R, et al. Adverse cerebral outcomes after coronary bypass surgery: Multicenter Study of Perioperative Ischemia Research Group and the Ischemia Research and Education Foundation Investigators. N Engl J Med 1996;335:1857.

20. Rohrer MJ, Natale AM. Effect of hypothermia on the coagulation cascade. Crit Care Med 1992;20:1402.

21. Robotham JL, Rabson J, Permutt S, Bromberger-Barnea B. Left ventricular hemodynamics during respiration. J Appl Physiol 1979;47:1295.

22. Ross J. Afterload mismatch in aortic and mitral valve disease: implications for surgical therapy (review). J Am Coll Cardiol 1985;5:811.

23. Ross J. Afterload mismatch and preload reserve: a conceptual framework for the analysis of ventricular function (review). Prog Cardiovasc Dis 1976;18:255.

S

1. Sheppard LC, Kouchoukos NT, Kurts MA, Kirklin JW. Automated treatment of critically ill patients following operation. Ann Surg 1968;168:596.

2. Sturtz GS, Kirklin JW, Burke EC, Power MH. Water metabolism after cardiac operations involving a Gibbon-type pump-oxygenator. II. Benign forms of water loss. Circulation 1957;16:1000.

3. Seguin JR, Loisance DY. Omental transposition for closure of median sternotomy following severe mediastinal and vascular infection. Chest 1985;88:684.

4. Sheppard LC, Shotts JF, Roberson NF, Wallace FD, Kouchoukos NT. Computer controlled infusion of vasoactive drugs in post cardiac surgical patients. Proc IEEE 1979: Frontiers of Engineering in Health Care (IEEE catalog no. 79CH1440-7).

5. Sheppard LC, Kouchoukos NT, Shotts JF, Wallace FD. Regulation of mean arterial pressure by computer control of vasoactive agents in postoperative patients. Computers in Cardiology (IEEE catalog no. 75CH1018-C). Rotterdam, The Netherlands, October 2-4, 1975, pp 91-94.

6. Stiegel RM, Beasley ME, Sink JD, Hester TR, Guyton RA, Perrella AM, et al. Management of postoperative mediastinitis in infants and children by muscle flap rotation. Ann Thorac Surg 1988;46:45.

7. Stenzl W, Rigler B, Tscheliessnigg KH, Beitzke A, Metzler H. Treatment of postsurgical chylothorax with fibrin glue. Thorac Cardiovasc Surg 1983;31:35.

8. Smith PL, Treasure T, Newman SP, Joseph P, Ell PJ, Schneidau A, et al. Cerebral consequences of cardiopulmonary bypass. Lancet 1986; 1:823.

9. Stone KS, Brown JW, Canal DF, King H. Long-term fate of the diaphragm surgically plicated during infancy and early childhood. Ann Thorac Surg 1987;44:62.

10. Smith CD, Sade RM, Crawford FA, Othersen HB. Diaphragmatic paralysis and eventration in infants. J Thorac Cardiovasc Surg 1986;91:490.

11. Sarr MG, Gott VL, Townsend TR. Mediastinal infection after cardiac surgery. Ann Thorac Surg 1984;38:415.

12. Stevenson LW, Child JS, Laks H, Kern L. Incidence and significance of early pericardial effusions after cardiac surgery. Am J Cardiol 1984;54:848.

13. Shumaker HB Jr, Mandelbaum I. Continuous antibiotic irrigation in the treatment of infection. Arch Surg 1963;86:384.

14. Shaw PJ, Bates D, Cartlidge NE, Heavisie D, French JM, Julian DG, et al. Neurological complications of coronary artery bypass graft surgery: six month follow-up study. Br Med J 1986;293:165.

15. Singer RB, Hastings AB. An improved clinical method for the estimation of disturbances of the acid-base balance of human blood. Medicine (Baltimore) 1948;27:223.

16. Snir E, Carotti A, Stark J. Management of major tracheal hemorrhage after repair of complex congenital heart defects. Ann Thorac Surg 1990;49:661.

17. Shaw PJ, Bates D, Cartlidge NE, French JM, Heaviside D, Julian DG, et al. Neurologic and neuropsychological morbidity following major surgery: comparison of coronary artery bypass and peripheral vascular surgery. Stroke 1987;18:700.

18. Sotamiemi KA, Mononen H, Hokkanen TE. Long-term cerebral outcome after open-heart surgery: a five-year neuropsychological follow-up study. Stroke 1986;17:410.

19. Savageau JA, Stanton B, Jenkins CD, Fraser RW. Neuropsychological dysfunction following elective cardiac operation. II. A six-month reassessment. J Thorac Cardiovasc Surg 1982;84:595.

20. Schoen FJ, Palmer DC, Bernhard WF, Pennington DG, Haudenschild CC, Ratliff NB, et al. Clinical temporary ventricular assist: pathologic findings and their implications in a multiinstitutional study of 41 patients. J Thorac Cardiovasc Surg 1986;92:1071.

21. Silverman NA, Wright R, Levitsky S. Efficacy of low-dose propranolol in preventing postoperative supraventricular tachyarrhythmias: a prospective, randomized study. Ann Surg 1982;196:194.

22. Schaff HV, Hauer JH, Bell WR, Gardner TJ, Donahoo JS, Gott VL, et al. Autotransfusion of shed mediastinal blood after cardiac surgery: a prospective study. J Thorac Cardiovasc Surg 1978;75:632.

23. Said SI. Peptides, endothelium, and pulmonary vascular reactivity. Chest 1985;88:207S.

24. Staub NC. Site of hypoxic pulmonary vasoconstriction. Chest 1985;88:210S.

25. Scannell JC. Discussion of McGoon DC, Mankin HT, Kirklin JW: Results of open heart operation for acquired aortic valve disease. J Thorac Cardiovasc Surg 1963;45:47.

26. Schulze-Neick I, Bultman M, Werner H, Gamillscheg A, Vogel M, Berger F, et al. Right ventricular function in patients treated with inhaled nitric oxide for congenital heart disease in newborns and children. Am J Cardiol 1997;80:360.

27. Suen WS, Mok CK, Chiu SW, Cheung KL, Lee WT, Cheung D, et al. Risk factors for development of acute renal failure (ARF) requiring dialysis in patients undergoing cardiac surgery. Angiology 1998; 49:789.

28. Salzman EW, Weinstein MJ, Weintraub RM, Ware JA, Thurer RL, Robertson L, et al. Treatment with desmopressin acetate to reduce blood loss after cardiac surgery. A double-blind randomized trial. N Engl J Med 1986;314:1402.

29. Schreiber GB, Busch MP, Kleinman SH, Korelitz JJ. The risk of transfusion-transmitted viral infections. N Engl J Med 1996;334:1685.

30. Salter DR, Dyke CM, Wechsler AS. Triiodothyronine (T3) and cardiovascular therapeutics: a review. J Cardiovasc Surg 1992;7:363.

31. Smedira NG, Moazami N, Golding CM, McCarthy PM, Apperson-Hansen C, Blackstone EH, et al. Clinical experience with 202 adults receiving extracorporeal membrane oxygenation for cardiac failure: survival at 5 years. J Thorac Cardiovasc Surg 2001;122:92.

32. Seghaye M, Grabitz R, Duchateau J, Dabritz S, Koch D, Alzen G, et al. Inflammatory reaction and capillary leak syndrome related to cardiopulmonary bypass in neonates undergoing cardiac operations. J Thorac Cardiovasc Surg 1996;112:687.

33. Sommers MS, Stevenson JS, Hamlin RL, Ivey TD, Russell AC. Mixed venous oxygen saturation and oxygen partial pressure as predictors of cardiac index after coronary artery bypass grafting. Heart Lung 1993;22:112.

34. Savage RM, Lytle BW, Aronson S, Navia JL, Licina M, Stewart WJ, et al. Intraoperative echocardiography is indicated in high-risk coronary artery bypass grafting. Ann Thorac Surg 1997;64:368.

35. Skoulargis J, Rothlisberger C, Skudicky D, Essop M, Wisebaugh T, Sareli P. Effectiveness of amiodarone and electrical cardioversion for chronic rheumatic atrial fibrillation after mitral valve surgery. Am J Cardiol 1993;72:423.

36. Suga H, Sagawa K, Kostiuk DP. Controls of ventricular contractility assessed by pressure–volume ratio, Emax. Cardiovasc Res 1976; 10:582.

37. Suga H. Cardiac mechanics and energetics—from Emax to PVA. Front Med Biol Eng 1990;2:3.

38. Suga H. Paul Dudley White International Lecture: cardiac performance as viewed through the pressure–volume window. Jpn Heart J 1994;35:263.

39. Smedira NG, Blackstone EH. Postcardiotomy mechanical support: risk factors and outcomes. Ann Thorac Surg 2001;71:S60.

40. Soloff LA, Zatuchui J, O'Neill TJ, Glover RP. Reactivation of rheumatic fever following mitral commissurotomy. Circulation 1953;8:481.

41. Stewart S III, Edmunds LH Jr, Kirklin JW, Allarde RR. Spontaneous breathing with continuous positive airway pressure after open intracardiac operations in infants. J Thorac Cardiovasc Surg 1973;65:37.

42. Stewart GN. Researches on the circulation time and on the influence which affects it. IV. The output of the heart. J Physiol 1897;22:159.

T

1. Tanaka J, Yasui H, Nakano E, Sese A, Matsui K, Takeda Y, et al. Predisposing factors of renal dysfunction following total correction of tetralogy of Fallot in the adult. J Thorac Cardiovasc Surg 1980;80:135.

2. Thurer RJ, Bognolo D, Vargas A, Isch JH, Kaiser GA. The management of mediastinal infection following cardiac surgery. An experience utilizing continuous irrigation with povidone-iodine. J Thorac Cardiovasc Surg 1974;68:962.

3. Thomas CS Jr, McGoon DC. Isolated massive chylopericardium following cardiopulmonary bypass. J Thorac Cardiovasc Surg 1971;61:945.

4. Townes BD, Bashein G, Hornbein TF, Coppel DB, Goldstein DE, Davis KB, et al. Neurobehavioral outcomes in cardiac operations: a prospective controlled study. J Thorac Cardiovasc Surg 1989; 98:774.

5. Tulla H, Takala J, Alhava E, Huttunen H, Kari A. Hypermetabolism after coronary artery bypass. J Thorac Cardiovasc Surg 1991;101:598.

6. Thurer RL, Lytle BW, Cosgrove DM, Loop FD. Autotransfusion following cardiac operations: a randomized, prospective study. Ann Thorac Surg 1979;27:500.

7. Tyson GS, Sladen RN, Spainhour V, Savitt MA, Ferguson TB Jr, Wolfe WG. Blood conservation in cardiac surgery. Ann Surg 1989;209:736.

8. Topol EJ, Humphrey LS, Borkon AM, Baumgartner WA, Dorsey DL, Reitz BA, et al. Value of intraoperative left ventricular microbubbles detected by transesophageal two-dimensional echocardiography in predicting neurologic outcome after cardiac operations. Am J Cardiol 1985;56:773.

9. Templeton AW, Almond CH, Seaber A, Simmons C, MacKenzie J. Postoperative pulmonary patterns following cardiopulmonary bypass. Am J Roentgenol Radium Ther Nucl Med 1966;96:1007.

10. Timek T, Vahl CF, Bonz A, Schäffer L, Rosenberg M, Hagl S. Triiodothyronine reverses depressed contractile performance after excessive catecholamine stimulation. Ann Thorac Surg 1998; 66:1618.

U

1. Ungerleider RM, Kisslo JA, Greeley WJ, Li JS, Kanter RJ, Kern FH, et al. Intraoperative echocardiography during congenital heart operations: experience from 1,000 cases. Ann Thorac Surg 1995;60:S539.

V

1. Venn GE, Sherry K, Klinger L, Newman S, Treasure T, Harrison M, et al. Cerebral blood flow during cardiopulmonary bypass. Eur J Cardiothorac Surg 1988;2:360.

2. Venn GE, Sherry K, Klinger L. Cerebral blood flow determinants and their clinical implications during cardiopulmonary bypass. Perfusion 1988;3:271.

3. Voelkel NF, Morganroth M, Feddersen OC. Potential role of arachidonic acid metabolites in hypoxic pulmonary vasoconstriction. Chest 1985;88:245S.

4. Vogt PR, Hauser M, Schwarz U, Jenni R, Lachat ML, Zund G, et al. Complete thromboendarterectomy of the calcified ascending aorta and aortic arch. Ann Thorac Surg 1999;67:457.

5. Vedrinne C, Bastien O, DeVarax R, Blanc P, Durand PG, DuGres B, et al. Predictive factors for usefulness of fiberoptic pulmonary artery catheter for continuous oxygen saturation in mixed venous blood monitoring in cardiac surgery. Anesth Analg 1997;85:2.

6. Van Onna IE, Metz R, Jekel L, Woolley SR, van de Wal HJ. Post cardiac surgery phrenic nerve palsy: value of plication and potential for recovery. Eur J Cardiothorac Surg 1998;14:179.

W

1. Wedley JR, Lunn HF, Vale RJ. Studies of temperature balance after open-heart surgery. Crit Care Med 1975;3:134.

2. Welling RE, Rath R, Albers JE, Glaser RS. Gastrointestinal complications after cardiac surgery. Arch Surg 1986;121:1178.

3. Waldo AL, Ross SM, Kaiser GA. The epicardial electrogram in the diagnosis of cardiac arrhythmias following cardiac surgery. Geriatrics 1971;26:108.

4. Waldo AL, MacLean WA, Karp RB, Kouchoukos NT, James TN. Sustained rapid atrial pacing to control supraventricular tachycardias following open heart surgery. Circulation 1975;51/52:II13.

5. Waldo AL, MacLean WA. Diagnosis and treatment of cardiac arrhythmias following open heart surgery: emphasis on the use of atrial and ventricular epicardial wire electrodes. Mount Kisco, N.Y.: Futura, 1980.

6. Williams GD, Seifen AB, Lawson NW, Norton JB, Readinger RI, Dungan TW, et al. Pulsatile perfusion versus conventional high-flow nonpulsatile perfusion for rapid core cooling and rewarming of infants for circulatory arrest in cardiac operation. J Thorac Cardiovasc Surg 1979;78:667.

7. Weller TH. The cytomegaloviruses: ubiquitous agents with protean clinical manifestations. N Engl J Med 1971;285:267.

8. Wood EH. Use of indicator-dilution technics. In Congenital heart disease. Washington, DC: American Association of Advanced Science, 1960, p. 209.

9. Wallach R, Karp RB, Reves JG, Oparil S, Smith LR, James TN. Pathogenesis of paroxysmal hypertension developing during and after coronary bypass surgery: a study of hemodynamic and humoral factors. Am J Cardiol 1980;46:559.

10. Weitzman LB, Tinker WP, Kronzon I, Cohen ML, Glassman E, Spencer FC. The incidence and natural history of pericardial effusion after cardiac surgery: an echocardiographic study. Circulation 1984;69:506.

11. Woods JE, Taswell HF, Kirklin JW, Owen CA Jr. The transfusion of platelet concentrates in patients undergoing heart surgery. Mayo Clin Proc 1967;42:318.

12. Williams ME, Rosa RM. Hyperkalemia: disorders of internal and external potassium balance. J Intensive Care Med 1988;3:52.

13. Wheller J, George BL, Mulder DG, Jarmakani JM. Diagnosis and management of postoperative pulmonary hypertensive crisis. Circulation 1979;60:1640.

14. Watanabe T, Trusler GA, William WG, Edmonds JF, Coles JG, Hosokawa Y. Phrenic nerve paralysis after pediatric cardiac surgery: retrospective study of 125 cases. J Thorac Cardiovasc Surg 1987;94:383.

15. Wilson AP, Treasure T, Gruneberg RN, Sturridge MF, Burridge J. Should the temperature chart influence management in cardiac operations? Result of a prospective study in 314 patients. J Thorac Cardiovasc Surg 1988;96:518.

16. Wilson AP, Livesey SA, Treasure T, Gruneberg RN, Sturridge MF. Factors predisposing to wound infection in cardiac surgery: a prospective study of 517 patients. Eur J Cardiothorac Surg 1987;1:158.

17. Walsh EP, Saul JP, Sholler GF, Triedman JK, Jonas RA, Mayer JE, et al. Evaluation of a staged treatment protocol for rapid automatic junctional tachycardia after operation for congenital heart disease. J Am Coll Cardiol 1997;29:1046.

18. Werner HA, Wensley DF, Lirenman DS, LeBlanc JG. Peritoneal dialysis in children after cardiopulmonary bypass. J Thorac Cardiovasc Surg 1997;113:64.

19. Wolman RL, Nussmeier NA, Aggarwal A, Kanchuger MS, Roach GW, Newman MF, et al. Cerebral injury after cardiac surgery: identification of a group at extraordinary risk. Multicenter Study of Perioperative Ischemia Research Group (McSPI) and the Ischemia Research Foundation (IRF) Investigators. Stroke 1999;30:514.

20. Wareing TH, Davila-Roman VG, Barzilai B, Murphy SF, Kouchoukos NT. Management of the severely atherosclerotic ascending aorta during cardiac operations: a strategy for detection and treatment. J Thorac Cardiovasc Surg 1992;103:453.

21. Warkentein TE, Kelton JG. Heparin and platelets. Hematol Oncol Clin North Am 1990;4:243.

Y

1. Yamaki S, Horiuchi T, Takahashi T. Pulmonary changes in congenital heart disease with Down's syndrome: their significance as a cause of postoperative respiratory failure. Thorax 1985;40:380.

Z

1. Zobel G, Stein JI, Kuttnig M, Beitzke A, Metzler H, Rigler B. Continuous extracorporeal fluid removal in children with low cardiac output after cardiac operations. J Thorac Cardiovasc Surg 1991;101:593.

6   Generating Knowledge from Information, Data, and Analyses

SECTION 1

Generating Knowledge from Information, Data, and Analyses

INTRODUCING THE CHAPTER

What It Is About

Cardiac surgical procedures, particularly coronary artery bypass grafting, have been the most completely and quantitatively studied therapies in the history of medicine.[A5] These studies have revealed a complex, multifactorial, and multidimensional interplay among patient characteristics, variability of the heart disease, effect of the disease on the patient, conduct of the procedure, and response of the patient to treatment. Because cardiac surgeons were "data collectors" from the beginning of the subspecialty, it was natural that efforts to improve the quality of medical care generally while containing costs found cardiac surgical results (outcomes) an easy target. The dawn of medical report cards made it evident that multiple factors influencing outcome must be taken into account to make fair comparisons of outcomes (see "Risk Stratification" and "Risk Adjustment" in Section 6). This scrutiny of results, often by the media, revealed that variability in performing the technical details of operations, coupled with environmental factors often not under direct control of cardiac surgeons, contributed to differences in results.

The propensity toward data collection in cardiac surgery was reinforced in the 1970s and early 1980s by challenges from cardiologists to demonstrate not simply symptomatic improvement from operative procedures, but improved survival and long-term quality of life (appropriateness). This resulted in one of the first large-scale, government-funded registries and an in-depth research database (Box 6-1) of patients with ischemic heart disease, and a rather small, restricted randomized trial (Coronary Artery Surgery Study[N5]). It stimulated subsequent establishment by the Society of Thoracic Surgeons (STS) of what has grown to be the largest registry of cardiac surgical data.

Thus, it has become important for all in the subspecialty of cardiac surgery, not just those engaged in bench, translational, or clinical research, to (1) understand how information generated from observations during patient care becomes transformed into data suitable for analysis, (2) appreciate at a high level what constitutes appropriate analyses of those data, (3) evaluate effectively the inferences drawn from those analyses, and (4) apply new knowledge to better care for individual patients.

It is our desire that the reader realize these goals and not conclude prematurely that this chapter is simply a treatise on biostatistics, outcomes research, epidemiology, biomathematics, or bioinformatics.[1]

Who Should Read It

This chapter should be read in whole or in part by (1) all cardiac surgeons, to improve their comprehension of the medical literature and to hone their skills in its critical appraisal; (2) young surgeons interested in becoming clinical investigators, who need instruction on how to pursue successful research (see "Technique for Successful Clinical Research" later in this section); (3) mature surgeon–investigators and other similar medical professionals and their collaborating statisticians, mathematicians, and computer scientists, who will benefit from some of the philosophical ideas included in this section and particularly from the discussion of emerging analytic methods for generating new knowledge; and (4) data managers of larger clinical research groups, who need to fully appreciate their pivotal role in successful research (Appendix 6A), particularly as described in Sections 1, 2, and 3 of this chapter.

The potential obstacle for all will be language. For the surgeon, the language of statistics, mathematics, and computer science may pose a daunting obstacle of symbols, numbers, and algorithms. For collaborators in statistics, mathematics, and computer science, the Greek and Latin language of medicine is equally daunting. This chapter attempts to surmount the language barrier by translating ideas, philosophy, and unfamiliar concepts into words, while introducing only sufficient statistics, mathematics, and algorithms to be useful for the collaborating scientist.

---

[1] In its narrowest definition, bioinformatics is a collection of methods devised to process genomic data, representing the reality that advances in genomics require sophisticated and often new computer algorithms. Some would say bioinformatics is the next frontier for statistics, others for machine learning. This is the narrow view. The National Institutes of Health (NIH) in the United States has provided a broader view. The NIH Biomedical Information Science and Technology Initiative Consortium agreed on the following definition of bioinformatics, "recognizing that no definition could completely eliminate overlap with other activities or preclude variations in interpretation by different individuals and organizations."

Bioinformatics is research, development, or application of computational tools and approaches for expanding the use of biological, medical, behavioral or health data, including those to acquire, store, organize, archive, analyze, or visualize such data. (http://grants1.nih.gov/grants/bistic/CompuBioDef.pdf)

They go on to define computational biology in a broader context than genomics as "the development and application of data-analytical and theoretical methods, mathematical modeling and computational simulation techniques to the study of biological, behavioral, and social systems."

Thus, they envision bringing together the quantitative needs in structural biology, biochemistry, molecular biology, and genomics at the microscopic level, and medical, health services, health economics, and even social systems disciplines at the macroscopic level, with analytic tools from computer science, mathematics, statistics, physics, and other quantitative disciplines to lead from information to new knowledge.

This vision transcends the current restrictiveness of traditional biostatistics in analysis of clinical information. This is why we have emphasized in this chapter that the material is not simply for surgeons, their clinical research team, and consulting and collaborating biostatisticians, but also for a wider audience of professionals in a variety of quantitative disciplines.

Lauer and Blackstone have reviewed various types and purposes of databases in cardiology and cardiac surgery.[L15] Among these are the following, each containing a different fraction of the information on the longitudinal health care of individual patients, and each constructed for differing purposes, although they at times overlap.

Registry

A database consisting of only a few core data elements (those likely to be needed for identifying patients according to diagnosis and procedure) on every patient in a defined population.

Typical registries would be all cardiac surgical patients for whom core Society of Thoracic Surgery (STS) or EuroSCORE variables are collected. The implication is that a registry is an ongoing activity that is broad, but thin in data content. It is enormously expensive to sustain and maintain a registry with in-depth variables.

Research Database

A database consisting of in-depth data about a defined subset of patients. A research database, in contrast to a registry, is narrow and deep. Williams and McCrindle have called such databases "academic databases," because they usually are constructed by those in academic institutions to facilitate clinical research.[W10]

Even with such a database, an individual study may use a fraction of the variables and then must add a number of new variables that are relevant to particular studies. Often the fixed structure of the database is not such that these additional variables can easily be assimilated, so they are often contained in ancillary databases. These ancillary databases may not be available as a resource to subsequent investigators (see Section 2).

Administrative Database

A database consisting of demographic variables, diagnostic codes, and procedural codes that are available electronically, generally from billing systems. Administrative databases are used by outcomes or health services research professionals for quality assessment.

National Database

A database consisting of completely de-identified data, generally of limited scope, but usually containing meaningful medical variables, including patient demography, past history, present condition, some laboratory and diagnostic data, procedure, and outcomes. National (and international) databases are intended to be used for general quality assessment; medical health quality improvement; government activities at a regional, national, or international level; and public consumption.

Because this chapter is intended for a mixed audience, it focuses on the most common points of intersection between cardiac surgery and quantitative science, with the goal of establishing sufficient common ground for effective and efficient collaboration.

How It Has Evolved

At least three factors have contributed to the evolution of Chapter 6 from edition to edition of this book: the increasing importance of computers in analyzing clinical data, the introduction of new and increasingly appropriate and applicable methods for analyzing those data, and the growing importance of nonstatistical methods for mining medical data.

Thus, the title of this chapter in Edition 1 was "Surgical Concepts, Research Methods, and Data Analysis and Use."

Its sections highlighted (1) surgical success and failure, (2) incremental risk factors, (3) research methods, (4) methods of data presentation and analysis and comparison, (5) decision-making for individual patients, and (6) improving results of cardiac surgery. All remain important, but progress in each of these areas warrants a fresh approach. In the first edition, considerable emphasis was placed on providing formulae for surgeons to implement on a new generation of *programmable calculators*. These calculator programs provided confidence limits and simple statistical tests that continue to be valuable, particularly in reading and evaluating the literature; however, the increasing sophistication and complexity of programmable calculators have taken implementation of the programs out of the reach of most surgeons.

In Edition 2, the germ of an organizing schema for clinical research was developed, and the name of the chapter was changed to reflect it: "The Generation of Knowledge from Information, Data, and Analyses." This schema did not lead at that time to a matching organizational format for the chapter, but paved the way for one. At the time of its writing there had been explosive progress in techniques for analyzing time-related events, so an important portion of the chapter was devoted to this topic. Effective analysis of time-related events was no longer possible with small calculators, but demanded powerful computer resources.

In this edition, we have exploited the idea of progressing from information to data to analyses to knowledge as an explicit organizing schema for the chapter. It will become evident to the reader that except for simple statistics, computers have become indispensable tools for clinical research. In addition, whereas the statistician was once the surgeon's primary collaborator in data analysis, experts in computer science and mathematics are now equally likely to fill that role.

Undoubtedly, evolution of this chapter will continue in subsequent editions, because new methods are constantly being developed to better answer clinical questions.[B39] For example, although analysis of time-related events is still emphasized in this edition, new methods of longitudinal analysis are now highlighted, as are new methods for nonrandomized comparisons and multivariable analysis.

How It Is Organized

The organizational basis for this chapter is the Newtonian *inductive method* of discovery.[N6] It begins with *information* about a microcosm of medicine, proceeds to translation of information into *data* and *analysis* of those data, and ends with new *knowledge* about a small aspect of nature. This organizational basis emphasizes the phrase, "let the data speak for themselves." It is that philosophy that dictates, for example, placing "Indications for Operation" after, not before, presentation of surgical results throughout this book.

Information

In health care, information is a collection of material, workflow documentation, and recorded observations (see Section 2). Information may be recorded in paper-based medical records or in electronic (computer) format.

Data

Data consist of organized values for variables, usually expressed symbolically (e.g., numerically) by means of a controlled vocabulary (see Section 3).[K16] Characterization of data includes descriptive statistics that summarize parts or all of the data and express their variability.

Analysis

Data analysis is a process, often prolonged and repeated (iterative), that uses a large repertoire of methods by which data are explored, important findings are revealed and unimportant ones suppressed, and relations are clarified and quantified (see Sections 4 and 6).

Knowledge

Knowledge is the synthesis of information, data, and analyses arrived at by inductive reasoning (see Section 5). However, generation of new knowledge does not occur in a vacuum; an important step is assimilating new knowledge within the body of existing knowledge.

New knowledge may take the form of *clinical inferences*, which are simple summarizing statements that synthesize information, data, and analyses, drawn with varying degrees of confidence that they are true. It may also include *speculations*, which are statements suggested by the data or by reasoning, often about mechanisms, without direct supportive data. Ideally, it also includes new *hypotheses*, which are statements to be tested that are suggested by reasoning or inferences from the information, data, and analyses.

New knowledge can be applied to a number of processes in health care, including (1) generating new concepts, (2) making individual patient care decisions, (3) obtaining informed consent from patients, (4) improving surgical outcomes, (5) assessing the quality and appropriateness of care, and (6) making regulatory decisions (see Section 5).

How to Read This Chapter

Unlike most chapters in this book, whose various parts can be read somewhat randomly and in isolation, Section 1 of this chapter should be read in its entirety before embarking on other parts of the text. It identifies the mindset of the authors; defends the rationale for emphasizing surgical success and failure; contrasts philosophies, concepts, and ideas that shape both how we think about the results of research and how we do research; lays out a technique for successful clinical research that parallels the surgical technique portions of other chapters; and, for collaborating statisticians, mathematicians, and computer scientists engaged in analyzing clinical data, lays the foundation for our recommendations concerning data analysis.

Much of the material in this introductory section is amplified in later portions of the chapter, and we provide cross-references to these to avoid redundancy.

THE DRIVING FORCES OF NEW KNOWLEDGE

Many forces drive the generation of new knowledge in cardiac surgery, including the economics of health care, need for innovation, clinical research, surgical success and failure, and increased awareness of medical error.

Economics

The economics of health care are driving changes in practice toward what is presumed to be less expensive, more efficient, and higher quality care. Interesting methods for testing the validity of these claims have become available in the form of *cluster randomized trials*.[B29,D5] In such trials (e.g., a trial introducing a change in physician behavior), patients are not randomized, physicians are (patients form the cluster being cared for by each physician)! This leads to inefficient studies that nevertheless can be effective with proper design and a large enough pool of physicians.[B28,D5] It is a study design in which the unit of randomization (physician) is not the unit of analysis (individual patient outcome).[D6] Such trials appear to require rethinking of traditional medical ethics.[E6]

Innovation

Just when it seems that cardiac surgery has matured, innovation intervenes and drives new knowledge both from proponents and opponents. Innovation occurs at several levels. It includes new devices; new procedures; existing procedures performed on new groups of patients, such as the elderly and the fetus; simplifying and codifying seemingly disparate anatomy, physiology, or operative techniques; standardizing procedures to make them teachable and reproducible; and introducing new concepts of patient care (the intensive care unit, automated infusion devices, automated care by computer-based protocols). Many of these innovations have had applications far beyond the boundary of cardiac surgery.

Yet, innovation is often at odds with cost reduction and is perceived as being at odds with traditional research. In all areas of science, however, injection of innovation is the enthalpy that prevents entropy, stimulating yet more research and development and more innovation. Without it cardiac surgery would be unable to adapt to changes in managing ischemic heart disease, potential reversal of the atherosclerotic process, percutaneous approaches to valvar and congenital heart disease, and other changes directed toward less invasive therapy.

What is controversial is (1) when and if it is appropriate to subject innovation to formal clinical trial and (2) the ethics of innovation in surgery for which standardization is difficult.[A3,E6,M4-M6]

Reducing the Unknown

New knowledge in cardiac surgery has been driven from its inception by a genuine quest to fill obvious voids of the unknown, whether by clinical research or laboratory research (which we do not emphasize in this chapter, although the principles and recipe for success are the same as for clinical research). This has included research to clarify both normal physiology and abnormal physiology, but also to characterize the abnormal state of the body supported on cardiopulmonary bypass.

Clinical research has historically followed one of two broad designs: randomized clinical trials and nonrandomized studies of cohorts of patients ("clinical practice"), as detailed later in this section under "Clinical Trials with Randomly Assigned Treatment" and "Clinical Studies with Nonrandomly Assigned Treatment," respectively. Increasing emphasis, however, is being placed on translational research, that is, bringing basic research findings to the bedside. John Kirklin called this the "excitement at the interface of disciplines." Part and parcel of the concept of incremental risk factor identification (see "Incremental Risk Factor Concept" in Section 4) is that it is an essential link in a feedback loop that may start with a surgical failure, proceed to identifying risk factors, draw inferences about specific gaps in knowledge that need to be addressed by basic science, generate fundamental knowledge by the basic scientists, and end by bringing these full circle to the clinical arena, testing and assessing the value of the new knowledge for improving medical care.[B18]

Surgical Success and Failure

Results of operative intervention in heart disease, particularly surgical failure, have driven much of the new knowledge generated by clinical research. In the late 1970s and early 1980s a perhaps oversimplified but useful concept arose about surgical failures. That is, in the absence of natural disaster or sabotage, there are two principal causes of failure of cardiac operations (or other treatments) to provide a desired outcome for an individual patient: (1) lack of scientific progress and (2) human error.

The utility of this concept was that it led to the programmatic strategies of *research* on the one hand and *development* on the other, in the business sense of "research and development." Thus, lack of scientific progress, the unknown, may be gradually minimized by generating new knowledge (research), and human error may be minimized in frequency and consequences by implementing available knowledge (development), a process as vital in cardiac surgery as it is in the transportation or manufacturing sectors.[E1,H5,L1,W2]

Error

Increased awareness of medical error is driving the generation of new knowledge just as it is driving increasing regulatory pressure and medico-legal litigation.[K14] The UAB group was one of the first not only to publish information about human error in cardiac surgery but also to place it into the context of cognitive sciences, human factors, and safety research.[R2] This interface of disciplines is essential for facilitating substantial reduction in injury from medical errors.

SURGICAL FAILURE

Surgical failure has been a strong stimulant of clinical research aimed at making scientific progress. It has not stimulated a quest for reduction of human error to the same degree, and rightly so, because we presume it is the unknown that has the greatest impact on surgical failure. Further, human error carries negative connotations that make it more difficult to discuss in a positive, objective way. It is too often equated with negligence or malpractice, and almost inevitably leads to blame of persons on the "sharp end" (caregivers), with little consideration of the decision-making, organizational structures, infrastructures,

or other factors that are remote in time and distance (blunt end).

Interestingly, although covered in some detail in the first edition of this book, discussion of human error was abbreviated in the second. However, release of the Institute of Medicine's report on medical errors in 1999,[K14] publication of James Reason's book *Human Error*[R3] and his close collaboration with Marc deLeval at Great Ormond Street Hospital for Children in the United Kingdom–wide study of human error during the arterial switch operation,[D7] and Gawande's series of articles in the *New Yorker* now collected in *Complications: A Surgeon's Notes on an Imperfect Science*[G33] have reestablished it as an important topic for this chapter. Thus, we begin with what might be called the failure to apply new knowledge as a prelude to generating new knowledge.

Human Error

As early as 1912, the need to eliminate "preventable disaster from surgery" was recognized.[R5] Human errors as a cause of surgical failure are not difficult to find,[R2] particularly if one is careful to include errors of diagnosis, delay in therapy, inappropriate operations, omissions of therapy, and breaches of protocol.

When we initially delved into what was known about human error in the era before Canary Island (1977), Three-Mile Island (1979), Bhopal (1984), Challenger (1986), and Chernobyl (1986), events that contributed enormously to knowledge of the nature of human error, we learned two lessons from the investigation of occupational and mining injuries.[L1,W2] First, successful investigation of the role of the human element in injury depends on establishing an environment of *non-culpable error.*[W2] The natural human reaction to investigation of error is to become defensive and to provide no information that might prove incriminating. An atmosphere of blame impedes investigating, understanding, and preventing error. How foreign this is from the culture of medicine! We take responsibility for whatever happens to our patients as a philosophic commitment.[B33,M10] Yet cardiac operations are performed in a complex and imperfect environment in which every individual performs imperfectly at times.[C12] It is too easy, when things go wrong, to look for someone to blame.[W9] Blame by 20/20 hindsight allows more fundamental circumstances and causes to be overlooked.

Second, we learned that errors of *omission* exceed errors of *commission.* This is exactly what we found in ventricular septal defect repair (Table 6-1), suggesting that the cardiac surgical environment is not so different from that of a gold mine and that we can learn from that literature.

These two lessons reinforced some surgical practices and stimulated introduction of others that were valuable in the early stages of growth of the UAB cardiac surgery program: using hand signals for passing instruments, minimizing distractions, replying simply to every command, reading aloud the protocol for the operation as it proceeds, standardizing apparently disparate operations, and focusing morbidity conferences candidly on human error and lack of knowledge in order to prevent the same failure in the future. To amplify, these practices might be enunciated as a "culture of clarity," the end result of which is a

■ **TABLE 6-1 Management Errors Associated with 30 Hospital Deaths Following Repair of Ventricular Septal Defect (UAB; 1967 to 1979; $n = 312$)**

Error	Number
Operation despite severe pulmonary vascular disease	3
Undiagnosed and overlooked VSDs	8
Despite heart block, no permanent pacing electrodes inserted at operation	1
Clots in oxygenator and heat exchanger (and Circle of Willis)	1
Extubation without reintubation within a few hours of operation in seriously ill infants	4
Self-extubation without reintubation in the face of low cardiac output	1
Transfusion of packed RBCs of wrong type	1

(Data from Rizzoli and colleagues.[R2])

Key: *RBC,* Red blood cell; *VSD,* ventricular septal defect.

reproducible and successful surgical endeavor. In the operating room, each individual on the surgical team is relaxed but alert:

- Hand signals serve to inform assistants and the scrub nurse of anticipated needs for a relatively small number of frequently utilized instruments or maneuvers.
- Spoken communication is reserved for those out of the field of sight, that is, the anesthesiologist and perfusionist. When verbalized, "commands" are acknowledged with a simple reply: "thank you," "roger," "yes." Even those individuals out of the field learn to anticipate these events or commands.
- Anticipated deviations from the usual are presented a few minutes to a day or two before the event. (In teaching settings, residents are encouraged to write an operative plan in the preoperative note.) Unanticipated deviations are acknowledged to all concerned as soon as possible.
- Successful routines are codified. These include chronology for anticoagulation and its reversal, myocardial management routines (induction of cardioplegia, intervals of cardioplegia reinfusion, controlled myocardial reperfusion before aortic clamp removal), and protocols controlled by the surgeon for commencing and weaning the patient from cardiopulmonary bypass.
- Technical intuitive concepts are articulated. For example, some think the ventricular septal defect in tetralogy of Fallot is a circular hole. Thus, closing such a hole would simply involve running a suture circumferentially to secure a patch. Kirklin and Karp were able to describe the suture line as having four different areas of transition in three dimensions and precisely articulated names for those transitions.[K25] Each had a defined anatomic relationship to neighboring structures, so the hole became infinitely more interesting!
- Discussion of surgical failure is planned for a time (usually Saturday morning) when distractions are at a minimum. The stated goal is improvement, measurable in terms of reproducibility and surgical success. The philosophy is that events do not simply occur but have antecedent associations. An attempt is made to determine if errors can be avoided and if scientific knowledge exists or does not exist to prevent future failure.

A major portion of the remainder of this chapter addresses the acquisition and description of this new knowledge.

Categories of Human Error

Slips are failures in execution of actions and are commonly associated with attention failures (Box 6-2). Some external stimulus interrupts a sequence of actions or in some other way intrudes into them so that attention is redirected. In that instance, the intended action is not taken. *Lapses* are failures of memory. A step in the plan is omitted, a place in a sequence of actions is lost, or the reason for what one is doing is forgotten. *Mistakes* relate to plans and so take two familiar forms: (1) misapplication to the immediate situation of a good plan (rule) appropriate for a different and more usual situation and (2) application of the wrong plan (rule).

Slips and lapses constitute *active errors.* They occur at the physician–patient interface.[C13] Mistakes, in addition, constitute many *latent errors.* These are indirect errors that relate to performance by leaders, decision-makers, managers, certifying boards, environmental services, and a host of activities that share a common trait: planning, decisions, ideas, and philosophy removed in time and space from the intermediate health care environment in which the error occurred (blunt end). These are a category of error over which the surgeon caring for a patient (sharp end) has little or no control or chance of modifying, because latent errors are embedded in the system. It is claimed by students of human error in other contexts that the greatest chance of preventing adverse outcomes from human error is in discovering and neutralizing latent error.[R3]

Inevitability of Human Error

If one considers all the possibilities for error in daily life, what is remarkable is that so few are made. We are surrounded with unimaginable complexity, yet we cope nearly perfectly because our minds simplify complex information. Think of how remarkably accident-free are our early morning commutes to the hospital driving complex machines in complex traffic patterns.

When this cognitive strategy fails us, it does so in only a few stereotypical ways.[R6] Because of this, models have been developed, based largely on observation of human error, that mimic human behavior by incorporating a fallible information handling device (our minds) that operates correctly nearly always, but is occasionally wrong. Central to the theory on which these models are based is that our minds can remarkably simplify complex information. Exceedingly rare imperfect performance is theorized to be the price we pay for being able to cope, probably nearly limitlessly, with complexity. The mechanisms of human error are purported to stem from three aspects of "fallible machines": downregulation, upregulation, and primitive mechanisms of information retrieval.

Downregulation. We call this habit formation, skill development, and "good hands." Most activities of life, and certainly those of a skillful surgeon, need to become automatic. If we had to think about every motion involved in either driving a car or performing an operation, the task would become nearly impossible to perform accurately. It would not be executed smoothly and thus would be error prone. It is hard to quantify surgical skill. It starts with a baseline of necessary sensory–motor eye–hand coordination that is likely innate. It becomes optimized by aggregation of correct "moves" and steps as well as by observation. It is refined by repetition of correct actions, implying identification of satisfactory and unsatisfactory immediate results (feedback). Then comes individual reflection and codification of moves and steps by hard analysis. Finally, motor skills are mastered by a synthesis of cognition and motor memory. The resulting automaticity and reproducibility of a skillful surgeon make a complex operation appear effortless, graceful, and flawless. However, automaticity renders errors inevitable.

Skill-based errors occur in the setting of routine activity.[R4] They occur when attention is diverted (distraction or preoccupation) or when a situation changes and is not detected in a timely fashion. Interestingly, they also occur as a result of overattention. Skill-based errors are ones that only skilled experts can make—beautiful execution of the wrong thing (slip) or failure to follow a complex sequence of actions (lapse). Skill-based errors tend to be easily detected and corrected.

Rule-based errors occur during routine problem-solving activities.[R4] Goals of training programs are to produce not only skillful surgeons but also expert problem solvers. Indeed, an expert may be defined as an individual with a wide repertoire of stored problem-solving plans or rules. Inevitable errors that occur take the form of either inappropriate application of a good rule or application of a bad rule.

Upregulation. Our mind focuses conscious attention on the problem or activity with which we are confronted and filters out distracting information. The price we pay for this powerful ability is susceptibility to both data loss and information overload. This aspect of the mind is also what permits distractions or preoccupations to capture the atten-

tion of the surgeon, who would otherwise be focused on the routine tasks at hand. In problem solving, there may be inappropriate matching of the patient's actual condition to routine rules for a somewhat different set of circumstances. Some of the mismatch undoubtedly results from the display of vast quantities of undigested monitored information about the patient's condition. Errors of information overload need to be addressed by more intelligent computer-based assimilation and display of data.

Primitive mechanisms of information storage and retrieval. The mind seems to possess an unlimited capacity for information storage and a blinding speed of information retrieval unparalleled by computers. In computer systems there is often a tradeoff between storage capacity and speed of retrieval; not so for the mind. The brain achieves this, apparently, not by storing facts, but by storing models and theories–abstractions–about these facts (i.e., it stores meaning, not the data behind the meaning). Further, the information is stored in finite packets along with other, often unrelated, information. (Many people use the latter phenomenon to recall names, for example, by associating them with more familiar objects, such as animals.) The implications for error are that our mental image may diverge importantly from reality.

The mind's search strategy for information achieves remarkable speed by having apparently just two tools for fetching information. First, it matches patterns. Opportunity for error arises because our interpretation of the present and anticipation of the future are shaped by patterns or regularities of the past. Second, if pattern matching produces multiple items, it prioritizes these by choosing the one that has been retrieved most often. This mechanism gives rise to rule-based errors, for example, in a less frequently occurring setting.

Conscious mind. When automatic skills and stored rules are of no help, we must consciously think. Unlike the automaticity we have just described, the conscious mind is of limited capacity, but possesses powerful computational and reasoning tools, all those attributes we ascribe to the thought process. However, it is a serial, slow, and laborious process that gives rise to *knowledge-based errors*.[R4] Unlike stereotypical skill- and rule-based errors, knowledge-based errors are less predictable. Further, there are far fewer opportunities in life for "thinking" than for automatic processes, and therefore the ratio of errors to opportunity is higher. Errors take the form of confirmation bias, causality versus association, inappropriate selectivity, overconfidence, and difficulties in assimilating temporal processes.

The unusual ordering of material presented in the clinical chapters of this book was chosen by its original authors to provide a framework for thinking with the conscious mind about heart disease and its surgical therapy that would assist in preventing knowledge-based errors. For example, an algorithm (protocol, recipe) for successfully managing mitral valve regurgitation is based on knowledge of morphology, etiology, and detailed mechanisms of the regurgitation; preoperative clinical, physiologic, and imaging findings; natural history of the disease if left untreated; technical details of operation; postoperative management; both early and long-term results of operation; and from all these considerations the indications for operation and type of operation. Lack of adequate knowledge results in inappropriate use of mitral valve repair, too many mitral valve replacements, or suboptimal timing of operation.

Reducing Errors

We have presented this cognitive model in part because it suggests constructive steps for reducing human error and, thus, surgical failure.[C11,L8,L9]

It affirms the necessity for intense apprentice-type training that leads to automatization of surgical skill and problem-solving rules. It equally suggests the value of simulators for acquiring such skills. It supports creation of an environment that minimizes or masks potential distractions. It supports a system that discovers errors and allows recovery from them before injury occurs. This requires a well-trained team in which each individual is familiar with the operative protocol and is alert to any departures from it. In this regard, deLeval and colleagues' findings are sobering.[D7] Major errors were often realized and corrected by the surgical team, but minor ones were not, and the number of minor errors was strongly associated with adverse outcomes. It was also sobering that self-reporting of intraoperative errors was of no value. Must there be a human factors professional at the elbow of every surgeon and physician?

James Reason suggested that other "cognitive prostheses" may be of value,[R3] some of which are being advocated in medicine. For example, there is much that computers can do to reduce medication errors. A prime target is knowledge-based errors. Reducing these errors may not be achievable through computer artificial intelligence but rather through more appropriate modes of information assembly, processing, and display for processing by the human mind. Finally, if latent errors are the root cause of many active errors, analysis and correction at the system level will be required. A cardiac surgery program may fail, for example, from latent errors traceable to management of the blood bank, postoperative care practices, ventilation systems, and even complex administrative decisions at the level of hospitals, universities with which they may be associated, and national health system policies and regulations within which they operate.

Lack of Scientific Progress

A practical consequence of categorizing surgical failures into two causes is that they fit the programmatic paradigm of "research and development": discovery on the one hand and application of knowledge to prevent failures on the other. The quest to reduce injury from medical errors that has just been described is what we might term "development." The remainder of this chapter focuses mainly on the portion of the paradigm that is research, but also more narrowly on *clinical research.*

PHILOSOPHY

Clinical research in cardiac surgery as emphasized in this chapter consists largely of patient-oriented investigations motivated by a serious quest for new knowledge to improve surgical results—that is, to increase survival, early and long term; to reduce complications; to be able to extend appro-

priate operations to more patients, such as high-risk subsets; and to devise and evaluate new beneficial procedures, such as the Fontan operation and its variants (see Chapter 27) and the Norwood operation (see Chapter 35), that have been generalized into a strategy of managing not so much individual malformations as a physiologic situation.

This inferential activity, aimed at improving clinical results, is in contrast to pure description of experiences. Its motivation also contrasts with those aspects of "outcomes assessment" motivated by regulation or punishment, institutional promotion or protection, quality assessment by outlier identification, and negative aspects of cost justification or containment. These coexisting motivations have stimulated us to identify, articulate, and contrast philosophies that underlie serious clinical research. It is these philosophies that inform our approach to analysis of clinical experiences.

Deduction versus Induction

"Let the data speak for themselves."

Arguably, Sir Isaac Newton's greatest contribution to science was a novel intellectual tool: a method for investigating the nature of natural phenomena.[G15] His contemporaries considered his method not only a powerful scientific investigative tool, but also a new way of philosophizing applicable to all areas of human knowledge. His method had two strictly ordered aspects that for the first time were truly systematically expressed: a first, and extensive, phase of data *analysis,* whereby observations of some small portion of a natural phenomenon are examined and dissected, followed by a second, less emphasized, phase of *synthesis,* whereby possible causes are inferred and a small portion of nature revealed from the observations and analyses.[N6] This was the beginning of the *inductive method* in science: valuing first and foremost the observations made about a phenomenon, then "letting the data speak for themselves" in suggesting possible natural mechanisms.

This represented the antithesis of the *deductive method* of investigation that had been so successful in the development of mathematics and logic. The deductive method begins with what is believed to be the nature of the universe (referred to by Newton as "hypothesis"), from which logical predictions are deduced and tested against observations. If the observations deviate from logic, the data are suspect, not the principles behind the deductions. The data do not speak for themselves.

Newton realized that it was impossible at any time or place to have complete knowledge of the universe. Therefore, a new methodology was necessary to examine just portions of nature, with less emphasis on synthesizing the whole. The idea was heralded as liberating in nearly all fields of science.

As the eighteenth century unfolded, the new method rapidly divided such diverse ideas as religion into those based on deduction (fundamentalism) and those based on induction (liberalism), roughly Calvinism versus Wesleyan-Arminianism. This philosophic dichotomy continues to shape not just the scientific but the social, economic, and political climate of the twenty-first century.

Determinism versus Empiricism

Determinism is the philosophy that everything—events, acts, diseases, decisions—is an inevitable consequence of causal antecedents: "Whatever will be will be." If disease and patients' response to disease and to disease treatment were clearly deterministic and inferences deductive, there would be no need to analyze clinical data to discover their general patterns. Great strides are being made in linking causal mechanisms to predictable clinical response (see "Classification Methods" in Section 6).[B38,C14,H15,L12,R8,Y3,Z1] Yet many areas of cardiovascular medicine remain nondeterministic and incompletely understood. In particular, the relation between a specific patient's response to complex therapy such as a cardiac operation and known mechanisms of disease appears to be predictable only in a probabilistic sense. For these patients, therapy is based on empirical recognition of general patterns of disease progression and observed response to therapy.

Generating new knowledge from clinical experiences consists, then, of inductive inference about the nature of disease and its treatment from analyses of ongoing, empirical observations of clinical experience that take into account variability, uncertainty, and relationships among surrogate variables for causal mechanisms.

Collectivism versus Individualism

To better convey how new knowledge is acquired from observing clinical experiences, we look back to the seventeenth century to encounter the proverbial dichotomy between collectivism and individualism, so-called lumpers and splitters or forests and trees.

In 1603, during one of its worst plague epidemics, the City of London began prospective collection of weekly records of christenings and burials. In modern language, this was an administrative database or registry (see Box 6-1). Those "who constantly took in the weekly bills of mortality made little use of them, than to look at the foot, how the burials increased or decreased; and among the casualties, what has happened rare, and extraordinary, in the week current," complained John Graunt.[H11] Unlike those who stopped at counting and relating anecdotal information, Graunt believed the data could be analyzed in a way that would yield useful inferences about the nature and possible control of the plague.

His ultimate success might be attributed in part to his being an investigator at the interface of disciplines. By profession he was a shopkeeper, so Graunt translated store inventory dynamics into terms of human population dynamics. He described the rate of goods received (birth rate) and the rate of goods sold (death rate); he then calculated the inventory on the store shelves (those currently alive).

Graunt then made a giant intellectual leap. In modern terms, he assumed that any item on the shelf was interchangeable with any other (collectivism). By assuming, no matter how politically and sociologically incorrect, that people are interchangeable, he achieved an understanding of the general nature of the birth-life-death process in the absence of dealing with specific, named individuals (indi-

vidualism). He attempted to discover, as it were, the general nature of the forest at the expense of the individual trees.

Graunt then identified general factors associated with variability of these rates (risk factors, in modern terminology; see "Multivariable Analysis" in Section 4). From the City of London Bills of Mortality, he found that the death rate was higher when ships from foreign ports docked, in the more densely populated areas of the city, and in households harboring domestic animals. Based on these observations, he made inferences about the nature of the plague—what it was and what it was not—and formulated recommendations for stopping its spread. They were crude, nonspecific, and empirical: Flee the night air brought in from foreign ships (which we now know is not night air but rats), go to the country, separate people from animal vectors, and quarantine infected individuals.[G9] Nevertheless, they were effective in stopping the plague for 200 years until its cause and mechanism of spread were identified.

Lessons based on this therapeutic triumph of clinical investigation conducted more than 300 years ago include the following: (1) empirical identification of patterns of disease can suggest fruitful directions for future research and eliminate some hypothesized causal mechanisms, (2) recommendations based on empirical observations may be effective until causal mechanisms and treatments are discovered, and (3) new knowledge is often generated by overview (synthesis), as well as by study of individual patients.

When generating new knowledge about the nature of heart disease and its treatment, it is important both to examine groups of patients (the forest) and to investigate individual therapeutic failures (the trees). This is similar to Heisenberg's uncertainty principle in chemistry, thermodynamics, and mechanics, in which physical matter and energy can be thought of as discrete particles on the microhierarchical plane (individualism, splitting, trees), and as waves (field theory) on the macrohierarchical plane (collectivism, lumping, forests). Both views give valuable insights into nature, but they cannot be viewed simultaneously. Statistical methods emphasizing optimum discrimination for identifying individual patients at risk tend to apply to the former, whereas those emphasizing probabilities and general inferences tend to apply to the latter.[C14,Y3]

Continuity versus Discontinuity in Nature

When we turn our focus from named individuals experiencing surgical failure to groups of patients, data analysis becomes mandatory to discover relationships between outcome and items that differ in value from patient to patient (variables). A challenge immediately arises: Many of the variables related to outcome are measured either on an ordered clinical scale (ordinal variables), such as New York Heart Association (NYHA) functional class, or on a more or less unlimited scale (continuous variables), such as age.

Three hundred years after Graunt, the Framingham Heart Disease Epidemiology Study investigators were faced with this frustrating problem.[G7,G14] Many of the variables associated with development of heart disease were continuously distributed ones, such as age, higher blood pressure, and higher cholesterol level. To examine the relationship of such variables to the development of heart disease, it was then accepted practice to categorize continuous variables coarsely and arbitrarily so that cross-tabulation tables could be made. Valuable information was lost this way. Investigators recognized that a 59-year-old's risk of developing heart disease was more closely related to a 60-year-old's than to that of the group of patients in the sixth versus seventh decade of life. They therefore insisted on examining the entire spectrum of continuous variables rather than subclassifying the information.

What they embraced is a key concept in the history of ideas, namely, *continuity in nature*. The idea has emerged in mathematics, science, philosophy, history, and theology.[B34] In our view, the common practice of stratifying age and other more or less continuous variables into a few discrete categories is lamentable, because it loses the power of continuity (some statisticians call this "borrowing power"). Focus on small, presumed homogeneous groups of patients also loses the power inherent in a wide spectrum of heterogeneous, but related, cases. After all, any trend observed over an ever-narrower framework looks more and more like no trend at all! Like the Framingham investigators, we therefore embrace continuity in nature unless it can be demonstrated that doing so is not valid, useful, or beneficial. (Modern methods of machine learning stumble at this point; see "Classification Methods" in Section 6.)

Single versus Multiple Dimensionality

The second problem the Framingham investigators addressed was the need to consider multiple variables simultaneously. Univariable statistics are attractive because they are simple to understand. However, most clinical problems are multifactorial. At the same time, clinical data contain enormous redundancies that somehow need to be taken into account (e.g., height, weight, body surface area, and body mass index are highly correlated and relate to the conceptual variable "body size").

Cornfield came to the rescue of the Framingham investigators with a new methodology called *multivariable logistic regression*[C9] (see "Logistic Regression Analysis" in Section 4). It permitted multiple factors to be examined simultaneously, took into account redundancy of information among variables, and identified a parsimonious set of variables for which the investigators coined the term *risk factors* (see "Parsimony versus Complexity" later in this section and "Multivariable Analysis" in Section 4).

Various forms of multivariable analysis, in addition to logistic regression analysis, have become available to clinical investigators. Their common theme is to identify patterns of relationships between outcome and a number of variables considered simultaneously. These are not deterministic cause–effect relations, but associations, surrogates for underlying causal mechanisms. The relationships that are found may well be spurious, fortuitous, hard to interpret, and even confusing because of the degree of correlation among variables. For example, women may be at a higher risk of mortality after certain cardiac procedures, but female gender may not be a "risk factor" because other factors, such as body mass index, may be the more general variable related to risk, whether in women or men. Even so, it is simultaneously true that (1) being female is not per se a risk factor, but (2) women are at higher risk by virtue of the fact that on average they are smaller than men.

This means that a close collaboration must exist between statistical experts and surgeons, particularly in organizing variables for analysis.

Linearity versus Nonlinearity

Risk factor methodology introduced another complexity besides increased dimensionality. The logistic equation is a symmetric S-shaped curve that expresses the relationship between a scale of risk, called logit units, and a corresponding scale of the absolute probability of experiencing an event (Fig. 6-1).[B9,K3] Because the relationship is not linear, it is not possible to simply add up scores for individual variables and come up with a probability of an event, a technique that has been attempted in other settings (see "Risk Stratification" in Section 6).[P10]

The nonlinear relationship between risk factors and probability of outcome makes an enormous amount of medical sense. Imagine a risk factor with a logit unit coefficient of 1.0 (representing an odds ratio of 2.7; Box 6-3 and Fig. 6-1). If all other things position a patient far to the left on the logit scale, a 1-logit-unit increase in risk results in a trivial increase in the probability of experiencing an event. But as other factors move a patient closer to the center of the scale (0 logit units, corresponding to a 50% probability of an event), a 1-logit-unit increase in risk makes a huge difference. This is consistent with the medical perception that some patients experiencing the same disease, trauma, or complication react quite differently. Some are robust, sitting far to the left on the logit curve before the event occurred. Others are fragile, sitting close to the center of the logit curve. For the latter, a 1-logit-unit increase in risk can be "the straw that breaks the camel's back." It is this kind of relation that makes it hard to demonstrate, for example, the benefit of bilateral internal thoracic artery grafting in relatively young adults followed for even a couple decades, but easy in patients who have other risk factors.[L10]

This type of sensible, nonlinear medical relation makes us want to deal with absolute risk rather than relative risk or risk ratios (see Box 6-3).[G32] Relative risk is simply a translation of the scale of risk, without regard to location on that scale. Absolute risk integrates this with the totality of other risk factors.

Raw Data versus Models of Data

Importantly, the Framingham investigators did not stop at risk factor identification. Because logistic regression generates an equation based on raw data, it can be solved for any given set of values for risk factors. The investigators even devised a cardboard slide rule for use by lay persons to determine their predicted risk of developing heart disease within the next 5 years.

Whenever possible and appropriate, the results of clinical data analyses should be expressed in the form of

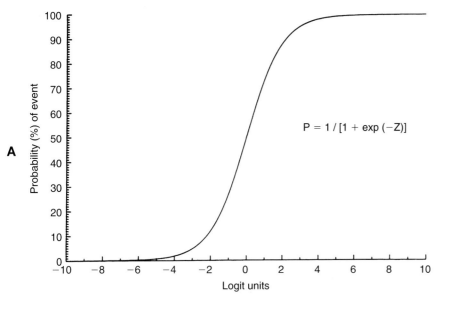

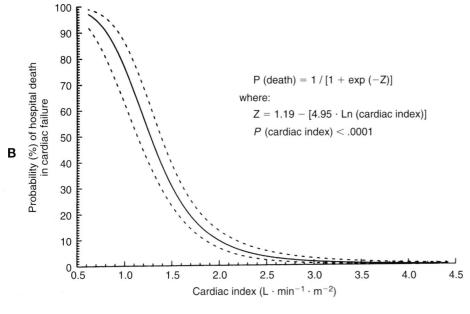

Figure 6-1   The fundamental logistic relation of a scale of risk (logit units) to absolute probability of an event. **A,** The logistic relation, shown when the risk factors are translated into logit units,[B9] is depicted along the horizontal axis and the probability of the outcome event along the vertical axis. The logistic equation is inserted where *exp* is the natural exponential function. **B,** Relation between cardiac index and probability of hospital death in cardiac failure determined by logistic regression analysis of data obtained in the intensive care unit (UAB). Cardiac index as $L \cdot min^{-1} \cdot m^{-2}$ is plotted along the horizontal axis. Z describes the transformation of cardiac index to logit units, where *Ln* is the natural logarithm. If the data were replotted with the transformation to logit units along the horizontal axis, the depiction would reflect *some portion* of the curve in *A.*

mathematical models that become equations. These can be solved after "plugging in" values for an individual patient's risk factors to estimate absolute risk and its confidence limits. Equations are compact and portable, so that with the ubiquitous computer, they can be used to advise individual patients (see "Decision-making for Individual Patients" in Section 5).

It can be argued that equations do not represent raw data. But in most cases, are we really interested in raw data? Archeologists are interested in the past, but the object of most clinical investigation is not to predict the past, but to draw inferences based on observations of the past that can be used in treating future patients. Thus, one might argue that equations derived from raw data about the past are more useful than raw, undigested data.

Nihilism versus Predictability

One of the important advantages of generating equations is that they can be used to predict future results for either groups of patients or individual patients. We recognize that when speaking of individual patients, we are referring to a prediction concerning the probability of events for that patient; we generally cannot predict exactly who will experience an event or when an event will occur. Indeed, whenever we apply what we have learned from clinical experience or the laboratory to a new patient, we are predicting. This motivated us to develop statistical tools that yield patient-specific estimates of absolute risk as an integral by-product.[B20] These were intended to be used for formal or informal comparison of predicted risks and benefits among alternative therapeutic strategies.

BOX 6-3   Expressions of Relative Risk

Proportion

Consider two groups of patients, A and B. Mortality in group A is 10 of 40 patients (25%); in B, it is 5 of 50 patients (10%). For the sake of illustrating the various ways these proportions (see Box 6-13), 0.25 and 0.10, can be expressed relative to one another, designate a as the number of deaths (10) in A and b as the number alive (30). The total in A is $a+b$ (40) patients, n_A. Designate c as the number of deaths (5) in B and d as the number alive (45). The total in B is $c+d$ (50) patients, n_B. Designate P_A as the proportion of deaths in A, $a/(a+b)$ or a/n_A, and P_B as the proportion in B, $c/(c+d)$ or c/n_B.

Relative Risk (Risk Ratio)

Relative risk is the ratio of two probabilities. In the example above, relative risk of A compared with B is $P_A/P_B = [a/(a+b)]/[c/(c+d)] = 0.25/0.10$ or 2.5. Equivalently, one could reverse the proportions, $P_B/P_A = 0.10/0.25 = 0.4$. If P_A were to exactly equal P_B, relative risk would be unity (1.0). Another way to express relative risk when comparing two treatments is by *relative risk reduction*, which for relative risks greater than 1 is 1 minus relative risk. This is mathematically identical to dividing the absolute difference in proportions by the higher of the two: $(P_B-P_A)/P_B$.

Odds

The odds of an event is the number of events divided by non-events. In the example above, the odds of death in A is $a/b = 10/30 = 0.33$; in B, it is $c/d = 5/45 = 0.11$. The mathematical interrelation of probability (P) of an event and odds (O) are these: $O = P/(1 - P)$ and $P = O/(1 - O)$. A probability of 0.1 is an odds of 0.11, but a probability of 0.5 is an odds of 1, of 0.8 an odds of 4, 0.9 an odds of 9, and 1.0 an odds of infinity. Often, it is interesting to examine the odds of the complement $(1 - P)$ of a proportion, $(1 - P)/P$, which is *gambler's odds*. Thus, a P value of .05 is equivalent to an odds of .053 and a gambler's odds of 19:1. A P value of .01 has a gambler's odds of 99:1, and a P value of .2 has a gambler's odds of 4:1.

Odds Ratio

The odds ratio is the ratio of odds. In the above example, the odds ratio of A compared with B is $(a/b)/(c/d) = ad/bc$, which is either $(10/30)/(5/45) = 3$ or $(10 \cdot 45)/(30 \cdot 5) = 3$.

Note that the logistic equation is $Ln[P/(1-P)]$. For A, $P_A/(1-P_B)$ is a/b, the odds of A. Thus, $Ln[P/(1-P)]$ is *log odds*. Logistic regression can, then, be thought of as an analysis of log odds. Exponentiation of a logistic coefficient for a dichotomous (yes/no) risk factor from such an analysis re-expresses it in terms of the odds ratio for those with versus those without the risk factor (see Box 6-5).

When the probability of an event is low, say less than 10%, *relative risk* (RR) and the *odds ratio* (OR) are numerically nearly the same. The mathematical relation is $OR = [(1 - P_A)/(1 - P_B)] \cdot RR$. In the above example, the relative risk was 2.5, but the odds ratio was 3, and the disparity increases as the probability of event increases to 50%.

Relative risk is easier for most physicians to grasp, because it is simply the ratio of proportions. It is unusual to encounter a physician without an epidemiology background who understands the odds ratio.

Expressing Relative Risk and Odds Ratios

Both relative risk and odds ratios are expressed on a scale of 0 to infinity. However, all odds ratios less than 1 are squeezed into the range 0 to 1, in contrast to those greater than 1, which are spread out from 1 to infinity. It is thus difficult to visualize that an odds ratio of 4 is equivalent to one of 0.25 if a linear scale is used. We recommend that a scale be chosen to express these quantities with equal distance above and below 1.0.[A5] This can be achieved, for example, by using a logarithmic or logit presentation scale.

Risk Difference (Absolute Risk Reduction)

The risk difference is the difference between two proportions. In the above example, $P_A - P_B$ is the risk difference. In many situations, risk difference is more meaningful than risk ratios (either relative risk or the odds ratio). Consider a low probability situation with a risk of 0.5% and another with a risk of 1%. Relative risk is 2. Yet risk difference is only 0.5%. In contrast, consider a higher probability situation in which one probability is 50% and the other 25%. Relative risk is still 2, but risk difference is 25%. These represent the proverbial statement that "twice nothing is still nothing." They reflect the relation between the logit scale and absolute probability (see Fig. 6-1, *A*), recalling that the logit scale is one of log odds.

An alternative way to express a difference in probabilities when the difference is arranged to be positive (e.g., $P_A - P_B$), and thus expresses absolute risk reduction, is as the inverse, $1/(P_A - P_B)$. This expression of absolute risk reduction is called *number to treat*. It is useful in many comparisons in which it is meaningful to answer the question, "How many patients must be treated by A (compared with B) to prevent one event (death)?" In our example, absolute risk reduction is $25\% - 10\% = 15\%$, and number needed to treat is $1/0.15 = 6.7$. Number needed to treat is particularly valuable for thinking about risks and benefits of different treatment strategies. If it is large, one may question the risk of switching treatments, but if it is small, the benefit of doing so becomes more compelling.

Hazard Ratio

In time-related analyses, it is convenient to express the model of risk factors in terms of a log-linear function (see Box 6-5 and "Cox Proportional Hazards Regression" in Section 4): $Ln(\lambda_t) = Ln(\lambda_t)$ $\beta_0 + \beta_1 x_1 \ldots \beta_k x_k$, where Ln is the natural logarithm and λ_t is the hazard function. The regression coefficients, β, for a dichotomous risk factor thus represent the logarithm of the ratio of hazard functions. Hazard ratios, as well as relative risk and the odds ratio, can be misleading in magnitude (large ratios, small risk differences) in some settings. Hazard comparisons, just like survival comparisons, often are more meaningfully and simply expressed as differences.

Of course, the nihilist will say, "You can't predict." However, in a prospective study of 3720 patients in Leuven, Belgium, we generated evidence that predictions from multivariable equations are generally reliable (see "Residual Risk" in Section 6).[S9] We compared observed survival, obtained at subsequent follow-up, with prospectively predicted survival. The correspondence was excellent in 92% of patients. However, it was poor in the rest (Fig. 6-2 and Table 6-2; see also "Residual Risk" in Section 6). A time-related analysis of residual risk identified circumstances leading to poor prediction and revealed the limitations of quantitative predictions: (1) When patients have important rare conditions that have not been considered in

the analysis risk is underestimated. (2) When large data sets rich in clinically relevant variables are the basis for prediction equations, prediction should be suspect in only a small proportion of patients with unaccounted-for conditions (see "Residual Risk" in Section 6 for details). Except for these limitations, multivariable equations appear capable of adjusting well for different case mixes.

This analysis has important implications for "report card" registries used in institutional comparisons.[H13] Surgeons often object to these comparisons on the basis that risk adjustment (see "Risk Adjustment" in Section 6) accounts for neither risk stratification (see "Risk Stratification" in Section 6) nor rare combinations of risk factors that

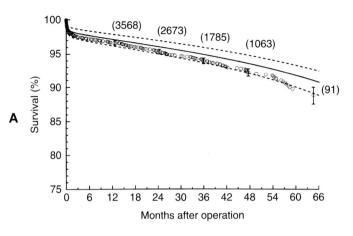

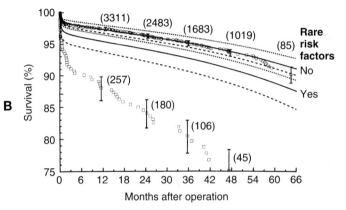

Figure 6-2   Predicted and observed survival after coronary artery bypass grafting, illustrating both the ability to predict from multivariable equations and the pitfalls in doing so. **A**, Observed overall survival among prospectively studied patients (*n* = 3720) compared with predicted survival. Each circle represents an observed death and is positioned at the time of death along the horizontal axis, and according to the Kaplan–Meier life-table method along the vertical axis; vertical bars are 70% confidence limits (CL). Solid line and its 70% CLs represent predicted survival. Notice the systematic underestimation of survival. Number of predicted deaths = 273 (5.7%) and observed deaths = 243 (6.5%), *P* = .03. **B**, Patients stratified by the presence *(open squares)* and absence *(circles)* of rare, unaccounted-for risk factors (malignancy, preoperative dialysis, atrial fibrillation, ventricular tachycardia, or aortic regurgitation). Otherwise, format is as in *A*. Note the excellent correspondence of predicted survival to observed survival in patients without these factors and the substantial underestimation of risk in patients with them.

defy prediction. They may be correct. Unfortunately, in advising patients about operation, we find that these are the very individuals whose risk is difficult to predict on clinical grounds and for whom we wish we had good prediction equations.

The amount of data necessary for generating new knowledge is much larger than that needed to use the knowledge in a predictive way. To generate new knowledge, data should be rich both in relevant variables and in variables eventually found not to be relevant. But for prediction, one needs to collect only those variables used in the equation

■ **TABLE 6-2   Predicted and Observed Number of Deaths after Primary Isolated Coronary Artery Bypass Grafting** *a*

| Rare Risk Factors | n | Total Deaths | | | | |
| | | Observed | | Predicted | | |
		No.	%	No.	%	P
No	3428	186	5.4	191	5.6	.7
Yes	292	57	20	22	7.5	<.0001

(Data from Sergeant and colleagues,[59] July 1987 to 1992; *n* = 3720.)

a The table illustrates both the ability to predict from multivariable equations and the pitfalls of doing so.

(see "Risk Adjustment" in Section 6), unless one is interested in investigating reasons for lack of prediction (see "Residual Risk" in Section 6).

Blunt Instruments versus Fine Dissecting Instruments

A related use of predictive equations is in comparing alternative therapies. Some would argue that the only comparisons that can be believed are those based on randomized trials, and that documented clinical experiences are irrelevant and misleading.[B3,B35] However, many randomized trials are homogeneous and focused and are analyzed as a blunt instrument. On the other hand, real-world clinical experience involves patient selection that is difficult to quantify, may be a single-institution experience with limited generality except to other institutions of the same variety, is not formalized unless there is prospective gathering of clinical information into registries, and is less disciplined. Nevertheless, analyses of clinical experiences can yield a fine dissecting instrument in the form of equations that are useful across the spectrum of heart disease for comparing alternative treatments and therefore for advising patients.

Parsimony versus Complexity

Although clinical data analysis methods and results may seem terribly complex at times, as in the large number of risk factors that must be assessed for comparing treatment strategies in ischemic heart disease, an important philosophy behind such analysis is parsimony (simplicity). We have discussed two reasons for this previously. One is that clinical data contain inherent redundancy, and one purpose of multivariable analysis is to identify that redundancy and thus simplify the dimensionality of the problem. A second reason is that assimilation of new knowledge is incomplete unless one can extract the essence of the information. Thus, clinical inferences are often even more digested and simpler than the multivariable analyses.

We must admit that simplicity is a virtue based on philosophic, not scientific, grounds. The concept was introduced by William of Ocken in the early fourteenth century as a concept of beauty—beauty of ideas and theories.[F12] Nevertheless, it is pervasive in science.

There are dangers associated with parsimony and beauty, however. The human brain appears to assimilate information in the form of models, not actual data (see "Human

A common misconception is that the larger the study group (called the *sample* because it is a sample of all patients, past, present, and future; see Box 6-13), the larger the amount of data available for analysis. However, in studies of outcome events, the effective sample size for analysis is proportional to the *number of events* that have occurred, not the size of the study group. Thus, a study of 200 patients experiencing 10 events has an *effective sample size* of 10, not 200.

Ability to detect differences in outcome is coupled with effective sample size. A statistical quantification of the ability to detect a difference is the *power* of a study. A few aspects of power that affect multivariable analyses of events are mentioned.

Many variables in a data set represent subgroups of patients, and some of them may be few in number. If a single patient in a small subgroup experiences an event, multivariable analysis may identify that subgroup as one at high risk when, in fact, the variable represents only a specific patient, not a common denominator of risk (see "Incremental Risk Factor Concept" in Section 4). The purpose of a multivariable analysis is to identify general risk factors, not individual patients experiencing events!

Thus, more than one event needs to be associated with every variable considered in the analysis. The rule of thumb in multivariable analysis is that the ratio of events to risk factors identified should be about 10 to 1.[H17,M14] For us, *sufficient data* means at least five events associated with every variable. This strategy could result in identifying up to one factor per five events. We get nervous at this extreme, but in small studies we are sometimes close to that ratio. However, bear in mind that variables may be highly correlated and subgroups overlap; thus, in the course of analysis, the number of unexplained events in a subgroup may effectively fall below five, which is *insufficient data*.

Thus, there is both an upper limit of risk factors that can be identified by multivariable analysis and a lower limit of events to allow a variable to be considered in the analysis. Sufficient data implies having enough events available to test for all relevant risk factors.

Error" earlier in this section).[R3] Thus, new ideas, innovations, breakthroughs, and new interpretations of the same data often hinge on discarding the paradigms of the past (thinking "outside the box").[H12] There are other dangers in striving for simplicity. We may miss important relations because our threshold for detecting them is too high. We may reduce complex clinical questions to simple but inadequate questions that we know how to answer.

For analyses whose primary purpose is comparison, it is important, when there is sufficient data (Box 6-4), to account for "everything known."[S10] In this way the residual variability that is attributed to the comparison is most likely to be correct.

New Knowledge versus Selling Shoes

The philosophies described so far focus on the challenge of generating new knowledge from clinical experiences. However, there are other uses made of clinical data.

Clinical data may be used as a form of advertising. Innovation stems less from purposefulness than from aesthetically motivated curiosity, frustration with the status quo, sheer genius, fortuitous timing, favorable circumstances, and keen intuition. With innovation comes the need to promote and indoctrinate. However, promotional records of achievement should not be confused with serious study of clinical efficacy, effectiveness, and long-range appropriateness.

Of growing importance is the use of clinical information for regulation or to gain institutional competitive advantage. Using clinical outcomes data to rank institutions or individual doctors has become popular in the United States (see "Risk Stratification" and "Risk Adjustment" in Section 6).[H13,M13] Many surgeons perceive clinical report cards as a means for punishment or regulation. What is troubling is that their use is based on a questionable quality-control model of outlier identification. Because doctors are people and not machines, this approach generates counterproductive ethical side effects, including defensiveness and hiding the truth.[B36] It hinders candid, non-accusatory (non-culpable), serious examination of medical processes for the express purpose of improving patient care (see "Human Error" earlier in this section).

Critics of clinical report cards charge that to improve their rankings, some institutions refuse to operate on sicker patients.[H14,O2,P11] In several studies of community hospitals by the UAB group, it was shown that they could indeed improve their risk-unadjusted rankings by restricting surgery to low-risk cases. However, their results were often inferior to those of institutions of excellence operating on similar low-risk patients. That is, their risk-adjusted mortality was high even for low-risk cases.

With the intense focus on institutional performance, another undesirable side effect of data analysis decried years ago has crept back in: undue emphasis on hospital mortality and morbidity. Studies of hospital events have the advantage of readily available data for extraction, but early events may be characterized incompletely. After repair of many congenital and acquired heart diseases, early risk of surgery extends well beyond the hospital stay.[O3] This has led to reflection on the effect of time frame on studies of clinical experiences. Use of intermediate-term data is likely to characterize the early events well, but requires cross-sectional patient follow-up.[O3] Long-term follow-up is essential to establish appropriateness of therapy, but it is expensive and runs the risk of being criticized as being of historical interest only.

Yet another reason for interest in clinical information is to use it for profit or corporate advantage. At present, the philosophies of scientific investigation and business are irreconcilable.[C15,C16,H16] One thrives on open dissemination of information, the other on proprietary information offering a competitive advantage. In an era of dwindling public resources for research and increasing commercial funding, we may be seeing the beginning of the end of open scientific inquiry.

Past versus Future

Is there, then, a future for quantitative analysis of the results of therapy, as there was in the developmental phase of cardiac surgery? Kirklin and Barratt-Boyes wrote in their preface to the second edition of this book:

The second edition reflects data and outcomes from an era of largely unregulated medical care, and similar data may be impossible to gather and freely analyze when care is largely regulated. This is not intended as an opinion as to the advantages or disadvantages of regulation of health care; indeed, as regulation proceeds, the data in this book, along with other data, should be helpful in establishing priorities and guidelines. As already noted, in both the first and second editions, the last section of each chapter is on indications for operation. In the future, regulations of policy makers may need to be added to the other variables determining indications.

On the horizon is the promise that medicine will become decreasingly empirical and more deterministic. However, as long as treatment of heart disease requires complex procedures, and as long as most are palliative in the life history of chronic disease, there will be a need to understand more fully the nature of the disease, its treatment, and its optimal management. This will require adoption of approaches to data that are inescapably philosophic.

CLINICAL RESEARCH

In response to the American Medical Association's Resolution 309 (I-98), a Clinical Research Summit and subsequently an ongoing Clinical Research Roundtable (Institute of Medicine) have sought to define and reenergize clinical research.[A7] The most important aspects of the definition of clinical research are that (1) it is but one component of medical and health research aimed at producing new knowledge; (2) the knowledge produced should be valuable for understanding the nature of disease, its treatment, and prevention; and (3) it embraces a wide spectrum of types of research. Here, we highlight only two broad examples of that spectrum: *clinical trials with randomly assigned treatment* and *clinical studies with nonrandomly assigned treatment.*

Clinical Trials with Randomly Assigned Treatment

Controlled trials date back at least to biblical times, when casting of lots was used as a fair mechanism for decision-making under uncertainty (Numbers 33:54). Solomon noted, "The lot causeth disputes to cease, and it decideth between the mighty" (Proverbs 18:18). An early clinical trial took place in the Court of Nebuchadnezzar, king of Babylon (modern Iraq). He ordered several gifted Hebrew youths ("well favored, skillful in all wisdom, cunning in knowledge, and understanding science") to reside at his palace for 3 years as if they were his own children. He purposed to train them in Chaldean knowledge and language. Among them were Daniel and the familiar Shadrach, Meshach, and Abednego. Daniel objected to the Babylonian diet and so proposed a 10-day clinical trial: The Hebrews would be fed a vegetarian diet with water, while the children of the king would be fed the king's meat and wine. After 10 days the condition of the Hebrews was determined to be better than that of the king's children, and they received permission to continue to eat their own diet (Daniel 1:1-15). (This is remarkably reminiscent of the contemporary controversy surrounding carbohydrate-rich versus protein-rich diets.)

The first modern placebo-controlled, double-blinded, randomized clinical trial was carried out in England by Sir Austin Bradford Hill on the effectiveness of streptomycin versus bed rest alone for treatment of tuberculosis.[S8]

Clinical trials in which cardiac surgical procedures and medical therapy have been randomly assigned have made major contributions to our knowledge of treatment and outcomes of heart disease.[Y2] Notable examples are the Veterans Administration (VA) study of coronary artery bypass grafting,[E7] the Coronary Artery Surgery Study (CASS) trial of coronary artery bypass grafting,[N5] and the European Coronary Surgery Study trials.[V1] Trials of coronary artery bypass grafting versus percutaneous coronary intervention have also been important (e.g., the Balloon Angioplasty Revascularization Investigation [BARI][F9]).

Randomization of treatment assignment has three valuable and unique characteristics:

- It eliminates selection factors (bias) in treatment assignment (although this can be defeated at least partially by enrollment bias).
- It distributes patient characteristics between the groups, whether they are measured or not, known or unknown (balance).
- It meets the assumptions of statistical tests used to compare outcomes.[B3]

Random assignment of treatment is a well-accepted method of risk adjustment.[B1-B3,W7] Randomized clinical trials are also characterized by concurrent treatment, excellent and complete compilation of data, and proper follow-up evaluation of patients; these operational by-products may have contributed nearly as much new knowledge as the random assignment of treatment.

Unfortunately, it has become ritualistic for some to dismiss out of hand all information, inferences, and comparisons relating to outcome events derived from experiences in which treatment was not randomly assigned.[B35] If this attitude is valid, then much of the information now used to manage patients with cardiac disease would need to be dismissed and ignored! Investigations concerning differences of outcome among different physicians, different institutions, and different time periods would have to be abandoned. However, moral justification may not be present for a randomized comparison of procedures and protocols that clinical experience strongly suggests have an important difference.[B2] (The difficulty of recruitment in BARI reflects this problem.) In fact, when Benson and Hartz[B31] investigated differences between randomized trials and observational comparisons over a broad range of medical and surgical interventions, they found "little evidence that estimates of treatment effects in observational studies reported after 1984 are consistently larger than or qualitatively different from those obtained in randomized controlled studies."[B40] (See, however, the rebuttal by Pocock and Elbourne.[P9]) These findings were confirmed by Concato and colleagues.[C10] Nevertheless, we acknowledge a hierarchy of clinical research study designs, and the randomized trial generates the most secure information about treatment differences.

Trials in which treatment is randomly assigned are testing a hypothesis, and hypothesis testing, in general, requires a yes or no answer unperturbed by uncontrollable factors. Thus, ideally, the study is of short duration, with all participants blinded and with a treatment that can be well standardized. However, in many clinical situations involving patients with congenital or acquired heart disease, the time-relatedness of freedom from an unfavorable outcome event is important and can jeopardize interpretation of the trial.[F8] This is because individual patients assign different values to different durations of time-related freedoms, in part because differing severities of disease (and corresponding differences in natural history) affect different time frames and in part because the longer the trial, the more likely there will be crossovers (such as from medical to surgical therapy).[F11,L7] Also, the greater the number of risk factors associated with the condition for which treatment is being evaluated, the greater the potential heterogeneity (number of subsets) of patients with that condition and the greater the likelihood that a yes–no answer will apply only to some subset of patients. In such situations, a randomized trial may have the disadvantage of including only a limited number of subsets. It may, in fact, apply to no subset, because the "average patient" for whom the answer is derived may not exist except as a computation. Trials have addressed this problem by basing the randomization on subsets[F10] or by later analyzing subsets by stratification.

These considerations, in addition to ethical concerns,[B30,M4,M7] have fueled the debate on whether surgery is an appropriate arena for randomized trials of innovation, devices, and operations.[B31,B32,G10,G12,G13,H10,L6]

Some argue strongly that randomization should be required at the outset of every introduction of new therapy.[M7] Steven Piantadosi of Johns Hopkins University describes a number of important methodological problems with conducting successful surgical trials, however (personal communication; November 2001):

- Operations are often not amenable to blinding or use of placebos (sham operations). This can introduce bias that may be impossible to control; however, thoughtful and creative study designs can often produce substantial blinding, such as of those assessing outcome.
- Selection bias is difficult to avoid. He notes that it is insufficient to compare operated and unoperated patients, no matter how similar the groups appear, unless every unoperated patient is completely eligible for surgical intervention. Judgment is a characteristic of a good surgeon, and the better the surgical judgment, the more likely bias will enter any trial of surgical versus nonsurgical therapy, even if it is the bias of selecting patients for the trial.
- Surgical therapy is skill-based. Therefore, any result obtained from a trial consists of the inextricable confounding of (1) procedure efficacy and (2) surgical skill.
- Surgery is largely unregulated. Every operation is different, and, particularly in treatment of complex congenital heart diseases, tailoring operations to the specific anomaly is expected and often necessary for patient survival. There is little uniformity from patient to patient to provide a basis for randomizing therapy.

Moses[M8] and others[B32,G10-G13] present the case for a balance between randomized clinical trials and observational clinical studies. However, observational studies are beset with these same problems of selection bias and skill variance; thus, not to be overlooked are the development and rapid introduction of powerful new methods for drawing causal inferences from nonrandomized trials (see "Causal Inferences" later in this section).[R9]

Clinical Studies with Nonrandomly Assigned Treatment

General Comments

Clinical studies with nonrandomly assigned treatment produce little knowledge when improperly performed and interpreted. Because this is often the case, many physicians have a strong bias against studies of this type. However, when properly performed and interpreted, and particularly when they are multiinstitutional or externally validated, clinical studies can produce secure knowledge.

This statement would be considered a hypothesis by some, a fact by others.[B40,P9] For those who consider it a hypothesis, the hypothesis could be tested as a separate project in a large randomized trial. Hypothetically, such a trial could have two parts: (1) a trial with randomly assigned treatment and (2) a registry with nonrandomly assigned treatment (a registry usually contains many more patients than a trial). For the test, multivariable analyses would be performed of patients in the registry, with propensity adjustment or matching (see "Propensity Score" later in this section).[R9] The resulting multivariable equations for various unfavorable events would then be used to predict the now-known outcomes of the patients randomly assigned to the alternative forms of therapy. The predicted outcomes would be compared with observed outcomes (see "Residual Risk" in Section 6); if they were the same, the validity of the technique of properly performed and analyzed studies with nonrandomly assigned treatment would, in that instance, be established. If they were not the same, the reason should be investigatable.

Causal Inferences

The fundamental objection to using observational clinical data for comparing treatments is that many uncontrolled variables affect outcome.[R17] Thus, attributing outcome differences to just one factor—alternative treatment—stretches credibility. Usually even a cursory glance at the characteristics of patients treated one way versus another reveals that they are different groups. This should be expected, because treatment has been selected by experts who believe they know what is best for a given patient. The accusation that one is comparing apples and oranges is well justified![B41]

Indeed, a consistent message since Graunt is that risk factors for outcomes from analyses of clinical experience (and these include treatment differences) are *associations,* not *causal relations.*[H11] Multivariable adjustment for differences is valuable but not guaranteed to be effective in eliminating selection bias as the genesis of a difference in outcome (a form of *confounding*).[D8,D9]

Over the years a number of attempts have been made to move "association" toward "causality." One such method is the case–control study.[C17,S11] The method seems logical and straightforward in concept. Patients in one treatment group (cases) are matched with one or more patients in the other treatment group (controls) according to variables such as age, sex, and ventricular function. However, case matching is rarely easy in practice. How closely matched must the pair of patients be in age? How close in ejection fraction? "We don't have anyone to match this patient in both age and ejection fraction!" The more variables that need to be matched, the more difficult it is to find a match in all specified characteristics. Yet matching on only a few variables may not protect well against apples and oranges comparisons.[J2,R11,R12] Diabolically, selection factor effects (called *bias*), which case matching is intended to reduce, may *increase* bias when unmatched cases are simply eliminated.[R13]

During the 1980s, federal support for complex clinical trials in heart disease was abundant. Perhaps as a result, few of us noticed the important advances being made in statistical methods for valid, nonrandomized comparisons. One example was the seminal 1983 *Biometrika* paper "The Central Role of the Propensity Score in Observational Studies for Causal Effects," by Rosenbaum and Rubin.[R9] In the 1990s, as the funding climate changed, interest in methods for making nonrandomized comparisons accelerated.[R10]

Balancing Scores

Apples-to-apples nonrandomized comparisons of outcome can be achieved, within certain limitations, by use of so-called *balancing scores,* of which the *propensity score* is the simplest (see "Propensity Score" later in this section).[R9] Balancing scores are a class of multivariable statistical methods that identify patients with similar chances of receiving one or the other treatment. Perhaps surprisingly, even astonishingly, patients with similar balancing scores are well balanced with respect to at least all patient, disease, and comorbidity characteristics taken into account in forming the balancing score. This balancing of characteristics permits the most reliable nonrandomized comparisons of treatment outcomes available today. Indeed, developers of balancing score methods claim that the difference in outcome between patients who have similar balancing scores but receive different treatments provides an unbiased estimate of the effect attributable to the comparison variable of interest.[R9] That is technical jargon for saying that the method can identify the apples from among the mixed fruit of clinical practice variance, transforming an apples-to-oranges outcomes comparison into an apples-to-apples comparison.[D10,L13,R14,R15]

Randomly assigning patients to alternative treatments in clinical trials balances both patient characteristics (at least in the long run) and number of subjects in each treatment arm. In a nonrandomized setting, neither patient character-

istics nor number of patients is balanced for each treatment. A balancing score achieves *local* balance in patient characteristics at the expense of unbalancing *n*. Tables 6-3 and 6-4 illustrate local balance of patient characteristics achieved by using a specific balancing score known as the *propensity score* (see "Propensity Score" later in this section for details on how it is derived from patient data). Table 6-3 demonstrates that patients on long-term aspirin therapy have dissimilar characteristics from those not on this therapy. Unadjusted comparison of outcomes in these two groups is invalid—an apples-to-oranges comparison.[B41] Therefore, multivariable logistic regression analysis (see "Logistic Regression Analysis" in Section 4) was performed to identify factors predictive of group membership (long-term aspirin users versus non-users).[G16] The resulting logistic equation was solved for each patient's probability of being on long-term aspirin therapy. This probability is one expression of what is known as a *propensity score* (in this case, the propensity to be on long-term aspirin therapy). Patients were then sorted according to the balancing (propensity) score and divided into five equal-size groups, called *quintiles,* from low score to high.[R9] Thus, patients in each quintile had similar balancing scores (Table 6-4).

Simply by virtue of having similar balancing scores, patients within each quintile were found to have similar

■ **TABLE 6-3   Selected Patient Characteristics According to Long-term Aspirin Use in Patients Undergoing Stress Echocardiography for Known or Suspected Coronary Artery Disease**[a]

Patient Characteristic	ASA	No ASA	P
n	2455	4072	
Men (%)	49	56	.001
Age (mean ± SD years)	62 ± 11	56 ± 12	<.0001
Smoker (%)	10	13	.001
Resting heart rate (beats/minute)	74 ± 13	78 ± 14	<.0001
Ejection fraction (%)	50 ± 9	53 ± 7	<.0001

(Data from Gum and colleagues.[G16])

Key: *ASA,* Long-term aspirin use; *SD,* standard deviation.

[a] Table shows that patient characteristics differ importantly, making direct comparisons of outcome invalid. As shown in the original article, a long list of other patient characteristics also differed between the two groups.

■ **TABLE 6-4   Selected Patient Characteristics According to Long-term Aspirin Use in Patients Undergoing Stress Echocardiography for Known or Suspected Coronary Artery Disease: Stratified by Propensity Score for Aspirin Use**[a]

Patient Characteristic	Quintile									
	I		II		III		IV		V	
	ASA	No ASA	ASA	No ASA	ASA	No ASA	ASA	No ASA	ASA	No ASA
n	113	1092	194	1111	384	922	719	586	1045	261
Men (%)	22	22	57	63	74	71	78	78	88	87
Age (years)	55	49	56	55	61	61	62	64	63	65
Smoker (%)	15	13	15	15	12	11	11	13	7	9
Resting heart rate (beats/minute)	84	83	79	79	76	76	76	76	71	73
Ejection fraction (%)	53	54	54	54	53	53	49	49	49	48

(Data from Gum and colleagues.[G16])

Key: *ASA,* Long-term aspirin use.

[a] Table illustrates that balancing patient characteristics by the propensity score comes at the expense of unbalancing number of patients within comparable quintiles.

characteristics (except for age in quintile I). As might be expected, patient characteristics differed importantly from one quintile to the next. For example, most patients in quintile I were women; most in quintile V were men. Except for unbalanced *n*, these quintiles look like five individual randomized trials with differing entry and exclusion criteria, which is exactly what balancing scores are intended to achieve! Thus, the propensity score balanced essentially all patient characteristics within *localized* subsets of patients, in contrast to randomized clinical trials that balance both patient characteristics and *n* globally within the trial.

To achieve this balance, a widely dissimilar number of patients *actually* received long-term aspirin therapy from quintile to quintile. Quintile I contained only a few patients who received long-term aspirin therapy, whereas quintile V had few *not* receiving aspirin. Thus, balance in patient characteristics was achieved by unbalancing *n*. Table 6-5 illustrates this unbalancing of *n* to achieve balanced patient characteristics in not only the long-term aspirin use study but also a study of atrial fibrillation in which nature is the selecting mechanism, and on- versus off-pump coronary artery bypass grafting.

Propensity Score

The most widely used balancing score is the propensity score.[R9] It provides for each patient an estimate of the propensity toward (probability of) belonging to one group versus another (*group membership*). Here we describe (1) constructing a propensity model, (2) calculating a propensity score for each patient using the propensity model, and (3) using the propensity score in various ways for effecting a balanced comparison.

Constructing a propensity model. For a two-group comparison, multivariable logistic regression is used to identify factors predictive of group membership (see "Logistic Regression Analysis" in Section 4).[R9] In most respects, this is what cardiac surgery groups have done for years—find correlates of an event. In this case, it is not risk factors for an event, but rather correlates of membership in one or the other comparison group of interest.

We recommend initially formulating a parsimonious multivariable explanatory model that identifies the common denominators of group membership (see "Multivariable Analysis" in Section 4). Once this traditional modeling is completed, a further step is taken to generate the *propensity model*, which augments the traditional model by other factors, even if not statistically significant. Thus, the propensity model is not parsimonious.[R14] The goal is to balance patient characteristics by whatever means possible, incorporating "everything" recorded that may relate to either systematic bias or simply bad luck, no matter the statistical significance.[R12] (However, this is not to say that the addition of nonsignificant variables is done carelessly; the same rigor in variable preparation described in "Multivariable Analysis" in Section 4 is mandatory.)

When taken to the extreme, forming the propensity model can cause problems because medical data tend to have many variables that measure the same thing. The solution is to pick one variable from among a closely correlated cluster of variables as a representative of the cluster. An example is to select one variable representing

■ **TABLE 6-5 Balance in Patient and Selection Characteristics Achieved by Unbalancing Number of Cases in Each Propensity-Ranked Group**

Study	Factor Present, *n*	Factor Absent, *n*
Long-Term Aspirin Use		
Quintile 1	113	1192
Quintile 2	194	1111
Quintile 3	384	922
Quintile 4	719	586
Quintile 5	1045	261
Natural Selection: Preoperative AF in Degenerative MV Disease		
Quintile 1	2	225
Quintile 2	13	214
Quintile 3	32	195
Quintile 4	78	149
Quintile 5	162	66
OPCAB versus PCAB		
Quintile 1	40	702
Quintile 2	71	671
Quintile 3	61	682
Quintile 4	90	652
Quintile 5	219	524

Key: *AF,* Atrial fibrillation; *MV,* mitral valve; *OPCAB,* off-pump coronary artery bypass; *PCAB,* on-pump coronary artery bypass.

body size from among height, weight, body surface area, and body mass index.

Calculating a propensity score. Once the propensity modeling is completed, a propensity score is calculated for each patient. A logistic regression analysis, such as used for the propensity model, generates a *coefficient* or numerical weight for each variable (Box 6-5). The coefficient maps the units of measurement of the variable into units of risk. Specifically, a given patient's value for a variable is transformed into risk units by multiplying it by the coefficient. If the coefficient is 1.13 and the variable is "male" with a value of 1 (for "yes"), the result will be 1.13 risk units. If the coefficient is 0.023 for the variable "age" and a patient is 61.3 years old, 0.023 times 61.3 is 1.41 risk units.

One continues through the list of model variables, multiplying the coefficient by the specific value for each variable. When finished, the resulting products are summed. To this sum is added the *intercept* of the model (see Box 6-5), and the result is the propensity score. Note that technically, the intercept of the model, which is constant for all patients, does not have to be added; however, in addition to using the propensity score in logit risk units as described here, it may be used as a probability, for which the intercept is necessary.

Using the propensity score for comparisons. Once the propensity model is constructed and a propensity score is calculated for each patient, three common types of comparison are employed: matching, stratification, and multivariable adjustment.

The propensity score can be used as the sole criterion for *matching* pairs of patients (Table 6-6).[D10,P13] Although a number of matching strategies have been used by statisticians for many years, new optimal matching algorithms have arisen within computer science and operations research. These have been motivated by the need to optimally match volume of intranet and internet traffic to computer network configurations.[L14]

BOX 6-5   Regression

Sir Francis Galton, cousin of Charles Darwin, explored the relation between heights of adult children and the average height of both parents (midparent height). He found that children born to tall parents were, in general, shorter than their parents and children born to short parents taller.[G29] He called this "regression towards mediocrity." He even generated a "forecaster" for predicting son and daughter height as a function of father and mother height. It is presented in an interesting way as pendulums of a clock, with chains around two different sized wheels equivalent to the different weights (regression coefficients) generated by the regression equation!

Today, any empirical relation of an outcome or dependent variable to one or more independent variables (see Box 6-18) is termed a *regression analysis*. Several of these are described below.

Linear

The form of a *linear regression equation* for a single dependent variable Y and a single independent variable x is

$$Y = a + bx$$

where a is called the *intercept* (the estimate of Y when x is zero) and b is the *slope* (the increment in Y for a one-unit change in x). More generally, when there are a number of x's:

$$Y = \beta_0 + \beta_1 x_1 + \cdots + \beta_k x_k$$

where β_0 is the intercept, x_1 through x_k are independent variables, and β_1 through β_k are weights, regression coefficients, or model parameters (see Box 6-13) that are multiplied by each x to produce an incremental change in Y.

It would be surprising if biologic systems behaved as a series of additive, weighted terms like this. However, this empirical formulation has been valuable under many circumstances in which there has been no basis for constructing a biomathematical model based on biologic mechanisms (computational biology).

An important assumption is that Y is distributed in Gaussian fashion (see Box 6-15), and this may require the raw data to be mathematically transformed.

Log-Linear

A *log-linear regression equation* has the following form:

$$\text{Ln}(Y) = \beta_0 + \beta_1 x_1 + \beta_2 x_2 + \cdots + \beta_k x_k$$

where Ln is the logarithm to base e. Such a format is used, for example, in the Cox proportional hazards regression model (see Section 4). However, in studies of events (see "Logistic Regression Analysis" and "Time-Related Events" in Section 4), the estimation procedure does not actually use a Y. Rather, just as in finding the parameter estimates called *mean* and *standard deviation* of the

Gaussian equation (see Box 6-15), parameter estimation procedures use the data directly. Once these parameters are estimated, a *predicted Y* can be calculated.

Logit-Linear

A *logit-linear regression equation*, representing a mathematical transformation of the logistic equation (see Fig. 6-1, *A* and Section 4), has the following form:

$$\text{Ln}[P/(1-P)] = \beta_0 + \beta_1 x_1 + \beta_2 x_2 + \cdots + \beta_k x_k$$

where Ln is the logarithm to base e and P is probability. The logit-linear equation is applicable to computing probabilities once the βs are estimated.

Model

A model is a representation of a real system, concept, or data, and particularly the functional relationships within these, that is simpler to work with, yet predicts real system, concept, or data behavior.

Mathematical Model

A mathematical model consists of one or more interrelated equations that represent a real system, concept, or data by mathematical symbols. These equations contain symbols that represent parameters (constants) whose values are estimated from data and an estimating procedure.

A mathematical model may be based on a theory of nature or mechanistic understanding of what the real system, concept, or data represent (biomathematical models or computational biology). It may also be empirical. The latter characterizes most models in statistics, as depicted above. The Gaussian distribution is an empirical mathematical model of data whose two parameters are called *mean* and *standard deviation* (see Box 6-15). All mathematical models are more compact than data, summarizing them by a small number of parameters in a ratio of 5 to 10 or more to 1.

Linear Equation

When applied to mathematical models, it is an equation that can be solved directly with respect to any of its parameter values by simple mathematical manipulation. A linear regression equation is a linear model.

Nonlinear Equation

When applied to mathematical models, it is an equation that cannot be solved directly with respect to its parameter values, but rather, must be solved by a sequence of guesses following a recipe (algorithm) that converges on the answer (iterative). The logistic equation is a nonlinear model.

Rarely does one find exact matches. Instead, a patient is selected from the *control* group whose propensity score is nearest to that of a patient in the *case* group. If multiple patients are close in propensity scores, optimal selection among these candidates can be used.[D10] Remarkably, problems of matching on multiple variables disappear by compressing all patient characteristics into a single score (compare Table 6-6 with unmatched data in Table 6-3).

Tables 6-4 and 6-6 demonstrate that such matching works astonishingly well. The comparison data sets have all the appearances of a randomized study! The average effect of the comparison variable of interest is assessed as the difference in outcome between the groups of matched pairs. However, unlike a randomized study, the method is unlikely to balance unmeasured variables well, and this may be fatal to the inference.

■ **TABLE 6-6   Comparison of Patient Characteristics According to Long-term Aspirin Use in Propensity-Matched Pairs** [a]

Patient Characteristic	ASA	No ASA
n	1351	1351
Men (%)	49	51
Age (years)	60	61
Smoker (%)	50	50
Resting heart rate (beats/minute)	77	76
Ejection fraction (%)	51	51

(Data from Gum and colleagues.[G16])

Key: *ASA*, Long-term aspirin use.

[a] Table illustrates ability of the propensity score to produce what appears to be a randomized study balancing both patient characteristics and n.

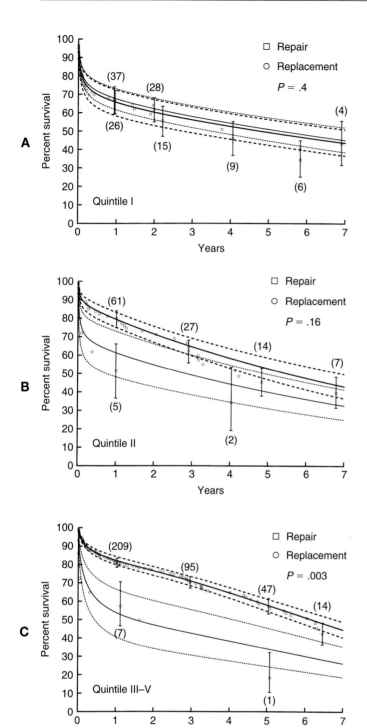

Figure 6-3   Demonstration of changing risk across propensity score for mitral valve repair versus replacement. Because of small numbers of patients with mitral valve replacement in quintiles III through V, these quintiles are grouped together. Patient profiles are similar in each quintile, but differ across quintiles. Each symbol represents a death according to the Kaplan–Meier estimator. Vertical bars enclose asymmetric 68% confidence limits (CL). Solid lines represent parametric survival estimates; these are enclosed within dashed 68% CLs. Numbers in parentheses are numbers of patients traced beyond that point. *P* values are for log-rank test. **A,** Quintile I. **B,** Quintile II. **C,** Quintiles III through V. (From Gillinov and colleagues.[G28])

Outcome can be compared within broad groupings of patients, called *strata* or *subclasses,* according to propensity score.[R14] After patients are sorted by propensity score, they are divided into equal-sized groups. For example, they may be split into five groups, or quintiles (see Tables 6-4 and 6-5), but fewer or more groups may be used, depending on the size of the study. Comparison of outcome for the comparison variable of interest is made within each stratum. If a consistent difference in outcome is not observed across strata, intensive investigation is required. Usually, something is discovered about the characteristics of the disease, the patients, or their clinical condition that results in different outcomes across the spectrum of disease. For example, in their study of ischemic mitral regurgitation, Gillinov and colleagues[G28] discovered that the difference in survival between those undergoing repair versus replacement progressively narrowed as complexity of the pattern of regurgitation increased and condition of the patient worsened (Fig. 6-3). Apparent anomalies such as this give important insight into the nature of the disease and its treatment.

The propensity score for each patient can be included in a *multivariable analysis* of outcome.[B55,C28,M9] Such an analysis includes *both* the comparison variable of interest and the propensity score. The propensity score adjusts the apparent influence of the comparison variable of interest for patient selection differences not accounted for by other variables in the analysis.

Occasionally the propensity score remains statistically significant in such a multivariable model. This constitutes evidence that adjustment for selection factors by multivariable analysis alone is ineffective, something that cannot be ignored.[D9] It may mean that not all variables important for bias reduction have been incorporated into the model, such as when one is using a simple set of variables. It may mean that an important modulating or synergistic effect of the comparison variable occurs across propensity scores as noted above (e.g., the mechanism of disease may be different within quintiles). It may mean that important interactions of the variable of interest with other variables have not been accounted for, leading to a systematic difference identified by the propensity score. The collaborating statistician must investigate and resolve these possibilities. Understanding aside, this statistically significant propensity score has performed its intended function of adjusting the variable representing the group difference.

In some settings in which the number of events is small, the propensity score can be used as the sole means of adjusting for the variable representing the groups being compared.[R12]

Oranges

The propensity score may reveal that a large number of patients in one group do not have scores close to patients in the other.[L10] Thus, some patients may not be matched. If stratification is used, quintiles of patients may have hardly any matches at one or the other, or both, ends of the propensity spectrum.

The knee-jerk reaction is to infer that these unmatched patients represent, indeed, apples and oranges unsuited for direct comparison.[R13] However, the most common reason for lack of matches is that a strong surrogate for the comparison group variable has been included inadvertently in the propensity score. This variable must be removed and the propensity model revised. For example, Banbury and colleagues studied blood usage with vacuum-assisted venous return (VAVR) by comparing two sequential VAVR configurations with gravity drainage.[B63] Because the three groups represented consecutive sequences of patients, date of operation was a strong surrogate for group membership. Further, physical configuration and size of tubing and cannulae varied systematically among groups. Thus, priming volume also was a strong surrogate for group. Neither could be used in forming propensity scores (multiple scores in this instance).

If this is not the case, the analysis may indeed have identified truly unmatchable cases (mixed fruit). In some settings, they represent a different end of the spectrum of disease for which different therapies have been applied systematically.[G28] Often the first clue to this "anomaly" is finding that the influence of the comparison variable of interest is inconsistent across quintiles.[G28]

Thus, when apples and oranges and other mixed fruit are revealed by a propensity analysis, investigation should be intensified rather than the oranges simply being set aside. After the investigations are over, comparisons among the well-matched patients can proceed while at the same time the reader can be provided with the boundaries within which a valid comparison was possible.

Limitations

Some investigators tell us that balancing score methods are valid only for large studies, citing Rubin.[R10] It is true that large numbers facilitate certain uses of these scores, such as stratification. Case–control matching is also better when a large group of controls far exceeding cases is available. However, we believe that there is considerable latitude in matching that still reduces bias; the method seems to "work" even for modest-sized data sets.

Another limitation is having few variables available for propensity modeling. The propensity score is seriously degraded when important variables influencing selection have not been collected.[D8] A corollary to this is that unmeasured variables cannot be reliably balanced. If these are influential on outcome, a spurious inference may be made.

The propensity score may not eliminate all selection bias.[H18] This may be attributed to limitations of the modeling itself imposed by the linear combination of factors in the regression analysis that generates the balancing score (see Box 6-5). If the comparison data sets are comparable in size, it may not be possible to match every patient in the smaller of the two data sets, simply because closely comparable patients have been "used up."

Perhaps the most important limitation is inextricable confounding. Suppose one wishes to compare on-pump coronary artery bypass grafting with off-pump operations. One designs a study to compare the results of institution A, which performs only off-pump bypass, with those of institution B, which performs only on-pump bypass. Even after careful application of propensity score methods, it remains impossible to distinguish between an institutional and a treatment difference because they are inextricably inter-

twined (confounded); that is, the values for institution and treatment are 100% correlated.

Extension

At times, one may wish to compare more than two groups, such as groups representing three different valve types. Under this circumstance, multiple propensity models are formulated.[L13] We prefer to generate fully conditional multiple logistic propensity scores (see "Polytomous and Ordinal Logistic Regression" in Section 4),[H19] although some believe this "correctness" is not essential.

Most applications of balancing scores have been concerned with dichotomous (yes–no) comparison group variables. However, balancing scores can be extended to a multiple-state ordered variable (ordinal) or even a continuous variable.[R16] An example of the latter is the use of correlates of prosthesis size as a balancing score to isolate the possible causal influence of valve size on outcome.

TECHNIQUE FOR SUCCESSFUL CLINICAL RESEARCH

Because of increasingly limited resources for conducting serious clinical research, a deliberate plan is needed for successfully carrying a study through from inception to publication. Here we outline such a plan for study of a clinical question for which clinical experience (a patient cohort) will provide the data.[2] This plan appears as linear *workflow* (Fig. 6-4); in reality, most research efforts do not proceed linearly but rather iteratively, with each step being ever more refined and usually more focused, right up to the last revision of the manuscript. As is true of most workflow, there are mileposts at which there need to be *deliverables,* whether a written document, data, analyses, tables and graphs, a manuscript, or page proofs.

Research Proposal

Because of the necessity for Institutional Review Board (Ethics Committee) oversight, but also because it is good science, every serious clinical study needs a formal proposal (Box 6-6). This proposal serves to clarify and bring into focus the *question* being asked. A common mistake is to ask questions that are unfocused. Brainstorming with fellow surgeons and collaborators is essential. The first deliverable is the research question, well debated.

The next step is to define clearly the inclusion and exclusion criteria for the *study group* (see "Identify Study Group" in Section 3). A common mistake is to define this group too narrowly, such that cases "fall through the cracks" or an insufficient spectrum is stipulated (see "Continuity versus Discontinuity in Nature" earlier in this section). The inclusive dates should be considered carefully. Readers will be suspicious if the dates are "strange"; did you stop just before a series of deaths? Whole years or at least half years dispel these suspicions. Similarly, suspi-

---

[2] Although the technique described is aimed at clinical studies of cohorts of patients, many aspects apply to randomized clinical trials, retrospective clinical studies, and even laboratory research.

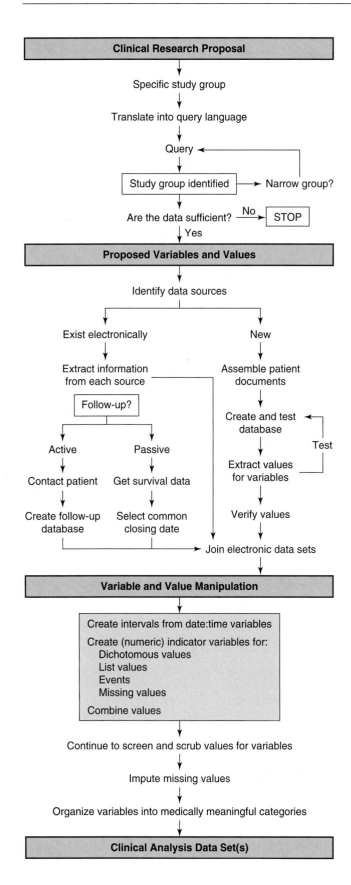

Figure 6-4 Linearized workflow for a clinical research study: transforming information to data suited for analysis.

cion arises when a study consists of some "nice" number of patients, such as "the first 100 or 1000 repairs."

In defining the study group, particular care should be taken to include the denominator. For example, a study may be made of postoperative neurologic events, but it is also important to have a denominator to put these events into context. Or one may study a new surgical technique, but be unable to compare it with the standard technique without a comparison group. A study of only numerators is the true definition of a *retrospective* study; if the denominator is included, it is a *prospective* or *cohort* study (Box 6-7).

End points (results, outcomes) must be clearly defined in a reproducible fashion. Generally, every event should be accompanied by its date of occurrence. A common failing is that repeated end points (e.g., thromboembolism or assessments of functional status) are recorded only the first or most recent time they occur. This should never be done. Techniques to analyze repeated end points are available (see "Longitudinal Outcomes" in Section 4).

Careful attention must be paid to the *variables* that will be studied. They should be pertinent to the study question (purpose, objective, hypothesis). A common failing is to collect values for too many variables such that quality suffers. This error usually arises in a reasonable and understandable way. The surgeon–investigator reasons that because the patient records must be reviewed, a number of other variables may as well be abstracted "while there." Or realizing the full complexity of the clinical setting, the surgeon–investigator feels compelled to collect information on all possible ramifications of the study, even if it is quite peripheral to the focus of the study. John Kirklin called this the "Christmas tree effect"—adding ornament upon ornament until they dominate what once was "just" a fine tree. There needs to be a balance between so sparse a set of variables that little can be done by way of risk factor identification or balancing characteristics of the group, and so rich a set of variables that the study flounders or insufficient care is given to the quality and completeness of relevant variables.

Study *feasibility* must then be assessed. A common failing is forgetting that if an outcome event is the end point, the effective sample size is the number of events (see Box 6-4). A study may have 1000 patients, but if there are only 10 events, one cannot find multiple risk factors for those events.

It is wise at the outset to plan the *data analysis*. Often, for example, the setup for the analysis data set is specific to the methods of analysis. This needs to be known by the data managers (see Appendix 6A).

A necessary step is review of the *literature*. Sifting through articles is often painful, but it should result in identifying those few key papers that are absolutely pertinent to the study. Unfortunately, the search is too often confined to recent literature, and this may result in "reinventing the wheel."

For executing the study, some realistic *time frame* should be established with collaborators. A common failing is not providing sufficient time for data verification and other aspects of data management that are the heart of a high-quality study. Actual analysis of data may consume one tenth the time of high-quality data preparation.

BOX 6-6   Clinical Research Proposal

Title
The title of a research proposal should reflect the question (topic) being addressed.

Investigators
Name the principal and collaborators. Just performing surgery should not confer investigator (or author) status. Often overlooked is inclusion of a collaborating scientist in quantitative sciences (such as biostatistics) from the outset of the study. This is an error that has increasing ramifications as the study progresses.

Background
Report what is unknown, or what is controversial, or the current state of knowledge, to indicate why a study is needed. "Background" answers the question, "So what?"

Research Question/Purpose
Clearly state the purpose (aim) of the study. Often this is best stated as a question. The statement must be well formulated and focused; it is the single most important ingredient for success. It should be revisited, revised, restated, and kept uppermost in mind throughout the study and its eventual presentation. The study cannot be initiated without this step, because the study group, end points, variables, and analyses all depend on it.

Study Group Definition
What is the appropriate study group pertinent to answering the research question? Define both inclusion and exclusion criteria and well-justified inclusive dates. If one proposes that outcome is improved or different, a comparison group is needed. If one proposes to study an *event*, this is a numerator; *both numerator and denominator are needed*.

End Points
End points are the study outcomes. Each must relate and contribute to answering the research question. State them specifically—their exact, reproducible, and unequivocal definitions—determine how they can be assessed in *each* individual in the study, and show how each relates to the study. One temptation is to specify many end points that are unrelated to the research question and spend too little time thinking about what end points are critical.

Variables from Electronic Sources
What variables can be obtained from electronic sources? Some aspects of these data may need to be verified. Of vital importance is determining the units of measurement for values from electronic sources. For example, in one source, height may be in inches and in another in centimeters!

Variables Specific to Study That Need Collecting
For many studies, at least some values for variables needed are not available electronically. This requires developing a database for their acquisition. Note that for successful data analysis, the vocabulary for these variables must be controlled, meaning that all possible values (including "unknown") for each variable must be explicitly specified at the outset (no "free text"). These will become "pick" lists for data entry.

Importantly, specify only those study-specific variables needed to answer the research question. The natural tendency is to collect data for too many variables with little thought given to how they might be used. This wastes scarce resources and compromises the quality of collecting relevant variables.

Sample Size
For any study, a minimum sample size is needed to detect an effect reliably. For events (e.g., death), sample size is dependent on the number of events, not size of the study group (see Box 6-4).

Feasibility
Successful projects are built on ascertaining that (1) the study population can be identified reliably (ideally from electronic databases), (2) the values for variables required are either already in electronic format (but may need to be verified) or can be obtained readily by review of medical documents, (3) the sample size is sufficient to answer the question (see Box 6-4), (4) clinical practice is not completely confounded with the question being asked (one cannot compare two techniques if only one is performed; one may not be able to unravel confounding of two techniques if one surgeon performs one and another the other), and (5) institutional resources are not available (one cannot assess PET scans if they are not performed). If the project is not feasible, the study should be abandoned or a long-range plan devised for prospectively obtaining and recording the needed data.

Limitations and Anticipated Problems
Every study has limitations and anticipated problems. These can be identified by a brief but serious investigation of the state of all the above. If any appear insurmountable or present fatal flaws that preclude later publication, the study should be abandoned. There are always more questions than can be addressed in cardiac surgery, so not being able to answer some specific research question is not an excuse to abandon the search for new knowledge!

Data Analysis
Details of analytic methodology should be formulated in collaboration with a statistician or other quantitative analyst (see Section 4). The surgeon–investigator often does not recognize or know the most appropriate methodology. Collaboration with a statistician or other quantitative professional should reveal appropriate methodology and whether the proposed manner in which data are to be collected will meet the requirements of the methodology. Unfortunately, the surgical literature is not a good resource for determining appropriate methods.

Key References
Identify key references. A study is not an exhaustive review. The few references that are most pertinent should be studied in detail as part of the planning process. However, just because another investigative team has performed a study in a certain way, or used a specific method of analysis, does not mean that it is appropriate to copy these if better methods are more applicable to your study.

Institutional Review Board (IRB)
Any proposal that does not use existing data already approved for use in research by an IRB requires study-specific IRB approval *before* any research is commenced.

Timetable
Develop a timetable for data abstraction, data set generation (see Fig. 6-3), data analysis, and reporting. If the timetable is beyond that tolerable, abandon the study. It is rare for a study to be completed in a year from start to finish. This emphasizes both the bottlenecks of research and the need for lifelong commitment. Although abstract deadlines often drive the timetable, this is a poor milepost (see "Presentations" in Section 5).

The completed formal research proposal becomes the second deliverable of a study. It is likely to be updated throughout the course of a study, and we advocate online tracking of each study, with periodic updates of the protocol as one of the tasks in project management.

Database Development and Verification

The next step for successful research is careful attention to the data themselves (see "Extract Values for Variables" in Section 3). If electronically available data are to be used, every variable must be defined both medically and at the

BOX 6-7 Retrospective, Prospective

When clinical data are used for research, some term this *retrospective research*; epidemiologists also perform what they call retrospective studies that bear no resemblance to typical clinical studies. Thus, confusion has been introduced by the use of both the word *retrospective* and *prospective* to designate interchangeably two antithetical types of clinical study. The confusion is perpetuated by institutional review boards and government agencies that believe one (prospective), but not the other (retrospective), constitutes "research" on human subjects. The confusion can be eliminated by differentiating between (1) the temporal direction of study design and (2) the temporal direction of data collection for a study.

Temporal Direction of Study Design

The temporal pursuit of patients may be *forward*. That is, a cohort (group) of patients is defined at some common time zero, such as operation, and this group is followed for outcomes. Some call this a *cohort study*.[F3,F13] It is the most typical type of study in cardiac surgery: A group of patients is operated on and outcome is assessed. Statisticians call this a *prospective clinical study design*; it moves from a defined time zero forward (which is what the word prospective means).

In contrast, temporal pursuit of patients may be *backward*. Generally, in such a study an outcome event occurs, such as death from a communicable disease. Starting from this event (generally, a group of such events), the study proceeds backward to attempt to ascertain its cause. Feinstein suggests calling such a study a *trohoc study* (cohort spelled backwards).[F13] For years, epidemiologists have called this a *retrospective clinical study design* because of its backward temporal direction of study.

Temporal Direction of Data Collection

Increasingly, "retrospective" is used to designate the temporal aspect of collecting data from existing clinical records for either a cohort or trohoc study. If charts or radiographs of past patients in a cohort study must be reviewed or echocardiographic features measured, the *data collection* is retrospective. Feinstein has coined the term *retrolective* for this to avoid use of the word retrospective, because of the previously well understood meaning of the latter in study design.[F13] If registry data are collected concurrently with patient care, this process is surely *prospective* data collection. Feinstein suggests calling such data collection *prolective* data collection.[F13]

database content level (see Section 2). If data are to be collected de novo, then an appropriate database must be developed (see Fig. 6-4). Every variable must be in a format of one value per variable. These variables must follow a controlled vocabulary for analysis, not free text. The deliverable at this stage is a database ready for data to be collected and entered.

Data Collection

Research on existing databases for which blanket Institutional Review Board (IRB) approval has been secured generally does not require separate approval of each study. However, before any de novo data are gathered from medical records or by patient follow-up, separate IRB approval must be sought.

There is generally a core set of variables that should be collected for each patient. In many cardiac surgical settings, these core elements are stipulated by regulatory agencies (e.g., the state of New York) or surgical societies (e.g., Society of Thoracic Surgeons National Database). They include demography (note that it is essential to record patients' date of birth rather than age because age can be calculated from date of birth to any chosen "time zero"), the cardiac procedure and possibly clinical symptoms and status at time of operation, past cardiac medical history (particularly prior cardiac procedures), disease etiology, coexisting cardiac defects, coexisting noncardiac morbidity (such as diabetes), laboratory measurements known to be consistently associated with clinical outcomes, findings of diagnostic testing, intraoperative findings, support techniques during operation, and factors related to experience (such as date of operation).

Beyond these core variables, there will likely be a need for variables specific to a particular study. These should be identified and reproducibly defined. The danger is specifying too many variables; however, a thoughtfully compiled list adds depth to a study. Further, experienced investigators realize that in the midst of a study, it occasionally becomes evident that some variables require refinement, others collecting de novo, others rechecking, and others redefining. It is important to understand that when this occurs, the variables must be refined, collected, rechecked, or redefined uniformly for *every* patient in the study.

Clinical studies are only as accurate and complete as the data available in patients' records.[F3] Therefore, cardiac surgeons and team members seriously interested in scientific progress must ensure their preoperative, operative, and postoperative records are clear, organized, precise, and extensive, so that information gathering from these records can be complete and meaningful. The records should emphasize description, and, although they may well contain the conclusions of the moment, it is the description of basic observations that becomes useful in later analyses.

Verification

The first step in data verification is to enter values for each data element (variable) for 5 to 10 patients only. These reveal problems of definition, incomplete "pick lists," missed variables, difficult-to-find variables that may not be worth the effort to locate, poor-quality variables/incomplete recording, lack of good definition, inconsistent recording, and questionable quality of observations. Once these issues are addressed, general data abstraction may proceed (see "Verify Data" in Section 3).

When all values for variables are in a computer database, formal verification commences. This can take two general forms: (1) value-by-value checking of recorded data against primary source documents or (2) random quality checking. If a routine activity of recording core data elements is used, it is wise to verify each element initially to identify those that are rarely in error (these can be "spot checked" by a random process) and those that are more often in error. The latter are usually a small fraction of the whole and are often values requiring interpretation. These may require element-by-element verification.

When it is believed that data are correct (this is an iterative process with the above), they are checked for reasonableness of ranges, including discovery of inconsistencies among correlated values. For example, the database may indicate that a patient had a quadrangular resection of the mitral valve, but someone had failed to record that the posterior leaflet was prolapsing and had ruptured chordae. Or the database records that a patient is 60 cm tall and weighs 180 kg; this is likely a problem of confused units of measurement (inches and pounds).

Data Conversion for Analysis

An often underappreciated, unanticipated, and time-consuming effort is the conversion of data residing in a database to a format suitable for data analysis (see "Analysis Data Set" in Section 3). Even if the day comes that all medical information is recorded as values for variables in a computer-based patient record,[D11] this step will be unavoidable. Statistical procedures require data to be arranged, generally in "columns and rows," with each column representing values for a single variable (often in numerical format), and each row either a separate patient or multiple records on a single patient (as in repeated-measures longitudinal data analysis).

Unfortunately, this conversion process may involve some redundancy, such as the necessity to again document all variables and provide a key to the possible values for each.

This process nearly always involves creating additional variables from a single variable, such as a separate variable for each mutually exclusive etiology of cardiomyopathy. These polytomous variables (lists) are then converted to a series of dichotomous variables (best expressed as 0 for absence and 1 for presence of the listed value).

Some categorical variables are ordinal, such as NYHA functional classes. These may need to be reformulated as an ordered number sequence (e.g., 1-4). Variables recorded with units (e.g., weight in kilograms, weight in pounds) must be converted to a common metric.

Calculated variables are also formed. These include body surface area and body mass index from height and weight, Z values (see Chapter 1) from measured cardiac dimensions, ejection fraction from systolic and diastolic ventricular volumes, intervals between date and time variables for which event indicator variables are created, and many other calculations. Because data conversion, creation of derived variables, and formation of calculated variables is time consuming and error prone, groups that conduct a large number of studies often store trusted, well-verified computer code to perform these operations on a repetitive basis.

Often, information is coalesced from multiple databases, and these queries, concatenations, and joining functions transpire in this phase of the process. These otherwise arduous functions can, under some circumstances, be automated. Alternatively, a data warehouse composed of multiple disparate electronic data sources can be implemented and maintained and appears to the investigator as a single data source.

An important activity is managing sporadic missing data. If too many data are missing, the variable may be unsuitable for analysis (see "Impute Values" in Section 3). Otherwise, missing value imputation is necessary so that entire patients are not removed from analyses, the default option in many analysis programs.

Data Analysis

Specific data analysis methods will be described in Section 4. Here, we simply indicate how this aspect of the research process leads to success.

First, the analysis process leads to understanding of the "raw data," often called *exploratory data analysis.*[T1] This understanding is gleaned from such analyses as simple descriptive statistics, correlations among variables, simple life tables for time-related events, cumulative distribution graphs of continuously distributed variables (see "Descriptive Statistics" in Section 3), and cluster analyses whereby variables with shared information content are identified. What is the relationship of one variable to another, either singly or as a set? How do values of variables form clusters of similarities?

Second, the analytic process attempts to extract meaning from the data by various methods akin to pattern recognition.[B38] Answers are sought for questions, for example: Which variables relate to outcome and which do not? What inference can be made about whether an association is or is not attributable to chance alone? Might there be a causal relationship? For what might a variable associated with outcome be a surrogate?

What will be discovered is that answering such questions in the most clinically relevant way often outstrips available statistical, biomathematical, and algorithmic methodology! Instead, *a* question is answered with available techniques, but not *the* question. Some statisticians, because of insufficient continuing education, lack of needed statistical software, lack of awareness, failure of communication, or lack of time, may explore the data less expertly than required. One of the purposes of this chapter is to stimulate effective collaboration between cardiac surgeons and data analysis experts so that data are analyzed thoroughly and with appropriate methodology.

Interpreting Analyses

It is one thing for a statistician to provide a statistical inference; it is quite another for the cardiac surgeon, using that information, to draw meaningful interpretations that affect patient care.

Kirklin and Blackstone empirically found that the most successful way to embark on this interpretive phase of clinical research is to write on a clean sheet of paper the truest two or three sentences that capture the essence of the findings (and no more!).[K15] This important exercise produces an ultramini-abstract for a paper (whether or not it is required by a journal) and provides the roadmap for writing the manuscript (see "Scientific Paper" in Section 5).[B37]

Communicating the Findings

A common error of the surgeon–investigator is to simply summarize the data instead of taking the important step of drawing meaningful clinical inferences from the data and analyses. He or she has not taken the vital step of asking (1) What new knowledge has been gleaned from the clinical investigation? (2) How can this new knowledge be incorporated into better patient care? (3) What do the data suggest in terms of basic research that needs to be stimulated? (4) How can I best communicate information to my local colleagues? (5) How can I best present this information to the cardiac surgical and cardiologic world at large?

Meaningful new knowledge may not be generated because the *statistical inferences* from data analyses are accepted as the final result. Instead, the results need to be studied carefully and many questions asked. Often, this will lead to additional analyses that increasingly illuminate the message the data are trying to convey. Graphical depictions are of particular importance in transforming mere numbers on computer printouts to insight. Depictions must lead beyond statistical inference to clinical inference. What have the data revealed about how to better care for patients? This question is the one best linked to the original purpose of the study. If the study has suggested ways to improve patient care, the next step is to put what has been learned into practice (see Section 5).

Most studies generate more new questions than they answer. Some of these new questions require additional clinical research. Others require the surgeon–investigator to stimulate colleagues in the basic sciences to investigate fundamental mechanisms of the disease process.

Because most surgeon–investigators are part of a group, an important facet of generating new knowledge is discussing with colleagues the results, statistical and clinical inferences, and implications of a study. Multiple points of view nearly always clarify rather than obscure their interpretation.

Finally, clinical research is not a proprietary activity. Yet, too often manuscripts fail to eventuate from research. One reason may be that an abstract was not accepted for a meeting, perhaps because the data were not thoroughly digested before its submission. Although abstract deadlines may be important mechanisms for wrapping up studies, they too often stifle a serious and contemplative approach to generating new knowledge. A second reason manuscripts do not get written is that the surgeon–investigator views the task as overwhelming. Possibly he or she has not developed an orderly strategy for writing. We provide some guidance for this in Section 5. A third barrier to writing is time demands on the surgeon–investigator. Usually, this results from not making writing a priority in one's professional life. This is a decision that should be made early in a surgical career. If dissemination of new knowledge is a desire, then writing must be made part of one's lifestyle.

SECTION 2

Information

Information is a collection of facts. The paper medical record is one such collection of facts about the health care of a patient. In it, observations are recorded for clinical documentation, for communication among health care professionals, and for workflow (orders). However, perhaps as much as 90% of the information communicated in the care of a patient is never recorded.[C18-C20] The attitude of health insurers—"If it is not recorded, it did not happen"—thus represents a sobering lack of appreciation of the way information about patient care is used and communicated. However, it is also an indictment of the way medical practice is documented. Too much is left out of written records, and too many operative reports are poorly organized and incomplete. Too often this reflects the kind of imprecise thinking that gives rise to medical errors (see "Human Error" earlier in this section). If important clinical observations are not recorded during patient care, preferably in a clear, complete, and well-organized (structured) fashion, they are unavailable subsequently for clinical research.

COMPUTER-BASED PATIENT RECORD

In 1991, the Institute of Medicine recognized the need not only for computerizing the paper medical record (as the electronic medical record [EMR]) but also for devising a radically different way to record, store, communicate, and use clinical information.[D11] They coined the term "computer-based patient record," or CPR, and distinguished it from the EMR by the fact that it would contain values for variables using a highly controlled vocabulary rather than free text (natural language).

More than a decade has passed since the Institute issued its initial report, which has now been updated.[D12] Still, there is no universally accepted definition of the CPR beyond that it contains electronically stored information about an individual's lifetime health status and health care. There is no accepted information (data) model, catalog of data elements, or comprehensive controlled medical vocabulary, all of which are fundamental to developing and implementing the envisioned CPR.

These issues aside, for the cardiac surgical group interested in serious clinical research, a CPR with a few specific characteristics could enormously facilitate clinical studies.[K16] Further, it could transform the results into dynamic patient-specific strategic decision support tools to enhance patient care.

First and foremost, the CPR must consist of *values for variables,* selected from a *controlled vocabulary.* This format for recording information is necessary because analysis now and in the foreseeable future must use information that is formatted in a highly structured, precisely defined fashion, not uncontrolled natural language. Extracting structural information from natural language is a formidable challenge and one that should be unnecessary. Second, the CPR must accommodate *time* as a fundamental attribute.[S15] This includes specific time (date:time stamps), inexact time (about 5 years ago), duration (how long an event lasted, including inexact duration), sequence (second myocardial infarction, before, after) and repetition (number of times, such as three myocardial infarctions). Third, the CPR must store information in a fashion that permits retrieval not only at the *individual* patient level but also at the *group* level, according to specified characteristics. Fourth, the CPR will ideally incorporate mechanisms for utilizing results of clinical studies in a patient-specific fashion for *decision support* in the broadest sense of the term, such as patient management algorithms and patient-specific predictions of outcome from equations developed by research (see "Use of Incremental Risk Factors" in Section 5).[A5,C22,S16]

There are many other requirements for CPRs, from human-user interfaces, to administrative and financial functions, to health care workflow, to human error avoidance systems, that are beyond the scope of the clinical research theme in this section.

Ontology

If medical information is to be gathered and stored as values for variables, a medical vocabulary and organizing syntax must be available.[J4] A technical term for this is *ontology.*

In Greek philosophy, ontology meant "the nature of things." Specifically, it meant what actually is (reality), not what is perceived (see "Human Error" in Section 1) or known (epistemology). In medicine of the seventeenth and eighteenth centuries, however, it came to mean a view of disease as real, distinct, classifiable, definable entities. This idea was adopted by computer science to embrace with a single term everything that formally *specifies the concepts and relationships* that can exist for some subject, such as medicine. An ontology permits sharing of information, such as a vocabulary of medicine (terms, phrases), variables, definitions of variables, synonyms, all possible values for variables, classification and relationships of variables (e.g., in terms of anatomy, disease, health care delivery), semantics, syntax, and other attributes and relationships.

An ontology for all of medicine does not yet exist. Efforts to develop a unified medical language, such as the Unified Medical Language System (UMLS) of the National Library of Medicine, are well under way and are becoming increasingly formalized linguistically as ontologies.[G19]

Ontology is familiar to clinical researchers, who must always have a controlled vocabulary for values for variables, well-defined variables, and explicit interrelations among variables. Without these, there is no way to accurately interpret analyses or relate results to the findings of other investigators. However, a clinical study is a microscopic view of medicine; scaling up to all of medicine is daunting.

Perhaps, then, the simplest way of thinking about an ontology for the researcher is as dictionaries of variables and values and their organizational structure, and some mechanism to develop and maintain them. These attributes have collectively been called metadata (data about data) or a knowledge base, and metadata-base or knowledge-base management systems, respectively.[K16]

Information (Data) Model

An information (data) model is a specification of the arrangement of the most granular piece of information according to specific relationships and the organization of all of these into sets of related information. The objective of an information model is to decrease entropy, that is, to decrease the degree of disorder in the information and thereby increase efficiency of information storage and retrieval (performance).

Object-Oriented Information Model

In 1993 at UAB, John Kirklin led a team effort to develop a CPR that would be ideal for clinical care as well as clinical research.[K16] The first step was an attempt to develop an object-oriented information model. These efforts failed. In object technology, only a few formal relationships can be established easily. Failure of the object data model was attributed to the realization that, in medicine, "everything is related to everything" on multiple hierarchical (polyhierarchical) levels. Indeed, medical linguistics forms a semantic network.[S12]

Relational Information Model

The most ubiquitous information model in business, the relational database model, was found to be even more unsuitable as a medical information model,[M15] just as it is now being found to be unsuitable in complex, rapidly changing, multidimensional businesses such as aircraft building and repair. In relational database technology, variables are arranged as columns of a table, sets of columns are organized as a table, individual patients are in rows, and a set of interrelated tables constitute the database. However, in medicine, information is multidimensional. A given value for a variable must carry with it time, who or what machine generated the value, the context of obtaining the value ("documentation"), format or units of measurement, and a host of attributes that give the value meaning within the context of health care delivery. Simply storing a set of values is insufficient. Further, when data must be analyzed, information relevant to the values, such as described earlier, may importantly affect the analysis and needs to be present even if it seems ancillary. The relational data model also poorly represents and retrieves sequences (in which retention of order is vital) and is difficult to maintain for complex data, because every change (addition, subtraction) in data structure requires the database to be updated.

Popularity of the relational model among clinical researchers stems from its simplicity in handling a microscopic corner of medical information. As soon as a new topic is addressed or new variables must be collected, the typical behavior of the research team is to generate a new specific database. Rarely do these multiple, independent, and to some extent redundant databases communicate with one another across studies. This attests to the inappropriateness of such a simplistic data model for a CPR, and even for a busy cardiac surgery research organization.[F14]

Semistructured Information Model

A different kind of information model emerged from an important conference at UAB of leaders in the development of several different types of database as part of the CPR project. After review of the strengths and profound limitations of various information models, a novel approach was suggested by Kirklin and then formalized. He proposed that all information that provided context and meaning to a value for a variable be packaged together. He envisioned that such a *complex data element* should be able to reside as an independent, self-sufficient entity.[K16] (In computer science terminology, this would be called a completely *flattened data model.*)

This idea has several meritorious implications. First, an *electronic container* for a collection of complex data elements could consist of a highly stable, totally generic repository for a CPR, because it would need to possess no

ID	SOURCE	SEX	NYHA	HX_MI	HX_DIALYSIS	CREAT_PR
22005	CCF	M	3	1	N	0.8
22006	UAB	F	2	0	Y	2.3

ID	DT_Echo	MR_PO
22005	1996-05-02	1+
22005	1998-08-26	1+
22005	2000-06-14	2+
22006	1999-01-19	3+

Source	Type	Location
CCF	MSC	CLEVELAND
UAB	UNIV	BIRMINGHAM

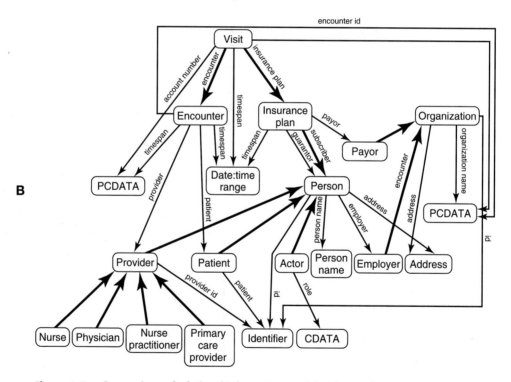

Figure 6-5   Comparison of *relational* information model with a *semistructured* one presented as an acyclic directed graph. **A,** Relational. Tables are related by ID and source. Note that the second table is many-to-one, that is, many postoperative echocardiograms were performed on one patient. **B,** Semistructured (from Jonathan Borden, *www.jonathanborden-md.com*).

knowledge of content of any data element. It could, therefore, manage important information storage and retrieval functions, implement data encryption for privacy and confidentiality, store knowledge bases used to construct the complex data elements and retrieve them, maintain audit trails, and perform all those functions of database management systems that are independent of data content. The second implication is that as medical knowledge increases, new entries would be made in the knowledge-base dictionaries. These would be updated, not the database structure.

Two illustrations of semistructured data are given in the format of XML. In the first, several observations made of the mitral valve at operation are recorded. The format is as a nested hierarchy within health care (indents). The deepest model would be an XML structure such as this for all of the patient's medical data in a single document. However, chunks of the size depicted are likely more easily retrieved and information extracted, and they permit richer data relations to be established for subsequent research.

In the second illustration, a single value for a single variable (the value *severe* for the variable *degree of mitral valve regurgitation*) is displayed as a maximally flattened data element. Process information as well as medical linguistic attributes are contained in a string of attributes called a *start tag*.

Such structures for medical data permit maximum flexibility for later research:

XML: Semistructured Format for Values of Nested Closely Related Variables
```
<PatientRecord PatientID="P-0024">
  <EpisodeOfCare EncounterID="2" EpisodeStartDate=
  "1997-02-03" EpisodeEndDate="1997-02-22">
    <Management>
      <TherapeuticProcedures>
        <Surgery SurgeryDate="1997-02-13">
          <ValveData Valve="Mitral" NativeOrProsthetic=
          "Native">
            <Disease>Yes</Disease>
            <Stenosis>No</Stenosis>
            <Regurgitation>Severe</Regurgitation>
            <Etiology>Calcific</Etiology>
            <Gradient Units="mmHg">5</Gradient>
            <Pathology>Dilated anulus</Pathology>
            <Pathology>Calcified leaflets</Pathology>
            <Pathology>Thickened leaflets</Pathology>
            <Pathology>Calcified anulus</Pathology>
          </ValveData>
        </Surgery>
      </TherapeuticProcedures>
    </Management>
  </EpisodeOfCare>
</PatientRecord>
```

XML: Semistructured Format for a Single Value for a Variable and Its Contextual Information
```
<CardiacValveRegurgitation Valve ="Mitral" NativeOrProsthetic=
"Native" Procedure="Cardiac Catheterization" CathNo=
"012345678" CathMethod="Femoral (Judkins)" CathType=
"Complete" TypeOfProcedure="Diagnostic" Purpose="Medical
Decision Making" DateEvent="1997-02-06" DateEntered=
"1997-02-22" Source="Cardiac Catheterization Report" Site=
"CCF" EpisodeOfCareEncounterID="2" EpisodeStartDate=
"1997-02-03" EpisodeEndDate="1997-02-22" PatientID=
"P-0024 "> Severe </CardiacValveRegurgitation>
```

Not only would this ease database maintenance, it would enforce documentation in the knowledge base. The third implication, and the one most important for clinical research, is that no a priori limitations would be placed on relations; they could be of any dimensionality considered useful at the time data elements were *retrieved* for analysis. Thus, the electronic container is a single variable–value pair augmented with contextual documentation and capable of being modified as new or more knowledge accrues.

The essential characteristics of such an information repository are

- Self-documentation at the level of individual values for a variable (complex data element)

- Self-reporting at the time of data element retrieval and potential
- Self-displaying in the human–computer interface
- Self-organizing

The latter is an important attribute for future implementation of what might be called "artificial intelligence" features of a CPR. These may be as simple as self-generation of alerts, solution of multivariable equations for decision support at the individual patient level,[A5] or intelligent data mining for undiscovered relations within the information.

About 1995, at the time these ideas were being developed at UAB, similar thinking was going on among computer scientists at Stanford University and the University of Pennsylvania, arising from different stimuli.[B43,M15] They termed an information model of complex data elements that carried with them all attributes intended for self-documentation, self-reporting, and self-organizing *semistructured data*. This phrase meant that the data elements were fully structured, but no necessary relation of one data element to another was presupposed. The culmination of these efforts was a database for storing complex data elements called Lore[M15] and a novel query language for retrieving complex data elements called Lorel.[A4]

In the 1990s, it was recognized that the information structure suggested by Kirklin and the University of Pennsylvania and Stanford computer scientists could be conceptualized as an acyclic directed graph (Fig. 6-5).[C21,E9,L2] At that time, another entity was also rapidly coming into existence with similar properties, but of global proportions: the World Wide Web (www). A web page is analogous to a complex data element, with an essential feature being that it is self-describing so that it can be retrieved. The www is the infrastructure for these pages. It has no need to be aware of web page content. The subject matter has no bounds. Not surprisingly, then, the tools developed for retrieving semistructured data were quickly adapted to what has become known as *search engines* for the www. Like Dr. Kirklin's vision of complex data elements, information retrieved by a search engine can become related in ways never envisioned by the person generating it because full structure is imposed only at the time of retrieval, not at the time of storage.

In 1998, the Lore scientists realized that the information model for semistructured data could be implemented in XML (extensible markup language). XML is a textual language for information representation and exchange, largely developed for document storage and retrieval but adaptable to values for variables.[D20,G17]

Thus, at least on a conceptual basis, we believe a CPR can be formulated using a semistructured information model that will facilitate clinical research by not imposing restrictions at the time of storage, as do relational and object models (Box 6-8).

TIME

The ability to manage that ubiquitous attribute of all medical data—*time*[S13,S15]—is not part of any widely available information retrieval system (generally called query languages). Some proposals have been tested in a limited fashion, such as the Tzolkin system developed at Stanford University,[N7] but the software is not generally available. The reason for needing to consider time is readily apparent.

Whenever we think about retrieving medical information along some time axis (e.g., sequence, duration, point in time), new logical relations must be generated to obtain reasonable results. For example, if we ask for all patients younger than 80 years of age who have undergone a second coronary artery bypass grafting (CABG) operation followed within 6 months by a myocardial infarction, a number of time-related logical steps must be formulated. What is meant by patients younger than 80? Younger than 80 when? At the time of the initial surgery, second surgery, myocardial infarction, or at the time of the inquiry? The sequence of CABG must be ascertained from data elements about each procedure a patient has undergone. Information about the myocardial infarction and its relation to the date of the second CABG must be retrieved. The process is even more complex if only approximate dates are available.

Perhaps a growing interest pertaining to the time axis in business[S14] may stimulate development of better tools for managing queries related to time in medical information.

SECTION 3
Data

Data consist of organized information. We add the following further constraints.

First, *data consist of values for variables.* These values have been selected from a list of all possible values for a variable, and this list is part of a constrained vocabulary. Natural language processing is too primitive at present to allow values to consist of free text, and that will not change in the foreseeable future. Our exploration with linguistics experts of the needed lexical parsing rules to determine from dictated medical notes whether a person experienced a hospital death after cardiac operation produced multiple pages of daunting logic. In part, the complexity arises because of the richness of language that includes euphemisms, synonyms, and misspellings; in part it is because one must also identify negating ("did not expire"), adjudicate probabilities ("may have died"), and examine indirect evidence (no mention of death in available dictated notes, but an autopsy was reported).

Second, *data consist of values for variables that have been accurately and precisely defined both at the level of the database and medically.* One of the important benefits of multicenter randomized trials, concurrent observational studies, or national registries is that these activities require establishing agreed-upon definitions at the outset. Coupled with this is often intensive and ongoing education of study coordinators and other data-gathering personnel about these definitions, exceptions, and evolution of definitions and standards. Further, there is a mechanism to monitor compliance with these definitions and standards throughout the study. The same should hold true for any registry. However, a mechanism to ensure similar adherence to definitions is essential even for individual clinical studies. Further, documentation must be in place to identify dates on which changes in definition have occurred, and these must be communicated to the individuals analyzing the data (generally, indicator variables are created that "flag" cases for which definitions of an individual variable have changed).

The rigor of establishing good definitions is considered distasteful by investigators who are impatient to collect data, but it is essential for successful research. It is also somewhat of an iterative process, which is why we suggest extracting data on the basis of initial definitions for a few patients scattered over the entire time frame of the study, then refining the definitions. One must also be aware of standards developed by national and international groups of cardiac surgeons and cardiologists assembled for this purpose.

Third, *data consist of values for variables that have been organized, generally using a database management system, into a database or data set(s) suitable for analysis.* There is an essential translation step in going from even organized information into data in a format that is compatible with the analytic technique to be employed. For example, if one is analyzing survival after a cardiac surgical procedure, one must define "time zero," construct the interval from time zero to occurrence of the event of interest from date:time data, generate an indicator variable for whether by the end of follow-up a patient has or has not experienced the event, impute values for additional variables if some of the data are known only inexactly, and manage the problem of possible missing values for some of these variables (see "Time-Related Events" in Section 4). These details will not be part of the medical information system, but must be created at the time of analysis (see "Analysis Data Set" later in this section). This is because at the present time, and for the foreseeable future, data analysis procedures presume that data will be organized in fully structured format, generally a relational one (tables with columns for each variable and rows for each separate observation, which may be a single patient or multiple measurements for a single patient). It is our view that the fully structured organization of data, probably in relational database format (see "Relational Information Model" in Section 2), should be imposed only at the point of extraction of values for variables from information (often called the "export" phase in a process termed "rectangularization"). This allows the input of data to be semistructured (see "Semistructured Information Model" in Section 2), maximally flexible, and with few imposed organizational constraints (outside of retrievability), so that the relations among variables is imposed by the research question being asked and not by a priori database constraints.

INFORMATION TO DATA

An idealized, linearized perspective on the process of transforming clinical information to data suitable for analysis requires three broad steps (see Fig. 6-4): (1) formulating a clinical research proposal that leads to identifying a suitable study group, (2) gathering proposed variables and values that lead to an electronic data set, and (3) manipulating the values and variables to create a data set in a format suitable for analysis. This is a linear process in theory only. In reality, it contains checks that cause the investigator to retrace steps.

Identify Study Group

The clinical research proposal (see Box 6-6) provides detailed specifications for the study group of interest. The medical specification must be translated into a formal query, generally using a query language, that will be used to identify patients in the study group. Query "engines" include the now-familiar Yahoo, Google, and AltaVista, and the search engines of the National Library of Medicine, including PubMed and Gateway. For data managers familiar with relational databases, the Structured Query Language (SQL) is a universal query language. At UAB for many years, the search "engine" was a person who maintained every surgical case classified by (1) procedure performed (such as CABG, Fontan operation), (2) cardiac diagnosis (such as endocarditis, ascending aortic aneurysm), and (3) date of operation (time frame of the study). Today, many cardiac surgery centers have a registry (see Box 6-1) of patients that can be queried at least by these same three attributes, and often in an even more specific fashion.

It is frequently true that electronic sources of registry data do not narrow the study group as much as desired. This may require investigating a larger group of candidate patients and selecting by medical records review those who meet the specifications of the study.

If the semistructured information model is adopted (see "Semistructured Information Model" in Section 2), as we advocate, then at the present time experts in query languages specific to this type of information must be consulted. However, because such information is stored in the same format as www documents, the increasing sophistication, accuracy, and usability of internet search engine technology will simplify this process.

The end result of a query is identification of a group of patients (or candidate patients) for the study. The major checks here are whether the patients indeed meet criteria for inclusion and exclusion and whether a sufficient number of patients (or a sufficient number of outcome events, as will be found in subsequent steps; see Box 6-4) are retrieved for a meaningful analysis.

Extract Values for Variables

A source, or sources, for obtaining values for the set of variables specified in the clinical research proposal must now be identified for the study group (see Fig. 6-4 and Box 6-6). Currently, these are contained either in some electronic format (such as the hospital information system) or in the paper record.

Export from Electronic Information Sources

If some or all of the variables specified are in electronic format, then the sources must be identified and a query made for the patients in the study to extract values for the variables. This often time-consuming step is facilitated by three factors. First, at the time the information system is created, procedures can be built in to ease extracting, formatting, and exporting values for variables. This is particularly feasible in a so-called metadata-driven system, in which "data about data" drives not only the data entry process but the data extraction process as well.[K16] It is also particularly feasible for relational databases that are electronically linked (e.g., portals) to the analysis system. Second, "standard" groups of core data elements can be identified that form the basis for at least a major portion of the variables needed for most studies. The advantage of this

strategy is that the queries can be assembled carefully and refined over time. Third, successful, accurate ad hoc queries can be stored so that when the same variables are again specified, these queries can be reused.

Often more than one electronic data source must be used. In this case, values for variables in common may need to be adjudicated if they do not match in value or in variable nomenclature. Ultimately, unique variables must be joined into a common database.

Extraction from Medical Records

Even if the majority of information is available electronically, there are nearly always some variables new to the study that must be gathered from paper records if a CPR is not available. A more arduous process must be put into place for extracting data from original documents.[F3] A precise methodology is necessary for assembling information to prevent repetitive handling of both the patient's record and the extracted information, as well as to ensure complete and accurate data retrieval.

All information should be recorded in clearly defined, objective terms. There may be a preference for using descriptive terms that have been clearly defined (e.g., absent, trivial, mild, moderate, severe). Alternatively, numerical coding may be used,[B19,F8] with each numeral clearly defined. Pedal pulses, for example, may be recorded as 0, 1, 2, 3, or 4, with 4 indicating normal. Either method is equally rigorous as long as values are picked from a controlled vocabulary.

At UAB, insofar as possible, key documents from which information is extracted are photocopied, organized into loose-leaf ring binders, and permanently stored for the study group identified from the registry. These documents may include the patient's admission slip for demographic data, any diagnostic reports (such as catheterization reports), operative notes, hospital discharge summaries, pathology reports, and follow-up questionnaires. Particular studies will require other documents, such as electrocardiograms and anesthesia or perfusion records. No attempt is made to organize these patient documents except by a noninformative master research patient index that is keyed to the hospital's master patient index in a way that protects patient privacy and confidentiality.[3] Any necessary shuffling or reordering of patient data is done later by computer sorting routines, not by reordering patient documents. Investigators use these notebooks in the initial stages of the

---

[3] Regulations regarding patient privacy and confidentiality are still in flux and surrounded by concerns about how clinical data can be used in the future for research. Some generalities can be made, however. First, during analysis of data, informative patient identifiers are unnecessary and should be eliminated from the analysis data set. Second, those who must verify data values for medical records, perform patient follow-up, and join disparate databases will need patient identifiers to accomplish these tasks. Because these activities take place within the confines of an institution, it is generally agreed at the present time that use of patient identifiers is appropriate under the purview of an Institutional Review Board (IRB). Third, communication with patients by IRB-approved mailed questionnaires or IRB-approved telephone scripts must begin with obtaining patient consent. Fourth, communication with medical professionals about follow-up status or documentation of events requires patient consent. Fifth, databases should conform to regulatory (HIPAA) standards.

study to purify the study group. If a patient does not fit into the study, his or her records are merely removed from the notebook without altering the numbering sequence. At the end of the study, the notebooks are permanently stored for future reference. Index tabs are used to conveniently separate each patient's documents from others. The tab bears the study number on front and back to provide viewing from both sides. Although this method may seem archaic, for many studies it is the most cost-effective and simplest one available.

The data are now formally entered into the computer database. This may involve direct data entry into either a database prepared especially for a particular study (the most expensive method) or a master research database (if semistructured technology becomes viable, this will likely be the best method), or transcription onto paper forms that are then entered by data entry personnel or scanning technology.

Accuracy of data entry is improved by recording only primary information (e.g., date of birth, date of operation) and not indexes derived or calculated from them (e.g., patient age at operation, body surface area). Such indexes can later be calculated quickly and reproducibly by computer. Data should also be coded in a way that is simple and self-documenting (using words or phrases from a constrained list of possible values for a variable, sometimes called "pick lists").

The process of gathering data is the most time-consuming step in a study. It is not unusual for it to consume months or years of work. Even if electronic sources of information are used, if values for variables were not entered at the point of care, the expense can be enormous. This is why the CPR, as the repository of all patient data and patient care workflow, is essential to increase the efficiency of clinical research.

For many institutions, identifying patients using a simple registry (such as the Society for Thoracic Surgery Database) and extracting more detailed data for a specific study is the most cost-effective method for clinical research. A major added benefit is gaining detailed knowledge and understanding of each patient's medical condition and management.

Verify Data

No matter what method of data export or extraction is used, experience dictates that one or more iterative data verification steps must be inserted before any analyses are performed. This process is long and tedious and can be boring. It usually reveals *many* errors. However, it also allows review of each patient's record to detect missed information. The data are then checked for reasonableness (range checks), a process greatly aided by computer. This can be accomplished quite simply by looking at the maximum, minimum, and average of each variable (although sometimes more sophisticated univariate analyses must be done, as described later in this section under "Descriptive Data Exploration") and by making simple scatter plots (e.g., age, height, and weight form a smooth scatter plot against one another) and cumulative distribution plots. Discrepancies and inaccurate outliers are found and the data corrected.

Importantly, if data errors are found, they should be corrected in the primary information repository and the data re-exported. This policy ensures upgrades of repository quality.

Although a controversial statistical point, the data should probably not be "doctored" by rejecting outliers, unless there is a reason to suspect they are less reliable than the values obtained for other patients. It is also useful to list all patients with missing data so that renewed efforts can be made to obtain them. Finally, a list is made to make sure that patients do not have duplicate records, particularly if the same patient was the subject of a preceding study or if the data were extracted from an electronic source in which patients may be entered multiple times.

Follow-up

Time-related events occurring after hospital discharge are often extracted simply from clinic visit records rather than by systematic patient contact. Patients not appearing for clinic visits are said to be untraced. This is a completely unacceptable method of follow-up.

Even with acceptable methods, however, some patients cannot be traced. It has been demonstrated that untraced adult patients have a high probability of being dead. In contrast, in the UAB experience, untraced infants usually were doing well; their parents, generally young and often highly mobile, had simply dropped contact with the pediatric cardiologist. Either way, a high prevalence of untraced patients introduces bias into the time-related analysis, leading to overestimating or underestimating survival or freedom from other events.[A2]

Follow-up may be *active* (direct patient contact) or *passive* (use of government death indices). In either case, most institutions require IRB (Ethics Committee) approval of the follow-up process, and often patient approval as well.

Active Follow-up

Active follow-up means that patients or their families are contacted directly by mailed questionnaire, telephone, or electronic means (e-mail, internet). If a patient is found to have died, nearest relatives are contacted in a sensitive, sympathetic fashion to document the circumstances of death and to ascertain all other pertinent cardiac events that occurred between the date of last active contact and death. There are two general methods of active follow-up: anniversary and cross-sectional.[B25]

Anniversary method. In the anniversary method, the patient is contacted yearly, on the anniversary of his or her entry into the study (or periodically if not yearly), or is given a set of forms to send to the investigators on the anniversary of entry. This method is perhaps ideal for sampling the time-varying condition of the patient, such as functional status, freedom from angina, and growth and developmental patterns. The anniversary method has the added advantage of maintaining at least yearly contact with the patient, an important consideration in a mobile society. It has also been demonstrated that non-lethal morbid events such as thromboembolism and hemorrhage after heart valve replacement are forgotten unless there is at least yearly contact.[B56] Yearly active contact also makes it more likely that patients will report events to their physicians during the course of the year.

Cross-sectional method. In the cross-sectional method, a specific follow-up inquiry of all patients known to be alive is initiated at a specific calendar date, with the goal of obtaining the status of all patients at a specific instant in time. In practice, of course, a finite period of time is necessary to conduct the follow-up. For example, a cross-sectional follow-up may be initiated on August 1 and questionnaires returned over the ensuing 2 months. During this time, telephone calls may be made to nonresponders or those whose questionnaires have been returned as undeliverable.

Two techniques are then used to manage the cross-sectional data. Theoretically, the best method is to choose a *common closing date.* In the example stated, this would be August 1. Alternatively, all events reported during follow-up are used, with the date of follow-up taken as the date the questionnaire was signed or the telephone call completed. This method was suggested by the Mayo Clinic group, which called it *date of last report.*[E4] Note that if a patient responds to the questionnaire but shortly thereafter experiences an event and contacts those performing the follow-up study, the new information is disregarded.

Restriction to initially reported events emphasizes a property of active follow-up: It is *systematic.* Any other method, be it physician office visits or voluntary contact, is, in contrast, opportunistic and nonsystematic. The problem with nonsystematic follow-up is that it captures numerators but not the denominator of a patient cohort. Thus, time-related events analyses are distorted.

Goodness of follow-up. In performing active follow-up, particularly in longitudinal studies that are conceived after considerable experience has accumulated, every effort should be made to contact every patient in as short a time as possible.[B12] Special assistance may be required to achieve 95% to 100% follow-up under these circumstances; this may be in the form of cross-reference indexes to former neighbors or contact of relatives and former physicians, churches, and other agencies.[B12]

There is no perfect way to describe and quantify goodness of follow-up. Traditionally, the mean and standard deviation of follow-up duration, including either all patients or only living patients, are given, as well as total patient-years of follow-up. Various percentiles of follow-up are also useful (see "Descriptive Statistics" later in this section), such as the 10th, 50th, and 90th. Alternatively, the percentage of patients traced beyond certain intervals (e.g., 5, 10, 15 years) may be given. We then recommend stating what percentage of patients have not been traced beyond hospital discharge (lost to follow-up) and how many could not be contacted by active follow-up at the latest inquiry.

Grunkemeier and Starr have described a patient-year method for estimating goodness of follow-up based on observed versus potential follow-up duration.[G31] For each patient the duration of potential follow-up is computed (this is the interval from study entry until death or, for the patient still alive at follow-up, common closing date or response date, anniversary date, or analysis date, depending on the type of follow-up study performed). The ratio of total observed follow-up duration to total potential follow-up duration is used as a measure of goodness of follow-up.

Neither of these methods of reporting adequately indicates the degree of information lost by incomplete follow-up. The traditional reporting method may be overly optimistic, and the Grunkemeier and Starr method has the same drawback as all patient-year methods in that it reflects loss of information accurately only when the hazard function for the event is reasonably constant. For example, if a patient has been traced for 10 years but has been lost for the past 5 years, the contribution to the goodness of follow-up statistic would be the same as that of five individuals who were lost just after study entry (e.g., after hospital discharge) 1 year ago. If the hazard function is steeply declining in the first year, as it often is, then is very low after 10 to 15 years, the information lost by failure to trace the five recent patients is greater than the information lost by failure to trace further the patient with a follow-up duration of 10 years.

It may be possible to devise a better expression of goodness of follow-up. For example, if a parametric estimate of the cumulative hazard function is made, then the difference in potential versus observed cumulative hazard experienced (expressed as a percentage) may better account for the time-related loss of information. However, the important thing is to expend great effort to obtain complete follow-up information.[B12] Failure to trace a substantial number of patients, however expressed, makes even the most sophisticated analysis suspect.

Follow-up instrument. The follow-up instrument may be a simple questionnaire mailed to the patient (with one or two remailings followed by telephone contacts to nonresponders). If so, it is wise not to exceed a single sheet in length, relying on the telephone or personal contact to obtain more details if events have occurred. Alternatively, the inquiry may be completely by telephone, using well-trained individuals, a script, and a form that is filled out during the conversation.

Patients rarely resent being followed up; to the contrary, periodic follow-up is useful not only in detecting medical trends in individual patients who may need attention, but also in generating goodwill between the patient and the medical system.

Passive follow-up. If vital status is the only outcome of interest, date of death may be obtainable from government death indices. In passive follow-up, only death and date of death are identified, not whether each individual in the study is alive or dead at the time of inquiry.[T7] However, usually there is a lag between death and reporting, so methods must be employed to determine the status of living patients at any given time. At The Cleveland Clinic Foundation, investigators have available a large registry of patients who are actively followed up. When passive follow-up is used, many patients known by active follow-up to be dead are purposely included. It is then determined when most of these actively followed patients were identified as dead by the passive United States Social Security Death Index. A common closing date is thereby selected for all passively followed patients in the study (this is often 6 months before the date of passive inquiry), and any events occurring after that date are ignored.

It is important to remember that nonfatal events cannot be determined by passive follow-up. If passive follow-up is used for only a fraction of patients, then a separate date for end of active follow-up may be retained for analysis of nonfatal events.

Analysis Data Set

The last step in transforming information into analyzable data is creating one or more analysis data sets in a format compatible with analytical procedures (see Fig. 6-4). This step includes (1) manipulating variables and values, (2) further screening and scrubbing of data, (3) imputing missing values, and (4) organizing a set of analysis variables into medically meaningful categories. The general process has been described under "Technique for Successful Clinical Research" in Section 1.

Manipulate Variables and Values

To interpret patient information meaningfully, an *index time for study entry* must be established for every patient. The reason is the central place of date:time in medicine. Thus, in a system of longitudinal data entry at the time of patient care, past, present, and future are defined in terms of this index time. For surgeons, fortunately, this is often the time of an operative procedure. It is more difficult in medical situations to define, say, onset of disease. Once index time for study entry has been determined, then, using dates for each data element, one can determine if there have been previous events such as myocardial infarctions, how many of these have occurred, and the interval from the most recent to the index time. All items in what we commonly think of as "past medical history" are defined in terms of this index time for study entry.

One of the most common requirements is to compute *intervals* between dates. For example, the age of a patient at index time is calculated from index time and date of birth. Follow-up intervals are similarly computed from dates. A common error is attempting to calculate intervals between dates and index time manually. This is rarely accurate and should be done by computer.

Indicator variables are always required. These may simply be the translation of a variable whose value has been coded as YES or NO into the numbers 1 and 0, respectively. A cardinal rule to avoid ambiguity, human error, and misinterpretation is that the computer variable name of an indicator variable must always be the one indicated by a "YES" or 1. Thus, in forming an indicator variable from a primary variable called SEX with values of MALE and FEMALE, one would name the indicator variable MALE with values of 0 for female and 1 for male. An indicator variable called SEX or GROUP is ambiguous and should never be used as an analysis variable, because it is not self-documenting.

Another common requirement is to form *multiple indicator variables* from a single variable containing values from a non-ordered list. These list variables often are represented by a set that allows selection of multiple items from the list. Typical list variables are diagnoses or type of operation. A non-ordered (polytomous) list variable is not interpretable in many types of data analysis (the exception is mutually exclusive lists, for which polytomous methods are useful; see "Polytomous and Ordinal Logistic Regres-

sion" in Section 4). Generally, a variable useful for data analysis from such list variables must take on one of three values: 0 (NO), 1 (YES), or blank (MISSING). However, in many cases the medical pick list would be so long that in general clinical practice, only positive findings have been recorded and all the rest (e.g., thousands of possible diagnoses) "dismissed" (Kirklin called these "dismissal lists").

When it comes to data analysis, however, we often need indicator variables for all list items that identify more than "yes" (1). Generally, the assumption is made that if a list item is not selected, the patient did not have that condition or procedure. However, it is possible that he or she did, but (1) the list item was added recently and so was not collected at index time, (2) the data abstractor could not find the item, forgot to look for it, or was distracted and did not return to find it, or (3) the item was recorded in a previous clinical record that was not retrieved by the criterion used to gather the electronic data set.

Such ambiguities can be avoided to some extent for a particular discipline by gathering important data elements using individual variables. For example, one may wish to have unambiguous information on the comorbidities diabetes (and its treatment); preoperative dialysis for chronic renal failure; history of prior myocardial infarction (perhaps with date or a count of the number experienced); history of cerebral vascular accident, carotid artery, and often peripheral vascular disease; chronic pulmonary disease, and the like. Rather than making them items in a long list variable, create individual variables whose values of YES or NO must be explicitly entered.

Screen and Scrub

As intervals and indicator variables are created, data screening is performed. Negative intervals are found and dates or times corrected in original sources. Impossible combinations of variables may be found, such as a "normal" aortic valve said to have a 100-mmHg gradient and valve area less than 1 cm^2. Parent–child relations are verified, particularly if the database has inadvertently not been set up properly to manage such relations.[4] For example, specifying an aortic valve prosthesis should be a child variable of a parent variable for "aortic valve replacement."

Inconsistencies are reported to the investigation team for resolution, and the iterative process is repeated. This process is often discouraging to the unknowledgeable investigator who assumes that all data (particularly those extracted by him or her) are flawless.

Just as important as improving the accuracy of the data set is evaluating the quality of each variable by this screening and scrubbing process. One may find that information is too often not available in medical records to trust

---

[4] In a hierarchical data structure, a *parent* variable (or node) is one level higher and directly associated with one or more *child* variables (or nodes). Thus, "duration of smoking" is a child variable to the parent variable "history of smoking." If history of smoking is positive, then duration is a child node associated with that positive response. Likewise, coronary artery bypass grafting is a child node of "cardiac procedures," which itself is a child node of "therapeutic interventions."

the variable, and it is dropped. One may also find that interpretation of the clinical condition has been so variable that the values gathered are not reproducible. Either a better surrogate needs to be found or the data element must be dropped from further consideration.

If an electronic repository of information is maintained by a research enterprise, it is important that corrections discovered in the information anywhere along the way be fed back to the original database and the data re-exported. Ideally, the change in the primary data will be documented (audit trail). In this way, database quality will be constantly improved.

Impute Values

In any study, there are likely to be values that have not been recorded. Most statistical procedures eliminate observations for which any data requested for analysis are missing. In medical data analysis, however, one is more likely to introduce bias by eliminating data on an entire patient than by substituting a value for the missing data that can be shown not to importantly bias the analysis. The process is called *missing value imputation.*

Although there is an extensive literature on managing missing data, much of it is directed toward survey investigations in which entire survey instruments have not been returned. The general directive for such data is to eliminate the records for nonresponders. In clinical research, missing data are most commonly sporadic or systematic for some specific time segment (e.g., missing magnetic resonance imaging data before the introduction of the technique). These common types of missing data should be managed in a different way from that of surveys.

Sporadic missing values. For sporadic values missing in a small proportion of patients, it is reasonable to substitute (impute) the mean value for all patients with non-missing data (called *noninformative imputation*).[C29] Thus, if 5% of patients are missing values for ejection fraction, the mean value is substituted.

If there are at least five outcome events associated with patients having sporadic missing values for a variable, a dichotomous (0,1) missing value indicator is created and forced into all models in which the primary variable is incorporated. If the indicator variable is not statistically significant, it is likely that the imputation has been noninformative with respect to outcome. If it is significant, the indicator variable both adjusts for this and serves as a warning that additional work must be done, such as use of informative imputation.

Informative imputation capitalizes on redundancy in medical information.[L3] A multivariable equation is generated (see "Multivariable Analysis" in Section 4) for the variable of interest, using, however, only patients for whom values are not missing. A value is predicted from this equation for the patient with the value missing, and this is the imputed value. Missing value indicators are just as germane for informative as for noninformative imputation.

Yet another strategy is *multiple imputation.*[L3,R7,R18] Briefly, a set of randomly chosen values is used for imputing missing values for each patient and analysis is performed, followed by another set of values and analysis.

This process may be repeated as many as 200 to 1000 times and the many analyses summarized.

Systematic missing values. Systematic missing values occur under two conditions that can be managed similarly. First, a value may be inapplicable. For example, in a study of mitral valve surgery, values for various repair techniques are inapplicable to patients receiving a prosthesis. Second, some test may come into use part way (in calendar time) through a study, or information may not have been collected about some variable until a certain calendar date. For such patients, we suggest that the missing data be managed as "interaction terms." By this we mean that systematic missing values be set to zero (0). Then a missing value indicator is generated—1 for patients with systematic missing values and 0 otherwise. Both variables are linked in all analyses. This makes interpretation of the models realistic, although it is a strategy that is computationally close to noninformative missing value imputation.

Organize Variables for Analysis

Once the aforementioned steps have been achieved, often iteratively, the result is a final data set in the format needed for analysis. However, one further step remains: organizing variables deemed suitable for analysis in a medically meaningful way. The reason for this is the importance we place on *informed data analysis.* Those analyzing the data must "know the data" just as the investigator knows the data. Not every variable has equal weight in analysis.

For example, quantitative ejection fraction is "better data" than a qualitative assessment of left ventricular function on a coarsely graded scale; creatinine level at surgery contains more data than a diagnosis of renal failure; individual components of leaflet morphology in atrioventricular septal defect contain higher information content than Rastelli type. Not every variable is of equal reliability.

Many variables are highly correlated, such as height, weight, body surface area, and body mass index (indeed, the latter two are calculated from the former two). Therefore, the data management team, in collaboration with the investigator, must compile a final list of *analyzable variables.* These are then grouped in a medically meaningful fashion that aids informal data analysis. A suggested grouping might be as follows, although it will vary from study to study:

- Demography (age, sex, size)
- Symptoms (functional status, angina class)
- Ventricular function (ejection fraction, number of previous myocardial infarctions, interval from last infarction to surgery)
- Pathophysiology and etiology (grade of mitral valve regurgitation, etiology of valvar regurgitation)
- Coronary artery anatomy and disease (degree of left main disease and that of each coronary system, dominance)
- Other cardiac comorbidity (previous cardiac operations, atrial fibrillation)
- Noncardiac comorbidity (smoking history, creatinine, chronic dialysis, diabetes, albumin level)
- Preoperative management (preoperative intraaortic balloon counterpulsation for hemodynamic instability, intravenous nitroglycerine and heparin for unstable angina)

- Cardiac procedure (CABG, bilateral internal thoracic artery grafts, quadrangular resection of mitral valve)
- Support techniques (duration of aortic clamping, use of warm substrate-enhanced induction cardioplegia, duration of circulatory arrest)
- Experience (date of operation, surgeon)
- Outcome, in-hospital events (length of postoperative stay, occurrence of various complications, hospital death)
- Outcome, time-related events (all-cause mortality, interval from surgery to death or censoring)
- Missing value indicator variables
- Interaction terms (organized according to above schema)

A practical way to implement this organizational structure is to isolate programming code in the form of a computer macro that contains the list of available variables for analysis and a place for those analyzing the data to insert code for missing value imputation, to transform the scale of variables, to form additional indicator variables, and to perform other useful data manipulations. This strategy guards against human error in data analysis by isolating all data manipulation to a single location useful for all analyses.

DESCRIPTIVE DATA EXPLORATION

After the analysis data set has been constructed, the data are explored by producing simple descriptive tables (sorting and tallying) and simple statistics about continuous variables, scatter plots of variables, and other exploratory data analyses.[T1] To understand this process, some appreciation of numerical data is necessary.

Numbers

Accuracy and Precision

Because both calculators and computers express numbers to many digits (Box 6-9), it is necessary to know a set of rules for compaction and expression (display) of numerical data. The format in which a numerical value is expressed has implications. The number 493, for example, implies that the

---

BOX 6-9   Expressing Numbers

Digit
A digit is one of the 10 Arabic number symbols, 0 through 9. Digits are also called numbers, numerals, or integers.

Number
Although *number* and *digit* are synonyms, a number is more generally applied to a series of digits, separators (commas, decimal points), and other notations (see "Scientific Notation" in this box) that together represent a numeric quantity.

Even Numbers
The Arabic numerals 0, 2, 4, 6, and 8. These numbers are all divisible by 2 without a remainder.

Odd Numbers
The Arabic numerals 1, 3, 5, 7, and 9. These are divisible by 2 with a remainder of exactly 1.

Decimal Format
Most numbers in scientific work are expressed in *decimal* format, that is, in a numerical system based on multiples of 10 as the fundamental unit, called the *base* of the numbering system. Other systems were prominent in antiquity, such as base 60 in Babylonian times, existing now only as the basis for clock time. Bases other than 10 are used in computer systems, such as base 2, 8, or 16. Yet others have been suggested as having better arithmetic properties; however, the fact that humans have 10 fingers has played a dominant role in popularizing the decimal system.

In decimal notation, each place is a multiple of 10 and is named. A symbol known as the *decimal point* (a period is used in the United States and throughout this book) separates what is known as the *units* or *ones* place from the "tenths" (1/10) place. Whole numbers are to the left of the decimal point and fractional ones to the right.

To the left of the decimal point, the first place is called the *units* (or ones) place, the second the *tens* place, the third the *hundreds* place, and the fourth *thousands* place. Commonly, a separator is inserted for each multiple of 1,000 (a comma in the United States, and period in Europe; see below). In the number 1,234, the 4 is in the units place, 3 in the tens place, 2 in the hundreds place, and 1 in the thousands place. Another way to express this number is as the sum of 4 + 30 + 200 + 1,000.

To the right of the decimal point, the first place is called the *tenths* (1/10) place, the second the *hundredths* (1/100) place, and the third the *thousandths* (1/1000) place. Thus, in 0.1234, the 1 is in the tenths place, 2 in the hundredths place, 3 in the thousandths place, and 4 in the ten thousandths place. Another way to express this number is as the sum of 0.0004 + 0.003 + 0.02 + 0.1.

Decimal Place
In the decimal system, decimal place is the position of digits immediately to the right of the symbol designating the decimal point. Location of the decimal point reflects the scale of measurement and is unrelated to *significant digits*.

Significant Digit
Digits of the decimal form of a number beginning with the leftmost nonzero digit and extending to the right, with the implicit implication that all digits to the right are *significant digits*. That is, they are warranted either by inherent properties of the measuring device used to generate the numbers or by statistical properties of a collection of such numbers.

Scientific Notation
A method of expressing (displaying) numbers from 1 to 9, followed by a *decimal point*, the remaining significant digits, if any, multiplied by a power of 10. For example, 0.00037 in scientific notation is 3.7×10^{-4}, where 10^{-4} is 0.0001. In general, the numeric value, here 3.7, is called the *mantissa*, 10 is called the *radix*, and −4 is called the *exponent*.

Leading Zero
Zero placed before a decimal point that is not considered a significant digit. It is generally used (1) when it is implied that a nonzero significant digit could replace it, or (2) to separate a negative sign (−), a positive sign (+), or a plus or minus sign (±) from the decimal point. Increasingly, numbers that are constrained to the range 0 to 1, such as probabilities (including *P* values), are expressed (displayed) without a leading zero.

truth is somewhere between 492.5 and 493.5 (accuracy) and that the scatter in repeated measurements of the number (precision) is no greater than that explicitly expressed (Box 6-10). The number 492.8 implies that the result is somewhere between 492.75 and 492.85, and 492.76 implies that the result is somewhere between 492.755 and 492.765. This last numeral to the right (right-most digit) explicitly indicates that the accuracy is much greater and the precision much less than when the number is 493.

Rounding

In computation and computer storage, all available digits of numbers should be retained. It is only at the last step of numerical presentation that numbers are rounded (Box 6-11). In presenting numeric information, numbers should be rounded in such a way as to reflect their precision or reproducibility, although consistency within tables is also important.[E2,K17]

Tabular Presentation

Numbers are often presented in tabular form, indicating the distribution of data between the extremes of a continuous variable (such as patient age).[K17] Such tables should be prepared so that the positioning of any point along the continuous variable can be *unambiguously* determined. In this text, intervals between extremes of a continuous variable are indicated by symbols of inequality (Table 6-7). This method of presentation of tabular information is mathematically conventional (Box 6-12), but not conventional for medical publications, where ambiguity often abounds.

Descriptive Statistics

Descriptive statistics are numbers used to summarize values for a specific variable recorded for a group of patients (*sample;* nomenclature is given in Box 6-13), such as age, presence or absence of coronary artery disease, and NYHA functional class. Variables fall into two broad categories for which different methods and expression of summarization are appropriate: (1) *categorical* and (2) *continuous.*

Categorical variables take on a small number of values. If they take on just two, such as "yes" and "no," they are called *dichotomous variables.* If they have values that are ordered, such as none, mild, moderate, and severe,

they are called *ordinal* variables. If they are just a list (such as type of valve prosthesis), they are called *polytomous variables.*

Continuous variables take on a theoretically limitless number of values, although these values may have natural constraints (such as age, which cannot be negative). Their degree of granularity may vary (e.g., age may be calculated in whole years in adults, but in days or even hours [higher granularity] in neonates).

BOX 6-11   Rounding Numbers

Certain generally agreed upon conventions for rounding numbers exist, although they are not easily found in print.

Step 1: Determine the Number of Digits to Save
This is suggested by precision of the measuring instrument for individual numbers and by the standard error of the mean value or proportion associated with a series of numbers (see Box 6-12). For the latter, the place of the first significant digit of the standard error is found, and the mean or proportion is then rounded to that place. The same place is saved in confidence limits. If the standard error is also being expressed, one additional place is saved in it (because the usual ± expression of the standard error is a form of shorthand, and saving the extra place helps in using the standard error to calculate confidence limits).

Step 2: Look for Exceptions
Exceptions to Step 1 are as follows: (1) if the first significant digit of the standard error is 1, then one additional place is saved; and (2) within a single contingency table, consistency in saving digits is desirable, so all numbers may be rounded to the place indicated by the majority of the numbers. In medical data, two significant digits (see Box 6-9) usually suffice.

Step 3: Round
Round the number by removing digits from its right side that falsely suggest a high degree of precision or accuracy. This is done as follows[C1]:
- If the digit in the first place beyond (to the right of) the digit to be rounded is greater than 5, add 1 to the right-most digit to be retained and drop all other digits to its right. This is called "rounding up."
- If the digit in the first place beyond the digit to be rounded is less than 5, simply drop it and all other digits to its right. This is called "rounding down."
- If the digit in the first place beyond the digit to be rounded is exactly 500 . . . 0, add 1 to the rightmost digit to be retained if the last significant digit is odd (that is, 1, 3, 5, 7, or 9), and leave the digit to be rounded as is if it is even (that is, 0, 2, 4, 6, or 8). This rule results after rounding in a rightmost digit that is always an even number.

BOX 6-10   Accuracy versus Precision

Accuracy
Absence of systematic error of measurement (bias) from the "truth." It is an expression of "rightness."

Precision
Ability to provide the same answer in repeated measurements. It is an expression of "exactness."
These terms are often interchanged, but in data analysis they are not synonymous! Repeated measurements of Po_2 in a blood gas machine may have a great deal of scatter on repeated readings (imprecise), but their average value may reflect faithfully the true Po_2 (accurate). Another blood gas machine may yield Po_2 with little scatter in repeat readings (precise), but may be uncalibrated, so the readings are inaccurate (*biased*). There is often a trade-off between accuracy and precision in medical measuring instruments.

■ **TABLE 6-7   Use of Symbols of Inequality: Illustration with *P* Values and Their Interpretation**[a]

≤ *P* <		Interpretation of Null Hypothesis	Inferences about the Difference
	.05	Almost certainly not true	Unlikely to be due to chance
.05	.1	Probably not true	Probably not due to chance
.1	.2	Possibly not true	Possibly not due to chance
.2		Nearly certainly true[b]	Likely to be due to chance

[a] Each *P* value can be unambiguously located in one of the four lines of the table. The top line contains all *P* values less than .05. The fourth, or bottom, line contains all *P* values greater than or equal to .2. The second line embraces all *P* values greater than or equal to .05 but less than .1.

[b] A small sample size also could account for this *P* value.

Categorical Variables

Dichotomous. Descriptive statistics for dichotomous categorical variables include simple counts; that is, a count of the number of times the variable was YES (or 1) or NO (or 0): How many cases were performed? How many men and women were in the study? How many patients died after operation? However, summary counts are of limited value because they do not reflect the size of the sample. Therefore, a summary statistic can be formulated that normalizes the counts to a standard denominator, commonly 100 (percent). This is a probability parameter estimate, so it not only reflects what is experienced within the sample but also begins to give insight into characteristics of the population (Box 6-14).

Ordinal. Each value of an ordinal variable bears a strictly increasing or decreasing (monotonic) relation to all other possible values. It may be tempting, for simplicity, to group some of these values together, such as forming a dichotomous variable that lumps NYHA classes I and II versus III and IV. This is an information-losing transformation of scale that should be done only if outcome is truly found by analysis not to follow the ordinal scale, but to suggest just two groups of patients.

When ordinal variables are analyzed with respect to outcome, it is important to use statistical methods that are appropriate for ordered values (trend statistics) rather than for lists (tests of independence of categories). This must be communicated to the biostatistician or other data analyst.

BOX 6-12 Inequalities

$<$
Less than. $3 < 4$ means "3 is less than 4."
$>$
Greater than. $5 > 3$ means "5 is greater than 3."
$\leq$
Less than or equal to. Systolic blood pressure ≤ 130 means systolic pressure is "less than or equal to 130."
$\geq$
Greater than or equal to. Diastolic blood pressure ≥ 80 means diastolic pressure is "greater than or equal to 80."
$30 \leq x < 40$
The number represented by x is greater than or equal to 30 (that is, 30 is less than or equal to x), but is less than 40. Note that x is strictly less than 40 (39.999...), not exactly equal to 40. This statement is unambiguous, whereas the statement that "x is between 30 and 40" is ambiguous, because it is unclear whether 30 or 40 is included by the word "between."

BOX 6-13 Words

Piantadosi, Kirklin, and Blackstone provided a glossary of statistical terms in the first edition of Pearson and colleagues' *Thoracic Surgery*.[P17]

Population
The entire set of things with specified attributes. For example, the population of patients with ischemic heart disease encompasses everybody with that disease, not only at the present time, but anyone in the past or future.

Sample
One or more things with specific attributes belonging to a population. Thus, my next patient, or a group of patients I have operated on with ischemic heart disease, represents a sample of the population of such individuals.

Proportion
A proportion is a part compared with the whole. Specifically, it is the number having some attribute value of interest, divided by the number in the sample. Ten deaths among 30 patients is a proportion of 0.3.

Percent
Percent is a part compared with the whole normalized to a sample size of 100. It is calculated by multiplying a proportion by 100.

Parameter
A constant used to characterize some attribute of a population. One generally uses a sample of patients to estimate such constants. These constants are commonly (but not always) designated by letters or symbols in mathematical equations called *models* (see Box 6-5).

Variable
An attribute about a thing that can take on different values from one thing to another. For example, systolic blood pressure is a variable because its value differs from patient to patient. The word *parameter* is often used incorrectly when the word *variable* is meant.

Prevalence, Incidence, Rate
Prevalence, incidence, and *rate* are often used interchangeably. Perhaps common usage should prevail (it rarely leads to confusion), but from the standpoint of correct usage, these are not interchangeable terms. We prefer selecting the specific word whose technical definition matches the context.

Prevalence
Frequency of occurrence of some factor, characteristic, event, or incident in a group. Of the three words being considered, it is the least commonly used but the most commonly meant! For example, if 78% of patients are men, then the prevalence of males in the sample is 78%; we would not use the phrase, "The incidence of males was...." Similarly, hospital mortality may be 1%. That is the prevalence or occurrence of hospital mortality; we would not use the phrase, "Hospital mortality rate was..." or "Incidence of hospital mortality was...." The word *occurrence* is often a suitable substitute for prevalence.

Incidence
Frequency of occurrence *per unit of time.* It is expressed on a scale of inverse time (cases per year, deaths per year), or *rate* of occurrence. The prevalence of mortality across time is expressed as survival; the incidence of mortality is expressed by the hazard function.

Rate
Quantity per unit time. Speed is a rate: $km \cdot h^{-1}$; cardiac output is a blood flow rate: $L \cdot min^{-1}$. In the context of events, rate is synonymous with incidence. The hazard function is a rate (mortality $\cdot$ year^{-1}) and incidence.
How, then, can we rephrase such common expressions as the following?
- Incidence of hospital mortality was....
- Hospital mortality rate was....
- Five-year survival rate was....
We could write "Prevalence of hospital mortality was...." However, in most instances, the words prevalence, incidence, and rate are superfluous. It is better to just write "Hospital mortality was..." or "Five-year survival was...."

Polytomous. Variables with values that are simply a list (complications after operation, type of valve prosthesis) can be counted, but special mention must be made as to whether the counts represent mutually exclusive categories. A list of types of prosthesis used is likely to be mutually exclusive (a patient can fall into only one category), but a table of complications is unlikely to be so (a patient can experience more than one complication). In presenting lists, all categories should be represented, including number of missing values and whether categories have been coalesced (such as under "other").

List variables are often useful for analysis if they are mutually exclusive (see "Polytomous and Ordinal Logistic Regression" in Section 4). Otherwise, the list needs to be decomposed into a set of dichotomous variables for each category.

Continuous Variables

The other broad category of variables is continuous, for which each patient in a study (sample) may have a different value (e.g., age, weight, ejection fraction). Thus, the raw data are rarely published because each patient or subject in a study is likely to be unique in regard to continuous variables, making any tabular presentation unwieldy unless the number of patients and number of variables are small. Summarizing statements may be made of the raw data by one of several techniques.

A commonly used summarization of raw data is a simple table with patients grouped into "nice" ordered categories. A *histogram* is a plot of such a table (Fig. 6-6, *A*). Another method of constructing a simple table is to sort patients into several groups of equal number, even if the width of the range of values in each group is different. Because the

number of such groups was originally 10, these are called *decile tables.*

Yet another alternative is to divide patients into *percentiles,* stating the value of the variable at these percentiles as follows. Patients or subjects are first sorted by (generally) increasing magnitude of the variable under consideration (for example, by increasing age). Then the number (or more commonly the proportion) of patients with values less than or equal to each value is calculated. For example, if there are 21 patients and each is a different age at operation, then patients are first sorted from youngest to oldest. No patient

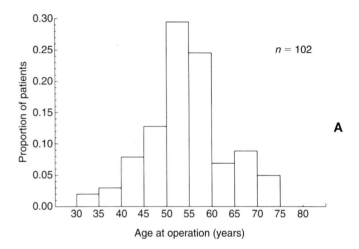

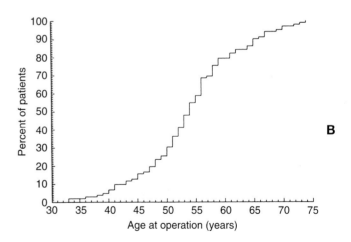

Figure 6-6   Distribution of a continuous variable, age at operation. **A,** Histogram of age at operation of 102 patients undergoing coronary artery bypass grafting. Approximately 30% were 50 to 55 years of age at operation, 25% were age 55 to 60, and lesser percentages of patients were older or younger. **B,** Cumulative distribution plot of age at operation in these 102 patients. Vertical axis shows the percentage of patients coming to operation at or younger than any given age on the horizontal axis. Vertical axis gives directly the percent of patients coming to operation by a given age. The median is the 50th percentile. S shape of this particular plot suggests a normal distribution; any other shape would suggest a different distribution.

---

is younger that the youngest one (0/21, 0%, or minimum); 1/21 are as young or younger than the youngest (4.8%), and for these data, this is also the 5th percentile; 2/21 (9.5%) are as young or younger than the second youngest patient, and this is also the 10th percentile. The middle value of age, that of the 11th patient in this list, is called the median or 50th percentile. All (21/21, 100%) are as young or younger than the oldest. A *cumulative distribution plot,* produced easily by computer but laboriously by hand, presents all the raw data in this percentile format (Fig. 6-6, *B*).

Alternatively (and more commonly), a value is found below which a stated proportion of patients have that value or a lesser one (100 times that proportion is the percentile). For example, the *median* is the 50th percentile. This means that half the patients have a value for the continuous variable below the median, and half have values greater. For consistency, one might also state the 15th and 85th percentiles, as they correspond to 70% confidence limits (see "Confidence Limits [Intervals]" in Section 4). More commonly, 25th and 75th percentiles (quartiles) or 10th and 90th percentiles are used.

This method of summarizing data is called *nonparametric* (see Box 6-14). Beyond such simple counting (percentages and percentiles), more abstract methods are often brought into play to describe continuous data. The methods have in common a process whereby raw data on a sample of patients are used to estimate values of *parameters* of mathematical equations. The most familiar of these is the *arithmetic average,* or *mean,* which is estimated as the summation of all values of the continuous variable (such as age or pulmonary artery pressure) divided by the number of people or observations *(n).* The rationale for using the arithmetic average is that it provides an estimate of the *central tendency* of the data and a characteristic of the population studied. If the data are distributed perfectly symmetrically in the form of a bell-shaped curve, the arithmetic average is exactly at the midpoint of the data range (Fig. 6-7). It is also the most frequently occurring number *(mode),* with half the patients above it and half below *(median).*

The derivation of averages, or means, was begun by astronomers centuries ago. They thought that the scatter in their data was from observational error or imprecision, and they used means, or averages, in an attempt to obtain true values (accuracy). Later, Gauss discussed and described the symmetric *normal distribution curve,*[G2] which actually was described earlier by DeMoivre[D2] (Box 6-15).

The mean is the easiest statistic to calculate. Unfortunately, it is not a robust measure of central tendency. If many infants and only one or two adults are in a study, average age is greatly exaggerated by the few adults. A more robust measure of central tendency is the median. Whether or not the sample data are distributed in a Gaussian-type bell-shaped curve (see Fig. 6-7 and Box 6-15) may be tested by such statistics as the Shapiro–Wilk W statistic[S1] for small n (say, 50 or less) and the Kolmogorov–Smirnov D statistic[S2] for larger samples. The skewness of the data (rightward or leftward asymmetric tail) and their kurtosis (unusual peakedness of the distribution of values) are also tested.

Thus, in addition to an estimation of the population mean, some measure of *dispersion* (variance, spread, scatter) of values is needed. One such measure is the *standard*

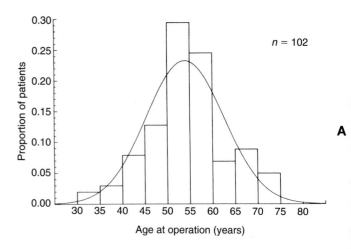

A

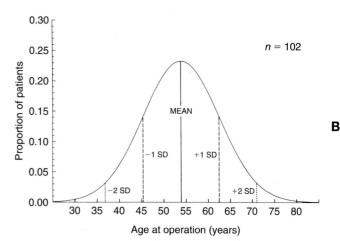

B

Figure 6-7 Gaussian bell-shaped distribution curve for age. **A,** Distribution curve *(smooth line)* fitted to the data in Fig. 6-6. **B,** Distribution with mean ±1 and 2 standard deviations (SD) marked by vertical lines. Point of inflection of the curve from concave to convex is 1 SD.

Key: *SD,* Standard deviation.

deviation. Standard deviation is the name of the second parameter of the Gaussian distribution equation (see Box 6-15).[G3] It refers to variability from subject to subject or variability of individuals within the sample. It is used to determine whether an individual is "within limits of normal" and is necessary for comparison statistics. For example, an individual's standard deviation from the mean regarding a particular measured variable (commonly called Z) is often useful. This is calculated from the difference between the measurement for the individual and the mean normal value divided by the standard deviation. Z may be negative or positive and has no units[5] (see "Standardization of Dimensions" under Dimensions of Normal Cardiac and Great Artery Pathways in Chapter 1).

Standard error is a measure of the reliability with which the population mean is estimated from the sample mean, and

---

[5] The standard deviation has the same units as the mean value (for example, the mean normal value may be 12 mm and one standard deviation 3 mm and two standard deviations 6 mm). However, the *number* of standard deviations (here one or two) has no units.

BOX 6-15 Gaussian Distribution

The equation of the bell-shaped *Gaussian (normal) distribution* curve is

$$y = \frac{1}{\sigma\sqrt{2\pi}}e^{-\frac{(x-\mu)^2}{2\sigma^2}}$$

where:
π is a constant, approximately 3.1415927..., pi.
e is a constant, approximately 2.7183..., the base of the natural logarithms.
σ is a parameter that represents the standard deviation of the variable.
μ is a parameter that represents the mean of the variable.
x represents a value of the variable X, generally graphed on the horizontal axis.
y represents the probability of occurrence of a particular value of x.

Because in medicine *normal* has several unrelated meanings, we have used the more technical term *Gaussian*.

Standard Deviation versus Standard Error

Standard deviation is the Gaussian distribution parameter representing the scatter or deviation of individual values from the mean. It is a descriptive statistic, the inflection point of the Gaussian distribution (see Fig. 6-7, *B*).

Standard error is the standard deviation of the mean, an estimate of the *precision* of the mean (see Box 6-10). Unlike the standard deviation, which is similar in value for large and small samples of data, the standard error decreases as approximately the square root of n increases.

Because the Gaussian curve is symmetric around the mean, the two parameters of the Gaussian distribution are expressed by the shorthand *mean ± SD*, where SD is 1 standard deviation. This means 68.3% of values for patient age fall between (mean – SD) and (mean + SD). This is one instance, not common in statistics, where the shorthand ± is used instead of *confidence limits* (see Box 6-16).

it is needed for comparing one group to another. It is more appropriately, but infrequently, called the *standard deviation of the mean* and is obtained simply by dividing the standard deviation by the square root of n (see Box 6-15).

Other methods are available for summarizing skewed data. One is to resort to a purely *nonparametric* (i.e., without equations, coefficients) description (e.g., using the median and its various percentiles).[F1,H1] Another is to *transform* the data into a more normally distributed variable.[T1] For example, a logarithmic transformation is often useful; the resultant mean is called a *geometric mean*.

SECTION 4
Analyses

HISTORICAL NOTE

Analysis, as expressed by Sir Isaac Newton, is that part of the inductive scientific process whereby a small part of nature (a phenomenon) is examined in the light of observations (data) so that inferences can be drawn about it that help explain the workings of nature.[N6]

The philosophies underpinning methods of data analysis have evolved rapidly over the past 100 years and may be at an important crossroad. Stimulated in large part by the findings of his cousin Charles Darwin, Sir Francis Galton, along with Karl Pearson and Francis Edgeworth, established in the latter part of the nineteenth century what has come to be known as *biostatistics*. Because of the Darwinian link, much of their thinking was directed toward an empirical study of genetics versus environmental influence on biological development. It stimulated development of the field of eugenics (human breeding) and study of mental and even criminal characteristics of humans as they relate to physical characteristics. The outbreak of World War I led to statistics of quality. Sir Ronald Fisher formalized a methodologic approach to experimentation, including randomized designs.[F5] The varying milieus of development led to several competing schools of thought within statistics, such as frequentist and Bayesian, with different languages and different methods. Formalization of the discipline occurred, and whatever the flavor of statistics, it came to dominate the analytic phase of inferential data analysis, perhaps because of its empirical approach and lack of underlying mechanistic assumptions.

Simultaneously, the discipline of biomathematics arose, stimulated in particular by the need to understand the growth of organisms and populations in a quantitative fashion. Biomathematical models became important in attempts to understand clearance of pharmaceuticals, enzyme kinetics, and blood flow dynamics. Biomathematicians specifically attempt to develop mathematical models of natural phenomena. These continue to be important today in understanding such altered physiology as cavopulmonary shunt flow. Many of the biomathematical models came to compete with statistical models for distributions, such as the distribution of times to events.

Advent of the fast Fourier transform in the mid-1960s[C30] led to important medical advances in filtering signal from noise and image processing. The impetus for this development came largely from the communications industry, so only a few noticed that concepts in communication theory coincided with those in statistics and mathematics.

As business use of computers expanded, and more recently as genomic data became voluminous, computer scientists developed methods for examining large stores of data (see footnote 1, p. 256).[B38] These included data mining in business and computational biology and bioinformatics in the life sciences. Problems of classification (such as of addresses for mail) led to such tools as neural networks,[R8] which have been superseded in recent years by an entire discipline of machine learning.[H15]

In the past quarter century, all these disciplines of mathematics, computer science, information modeling, and digital signal processing have been vying for a place in the analytic phase of clinical research that in the past has largely been dominated by biostatistics (see footnote 1, p. 256). Fortunately for those of us in cardiac surgery, we need not be threatened by these alternative voices, but rather can seize the opportunity to discover how each can help us understand the phenomena we are trying to understand.

OVERVIEW

This section highlights (1) the important statistical concept of dealing with *uncertainty*, illustrating it with confidence limits and *P* values, (2) the increasingly important signal processing concept, *multivariable analysis,* illustrating it with logistic regression of early postoperative events, and (3) the *analysis of time-related and longitudinal events,* which we believe should be thought of in terms of biomathematical concepts. In Section 6, other specialized methods are highlighted, including some that are only peripherally related to serious clinical research but importantly affect cardiac surgeons.

UNCERTAINTY

Publication of an experience with mitral valve repair in 438 patients, among whom 8 (1.8%) died in-hospital, is in isolation a record of past achievement. Assuming honest reporting, there is no uncertainty about this result, but in and of itself, except for inviting applause or criticism, it has only historical value. Yet most persons expect past experience to be useful in predicting what can be accomplished in the present or the future, or in comparing outcome with that of other surgical options or continued medical therapy (see "Nihilism versus Predictability" in Section 1). That is, they recognize that the future is uncertain, but they are not nihilists; they assume there is continuity in nature (see "Continuity versus Discontinuity in Nature" in Section 1). There are well-tested theories and methods that quantify the degree of uncertainty of inferring from the past the probable results in the future, assuming nothing changes, expressed as a degree of uncertainty. Quantifying the degree of uncertainty is a major part of making results of past experience truly useful.

Point Estimates

Point estimates usually represent the central tendency of a set of numbers that describe the characteristics or state of a sample (such as a group of patients). The previously mentioned 1.8% hospital mortality is a point estimate. So are the mean value of age in a group of patients and the percent survival (survivorship) 1 or 20 years after an operation.

Such numbers are generally derived from a study of a *sample* (see Box 6-13) of all members of a *population* (e.g., everyone everywhere undergoing mitral valve repair). Yet the clinical study is nearly always performed to generalize beyond the sample examined.

Generalizing from a sample to the population is fraught with uncertainty. For example, recorded, unrecorded, or unrecognized patient characteristics may occur at a different frequency in the sample than in the population (including your future patients). Surgeons use expert clinical judgment in decision-making, and this introduces selection bias into the sample. There is well-recognized variance in institutional policies, processes, procedures, skill, and experience that influences outcome in ways that are difficult to dissect and that are confounded inextricably with both outcomes and interpretation of outcomes. These all suggest that inferences from sample point estimates alone are unlikely to be predictive of results in either the population or future samples.

Despite this admonition, over the past quarter century we have observed fewer and fewer cardiac surgery publications that accompany point estimates with a measure of uncertainty. Although it is speculation, the cause may be in part the complexity of programming the present generation of programmable calculators and handheld computers to generate confidence limits (Appendix 6B). In part it is the unfortunate fact that it is unusual for currently available statistical analysis packages—either those accessible to surgeons or those used by professional statisticians—to provide measures of uncertainty automatically, particularly for proportions (such as hospital mortality).

Confidence Limits (Intervals)

Confidence limits, the extremes of a confidence interval (Box 6-16) are the fundamental statistics that quantify the uncertainty of point estimates. It is not the underlying data that are uncertain (such as how many hospital deaths occurred in a well-defined group of patients), but inferences about the future based on known data from the past.

For example, if there was one hospital death in three operations for postinfarction ventricular septal defect (VSD), the proportion of hospital deaths (hospital mortality) was .33 (1/3, 33% hospital mortality). This *was* the mortality in that experience, looking at it solely as a record of achievement. Likewise, if 10 deaths occurred among 30 such operations, or 100 occurred among 300, the mortality was also 33%. Intuitively, there would be more confidence that the risk in an entire population, not just in the small sample studied, was near 33% on the basis of the experience with 300 operations than on the basis of three operations. Yet, also intuitively, one suspects *something* has been learned about the risk in an entire population from only three operations. For example, the true risk cannot be exactly 0% or exactly 100%.

Historical Development

The questions "What is the risk of repair of postinfarction VSD in general?" and "Is risk with the method of repair I used higher or lower than that with the method another surgeon is using?" are similar to questions put to Galileo about the nature of chance, and particularly games of chance, by seventeenth century gamblers.[D17,H11] From those questions emerged the Laws of Chance, now known as the theory of probability.[G1] These laws are believed to apply to all things that can have more than one possible result; things with exactly one result are the limiting case of this theory, having a probability equal to 1, or certainty. More and more scientists believe that all natural phenom-

---

BOX 6-16   Confidence Limits, Confidence Intervals

Confidence Limits
   Numbers at the two extremes of an interval that encompasses a stated percentage of the variability of a point estimate. In this book, we use confidence limits (CL) rather than confidence intervals (CI) to avoid confusion with cardiac index (CI), a familiar abbreviation used by cardiac surgeons.

Confidence Interval
   Interval encompassing a stated percentage of the variability of a point estimate. Confidence limits for proportions can be calculated to a reasonable degree of accuracy with a simple programmable calculator (see Appendix 6B).

ena, including those of the physical world, behave in accordance with the theory of probability.[B14,H4] Events and phenomena of cardiac surgery can also be considered to behave in accordance with this theory.

Galileo showed that there is variability in sample point estimates. To illustrate, if the risk of death in the entire population of patients undergoing repair of postinfarction VSD by a given method is 33%, and samples of three patients are taken repeatedly, zero deaths among the three would be experienced in 30% of samples, one death in 44% of samples, two deaths in 22% of samples, and three deaths in 4% of samples. In larger samples, results are less variable. For example, with samples of size 300, although the number of deaths experienced may still be quite variable, the proportion dying will be 30% to 36% in 70% of samples taken.

Because of this random variability in the sample estimates of risk, it is impossible to estimate the population parameter (see Box 6-13) with certainty (i.e., to know the risk in the entire population) from sample information. However, the pattern of variability in repeated sampling is well understood, and in most situations it is possible to derive a formula to calculate the range of values that would contain the parameter for a specified percentage (e.g., 70%) of samples taken.

Users of confidence limits should be aware that this range of values (confidence limits) for all proportions except .5 (50%) is asymmetric, in contrast to standard deviations, which are symmetric. Thus, we must report both the point estimate (probability) and lower and upper confidence limits.

As the sample size increases and more information becomes available, width of the confidence interval decreases. That is, a more precise estimate is obtained. With a more precise estimate, the investigator is less uncertain where the population parameter lies, or, in other words, what the "true" risk is. With a less precise estimate, the investigator is more uncertain.[D1,J1,N1,N2]

Computational Methods

Methods have been developed to calculate confidence limits for proportions.[B7,B13,W3] These methods are best left to computers. However, confidence limits that closely approximate these can be easily and rapidly obtained with a small programmable calculator (see Appendix 6B).

Bootstrapping[6] is a generalized method for obtaining confidence limits for any statistic.[D16] The original sample of data is randomly sampled in such a way that the patient can be sampled again (sampled with replacement) to form a data set equal in size to the original. Because of replacement, some patients will appear more than once in this bootstrap sample and others will not appear at all. The point estimate (such as hospital mortality) is estimated in this sample. Then another sample is drawn in the same fashion,

and this process is repeated as many as 1000 times. All the point estimates from each sample are sorted from smallest to largest, as in forming a cumulative frequency distribution (see "Descriptive Data Exploration" in Section 3). The "best" estimate of the point estimate is the median value (50% above and 50% below). If 70% confidence limits are desired, then the 15th percentile is the lower confidence limit and the 85th percentile is the upper limit (if 68.3% limits are desired, the numbers would be approximately the 16th and 84th percentiles).

What Level of Confidence?

Any desired confidence limit (CL) can be derived, such as 50%, 70%, 90%, 95%, or 97.5%. Choice of confidence limits to be expressed (called the *confidence coefficient*) depends on the use to be made of them, on consistency, or on convention, in that order of preference.

Most often in cardiac surgery, CLs are used as scanning tools to aid predictions and comparisons, either of proportions or of time-related depictions (see "Scanning Tool" later in this section). If great certainty is desired in the inference that there is a difference between two proportions of time-related depictions, 95% confidence intervals may be chosen for the comparisons. If only moderate certainty is required that the evident difference is a true difference and would be found in larger samples, 50% confidence intervals might be chosen.

Most situations in cardiac surgery seem to lie somewhere between these extremes; thus, use of 70% CLs for most comparisons is reasonable. The interval is relatively narrow (specific), and although it is reasonably certain that the truth lies within the confidence limits, there is a 15% chance it will be higher and 15% chance it will be lower.

Seventy percent CLs (actually 68.3%) are equivalent to 1 standard deviation (SD), and 95% CLs are consistent with 2 SDs. For consistency, if other numerical estimates are presented to 1 SD, then 70% CLs should be used, and if 2 SDs are presented, then 95% CLs should be used. We emphasize consistency because we believe that surgeons should become familiar with using confidence limits as a scanning tool. To use a tool effectively, it is helpful to be consistent among all measures of uncertainty. Conventionally, many statisticians use 95% CLs, even in the context of using 1 SD for everything else. This makes no sense and is simply a habit, not a product of reflective thinking about the inferences nor about consistency.

In numeric presentation of differences, such as difference in survival curves (see Box 6-3), 90% CLs are equivalent in comparative inference to individual 70% confidence limits, a largely empirical finding.[A5] The reason is that a one-sided confidence interval of a difference between two estimates is narrower than the sum of the 70% upper and lower CLs that just touch. This narrowness is compensated for by use of somewhat wider CLs (90%) of the difference.

Scanning Tool

Overlapping or nonoverlapping of confidence limits around two or more point estimates can be used as a simple and intuitive scanning method for determining whether the difference in point estimates is unlikely to be due to chance alone.[B18] They delimit the effect, and because they are

---

[6] Bootstrapping is a word chosen by Efron and his colleagues to reflect the idea of "pulling yourself up by your own bootstraps." That is, the statistics are generated by the set of data itself rather than by an estimation procedure that makes assumptions about the data (such as its being distributed in Gaussian fashion). The historical background is discussed in more detail under "Variable Selection" later in this section.

accompanied by the magnitude of the effect, there is no confusion between statistical significance and magnitude of the effect, as there may be if *P* values are used (see "*P* Values" later in this section). When confidence limits are not overlapping, the difference is unlikely to be due to chance alone.

Because the phrase "nonoverlapping confidence limits suggests with a stated degree of uncertainty that a difference exists" is cumbersome, the phrase *evident difference* may be used to express the same idea (Appendix 6C). Nonoverlapping confidence limits are easily visualized in a nomogram in which the confidence limits are displayed around the point estimate expressing the association between variables. Within this context, it can be said with a stated degree of uncertainty that the effect of the independent variable compared with a baseline value becomes evident at the point at which the confidence limits just separate. However, in contrast to evident differences in a contingency table, this point is not easily seen in a nomogram, and it does not appear in an equation. The point at which evident differences appear in equations can, however, be calculated mathematically (see Appendix 6C).

We stress that comparing confidence limits in this way is a *scanning tool*. The classic method using *P* values involves computing the difference between the two proportions and testing the hypothesis that the difference is zero. Experience with scanning and *P* value methods has taught that when the lower 70% confidence limit of one estimate just touches the upper 70% confidence of the other, the *P* value for the difference is between .08 and .1; when similar 95% confidence limits just touch, the *P* value is about .01.

P Values

The phrase "statistically significant," generally referring to *P* values, has done disservice to the understanding of truth, proof, and uncertainty. This is in part because of fundamental misunderstandings, in part because of failure to appreciate that all test statistics are specific in their use, and in part because *P* values are frequently used for their effect on the reader rather than as one of many tools useful for promoting understanding and framing inferences from data.

In fact, *P* values are deemed by some to be unnecessary statistics and not worth the risk of misinterpreting or misusing them. They prefer confidence limits.[G30]

Definition

In the context of hypothesis (or significance) testing, the *P* value is the probability of observing the data we have, or something even more extreme, if a so-called *null hypothesis* is true (Box 6-17).[W13]

Historically, hypothesis testing is a formal expression of English common law. The null hypothesis represents "innocent until proven guilty beyond a reasonable doubt." Clearly, two injustices can occur: a guilty person can go free or an innocent person can be convicted. These possibilities are termed type I error and type II error, respectively (see Box 6-17). Evidence marshaled against the null hypothesis is called a *test statistic,* which is based on the data themselves (the exhibits) and *n*. The probability of guilt (reasonable doubt) is quantified by the *P* value or its inverse, the odds $[(1/P) - 1]$ (see Box 6-3).

BOX 6-17 Hypothesis (Significance) Testing

Statistical Hypothesis
A claim about the value of one or more parameters. For example, the claim may be that the mean for some variable, such as creatinine, is greater than some fixed value or than some value obtained under different conditions or in a different sample of patients. It can be calculated only if the distribution of the data is known.

Null Hypothesis
A claim that the difference between one or more parameters is zero or no change (written H_0). It is the claim the investigator is arguing against. When a statistician infers that there is "statistical significance," it means that by some criteria (generally a *P* value) this null hypothesis has been rejected. Some argue that the null hypothesis can never be true and that sample size is just insufficient to demonstrate this fact. They emphasize that the magnitude of *P* values is highly dependent on *n*, so other "measures of surprise" need to be sought.

Alternative Hypothesis
This is the "investigator's claim" and is sometimes called the *study hypothesis*. The investigator would like for the data to support the alternative hypothesis.

Test Statistic
A number, computed from the distribution of the variable to be tested in the sample of data, that is used to test the merit of the null hypothesis.

Type I Error
Rejecting the null hypothesis when it is true (false negative). The probability of a type I error is designated by the Greek letter alpha (α).

Type II Error
Not rejecting the null hypothesis when it is false (false positive). The probability of type II error is designated by the Greek letter beta (β).

Had the originators been raised under a different judicial system, perhaps a different pattern for testing hypotheses might have arisen. Specifically, the system does not judge how innocent a person is (the "alternative hypothesis"; see Box 6-17), nor does it test for equivalence, a very important matter for comparing pharmaceuticals and even alternative surgical therapies.[B59-61,P15,S24]

Some statisticians believe that hypothesis or significance testing and interpretation of the *P* value by this system of justice is too artificial and misses important information.[B57,K4,S23] For example, it is sobering to demonstrate the distribution of *P* values by bootstrap sampling. Further, the magnitude of the *P* value is dependent on two factors: the magnitude of difference and sample size. These individuals would prefer that *P* values be interpreted simply as "degree of evidence," "degree of surprise," or "degree of belief."[B58] We agree with these ideas and suggest that rather than using *P* values for judging guilt or innocence (accepting or rejecting the null hypothesis), the *P* value itself should be reported as degree of evidence.

Calculating the P Value

All methods for calculating *P* values have in common one or more point estimates, some measure of variability for each, some comparison statistic related to the point estimates (e.g., the difference or a ratio), an estimate of the variability of the comparison statistic, and size of the groups.

The test to be used is selected. This must be appropriate for the comparison. It is crucial that a biostatistician familiar with the data and the comparison be the one to select this test and interpret the results. In general terms, this demands that a specific distribution of the difference or ratio be selected. From the difference or ratio, some measure of its variability,[W4,W5] and *n*, a number is computed for the particular distribution selected, called the *test statistic* (see Box 6-17). There are a number of test statistics, which means there are a number of prescribed, defined, specific methods (tests) for calculating the test statistic. The statistician selects the test statistic to be used on the basis of the fit of the data to the assumptions underlying the test.

The magnitude of the computed test statistic among the hypothetically determined distribution of values for the test chosen is determined. The area under the distribution curve (proportion of the total area) occupied by more extreme values of the test statistic is the *P value,* a number ranging from 0 to 1.

In the case of many test statistics, a family of distribution curves exists, and to determine the *P* values, one of these must be selected. The selection is based, more or less, on the sample size (*n*).[S3] By "more or less," we mean that some information content in the *n* may already have been "used up" in other calculations in the process and may not be available for computation of the *P* value. What is left, called *degrees of freedom,* determines the distribution curve selected.

The phrases *one-tailed P value* and *two-tailed P value* are commonly used. Which is appropriate depends on the research hypothesis being tested. When the hypothesis relates to differences in either direction ("different from zero"), a two-tailed *P* value is used; when it relates to differences in only one direction ("less than," for example), a one-tailed *P* value is used. A two-tailed *P* value is always the same as, or larger than, a one-tailed *P* value. Generally, in the work described in this book, two-tailed *P* values are used.

Use of Expressions of Degree of Uncertainty

Whether one uses confidence limits or *P* values, a decision must be made concerning the degree of certainty desired in the inference that *A* is different from *B*. Some have a slavish attachment to a certain *P* value, such as .05, or a certain width of confidence limits, such as 95%, as the yardstick for all situations. Sir Ronald Fisher wrote, "No scientific worker has a fixed level of significance at which from year to year, and in all circumstances, he rejects hypotheses; he rather gives his mind to each particular case in the light of his evidence and his ideas."[F6] This admonition is particularly germane in cardiac surgery, wherein the investigator often has available a smaller sample size than is desirable, yet wishes to infer at least something from it.

This discussion would be unnecessary if all sample sizes were moderately large and the number of events ample, providing adequate power (information content) for all computations (see Box 6-4). In many clinical investiga-

tions, a large sample is simply not available, yet important decisions must be made on the basis of the inference generated. Then the cost of making a wrong decision based on an analysis, and the risk of overlooking or not finding a relation between two variables that in fact exists, plays importantly in the decision regarding what *P* value to use (see Table 6-7 and Box 6-17).[K4] The greater the cost, the smaller the *P* value demanded.

An apparent contradiction to the foregoing discussion is the setting of so-called "humongous" databases of hundreds of thousands or millions of patients.[M11] In this setting, the dependence of *P* values on *n* becomes glaringly apparent. Essentially in every comparison, no matter how small the clinical difference, *P* values are small.[7] "All null hypotheses are false."[M12] In this circumstance, other measures of surprise must be devised for testing differences that take into account the magnitude of the difference.

MULTIVARIABLE ANALYSIS
The Necessity

Surgeons have intuitively understood that surgical outcome, such as hospital mortality, may be related to a number of explanatory variables, such as renal and hepatic function.[L5] However, when presenting a risk factor analysis of outcome for a group of patients, two reactions are heard, often from the same critic: (1) "Your analyses are much too complex, far beyond the comprehension of ordinary cardiac surgeons," and (2) "This is a very complex, multifactorial situation, and you have not begun to take all the things that could have influenced outcome into consideration." This contradiction reflects the cognitive structure of the human mind, as discussed in Section 1. On the one hand, we perceive, understand, and store in our brains simplified models of reality. On the other hand, our conscious minds recognize that "things are often less simple than they seem."

To complicate matters, we generally know neither the cause nor the causal sequence that leads to a surgical failure, and that is what we want to know to make progress toward preventing future failures. The cause may in fact be buried in the clinical information and the data we have extracted therefrom, but we do not know this is true and suspect we are ignorant of the real cause. Extensive cautionary literature on surrogate end points for clinical trials and how they can lead us astray fuel this anxiety (Fig. 6-8).[F16,T6] We need, perhaps, to be reminded that public health recommendations based on the crude risk factors for the plague were effective in halting it and preventing its recurrence for 200 years while the causative organism and vector were being discovered.[H11]

Faced with hundreds, perhaps thousands, of variables, the investigator, too, seeks to find simple, or dominant, or stratospheric comprehension of the data. He or she wants to discover the forest, not necessarily the trees (or branches and leaves, for that matter). Multivariable analysis

---

[7] Thus, GUSTO-I demonstrated a statistically significant ($P = .01$) benefit of accelerated TPA over streptokinase plus subcutaneous heparin, but difference in 1-year mortality was only 1 percentage point, and number of lives saved per 1000 treated was 10 (see Box 6-3).[C33]

Time

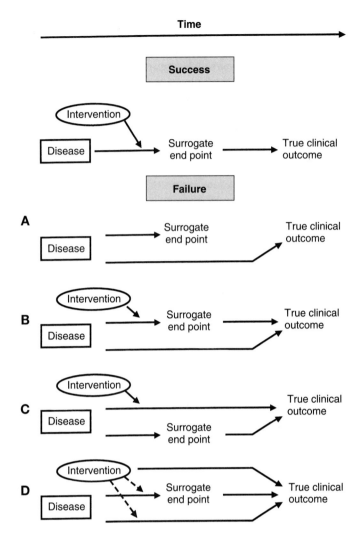

Figure 6-8   *Success and failure of surrogate end points. Success:* Setting that provides the greatest potential for the surrogate end point to be valid. *Failure:* Four reasons for failure of surrogate end points. **A,** Surrogate is not in the causal pathway of the disease process. **B,** Of several causal pathways of disease, the intervention affects only the pathway mediated through the surrogate. **C,** Surrogate is not in the pathway of the intervention's effect or is insensitive to its effect. **D,** Intervention has mechanisms of action independent of the disease process. Dotted lines represent mechanisms of action that might exist. (Redrawn from Fleming and DeMets.[F16])

(Box 6-18) is a set of methods for considering multiple variables simultaneously and for (1) identifying those that by some criteria are associated with an outcome, (2) estimating the magnitude of each variable's influence in light of all others, (3) quantifying the degree of uncertainty of those estimates, and (4) revealing the relation among the set of variables so identified while (5) dismissing others either as noise, or as so correlated with variables associated with outcome that they either do not contribute further information or are so lacking in information (sparse) that their association cannot be determined.

Multivariable analysis is an analysis of a set of explanatory variables with respect to a *single outcome* variable. *Multivariate analysis* is an analysis of *several outcome variables simultaneously* with respect to explanatory variables. Before modern multivariable analysis was possible, the terms most used for a multivariable analysis were "multiple" or "multivariate." Since the advent of methods to analyze multiple outcomes simultaneously, *multivariable* has come to be associated with single outcomes analysis. Some statisticians argue, however, that *multivariate* is still the correct word to use, because multivariable analysis is the degenerate form of multivariate analysis when number of outcomes accounted for simultaneously is one.

Explanatory Variables

The set of variables examined in relation to an outcome is called *explanatory variables, independent variables, correlates, risk factors, incremental risk factors, covariables,* or *predictors.* These alternative names distinguish this set of variables from outcomes. No statistical properties are implied. The least understood name is *independent variable* (or *independent risk factor*). Some mistakenly believe it means the variable is uncorrelated with any other risk factor. All it actually describes is a variable that by some criterion has been found (1) to be associated with outcome and (2) to contribute information about outcome in addition to that provided by other variables considered simultaneously. The least desirable of these terms is "predictor," because it implies causality rather than association.

Dependent Variable

In ordinary regression, this meant the variable on the left side of the equals sign and therefore was distinguished from independent variables on the right side (see Box 6-5). In analysis of non–time-related outcome events, it is synonymous with an indicator variable for occurrence of the event. It is sometimes called the response variable or end point. In time-related analysis, the dependent variable is actually the entire distribution of times to an event, although the indicator variable (such as death) is often cited inaccurately as the dependent variable.

Historical Note

Fisher understood the relation of outcome to possibly multiple explanatory variables when he wrote that the behavior of a sample could be considered characteristic of the population only when no subsets within the population behaved differently.[F6] Yet the use of these ideas in a formal way in medicine emerged only during the last half of the twentieth century. This is because multivariable analysis, particularly of events after cardiac procedures and more especially time-related outcomes, involves considerable computational power. The mathematical models are nonlinear (see Box 6-5), so solving for their parameters is (1) *an iterative process,* that is, a series of systematically directed mathematical steps that follow an algorithm or plan, to find the best value of the coefficient and its variability by gradually closing in on it, and (2) a *mathematical process,* in which computations for explanatory variables are performed simultaneously. Because the computational challenge is considerable, use of multivariable analysis had to await the development of computers.

The first use of multivariable analysis to identify risk factors for *outcome events* in humans was probably the Framingham epidemiologic study of coronary artery disease.[G14] Two papers are landmarks in this regard. In 1967, Walker and Duncan published their paper on multivariable analysis in the domain of logistic regression analysis, stating that "the purpose of this paper is to develop a method for estimating from dichotomous (quantal) or polytomous data the probability of occurrence of an event as a function of a relatively large number of independent variables."[W1] Then in 1976, Kannel and colleagues coined the term "risk factors," noting that (1) "a single risk factor is neither a logical nor an effective means of detecting persons at high risk" and (2) "the risk function . . . is an effective instrument . . . for assisting in the search for and care of persons at high risk for cardiovascular disease."[K8] In 1979 the phrase "incremental risk factors" was coined at UAB to emphasize that risk factors add in a stepwise, or incremental, fashion to the risk present in the most favorable situation.[K3]

Before the advent of multivariable analysis, stratification of the values of one or more potential risk factors was often used to search for association of risk with outcome. Although this is still of interest as a scanning method, it has serious disadvantages, including (1) loss of information by coarseness of stratification and (2) possibly erroneous inferences from the necessarily arbitrary nature of stratification. These dangers were well summarized by Kannel and colleagues, who stated that "while there is some convenience in dichotomizing a continuous variable like blood pressure into high and low, one would prefer some method to take into account the exact value."[K8]

Carrier of Risk Factors: Underlying Mathematical Model

Multivariable analysis requires a model (equation) that relates a placeholder for explanatory variables (generally one or more of the model parameters) to the dependent (outcome) variable. The equation may be a completely *linear* one; for these, iterative techniques are not required, but the computations are large and for all practical purposes require a computer. The general term for such a model is a *regression equation* (see Box 6-5).

Logistic multivariable regression analysis is a special type of *nonlinear* model that can be used as a prototype to understand the nature of the relation of risk factors to outcome in a medically rational fashion. Fig. 6-1, *A*, illustrates the relation between the absolute probability of an event on the vertical axis and an expression of risk measured in logit units along the horizontal axis. The horizontal axis is the one related to risk factors. The relation is sigmoidal (S-shaped). Notice that an increment of risk along the horizontal axis, if far to the left or right of the curve, is not associated with a perceptible increase or decrease along the probability scale. However, a small increment near 0 logit units is associated with a large change in probability.

To illustrate, imagine two patients. One is a strapping football player who is mugged on his way to a pharmacy late at night. He is stabbed in the abdomen, and his inferior vena cava is lacerated. Fortunately, a trauma center is nearby, and he is rushed to surgery. His anxious parents arrive at the hospital about an hour after the incident and

want to know, "What are his chances, doctor?" Let us say that the injury moves the football player's risk two units to the right on the logit scale. Before the incident, this robust individual was positioned far to the left on the logit curve, so his chances of recovery are good.

A week later, the second patient, a frail, elderly diabetic man, is walking to the same pharmacy for his insulin when he is stabbed in the abdomen, and his inferior vena cava is lacerated. He, too, is rushed to the trauma center and into the operating room. An hour later, his anxious daughter arrives at the hospital and wants to know, "What are his chances, doctor?" The fragile patient may already have been sitting near the center of the logit curve, say at –1 logit units, before the incident. Two logit units of acute risk greatly increase his probability of hospital mortality.

These anecdotes emphasize that the models underlying risk make good medical sense. They reflect what we mean by a robust patient, a fragile patient, and an unsalvageable patient. They reflect the reality that the identical risk factor may operate with respect to absolute risk differently, depending on the presence or absence of other risk factors.

Risk Factor Identification

Given a mathematical model to carry risk factors (see Box 6-5), the next task is risk factor identification. It requires (1) screening of candidate variables for suitability in the analysis, (2) calibrating continuous and ordinal variables to outcome, (3) selecting variables related to outcome, and (4) presenting results in the format of incremental risk factors.

Screening

Screening candidate variables has two purposes: (1) to determine whether there are sufficient data (see Box 6-4) to be suitable in the analysis and (2) to understand a variable in relation to other candidate variables. Because for outcome events the effective sample size for analysis is the number of events, not the number of patients, a variable may not be suitable for analysis when it represents a subgroup of patients with too few events to evaluate. This represents a limitation of the study, not of methodology. Indeed, one is generally happy with a therapy associated with few events[G22]; however, it then makes sense that risk factors cannot be identified.

We do not screen variables to discover which ones relate individually to outcome. It is a common practice of many groups to ignore variables that are not univariably associated with outcome. However, there is a long history of occurrence of so-called *lurking variables* (Box 6-19) that are found to relate to outcome only when (1) other variables that mask their importance are accounted for in the analysis or (2) they are suitably transformed (or coupled with nonlinear rescaling of themselves), indicating a complex association with outcome.[G16,J5]

It is valuable to determine the pair-wise correlation of variables. This will help one understand why many variables may be associated with outcome, but only a few are selected as risk factors. Medical data are highly redundant, sharing a great deal of information.

Lurking variables are those found to relate to some outcome or dependent variable (see Box 6-5) only after (1) other variables masking their importance are taken into account either by multivariable analysis or matched-type analyses (e.g., using balancing scores) or (2) the lurking variable (if continuous or ordinal) is properly rescaled (e.g., transformed) so that complex relations are revealed, such as higher risk of mortality at both old and young age.

Fig. 6-9, *A*, shows survival in patients after exercise stress testing stratified according to long-term aspirin use.[G16] Apparently there is no relation to survival. However, Table 6-3 shows that there are multiple differences in patient characteristics between these two groups of patients, with those taking aspirin being older, for example. Indeed, in multivariable analysis, the moment age is taken into account, a beneficial effect of long-term aspirin is revealed. Fig. 6-9, *B*, shows survival in propensity-matched pairs of patients (see "Clinical Studies with Nonrandomly Assigned Treatment" in Section 1). The lurking benefit of long-term aspirin use is clearly revealed.

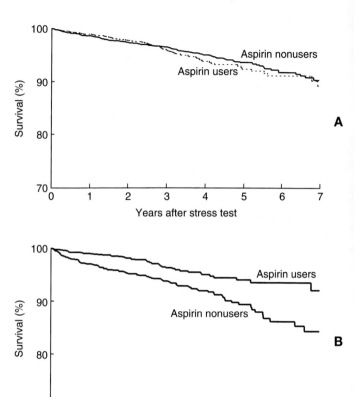

Figure 6-9   Demonstration of a lurking variable. Survival after stress testing is shown on an expanded scale and is stratified according to use and non-use of long-term aspirin therapy. **A,** Risk-unadjusted survival in entire cohort. Note the similarity of survival. **B,** Survival in propensity-matched patients. Note the dissimilarity of survival revealed when risk factors for death are balanced between the groups. (From Gum and colleagues.[G16])

Calibration

Continuous variables contain unique values for each patient and so are particularly valuable in analyses. For unclear reasons (statisticians uniformly decry the practice), many investigators stratify continuous variables into two or a few arbitrary categories, throwing away valuable information. This flies in the teeth of a fundamental philosophy of data analysis: continuity in nature (see "Continuity versus Discontinuity in Nature" in Section 1). Further, to better understand the phenomenon we are studying, it is important to determine the shape of the relation of continuous variables (such as age, birth weight, or creatinine) to outcome.

However, the scale on which a continuous variable has been measured or expressed may not coincide with the outcome.[G32] Nature does not know about our rulers! Therefore, the appropriate calibration of the variable to outcome must be discovered. One method to accomplish this is to examine various *linearizing transformations* (Fig. 6-10). However, the "perfect" transformation of scale may not coincide with the best one after other factors have been considered in a multivariable model. Thus, we rely on graphical methods, as in the figure, to obtain a set of similar transformations, and then include all transformed variable candidates in the selection process to be described.

Variable Selection

A seminal contribution of the Framingham Study investigators was the idea that in the absence of identified mechanisms of either disease or treatment failure, useful inferences for medical decision-making, for lifestyle modification, and for programmatic decisions about avenues of further research can be gleaned by nonspecific risk factor identification.[G14] A direct consequence of the idea, however, is that for any set of potential variables that may be associated with outcome, there is no unique set of risk factors that constitute the best common denominators of disease or treatment failure. Therefore, different persons analyzing the same data may generate different sets of risk factors.[N11]

As a consequence, multivariable identification of risk factors has become an art that depends on expert medical knowledge of the entity being studied, understanding the goals of the research, knowledge of the variables and how they may relate to the study goals as well as to one another, identification of the quality and reliability of each variable, and development of different, often sequential, analysis strategies appropriate to each research question.[B16,B37,H7,H17] Not all these issues of art or expertise will disappear, but there are substantial aspects of multivariable analysis that are yielding to science.

Naftel, in an important 1994 letter to the editor, addressed nine aspects of multivariable analysis that contribute to obtaining different models (sets of risk factors).[N11] He called these "steps and decisions that may influence the final equation":

- Differing statistical models. For example, if time-related events are being modeled, results using a Cox proportional hazards model (see "Cox Proportional Hazards Regression" later in this section) will differ from those using a multiphase nonproportional hazards model (see "Parametric Hazard Function Regression" later in this section).

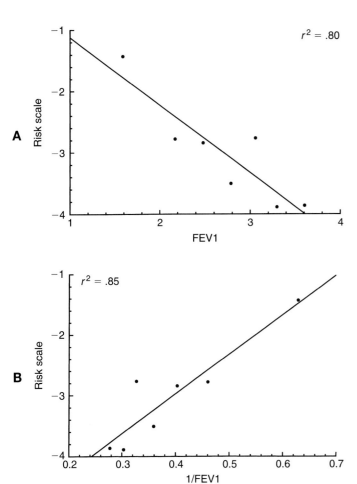

Figure 6-10   Calibration of 1-second forced expiratory volume (FEV1) to risk of hospital mortality. A scale of risk is given on the vertical axis (akin to the logit units of Fig. 6-1) and eight groups of equal numbers of patients according to the value for FEV1 along the horizontal axis. Their mortality, converted to the risk scale, is shown by each closed circle. (The eighth closed circle cannot be shown because there were no deaths in the eighth group with the highest FEV1s.) **A,** Linear scale of FEV1. Clearly, there is a decreasing (more negative) value of risk at higher FEV1 (simple regression line shown, with explained scatter for these points of 80%). **B,** Inverse scale of FEV1. Because of the inverse transformation, the lower FEV1s are to the right of the scale and the higher FEV1s to the left. Risk falls from left to right, unlike in *A*. There is now tighter correspondence of risk to this rescaling of FEV1 (85% of scatter explained) than in the conventional scale of *A*. (From Blackstone and Rice.[B37])

Key: *FEV1*, 1-second forced expiratory volume.

- Differing approaches to missing data (see "Impute Values" in Section 3).
- Differing approaches to minimal information (see Box 6-4).
- Differing approaches to correlated data. Variables with similar information content should be chosen for maximal insight by the clinical investigator, not necessarily the statistician.
- Differing coding of data. Some may pay more attention than others to linearizing transformation of continuous variables, to whether continuous or ordinal

variables should be dichotomized or in other ways collapsed, or to management of interaction (multiplicative) variables.
- Differing approach to apparently incorrect data. True data outliers, handling of clearly imperfect data, improbable combinations of variables (such as apparently exceedingly short, very heavy patients as a result of misplaced decimal points), and attitude toward whether or not a large sample negates errors are all decisions made during the screening process for multivariable analysis.
- Differing variable selection methods and *P* value criteria. This area is undergoing complete change through introduction of machine learning algorithmic methods.[B38] Even with new methods, however, a criterion must be arbitrarily established to differentiate what is signal from what is noise (*P* values, for example).
- Differing computer resources. Although even desktop computers rival the computational capacity of large-scale computers of a decade ago, computer-intensive methods will soon require entire networks of computers.
- Differing appreciations of the science. Unless data analysts work collaboratively with the surgeon–investigator, analysis may be unrevealing. One cannot divorce the underlying clinical science from data analysis.

In all these areas but one, new knowledge has been generated that is beginning to differentiate inadequate techniques from reasonable techniques and optimal techniques. That one area remaining is "differing variable selection methods," and it is an important one.

Part of the challenge is that variables may be thought to be risk factors because they are associated with a small *P* value, and other factors may be thought not to be risk factors because of larger *P* values, but both opinions may be erroneous (type I and type II statistical errors, respectively; see Box 6-17). There is therefore a need for a method that balances these two types of error. Closely coupled with this is the need for a statistic that measures the reliability with which a risk factor has been identified. Because one is analyzing only a single set of data rather than many sets of data about the same subject, determining this reliability has been elusive.

There is new thinking about what risk factor identification is. In thinking anew, we leave traditional statistical methodology out of the picture, and risk factor identification becomes an attempt to find *signal* (risk factors) in *noise* (other candidates). Important advances in pure mathematics *(logical analysis)*[A6,L21] and machine learning *(algorithmic analysis)*[B38] are proving valuable for such diverse signal detection challenges as handwriting identification, genomic identification, and now risk factor identification. These techniques are evolving rapidly, and we will describe only the most primitive here: bootstrap bagging.[A8,B53,C5,S25]

Bootstrap bagging belongs to a class of new methods that has developed over the past 20 years. In 1983, an astonishing article entitled "Computer-Intensive Methods in Statistics" appeared in the popular scientific literature.[D16] Its authors, Persi Diaconis and Bradley Efron from Stanford University, indicated that "most statistical methods in common use today were developed between 1800 and 1930, when computation was slow and expensive. Now, computation is fast and cheap. . . .The new methods are fantastic computational spendthrifts. . . .The payoff for such intensive computation is freedom from two limiting factors that have dominated statistical theory since its beginnings: the assumption that the data conform to a bell-shaped curve and the need to focus on statistical measures whose theoretical properties can be analyzed mathematically."

Efron and his group demonstrated that random sampling with replacement[8] from a data set to create a new data set, resampling to produce perhaps thousands of new data sets, and combining the information generated from these many data sets can produce robust and accurate statistics without assumptions. His group called this technique *bootstrapping,* after the expression "pulling yourself up by your own bootstraps," because it reflected the fact that one could develop all the statistical testing necessary directly from the actual data simply by repeatedly sampling them (see footnote 6, p. 297).

These techniques have been applied to entire analytical processes, including multivariable analysis.[A8,B53,C5,S25] In fact, one still has to pay attention to appropriate models, missing data, variable considerations, correlated variables, appropriate strategy, and so forth, that remain part of a disciplined, informed approach to the data. However, the variable selection process is bootstrapped.

In practice, a carefully crafted set of variables is formulated that will be subjected to simple automated variable selection, such as forward stepwise selection, whereby the most significant variables are entered one by one into a multivariable model. A specific *P* value criterion for entering and retaining these variables is specified. Then, a random sample of cases is selected, generally of the same sample size as the original *n*. A complete automated analysis is performed, and its results are stored. Then, another random set of cases is drawn from the original data set, and analysis is performed. This resampling of the original data set followed by analysis continues perhaps hundreds and even thousands of times. Then, the frequency of occurrence of risk factors among these many models is summarized. The frequency of occurrence generally stabilizes after about 100 bootstrap analyses. The many models

are also analyzed by cluster techniques to detect closely related variables that in the final model will be represented by the most commonly occurring representative. All this information is used to select variables for the final multivariable model.

Of interest, the variables identified for every bootstrap data set are usually different, a sobering revelation. However, it becomes evident that some variables never are selected and others are seldom selected; these constitute "noise." Variables that appear in 50% or more of models are claimed to be reliable and are considered "signal" for inclusion in the final model.

This phenomenon is illustrated in Table 6-8. Fifteen variables were selected from among many being analyzed for the late hazard phase of death following mitral valve repair or replacement for degenerative disease. In analysis of the first bootstrap sample, eight of these 15 variables were selected (only five were ultimately found to be reliable risk factors). By 100 analyses, although every variable had been identified as a risk factor in at least two analyses, five variables dominated the analyses (we considered these reliable risk factors), eight rarely appeared, and two appeared in 22% to 32% of analyses.

What happens in bootstrap bagging is similar to what is seen in signal averaging, such as in visual evoked potentials: Noise becomes canceled out and signal becomes amplified. In the same way, many variables appear rarely in models, but a few show up time and time again. One therefore can express the reliability of identification of a given risk factor.

Bootstrap bagging, although demanding a huge number of computer cycles, removes much of the human arbitrariness from multivariable analysis and provides another important statistic: a measure of reliability of each risk factor. Thus, increasingly we have been reporting not only the magnitude of the effect, its variance, and its *P* value, but also its bootstrap reliability. The technique appears to provide a balance between selecting risk factors that are not reliable (type I error) and overlooking variables that are reliable (type II error).

Verification

The ideal verification of a multivariable analysis is to demonstrate its accuracy in predicting results of a new set of patients, preferably extramurally.[B62,P16] Another popular method, if the data set or number of events is large, is to split the data set randomly into a training data set and testing data set. Modeling is performed on the former and verification on the latter. Whether this is an efficient and effective strategy has been debated.[C31] One of the first applications of bootstrapping was to address this issue by generating multiple training and testing sets.[E15] Within the domain of the primary multivariable analysis itself, there are, as it were, internal validity diagnostics. For example, in linear regression (see Box 6-5), a measure of explained scatter is the r^2 value (square of the familiar correlation coefficient). It is desirable that the value of r^2 be high (closer to 1 than 0); however, if a model is overdetermined by having in it either too many factors or surrogates for the outcome-dependent variable, a high r^2 may be spurious.

In logistic regression (see "Logistic Regression Analysis" later in this section), there are a number of diagnostic

---

[8] *Sampling with replacement:* Imagine a data set having 869 patients and 30 variables. A uniform random number generator produces at random a number between 0 and 1 (the numbers chosen at random are, in the long run, equally likely across that range). The random number is multiplied by 869, and the product is rounded to the nearest integer from 1 to 869. All the variables and their values for the patient with that observation number are copied to a new data set. Importantly, the patient is *not* removed from the original data set and is available to be selected at random again. This is what is meant by "sampling with replacement"; the patient is chosen but not removed from the possibility of being chosen again.

In bootstrapping, the random selection continues until a new data set is built with the same *n* as the original. However, because patients were never removed from the original data set, the new data set likely contains many duplicate observations and does not contain patients who were never chosen.

When hundreds or even thousands of such data sets are built by this sampling with replacement mechanism, it is rare that any two are alike; it is also extremely rare that one of the data sets will, by chance, have the exact composition of the original data set (each patient selected only once).

■ **TABLE 6-8   Frequency of Occurrence (%) of Variables Selected in Bootstrap Analyses of the Late Hazard Phase of Death after Mitral Valve Repair or Replacement for Degenerative Disease**

Variable	Number of Bootstrap Analyses							
	1	5	10	55	100	250	500	1000
Demography								
Age	100	100	100	100	99	99	99	99
Women	0	0	0	6	7	4	3	5
Noncardiac Comorbidity								
Bilirubin	0	40	20	16	12	10	10	10
BUN	100	40	60	72	76	78	77	78
Hypertension	0	0	10	6	6	5	6	6
Peripheral vascular disease	0	0	0	4	2	4	3	3
Smoker	0	0	0	6	8	9	11	10
Ventricular Function								
Ejection fraction	0	0	0	18	22	22	24	25
Left ventricular dysfunction (grade)	100	60	70	70	66	66	68	68
Right ventricular systolic pressure	100	20	10	10	8	8	8	8
Cardiac morbidity								
Coronary artery disease	100	100	100	96	94	92	92	91
Anterior leaflet prolapse	100	80	90	82	82	84	85	85
Preoperative Condition								
NYHA class	100	20	20	30	32	34	33	36
Hematocrit	0	0	20	16	17	14	16	17
Experience								
Date of operation	100	20	10	14	15	14	13	14

Key: *BUN,* Blood urea nitrogen; *NYHA,* New York Heart Association.

tools available. One of the earliest was the decile table, often attributed to Hosmer and Lemeshow,[H19] but used much earlier by the Framingham investigators and others. By solving the multivariable equation for each patient, patients are ordered with respect to their estimated probability of experiencing an event. They are then stratified in up to 10 groups (thus "decile"), and within each group the estimated probabilities summed. This sum represents expected events; it is compared with observed events in each decile. The *Hosmer-Lemeshow statistic* is a general test of the differences between observed and predicted events.

Borrowing from classification theory, which deals with false and true positives and false and true negatives, an analysis of *sensitivity* and *specificity* can be performed, varying the cut point from 0 to 1 of what probability is considered predictive of an event's occurring. The number of correctly predicted events (true positives) divided by the number of true positives plus false negatives is sensitivity. The number of correctly predicted nonevents (true negatives) divided by the number of true negatives plus false positives is specificity. A graph of 1-specificity on the horizontal axis and sensitivity on the vertical axis is then constructed—the *receiver operating characteristic* (ROC) curve (Fig. 6-11). The area beneath this curve is a measure of goodness of fit.[H24,Z2] (Harrell and colleagues called this the c index of concordance.[H23]) It varies from .5 to 1. A concordance index between .8 and .9 is desirable for prediction purposes.

In addition, for all varieties of multivariable models, a number of regression diagnostic procedures are used, including formal testing of goodness of fit, identification of observations that particularly influence the results, and analysis of residuals (difference between observed and predicted values) in linear regression.[C32,H25,P4,P5]

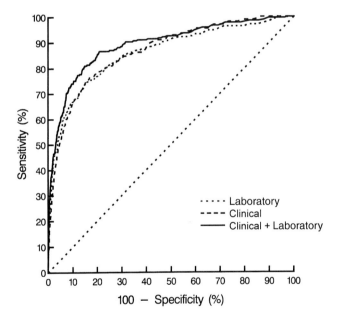

Figure 6-11   Illustration of receiver operating characteristic (ROC) curves. These are for renal failure after either coronary artery bypass grafting or cardiac valve procedures in 15,844 patients operated on at The Cleveland Clinic Foundation from 1986 to 2000. Three ROC curves are shown. One is based on preoperative laboratory measurements alone, the second on extensive clinical data alone, and the third combines the two. The diagonal dashed line is the line of random prediction.

Presentation

A multivariable analysis generates an enormous amount of information, including:

- The structure of the model and estimates of parameters related to that structure
- A list of the risk factors identified
- Magnitude of the association of each risk factor with outcome as adjusted for all other variables in the model (these multipliers may be expressed either as the parameter estimates themselves—called model coefficients—or as some reformatted relative risk expression; see Box 6-3)
- Direction of each relation, positive or negative
- Uncertainty of the associations, generally expressed as standard deviations of the coefficients
- A statistical score on which a P value is based
- P values
- A set of numbers indicating quantitative interrelation of all parameter estimates in the model (the variance–covariance matrix)
- Bootstrap reliability of each risk factor identified

There is some controversy about which of these nine sets of numbers should be reported in a manuscript. It may be sufficient for understanding the relations to simply list the risk factors and place in an appendix some of the numeric data. If the model is intended to be used fully for prediction, including confidence limits, then the entire list must be reported or provided electronically.

None of the nine, however, addresses directly the way a final multivariable model is formulated to reveal incremental risk factors (see "Incremental Risk Factor Concept" later in this section). The incremental risk factor concept was developed to facilitate medical interpretation of a multivariable analysis. Any dichotomous risk factor in a multivariable analysis can be complemented to allow it to have a positive sign.[B27] This is desirable, because we think of variables in the model as risk factors, and usually we consider risk to be increasing (positively valued) with increasing value of the risk factor. Generally, continuous and ordinal variables cannot be formulated this way, so we recommend that each of these be accompanied by an indication of the direction of greater risk (younger age, lower ejection fraction, higher functional impairment, higher bilirubin).

Incremental Risk Factor Concept

An incremental risk factor is a variable identified by multivariable analysis that is associated with an increased risk of an adverse outcome (surgical failure).[B18,K3] The surgical failure may be an *event,* such as early postoperative stroke, and risk is expressed in terms of probability. It may be a *time-related event,* and risk is expressed in terms of a shorter interval to the event, such as premature death. It may be a *longitudinal outcome,* and risk is expressed as increased prevalence, higher grade of failure, or elevated or lowered quantitative level. In the context of other simultaneously identified factors, the *magnitude* (strength) and *certainty* (P value) of an incremental risk factor represent its contribution over and above those of all other factors. Thus, it is incremental in two ways: (1) with respect to being associated with increased risk and (2) with respect to other factors simultaneously incorporated into a risk factor equation.

There are a number of possible interpretations of an incremental risk factor, all of which should be assessed in drawing inferences.

- Incremental risk factors are variables that reflect increased difficulty in achieving surgical success. This original definition addressed the reality of *surgical complexity.* Complexity may be expressed in terms of morphologic features, such as those of an atrioventricular septal defect.[S4] It may also relate to duration of operation, such as reflected in longer myocardial ischemic time; to both the operation and components of it[J3,S26]; to presence of associated cardiac or noncardiac diseases[S4]; to demography, such as young age,[K13] low birth weight,[C4] gender,[S19] or socioeconomic status[D18]; or to conditions that increase difficulty of access (reoperations) or add a potential for complication, such as a religious preference that precludes administration of blood products or administration of thrombolytics shortly before operation.
- Incremental risk factors are *common denominators* of surgical failure. Framingham investigators of the risk factor concept were initially disappointed that they did not discover mechanistic (deterministic) causes of heart disease, only weak associations. These weak associations are what we call common denominators. They are general factors associated with increased or decreased risk of an outcome. Sufficient data (see Box 6-4) are necessary to keep them from becoming identifiers of specific patients.
- Some incremental risk factors reflect *disease acuity.* Need for emergency or urgent operation[S19] in patients with severely impaired functional status, such as NYHA Class IV or V (the latter designating severe hemodynamic instability or cardiogenic shock), low pH,[S26] or short interval from myocardial infarction to ruptured ventricular septum, represent risk factors that increase acuity.
- Some incremental risk factors reflect *immutable conditions* that increase risk. These include the extremes of age, extremes of body size, genetic disorders, gender, and ethnicity.
- Some incremental risk factors reflect influential coexisting *noncardiac diseases* that shorten life expectancy in the absence of cardiac disease. These include chronic renal disease, diabetes, malignancies, atherosclerosis, and infectious diseases.
- Incremental risk factors are usually *surrogates* for true, but unmeasured or unrecognized, sources of surgical failure. It is tempting to misinterpret *associations* as *causes.* Studies of surrogate end points to decrease sample size for randomized clinical trials are instructive.[F16,T6] They demonstrate a number of circumstances under which such surrogates may be misleading (see Fig. 6-8).[F16] On the other hand, if unknown cause and measurable surrogate are strongly mechanistically linked, interim neutralization of the surrogate may neutralize the cause (Appendix 6D). The Framingham investigators classified most risk factors as rather general, insensitive, but useful surrogates for underlying mechanisms.[G14]
- Incremental risk factors may be *spurious associations* with risk. One of our motivations to base risk factor identification on algorithmic methods such as bootstrap

bagging is that in simulations, these methods balance very nearly 50:50 the probability of overlooking a risk factor and identifying a spurious association.

■ An incremental risk factor may be a cause or mechanism of *surgical failure*. It is difficult to establish a causal mechanism outside the scope of a randomized, well-powered, and well-conducted generalizable clinical trial. This is a because of confounding between selection factors influencing treatment recommendations and decisions and outcome. Balancing score methods (such as propensity score) attempt to remove such confounding and approach more closely causal inferences (see "Balancing Scores" in Section 1).[B4]

In addition, we must acknowledge that "association," "cause," and "mechanism" may be simply levels of granularity in the pathway of cause to effect. As more becomes known at the molecular level, it may be assumed that at that level of fine granularity, a clear understanding of mechanisms may emerge. However, a macroscopic event, such as death or a complication after a cardiac operation, may not be completely understood by knowledge of the many individual events taking place at the microscopic level, which probably interact in a complex fashion.

■ Some incremental risk factors reflect *temporal experience*. The "learning curve" idea is intended to capture variables relating to experience of the surgical team, but also those representing temporal changes in approach or practice (such as addition of retrograde cardioplegia to myocardial management or preservation of chordae in mitral valve replacement). It is more helpful to identify specific temporal changes in management as separate variables than to lump them into a "date of operation" variable.[B37] To do so may require initially suppressing date of operation in the analysis to allow entry of such identifiers of management changes.

■ Some incremental risk factors reflect *quality of care* and, as such, "blunt end" ramifications of institutional policies and practices, health care systems, and national and political decisions. Just like temporal experience, however, it is more helpful to identify the specific factors reflected in institutional variance than simply to state that some institutions are high risk and others low risk.[K22] If these can be identified and institutions no longer enter an analysis as risk factors, it becomes important to quantify their frequency of occurrence in each institution. If the prevalence is high, and if associations are strongly linked to mechanisms of failure, then institutional protocols to lower the prevalence are warranted. Although quality of care is measured by outcomes, factors influencing it are identified in risk factor assessment and serve as important information for quality monitoring, quality improvement, quality comparison, and assessment of strategies implemented. (Institutional variance is addressed in more detail under "Risk Stratification" in Section 6.)

■ Incremental risk factors reflect individual patient *prognosis*. They cannot be used to identify *which* patient will suffer a surgical failure, but they can be used to predict the *probability* of failure. Surgeons make recommendations and decisions every day that reflect conscious or unconscious assessment of probabilities. *Patient selection* requires weighing the probabilities of risks and benefits (value) of intervention versus nonintervention or an alternative management strategy. *Indications for operation* is the same. Analysis of clinical experience transforms generalities of patient selection and indication guidelines into quantitative probabilities for an individual patient's characteristics (see "Decision-making for Individual Patients" in Section 5).

EARLY EVENTS
Method of Expression

Early mortality is often expressed as *hospital mortality,* which includes all deaths that occur after operation but before discharge. The disadvantage of using hospital mortality is that the relatively high but rapidly declining early phase of risk after cardiac operation nearly always extends beyond the hospital period, often out to 3 months and occasionally out to 6 months.[O3] The degree of extension, even after such safe operations as CABG, appears to increase as risk factors increase. Thus, hospital mortality underestimates the true early risk of operation and gives an incomplete picture of this measure of quality of care. It also covers a variable time period.

An alternative is to use *30-day mortality.* However, this requires patient follow-up, either active (and expensive) or passive (and delayed). The hybrid of these, *operative mortality,* is all hospital deaths plus those that occur in the first 30 days.[E14] Actually, the most appropriate way to depict early mortality (or any other outcome event) after a procedure or decision is in a time-related manner, beginning at time zero (see "Time-Related Events" later in this section).

If simple percentages are used, at least the confidence intervals around that percentage need to be stated (see "Uncertainty" earlier in this section and Appendix 6B), and ideally some information about the heterogeneity of the patient group. Often the patient group is stratified in some manner to demonstrate the effects of heterogeneity on outcomes.

Logistic Regression Analysis

The logistic regression model is used for multivariable analysis of hospital outcomes (events) that are dichotomous (yes/no).

Historical Note

The logistic equation was introduced by Verhulst between 1835 and 1845 to describe population growth in France and Belgium.[V2,V3] Thus, it belongs to a large class of "growth equations." The logistic equation is the simplest of these, resulting in a symmetric S-shaped curve when plotted (see Fig. 6-1, *A*).[T2] The model reappeared in the work of Pearl and Reed in 1920[P6] while they were at Johns Hopkins University. They recognized in the characteristic pattern of the logistic equation for populations the pattern of an autocatalytic reaction; this was earlier suspected by Pearl in 1909 while he was reflecting on the relation of these curves to organic laws of change.[P7] The equation is characterized by an initial phase of increasingly rapid chemical conversion catalyzed by the products produced, followed by a decelerating phase as reactants are consumed (hydrolysis of ethyl acetate to acetic acid and ethyl alcohol).

Also at Johns Hopkins University during the late 1920s, Berkson and colleagues found that the logistic equation represented kinetics between enzymes and certain substrates.[B21,B22,R1] At the Mayo Clinic in the 1940s, Berkson found a logistic relation between dosage of drug and proportion of small experimental animals killed (binary).[B8,B10] In his studies, the outcome variable was a probability. Unlike population or biochemical kinetics in which not only the rate but also the initial (base) level and the final (asymptotic, limiting) level must be estimated, when the logistic equation is used to estimate the probability of an event, the values are constrained within a base of 0 and asymptotic level of 100% (or unity), simplifying the equation and leaving a single parameter to estimate from the data, Z.

In 1955, Berkson dubbed the units of the logistic nomogram *logit units*, parallel to the *probit units* of another method of bioassay.[B9] Thus, certain aspects of the nature of population behavior, enzyme kinetics, lethality of drugs, and risk factors for human outcomes found common ground in this fundamental logistic expression. The logistic equation was made multivariable in the 1960s by Cornfield and colleagues[C9] and Walker and Duncan.[W1]

Logistic Regression Equation

Multivariable logistic regression generalizes the discriminant analysis of Fisher[F7] by embedding it within the logistic equation.[W1] Z, the logistic parameter expressed in logit units, is assumed to be related to a logit-linear combination of incremental risk factors (see Box 6-5):

$$z = \beta_0 + \beta_1 x_1 + \beta_2 x_2 + \cdots + \beta_k x_k$$

$$(6\text{-}1)$$

where β_0 is the intercept term (logit units when all $\mathbf{x} = 0$), x_1 through x_k are the numeric values of the independent variables, and β_1 through β_k are coefficients, estimated from the data, that translate the values of the independent variables (see Box 6-18) to logit units. Logit units are related to probabilities (P) by the logistic relationship

$$z = \mathsf{Ln}\left(\frac{P}{1-P}\right)$$

$$(6\text{-}2)$$

where Ln is the natural logarithm. This form of the logistic equation makes clear why "log" is part of its name. Notice, also, that z is a function of the ratio of P, the probability of an event, and $1 - P$, the complementary probability of the event's not occurring. Such a ratio has been called the *odds ratio* (see Box 6-3), and Equation 6-2 has been referred to as *log odds*.[C6] Equation 6-2 is not computationally applicable to raw clinical data for which P is exactly 0 or 1 for each patient (such as in analysis of a dichotomous variable like mortality; see Box 6-5). Thus, the computational form is a nonlinear equation obtained by exponentiating Equation 6-2:

$$P = \frac{1}{1+e^{-z}}$$

$$(6\text{-}3)$$

where P is the estimated probability using the maximum likelihood principle, and e is the base of the natural logarithms.[W1] In practice, the dependent variable is a dichotomous variable with value 0 (no event) or 1 (event),

and the independent variables are potential incremental risk factors (see Box 6-18). In this form, no restrictions are made on the distribution of the risk factors ($\mathbf{x}$); they may be any mix of continuous, dichotomous, or ordinal variables.

Polytomous and Ordinal Logistic Regression

Polytomous logistic regression. The "event" whose probability is being calculated does not always take the simple form of 0 and 1; sometimes, it is a list of possible dichotomous outcomes. Consider hospital mortality. It may occur in a multiplicity of modes (e.g., acute cardiac failure, death from hemorrhage, death in renal failure). The data may need to be analyzed for more than one mode of death. Such analysis leads to the coding of multiple so-called competing events[B25,D4]: alive, acute cardiac failure, death in renal failure, and so forth. These are *unordered lists* of modes of death for which polytomous logistic regression might be considered.

One option for polytomous variables is to analyze each event category independently, determining its incremental risk factors using logistic regression for dichotomous outcomes as previously described. It is important to note that for such analyses, the entire data set is used.

Another option is to analyze each variable in the same fashion as time-related competing risks (see "Competing Risks" under Time-Related Events later in this section). The assumption is that all items in the list are independent. As in temporal competing risks analysis, patients experiencing events in any other category are eliminated (e.g., all patients dying in other modes) in these separate analyses. Thus, the data set used to analyze each event in the list contains all patients experiencing each successive event in the list. The entire data set is not used. The analysis is performed and the results interpreted as a conditional probability; that is, the probability of an event of one type, conditional on the absence of another type (e.g., the probability of cardiac death given the absence of any other mode of death.)

An important feature of this type of conditional probability analysis is that event categories must be strictly mutually exclusive. This means that a patient can be assigned only one mode of death, for example. If one were analyzing morbid events such as hospital complications, this should be the earliest occurring complication (in which case one would normally use time-related techniques, of course). This introduces a certain arbitrariness into the analysis. Further, if one adds another category of morbid event to the list, the probabilities of the remaining new ones will not be the same because the "denominator" (all those not experiencing an event), plus the patients in each successive category, will change.

On the other hand, if one then uses the logistic regression equation to predict the occurrence of each event category, the method of conditional probability guarantees these will add to 100% (including the category "no event") as long as the same risk factors are used for each analysis, and approximately so if a different set is used. This property of polytomous logistic regression, then, distinguishes it from ordinary logistic regression. In ordinary logistic regression in which the entire patient sample is used for each event, it is unlikely that the probabilities for a list of events will add to 100%.

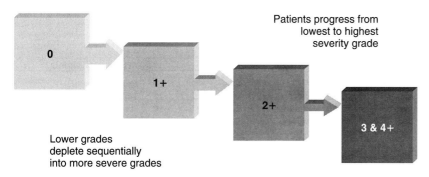

Figure 6-12   Illustration of ordinal longitudinal outcomes. Diagram illustrates the assumption that aortic regurgitation across stented bovine pericardial aortic valve prostheses progresses from grade 0 to grade 1+, then to grade 2+, and finally to grades 3+ and 4+. (Redrawn from Blackstone.[B39])

This leads us to reflect that ordinary logistic regression examines an event in isolation of any other kind of event. It is ideal for answering the question "What is the nature of this outcome phenomenon?" Polytomous logistic regression, by considering the entire list of events that make up a more global event (such as death or complication), answers the question, "What are the probabilities of each kind of event conditional on none of the others occurring?" All these will add up to the total probability of the overall event.

Hosmer and colleagues described the equations and programmed the software for performing a multiple (polytomous) logistic regression simultaneously on multiple events,[H8] and these algorithms are incorporated into most modern logistic regression computer software. Generally, all items in the polytomous list are analyzed simultaneously, with multiple streams of the same set of risk factors. This allows assessment of the sometimes complex interplay of risk factors among the various list items.

An important limitation of polytomous logistic regression is that the number of risk factors must be such that the category with the fewest events does not become overdetermined. When there is wide difference among the categories in number of events, perhaps one or two orders of magnitude, this can limit the model considerably, permitting little insight into the most commonly occurring category and jeopardizing the least commonly occurring. Some coalescence of categories may be necessary.

Assumptions of polytomous logistic regression include that of noninformative censoring (just as for time-related events); that is, occurrence of one item in the list is unrelated to the possible occurrence of another had the first not happened first. In cardiac operations, in which multiorgan system failure often leads to death, independence of modes of death such as from renal failure or hepatic failure is hard to accept.

Ordinal logistic regression. A generalization of logistic regression is to an ordinal response (dependent) variable such as NYHA functional status after operation.[H19,W1] The logistic equation, by means of multiple intercept terms, then predicts the probability for each ordinal level, all of which sum to 100%. We have found the widest application of this method in examining repeated assessment of time-related patient status (NYHA class or degree of regurgitation of a cardiac valve after repair[B39]); thus, this topic is discussed in more depth under "Longitudinal Outcomes" later in this section.

The primary assumption of ordinal logistic regression is that there is an orderly relation between increasing risk and increasing ordinal level of the outcome variable.[B39] Patients "flow," as it were, into states of greater severity, and states of lesser severity empty (Fig. 6-12). This assumption may be violated, so testing the *proportional odds* assumption is mandatory during analysis. The most common reason for violation of the proportional odds assumption is too few patients in some categories. This requires coalescence of categories until the proportional odds assumption is met.

A practical note is that a naive solution of an ordinal logistic equation generates cumulative probabilities. What one generally is interested in is the actual probabilities of each level of the ordinal variable. These must be obtained by subtraction and the confidence limits calculated for each such conditional probability.

TIME-RELATED EVENTS

The interval between an intervention such as a cardiac procedure and an unfavorable outcome event such as death is of obvious importance.

The usual outcome events considered, such as death, are called *terminating events;* that is, they can occur only once. Other morbid events, such as thromboembolism and transplant rejection, may occur a number of times and are called *repeated morbid events.*[B26] Yet others are not dichotomous events but events associated with a severity scale; these are called *weighted morbid events.* Terminating, repeated, and weighted events have in common one attribute or assumption: They occur instantly in time distant from some starting time (such as a cardiac operation).

Depictions of time-related events have been called by many names that reflect their origin in the discipline from which they arose (economics, government, industrial reliability testing, biologic sciences).[B47] In this book, estimates based on counting theory alone (nonparametric estimates; see Box 6-14) are termed *actuarial estimates* or *life-table estimates,* for which there is strong historical precedence.[B47] These terms do not imply for us the specific theoretical underpinnings or method of calculation, of which there are many.

Historical Note

The word *actuarial* comes from the Latin *actuarius,* meaning secretary of accounts. The most notable actuarius was the Praetorian Prefect Domitius Ulpianus, who produced a table of annuity values in the early third century AD.[H11] This table continued to be used in Europe into the early nineteenth century. With emergence of both definitive population data and the science of probability, modern actuarial tables arose, produced first by Edmund Halley (of comet fame) in 1693.[H2] He was motivated, as was Ulpianus, by economics related to human survival, because governments sold annuities to finance public works.[H11] Workers in this combined area of demography and economics came to be known as *actuaries* in the late eighteenth century. Importantly for this discussion, the methodology of the actuary varied widely. In the nineteenth century the actuary of the Alliance Assurance Company of London, Benjamin Gompertz, developed mathematical models of the dynamics of population growth (birth and death) to characterize survival.[G8] This model-based, completely parametric (equations with constants estimated from data) methodology (see Box 6-14) was substantially different from the simple empirical counting methodology (nonparametric) of Halley.

In the more than 300 years since Halley, a multitude of methods have been developed, and often reinvented, in actuarial science, demography, statistics, industry, and medical science. They all have the common goal of estimating the distribution of intervals between a designated time zero and occurrence of an event. In medicine, an ad hoc *direct method* of survival estimation was developed in which nth-year survival (such as 5-year survival) excluded all patients whose follow-up interval was less than n years.[B23] Life tables constructed in this fashion were not guaranteed to be monotonically decreasing, nor did they use all patients with all available information for each time-related estimate.

The direct method highlights a unique problem with time-related events data: *incomplete* (not missing) *data* (Box 6-20). Rarely are we patient enough to observe a group of patients until all have died. Rather, at a given point in time we know the duration of survival for some patients and therefore have *complete data* with respect to vital status. For others we know only that they are still living after a certain interval of time; we know something (they have not died within that interval), but information about when they will eventually die is *incomplete*. A method was needed to use both complete and incomplete data. The latter is called *censored* data (see Box 6-20).

In 1950, Berkson and Gage published their landmark medical paper on the life-table (actuarial) method for censored data, which they stated was no different from that used by others as early as at least 1922.[B23,M1] Estimates of percent survival and censoring were made at arbitrarily determined intervals (such as yearly), although the original papers Berkson cites also address a method of generating a new estimate at every unique death interval that went unrecognized even after the work by Kaplan and Meier.

In 1952, Paul Meier at Johns Hopkins University and, in 1953, Edward Kaplan at Bell Telephone Laboratories submitted to the *Journal of the American Statistical Association* a new method for survival analysis, the product-limit method, that used more of the data. Estimates were generated at the time of each occurrence of an event. Further, the basis for the estimates was grounded in sound statistical theory. Meier was interested in the survival of cancer patients; Kaplan was interested in the lifetime of vacuum tubes in repeaters in telephone cables buried in the ocean.

BOX 6-20 Censored Data

In survival analysis, time to an event is often not known. The data with respect to time of event is *incomplete*. It is as if some information has been "cut off," resulting in *censored data*.

In contrast, an *uncensored observation* is one for which (1) the event of interest has occurred and (2) the exact time the event occurred, X, is known. Some call such an observation *complete data*.

The most commonly encountered instance of incomplete (censored) data is the finding at follow-up of a patient who is still alive or has not experienced the event of interest. If t is the interval between time zero ($T = 0$) and time of follow-up, $T = t$, and X is the exact (future and unknown) time the event occurs, X is to the right of t on the time line (time is presumed to progress from left to right). This form of censoring is called *right censored data*. Other examples of right censored data are morbid events that do not occur before the patient dies, and death (rather than follow-up) is the censoring mechanism.

Occasionally, we know that a patient has experienced the event, but do not know exactly when. We may know it occurred between time t_1 at the earliest and t_2 at the latest, that is, $t_1 \leq x \leq t_2$ (see Box 6-12). This form of inexact timing of the event is called *interval censored data*. An extreme variant of interval censored data is the situation in which the event is known to have occurred before the date of follow-up, but no information is known as to when. In this case, the interval is between time zero and follow-up. Such data are called *left censored*.

An assumption of most methods for analyzing time-related events is that the mechanism of censoring is unrelated to occurrence leading to an event. Such mechanisms are said to result in noninformative censoring. Under some circumstances, however, it is intuitive that this is a poor assumption. For example, if transplantation is a censoring mechanism for death after a patient is placed on a waiting list, it is possible that informative censoring has occurred, because transplants may preferentially be triaged to the patients thought least likely to survive. Methods for identifying and managing informative censoring are not yet in widespread use.[K21,W11]

The journal editor, John Tukey, believed the two had discovered the same method, although presented differently, and insisted they join forces and produce a single publication. For the next 5 years, before its publication in 1958,[K2] the two hammered out their differences in terminology and thinking, fearing all the while they would be scooped. The product-limit method (usually known as the Kaplan–Meier method), after considerable delay awaiting the advent of high-speed computers to ease the computation load, became the gold standard of nonparametric analysis.

Until 1972, only crude methods were available to *compare survival curves* according to different patient characteristics.[G4,L4,M2,M3,O1,P1,P2,W6] The introduction by Cox of a proposal for multivariable survival analysis revolutionized the field.[C3] From then through the 1980s, survival analysis became the subject of thousands of practical and theoretical papers and scores of textbooks. These explored both parametric and nonparametric methods and identified limitations and assumptions, such as the effect of informative censoring. Much of the development was in the field of medicine.

Important developments also took place in industrial reliability. Wayne Nelson[N3] at General Electric developed a method for analyzing time-related events in the *cumulative hazard function* rather than the survivorship domain (see "Fundamentals" under Time-Related Events later in this section) because he was interested in the rate at which events occurred (hazard function). The estimation procedure differed, therefore, from that of Kaplan and Meier, but the two methods converge as the number of events increases (see "Repeated Events" and "Weighted Events" later in this section). Importantly, by not "thinking" in the probability domain but rather the hazard function domain, he extended his method to repeated events, and then extended this further to weighted events.[N4,N9] He called the latter *time-related cost functions,* recognizing that recurrence of the same event, such as a machine repair, may be associated with different costs. (We have used this, for example, to analyze the grade of medical impairment from repeated episodes of thromboembolism following heart valve replacement.[B24,B26])

Fundamentals

Time-related events are those presumed to occur at an instant in time after a defined starting time. Time of occurrence generally differs from patient to patient. Information about occurrence of the event and when it occurred is obtained by patient follow-up, as detailed under "Follow-up" in Section 3.

Essential Data

Successful analysis of time-related events requires answers to three fundamental questions:
- What is the event?
- When is time zero?
- Who is at risk?

Event. Defining the *event* for an analysis may be straightforward, such as death from any cause. Events that are not uniformly fatal are called *nonterminating* or *morbid events.* Examples include brain abscesses, reoperations, degeneration of a xenograft valve, and development of angina. A clear, uniformly applied definition of the event is vital and has two components: (1) It defines an *uncensored* patient who experiences the event, and (2) it defines a *censored* patient who at some point in time becomes untraced as regards the event.

Caution must be exercised in considering the time-relatedness of some events. For example, degeneration of a porcine xenograft is a time-related *process,* not an event. Timing of reoperation for structural valve deterioration of the xenograft, therefore, depends on the rate of a process, the patient's response to that process, and medical decision-making. Processes that can be measured at multiple times are best studied by the methods described under "Longitudinal Outcomes" later in this section.

Time zero. The moment a patient becomes at risk of experiencing the event of interest is called *time zero* (Fig. 6-13). For patients who undergo interventions such as a cardiac procedure, time zero is often the time of the procedure. Under many circumstances, however, defining time zero is not so simple. For example, it is not easy to date the onset of ischemic heart disease, although it may be easy to identify the date of first myocardial infarct.

At risk. Patients remain *at risk* of experiencing the event from time zero to either the occurrence of the event or the time at which they no longer can experience the event (censoring; see Box 6-20). Defining who is at risk demands thought. For example, if the event is reoperation for bioprosthetic structural valve deterioration, then patients receiving a mechanical prosthesis are never at risk! This distinction may not be obvious to a statistician asked to analyze structural valve deterioration unless the surgeon–investigator explains it in detail. In this example, patients receiving a bioprosthesis also become no longer at risk of this event the moment the bioprosthesis is explanted for other indications. They are permanently censored at that point. Note that if a repeated morbid event is being analyzed, such as transplant rejection or thromboembolism, patients continue to remain at risk after each occurrence of the event until they are censored by death, end of follow-up, or, for these examples, retransplantation or removal of the valve prosthesis.

Granularity of Time

The basic data required for the simplest time-related analyses are (1) the interval from time zero to either occurrence of the event or censoring (usually the interval to end of follow-up) and (2) an indicator variable specifying that the event occurred (uncensored) or did not (censored). Granularity of this interval is important, particularly for parametric models (see "Parametric Survival Estimation" later in this section). The shorter the interval from time zero to the event, the finer the granularity required. In cardiac surgery, calculating the interval for a patient dying on the day of operation or experiencing a complication may require use of clock time (hours and minutes) of time zero (generally the first time that an attempt is made to wean the patient from CPB or that the operation is declared to be completed) and clock time of death or the complication. When the interval is long, simply subtracting the calendar date of the event from that of surgery is sufficiently granular.

Time-to-Event Model

There are two distinctly different ways to think about time-related events, and this difference must be understood for effective communication between the surgeon–investigator and the statistician. First, time-to-event data may be thought of as simply the *distribution of intervals* to an event (martingale or counting theory). This will be the framework with which most statisticians are familiar. Second, time-to-event data may be thought of in terms of the mathematics of mass transport from one state (such as alive) to another (death) (Markov process theory). This is the framework more familiar to a surgeon, who has training in such mass transport phenomena as diffusion, heat transfer, blood flow, and other dynamic transport processes involving rates.

Distribution framework (counting process). Intervals to event are thought of like any other continuous, positive-valued variable. They can be expressed as a *cumulative distribution* graph (see Fig. 6-6, *B*), just like age. The only nuance is that by convention, the graph is turned upside down (its *complement*) so that it starts at 100% and falls as the interval lengthens. This is called the *survivorship function.* A common alternative expression for a cumulative distribution function is its slope (derivative), the *probability density function,* which is analogous to an ordinary histogram (see Fig. 6-6, *A*). Typically, this function is not useful

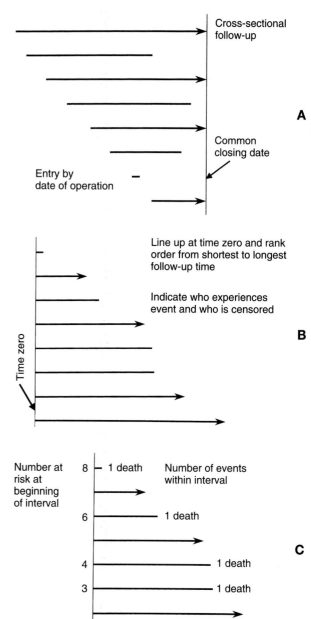

Figure 6-13   Right censored time-related events data. Conceptual graph of incomplete data in a group (cohort) of patients followed after operation cross-sectionally (see "Follow-up" in Section 3). **A,** Calendar date is along the horizontal axis, and each patient enters at a different date, ordered from earliest date of operation to most recent, top to bottom. Systematic active follow-up has a common closing date. Patients still alive at follow-up are depicted by arrowheads indicating that they will continue to be followed. Terminated lines are deaths. **B,** Patients are now aligned at *time zero,* when operation was performed. They have also been sorted from shortest interval to longest (called *rank order*). Patients who are still alive are depicted by lines with arrowheads. The time of their death is unknown and in the future. However, we at least know they have lived as long as is indicated by the length of their follow-up line. This is called *incomplete data* with respect to death, or *censored data.* Because the arrow of time is presumed to proceed from left to right, the data are called *right censored.* The four lines that terminate without an arrow are deaths. **C,** Basic counting needed to estimate survival. Along the left is the number of patients at risk. Thus, at the time of shortest follow-up, all eight patients were at risk. The number decreases progressively as patients either die or are no longer traced. On the right is the count of deaths at that interval (here, as is usually the case, the number is 1).

in survival analysis. What is useful is the ratio of the probability density function to the survivorship function (the conditional probability density function), because it represents the risk of the event in patients who have not yet experienced it. This ratio is the *hazard function* in survival analysis.

If $S(t)$ is the survivorship function across time t, $h(t)$ the probability density function, and $\lambda(t)$ the hazard function, the following mathematical equations express the above relations:

$$h(t) = \frac{\partial S(t)}{\partial t}$$

(6-4)

where $\partial S(t)/\partial t$ is the slope (derivative) of $S(t)$, and

$$\lambda(t) = h(t)/S(t)$$

(6-5)

Mass transport framework (hazard function). A force of mortality, called the *hazard function* or $\lambda(t)$, transports patients from the state of being alive, $S(t)$, to the state of death $F(t)$ (Fig. 6-14). This framework of thinking was initially suggested by John Graunt in the mid-1600s.[G9] Exactly the same equations, 6-4 and 6-5, hold for this dynamic process.

Useful Mathematical Relations

The area beneath the hazard function accumulates exposure to risk across time and is called the cumulative hazard function, $\Lambda(t)$:

$$\Lambda(t) = \int_0^t \lambda(u)du$$

(6-6)

This relation yields other useful relationships:

$$S(t) = e^{-\Lambda(t)}$$

(6-7)

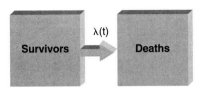

Figure 6-14   Compartmental mass-balance analog of a time-related terminating event such as death. The decrease in survivors as the interval (time t) after operation increases is proportional to the hazard rate $\lambda(t)$ (the instantaneous risk) for death multiplied by the number of individuals remaining at risk at time t.

where e is the base of the natural logarithms, and

$$Ln\left[S(t)\right] = \Lambda(t)$$

$$(6\text{-}8)$$

where Ln is the natural logarithm. Thus, the cumulative hazard function is easily calculated from estimates of $S(t)$, and its shape reflects the shape of $\lambda(t)$.

Nonparametric Survival Estimation

The nonparametric *Kaplan–Meier method*[K2] is the most commonly used method for estimating the survivorship function in medicine, although a number of others have been proposed.[C2] Each Kaplan–Meier estimate incorporates the number of patients experiencing an event since the last event occurred and the number of patients at risk in that interval, taking into account censoring (see Fig. 6-13, *C*). Computing Kaplan–Meier survival estimates is relatively straightforward. The basic idea is to first calculate the probability of surviving (being event-free) in the interval since the last event occurred (the ratio of events, generally 1, to number at risk). This probability is then multiplied by the probability of surviving up to that time, a product called a *conditional probability*. This successive multiplication of individual probabilities by preceding ones is what gave rise to the generic description of this method, the *product-limit* method. It also guarantees that the estimates of survival decrease monotonically.

As can be imagined, at the longest intervals, few patients remain at risk and individual survival estimates make large jumps. For example, if four patients are alive and one dies, the probability of survival in that interval is only 75%. This phenomenon results in systematic bias downward, underestimating the survivorship function. This is called the *completion effect*.[C8]

Each Kaplan–Meier estimate has an expressed degree of uncertainty.[G5,G6,K5] Often this is reported as the standard error (essentially the 68% symmetric confidence intervals). Preferably, however, the degree of uncertainty is expressed using asymmetric confidence units. When plotted, a symbol positioned on the horizontal axis at the time of each event and on the vertical axis at the Kaplan–Meier estimate graphically displays the information (Fig. 6-15, *A*).

There is controversy about (1) whether or not Kaplan–Meier estimates should be connected and (2) if they are connected, in what fashion. If parametric estimates are also generated, the obvious solution is to compare nonparametric and parametric estimates, with nonparametric estimates unconnected (Fig. 6-15, *B*). If this is not the case and

connection is desired, most statisticians connect estimates with a horizontal straight line at the level of the previous estimate. This is technically called "zero order" interpolation with a left step. It can be proven that this practice is the worst possible means of connecting estimates. Therefore, some statisticians connect the estimates by straight line segments (first-order interpolation), as did Berkson and Gage,[B4] but others use yet higher-order interpolation methods that approach the smoothness of parametric estimates.

Kaplan–Meier and other nonparametric life-table estimates are not "raw data" (descriptions of actual events). The time of death actually "happened," but the proportion, or percentage, is a computation and thus an estimate.

Parametric Survival Estimation

Unlike nonparametric survival estimation that arose from the theory of counting, model-based or parametric survival estimation (see Box 6-14) arose out of biomathematical consideration of the force of mortality, the hazard function.[G9] Unlike survival, which depicts *prevalence* of an event (or freedom therefrom) across time, the hazard function depicts the *rate* of occurrence, or *incidence,* of an event across time (see Box 6-13).

General Comments

During the Great Plague, John Graunt assumed a constant risk of mortality (the mortality rate or force of mortality). He called it the *hazard function* after a technical term for a form of dicing that had, by the mid-seventeenth century, come into common usage to mean "calamity," much as "crap shoot" has taken on the connotation of the losing throw in craps.[G9] Because a constant hazard rate presumes a mathematical model of survival, his was a *parametric method*. Graunt's colleague, William Petty, believed instead that the hazard rate was age related (time varying).[H11]

Thereafter, the hazard function essentially disappeared from the medical world until the 1980s, although it remained in use in industry and in government depictions of population behavior.[G8,W8] This is possibly because the hazard function, unlike the survivorship function, appears to have no well-understood statistical counterpart, as do the Kaplan–Meier estimator and death density function. It may also be related to the difficulty of relating intuitively a series composed of almost an infinite number of instantaneous estimates of risk to the easily perceived accumulated risk expressed as freedom from the event. Also, the inherently mathematical nature of the hazard function makes it difficult and forbidding to many physicians whose statistical collaborators may not have thought to introduce it to them in terms of biochemical reaction rates or other familiar physiologic rates. For those who need a visceral sense of the hazard function, think of its magnitude in terms of the sudden change from a sense of well-being to one of danger, as when screeching tires are heard close by.

Linearized rate. The most common expression of hazard is the *linearized rate*. It was linearized rates that John Graunt used when exploring risk factors for the plague.[G9] A linearized rate means the hazard function is constant across time. The analogy is radioactive decay: A constant rate of decay leads to exponential decay. Likewise, a constant hazard leads to an exponentially decreasing survivorship

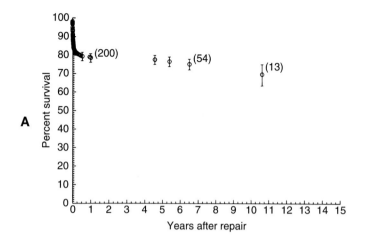

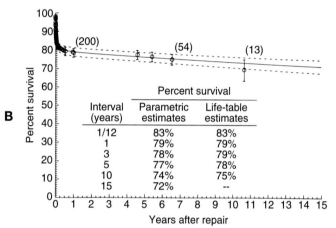

Figure 6-15 Nonparametric and parametric depictions of survival after repair of atrioventricular septal defects. Nonparametric estimates are represented by individual circles and their 70% confidence limits (CL) by vertical bars; parametric depictions are represented by the solid line and their 70% CLs by dashed lines. Numbers in parentheses are the number remaining at risk at various times. **A,** Nonparametric depiction. **B,** Parametric depiction. Note the excellent correspondence between parametric and nonparametric estimates, each obtained independently of the other. (From Studer and colleagues.[S4])

function. When hazard is constant, the cumulative hazard is linearly increasing: $\Lambda(t) = at$; that is, it increases linearly with increasing time with constant hazard slope a. Then $S(t) = exp(-at)$, where exp is the exponential function, and thus survival decreases exponentially.

The linearized rate is easily computed by simply counting the number of events and dividing by the total follow-up time of a group of patients.

$$\hat{\lambda} = \frac{n_d}{\sum_{i=1}^{n} t_i}$$

(6-9)

where $\hat{\lambda}$ is estimated constant hazard, n_d is number of events, n is total number of patients, and t_i is individual (i) time to the event.

Importantly, if there are multiple events per patient, such as thromboembolic events, all occurrences are counted. Confidence limits of linearized rates are also easily calculated (see "Repeated Events" later in this section).[G22,L19] However, there are a number of different, although roughly equivalent, formulae for these confidence limits. For example, Cox and Oakes[C8] present a simple formula:

$$S_D\left[Ln(\hat{\lambda})\right] = \sqrt{\frac{1}{n_d}}$$

(6-10)

and the upper confidence limit of $\hat{\lambda}$, $\hat{\lambda}^+$, is

$$\hat{\lambda}^+ = e^{Ln(\hat{\lambda}) + z\sqrt{1/n_d}}$$

(6-11)

and the lower confidence limit, $\hat{\lambda}^-$, is

$$\hat{\lambda}^- = e^{Ln(\hat{\lambda}) - z\sqrt{1/n_d}}$$

(6-12)

where z is the confidence coefficient (1 for 68% CL, 1.96 for 95% CL), and e is the base of the natural logarithms.

Time-varying rate. Although linearized rates have frequently been used for cardiac surgery data, particularly by regulatory agencies, it is uncommon for hazard to be constant.[G10] Rather, cardiac procedures, perhaps more than many other therapies, impose on patients a time-related course composed of highly variable and sometimes rapidly changing instantaneous risks of death modulated by multiple risk factors of varying strength and times of influence. Certainly the hazard function is greater 1 hour after operation than it is 1 week, 1 month, or 1 year after operation. Thus, a great deal of practical importance is attached to the time-varying hazard function after operation.

Visual examination of life-table depictions of events after cardiac operation in cohorts of well-followed patients reveals simple, smoothly time-varying patterns (see Fig. 6-15). These patterns suggest that the intervals between events are closely spaced immediately after the operation (usually time zero) and become more widely spaced in the hours and days that follow. Some days, weeks, or even months later, they merge into a sparse, random spacing of events. If follow-up evaluation is extended considerably, the time interval between events may again begin to shorten, representing accelerated risk. Nevertheless, under most circumstances the majority of patients are free of the event even after many years, making censoring prevalence high in the cardiac surgical setting.

The stereotypical patterns observed in analysis of several thousand life tables of freedom from an unfavorable outcome event after cardiac operation led the UAB group to believe that a mathematical model for time-related events could be developed.[B25] In this development,[H3,T2,T3] it was thought likely that risk factors for late-occurring events would differ at least in strength from those in the acute phase of recovery after operation, and that their prevalence might be different in different time frames. Further, the ability to graph patient-specific risk and survival estimates became increasingly important to development of new knowledge in cardiac surgery. Finally, these depictions required confidence limits. Therefore, the UAB group introduced a hazard function modeling method that produced not only time-related freedom from an event but also time-varying risk (hazard function) for an event.[B20] The method is analogous to using a prism to decompose white light into its various colors. It decomposes time-varying hazard into as many as three simple, additive hazard phases as shown in Fig. 6-16 (a more generalized method would allow more than three phases for unusual situations).

The mathematical model is as follows[B20]:

$$\Lambda(t,x) = \sum_{j=1}^{k} \mu_j(x_j,\beta_j) \cdot G_j(t,\Theta_j)$$

(6-13)

where $\Lambda(t,x)$ is the cumulative hazard function, $\mu_j(x_j,\beta_j)$ is a function of risk factors for the jth phase, $G_j(t,\Theta_j)$ is a shaping function unique for each phase, and Σ is the sum of the individual components (phases) j through k. Such a formulation places Equation 6-9 into the class of mixture distribution and competing risk models (see "Competing Risks" later in this section), with each hazard phase competing for the event.[E5,K12]

The shaping functions $G_j(t,\Theta_j)$ are based on a collection of biomathematical models of risk that were assembled into generic equations. They permit great flexibility in shape of the short- and long-term hazard.[H3,T2,T3] Shape of the early hazard phase of short-term risk originated as an assembly of a large number of nested mathematical models describing biochemical reactions, ecology, and population growth.[H3,T2,T3] The early hazard function can begin at infinity after time zero, it can start at zero and peak, or it can start at a finite value and decline from there. Shape of the constant hazard phase, as its name implies, is a constant value (horizontal line) across time. Shape of the late hazard function is based on a generalization of the Weibull model of risk used widely in industrial settings.[9]

Although early and late hazard phases can have several of their shaping parameters estimated, in practice they usually reduce from four down to one or two parameters, resulting in simple, special-case forms of their respective generic mathematical constructs.

Each phase also has a scaling function μ_j that can carry risk factors. This parameter was selected by sensitivity analyses and was not arbitrary. The form of the regression model may be either logit-linear or log-linear (see Box 6-5); they yield nearly identical coefficients and shapes.

All phases of the model are defined from time 0 to infinity. Thus, the phases are overlapping and additive across time (see Fig. 6-16, *B*). However, the nature of the

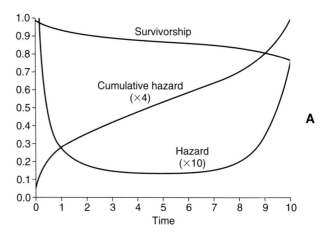

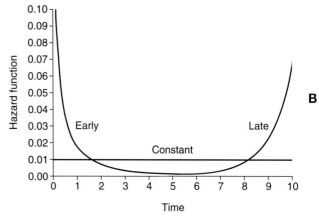

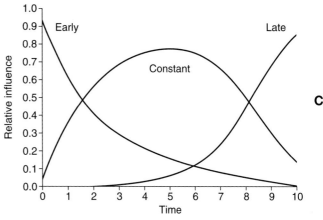

Figure 6-16   Conceptual depiction of time-varying patterns of hazard. **A,** Survivorship (proportion event free), its corresponding cumulative hazard function, and hazard function (time-related instantaneous risk of the event and the slope of cumulative hazard). **B,** Hazard function from *A,* shown decomposed into three simpler components, or phases, that when added together yield total hazard: (1) a rapidly declining early hazard phase, (2) a constant hazard phase, and (3) a late rising hazard phase. **C,** Relative influence of each hazard phase across time as a proportion of total hazard shown in *A.* Initially, the early hazard phase predominates, at 2 to about 8 years the constant hazard phase predominates, and thereafter the late hazard phase predominates. It is the temporal separation of components (decomposition) that permits separate sets of risk factors to essentially independently modulate each hazard phase.

---

[9] Under most circumstances the late hazard phase equation is constrained such that hazard increases monotonically, that is, without decreasing at any point. In reality, the equation is more flexible than this and can conform to late hazards that may at some point diminish. For example, the hazard function for the population of the United States has an early declining hazard phase reflecting infant mortality, a constant hazard phase that over the past century has practically disappeared, and a generally rising late hazard phase. However, this phase is interrupted by a small peaking hazard phase during late teenage and early adulthood years, representing, among other causes, accidental deaths. Further, at the extreme of old age, hazard may not increase to the extent predicted by a Weibull relation, perhaps because these elderly individuals are a highly select robust group.

shaping functions allows a phase to predominate more at one time than another (see Fig. 6-16, *C*). This property permits the model to accommodate risk factors not displaying proportional hazard properties across all time (see "Cox Proportional Hazards Regression" later in this section).

A computer software program interfaced to the SAS system[S5] is available at *http://www.clevelandclinic.org/ heartcenter/hazard*.

Estimating the time-related hazard function. The first step in developing a model specific to a set of event-time data is to determine the overall hazard function across time (without considering risk factors). This is the step, sometimes a time-consuming one, that differs from the work required in using the Cox model described later in this section. The work is best done in the cumulative hazard domain by taking the logarithm of the life-table estimates[N3] (Fig. 6-17). This depiction makes evident the early phase of hazard, the duration of its predominance, and the point at which it levels off (its asymptotic value). Slope of the intermediate phase of risk yields an estimate of the constant hazard scaling parameter. Departures late from the constant hazard slope yield information about the late rising phase of hazard if it is present. Such plots also reveal whether one or two of the three phases may be completely absent, given the duration of follow-up and distribution of observed events.

The method of maximum likelihood is used to estimate values for the parameters of the proposed model, which includes exploring various mathematical forms of the early and late generic shaping equations, defined by the sign of their exponents, and reducing the model to its simplest form (parsimony).[K1] The only input to this process is the sequence of events and censoring intervals. No arbitrary assignment of events to early, constant, or late hazard phase is required. The model simply attempts to best represent the distribution over time of these intervals. An iterative (optimization) procedure is used to estimate the parameter values. Once estimated, these values can be used to solve the resulting equation for time-related freedom from the event and the hazard function (Fig. 6-18).

Absence of some phases may be related to duration of follow-up or to the number of events observed and their intervals, which may make it difficult to identify statistically the existence of a phase. Most commonly, one or two phases are found.

At this juncture, investigation is made of model validity. The calculated (parametric) event-free curves are superimposed on the Kaplan–Meier estimates and examined for lack of correspondence (see Figs. 6-15 and 6-17).

Multivariable Analysis

Feigl and Zelen introduced multivariable analysis of constant hazards using a log-linear model (see Box 6-5).[F15] This formalized the method used 300 years earlier by Graunt,[G9] but it is inapplicable to data with time-varying hazards.

A number of methods were used in a limited way in demography and industry, but in 1972 everything changed.[B6,G8,W8] That year, D.R. Cox proposed a multivariable method that did not require estimating the hazard

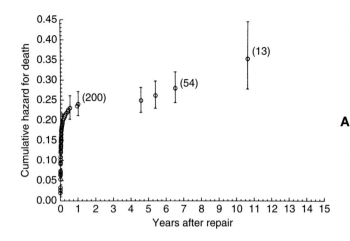

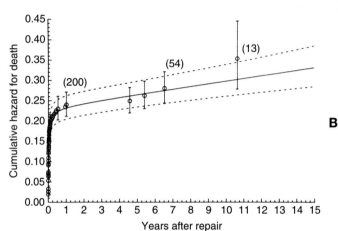

Figure 6-17 *Cumulative hazard depiction of the data set used in Fig. 6-15. An early phase component is apparent. Thereafter it is not clear whether there is a constant hazard phase or a rising one. This must be tested by statistical analysis. Nonparametric depiction is as in Fig. 6-15. **A**, Nonparametric estimates. **B**, Superimposed nonparametric and parametric estimates. Note the good correspondence between the two sets of estimates. (From Studer and colleagues.[S4])*

function.[C3] Rather, it assumed that an unspecified underlying hazard function of any shape was modulated in a regular way by a set of risk factors. This is called a *semiparametric* method because the model for risk factors was parametric, but the underlying hazard was unspecified.[B5]

Cox Proportional Hazards Regression

The log-linear (see Box 6-5) form of the Cox model of risk factors is

$$Ln[\lambda(t)] = Ln[\lambda_0(t)] + \beta_1 x_1 + \beta_2 x_2 + \cdots + \beta_k x_k$$

$$(6\text{-}14)$$

where $\lambda_0(t)$ is the underlying unspecified hazard that is modified by risk factors (**x**) that are weighted by coefficients **β** and *Ln* is the natural logarithm. The importance of the log-linear form is that the scale of both **β** and **x** can span the entire number line, and still the hazard function will be positive when $Ln[\lambda(t)]$ is exponentiated, which must be the case.

Another way to express the Cox model is in the cumulative hazard domain. Let us say there is one dichotomous risk factor, x_1, and coefficient β_1. Then:

$$\Lambda(t) = \Lambda_0(t)e^{\beta_1 x_1}$$

(6-15)

where $\Lambda(t)$ is the cumulative hazard function, $\Lambda_0(t)$ is the underlying cumulative hazard, and e is the base of the natural logarithms. The ratio of cumulative hazard with the factor present ($x_1 = 1$) to that with it absent ($x_1 = 0$) is

$$\frac{\Lambda(t, x_1 = 1)}{\Lambda(t, x_1 = 0)} = e^{\beta_1}$$

(6-16)

Taking logarithms and rearranging:

$$\beta_1 = Ln[\Lambda(t, x_1 = 1)] - Ln[\Lambda(t, x_1 = 0)]$$

(6-17)

Notice that the logarithm of the two cumulative hazard curves is separated across all time by a constant distance β_1 (Equation 6-17), and the exponential of β_1 (Equation 6-16) represents a constant ratio of cumulative hazards. This idea of a constant distance of separation or constant ratio is known as the *proportional hazards assumption* of the Cox method.[K11] Recall that cumulative hazard is estimated from the survival curve $S(t)$ by taking the logarithm (Equation 6-8). Therefore, if logarithms are taken of cumulative hazard using either Kaplan–Meier or Nelson estimates, or a single logarithm of Nelson cumulative hazard estimates, the proportionality assumption can be checked. If the proportional hazards assumption does not hold, nonproportional hazard methodology must be used.[P8]

Often β is expressed in a fashion to reflect relative risk as hazard ratios and their confidence limits (see Box 6-3). This can be seen from Equation 6-16, where the β_1 is exponentiated, showing a ratio of hazards with and without the risk factor. Confidence limits are asymmetric, obtained from the variance of β. The hazard ratio makes sense for dichotomous variables, but less sense for continuous ones, particularly if transformation of scale has been necessary.

Parametric Hazard Function Regression

Multivariable analysis of risk factors is no more (or less) difficult in the totally parametric hazard function domain than in the logistic or Cox regression domain (see "Multivariable Analysis" earlier in this section). The only intellectual (not computational) complexity is that risk factors are estimated simultaneously in all phases of hazard.[B21] Within each hazard phase, risk factors are assumed to obey a proportional hazards assumption (see "Cox Proportional Hazards Regression" earlier in this section). However, the entire model need not (and generally does not) obey the proportional hazards assumption. It therefore has been classified as a model of nonproportional hazards.[G23]

The main additional work in using a multiphase hazard method is obtaining the underlying, specified hazard function. Among the diagnostics for such a model is the general depiction of the time frame during which each hazard phase

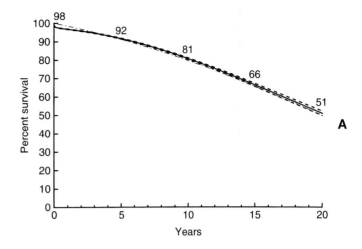

A

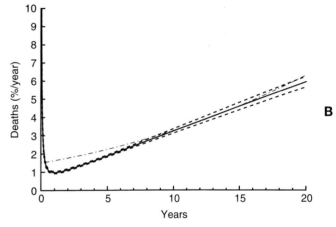

B

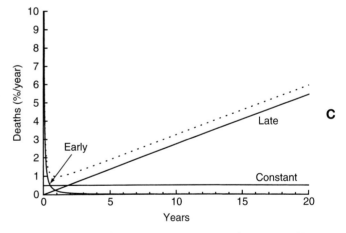

C

Figure 6-18   Death after coronary artery bypass grafting (CABG), illustrating survivorship and hazard functions and decomposition of hazard into phases. **A,** Survival. Solid line is survival estimate, and dashed lines enclose confidence limits (CL) equivalent to 1 standard error. Numbers are percent survival at 30 days, 5, 10, 15, and 20 years after operation. Dot-dash-dot line is survival in an age–sex–ethnicity–matched population life table.[A1,C7,E3] **B,** Hazard. Solid line is hazard estimate, and dashed lines enclose CLs equivalent to 1 standard error. Dot-dash-dot line is hazard in an age–sex–ethnicity–matched population life table. **C,** Components of instantaneous risk of death (hazard). Three are depicted: (1) an early rapidly falling hazard phase, (2) a constant hazard phase, and (3) a late rising hazard phase. These components sum across time to the overall hazard function shown by the dotted line. (From Sergeant and colleagues.[S22])

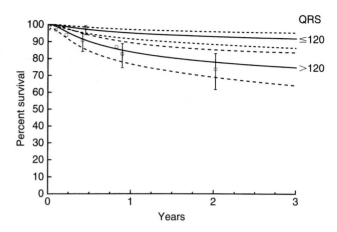

Figure 6-19 Validation of time-related multivariable equation. A multivariable equation for time-related death after left ventricular reconstruction (Dor operation) was solved for each patient in the study. Patients were then stratified by duration of preoperative QRS and the curves averaged within strata (solid lines with dashed confidence limits [CL] equivalent to ±1 standard deviation of the estimates). Superimposed on these predictions are Kaplan–Meier survival estimates, shown by the open circle (QRS duration = 120 ms) and open squares (QRS duration >120 ms); vertical bars represent 70% CLs. Note the good correspondence between model-based predictions and observed survival estimates. (From The Cleveland Clinic Foundation, 1997 to 2002, n = 84.)

dominates (see Fig. 6-16, *C*). The data can be examined within these separate time frames for screening and for transformation that may be necessary for continuous and ordinal variables.

After risk factors have been identified in each hazard phase, a final check on which phase a risk factor properly belongs to is performed. Occasionally a risk factor will be found with similar strength in each hazard phase, and such a variable indeed meets the proportional hazards assumption across the entire span of follow-up represented in the data.

A complete description of the final equation that emerges from the hazard function multivariable analysis includes a model specification, coefficients for all variables (incremental risk factors) in each phase of the equation (recall that a risk factor can occur in more than one phase), intercept for each phase, shaping parameter estimates, and a variance–covariance matrix. Because the equation is by definition completely parametric, prediction of an event-free curve and its corresponding hazard function, each accompanied by confidence limits, is possible for any desired combination of values for the risk factors by substituting values for each variable in the equation and solving it for any time interval(s) desired.

Validating the multivariable analysis. Validation of the multivariable analysis in a specific study is accomplished by comparing the computed time-related survival of a stratified life-table depiction of the entire study group with that predicted by the multivariable equation (Fig. 6-19). This process can be extended to subgroups in order to check the adequacy of modeling efforts. The process is similar to that for risk adjustment (see "Risk Stratification" in Section 6) and is accomplished in the following manner.[F4] For each patient, the survivorship function is estimated across time $\hat{S}(t;x_i,\Theta,\beta)$ from each individual's specific values for the risk factors in the equation.[S5] In the above notation, t is the time interval after time zero, Θ is the vector (column of numbers) of shaping parameter estimates, β is the vector of regression coefficient estimates, and x_i is the corresponding vector of risk factor values for individual i. For clarity, this is abbreviated to notation $\hat{S}(t;x_i)$. In addition, the upper and lower confi-

dence limits for $\hat{S}(t;x_i)$ are calculated using the variance–covariance matrix from the multivariable analysis.[K6]

The predicted value of time-related survival in a group of n individuals is then calculated as the average at each point in time of the individual survival estimates:

$$\tilde{S}(t) = \sum_{i=1}^{n} \tilde{S}(t;x_i)/n$$

(6-18)

The theoretical justification for this is that the individual $\hat{S}(t;x_i)$ represents proper cumulative distribution functions, and these should sum to another proper cumulative distribution function.[E5] On the other hand, specific theory underlying the formulation of confidence limits for this estimate in a straightforward manner has not been available. However, a conservative estimate has been made by averaging the upper confidence limits for each individual to form an upper confidence limit for $\tilde{S}(t)$, and similarly for the lower confidence limit. The error, if present, is that the confidence intervals are too wide. These confidence intervals have been found to be roughly equivalent to those obtained by averaging the variance of the logistic transform of $\tilde{S}(t)$, but they are somewhat more stable.

For the validation, time-related freedoms from the event of stratified groups of the cohort are determined nonparametrically as well and plotted according to the Kaplan–Meier estimator. For example, Fig. 6-20 shows tetralogy data stratified according to presence or absence of a transanular patch. This variable was not identified as a "significant" risk factor in the multivariable analysis. Nonetheless, averaged parametric survival values for the patients in the subset compare well with stratified Kaplan–Meier survival. (This validation study also indicates that the difference in prevalence of risk factors in patients with and without transanular patching, not the patching itself, appears to account for the difference in mortality.) Propensity score matching would provide the most reliable support for this inference (see "Propensity Score" in Section 1).

In a fashion akin to the logistic model, an overall assessment of validity within each stratum also may be obtained by calculating the number of expected events and comparing that with the number of observed events. In the

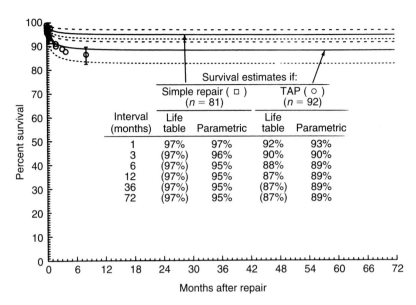

Figure 6-20   Internal validation of a parametric multivariable analysis of death after repair of tetralogy of Fallot. Transanular patching versus simple repair is not a risk factor in the multivariable equation. Patients have, however, been stratified according to this variable. Nonparametric estimates (*circles* and *squares*) are Kaplan–Meier depictions for these strata. Solid parametric lines represent the average of individual parametric curves calculated for each patient in the stratum, obtained as described in the text. The close agreement of predicted and observed survival indicates that prevalence of other risk factors differs in these two groups, leading to an apparent difference in survival. (From Kirklin and colleagues.[K13])

Key: *TAP*, Transanular patching.

domain of time-related events, conservation of events is attributed to the cumulative hazard function rather than to the probability domain. Thus, for each individual's specific follow-up interval (t_i), the cumulative hazard, $\hat{\Lambda}(t_i; x_i)$, is calculated. These are summed to estimate the expected number of events (E):

$$E = \sum_{i=1}^{n} \hat{\Lambda}(t_i; x_i)$$

$$(6\text{-}19)$$

The expected number of events is compared with the observed number of events by a chi-square goodness-of-fit test.

Expressing Degree of Uncertainty in Time-Related Depictions of Freedom from an Event

There is conflict (or at least difference of opinion) between (1) those who focus on a single overall P value for the difference between two time-related freedom-from-event depictions (life tables) and (2) those who use time-related depictions as one basis for their work with individual patients in the realm of clinical care (see "Time-Related Events" earlier in this section). This stems from their differing needs. Studies involving testing hypotheses, such as clinical trials in which treatment is randomly assigned, usually require a yes–no (true–false) answer to a hypothesis, and a single overall P value may be appropriate. The clinician, on the other hand, lives daily with the reality that in an individual patient, occurrence of an unfavorable outcome event at one point in time (interval after time zero) is often considerably less disadvantageous than occurrence of the same event at another point in time; the clinician also understands that there is considerable variability among patients as to the time of greatest disadvantage.

Mantel recognized in 1966, as no doubt did others, that time-related variability occurs in the relation between survival curves of two different treatments or between groups

of patients.[M3] He noted that in some cases the difference may be similar throughout time; that in others the relation between the two may be similar at some times but not at others; and that in still others one survival curve may cross another. He also recognized that varying hazard phases are present after surgical procedures, and he understood the variability in the "utility function," or value, ascribed by different individuals to the same survival curve.

These matters posed difficulties for those seeking a simple yes–no answer to a hypothesis. In response to this, Mantel and others set about to devise tests that would generate a single overall P value.[G4,M2,M3,P1,P2,W6] These tests make different assumptions, each attempting to overcome some difficulty posed by the differing patterns of survival. In contrast, clinicians wish to compute, examine, and understand the variability in the time-related comparisons between curves in order to best inform and advise patients. Thus, they wish to know the *time-related certainty* of differences that may exist.

The scanning method of comparing confidence intervals, as well as methods involving P values, can be applied to develop time-related estimates of the degree of uncertainty in comparing survival and other event-free curves. A depiction of time-related survival is in actuality a series of proportions; the proportions are discrete when determined by the Kaplan–Meier life-table method[K2] and are continuously variable when determined by the hazard function regression analysis method.[B20] Thus, the overlapping or nonoverlapping of confidence intervals around each of two survival curves can be used to scan the possibility, at various specific intervals after time zero, that the difference between the curves is or is not likely to be due to chance alone (Fig. 21, *A*). Also, based on classic statistical principles, the time-related confidence intervals around the *difference* between the two proportions can be determined and their relation to zero computed and visualized in a continuous, time-related depiction (Fig. 6-21, *B*). An equivalent expression of absolute difference is *absolute risk*

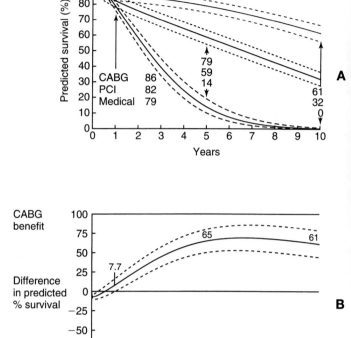

Figure 6-21   Survival estimates for a cachectic diabetic man with unstable angina according to different initial treatment strategy for his ischemic heart disease (see Appendix B in Chapter 7). **A,** Survival. Solid lines enclosed within dashed confidence limits (CL) are point estimates for (1) natural history (medical), (2) percutaneous coronary intervention *(PCI)*, and (3) coronary artery bypass grafting *(CABG)*. These predictions are based on patient-specific solutions of the multivariable equations presented in Appendix B of Chapter 7. Within the first year, procedure mortality results in a survival advantage for medical therapy, but after 2 years, non-overlapping CLs indicate an advantage for intervention. **B,** Difference in predicted percent survival *(solid curve)* between CABG and natural history (medical) with dashed 90% CLs. Initially, there is a medical benefit (negative difference), but after 1 year, a CABG benefit.

Key: *CABG,* Coronary artery bypass grafting.

Continued

reduction, the inverse of this difference, often expressed as *number to treat* to save one life (see Box 6-3). The time-related relation of the difference compared to zero difference can be depicted continuously in terms of the *P* value[F2,K7] (Fig. 6-21, *C*).

The relation between two time-related expressions of freedom from an event can also be expressed by comparing the confidence intervals of the *hazard function* (Fig. 6-21, *D*). They may also be compared using the confidence limits around the hazard ratio (see Fig. 6-21, *E*). Alternatively, the area between survival curves—the lifetime function—can be computed (Fig. 6-21, *F*). We prefer the lifetime function to the alternative statistic, *expected lifetime,* because the complete hazard function beyond the follow-up information available affects the value of this extrapolated statistic, and its trajectory may not be well characterized.

Repeated Events

Unlike death, morbid events such as thromboembolism or important bleeding after heart valve replacement may recur. Further, the consequences of these events may be variable, from apparently "no functional residual" from a transient ischemic attack to a fatal outcome (Fig. 6-22).

If the hazard function is truly constant, the method of linearized rates, as described earlier in this section under "Parametric Survival Estimation," may be used. The esti-

mation procedure is simple but rarely appropriate, because most hazard functions are not constant.

When the hazard function is not constant, three general approaches to display and analysis of morbid events have been used: analysis as a terminating event, repeated events analysis, and modulated renewal process analysis.

Terminating Events Approach

The most common method of display and analysis of repeated morbid events is to focus only on the first occurrence, ignoring any further information beyond that point for the patients experiencing the event. It thus becomes a terminating event analysis, with Kaplan–Meier estimation of freedom from occurrence of the event.

Repeated Events Approach

True repeated events analysis can be performed; however, generally this requires abandoning the Kaplan–Meier estimator and turning to the Nelson estimator. The Nelson method is formulated in the cumulative hazard domain (see "Fundamentals" under "Time-related Events" earlier in this section). Patients continue to be followed after each occurrence of the event until end of follow-up or death or some other appropriate censoring mechanism (see Fig. 6-22). Estimates are made at the time of each occurrence, with the hazard estimated as 1/number at risk, and the cumulative hazard as the sum of all these hazards. Graphical depiction of Nelson estimates is as cumulative hazard across

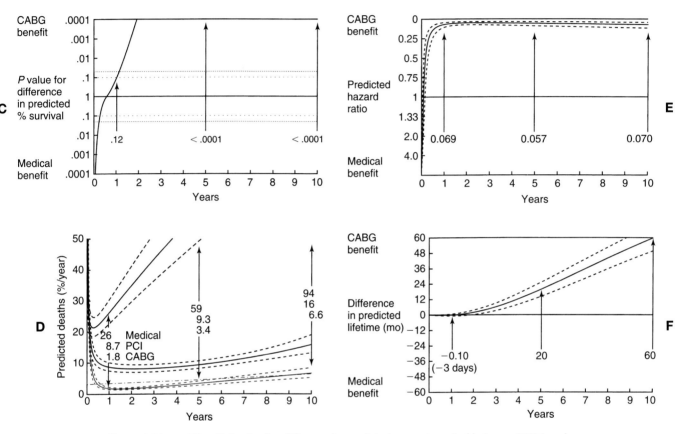

Figure 6-21, cont'd   **C**, *P* value for difference in predicted percent survival between CABG and natural history (medical). Difference in benefit shown by overlap and non-overlap of CLs in *B* is depicted in terms of *P* value; note that *P* value is shown symmetrically above and below 1, reflecting a change in direction of benefit. **D**, Hazard function *(solid curves)* for death from natural history (medical), PCI, and CABG with dashed 70% CLs. Note that instantaneous risks diverge considerably earlier than do survival estimates *(A)* and lifetime estimates *(F)*, because rates must both change and remain changed sufficiently long to produce a survival or lifetime difference. **E**, Hazard ratio *(solid curve)* of CABG and natural history (medical) with dashed 90% CLs. Initially, the hazard ratio favors medical therapy, but then CABG. Note that hazards become proportional after about 6 months (flat portion of ratio), but are nonproportional before then. Vertical axis has been arranged to give equal weight to a 2-fold increase in risk and a 0.5-fold decrease in risk. **F**, Difference in predicted lifetime *(solid curve)* between CABG and natural history (medical) with dashed 90% CLs. The lifetime difference is the area between the two corresponding survival curves depicted in *A*.

Key: *CABG,* Coronary artery bypass grafting; *PTCA,* percutaneous coronary intervention.

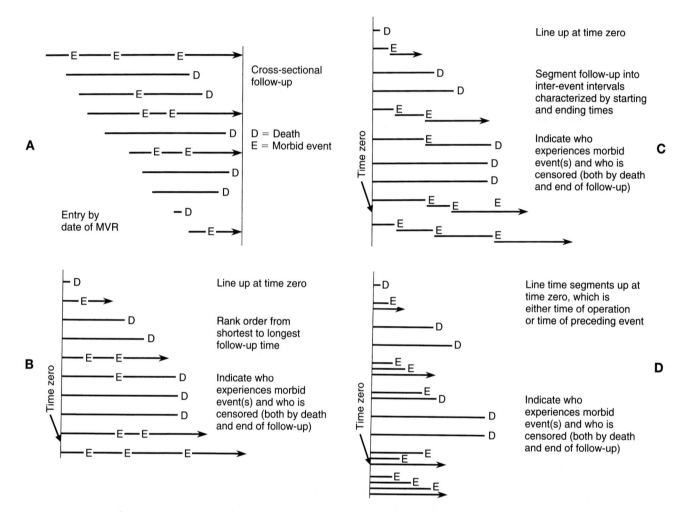

Figure 6-22 Repeated morbid events data. Conceptual graph of incomplete data in a group (cohort) of patients followed cross-sectionally after mitral valve replacement (MVR) with a mechanical prosthesis, depicting repeated morbid events. Deaths are depicted by *D*, and the morbid event thromboembolism is depicted by *E*. Censored patients (alive at follow-up) are indicated by arrows. **A**, Calendar date is along the horizontal axis, and each patient enters on a different date of operation, similar to the depictions in Fig. 6-13. Five patients have experienced the morbid event, and two of these have experienced two events, and one has experienced three events. However, note that follow-up continues beyond these events. **B**, Patients are again ordered for analysis by aligning them at time zero. **C**, From a purely practical point of view, the longitudinal record of each patient is broken into segments, each with a starting and ending time. **D**, In a modulated renewal process analysis, all the segments are moved back to time zero (and for analysis, they would also be reordered from shortest to longest interval, which is not depicted here).

time, with the vertical axis being the number of repetitions of the event expected per patient (Fig. 6-23). Thus,

$$\Lambda(t_i) = \sum_{k=1}^{i} \frac{n_{dk}}{n_{rk}}$$

(6-20)

where n_{dk} is the number experiencing the event (generally 1) at time t_i, and n_{rk} is number at risk.[10]

The Blackstone–Naftel–Turner parametric hazard methodology is designed to analyze repeated morbid events. An interesting but useful technical detail of such an analysis is that each patient's follow-up history is recorded as a sequence of intraevent segments: time zero to first event, first event to second, etc., last event to censoring mechanism. Each segment has a beginning and ending time. Kalbfleisch and Prentice point out that this approach to the data simplifies what might otherwise appear to be a daunting analytical challenge.[K1]

Modulated Renewal Process Approach

The hazard function for repeated events such as cardiac rejection episodes may follow a similar pattern after each repeated episode, only modulated to some degree (higher or lower) in its intensity. Such a phenomenon, commonly observed in the industrial setting, is called a *modulated renewal process* (see Fig. 6-22, *D*).[K1]

The idea behind a modulated renewal process is that the industrial machine (or patient) is restarted at a new time zero each time the event occurs. This permits (1) ordinary Kaplan–Meier methods to be employed, (2) the number of occurrences and intervals between each recurrence to be used in multivariable analyses, and (3) change in patient characteristics at each new time zero to be used in analyses. Thus, if the modulated renewal assumption can be shown to be valid, it increases the power and utility of the analysis tremendously. For example, Hickey and colleagues demonstrated that each repeated episode of thromboembolism following mitral valve commissurotomy increased the risk (shortened the interval) of the next (Fig. 6-24).[H8] Kubo, Naftel, and colleagues demonstrated that rejection after cardiac transplantation behaved as a modulated renewal process, and among other factors, number of previous rejection episodes was a risk factor for subsequent episodes (Fig. 6-25).[K24] Blackstone and colleagues exploited the

---

[10] *Comparison of Kaplan–Meier and Nelson estimators.* The Kaplan–Meier estimator for survival at time t_i, $S(t_i)$, is

$$S(t_i) = \prod_{k=1}^{i} \left(1 - \frac{n_{dk}}{n_{rk}}\right).$$

Transforming $S(t_i)$ to cumulative hazard:

$$\Lambda(t_i) = -\sum_{k=1}^{i} \text{Ln}\left(1 - \frac{n_{dk}}{n_{rk}}\right).$$

If $n_{rk} = 100$ and $n_{dk} = 1$, the logarithmic term $1 - n_{dk}/n_{rk} = 0.99$ and its logarithm is 0.01005. Compare this to the Nelson estimate of cumulative hazard, n_{dk}/n_{rk}, which in this case is $1/100 = 0.01$. Thus, for all practical purposes, the two estimates are equivalent. The advantage of the Nelson estimator is that it can be extricated from the probability domain $S(t_i)$ so that repeated and weighted events can be evaluated, neither of which has a probability domain counterpart.

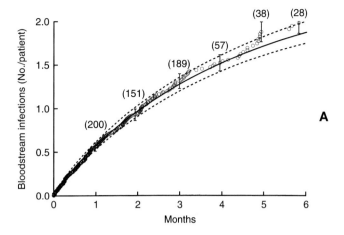

A

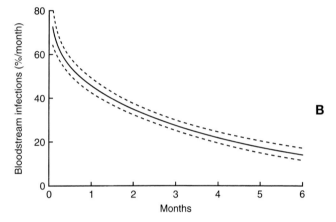

B

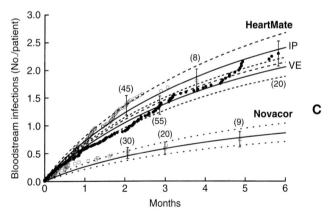

C

Figure 6-23   Illustration of repeated events data. Repeated bloodstream infections after left ventricular assist device (LVAD) insertion are shown. **A,** Cumulative number of bloodstream infections, expressed on the vertical axis as number per patient (repeating events analysis). Each circle represents an infection, vertical bars represent asymmetric 68% confidence limits (CL), and numbers in parentheses are number of patients remaining at risk. Solid line enclosed by dashed 68% CLs is the parametric estimate of bloodstream infections from which the hazard for the event was derived. **B,** Hazard function for bloodstream infections expressed on the vertical axis as percent per month (solid line enclosed by 68% CLs). **C,** Cumulative number of bloodstream infections according to type of LVAD. Open circles represent events experienced by patients receiving implantable pneumatic HeartMate devices (IP), solid circles vented electric HeartMate devices (VE), and open squares Novacor devices. (From Navia and colleagues.[N12])

Figure 6-24 Freedom (risk-adjusted) from a postcommissurotomy thromboembolic event, illustrating analyses of repeated morbid events as a modulated renewal process. The top curve represents freedom from the first thromboembolic event, and time zero is the time of operation. The middle curve represents freedom from a second thromboembolic event among 33 patients who had a first thromboembolic event after commissurotomy, and time zero for this depiction is the time of the first thromboembolic event. The lowest curve represents freedom from the third thromboembolic event among the patients who already had experienced two, and time zero is the time of the second episode. (From Hickey and colleagues.[H8])

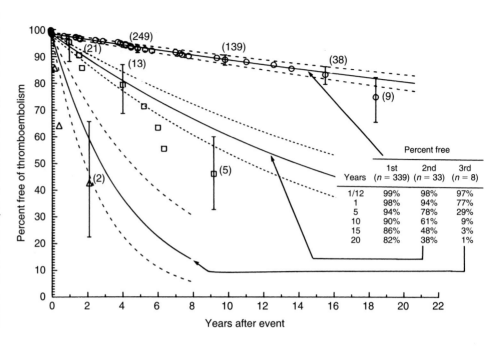

	Percent free		
	1st	2nd	3rd
Years	(n = 339)	(n = 33)	(n = 8)
1/12	99%	98%	97%
1	98%	94%	77%
5	94%	78%	29%
10	90%	61%	9%
15	86%	48%	3%
20	82%	38%	1%

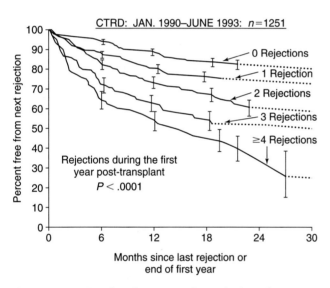

Figure 6-25 Freedom from transplant rejection after 1 year or any rejection episode later than 1 year, stratified according to number of rejection episodes during first year after transplantation. Data illustrate a repeated event analyzed as a modulated renewal process. Vertical bars represent 70% confidence limits. (Redrawn from Kubo and colleagues.[K24])

Key: *CTRD,* Cardiac Transplant Research Database.

modulated renewal process methodology for reoperations, periprosthetic leakage, and replacement device endocarditis after valve replacement.[B48]

From a data handling perspective, the patient's follow-up record is segmented just as described earlier in this section for the "Repeated Events Approach," but the starting time of each segment is set to zero and the ending time to duration of the segment.[K1]

Weighted Events

When a machine is repaired, there is a cost associated with the repair. Thus, in industrial settings it is important not just to estimate the risk (hazard) of repair but also to weight those risks by the cost of repair (Fig. 6-26).[N4,N9] Mathematically, cost is taken into account by what is termed "weighting" of the hazard estimate. This simply means the hazard is multiplied by the cost.

Medically, there are a number of cost scales that can be used to quantify, or at least grade, severity of an event. The UAB group, for example, used a simple five-point scale for residual neurologic consequences of a thromboembolic episode, with 0 being no consequences and 4 being death.[B26]

Nonparametric estimation is in the cumulative cost domain, and Nelson's method is used.[N4,N9] The Blackstone–Naftel–Turner parametric hazard function method also accommodates weighted events and complete multivariable analysis.[B20]

Competing Risks

Competing risks analysis is a method of time-related data analysis in which multiple, mutually exclusive events are considered simultaneously.[D4,P3] It is the simplest form of continuous-time Markov process models of transition among states.[A9] In this simplest case, patients make a transition from an initial state (called event-free survival) to at most one other state that is considered to be terminating (Fig. 6-27). Thus, there is a single set of intervals from time zero to the earliest occurring of each event for a given patient. Rates of transition from the initial state to one of the events (called an *end state*) are individual, independent functions. One way to think about this is that the initial state is represented by a bucket of water (Fig. 6-28). The transition rates are holes in the bucket of varying size. If all but one hole is blocked, the amount of water filling a

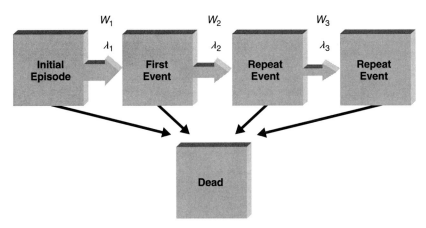

Figure 6-26 Weighted repeated events. This compartmental analog shows patients experiencing an initial episode such as a cardiac valve replacement, at time zero. A repeating morbid event is then shown, such as thromboembolism. The rate at which these occur is depicted by λs (which may differ after each event). In addition, the medical cost of each episode is depicted by a severity weight (Ws). From each compartment (after each event), the patient may die, an eventuality governed by another set of hazard rates not depicted.

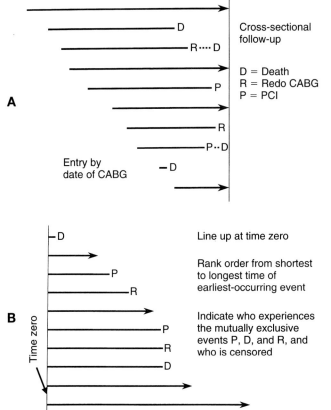

Figure 6-27 Competing risks data. Conceptual graph of incomplete data in a group (cohort) of patients followed after coronary artery bypass grafting (CABG) for death (*D*), redo CABG, or percutaneous coronary intervention (PCI). The depiction is similar to that of Fig. 6-13. **A,** Calendar date is along the horizontal axis, and patients are operated upon on various dates. They are systematically followed and their status ascertained as of a common closing date, shown by the vertical line. Notice that one patient died a while after redo CABG and another after PCI. Four patients experienced no events and are censored. **B,** Patients are aligned at time zero and rank ordered from shortest to longest follow-up time. The first occurring event is shown. Thus, the two patients who died after redo CABG or PCI are depicted only to their intervention (other analyses of events following redo CABG and PCI should also be performed). In this way, each patient falls into exactly four mutually exclusive categories: PCI, redo CABG, death before either of these interventions, and event-free survival. Notice that each patient has in this depiction, unlike *A*, a single follow-up interval. This common follow-up interval to all events is characteristic of this simplest form of competing risks analysis.

Key: CABG, Coronary artery bypass grafting; *PCI,* percutaneous coronary intervention.

container beneath the hole is identical to an ordinary survival function turned upside down. In a competing risks analysis, one is interested in discovering the amount of water in each of several containers when all the holes are unblocked simultaneously.

Motivation

Analysis of a single time-related event is performed in isolation of any other event. This is ideal for understanding that specific phenomenon. In contrast, competing risks analysis considers multiple outcomes in the context of one another. It is thus an integrative analysis.

Fig. 6-29 shows three events following coronary artery bypass grafting: death before reintervention, reintervention by percutaneous methods, and operative reintervention. At time zero, all patients are alive and without reintervention. They then migrate at different rates into the above various end states (see Fig. 6-29, *A*). The consequence of these migrations is that the initial state is gradually emptied and the reintervention states and death state fill (see Fig. 6-29, *B*).

The nature of migration into each of these end states is itself an important phenomenon. Results from the Cardiac Transplant Research Database[B64] and the UAB group[M20] show the provocative difference in the various competing hazard functions for modes of death after transplantation, just as the UAB group had shown for modes of death after valve replacement.[B48]

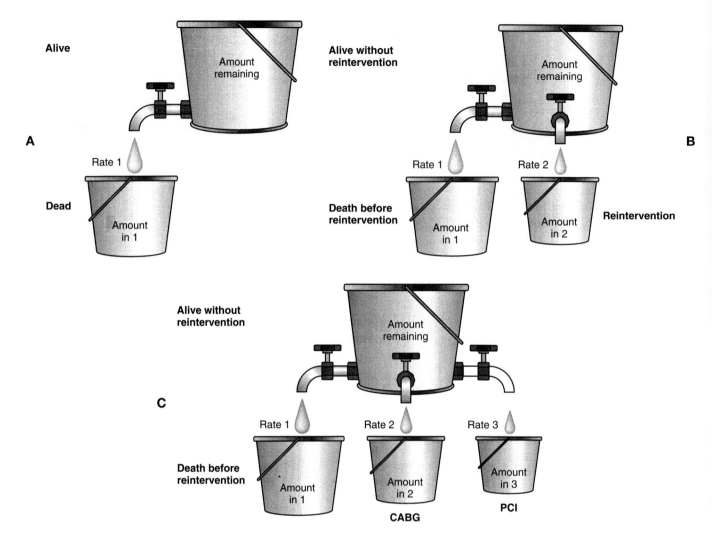

Figure 6-28 Competing risks cartoon using a bucket and water analogy. In each case, the large bucket is initially filled with water at time zero and represents event-free survival. Each spigot represents a route of exit of water from the main bucket to smaller, initially empty, containers. Rate of flow is governed by position of the tap. **A,** In ordinary analysis of single time-related events, there is only one tap. In competing risks analysis, this is analogous to closing all but one tap to permit estimation of its properties (called the hazard function). **B,** In the simplest competing risks analysis, two taps are opened simultaneously, and each water molecule (representing patients) must flow into only one container through one of the spigots. Level of water across time as each container fills (and the main bucket empties) is quantified by the cumulative incidence function. **C,** A more complex competing risks case with three taps opened. Reintervention is broken down into the two mutually exclusive components of percutaneous coronary intervention and repeat coronary artery bypass grafting.

Key: *CABG,* Coronary artery bypass grafting; *PCI,* percutaneous coronary intervention.

Because many possible paths of migration exist, it is important for understanding each phenomenon to isolate it from all others, much as one would perform a controlled experiment with all other factors held constant. If one assumes that the rates of migration (hazard functions) are independent of one another, factors influencing those rates (incremental risk factors) can be discovered and their influence explored. As long as it is reasonable to assume independence of events, such analyses are valuable to estimate matters like how often death would occur in the absence of reintervention.

However, individual analyses do not address the question of how often an event might occur in the presence of competing risks of other events. For example, it is valuable to know the influence of age and extent of grafting on reintervention or death. "How often will elderly patients need reoperation given the risk of mortality from old age itself?"

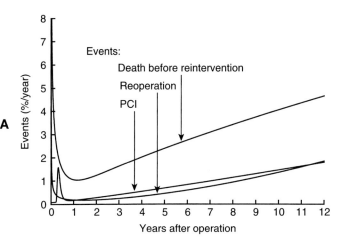

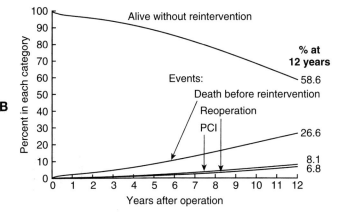

Figure 6-29   Illustration of competing risks. The figure depicts time-related competing events after coronary artery bypass grafting. **A,** Risk–unadjusted migration rates (hazard functions) into each of three mutually exclusive event categories: death before reintervention, reintervention by reoperation, and reintervention by percutaneous coronary intervention (PCI). **B,** Competing risks depiction of the consequences of the three migration rates shown in *A*. Units along the vertical axis are cumulative incidence. Rates shown in *A* deplete the proportion (%) of patients "alive, without reintervention" and increase the proportion dying before reintervention or experiencing reintervention by reoperation or PCI. At all points in time, the percentage of patients in all categories sums to 100%, as shown in the percentages at 12 years in the right margin of the figure. (From Blackstone and Lytle.[B17])

Key: *CABG,* Coronary artery bypass grafting; *PCI,* percutaneous coronary intervention.

Historical Note

In the early eighteenth century, some progress was made in the war against smallpox by inoculating people with small doses of the virus to establish immunity to the full-blown disease. The technique was 10% fatal in otherwise healthy individuals! The search for reliable low-risk protection became intense. Because governments at that time were supported in part by annuities, it was of considerable economic importance to know the consequences a cure of smallpox might bring upon the government's purse! Daniel Bernoulli tackled this question by classifying deaths into mutually exclusive categories, one of which was death from smallpox.[B54] For simplicity, he assumed that modes of death were independent of one another. He then developed kinetic equations for the rate of migration from the state of being alive to any one of several categories of being dead, including from smallpox. It was like hanging a bucket of water with multiple different sizes of holes in the bottom (see Fig. 6-28) and assuming no interactions between the holes. He could then compute how stopping up one large hole, smallpox, would influence both the number of people still alive and the redistribution of deaths into the other categories.

The triumph of the "war on smallpox" came in 1796, just 36 years after his publication.

What's in a Name?

Competing risks analysis has many names, which makes communication between disciplines, as well as assembly of a common body of methodologic knowledge, difficult. In vital statistics, competing risks are often called *disease-specific event rates.* In actuarial statistics, they may be called *multiple decrement analyses.* In statistics, they are usually called *competing risks,* but also *cumulative incidence functions* or *marginal* or *conditional survival analyses.* In demography, they may be called *crude* versus *net* versus *partial crude survival functions.* In medicine, and heart valve procedures specifically, the terms *cumulative events,*[G25] *multiple decrement,*[B49] *competing risks,*[C27,M18] and *mode-specific survival*[B48] have been used. The most recent entry into "competing names" was the introduction of *actual* versus *actuarial analysis* by Grunkemeier and colleagues.[G24,G26,G27] Competing risks are called *actual* and single-event analyses *actuarial.*

These methods are contrasted as if they were competing methods, or, indeed, as if one were right and the other wrong. We must emphasize that each answers different questions, and, assuming independence, the hazard functions are the same. Had one of them not yet been invented, the other surely would have because of the different questions answered. Individual event analyses (actuarial) using the entire patient cohort answer the question, "What is the probability of this event among patients still exposed to risk of the event, and what are its risk factors?" It is an unconditional probability. It is relevant to the investigation of a phenomenon. Such an investigation needs to be conducted as best possible free of confounding from occurrence of other outcomes. In contrast, competing risks analyses address the question, "How many patients are expected to experience a certain event before they experience another (specified) event?" Thus, individual event analyses indicate the probability of reoperative CABG as a function of age; competing risks analyses may indicate that few elderly patients will survive to have such a reoperation.[L10]

We caution against direct display of actual and actuarial estimates on the same graph. In fact, each has a different scale (the probability scale for individual events, the cumulative incidence scale for competing risks). Two aspects of scale are noted by Grunkemeier and colleagues.[G24] First, actuarial estimates of multiple different events do not sum to 100%. They should not; this is not a defect but a property of unconditional, independent events. Competing risks are conditional, which implies *multiplication* rather than *addition*. Indeed, it is easy to show that multiplication of independent survivorship functions yields event-free survival. Second, they note that the complement of the cumulative incidence function of competing risks is usually a higher number than actuarial estimates. Again, this is guaranteed, because competing risks must all sum to 100%, and this number is "adjusted" for occurrence of several risks that are competing. The more events considered to be competing, the higher the number will be. This "instability" is not a defect of competing risks analysis but rather a fundamental property. In the water bucket analogy, if more holes are punched in the bucket, there are more routes of exit, and each container under each hole will be filled less than when there were fewer holes. Because Grunkemeier and colleagues turn cumulative incidence curves upside down, "less filling" is equivalent to their "higher number."

Ideally, because competing risks estimates are of the number of patients (or percentage of all patients) in each end state, they should be plotted on the scale of cumulative incidence. In such a plot, the initial state empties (decreases) and all other states fill (increase) (see Fig. 6-29, *B*).

Limitations and Assumptions

An important assumption of time-related analyses is *noninformative censoring.*[C26] Either systematic anniversary or cross-sectional follow-up methods help with this assumption. However, in analysis of morbid events, death is a censoring mechanism, and it may not be independent of morbidity. In competing risks analysis, all events cause censoring of one another, and the possibility of informative censoring multiplies.

The number of hazard phases resolved in parametric hazard estimation depends on length of follow-up. Therefore, their ability to extrapolate beyond the length of follow-up is limited.

The number of events limits the number of risk factors that can be identified in either Cox proportional hazards analysis or hazard function multivariable analysis (see Box 6-5). If the latter is performed, this limitation is true within each hazard phase.

LONGITUDINAL OUTCOMES

In analysis of time-related events, the event is assumed to be a point process; that is, it is assumed to occur at some specific point in time, and the analysis focuses on the distribution of times until that event occurs. A number of phenomena of equal importance to the cardiac surgeon are not point processes but rather outcomes that continually *evolve* across time. That evolution may be assessed on a continuous, ordinal, or polytomous scale (list of possible outcomes).

Examples include time-related change in NYHA functional class after a Dor procedure, degree of return of valvar regurgitation and its progression after mitral valve repair, change in ventricular volume after myocardial infarction, sensitization after left ventricular assist device insertion, change in pulmonary function after single or double lung transplantation, and electrocardiographic status after a Maze procedure. For all these phenomena, information generally is obtained from patients periodically, usually at irregular intervals that differ from patient to patient. These are *longitudinal outcomes.*[D13]

Assessment of longitudinal outcome may be interrupted (censored) permanently by death, temporarily at active cross-sectional follow-up, or by other events that remove patients from risk, just as in time-related events studies (see "Fundamentals" under Time-related Events earlier in this section). One would like to use the data up to the time of censoring. Further, the clinical investigator is interested in factors that affect longitudinal evolution of these phenomena.

Historical Note

Severe technologic barriers to comprehensive analysis of these types of data existed before the late 1980s.[B39] Repeated-measures analysis of variance for continuous variables had restrictive requirements, including fixed time intervals of assessment and no censored data. Ordinal logistic regression for assessment of functional status was useful for assessments made at cross-sectional follow-up,[F17,H6] but not for repeated assessment at irregular time intervals with censoring.

In the late 1980s, Zeger and his students and colleagues at Johns Hopkins University incrementally, but rapidly, evolved the scope, generality, and availability of what they termed "longitudinal data analysis."[D13] Their methodology accounts for correlation among repeated measurements in individual patients and variables that relate to both the average effect and the nature of the variability. Because average response and variability are analyzed simultaneously, the technology has been called "mixed modeling." The technique has been extended to continuous, dichotomous, ordinal, and polytomous outcomes using both linear and nonlinear modeling.

Because of its importance in many fields of investigation, the methodology acquired different names. In 1982, Laird and Ware published a *random effects model* for longitudinal data from a frequentist school of thought.[L16] In 1983, Morris presented his idea on *empirical Bayes* from a Bayesian school of thought.[M16] The *generalized estimating equation* (GEE) approach was popularized in the late 1980s by members of Zeger's department at Johns Hopkins University.[D13]

Goldstein's addition to the Kendall series in 1995 emphasized the hierarchical structure of these models.[G18] His is a particularly apt description. The general idea is that such analyses need to account for covariables that are measured or recorded at different hierarchical levels of aggregation. In the simplest cases, time is one level of aggregation and individual patients with multiple measurements is another level. These levels have their corresponding parameters that are estimated, and each may require different assumptions about variability (random versus fixed effects distributions).

Except under exceptional circumstances, these techniques have replaced former restrictive varieties of repeated-measures analysis, which we now consider of historical interest except for controlled experiments designed to exactly meet its assumptions.

Concept

One way to think about the concepts underlying longitudinal data analysis is to consider it as a method that summarizes the results of individual regression analyses for each individual. The completely hypothetical data shown for pressure gradient across time in Fig. 6-30, *A*, would lead one to think that there is a gradual decrease. However, Fig. 6-30, *B*, shows that this apparent decrease is an artifact. It turns out that two pressure gradients were determined in each hypothetical patient. The measurements were made a few months to about a year apart in a cross-sectional manner for a group of hypothetical patients operated on at different times. Nearly all patients experienced an *increase* in pressure gradient. Thus, at the patient level of data aggregation, there is a temporal increase, not decrease, in pressure. On another hierarchical level, another phenomenon, such as change in operative technique, may account for the lower pressures in patients operated on earlier in the series. Fig. 6-30, *C*, shows the same data points as Fig. 6-30, *A*, but this time hypothetical individual patients are following a *downward* trend in pressure gradient. Here, the initial impression from the scattergram of Fig. 6-30, *A*, is confirmed. In fact, real data could be an admixture of panels *B* and *C*.

Thus, naive examination of the pattern of scatter of multiple measurements in patients does not guarantee that the trends imagined hold at the individual patient level. Individual data points cannot be treated as independent observations. Instead, trends and variability must be analyzed at each successive level of aggregation.

Implications

Cardiac surgeons have often collected information on longitudinal outcomes only at the time of last follow-up: most recent NYHA functional class,[H6] most recent echocardiographic assessment of valve regurgitation after repair, or degree of sensitization at transplant after implanting a permanent left ventricular assist device. Such a strategy cripples establishing time trends, because each patient contributes only one data point, preventing trends from being identified at the individual patient level. Therefore, it is imperative that every observation of longitudinal outcome be gathered and included in the analysis as part of the follow-up process.

A further cautionary note is that one-time survey of patients at follow-up (for example, a quality of life questionnaire) also represents a single observation per patient. Yet often, inferences are desired of a longitudinal nature. It is a huge assumption that *ensemble averages* based on one point per patient will reflect what multiple longitudinal measurements per patient would tell you (although repeated testing bias must also be considered).

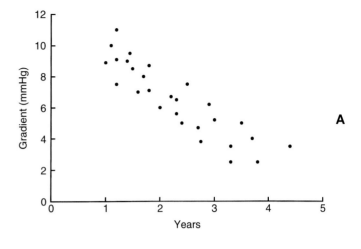

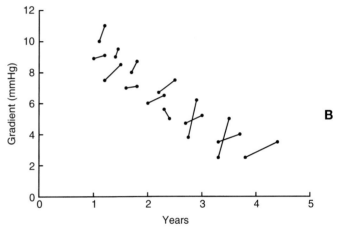

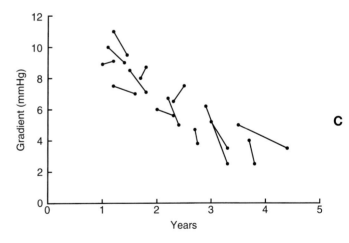

Figure 6-30   Hypothetical illustration of longitudinal data. Pressure gradient, determined by echocardiography, is shown on the vertical axis and years after operation on the horizontal axis. Measurements were obtained at two cross-sectional follow-up studies about 6 months apart in 14 patients. **A,** Scattergram of all measurements. **B,** One hypothetical set of measurements in individual patients, with their two measurements connected by the solid lines. In most cases, gradient increased between successive measurements. **C,** Another hypothetical set of measurements in individual patients, connected by the solid lines. In most cases, gradient decreased in between successive measurements. In both *B* and *C,* data points are identical to those shown in *A.*

Assumptions

Assumptions underlying longitudinal models are important to understand. At one time, mixed models demanded repeated values to be measured at identical times for all subjects. As mathematical and statistical developments progressed, flexibility increased. Thus, today, longitudinal data analyses can be employed for data

- observed at haphazard intervals,
- with a differing number of observations (including one) per patient,
- encompassing an observation period of variable length,
- containing missing observations in a sequence of observations, and
- having sequences interrupted by a censoring mechanism, such as death.

This flexibility comes at a price.

The most important price is the assumption that censoring for any reason is noninformative with respect to the outcome being assessed. Although this assumption is similar to that for time-related events, some aspects of longitudinal data make them even more susceptible to bias.[S18] First, it is not hard to imagine settings in which various factors "deplete" availability of longitudinal outcomes in a systematic fashion. For example, if the outcome is NYHA functional status, death interrupts assessment, and it is likely that the sickest patients with highest NYHA class die; the remaining patients may be more robust, leading to the possible inference that results are improving with time. Immunologic sensitization during permanent left ventricular assist device operation may be interrupted by availability of a donor heart sooner than if patients are doing well, or it may postpone transplant longer than usual; thus, degree of sensitization in remaining patients may skew the ensuing estimates up or down. If patients are being followed longitudinally for rhythm after a Maze operation, those with return of atrial fibrillation may be assessed more often than those in sinus rhythm; prevalence of atrial fibrillation may, therefore, appear higher than it actually is. Patients assessed by coronary angiography for recurrent angina often become the basis for assessing longitudinal patency of coronary artery bypass conduits; these patients may not be representative of all patients (estimates are likely to be overly pessimistic). It is questionable whether patients remaining after these mechanisms of censoring are representative of the original group. Biased inferences could result from this *informative censoring.*

Just as Berkson and Gage in the early 1950s found that one should ignore follow-up intervals beyond the point at which about 10% of the original group was followed, we believe that a similar truncation of longitudinal data should be considered.[B4] This does not address, however, an important bias of ascertainment. For example, patients being monitored longitudinally for a disease, or because of a recurrent event (such as return of atrial fibrillation after ablation or recurrent angina after CABG), may be observed more frequently than patients who are deemed to be disease- or symptom-free.

Modulators

Factors modulate longitudinal outcomes just as they do any other type of outcome. Thus, multivariable analysis within the longitudinal analysis domain is necessary. Currently, the facility for such analyses is limited in available statistical software. However, this provides an opportunity to utilize newer algorithmic techniques for risk factor identification, such as random forests.[B38,H15] To temporarily overcome these limitations, at present we perform preliminary analyses under the assumption of independence of observations using available multivariable analysis tools. We then construct the longitudinal models "by hand."

It would also not be surprising if, just as in analysis of time-related events after cardiac surgery, different factors modulate different time frames of longitudinal evolution. To date, a time-decomposition method to accomplish this has not been formulated. Therefore, while such a method is being developed, in attempting to identify factors modulating the longitudinal evolution, interaction between follow-up time and each factor must be examined.

Example

For illustration, Fig. 6-31, *A* is a scattergram of mean pressure gradient measurements from echocardiography across aortic pericardial valves.[B42] Questions asked include (1) What is the behavior pressure gradient across time? (2) What is the influence of prosthesis size? (3) What other factors relate to the gradient? These were opportunistically acquired data points that may contain biases of ascertainment. Further, most patients were dead by 18 years, and some had their prosthesis explanted (censoring mechanisms). Importantly, Fig. 6-31, *B* illustrates that pressure gradients were measured multiple times in some patients. How do we make sense of such data?

Conceptually, imagine modeling each patient's gradient pattern across time, then averaging the individual model parameters to obtain a global pattern. This is a simplistic but useful notion of what the analysis is doing in a more sophisticated fashion. Fig. 6-31, *C,* shows the average response, illustrating the general evolution of mean gradient from the data and the expected differences according to valve size.[B42]

A second example is an ordered categorical outcome in these same valve prosthesis patients: aortic valve regurgitation.[B42] The assumption is that patients progress across time from lower to higher grades of regurgitation (see Fig. 6-12). Think of progression as a series of cascading, leaking containers. Now imagine the first container (grade 0) gradually emptying into the grade 1+ container, which in turn leaks into grade 2+, which leaks into grades 3+ and 4+. Then imagine graphing the level of water in each container as time progresses. This is the conceptual idea behind an ordinal outcome assessment. Aortic regurgitation was assessed at the same time that mean pressure gradients were measured for the patients shown in Fig. 6-31. Some had a single echocardiogram, but many had two or more. Longitudinal data analyses for ordinal outcomes were used to construct the average evolution of aortic regurgitation shown in Fig. 6-32. To provide a sense of visual validation, the proportion of observations in each regurgitation grade for broad time intervals has been superimposed. (For this visual validation, the fact that multiple observations may have been made in the same patient has been ignored, but the analysis shown by the solid lines takes multiple observations into account.)

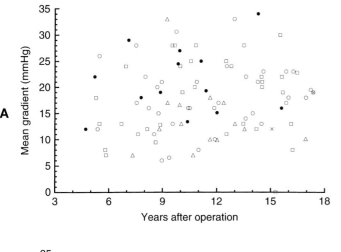

A

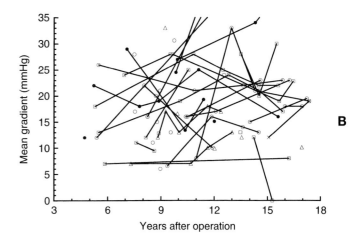

B

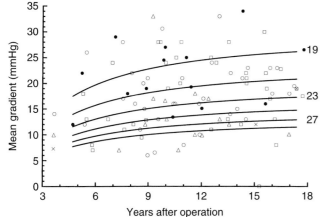

C

Figure 6-31   Mean pressure gradient across stented bovine pericardial aortic valve prostheses estimated by serial echocardiograms, illustrating longitudinal data and their analysis. **A,** Scattergram of individual measurements. Closed circles are for size 19 valves, open circles for size 21, squares for size 23, triangles for size 25, and x for size 29. Mean gradients were not measured for size 27 valves. **B,** Same depiction as in A, but repeated assessments in individual patients are connected. **C,** Average evolution of mean gradient by valve size using longitudinal data analysis. Symbols are as in A. (From Banbury and colleagues.[B42])

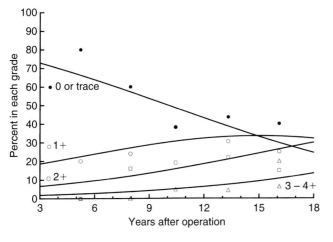

Figure 6-32   Evolution of grade of aortic valve regurgitation across stented bovine pericardial aortic valve prostheses during follow-up, illustrating ordinal longitudinal outcomes data. Symbols for each regurgitation grade represent summary raw data within intervals, ignoring repeated measurements within patients. Closed circles are for grade 0, open circles for grade 1+, squares for grade 2+, and triangles for grades 3+ and 4+ (combined because of sparse information). The smooth lines are model predictions for each regurgitant grade. (From Banbury and colleagues.[B42])

Although the graph has multiple lines and so is somewhat intimidating, the picture portrays how the proportion of patients with a competent prosthesis decreases across time as the number of patients in grade 1+ builds up. Grade 1+ is just beginning to peak at 15 years because few patients remain in grade 0 to enter grade 1+ and other patients are progressing to grade 2+ regurgitation. More severe grades have already begun to develop in a few patients.

A third example from this same data set is progression of ordinal NYHA functional class recorded at yearly follow-up (Fig. 6-33). Note that this depiction censors patients at death; a more reasonable strategy may be to incorporate death as another ordinal category. Other data illustrating the need for the type of analyses just described include NYHA functional class after mitral valve repair (see Fig. 11-24 in Chapter 11) and assessment of mitral transvalvar gradient (see Fig. 11-25 in Chapter 11).

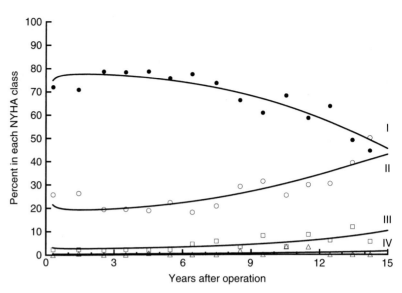

Figure 6-33 Evolution of New York Heart Association (NYHA) functional class across time in the Premarket Approval cohort (*n* = 267) of a bovine pericardial aortic valve prosthesis, illustrating ordinal longitudinal data. Symbols represent the percentage of patients in each class in 1-year intervals. Closed circles = NYHA class I, open circles = class II, squares = class III, and triangles = class IV. In this depiction, death is a censoring mechanism. Solid lines are the solution for an ordinal logistic longitudinal repeated-measures model with only time as a variable. (From Banbury and colleagues.[B42])

Key: *NYHA,* New York Heart Association.

SECTION 5
Use of Knowledge

TRANSFORMING STATISTICAL INFERENCES INTO CLINICAL INFERENCES

Statistical inferences focus on interpreting the magnitude and variability of parameter estimates, reliability of numeric results, summary statistics, behavior of confidence limits, *P* values, and many other numeric results. The data truly speak through these results, often revealing what is important and what is not. However, numeric information often does not lead to the kind of mental picture or overview of the data that is needed to generate new knowledge. There must be a view of the forest. Something further is therefore needed to translate statistical inferences into clinical inferences and new knowledge.

One of the most powerful tools to accomplish this is graphics.[K18] An important reason for our using and even developing completely parametric models was that they so easily allow graphics to be generated in the form of *nomograms,* as advocated by the Framingham investigators.[G32] For example, if an analysis indicates an association of survival with age, we want to know what the shape of that relationship is. Is it relatively flat for a broad spectrum of age and then rapidly increasing at either extreme of age? Or does risk increase rather linearly with age? Although the answers to these questions are contained within the numbers on computer printouts, these numbers are not easily assimilated by the mind. However, they can be used to demonstrate graphically the shape of the age relation with all other factors held constant (see "Risk Adjustment" in Section 6).

Because graphics are so powerful in the process of generating new knowledge, an important responsibility is placed on the statistician to be sure that relations are correct. Often, variables are examined and statistical inferences made simply to determine whether a continuous variable is a risk factor, without paying particular attention to what the data convey regarding the shape of the relationship to outcome. Instead, the statistician needs to focus during analysis on transformations of scale that may be needed to faithfully depict the relationship (see "Multivariable Analysis" in Section 4). Our experience indicates that most relations of continuous variables with outcome are smooth. They do not show sharp cut-offs (see "Continuity versus Discontinuity in Nature" in Section 1), although they may well show evident differences (see Appendix 6C).

Use of Incremental Risk Factors

Multivariable analysis identifies *incremental risk factors* for *outcomes,* and this provides one form of new knowledge. The risk factors identified are sometimes proclaimed by cardiac surgeons and others to be "truly independent," suggesting that such a risk factor is independent of the action of any other risk factor in exerting its influence. Such is not the case, and this idea is not the origin of the use of the adjective "independent." An independent variable is simply one that may be associated with the dependent (outcome) variable (see Box 6-18). Draper and Smith state, "The words 'independent variables' must not be too literally interpreted. In a particular body of data, two or more independent variables may vary together in some definite way."[D3]

In addition to generating specific new knowledge by identifying risk factors for an outcome, multivariable analysis (see Box 6-18) can be used for *patient-specific predictions and comparisons* of outcomes after competing forms of therapy[K9] (see "Patient-Specific Predictions and Comparisons in Ischemic Heart Disease," Appendix B in Chapter 7). Risk-adjusted comparisons can be made of the results of different surgeons, different interventional cardiologists, different methods, and different institutions (see "Risk Adjustment" in Section 6).[H9,K9,K10] Multivariable analysis for these purposes is usually best performed in a parsimonious manner.

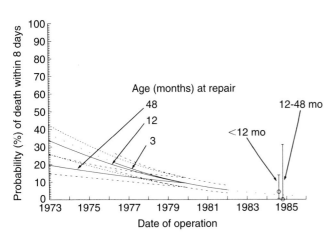

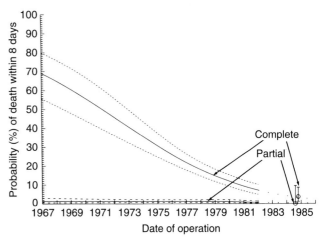

Figure 6-34   Illustration of prediction from multivariable models. Observed hospital mortality after repair (1984 to September 1985) of isolated complete atrioventricular septal defects in patients younger than age 12 months (*n* = 23, deaths = 1) and in those age 12 to 48 months (*n* = 5, deaths = 0). Note that both observed mortalities (circles) and their confidence limits (CL; vertical bars) lie within the 70% CLs of the mortality predicted for the repair by the multivariable equation derived from the 1967 to 1982 experience. (From Kirklin and colleagues.[K23])

Figure 6-35   Illustration of prediction when risk factors modulate and neutralize one another. Observed hospital mortality after repair (1984 to September 1985) of complete and partial atrioventricular septal defects with or without major associated cardiac anomalies; observed mortality is shown as open circles, and vertical bars represent 70% confidence limits (CL). Note that these observed mortalities lie on the nomogram lines representing a solution of the multivariable equation. Solid line represents 8-day mortality, and dashed lines enclose 70% CLs. The widely dotted depiction extends the solid line of probability estimate into a time period (1982 to 1986) not included in the experience used for derivation of the equations and coefficients. (From Kirklin and colleagues.[K23])

Multivariable analysis of clinical experiences can also be used to investigate the nature of cardiac surgery for a specific situation, such as transposition of the great arteries or the postcardiopulmonary bypass state. For such purposes a series of *sequential analyses* are often useful, rather than a single analysis performed in a parsimonious manner. In sequential analysis, often the patient-specific potential risk factors are first examined and the multivariable equation for the outcome event generated.[B37,K22] Then, the procedural variables may be entered and their effect on the certainty and strength of the patient-specific variables studied. New ideas then generate reanalyses, reevaluation of the correlations between risk factors, and additional new analyses.

Multivariable analysis can also be used to examine and interpret the way one risk factor *modulates influence* on outcome of another. One such use is to determine if a risk factor, such as age, is neutralized with experience (Fig. 6-34; see Appendix 6D). Another is to determine if treatments modulate some risk factor differently from another (interaction terms) (Fig. 6-35).

All of this emphasizes the care with which all multivariable analyses must be made.[B24] Good, reliable, and valid analyses are not made by computers alone, but by people using computers expertly as just one tool of analysis and synthesis.

SCIENTIFIC PAPER

A scientific paper is a formal communication of new knowledge generated by a scientific study. Unlike most other forms of communication, it has all the following elements:

- It is in the public domain and not proprietary.
- It is objective.
- It presents sufficient information to allow verification elsewhere.
- It builds on what has been previously discovered.
- It predicts what should subsequently transpire in an orderly universe.
- It is not written with just authority as its basis, but rather, with information, data, and analyses at its core.
- It does not intuit or pass along traditions, but draws inferences and relates these to the context of past investigations.
- It is a formally structured communication.

The structure of a scientific paper is said to have been formalized by Louis Pasteur, who established the "IMRD" format for reporting scientific information: *Introduction, Methods, Results, Discussion.*[D14,H20,U1] This format has been codified into requirements of all scientific journals.[U1] It provides a valuable structure for thinking about, and expressing clearly, the findings of one's research.

Rarely is the progress from research proposal (see Box 6-6) to scientific paper (formatted according to this formal structure) linear.[B37] That is, the paper, written on the basis of what has been discovered from the investigation, likely cannot simply reflect the original study proposal. The best way, then, to begin writing a scientific paper is to study intently the descriptive statistics, results of the various analyses, tabular results, and graphical depictions from the analyses, allowing "the data to speak for themselves."

One should then write the truest two or three sentences (50 words maximum) that capture the essence of the findings.[K15] Only if one can simply and succinctly state the findings and what they mean will one be able to convey them clearly to the reader. By experimentation, we found that if the essence can be stated adequately in fewer than 25 words, the paper may have low information content and should be conveyed as a brief communication or letter to the editor. If it cannot be stated in 25 to 50 words, there may be information overload, and the study should be split into more than one manuscript, each focused on a different aspect of the results.

Once the essence is written, the entire manuscript—tables, figures, and text—should be sharply focused on those results that are supportive. Other information should be either relegated to appendices (for the aficionado) or eliminated altogether.[K17,K18,K20] This process has been termed "boiling and distilling." We recommend assembling all this material into a small notebook, with tabs for notes, the original research protocol, key literature, reports of analyses, tables, figures, manuscript, revised manuscript, and presentation.

The next step is to write a clear statement of purpose of the study. Although this has been the most important aspect of the original research proposal, it now must be refined and either limited or expanded to include the one, two, or three aspects of the study that led to the essence of the findings.[K19] For example, your original research purpose may have been to discover any possible adverse effect of reoperation for bleeding on hospital outcomes. However, to investigate this properly, you likely would have determined the prevalence of postoperative bleeding and incremental risk factors associated with bleeding, perhaps then using these to develop a propensity score so that an apples-to-apples comparison could be made of outcomes in patients who did and did not require reoperation. Thus, for the manuscript, the stated purpose may be (1) to determine the prevalence of postoperative bleeding, (2) to identify incremental risk factors for postoperative bleeding, and (3) to compare the prevalence of hospital complications between those who experienced bleeding and those who did not. These purposes would constitute the last part of the introduction, preceded by a paragraph simply setting the context of the study or stating the controversy. (A mistake many writers make is to confuse the function of an introduction with that of a discussion or an exhaustive review of the literature.[K19])

Given a clear message for the paper (the 50-word essence) and a clear statement of purpose or purposes that will support that essential message, it becomes rather easy to organize subsequent sections of the paper (Patients and Methods, Results, and Discussion) to exactly follow the organization suggested by the purposes (using identical words each time).[B37] In this way, the manuscript stays focused, supporting material is highlighted, and triage of extraneous information is facilitated.

Coupled with initial manuscript writing, a decision should be made regarding the appropriate audience and, therefore, journal for the paper. As general rules, manuscripts of interest to a broad spectrum of medicine should be targeted to general medical journals; those that should be read by both cardiologists and cardiac surgeons should be targeted to general cardiologic journals; those that

should be read by cardiac surgeons should be targeted to cardiac surgical journals.

When the manuscript has been completed, one may be tempted to send it to a journal immediately. The quality of the manuscript, however, can be improved considerably by allowing it to sit on the shelf for a time. After a few weeks, review the manuscript afresh from beginning to end, along with comments that may have been made by co-authors. By this time, three things have happened. First, you have distanced yourself just a bit from the manuscript and can see its possible deficiencies more clearly. Second, the passage of time has allowed your unconscious mind to work on the material, and by the time the manuscript is revisited, this process has provided further insights and clarity. Third, you have had the opportunity to present the material intramurally and have received valuable feedback. In other words, the work has matured. (In addition, the manuscript shelf provides the best possible resource for abstracts for upcoming scientific meetings.)

The next important step is to respond to peer review of the manuscript. Some authors become despondent and never revise and return their paper. Others decide to send the original manuscript to another journal, ignoring the peer review, which is wasteful of reviewers' time and expertise. Others respond defensively, making little change in the manuscript. Instead, this important phase of generating new knowledge should be viewed as an essential exercise to improve the manuscript. Sometimes it will require performing new analyses or gathering new information. If some point is confusing to a reviewer, and particularly if it is confusing to more than one, or if the reviewers have completely missed the point, simplification and clarity are needed. Rethink the purposes, structure the paper anew, move overly detailed material from the text to appendices, construct new tables and simplify others, prepare more intuitive graphics, or state things more clearly and logically. The peer review process may delay publication for some days to weeks, but as a whole, it functions superbly to improve the quality of papers.

Presentations

The best possible preparation for writing and submitting a meeting abstract and for subsequently presenting the findings is to have completed a well-crafted manuscript. There is no substitute for this.

If it is not possible to complete all analyses and to prepare a manuscript, at least enough of this must be done so that the essence of the findings is known, the purpose of the study is clear, and the conclusions are supported.

It is common practice to use meeting abstract deadlines either to drive the research process or to serve as a triage function for bouncing half-formulated and partially analyzed data off reviewers; if the paper is not accepted, the research is not pursued. This is not serious clinical research. It also represents a lack of understanding of the process whereby papers are accepted for presentations at meetings. For example, if there are two excellent abstracts submitted by two groups on the same subject, one may be taken and the other not; it would be a mistake for the submitter of the rejected abstract to conclude that the work is unworthy! A poor abstract may be the only abstract submitted on a subject that is deemed to be needed for a well-rounded meeting, so it is accepted. An entire category of abstracts may be jettisoned because there is no room for them on the program. Other abstracts, because of the excellent way they are crafted, are accepted, but the work is of less than stellar quality when presented.

A meeting abstract does not serve the same function as the abstract for a scientific paper. Its purpose is to get the work onto a program. Thus, crafting a meeting abstract is an art. The title must be eye-catching. Such a title may not be appropriate for a manuscript, but it is the first thing the graders will see. Second, the purposes and conclusions of the abstract must be clear and must match one to one. The purposes and conclusions may be all that is read before the abstract is discarded! If there is a gripping title, clear and interesting purposes, and new conclusions, the abstract graders will read the methods and results sections. There is no sense in including detailed methods that are well known; instead, focus on those that (1) succinctly define the patient sample, (2) address each purpose, and (3) make the study novel or more valid than other work in the field. Results are usually less detailed than for a manuscript abstract, highlighting just those numeric findings that relate to the purposes. A well-crafted table, or especially a seminal figure, often speaks louder than words and may constitute nearly the entire results section. Clearly, then, a well-crafted meeting abstract is inappropriate as the abstract for the manuscript itself. Never confuse the two.

If the presentation is accepted, the most important preparation is to remember that the listener will hear it serially. He or she cannot go back to review the material; there is no second chance to determine if your progression of thought is logical or to study a table or figure in detail. The classic IMRD format for a scientific paper is not conducive to serial aural disclosure!

Elements, then, of a good presentation are more like those of a good speech than a good scientific paper.[P14] At the outset, you must *capture the attention of the audience*. This can be accomplished, for example, by illustrating the nature of the problem that is the object of the presentation. This may be a clinical example, an echocardiogram, a picture of a pathologic specimen, or a statement of controversy. The *purposes* of the research can then be presented, followed by a simple depiction of the characteristics of the patients being studied. The temptation will now be to present methods, followed by results and discussion. This should be resisted. Instead, as you *present evidence* ("let the data speak for themselves"), weave in methodology for obtaining the data and results of analysis if essential. Generally, however, very little presentation of methodology is necessary for clinical studies, and the time restrictions preclude lengthy description. Results should be presented *extraordinarily simply*. Typically, slides (generally computer-generated presentation frames) should contain only one idea and as few words as possible. Graphics should be clean, clear, with a cryptic descriptive title, large numerals on axes, and simple lines. They must be *seen clearly* in the back of the room, and these days they must survive the severe pixelation of internet broadcast.

At the end of the presentation, it is common for speakers simply to summarize the results. But if the presentation has been logical and has focused primarily on results, there is *little need for recapitulation*. It is better to spend the last portion of the presentation on the *clinical inferences* that you have drawn from the study. Leave the audience with the essence of your findings ("the message") and what it should mean to them and to their patients.

Finally, never plan to give a presentation without writing the manuscript, preferably prior to submission of the abstract. Presentations are soon forgotten, or are remembered but not retrievable, because the presenter has never pushed the study through to publication.

DECISION SUPPORT

Publication is a static medium. However, most analyses generate mathematical models that, at least in theory, can be solved for the characteristics of a specific patient (*patient-specific predictions*), complete with confidence limits. Figures in Appendix 7B in Chapter 7 illustrate how these equations can be used to predict survival for specific patients were they to be initially managed medically, surgically, or by percutaneous intervention. Used in this way, static presentation of "risk factors" becomes a basis for dynamic decision support for individual patients.

The most important impediment to using equations resulting from clinical research data analysis is lack of the CPR (see "Computer-based Patient Record" in Section 2). If such systems were in place to provide values for variables in the course of working up a patient, they could be automatically inserted into appropriate equations, the equations solved, and the solutions displayed. These results could then be used by physicians for making recommendations about the most appropriate course of treatment, and also by patients as a best basis for informed consent.

It will be argued that medical and surgical treatment are changing so rapidly that no data from the past are relevant for today's decision support; at best, general guidelines and judgment are all that is available. However, this gives more credit to new therapy than most medical and surgical innovations deserve. Further, a decision must be made, and making it on the basis of past data is likely to be less faulty than using no data at all.

In most places in the world today, the resources available for cardiac operations are insufficient to treat every patient potentially amenable to this kind of intervention. Thus, a process of *triage* (the sorting process used by military surgeons during combat) is consciously or unconsciously used to allocate resources among the patients most likely to benefit.[B11] Again, such decisions are best made when the potential benefits can be described factually and with knowledge of the degree of uncertainty attached to the conclusions. The special circumstances of each patient and the need for continued probing into the possibility and methods of extending and improving the results of cardiac surgery must also form part of each patient care decision.

To improve surgical outcome, errors (both active and latent) must be reduced and scientific progress made. Errors can be reduced by various mechanisms of decision support, particularly obvious pharmaceutical errors. Error reduction in the operating room may be reduced by the vigilance suggested in "Human Error" in Section 1.

Some surgical failures are related to inadequacies in the decision-making process for an individual patient, either as a result of human error or lack of scientific progress. For example, deciding not to operate on a patient whose risks without operation are known to be significantly greater than those with operation is a human error; deciding to operate on a patient whose risk of an early fatal outcome is known with considerable certainty is also an error.

Analysis of clinical information, either by use of risk-adjusted information from applying benchmarks (see "Risk Stratification" in Section 6) or by formal analysis of surgical experience, yields risk factors that may be amenable to neutralization (see Appendix 6D).

Decision-Making for Individual Patients

When cardiac operation is advised, it is in anticipation of cure or palliation. In either case, operation should be recommended only when life expectancy and functional capacity are predicted to be better with operation than without. Thus, each patient care decision involves a comparison, and the comparison should be made with full knowledge of the degree of uncertainty imposed by the available data and their analysis.[B18] In fact, one goal of research is providing this information for decision-making in as many areas of cardiac surgery as possible and with as high a degree of certainty as possible.

When patients fall into defined categories for which reliable information is available, individual patient care decisions can be made largely on the basis of prior appropriate comparisons of the options. That is, the option can be chosen that has been shown to result in the lowest hospital mortality, the highest long-term survival, and the least incidence of reoperation in similar patients. One of the goals of this book is to present data in sufficient detail to be useful for most individual patient care decisions. However, decision-making is not always easy. Indeed, some decisions that may appear easy in fact are not. This is when solution of equations using a patient's specific characteristics becomes valuable.

When reliable information is not available or the options being considered are different from those that have been studied, the same principles can be used, but only anecdotal information, judgments, and general knowledge of the area are available as a basis for the decision. Obviously, the degree of uncertainty is considerably greater. In such situations, a proper clinical study of some type is needed to generate the information desired.

SECTION 6 ▊▊▊▊▊▊
Special Methods and Controversies

RISK STRATIFICATION

The goal of risk stratification is to account broadly for differences in patient characteristics that affect outcomes of interest. These include cost of health care services and outcomes that have been selected to reflect institutional

quality[S6,S7] (clinical report cards[D19,I2,S21]). Risk stratification can be used for profiling practices or to develop guidelines and indications for procedures.

There are two general approaches to risk stratification: risk scores and risk equations.

Risk Scores

Primarily in the older literature, risk scores were reported that were based partly on data and partly on expert opinion.[H21,P10] These have a common feature: *addition of risks*. Those that understand probability theory will immediately notice that the logistic equation, by virtue of the exponential function, is a *multiplicative function* of risk factors (see Fig. 6-1, *A* and Box 6-5).[H22] Even today, investigators attempt to develop "modern" additive risk scores, claiming that busy physicians can add but not multiply![H22]

Unless a score is specifically calibrated to outcome, it is useful merely for risk stratification, not for calculation of absolute risk.

The initial use of risk scores was to broadly classify patient mix according to outcome, usually into a small number of groups with increasing risk (see "Classification Methods" later in this section). Subsequently, however, they have been used as a basis for reimbursement, quality assessment, and institutional comparisons rather than generation of new knowledge. Therefore, they have been simultaneously welcomed and distrusted. What is likely true is that they perform well for risk stratifying typical patients, but poorly for patients at the extremes of low and high risk.

Risk Equations

Multivariable analysis is used to develop risk equations, usually by logistic regression. The equation is used to calculate absolute risk of events in a group of patients (such as those from an institutional experience), or the calculation may be left in terms of logit units as a type of quantitative score. Patients can then be sorted according to increasing probability score for risk stratification.

Use of multivariable analysis for risk stratification was anticipated by Gordon and Kannel in the Framingham study when they wrote, "In the multivariate case it is possible to make statements for one variable which are invariant whatever the values assumed by the other variables. This makes it possible to estimate the net effect of one variable taking into account the effect of other related variables."[G7]

If equations are used, the distinction between risk stratification (grouping) and risk adjustment (placing patients on a level playing field) becomes blurred.

RISK ADJUSTMENT

Risk adjustment has been used in two senses. In both, a formal statistical multivariable model has been generated and then used in a predictive fashion. In the first, predictions are made in which a single variable is explored in relation to outcome while all other variables are held constant. This technique is an essential part of clinical research, and we have termed such depictions *nomograms*.

The second use is part of a process whereby two or more protocols, procedures, surgeons, physicians, or institutions with patient populations that are to some extent heterogeneous are *compared with regard to outcome*. A multivariable risk factor equation is used to generate hypothetical patient populations that are identical except for the variables being compared (leveling the playing field).

To generate the risk factor equation, a large group of patients representing all the subgroups being compared (such as institutions) are pooled, and a multivariable analysis of the pooled data is performed in which the subgroups themselves may or may not be variables. From a statistical point of view, it would seem ideal to assess subgroups such as institutions within the context of the analysis. This could include exploration of specific interaction of subgroups with other variables, and other investigations that might yield important insight into institutional variance. This has been done, for example, in the context of the Congenital Heart Surgeons Society.[K10] More commonly, subgroups are ignored completely when generating a generic overall equation that will be applied to them subsequently. This is the strategy behind the Society of Thoracic Surgeons Database[S19] and the EuroSCORE.[N10]

Technique of Risk Adjustment

After the risk factor equation is generated, it is typically used as follows. Characteristics of each patient in a subgroup (institution, country) are inserted into the regression equation, and the equation is solved to yield the absolute predicted risk of the outcome of interest for each patient. These individual probabilities are added to yield *expected outcome*. Expected outcome is then compared to *actual outcome*.

The theory behind this technique is this. When estimates of the weights (the βs, coefficients, or parameter estimates; see Box 6-5) are generated by maximum likelihood estimation, events are conserved. *Conservation of events* is, in statistics, analogous to conservation of mass in biochemistry. Specifically, if, for the patients used to generate the equation, the probability of the event is calculated, the sum is guaranteed to equal the total number of events that actually occurred. If for some subgroup of patients this sum deviates from actual, then either unaccounted-for factors have not been included in the risk factor equation or the subgroup is behaving differently from the average.[H8]

Comparison Statistic

One statistic that may be used to compare observed (O) and expected (E) number of events in a subgroup of n patients is the chi-square goodness-of-fit test. A value for chi-square (χ^2) is obtained from the formula:

$$\chi_1^2 = \frac{n(O-E)^2}{E(n-E)}$$

$$(6\text{-}20)$$

A P value is obtained from a chi-square table or computer program equivalent.

DeLong and colleagues have studied eight methods for comparing observed and expected outcomes, focusing particularly on fairness in judging a subgroup to be an "outlier."[D15] Treasure and colleagues have developed a highly sophisticated method of using risk-adjusted CUSUM charts to continuously monitor deviation of individual institution programs from the norm.[L20,S20]

Illustrations of Risk Assessment

Risk adjustment by multivariable analysis can be illustrated as follows. Hospital A experienced 18 (8.3%) hospital deaths among 205 patients undergoing mitral valve replacement, while hospital B experienced 16 (2.6%) hospital deaths among 612 patients undergoing the same operation. The P *value* for the difference is <.0001, so the difference is unlikely to be due to chance alone.

Hospital A believes the difference is attributable to a more severe case mix, while hospital B believes it reflects a difference in expertise. Using a risk-adjustment equation that accounts for NYHA functional class, age, left ventricular size, and other factors, a probability of death is computed for each patient by solving the logistic equation, using the patient's specific values for each of the risk factors. The 205 probabilities for hospital A are summed and found to total 11.07, the number of expected deaths (if divided by 205, this yields 5.4%). The difference between expected deaths (11.07) and observed deaths (18) is unlikely to be due to chance alone, $P = .03$.

This is equivalent to saying that if the patients in hospital A had been operated on in hospital B, their mortality would have been 5.4%, not 8.3%. We could ask for the hospital mortality had B's patients been operated on at hospital A. We already know that hospital A had a higher actual than expected mortality and that actual divided by expected mortality equals 1.6. This ratio quantifies the difference in what could be called the expertise of the two institutions. This means that had hospital B's patients been operated on at hospital A, there would have been more deaths, specifically, 1.6 times 16, or 26 deaths; 26 deaths among 612 patients is a mortality of 4.3%. This is what the state of New York has termed *risk-adjusted mortality* (the state as a whole is analogous to hospital B), an index it uses to rank hospitals.[H9]

Controversies

Naturally, different risk adjustment equations yield different estimates of expected events.[B50,W12] In addition, the variables used in developing the risk equation—administrative, laboratory, or clinical—make a difference.[I1] Even more important is the number of risk factors in the risk equation (richness, depth).[S9,T5] Probabilities for patients with a large number or unusual combination of risk factors—the very patients for whom we want risk adjustment—are systematically underestimated.[S9]

Residual Risk

A valuable adjunct to risk adjustment methodology is *analysis of residual risk*. In analysis of residual risk, the risk score for each patient is calculated. For logistic regression, this is the logit of the probability of the event; for Cox proportional hazards modeling, it is the sum of the weighted risk factors; for hazard function regression, it is the sum of the weighted factors in each hazard phase (see Box 6-5). These are forced into the model, and a search is made for risk factors not accounted for by the risk score or for factors in the risk score that are either underweighted or overweighted.[S9]

For example, Sergeant and colleagues studied 3720 patients prospectively, applying a previously published time-related equation to generate a survival curve for each.[A5,S9,S22] The patients were subsequently followed up and comparison made of actual and expected survival (see Fig. 6-2, *A*). Estimated survival was too optimistic. Therefore, an analysis of residual risk was performed. Five residual risk factors were found, falling into three categories:

- Two factors had been suspected in the original analysis, but they occurred so infrequently that reliable parameter estimates could not be computed.
- Two variables were related to preoperative atrial and ventricular rhythm disturbances. These data had been available for the original analysis, but the investigator ignored them because he thought they were unimportant.
- The fifth variable identified a patient subset that had not been represented at all (extended indication) in the original data set.

These residual risk factors accounted for only a small fraction of the new patient group, but a group whose risk was vastly underestimated (see Fig. 6-2, *B,* and Table 6-2).

This experience has driven us to the opinion that clinically rich models, rather than simple ones, are required for accurate risk adjustment. The factors liable to lead to risk underestimation are (1) rare factors, (2) factors that are important but not included in models, and (3) factors related to subgroups for whom indication for operation has been extended beyond that of patients included in developing the models.

META-ANALYSIS

Definition

Meta-analysis combines or integrates the results of multiple independently conducted clinical trials, observational clinical studies, or sets of individual patient data that are deemed combinable with respect to a common research question, then analyzes them statistically.[G20] Other terms for meta-analysis are *quantitative overview, pooling studies, systematic review,* and *quantitative synthesis.* The root of the prefix "meta" means *later in time.*

Historical Note

There is a nearly 300-year history of using statistical methods to draw inferences broader than any individual study from a combined analysis of results. In 1722, Cotes used weighted averages to combine measurements of different astronomical observers.[C23] In 1805, Legendre introduced the now familiar method of least squares, used in linear regression (see Box 6-5), for similar synthesis. In 1904, Pearson averaged five different estimates of *correlation* because "many of the groups . . . are far too small to allow any definite opinion being formed."[P12] In 1931, Trippett combined

P values.[T4] In 1937 and 1938, Cochran and Yates combined results of agricultural experiments.[C24,Y1]

Beecher is credited as having performed the first medical meta-analysis in 1955, but the appropriate methodology developed primarily in educational research.[B46] In 1976, Glass coined the term meta-analysis to mean "the analysis of analyses."[G20] Most of the statistical procedures used today were introduced at that time in the social sciences.

In 1993, clinicians, epidemiologists, statisticians, and other professionals joined together to prepare, maintain, and discriminate comprehensive and systematic reviews of health-related questions. This was called the Cochran collaboration.[B45,C25]

Motivation

Motivations for meta-analysis are to

- Increase sample size and thereby better protect against either (1) misplaced enthusiasm for positive results (type I error) or (2) failure to find a beneficial effect (type II error)
- Detect small effects (or exclude small effects more definitively)
- Detect bias of reporting multiple, possibly underpowered, trials (positive results of trials tend to be reported more frequently than negative ones)
- Make better use of studies performed independently by synthesizing the results
- Suggest the most promising avenue for future research on a subject and the sample size likely needed to study the question definitively
- Formalize the review process of past studies, including independent assessment of study quality by individuals not associated with the original studies
- Determine whether "enough is enough" and no further corroborative studies are needed to establish a relation
- Corroborate, refute, or modify evidence-based medical guidelines that emanate from expert opinion and literature review rather than from statistical analysis of data

Types

Meta-analyses may be categorized according to (1) type of analyses assembled and (2) type of data gathered. The types of analyses assembled may be only randomized clinical trials, only observational clinical studies, or a combination of the two.[E13] Just as any clinical study, there is a presumed hierarchy of quality; generally, preference is given to randomized clinical trials.

Type of data used in a meta-analysis may be (1) summary (aggregated) statistics or (2) raw individual patient data from each trial or study, the highest level of quality.[O4] The latter is considered to be the most time-consuming and politically most difficult to perform, because investigators are often wary (and rightly so) of relinquishing their raw data to a third party.[S17]

Conduct

Because the design of a meta-analysis is that of an *observational study of accumulated evidence* from prior investigations, a rigorous plan for conducting the study must be put into place.[G21] Elements of conduct include the following:

- Formulating the question to be addressed, without which comparability of studies cannot be assessed
- Establishing criteria for studies to be included and excluded
- Identifying all relevant studies
- Assessing the quality of each study
- Establishing a rigorous protocol for data extraction, including calculations necessary for putting all data into a standard format on a uniform scale
- Extracting and verifying data
- Diagnosing bias and sensitivity to inclusion and exclusion criteria to be sure the analysis should proceed further
- Analyzing the analyses, generally using mixed (hierarchical) models that account for fixed and random effects at various levels of aggregation (see "Longitudinal Outcomes" in Section 4)

In calculating an overall effect from multiple studies, the simple arithmetic average gives misleading results. Specifically, small studies have more scatter by chance alone and should be weighted less than large studies. Proper analyses can be broadly grouped into two approaches that differ only in the way variability among studies is managed: (1) fixed effects models that assume variability is simply random variation and (2) random effects models that assume a different mechanism of variation for each study. Tests of heterogeneity of variation may be used to assess which model may be more applicable. Ideally, features of each study, such as gender ratio, publication date, patient status, and age, can be incorporated into the analysis. Such a model has both fixed and random effects.[L18] Details of these and other considerations are found in the now abundant literature on the topic.[B15]

We enumerate these points of study conduct to emphasize that meta-analysis is a disciplined, rigorous, and often statistically challenging type of observational study. In the cardiac surgical literature, including some publications cited in this book, less rigorous methods have been used to synthesize multiple independent, but related, analyses. In the future, attention to meta-analytic techniques will be necessary to raise the quality of such syntheses.

Limitations

Shortly after its introduction, Eysenck declared meta-analysis "mega-silliness."[E11] Similar skepticism or outright disdain has been voiced in medicine.[B44,M17] These attitudes are based on such findings as two separate meta-analyses of the same subject coming to diametrically opposite conclusions[L17,N8] and the contradiction of meta-analysis results by a large randomized trial.[E10,E12]

Perhaps surprisingly, limitations of meta-analyses are not different in kind from those of observational clinical studies. First, they require an extremely focused question, without which it is not possible to assess combinability of studies. It may be found that, in fact, there are no truly combinable studies for some topics of interest, or that there are too few studies to achieve sufficient statistical power to

determine from diagnostic testing whether the studies are combinable (heterogeneity).

Second, it may be difficult to assemble the entire literature on a well-framed question. Medical libraries are generally more successful in doing this than physicians using search engines. References in identified articles must be found. In the process, it is common to uncover either wholly duplicate publications or some overlap that may be challenging to pull apart. Even a thorough search will not correct for confounding from publication bias that favors large studies, positive results, and mainstream topics.

Third, different meta-analyses may produce conflicting results, depending on thoroughness of the search and evaluation of applicability and combinability. These represent forms of selection bias over and above publication bias.

Fourth, there are limitations of data. One would like to adjust the analysis for multiple variables, but often the number of variables in common across studies is small. This is why combining individual data with many variables in common leads to the most robust estimates.[B15,O4]

Finally, there are limitations in methodology, variance in professional skill and experience in using the methodology, and potential problems in both data presentation and interpretation.

CLASSIFICATION METHODS

Classification methods encompass a group of mathematical, computer science, and statistical methods that will become of increasing importance in analysis of clinical experiences. Classification methods can be used in a number of ways for the following:

- Predicting outcome
- Identifying risk factors
- Classifying disease

Predicting Outcome

One motivation for using classification methods to predict outcome is to answer the question, "Who will experience the event (and when)?" Conventional methodology is focused on probabilities, not "who" and "when." Nevertheless, any method that more accurately identifies patients at risk is valuable. The methods include neural networks,[L11,R8] which have largely been replaced by a host of machine learning techniques,[H15] multivariable optimal discriminant analysis,[Y3] and more recent additions to the arsenal such as logical analysis of data (LAD), which is a purely mathematical technique.[A6] However, to date it is not clear that these methods outperform the standard regression approaches outlined in this chapter.[E8,L21]

Identifying Risk Factors

Risk factor identification is surely a classification problem: A variable is a risk factor or it is not. Enormous strides have been made in machine learning (see "Multivariable Analysis" in Section 4) for this and other classification problems.[H15] Prominent among current researchers in this area are Jerome Friedman and colleagues at Stanford University and Leo Brieman at the University of California, Berkeley.[B38,B51,B52,H15] Their work addresses the instability of a single multivariable analysis of a single set of data, using resampling and other adaptive methods to arrive at a believable set of variables that can be claimed as risk factors.

Classifying Disease

Classification and regression tree (CART)[B52] and recursive partitioning analyses[Z1] have been particularly useful in devising simple classifications for cancer. Thus, they would seem ideal for risk stratification, not just disease classification. Their limitation until recently has been their two-dimensionality, which has changed with introduction of a much wider spectrum of machine learning techniques, such

as *random forests*.[B38] In particular, these techniques will be important for identifying genomic footprints of heart disease, as detailed by Brieman.[B38]

Limitations

A temporary limitation of many machine learning techniques is that they either require data in dichotomous format or split continuous variables into optimal classes, rather than treating them as a continuum. This, and certain assembly of forests, trees, and leaves, at times produces results that defy continuity in nature and represents local properties of a specific data set and not generalizable information, in part because it may be assumed that the leaves are independent. Thus, interpreting the result to generate new knowledge may be complex.

APPENDIXES

APPENDIX 6A
Knowledge Generating Team

Serious clinical research in cardiac surgery can be accomplished, no doubt, by the cardiac surgeon alone. Individual cases can be reported (case reports) with keen insight. Data can be entered and tallied with both simple calculators and user-friendly statistical software such as SPSS *(http://www.spss.com)*.

More commonly, though, a surgeon or full-time clinical investigator will be either the leader of, or the medical expert for, a small to medium-sized research team. With the growing sophistication of data management and analytic tools, it becomes necessary to assemble a research group with varied roles and expertise, all focused on the goals of clinical investigation.

Structure
Regardless of whether the same individuals are involved, clinical research generally includes two fundamentally different activities: (1) continuous registry and database activity (see Box 6-1) and (2) individual clinical studies activity. The *registry activity* involves gathering and entering data for a prescribed set of core data elements for every case. Until the advent of effective computer-based patient record (CPR) systems in the form of values for variables (rather than narrative) that contain the life history of a patient, at least some portions of a registry or database will have to be extracted from medical records (see "Computer-based Patient Record" in Section 2).[D11] *Individual clinical studies activity* can be categorized roughly into two classes that require different skill sets: (1) clinical trials (either intramurally funded or extramurally sponsored by government or industry) and (2) studies of clinical experience (cohort studies).

Roles
Surgeon–investigator
The surgeon (clinical) investigator, with collaboration of key individuals in data management, statistics, and study coordination, must develop the clinical question (aims, objectives), define the study group of interest, identify variables and end points (outcomes) of interest, review the literature, and develop all elements of a study protocol (see "Technique for Successful Clinical Research" in Section 1). He or she must adjudicate data quality, often gather values for variables in addition to the core data elements, help interpret the analyses performed, present the findings to colleagues, and write manuscripts.

Data manager
There is no more key support person than the data manager. He or she is at the interface between data gathering and data analysis. Assembly of data for meaningful analysis is often complex, requiring information to be retrieved from a variety of electronic sources. Data managers usually need formal training in computer science and specifically in database construction and management. They must master an effective data query language.

Their most valuable skill, however, perhaps inborn rather than developed, is attention to the smallest detail of the data. Surgeons are usually not of the temperament for this kind of work, and statisticians by training are "big-picture" oriented; if surgeons see the forest, data managers must see the trees. Thus, data management is not simply skill in formulating databases, writing and executing query logic, and documenting these in detail (although these are important); rather, it is skill in examining the actual data, finding errors in them, finding inconsistencies and deviation from the norm that should be verified, verifying what appear as outliers, and assessing the quality of data for every variable.

The surgeon and data manager then together organize the variables in a way that is meaningful for analysis. If time-related or longitudinal outcomes are being assessed, we recommend that the data manager become expert in forming intervals and assessing time-related data (time zero, events, intervals), two of the most demanding and essential tasks for such analyses.

Part of the data management team is the statistical programmer, who must convert data from database format into analysis data sets that make sense to the statistician.

Data gatherers
Persons skilled in data gathering for data entry fall into a hierarchy of individuals. For gathering some variables, expert medical domain knowledge as possessed by the surgeon or a knowledgeable research nurse is essential. Other data elements can be extracted by individuals with little formal training other than medical terminology. Essential ingredients are accuracy and integrity. Accuracy may be inborn and is indispensable; it can be assessed prospectively by testing and maintained by quality management and education.

Education/quality
If large quantities of data are maintained, one or more individuals must assess the quality of the data and from these findings educate the data gatherers. Such individuals must have expert medical domain knowledge, for example, the surgeon or a research and education

nurse. In large organizations, this role includes maintaining clinical documentation of the database, keeping current with new surgical trends, and pruning variables that no longer are of value or are of questionable quality.

Statistician

Most serious clinical research efforts require equally serious collaboration with one or more statisticians. The applied statistician needs to become expert, facile, and experienced in many methods. This chapter provides a compendium of such areas of expertise (see Sections 4 and 6): time-related events analysis, binary, ordinal, and polytomous regression, longitudinal mixed-model (hierarchical) data analysis, multivariable analysis, case-matching analysis, cluster randomized trials, diagnostic accuracy, and classification algorithms, to name a few. Backing such applied efforts must be ongoing statistical methodologic research. Many studies, perhaps most, use analytic methods that answer specific questions, but the questions answered may not precisely match the ones that are medically relevant (because of assumptions or lack of more appropriate methods). Encountering these difficulties should stimulate development of more appropriate methodology.

Other professionals

Other professionals that may be part of a team, depending on the nature of the surgeon's research interests, include mathematicians (who develop mathematical models that attempt to capture known mechanistic relations within the data, in contrast to the statistician, who takes a more generic and empirical approach), computer scientists (such as those in bioinformatics, computational biology, data mining, or algorithmic data analysis), human factors psychologists (for investigation of human error), and many others. Indispensable is the editorial assistant who assists in manuscript preparation, ensures proper grammar and style, and manages references.

Infrastructure

Some individuals are shared by several groups. They maintain computer networks, computers, and software, enter and verify data, perform patient follow-up, do financial analysis, write grants, produce medical illustrations or computer graphics, and engage in many other support roles.

It may be more comfortable and convenient for the surgeon to have a single point of contact among these individuals. However, today it is a collaborative team with a multitude of skills that is often needed, with data flowing progressively (often iteratively) from the information through analysis phases, forcing the surgeon to leave comfort and convenience behind and become immersed in a multidisciplinary effort!

APPENDIX 6B

Confidence Limits for Proportions

Reasonably accurate confidence limits (CL) can be obtained quickly and easily with small programmable calculators. This versatile tool is helpful not only for clinical and laboratory research, but also for calculating CLs (if not given) while reading the literature.

A simple quadratic normal approximation to the binomial distribution containing a correction for continuity has been found to yield CLs nearly as accurate as those obtained using more complex F-ratios,[B13] even when n is small.[B13]

Continuity correction (p') for the upper CL of a proportion (p) is

$$p' = p + \frac{1}{2n}$$

$$(6B-1)$$

and the sign of $\pm$ in Equation 6B-3 is positive.

Continuity correction for the lower CL of the proportion is

$$p' = p - \frac{1}{2n}$$

$$(6B-2)$$

and the sign of $\pm$ in Equation 6B-3 is negative.

The upper (p_U) and lower (p_L) CLs are successively solved by substituting p' and K into the following quadratic equation:

$$CL = \frac{2np' + K[K \pm \sqrt{K^2 + 4np'(1-p')}]}{2(n+1)}$$

$$(6B-3)$$

Choice of K depends on the confidence coefficient desired. For 70% CLs, $K = 1.03643$; for 50% CLs, $K = 0.67449$; for 90% CLs, $K = 1.64485$; for 95% CLs, $K = 1.95996$; and for 68.3% CLs, corresponding exactly to ± 1 standard deviation of p, $K = 1.0$. When $K = 1$, Equation 6B-3 reduces to

$$CL = \frac{2np' + 1 \pm \sqrt{1 + 4np'(1-p')}}{2(n+1)}$$

$$(6B-4)$$

The error in CLs using this simple approximation is at maximum 1 percentage point when n is small. As n becomes large (>10), the difference approaches zero.

Although not useful in and of itself, the standard deviation (SD) of a proportion can be used as a guideline for rounding proportions and their CLs to reflect appropriate precision (see Box 6-10):

$$SD = \sqrt{\frac{p(1-p)}{n}}$$

$$(6B-5)$$

The guideline is to round the proportion and its CLs to the place of the first significant digit of the standard deviation (see Box 6-11). For the most part, this will be found to be to a whole percent except for small ($<10\%$) or large ($>90\%$) proportions, for which another significant digit is often required. Thus, as a general rule, proportions and their CLs can be presented to two significant digits.

APPENDIX 6C

Equations for Calculating Evident Differences

Nonoverlapping Confidence Limits

To find the point at which the effect of a variable is evident using nonoverlapping confidence limits (CL), consider a simple linear relationship between effect x and outcome z:

$$z = \beta_0 + \beta_1 x_1$$

$$(6C-1)$$

where coefficients β_0, the intercept, and β_1, the slope, are determined from a regression analysis (see Box 6-5). The first requisite is to select a reference value of x; call it x_1. The object is to find a different x, call it x_2, at and beyond which the effect is evident, that is, different from that at x_1.

The CLs for z at x_1, calculated from the variance of z, $Var[z(x_1)]$, and a confidence coefficient transformed to an appropriate t (e.g., $t = 1$ for 68.3% CLs; see Appendix 6B), are calculated as follows:

$$Var[z(x_1)] = V_0 + V_1 x_1^2 + 2Cov_{0,1} x_1$$

$$(6C-2)$$

and

$$CL[z(x_1)] = z(x_1) \pm t\sqrt{Var[z(x_1)]}$$

$$(6C-3)$$

where V_0 and V_1 are the variances of β_0 and β_1 (variance being the square of the standard deviation, SD) and $Cov_{0,1}$ is the covariance term between β_0 and β_1 ($Cov_{0,1}$ is related to the correlation r between β_0 and β_1 by the expression $SD_0 SD_1 r$). The CLs of the unknown x_2 are given by Appendix Equations 6C-2 and 6C-3, with x_2 substituted for x_1.

Because CLs of $z(x_2)$ must exactly equal either the upper or lower CLs of $z(x_1)$, we can write, using Equations 6C-2 and 6C-3,

$$CL\,[z(x_1)] = CL\,[z(x_2)] = z(x_2) \pm t\,\sqrt{\mathrm{Var}[z(x_2)]}$$

(6C-4)

or

$$CL\,[z(x_1)] = \beta_0 + \beta_1 x_2 \pm t\,\sqrt{V_0 + V_1 {x_2}^2 + 2\mathrm{Cov}_{0,2} x_2}$$

(6C-5)

The only unknown in Equation 6C-5 is x_2, which, in this case, can be found using the general solution for roots of a quadratic equation. For uncomplicated situations that reduce to Equation 6C-5, the four roots (two each for the $\pm$ expression) can be calculated using a handheld calculator program. Two of the roots will simply yield x_1. Which of the other two roots is the desired x_2 is easily selected by inspection. For more complex multivariable cases, the equation must be solved for explicit values of all variables except x_2; thus, even a complex set of coefficients often can be reduced to the form of Equation 6C-5. However, if higher-order terms in x (higher powers) are involved, it is probably easier to solve the equation using an iterative method for solving nonlinear equations.

P Values

If, instead of (or in addition to) determining an evident difference using nonoverlapping CLs, one wishes to detect an evident difference at some level of significance (*P value*), then Equations 6C-1 and 6C-2 are used to define $z(x_1)$, $z(x_2)$, $\mathrm{Var}[z(x_1)]$, and $\mathrm{Var}[z(x_2)]$. Then the general equation for a test of significance is used:

$$t = \frac{z(x_1) - z(x_2)}{\sqrt{\mathrm{Var}[z(x_1)] + \mathrm{Var}[z(x_2)]}}$$

(6C-6)

where t is the number of standard deviations represented by the selected significance level (*P value*). Expanding Equation 6C-6:

$$t = \frac{z(x_1) - (\beta_0 + \beta_1 x_2)}{\sqrt{\mathrm{Var}[z(x_1)] + (V_0 + V_1 {x_2}^2 + 2\mathrm{Cov}_{0,1} x_2)}}$$

(6C-7)

yields an equation with only one unknown, x_2. In the simplest cases, Equation 6C-7 can be solved using a solution for roots of a quadratic equation. Higher-order terms of x require use of iterative methods.

Note that if Equation 6C-2 represents a logistic equation, solving for evident differences is performed in the logit domain, not the probability domain. Similarly, if time-related evident differences are desired, calculations are performed in the domain in which estimation of the parameters is performed.

APPENDIX 6D

Neutralization of Incremental Risk Factors

Multivariable analysis (see Box 6-18) can be used to discover if an incremental risk factor has been neutralized with experience (see "Incremental Risk Factor Concept" in Section 4). Date of operation (expressed on a "continuous" scale from, for example, the beginning of a program or beginning of a calendar year) is multiplied by the risk factor to form a new variable, called an *interaction term,* and the risk factor, date of operation (both called *main effects*), and interaction term are forced into the multivariable model. If a risk factor has been completely neutralized, the magnitude of the interaction term should have a sign opposite that of the main effect and be of equal magnitude. Of course, the risk factor may be only partially neutralized.

Interaction

A note on *interaction terms* and their interpretation in general is in order. Interaction can be found between factors x_1 and x_2 in the following ways, particularly if one (say x_2) is dichotomous:

- $x_1, x_2, x_1 \cdot x_2$
- $x_1, x_1 \cdot x_2, x_1 \cdot (1 - x_2)$
- $x_1, 1 - x_2, x_1 \cdot (1 - x_2)$

Note that the interaction term is the one that multiplies one x by another. Depending on the signs and magnitude of these factors, they provide equivalent model fit but different insights. Specifically, they may identify possible neutralization of an effect. In another setting, they examine the relation when a factor is present, and the same relation when it is not. Finally, the increment of risk from interaction can be quantified. Thus, simply multiplying two factors should not be done blindly but in several ways, to explore each aspect of interaction.

REFERENCES

A

1. Axtell LM. Computing survival rates for chronic disease patients: a simple procedure. JAMA 1963;186:1125.
2. Austin MA, Berreyesa S, Elliott JL, Wallace RB, Barrett-Connor E, Criqui MH. Methods for determining long-term survival in a population based study. Am J Epidemiol 1979;110:747.
3. Antman K, Lagakos S, Drazen J. Designing and funding clinical trials of novel therapies. N Engl J Med 2001;344:762.
4. Abiteboul S, Quass D, McHugh J, Widom J, Weiner J. The Lorel query language for semistructured data. Int J Digital Libraries 1997;1:68.
5. ACC/AHA guidelines and indications for coronary artery bypass graft surgery. A report of the American College of Cardiology/American Heart Association Task Force on Assessment of Diagnostic and Therapeutic Cardiovascular Procedures (Subcommittee on Coronary Artery Bypass Graft Surgery). Circulation 1991;83:1125.
6. Alexe S, Hammer PL, Blackstone EH, Ishwaran H, Lauer MS, Pothier Snader CE. Coronary risk prediction by logical analysis of data. Ann Operations Res 2003;119:15.
7. Association of American Medical Colleges Task Force on Clinical Research. For the health of the public: ensuring the future of clinical research, Vol. 1. Washington, DC: AAM, 1999, p. 16.
8. Altman DG, Andersen PK. Bootstrap investigation of the stability of a Cox regression model. Stat Med 1989;8:771.

9. Andersen PK, Hansen LS, Keiding N. Assessing the influence of reversible disease indicators on survival. Stat Med 1991;10:1061.

B

1. Burdette WJ, Gehan EA. Planning and analysis of clinical studies. Springfield, Ill.: Charles C Thomas, 1970.
2. Birnbaum Memorial Symposium. Medical research: statistics and ethics. Science 1977;198:677.
3. Byar DP, Simon RM, Friedewald WT, Schlesselman JJ, DeMets DL, Ellenberg JH, et al. Randomized clinical trials: perspectives on some recent ideas. N Engl J Med 1976;295:74.
4. Berkson J, Gage RP. Calculation of survival rates for cancer. Mayo Clin Proc 1950;25:270.
5. Breslow NE. Analysis of survival data under the proportional hazards model. Int Stat Rev 1975;43:45.
6. Buckland WR. The life characteristic. London: Charles Griffin, 1964.
7. Breslow N. Covariance analysis of censored survival data. Biometrics 1974;30:89.
8. Berkson J. Application of the logistic function to bioassay. J Am Stat Assoc 1944;39:357.
9. Berkson J. Why I prefer logits to probits. Biometrics 1951;7:327.
10. Berkson J. A statistically precise and relatively simple method of estimating the bioassay with quantal response, based on the logistic function. J Am Stat Assoc 1953;48:565.

11. Bunker JP, Barnes BA, Mosteller F, eds. Costs, risks, and benefits of surgery. New York: Oxford University Press, 1977.

12. Boice JD Jr. Follow-up methods to trace women treated for pulmonary tuberculosis, 1930–1954. Am J Epidemiol 1978;107:127.

13. Brownlee KA. Statistical theory and methodology in science and engineering, 2nd Ed. New York: John Wiley & Sons, 1965, pp. 91, 148.

14. Bartlett MS. Essays on probability and statistics. New York: John Wiley & Sons, 1962.

15. Berry DA, Stangl DK. Meta-analysis in medicine and health policy. New York: Marcel Dekker, 2000.

16. Baskerville JC, Toogood JH. Guided regression modeling for prediction and exploration of structure with many explanatory variables. Technometrics 1982;24:9.

17. Blackstone EH, Lytle BW. Competing risks after coronary bypass surgery: the influence of death on reintervention. J Thorac Cardiovasc Surg 2000;119:1221.

18. Blackstone EH, Kirklin JW. Rational decision-making in pediatric cardiac surgery. In Godman M, ed. Pediatric cardiology, Vol. 4. Edinburgh: Churchill Livingstone, 1981, p. 334.

19. Bryant GD, Norman GR. Expressions of probability: words and numbers (letter). N Engl J Med 1980;302:411.

20. Blackstone EH, Naftel DC, Turner ME Jr. The decomposition of time-varying hazard into phases, each incorporating a separate stream of concomitant information. J Am Stat Assoc 1986;81:615.

21. Berkson J, Flexner LB. On the rate of reaction between enzyme and substrate. J Gen Phys 1928;11:433.

22. Berkson J, Hollander F. Chemistry—on the equation for the reaction between invertase and sucrose. J Wash Acad Sci 1930;20:157.

23. Berkson J, Gage RP. Calculation of survival rates for cancer. Mayo Clin Proc 1950;25:270.

24. Blackstone EH. Methods and limitations of follow-up assessment of replacement heart valves. In Bodnar E, Frater RW, eds. Replacement cardiac valves. New York: Pergamon, 1991, p. 391.

25. Blackstone EH. Analysis of death (survival analysis) and other time-related events. In Macartney FT, ed. Current status of clinical cardiology: congenital heart disease. Lancaster, UK: MTP Press, 1986, p. 55.

26. Blackstone EH. Research methods for decision-making in cardiac surgery. Inferences from repeating morbid events. In D'Alessandro, LC, ed. Heart surgery 1989. Rome: Casa Editrice Scientifica Internazionale, 1989, p. 301.

27. Blackstone EH, Kirklin JW. Incremental risk factors of open cardiac surgery. In Marcelletti C, Anderson RH, Becker AE, Corno A, diCarlo D, Mazzera E, eds. Pediatric cardiology, Vol. 6. New York: Churchill Livingstone, 1986, p. 281.

28. Bland JM. Sample size in guidelines trials. Fam Pract 2000;17:S17.

29. Bland JM, Kerry SM. Statistics notes. Trials randomized in clusters. Br Med J 1997;315:600.

30. Bonchek LI. Are randomized trials appropriate for evaluating new operations? N Engl J Med 1979;301:44.

31. Benson K, Hartz AJ. A comparison of observational studies and randomized, controlled trials. N Engl J Med 2000;342;1878.

32. Blackstone EH. In response to: Grunkemeier GL, Starr A. Alternatives to randomization in surgical studies. J Heart Valve Dis 1993;2:119.

33. Berwick DM, Leape LL. Reducing errors in medicine. Qual Health Care 1999;8:145.

34. Bochner S. Continuity and discontinuity in nature and knowledge. In Wiener PP, ed. Dictionary of the history of ideas: studies of selected pivotal ideas, Vol. 1. New York: Charles Scribner's Sons, 1968, p. 492.

35. Byar DP. Problems with using observational databases to compare treatments. Stat Med 1991;10:663.

36. Burack JH, Impellizzeri P, Homel P, Cunningham JN Jr. Public reporting of surgical mortality: a survey of New York State cardiothoracic surgeons. Ann Thorac Surg 1999;68:1195.

37. Blackstone EH, Rice TW. Clinical-pathologic conference: use and choice of statistical methods for the clinical study, "Superficial adenocarcinoma of the esophagus." J Thorac Cardiovasc Surg 2001; 122:1063.

38. Breiman L. Statistical modeling: the two cultures. Stat Sci 2001; 16:199.

39. Blackstone EH. Breaking down barriers: helpful breakthrough statistical methods you need to understand better. J Thorac Cardiovasc Surg 2001;122:430.

40. Benson K, Hartz AJ. A comparison of observational studies and randomized, controlled trials. N Engl J Med 2000;342:1878.

41. Blackstone EH. Comparing apples and oranges. J Thorac Cardiovasc Surg 2002;123:8.

42. Banbury MK, Cosgrove DM III, Thomas JD, Blackstone EH, Rajeswaran J, Okies JE, et al. Hemodynamic stability during 17 years of the Carpentier-Edwards aortic pericardial bioprosthesis. Ann Thorac Surg 2002;73:1460.

43. Buneman P, Davidson S, Fan W, Hara C, Tan WC. Keys for XML. Proceedings of the Tenth International Conference on World Wide Web. New York: AMC Press, 2001.

44. Boden WE. Meta-analysis in clinical trials reporting: has a tool become a weapon? Am J Cardiol 1992;69:681.

45. Bero L, Rennie D. The Cochrane Collaboration. Preparing, maintaining, and disseminating systematic reviews of the effects of health care. JAMA 1995;274:1935.

46. Beecher HK. The powerful placebo. JAMA 1955;159:1602.

47. Blackstone EH. Actuarial and Kaplan–Meier survival analysis: there is a difference. J Thorac Cardiovasc Surg 1999;118:973.

48. Blackstone EH, Kirklin JW. Death and other time-related events after valve replacement. Circulation 1985;72:753.

49. Bodnar E, Haberman S, Wain WH. Comparative method for actuarial analysis of cardiac valve replacements. Br Heart J 1979;42:541.

50. Bridgewater B, Neve H, Moat N, Hooper T, Jones M. Predicting operative risk for coronary artery surgery in the United Kingdom: a comparison of various risk prediction algorithms. Heart 1998; 79:350.

51. Breiman L. Heuristics of instability and stabilization in model selection. Ann Stat 1996;24:2350.

52. Breiman L, Friedman JH, Olshen RA, Stone CJ. Classification and regression trees. Belmont: Wadsworth International, 1984.

53. Breiman L. Bagging predictors. Machine Learning 1996;24:123.

54. Bernoulli D. Essai d'une nouvelle analyse de la mortalité causée par la petite vérole, et des avantages de l'inoculation pour la prévenir." Histoires et Mémoires de l'Académie Royale des Sciences de Paris, 1766, p. 1.

55. Barker FG II, Chang SM, Gutin PH, Malec MK, McDermott MW, Prados MD, et al. Survival and functional status after resection of recurrent glioblastoma multiforme. Neurosurgery 1998;42:709.

56. Bodnar E, Horstkotte D. Potential flaws in the assessment of minor cerebrovascular events after heart valve replacement. J Heart Valve Dis 1993;2:287.

57. Barnard GA. Must clinical trials be large? The interpretation of *P*-values and the combination of test results. Stat Med 1990;9:601.

58. Burton PR, Gurrin LC, Campbell MJ. Clinical significance not statistical significance: a simple Bayesian alternative to p values. J Epidemiol Community Health 1998;52:318.

59. Blackwelder WC. "Proving the null hypothesis" in clinical trials. Control Clin Trials 1982;3:345.

60. Bartko J. Proving the null hypothesis. Am Psychol 1991;46:1089.

61. Berger RL, Hsu JC. Bioequivalence trials, intersection–union tests, and equivalence confidence sets. Stat Sci 1996;11:283.

62. Berk KN. Validating regression procedures with new data. Technometrics 1984;26:331.

63. Banbury MK, White JA, Blackstone EH, Cosgrove DM. Vacuum-assisted venous return reduces blood usage. J Thorac Cardiovasc Surg (in press).

64. Bourge RC, Kirklin JK, Naftel DC, McGiffin DC. Predicting outcome after cardiac transplantations: lessons from the Cardiac Transplant Research Database. Curr Opin Cardiol 1997;12:126.

C

1. Croxton FE. Elementary statistics with applications in medicine and the biological sciences. New York: Dover, 1953.

2. Chiang CL. The life table and its applications. Malabar, Fla.: Krieger, 1984.

3. Cox DR. Regression models and life tables. JR Stat Soc B 1972;34:187.

4. Castaneda AR, Trusler GA, Paul MH, Blackstone EH, Kirklin JW, and the Congenital Heart Surgeons Society. The early results of treatment of simple transposition in the current era. J Thorac Cardiovasc Surg 1988;95:14.

5. Collett D, Stepniewska K. Some practical issues in binary data analysis. Stat Med 1999;18:2209.

6. Cox DA. The analysis of binary data. London: Methuen, 1970.

7. Califf RM, Lee KL, Harrell FE Jr, Kimm SY, Grufferman S, Rosati RA. Assessment of the use of the age- and sex-specific United States population as a control group for analysis of survival in coronary artery disease. Am J Cardiol 1982;50:1279.

8. Cox DR, Oakes D. Analysis of survival data. London: Chapman & Hall, 1984, p. 56.

9. Cornfield J, Gordon T, Smith WS. Quantal response curves for experimentally uncontrolled variables. Bull Int Stat Inst 1961;3:97.

10. Concato J, Shah N, Horwitz RI. Randomized, controlled trials, observational studies, and the hierarchy of research designs. N Engl J Med 2000;342:1887.

11. Cooper JB, Newbower RS, Kitz RJ. An analysis of major errors and equipment failures in anesthesia management: considerations for prevention and detection. Anesthesiology 1984;60:34.

12. Christensen JF, Levinson W, Dunn PM. The heart of darkness: the impact of perceived mistakes on physicians. J Gen Intern Med 1992;7:424.

13. Cook RI, Woods DD. Operating at the sharp end: the complexity of human error. In Bogner MS, ed. Human error in medicine. Hillside, N.J.: Lawrence Erbaum, 1994, p. 255.

14. Chipman HA, George EI, McCulloch RE. Bayesian CART model search. J Am Stat Assoc 1998;93:935.

15. Coyle SL. Physician–industry relations. Part 1: individual physicians. Ann Intern Med 2002;136:396.

16. Coyle SL. Physician–industry relations. Part 2: organizational issues. Ann Intern Med 2002;136:403.

17. Cologne JB, Shibata Y. Optimal case–control matching in practice. Epidemiology 1995;6:271.

18. Coiera EW, Jayasuriya RA, Hardy J, Bannan A, Thorpe ME. Communication loads on clinical staff in the emergency department. Med J Aust 2002;176:415.

19. Coiera E. Clinical communication: a new informatics paradigm. Proc AMIA Annu Fall Symp 1996;:17.

20. Coiera E. When conversation is better than computation. J Am Med Inform Assoc 2000;7:277.

21. Cimino JJ, Clayton PD, Hripcsak G, Johnson SB. Knowledge-based approaches to the maintenance of a large controlled medical terminology. J Am Med Inform Assoc 1994;1:35.

22. Coiera E. Guide to medical informatics, the internet, and telemedicine. London: Oxford University Press, 1997.

23. Cotes R. Aestimatio Errorum in Mixta Mathesi, per Variationes Partium Trianguli Plani et Sphaerici [Part of Cotes's Opera Miscellanea, published with Harmonia Mensurarum, Robert Smith, ed.; Cambridge], 1722.

24. Cochran WG. Problems arising in analysis of a series of similar experiments. J Royal Stat Soc 1937;4:102.

25. Chalmers I, Dickersin K, Chalmers TC. Getting to grips with Archie Cochrane's agenda. Br Med J 1992;305:786.

26. Crowder M. On assessing independence of competing risks when failure times are discrete. Lifetime Data Anal 1996:2:195.

27. Cornfield J. The estimation of the probability of developing a disease in the presence of competing risk. Am J Public Health 1957;47:601.

28. Cook EF, Goldman L. Performance of tests of significance based on stratification by a multivariate confounder score or by a propensity score. J Clin Epidemiol 1989;42:317.

29. Curran D, Bacchi M, Schmitz SF, Molenberghs G, Sylvester RJ. Identifying the types of missingness in quality of life data from clinical trials. Stat Med 1998;17:739.

30. Cooley JW, Tukey JW. An algorithm for machine calculation of complex Fourier series. Math Computation 1965;19:297.

31. Cox DR. A note on data-splitting for the evaluation of significance levels. Biometrika 1975;62:441.

32. Cook RD, Weisberg S. Residuals and influence in regression. New York: Chapman and Hall, 1982.

33. Califf RM, White HD, Van de Werf F, Sadowski Z, Armstrong PW, Vahanian A, et al. One-year results from the Global Utilization of Streptokinase and TPA for Occluded Coronary Arteries (GUSTO-I) trial. GUSTO-I Investigators. Circulation 1996;94:1233.

D

1. Dixson WJ, Massey FJ Jr. Introduction to statistical analysis, 2nd Ed. New York: McGraw-Hill, 1957.

2. DeMoivre A. The doctrine of chances. 1756. Reprint, 3rd Ed. New York: Chelsea, 1967.

3. Draper NR, Smith H. Applied regression analysis, 2nd Ed. New York: John Wiley & Sons, 1981.

4. David HA, Moeschberger ML. The theory of competing risks. New York: Macmillan, 1978.

5. Donner A, Klar N. Design and analysis of cluster randomization trials in health research. London: Arnold, 2000.

6. Divine GW, Brown JT, Frazier LM. The unit of analysis error in studies about physicians' patient care behavior. J Gen Intern Med 1992;7:623.

7. de Leval MR, Carthey J, Wright DJ, Farewell VT, Reason JT. Human factors and cardiac surgery: a multicenter study. J Thorac Cardiovasc Surg 2000;119:661.

8. Drake C. Effects of misspecification of the propensity score on estimators of treatment effect. Biometrics 1993;49:1231.

9. Drake C, Fisher L. Prognostic models and the propensity score. Int J Epidemiol 1995;24:183.

10. D'Agostino RB Jr. Propensity score methods for bias reduction in the comparison of a treatment to a non-randomized control group. Stat Med 1998;17:2265.

11. Dick RS, Steen EB, eds. The computer-based patient record: an essential technology for health care. Washington, DC: The National Academy Press, 1991.

12. Dick RS, Steen EB, Detmer DE, eds. The computer-based patient record: an essential technology for health care, 2nd Ed. Washington, DC: The National Academy Press, 1997.

13. Diggle PJ, Heagerty P, Liang KY, Zeger SL. Analysis of longitudinal data. New York: Oxford University Press, 2002.

14. Day RA. How to write and publish a scientific paper, 5th Ed. Westport, Conn.: Greenwood, 1998.

15. DeLong ER, Peterson ED, DeLong DM, Muhlbaier LH, Hackett S, Mark DB. Comparing risk-adjustment methods for provider profiling. Stat Med 1997;16:2645.

16. Diaconis P, Efron B. Computer-intensive methods in statistics. Sci Amer 1983;248:116.

17. David FN. Games, gods & gambling: a history of probability and statistical ideas. London: Charles Griffin, 1962.

18. Diethelm AG, Blackstone EH. Cadaveric renal preservation with hyperosmolar, intracellular hypothermic washout solution and cold storage. Surg Gynecol Obstet 1978;147:56.

19. Davies HT, Washington AE, Bindman AB. Health care report cards: implications for vulnerable patient groups and the organizations providing them care. J Health Polit Policy Law 2002;27:379.

20. Daum B, Merten U. System architecture with XML. New York: Morgan Kaufmann, 2003.

E

1. Eidelman D. Fatigue. Towards an analysis and a unified definition. Med Hypoth 1980;6:517.

2. Eisenhart C. Expression of the uncertainties of final results. Science 1968;160:1201.

3. Elandt-Johnson RC, Johnson JL. Survival models and data analysis. New York: John Wiley & Sons, 1980.

4. Elveback L. Estimation of survivorship in chronic disease: the "actuarial" method. Am Stat Assoc J 1958;420.

5. Everitt BS. Mixture distributions. In Kotz S, Johnson NL, Read CB, eds. Encyclopedia of statistical sciences, Vol. 5. New York: John Wiley & Sons, 1985, p. 559.

6. Edwards SJ, Braunholtz DA, Lilford RJ, Stevens AJ. Ethical issues in the design and conduct of cluster randomized controlled trials. Br Med J 1999;318:1407.

7. Eleven-year survival in the Veterans Administration randomized trial of coronary bypass surgery for stable angina. The Veterans Administration Coronary Artery Bypass Surgery Cooperative Study Group. N Engl J Med 1984;311:1333.

8. Ennis M, Hinton G, Naylor D, Revow M, Tibshirani R. A comparison of statistical learning methods on the GUSTO database. Stat Med 1998;17:2501.

9. Ezquerra N, Capell S, Klein L, Duijves P. Model-guided labeling of coronary structure. IEEE Trans Med Imaging 1998;17:429.

10. Egger M, Davey Smith G, Schneider M, Minder C. Bias in meta-analysis detected by a simple, graphical test. Br Med J 1997;315:629.

11. Eysenck HJ. An exercise in mega-silliness. Am Psychol 1978;33:517.

12. Egger M, Smith GD. Misleading meta-analysis. Br Med J 1995; 310:752.

13. Egger M, Schneider M, Davey Smith G. Spurious precision? Meta-analysis of observational studies. Br Med J 1998;316:140.

14. Edmunds LH Jr, Clark RE, Cohn LH, Grunkemeier GL, Miller DC, Weisel RD. Guidelines for reporting morbidity and mortality after cardiac valvular operations. J Thorac Cardiovasc Surg 1996;112:708.

15. Efron B. Censored data and the bootstrap. J Am Stat Assoc 1981; 76:312.

F

1. Fraser DA. Nonparametric methods in statistics. New York: John Wiley & Sons, 1957.

2. Forsythe AB, Frey HS. Tests of significance from survival data. Comput Biomed Res 1970;3:124.

3. Feinstein AR. Clinical biostatistics XX: The epidemiologic trohoc, the ablative risk ratio and "retrospective" research. Clin Pharmacol Ther 1973;14:291.

4. Ferrazzi P, McGiffin DC, Kirklin JW, Blackstone EH, Bourge RC. Have the results of mitral valve replacement improved? J Thorac Cardiovasc Surg 1986;92:186.

5. Fisher RA. Statistical methods for research workers. 1925. Reprint, 14th Ed. New York: Hafner, 1970.

6. Fisher RA. Statistical methods and scientific inference, 3rd Ed. New York: Hafner, 1973, p. 45.

7. Fisher RA. The use of multiple measurements in taxonomic problems. Ann Eugen 1936;7:179.

8. Feinstein AR. The Jones criteria and the challenges of clinimetrics. Circulation 1982;66:1.

9. Frye RL, Sopko G, Detre KM. The BARI trial: baseline observations. The BARI Investigators. Trans Am Clin Climatol Assoc 1992;104:26.

10. Feinstein AR, Landis JR. The role of prognostic stratification in preventing the bias permitted by random allocation of treatment. J Chronic Dis 1976;29:277.

11. Frye RL, Fisher L, Schaff HV, Gersh BJ, Vlietstra RE, Mock MB. Randomized trials in coronary artery bypass surgery. Prog Cardiovasc Dis 1987;30:1.

12. Formigari L. Chain of being. In Wiener PP, ed. Dictionary of the history of ideas: studies of selected pivotal ideas, Vol. 1. New York: Charles Scribner's Sons, 1968, p. 325.

13. Feinstein AR. XXXII. Biologic dependency, "hypothesis testing," unilateral probabilities, and other issues in scientific direction vs. statistical duplexity. Clin Pharmacol Ther 1975;17:498.

14. French JC, Jones AK, Pfaltz JL. Report of the first invitational NSF workshop on scientific database management. Technical report 90-21, Department of Computer Science, University of Virginia Charlottesville, August 1990.

15. Feigl P, Zelen M. Estimation of exponential survival probabilities with concomitant information. Biometrics 1965;21:826.

16. Fleming TR, DeMets DL. Surrogate end points in clinical trials: are we being misled? Ann Intern Med 1997;126:667.

17. Fontan F, Kirklin JW, Fernandez G, Costa F, Naftel DC, Tritto F, et al. Outcome after a "perfect" Fontan operation. Circulation 1990;81:1520.

G

1. Galilei G. Sopra le scoperte dei dadi, as summarized in R Langley: Practical statistics simply expanded. New York: Dover, 1970.

2. Gauss CF. Theory of motion of the heavenly bodies moving about the sun in conic sections. 1809. Reprint. New York: Dover, 1963.

3. Gauss's work (1803–1826) on the theory of least squares, Trotter F, trans. Statistical Techniques Research Group, Technical Report No. 5. Princeton, N.J.: Princeton University Press, 1957.

4. Gehan EA. A generalized Wilcoxon test for comparing arbitrarily singly-censored samples. Biometrika 1965;52:203.

5. Greenwood M. The natural duration of cancer. Rep Public Health Medi Subjects 1926;33:1.

6. Goodman LA. The variance of the product of k random variables. J Am Stat Assoc 1962;57:54.

7. Gordon T, Kannel WB. Predisposition to atherosclerosis in the head, heart, and legs. The Framingham study. JAMA 1972;221:661.

8. Gompertz B. On the nature of the function expressive of the law of human mortality. Philos Trans R Soc Lond 1825;115:513.

9. Graunt J. Natural and political observations made upon the Bills of Mortality. 1662. Reprint. Baltimore: Johns Hopkins University Press, 1939.

10. Grunkemeier GL, Thomas DR, Starr A. Statistical considerations in the analysis and reporting of time-related events: application to analysis of prosthetic valve-related thromboembolism and pacemaker failure. Am J Cardiol 1977;39:257.

11. Grunkemeier GL, Starr A. Alternatives to randomization in surgical studies. J Heart Valve Dis 1992;1:142.

12. Grunkemeier, GL, Starr A. Reply to correspondence on randomization in surgical studies. J Heart Valve Dis 1993;2:359.

13. Grunkemeier GL. Will randomized trials detect random valve failure? Reflections on a recent FDA workshop. J Heart Valve Dis 1993;2:424.

14. Gordon T. Statistics in a prospective study: the Framingham Study. In Gail MH, Johnson NL, eds. Proceedings of the American Statistical Association: sesquicentennial invited paper sessions. Alexandria, Va.: ASA, 1989, p. 719.

15. Guerlac H. Theological voluntarism and biological analogies in Newton's physical thought. J Hist Ideas 1983;44:219.

16. Gum PA, Thamilarasan M, Watanabe J, Blackstone EH, Lauer MS. Aspirin use and all-cause mortality among patients being evaluated for known or suspected coronary artery disease: a propensity analysis. JAMA 2001;286:1187.

17. Goldman R, McHugh J, Widom J. From semistructured data to XML: migrating the Lore data model and query language. Proceedings of the 2nd International Workshop on the Web and Databases, 1999, Philadelphia.

18. Goldstein H. Multilevel statistical models, 2nd Ed. London: Arnold, 1995.

19. Gangemi A, Pisanell DM, Steve G. Formal ontology in information systems. Ontology integration: experiences with medical terminologies. Amsterdam: IOS Press, 1998, p. 163.

20. Glass G. Primary, secondary and meta-analysis of research. Education Res J 1976;5:3.

21. Greenhalgh T. Papers that summarise other papers (systematic reviews and meta-analyses). Br Med J 1997;315:672.

22. Grunkemeier GL, Anderson WN Jr. Clinical evaluation and analysis of heart valve substitutes. J Heart Valve Dis 1998;7:163.

23. Gail MH. A bibliography and comments on the use of statistical models in epidemiology in the 1980s. Stat Med 1991;10:1819.

24. Grunkemeier GL, Anderson RP, Miller DC, Starr A. Time-related analysis of nonfatal heart valve complications. Circulation 1997; 96:70.

25. Grunkemeier GL, Lambert LE, Bonchek LI, Starr A. An improved statistical method for assessing the results of operation. Ann Thorac Surg 1975;20:289.

26. Grunkemeier GL, Jamieson WR, Miller DC, Starr A. Actuarial versus actual risk of porcine structural valve deterioration. J Thorac Cardiovasc Surg 1994;108:709.
27. Grunkemeier GL, Wu Y. Actual versus actuarial event-free percentages. Ann Thorac Surg 2001;72:677.
28. Gillinov AM, Wierup PN, Blackstone EH, Bishay ES, Cosgrove DM, White J, Lytle BW, et al. Is repair preferable to replacement for ischemic mitral regurgitation? J Thorac Cardiovasc Surg 2001;122: 1125.
29. Galton F. Regression towards mediocrity in hereditary stature. J Anthropolog Inst 1886;15:246.
30. Gardner MJ, Altman DG. Confidence intervals rather than P values: estimation rather than hypothesis testing. Br Med J (Clin Res Ed) 1986;292:746.
31. Grunkemeier GL, Starr A. Actuarial analysis of surgical results: rationale and method. Ann Thorac Surg 1977;24:404.
32. Gordon T, Kannel WB. Multiple risk functions for predicting coronary heart disease: the concept, accuracy, and application. Am Heart J 1982;103:1031.
33. Gawande A. Complications: a surgeon's notes on an imperfect science. New York: Metropolitan Books, 2002.

H

1. Hollander M, Wolfe DA. Non-parametric statistical methods. New York: John Wiley & Sons, 1973.
2. Halley E. An estimate of the degrees of the mortality of mankind, drawn from curious tables of the births and funerals of the city of Breslau. Philos Trans R Soc Lond 1693;17:596.
3. Hazelrig JB, Turner ME, Blackstone EH. Parametric survival analysis combining longitudinal and cross-sectional censored and interval censored data with concomitant information. Biometrics 1982;38:1.
4. Heisenberg W. Physics and philosophy: the revolution in modern science. New York: Harper, 1958.
5. Haddon W. The prevention of accidents. In Clark DW, McMahon B, eds. Textbook of preventive medicine. Boston: Little, Brown, 1967, p. 591.
6. Hickey MS, Blackstone EH, Kirklin JW, Dean LS. Outcome probabilities and life history after surgical mitral commissurotomy: implications for balloon commissurotomy. J Am Coll Cardiol 1991;17:29.
7. Harrell FE Jr, Lee KL, Matchar DB, Reichert TA. Regression models for prognostic prediction: advantages, problems, and suggested solutions. Cancer Treat Rep 1985;69:1071.
8. Hosmer DW Jr, Wang CY, Lin IC, Lemeshow S. A computer program for stepwise logistic regression using maximum likelihood estimation. Comput Programs Biomed 1978;8:121.
9. Hannan EL, O'Donnell JF, Kilburn H Jr, Bernard HR, Yazici A. Investigation of the relationship between volume and mortality for surgical procedures performed in New York State hospitals. JAMA 1989;262:503.
10. Horton R. The clinical trial: deceitful, disputable, unbelievable, unhelpful, and shameful—what next? Control Clin Trials 2001;22:593.
11. Hacking I. The emergence of probability. Cambridge: Cambridge University Press, 1975, p. 102.
12. Hrushkey WJ. Triumph of the trivial. Perspectives Biol Med 1998; 41:341.
13. Hannan EL, Kumar D, Racz M, Siu AL, Chassin MR. New York State's Cardiac Surgery Reporting System: four years later. Ann Thorac Surg 1994;58:1852.
14. Hannan EL, Siu AL, Kumar D, Racz M, Pryor DB, Chassin MR. Assessment of coronary artery bypass graft surgery performance in New York. Is there a bias against taking high-risk patients? Med Care 1997;35:49.
15. Hastie T, Tibshirani R, Friedman JH. The elements of statistical learning: data mining, inference, and prediction. New York: Springer-Verlag, 2001.
16. Horrobin DF. Evidence-based medicine and the need for non-commercial clinical research directed towards therapeutic innovation. Exp Biol Med (Maywood) 2002;227:435.

17. Harrell FE Jr, Lee KL, Califf RM, Pryor DB, Rosati RA. Regression modeling strategies for improved prognostic prediction. Stat Med 1984;3:143.
18. Heckman JJ, Ichimura H, Smith J, Todd P. Sources of selection bias in evaluating social programs: an interpretation of conventional measures and evidence on the effectiveness of matching as a program evaluation method. Proc Natl Acad Sci U S A 1996;93:13416.
19. Hosmer D, Lemeshow S. Applied logistic regression. New York: John Wiley & Sons, 1989.
20. Hamilton CW. How to write and publish scientific papers: scribing information for pharmacists. Am J Hosp Pharm 1992;49:2477.
21. Higgins TL, Estafanous FG, Loop FD, Beck GJ, Blum JM, Paranandi L. Stratification of morbidity and mortality outcome by preoperative risk factors in coronary artery bypass patients. JAMA 1992;267:2344.
22. Harrell F. Regression coefficients and scoring rules. J Clin Epidemiol 1996;49:819.
23. Harrell FE Jr, Califf RM, Pryor DB, Lee KL, Rosati RA. Evaluating the yield of medical tests. JAMA 1982;247:2543.
24. Hanley JA. Receiver operating characteristic (ROC) methodology: the state of the art. Crit Rev Diagn Imaging 1989;29:307.
25. Hadorn DC, Draper D, Rogers WH, Keeler EB, Brook RH. Cross-validation performance of mortality prediction models. Stat Med 1992;11:475.

I

1. Iezzoni LI, Ash AS, Shwartz M, Landon BE, Mackiernan YD. Predicting in-hospital deaths from coronary artery bypass graft surgery. Do different severity measures give different predictions? Med Care 1998;36:28.
2. Ireson CI, Ford MA, Hower JM, Schwartz RW. Outcome report cards: a necessity in the health care market. Arch Surg 2002;137:46.

J

1. Jaynes ET. Prior probabilities. Trans Syst Sci Cybernet 1968;SSC-4:227.
2. Joffe MM, Rosenbaum PR. Invited commentary: propensity scores. Am J Epidemiol 1999;150:327.
3. Jenkins KJ, Gauvreau K, Newburger JW, Spray TL, Moller JH, Iezzoni LI. Consensus-based method for risk adjustment for surgery for congenital heart disease. J Thorac Cardiovasc Surg 2002;123:110.
4. Johnson SB. Generic data modeling for clinical repositories. J Am Med Inform Assoc 1996;3:328.
5. Joiner BL. Lurking variables: some examples. Am Stat 1981;35:227.

K

1. Kalbfleisch JD, Prentice RL. The statistical analysis of failure-time data, 2nd ed. New York: John Wiley & Sons, 2002.
2. Kaplan EL, Meier P. Nonparametric estimation from incomplete observations. J Am Stat Assoc 1958;53:457.
3. Kirklin JW. A letter to Helen. J Thorac Cardiovasc Surg 1979;78:643.
4. Kempthorne O. Of what use are tests of significance and tests of hypotheses? Commun Statist Theor Method A 1976;5:763.
5. Kuzma J. A comparison of two life table methods. Biometrics 1967;23:51.
6. Ku HH. Notes on the propagation of error formulas. J Res Nat Bur Stds 1966;70C:263.
7. Kirklin JW, Kouchoukos NT, Blackstone EH, Oberman A. Research related to surgical treatment of coronary artery disease. Circulation 1979;60:1613.
8. Kannel WB, McGee D, Gordon T. A general cardiovascular risk profile: the Framingham Study. Am J Cardiol 1976;38:46.
9. Kirklin JW, and the ACC/AHA Task Force Subcommittee on Coronary Artery Bypass Graft Surgery. Guidelines and indications for the coronary artery bypass graft operation. J Am Coll Cardiol 1991;17: 543; Circulation 1991;83:1125.
10. Kirklin JW, Blackstone EH, Tchervenkov CI, Castaneda AR, and the Congenital Heart Surgeons Society. Clinical outcomes after the arterial switch operation for transposition. Patient, support, procedural, and institutional risk factors. Circulation 1992;86:1501.

11. Kay R. Proportional hazard regression models and the analysis of censored survival data. Appl Stat 1977;26:227.

12. Kodlin D. A new response time distribution. Biometrics 1967; 23:227.

13. Kirklin JW, Blackstone EH, Jonas RA, Shimazaki Y, Kirklin JK, Mayer JE Jr, et al. Morphologic and surgical determinants of outcome events after repair of tetralogy of Fallot and pulmonary stenosis: a two-institution study. J Thorac Cardiovasc Surg 1992;103:706.

14. Kohn LT, Corrigan JM, Donaldson M, eds. To err is human: building a safer health system. Washington, DC: Institute of Medicine, 1999.

15. Kirklin JW, Blackstone EH. Notes from the editors: ultramini-abstracts and abstracts. J Thorac Cardiovasc Surg 1994;107:326.

16. Kirklin JW, Vicinanza SS. Metadata and computer-based patient records. Ann Thorac Surg 1999;68:S23.

17. Kirklin JW, Blackstone EH. Notes from the editors: tables. J Thorac Cardiovasc Surg 1994;107:969.

18. Kirklin JW, Blackstone EH. Notes from the editors: figures. J Thorac Cardiovasc Surg 1994;107:1175.

19. Kirklin JW, Blackstone EH. Notes from the editors: the format of a paper. J Thorac Cardiovasc Surg 1994;108:196.

20. Kirklin JW, Blackstone EH. Notes from the editors: the section entitled "Results." J Thorac Cardiovasc Surg 1994;108:398.

21. Kent JT, O'Quigley J. Measures of dependence for censored survival data. Biometrics 1988;75:525.

22. Kirklin JW, Blackstone EH, Tchervenkov CI, Castaneda AR, and the Congenital Heart Surgeons Society. Clinical outcomes after the arterial switch operation for transposition. Patient, support, procedural, and institutional risk factors. Circulation 1992;86:1501.

23. Kirklin JW, Blackstone EH, Bargeron LM Jr, Pacifico AD, Kirklin JK. The repair of atrioventricular septal defects in infancy. Int J Cardiol 1986;13:333.

24. Kubo SH, Naftel DC, Mills RM Jr, O'Donnell J, Rodeheffer RJ, Cintron GB, et al. Risk factors for late recurrent rejection after heart transplantation: a multiinstitutional, multivariable analysis. J Heart Lung Transplant 1995;14:409.

25. Kirklin JW, Karp RB. The tetralogy of Fallot, from a surgical point of view. Philadelphia: W. B. Saunders, 1970.

L

1. Lawrence AC. Human error as a cause of accidents in gold mining. J Safety Res 1974;6:78.

2. Larkin JH, Simon HA. Why a diagram is (sometimes) worth ten thousand words. Cognitive Sci 1987;11:65.

3. Little RJ, Rubin DB. Statistical analysis with missing data. New York: John Wiley & Sons, 1987.

4. Lilienfeld DE, Pyne DA. On indices of mortality: deficiencies, validity, and alternatives. J Chronic Dis 1979;32:463.

5. Lew RA, Day CL Jr, Harrist TJ, Wood WC, Mihm MC Jr. Multivariate analysis: some guidelines for physicians. JAMA 1983;249:641.

6. Love JW. Drugs and operations. Some important differences. JAMA 1975;232:37.

7. Lee YJ, Ellenberg JH, Hirtz DG, Nelson KB. Analysis of clinical trials by treatment actually received: is it really an option? Stat Med 1991;10:1595.

8. Leape LL. Error in medicine. JAMA 1994;272:1851.

9. Leape LL, Lawthers AG, Brennan TA, Johnson WG. Preventing medical injury. Qual Rev Bull;1993;8:144

10. Lytle BW, Blackstone EH, Loop FD, Houghtaling PL, Arnold JH, Akhrass R, et al. Two internal thoracic artery grafts are better than one. J Thorac Cardiovasc Surg 1999;117:855.

11. Lippmann RP, Shahian DM. Coronary artery bypass risk prediction using neural networks. Ann Thorac Surg 1997;63:1635.

12. Loh WY, Vanichsetakul N. Tree-structured classification via generalized discriminant analysis. J Am Stat Assoc 1998;83:715.

13. Little RJ, Rubin DB. Causal effects in clinical and epidemiological studies via potential outcomes: concepts and analytical approaches. Annu Rev Public Health 2000;21:121.

14. Li YP. Balanced risk set matching. J Am Stat Assoc 2001;96:870.

15. Lauer MS, Blackstone EH. Databases in cardiology. In Topol EJ, ed. Textbook of cardiovascular medicine, 2nd Ed. Philadelphia: Lippincott Williams & Wilkins, 2002, p. 981.

16. Laird NM, Ware JH. Random-effects models for longitudinal data. Biometrics 1982;38:963.

17. Leizorovicz A, Haugh MC, Chapuis FR, Samama MM, Boissel JP. Low molecular weight heparin in prevention of perioperative thrombosis. Br Med J 1992;305;913.

18. Lau J, Ioannidis JP, Schmid CH. Quantitative synthesis in systematic reviews. Ann Intern Med 1997;127:820.

19. Lao CS. Statistical considerations for survival analysis from medical device clinical studies. J Biopharm Stat 1995;5:159.

20. Lovegrove J, Valencia O, Treasure T, Sherlaw-Johnson C, Gallivan S. Monitoring the results of cardiac surgery by variable life-adjusted display. Lancet 1997;350:1128.

21. Lauer MS, Alexe S, Pothier-Snader CE, Blackstone EH, Ishwaran H, Hammer PL. Use of the logical analysis of data method for assessing long-term mortality risk after exercise electrocardiography. Circulation 2002;106:685.

M

1. Murphy RD, Papps PC. Construction of mortality tables from the records of insured lives. New York: The Actuarial Society of America, 1922.

2. Mantel N, Haenszel W. Statistical aspects of the analysis of data from retrospective studies of disease. J Natl Cancer Inst 1959;22:719.

3. Mantel N. Evaluation of survival data and two new rank order statistics arising in its consideration. Cancer Chemother Rep 1966; 50:163.

4. Margo CE. When is surgery research? Towards an operational definition of human research. J Med Ethics 2001;27:40.

5. McKneally MF. A bypass for the Institutional Review Board: reflections on the Cleveland Clinic study of the Batista operation. J Thorac Cardiovasc Surg 2001;121:837.

6. McCarthy PM, Franco-Cerceda A, Blackstone EH, Hoercher K, White JA, Young JB, et al. A question of terminology (letter). J Thorac Cardiovasc Surg 2002;123:830.

7. Meier P. Statistics and medical experimentation. Biometrics 1975; 31:511.

8. Moses LE. Measuring effects without randomized trials? Options, problems, challenges. Med Care 1995;33:AS8.

9. Mark DB, Nelson CL, Califf RM, Harrell FE Jr, Lee KL, Jones RH, et al. Continuing evolution of therapy for coronary artery disease: initial results from the era of coronary angioplasty. Circulation 1994;89:2015.

10. McIntyre N, Popper K. The critical attitude in medicine: the need for a new ethics. Br Med J (Clin Res Ed) 1983;287:1919.

11. McDonald CJ, Hui SL. The analysis of humongous databases: problems and promises. Stat Med 1991;10:511.

12. Moses LE. Innovative methodologies for research using databases. Stat Med 1991;10:629.

13. Malcolm JA Jr. Plans proceed to publish physician-specific data. Pa Med 1992;95:18.

14. Marshall G, Grover FL, Henderson WG, Hammermeister KE. Assessment of predictive models for binary outcomes: an empirical approach using operative death from cardiac surgery. Stat Med 1994;13:1501.

15. McHugh J, Abiteboul S, Goldman R, Quass D, Widom J. A database management system for semistructured data. SIGMOD Rec 1997; 26:54.

16. Morris CN. Parametric empirical Bayes inference: theory and applications. J Am Stat Assoc 1983;78:47.

17. Mann C. Meta-analysis in the breech. Science 1990;249:476.

18. McGiffin DC, Galbraith AJ, O'Brien MF, McLachlan GJ, Naftel DC, Adams P, et al. An analysis of valve re-replacement after aortic valve replacement with biologic devices. J Thorac Cardiovasc Surg 1997; 113:311.

19. Miller ME, Hui SL, Tierney WM. Validation techniques for logistic regression models. Stat Med 1991;10:1213.

20. McGiffin DC, Kirklin JK, Naftel DC, Bourge RC. Competing outcomes after heart transplantation: a comparison of eras and outcomes. J Heart Lung Transplant 1997;16:190.

N

1. Neyman J. On the problem of confidence intervals. Ann Math Stat 1935;6:111.
2. Neyman J. Outline of a theory of statistical estimation based on the classical theory of probability. Philos Trans Ser 1937;236:333.
3. Nelson W. Theory and applications of hazard plotting for censored failure data. Technometrics 1972;14:945.
4. Nelson W. Graphical analysis of system repair data. J Qual Technol 1988;92:186.
5. National Heart, Lung, and Blood Institute Coronary Artery Surgery Study. A multicenter comparison of the effects of randomized medical and surgical treatment of mildly symptomatic patients with coronary artery disease, and a registry of consecutive patients undergoing coronary angiography. Circulation 1981;63:I1.
6. Newton I. Philosophiæ Naturalis Principia Mathematica, 1687.
7. Nguyen J, Shahar Y, Tu SW, Das AK, Musem MA. Integration of temporal reasoning and temporal-data maintenance into a reusable database mediator to answer abstract, time-oriented queries: the Tzolkin System. J Intelligent Information Systems 1999;13:121.
8. Nurmohamed MT, Rosendaal FR, Buller HR, Dekker E, Hommes DW, Vandenbroucke JP, et al. Low-molecular-weight heparin versus standard heparin in general and orthopaedic surgery: a meta-analysis. Lancet 1992;340:152.
9. Nelson W. Confidence limits for recurrence data-applied to cost or number of product repairs. Technometrics 1995;37:147.
10. Nashef SA, Roques F, Michel P, Gauducheau E, Lemeshow S, Salamon R. European system for cardiac operative risk evaluation (EuroSCORE). Eur J Cardiothorac Surg 1999;16:9.
11. Naftel DC. Do different investigators sometimes produce different multivariable equations from the same data? J Thorac Cardiovasc Surg 1994;107:1528.
12. Navia JL, McCarthy PM, Hoercher KJ, Smedira NG, Banbury MK, Blackstone EH. Do left ventricular assist device (LVAD) bridge-to-transplantation outcomes predict the results of permanent LVAD implantation? Ann Thorac Surg 2002;74:2051-63.

O

1. O'Neill TJ. Distribution-free estimation of cure time. Biometrika 1979;66:184.
2. Omoigui NA, Miller DP, Brown KJ, Annan K, Cosgrove D III, Lytle B, et al. Outmigration for coronary bypass surgery in an era of public dissemination of clinical outcomes. Circulation 1996;93:27.
3. Osswald BR, Blackstone EH, Tochtermann U, Thomas G, Vahl CF, Hagl S. The meaning of early mortality after CABG. Eur J Cardiothorac Surg 1999;15:401.
4. Olkin I. Statistical and theoretical considerations in meta-analysis. J Clin Epidemiol 1995;48:133.

P

1. Prentice RL, Marek P. A qualitative discrepancy between censored data rank tests. Biometrics 1979;35:861.
2. Peto R, Peto J. Asymptotically efficient rank invariant test procedures. J R Stat Soc A 1972;135:185.
3. Prentice RL, Kalbfleisch JD, Peterson AV Jr, Flournoy N, Farewell VT, Breslow NE. The analysis of failure times in the presence of competing risks. Biometrics 1978;34:541.
4. Pregibon D. Logistic regression diagnostics. Ann Stat 1981;9:705.
5. Pregibon D. Goodness of link tests for generalized linear models. Appl Stat 1980;29:15.
6. Pearl R, Reed LT. On the rate of growth of the population of the United States since 1790 and its mathematical representation. Proc Natl Acad Sci 1920;6:275.
7. Pearl R. Some recent studies on growth. Am Nat 1909;43:302.

8. Peduzzi P, Detre K, Wittes J, Holford T. Intent-to-treat analysis and the problems of crossovers. An example from the Veterans Administration Coronary Bypass Surgery Study. J Thorac Cardiovasc Surg 1991;101:481.
9. Pocock SJ, Elbourne DR. Randomized trials or observational tribulations? N Engl J Med 2000;342:1907.
10. Parsonnet V, Dean D, Bernstein AD. A method of uniform stratification of risk for evaluating the results of surgery in acquired adult heart disease. Circulation 1989;79:I3.
11. Peterson ED, DeLong ER, Jollis JG, Muhlbaier LH, Mark DB. The effects of New York's bypass surgery provider profiling on access to care and patient outcomes in the elderly. J Am Coll Cardiol 1998;32:993.
12. Pearson K. Report on certain enteric fever inoculation statistics. Br Med J 1904;3:1243.
13. Parsons LS. Reducing bias in a propensity score matched-pair sample using greedy matching techniques. Proceedings of the twenty-sixth annual SAS Users Group international conference. Cary: N.C.: SAS Institute, 2001.
14. Perlman AM. Writing great speeches: professional techniques you can use. Boston: Allyn and Bacon, 1998.
15. Patel H, Gupta G. A problem of equivalence in clinical trials. Biometric J 1984;26:471.
16. Phillips AN, Thompson SG, Pocock SJ. Prognostic scores for detecting a high risk group: estimating the sensitivity when applied to new data. Stat Med 1990;9:1189.
17. Piantadosi S, Kirklin J, Blackstone E. Statistical terminology and definitions. In Pearson FG, Deslauriers J, Ginsberg RJ, Hiebert CA, McKneally MF, Urschel HC Jr, eds. Thoracic surgery, 1st Ed. New York: Churchill Livingstone, p. 1649.

R

1. Reed LJ, Berkson J. The application of the logistic function to experimental data. J Phys Chem 1929;33:760.
2. Rizzoli G, Blackstone EH, Kirklin JW, Pacifico AD, Bargeron LM Jr. Incremental risk factors in hospital mortality rate after repair of ventricular septal defect. J Thorac Cardiovasc Surg 1980;80:494.
3. Reason JT. Human error. Cambridge: Cambridge University Press, 1990.
4. Rasmussen J. Skills, rules, knowledge: signals and symbols and other distinctions in human performance models. IEEE Transactions: Systems, Man & Cybernetics, 1983;13:257.
5. Richardson MH. The gradual elimination of the preventable disaster from surgery. Thorac Med Assoc 1912;:181.
6. Rouse WB. Analysis and classification of human error. IEEE Transactions: Systems, Man & Cybernetics 1983;13:539.
7. Rubin DB. Multiple imputation. J Am Stat Assoc 1996;434:473.
8. Ripley BD. Neural networks and related methods for classification. J Royal Stat Soc 1994;56:409.
9. Rosenbaum PR, Rubin DB. The central role of the propensity score in observational studies for causal effects. Biometrika 1983;70:41.
10. Rubin DB. Estimating causal effects from large data sets using propensity scores. Ann Intern Med 1997;127:757.
11. Rubin DB. Bias reduction using Mahalanobis metric matching. Biometrics 1980;36:393.
12. Rosenbaum PR. Optimal matching for observational studies. J Am Stat Assoc 1989;84:1024.
13. Rosenbaum PR, Rubin DB. The bias due to incomplete matching. Biometrics 1985;41:103.
14. Rosenbaum PR, Rubin DB. Reducing bias in observational studies using subclassification on the propensity score. J Am Stat Assoc 1984;79:516.
15. Rosenbaum PR. From association to causation in observational studies: the role of tests of strongly ignorable treatment assignment. J Am Stat Assoc 1984;79:41.
16. Robins JM, Mark SD, Newey WK. Estimating exposure effects by modelling the expectation of exposure conditional on confounders. Biometrics 1992;48:479.

17. Rosenbaum PR. Observational studies. New York: Springer-Verlag, 1995.
18. Rubin DB. Multiple imputation after 18+ years. J Am Stat Assoc 1996;91:473.

S

1. Shapiro SS, Wilk MB. An analysis of variance test for normality (complete samples). Biometrika 1965;52:591.
2. Stephens MA. Use of the Kolmogorov-Smirnov, Cramer-Von Mises and related statistics without extensive tables. J Am Stat Assoc 1974;69:730.
3. "Student." The probable error of a mean. Biometrika 1908;6:1.
4. Studer M, Blackstone EH, Kirklin JW, Pacifico AD, Soto B, Chung GK, et al. Determinants of early and late results of repair of atrioventricular septal (canal) defects. J Thorac Cardiovasc Surg 1982;84:523.
5. SAS Institute, Inc. SAS technical report P-175: changes and enhancements to the SAS system, release 5.18, under OS and CMS. Cary, N.C.: SAS Institute, 1988, p. 261.
6. Silber JH, Williams SV, Krakauer H, Schwartz JS. Hospital and patient characteristics associated with death after surgery. Med Care 1992;30:615.
7. Silber JH, Rosenbaum PR, Schwartz JS, Ross RN, Williams SV. Evaluation of the complication rate as a measure of quality of care in coronary artery bypass graft surgery. JAMA 1995;274:317.
8. Streptomycin treatment of pulmonary tuberculosis: a Medical Research Council investigation. Br Med J 1948;2:769.
9. Sergeant P, Blackstone E, Meyns B. Can the outcome of coronary bypass grafting be predicted reliably? Eur J Cardiothorac Surg 1997;11:2.
10. Steyerberg EW, Eijkemans MJ, Harrell FE Jr, Habbema JD. Prognostic modelling with logistic regression analysis: a comparison of selection and estimation methods in small data sets. Stat Med 2000; 19:1059.
11. Schlesselman J. Case–control studies. New York, Oxford University Press, 1982.
12. Sacco GM. Dynamic taxonomies: a model for large information bases. IEEE Trans Knowledge Data Eng 2000;12:468.
13. Shahar Y. Dimensions of time in illness: an objective view. Ann Intern Med 2000;132:45.
14. Snodgrass R. Developing time-oriented database applications in SQL. San Francisco: Morgan Kauffmann, 2000.
15. Samet JM. Concepts of time in clinical research. Ann Intern Med 2000;132:37.
16. Shortliffe EH, Perreault LE, Wiederhold G, Fagan LM, eds. Medical informatics: computer applications in health care and biomedicine, 2nd Ed. New York: Springer-Verlag, 2000.
17. Stewart LA, Clarke MJ. Practical methodology of meta-analyses (overviews) using updated individual patient data. Cochrane Working Group. Stat Med 1995;14:2057.
18. Smith FB, Helms RW. EM mixed model analysis of data from informatively censored normal distributions. Biometrics 1995;51:425.
19. Shroyer AL, Plomondon ME, Grover FL, Edwards FH. The 1996 coronary artery bypass risk model: the Society of Thoracic Surgeons Adult Cardiac National Database. Ann Thorac Surg 1999;67:1205.
20. Steiner SH, Cook R, Farewell V, Treasure T. Monitoring surgical performance using risk adjusted cumulative sum charts. Biostatistics 2000;1:441.
21. Shahian DM, Normand SL, Torchiana DF, Lewis SM, Pastore JO, Kuntz RE, et al. Cardiac surgery report cards: comprehensive review and statistical critique. Ann Thorac Surg 2001;72:2155.
22. Sergeant P, Blackstone E, Meyns B. Validation and interdependence with patient-variables of the influence of procedural variables on early and late survival after CABG. K.U. Leuven Coronary Surgery Program. Eur J Cardiothorac Surg 1997;12:1.
23. Salsburg D. Hypothesis versus significance testing for controlled clinical trials: a dialogue. Stat Med 1990;9:201.
24. Sheiner LB. Bioequivalence revisited. Stat Med 1992;11:1777.
25. Sauerbrei W, Schumacher M. A bootstrap resampling procedure for model building: application to the Cox regression model. Stat Med 1992;11:2093.
26. Sell JE, Jonas RA, Mayer JE, Blackstone EH, Kirklin JW, Castaneda AR. The results of a surgical program for interrupted aortic arch. J Thorac Cardiovasc Surg 1988;96:864.

T

1. Tukey JW. Exploratory data analysis. Reading, Mass.: Addison-Wesley, 1977.
2. Turner ME, Pruitt KM. A common basis for survival, growth, and autocatalysis. Math Biosci 1978;39:113.
3. Turner ME, Hazelrig JB, Blackstone EH. Bounded survival. Math Biosci 1982;59:33.
4. Trippett LH. The methods of statistics. London: Williams & Norgate, 1931.
5. Tu JV, Sykora K, Naylor CD. Assessing the outcomes of coronary artery bypass graft surgery: how many risk factors are enough? J Am Coll Cardiol 1997;30:1317.
6. Temple R. Are surrogate markers adequate to assess cardiovascular disease drugs? JAMA 1999;282:790.
7. Tallis GM, Leppard P, O'Neill TJ. The analysis of survival data from a central cancer registry with passive follow-up. Stat Med 1988;7:483.

U

1. Uniform requirements for manuscripts submitted to biomedical journals. International Committee of Medical Journal Editors. N Engl J Med. 1997;336:309.

V

1. Varnauskas E. Twelve-year follow-up of survival in the randomized European Coronary Surgery Study. N Engl J Med 1988;319:332.
2. Verhulst PF. Notice sur Ia loi que la population suit dans son accroissement. Math Phys 1838;10:113.
3. Verhulst PF. Recherches mathematiques sur la loi d'accroissement de la population. Nouv Mem Acad R Sci Belleslett Brux 1845;18:1.

W

1. Walker SH, Duncan DB. Estimation of the probability of an event as a function of several independent variables. Biometrika 1967;54:167.
2. Wigglesworth EC. A teaching model of injury causation and a guide for selecting countermeasures. Occup Psychol 1972;46:69.
3. Weast RC, Selby SM, eds. Handbook of tables for mathematics. Boca Raton, Fla.: CRC Press, 1975.
4. Welch BL. The significance of the difference between two means when the population variances are unequal. Biometrika 1937;29:350.
5. Welch BL. The generalization of "Student's" problem when several different population variances are involved. Biometrika 1947;34:28.
6. Wilcoxon F. Individual comparisons by ranking methods. Biomet Bull 1947;1:80.
7. Weinstein MC. Allocation of subjects in medical experiments. N Engl J Med 1974;291:1278.
8. Weibull W. A statistical theory of the strength of materials. Ing Vetenskaps Akad Handl 1939;151:1.
9. Wu AW, Folkman S, McPhee SJ, Lo B. Do house officers learn from their mistakes? JAMA 1991;265:2089.
10. Williams WG, McCrindle BW. Practical experience with databases for congenital heart disease: a registry versus an academic database. Semin Thorac Cardiovasc Surg Pediatr Card Surg Annu 2002;5:132.
11. Wu MC, Carroll RJ. Estimation and comparison of changes in the presence of informative right censoring by modeling the censoring process. Biometrics 1988;44:175.
12. Weightman WM, Gibbs NM, Sheminant MR, Thackray NM, Newman MA. Risk prediction in coronary artery surgery: a comparison of four risk scores. Med J Aust 1997;166:408.

13. Ware JH, Mosteller F, Delgado F, Donnelly C, Ingelfinger AJ. *P* values. In Bailar JC 3rd, Mosteller F, eds. Medical uses of statistics, 2nd Ed. Boston: NEJM Books, 1992, p. 181.

Y

1. Yates F, Cochran WG. The analysis of groups of experiments. J Agricultural Sci 1938;28:556.
2. Yusuf S, Zucker D, Peduzzi P, Fisher LD, Takaro T, Kennedy JW, et al. Effect of coronary artery bypass graft surgery on survival: overview of 10-year results from randomized trials by the Coronary Artery Bypass Graft Surgery Trialists Collaboration. Lancet 1994; 344:563.

3. Yarnold PR, Soltysik RC, Lefevre F, Martin GJ. Predicting in-hospital mortality of patients receiving cardiopulmonary resuscitation: unit-weighted MultiODA for binary data. Stat Med 1998;17:2405.

Z

1. Zhang HP, Singer B. Recursive partitioning analysis in the health sciences. New York: Springer-Verlag, 1999.
2. Zhou XH, Obuchowski NA, McClish DK. Statistical methods in diagnostic medicine. New York: John Wiley & Sons, 2002.

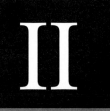

II   Ischemic Heart Disease

7

Stenotic Atherosclerotic Coronary Artery Disease

DEFINITION

Stenotic atherosclerotic coronary artery disease (CAD) is a narrowing of the coronary arteries caused by thickening and loss of elasticity of their arterial walls (arteriosclerosis) that, when sufficiently severe, limits blood flow to the myocardium. Initially, the disease limits only coronary flow reserve (increase in flow that normally accompanies increased myocardial oxygen demands), but when sufficiently advanced, CAD reduces blood flow through the affected artery even at rest. In its most severe form, atherosclerotic CAD occludes the coronary artery.

HISTORICAL NOTE

Development of coronary cineangiography by Sones and Shirey at the Cleveland Clinic during the early 1960s made possible direct identification of stenotic and occlusive atherosclerotic lesions in the coronary arteries during life and laid the foundation for coronary artery surgery.[S1] Sporadic surgical attempts to improve coronary blood flow had previously been made, but these efforts were ineffective because of lack of precise anatomic diagnosis. In 1951 in Montreal, Vineberg and Miller reported direct implantation of an internal thoracic artery (ITA), also known as the internal mammary artery (IMA), into the myocardium.[V1] More than a decade later, the Cleveland Clinic group demonstrated that this procedure brought new blood to the left ventricular (LV) myocardium.[E4] However, the new blood flow was too limited in quantity and distribution to be effective. In 1954, Murray and colleagues were considering a direct surgical approach to CAD when they reported experimental studies of anastomosing the ITA to a coronary artery.[M7] Shortly thereafter, Longmire and colleagues at the University of California in Los Angeles reported a series of patients in whom direct-vision coronary endarterectomy was performed without cardiopulmonary bypass (CPB).[L9] Subsequently, CPB was used to facilitate the operation, and Senning reported patch grafting of a stenotic coronary artery in 1961.[S16] At about this time, Effler and colleagues at the Cleveland Clinic began their pioneering efforts to achieve myocardial revascularization by a direct surgical attack on stenotic coronary lesions, as demonstrated by Sones using coronary angiography.[E2,S15]

Largely overlooked is the first operation for CAD in which the ITA was anastomosed to the left anterior descending coronary artery (LAD) by Kolesov in Leningrad in 1964.[K22,K24] Probably without knowledge of this contribution, in May 1967, Favaloro and Effler at the Cleveland Clinic began performing reversed saphenous vein bypass grafting,[F4] and by January 1971, this group had performed 741 such operations.[L3] Even earlier, Garrett, at that time working with DeBakey in Houston, successfully performed a reversed saphenous vein coronary artery bypass graft to the LAD in an unplanned way[G6]; at restudy 7 years later the vein graft was patent.

Progress was rapid after this early era. In 1968 in New York, Green and colleagues re-reported anastomosing the distal end of the left ITA to the LAD[G7] using a dissecting microscope, and Edwards and colleagues began using this procedure at UAB in 1969.[E3] In Milwaukee in 1971, Flemma, Johnson, and Lepley described the technique and advantages of *sequential grafting,* in which one vein was used for several distal anastomoses.[F6] Advantages of this technique were further amplified by the reports of Bartley, Bigelow, and Page[B2] in 1972 and Sewell in 1974.[S2] Bilateral ITA grafting was performed at least by 1972 and probably as early as 1968.[K28] Thus, within a very short time, the foundations were laid for the rapid worldwide spread of *coronary artery bypass grafting* (CABG).

MORPHOLOGY

Development of Coronary Artery Stenosis

Atherosclerosis, the most common form of arteriosclerosis, is a process that in coronary arteries, as in other blood vessels, consists of focal intimal accumulations of lipids, complex carbohydrates, blood and blood products, fibrous tissue, and calcium deposits, and associated changes in the media. Lipoid foci are associated with or converted into plaques of fibrous or hyaline connective tissue, although at least some atherosclerotic plaques may result from organization of thrombi.[R7]

Fibrolipoid plaques may become thick enough to encroach on the lumen of the artery, producing a stenotic lesion. Probably episodically and at times over years, new layers develop on the luminal side of the plaque, resulting in further narrowing and sometimes complete coronary occlusion. Newly formed, small blood vessels form around and within the plaque. Gradual regression of plaque enlargement, seen clinically as regression of stenoses in a few patients,[S35] and development of collateral coronary blood flow can result in at least partial spontaneous restoration of antegrade regional myocardial blood flow.

Hemorrhage may occur suddenly within a plaque (see "Atherosclerotic Plaque Rupture and Thrombosis" later in chapter), and occasionally this may suddenly increase the degree of coronary stenosis and precipitate acute myocardial infarction (MI) or unstable angina pectoris. *Thrombosis* occasionally complicates the coronary atherosclerotic process, generally when there is luminal narrowing. Sudden complete obstruction may result, and it is generally agreed that acute thrombotic occlusion is the genesis of acute MI in most patients. Rapid recanalization frequently follows this process. *Platelet aggregation* within the lumen of an already narrowed coronary artery may induce the thrombosis or suddenly narrow the lumen and provoke an acute MI or unstable angina, and it may play a role in development of the atherosclerotic plaque itself. Platelet aggregation releases thromboxane A_2, an extremely potent vasoconstrictor. Thus, interrelationships among atherosclerotic narrowing, platelet aggregation, and coronary spasm are important.

The atherosclerotic process usually affects multiple coronary arteries. In 1975, Gensini reported that 40% of patients with CAD sufficient to lead to cineangiographic study had important stenoses in all three major coronary arteries, and in 30% two vessels were involved.[G9] Ninety-five percent of patients with complete occlusion of one artery had important stenoses in at least one of the other two arteries.

Atherosclerotic CAD usually involves the proximal portion of the larger coronary arteries, particularly at or just beyond sites of branching. Thus, stenoses in the main trunks of the LAD, circumflex (Cx) coronary artery, and right coronary artery (RCA) often involve the first of the secondary branches (first diagonal branch of LAD, obtuse marginal branch of Cx artery, and posterior descending branch of RCA). When CAD is more extensive in the main trunks, origins and first portions of secondary branches may be involved. Diffuse distal disease severe enough to render the patient unsuitable for CABG is uncommon. In 10% to 20% of patients with atherosclerotic CAD, the left main coronary artery is importantly stenotic.

Occasionally a major coronary artery may lie beneath a muscle bridge. This is most common in the middle third of the LAD, but sometimes one or all of the obtuse marginal branches of the Cx artery are buried in muscle throughout their course. These portions of artery are typically free of atherosclerotic changes.

Myocardial Infarction and Morphologic Sequelae

When myocardial blood flow is sufficiently impaired in relation to myocardial oxygen demands, myocardial necrosis occurs. The resultant infarction may be *subendocardial,* that is, not involving the entire thickness of the ventricular wall. In its most extreme form, subendocardial infarction may be diffuse and result from multiple-system disease. More often, however, subendocardial infarcts are regional and result primarily from a stenotic lesion in one or two systems. These infarcts are generally less extensive than so-called transmural infarcts, but still have serious implications. A *transmural* MI involves the entire thickness of the ventricular wall. Transmural infarction usually results from a sudden increase in luminal narrowing or complete obstruction of the artery supplying that area, or a sudden generalized increase in myocardial oxygen demand in the presence of a severely stenotic coronary artery. Although categorization of acute infarctions as subendocardial or transmural is convenient, most transmural MIs are not homogeneous, but contain islands of viable muscle of varying number and size.

The process of infarction is complex. Animal studies indicate that some myocardial cells die after 20 minutes of complete coronary artery occlusion, and that extensive myocardial cell death occurs after 60 minutes.[S13] Although these time frames may vary, some reperfusion generally occurs within the ischemic area of myocardium within minutes of onset of acute ischemia, particularly in the zone between ischemic and nonischemic myocardium (border zone). If this spontaneous reperfusion occurs within 3 to 4 hours, the amount of necrosis is restricted, at times substantially,[T3] infarct size is reduced, and mortality is decreased.[B26] The process is complex because, in addition to these beneficial effects, spontaneous reperfusion can result in hemorrhage, edema, and ventricular electrical instability.[C14,K14]

Healing of the acute MI leaves a scarred area of myocardium. In most cases this area is a mixture of fibrous tissue and viable myocardial cells in varying proportions. Such scarring is evident from (1) intraoperative inspection of areas of previous infarction at the time of CABG and (2) change from akinesia or dyskinesia to hypokinesia or normal wall motion in some LV wall segments when patients go from a symptomatic to an asymptomatic state after percutaneous coronary intervention (PCI) or CABG. When the scar is almost all fibrous tissue, it is usually large, and the LV wall may become akinetic or aneurysmal (see Chapter 8).

These morphologic changes may be self-aggravating because of their effect on circulation to the subendocardial layer. Repeated infarctions may occur and add still more scarring. In the aggregate, myocardial scarring leads to LV systolic and diastolic dysfunction and, ultimately, if the patient survives long enough, to the syndrome of chronic heart failure with elevated right atrial and jugular venous pressure, hepatomegaly, and fluid retention. More often, however, patients with severe ischemic LV dysfunction die of another infarction or of ventricular fibrillation.

Atherosclerotic Plaque Rupture and Thrombosis

Recent studies emphasize the dynamic nature of coronary atherosclerotic plaque as a fundamental feature of CAD.[D7,F14] *Fissuring,* or rupture, of atherosclerotic plaques is probably the genesis of the acute coronary syndromes termed *unstable angina* and *acute myocardial infarction.*

When this occurs, mural or occlusive coronary thrombi often coexist and contribute further to development of the unstable states.[F13]

Coronary stenoses that produce less than 50% reduction in lumen diameter are usually the site of the atherosclerotic plaque rupture that precipitates unstable angina or acute MI.[F15,L21,M13] More severe stenoses also undergo plaque rupture, and total vessel occlusion may occur. However, an acute ischemic episode does not always develop, possibly because severely stenotic lesions are long-standing and have stimulated development of a protective collateral circulation.

Certain atherosclerotic plaques appear to have a higher risk of rupture than others. These plaques are characterized by relative softness, a high concentration of cholesterol and cholesterol esters, and a lipid pool that tends to be situated eccentrically.[M13] Rupture is through the cap of the plaque, and areas in which the cap lacks underlying collagen support seem particularly vulnerable.[D7,R21]

CLINICAL FEATURES AND DIAGNOSTIC CRITERIA

Routine Methods

CAD is usually first suspected with development of the symptom complex of angina pectoris or of an acute myocardial infarction, occasionally because of electrocardiographic (ECG) evidence of a silent acute MI, because of a positive ECG response to a graded exercise test, or because of sudden death with resuscitation. Occasionally, CAD is first suspected because of cardiomegaly and symptoms of chronic heart failure without any other obvious cause.

The precise nature, location, duration, and severity of any chest pain are determined by carefully questioning the patient. Precipitating causes and maneuvers that relieve the pain are noted, as are any recent changes in pain pattern. Findings on physical examination are usually not specific.

Many *noninvasive* tests, beginning with a chest radiograph and an electrocardiogram at rest and during exercise, and proceeding to more complex studies, are currently used to identify and quantify CAD and its sequelae.[J11,M21,S7,S62] Such tests cannot yet define extent or distribution of anatomic coronary disease with great accuracy. From a surgical standpoint, therefore, properly performed coronary angiography remains the definitive diagnostic procedure (see "Coronary Angiography" in text that follows).[F9] This situation could change as new noninvasive methods and techniques that enable the surgeon to define stenotic lesions in the operating room with reasonable accuracy are perfected.

Methods of evaluating LV function are also necessary. These may be based in part on historical data, physical findings, and chest radiography. Noninvasive and invasive special study methods may be used. Even when complex study methods are employed, results must be interpreted with knowledge of the simple but reliable clinical data. An ejection fraction (EF) of 0.35 has a different implication when accompanied by minimal LV enlargement, as seen on a chest radiograph, than when enlargement is marked. An EF of 0.30 is much more ominous when accompanied by important elevation of jugular and right atrial pressure with hepatomegaly and fluid retention than when these pressures

are normal. Exercise capacity may be variable in patients with similar EFs, and the variations are prognostically important. It should be emphasized, however, that heart size can be deceptive because it can remain normal in the presence of severe LV dysfunction.

Such important associated conditions as hyperlipidemia, arterial hypertension, and diabetes, and a history of MI, smoking, or a particularly stressful occupation or lifestyle should be noted. Because atherosclerosis is the cause of CAD, its presence elsewhere in the circulatory system should be sought. A history suggesting transient cerebral ischemic attacks or stroke and the finding of carotid bruits must be carefully pursued. A history of intermittent claudication and presence of diminished femoral, popliteal, or pedal pulses are indicative of peripheral vascular occlusive disease. The thoracic and abdominal aorta are examined for possible aneurysm or occlusive disease. Renal function should also be evaluated.

Coronary Angiography

Coronary angiograms provide important information. Their quality must be sufficient to permit detailed assessment from several angles of both coronary ostia and all major and minor branches of both the left and right coronary arterial systems. However, angiography currently remains an imperfect method. Severity of a visualized stenotic lesion may be underestimated and diameter of vessels distal to a stenosis is often underestimated.

Assessment of coronary arteries at operation by external palpation or probing of the open vessel cannot substitute for coronary angiography. When the arteries cannot be adequately filled by contrast media, however, or the available study is incomplete and cannot be repeated (this should be uncommon), intraoperative observations can be used to supplement angiographic findings. The surgeon should assess all coronary arterial branches carefully at the time of operation, rather than assume the coronary angiogram is a totally accurate diagnostic tool.

Recording and Reporting Data

Whatever the techniques used for coronary angiography, methods of recording and analyzing the data are crucial. A 75% cross-sectional area loss (50% diameter) is considered an important but moderate stenosis, and a 90% cross-sectional area loss (67% diameter) is considered severe (Fig. 7-1). Some groups consider only those lesions with 70% or more diameter loss (90% or more cross-sectional area loss) as important,[H8,K17,W7] but an appropriately documented basis for this has not been established.

Extent of important coronary artery stenoses has conventionally been summarized as "single-vessel," "double-vessel," or "triple-vessel" disease, usually with left main coronary artery disease as a separate category. This chapter uses the terms *single-system, two-system,* and *three-system* disease because each coronary system (LAD, Cx, and RCA) consists of several vessels. Use of the term "system" is, therefore, more accurate than vessel.

These classifications have been criticized[G21,S30] because they give no indication of the amount of LV myocardium rendered ischemic by the lesions. For example, a stenosis in the LAD system has a different significance when it lies at

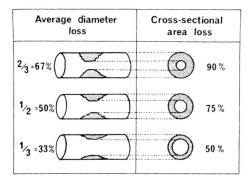

Figure 7-1   Diagrammatic representation of relationship between two methods of estimating severity of coronary artery stenosis. (From Brandt and colleagues.[B32])

the origin of a large first diagonal artery than when it involves the middle one third of the LAD beyond its major septal and diagonal branches, or only the first portion of a large first diagonal branch. A single stenosis in the proximal portion of the Cx artery varies in significance depending on whether this artery is dominant. Single-system disease involving the proximal RCA has a different implication from that involving only the posterior descending branch of the RCA. Many other examples can be given of the inadequacies of these classifications.

Relating results of medical or surgical treatment to the distribution and severity of CAD will remain imprecise until the simpler terms are abandoned in favor of a more precise method of recording and quantifying obstructions to myocardial perfusion by some type of myocardial perfusion score.

A few classification systems have been described to obviate these shortcomings. These include Gensini's old and rather complex scheme, which takes into account severity of the stenoses, the various segments of the coronary artery tree involved, and the area of myocardium usually perfused by them[G21-G23]; a simple scheme from the Massachusetts General Hospital[J7]; and the incomplete method of the Coronary Artery Surgery Study (CASS) of the United States National Heart, Lung, and Blood Institute (NHLBI), dividing the coronary arteries into a total of 27 specified segments.[C6] Some *myocardial jeopardy scores* have attempted to provide the same information, but are limited by the assumption that akinetic areas cannot be revascularized.[R10]

A myocardial perfusion scoring system has been in continuous use at GLH since 1972 (see Appendix 7A).[B32] A diagram made by the reporting cardiologist or radiologist is displayed at the time of operation, when it functions as an accurate guide for the surgeon. The diagram can also be used for computer storage of arteriographic information.

Whatever the recording and reporting methods, they are not a substitute for the surgeon personally reviewing the cineangiograms before deciding for or against operation and again immediately before operation.

Left Ventricular Function Testing

Tests of LV function continue to evolve. Some general concepts underlying all such tests are important.

■ **TABLE 7-1   General Interrelations among Modifiers Describing Left Ventricular Dysfunction, Ejection Fraction, and Coronary Artery Surgery Study Score**

LV Dysfunction	EF		CASS Score (Normal = 5)	
	< Ratio ≤		< Score ≤	
None	.60			5
Mild	.50	.60	5	9
Moderate	.35	.50	9	15
Severe		.35	15	

Key: *CASS,* Coronary Artery Surgery Study; *EF,* ejection fraction; *LV,* left ventricular.

Resting and Exercise Tests

Resting LV function is presumed to depend on the amount of myocardium that is free of scar. Thus, severity of LV dysfunction at rest is a good surrogate for amount of myocardial scar. This may not be entirely accurate in patients with ischemic heart disease, because ischemia may result in myocardial stunning or hibernation and reversible depression of at least systolic LV function (see "Myocardial Cell Stunning" in Chapter 3). CABG and PCI cannot favorably affect myocardial scarring. Increase in EF of about 0.10 often seen after CABG probably results from disappearance of the hibernating component of the preoperatively depressed resting LV function.

Exercise LV function in patients with ischemic heart disease is characteristically depressed compared with resting function. The depression with exercise reflects loss of coronary flow reserve imposed by the distribution and severity of CAD. Amount of decrease in EF or of other measures of the heart's response to stress is a good surrogate for the distribution and severity of coronary arterial stenoses.

Systolic and Diastolic Function

LV function can be expressed as systolic function or diastolic function. *Systolic function* is determined by *contractility* of the ventricle (see "Cardiac Output and Its Determinants" in Section 1 of Chapter 5). *Diastolic function* describes compliance, or *extensibility,* of the ventricle, which is related to preload.

Global and Segmental Function

Global LV function is usually described by an index of overall ventricular systolic function, most often EF. EF is not independent of preload or afterload and therefore is not an ideal index, but it is the most frequently used index and is reasonably satisfactory. EF is obtained most often and least accurately by visual estimation from a cineangiographically recorded left ventriculogram, more accurately (and originally) by quantitative angiography, and also by noninvasive methods such as radioisotopic imaging and echocardiography.

The CASS score was developed by CASS investigators as a measure of global LV function and actually is a summation of five segmental wall scores based on wall motion observed in the right anterior oblique (RAO) projection of the cineangiogram.[C6] Table 7-1 shows the relationship between EF and CASS scores. Other scoring systems have also been developed.

Segmental wall function refers to function, usually systolic, of segments of the LV wall. Methods usually depend on observation of wall motion or wall thickening throughout the cardiac cycle. Analysis of segmental wall motion is particularly informative in patients who have previously sustained MIs.

Load-Independent Function

High LV afterload tends to depress LV systolic function and therefore cardiac output, and high LV preload generally increases cardiac output (see "Cardiac Output and Its Determinants" in Section 1 of Chapter 5). Methods previously discussed generally do not reflect load-independent LV function and are therefore suboptimal.

NATURAL HISTORY

Great gaps exist in knowledge of the natural history of persons with atherosclerotic CAD. Many of these gaps will be permanent because withholding treatment is no longer justifiable. The closest approach to natural history comes from data gathered in patients seen and treated medically before about 1970. Unfortunately, many studies from that era have the disadvantage that patients were not categorized according to anatomic extent of their disease and LV function.

A further complexity is that in nearly all studies since 1970, patients initially undergoing no treatment or medical treatment have properly been allowed thereafter to cross over to interventional treatment (PCI or CABG). This has made it even more difficult to generate accurate information about the natural history of CAD.

Stenotic Coronary Artery Disease

The natural history of patients with a given severity and distribution of CAD depends in part on the rate of progression of both. As an added complexity, regression of some lesions also occurs.[B54,W14] In general, however, both severity and distribution of coronary artery stenoses tend to increase with time,[B31,M9] although the rate of increase is highly variable and difficult to predict.[S35] In general, over a 2-year period, in patients with already important stenoses, 20% of the stenoses increase in severity, and about half the patients develop important new lesions.[B30,S35] The mechanism of increase in severity is variable, but atherosclerotic plaque rupture and thrombosis clearly play important roles in some cases (see "Atherosclerotic Plaque Rupture and Thrombosis" earlier in this chapter).

Of the usually accepted risk factors for *presence* of stenotic CAD, not all have been helpful in predicting its rate of *progression*.[B30,K16,S35] *Aggressiveness of the atherosclerotic process* seems to be a risk factor for progression; surrogates for it include young age at presentation with symptomatic CAD,[B31,K16,M9] peripheral vascular disease, diabetes, and hyperlipidemia.[B56] *Nature of the atherosclerotic plaque* is a risk factor because plaque rupture is frequently the inciting incident leading to progression in severity of coronary artery stenosis. Eccentric positioning of the lipid pool within the plaque appears to predispose to rupture[F13] and thus progression in severity of stenosis. *Rheologic factors* play a role; the more severe the steno-

sis, the more rapid is the progression toward total occlusion.[B30,K25,W2]

Left Ventricular Dysfunction
Stress-Induced Dysfunction

First indications of LV dysfunction in patients with ischemic heart disease are localized abnormalities of regional wall motion (LV systolic function) during exercise or other forms of stress.[S3] These abnormalities are the result of transient myocardial ischemia, which can be demonstrated as myocardial perfusion defects during exercise.[S4,S5]

Global LV systolic function improves during exercise in normal persons, except in old age. By contrast, when initially localized regional areas of myocardial ischemia become sufficiently extensive, global LV systolic function declines during exercise.[B38,H1,J1,R2,S4] Exercise-induced ECG changes also reflect these reversible myocardial perfusion abnormalities, which may be so severe as to cause hypotension during exercise testing.[B33] Related to this exercise-induced decrease in function in some patients, LV end-diastolic volume responds abnormally to exercise by increasing, often to more than 50% above resting value.[B3,H1,J1,R2] These reversible abnormalities of regional myocardial perfusion and wall motion occasionally occur at rest, most often in patients with unstable angina.[K3]

Abnormalities of LV diastolic function during stress can be demonstrated in most patients with extensive CAD.[M20,R14] These abnormalities take the form of reduced peak LV filling rate and increased time to peak filling rate.[B40,R14] These phenomena are the clinical reflection of the laboratory demonstration that ischemia impairs rate of diastolic relaxation of papillary muscle, related to the fact that myocardial relaxation during early diastole is an active, energy-dependent process. Diastolic abnormalities in patients with coronary artery stenoses may also reflect lack of an increase in early diastolic coronary blood flow.

In the aggregate, these purely ischemic abnormalities of LV systolic and diastolic function may be severe enough during stress to result in a considerable increase in LV end-diastolic pressure. This may produce dyspnea and even transient paroxysmal nocturnal dyspnea and pulmonary edema, as well as angina, during severe ischemic episodes. Further evidence that these abnormalities of LV systolic and diastolic function can result from myocardial ischemia alone is provided by their reversal after successful PCI[B39,B46] or CABG.

Dysfunction at Rest

LV dysfunction with the patient at rest and under no stress has been considered the result of myocardial scar. Therefore, it can be expected that it will not improve after neutralization of the coronary arterial stenoses by CABG or PCI. However, there is evidence that myocardial stunning or hibernation, or both, may be responsible at times for considerable LV dysfunction, and that this element of resting LV dysfunction can be relieved by revascularization.

Myocardial scars from previous MIs also result in abnormalities of LV diastolic function.[S32] Both clinical and experimental studies indicate that increase in LV end-diastolic volume, which results from both diastolic and systolic abnormalities of function, is directly related to the amount of scar in the ventricle.

Patients whose LV function is depressed from myocardial scarring exhibit morphologic, physiologic, and functional variability. Some have moderately increased LV end-diastolic pressure at rest and a considerably reduced exercise capacity, but only a mildly increased cardiac size on chest radiography. These patients have moderate scarring and marked ischemic dysfunction in scarred or nonscarred parts of the ventricles that can often be improved by revascularization. Some have chronic symptoms of pulmonary venous hypertension and may still be helped by revascularization. A few have moderate or severe cardiomegaly, reduced cardiac output, importantly elevated right atrial and jugular venous pressure, hepatomegaly, and fluid retention. Patients in the latter group have advanced LV dysfunction from extensive myocardial scarring, and it generally cannot be improved by operation unless the scar is discrete, is full thickness (aneurysmal or akinetic), and can be resected (see Chapter 8).

Unfavorable Outcome Events

Stable Angina

Development of chest discomfort or pain on exertion is common in patients with coronary artery stenosis.[C15] However, chest discomfort is not an inevitable accompaniment of even important CAD. Severity of angina is typically categorized by the Canadian class system, which differs from the New York Heart Association (NYHA) classification for heart failure.[C19]

- *Class 1: Angina* occurring only with strenuous or prolonged exertion at work or recreation and *not* with ordinary physical activity (thus, Class 0 means no angina under any circumstance).
- *Class 2:* Angina occurring with walking rapidly on level ground or a grade and with rapidly walking up stairs. Ordinary walking for fewer than two blocks on level ground or climbing one flight of stairs does *not* cause angina except during the first few hours after awakening, after meals, under emotional stress, in the wind, or in cold weather. This implies slight limitation of ordinary activity.
- *Class 3:* Angina occurring when walking fewer than two blocks on level ground at a normal pace, under normal conditions, or when climbing one flight of stairs. This implies marked limitation of ordinary physical activity.
- *Class 4:* Angina occurring with even mild activity. It may occur at rest but must be brief (less than 15 minutes) in duration. (If the angina is of longer duration, it is called "unstable angina.") This implies inability to carry out even mild physical activity.

Angina generally results from reduction in coronary flow reserve in a portion of the myocardium. The more severe the reduction, the greater is the severity of angina. However, severity of angina also depends on amount of stress or exercise, which increases myocardial oxygen demand in proportion to the intensity of the activity. Standardization of demand gives graded exercise testing its advantage in quantifying, to some extent, the amount of "reversible ischemia" (more properly, the amount of reduction of coronary flow reserve). Absence of angina does not elimi-

nate the possibility that the patient has "reversible ischemia." Although angina tends to become more severe as time passes, a number of patients do not experience this trend.

Unstable Angina

Unstable angina undoubtedly signifies a prognostically important change in the coronary circulation, but the syndrome takes so many different forms that its precise definition has been difficult. Not surprisingly, different practitioners and even different randomized trials have used different definitions.[B34,R3] In 1989, Braunwald devised a classification system to ensure uniformity of categorization and provide diagnostic and prognostic information.[B13]

Although "unstable angina" implies several syndromes, no differences in outcome have been identified among the subgroups. The term applies to patients with severe and persisting angina on presentation to the physician or hospital, with ECG evidence of ischemia and only minor enzymatic evidence (available only later) of MI. The syndrome is considered more ominous if it occurs in the absence of stimuli that increase total body oxygen consumption or catecholamine release (e.g., unusual emotional stress, fever, infection, hypotension or uncontrolled hypertension, tachyarrhythmia, hypoxemia). Unstable angina also applies to patients who have onset of severe angina (Canadian class 4) within 2 months of presentation or who have recurring or prolonged (more than 15 minutes) severe angina within 10 days of presentation, whether or not it is of new onset. The term is also appropriate for patients who develop (or continue with) severe angina in the first 2 weeks after an acute MI. All subsets usually demonstrate ECG evidence of myocardial ischemia during the severe pain and no enzymatic evidence of more than minimal myocardial necrosis.

The cause of unstable angina is now considered to be an acute change in coronary circulation with or without changes in related neurohumoral responses. Unstable atherosclerotic plaque, which may fissure and rupture, is the genesis of unstable angina in many patients (see "Atherosclerotic Plaque Rupture and Thrombosis" earlier in this chapter).[F13] However, superimposed thrombosis and platelet aggregation complicate local situations,[G31,V5] and the clinical state largely depends on activity of the patient's thrombolytic state and mechanisms for reversing platelet aggregation. The process is reversible, but tends to recur either as another episode of unstable angina or as an acute MI.

Acute Myocardial Infarction

Prevalence of acute MIs in patients with coronary artery stenoses is not known precisely, but it is surely affected by prevalence of risk factors. For example, patients with severe proximal LAD lesions have a particular tendency to develop acute and often fatal MI.[S26] Among patients who are sufficiently symptomatic that they undergo coronary angiography, at least 10% have an acute MI within 1 year, 30% within 5 years, 40% within 10 years, and 50% within 15 years, as determined from patients assigned to initial medical treatment in the Veterans Administration (VA) randomized trial of stable angina.[B56]

Acute MI is usually caused by acute subtotal or total occlusion of the vessel supplying the infarcted region, and the vessel usually does not have well-formed collateral arteries. This fact has been suspected for many years and gave rise to the early phrase "coronary thrombosis," but thrombosis was first convincingly demonstrated by De-Wood and colleagues in Spokane, Washington, in a series of patients undergoing emergency CABG for acute infarction.[D5] Often the acutely occluded vessel has not previously had a severe stenosis, which is consistent with the concept that the myocardium supplied by the diseased vessel is usually devoid of important collateral vessels. Current information suggests that rupture of an unstable atheromatous plaque is the genesis of the acute reduction in luminal diameter, often accompanied by thrombosis and platelet aggregation (see "Atherosclerotic Plaque Rupture and Thrombosis" earlier in this chapter).[F15,T2]

The greater the number of myocardial infarctions, the greater is the likelihood that the patient will have another one, which may indicate that some people generate more unstable plaques than others. Also, the more coronary artery systems (LAD, Cx, RCA) that contain important stenoses, the greater is the probability of an acute MI.[B56] This may result simply from the increased number of coronary atherosclerotic plaques available to undergo rupture.

Early (3-month) mortality after acute MI is difficult to define for the current era. Hospital mortality is usually described, but the early phase of the hazard function continues for about 3 months. Until recently, hospital mortality in a heterogeneous group of patients admitted with acute MI has been 10% to 50%, depending on prevalence of risk factors. Death was usually in acute or subacute cardiac failure, or suddenly with ventricular fibrillation.[B37] Size of the infarct was an important risk factor; hospital mortality was 5% for patients with small infarcts versus 50% for those with large infarcts (involving 40% or more of LV mass).[B19,P4] Reserve in the adjacent "non-ischemic" myocardium appeared also to relate to probability of surviving an acute MI, indicating the importance of metabolically supporting this area and revascularizing it even if the stenoses are not severe.[B52,B53] Overall probability of death was higher after the second infarction and still higher after the third, related to scarring imposed by the previous infarctions.[B65] Development of pulmonary edema soon after acute MI increased the risk of death, but 1-year mortality was as low as 10% when other risk factors were favorable.[D12]

Now, therapy is directed toward use of inhibitors of platelet aggregation, thrombolytic agents, heparin, and PCI as soon as possible after onset of infarction. Although the optimal protocol may be arguable, effectiveness of this therapy is not. Hospital mortality has been reduced to about 7% to 10% by these measures. When cardiogenic shock develops, emergency PCI or CABG with maximal measures for myocardial management can salvage many patients (see "Cold Cardioplegia, Controlled Aortic Root Reperfusion, and [When Needed] Warm Cardioplegic Induction" in Chapter 3).[A2,A11,G8,H29,H30,L27]

Death

Probably 70% to 80% of a heterogeneous group of patients with CAD of sufficient severity to cause them to seek medical advice ultimately die a *cardiac death.* The remaining 20% to 30% die of unrelated causes. However, time-related probability of death in a group of CAD patients is so related to prevalence of risk factors that overall estimates are of little value.

Most often, death occurs with acute or subacute cardiac failure, often within a few months of an acute MI and sometimes precipitated by a ventricular arrhythmia.[B56] Infrequently, death is attributable to chronic heart failure, either late after one or more infarctions or without any identifiable earlier episode of infarction. This mode of death is generally characterized by a slow downhill course, eventually leading to hepatomegaly, ascites, and ultimately death. Death in this mode is usually the direct result of myocardial scarring.

About 20% of patients with important CAD who have had no interventional therapy die suddenly.[B56] CAD is not the only cause of sudden death. Presumably, sudden cardiac death in patients with ischemic heart disease can result from acute, severe myocardial ischemia, resulting in ventricular fibrillation, asystole, or acute severe depression of ventricular function.[B36]

Overall survival for a heterogeneous group of patients with clinically evident CAD is 75% at 5 years after initiation of medical treatment, 60% at 10 years, and 45% at 15 years.[B56]

Incremental Risk Factors for Unfavorable Outcome Events

Understanding the benefit of interventional therapy, whether CABG or PCI, demands a knowledge of the incremental risk factors for unfavorable outcome events in patients treated medically for CAD.

Multivariable analysis is used to generate incremental risk factors for various unfavorable events after CABG, PCI, or medical treatment. However, those identified are often surrogates for more basic risk factors, and at times several surrogates for the same basic risk factors appear. Box 7-1 presents the basic risk factors as currently perceived. In the future these factors themselves may become more clearly identifiable.

Reduced Regional Coronary Flow Reserve

Reduced regional flow reserve results from severity of the coronary arterial stenoses and number of coronary arterial systems with important stenoses. The left main coronary artery is an additional "system."

Time-related survival for a heterogeneous group of patients with *single-system stenosis* is high, approximately 90% to 95% at 5 years (Fig. 7-2, *A*). Even at 15 years, survival is about 50%. Additional risk factors relating to reduction in regional coronary flow reserve include (1) specific vessel(s) diseased, (2) location of the stenosis within the vessel, and (3) severity of the stenosis. Because time-related mortality from single-system disease is relatively low, the differences attributable to further refinements in this category will be small and therefore difficult to identify. Also, inferences from the analyses are only as good as reliability of the cineangiogram.

In any event, single-system disease with stenosis in the RCA appears to confer better survival than can be expected with LAD disease, at least for 5 years (RCA 96%, LAD

BOX 7-1   Incremental Risk Factors for Death and other Unfavorable Outcome Events in Patients with Stenotic Atherosclerotic Coronary Artery Disease [a]

Severity of Reduction in Regional Coronary Flow Reserve [b]
- Angina severity (Canadian class 0 to 4)
- Degree of positive response to stress testing
- Severity and number of stenoses

Number of Myocardial Regions with Reduced Coronary Flow Reserve [b]
- Left main stenosis and severity
- Distribution and severity of coronary stenoses
- Myocardial score

Nature of Coronary Atherosclerotic Plaque
- Number of previous myocardial infarctions
- Acute myocardial infarction
- Distribution of coronary stenoses

Internal Milieu (thrombotic or fibrinolytic)
- Number of previous myocardial infarctions
- Acute myocardial infarction
- Distribution of coronary stenoses

Aggressiveness of Atherosclerotic Process
- Diffusely narrowed coronary arteries
- Peripheral vascular disease
- Cerebrovascular disease
- Hyperlipidemia
- Diabetes
- Hypertension
- Younger age at intervention

Rate of Progression of Coronary Arterial Stenoses

Amount and Distribution of Myocardial Scar
- Number of previous acute myocardial infarctions
- Left ventricular ejection fraction
- Left ventricular Coronary Artery Surgery Study (CASS) score
- Left ventricular end-diastolic pressure
- Defects identified by exercise or resting thallium-201 scintigraphy (delayed or after reinjection)

Secondary Conditions
- Hemodynamic instability
- Cardiogenic shock
- Ischemic instability (unstable angina)
- Ventricular electrical instability

Coexisting Conditions (comorbidity)
- Older and younger age
- Larger and smaller body size
- Ethnicity
- Diabetes
- Hyperlipidemia
- Hypertension
- Chronic pulmonary disease
- Chronic renal disease
- Smoking
- Previous stroke

[a] Factors/events listed are not the result of a formal multivariable analysis, but rather a composite of many such analyses.
[b] These categories constitute *reversible ischemia.*

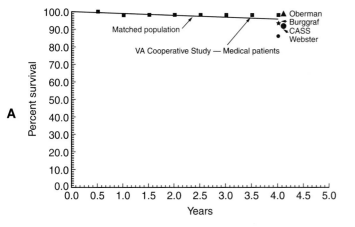

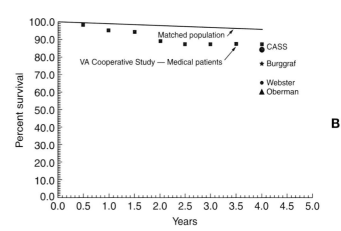

A

B

Figure 7-2   Survival of medically treated men with coronary artery disease, stable angina of at least 6 months' duration, and less than severe left ventricular dysfunction enrolled in the U.S. Veterans Administration *(VA)* Cooperative Study *(solid squares).*[R5] For comparison, survival is shown of a population matched for age and gender from the 1976 U.S. life tables *(solid line).* Data for other groups of medically treated patients published earlier by Burggraf,[B14] and by Oberman[O2] and Webster[W3] and their colleagues are also shown. Lower survival in the last three groups may have been the result of less restrictive selection of patients than for the VA group and better medical treatment in the more recent VA group. Data from the Coronary Artery Surgery Study *(CASS),* in which important stenosis meant a 70% diameter reduction, are also presented.[M18] These data include patients treated medically in the current era with all types of ventricular function. Left main coronary artery data from CASS refer to left main coronary artery plus triple-system disease. **A,** Single-system disease. **B,** Double-system disease.

Key: *CASS,* Coronary Artery Surgery Study; *VA,* Veterans Administration.   *Continued*

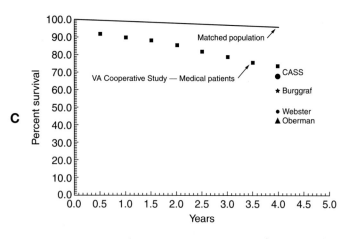

C

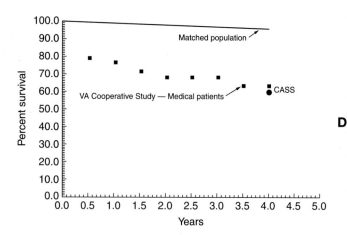

D

Figure 7-2, cont'd   C, Triple-system disease. **D,** Left main coronary artery disease. (From Kirklin and colleagues.[K7])

Key: *CASS,* Coronary Artery Surgery Study; *VA,* Veterans Administration.

92%).[C25] When the single-system stenosis is in the LAD, a very proximal location (proximal to the large septal branch) imposes less favorable survival than do more distal lesions (proximal 90% at 5 years, distal 98%).[C25] Although not conclusively demonstrated, more severe stenoses (greater than 90%), especially those proximal in the artery, probably impose higher time-related mortality than do less severe stenoses.

Patients with *two-system stenoses* as a heterogeneous group have lower survival than do those with single-system stenoses, with 5-year survival of about 88% (Fig. 7-2, *B*). At 15 years, survival is about 56%. When the LAD is one of the two systems, the same effects of location and severity as mentioned above pertain.[V6] Differences in outcome between one- and two-system stenoses are not as great as those between two- and three-system stenoses.

As a heterogeneous group, patients with *three-system stenoses* have a 5-year survival without interventional treatment of about 70% (Fig. 7-2, *C*) and a 10- and 15-year survival of about 60% and 40%, respectively.[B14] Factors affecting survival in patients with important single-system stenosis involving the LAD also affect survival in patients with three-system stenosis. Also, the greater the number of systems with important proximal stenoses, the lower is survival: at 5 years, survival with no, one, two, and three systems with proximal stenoses is 71%, 64%, 51%, and 45%, respectively.[M11]

Important *left main coronary artery stenoses* impose an even lower survival: 40% to 60% at 5 years (Fig. 7-2, *D*). Survival falls to about 10% to 26% by 15 years (Fig. 7-3).

Severity of angina is a surrogate for the basic risk factor of severity of reduction in coronary blood flow reserve (Fig. 7-4). Also, *results of graded exercise testing* (GXT) is a surrogate for the basic risk factor of severity of reduced coronary blood flow reserve and is related to outcome events in CAD patients. For example, in the heterogeneous group of patients randomly assigned to initial medical treatment in the European Coronary Surgery Study Group randomized trial, 1-, 5-, and 10-year survival was 94%, 83%, and 71% in patients with a mildly positive GXT but 92%, 77%, and 62% in those with a strongly positive GXT.[V6] Similarly, in a study from the CASS Registry,

survival at 12 years after medical treatment was substantially lower among patients with a strongly positive GXT (55% for men, 62% for women) than among those with a mildly positive test (75% for men, 82% for women).[W5]

Progression of Coronary Atherosclerosis

Rate of progression of coronary atherosclerosis, which could also be termed *aggressiveness of the atherosclerotic process,* cannot as yet be examined directly in multivariable risk factor analyses. Its surrogates have appeared in a number of such analyses. The surrogates may be a substitute not solely for one basic risk factor but at times for several factors. Among them are young age at presentation, diabetes, hypertension, and hyperlipidemia.

An important advance has been the demonstration that progression of atherosclerotic CAD can be slowed, and that regression of some lesions in some circumstances can be initiated by intensive lipid-lowering therapy.[B54,W14]

Coronary Atherosclerotic Plaques

Number of previous episodes of acute MI may be a surrogate for coronary atherosclerotic plaques as well as for total area (or number) of atherosclerotic plaques within the coronary arterial tree. Presence of unstable angina and number of recent episodes may likewise be surrogates. In this regard, however, status of the patient's fibrinolytic and disaggregating systems also plays a role. During very active periods, these systems may neutralize the effects of plaque rupture and minimize the severity and frequency of unstable angina and acute MI.

Myocardial Scar

To the extent that resting LV dysfunction in patients with CAD is related directly to amount of scar in the myocardium, surrogates for presence and extent of this basic risk factor include number of prior episodes of acute MI; resting LV systolic and diastolic dysfunction (presence and severity), as determined by any of several methods; and a history of chronic heart failure.

Reversible ischemia is capable of producing *resting* LV dysfunction. Myocardial stunning may persist after revers-

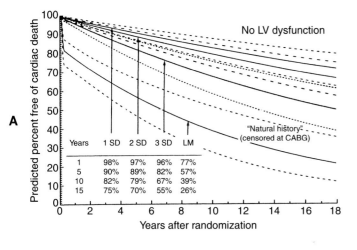

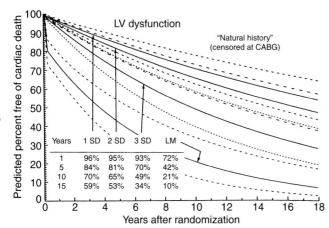

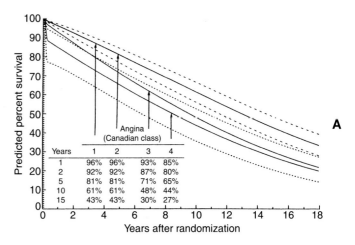

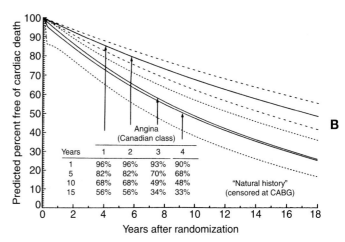

Figure 7-3   Nomograms of specific solutions of multivariable risk factor equations illustrating effect of number of coronary artery systems with important stenoses on time-related freedom from cardiac death in patients randomly assigned to initial medical treatment in Veterans Administration randomized trial of chronic stable angina. For this depiction, patients were censored if they crossed over to coronary artery bypass grafting. Values for each risk factor in the specific solutions of the multivariable equation represented by these nomograms are provided in the ACC/AHA Joint Task Force Subcommittee on Coronary Artery Bypass Graft Surgery.[A20] **A,** Patients with normal left ventricular *(LV)* function. **B,** Patients with importantly impaired LV function.

Key: *ACC,* American College of Cardiology; *AHA,* American Heart Association; *CABG,* coronary artery bypass grafting; *LM,* left main coronary artery disease; *LV,* left ventricular; *SD,* systems diseased.

Figure 7-4   Nomograms illustrating effect of severity of angina (expressed as Canadian class) on survival in patients randomly assigned to initial medical treatment in the Veterans Administration randomized trial of chronic stable angina (same equation as in Fig. 7-3). **A,** Survival, leaving patients in follow-up evaluation after crossover to coronary artery bypass grafting (CABG) ("intent to treat" analysis). **B,** Freedom from cardiac death, censoring patients at time of crossover to CABG.

Key: *CABG,* Coronary artery bypass grafting.

stantially reduces it. Thus, other factors being equal, 1- and 5-year survival in patients with mild LV dysfunction is about 95% and 80%, respectively, whereas with severe dysfunction it is about 70% and 40%.[C17,M11] Good LV function is found more frequently in patients with single-system disease than those with three-system disease (Table 7-2).

Secondary Conditions

Certain conditions develop secondary to ischemic heart disease and are additional incremental risk factors for death and other unfavorable events.

Hemodynamic instability.   Grade 1 hemodynamic instability is mild and responds to catecholamine infusion. Grade 2 is more severe and responds only when intraaortic balloon pumping is added. Grade 3 is unresponsive even to addition of intraaortic balloon pumping and requires cardiopulmonary support (cardiopulmonary bypass) or a ventricular

ible ischemia has disappeared and may result in LV dysfunction. Unfortunately, methods for distinguishing between scar and reversible ischemia, although useful, are neither entirely accurate nor precise. The frequent finding of only a 0.05 to 0.10 increase in preoperatively depressed EF in many patients after CABG suggests that the proportion of LV dysfunction not attributable to myocardial scarring is small.

In CAD patients treated noninterventionally, mild resting LV dysfunction (EF 35% to 50%) minimally affects survival, but severe dysfunction (EF less than 35%) sub-

assist device. Because hemodynamic instability in patients with ischemic heart disease typically reflects acute myocardial necrosis and produces secondary deleterious effects throughout the body, it adversely affects outcome.

Ischemic instability. Ischemic instability is a state of unstable angina and implies acute myocardial ischemia. It carries the risk that severe myocardial stunning and necrosis or ischemic ventricular electrical instability can develop acutely.

Ventricular electrical instability. Either ischemic or secondary to phenomena associated with myocardial scarring, ventricular electrical instability is a risk factor incremental to that of the basic milieu that gives rise to it.

Coexisting Conditions

Older age. Older age at presentation is a risk factor for death in patients with ischemic heart disease. Older age probably acts as a coexisting condition rather than affecting CAD directly.

Diabetes. Diabetes is a strong risk factor for death in CAD patients because of its effect as a coexisting condition and its accelerating effect on the atherosclerotic process. Fig. 7-5 illustrates the powerful effect of diabetes in elderly patients who have undergone PCI.

Hypertension. The strong effect of hypertension as a risk factor for death in CAD patients is related to kidney damage, intracranial complications, and LV hypertrophy, as well as acceleration of the atherosclerotic process (Fig. 7-6).

Gender. Although overall mortality is lower in women with angina than in men, among subjects over age 65, relative risks are similar (2.7 versus 2.4, respectively).[L28,M22]

Other comorbidity. Any serious coexisting disease adversely affects survival in patients with CAD. Of particular importance, because of their prevalence in this group of patients, are *chronic obstructive pulmonary disease* and *chronic renal disease. Smoking* can be considered an important coexisting condition.

■ **TABLE 7-2**   **Association of Left Ventricular Systolic Function and Extent of Severe Coronary Artery Disease with 4-Year Survival in Patients Treated Medically** [a]

Ejection Fraction			Single-System Disease				Double-System Disease				Triple-System Disease				$P[\chi^2]$ [b]
≤ Ratio	<		n	No.	%	CL (%)	n	No.	%	CL (%)	n	No.	%	CL (%)	
0.50			761	723	95	94-96	415	386	93	91-94	227	186	82	79-85	<.0001
0.35	0.50		184	167	91	88-93	144	120	83	79-87	88	62	70	65-76	.0001
	0.35		57	42	74	66-80	57	32	56	48-64	69	35	51	44-58	.03
$P[\chi^2]$			<.0001				<.0001				<.0001				

(Recalculated from CASS Registry by Mock and colleagues.[M18])

Key: *n*, Total patients; *No.*, patients with disease; *CL*, 70% confidence limits.

[a] In current era, as estimated by global ejection fraction. Severe disease is 70% or greater reduction in diameter. These data must be interpreted in light of the fact that during the study period, approximately 20%, 30%, and 45% of patients with single-, double-, and triple-system disease, respectively, crossed over to surgical treatment.

[b] P values for difference in predicted survival.

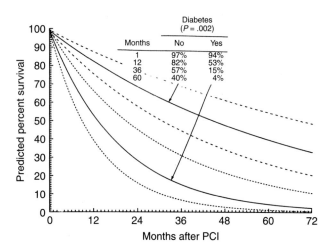

Figure 7-5   Nomogram illustrating effect of diabetes on survival after percutaneous coronary intervention in elderly patients (same equation as in Fig. 7-3). (Equation from Garrahy and colleagues.[G17])

Key: *PCI*, Percutaneous coronary intervention.

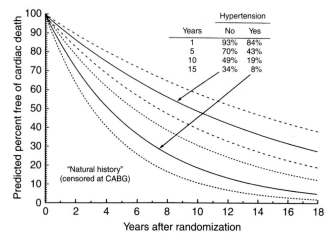

Figure 7-6   Nomogram illustrating effect of hypertension on time-related probability of freedom from cardiac death in patients randomly assigned to initial medical treatment in the Veterans Administration randomized trial of chronic stable angina (same equation as in Fig. 7-3).

Key: *CABG*, Coronary artery bypass grafting.

TECHNIQUE OF OPERATION

Most patients undergoing CABG have extensive three-system disease, often with important stenoses in four, five, or six arteries. Many have substantial impairment of LV function. This discussion focuses on operation under these circumstances and on tactics for accomplishing optimal revascularization and optimal intraoperative management of the myocardium.

Surgical management of atherosclerotic CAD has evolved from treatment primarily of patients with stable coronary syndromes undergoing elective operation to treatment of more heterogeneous groups of patients with various clinical syndromes who are older and have more comorbid conditions, including patients who require urgent or emergent operation.[A10] Economic and other external pressures often result in CABG being performed within hours after diagnostic coronary angiography or PCI.

At present, CABG with use of total CPB through a full sternotomy remains the most widely used surgical technique. Because of extensive experience, this approach is the technique to which all others must be compared. Other techniques currently in use include CABG through a full sternotomy but without use of CPB (OPCAB) and operations through smaller sternal, parasternal, or thoracotomy incisions with or without use of CPB (MIDCAB) (see Fig. 2-22).

Here, the conventional operation with CPB, as well as the OPCAB procedure, are presented. Other procedures are discussed under "Special Situations and Controversies" later in this chapter.

Preoperative Preparation

Many patients come to CABG taking β-adrenergic receptor or calcium channel blocking agents, angiotensin converting enzyme (ACE) inhibitors, digitalis preparations, antiarrhythmic agents, and platelet antiaggregating drugs. Some are receiving intravenous heparin and nitroglycerin. It is advisable, in most circumstances, to continue β-adrenergic receptor blocking and calcium channel blocking agents, as well as ACE inhibitors, up to the time of operation. Several studies have shown a tendency toward development of acute MI in patients in whom β-adrenergic receptor agents are discontinued. Boudoulas and colleagues demonstrated an important increase in adrenergic tone in most patients the day before operation that could be reduced by propranolol.[B28] Propranolol has also been shown to lessen prevalence of intraoperative ventricular arrhythmias[S18] without compromising LV function in low or moderate dosages.[R6] Patients receiving β-adrenergic receptor agents, amiodarone, or sotalol preoperatively are less likely to develop atrial fibrillation postoperatively.[D17,G36,K9]

Digitalis preparations can be discontinued preoperatively unless atrial fibrillation is present (see Chapter 4). They can be administered intraoperatively and postoperatively for control of heart rate if atrial fibrillation or other atrial arrhythmias are present.

Platelet antiaggregating drugs such as abciximab (ReoPro), eptifibatide (Integrilin), tirofiban (Aggrastat), and clopidogrel (Plavix) bind to the glycoprotein IIb/IIIa platelet receptors. When feasible, these drugs as well as aspirin should be discontinued at the appropriate time interval before operation (each has a different half-life) if the patient has a stable coronary syndrome, because their use is associated with increased postoperative bleeding.[G34,G37]

Patients who have received plasminogen-activating (fibrinolytic) agents such as steptokinase, alteplase, and releplase preoperatively require careful attention intraoperatively and postoperatively to manage excessive bleeding.

Operating Room Preparation

Anesthetic methods for CABG are described in Chapter 4. After inserting an endotracheal tube and appropriate monitoring devices (see Chapter 2), the skin is prepared over the chest, abdomen, groin, one or both arms if indicated, and the complete circumference of both legs, including the feet. Draping includes isolating the feet, genitalia, and pubis and placing sterile waterproof drapes beneath the legs.

Surgical Strategy

The prime objective of CABG is to obtain *complete revascularization* by bypassing all severe stenoses (at least 50% diameter reduction) in all coronary arterial trunks and branches having a diameter of about 1 mm or more.[B44,J9] Because five or more individual conduits cannot be conveniently used in most patients, at least some of the grafts must have sequential (side-to-side) anastomoses. To increase the likelihood that the entire graft will remain patent, the distal end-to-side anastomosis of a sequential graft should be made, whenever possible, to a relatively large artery with a substantial proximal stenosis and good runoff. It is not clearly established whether grafts with more than one distal anastomosis have the same, higher, or lower patency rates than those with only a single distal anastomosis. As a general principle, conservation of conduit by employing sequential grafting is prudent because of the likelihood of subsequent CABG.

A widely used strategy involves routine use of the left ITA to the LAD and segments of saphenous vein to the remaining coronary arteries requiring revascularization. The right ITA, one or both radial arteries, and the right gastroepiploic artery can also be used in combination with the left ITA. Sequential anastomoses with the ITA and radial artery can be performed with satisfactory results.[B58,C35,D10,S47,T8] Figs. 7-7 and 7-8 show the most widely used combinations and configurations of bypass grafts. Details of graft placement are often individualized according to location and severity of the atherosclerotic disease, surgeon preference, availability of suitable conduit, and knowledge of the long-term function of various conduits.

The cineangiogram provides key information for planning CABG. However, the surgeon may elect to open vessels suspected of having important stenosis, as determined from the cineangiogram or from observations made at operation. A few errors will inevitably be made regarding which vessels should be grafted. The surgeon must decide which error is more acceptable: opening and grafting an artery that does not need it or failing to open and graft a vessel with an important stenosis. The latter is generally considered a more serious error.

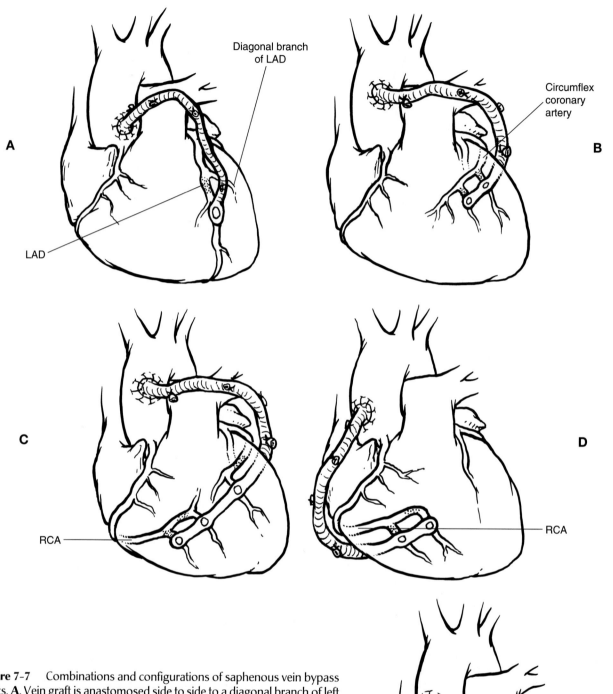

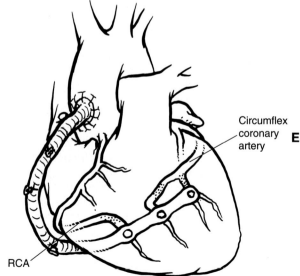

Figure 7-7   Combinations and configurations of saphenous vein bypass grafts. **A,** Vein graft is anastomosed side to side to a diagonal branch of left anterior descending coronary artery *(LAD)* and end to side to LAD. **B,** In circumflex system, vein graft is anastomosed side to side to one or more proximal marginal branches and end to side to most distal marginal branch. **C,** Sequential grafts to circumflex system (Cx) can be extended to include branches of right coronary artery *(RCA)*. **D,** In RCA system, vein graft can be anastomosed side to side to posterior descending coronary artery and end to side to one or more left ventricular branches of RCA. **E,** Sequential grafts to RCA system can be extended to include branches of Cx artery. Direction of a sequential graft to RCA and Cx artery systems (configuration *C* or *E*) is chosen so that the largest coronary artery branch is placed at end of sequence.

Key: *LAD,* Left anterior descending coronary artery; *RCA,* right coronary artery.

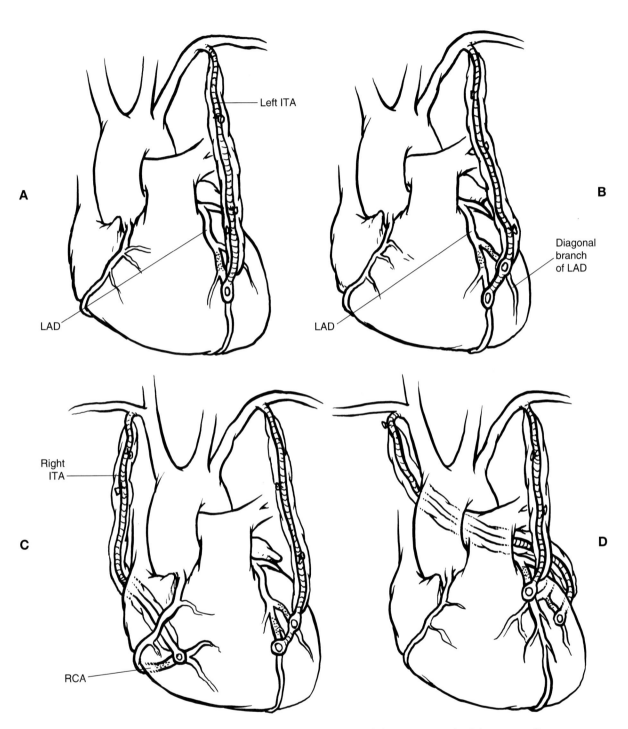

Figure 7-8 Combinations and configurations of internal thoracic artery (ITA) bypass grafts. **A,** Left *ITA* is most often used to bypass the left anterior descending coronary artery *(LAD).* **B,** Sequential grafting using left ITA may include a diagonal branch of LAD. **C,** Right ITA can be used to bypass right coronary artery alone or in combination with an ITA graft to LAD system. **D,** Alternatively, right ITA can be passed through transverse sinus and anastomosed to one or more marginal branches of left circumflex coronary artery.

Key: *ITA,* Internal thoracic artery; *LAD,* left anterior descending coronary artery; *RCA,* right coronary artery. *Continued*

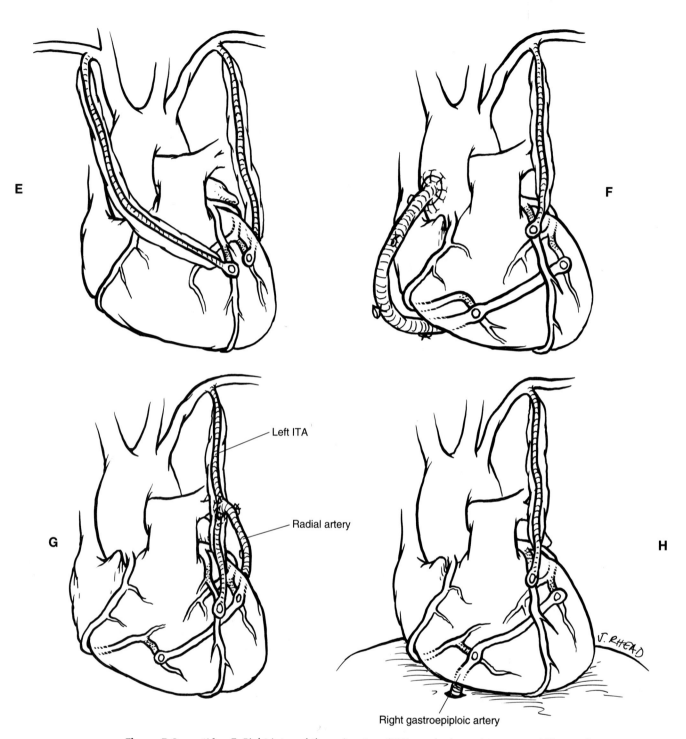

E

F

Left ITA

Radial artery

G

H

Right gastroepiploic artery

Figure 7-8, cont'd   **E,** Right internal thoracic artery (ITA) can be brought across midline and used to bypass left anterior descending coronary artery (LAD), and if indicated, left ITA can be anastomosed to one or more marginal branches of left circumflex coronary artery. **F,** When extensive revascularization of posterior wall of left ventricle (LV) is required, a posteriorly positioned sequential vein graft (or radial artery) in combination with a left ITA graft to the LAD is typically used. **G,** Radial artery graft may be used as a sequential graft to bypass arteries on lateral and posterior surfaces of LV. Radial artery can be anastomosed proximally to left ITA, which is used to bypass the LAD. Alternatively, radial artery can be anastomosed directly to ascending aorta. **H,** Right gastroepiploic artery or splenic artery may be used to bypass branches of right and circumflex coronary arteries in combination with ITA or other grafts to LAD circulation.

Key: *ITA,* Internal thoracic artery.

Coronary Artery Bypass Grafting

With Cardiopulmonary Bypass

A median sternotomy is made, and at the same time a segment of greater saphenous vein (or radial artery or other conduit) is removed. Before the pericardium is opened, the left ITA (and the right, if indicated) is completely mobilized. Heparin is administered as dissection of the ITA is being completed. The ITA is then divided. A bulldog clamp is placed on the artery near the open end, and the distal segment of the artery on the chest wall is ligated or clipped. The pericardium is opened, and pericardial stay sutures are placed. Purse-string sutures are placed at the sites for cannulation and in the ascending aorta and right atrial wall for controlled aortic root perfusion and delivery of cardioplegia into the coronary sinus (see Fig. 2-21). Because atherosclerosis is frequently present in the ascending aorta and proximal aortic arch in patients with CAD, particularly elderly patients, epiaortic ultrasonographic scanning of the aorta is advisable before aortic cannulation to obtain information that can lead to safe positioning of cannulae and aortic clamps (see "Epiaortic Ultrasonography" in Chapter 53).[B51,C12,F8,G26,W15]

CPB is established using a single venous cannula. Catheters for administering cardioplegic solution are placed into the ascending aorta and coronary sinus through the previously placed purse-string sutures and secured with tourniquets. The aorta is clamped and cardioplegic solution infused (see "Cold Cardioplegia, Controlled Aortic Root Reperfusion, and [When Needed] Warm Cardioplegic Induction" in Chapter 3). The heart is covered with cold saline during administration of cold cardioplegia.

With the heart retracted out of the pericardial cavity and toward the head of the patient by an assistant standing to the surgeon's left or by traction sutures placed on the acute margin of the heart, the first anastomosis of the conduit that has been selected is made to the distal RCA or to the posterior descending artery (PDA) (Fig. 7-7, *D*). (See "Distal Anastomosis" later in this chapter.) Sequential anastomoses of the conduit can be performed to more distal branches of the RCA or to the marginal branches of the Cx coronary artery (Fig. 7-7, *E*). The graft is then distended gently with cardioplegic solution, positioned along the right atrium up to the right side of the ascending aorta, and transected at the point that will permit a smooth course of the conduit without kinking or tension. The free end of the graft is spatulated.

The heart is then retracted to the right by the assistant. A separate conduit is anastomosed to one or more of the marginal branches of the Cx artery (Fig. 7-7, *B*). The graft is properly oriented to avoid twisting, and the heart is repositioned in the pericardial cavity. The graft is distended by infusing cardioplegic solution, cut to the appropriate length, and spatulated. This graft can be positioned anterior to the pulmonary artery or passed through the transverse sinus for anastomosis to the right side of the aorta.[G12] A third segment of conduit can be anastomosed to one or more diagonal branches of the LAD. This segment can be brought anterior to the pulmonary artery or through the transverse sinus.

The ITA is cut to the appropriate length and a bulldog clamp placed on the proximal portion. If the operation has been performed using hypothermia, rewarming is begun at this time. The pericardium is incised widely to permit proper alignment of the ITA with the LAD and its diagonal branches, taking care to avoid injury to the left phrenic nerve. A pad is placed beneath the LV, and the LAD is isolated and incised. The distal end of the ITA is spatulated and sutured to the LAD and sequentially to a diagonal branch of the LAD, if indicated (Fig. 7-8, *A* and *B*).

The aortic clamp is removed, a partially occluding clamp is placed on the ascending aorta, and two or three openings are made with a punch in the isolated aortic segment. The grafts are sutured to the aorta so that they are free of kinking or tension. If grafts have been passed through the transverse sinus, they are anastomosed to openings made on the right lateral surface of the ascending aorta. Because of increasing evidence implicating the atherosclerotic ascending aorta as an important source of emboli to the brain and other organs, it may be preferable to avoid placing the partially occluding clamp on it and to perform the proximal anastomoses during a single period of aortic clamping with the heart arrested.[A9]

The partially occluding clamp (or the aortic clamp if a partially occluding clamp has not been used) is then removed. Air is evacuated from the ascending aorta, and controlled aortic reperfusion, if indicated, is begun. Once rewarming has been completed and the heart is beating well, CPB is discontinued and the cannulae are removed. Temporary atrial and ventricular pacing wires and chest drainage tubes are placed. The remainder of operation is completed in the standard manner (see "Completing Cardiopulmonary Bypass" in Section 3 of Chapter 2).

Without Cardiopulmonary Bypass

Perfection of techniques and equipment for stabilizing the beating heart has resulted in an increased number of CABG procedures performed without use of CPB. Procedures involving placement of grafts to more than one of the three major coronary arteries are generally performed through a median sternotomy (OPCAB). With development of stabilization devices that permit adequate and safe exposure of all surfaces of the LV, OPCAB can be safely performed in patients with three-system disease and with left main coronary artery disease.[C24,K2,P11,Y2]

In contrast to CABG performed with CPB, methodology for OPCAB continues to evolve, and many issues relating to preoperative selection and preparation of patients, their anesthetic management, and conduct of the operation remain incompletely defined and unresolved. The following discussion presents a generalized representation of OPCAB, with schematic illustrations of the techniques and equipment for exposing and stabilizing surfaces of the LV.

Anesthetic management of patients undergoing CABG without CPB is discussed in Section 1 of Chapter 4. Close communication between the surgeon and anesthesiologist is essential during OPCAB. The surgeon must inform the anesthesiologist when and how the heart is being displaced, when a coronary artery is occluded, and when a shunt or other perfusion device is used. The anesthesiologist must keep the surgeon informed of ischemic changes detected by the electrocardiogram, occurrence of arrhythmias, and the patient's overall hemodynamic status. When the heart is displaced, amplitude of the ECG signal may be greatly decreased, and thus severity of ST-segment changes indicative of ischemia may be underestimated. Transesophageal echocardiography is used to monitor regional wall motion and right and left ventricular volumes.

A median sternotomy is made, and at the same time a segment of the greater saphenous vein (or a radial artery or other conduit) is removed (see "Vein Graft" in text that follows). Before the pericardium is opened, the left ITA and right ITA (if indicated) are completely mobilized (see "Internal Thoracic Artery" later in this chapter). Heparin is administered as dissection of the ITA is being completed. The ITA is then divided. A bulldog clamp is placed on the artery near the open end, and distal segment of the artery on the chest wall is ligated or clipped. The pericardium is opened and pericardial stay sutures placed. Epiaortic ultrasonographic scanning of the ascending aorta to detect severe atherosclerosis that may affect the conduct of the operation is advisable in older patients (see Chapter 53).[B51,C12,F8,G26,W15]

Heparin, dose optimal activated clotting time (ACT), and protocol for administering protamine vary from institution to institution. Heparin dose varies from a minimum of 5000 units to full heparinization ($3 \text{ mg} \cdot \text{kg}^{-1}$). Protocols to reverse heparin activity with protamine range from no administration to partial or full doses.

Hypothermia should be avoided. Normothermia can be maintained by use of warm intravenous and irrigating fluids, a heated mattress or blanket, humidification of the airway, and by maintaining a warm temperature in the operating room.

Hemodynamic stability during manipulation of the heart can be preserved by several maneuvers. These include placing the patient in the head-down (Trendelenburg) position, which increases preload by redistributing blood volume; rotating the operating table; and opening the right pleural space by incising the pericardium vertically. The latter two maneuvers minimize the manipulation required to create optimal exposure of the lateral wall of the LV. Placing and using temporary ventricular pacing wires will prevent prolonged periods of bradycardia. Preoperative insertion of an intraaortic balloon pump in high-risk patients may increase tolerance of the heart to manipulation.

Exposure of the LV surfaces containing the arteries to be bypassed is achieved by different combinations of elevation (apex of heart toward ceiling) and lateral displacement (apex of heart to right or left). To facilitate these maneuvers, a heavy suture (No. 0 silk or polyester) is placed in the posterior pericardium opposite the oblique sinus and midway between the right and left inferior pulmonary veins (Fig. 7-9, *A*), the most dependent portion of the pericardial cavity.[R22] This should be done quickly to avoid prolonged hypotension. The suture should not be placed deeply because this may result in injury to the descending aorta or esophagus. The suture is passed through a wide strip of cloth tape (Fig. 7-9, *B*), and a snare is placed over both ends of the suture and tightened (Fig. 7-9, *C*). By adjusting orientation of the snare and tape sling and the traction placed on them, adequate exposure of the coronary arteries requiring bypass grafting can be accomplished in nearly all patients.[R22] Circumferential pressure on the heart should be avoided.

Next, the artery to be grafted is stabilized with a device that depresses the myocardium to expose the segment to

be grafted (Fig. 7-10, *A*). Alternatively, a device that elevates the myocardium on both sides of the segment of artery to be grafted (typically a suction device) can be used (Fig. 7-10, *B*).

Exposure of the posterior descending branch of the RCA is achieved by marked elevation of the apex of the heart with minimal lateral displacement. This is facilitated by applying traction on the ends of the cloth tape upward toward the head and to the left (avoiding compression of the heart) and using downward traction on the snare (Fig. 7-11, *A*). A stabilizing device is then applied.

Exposure of the distal RCA is obtained by leftward traction on the ends of the cloth tape, downward traction on the snare, rotation of the table to the left, and use of the Trendelenburg position.

The LAD is exposed by traction on the ends of the cloth tape to the left and upward toward the head and gentle downward traction on the snare. A stabilizing device is then applied (Fig. 7-11, *B*). These maneuvers are applied more forcefully to obtain exposure of diagonal branches of the LAD.

Exposure of the marginal branches of the Cx artery requires a combination of elevation of the apex of the heart and substantial lateral displacement to the right. This can be accomplished by pulling the ends of the cloth tape upward and to the left and applying rightward traction on the snare. Lateral displacement of the heart to the right can be facilitated by incising the right side of the pericardium and right pleura vertically to allow positioning the apex of the heart in the right pleural cavity, rotating the operating table rightward, and using the Trendelenburg position.[R22]

After exposing the appropriate wall of the LV, the artery to be grafted is encircled proximal to the site of the arteriotomy with a fine suture, an elastic vessel loop, or a tourniquet. Encircling the artery distal to the arteriotomy site is not always necessary and should be avoided when possible. After the stabilization device is applied, the artery is incised, and anastomosis to the appropriate conduit is performed using techniques described later in this chapter (see "Distal Anastomoses"). Performing the anastomosis can be facilitated by use of a blowing device that disperses humidified carbon dioxide over the anastomotic site to remove blood. This device should be directed at the anastomotic site only during actual placement of sutures to minimize injury to the endothelium of the coronary artery. An intracoronary shunt may also facilitate performing the anastomosis, although it also may result in injury to the endothelium (Fig. 7-12). When the anastomosis is performed on a distal RCA that is not critically narrowed or occluded proximally, a shunt may be particularly valuable because bradycardia and hypotension may occur when the artery is occluded. A shunt may also provide sufficient distal flow to an arterial segment that may be an important source of collateral blood flow to other segments of the LV that have not been bypassed, thus preventing hypotension and cardiac decompensation.[P12]

Proximal anastomoses of vein grafts, radial arteries, or free ITA grafts to the ascending aorta are performed after placing a partially occluding clamp on the aorta (see "Proximal Anastomoses" later in this chapter). These can be performed before or after the distal anastomoses. Temporary atrial and ventricular pacing wires (if not already in

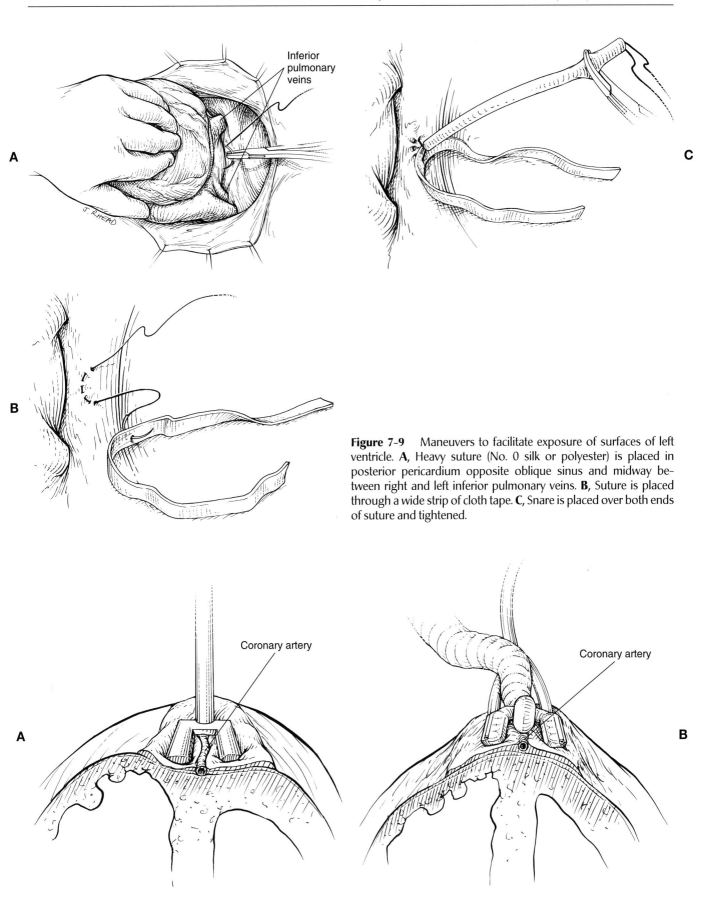

Figure 7-9   Maneuvers to facilitate exposure of surfaces of left ventricle. **A,** Heavy suture (No. 0 silk or polyester) is placed in posterior pericardium opposite oblique sinus and midway between right and left inferior pulmonary veins. **B,** Suture is placed through a wide strip of cloth tape. **C,** Snare is placed over both ends of suture and tightened.

Figure 7-10   Stabilization devices to facilitate exposure of segment of artery to be grafted. **A,** Generic device that depresses myocardium on both sides of the artery. **B,** Generic device that elevates myocardium on both sides of the artery using suction.

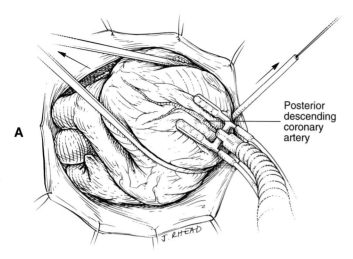

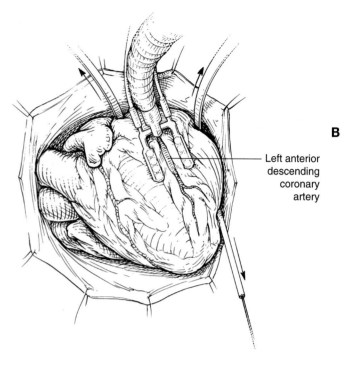

Figure 7-11 Exposure of posterior and anterior descending coronary arteries. **A,** Posterior descending coronary artery. Heart is elevated with minimal lateral displacement by upward traction toward the head on ends of tape and downward traction on the snare. A stabilizing device is then applied. **B,** Anterior descending coronary artery. Ends of tape are pulled upward and slightly to patient's left, and downward traction in the opposite direction is exerted on the snare. A stabilization device is then applied.

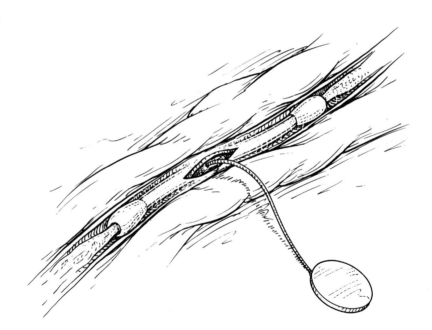

Figure 7-12 An intracoronary shunt can be used to facilitate performing the distal anastomosis.

place) and chest drainage tubes are placed. The remainder of the operation is completed in the standard manner (see Chapter 2).

When OPCAB is used in patients with multisystem disease, sequence of performing the distal anastomoses becomes important. As a general rule, it is advisable to first graft the artery or arteries that have evidence for collateral blood supply to the distal arterial bed. If an ITA graft is used, the clamp on the ITA pedicle is released as soon as the distal anastomosis to the coronary artery is completed. If a vein graft or another conduit is used, the proximal anastomosis of this conduit to the aorta is performed before the distal anastomosis. Flow is thus established to the distal arterial bed as soon as the distal anastomosis is completed. Vessels without demonstrable collateral blood supply are then grafted. With this approach, important collateral flow is not interrupted before flow through the grafts is established.

The common practice of performing the left ITA to LAD anastomosis first is based on the principle of restoring flow to the anterior wall and septum of the LV before substantial manipulation of the heart is performed to expose the Cx arterial branches. This approach may be valid in many patients, but is not advised if the LAD provides substantial collateral flow to the remainder of the LV.[P12]

Vein Graft

After preoperative examination of both legs with the patient erect, and with ultrasonic imaging when indicated, the right or left greater saphenous vein is chosen for removal. Presence of superficial varicosities does not indicate an unusable vein. However, wound healing may be poor in such extremities so if possible, a leg without varicosities is chosen. Multiple large varicosities in the saphenous vein render it unsuitable. If vein from one leg is too short or too abnormal for use, an additional segment of appropriate length is removed from the other leg. Occasionally, particularly during reoperations, suitable segments of greater saphenous vein cannot be found, and the lesser saphenous vein can be used if it is of adequate diameter. If suitable segments of vein cannot be found in the legs by any method, use of alternative conduits becomes necessary. These include the right ITA, one or both radial arteries, right gastroepiploic artery, inferior epigastric artery, and in rare circumstances splenic or ulnar artery. The cephalic vein can be taken from wrist to shoulder, but its walls are usually thinner than those of leg veins, and its late patency is less.[W13]

For removal of the greater saphenous vein, the leg is abducted and the knee is flexed about 45° and supported (Fig. 7-13, *A*). If the vein from the lower leg is to be used, the initial skin incision is made just anterior to the medial malleolus. If the upper portion of the vein will be used, the initial skin incision is made in the groin. The desired plane is accessed by blunt dissection with scissors down to the level of the vein. Skin and subcutaneous fat are undermined with the scissors, staying just superficial to the saphenous vein and spreading the tips of the scissors over the vein. A continuous incision or multiple small incisions over the length of the vein may be used (Fig. 7-13, *B* and *C*). Creation of flaps is avoided. Care is taken to preserve the saphenous nerve. The vein may divide just above the knee, becoming confluent again just below the knee. Either of the two branches may be the larger vessel and is preserved. The saphenous vein usually becomes too large and unsuitable for bypass purposes just before it penetrates the fascia lata and joins the femoral vein. Therefore, dissection is usually not performed in this area.

Whenever possible, a single long segment (usually 50 to 65 cm) of the greater saphenous vein is removed. About 12 to 15 cm may be needed for diagonal branches of the LAD, about 20 to 24 cm for marginal Cx branches, and about 18 to 22 cm for RCA and its branches. As long as the external diameter of the vein is greater than about 3.0 to 3.5 mm, vein width is probably not an important consideration. Large veins reduce in size with time after insertion, and thus adaptation to function seems to occur.[S28] Veins of

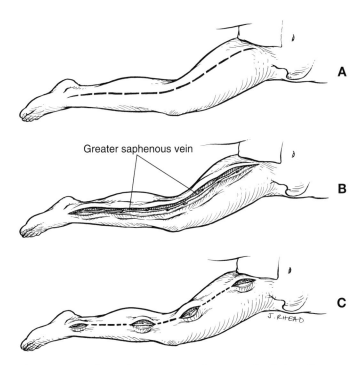

Figure 7-13   Removing greater saphenous vein. **A**, Location of greater saphenous vein and line of incision. **B**, Continuous incision over entire length of saphenous vein. **C**, Multiple small incisions over saphenous vein.

overall poor quality should be avoided whenever possible; experience in peripheral vascular surgery indicates they are prone to failure.

When the usable vein has been exposed and its length measured, the proximal (femoral) end is isolated and divided between ligatures. A vascular clamp is placed on the vein to mark what will become the *distal* end of the graft. The vein is then removed, retracting it upward so that just enough tension exists to expose, but not to tear, the branches. Branches may be ligated with fine sutures and divided, or divided between hemostatic clips (Fig. 7-14, *A*). The saphenous vein must not be narrowed by ligating or clipping the branches too close to it. (Fig. 7-14, *A* [*upper inset*]). The branches should be ligated or clipped just flush with the saphenous vein to avoid creating diverticula, which can be the nidus for thrombus formation (Fig. 7-14, *A* [*lower inset*]). After division of all branches and removal from its bed, the vein is divided between ligatures at its peripheral end (*proximal* end of the graft) and removed.

Alternatively, the greater saphenous vein can be removed endoscopically. Using small transverse or vertical incisions, a lighted dissector is introduced into the wounds (Fig. 7-15, *A*). A plane of dissection anterior to the vein is established with a balloon-tipped dilator (Fig. 7-15, *B*) and the dissector used to isolate the vein and its branches (Fig. 7-15, *C*). The branches are clipped and divided with a cautery, and after ligating its proximal and distal ends, the vein is removed. Although long-term patency of grafts removed with this technique is not available, short-term follow-up studies suggest satisfactory function.[C34] The time required to remove veins with this technique is longer than

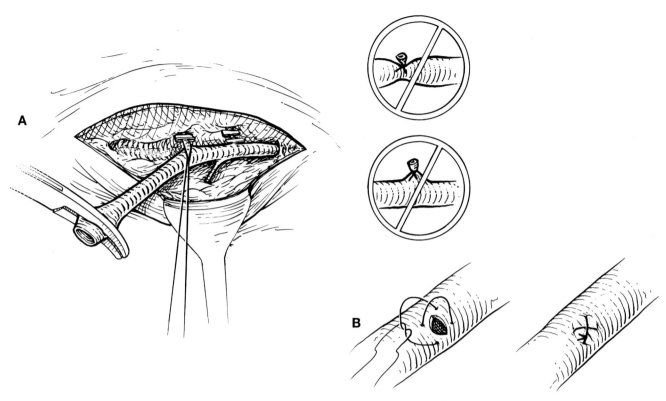

Figure 7-14   Division of side branches of saphenous vein using fine ligatures or hemostatic clips. **A,** Venous branches should be secured just flush with the saphenous vein to avoid narrowing *(upper inset)* or creating diverticula *(lower inset),* which can be a nidus for thrombus formation. **B,** Avulsed branches are secured with a double-loop suture of No. 7-0 polypropylene.

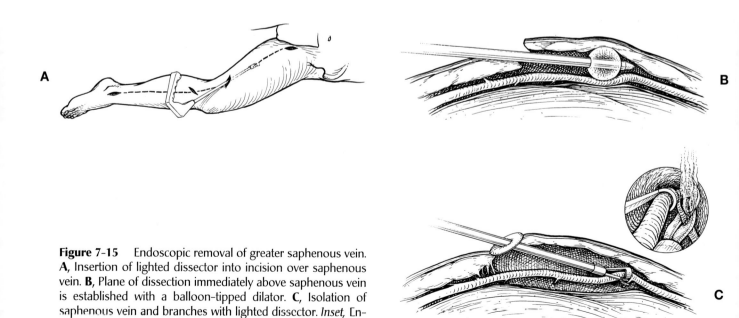

Figure 7-15   Endoscopic removal of greater saphenous vein. **A,** Insertion of lighted dissector into incision over saphenous vein. **B,** Plane of dissection immediately above saphenous vein is established with a balloon-tipped dilator. **C,** Isolation of saphenous vein and branches with lighted dissector. *Inset,* Endoscopic view.

with the conventional method. However, a lower prevalence of leg wound complications has been observed.[A8,C34]

If the *lesser saphenous vein* is to be used, it can be removed with the patient in the prone or supine position with the leg either straightened and elevated or flexed at the knee and rotated medially. If the prone position is used, the patient is subsequently repositioned and redraped in the supine position. The initial skin incision is made posterior to the lateral malleolus and extended superiorly toward the popliteal fossa. The vein is divided at the level where it penetrates the deep fascia to join the greater saphenous vein. The sural nerve lies parallel to the vein and is preserved. Branches of the vein are secured and divided as described for the greater saphenous vein.

Leg incisions are closed with continuous absorbable suture in the subcutaneous layers. A small drainage catheter is placed beneath these layers in the thigh, and the skin is closed with a continuous subcuticular suture or with metal clips. This can be done immediately after the vein is removed or deferred until after CPB has been discontinued and protamine administered.

The vein is removed to a preparation table, and a small adaptor is inserted into the open peripheral end and secured with a ligature. The previously placed clamp on the central end of the graft is removed. The vein is flushed with a room-temperature, heparinized, balanced salt solution (500 mL) to which a small amount of heparinzed blood (30 mL) has been added. The vein is gently distended (less than 150 mmHg) with the solution. Any remaining unsecured branches are ligated or clipped and any constricting adventitial bands removed. Branches that have been avulsed are secured with No. 7-0 polypropylene sutures (see Fig. 7-14, *B*). The vein is then gently distended and clamped at the end, and a straight line is drawn along its length with an indelible surgical pencil. The vein is placed in the heparinized solution at room temperature until used.

It is generally agreed that details of removing and storing saphenous veins until their insertion are important in minimizing damage, which may include intimal disruption, deposition of platelets and leukocytes on the intimal surface, damage to smooth muscle, and disruption of the extracellular matrix.[C20,G10,G15,L10,L15,L17,S33] Despite this general agreement, opinions differ as to which maneuvers or interventions result in the least injury. Overdistention of the vein[H14] and venous spasm[L15] are surely disadvantageous. No consensus exists as to the optimal temperature to maintain the graft or the optimal solution to flush and distend the graft before its insertion.

Arterial Grafts
Internal Thoracic Artery

The ITA is usually mobilized immediately after dividing the sternum, before incising the pericardium and before administering heparin. A standard sternal retractor can be used to widely separate the divided sternal edges, tilting the retractor to elevate the left half of the sternum and expose the ITA. Alternatively, an externally positioned retractor, such as that developed by Favaloro, can be used. With either type of retractor, the table is elevated and rotated to optimally expose the undersurface of the left sternal segment and left ITA. The ITA can be *skeletonized* or removed

as a *pedicle* with the internal thoracic veins, fat, muscle, and pleura. Skeletonization better preserves blood supply of the sternum and may be preferable in situations in which risk of sternal infection may be increased (e.g., obese patients, diabetic patients, use of both ITAs).

Fig. 7-16 shows the technique for removing the ITA with a pedicle. An incision using the electrocautery at low power is made in the parietal pleura and muscle on the medial side of the ITA, several millimeters from the accompanying internal thoracic vein (Fig. 7-16, *A*). The incision is extended along most of the length of the vessel down to the sixth intercostal space. A parallel incision lateral to the ITA and the accompanying lateral internal thoracic vein (if present) is made. Dissection is begun in the sixth intercostal space, where there are usually no branches. Using the tip of the electrocautery blade without current, the pedicle is freed from the sixth costal cartilage. With the pedicle gently retracted downward and with gentle blunt dissection, the intercostal arteries are identified and either occluded with small metal clips and divided, or simply divided with the electrocautery (Fig. 7-16, *B*). The ITA should not be grasped with instruments.

The pedicle is dissected up to the level of the second or first rib (Fig. 7-16, *C*), and the left phrenic nerve is identified and protected. If there is sufficient length, the internal thoracic vein is preserved at its junction with the innominate vein; if not, the vein is ligated or clipped and divided. It is not necessary to routinely divide the proximal branches of the ITA, although it is recognized that such branches, if not divided, can result in "steal" of blood from the LAD in some situations.[S45]

After proximal dissection is completed, heparin is administered and the ITA divided in the sixth or seventh intercostal space (Fig. 7-16, *D*). The proximal end is controlled with a small bulldog clamp and the distal end ligated or clipped. The ITA is wrapped in a sponge saturated either with a balanced salt solution containing papaverine (20 mg) dissolved in 20 mL of saline solution, or with 500 mL of lactated Ringer's solution to which 50 mg of sodium nitroprusside and 30 mL of heparinized blood have been added. If the ITA bleeds freely, even though not briskly, the graft is generally considered satisfactory for use. The ITA is not probed or injected with fluid unless there is no flow; probing or injecting may produce endothelial damage and dysfunction.[J3] If the right ITA is to be used, it is prepared in the same manner. The internal thoracic vein leaves the chest wall to enter the innominate vein at a lower level on the right than on the left, and it is usually divided.

The left ITA pedicle is brought into the surgical field after the LAD has been opened, usually through a wide incision in the pericardium. The ITA is cut obliquely at the site for anastomosis and freed from adjacent tissue for a short distance (Fig. 7-16, *E*). It is then incised at the bottom of the bevel for the appropriate distance to correspond to the size of the opening in the artery (Fig. 7-16, *F*). It is anastomosed to the artery with a continuous No. 7-0 or 8-0 polypropylene suture. The ITA is not dilated or otherwise manipulated, and only the adventitia is grasped with forceps. After anastomosis is completed, the pedicle is tacked to the epicardium with a fine suture on both sides of the artery.

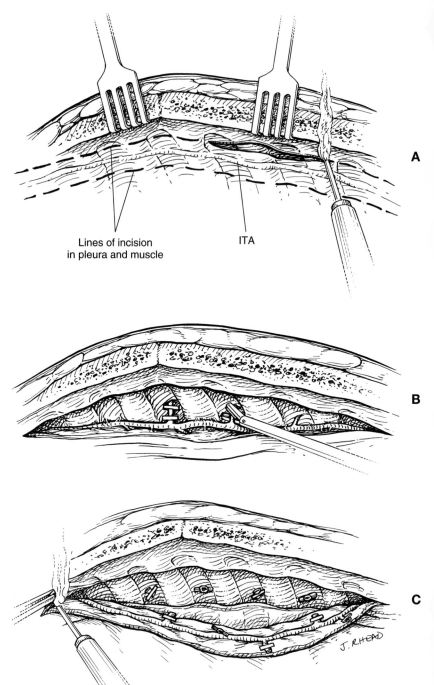

Lines of incision
in pleura and muscle

ITA

A

B

C

Figure 7-16   Preparation of internal thoracic artery *(ITA)* pedicle. **A,** Using electrocautery, pleura and muscle are incised on either side of ITA and its accompanying veins. **B,** Branches of ITA and accompanying veins are divided between clips or with electrocautery. **C,** Dissection is continued to level of second or first rib.

Key: *ITA,* Internal thoracic artery.   *Continued*

J. RHEAD

If the ITA is to be anastomosed to a diagonal branch of the LAD as well as to the LAD itself, anastomosis to the diagonal artery is performed first. The pleura is incised over the ITA at the site of the anastomosis (Fig. 7-16, *G*). The anastomosis is completed with a No. 7-0 or 8-0 polypropylene suture (Fig. 7-16, *H*). Anastomosis to the LAD is then performed.

When the left ITA does not reach the LAD but is patent, it can be used as a free graft. The proximal end of the ITA can be anastomosed directly to the aorta, to the right ITA, or to a segment of vein that has been used to bypass other coronary arteries. Patency of free ITA grafts is almost as good as in situ ITA grafts.[L11] If the ITA has been used as a pedicle graft and is under tension after CPB is discontinued, it can be lengthened by completely dividing the tissues of the pedicle at several sites.

Radial Artery

Before operation, an Allen's test is performed on the nondominant hand. The radial and ulnar arteries are compressed at the wrist while the patient opens and closes the fist vigorously (five to ten times), to produce blanching of the skin on the palm of the hand. Pressure on the ulnar artery is then released while the radial artery remains

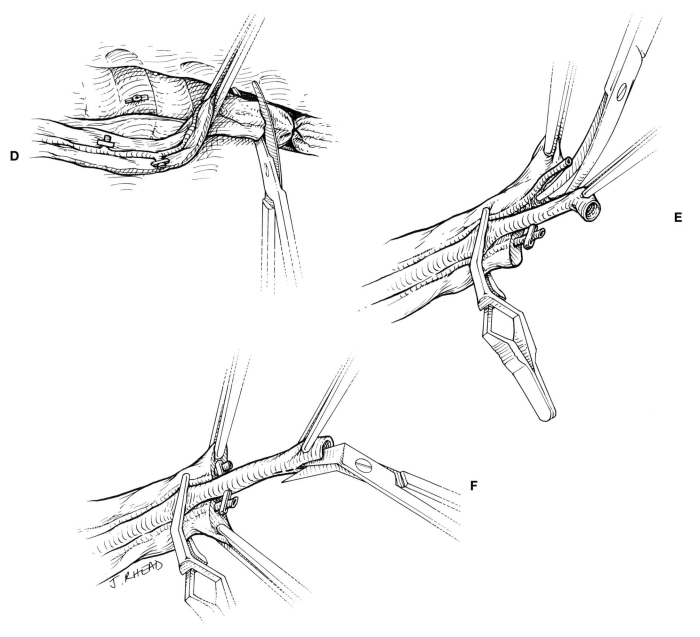

Figure 7-16, cont'd   **D**, Internal thoracic artery (ITA) pedicle is divided at level of sixth or seventh intercostal space. **E**, End of ITA is freed from adherent fascia, muscle, and veins. **F**, ITA is incised to appropriate length.   *Continued*

compressed. The skin of the palm of the hand should immediately become flushed as flow is restored to the palmar arch from the ulnar artery. If the test is equivocal, ultrasonic imaging may be necessary to establish the safety of removing the radial artery.

The arm is positioned on an arm board at the side of the patient. An incision is made in the forearm beginning over the radial pulse at the wrist (Fig. 7-17, *A*). It is then extended proximally over the belly of the brachioradialis. The lateral antebrachial cutaneous nerve is located lateral to the incision and retracted. The deep fascia is opened at the

wrist, exposing the radial vascular pedicle. Incision in the fascia is extended proximally, exposing the muscles of the forearm (Fig. 7-17, *B*). The superficial radial nerve is also lateral to the incision and should be preserved.

The vascular pedicle containing the radial artery and accompanying veins is mobilized in the middle of the forearm, then encircled in this area with an elastic vessel loop for retraction (Fig. 7-17, *C*). Dissection proceeds proximally up to the origin of the recurrent radial artery and distally to the tendons at the wrist. Branches of the artery and accompanying veins are controlled with small hemo-

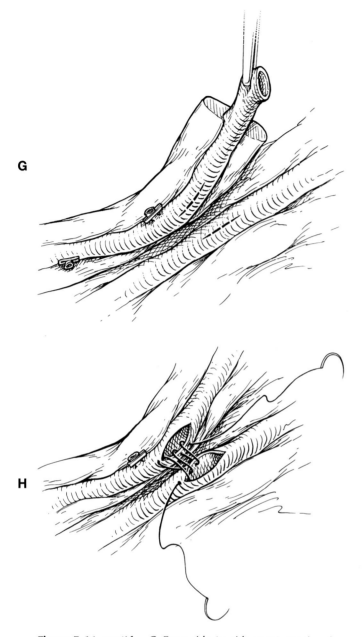

Figure 7-16, cont'd G, For a side-to-side anastomosis using the internal thoracic artery, pleura is incised over artery at site of anastomosis. **H,** Anastomosis is completed using a continuous No. 7-0 or 8-0 polypropylene suture.

static clips and are divided lateral to the accompanying veins. Proximal and distal ends of the artery are ligated, and the artery is removed.

A small olive-tipped catheter is inserted into the distal end of the artery. The artery is gently irrigated and dilated with heparinized whole blood or a solution of lactated Ringer's solution (500 mL) to which 50 mg of sodium nitroprusside and 30 mL of heparinized blood have been added. The graft is then immersed in this solution until it is used. The incision in the arm is closed with two continuous absorbable sutures in the subcutaneous and subcuticular layers. A compression dressing is applied, and the arm is

repositioned parallel to the patient's trunk before proceeding with the remainder of the operation.

When the graft is anastomosed to the coronary arteries, it is positioned so that the smooth (posterior) surface of the radial artery lies on the surface of the heart and the anterior surface, which contains most of the branches, is visible. This surface can also be marked with an indelible surgical pencil for proper orientation.

Right Gastroepiploic Artery

To expose the right gastroepiploic artery, the midline incision over the sternum is extended over the upper abdomen, and the linea alba is divided halfway from the tip of the xiphoid to the umbilicus (Fig. 7-18, *A [inset]*). With the sternum divided, excellent exposure of the upper abdomen can be obtained. The triangular ligament of the liver is divided, and the liver is retracted superiorly and to the right. Branches of the right gastroepiploic artery to the stomach and omentum are ligated or clipped and divided, creating a pedicle (Fig. 7-18, *A*). Dissection extends from the pylorus along the greater curvature of the stomach until sufficient length is achieved. After the distal end is divided, the arterial pedicle is wrapped in a sponge saturated with a solution containing 50 mg of sodium nitroprusside and 30 mL of heparinized blood dissolved in 500 mL of lactated Ringer's solution.

The prepared pedicle can be positioned either anterior or posterior to the duodenum and stomach, depending on anatomic conditions (Fig. 7-18, *B*). The pedicle should be positioned where there is the least amount of tension and distortion. A circular opening is made in the diaphragm medial to the inferior vena cava, and the pedicle is passed through this opening into the pericardial cavity.

The right gastroepiploic artery can be used to bypass most coronary arteries, but it is usually anastomosed to the distal RCA or PDA (see Fig. 7-8, *H*) because these arteries are closer to the proximal portion of the gastroepiploic artery than other vessels. This approach allows creation of an anastomosis with a relatively large diameter. Anastomoses can be performed to the LAD or its diagonal branches by bringing the pedicle anteriorly over the acute margin of the heart. The pedicle can also be positioned adjacent to the atrioventricular groove posteriorly and anastomosed to a marginal branch of the Cx coronary artery (see Fig. 7-8, *H*).

Inferior Epigastric Artery

The inferior epigastric artery (IEA) originates from the medial side of the external iliac artery posterior to the inguinal ligament. The IEA pursues a course along the medial edge of the deep inguinal ring, encircling the vas deferens in men and the round ligament in women. It then ascends obliquely toward the umbilicus. In an angiographic study of 100 right IEAs by Schroeder and colleagues, 96 were considered suitable as conduits for CABG.[S46] The mean length in situ from the origin to the distal bifurcation was 13.1 ± 1.3 cm, and the mean diameter, measured 5 cm from its origin, was 2.4 ± 0.4 mm.

The IEA is removed through a paramedian incision beginning at the umbilicus. Incision follows the external edge of the rectus muscle and ends 2 to 3 cm above the inguinal ligament. The anterior sheath of the rectus muscle

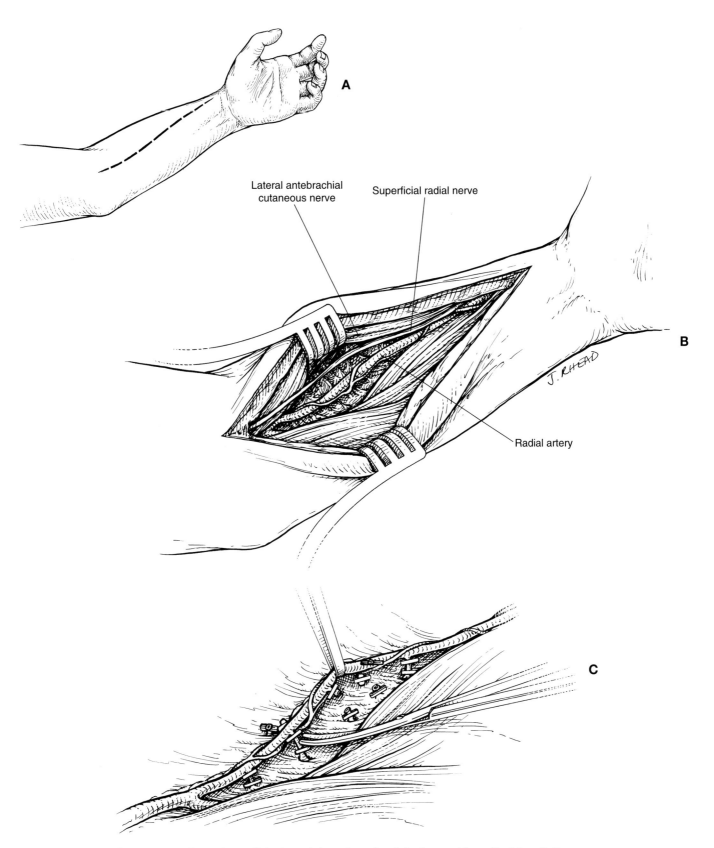

Figure 7-17   Removing radial artery. **A,** Location of radial artery and line of incision. **B,** Deep fascia is divided over vascular pedicle, which contains radial artery and accompanying veins. **C,** Elastic vessel loop is passed around pedicle and branches of radial artery and accompanying veins are doubly clipped and divided.

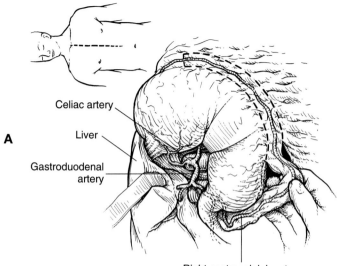

A

Celiac artery

Liver

Gastroduodenal artery

Right gastroepiploic artery

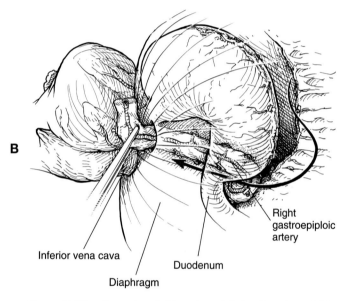

B

Inferior vena cava

Diaphragm

Duodenum

Right gastroepiploic artery

Figure 7-18   Preparing right gastroepiploic artery. *Inset,* Midline sternotomy is extended onto abdomen, and linea alba is divided halfway from tip of xiphoid to umbilicus. **A,** Triangular ligament of liver is divided, and liver is retracted superiorly and to the right. Branches of right gastroepiploic artery to stomach and omentum are ligated or clipped and divided. **B,** Prepared pedicle can be positioned anterior or posterior to duodenum. It is then passed through opening in diaphragm medial to inferior vena cava.

is divided and the muscle retracted medially. The artery is mobilized with accompanying veins, and branches of the IEA and accompanying veins are clipped and divided. The pedicle containing the artery is divided at its origin and at the level of the first major bifurcation. The IEA is removed and wrapped in a gauze sponge soaked with a solution containing papaverine or sodium nitroprusside and immersed in this solution until it is used (see "Radial Artery" earlier in this chapter). The abdominal wound is packed with a gauze sponge and closed in two layers with

absorbable suture after discontinuing CPB. A suction drain can be positioned behind the rectus muscle and removed 24 to 48 hours postoperatively.

Splenic Artery

When no other conduit is available, the splenic artery can be used. It is exposed through a midline extension of the median sternotomy. The lesser peritoneal sac is opened to gain access to the splenic artery, which courses along the superior margin of the pancreas. Branches of the artery to the pancreas are ligated or clipped and divided, and then the artery is mobilized in the hilum of the spleen, where it is ligated and divided. It is not necessary to remove the spleen because it is also supplied with blood from short gastric branches of the left gastric artery. The splenic artery is passed into the pericardial cavity through a circular opening in the diaphragm medial to the inferior vena cava. The splenic artery can be anastomosed to branches of the RCA and Cx coronary artery.

Distal Anastomoses

The technique for anastomosing the ITA to the LAD and its diagonal branches is described earlier (see Fig. 7-16, *E* to *H*). Here, techniques for anastomosis of a segment of vein are described. Although the description is explicitly for vein grafts, the techniques are applicable to anastomosis of ITA, radial artery, and other conduits to a coronary artery.

The epicardium is incised over the area of the coronary artery that has been selected for anastomosis using a scalpel blade with a rounded end or small scissors. The anterior surface of the artery can be cleared by gentle brushing with the scalpel blade. Even when crystalloid cardioplegic solution has been infused, careful inspection of the artery usually reveals a thin central line that is red or translucent, indicating the location of the lumen. The anterior wall of the artery is opened longitudinally in this area with a pointed scalpel blade to avoid injury to the posterior wall (Fig. 7-19, *A*). The blade must enter the artery obliquely to avoid this injury. The incision is enlarged with fine angled scissors to a length of 4 to 6 mm (Fig. 7-19, *B* and *C*). The incision in the epicardium must extend beyond each end of the arteriotomy to facilitate the anastomosis. The artery is sized by passing calibrated probes into it, and patency of the proximal and distal segments is assessed.

When the end of the vein (or other conduit) is being prepared for the most distal anastomosis, it is beveled so that the circumference of the opening is slightly larger than the opening of the artery. The incision is made about 10% to 20% longer than that in the artery, and sutures in the vein are placed slightly farther apart than those in the artery to create the desired "cobra head" of the vein. If the vein is small, a larger vertical incision provides a larger hood over the distal anastomosis.

The technique of anastomosis uses one double-armed No. 6-0 or 7-0 polypropylene suture placed as a continuous stitch (Fig. 7-20, *A*). Stitches in the coronary artery generally are placed from intima to adventitia (inside to outside). The stitch pierces the intima near the vessel edge, but often emerges through periarterial tissue several millimeters away from the edge. Stitches in the vein are passed from outside to inside. The stitches are generally placed sepa-

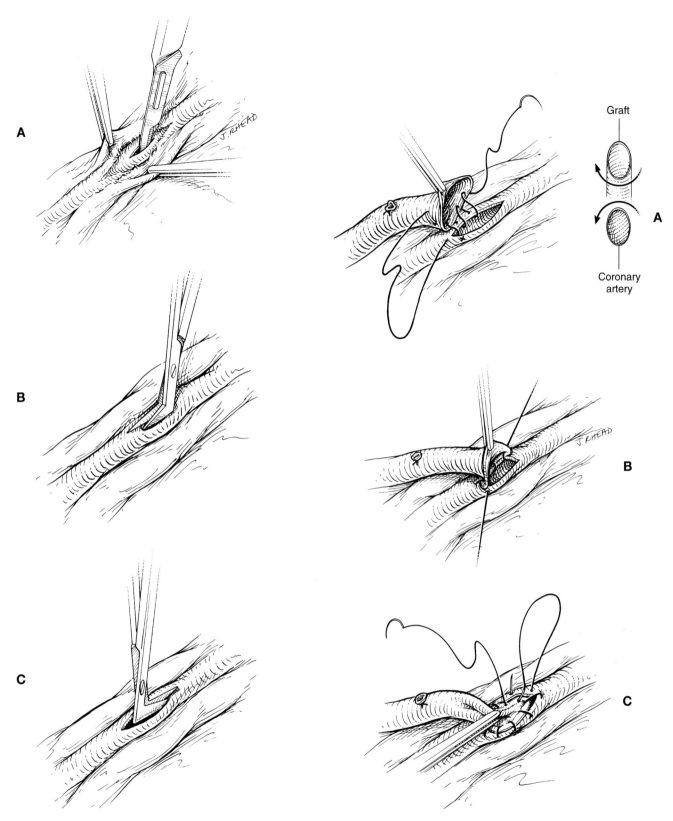

Figure 7-19   Distal anastomosis in coronary artery bypass grafting. **A,** Anterior wall of coronary artery is opened with a scalpel. **B** and **C,** Incision is enlarged to the appropriate length with angled scissors.

Figure 7-20   Technique of anastomosis for left coronary system grafts. **A,** Suture is passed through artery and continued to heel of anastomosis. *Inset,* Direction of suture placement. **B,** Vein is approximated to artery. **C,** Suture line is continued around toe of anastomosis and ends of suture tied.

rately through the artery and the vein unless it is convenient to place them with one pass of the needle holder. Even then, the vein and artery should be held apart so that the needle is visualized after it has pierced the vein and before it pierces the artery (Fig. 7-20, *A*). This maneuver ensures that the stitch is placed accurately and that no extraneous tissue has been incorporated.

The sequence of stitching varies from one location on the heart to another and may vary in the same location because of special conditions of exposure or arterial pathology. For anastomoses to the *left coronary circulation,* the suture is passed first through the vein (outside to inside) near the midpoint of the arterial wall opposite the surgeon for the LAD system (Fig. 7-20, *A*) and to the surgeon's right for branches of the Cx system. The suture is then passed through the artery (inside to outside) and continued to the heel of the anastomosis. The vein is approximated to the artery by tension on both ends of the suture (Fig. 7-20, *B*). The suture line is then continued around the toe of the anastomosis, and the two ends of the suture are tied (Fig. 7-20, *C*).

For anastomoses to the *right coronary circulation,* the suture is passed first through the vein (outside to inside) near the midpoint of the wall of the artery opposite the surgeon (Fig. 7-21, *A*). It is then passed through the artery (inside to outside) and continued to the toe of the anastomosis. The vein is approximated to the artery, and the suture line is completed around the heel of the anastomosis and remaining far wall of the artery (Fig. 7-21, *B*). The two ends of the suture are then tied (Fig. 7-21, *C*).

For sequential anastomoses in which the vein or other conduit will lie perpendicular to the arterial branches, the conduit can be opened perpendicular to its long axis for the *side-to-side anastomosis* if it is of sufficient diameter (Fig. 7-22, *A*). The incision should not exceed one third of the circumference of the conduit. The anastomosis is begun at the midpoint of the arteriotomy on the right side. The suture is passed inside to outside on the artery and then through the vein at the midpoint of the incision on its right side (Fig. 7-22, *B*). The suture is continued across the heel of the anastomosis, along the left side, and across the toe of the anastomosis and completed at the midpoint on the right side. If the vein is small or if the radial artery or ITA is used, the conduit is incised parallel to its long axis (Fig. 7-22, *C*), the *diamond anastomosis.*[G41] The anastomosis is begun close to the midpoint of the arteriotomy on the right side, and the suture is passed through the graft close to the right end of the longitudinal incision (Fig. 7-22, *D*). The suture line is continued leftward across the heel of the anastomosis and completed as already described.

For terminal *end-to-side anastomosis,* the conduit is beveled and the suture line begun at the midpoint of the arteriotomy on the left side (Fig. 7-22, *E*). The suture line is continued to the right across the proximal end of the arteriotomy and along the right side of the artery to its midportion. Using the other end of the suture, the anastomosis is completed by continuing the suture line across the distal end of the arteriotomy and completing it at the midpoint on the right side.

If the conduit and artery are parallel rather than perpendicular, a side-to-side anastomosis is performed (Fig. 7-22, *F* and *G*). The technique is identical to that for side-to-side

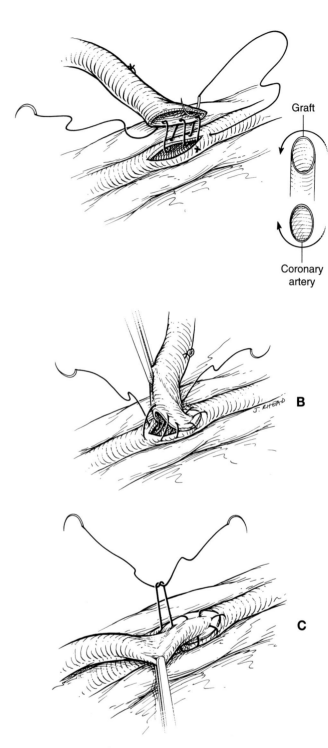

Figure 7-21   Technique of anastomosis for right coronary system grafts. **A,** Suture line begins near midpoint of arterial wall and is continued to toe of anastomosis. *Inset,* Direction of suture placement. **B,** Vein is approximated to artery, and suture line is continued around heel of anastomosis. **C,** Suture ends are tied.

anastomosis of the ITA to the LAD (see Fig. 7-16, *G* and *H*). After each sequential anastomosis is completed, the conduit is gently distended by injection of cardioplegic solution or a balanced salt solution to avoid excessive length or tension between sequential anastomoses.

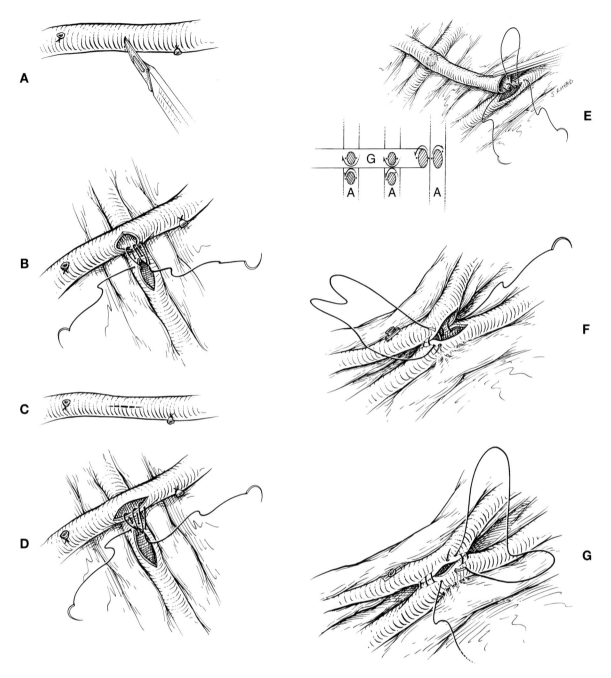

Figure 7-22   Technique of sequential grafting. **A,** Vein graft is opened perpendicular to its long axis. **B,** Anastomosis is begun at midpoint of arteriotomy on its right side. **C,** Alternatively, vein is incised parallel to its long axis. **D,** In alternative approach (diamond anastomosis with longitudinal incision in graft), suture is passed through graft close to right end of incision and continued across heel of anastomosis. **E,** End-to-side anastomosis. *Inset,* Direction of suture placement for side-to-side and end-to-side anastomoses. **F** and **G,** Side-to-side anastomosis. Technique is identical to that in Fig. 7-16, *G* and *H.*

Key: *A,* Coronary artery; *G,* graft.

Coronary Artery Endarterectomy

Endarterectomy is most often performed on the distal RCA and its major branches and only infrequently on branches of the Cx artery and LAD. If the distal RCA and its branches are diffusely diseased or occluded, endarterectomy is an alternative to bypass of the branches.

A common procedure involves incising the distal RCA just proximal to the origin of the PDA (Fig. 7-23, *A*). An endarterectomy plane in the outer third of the medial layer of the artery is developed with a dissector (Fig. 7-23, *B*). A small curved clamp is placed beneath the isolated atheromatous core, which is divided (Fig. 7-23, *C*). Using the

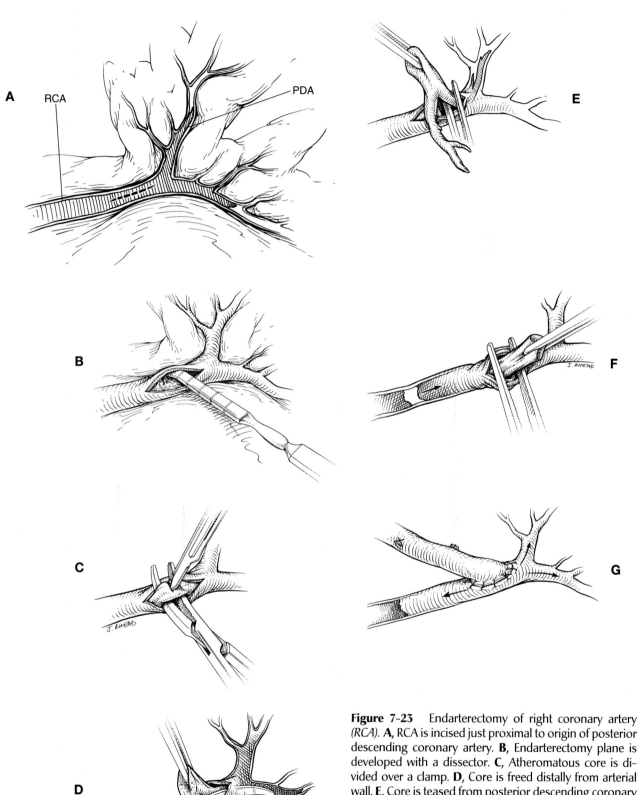

Figure 7-23   Endarterectomy of right coronary artery *(RCA)*. **A**, RCA is incised just proximal to origin of posterior descending coronary artery. **B**, Endarterectomy plane is developed with a dissector. **C**, Atheromatous core is divided over a clamp. **D**, Core is freed distally from arterial wall. **E**, Core is teased from posterior descending coronary artery and distal right coronary artery (RCA). **F**, Core is removed from proximal RCA. **G**, Vein graft is sewn to edges of artery (see Fig. 7-21).

Key: *PDA*, Posterior descending coronary artery; *RCA*, right coronary artery.

dissector, the core is freed distally from the arterial wall (Fig. 7-23, *D*). The core is then teased from the PDA and distal RCA using a clamp and exerting pressure on the core in the opposite direction from the clamp (Fig. 7-23, *E*). The core usually separates cleanly from the distal vessels and is then removed from the proximal RCA using the same technique (Fig. 7-23, *F*). A saphenous vein or other conduit is then sewn to the edges of the artery with No. 6-0 or 7-0 polypropylene suture (Fig. 7-23, *G*).

Proximal Anastomoses

After completing the last distal anastomosis, and when the procedure is being performed with CPB, the proximal anastomoses are performed. Usually the aortic clamp is removed, and a partially occluding, side-biting clamp is placed on the ascending aorta. This permits reperfusion of the heart and resumption of cardiac contractions as rewarming is completed. However, the side-biting clamp is not necessary and is not used when there is important atherosclerosis of the ascending aorta (see "Surgical Strategy" earlier in this chapter). In this situation the aortic clamp is left in place and the heart remains arrested.

Using a punch, two or three openings are made in the ascending aorta. Vein grafts or other conduits are positioned so that they will be free of kinking or tension when the heart is filled with blood. They are aligned properly using the mark previously placed on the conduit to avoid twisting. The vein is cut obliquely and incised to create a circumference that is 10% to 20% larger than that of the circular opening in the aorta, resulting in a "cobra head." A double-armed No. 5-0 or 6-0 polypropylene suture line is begun in the middle of the right edge of the vein graft, passing the suture from outside to inside on the vein and then inside to outside on the aorta (Fig. 7-24, *A*). This suture line is continued leftward across the heel of the anastomosis. The vein is approximated to the aorta by exerting tension on both ends of the suture. The suture line is continued across the toe of the anastomosis (Fig. 7-24, *B*), and the ends of the suture are tied on the right side of the anastomosis (Fig. 7-24, *C*).

When CPB is not used, these proximal anastomoses are generally performed before the distal anastomoses using a partially occlusive, side-biting clamp (see "Without Cardiopulmonary Bypass" under Coronary Artery Bypass Grafting earlier in this chapter). When CPB is used, proximal anastomoses can be performed before or after CPB is established, but before the aorta is occluded and cardioplegic solution is administered. Use of CPB facilitates performing proximal anastomoses because of lower pressure in the ascending aorta.

Emergency Operation for Cardiogenic Shock

If the patient is hemodynamically unstable at the time of operation, an intraaortic balloon pump is inserted, if not already in place. Appropriate monitoring devices are inserted, the sternum is quickly opened, and CPB expeditiously established. The left ITA can be mobilized after CPB is established, with the heart decompressed but still beating. Saphenous vein is removed from one or both legs as needed. Optimal myocardial management is essential

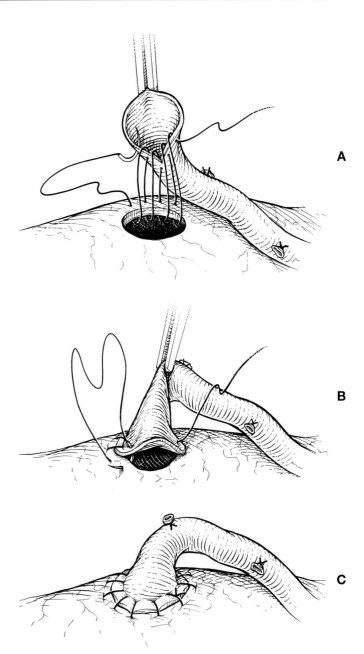

A

B

C

Figure 7-24   Proximal anastomosis in coronary artery bypass grafting. **A**, After incising conduit on its undersurface and creating an opening in aorta, suture line is passed from outside to inside on conduit and then inside to outside on aorta. **B**, Conduit is approximated to aorta. **C**, Suture line is continued across toe of anastomosis and completed.

under these circumstances, and use of warm cardioplegic induction and controlled aortic reperfusion may be advantageous (see "Methods of Myocardial Management during Cardiac Surgery" in Chapter 3). Operation is completed as described under "Surgical Strategy" earlier in this chapter. If intraaortic balloon pumping is not sufficient to permit safe discontinuation of CPB, use of extracorporeal membrane oxygenation (ECMO) or a temporary ventricular assist device may be necessary (see "Temporary Ventricular Assistance" in Section 1 of Chapter 5).

Reoperation

Secondary Median Sternotomy

The technique of many (but not all) CABG reoperations is similar to that of the original operation, with a few important differences. Sternotomy is most often made with an oscillating saw (see Section 3 of Chapter 2 for technique). Vein grafts are obtained from the leg, and one or both ITAs can be mobilized if they were not used at the initial operation. The radial artery can also be used. If difficulties are anticipated with mobilizing the heart, ascending aorta, or previously inserted vein grafts (i.e., they are adherent to the undersurface of the sternum), provisions are made for peripheral cannulation such as through the femoral artery and vein (see "Cardiopulmonary Bypass Established by Peripheral Cannulation" in Section 3 of Chapter 2). CPB can be established before dividing the sternum and then temporarily discontinued until the heart has been mobilized, or it can be established and maintained until the operation is completed.

After the sternum is divided, and if peripheral cannulation is not used, the right atrium and ascending aorta are mobilized to permit placing of cannulae and clamps. Mobilization of the ventricles is begun only after CPB is initiated.[L14] The heart must be completely mobilized. If the left or right ITA was used at the initial operation and is patent, the pedicle must be sufficiently mobilized to permit placing small clamps across it. Manipulating previously placed vein grafts must be minimized to avoid dislodging atheromatous debris into the distal coronary circulation.

The aorta is occluded immediately after CPB is established and cardioplegic solution is administered into the aortic root. Subsequent infusions are given retrogradely into the coronary sinus (see "Technique of Retrograde Infusion" in Chapter 3). Severely narrowed or diffusely atherosclerotic vein grafts are divided and ligated immediately after the first dose of antegrade cardioplegia. If there is concern about possible dislodgement of atheromatous debris into the distal coronary circulation as a result of manipulating a diseased graft, it is divided and ligated proximally, and retrograde cardioplegia is then administered. This may permit washout of debris from the opened graft. The distal end of the divided graft is then ligated.

Management of vein grafts having no or minimal evidence of atherosclerosis, as determined by angiography, and that are soft and relatively normal in appearance is controversial. Some centers favor complete removal of grafts that have been in place for more than 5 or 6 years; other centers leave such grafts in place. If a diseased graft is removed and there is no important obstruction in the coronary artery distal to the site of attachment, it is possible in some circumstances to leave a small cuff of this graft adjacent to the artery, which can then be anastomosed to the new graft. If there is important occlusive disease in the coronary artery distal to the site of the previous anastomosis, a new vein graft should be anastomosed directly to the artery beyond the obstruction. If an ITA is to be attached to the LAD previously bypassed by a vein graft that is not occluded or critically stenotic, the vein graft should not be ligated because the ITA may not initially provide sufficient flow to prevent serious myocardial ischemia.[J6]

A diligent search should be made for all graftable vessels. After completion of distal anastomoses, proximal anastomoses to the ascending aorta are completed. In general, it is preferable to perform these anastomoses with the aortic clamp in place, thus avoiding need for placing a partially occluding clamp on the aorta. After completing the proximal anastomoses, the aortic clamp is removed and the operation completed as previously described.

Reoperations can be performed without use of CPB, employing the OPCAB technique described previously in this chapter.[S48,S49]

Left Thoracotomy

An alternative approach through a left thoracotomy is a convenient and safe method for reoperation[B55,B59,C32,G32,U2] and is frequently chosen when the branches of the Cx artery and diagonal branches of the LAD are to be revascularized. Occasionally, branches of the posterolateral segment of the RCA are accessible through this approach. It is particularly useful in the presence of a patent and functioning ITA graft to the LAD. It may also have value when the ascending aorta is heavily calcified and therefore hazardous to manipulate.

It is sometimes necessary to remove the needed segment of saphenous vein with the patient supine. After rotating the patient to a near right lateral decubitus position, a left thoracotomy is made through the bed of the resected or nonresected fifth rib. The left femoral artery and vein are simultaneously exposed through a vertical or oblique groin incision after rotating the patient's hips back toward the surgeon. The femoral artery and vein are cannulated, making certain the 28, 30, or 32 French long venous cannula passes over the promontory of the sacrum and into the inferior vena cava (see "Cardiopulmonary Bypass Established by Peripheral Cannulation" in Section 3 of Chapter 2). CPB is established in the usual manner, and the patient's body temperature is reduced to about 22°C with the perfusate. If an additional route of venous return is necessary, the pulmonary artery is cannulated with an angled cannula (28, 30, or 32 French size) positioned across the pulmonary valve into the right ventricle. Usually the heart spontaneously fibrillates, but if not, it is electrically fibrillated. Once the patient's nasopharyngeal temperature is below about 25°C, CPB flow can be reduced to about $1.0 \ L \cdot min^{-1} \cdot m^{-2}$. A left-sided heart vent may be needed and can be inserted into the left atrial appendage or through the left inferior pulmonary vein. Distal anastomoses are made as usual, using fine sutures or elastic tourniquets around the coronary artery.

When these maneuvers have been completed, rewarming is begun, and the heart usually spontaneously defibrillates. Proximal anastomoses performed with a side-biting clamp, are made to the proximal descending thoracic aorta or to left subclavian artery. Remainder of operation is completed in the usual manner.

Reoperations using the left thoracotomy approach can also be performed without CPB.[B59,S50]

SPECIAL FEATURES OF POSTOPERATIVE CARE

Early Postoperative Care

Most patients are extubated either in the operating room or a few hours postoperatively and are discharged from the intensive care unit the following morning. Discharge from the hospital to outpatient supervision may occur on the third or fourth postoperative day. Thus, postoperative care is simple in most patients (see Chapter 5).

Occasionally, 8 to 12 hours after operation, arterial blood pressure falls to levels 10% to 20% below normal, whereas pedal pulses remain full and cardiac index is greater than 2.0. No treatment or a low-dose (2.5 μg · kg^{-1} · min^{-1}) infusion of dopamine is indicated.

Oral β-adrenergic receptor blocking agents may be given beginning 4 to 6 hours postoperatively. This regimen is continued until discharge as prophylaxis against supraventricular tachyarrhythmias.[F18,W9] Alternatively, no prophylactic medication is given, although a case can be made for prophylaxis in elderly patients, who are more susceptible to postoperative atrial fibrillation.[F18,H25] Digitalis is not routinely used prophylactically because it may produce atrial and ventricular arrhythmias and is less effective than other drugs.[K8] Other drugs or combinations of drugs are recommended by some authors.[G36,K8,K9,P13,R15] Biatrial pacing may reduce the prevalence of postoperative atrial fibrillation.[D18,F10,G38,L29]

Currently, warfarin is not routinely administered. A modification of the aspirin-dipyridamole protocol evolved by Chesebro and colleagues is used to enhance vein graft patency because of its antiplatelet effect.[C13,C16] In this modified protocol, aspirin (325 mg) is administered through a nasogastric tube 1 hour after operation. Another 325 mg is given by nasogastric tube 7 hours postoperatively and is continued by mouth once daily thereafter.[G13,G16] Although perioperative bleeding may increase with this protocol, major complications are not encountered. The patient is advised to continue this protocol for at least 1 year.[P7] Aspirin in a dose of 80 mg daily may be sufficient for maintenance except in large patients. In patients with a history of aspirin intolerance, dipyridamole (Persantine), clopidogrel (Plavix), or ticlopidine (Ticlid) may be substituted. Heparin may be administered subcutaneously as prophylaxis against deep venous thrombosis and pulmonary embolism in the first 48 to 72 hours postoperatively.

Occasionally, intraaortic balloon pumping is required for a few hours to a few days after operation (see Chapter 5). The indication is usually low cardiac output with high left atrial pressure or occasionally occurrence of intractable ventricular arrhythmias intraoperatively or early postoperatively. If this is not effective, placing temporary left and right ventricular assist devices may be necessary (see "Temporary Ventricular Assistance" in Section 1 of Chapter 5).

Late Postoperative Care

In contrast to many surgical procedures, CABG is simply one facet of treatment of patients with atherosclerotic CAD. Thus, late postoperative care relative to the basic disease, atherosclerosis, is as important as late postoperative care relative to the bypassing conduits. This has been discussed in considerable detail in reports by the American College of Cardiology/American Heart Association (ACC/AHA) Joint Task Force Subcommittee on Coronary Artery Bypass Graft Surgery.[A20,E9]

Facilitation of Complete Recovery

During the first 6 to 8 weeks of convalescence from CABG, patients often have a poor appetite; insomnia; emotional depression; visual, memory, or intellectual deficits; loss of sexual ability; lack of desire to return to work; and other potentially disabling manifestations of the postoperative state. Studies have documented the transient nature of most of these phenomena. The responsible physician and staff should reassure the patient in this regard and help him or her return to usual activities as rapidly as possible. During this period, excessive medications may predispose the patient to symptoms, and their minimization is frequently beneficial.

A program of daily exercise should be started as soon as the patient leaves the hospital, with emphasis on regular walking for progressively longer periods. This program should be individualized, based primarily on knowledge of completeness of the operation and LV function. Formal programs of rehabilitation can be helpful in guiding some patients through this resumption of physical activity. Ultimately, and unless specifically contraindicated, patients should be encouraged to obtain some form of regular physical activity daily and to increase this over the months after operation. Patients who were active and gainfully employed before surgery are urged to return to full activity and employment as soon as possible and, except in unusual circumstances, no later than 2 to 3 months postoperatively.

Promotion of Graft Patency

The most powerful promoter of graft patency is use of the ITA to the LAD. Whether overall graft patency is enhanced by use of both ITAs remains to be proven (see "Internal Thoracic Arteries" under Graft Patency later in this chapter).

Aspirin (325 mg · day^{-1}) should be administered immediately after operation and continued for at least 1 year postoperatively. Efficacy of this regimen has been well established,[F11,G13,G16,G35,P7] particularly when anastomoses have been made to smaller coronary arteries (Table 7-3). However, recent studies indicate that a lower dose of 80 to 100 mg daily appears to be as effective as 325 mg. Addition of dipyridamole postoperatively provides no additional protection.

Preoperative aspirin therapy likewise offers no further protection and increases bleeding.[G34] Ticlopidine (Ticlid) or clopidogrel (Plavix) can be used in patients who are sensitive or allergic to aspirin.

Control of risk factors for atherosclerosis probably retards and may even reverse to some extent development of atherosclerosis in vein grafts.[B25,C27,C36,K12,P3,P17,S14,S37,S38] This is an added reason for recommendations in the text that follows.

Control of Risk Factors for Atherosclerosis

A well-developed body of knowledge exists concerning risk factors for atherosclerosis. The general consensus is that this knowledge should be focused on patients who have established CAD and who undergo CABG. Smoking must be stopped, and cessation must be emphasized to the patient even before operation. An appropriate body weight should be maintained, even if special dieting is required. Hypertension and saturated fats in the diet must be controlled, and serum lipids should be kept within proper levels through dietary measures and administration of specific medication if required.[A20,B54,C33,K30,W14]

■ **TABLE 7-3 Association of Late (1-Year) Graft Patency after Coronary Artery Bypass Grafting with Regimen of Pre/Postoperative Dipyridamole/Aspirin and with Coronary Artery Size**

Coronary Artery Internal Diameter			DIP and Aspirin				Placebo				
				Anastomosis Patent				Anastomosis Patent			
≤	mm	<	n	No.	%	CL (%)	n	No.	%	CL (%)	$P[\chi^2]$
		1	9	6	67	44-85	15	6	40	25-57	.21
1		1.5	128	120	94	91-96	113	80	71	66-75	<.0001
1.5		2.0	98	90	92	88-95	38	20	53	43-62	<.0001
2.0			15	14	93	79-99	19	18	95	83-99	.9
	$P[\chi^2]$				.04				.001		

(Modified from Chesebro and colleagues.[C18])

Key: *CL,* 70% confidence limits; *DIP,* dipyridamole.

Surveillance for Recurrent Myocardial Ischemia

ECG stress testing should be performed 6 weeks to 3 months after operation to obtain a baseline and to prescribe an appropriate cardiac rehabilitation program. When a postoperative patient with an initially negative post-CABG stress test later develops a positive one, this is usually a reliable indicator of either graft closure or progression of disease in the native circulation.[A4,M3] In addition, myocardial perfusion imaging with either exercise stress or dipyridamole infusion can enhance detection of recurrent myocardial ischemia in patients with resting ST–T wave abnormalities.[M3]

RESULTS

Because CABG is probably the most completely studied operation in history, an enormous amount of information is available about outcomes. There is minimal value in presenting outcome simply as "survival" or "freedom from some unfavorable event" of a heterogeneous group of patients. Only risk-adjusted depictions are truly informative, as emphasized early by DeRouen, Detre, Green, Kouchoukos, and their colleagues.[D2,D6,G18,K10]

This section makes no comparisons of outcomes after medical treatment or PCI. Instead this information is presented later in this chapter under "Indications for Operation," because such comparisons are the basis for these indications. Where appropriate, comparisons between CABG performed with and without CPB are presented.

Early (Hospital) Death

Risk of early (hospital) death has been extensively studied over the past three decades. Risk stratification models have been created to provide accurate prediction of operative risk for groups of patients undergoing CABG (see "Risk Stratification" in Section 6 of Chapter 6). Large databases have been established in single institutions and in multicenter studies, and analyses of these data have established the predictive power of certain preoperative variables. In an analysis of seven large datasets representing more than 172,000 patients, Jones and colleagues identified seven variables most predictive of early mortality[J8]:

■ Older age (Fig. 7-25)[E9,H28]
■ Female gender[E11]
■ Previous CABG

■ Urgency of operation
■ Increasing LV dysfunction
■ Left main disease
■ Increasing extent of coronary artery disease

The relative mortality risks of these variables are shown in Table 7-4 for six of the data sets.

Older age has consistently predicted operative risk after CABG (see Fig. 7-25).[E9,H28] Female gender is also independently associated with increased operative risk.[E11] Previous CABG and emergent operation are associated with substantial increases in relative risk (2.0 or greater). Other variables associated with increased early mortality are recent (less than 30 days) Q-wave myocardial infarction and comorbidities (e.g., diabetes, end-stage renal disease, valvar heart disease, chronic obstructive pulmonary disease, severe peripheral vascular disease),[E9] and perhaps lack of use of the ITA.[A7]

In two randomized clinical trials that compared on-pump and off-pump procedures in 361 patients, no difference in early mortality was observed.[B60,V8]

Time-Related Survival

In general, after isolated CABG, approximately 98% of heterogeneous groups of patients survive at least 1 month, and 97%, 92%, 81%, and 66% survive 1, 5, 10, and 15 years or more, respectively (Fig. 7-26, *A*).[S20]

The hazard function for death has an early and rapidly declining phase that merges with a constant hazard phrase at about 6 months, and this gives way to a gradually rising phase of hazard at about 1 year (Fig. 7-26, *B*). This rising phase of hazard probably results from closure of grafts, progression of native arterial disease, but mostly from comorbidities. This phase of hazard is particularly favorably affected by use of ITA grafts.[A6,C37,K21,L6]

Morbidity

Common postoperative complications that result in substantial morbidity and their management are discussed in Chapter 5. Several of these morbidities deserve special emphasis.

Adverse Cerebral Outcomes

Postoperative neurologic deficits are an important cause of postoperative morbidity and mortality after CABG. Important neurologic injury occurs in up to 5% to 6% of patients

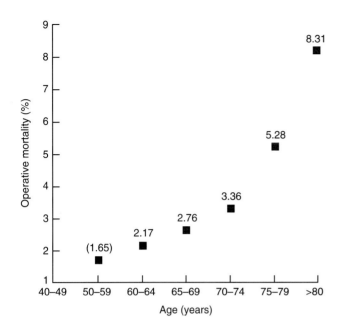

Figure 7-25   Operative mortality for coronary artery bypass grafting in various age cohorts in New York State Cardiac Surgery Reporting System for 1991-1992 (*n* = 30,972). (From Eagle and colleagues.[E9])

■ TABLE 7-4   **Relative Risks for Early Mortality after Coronary Artery Bypass Grafting in Six Large Data Sets**

	NNE[03]	VA[G39]	STS[E10]	NYS[H26]	CC[H27]	AGH[M23]
Number of patients	3055	12,712	332,064	57,187	5051	1567
Year of publication	1992	1993	1997	1994	1992	1996
Years included	1987-1989	1987-1990	1990-1994	1989-1992	1986-1988	1991-1992
Type	Vol reg	Man nat	Vol nat	Man state	SI	SI
Database Variables						
Age (years)[a]	1.04	1.04	1.05	1.04	1.05	NA
Female gender	1.2	NA	1.5	1.52	1.63	1.48
Prior heart surgery	3.6	3.2	3.0 3.5 (multireops)	3.73	1.72	1.39
Left main disease (≥70%)	NS	NA	1.3	1.43 (>90%)	NA	NA
Number of Diseased Systems						
One	1.0	NA	1.0	NA	NA	NA
Two	1.3	NA	1.0	NA	NA	NA
Three	1.6	NA	1.2	NA	NA	NA
Urgency of Operation[b]						
Elective	1.0	1.0	1.0	1.0	1.0	1.0
Urgent	2.1	2.4	1.2	1.42	NA	3.5
Emergent	4.4	3.8	2.0	3.98	5.07	7.14
Salvage	NA	NA	6.7	NA	NA	29.9
Ejection Fraction						
≥0.60	1.0	NA	NA	1.0 (>40%)	NA	NA
0.50-0.59	1.4	NA	NA	NA	NA	NA
0.40-0.49	1.6	NA	NA	NA	NA	NA
0.30-0.39	1.9 (<40%)	NA	NA	1.63	NA	2.89 (<30%)
0.20-0.29	NA	NA	NA	2.21	NA	NA
<0.20	NA	NA	NA	4.06	NA	NA

(Data from Eagle and colleagues.[E9])

Key: *NNE,* Northern New England Cardiovascular Disease Study Group; *VA,* Veterans Affairs Cardiac Surgery Database; *STS,* Society of Thoracic Surgeons National Cardiac Surgery Database; *NYS,* New York State's Cardiac Surgery Reporting System; *CC,* Cleveland Clinic; *AGH,* Allegheny General Hospital; *Vol,* voluntary; *reg,* regional; *Man,* mandatory; *nat,* national; *state,* single state; *SI,* single institution; *NA,* not available; *NS,* not significant.

[a] Relative risk coefficient for age indicates additional mortality risk per year of age > 50 years.

[b] *Urgent* indicates that patients are required to stay in hospital but may be scheduled and operated on within a normal scheduling routine; *emergent,* ongoing refractory cardiac compromise unresponsive to other forms of therapy except for cardiac surgery; *salvage,* ongoing cardiopulmonary resuscitation en route to operating room.

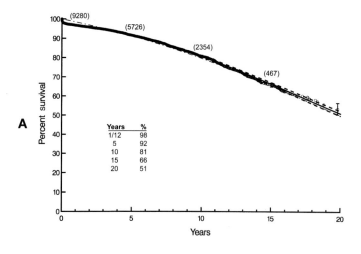

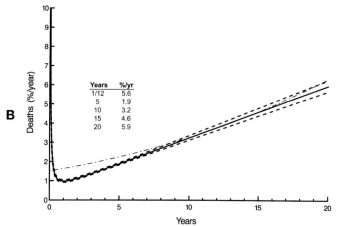

Figure 7-26 Survival after coronary artery bypass grafting (CABG). **A,** Time-related survival in a heterogeneous group of patients. *Circles,* Individual deaths, positioned along horizontal axis at time of death and along vertical axis according to Kaplan–Meier estimator; *vertical bars,* 70% confidence limits; *(parentheses),* number of patients still being traced; *solid line* (not visible in some areas because of density of circles), nomogram of separately determined parametric survival; *dashed lines* enclose 70% confidence limits; *dot-dash-dot line,* survival of age–gender–ethnicity–matched general population. **B,** Hazard function for death in same group of patients. Note (1) early, rapidly declining phase; (2) constant phase, which elevates entire hazard function above baseline; and (3) slowly rising third phase. (Modified from Sergeant and colleagues.[S20])

who undergo CABG with CPB. Because of lack of large randomized trials, it has not been conclusively proved that use of off-pump procedures is associated with a lower prevalence of neurologic injury.

A multicenter study by Roach and colleagues of 2108 patients undergoing CABG with CPB documented adverse cerebral outcomes in 129 patients (6.1%).[R23] *Type 1 deficits* (major focal deficits, stupor, and coma) occurred in 3.1% and *type 2 deficits* (deterioration in intellectual function or memory) in 3.0% of the patients. In addition to increased early mortality in these groups (21% for type 1 and 10% for type 2 deficits), hospital length of stay and likelihood of discharge

to a nursing home were substantially increased compared with the remaining patients. Predictors of type 1 deficits included presence of proximal aortic atherosclerosis, history of prior neurologic disease, use of intraaortic balloon pump, diabetes, hypertension, unstable angina, and older age.

Mediastinitis

Deep sternal wound infection occurs in 1% to 4% of patients after CABG with CPB and is associated with increased mortality.[E9,L30] Obesity is a risk factor for mediastinitis.[M24,N7] Other factors associated with an increased prevalence of deep wound infection include diabetes, previous CABG, use of both ITAs, and duration of operation.[K20,M24,N7] Two randomized trials showed that off-pump CABG was not associated with a lower prevalence of sternal wound infection.[B60,V8]

Renal Dysfunction

In a multicenter study of renal dysfunction after CABG with CPB in 2222 patients, "dysfunction" was defined as a postoperative serum creatinine level of $2.0 \text{ mg} \cdot \text{dL}^{-1}$ or greater, or an increase of $0.7 \text{ mg} \cdot \text{dL}^{-1}$ or more from preoperative level.[M29] Renal dysfunction occurred in 171 (7.7%) patients, and 30 (1.4%) required dialysis. Early mortality was 0.9% among patients who did not develop renal dysfunction, 19% in those with renal dysfunction who did not require dialysis, and 63% among those who required dialysis. Preoperative risk factors for renal dysfunction included advanced age, moderate to severe cardiac failure, previous CABG, diabetes, and preexisting renal disease.[M29] In two randomized trials, prevalence of postoperative renal failure was similar in on-pump and off-pump groups.[B60,V8]

Modes of Death

Most deaths early and late after CABG are from cardiac failure, which could be termed *cardiac death* (Table 7-5). A smaller proportion of deaths (about 15%) are sudden, considerably less than in the natural history of patients with CAD. Although it is difficult to be certain, about 25% of all deaths early and late after CABG are unrelated to the ischemic heart disease or the operation.

Incremental Risk Factors for Premature Death

Many patient-specific risk factors for death in patients with atherosclerotic heart disease pertain to patients who have undergone CABG (see Box 7-1). In addition, procedural and institutional incremental risk factors affect outcome (Table 7-6).

The Califf-Harrell nomogram and its conceptual bases are fundamental to understanding risk factors and outcome after interventional therapy (Fig. 7-27).[C17] Only patient risk factors summarized as "reversible ischemia" (see Box 7-1) can be neutralized by CABG (or PCI) and, when neutralized, outcome is determined in large part by other risk factors. "Vessel stenoses neutralized" (Fig. 7-27) depicts *potential* for improvement ("comparative benefit") by interventional therapy because this possibility is determined by number of systems (vessels) stenosed. *Actual* improvement, or "comparative benefit," is determined by the *actual*

■ **TABLE 7-5   Modes of Death after Coronary Artery Bypass Grafting** [a]

Mode	All Deaths after CABG	
	No.	Percent of 545
Cardiac	298	55
Failure [a]	216	40
Acute	145	27
Subacute	35	6
Chronic	36	7
Sudden	78	14
Arrhythmia	4	0.7
Cancer	90	17
Neurologic	53	10
Trauma	27	5
Pulmonary failure	19	3
Pulmonary thromboembolism	10	2
Hemorrhage	10	2
Acute intraabdominal catastrophe	6	1
Hepatic failure	6	1
Infection	5	0.9
Renal failure	3	0.6
Miscellaneous	8	1
Uncertain	10	2
TOTAL	545	100.7

(Data from Sergeant and colleagues.[S11])

[a] Cardiac failure, which could be termed *cardiac death*, is considered *acute* when it occurs within 3 days of an operation or a new myocardial infarction; *subacute* when it occurs between 3 days and 6 weeks of such events; and *chronic* when it occurs more than 6 weeks after an event that appears responsible for it, or when death is in the syndrome of chronic heart failure but is not preceded by an identified proximal previous event.

■ **TABLE 7-6   Procedural Risk Factors for Death after Coronary Artery Bypass Grafting** [a]

	Incomplete revascularization
	Nonuse of internal thoracic artery to left anterior descending artery
(Longer)	Global myocardial ischemic time interacting with method of myocardial management
(Longer)	Cardiopulmonary bypass time
	Surgeon
(Earlier)	Date of operation

[a] *Institution* in which procedure is performed may also be a risk factor.

number of systems with important stenoses that are in fact neutralized by interventional therapy.

The depiction emphasizes that the greater the number and severity of patient-specific risk factors, the greater is the comparative benefit (in terms of survival) of interventional therapy. At the same time, 5- or 10-year survival is less when patient risk factors are numerous. It also illustrates that the favorable effect of interventional therapy is difficult to demonstrate, even though present on conceptual grounds, in most patients with good LV function and few unfavorable risk factors.

A classic parsimoniously derived multivariable risk factor equation for death after CABG has been derived by Blackstone, working with Sergeant and colleagues (Table 7-7).[K21,S11,S20] Actual risk factors are similar to those derived from other experiences.

Strength and *shape* (time of maximal effect) of risk factors are best determined by nomograms, which also have the advantage of presenting risk-adjusted depictions (see Chapter 6). *Number* of systems with important stenoses is a weak risk factor for death after CABG in the first 5 years

■ **TABLE 7-7   Incremental Risk Factors for Death after Primary Isolated Coronary Artery Bypass Grafting**

	Risk Factors	Hazard Phase		
		Early	Constant	Late
	Patient Risk Factors			
	Demographic			
(Older)	Age	•	•	•
(Younger)	Age		•	•
(Lighter)	Weight	•		
(Higher)	Weight/height ratio		•	
	Symptoms of reversible ischemia			
(Higher)	Canadian angina class	•		•
	No angina		•	
(Higher)	Unstable angina grade	•		
	Cardiac comorbidity			
	Mitral regurgitation (mild)	•		
	Aortic regurgitation			•
	Chronic atrial fibrillation		•	•
	Ventricular tachycardia/fibrillation		•	
	Cardiac pacemaker			•
	Noncardiac comorbidity			
	Overweight			•
	History of vascular disease	•		•
	History of cerebrovascular disease		•	
	Previous vascular surgery (noncarotid)		•	
	History of smoking			•
(Lower)	1-second expiratory rate (% of normal)	•	•	•
	History of renal failure			•
	On renal dialysis	•		
	Serum creatinine higher than 2.5 mg/dL			•
	Hypertensive			•
(Higher younger)	Grade of diabetes and age		•	•
	History of malignancy		•	
	History of hepatic disease		•	
(Higher)	Triglyceride level			•
	Left ventricular function			
	Cardiogenic shock	•		
(Better)	Clinical status		•	
(Lower)	Ejection fraction (lower)	•	•	•
(Earlier)	and date of operation (earlier)			•
(Greater)	Limitation by heart failure		•	
	Coronary disease			
(Earlier)	90% left main stenosis	•		
	and date of operation	•		
(Greater)	Number of diseased systems			•
	Three-system disease	•		
	Procedural Risk Factors			
	Coronary operation			
	Grafting to LAD			•
	Use of arterial grafts			•
	Use of only arterial grafts in single-system disease		•	•
	Use of patch grafts			•
(Higher)	Ratio of distals to conduits	•		•
(More)	Coronary endarterectomies	•		
(Higher)	Proportion of distals to small vessels	•		•
	Incomplete revascularization	•		•
	Concomitant procedures			
	Left ventricular incision or plication	•		
	Institutional experience			
	One surgeon	•		
(Lower)	Preceding year per surgeon volume	•		

(Data from Sergeant and colleagues[S20]; KU Leuven, 1971 to 1992; n = 9600.)

Key: *LAD*, Left anterior descending coronary artery.

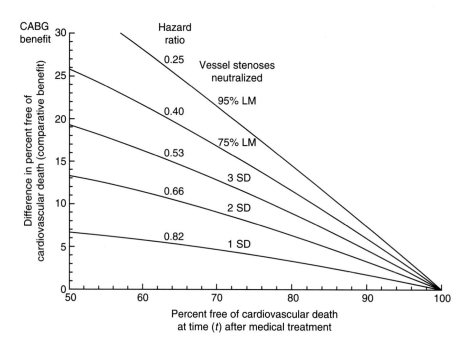

Figure 7-27 Nomogram of an equation describing comparative benefit of coronary artery bypass grafting (CABG) or percutaneous coronary intervention (PCI) over medical treatment. *Comparative benefit* is difference in percent freedom from cardiovascular deaths after two treatments at some time *(t)*. Patient's position on horizontal axis conceptually is determined by sum of all patient risk factors, such that the higher the percent freedom from cardiovascular death, the fewer the risk factors in the particular patient. Comparative benefit, along vertical axis, is determined by interrelationship between patient's position along horizontal axis and number of coronary arteries with stenoses completely neutralized by interventional therapy *(isobars)*. Values of isobars are, in fact, *hazard ratios*, which represent effect on comparative benefit of number of arteries with important stenosis in patients undergoing CABG, assuming all stenoses are neutralized by interventional therapy. Nomogram pertains when time *(t)* is 2 to 7 years (time of approximately proportional hazards) after CABG (or PCI) and when early risks of intervention (CABG or PCI) are negligible. Abstract equation is as follows:

$$\text{Comparative benefit} = S_{CABG}(t) - S_M(t)$$

$$S_M(t)^h = S_{CABG}(t)$$

Key: *CABG,* Coronary artery bypass grafting; *h,* hazard ratio; *LM,* left main coronary artery; S_{CABG}, survival after CABG; *SD,* vessels diseased (stenosis ≥50%); S_M, survival with medical treatment; *t,* time. (Modified from Califf and colleagues,[C17] and from Califf RM, Harrell FE Jr: personal communication; 1990.)

(Fig. 7-28, *A*) when revascularization is complete and the ITA is used for the LAD graft. Also, number of diseased vessels and even left main coronary artery stenosis, as well as number of distal anastomoses, are not risk factors for hospital death when an adequate operation has been performed.

Pre-CABG LV function, expressed as *ejection fraction,* has a powerful effect on time-related outcome (Fig. 7-28, *B* and *C*), particularly when it is low.[C22] Surprisingly, some patients with low EF have none of the symptoms of *chronic heart failure.* Presence of this syndrome, often associated with secondary mitral regurgitation, increases the risk above that for low EF alone.[W12]

Unstable angina has a minimally unfavorable effect on survival (Fig. 7-28, *D*).

Some patients undergo CABG soon after an acute MI. Use of CABG for primary reperfusion during Q-wave MI

has been largely superseded by thrombolysis and PCI. Early risks of CABG are increased only when operation is performed for acute hemodynamic deterioration after an acute (usually Q-wave) MI or for any reason within about 8 days of a Q-wave infarction.[K21,K26] Early mortality in patients operated on for cardiogenic shock after an acute MI also depends on other risk factors and largely on methods of treatment. When intense resuscitative measures such as intraaortic balloon pumping stabilize the hemodynamic state before operation, early mortality may be as low as 5%.[G28] When cardiogenic shock is present until operation or until establishment of CPB, mortality is higher.[A12] However, using best available methods of myocardial management intraoperatively (see "Cold Cardioplegia, Controlled Aortic Root Reperfusion, and [When Needed] Warm Cardioplegic Induction" in Chapter 3) and with intensive postoperative care, including ventricular assist devices

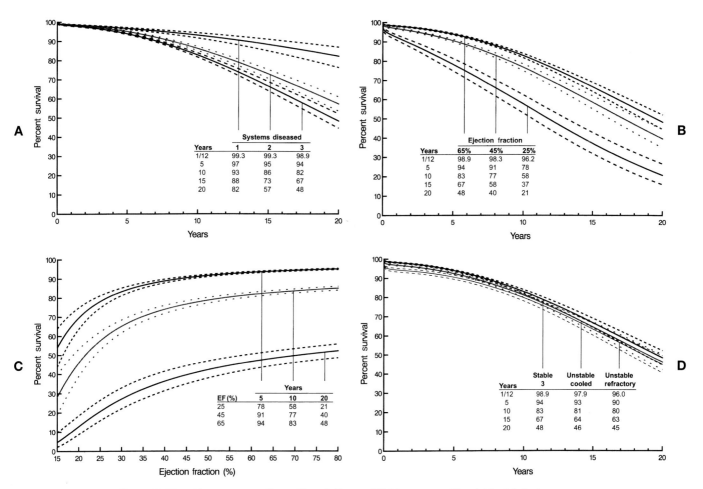

Figure 7-28   Nomograms of specific solutions of KU Leuven multivariable risk factor equation for death after coronary artery bypass grafting (CABG), illustrating strength and shape of certain risk factors for death (see Table 7-7).[S20] In all figures, dashed lines represent 70% confidence limits. **A,** Risk-adjusted effect on survival after CABG of number of stenosed systems. **B,** Risk-adjusted effect of moderate and severe left ventricular dysfunction. **C,** Risk-adjusted effect of left ventricular ejection fraction (continuously represented along horizontal axis) on survival to 5, 10, and 20 years after operation. **D,** Risk-adjusted effect of pre-CABG unstable angina, both after "cooling" and when refractory to treatment, compared with moderately severe but stable angina.

Key: *EF,* Ejection fraction.

when needed (see "Treatment of Low Cardiac Output" in Section 1 of Chapter 5), at least 50% of patients survive the early postoperative period.[A11,L27,N4] Late survival depends on prevalence of other risk factors.

Nonuse of the ITA as a bypass graft to the LAD is a strong procedural risk factor and the basis for its near-routine use (Fig. 7-29) (see "Internal Thoracic Arteries" under Graft Potency later in this chapter). Older age at operation does not contraindicate use of the ITA because its use decreases early risks, even in elderly patients.[G29,K21,N3,S22] Whether bilateral ITA grafting has a beneficial effect on survival remains controversial,[J4,K21,S11] but recent studies suggest that it does.[E12,L31,L32] Risk of sternal wound complication is increased by the double-ITA procedure in obese or diabetic patients.[K20]

Older age as a risk factor for death is receiving increasing attention as the population ages. Although hospital stay

is longer and early complications more frequent in elderly patients, highly favorable results can be obtained with CABG, even in those over age 75.[A7,H23,I3,S42,U3] This situation has been well summarized in the reports by the ACC/AHA Joint Task Force Subcommittee on Coronary Artery Bypass Graft Surgery.[A20,E9]

Return of Angina

Evidence from evaluation of symptoms and from graded exercise testing shows that CABG usually relieves angina.[K32,M28] However, return of angina is the most common post-CABG ischemic event. In a heterogeneous group of patients, only about 60% were free of angina 10 years after CABG (Fig. 7-30, *A*).[C8,K21,S11,S22]

The hazard function for return of angina, although also having a constant phase, is dominated by an early phase

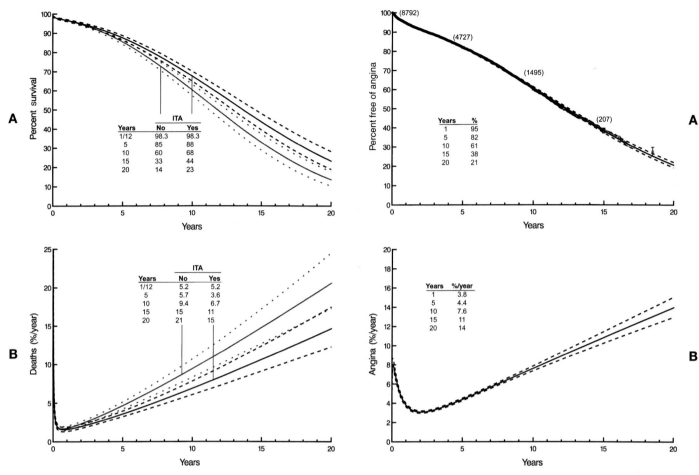

Figure 7-29   Nomograms illustrating advantage in terms of **A**, survival, and **B**, hazard function, of using internal thoracic artery *(ITA)* in coronary artery bypass grafting for an elderly patient in current era. Note that advantage of an ITA is not apparent before about 4 years after operation. (From Sergeant and colleagues.[S22])

Key: *ITA,* Internal thoracic artery.

Figure 7-30   Freedom from return of angina after coronary artery bypass grafting (CABG); representations as in Fig. 7-26. **A,** Time-related probability of freedom from angina after CABG in a heterogeneous group of patients. **B,** Hazard function for return of angina in the same group of patients. (From Sergeant and colleagues.[S22])

that peaks at about 3 months after operation and by a late, steadily rising phase that becomes evident about 3 years postoperatively (Fig. 7-30, *B*). The early, peaking phase probably most often results from incomplete revascularization as well as early graft closure. Therefore, return of angina early after CABG is an indication for restudy of the coronary circulation. The late, rising phase of hazard for return of angina is caused by progression of native vessel disease and narrowing or closure of one or more grafts.

The most interesting aspect of risk factors for return of angina is that nonuse of the ITA has only a mild effect, at least in the KU Leuven (Katholieke Universiteit, Leuven, Belgium) experience (Table 7-8).[S22,S43] This appears to be limited to the early hazard phase, however (Fig. 7-31). This finding suggests that survival depends greatly on a continuing blood supply to the LAD with its septal branches. Also, angina may return from recurrent or new ischemia in the myocardial regions supplied by the Cx artery or RCA as well as from recurrent or new ischemia in the distribution of the LAD. In fact, as best as can be determined, patients

who experience return of angina have nearly the same survival thereafter as do other patients (Fig. 7-32).

Patient incremental risk factors for return of angina are not powerful compared with those for death. This implies that return of angina is inherent in stenotic atherosclerotic CAD.

Procedural risk factors for return of angina are likewise not very powerful, as seen in the case of the ITA. The inference again may be that the process leading to return of angina is inherent in atherosclerotic CAD.

Myocardial Infarction

Perioperative MI, usually defined by appearance of new Q waves in the electrocardiogram or by elevation of serum levels of myocardial biomarkers, is most often related to inappropriate myocardial management, but can also result from technical problems or incomplete revascularization. Prevalence of MI is highly variable and depends on the criteria used, but it is approximately

■ **TABLE 7-8   Incremental Risk Factors, Based on Patient, Procedure, and Institutional Variables, for the Return of Angina, without Infarct or Death the Same Day, after Primary Isolated Coronary Artery Bypass Grafting**

Risk Factors	Hazard Phase	
	Early	Late
Patient Risk Factors		
Demographic		
Younger age	●	●
Female	●	●
Anginal status		
Longer duration of angina history	●	●
Higher angina class		●
Unstable ST segment at operation	●	
Clinically positive cycloergometric test and	●	
electrocardiogram negative exercise test	●	
(interaction)		
Left ventricular function		
Absence of preoperative anterior or septal infarct		●
Coronary disease distribution		
Lesser stenosis of left main coronary artery	●	●
Multisystem coronary artery disease		●
Comorbidity (cardiac)		
Left ventricular hypertrophy		●
Aortic valve stenosis (mild)		●
Comorbidity (vascular)		
History of peripheral vascular disease	●	
History of noncarotid vascular operation		●
Calcified ascending aorta		●
Comorbidity (noncardiac, nonvascular)		
Hypertensive		●
Higher diabetic grade		●
Absence of overweight now or previously and age		●
(interaction)		
Higher preoperative triglyceride level		●
History of renal failure		●
Procedural Risk Factors		
Details of the conduit used		
Nonuse of vein grafts only	●	
Use of vein grafts to the LAD system		●
Use of patch grafts	●	
Details of the distal anastomoses		
Proportion of total distal anastomoses to anastomosed	●	
vessels ≤1 mm		
Nongrafting to the LAD	●	
Ratio of number of arterial anastomoses to total	●	
number of distal anastomoses		
Completeness of revascularization		
Incomplete revascularization and use of internal	●	
thoracic artery grafts only (interaction)	●	
Other surgical details		
Number of coronary endarterectomies	●	
Institutional Risk Factors		
Surgeons		
High risk for angina return surgeon	●	
Low risk for angina return surgeon	●	
Experience		
Later date of operation		●

(Data from Sergeant and colleagues[S22]; KU Leuven, 1971 to 1992; *n* = 9600.)

Key: *LAD*, Left anterior descending coronary artery.

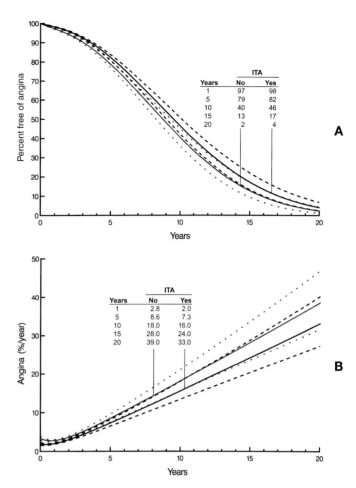

Figure 7-31   Effect of use of internal thoracic artery on return of angina after coronary artery bypass grafting, illustrated in nomograms of specific solutions of multivariable risk factor equations represented by Table 17-8. **A,** Time-related, risk-adjusted freedom from return of angina. **B,** Hazard function for return of angina. (From Sergeant and colleagues.[S22])

Key: *ITA,* Internal thoracic artery.

2.5% to 5%.[C26,C38,K13,O1,S12] Perioperative infarction, when quantitatively more than trivial, is a risk factor for later death.[B49,N6,S12]

Including perioperative cases, MI is relatively uncommon after CABG, with 94% of patients in the KU Leuven experience free of infarction for at least 5 years and 73%

for at least 15 years (Fig. 7-33). However, the hazard function for MI begins to increase at about 4 years postoperatively. Risk factors for the first post-CABG infarction (excluding those that occur perioperatively) are relatively few (Table 7-9).

Survival appears to be considerably adversely affected by occurrence of post-CABG MI (Fig. 7-34).[C10,S36] Furthermore, time-related freedom from subsequent post-CABG MI declines with each MI episode (Fig. 7-35).

Sudden Death

Time-related prevalence of sudden death is low after CABG; this may be an important factor in the survival benefit derived from CABG.[E8] In the KU Leuven experience, 97% of patients were free of sudden death 10 years after CABG (Fig. 7-36, *A*). The late phase of the hazard function rises more slowly than in other post-CABG ischemic events (Fig. 7-36, *B*).[S43] Not unexpectedly, poor LV function before CABG is statistically the most significant

Figure 7-32 Survival after return of angina after coronary artery bypass grafting, represented by depiction labeled *Actual* (circle), compared with that predicted for an equal number of patients (smooth line enclosed within 70% confidence limits), each individually identical to a patient in the Actual group but without return of angina. Probability of death within 1 year after angina return is twice that predicted for those without return, but survival still is 95%. (Predictions based on method of Ferrazzi and colleagues,[F1] using risk factor equation from KU Leuven experience.[S20,S22])

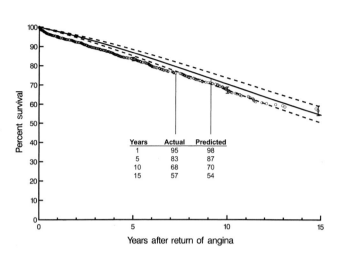

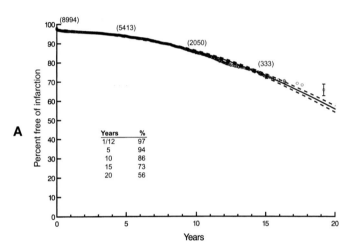

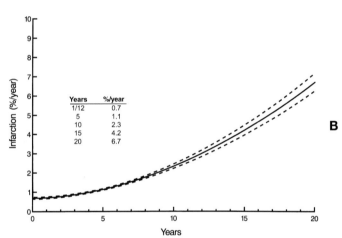

A

B

Figure 7-33 Freedom from first myocardial infarction after coronary artery bypass grafting, including those occurring perioperatively. Format is as in Fig. 7-26. **A**, Time-related probability of freedom from first myocardial infarction. **B**, Hazard function for first myocardial infarction. (From Sergeant and colleagues.[S36])

Figure 7-34 Survival after first post-bypass myocardial infarction. Format is as in Fig. 7-26. (From Sergeant and colleagues.[S36])

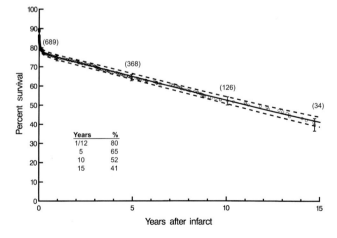

■ TABLE 7-9   Incremental Risk Factors, Based on Patient, Procedure, and Institutional Variables, for Freedom from First Infarct after Primary Isolated Coronary Artery Bypass Grafting

	Risk Factors	Hazard Phase		
		Early	Constant	Late
	Patient Risk Factors			
	Demographic			
(Younger)	Age		●	
	Blood group A			●
(Taller)	Height of patient			●
(Shorter)	Height of patient	●	●	
	Anginal status			
(Higher)	Previous infarct within 30 days of operation			●
(Lower)	Previous infarct within 30 days of operation	●		
(Lower)	Stable angina before operation		●	
(Lower)	Clinic or ECG + result of preop cycloergometric test		●	
	Unstable ST segment but not acute infarct	●		
	Left ventricular function			
(Lower)	Previous inferior infarct	●		
	Coronary disease distribution			
	Two- or three-system disease			●
(Lower)	Higher percent stenosis of left main		●	
	Comorbidity (cardiac)			
	Aortic valve regurgitation		●	
	Concomitant planned pacemaker insertion	●		
	Comorbidity (vascular)			
	History of peripheral vascular disease	●		●
	History of abdominal aortic disease		●	
	Cerebral, noncarotid, vessel disease			●
	Comorbidity (noncardiac, nonvascular)			
	BUN > 50 mg/dL		●	
(Lower)	Pulmonary vital capacity as percent of normal	●		●
(Higher)	Grade of diabetes			●
(Higher)	Preoperative cholesterol level			●
	Procedural Risk Factors			
	General technical aspects			
	Patch graft		●	
	Coronary endarterectomy	●		
	Incomplete revascularization	●	●	
	Arterial grafting			
	Absence of at least one arterial graft	●	●	
	Absence of only arterial grafts and single-system disease		●	
	Nonarterial graft to the LAD			●
	Institutional Risk Factors			
	Surgeons			
	Lower risk surgeons for first infarct	●		

(Data from Sergeant and colleagues[S36]; KU Leuven, 1971 to 1992; $n = 9600$.)

Key: *BUN*, Blood urea nitrogen; *ECG*, electrocardiogram; *LAD*, left anterior descending coronary artery.

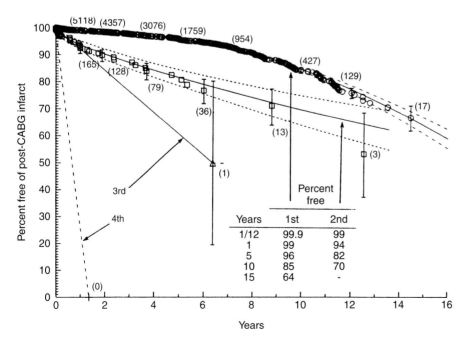

Figure 7-35   Freedom from myocardial infarction after coronary artery bypass grafting *(CABG)*, exclusive of perioperative infarction, according to number of previous post-CABG episodes of infarction. Time zero is time of CABG in depiction of freedom from *first* post-CABG infarction; it is time of first post-CABG infarction in depiction of time-related probability of a second post-CABG infarction; and so on. Format is as in Fig. 7-26. (Depictions from analyses of KU Leuven experience, 1971 to July 1987; $n = 5880$.[A20,K21,S11])

Key: *CABG*, Coronary artery bypass grafting.

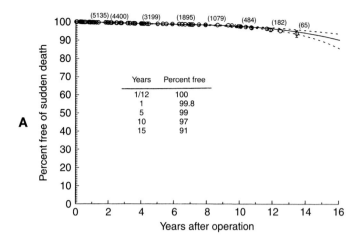

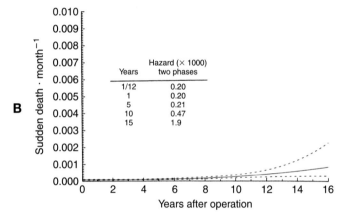

Figure 7-36   Sudden death after coronary artery bypass grafting. Format is as in Fig. 7-26. **A,** Freedom from sudden death. **B,** Hazard function. (From Sergeant and colleagues.[S43])

risk factor for sudden death (Table 7-10). A patient with a preoperative EF of 0.65 has only a small probability of dying suddenly within 15 years, whereas a patient with EF of 0.25 before CABG has a 15% probability of sudden death within 15 years (Fig. 7-37)[S43]

Failure to Work

Time-related freedom from failure to work has been less well documented than for other outcome events. Its time course is probably similar to that of freedom from angina. Patients who are free of angina after CABG are more likely to be working than those with angina.[S10]

A common belief is that CABG does not improve prevalence of gainful employment among patients with ischemic heart disease,[B10,C9,R4,S6] but this has not been a universal finding.[A1,B22] Failure to take into account the differing prevalences of risk factors for failure to work after CABG explains many of the discrepancies in results.[B22] Patients working before CABG have the highest probability of continued employment after operation.[B10,S10] Under "favorable circumstances" (as defined by risk factors listed in Table 7-11), more than 80% of patients not working at the time of CABG are working 1 year later; 20% or fewer are working after CABG when the risk factors are "unfavorable."[H17,R13]

■ **TABLE 7-10   Incremental Risk Factors for Sudden Death after Primary Isolated Coronary Artery Bypass Grafting (Events = 78)**

	Risk Factors	Hazard Phase	
		Constant	Late
	Patient Risk Factors		
	Angina		
	Other than stable angina	●	
(Longer)	Duration of anginal symptoms	●	
	Distribution of coronary artery disease		
	Triple-system disease	●	
	Absence of left main disease >50%	●	
	Atherosclerotic disease		
	Peripheral vascular disease	●	
(Poorer)	Quality of aortic anastomotic sites	●	
	Left ventricular function		
(Lower)	Ejection fraction	●	
	Procedural risk factor		
	Incomplete revascularization		●

(Data from Sergeant and colleagues[S43]; KU Leuven, 1971 to July 1987; n = 5880.)

Unsatisfactory Quality of Life

Even though unsatisfactory quality of life after CABG is one of the most important unfavorable outcome events, quantifying it is difficult because it is a composite of at least three factors: (1) freedom from limiting angina or heart failure, (2) reasonable freedom from need for medication, rehospitalization, and reintervention, and (3) preservation of a reasonable exercise capacity. Most surviving patients have a satisfactory quality of life early after CABG, but the probability of retaining this gradually begins to decline after about 5 years.[B23] Rate of decline is probably similar to that of freedom from angina.

Neurobehavioral and Neurologic Outcomes

Unrelated to cardiac aspects of CABG, the damaging effects of CPB usually required for operation are postulated to result in neurobehavioral disturbances and decline in cognitive function in some patients (see "Neuropsychological Subsystem" in Section 1 of Chapter 5). These disturbances are sufficiently mild that they might not be apparent unless patients are tested specifically for them; their prevalence has been reduced by incorporating appropriate filters into the arterial tubing from the pump-oxygenator to the patient. As many as 75% of patients may exhibit these subtle defects when tested 8 days after CABG, but by 3 to 6 months postoperatively that proportion drops to only about 10% to 30%.[H13,N8,R19] Prevalence is unfavorably affected by preoperative and postoperative anxiety and depression and by older age.[T4] Only rarely are patients aware of or handicapped by these defects.[S24] Of interest, decline in cognitive function occurs in up to 45% of patients who undergo major noncardiac operations.[G40]

Gross neurologic defects, usually in the form of transient or permanent sequelae of strokes, are more serious but fortunately less common.[R23] Gross defects most likely result from embolization of atherosclerotic debris from the ascending aorta or from air and intracardiac thrombus

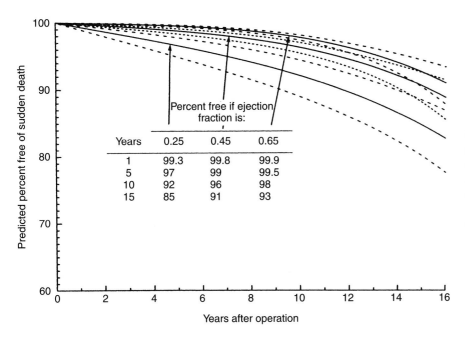

Figure 7-37 Nomogram of specific risk-adjusted solution of multivariable equation for sudden death after coronary artery bypass grafting (CABG), illustrating effect of pre-CABG ejection fraction. Format is as in Fig. 7-28. (From Sergeant and colleagues.[S43])

Years	Percent free if ejection fraction is:		
	0.25	0.45	0.65
1	99.3	99.8	99.9
5	97	99	99.5
10	92	96	98
15	85	91	93

■ **TABLE 7-11   Risk Factors for Time-Related Failure to Work after Coronary Artery Bypass Grafting**

Demographic	
(Older)	Age at operation
(Less)	Educational time
Preoperative Work Conditions	
(More)	Physical effort in job
(Longer)	Preoperative absence from work
(Lower)	Income from work
Clinical Status	
(Longer)	Duration of preoperative angina
(Greater)	Severity of preoperative angina
Aggressiveness of Atherosclerotic Process	
(More)	Peripheral vascular disease
Coexisting Disease	
(More)	Alcohol intake
Surgical Factor	
(Earlier)	Date of operation
Postoperative Factors	
(Shorter)	Duration of absence of angina
(Absence)	Cardiac rehabilitation program

(Data from Boulay and colleagues[B22] and Varnauskas.[V4])

rather than from damaging effects of CPB.[K31] Prevalence is about 0.5% in relatively young patients, but rises to about 5% in patients over age 70 and to about 8% in those over age 75.[C23,G26] Two randomized trials comparing on-pump and off-pump procedures showed similar prevalence of adverse neurologic outcomes.[B60,V8]

Use of Medication

Almost all studies report a decrease in use of vasodilators and β-blocking agents after CABG. The cooperative ran-domized study by the European Coronary Surgery Study Group, for example, found about 70% of patients randomized to medical treatment taking β-blockers during the first 3 years of follow-up in contrast to 25% of surgical patients.[V2] In the CASS trial, also randomized, surgically treated patients used fewer antianginal medications at 5 years than patients treated medically.[R13] By 10 years, however, the difference was likely due to chance.

Functional Capacity

Maximal exercise capacity of patients is improved by CABG,[B11,B12,F3,H19,K11,L7,S8,S9] and ECG abnormalities during exercise are usually importantly reduced.[S8] Degree of recovery and ultimate exercise capacity reached depend on preoperative LV function, graft patency, and completeness of revascularization. Increase in functional capacity, as evidenced by an increase in cardiac output with exercise postoperatively, is greater in patients with complete revascularization (26% versus 6%; $P = .0001$).[H18] Maximal exercise capacity generally is improved more by CABG than by medical treatment, at least for 3 to 10 years.[M12,V2]

The mechanisms of improvement in functional capacity after CABG are complex.[H15] Improvements in resting and stress LV function greatly contribute to the improved functional capacity (see next subheading). However, Serruys and colleagues found that an increase in maximal heart rate, presumably secondary to increased myocardial blood flow, is also an important determinant of increased functional capacity.[S8]

Left Ventricular Function
Resting Perfusion

Resting regional perfusion defects (at least in patients with unstable angina) are improved after CABG in at least 65% of patients,[K3,R12] indicating that preoperative resting perfusion defects were caused at least in part by ischemia; that is, the scarred areas contained considerable amounts of viable muscle.[C2,K3,Z1] Most patients who show no improvement have occluded grafts to the area. Wainwright and colleagues demonstrated that resting regional myocardial perfusion defects usually persist in areas supplied by ungrafted vessels (incomplete revascularization).[W4]

Left ventricular wall segments that are hypokinetic, akinetic, or even dyskinetic at rest preoperatively often have improved systolic function after CABG.[C4,C21,L19,W6,Z2] This is associated with increased regional myocardial perfusion.[K3] Improvement in segmental wall motion 12 months after CABG has been observed even in areas of scarring from previous MI.[M17] Brundage and colleagues showed that 19 of 29 LV wall segments with asynergy at rest preoperatively had improved function, and some even had normal function late postoperatively.[B50] This finding supports the concept that viable muscle cells, which may be hibernating, are scattered through hypokinetic and, at times, even akinetic and dyskinetic segments, and that wall motion in such segments can be improved by CABG.[D19] When segmental wall contraction does not occur after CABG, incomplete revascularization is the cause in some patients.[C21]

When preoperative global LV dysfunction is severe (EF less than 0.30), myocardial scarring is usually greater and usually limits recovery of LV function. In some patients, however, improvement in regional and global LV function occurs with CABG, and symptoms of pulmonary venous hypertension may regress.[A3,E13]

Several studies confirm that preoperatively depressed resting global LV systolic function (estimated by EF or dP/dt) is less depressed as early as 2 weeks after CABG.[B4,C4,H4] When this improvement fails to occur, incomplete revascularization is usually found.[H1,H4] Hellman and colleagues have demonstrated, in a slightly different setting, that 16 of 19 post-CABG patients with preoperative resting EFs of less than 0.40 showed similar or increased EFs with exercise early postoperatively (±2 weeks) and no deterioration of regional wall motion.[H4] Coronary angiography showed that three of four patients with persistence of an abnormal response to exercise had incomplete revascularization. Five years or more after operation, resting global LV function continues to be improved in some patients, whereas in others it is again depressed and may be even worse than preoperatively.[T1] Patients with worsened LV function usually have lower graft patency.[T1]

LV diastolic function, more specifically LV "relaxation," is also improved by successful CABG, and improvement may be immediate.[H7] This contributes to overall improvement in resting LV function that often promptly follows CABG.[C4,T5]

Exercise

The decrease in EF with exercise that is characteristic of ischemic heart disease is absent 2 weeks after operation in most patients, with EF rising normally with exercise.[H1,K15,N2] This favorable response to stress can be brought about only by CABG or PCI[S31] and does not result from collateral circulation alone, even when extensive.[S17] Further, patients who continue to experience angina postoperatively (presumably from incomplete revascularization) do not have this favorable response.[N2] When global and segmental function during exercise is not improved early (3 months) after operation, one or more bypass grafts are usually occluded or stenosed.[L18]

Most patients with preoperative exercise-induced abnormal increases in LV end-diastolic volume greater than 50% have a normal increase with exercise 2 weeks after operation.[H1] Presumably, these favorable early postoperative responses continue until the native CAD progresses or graft closure occurs.

Exercise-induced regional wall motion dysfunction, typically present preoperatively (even in the presence of normal LV function at rest) disappears within 2 weeks of operation in most patients.[H1,M1]

Ventricular Arrhythmias

Successful CABG, with relief of myocardial ischemia and its symptoms, generally does not decrease the frequency or severity of exercise-induced or resting ventricular arrhythmias,[D1,G1,L1] including ventricular tachycardia and fibrillation, although reports to the contrary exist.[B1,C1,E1,R1] This lack of favorable effect occurs because areas of ventricular scarring, rather than areas of myocardial ischemia, appear to be essential to arrhythmia development.

Failure of simple CABG to abolish serious ventricular electrical instability in most patients is particularly unfortunate because exercise-induced ventricular tachycardia or ventricular fibrillation carries a poor prognosis in patients with CAD.[L1] Sudden death is one mode of death late postoperatively. Therefore, when operation is contemplated in patients with important intractable ventricular tachyarrhythmias, consideration should be given to implantation of a cardioverter-defibrillator or procedures directed specifically at the ventricular arrhythmia, even in the absence of LV aneurysm.

Exceptions to these general statements are the few patients without ventricular scars or aneurysm in whom life-threatening ventricular arrhythmias occur purely from reversible LV myocardial ischemia. CABG can relieve the arrhythmic tendency in these patients.

A study of 900 patents with depressed LV function (EF less than 36%) and abnormalities on resting signal-averaged electrocardiograms suggested increased risk for postoperative ventricular arrhythmias.[B61] In the Coronary Artery Bypass Graft Patch Trial, 454 patients were randomized to CABG and 446 to CABG plus implantation of a cardioverter-defibrillator.[B61] During an average follow-up of 32 months, there was no evidence of improved survival among the patients in whom a cardioverter-defibrillator was implanted.

Coronary Flow Reserve

CABG is usually successful in improving coronary flow reserve (ability to increase flow in response to increased myocardial oxygen demand or pharmacologic vasodilatation). Surprisingly, coronary flow reserve returns to normal levels in many patients. This subject has been reviewed in detail by Wilson and colleagues.[W10,W11] Flow reserve has been obtained from measurements made in the operating room after CABG[B45,G25,S23] and has been confirmed in postoperative patients.[B9] Ability to increase coronary flow is absent when there is a stenotic coronary lesion beyond the graft.

In general, a patent anastomosis between a graft and a coronary artery perfuses only that segment of myocardium to which the native artery has supplied blood.[K4] However, about 25% of grafts distribute blood well beyond the segment of myocardium that would have been expected to be supplied by the native vessel.[M4] Often the area unexpectedly perfused by the graft is in the distribution of an occluded native vessel to which there is an obstructed graft. Importantly, segmental contractility is often improved postoperatively in the unexpectedly perfused area.[D15] This phenomenon probably explains the rather frequent finding of a functionally excellent result despite presence of one or two occluded grafts.

Not unexpectedly, in the few studies done late postoperatively, flow is greatest in vein grafts to the LAD system. Thus, using a radiographic densitometric method, Hamby and colleagues found at 2 weeks after operation a mean flow of 79 mL · min⁻¹ in grafts to the LAD (range 39 to 179) and 65 and 68 mL · min⁻¹ in those to the RCA and Cx artery, respectively.[H2] Flow through patent grafts during the early postoperative period is not related to graft size measured by cineangiographic techniques, and is presumably determined primarily by size of the arterial bed distal to the anastomosis.[W1]

An average of 2.5 years later, about 35% of vein grafts showed an important (average 45%) reduction in flow compared with early postoperatively. Thirty-five percent showed only a mild decrease during this period, and 30% showed no change. Such reductions of flow probably result largely from morphologic changes in the graft; thus, Weisz and colleagues found that change in graft flow was associated with a similar directional change in graft caliber[W1] (Fig. 7-38).

Concern has been expressed about flow capabilities of the ITA as a bypass graft. Although opinions differ,[F2,H6,M8] the bulk of evidence supports the ability of the ITA to supply a normal coronary flow reserve to an LAD with distal branches that are free of disease. This evidence has been well summarized by Hodgson and colleagues, who have also shown that adequate coronary flow reserve is provided when the ITA is used for sequential grafting.[H3] Separate ITA grafts can provide adequate flow to the entire left coronary system.[B57]

Graft Patency

Internal Thoracic Arteries

The ITA has proved an excellent conduit for use in CABG. About 90% of left ITAs whose distal end has been anastomosed end-to-side to the LAD are patent 10 to 20 years after operation (Fig. 7-39), and closure after that time is uncommon.[A6,A7,B47,G27,I2,L6,L13,T8,V9] However, 5% to 10% of patent grafts have stenoses late postoperatively.[I2] Accumulated information strongly suggests that most of the stenoses do not progress to occlusion. Use of the ITA as a free graft from aorta to LAD provides patency almost as high as with an in situ graft.[L11]

Favorable performance of the ITA when anastomosed to the LAD partly results from the continued function of its endothelial cells. Endothelium-derived relaxing factor and prostacyclin have been shown to be produced by human ITAs, which may be an important factor in the high patency of ITAs and their excellent function as bypassing conduits.[C11,L12] In addition, the ITA, when used for CABG as well as in its native position, has been shown to resist

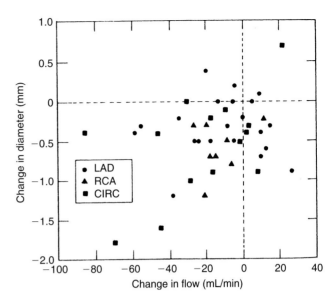

Figure 7-38   Relationship between change in saphenous vein bypass graft flow and change in diameter between early (2 weeks) and late (average 1.5 years) postoperative study by radiographic methods. In general, decrease in diameter correlates with decrease in flow. (From Weisz and colleagues.[W1])

Key: *CIRC,* Circumflex coronary artery; *LAD,* left anterior descending coronary artery; *RCA,* right coronary artery.

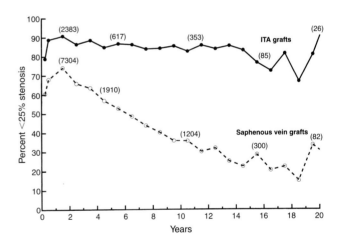

Figure 7-39   Patency of internal thoracic artery and saphenous vein grafts at 1-year intervals after coronary artery bypass grafting. Numbers in parentheses are the number of observations. (From Cleveland Clinic data, 1972 to 1999).

Key: *ITA,* Internal thoracic artery.

development of atherosclerosis.[B48,S19] Intimal hyperplasia develops in the ITA graft, however, and may be a cause of stenosis.[S19]

Another factor favorable to ITA patency is its grafting to the LAD, which has large runoff through the diagonal and septal branches. In support of this factor, ITA grafts to vessels other than the LAD appear to have lower patency that does not seem to be substantially different from that of vein grafts.[H31]

Use of bilateral ITA grafts has been favored by some groups, and the issue remains controversial.[G24,J4,K21,L26,S11]

Increasing evidence, however, indicates that use of both ITAs enhances survival in many subgroups of patients.[C37,E12,L31,L32,T6] Wound complications may be more prevalent when bilateral ITA grafting is used, particularly in obese and diabetic patients.[K20,L30] Wound problems tend to be serious, may require extensive procedures, and are associated with well-demonstrated devascularization of the sternum, which results from mobilization of even one ITA.[S39]

Other Arterial Grafts

The radial artery,[A13,B58,C35,R24,W16] right gastroepiploic artery,[C31,L25,M15,P2,S25,S51,S52] and inferior epigastric artery[G2,P9,P14] are currently used by a number of surgeons in combination with one or both ITA grafts or vein grafts and when an ITA graft is not available. Early (less than 13 months) patency of radial artery grafts exceeds 90% and does not differ from ITA patency.[R24,W16] A native coronary stenosis of less than 70% is associated with lower patency of a radial artery graft than if the stenosis is 70% or greater.[M25,R24] Acar and colleagues found late (4 to 7 years) patency of 64 radial artery grafts was 83%, and patency of 47 left ITA grafts was 91%.[A13]

In a study by Suma and colleagues of gastroepiploic artery grafts in 685 patients who underwent postoperative angiographic evaluation, patency was 94% within 1 year in all 685 patients, 88% between 1 and 5 years in 102 patients, and 83% between 5 and 10 years in 102 patients.[S52] Time-related patency at 1 month, 1 year, 5 years, and 10 years was 96%, 91%, 80%, and 62%, respectively. Principal causes of late occlusion were anastomotic stenoses and anastomoses to less critically stenosed coronary arteries.

Less information is available for the inferior epigastric artery. Gurne and colleagues performed postoperative angiography in 122 patients early (11 ± 5 days) and in 72 patients late (11 ± 6 months) after operation.[G2] Early patency was 98%, and late patency was 93%. Of 14 grafts that were occluded or threadlike at the late study, eight were anastomosed to arteries with a stenosis of 60% or less.

Saphenous Vein Grafts

Saphenous veins used as free aortocoronary grafts develop a unique disease complex.[U1] The condition begins with diffuse intimal thickening, so-called intimal hyperplasia, which is a universal finding in vein grafts that have been in place for more than 1 month.[B6,B17,B18,K6,M5,S29,V3] This process is not progressive.[S29] Thickness of the intimal hyperplasia seems to be inversely related to flow in the graft, and the process appears to result in a matching of vein lumen size to that of the coronary arteries supplied by the graft. Intimal hyperplasia is thus best considered as a remodeling process.[S29,V3]

As a result of these changes, most grafts show an angiographically detectable diffuse reduction in diameter; by 1 year after implantation, the diameter tends to approximate that of the recipient coronary artery. This diffuse smooth narrowing is not related to occlusion rates.[S29] Indeed, by increasing velocity of flow, remodeling may be beneficial, particularly when the vein is large initially.[B35,S28]

Of greater importance is development of lesions in the vein graft that are indistinguishable morphologically from the fibrous plaques of atherosclerosis.[B6-B8,C7,G3] These ath-

erosclerotic lesions are rarely found in saphenous vein grafts that have been in place for less than 3½ years.[S29] By 10 years after CABG, however, most saphenous vein grafts have undergone at least some atherosclerotic changes that are sometimes severe.[C27,C28,G5,S29] Whether this acceleration is related solely to morphologic damage to the graft caused by its removal and insertion into the arterial system, or whether it is caused by the patient's tendency to develop atherosclerosis, or whether both occur, is uncertain. Both factors probably play a role, because hyperlipidemia is a risk factor for extensive vein graft atherosclerosis.[C27,P3,S14,S37,S38] Also, aggressive efforts at controlling cholesterol levels retard progression of vein graft atherosclerosis.[B25,C36]

About 20% of vein grafts have proximal suture line stenosis within 1 year; about one fourth of these are found to be occluded 5 years later.[G4] Almost 50% of patients have some narrowing of the distal anastomosis within 1 year, but most have not progressed by 5 years after CABG.[G4] Unfortunately, minimal information is available on the relationship of type of anastomosis (e.g., end-to-side, side-to-side) to frequency and severity of anastomotic strictures. Anastomotic strictures may result from a localized separate process or may be a local manifestation of atherosclerosis.

Thrombosis, another process that can reduce graft patency, may develop early postoperatively. Endothelial cell loss and exposure of the basement membrane and collagen to blood tend to appear early after inserting the vein graft, predisposing it to early accumulation of platelets, fibrin, and thrombus on its luminal surface.[B6,B18,F5,J5,R9] More often, thrombosis develops later in heavily atherosclerotic areas.

Related to all these processes, about 10% of vein grafts close within the first few postoperative weeks, at least when antiplatelet therapy is not used. Late patency is highly variable, but only 50% to 60% of grafts are patent in heterogeneous groups of patients.[B16,G20,K5] However, patency has been about 80% when the greater saphenous vein has been used to bypass the LAD, which has a large runoff.[L6]

Other Vein Grafts

Patency of lesser saphenous vein grafts appears to approach that for the greater saphenous vein.[C39] Patency is lower when the bypass graft is to a particularly small coronary artery or one that supplies a heavily scarred area, perhaps because in both circumstances there is low graft flow. Upper extremity veins have even lower patency.[S21,W13] Cryopreserved allograft veins may be used when no other suitable autologous graft is available; late patency is substantially less than that of ITA and saphenous vein grafts.[L33]

Postoperative Progression of Native Coronary Artery Disease

Most important native vessel coronary artery stenoses proximal to a bypass graft become more severe or totally obstructive within 5 years of CABG.[B5,G4,H21,L2] Rates of progression of lesser stenoses proximal to a bypass graft remain uncertain. Important stenoses distal to the anastomosis also have a strong tendency to obstruct within

5 years.[G4,N1] Lesser stenoses distal to a functioning bypass graft tend to remain unchanged.[G4,I1] However, one study reported considerable progression of lesser distal arterial stenoses when the bypass graft to the artery was nonfunctioning.[N1]

Lesser stenoses in ungrafted arteries progress in severity with less frequency than do important stenoses, but 25% to 50% of such lesions progress within 5 years.[G4,L2] Thus, in a group of patients undergoing CABG, Laks and colleagues found progression of proximal stenosis in 16 (27%; CL 20%-34%) of 60 nonbypassed RCAs with less than 50% narrowings at a mean follow-up of 20 months.[L2] Two (3%; CL 1%-8%) of the 60 had progressed to complete obstruction.

Important stenoses in ungrafted vessels progress after operation, presumably at about the same rate as in the natural history of CAD (see "Stenotic Coronary Artery Disease" earlier in this chapter). Controversy continues as to whether important stenoses progress less rapidly in ungrafted than in grafted vessels.[E7,N1] Some information suggests that the rate is the same in both.[B5,G4,P5]

New stenoses appear in apparently nonstenotic arteries that were not grafted.[B5,H2] In following patients randomized to surgical versus medical treatment, Palac and colleagues found new lesions within 5 years in about 15% of both groups.[P5] These figures may be different in patients and populations in whom risk factors for atherosclerosis are altered.

Subsequent Reintervention

Prevalence of reintervention (repeat CABG or PCI), as with other outcome events, varies according to the patient's characteristics before the first CABG, details of the first CABG itself, and, to a lesser extent, management of the patient after the first operation. In a heterogeneous group of patients, freedom from reintervention is about 97% 5 years after the initial operation, 89% at 10 years, and about 72% at 15 years[S41] (Fig. 7-40, *A*). Instantaneous rate of reoperation begins to rise appreciably after about 5 years (Fig. 7-40, *B*).

Vein graft atherosclerosis is the most common cause of reintervention, with progression of native vessel disease the second most common.[J2,L14] Thus, more frequent use of the ITA to the LAD has reduced the frequency of reoperation and lengthened the interval between the first and second coronary operation.[L6,L14,L24,S34] Use of both ITAs may further reduce prevalence of reintervention.[E12,L31]

Results of a formal risk factor analysis for reintervention in the KU Leuven experience showed that younger age at first CABG clearly increased risk of reoperation (Table 7-12 and Fig. 7-41, *A*). Young age as a risk factor is also evident in other studies[F12,K21,S34,S41] and is a surrogate for "aggressiveness of the atherosclerotic process." In contrast to most other experiences, at KU Leuven use of the ITA did not reduce reoperations appreciably (Fig. 7-41, *B*).

Operative risk of a second CABG is about twice that of the first.[F12,L14,L20,Q1,S34] Higher prevalence of risk factors in patients undergoing repeat CABG, rather than the procedure itself, is the more important reason for this increased early risk. Including hospital deaths, 10-year survival in a heterogeneous group of patients is about 65%.[L14,S34] Con-

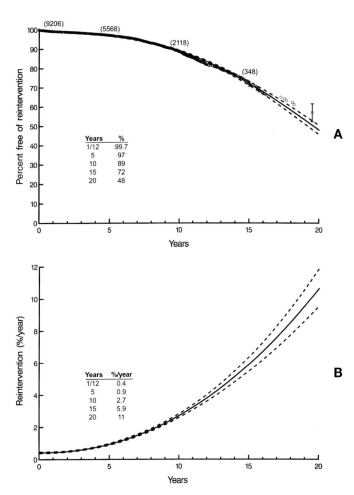

Figure 7-40 Reintervention after coronary artery bypass grafting. **A**, Freedom from reintervention. **B**, Hazard function. Format is as in Fig. 7-26. (From Sergeant and colleagues.[S41])

sidering deaths both early and late after repeat CABG, important left main coronary artery disease, three-system involvement, and severity of LV dysfunction are the most important risk factors.[L14]

Symptomatic improvement is usual in surviving patients, particularly when symptoms are severe before reoperation. Thus, in the Cleveland Clinic experience, 89% of those with severe angina before reoperation experienced either no angina or only mild angina postoperatively.[L14]

Transmyocardial revascularization, using a laser to create transmural channels, has been applied to patients with severe angina after CABG (see "Special Situations and Controversies" later in this chapter).[F16] It can be used as sole therapy or in combination with repeat CABG.

Percutaneous coronary interventions (PCIs) are being used with increasing frequency in symptomatic patients after CABG. Compared with balloon angioplasty, stenting of vein graft stenoses results in higher procedural efficacy (92% versus 69%) and greater increase in luminal diameter early after the procedure.[S53] Freedom from death, MI, repeat CABG, or revascularization of the targeted vessel are importantly better in the stent group (73% versus 58%).

■ **TABLE 7-12   Incremental Risk Factors for Reintervention after Coronary Artery Bypass Grafting** [a]

	Risk Factors	Early	Constant	Late
	Patient Risk Factors			
	Demographic			
	Female		•	
(Younger)	Age and female	•		
(Lesser)	Weight and female	•		
(Greater)	Height			•
(Younger)	Age		•	•
	Symptoms of reversible ischemia			
(Longer)	Anginal history		•	
(Higher)	Unstable angina grade (not infarct)	•	•	
	Cardiac comorbidity			
	Preoperative left or right bundle branch block		•	
	Aortic valve stenosis (moderate)		•	
	Left ventricular hypertrophy			•
	Noncardiac comorbidity			
	History of peripheral vascular disease			•
(Higher)	1-second forced expiratory volume/vital capacity		•	
(Higher)	Triglyceride level			•
	Left ventricular function			
	Preoperative anterior and septal infarct	•		
	Coronary disease			
(Lesser)	Left main stenosis (%)		•	
	No left main stenosis >90%			•
	One- or two-system disease		•	
	Procedural Risk Factors			
	Coronary operation			
	No graft to LAD		•	
	Venous graft to LAD			•
(Absence)	Two or more mammary anastomoses			•
(More)	Distals from venous grafts			•
	Incomplete revascularization	•		
	Institutional experience			
(Recent)	Date of surgery			•
	One surgeon		•	
(Lower)	Preceding year per surgeon volume	•		

(Data from Sergeant and colleagues[S41]; KU Leuven, 1971-1992; n = 9600.)

Key: *LAD,* Left anterior descending coronary artery.

[a] Includes only variables present before first CABG and procedural variables at first CABG.

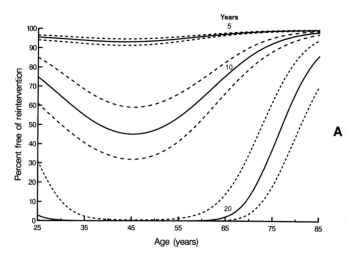

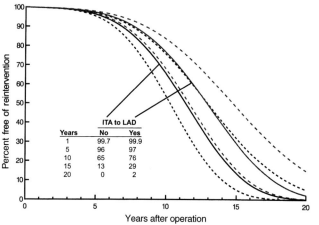

Figure 7-41   Nomograms illustrating strength and shape of risk factors for reintervention after coronary artery bypass grafting (CABG) in KU Leuven experience. **A,** Effect of age at initial CABG, depicted along horizontal axis. Predicted percent freedom is along vertical axis. Isobars represent interval between time of first CABG and time of estimation of prevalence of reintervention. **B,** Effect of using internal thoracic artery as a conduit to left anterior descending coronary artery at first CABG. (From Sergeant and colleagues[S41]; KU Leuven, 1971-1992; n = 9600.)

Key: *ITA,* Internal thoracic artery; *LAD,* left anterior descending coronary artery.

INDICATIONS FOR OPERATION

The bases of the indications for CABG involve comparative benefits of operation relative to those of no treatment (natural history), medical treatment, or treatment by PCIs. A complexity of these apparently simple propositions is that comparative benefit of CABG may be greater in one circumstance (e.g., severe versus mild LV dysfunction) compared with another, yet the actual time-related survival after CABG is less (Fig. 7-42).[C17] (The manner by which addition of the risk factors appears to amplify the contribution of another is explained under "Multivariable Analysis" in Chapter 6.)

Operation and other interventional therapies should increase regional coronary flow reserve. Small reductions in flow reserve are minimally life threatening; large reductions are life threatening. As techniques are perfected for quantifying these reductions, such as thallium-201 single-photon emission computed tomography and dobutamine stress echocardiography, predictions and comparisons of outcomes should become more accurate and precise, and patients will likely be better served.[M21]

Traditionally, physicians and surgeons have talked with patients about "your chances" of "being alive" or "without pain" 1 year from now, or 5 years or 15 years from now. A phrase such as "you have 95 chances out of a 100 of being

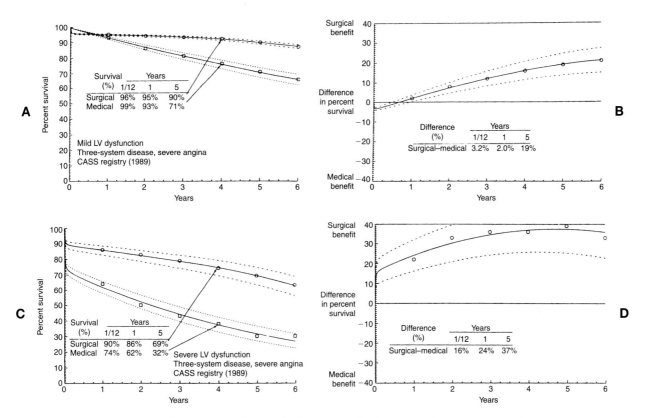

Figure 7-42 Comparison of survival after nonrandomly assigned coronary artery bypass grafting (CABG, "Surgical") with initial medical treatment in patients with triple-system disease and severe angina, according to severity of left ventricular (LV) dysfunction.[M11] Symbols represent published nonparametric estimates. Solid line enclosed within dashed confidence limits (CL) are parametric estimates. For survival estimates, CLs are 70%; for survival differences, CLs are 90%. **A,** Survival in patients with mild LV dysfunction. **B,** Comparative benefit, indicating that surgical benefit is unlikely to be caused by chance alone. **C,** Depiction similar to *A,* but in patients with severe LV dysfunction. Survival 1 month and 5 years after CABG is less than when LV dysfunction is mild, whereas survival after initial medical treatment is much less when LV dysfunction is severe. **D,** Depiction similar to *B,* but in patients with severe LV dysfunction. This emphasizes that surgical benefit is greater when LV dysfunction is severe than when it is mild, even though 1-month and 5-year survival after CABG are lower than when dysfunction is mild. (From ACC/AHA Guidelines and Indications for Coronary Artery Bypass Graft Surgery.[A20])

Key: *CASS,* Coronary Artery Surgery Study; *LV,* left ventricular.

---

alive for at least 10 more years" is frequently used, but such estimates have often been made on a qualitative basis. However, in an era when several different treatments are available, these types of predictions and comparisons for an individual patient with ischemic heart disease are often difficult to make. Fortunately, an enormous amount of information has been developed about effects of various risk factors on outcomes after different treatments for ischemic heart disease. Contrary to the belief of some, almost all this information is harmonious rather than internally conflicting. The problem is the efficient use of the data for (1) predicting and comparing for individual patients and (2) retrospectively evaluating quality of care and appropriateness of intervention.[A20,E9]

For most patients with congenital heart disease and for some with other diseases, the condition that requires surgical treatment is similar from patient to patient and is the dominant risk factor. This fact makes predicting and com-

paring for individual patients straightforward. In contrast, stenotic atherosclerotic CAD varies enormously from patient to patient, and the variations themselves are powerful risk factors. Therefore, recommendations to patients on the basis of predictions and comparisons of outcomes in heterogeneous groups of patients are of little value. Patient-specific predictions and comparisons are required (see Appendix 7B). General indications for CABG are discussed in the text that follows.

Stable Angina

Stable angina is usually well relieved by CABG, even though not permanently so; it can also be favorably influenced by modern medical treatment and under many circumstances by PCI.[E9,G14,H16,K19] Furthermore, it is now clearly established that CABG can accomplish considerably more than simple relief of angina. Thus, presence of chronic stable angina "unrelieved by medical treatment" is no longer an automatic indication for CABG. Rather, duration of relief of angina and effect on time-related probability of survival must be the major considerations. These factors depend not only on presence of angina, but also on all the patient-specific risk factors for unfavorable outcome events in patients with ischemic heart disease (see Box 7-1) and on the procedural risk factors for the various interventions.

Patients with *mild* chronic stable angina (Canadian class 1 or 2) can be considered to have mild "reversible ischemia," which, if confirmed by noninvasive testing, is not per se an indication for CABG or other forms of interventional therapy. However, severity and number of coronary stenoses and severity of LV dysfunction may combine to give these patients better survival and relief of angina with operation (see Fig. 7-3). When a clear comparative benefit of CABG over PCI or medical treatment can be predicted for an individual patient with mild reversible ischemia, such as when important stenoses in all three systems and LV dysfunction are present, operation is usually indicated.

When chronic stable angina is *moderate* or *severe* (Canadian class 3 or 4) despite good medical treatment, interventional therapy is usually advisable. When important stenoses are present in only one system, PCI often suffices.[P10] When important stenoses are present in three systems, or if left main coronary stenosis is present, CABG is preferable.[E9] There is consensus that left main equivalent disease (70% or more stenosis of proximal LAD and proximal left Cx artery), two-system disease with important proximal LAD stenosis (with EF less than 0.50 or demonstrable ischemia on noninvasive testing), and single-system or two-system disease without important proximal LAD stenosis but with a large area of viable myocardium and high-risk criteria on noninvasive testing, are indications for CABG.[E9]

Number of Systems with Important Stenoses

Left Main Stenosis

In general, stenosis of at least 50% in the left main coronary artery, either alone or in combination with stenoses in other coronary arteries, confers a sufficiently poor survival prognosis with medical treatment and is sufficiently hazardous to treat by PCI that CABG is indicated.[C29,L5] This is true even when the angina is well controlled by medical treatment or the patient is asymptomatic.[T7] The more severe the left main stenosis, the more urgent is the need for CABG.

Three-System Disease

In general, patients with good LV function and mild or moderate reversible ischemia have a sufficiently good outlook with noninterventional therapy that CABG need not be advised as initial therapy, even with three-system disease (Fig. 7-43, *A*). Periodic reevaluation is clearly indicated, however, because change in any one of a number of variables may make CABG advisable. If patients in this category have impaired LV function, their long-term prognosis with medical treatment is sufficiently poor and the prognosis after CABG sufficiently good that CABG is

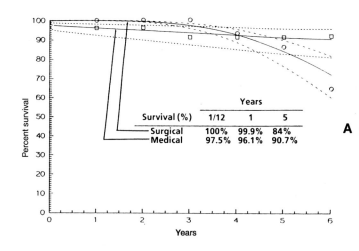

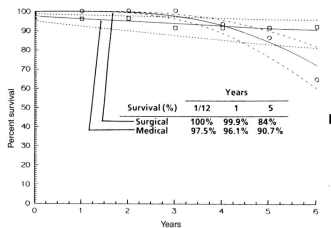

Figure 7-43   Survival after medical treatment and after coronary artery bypass grafting ("surgical") in a group of patients who are heterogeneous except for all having three-system coronary artery disease (generalizations from Fig. 7-42 pertain). Format is as in Fig. 7-42. **A,** Patients with normal left ventricular (LV) function. **B,** Patients with moderate LV dysfunction. (Modified from Myers and colleagues.[M10])

indicated, even though survival is not different at 5 years (Fig. 7-43, *B*).

When one or more important proximal stenoses are part of the three-system disease, particularly when one is in the LAD, in general the prognosis with noninterventional therapy becomes less favorable, whereas that after CABG is not adversely affected.[M10,V6] Thus, even with mild angina and good LV function, CABG is indicated when one or more important proximal stenoses coexist with three-system disease.[E9]

Two-System Disease

In general, PCI appears to be effective interventional therapy for many patients with important (at least 50% stenoses) two-system CAD.[G17] Also, prognosis with medical treatment is considerably better in patients with two-system disease than in those with three-system disease.[V11] Thus, CABG is not indicated in the majority of patients with mild angina and two-system disease. However, when such patients have left main equivalent disease, a severe proximal stenosis in the LAD, or impaired LV function, CABG is indicated.[E9]

Indications for CABG are stronger when angina is more severe (Canadian class 3 or 4). These indications are in addition to those described for patients with two-system disease without proximal LAD stenosis, but with a large area of viable myocardium and high-risk criteria on noninvasive testing.[E9]

Single-System Disease

CABG is infrequently indicated for patients with single-system disease. Results of CABG in this setting are excellent,[L8] but results of medical treatment and of PCI are also good, although probably not as long lasting.[F20] Bypass of the LAD with the ITA is an appropriate option in asymptomatic and symptomatic patients with proximal LAD stenosis and evidence of extensive ischemia on noninvasive testing or depressed EF (less than 50%).[B62,E9]

Left Ventricular Function

Patients with good LV function have a good prognosis with medical treatment even in the presence of important three-system disease, and in many patients, survival is not improved by immediate CABG (Fig. 7-43, *A*). Depressed LV function adversely affects outcome after CABG, even though in general the *comparative* benefit of CABG (vis-à-vis medical treatment) is greater the more depressed the LV function, and the indications for operation are more compelling (Fig. 7-44).[F7] However, risks and benefits of CABG become more uncertain when the resting LV EF is less than 0.30, and particularly when it is less than 0.20 (see "Left Ventricular Dysfunction" under Natural History earlier in this chapter). In some circumstances, risks of CABG may outweigh potential benefits when EF is less than 0.20. In some patients, even severe reductions in resting EF can result from myocardial "hibernation," and evidence indicates they benefit from CABG.[A3,E13] Exercise or resting thallium-201 scintigraphy, especially using the technique of enhancement by reinjection of thallium,[D16] may be particularly helpful in distinguishing between scar (which would contraindicate interventional therapy) and ischemia. Dobutamine stress echocardiography and positron emission tomographic (PET) scanning can also distinguish ischemic or hibernating myocardium from scar.

Performing CABG "prophylactically" in asymptomatic patients without noninvasive evidence for ischemia who have preserved LV function is undesirable from several standpoints. Medical treatment, including specific measures against unfavorable lipid profiles, may considerably or even indefinitely delay need for interventional therapy. Duration of the favorable effect of CABG appears to be finite, and for this reason alone, CABG should be delayed as long as is safe for the patient. Ideally, methods for prediction of the imminence of acute MI (the sequelae of which are the usual causes of depressed LV function) should be perfected so that CABG can be performed at the most appropriate time.

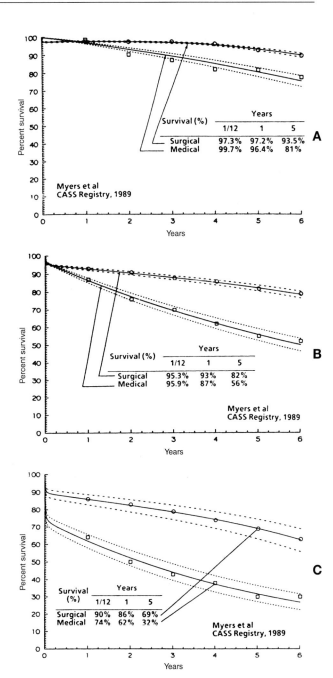

Figure 7-44   Survival after nonrandomly assigned medical treatment and coronary bypass grafting ("Surgical") treatment in patients with three-system coronary artery disease and severe angina. Format is as in Fig. 7-42. **A**, Patients with normal left ventricular (LV) function. **B**, Patients with moderate LV dysfunction (Coronary Artery Surgery Study [CASS] LV score = 10 to 15). **C**, Patients with severe LV dysfunction (CASS LV score = 16 to 30). (Modified from Myers and colleagues.[M10])

Key: *CASS,* Coronary Artery Surgery Study.

Unstable Angina

Unstable angina is usually best managed initially by intense medical treatment; surgical intervention in the presence of ongoing ischemic instability is rarely required.[B43,Y3] (In this discussion the description of "unstable angina" in the ACC/AHA Joint Task Force Subcommittee report is used.[A20])

Once the unstable state is controlled and the patient has been evaluated with noninvasive and invasive studies, the usual indications for CABG pertain. In some situations, however, indications for interventional therapy of some type become stronger than in patients with stable angina.[C30] Indications are particularly strong in patients with left main or left main equivalent disease, three-system disease, LV dysfunction, ongoing ischemia, or angina at rest.[E9,P6,S44] Indications are less strong in the subset of patients with unstable angina who have "new-onset angina."[W8]

Uncomplicated Non–Q-Wave Myocardial Infarction

In general, patients with non–Q-wave MI have the same indications for CABG, and for the same reasons, as do patients with unstable angina.

Uncomplicated Q-Wave Myocardial Infarction

In an era of increasing success with thrombolytic therapy for acute MI,[G19,M14,R8,R17,R18,R21] and more recently with PCI, CABG has little place in treating uncomplicated Q-wave MI. However, contrary opinions exist.[B41,D3,D4,S27]

When important angina persists early after an episode of acute MI, indications for operation are identical to those for unstable angina,[G30,J12,J13,K29] and results are almost as good. Because early risks of undertaking CABG after acute MI are less the longer the interval since onset of the episode, delaying the procedure for a minimum of 48 hours is often advisable.[B63,C40,H24]

Myocardial Infarction with Hemodynamic Deterioration

Acute hemodynamic deterioration is a serious and often fatal complication of ongoing MI, and delay in interventional therapy is probably disadvantageous. There is little doubt that more than 50% of patients with this complication can be salvaged by emergency CABG.[A2,B27,B29,K1,L27,N4] However, PCI is also effective in this setting.[G8,H29,H30,L4]

When CABG is used for patients with acute hemodynamic deterioration during ongoing MI, an effective regimen of myocardial management is essential[A2,A11] (see "Cold Cardioplegic, Controlled Aortic Root Reperfusion, and [When Needed] Warm Cardioplegic Induction" in Chapter 3). Even then, recovery of some patients may not be possible, because most patients in whom cardiogenic shock develops during an episode of acute MI are elderly, have a low EF on admission and a history of previous infarctions, and have a particularly large area of acute infarction. These are all important risk factors for death in this setting.[A12,H22]

Acute Complications during Percutaneous Coronary Intervention

Emergency CABG is indicated after unsuccessful PCI when hemodynamic compromise occurs or when there is evidence of ongoing ischemia or threatened occlusion of a major coronary artery with substantial myocardium at risk. Removal of a fractured guide wire or an undeployed stent may occasionally be required.[E9] If the hemodynamic state is severely compromised, CPB can be initiated in the catheterization laboratory (see "Cardiopulmonary Bypass Established by Peripheral Cannulation" in Section 3 of Chapter 2). When CABG is performed under these conditions, myocardial management should be that described under "Myocardial Infarction with Hemodynamic Deterioration" earlier in this chapter.

Emergency CABG under the circumstances just described is associated with a higher mortality and occurrence of perioperative infarction than is elective CABG.[B64,C41,L34] Factors that affect outcome include presence of cardiogenic shock, older age, LV dysfunction, previous infarction, and previous CABG. With increasing use of intracoronary stents, frequency of emergency CABG after PCI has declined.[L16]

Recurring Myocardial Ischemia

Evidence of return of important myocardial ischemia and symptoms may require consideration of repeat CABG. When these symptoms develop, and cineangiographic study shows that progression of native vessel disease is etiologic, PCIs are indicated. PCI to the native vessel disease for which bypass grafting was originally performed is occasionally possible, but in many cases these vessels have occluded by the time reintervention is under consideration.

When the cause of the recurring myocardial ischemia is graft disease, PCI is less effective and risks distal embolization of debris. Stenting of vein grafts is more effective in this setting than balloon angioplasty.[S53]

If PCI is not feasible, CABG is indicated in patients with moderate or severe angina despite optimal medical treatment if bypassable vessels are present in at least one system with noninvasive evidence for myocardium at risk (but preferably two or more systems). CABG may be the sole therapy or may be combined with transmyocardial laser revascularization.[F16]

SPECIAL SITUATIONS AND CONTROVERSIES

Coronary Artery Bypass Surgery versus Percutaneous Coronary Intervention

PCI is now an established method of management for many patients with atherosclerotic CAD. Although initially used for treating single-system disease,[G14] PCI is currently being applied to patients with multisystem disease. In addition to being less invasive, the advantages of PCI over CABG include shorter period of initial hospitalization and shorter recovery time. Disadvantages of PCI as the initial intervention include restenosis of the treated arteries and, in general, a lesser degree of revascularization than can be accomplished with CABG in comparable patients.

During the 1990s, results of nine randomized clinical trials comparing PCI and CABG were published. Outcomes with respect to the major end points examined were summarized in a document jointly published by the American College of Cardiology and American Heart Association (Table 7-13).[E9] Several inferences can be drawn from these

■ **TABLE 7-13   Comparison between Coronary Artery Bypass Grafting and Percutaneous Coronary Intervention in Nine Randomized Controlled Trials**

Trial [a]	Age (% Female)	CAD	n	Primary End Point	Follow-up (Years)	Intervention	Acute Outcome (5)			Late Outcome (%)				Primary End Point (%)
							Death	Q-Wave MI	Hosp CABG	Early and Late Death	Q-Wave MI	Angina	Reintervention (%)	
BARI[B4]	61 (26)	MV	1792	D	5[c]	CABG	1.3	4.6		10.7	19.6		8	10.7
						PCI	1.1	2.1	6.3	13.7	21.3		54	13.7
EAST[K18]	61 (26)	MV	392	D+MI+T	3	CABG	1.0	10.3		6.2	19.6	12	13	27.3
						PCI	1.0	3.0[b]	10.1	7.1	16.6	20	54	28.8
GABI[I9]	(20)	MV	359	A	1	CABG	2.5	8.0		6.5	9.4	26	6	26.0
						PCI	1.1	2.3[b]	8.5	2.6	4.5	29	44	29.0
Toulouse[C18]	67 (23)	MV	152	A	5	CABG	1.3	6.6		10.5	1.3	5.3	9	5.2
						PCI	1.3	3.9	3.9	13.2	5.3	21.1[b]	29	21.1[b]
RITA[C5]	57 (19)	SV+MV[c]	1011	D+MI	2½[d]	CABG	1.2	2.4		3.6	5.2	21.5	4	8.6
						PCI	0.8	3.5	4.5	3.1	6.7	31.3	31	9.8
ERACI[R11]	58 (13)	MV	127	D+MI+A+RR	1	CABG	4.6	6.2		4.7	7.8	3.2	6	23
						PCI	1.5	6.3	1.5	9.5	7.8	4.8	37	53[b]
MASS[H10]	56 (42)	SV (LAD)	142	D+MI+RR	3	CABG	1.4	1.4				2	0	3.0
						PCI	1.4	0	11			18	22	24[b]
Lausanne[G11]	56 (20)	SV (LAD)	134	D+MI+RR	2[d]	CABG	0	0		1.5	1.5	5	3	7.6
						PCI	0	0	2.9	0	2.9	6	25	36.8[b]
CABRI[F17]	60 (22)	MV	1054	D	1	CABG	1.3			2.7	3.5	10.1	9	2.7
						PCI	1.3			3.9	4.9	13.9[b]	36	3.9
Weighted average	60 (23)					CABG	1.3	4.1		6.5	11.3	10.4	7.3	
						PCI	1.0	2.3	5.9	7.7	11.0	15.5	42.3	

(Data from Eagle and colleagues.[E9])

Key: *A*, Angina; *BARI*, Balloon Angioplasty Revascularization Investigation; *CABRI*, Coronary Angioplasty versus Bypass Revascularisation Investigation; *CAD*, coronary artery disease; *D*, death; *EAST*, Emory Angioplasty versus Surgery Trial; *ERACI*, Estudio Randomizado Argentino de Angioplastia versus Cirugia; *GABI*, German Angioplasty Bypass Surgery Investigation; *Hosp CABG*, required CABG after PCI and before hospital discharge; *LAD*, left anterior descending coronary artery; *MASS*, Medicine, Angioplasty, or Surgery Study; *MI*, myocardial infarction; *MV*, multivessel; *PCI*, percutaneous coronary intervention; *RITA*, Randomised Intervention Treatment of Angina; *RR*, repeated revascularization; *SV*, single vessel; *T*, thallium defect.

[a] *P* <.05 comparing CABG and PCI cohorts.

[b] *P* <.05 comparing CABG and PCI cohorts.

[c] Included total occlusion.

[d] Planned 5-year follow-up (interim results).

studies. Early mortality is comparable for the two interventions. Prevalence of early Q-wave MI is generally higher among the CABG patients, but this was unlikely due to chance in only two of the trials. Using a weighted average, prevalence was 4.1% among the CABG patients and 2.3% among the PCI patients. Initial costs and length of stay are lower for PCI than for CABG. Patients with PCI are able to exercise more at 1 month and return to work sooner.[P15] In the Balloon Angioplasty Revascularization Investigation (BARI) and the Emory Angioplasty versus Surgery Trial (EAST), extent of revascularization achieved with CABG was higher than with PCI.[B4,K18]

When late results were examined, there was no statistically significant difference in survival in any of the nine trials at follow-up periods ranging from 1 to 5 years (see Table 7-13).[E9] In the subset of patients with diabetes, however, all-cause mortality and cardiac mortality were higher in those treated with PCI in BARI (34.7% versus 19.1% and 10.6% versus 5.8%, respectively).[E9] A similar finding in diabetic patients was observed in the Coronary Angioplasty versus Bypass Revascularisation Investigation (CABRI),[F17] but not in EAST.[K18]

No difference in prevalence of Q-wave MI or the combined end point of death and MI was demonstrated in any of the trials (see Table 7-13) or in subsequent meta-analyses.[P16,S54] Most of the trials found that CABG resulted in greater freedom from angina.

The most striking difference between CABG and PCI was need for subsequent procedures. Prevalence was 4 to 10 times higher for PCI in every trial (see Table 7-13).[E9]

In several studies that examined quality of life and cost, physical activity and employment were similar for both procedures after 3 years, and functional status was equivalent at 5 years in BARI.[H5,P15] Employment and emotional health were also similar.[E9,W17] The early cost benefit of PCI decreased during follow-up because of more frequent need for repeat procedures and hospitalization.[E9,H5,P16,S55,W17]

It must be emphasized that, for the most part, these trials excluded patients in whom survival had previously been shown to be better with CABG compared with medical therapy (i.e., patients with left main CAD, patients with multisystem disease and impaired LV function). To achieve a high degree of validity, randomized trials of this type must have high compliance with the original treatment, and only a small percentage of patients should "cross over" to the other form of therapy. Patients who are randomized must also be similar to those patients who are not enrolled to permit generalization of the findings. Many of the randomized trials conducted to date have been deficient in one or more of these categories.[E9] In addition, major technologic advances have occurred with both forms of treatment since these trials were completed, most notably use of intracoronary stents in PCI patients and multiple arterial grafts in patients undergoing CABG. Use of stents has substantially reduced need for urgent CABG and subsequent interventions, including repeat CABG.[M26] Nevertheless, results of these randomized trials, meta-analyses based on them, and results of large observational studies provide useful information that permits selection of the most appropriate form of interventional therapy for the individual patient with coronary atherosclerotic heart disease.

Endarterectomy

Although some surgeons use endarterectomy frequently, particularly in the distal RCA, most prefer to use the more distal branches of this artery for anastomosis to a bypass graft rather than to endarterectomize the parent trunk and graft to it. Some surgeons continue to employ long endarterectomies, even in the LAD, and report good results.[B20,P1,Q2]

Lower patency of grafts to endarterectomized arteries has been reported. Yeh and colleagues reported graft patency of 64% when endarterectomy was done to the artery grafted, compared with 92% when endarterectomy was not done.[Y1] However, many studies suggest that patency and flow in grafts to endarterectomized arteries compare favorably with those to nonendarterectomized arteries. Whether perioperative MI is more likely to occur when endarterectomy is employed is controversial,[M6] as is the relative completeness of revascularization that can be achieved with the two techniques.

Surgical Angioplasty

Surgical angioplasty of major coronary artery branches was abandoned years ago. However, some surgeons have successfully used angioplasty for the left main coronary artery and to a lesser extent for ostial lesions of the RCA.[D13,D14,S40]

For the left main coronary artery the anterior approach is preferable. With CPB and appropriate myocardial management, the pulmonary trunk is dissected away from the ascending aorta, and the left main coronary artery is exposed. An incision in the aorta just anterior to the left main coronary artery is extended a variable distance onto the left main artery. After excising atherosclerotic debris, patch-graft enlargement is performed using saphenous vein or autologous pericardium.[D13] Contraindications to this approach include extensive calcification of the left main coronary artery, involvement of the bifurcation, and older age.

Small Distal Vessels

Small distal size does not represent a contraindication to operation. Levin and colleagues found that bypass grafts could be successfully placed in 73% of vessels considered to be inadequate because of severe distal narrowing or absence of filling on the angiogram.[L23]

Transmyocardial Laser Revascularization

In the 1950s, Goldman and colleagues[G33] and Massimo and Boffi[M27] proposed that conduits could be created in the subendocardium through the LV cavity to direct blood through the coronary sinusoids and into ischemic areas of the myocardium. Subsequently, Sen and colleagues used direct needle acupuncture to create communicating channels in ischemic myocardium.[S56] Mihroseini and Cayton[M2] and Okada and colleagues[O4] used a laser to create transmyocardial channels. Initial observational studies in patients with severe angina who underwent transmyocardial laser revascularization (TMLR) showed that the procedure improved symptoms.[H11,H12]

Currently, TMLR is performed with a carbon dioxide or holmium laser. In a typical procedure, 10 to 50 channels are created in areas of ischemic myocardium. If TMLR is the sole therapy, a left anterior thoracotomy is made, and the procedure is performed without use of CPB. TMLR can also be performed in conjunction with primary or repeat CABG using CPB or with OPCAB. Laser channels are created in ischemic areas that are not amenable to bypass grafting.

Four randomized clinical trials compared TMLR with medical therapy in patients with severe angina refractory to medical treatment, reversible ischemia of the LV wall, and CAD not amenable to CABG or PCI. Findings indicated that TMLR results in substantial improvement in symptoms.[A14,A15,F16,S57] Exercise tolerance was not improved in the two studies that evaluated this factor.[A15,S57] In two of the three trials in which myocardial perfusion was assessed at rest and during stress, TMLR did not improve myocardial perfusion.[A14,S57] In the third study the magnitude of improvement in symptoms was disproportionate to the improvement in perfusion.[F16] TMLR was not associated with improvement in LV systolic function or survival 1 year after enrollment.

Mechanisms of action for TMLR remain unclear. These include placebo effect, creation of channels that provide increased blood flow to the ischemic myocardium, proliferation of new blood vessels (angiogenesis), denervation of ischemic myocardium, and infarction of ischemic myocardium.

TMLR can be performed with hospital mortality not exceeding 5% to 10% in properly selected patients.[A14,A16,B15,F16,H11,S57]

Gene Therapy

Enhanced understanding of the molecular biology of vascular cell activation and proliferation has resulted in development of interventions at the level of gene expression to enhance the microcirculation of ischemic muscle and alter the course of vein graft atherosclerosis. *Vascular endothelial growth factor* (VEGF) has been administered to patients with ischemic myocardium as sole therapy by direct injection using a minithoracotomy or as an adjunct to CABG.[L22,R16,V10] *Human fibroblast growth factor* (FGF) has been used for a similar purpose.[P8,S58] These studies have demonstrated evidence for improved myocardial perfusion in treated areas of the LV and improvement in symptoms early after treatment.

Ehsan and colleagues have demonstrated that a single intraoperative tranfection of vein grafts with a decoy oligonucleotide that blocks cell-cycle gene transactivation provides long-term resistance to neointimal hyperplasia and atherosclerosis.[E14] This has resulted in a reduction in primary graft failure unlikely to be due to chance when used in high-risk patients having CABG or peripheral arterial occlusions.[M16]

Combined Carotid and Coronary Artery Disease

Carotid artery disease is an important risk factor for stroke (cerebrovascular accident) after CABG.[D8,F19,R23] Hemodynamically significant carotid artery stenoses are associated with as many as 30% of the strokes occurring after CABG.[D8] Prevalence of hemodynamically significant carotid artery disease among patients undergoing CABG increases with increasing age. In a nonconsecutive series of 1087 patients 65 years of age and older undergoing cardiac surgical procedures (91% with CAD) who had preoperative carotid duplex ultrasonography, prevalence of a 50% or greater stenosis of one or both carotid arteries was 17%; for an 80% or greater stenosis, it was 5.9%.[B21] Prevalence of a 50% or greater stenosis was 8% in patients between ages 65 and 69, increasing to 17% for patients age 80 and older. Incremental risk factors for presence of an 80% or greater stenosis were a previous history of transient ischemic attack or stroke, female gender, left main coronary artery disease, peripheral vascular disease, and history of smoking.

Presence or absence of a cervical bruit is poorly predictive of high-grade stenosis even in the setting of known symptomatic carotid artery disease (sensitivity 63%, specificity 61%).[S59] Carotid duplex ultrasonography is currently the most widely used technique for preoperative screening to detect important carotid artery disease in patients undergoing CABG. It is used selectively in some centers and routinely in others to detect disease in older patients. If the preoperative carotid duplex study demonstrates high-grade (greater than 75% to 80%) stenosis and the patient's hemodynamic state is stable with no critically stenotic coronary arteries, carotid angiography is usually performed. Carotid and CABG procedures are staged, performing the carotid endarterectomy first. If the patient is hemodynamically unstable, or if there is high-grade left main coronary artery or proximal LAD disease, the carotid angiogram is often omitted, and a combined carotid and CABG procedure is performed.[M19] This approach is justified because prophylactic carotid endarterectomy has been shown to be superior to conservative therapy for preventing stroke in symptomatic or asymptomatic patients with high-grade stenosis, and carotid artery disease is an important risk factor for stroke in patients with CAD.[E15,E16,N5]

When a combined procedure is performed, carotid endarterectomy may be done before CPB is established. Alternatively, endarterectomy can be performed during hypothermic CPB, which may provide additional brain protection during occlusion of the carotid artery. In patients with severe stenosis of one carotid artery and severe stenosis or occlusion of the contralateral carotid artery, deep hypothermia with or without a brief interval of circulatory arrest may be advantageous.[K23]

Superiority of the combined versus staged approach has not been established by prospective trials. An individualized, patient-specific approach, with the decision based on symptoms and relative severity of the carotid and coronary artery disease, appears prudent and is used in many institutions.[E9] In experienced centers, staged or concomitant carotid endarterectomy and CABG can be accomplished with an early mortality that does not exceed 4%, stroke occurrence of less than 4%, and 10-year freedom from stroke of 88% to 96%.[A17,C5,F19,R20,V7,W18]

Coronary Artery Aneurysm and Dissection

Coronary artery aneurysm is a localized dilatation that is saccular or fusiform in shape and exceeds the diameter of normal adjacent segments or the diameter of the patient's largest coronary artery by 1.5 times. In patients undergoing coronary angiography, prevalence ranges from 0.4% to 4.9%.[S60] The majority of coronary aneurysms are atherosclerotic in origin. These aneurysms may also be congenital, result from Kawasaki disease, or develop after PCI. Aneurysms occur most often in the RCA; the left main coronary artery is involved infrequently.

No clinical features distinguish coronary aneurysms, and the natural history is largely unknown. Diagnosis is usually made by coronary angiography. Rupture was reported in 12% of a series of 53 autopsied cases reported by Daoud and colleagues in 1963.[D9] In CASS, however, which included more than 20,000 patients who underwent coronary angiography, no case of rupture was observed among 978 patients in whom coronary artery aneurysms were detected.[S61] Thrombus develops in these aneurysms and may be a source for distal embolization.[B24] Bypass grafting

of an artery containing an aneurysm with or without ligation of the artery distal to the aneurysm may be indicated in patients who have important occlusive disease in the artery or evidence of distal embolization in the absence of occlusive disease.[A5,A18,A19,E5]

Coronary artery dissection is a rare cause of ischemic heart disease and sudden death. Coronary dissection can occur spontaneously or result from aortic dissection, blunt chest trauma, cardiac catheterization, coronary angioplasty, or CABG.[B42,D11] Dissection has been observed after intense physical exercise and cocaine abuse.[E6,J10] Predisposing factors include atherosclerotic CAD and pregnancy. Sudden death is the most frequent clinical presentation. In patients who survive the initial event, medical therapy is appropriate for those without ongoing ischemia. Stenting or CABG is advisable for symptomatic patients.[D11,H20,K27] Patients with dissection of the left main coronary artery should undergo CABG.[T9]

APPENDIXES

APPENDIX 7A

Myocardial Perfusion Scoring System for Coronary Angiography

A preprinted background for a myocardial perfusion scoring system developed at GLH views the heart from the apex. The free wall of the left ventricle (LV) is flattened into a semicircle so that the curved perimeter represents the atrioventricular groove, and the septum is drawn as a central oblong. The LV free wall is divided into diagonal, obtuse marginal, and inferior (diaphragmatic or posterolateral) segments of fixed size and the septum into anterior and posterior portions of variable size (Fig. 7A-1). Each LV myocardial segment is given a numerical value, for a total of 15.[F9] When, for example, two equal-sized arteries go to a segment, half the numerical value of that segment is assigned to each artery as its *myocardial value*. The right ventricle is shown as a triangular area divided into conal, anterior, and inferior segments.

A 75% cross-sectional area (50% diameter) loss is considered an important but moderate stenosis, and a 90% cross-sectional area (67% diameter) loss is considered severe (Figs. 7A-2 and 7A-3). Some clinicians have considered only those lesions with a 70% or more diameter loss (greater than 90% cross-sectional area loss) important.[H8,K17,W7]

For scoring purposes, grade of severity of arterial obstruction is related to myocardial value of the particular branch (Table 7A-1). The total score for each patient is recorded. A score of less than 5 corresponds approximately to single-system disease; 5 to 10, double-system disease; and 10 to 15, triple-system disease.

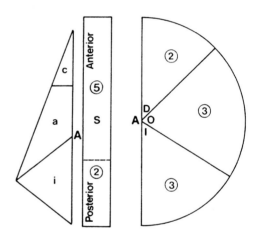

Figure 7A-1 Diagrammatic representation of segments of left and right ventricles, including ventricular septum. Myocardial value of each left ventricular segment is indicated by encircled numbers.

Key: *A*, Apex; *a*, right ventricular (RV) anterior area; *c*, RV conus area; *D*, left ventricular (LV) diagonal areas; *I*, LV inferior (diaphragmatic area); *i*, RV inferior area; *O*, LV obtuse marginal area; *S*, septum; *anterior*, portion of septum supplied by left anterior descending artery; *posterior*, portion of septum supplied by posterior descending artery.

■ **TABLE 7A-1   Computation of Myocardial Score of Stenosed Coronary Artery According to Grade of Arterial Obstruction and Myocardial Value**

| Score | Obstructional Grade (% Loss) | | | | Myocardial Value[a] | | | | | | | | | |
| | Cross-Sectional Area | | Cross-Sectional Diameter | | | | | | | | | | | |
	≤ % <		≤ % <											
A	100		100		1	2	3	4	5	6	7	8	9	10
B	90	100	67	100	0.8	1.6	2.4	3.2	4	4.8	5.6	6.4	7.2	8
C	75	90	50	67	0.6	1.2	1.8	2.4	3	3.6	4.2	4.8	5.4	6
D	50	75	33	50	0.4	0.8	1.2	1.6	2	2.4	2.8	3.2	3.6	4
E		50		33	0.2	0.4	0.6	0.8	1	1.2	1.4	1.6	1.8	2

[a] Myocardial value is directly proportional to the amount of left ventricular myocardium perfused by (assigned to) each artery if it were unobstructed. If two similar stenoses are present in series, or if a stenosis is more than 1 cm long, grade is increased by 1 but not to grade A. Score for each artery is entered separately in boxes provided beneath diagram (see Figs. 7A-1, 7A-2, and 7A-3) and summed to give total myocardial score. The higher the score, the greater is the amount of potentially ischemic myocardium. By this system, the score cannot exceed 15.

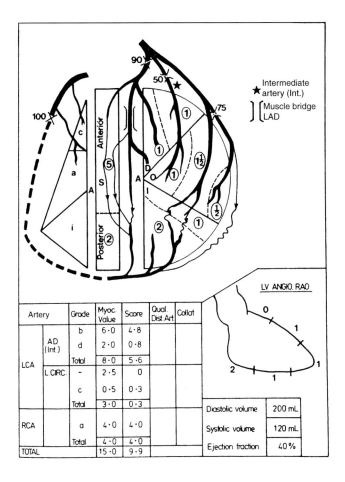

Artery		Grade	Myoc. Value	Score	Qual. Dist.Art	Collat
LCA	AD (Int.)	b	6·0	4·8		
		d	2·0	0·8		
		Total	8·0	5·6		
	L CIRC.	–	2·5	0		
		c	0·5	0·3		
		Total	3·0	0·3		
RCA		a	4·0	4·0		
		Total	4·0	4·0		
TOTAL			15·0	9·9		

Diastolic volume	200 mL
Systolic volume	120 mL
Ejection fraction	40%

Figure 7A-2 Diagrammatic representation of a coronary angiogram in a right dominant coronary tree. Myocardial areas are subdivided as shown in Fig. 7A-1. Distribution of arteries supplying these segments is sketched in to facilitate assessment of myocardial value of each artery or group of arteries. In this example, the proximal right coronary artery is occluded. Its distal branches, distributed to an average amount of the posterior septum (myocardial value = 2) and two thirds of the inferior left ventricular area (*posterolateral segment* area with myocardial value = 2, total value = 4) fill by collateral arteries from left coronary branches (*finer interconnecting lines,* with *arrows* indicating direction of flow). An intermediate (or first diagonal) artery supplies basal half of diagonal area and apical one third of obtuse marginal area (total myocardial value = 2). First marginal branch supplies most of the obtuse marginal segment (1½) but also left one third of the inferior area (*1*). Sites of stenosis are indicated by a cross, and degree of stenosis (cross-sectional area loss) by an adjacent number. Beneath diagram, score is calculated according to grade of stenosis and myocardial value of each branch (see Table 7A-1). In addition to myocardial score, the left ventricular, right anterior oblique angiogram *(LV ANGIO RAO)* is also recorded, dividing profile into five segments; segmental wall motion is indicated by number alongside each segment.

Key: *AD,* Anterior descending coronary artery; *Int,* intermediate (first diagonal) artery; *L CIRC,* left circumflex artery; *LAD,* left AD; *LCA,* left coronary artery; *O,* normal contraction; *RCA,* right coronary artery; *1,* hypokinesis; *2,* akinesis; *3,* dyskinesis.

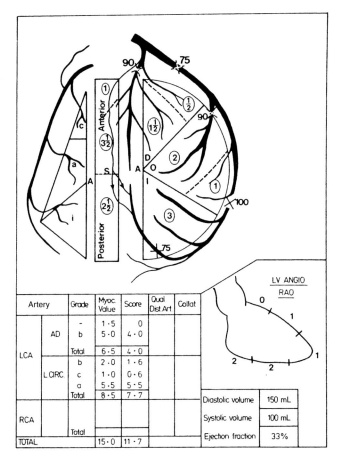

Artery		Grade	Myoc. Value	Score	Qual Dist Art	Collat
LCA	AD	–	1·5	0		
		b	5·0	4·0		
		Total	6·5	4·0		
	L CIRC.	b	2·0	1·6		
		c	1·0	0·6		
		a	5·5	5·5		
		Total	8·5	7·7		
RCA						
		Total				
TOTAL			15·0	11·7		

Diastolic volume	150 mL
Systolic volume	100 mL
Ejection fraction	33%

Figure 7A-3 Diagrammatic representation in a diseased left dominant coronary tree. Left anterior descending coronary artery is shorter than average, whereas posterior descending artery is correspondingly longer and arises from circumflex artery (value = 2.5). Right coronary artery *(RCA)* is small and does not supply left ventricle. Even severe narrowing or occlusion of RCA would not affect myocardial score. (See Fig. 7A-2.)

A diagram of each patient's coronary tree is drawn freehand on a preprinted background by the reporting radiologist. Stenoses are then indicated by crosses and degree of stenosis by an adjacent number (see Fig. 7A-2).

APPENDIX 7B

Patient-Specific Predictions and Comparisons in Ischemic Heart Disease

Bases for Predictions and Comparisons
One purpose of this book is to present indications for various cardiac surgical procedures and rationale for these indications. As already discussed under "Indications for Operation," the indications are based in large part on the predicted time-related probability of a good outcome after operation, as well as comparisons of this outcome with that after alternative forms of treatment, including no treatment.

More quantitatively, the indications are based on predicted, absolute, *time-related probability of freedom* from unfavorable outcome events (e.g., death); the predicted *time-related comparative benefit*[C17] of coronary artery bypass grafting (CABG) versus those of alternative forms of treatment; and degree of certainty in predictions and comparisons. Degree of certainty can be expressed in the usual way by *P* values and confidence intervals (see Chapter 6). Arbitrarily, and subject to decisions of society, when patient-specific predicted probability of freedom from specified unfavorable outcome events (e.g., death at 5 years) is at least 5% higher after CABG than after competing forms of therapy and at least 10% higher at 10 years, and if the difference can be shown to be unlikely due to chance alone, a useful comparative benefit of CABG can be considered to be established. The greater the comparative benefit, the longer is the duration of comparative benefit; and the greater the absolute probability of freedom from unfavorable events, the more compelling are indications for CABG.

Predictions and comparisons are complex in the case of CABG. Ideally, comparisons would be with percutaneous coronary intervention (PCI), with current medical treatment, and with no treatment (natural history). Further, there are many patient-related incremental risk factors of importance in patients with ischemic heart disease (see Box 7-1), as well as many procedural and institutional risk factors for surgical, percutaneous, and medical interventions. Thus, advice to a specific patient must be based on his or her unique combination of risk factors and those of the treatments being considered.

At an unrealistic minimum, risk factors to be considered in predicting and comparing outcomes of an individual patient with ischemic heart disease are (1) number of systems with important stenosis (four possible values), (2) left ventricular function (four possible values), (3) severity of reversible ischemia (five possible values), and (4) presence or absence of acute infarction (two possible values), making already 160 possible combinations. Other important risk factors, such as presence or absence of diabetes, hypertension, hemodynamic instability, and hyperlipidemia, are not yet included in this count. Furthermore, because there are currently four treatment options for patients with ischemic heart disease, the 160 (plus other factors) must be multiplied by 4, giving at least 640 different depictions of freedom from just one unfavorable event to be considered in making a recommendation about treatment. And procedural risk factors are not yet accounted for!

The only reliable way, arguably, in which patient-specific predictions and comparisons can be made in this setting is by using equations based on multivariable risk factor analysis, describing time-related probability of freedom from important unfavorable outcome events after various available interventions, including no treatment. After entering values for characteristics of the patient at hand, each equation is solved to obtain predicted time-related probability of freedom from the event and its confidence intervals (variability). Solutions for alternative treatments are compared, taking note not only of the predicted probabilities but also of the magnitude of any differences and degree of certainty that any differences are not due to chance alone.

Therefore, computer software is required for making patient-specific predictions and comparisons, and in this text only a few examples can be given of the types of output that are obtainable using such techniques. Currently, limitations to this approach are imposed by lack of detail of portions of the databases used for the multivariable analyses[S68] and the nonavailability for analysis of potentially important risk factors. These limitations must be described for each analysis and communicated to physicians using them.

Examples
Patient-specific predictions and comparisons are presented for one time-related outcome event: survival. These require (1) a risk factor equation for each alternative therapy and (2) values for all variables in those equations for each patient.

Equations for Survival
The multiphase multivariable risk factor equation for death after CABG comes from Sergeant and colleagues.[S20] Risk factors, regression coefficients and their standard deviations, and level of statistical significance in each hazard phase are presented in Table 7B-1.

The multivariable risk factor equation for PCI, performed in an era prior to extensive stenting and rapidly evolving adjunctive treatments to reduce restenosis, is from a study of 6209 patients undergoing primary balloon percutaneous transluminal coronary angioplasty (PTCA) at the Mid America Heart Institute between June 1980 and July 1991 (McCallister BD: personal communication; 1992). (The data, analyzed at UAB using multiphase hazard function methodology, formed the basis for comparing therapy in diabetics.[O5]) Table 7B-2 depicts in detail the risk factor equation for death.

The equation used to depict natural history of ischemic heart disease, albeit after availability of beta-blocking agents, is derived from the Coronary Artery Surgery Study (CASS) Registry.[N9] Eighteen-year follow-up data were analyzed at UAB using multiphase hazard function technology. The equation for death is given in Table 7B-3.

Limitations of Equations
Each equation has limitations. An overall limitation is that they come from disparate settings. It would have been better had data elements with identical definitions come from a common data set and analysis were performed on the combined data set. Another limitation is that both CABG and PCI information came from single-institution studies. Survival after CABG at KU Leuven and survival after PCI at Mid America Heart Institute seem, however, to be representative of patients undergoing these procedures in the modern era.

The CASS natural history data are, and must be, dated. They are valuable from the perspective that if outcomes of intervention are predicted to be worse than CASS natural history, then intervention is not appropriate. In contrast, present-day medical management of ischemic heart disease is confounded with interventional treatment and follow-up is short. This precludes using current information to depict medical treatment as a therapeutic option.

Use of Equations
In the examples that follow, predictions are shown at the time the patient presents for decision making. Decision making in the course of a chronic disease, such as ischemic heart disease, is not made at one point in time but during a series of evaluations. Risk factors are likely to change across time requiring use of the equations at each evaluation. The new calculations may lead to different decisions as the disease and other factors evolve.

Example 1: Athletic Woman with Mild Symptoms
An athletic 50-year-old normotensive, nonsmoking lady complains to her physician about chest tightness after strenuous tennis matches. Cineangiography reveals 35% diameter narrowing of the proximal left anterior descending coronary artery (LAD), 60% stenosis of the first diagonal, 30% stenosis of the proximal right coronary artery (RCA), and 40% stenosis of the obtuse marginal. Ejection fraction on left ventriculogram is 64%. Her past medical history is unremarkable except for mastectomy for in situ cancer 10 years earlier.

Her predicted survival is excellent no matter how her mild coronary disease is managed (Fig. 7B-1). Indeed, her chances are best without intervention at this time according to the natural history (medical) curve.

Unfortunately, recommendation against intervention is not reassuring. She subsequently undergoes PCI, 3 months later another PCI for restenosis, and eventually left internal thoracic artery to LAD grafting for occlusion of the LAD.

When survival according to natural history is predicted to be better than after intervention, it is prudent to manage symptoms conservatively.

■ TABLE 7B-1   Incremental Risk Factors for Death after Coronary Artery Bypass Grafting, Including Patient, Procedure, and Institutional Experience Variables [a]

| | | Hazard Phase | | | | | |
| | | Early | | Constant | | Late | |
	Risk Factors	Coefficient ± SD	P	Coefficient ± SD	P	Coefficient ± SD	P
	Patient Risk Factors						
	Demographic						
(Older)	Age [b]	0.5172 ± 0.132	<.0001	3.698 ± 0.66	<.0001	9.520 ± 2.1	<.0001
(Younger)	Age [c]			1.086 ± 0.37	.003	6.987 ± 2.1	.001
(Lighter)	Weight [d]	2.105 ± 0.56	.0001				
(Higher)	Weight/height ratio			8.680 ± 2.4	.0003		
	Symptoms of reversible ischemia						
(Higher)	Angina class	0.3467 ± 0.121	.004			0.01539 ± 0.0078	.05
	No angina			0.8158 ± 0.26	.002		
(Higher)	Unstable angina grade [e]	0.5112 ± 0.175	.004				
	Left ventricular function						
	Cardiogenic shock	2.743 ± 0.34	<.0001				
(Better)	Clinical status [f]			-0.9604 ± 0.48	.05		
(Lower)	Ejection fraction [g]	-1.295 ± 0.24	<.0001	-2.198 ± 0.35	<.0001	-3.475 ± 0.46	<.0001
(Earlier)	and date of operation [h]					1.016 ± 0.179	<.0001
(Greater)	Functional limitation by heart failure [i]			0.6096 ± 0.20	.002		
	Coronary disease						
(Greater)	Number of diseased systems [j]					0.2975 ± 0.075	<.0001
	Three-system disease	0.3925 ± 0.164	.02				
	90% left main disease	3.465 ± 0.93	.0002				
(Earlier)	and date of operation [k]	-1.184 ± 0.37	.002				
	Comorbidity (cardiac)						
	Mitral regurgitation (mild)	0.4655 ± 0.199	.02				
	Aortic regurgitation					1.309 ± 0.28	<.0001
	Atrial fibrillation			1.056 ± 0.51	.04	1.014 ± 0.32	.002
	Ventricular tachycardia/fibrillation			1.663 ± 0.46	.0003		
	Cardiac pacemaker					1.220 ± 0.51	.02

(Data from Sergeant and colleagues.[S20])

Key: *exp*, Natural exponential function; *Ln*, natural logarithm; *SD*, standard deviation.

[a] KU Leuven, 1971 to 1992; $n = 9600$.

[b] In early hazard phase, exp[age(years)/50] exponential transformation; in constant hazard phase, Ln{100/[100−age(years)]} logistic transformation; in late hazard phase, Ln[age(years)/10] − 1.7 logarithmic transformation.

[c] [50/age (years)] − 1 inverse transformation.

[d] [70/weight (kg)] − 1 inverse transformation.

[e] 0, No unstable angina; 1, unstable angina controlled by medication; 2, changing ST segment in the hours before surgery despite maximal intravenous medication.

[f] 0, Stable; 1, unstable angina with ongoing ST changes or acute myocardial infarction; 2, cardiogenic shock.

[g] Expressed as a fraction, with any value less than 0.15 set to 0.15, and the logarithmic transformation Ln[ejection fraction].

[h] Product (interaction) of ejection fraction (expressed in logarithmic form as Ln[ejection fraction]) and date of operation (expressed in logarithmic form as Ln[number of years since January 1971]).

[i] Degree by which functional limitation by symptoms of heart failure exceeds that by symptoms of angina (0, None; 1, mildly greater than angina; 2, moderately greater than angina; 3, severely greater than angina).

[j] By 70% diameter reduction criterion.

[k] Product (interaction) of 90% left main disease (*no*, 0; *yes*, 1) and date of operation (expressed in logarithmic form as Ln[number of years since January 1971]).

Continued

Example 2: Coal Miner with Chronic Stable Angina

A 55-year-old male coal miner and one-pack-per-day smoker with 85% of expected 1-second forced expiratory volume presents with a 2-year history of moderate-intensity stable angina. Coronary angiography reveals 85% proximal LAD stenosis, 60% first diagonal stenosis, 40% proximal circumflex stenosis, 40% obtuse marginal disease, and 60% RCA stenosis. He is in atrial fibrillation and has mild cardiomegaly, an ejection fraction of 0.48, and a history of surgery for peripheral vascular disease.

His predicted survival is good over the next 10 years (Fig. 7B-2, *A*). However, it is predicted to be better with intervention, either PCI or CABG, than natural history. PCI, followed by CABG if eventually required, appears to be the appropriate therapy at this time for his two-system coronary artery disease. Difference in predicted survival for PCI versus CABG is shown in Fig. 7B-2, *B*. The higher early risk of CABG is predicted to result in a PCI benefit until about 2 years, after which confidence limits (CL) for the difference in percent survival overlap zero. In contrast, Fig. 7B-2, *C* shows that PCI yields progressively better survival across time than natural history, and this benefit is unlikely to be due to chance (Fig. 7B-2, *C*). The hazard ratio of PCI and natural history is nearly flat, indicating a proportional hazards relationship except for the small early risk of PCI (Fig. 7B-2, *E*). However, lowering of overall risk for PCI contributes only 9.4 additional months of life over the 10 years following intervention (see Fig. 7B-2, *D*), although this added lifetime is unlikely to be due to chance (see Fig. 7B-2, *E*).

■ TABLE 7B-1   **Incremental Risk Factors for Death after Coronary Artery Bypass Grafting, Including Patient, Procedure, and Institutional Experience Variables** [a]—cont'd

		Hazard Phase					
		Early		Constant		Late	
	Risk Factor	Coefficient ± SD	P	Coefficient ± SD	P	Coefficient ± SD	P
	Comorbidity (noncardiac)						
	Overweight now or previously[l]					0.1876 ± 0.080	.02
	History of vascular disease	0.5286 ± 0.159	.0009			0.6059 ± 0.95	<.0001
	Cerebrovascular disease[m]			1.063 ± 0.27	<.0001		
	Previous vascular surgery (noncarotid)			1.255 ± 0.31	<.0001		
	History of smoking					0.2741 ± 0.097	.004
(Lower)	1-second forced expiratory volume (% of normal)[n]	0.6642 ± 0.21	.001	-0.01282 ± 0.0060	.03	0.5546 ± 0.137	<.0001
	Serum creatinine >2.5 mg/dL					1.773 ± 0.29	<.0001
	History of renal failure[o]					1.273 ± 0.36	.0004
	On renal dialysis	1.881 ± 0.43	<.0001				
	Hypertensive[p]					0.1849 ± 0.077	.02
(Higher)	Diabetic grade[q]					1.278 ± 0.47	.007
	and age[r]					-0.5611 ± 0.27	.04
	History of malignancy			1.502 ± 0.27	<.0001		
	History of hepatic disease[s]			1.170 ± 0.33	.0004		
(Higher)	Triglyceride level[t]					0.1072 ± 0.035	.002
	Procedural Risk Factors						
	Coronary operation						
	Grafting to LAD					0.5398 ± 0.153	.0004
	Use of arterial grafts to any location					-0.3632 ± 0.085	<.0001
	Nonuse of only arterial grafts in single-system coronary disease			1.410 ± 0.33	<.0001	1.146 ± 0.61	.01
	Use of patch grafts					1.470 ± 0.54	.006
(Higher)	Ratio of distals to conduits[u]	0.1016 ± 0.029	.0006			1.318 ± 0.52	.01
(More)	Coronary endarterectomies	0.5305 ± 0.24	.03				
(Higher)	Proportion of distals to small vessels[v]	0.9605 ± 0.32	.002			0.4640 ± 0.196	.02
	Incomplete revascularization	0.4754 ± 0.165	.004			0.2901 ± 0.097	.003
	Concomitant procedures						
	Left ventricular incision or plication	1.092 ± 0.36	.002				
	Institutional Experience						
	Surgeon Z	0.6833 ± 0.172	<.0001				
(Lower)	Surgeon's volume in previous year[w]	-0.3971 ± 0.141	.005				
	Intercepts	-8.638		-13.70		-10.79	

(Data from Sergeant and colleagues.[S20])

Key: *exp*, Natural exponential function; *LAD*, left anterior descending coronary artery; *Ln*, natural logarithm; *SD*, standard deviation.

[l] More than 10 kg over ideal weight. Ideal weight is [height(cm) − 100] for males and [height(cm) − 110] for females.

[m] Disease in the extracranial portion of vessels supplying the brain.

[n] [100/(1-second normalized expiratory rate)] inverse transformation in early and late hazard phases, untransformed in constant hazard phase. The normalized rate is expressed as percent of normal based on body surface area.

[o] Patients on dialysis or having received renal transplantation.

[p] Defined as systolic blood pressure greater than 160 mmHg or diastolic blood pressure greater than 100 mmHg, or being medicated for hypertension by history.

[q] *Grade 0*, No diabetes; *grade 1*, oral hypoglycemic-treated diabetes; *grade 2*, insulin-treated diabetes. The squared transformation of diabetic grade is used.

[r] Product (interaction) of age (expressed in logarithmic form as Ln[age (years)/10]) and grade of diabetes (expressed as the squared transformation).

[s] Hepatitis or clinical hepatic dysfunction.

[t] [Triglyceride level/100] − 1.75 scaling transformation.

[u] In the early phase [total number of distal anastomoses divided by total number of proximal conduits − 1]^2 squared transformation; in the late hazard phase, exp[total number of distal anastomoses divided by total number of proximal conduits − 1]/100 exponential transformation.

[v] 1 mm or smaller.

[w] [Number of CABG operations performed in previous calendar year by that surgeon]/200 scaling transformation.

Shaping parameters: Early hazard phase δ, 0; ρ, 0.01539; ν, 2.233; *m*, 0; late hazard phase τ, 1; α, 1; η, 1; γ, 2.229.

■ **TABLE 7B–2   Incremental Risk Factors for Death after Primary Percutaneous Coronary Intervention without Previous Coronary Artery Bypass Grafting, Including Patient, Procedure, and Experience Variables** [a]

		Hazard Phase					
		Early		Constant		Late	
	Risk Factors	Coefficient ± SD	P	Coefficient ± SD	P	Coefficient ± SD	P
	Patient Risk Factors						
	Demographic						
(Older)	Age [b]	−3.448 ± 0.73	<.0001	1.265 ± 0.24	<.0001	−7.869 ± 1.39	<.0001
(Younger)	Age [c]			1.709 ± 0.73	.02		
	Female	0.5069 ± 0.171	.003	0.4100 ± 0.126	.001		
	Symptoms of reversible ischemia						
(Higher)	Angina severity [d]	0.1313 ± 0.031	<.0001				
(Higher)	No angina symptoms [e]			0.9205 ± 0.24	.0001		
	Angina at rest			0.3241 ± 0.108	.003		
	Left ventricular function						
	Acute transmural myocardial infarct	1.335 ± 0.34	.0001				
	Cardiogenic shock	0.7740 ± 0.31	.01				
(Greater)	Number of previous myocardial infarcts			0.1591 ± 0.065	.01		
(Lower)	Ejection fraction [f]	1.308 ± 0.54	.01	3.536 ± 0.38	<.0001		
	Coronary disease						
(Greater)	Number of diseased systems (≥50% stenosis)	0.6450 ± 0.136	<.0001				
	Proximal LAD stenosis ≥50%	0.9498 ± 0.185	<.0001				
	Complete occlusion					0.8387 ± 0.37	.02
	Proximal RCA stenosis ≥70%			0.2732 ± 0.127	.03		
	Mid RCA stenosis ≥50%	0.5914 ± 0.196	.003				
(Greater)	Distal RCA stenosis [g]	0.9167 ± 0.26	.0004				
	Complete occlusion of PDA	1.139 ± 0.48	.02				
	Right posterolateral segment stenosis ≥95%	1.176 ± 0.36	.001				
	Proximal circumflex stenosis ≥50%			0.2893 ± 0.135	.03		
	Coexisting conditions						
	History of smoking			0.5319 ± 0.135	<.0001		
	History of hypertension					0.4904 ± 0.25	.05
	Treated diabetes			0.6043 ± 0.148	<.0001	1.071 ± 0.30	.0004
(Higher)	Serum creatinine level [h]	1.371 ± 0.196	<.0001	1.526 ± 0.197	<.0001	1.647 ± 0.44	.0002
(Lower)	Serum creatinine level [i]			0.6760 ± 0.21	.001		
	Procedure priority						
	Nonelective PCI	1.335 ± 0.27	<.0001				
	Procedural Risk Factors						
	PCI of left main coronary artery	1.866 ± 0.44	<.0001	1.647 ± 0.49	.0007		
	PCI of occluded distal LAD	2.310 ± 0.85	.007				
	PCI of occluded proximal circumflex coronary artery	1.083 ± 0.55	.05				
	Nondilatation of chronic total occlusion	0.7493 ± 0.183	<.0001				
	Experience						
(Earlier)	Date of PCI [j]	−0.3849 ± 0.136	.004				
	Intercepts	−4.043		−9.982		−3.699	

Key: *LAD*, Left anterior descending coronary artery; *Ln*, natural logarithm; *PCI*, percutaneous coronary intervention; *PDA*, posterior descending coronary artery; *RCA*, right coronary artery; *SD*, standard deviation.

[a] Mid America Heart Institute, June 1980 to July 1991; $n = 6209$.

[b] In early and late hazard phases, [50/age (years)] inverse transformation; in constant hazard phase, [age/50]^2 squared transformation.

[c] [50/age (years)] inverse transformation.

[d] [Angina severity]^2 squared transformation, where angina severity is graded as: *0*, no angina or acute infarction; *1*, angina with extreme exertion; *2*, angina with slight exertion; *3*, angina at rest.

[e] In patients without a history of prior myocardial infarction.

[f] [1−ejection fraction (decimal fraction)]^2 squared complementary transformation.

[g] Stenosis scaled to a decimal fraction.

[h] Ln[serum creatinine (mg/dL)] logarithmic transformation.

[i] [1/serum creatinine (mg/dL)] inverse transformation.

[j] Ln[date of PCI (years since 1 June 1980)] logarithmic transformation.

■ **TABLE 7B-3**　　**Incremental Risk Factors for Death in Medically Treated Patients in the Coronary Artery Surgery Study (CASS) Registry** [a]

	Risk Factors	Hazard Phase			
		Early		**Late**	
		Coefficient ± SD	**P**	**Coefficient ± SD**	**P**
	Patient Risk Factors				
	Demographic				
(Older)	Age [b]	0.3016 ± 0.129	.02	3.015 ± 0.56	<.0001
(Younger)	Age [c]			0.9480 ± 0.34	.005
(Lighter)	Weight [d]	1.916 ± 0.52	.0002		
(Higher)	Weight/height ratio			7.666 ± 2.0	.0001
	Symptoms of reversible ischemia				
(Higher)	Angina class	0.3003 ± 0.121	.01		
	No angina			0.5760 ± 0.22	.008
(Longer)	Duration of angina history [e]	0.1074 ± 0.048	.03		
(Higher)	Unstable angina grade [f]	0.6026 ± 0.176	.0006		
	Left ventricular function				
(Greater)	Number of prior infarcts				
	Cardiogenic shock	2.538 ± 0.34	<.0001		
(Lower)	Ejection fraction [g]	-1.370 ± 0.24	<.0001	-1.791 ± 0.30	<.0001
	and age [h]				
(Greater)	Functional limitation by heart failure [i]			0.5788 ± 0.177	.001

Key: *exp,* Natural exponential function; *Ln,* natural logarithm; *SD,* standard deviation.

[a] 1 July 1994 to 1 May 1979; $n = 24,959$; without previous intervention $= 23,723$.

[b] In early hazard phase, exp[age (years)/50] exponential transformation; in constant hazard phase, Ln{100/[100–age (years)]} logistic transformation; in late hazard phase, Ln[age (years)/10] – 1.7 logarithmic transformation.

[c] [50/age (years)] – 1 inverse transformation.

[d] [70/weight (kg)] – 1 inverse transformation.

[e] Ln[duration (months)] logarithmic transformation.

[f] *0,* No unstable angina; *1,* unstable angina controlled by medication; *2,* changing ST segment in the hours before surgery despite maximal intravenous medication.

[g] Expressed as a fraction, with any value less than 0.15 set to 0.15, and the logarithmic transformation Ln[ejection fraction].

[h] Product (interaction) of ejection fraction (expressed in logarithmic form as Ln[ejection fraction]) and age (expressed in logarithmic form as Ln[age (years)/10]).

[i] Degree by which functional limitation by symptoms of heart failure exceeds that by symptoms of angina (*0,* None; *1,* mildly greater than angina; *2,* moderately greater than angina; *3,* severely greater than angina.

Shaping parameters: Early hazard phase δ, 0; ρ, 0.01293; ν, 2.114; *m,* 0; late hazard phase τ, 1; α, 1; η, 1; γ, 2.607.

Continued

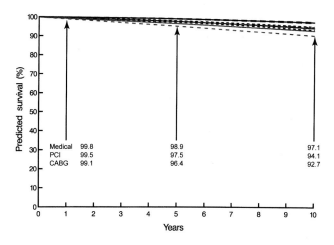

Figure 7B-1　　Example 1: Athletic woman with mild symptoms. Shown are three solid curves enclosed within dashed 70% confidence limits for (a) natural history (medical), (b) percutaneous coronary intervention, and (c) coronary artery bypass grafting. These predictions are based on patient-specific solutions of the three equations outlined in Tables 7B-1 through 7B-3.

Key: *CABG,* Coronary artery bypass grafting; *PCI,* percutaneous coronary intervention.

■ TABLE 7B-3   **Incremental Risk Factors for Death in Medically Treated Patients in the Coronary Artery Surgery Study (CASS) Registry** [a]—cont'd

| | | Hazard Phase | | | |
| | | Early | | Late | |
	Risk Factors	Coefficient ± SD	P	Coefficient ± SD	P
(Greater)	**Coronary disease**				
	Number of diseased systems[j]				
	Three-system disease	0.4147 ± 0.167	.01		
	Comorbidity (cardiac)				
	Mitral regurgitation (mild)	0.4096 ± 0.20	.04		
	Aortic regurgitation				
	Ventricular tachycardia/fibrillation			0.9128 ± 0.42	.03
	Atrial fibrillation			0.9840 ± 0.50	.05
	Cardiac pacemaker				
	Comorbidity (noncardiac)				
	Overweight now or previously[k]				
	History of vascular disease	0.5703 ± 0.160	.0004		
	Cerebrovascular disease[l]			0.9438 ± 0.24	<.0001
	Previous vascular surgery (noncarotid)			0.7582 ± 0.36	.03
	History of smoking				
	History of pulmonary disease[m]				
(Lower)	1-second forced expiratory volume (% of normal)[n]	0.8044 ± 0.20	<.0001	-0.01450 ± 0.0050	.004
	Serum creatinine >2.5 mg/dL				
	History of renal failure[o]				
	History of nephrectomy				
	On renal dialysis	1.673 ± 0.42	<.0001		
	Hypertensive[p]				
(Higher)	Diabetic grade[q]				
	and age[r]				
	History of malignancy			1.336 ± 0.24	<.0001
	History of hepatic disease[s]			0.8418 ± 0.28	.003
(Higher)	Triglyceride level[t]				
	Intercepts	-8.312		-11.66	

Key: *Ln,* Natural logarithm; *SD,* standard deviation.

[j] By 70% diameter reduction criterion.

[k] More than 10 kg over ideal weight. Ideal weight is [height (cm) − 100] for males and [height (cm) − 110] for females.

[l] Disease in the extracranial portion of vessels supplying the brain.

[m] Incapacitating anthracosilicosis, chronic obstructive pulmonary disease, or asthmatic bronchitis.

[n] [100/(1-second normalized expiratory rate)] inverse transformation in early and late hazard phases, and untransformed in constant hazard phase. Normalized rate is expressed as percent of normal based on body surface area.

[o] Patients on dialysis or having received renal transplantation.

[p] Defined as systolic blood pressure greater than 160 mmHg or diastolic blood pressure greater than 100 mmHg, or being medicated for hypertension by history.

[q] *Grade 0,* No diabetes; *grade 1,* oral hypoglycemic-treated diabetes; *grade 2,* insulin-treated diabetes. The squared transformation of diabetic grade is used.

[r] Product (interaction) of age (expressed in logarithmic form as Ln[age (years)/10] and grade of diabetes (expressed as squared transformation.)

[s] Hepatitis or clinical hepatic dysfunction.

[t] [Triglyceride level/100] − 1.75 scaling transformation.

Shaping parameters: Early hazard phase δ, 0; ρ, 0.01293; ν, 2.114; m, 0; late hazard phase τ, 1; α, 1; η, 1; γ, 2.607.

Example 3: Cachectic Retired Diabetic with Unstable Angina

A frail 65-year-old African-American insulin-treated diabetic man with a history of previous myocardial infarction and an 18-month history of moderate angina presents to the emergency room with accelerating angina symptoms. Cardiac-specific enzymes are not diagnostic of acute myocardial infarction, and the unstable angina is controlled by intravenous nitroglycerin. Echocardiography reveals mild to moderate ischemic mitral valve regurgitation and an ejection fraction of 0.35. Urgent coronary angiography reveals 90% proximal LAD disease, 70% diagonal stenosis, 40% proximal circumflex lesions with 70% obtuse marginal stenosis, 80% mid-RCA stenosis, and a 40% lesion of the posterior lateral artery.

His predicted survival according to various treatment strategies is presented in Fig. 7B-3, *A.* Although urgent intervention is encouraged, if it is important to postpone operation for a few days or weeks so that the patient can put his affairs in order or watch his granddaughter graduate from college, his best chance of surviving for that short period is intensive medical therapy. This is because the survival curves "cross," posing the realistic dilemma that long-term benefit of appropriate risk-lowering therapy may come at the expense of short-term higher risk. Thus, an early medical benefit in percent survival is later supplanted by a large and sustained benefit of CABG (Fig. 7B-3, *B*) that becomes statistically significant after about 1 year (Fig. 7B-3, *C*).

The individual hazard curves are shown in Fig. 7B-3, *D,* illustrating how the risk of natural history is reduced by intervention. Also, after the period of high risk early after CABG, risk continues at a level about commensurate with that for the general population of African-American 65-year-old males. The hazard ratio between CABG and natural history also has nearly a constant proportional hazards relationship after about 1 year (Fig. 7B-3, *E*).

Benefit of operation (appropriateness) is shown in Fig. 7B-3, *F.* Notice that over a period of 10 years, this patient is expected to gain 60 months of life from intervention.

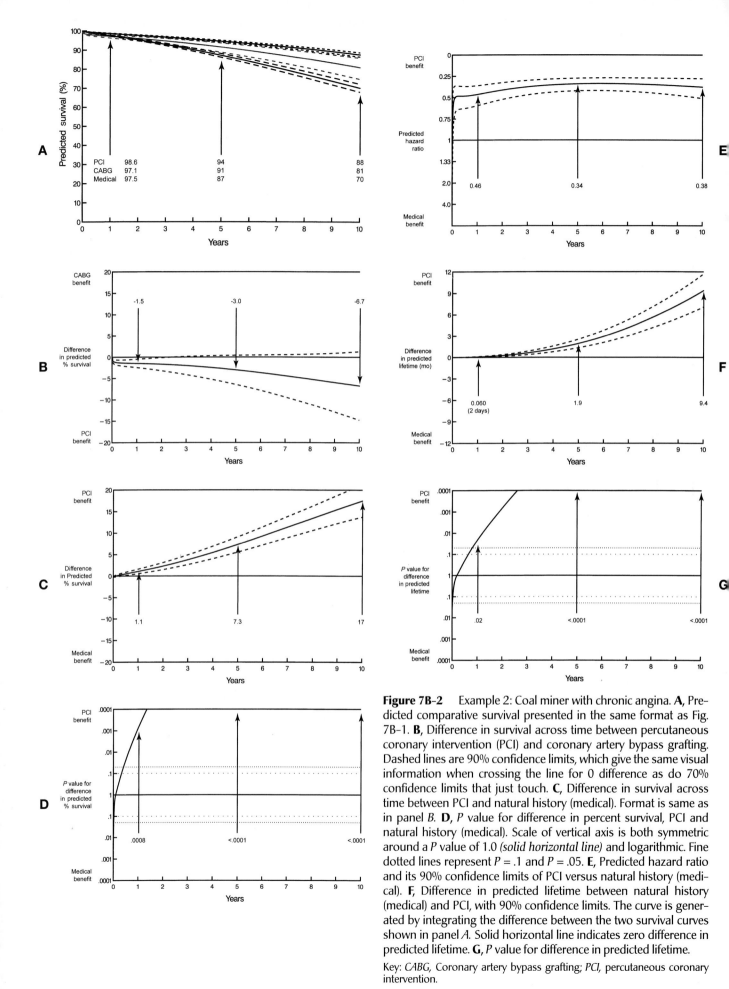

Figure 7B-2 Example 2: Coal miner with chronic angina. **A,** Predicted comparative survival presented in the same format as Fig. 7B-1. **B,** Difference in survival across time between percutaneous coronary intervention (PCI) and coronary artery bypass grafting. Dashed lines are 90% confidence limits, which give the same visual information when crossing the line for 0 difference as do 70% confidence limits that just touch. **C,** Difference in survival across time between PCI and natural history (medical). Format is same as in panel *B.* **D,** *P* value for difference in percent survival, PCI and natural history (medical). Scale of vertical axis is both symmetric around a *P* value of 1.0 *(solid horizontal line)* and logarithmic. Fine dotted lines represent *P* = .1 and *P* = .05. **E,** Predicted hazard ratio and its 90% confidence limits of PCI versus natural history (medical). **F,** Difference in predicted lifetime between natural history (medical) and PCI, with 90% confidence limits. The curve is generated by integrating the difference between the two survival curves shown in panel *A.* Solid horizontal line indicates zero difference in predicted lifetime. **G,** *P* value for difference in predicted lifetime.

Key: *CABG,* Coronary artery bypass grafting; *PCI,* percutaneous coronary intervention.

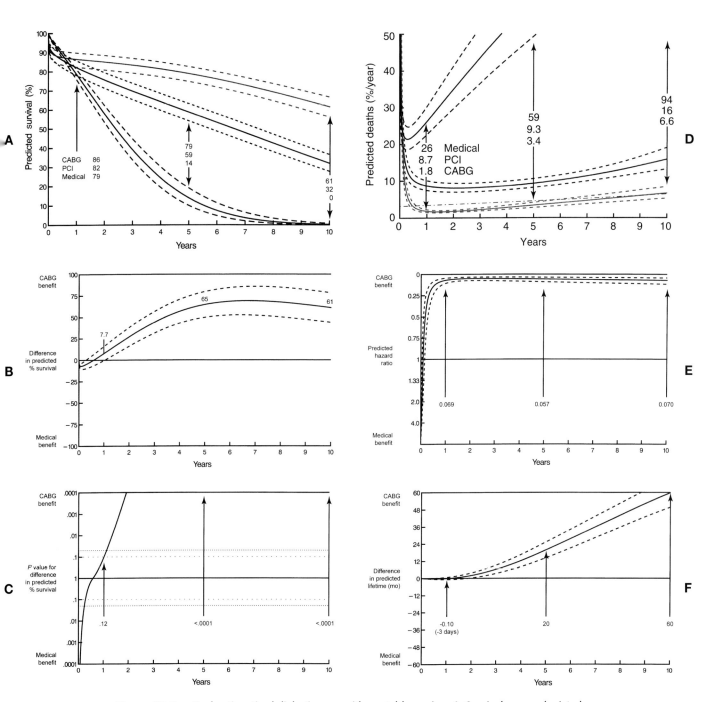

Figure 7B-3   Cachectic retired diabetic man with unstable angina. **A,** Survival curves depicted as in Fig. 7B-1. **B,** Difference in predicted percent survival between coronary artery bypass grafting (CABG) and natural history (medical). Depiction is as in Fig. 7B-2, *B.* **C,** *P* value for difference in percent survival between CABG and natural history (medical). Depiction is as in Fig. 7B-2, *C.* **D,** Hazard function for death from natural history (medical), percutaneous coronary intervention, and CABG. The dash-dot-dash line is hazard in the general population of 65-year-old African-American men. **E,** Hazard ratio of CABG and natural history (medical). **F,** Difference in predicted lifetime between CABG and natural history (medical). Depiction is as in Fig. 7B-2, *F.*

Key: *CABG,* Coronary artery bypass grafting; *PCI,* percutaneous coronary intervention.

REFERENCES

A

1. Anderson AJ, Barboriak JJ, Hoffmann RG, Mullen DC. Retention or resumption of employment after aortocoronary bypass operations. JAMA 1980;243:543.

2. Allen BS, Rosenkranz E, Buckberg GD, Davtyan H, Laks H, Tillisch J, et al. Studies on prolonged acute regional ischemia. VI. Myocardial infarction with left ventricular power failure: a medical/surgical emergency requiring urgent revascularization with maximal protection of remote muscle. J Thorac Cardiovasc Surg 1989;98:691.

3. Alderman EL, Fisher LD, Litwin P, Kaiser GC, Myers WO, Maynard C, et al. Results of coronary artery surgery in patients with poor left ventricular function (CASS). Circulation 1983;68:785.

4. Assad-Morell JL, Frye RL, Connolly DC, Davis GD, Pluth JR, Wallace RB, et al. Aorta-coronary artery saphenous vein bypass surgery: clinical and angiographic results. Mayo Clin Proc 1975;50:379.

5. Aintablian A, Hamby RI, Hoffman I, Kramer RJ. Coronary ectasia: incidence and results of coronary bypass surgery. Am Heart J 1978;96:309.

6. Acinapura AJ, Rose DM, Jacobowitz IJ, Kramer MD, Robertazzi RR, Feldman J, et al. Internal mammary artery bypass grafting: influence on recurrent angina and survival in 2,100 patients. Ann Thorac Surg 1989;48:186.

7. Azariades M, Fessler CL, Floten HS, Starr A. Five-year results of coronary bypass grafting for patients older than 70 years: role of internal mammary artery. Ann Thorac Surg 1990;50:940.

8. Allen KB, Griffith GL, Heimansohn DA, Robison RJ, Matheny RG, Schier JJ, et al. Endoscopic versus traditional saphenous vein harvesting: a prospective, randomized trial. Ann Thorac Surg 1998;66:26.

9. Aranki SF, Rizzo RJ, Adams DH, Couper GS, Kinchla NM, Gildea JS, et al. Single-clamp technique: an important adjunct to myocardial and cerebral protection in coronary operations. Ann Thorac Surg 1994;58:296.

10. Abramov D, Tamariz MG, Fremes SE, Guru V, Borger MA, Christakis GT, et al. Trends in coronary artery bypass surgery results: a recent, 9-year study. Ann Thorac Surg 2000;70:84.

11. Allen BS, Buckberg GD, Fontan FM, Kirsh MM, Popoff G, Beyersdorf F, et al. Superiority of controlled surgical reperfusion versus percutaneous transluminal coronary angioplasty in acute coronary occlusion. J Thorac Cardiovasc Surg 1993;105:864.

12. Applebaum R, House R, Rademaker A, Garibaldi A, Davis Z, Guillory J, et al. Coronary artery bypass grafting within thirty days of acute myocardial infarction. Early and late results in 406 patients. J Thorac Cardiovasc Surg 1991;102:745.

13. Acar C, Ramsheyi A, Pagny JY, Jebara V, Barrier P, Fabiani JN, et al. The radial artery for coronary artery bypass grafting: clinical and angiographic results at five years. J Thorac Cardiovasc Surg 1998;116:981.

14. Allen KB, Dowling RD, Fudge TL, Schoettle GP, Selinger SL, Gangahar DM, et al. Comparison of transmyocardial revascularization with medical therapy in patients with refractory angina. N Engl J Med 1999;341:1029.

15. Aaberge L, Nordstrand K, Dragsund M, Saatvedt K, Endresen K, Golf S, et al. Transmyocardial revascularization with CO_2 laser in patients with refractory angina pectoris. Clinical results from the Norwegian randomized trial. J Am Coll Cardiol 2000;35:1170.

16. Allen KB, Dowling RD, DelRossi AJ, Realyvasques F, Lefrak EA, Pfeffer TA, et al. Transmyocardial laser revascularization combined with coronary artery bypass grafting: a multicenter, blinded, prospective, randomized, controlled trial. J Thorac Cardiovasc Surg 2000;119:540.

17. Akins CW, Moncure AC, Daggett WM, Cambria RP, Hilgenberg AD, Torchiana DF, et al. Safety and efficacy of concomitant carotid and coronary artery operations. Ann Thorac Surg 1995;60:311.

18. Alford WC Jr, Stoney WS, Burrus GR, Frist RA, Thomas CS Jr. Recognition and operative management of patients with arteriosclerotic coronary artery aneurysms. Ann Thorac Surg 1976;22:317.

19. Anabtawi IN, deLeon JA. Coronary ectasia: incidence and results of coronary bypass surgery. Am Heart J 1978;96:309.

20. ACC/AHA Joint Task Force Subcommittee on Coronary Artery Bypass Graft Surgery. Guidelines and indications for coronary artery bypass graft surgery. Circulation 1991;83:1125.

B

1. Bryson AL, Parisi AF, Schechter E, Wolfson S. Life-threatening ventricular arrhythmias induced by exercise: cessation after coronary artery bypass surgery. Am J Cardiol 1973;32:995.

2. Bartley TD, Bigelow JC, Page US. Aortocoronary bypass grafting with multiple sequential anastomoses to a single vein. Arch Surg 1972;105:915.

3. Berger HJ, Reduto LA, Johnstone DE, Borkowski H, Sands JM, Cohen LS, et al. Global and regional left ventricular response to bicycle exercise in coronary artery disease. Am J Med 1979;66:13.

4. Bypass Angioplasty Revascularization Investigation (BARI) Investigators. Comparison of coronary bypass surgery with angioplasty in patients with multivessel disease. N Engl J Med 1996;335:217.

5. Bourassa MG, Lesperance JJ, Corbara F, Saltiel J, Campeau L. Progression of coronary disease 5 to 7 years after aortocoronary bypass surgery. Cleve Clin Q 1978;45:175.

6. Bulkley BH, Hutchins GM. Accelerated "atherosclerosis": a morphologic study of 97 saphenous vein coronary artery bypass grafts. Circulation 1977;55:163.

7. Barboriak JJ, Pintar K, Korns ME. Atherosclerosis in aortocoronary vein grafts. Lancet 1974;2:621.

8. Barboriak JJ, Pintar K, Van Horn DL, Batayias GE, Korns ME. Pathologic findings in the aortocoronary vein grafts: a scanning electron microscopic study. Atherosclerosis 1978;29:69.

9. Bates ER, Vogel RA, LeFree MT, Kirlin PC, O'Neill WW, Pitt B. The chronic coronary flow reserve provided by saphenous vein bypass grafts as determined by digital coronary radiography. Am Heart J 1984;108:462.

10. Barnes GK, Ray MJ, Oberman A, Kouchoukos NT. Changes in working status of patients following coronary bypass surgery. JAMA 1977;238:1259.

11. Bartel AG, Behar VS, Peter RH, Orgain ES, Kong Y. Exercise stress testing in evaluation of aortocoronary bypass surgery. Circulation 1973;48:141.

12. Balcon R, Honey M, Rickards AF, Sturridge MF, Walsh W, Wilkinson RK, et al. Evaluation by exercise testing and atrial pacing of results of aorto-coronary bypass surgery. Br Heart J 1974;36:841.

13. Braunwald E. Unstable angina. A classification. Circulation 1989;80:410.

14. Burggraf GW, Parker JO. Prognosis in coronary artery disease: angiographic, hemodynamic, and clinical factors. Circulation 1975;51:146.

15. Burkhoff D, Wesley MN, Resar JR, Lansing AM. Factors correlating with risk of mortality after transmyocardial revascularization. J Am Coll Cardiol 1999;34:55.

16. Bourassa MG, Fisher LD, Campeau L, Gillespie MJ, McConney M, Lesperance J. Long-term fate of bypass grafts: the coronary artery surgery study (CASS) and Montreal Heart Institute experiences. Circulation 1985;72:V71.

17. Brody WR, Angeli WW, Kosek JC. Histologic fate of the venous coronary artery bypass in dogs. Am J Pathol 1972;66:111.

18. Barboriak JJ, Batayias GE, Pintar K, Tieu TM, Van Horn DL, Korns ME. Late lesions in aorta-coronary artery vein grafts. J Thorac Cardiovasc Surg 1977;73:596.

19. Bigger JT, Heller CA, Wenger TL, Weld FM. Risk stratification after acute myocardial infarction. Am J Cardiol 1978;42:202.

20. Brenowitz JB, Kayser KL, Johnson WD. Triple vessel coronary artery endarterectomy and reconstruction: results in 144 patients. J Am Coll Cardiol 1988;11:706.

21. Berens ES, Kouchoukos NT, Murphy SF, Wareing TH. Preoperative carotid artery screening in elderly patients undergoing cardiac surgery. J Vasc Surg 1992;15:313.

22. Boulay FM, David PP, Bourassa MG. Strategies for improving the work status of patients after coronary artery bypass surgery. Circulation 1982;66:III43.

23. Booth DC, Deupree RH, Hultgren HN, DeMaria AN, Scott SM, Luchi RJ. Quality of life after bypass surgery for unstable angina. 5-year follow-up results of a Veterans Affairs Cooperative Study. Circulation 1991;83:87.

24. Berkoff HA, Rowe GG. Atherosclerotic ulcerative disease and associated aneurysms of the coronary arteries. Am Heart J 1975;90:153.

25. Blankenhorn DH, Nessim SA, Johnson RL, Sanmarco ME, Azen SP, Cashin-Hemphill L. Beneficial effects of combined colestipol-niacin therapy on coronary atherosclerosis and coronary venous bypass grafts. JAMA 1987;257:3233.

26. Baughman KL, Maroko PR, Vatner SF. Effects of coronary artery reperfusion on myocardial infarct size and survival in conscious dogs. Circulation 1981;63:317.

27. Berg R Jr, Kendall RW, Duvoisin GE, Ganji JH, Rudy LW, Everhart FJ. Acute myocardial infarction: a surgical emergency. J Thorac Cardiovasc Surg 1975;70:432.

28. Boudoulas H, Snyder GL, Lewis RP, Kates RE, Karayannacos PE, Vasko JS. Safety and rationale for continuation of propranolol therapy during coronary bypass operation. Ann Thorac Surg 1978;26:222.

29. Bolooki H. Myocardial revascularization after acute infarction. Am J Cardiol 1975;36:395.

30. Bruschke AV, Wijers TS, Kolsters W, Landmann J. The anatomic evolution of coronary artery disease demonstrated by coronary arteriography in 256 nonoperated patients. Circulation 1981;63:527.

31. Bemis CE, Gorlin R, Kemp HG, Herman MV. Progression of coronary artery disease: a clinical arteriographic study. Circulation 1973;47:455.

32. Brandt PW, Partridge JB, Wattie WJ. Coronary arteriography: a method of presentation of the arteriogram report and a scoring system. Clin Radiol 1977;28:361.

33. Bruce RA, DeRouen TA, Hammermeister KE. Noninvasive screening criteria for enhanced 4-year survival after aortocoronary bypass surgery. Circulation 1979;60:638.

34. Bertolasi CA, Tronge JE, Riccitelli MA, Villamayor RM, Zuffardi E. Natural history of unstable angina with medical or surgical therapy. Chest 1976;70:596.

35. Bourassa MG, Campeau L, Lesperance J, Grondin CM. Changes in grafts and coronary arteries after saphenous vein aortocoronary bypass surgery: results at repeat angiography. Circulation 1982;65:90.

36. Baum RS, Alvarez H 3rd, Cobb LA. Survival after resuscitation from out-of-hospital ventricular fibrillation. Circulation 1974;50:1231.

37. Borer JS, Rosing DR, Miller RH, Stark RM, Kent KM, Bacharach SL, et al. Natural history of left ventricular function during 1 year after acute myocardial infarction: comparison with clinical, electrocardiographic and biochemical determinations. Am J Cardiol 1980;46:1.

38. Borer JS, Bacharach SL, Green MV, Kent KM, Epstein SE, Johnston GS. Real-time radionuclide cineangiography in the noninvasive evaluation of global and regional left ventricular function at rest and during exercise in patients with coronary artery disease. N Engl J Med 1977;296:839.

39. Bonow RO, Kent KM, Rosing DR, Lipson LC, Bacharach SL, Green MV, et al. Improved left ventricular diastolic filling in patients with coronary artery disease after percutaneous transluminal coronary angioplasty. Circulation 1982;66:1159.

40. Bonow RO, Bacharach SL, Green MV, Kent KM, Rosing DR, Lipson LC, et al. Impaired left ventricular diastolic filling in patients with coronary artery disease: assessment with radionuclide angiography. Circulation 1981;64:315.

41. Berg R Jr, Selinger SL, Leonard JJ, Grunwald RP, O'Grady WP. Immediate coronary artery bypass for acute evolving myocardial infarction. J Thorac Cardiovasc Surg 1981;81:493.

42. Basso C, Morgagni GL, Thiene G. Spontaneous coronary artery dissection: a neglected cause of acute myocardial ischaemia and sudden death. Heart 1996;75:451.

43. Brown CA, Hutter AM, DeSanctis RW, Gold HK, Leinbach RC, Roberts-Niles A, et al. Prospective study of medical and urgent surgical therapy in randomizable patients with unstable angina pectoris: Results of in-hospital and chronic mortality and morbidity. Am Heart J 1981;102:959.

44. Buda AJ, Macdonald IL, Anderson MJ, Strauss HD, David TE, Berman ND. Long-term results following coronary bypass operation: importance of preoperative factors and complete revascularization. J Thorac Cardiovasc Surg 1981;82:383.

45. Bittar N, Kroncke GM, Dacumos GC Jr, Rowe GG, Young WP, Chopra PS, et al. Vein graft flow and reactive hyperemia in the human heart. J Thorac Cardiovasc Surg 1972;64:855.

46. Bonow RO, Vitale DF, Bacharach SL, Frederick TM, Kent KM, Green MV. Asynchronous left ventricular regional function and impaired global diastolic filling in patients with coronary artery disease: reversal after coronary angioplasty. Circulation 1985;71:297.

47. Barner HB, Swartz MT, Mudd JG, Tyras DH. Late patency of the internal mammary artery as a coronary bypass conduit. Ann Thorac Surg 1982;34:408.

48. Boerboom LE, Olinger GN, Tie-Zhu L, Rodriquez ER, Ferrans VJ, Kissebah AH. Histologic, morphometric, and biochemical evolution of vein bypass grafts in a nonhuman primate model. III. Long-term changes and their modification by platelet inhibition with aspirin and dipyridamole. J Thorac Cardiovasc Surg 1990;99:426.

49. Brindis RG, Brundage BH, Ullyot DJ, McKay CW, Lipton MJ, Turley K. Graft patency in patients with coronary artery bypass operation complicated by perioperative myocardial infarction. J Am Coll Cardiol 1984;3:55.

50. Brundage BH, Massie BM, Botvinick EH. Improved regional ventricular function after successful surgical revascularization. J Am Coll Cardiol 1984;3:902.

51. Barzilai B, Marshall WG Jr, Saffitz JE, Kouchoukos N. Avoidance of embolic complications by ultrasonic characterization of the ascending aorta. Circulation 1989;80:I275.

52. Beyersdorf F, Acar C, Buckberg GD, Partington MT, Sjostrand F, Young HH, et al. Studies on prolonged acute regional ischemia. III. Early natural history of simulated single and multivessel disease with emphasis on remote myocardium. J Thorac Cardiovasc Surg 1989;98:368.

53. Beyersdorf F, Acar C, Buckberg GD, Partington MT, Okamoto F, Allen BS, et al. Studies on prolonged acute regional ischemia. V. Metabolic support of remote myocardium during left ventricular power failure. J Thorac Cardiovasc Surg 1989;98:567.

54. Brown G, Albers JJ, Fisher LD, Schaefer SM, Lin JT, Kaplan C, et al. Regression of coronary artery disease as a result of intensive lipid-lowering therapy in men with high levels of apolipoprotein B. N Engl J Med 1990;323:1289.

55. Burlingame MW, Bonchek LI, Vazales BE. Left thoracotomy for reoperative coronary bypass. J Thorac Cardiovasc Surg 1988;95:508.

56. Blackstone EH, Takaro T, Hultgren H, Peduzzi P, Detre K, Kirklin JW. Unpublished study, 1990.

57. Barner HB, Naunheim KS, Willman VL, Fiore AC. Revascularization with bilateral internal thoracic artery grafts in patients with left main coronary stenosis. Eur J Cardiothorac Surg 1992;6:66.

58. Brodman RF, Frame R, Camacho M, Hu E, Chen A, Hollinger I. Routine use of unilateral and bilateral radial arteries for coronary artery bypass graft surgery. J Am Coll Cardiol 1996;28:959.

59. Byrne JG, Aklog L, Adams DH, Cohn LH, Aranki SF. Reoperative CABG using left thoracotomy: a tailored strategy. Ann Thorac Surg 2001;71:196.

60. Bull DA, Neumayer LA, Stringham JC, Meldrum P, Affleck DG, Karwande SV. Coronary artery bypass grafting with cardiopulmonary bypass versus off-pump cardiopulmonary bypass grafting: does eliminating the pump reduce morbidity and cost? Ann Thorac Surg 2001;71:170.

61. Bigger JT Jr. Prophylactic use of implanted cardiac defibrillators in patients at high risk for ventricular arrhythmias after coronary-artery bypass graft surgery. Coronary Artery Bypass Graft (CABG) Patch Trial Investigators. N Engl J Med 1997;337:1569.

62. Boylan MJ, Lytle BW, Loop FD, Taylor PC, Borsh JA, Goormastic M, et al. Surgical treatment of isolated left anterior descending coronary stenosis. Comparison of left internal mammary artery and venous autograft at 18 to 20 years of follow-up. J Thorac Cardiovasc Surg 1994;107:657.

63. Braxton JH, Hammond GL, Letsou GV, Franco KL, Kopf GS, Elefteriades JA, et al. Optimal timing of coronary artery bypass graft surgery after acute myocardial infarction. Circulation 1995;92:II66.

64. Borkon AM, Failing TL, Piehler JM, Killen DA, Hoskins ML, Reed WA. Risk analysis of operative intervention for failed coronary angioplasty. Ann Thorac Surg 1992;54:884.

C

1. Cline RE, Armstrong RG, Stanford W. Successful myocardial revascularization after ventricular fibrillation induced by treadmill exercise. J Thorac Cardiovasc Surg 1973;65:802.

2. Conde CA, Meller J, Espinoza J, Donoso E, Dack S. Disappearance of abnormal Q waves after aortocoronary bypass surgery. Am J Cardiol 1975;36:889.

3. Coronary angioplasty versus coronary artery bypass surgery: the Randomized Intervention Treatment of Angina (RITA) trial. Lancet 1993;341:573.

4. Chatterjee K, Swan HJ, Parmley WW, Sustaita H, Marcus HS, Matloff J. Influence of direct myocardial revascularization on left ventricular asynergy and function in patients with coronary artery disease, with and without previous myocardial infarction. Circulation 1973;47:276.

5. Cebul RD, Snow RJ, Pine R, Hertzer NR, Norris DG. Indications, outcomes, and provider volumes for carotid endarterectomy. JAMA 1998;279:1282.

6. CASS Principal Investigators: The National Heart, Lung, and Blood Institute Coronary Artery Surgery Study. A multicenter comparison of the effects of randomized medical and surgical treatment of mildly symptomatic patients with coronary artery disease, and a registry of consecutive patients undergoing coronary angiography. Circulation 1981;63:I1.

7. Campeau L, Lesperance J, Corbara F, Hermann J, Grondin CM, Bourassa MG. Aortocoronary saphenous vein bypass graft changes 5 to 7 years after surgery. Circulation 1978;58:I170.

8. Campeau L, Lesperance J, Hermann J, Corbara F, Grondin CM, Bourassa MG. Loss of the improvement of angina between 1 and 7 years after aortocoronary bypass surgery. Circulation 1979;60:1.

9. CASS Principal Investigators and their Associates. Coronary Artery Surgery Study (CASS): a randomized trial of coronary artery bypass surgery. Quality of life in patients randomly assigned to treatment groups. Circulation 1983;68:951.

10. CASS Principal Investigators and Their Associates. Myocardial infarction and mortality in the coronary artery surgery study (CASS) randomized trial. N Engl J Med 1984;310:750.

11. Chaikhouni A, Crawford FA, Kochel PJ, Olanoff LS, Halushka PV. Human internal mammary artery produces more prostacyclin than saphenous vein. J Thorac Cardiovasc Surg 1986;92:88.

12. Culliford AT, Colvin SB, Rohrer K, Baumann G, Spencer FC. The atherosclerotic ascending aorta and transverse arch: a new technique to prevent cerebral injury during bypass: experience with 13 patients. Ann Thorac Surg 1986;41:27.

13. Chesebro JH, Fuster V, Elveback LR, Clements IP, Smith HC, Holmes DR Jr, et al. Effect of dipyridamole and aspirin on late vein-graft patency after coronary bypass operations. N Engl J Med 1984;310:209.

14. Corbalan R, Verrier RL, Lown B. Differing mechanisms for ventricular vulnerability during coronary artery occlusion and release. Am Heart J 1976;92:223.

15. Cohn PF, Harris P, Barry WH, Rosati RA, Rosenbaum P, Waternaux C. Prognostic importance of anginal symptoms in angiographically defined coronary artery disease. Am J Cardiol 1981;47:233.

16. Chesebro JH, Clements IP, Fuster V, Elveback LR, Smith HC, Bardsley WT, et al. A platelet-inhibitor-drug trial in coronary-artery bypass operations. Benefit of perioperative dipyridamole and aspirin therapy on early postoperative vein-graft patency. N Engl J Med 1982;307:73.

17. Califf RM, Harrell FE Jr, Lee KL, Rankin JS, Hlatky MA, Mark DB, et al. The evolution of medical and surgical therapy for coronary artery disease. A 15-year perspective. JAMA 1989;261:2077.

18. Carrie D, Elbaz M, Puel J, Fourcade J, Karouny E, Fournial G, et al. Five-year outcome after coronary angioplasty versus bypass surgery in multivessel coronary artery disease: results from the French Monocentric Study. Circulation 1997;96:II1.

19. Campeau L. Grading of angina pectoris. Circulation 1976;54:522.

20. Catinella FP, Cunningham JN Jr, Srungaram RK, Baumann FG, Nathan IM, Glassman EA, et al. The factors influencing early patency of coronary artery bypass vein grafts: correlation of angiographic and ultrastructural findings. J Thorac Cardiovasc Surg 1982;83:686.

21. Chesebro JH, Ritman EL, Frye RL, Smith HC, Connolly DC, Rutherford BD, et al. Videometric analysis of regional left ventricular function before and after aortocoronary artery bypass surgery. J Clin Invest 1976;58:1339.

22. Coles JG, Del Campo C, Ahmed SN, Corpus R, MacDonald AC, Goldbach MM, et al. Improved long-term survival following myocardial revascularization in patients with severe left ventricular dysfunction. J Thorac Cardiovasc Surg 1981;81:846.

23. Cosgrove DM, Loop FD, Lytle BW, Baillot R, Gill CC, Golding LA, et al. Primary myocardial revascularization. J Thorac Cardiovasc Surg 1984;88:673.

24. Czerny M, Baumer H, Kilo J, Zuckermann A, Grubhofer G, Chevtchik O, et al. Complete revascularization in coronary artery bypass grafting with and without cardiopulmonary bypass. Ann Thorac Surg 2001;71:165.

25. Califf RM, Tomabechi Y, Lee KL, Phillips H, Pryor DB, Harrell FE Jr, et al. Outcome in one-vessel coronary artery disease. Circulation 1983;67:283.

26. Chaitman BR, Alderman EL, Sheffield LT, Tong T, Fisher L, Mock MB, et al. Use of survival analysis to determine the clinical significance of new Q waves after coronary bypass surgery. Circulation 1983;67:302.

27. Campeau L, Enjalbert M, Lesperance J, Bourassa MG, Kwiterovich P Jr, Wacholder S, et al. The relation of risk factors to the development of atherosclerosis in saphenous-vein bypass grafts and the progression of disease in the native circulation. N Engl J Med 1984;311:1329.

28. Campeau L, Enjalbert M, Lesperance J, Vaislic C, Grondin CM, Bourassa MG. Atherosclerosis and late closure of aortocoronary saphenous vein grafts: Sequential angiographic studies at 2 weeks, 1 year, 5 to 7 years, and 10 to 12 years after surgery. Circulation 1983;68:II1.

29. Chaitman BR, Fisher LD, Bourassa MG, Davis K, Rogers WJ, Maynard C, et al. Effect of coronary bypass surgery on survival patterns in subsets of patients with left main coronary artery disease. Am J Cardiol 1981;48:765.

30. Cobanoglu A, Freimanis I, Grunkemeier G, Lambert L, Anderson V, Nunley D, et al. Enhanced late survival following coronary artery bypass graft operation for unstable versus chronic angina. Ann Thorac Surg 1984;37:52.

31. Carter MJ. The use of the right gastro-epiploic artery in coronary artery bypass grafting. Aust N Z J Surg 1987;57:317.

32. Cheung D, Flemma RJ, Mullen DC, Lepley D Jr. An alternative approach to isolated circumflex coronary bypass reoperations. Ann Thorac Surg 1982;33:302.

33. Cashin-Hemphill L, Mack WJ, Pogoda JM, Sanmarco ME, Azen SP, Blankenhorn DH. Beneficial effects of colestipol-niacin on coronary atherosclerosis. A 4-year follow-up. JAMA 1990;264:3013.

34. Crouch JD, O'Hair DP, Keuler JP, Barragry TP, Werner PH, Kleinman LH. Open versus endoscopic saphenous vein harvesting: wound complications and vein quality. Ann Thorac Surg 1999;68:1513.

35. Chen AM, Brodman RF, Frame R, Graver LM, Tranbaugh RF, Banks T, et al. Routine myocardial revascularization with the radial artery: a multicenter experience. J Card Surg 1998;13:318.

36. Campeau L, Hunninghake DB, Knatterud GL, White CW, Domanski M, Forman SA, et al. Aggressive cholesterol lowering delays saphenous vein graft atherosclerosis in women, the elderly, and patients with associated risk factors. NHLBI post coronary artery bypass graft clinical trial. Post CABG Trial Investigators. Circulation 1999; 99:3241.

37. Cameron A, Davis KB, Green G, Schaff HV. Coronary bypass surgery with internal-thoracic-artery grafts—effects on survival over a 15-year period. N Engl J Med 1996;334:216.

38. Chaitman BR, Rosen AD, Williams DO, Bourassa MG, Aguirre FV, Pitt B, et al. Myocardial infarction and cardiac mortality in the Bypass Angioplasty Revascularization Investigation (BARI) randomized trial. Circulation 1997;96:2162.

39. Chang BB, Paty PS, Shah DM, Leather RP. The lesser saphenous vein: an underappreciated source of autogenous vein. J Vasc Surg 1992;15:152.

40. Creswell LL, Moulton MJ, Cox JL, Rosenbloom M. Revascularization after acute myocardial infarction. Ann Thorac Surg 1995;60:19.

41. Craver JM, Weintraub WS, Jones EL, Guyton RA, Hatcher CR Jr. Emergency coronary artery bypass surgery for failed percutaneous coronary angioplasty. A 10-year experience. Ann Surg 1992;215:425.

D

1. de Soyza N, Murphy ML, Bissett JK, Kane JJ, Doherty JE 3rd. Ventricular arrhythmias in chronic stable angina pectoris with surgical or medical treatment. Ann Intern Med 1978;89:10.

2. DeRouen TA, Hammermeister KE, Dodge HT. Comparisons of the effects of survival after coronary artery surgery in subgroups of patients from the Seattle Heart Watch. Circulation 1981;63:537.

3. DeWood MA, Notske RN, Berg R Jr, Ganji JH, Simpson CS, Hinnen ML, et al. Medical and surgical management of early Q-wave myocardial infarction. I. Effects of surgical reperfusion on survival, recurrent myocardial infarction, sudden death and functional class at 10 or more years of follow-up. J Am Coll Cardiol 1989;14:65.

4. DeWood MA, Spores J, Notske RN, Lang HT, Shields JP, Simpson CS, et al. Medical and surgical management of myocardial infarction. Am J Cardiol 1979;44:1356.

5. DeWood MA, Spores J, Notske R, Mouser LT, Burroughs R, Golden MS, et al. Prevalence of total coronary occlusion during the early hours of transmural myocardial infarction. N Engl J Med 1980; 303:897.

6. Detre K, Peduzzi P, Murphy M, Hultgren H, Thomsen J, Oberman A, et al. Effect of bypass surgery on survival in patients in low- and high-risk subgroups delineated by the use of simple clinical variables. Circulation 1981;63:1329.

7. Davies MJ, Thomas AC. Plaque fissuring—the cause of acute myocardial infarction, sudden ischemic death, and crescendo angina. Br Heart J 1985;53:363.

8. D'Agostino RS, Svensson LG, Neumann DJ, Balkhy HH, Williamson WA, Shahian DM. Screening carotid ultrasonography and risk factors for stroke in coronary artery surgery patients. Ann Thorac Surg 1996;62:1714.

9. Daoud AS, Pankin D, Tulgan H, Florentin RA. Aneurysms of the coronary artery. Report of ten cases and review of literature. Am J Cardiol 1963;11:228.

10. Dion R, Verhelst R, Rousseau M, Goenen M, Ponlot R, Kestens-Servaye Y, et al. Sequential mammary grafting. Clinical, functional, and angiographic assessment 6 months postoperatively in 231 consecutive patients. J Thorac Cardiovasc Surg 1989;98:80.

11. DeMaio SJ Jr, Kinsella SH, Silverman ME. Clinical course and long-term prognosis of spontaneous coronary artery dissection. Am J Cardiol 1989;64:471.

12. Dwyer EM Jr, Greenberg HM, Steinberg G, and the Multicenter Postinfarction Research Group. Clinical characteristics and natural history of survivors of pulmonary congestion during acute myocardial infarction. Am J Cardiol 1989;63:1423.

13. Dion R, Verhelst R, Matta A, Rousseau M, Goenen M, Chalant C, et al. Surgical angioplasty of the left main coronary artery. J Thorac Cardiovasc Surg 1990;99:241.

14. Deuvaert FE, De Paepe J, Van Nooten G, Peperstraete B, Primo G. Transaortic saphenous patch angioplasty for left main coronary artery stenosis. J Cardiovasc Surg 1988;29:610.

15. Dilsizian V, Cannon RO 3rd, Tracy CM, McIntosh CL, Clark RE, Bonow RO. Enhanced regional left ventricular function after distant coronary bypass by means of improved collateral blood flow. J Am Coll Cardiol 1989;14:312.

16. Dilsizian V, Rocco TP, Freedman NM, Leon MB, Bonow RO. Enhanced detection of ischemic but viable myocardium by the reinjection of thallium after stress-redistribution imaging. N Engl J Med 1990;323:141.

17. Daoud EG, Strickberger SA, Man KC, Goyal R, Deeb GM, Bolling SF, et al. Preoperative amiodarone as prophylaxis against atrial fibrillation after heart surgery. N Engl J Med 1997;337:1785.

18. Daoud EG, Dabir R, Archambeau M, Morady F, Strickberger SA. Randomized, double-blind trial of simultaneous right and left atrial epicardial pacing for prevention of post-open heart surgery atrial fibrillation. Circulation 2000;102:761.

19. Dilsizian V, Bonow RO, Cannon RO, Tracy CM, Vitale DF, McIntosh CL, et al. The effect of coronary bypass grafting on left ventricular systolic function at rest: evidence for preoperative subclinical myocardial ischemia. Am J Cardiol 1988;61:1248.

E

1. Ecker RR, Mullins CB, Grammer JC, Rea WJ, Atkins JM. Control of intractable ventricular tachycardia by coronary revascularization. Circulation 1971;44:666.

2. Effler DB, Sones FM Jr, Favaloro R, Groves LK. Coronary endarterectomy with patch-graft reconstruction: clinical experience with 34 cases. Ann Surg 1965;162:590.

3. Edwards WS, Jones WB, Dear HD, Kerr AR. Direct surgery for coronary artery disease: techniques for left anterior descending coronary artery bypass. JAMA 1970;211:1182.

4. Effler DB, Sones FM Jr, Groves LK, Suarez E. Myocardial revascularization by Vineberg's internal mammary artery implant: evaluation of postoperative results. J Thorac Cardiovasc Surg 1965;50:527.

5. Ebert PA, Peter RH, Gunnells JC, Sabiston DC Jr. Resecting and grafting of coronary artery aneurysm. Circulation 1971;43:593.

6. Ellis CJ, Haywood GA, Monro JL. Spontaneous coronary artery dissection in a young woman resulting from an intense gymnasium "work-out." Int J Cardiol 1994;47:193.

7. Enjalbert M, Campeau L, Lesperance J, Bourassa MG. Progression of coronary artery disease 10 years after aortocoronary bypass surgery. Circulation 1982;66:II246.

8. Every NR, Fahrenbruch CE, Hallstrom AP, Weaver WD, Cobb LA. Influence of coronary bypass surgery on subsequent outcome of patients resuscitated from out of hospital cardiac arrest. J Am Coll Cardiol 1992;19:1435.

9. Eagle KA, Guyton RA, Davidoff R, Ewy GA, Fonger J, Gardner TJ, et al. ACC/AHA Guidelines for Coronary Artery Bypass Graft Surgery: A Report of the American College of Cardiology/American Heart Association Task Force on Practice Guidelines (Committee to Revise the 1991 Guidelines for Coronary Artery Bypass Surgery). American College of Cardiology/American Heart Association. J Am Coll Cardiol 1999;34:1262.

10. Edwards FH, Grover FL, Shroyer AL, Schwartz M, Bero J. The Society of Thoracic Surgeons National Cardiac Surgery Database: current risk assessment. Ann Thorac Surg 1997;63:903.

11. Edwards FH, Carey JS, Grover FL, Bero JW, Hartz RS. Impact of gender on coronary artery bypass operative mortality. Ann Thorac Surg 1998;66:125.

12. Endo M, Nishida H, Tomizawa Y, Kasanuki H. Benefit of bilateral over single internal mammary artery grafts for multiple coronary artery bypass grafting. Circulation 2001;104:2164.

13. Elefteriades JA, Morales DL, Gradel C, Tollis G Jr, Levi E, Zaret BL. Results of coronary artery bypass grafting by a single surgeon in patients with left ventricular ejection fractions < or = 30%. Am J Cardiol 1997;79:1573.

14. Ehsan A, Mann MJ, Dell'Acqua G, Dzau VJ. Long-term stabilization of vein graft wall architecture and prolonged resistance to experimental atherosclerosis after E2F decoy oligonucleotide gene therapy. J Thorac Cardiovasc Surg 2001;121:714.

15. Endarterectomy for asymptomatic carotid artery stenosis. Executive Committee for the Asymptomatic Carotid Atherosclerosis Study. JAMA 1995;273:1421.

16. Endarterectomy for moderate symptomatic carotid stenosis: interim results from the MRC European Carotid Surgery Trial. Lancet 1996;347:1591.

F

1. Ferrazzi P, McGiffin DC, Kirklin JW, Blackstone EH, Bourge RC. Have the results of mitral valve replacement improved? J Thorac Cardiovasc Surg 1986;92:186.

2. Flemma RJ, Singh HM, Tector AJ, Lepley D Jr, Frazier BL. Comparative hemodynamic properties of vein and mammary artery in coronary bypass operations. Ann Thorac Surg 1975;20:619.

3. Frick MH, Harjola PT, Valle M. Work status after coronary bypass surgery: a prospective randomized study with ergometric and angiographic correlations. Acta Med Scand 1979;206:61.

4. Favaloro RG. Saphenous vein graft in the surgical treatment of coronary artery disease: operative technique. J Thorac Cardiovasc Surg 1969;58:178.

5. Ferrans VJ, Jones M, Roberts WC. The pathology of saphenous vein aortocoronary bypass grafts. In Gallucci V, Bini RM, Thiene G, eds. Proceedings of the International Symposium on Selected Topics in Cardiac Surgery. Bologna, Italy: Patron Editore, 1980, p. 423.

6. Flemma RJ, Johnson WD, Lepley D Jr. Triple aorto-coronary vein bypass as treatment for coronary insufficiency. Arch Surg 1971; 103:82.

7. Faulkner SL, Stoney WS, Alford WC, Thomas CS, Burrus GR, Frist RA, et al. Ischemic cardiomyopathy: medical versus surgical treatment. J Thorac Cardiovasc Surg 1977;74:77.

8. Furlan AJ, Breuer AC. Central nervous complications of open heart surgery. Stroke 1984;15:912.

9. Friesinger GC, Page EE, Ross RS. Prognostic significance of coronary arteriography. Trans Assoc Am Physicians 1970;83:78.

10. Fan K, Lee KL, Chiu CS, Lee JW, He GW, Cheung D, et al. Effects of biatrial pacing in prevention of postoperative atrial fibrillation after coronary artery bypass surgery. Circulation 2000;102:755.

11. Fuster V, Chesebro JH. Role of platelets and platelet inhibitors in aortocoronary artery vein-graft disease. Circulation 1986;73:227.

12. Foster ED, Fisher LD, Kaiser GC, Myers WO. Comparison of operative mortality and morbidity for initial and repeat coronary artery bypass grafting: The Coronary Artery Surgery Study (CASS) registry experience. Ann Thorac Surg 1984;38:563.

13. Fuster V, Stein B, Ambrose JA, Badimon L, Badimon JJ, Chesebro JH. Atherosclerotic plaque rupture and thrombosis. Evolving concepts. Circulation 1990;82:II47.

14. Falk E. Plaque rupture with severe pre-existing stenosis precipitating coronary thrombosis. Characteristics of coronary atherosclerotic plaques underlying fatal occlusive thrombi. Br Heart J 1983;50:127.

15. Falk E. Unstable angina with fatal outcome: dynamic coronary thrombosis leading to infarction and/or sudden death. Autopsy evidence of recurrent mural thrombosis with peripheral embolization culminating in total vascular occlusion. Circulation 1985;71:699.

16. Frazier OH, March RJ, Horvath KA. Transmyocardial revascularization with a carbon dioxide laser in patients with end-stage coronary artery disease. N Engl J Med 1999;341:1021.

17. First-year results of CABRI (Coronary Angioplasty versus Bypass Revascularisation Investigation). CABRI Trial Participants. Lancet 1995;346:1179.

18. Fuller JA, Adams GG, Buxton B. Atrial fibrillation after coronary artery bypass grafting. Is it a disorder of the elderly? J Thorac Cardiovasc Surg 1989;97:821.

19. Faggioli GL, Curl GR, Ricotta JJ. The role of carotid screening before coronary artery bypass. J Vasc Surg 1990;12:724.

20. Frierson JH, Dimas AP, Whitlow PL, Hollman JL, Marsalese DL, Simpendorfer CC, et al. Angioplasty of the proximal left anterior descending coronary artery: initial success and long-term follow-up. J Am Coll Cardiol 1992;19:745.

G

1. Guinn GA, Mathur VS. Surgical versus medical treatment for stable angina pectoris: prospective randomized study with 1- to 4-year follow-up. Ann Thorac Surg 1976;22:524.

2. Gurne O, Buche M, Chenu P, Paquay JL, Pelgrim JP, Louagie Y, et al. Quantitative angiographic follow-up study of the free inferior epigastric coronary bypass graft. Circulation 1994;90:II148.

3. Griffith LS, Bulkley BH, Hutchins GM, Brawley RK. Occlusive changes at the coronary artery-bypass graft anastomosis: morphologic study of 95 grafts. J Thorac Cardiovasc Surg 1977;73:668.

4. Guthaner DF, Robert EW, Alderman EL, Wexler L. Long-term serial angiographic studies after coronary artery bypass surgery. Circulation 1979;60:250.

5. Grondin CM, Campeau L, Lesperance J, Solymoss BC, Vouhe P, Castonguay YR, et al. Atherosclerotic changes in coronary vein grafts six years after operation: angiographic aspect in 110 patients. J Thorac Cardiovasc Surg 1979;77:24.

6. Garrett HE, Dennis EW, DeBakey ME. Aortocoronary bypass with saphenous vein graft: seven-year follow-up. JAMA 1973;223:792.

7. Green GE, Stertzer SH, Reppert EH. Coronary arterial bypass grafts. Ann Thorac Surg 1968;5:443.

8. Goldberg RJ, Samad NA, Yarzebski J, Gurwitz J, Bigelow C, Gore JM. Temporal trends in cardiogenic shock complicating acute myocardial infarction. N Engl J Med 1999;340:1162.

9. Gensini GG. Coronary arteriography. Mount Kisco, N.Y.: Futura, 1975.

10. Gundry SR, Jones M, Ishihara T, Ferrans VJ. Intraoperative trauma to human saphenous veins: scanning electron microscopic comparison of preparation techniques. Ann Thorac Surg 1980;30:40.

11. Goy JJ, Eeckhout E, Burnand B, Vogt P, Stauffer JC, Hurni M, et al. Coronary angioplasty versus left internal mammary artery grafting for isolated proximal left anterior descending artery stenosis. Lancet 1994;343:1449.

12. Grondin CM, Limet R. Vein grafts to left-sided coronary arteries: passage through the transverse sinus. Ann Thorac Surg 1976; 21:348.

13. Goldman S, Copeland J, Moritz T, Henderson W, Zadina K, Ovitt T, et al. Saphenous vein graft patency 1 year after coronary artery bypass surgery and effects of antiplatelet therapy. Results of a Veterans Administration Cooperative Study. Circulation 1989;80:1190.

14. Grüntzig AR, Senning A, Siegenthaler WE. Nonoperative dilation of coronary artery stenosis: percutaneous transluminal coronary angioplasty. N Engl J Med 1979;301:61.

15. Gundry SR, Jones M, Ishihara T, Ferrans VJ. Optimal preparation techniques for human saphenous vein grafts. Surgery 1980;88:785.

16. Goldman S, Copeland J, Moritz T, Henderson W, Zadina K, Ovitt T, et al. Improvement in early saphenous vein graft patency after coronary artery bypass surgery with antiplatelet therapy: results of a Veterans Administration Cooperative Study. Circulation 1988; 77:1324.

17. Garrahy PJ, Cox DA, Cavender JB, Dean LS, Blackstone EH, Kirklin JW. Survival following coronary angioplasty in elderly patients: comparison with bypass surgery (abstract). Circulation 1990; 82:III618.

18. Greene DG, Bunnell IL, Arani DT, Schimert G, Lajos TZ, Lee AB, et al. Long-term survival after coronary bypass surgery: comparison of various subsets of patients with general population. Br Heart J 1981;45:417.

19. Ganz W, Buchbinder N, Marcus H, Mondkar A, Maddahi J, Charuzi Y, et al. Intracoronary thrombolysis in evolving myocardial infarction. Am Heart J 1981;101:4.

20. Grondin CM, Campeau L, Lespérance J, Enjalbert M, Bourassa MG. Comparison of late changes in internal mammary artery and saphenous vein grafts in two consecutive series of patients 10 years after operation. Circulation 1984;70:I208.

21. Gensini GG. A more meaningful scoring system for determining the severity of coronary heart disease. Am J Cardiol 1983;51:606.

22. Gensini G, Giambartolomei A, Esente P, Archambault T, Shaw C. Natural history of coronary artery disease, angiographic findings in 830 patients: importance and significance of the angiographic coronary score (abstract). Circulation 1982;66:II369.

23. Gensini GG. Coronary arteriography. In Braunwald E, ed. Heart disease: a textbook of cardiovascular medicine. Philadelphia: WB Saunders, 1980, p. 308.

24. Galbut DL, Traad EA, Dorman MJ, DeWitt PL, Larsen PB, Kurlansky PA, et al. Seventeen-year experience with bilateral internal mammary artery grafts. Ann Thorac Surg 1990;49:195.

25. Greenfield JC Jr, Rembert JC, Young WG Jr, Oldham HN Jr, Alexander JA, Sabiston DC Jr. Studies of blood flow in aorta-to-coronary venous bypass grafts in man. J Clin Invest 1972;51:2724.

26. Gardner TJ, Horneffer PJ, Manolio TA, Pearson TA, Gott VL, Baumgartner WA, et al. Stroke following coronary artery bypass grafting: a ten-year study. Ann Thorac Surg 1985;40:574.

27. Greene GE. Internal mammary artery-to-coronary artery anastomosis: three-year experience with 165 patients. Ann Thorac Surg 1972; 14:260.

28. Guyton RA, Arcidi JM Jr, Langford DA, Morris DC, Liberman HA, Hatcher CR Jr. Emergency coronary bypass for cardiogenic shock. Circulation 1987;76:V22.

29. Gardner TJ, Greene PS, Rykiel MF, Baumgartner WA, Cameron DE, Casale AS, et al. Routine use of the left internal mammary artery graft in the elderly. Ann Thorac Surg 1990;49:188.

30. Gardner TJ, Stuart RS, Greene PS, Baumgartner WA. The risk of coronary bypass surgery for patients with postinfarction angina. Circulation 1989;79:I79.

31. Grande P, Grauholt AM, Madsen JK. Unstable angina pectoris. Platelet behavior and prognosis in progressive angina and intermediate coronary syndrome. Circulation 1990;81:I16.

32. Gandjbakhch I, Acar C, Cabrol C. Left thoracotomy approach for coronary artery bypass grafting in patients with pericardial adhesions. Ann Thorac Surg 1989;48:871.

33. Goldman A, Greenstone SM, Preuss FS, Strauss SH, Chang ES. Experimental methods for producing a collateral circulation to the heart directly from the left ventricle. J Thorac Surg 1956;31:364.

34. Goldman S, Copeland J, Moritz T, Henderson W, Zadina K, Ovitt T, et al. Starting aspirin therapy after operation. Effects on early graft patency. Department of Veterans Affairs Cooperative Study Group. Circulation 1991;84:520.

35. Gavaghan TP, Gebski V, Baron DW. Immediate postoperative aspirin improves vein graft patency early and late after coronary artery bypass graft surgery. A placebo-controlled, randomized study. Circulation 1991;83:1526.

36. Gomes JA, Ip J, Santoni-Rugiu F, Mehta D, Ergin A, Lansman S, et al. Oral *d,l* sotalol reduces the incidence of postoperative atrial fibrillation in coronary artery bypass surgery patients: a randomized, double-blind, placebo-controlled study. J Am Coll Cardiol 1999;34:334.

37. Gammie JS, Zenati M, Kormos RL, Hattler BG, Wei LM, Pellegrini RV, et al. Abciximab and excessive bleeding in patients undergoing emergency cardiac operations. Ann Thorac Surg 1998;65:465.

38. Greenberg MD, Katz NM, Iuliano S, Tempesta BJ, Solomon AJ. Atrial pacing for the prevention of atrial fibrillation after cardiovascular surgery. J Am Coll Cardiol 2000;35:1416.

39. Grover FL, Johnson RR, Marshall G, Hammermeister KE. Factors predictive of operative mortality among coronary artery bypass subsets. Ann Thorac Surg 1993;56:1296.

40. Grichnik KP, Ijsselmuiden AJ, D'Amico TA, Harpole DH Jr, White WD, Blumenthal JA, et al. Cognitive decline after major noncardiac operations: a preliminary prospective study. Ann Thorac Surg 1999; 68:1786.

41. Grow JB Sr, Brantigan CO. The diamond anastomosis: a technique for creating a right angle side-to-side vascular anastomosis. J Thorac Cardiovasc Surg 1975;69:188.

H

1. Hellman CK, Kamath ML, Schmidt DH, Anholm J, Blau F, Johnson WD. Improvement in left ventricular function after myocardial revascularization: assessment by first-pass rest and exercise nuclear angiography. J Thorac Cardiovasc Surg 1980;79:645.

2. Hamby RI, Aintablian A, Handler M, Voleti C, Weisz D, Garvey JW, et al. Aortocoronary saphenous vein bypass grafts: long-term patency, morphology and blood flow in patients with patent grafts early after surgery. Circulation 1979;60:901.

3. Hodgson JM, Singh AK, Drew TM, Riley RS, Williams DO. Coronary flow reserve provided by sequential internal mammary artery grafts. J Am Coll Cardiol 1986;7:32.

4. Hellman C, Schmidt DH, Kamath ML, Anholm J, Blau F, Johnson WD. Bypass graft surgery in severe left ventricular dysfunction. Circulation 1980;62:I103.

5. Hlatky MA, Rogers WJ, Johnstone I, Boothroyd D, Brooks MM, Pitt B, et al. Medical care costs and quality of life after randomization to coronary angioplasty or coronary bypass surgery. Bypass Angioplasty Revascularization Investigation (BARI) Investigators. N Engl J Med 1997;336:92.

6. Hamby RI, Aintablian A, Wisoff BG, Hartstein ML. Comparative study of the postoperative flow in the saphenous vein and internal mammary artery bypass grafts. Am Heart J 1977;93:306.

7. Humphrey LS, Topol EJ, Rosenfeld GI, Borkon AM, Baumgartner WA, Gardner TJ, et al. Immediate enhancement of left ventricular relaxation by coronary artery bypass grafting: intraoperative assessment. Circulation 1988;77:886.

8. Hammermeister KE, DeRouen TA, Dodge HT. Comparison of survival of medically and surgically treated coronary disease patients in Seattle Heart Watch: a nonrandomized study. Circulation 1982; 65:II53.

9. Hamm CW, Reimers J, Ischinger T, Rupprecht HJ, Berger J, Bleifeld W. A randomized study of coronary angioplasty compared with bypass surgery in patients with symptomatic multivessel coronary disease. German Angioplasty Bypass Surgery Investigation (GABI). N Engl J Med 1994;331:1037.

10. Hueb WA, Bellotti G, de Oliveira SA, Arie S, de Albuquerque CP, Jatene AD, et al. The Medicine, Angioplasty or Surgery Study (MASS): a prospective, randomized trial of medical therapy, balloon angioplasty or bypass surgery for single proximal left anterior descending artery stenoses. J Am Coll Cardiol 1995;26:1600.

11. Horvath KA, Cohn LH, Cooley DA, Crew JR, Frazier OH, Griffith BP, et al. Transmyocardial laser revascularization: results of a multicenter trial with transmyocardial laser revascularization used as sole therapy for end-stage coronary artery disease. J Thorac Cardiovasc Surg 1997;113:645.

12. Horvath KA, Aranki SF, Cohn LH, March RJ, Frazier OH, Kadipasaoglu KA, et al. Sustained angina relief 5 years after transmyocardial laser revascularization with a CO_2 laser. Circulation 2001;104:I81.

13. Harrison MJ, Schneidau A, Ho R, Smith PL, Newman S, Treasure T. Cerebrovascular disease and functional outcome after coronary artery bypass surgery. Stroke 1989;20:235.

14. Hasse J, Graedel E, Hofer H, Guggenheim R, Amsler B, Mihatsch MJ. Morphologic studies in saphenous vein grafts for aorto-coronary bypass surgery. II. Influence of a pressure-limited graft dilation. Thorac Cardiovasc Surg 1981;29:38.

15. Higginbotham MB, Morris KG, Conn EH, Coleman RE, Cobb FR. Determinants of variable exercise performance among patients with severe left ventricular dysfunction. Am J Cardiol 1983;51:52.

16. Hartzler GO, Rutherford BD, McConahay DR, McCallister SH. Simultaneous multiple lesion coronary angioplasty: a preferred therapy for patients with multiple vessel disease. Circulation 1982;66:II5.

17. Hultgren HN, Peduzzi P, Detre K, Takaro T. The 5 year effect of bypass surgery on relief of angina and exercise performance. Circulation 1985;72:V79.

18. Hossack KF, Bruce RA, Ivey TD, Kusumi F. Changes in cardiac functional capacity after coronary bypass surgery in relation to adequacy of revascularization. J Am Coll Cardiol 1984;3:47.

19. Hossack KF, Bruce RA, Ivey TD, Kusumi F, Kannagi T. Improvement in aerobic and hemodynamic responses to exercise following aortacoronary bypass grafting. J Thorac Cardiovasc Surg 1984;87:901.

20. Huber MS, Mooney JF, Madison J, Mooney MR. Use of a morphologic classification to predict clinical outcome after dissection from coronary angioplasty. Am J Cardiol 1991;68:467.

21. Hwang MH, Meadows WR, Palac RT, Piao ZE, Pifarre R, Loeb HS, et al. Progression of native coronary artery disease at 10 years: insights from a randomized study of medical versus surgical therapy for angina. J Am Coll Cardiol 1990;16:1066.

22. Hands ME, Rutherford JD, Muller JE, Davies G, Stone PH, Parker C, et al. The in-hospital development of cardiogenic shock after myocardial infarction: incidence, predictors of occurrence, outcome and prognostic factors. J Am Coll Cardiol 1989;14:40.

23. Horvath KA, DiSesa VJ, Peigh PS, Couper GS, Collins JJ Jr, Cohn LH. Favorable results of coronary artery bypass grafting in patients older than 75 years. J Thorac Cardiovasc Surg 1990;99:92.

24. Hake U, Iversen HG, Jakob HG, Schmid FX, Erbel R, Pop T, et al. Influence of incremental preoperative risk factors on the perioperative outcome of patients undergoing emergency versus urgent coronary artery bypass grafting. Eur J Cardiovasc Surg 1989;3:162.

25. Hashimoto K, Ilstrup DM, Schaff HV. Influence of clinical and hemodynamic variables on risk of supraventricular tachycardia after coronary artery bypass. J Thorac Cardiovasc Surg 1991;101:56.

26. Hannan EL, Kumar D, Racz M, Siu AL, Chassin MR. New York State's Cardiac Surgery Reporting System: four years later. Ann Thorac Surg 1994;58:1852.

27. Higgins TL, Estafanous FG, Loop FD, Beck GJ, Blum JM, Paranandi L. Stratification of morbidity and mortality outcome by preoperative risk factors in coronary artery bypass patients. A clinical severity score. JAMA 1992;267:2344.

28. Hannan EL, Burke J. Effect of age on mortality in coronary artery bypass surgery in New York, 1991–1992. Am Heart J 1994;128:1184.

29. Hochman JS, Sleeper LA, Webb JG, Sanborn TA, White HD, Talley JD, et al. Early revascularization in acute myocardial infarction complicated by cardiogenic shock. SHOCK Investigators. N Engl J Med 1999;341:625.

30. Hochman JS, Sleeper LA, White HD, Dzavik V, Wong SC, Menon V, et al. One-year survival following early revascularization for cardiogenic shock. JAMA 2001;285:190.

31. Huddleston CB, Stoney WS, Alford WC, Burrus GR, Glassford DM, Lea LW, et al. Internal mammary artery grafts: technical factors influencing patency. Ann Thorac Surg 1986;42:543.

I

1. Itscoitz SB, Redwood DR, Stinson EB, Reis RL, Epstein SE. Saphenous vein bypass grafts: long-term patency and effect on the native coronary circulation. Am J Cardiol 1975;36:739.

2. Ivert T, Huttunen K, Landou C, Bjork VO. Angiographic studies of internal mammary artery grafts 11 years after coronary artery bypass grafting. J Thorac Cardiovasc Surg 1988;96:1.

3. Ivert T, Lindblom D, Welti R. Coronary artery bypass grafting in patients 70 years of age and older. Early and late results. Eur J Cardiothorac Surg 1989;3:52.

J

1. Jengo JA, Oren V, Conant R, Brizendine M, Nelson T, Uszler JM, et al. Effects of maximal exercise stress on left ventricular function in patients with coronary artery disease using first-pass radionuclide angiocardiography. Circulation 1979;59:60.

2. Janardhan T, Ross JK, Shore DF, Lamb RK, Monro JL. Reoperation for recurrent angina after aortocoronary bypass surgery. Eur J Cardiothorac Surg 1990;4:29.

3. Johns RA, Peach MJ, Flanagan T, Kron IL. Probing of the canine mammary artery damages endothelium and impairs vasodilation resulting from prostacyclin and endothelium-derived relaxing factor. J Thorac Cardiovasc Surg 1989;97:252.

4. Johnson WD, Brenowitz JB, Kayser KL. Factors influencing long-term (10-year to 15-year) survival after a successful coronary artery bypass operation. Ann Thorac Surg 1989;48:19.

5. Jones M, Conkle DM, Ferrans VJ, Roberts WC, Levine FH, Melvin DB, et al. Lesions observed in arterial autogenous vein grafts: light and electron microscopic evaluation. Circulation 1973;4748:III198.

6. Jones EL, Lattouf OM, Weintraub WS. Catastrophic consequences of internal mammary artery hypoperfusion. J Thorac Cardiovasc Surg 1989;98:902.

7. Johnson RA, Zir LM, Harper RW, Leinbach RC, Hutter AM Jr, Pohost GM, et al. Patterns of haemodynamic alteration during left ventricular ischaemia in man: relation to angiographic extent of coronary artery disease. Br Heart J 1979;41:441.

8. Jones RH, Hannan EL, Hammermeister KE, Delong ER, O'Connor GT, Luepker RV, et al. Identification of preoperative variables needed for risk adjustment of short-term mortality after coronary artery bypass graft surgery. The Working Group Panel on the Cooperative CABG Database Project. J Am Coll Cardiol 1996;28:1478.

9. Jones EL, Craver JM, Guyton RA, Bone DK, Hatcher CR Jr, Reichwald N. Importance of complete revascularization in performance of the coronary bypass operation. Am J Cardiol 1983;51:7.

10. Jaffe BD, Broderick TM, Leier CV. Cocaine-induced coronary-artery dissection. N Engl J Med 1994;330:510.

11. Jain D, Thompson B, Wackers FJ, Zaret BL. Relevance of increased lung thallium uptake on stress imaging in patients with unstable angina and non-Q wave myocardial infarction: results of the Thrombolysis in Myocardial Infarction (TIMI)-IIIB Study. J Am Coll Cardiol 1997;30:421.

12. Jones EL, Waites TF, Craver JM, Bone DK, Hatcher CR Jr, Thompkins T. Unstable angina pectoris: comparison with the national cooperative study. Ann Thorac Surg 1982;34:427.

13. Jones EL, Craver JM, Michalik RA, Murphy DA, Guyton RA, Bone DK, et al. Combined carotid and coronary operations: when are they necessary? J Thorac Cardiovasc Surg 1984;87:7.

K

1. Kirklin JK, Blackstone EH, Zorn GL Jr, Pacifico AD, Kirklin JW, Karp RB, et al. Intermediate-term results of coronary artery bypass grafting for acute myocardial infarction. Circulation 1985;72:II175.
2. Kshettry VR, Flavin TF, Emery RW, Nicoloff DM, Arom KV, Petersen RJ. Does multivessel, off-pump coronary artery bypass reduce postoperative morbidity? Ann Thorac Surg 2000;69:1725.
3. Kolibash AJ, Goodenow JS, Bush CA, Tetalman MR, Lewis RP. Improvement of myocardial perfusion and left ventricular function after coronary artery bypass grafting in patients with unstable angina. Circulation 1979;59:66.
4. Kolibash AJ, Lewis RP, Goodenow JS, Bush CA, Tetalman MR. Extensive myocardial blood flow distribution through individual coronary artery bypass grafts. Chest 1980;77:17.
5. Kouchoukos NT, Karp RB, Oberman A, Russell RO Jr, Allison HW, Holt JH Jr. Long-term patency of saphenous veins for coronary bypass grafting. Circulation 1977;56:III189.
6. Kern WH, Dermer GB, Lindesmith GG. The intimal proliferation in aortic-coronary saphenous vein grafts: light and electron microscopic studies. Am Heart J 1972;84:771.
7. Kirklin JW, Kouchoukos NT, Blackstone EH, Oberman A. Research related to surgical treatment of coronary artery disease. Circulation 1979;60:1613.
8. Kowey PR, Taylor JE, Rials SJ, Marinchak RA. Meta-analysis of the effectiveness of prophylactic drug therapy in preventing supraventricular arrhythmia early after coronary artery bypass grafting. Am J Cardiol 1992;69:963.
9. Katariya K, DeMarchena E, Bolooki H. Oral amiodarone reduces incidence of postoperative atrial fibrillation. Ann Thorac Surg 1999;68:1599.
10. Kouchoukos NT, Oberman A, Kirklin JW, Russell RO Jr, Karp RB, Pacifico AD, et al. Coronary bypass surgery: analysis of factors affecting hospital mortality. Circulation 1980;62:I84.
11. Knoebel SB, McHenry PL, Phillips JF, Lowe DK. The effect of aortocoronary bypass grafts on myocardial blood flow reserve and treadmill exercise tolerance. Circulation 1974;50:685.
12. Knatterud GL, Rosenberg Y, Campeau L, Geller NL, Hunninghake DB, Forman SA, et al. Long-term effects on clinical outcomes of aggressive lowering of low-density lipoprotein cholesterol levels and low-dose anticoagulation in the post coronary artery bypass graft trial. Post CABG Investigators. Circulation 2000;102:157.
13. Klatte K, Chaitman BR, Theroux P, Gavard JA, Stocke K, Boyce S, et al. Increased mortality after coronary artery bypass graft surgery is associated with increased levels of postoperative creatine kinase-myocardial band isoenzyme release: results from GUARDIAN trial. J Am Coll Cardiol 2001;38:1070.
14. Kowey PR, Verrier RL, Lown B, Handin RI. Influence of intracoronary platelet aggregation on ventricular electrical properties during partial coronary artery stenosis. Am J Cardiol 1983;51:596.
15. Kent KM, Borer JS, Green MV, Bacharach SL, McIntosh CL, Conkle DM, et al. Effects of coronary artery bypass on global and regional left ventricular function during exercise. N Engl J Med 1977;298:1434.
16. Kramer JR, Matsuda Y, Mulligan JC, Aronow M, Proudfit WL. Progression of coronary atherosclerosis. Circulation 1981;63:519.
17. Kennedy JW, Kaiser GC, Fisher LD, Maynard C, Fritz JK, Myers W, et al. Multivariate discriminant analysis of the clinical and angiographic predictors of operative mortality from the Collaborative Study in Coronary Artery Surgery (CASS). J Thorac Cardiovasc Surg 1980;80:876.
18. King SB 3rd, Lembo NJ, Weintraub WS, Kosinski AS, Barnhart HX, Kutner MH, et al. A randomized trial comparing coronary angioplasty with coronary bypass surgery. Emory Angioplasty versus Surgery Trial (EAST). N Engl J Med 1994;331:1044.
19. Kent KM, Bentivoglio LG, Block PC, Cowley MJ, Dorros G, Gosselin AJ, et al. Percutaneous transluminal coronary angioplasty: report from the Registry of the National Heart, Lung, and Blood Institute. Am J Cardiol 1982;49:2011.
20. Kouchoukos NT, Wareing TH, Murphy SF, Pelate C, Marshall WG Jr. Risks of bilateral internal mammary artery bypass grafting. Ann Thorac Surg 1990;49:210.
21. Kirklin JW, Naftel CD, Blackstone EH, Pohost GM. Summary of a consensus concerning death and ischemic events after coronary artery bypass grafting. Circulation 1989;79:181.
22. Kolesov VI, Potashov LV. Surgery of coronary arteries. Eksp Khir Anesteziol 1965;10:3.
23. Kouchoukos NT, Daily BB, Wareing TH, Murphy SF. Hypothermic circulatory arrest for cerebral protection during combined carotid and cardiac surgery in patients with bilateral carotid artery disease. Ann Surg 1994;219:699.
24. Kolessov VI. Mammary artery-coronary artery anastomosis as method of treatment for angina pectoris. J Thorac Cardiovasc Surg 1967;54:535.
25. Kroncke GM, Kosolcharoen P, Clayman JA, Peduzzi PN, Detre K, Takaro T. Five-year changes in coronary arteries of medical and surgical patients of the Veterans Administration randomized study of bypass surgery. Circulation 1988;78:I144.
26. Kennedy JW, Ivey TD, Misbach G, Allen MD, Maynard C, Dalquist JE, et al. Coronary artery bypass graft surgery early after acute myocardial infarction. Circulation 1989;79:173.
27. Klutstein MW, Tzivoni D, Bitran D, Mendzelevski B, Ilan M, Almagor Y. Treatment of spontaneous coronary artery dissection: report of three cases. Cathet Cardiovasc Diagn 1997;40:372.
28. Kay EB. Internal mammary artery grafting. J Thorac Cardiovasc Surg 1987;94:312.
29. Kouchoukos NT, Murphy S, Philpott T, Pelate C, Marshall WG Jr. Coronary artery bypass grafting for postinfarction angina pectoris. Circulation 1989;79:I68.
30. Kane JP, Malloy MJ, Ports TA, Phillips NR, Diehl JC, Havel RJ. Regression of coronary atherosclerosis during treatment of familial hypercholesterolemia with combined drug regimens. JAMA 1990;264:3007.
31. Katz ES, Tunick PA, Rusinek H, Ribakove G, Spencer FC, Kronzon I. Protruding aortic atheromas predict stroke in elderly patients undergoing cardiopulmonary bypass: experience with intraoperative transesophageal echocardiography. J Am Coll Cardiol 1992;20:70.
32. Kloster FE, Kremkau EL, Ritzmann LW, Rahimtoola SH, Rosch J, Kanarek PH. Coronary bypass for stable angina: a prospective randomized study. N Engl J Med 1979;300:149.

L

1. Lehrman KL, Tilkian AG, Hultgren HN, Fowles RE. Effect of coronary arterial bypass surgery on exercise-induced ventricular arrhythmias: long-term follow-up of a prospective randomized study. Am J Cardiol 1979;44:1056.
2. Laks H, Kaiser GC, Mudd JG, Halstead J, Pennington G, Tyras D, et al. Revascularization of the right coronary artery. Am J Cardiol 1979;43:1109.
3. Loop FD, Cosgrove DM, Lytle BW, Thurer RL, Simpfendorfer C, Taylor PC, et al. An 11 year evolution of coronary arterial surgery (1968–1978). Ann Surg 1979;190:444.
4. Lee L, Bates ER, Pitt B, Walton JA, Laufer N, O'Neill WW. Percutaneous transluminal coronary angioplasty improves survival in acute myocardial infarction complicated by cardiogenic shock. Circulation 1988;78:1345.
5. Loop FD, Lytle BW, Cosgrove DM, Sheldon WC, Irarrazaval M, Taylor PC, et al. Atherosclerosis of the left main coronary artery: 5 year results of surgical treatment. Am J Cardiol 1979;44:195.
6. Loop FD, Lytle BW, Cosgrove DM, Stewart RW, Goormastic M, Williams GW, et al. Influence of the internal mammary artery graft on 10-year survival and other cardiac events. N Engl J Med 1986;314:1.
7. Lapin ES, Murray JA, Bruce RA, Winterscheid L. Changes in maximal exercise performance in the evaluation of saphenous vein bypass surgery. Circulation 1973;47:1164.

8. Lytle BW, Loop FD, Thurer RL, Groves LK, Taylor PC, Cosgrove DM. Isolated left anterior descending coronary atherosclerosis: long-term comparison of internal mammary artery and venous autografts. Circulation 1980;61:869.

9. Longmire WP Jr, Cannon JA, Kattus AA. Direct-vision coronary endarterectomy for angina pectoris. N Engl J Med 1958;259:993.

10. Lawrie GM, Lie JT, Morris GC Jr, Beazley HL. Vein graft patency and intimal proliferation after aortocoronary bypass: early and long-term angiopathologic correlations. Am J Cardiol 1976;38:856.

11. Loop FD, Lytle BW, Cosgrove DM, Golding LA, Taylor PC, Stewart RW. Free (aorta-coronary) internal mammary artery graft. Late results. J Thorac Cardiovasc Surg 1986;92:827.

12. Luscher TF, Diederich D, Siebenmann R, Lehmann K, Stulz P, von Segesser L, et al. Difference between endothelium-dependent relaxation in arterial and in venous coronary bypass grafts. N Engl J Med 1988;319:462.

13. Lytle BW, Loop FD, Cosgrove DM, Ratliff NB, Easley K, Taylor PC. Long-term (5 to 12 years) serial studies of internal mammary artery and saphenous vein coronary bypass grafts. J Thorac Cardiovasc Surg 1985;89:248.

14. Loop FD, Lytle BW, Cosgrove DM, Woods EL, Stewart RW, Golding LA, et al. Reoperation for coronary atherosclerosis. Changing practice in 2509 consecutive patients. Ann Surg 1990;212:378.

15. LoGerfo FW, Quist WC, Cantelmo NL, Haudenschild CC. Integrity of vein grafts as a function of initial intimal and medial preservation. Circulation 1983;68:II117.

16. Lindsay J, Hong MK, Pinnow EE, Pichard AD. Effects of endoluminal coronary stents on the frequency of coronary artery bypass grafting after unsuccessful percutaneous transluminal coronary vascularization. Am J Cardiol 1996;77:647.

17. LoGerfo FW, Quist WC, Crawshaw HM, Haudenschild C. An improved technique for preservation of endothelial morphology in vein grafts. Surgery 1981;90:1015.

18. Lim YL, Kalff V, Kelly MJ, Mason PJ, Currie PJ, Harper RW, et al. Radionuclide angiographic assessment of global and segmental left ventricular function at rest and during exercise after coronary artery bypass graft surgery. Circulation 1982;66:972.

19. Lazar HL, Plehn JF, Schick EM, Dobnick D, Shemin RJ. Effects of coronary revascularization on regional wall motion. J Thorac Cardiovasc Surg 1989;98:498.

20. Loop FD, Cosgrove DM, Kramer JR, Lytle BW, Taylor PC, Golding LA, et al. Late clinical and arteriographic results in 500 coronary artery reoperations. J Thorac Cardiovasc Surg 1981;81:675.

21. Little WC, Constantinescu M, Applegate RJ, Kutcher MA, Burrows MT, Kahl FR, et al. Can coronary angiography predict the site of a subsequent myocardial infarction in patients with mild-to-moderate coronary artery disease? Circulation 1988;78:1157.

22. Losordo DW, Vale PR, Symes JF, Dunnington CH, Esakof DD, Maysky M, et al. Gene therapy for myocardial angiogenesis: initial clinical results with direct myocardial injection of phVEGF$_{165}$ as sole therapy for myocardial ischemia. Circulation 1998;98:2800.

23. Levin DC, Cohn LH, Koster JK Jr, Collins JJ Jr. Accuracy of angiography in predicting quality and caliber of the distal coronary artery lumen in preparation for bypass surgery. Circulation 1982;66:II93.

24. Laird-Meeter K, Van Den Brand MJ, Serruys PW, Penn OC, Haalebos MM, Bos E, et al. Reoperation after aortocoronary bypass procedure: results in 53 patients in a group of 1041 with consecutive first operations. Br Heart J 1983;50:157.

25. Lytle BW, Cosgrove DM, Ratliff NB, Loop FD. Coronary artery bypass grafting with the right gastroepiploic artery. J Thorac Cardiovasc Surg 1989;97:826.

26. Lytle BW, Cosgrove DM, Saltus GL, Taylor PC, Loop FD. Multivessel coronary revascularization without saphenous vein: long-term results of bilateral internal mammary artery grafting. Ann Thorac Surg 1983;36:540.

27. Laks H, Rosenkranz E, Buckberg GD. Surgical treatment of cardiogenic shock after myocardial infarction. Circulation 1986;74:III11.

28. LaCroix AZ, Guralnik JM, Curb JD, Wallace RB, Ostfeld AM, Hennekens CH. Chest pain and coronary heart disease mortality among older men and women in three communities. Circulation 1990;81:437.

29. Levy T, Fotopoulos G, Walker S, Rex S, Octave M, Paul V, et al. Randomized controlled study investigating the effect of biatrial pacing in prevention of atrial fibrillation after coronary artery bypass grafting. Circulation 2000;102:1382.

30. Loop FD, Lytle BW, Cosgrove DM, Mahfood S, McHenry MC, Goormastic M, et al. J. Maxwell Chamberlain memorial paper. Sternal wound complications after isolated coronary artery bypass grafting: early and late mortality, morbidity, and cost of care. Ann Thorac Surg 1990;49:179.

31. Lytle BW, Blackstone EH, Loop FD, Houghtaling PL, Arnold JH, Akhrass R, et al. Two internal thoracic artery grafts are better than one. J Thorac Cardiovasc Surg 1999;117:855.

32. Lytle BW, Loop FD. Superiority of bilateral internal thoracic artery grafting: it's been a long time comin'. Circulation 2001;104:2152.

33. Laub GW, Muralidharan S, Clancy R, Eldredge WJ, Chen C, Adkins MS, et al. Cryopreserved allograft veins as alternative coronary artery bypass conduits: early phase results. Ann Thorac Surg 1992;54:826.

34. Ladowski JS, Dillon TA, Deschner WP, DeRiso AJ 2nd, Peterson AC, Schatzlein MH. Durability of emergency coronary artery bypass for complications of failed angioplasty. Cardiovasc Surg 1996;4:23.

M

1. Marshall RC, Berger HJ, Costin JC, Freedman GS, Wolberg J, Cohen LS, et al. Assessment of cardiac performance with quantitative radionuclide angiography: sequential left ventricular ejection fraction, normalized left ventricular ejection rate, and regional wall motion. Circulation 1977;56:820.

2. Mirhoseini M, Cayton MM. Revascularization of the heart by laser. J Microsurg 1981;2:253.

3. McConahay DR, Valdes M, McCallister BD, Crockett JE, Conn RD, Reed WA, et al. Accuracy of treadmill testing in assessment of direct myocardial revascularization. Circulation 1977;56:548.

4. McNamara JJ, Bjerke HS, Chung GK, Dang CR. Blood flow in sequential vein grafts. Circulation 1979;60:33.

5. Minick CR, Stemerman MB, Insull W Jr. Role of endothelium and hypercholesterolemia in intimal thickening and lipid accumulation. Am J Pathol 1979;95:131.

6. Miller DC, Stinson EB, Oyer PE, Reitz BA, Jamieson SW, Moreno-Cabral RJ, et al. Long-term clinical assessment of the efficacy of adjunctive coronary endarterectomy. J Thorac Cardiovasc Surg 1981;81:21.

7. Murray G, Porcheron R, Hilario J, Roschlau W. Anastomosis of a systemic artery to the coronary. Can Med Assoc J 1954;71:594.

8. McBride LR, Barner HB. The left internal mammary artery as a sequential graft to the left anterior descending system. J Thorac Cardiovasc Surg 1983;86:703.

9. Marchandise B, Bourassa MG, Chaitman BR, Lesperance J. Angiographic evaluation of the natural history of normal coronary arteries and mild coronary atherosclerosis. Am J Cardiol 1978;41:216.

10. Myers WO, Gersh BJ, Fisher LD, Mock MB, Holmes DR, Schaff HV, et al. Medical versus early surgical therapy in patients with triple-vessel disease and mild angina pectoris: a CASS registry study of survival. Ann Thorac Surg 1987;44:471.

11. Myers WO, Schaff HV, Gersh BJ, Fisher LD, Kosinski AS, Mock MB, et al. Improved survival of surgically treated patients with triple vessel coronary artery disease and severe angina pectoris. A report from the Coronary Artery Surgery Study (CASS) Registry. J Thorac Cardiovasc Surg 1989;97:487.

12. Mathur VS, Guinn GA. Prospective randomized study to evaluate coronary bypass surgery: 10 year followup. Circulation 1982;66:II219.

13. Moise A, Lesperance J, Theroux P, Taeymans Y, Goulet C, Bourassa MG. Clinical and angiographic predictors of new total coronary occlusion in coronary artery disease: analysis of 313 nonoperated patients. Am J Cardiol 1984;54:1176.

14. Markis JE, Malagold M, Parker JA, Silverman KJ, Barry WH, Als AV, et al. Myocardial salvage after intracoronary thrombolysis with streptokinase in acute myocardial infarction. N Engl J Med 1981;305:777.

15. Mills NL, Everson CT. Right gastroepiploic artery: a third arterial conduit for coronary artery bypass. Ann Thorac Surg 1989;47:706.

16. Mangi AA, Dzau VJ. Gene therapy for human bypass grafts. Ann Med 2001;33:153.

17. Mintz LJ, Ingels NB Jr, Daughters GT 2nd, Stinson EB, Alderman EL. Sequential studies of left ventricular function and wall motion after coronary arterial bypass surgery. Am J Cardiol 1980;45:210.

18. Mock MB, Ringqvist I, Fisher LD, Davis KB, Chaitman BR, Kouchoukos NT, et al. Survival of medically treated patients in the Coronary Artery Surgery Study (CASS) Registry. Circulation 1982;66:562.

19. Marshall WG Jr, Kouchoukos NT, Murphy SF, Pelate C. Carotid endarterectomy based on duplex scanning without preoperative arteriography. Circulation 1988;78:I1.

20. Mann T, Goldberg S, Mudge GH Jr, Grossman W. Factors contributing to altered left ventricular diastolic properties during angina pectoris. Circulation 1979;59:14.

21. Madsen JK, Stubgaard M, Utne HE, Hansen JF, van Duijvendijk K, Reiber JH, et al. Prognosis and thallium-201 scintigraphy in patients admitted with chest pain without confirmed acute myocardial infarction. Br Heart J 1988;59:184.

22. Murabito JM, Evans JC, Larson MG, Levy D. Prognosis after the onset of coronary heart disease. An investigation of differences in outcome between the sexes according to initial coronary disease presentation. Circulation 1993;88:2548.

23. Magovern JA, Sakert T, Magovern GJ, Benckart DH, Burkholder JA, Liebler GA, et al. A model that predicts morbidity and mortality after coronary artery bypass graft surgery. J Am Coll Cardiol 1996;28:1147.

24. Milano CA, Kesler K, Archibald N, Sexton DJ, Jones RH. Mediastinitis after coronary artery bypass graft surgery. Risk factors and long-term survival. Circulation 1995;92:2245.

25. Moran SV, Baeza R, Guarda E, Zalaquett R, Irarrazaval MJ, Marchant E, et al. Predictors of radial artery patency for coronary bypass operations. Ann Thorac Surg 2001;72:1552.

26. Moussa I, Reimers B, Moses J, Di Mario C, Di Francesco L, Ferraro M, et al. Long-term angiographic and clinical outcome of patients undergoing multivessel coronary stenting. Circulation 1997;96:3873.

27. Massimo C, Boffi L. Myocardial revascularization by a new method of carrying blood directly from the left ventricular cavity into the coronary circulation. J Thorac Surg 1957;34:257.

28. Mathur VS, Guinn GA. Prospective randomized study of coronary bypass surgery in stable angina pectoris: the first 100 patients. Circulation 1975;52:I133.

29. Mangano CM, Diamondstone LS, Ramsay JG, Aggarwal A, Herskowitz A, Mangano DT. Renal dysfunction after myocardial revascularization: risk factors, adverse outcomes, and hospital resource utilization. Ann Intern Med 1998;128:194.

N

1. Nitter-Hauge S, Levorstad K. Does aortocoronary saphenous vein bypass surgery change the native coronary arteries? Acta Med Scand 1980;207:189.

2. Newman GE, Rerych SK, Jones RH, Sabiston DC Jr. Noninvasive assessment of the effects of aorto-coronary bypass grafting on ventricular function during rest and exercise. J Thorac Cardiovasc Surg 1980;79:617.

3. Noyez L. The use of the internal mammary artery for myocardial revascularization in patients 70 years of age and older. Does it complicate the early post-operative period? Thorac Cardiovasc Surg 1989;37:305.

4. Naunheim KS, Kesler KA, Kanter KR, Fiore AC, McBride LR, Pennington DG, et al. Coronary artery bypass for recent infarction: predictors of mortality. Circulation 1988;78:I122.

5. North American Symptomatic Carotid Endarterectomy Trial: methods, patient characteristics, and progress. Stroke 1991;22:711.

6. Namay DL, Hammermeister KE, Zia MS, DeRouen TA, Dodge HT, Namay K. Effect of perioperative myocardial infarction on late survival in patients undergoing coronary artery bypass surgery. Circulation 1982;65:1066.

7. Nagachinta T, Stephens M, Reitz B, Polk BF. Risk factors for surgical-wound infection following cardiac surgery. J Infect Dis 1987;156:967.

8. Newman MF, Kirchner JL, Phillips-Bute B, Gaver V, Grocott H, Jones RH, et al. Longitudinal assessment of neurocognitive function after coronary-artery bypass surgery. N Engl J Med 2001;344:395.

9. National Heart, Lung, and Blood Institute Coronary Artery Surgery Study. American Heart Association Monograph No. 79. Circulation 1981; 63:I.

O

1. Oberman A, Kouchoukos NT, Makar YN, Russell RO Jr, Sheffield LT, Ray M, et al. Perioperative myocardial infarction after coronary bypass surgery. Cleve Clin Q 1978;45:172.

2. Oberman A, Jones WB, Riley CP, Reeves TJ, Sheffield LT. Natural history of coronary artery disease. Bull N Y Acad Med 1972;48:1109.

3. O'Connor GT, Plume SK, Olmstead EM, Coffin LH, Morton JR, Maloney CT, et al. Multivariate prediction of in-hospital mortality associated with coronary artery bypass graft surgery. Northern New England Cardiovascular Disease Study Group. Circulation 1992; 85:2110.

4. Okada M, Ikuta H, Shimizu K, Horii H, Nakamura K. Alternative method of myocardial revascularization by laser: experimental and clinical study. Kobe J Med Sci 1986;32:151.

5. O'Keefe JH, Blackstone EH, Sergeant P, McCallister BD. The optimal mode of coronary revascularization for diabetics. A risk-adjusted long-term study comparing coronary angioplasty and coronary bypass surgery. Eur Heart J 1998;19:1696.

P

1. Parsonnet V, Gilbert L, Gielchinsky I, Bhaktan EK. Endarterectomy of the left anterior descending and mainstem coronary arteries: a technique for reconstruction of inoperable arteries. Surgery 1976;80:662.

2. Pym J, Brown PM, Charrette EJ, Parker JO, West RO. Gastroepiploic-coronary anastomosis: a viable alternative bypass graft. J Thorac Cardiovasc Surg 1987;94:256.

3. Palac RT, Meadows WR, Hwang MH, Loeb HS, Pifarre R, Gunnar RM. Risk factors related to progressive narrowing in aortocoronary vein grafts studied 1 and 5 years after surgery. Circulation 1982; 66:I40.

4. Page DL, Caulfield JB, Kastor JA, DeSanctis RW, Sanders CA. Myocardial changes associated with cardiogenic shock. N Engl J Med 1971;285:133.

5. Palac RT, Hwang MH, Meadows WR, Croke RP, Pifarre R, Loeb HS, et al. Progression of coronary artery disease in medially and surgically treated patients 5 years after randomization. Circulation 1981;64:II17.

6. Parisi AF, Khuri S, Deupree RH, Sharma GV, Scott SM, Luchi RJ. Medical compared with surgical management of unstable angina. 5-year mortality and morbidity in the Veterans Administration Study. Circulation 1989;80:1176.

7. Pfisterer M, Burkart F, Jockers G, Meyer B, Regenass S, Burckhardt D, et al. Trial of low-dose aspirin plus dipyridamole versus anticoagulants for prevention of aortocoronary vein graft occlusion. Lancet 1989;2:1.

8. Pecher P, Schumacher BA. Angiogenesis in ischemic human myocardium: clinical results after 3 years. Ann Thorac Surg 2000;69:1414.

9. Puig LB, Ciongolli W, Cividanes GV, Dontos A, Kopel L, Bittencourt D, et al. Inferior epigastric artery as a free graft for myocardial revascularization. J Thorac Cardiovasc Surg 1990;99:251.

10. Parisi AF, Folland ED, Hartigan P, the Veterans Affairs ACME Investigators. A comparison of angioplasty with medical therapy in the treatment of single-vessel coronary artery disease. N Engl J Med 1992;326:10.

11. Puskas JD, Thourani VH, Marshall JJ, Dempsey SJ, Steiner MA, Sammons BH, et al. Clinical outcomes, angiographic patency, and resource utilization in 200 consecutive off-pump coronary bypass patients. Ann Thorac Surg 2001;71:1477.

12. Puskas JD, Vinten-Johansen J, Muraki S, Guyton RA. Myocardial protection for off-pump coronary artery bypass surgery. Semin Thorac Cardiovasc Surg 2001;13:82.

13. Parikka H, Toivonen L, Heikkila L, Virtanen K, Jarvinen A. Comparison of sotalol and metoprolol in the prevention of atrial fibrillation after coronary artery bypass surgery. J Cardiovasc Pharmacol 1998;31:67.

14. Perrault LP, Carrier M, Hebert Y, Cartier R, Leclerc Y, Pelletier LC. Early experience with the inferior epigastric artery in coronary artery bypass grafting. A word of caution. J Thorac Cardiovasc Surg 1993;106:928.

15. Pocock SJ, Henderson RA, Clayton T, Lyman GH, Chamberlain DA. Quality of life after coronary angioplasty or continued medical treatment for angina: three-year follow-up in the RITA-2 trial. Randomized Intervention Treatment of Angina. J Am Coll Cardiol 2000;35:907.

16. Pocock SJ, Henderson RA, Rickards AF, Hampton JR, King SB 3rd, Hamm CW, et al. Meta-analysis of randomised trials comparing coronary angioplasty with bypass surgery. Lancet 1995;346:1184.

17. Post–Coronary Artery Bypass Graft Trial Investigators. The effect of aggressive lowering of low-density lipoprotein cholesterol levels and low-dose anticoagulation on obstructive changes in saphenous-vein coronary-artery bypass grafts. N Engl J Med 1997;336:153.

Q

1. Qazi A, Garcia JM, Mispireta LA, Corso PJ. Reoperation for coronary artery disease. Ann Thorac Surg 1981;32:16.

2. Qureshi SA, Halim MA, Pillai R, Smith P, Yacoub MH. Endarterectomy of the left coronary system. Analysis of a 10 year experience. J Thorac Cardiovasc Surg 1985;89:852.

R

1. Ricks WB, Winkle RA, Shumway NE, Harrison DC. Surgical management of life-threatening ventricular arrhythmias in patients with coronary artery disease. Circulation 1977;56:38.

2. Rerych SK, Scholz PM, Newman GE, Sabiston DC Jr, Jones RH. Cardiac function at rest and during exercise in normals and in patients with coronary artery disease: evaluation by radionuclide angiography. Ann Surg 1978;187:449.

3. Russell RO Jr and Unstable Angina Study Associates. Unstable angina pectoris: National Cooperative Study Group to Compare Surgical and Medical Therapy. II. In-hospital experience and initial follow-up results in patients with one, two and three vessel disease. Am J Cardiol 1978;42:839.

4. Rimm AA, Barboriak JJ, Anderson AJ, Simon JS. Changes in occupation after aortocoronary vein-bypass operation. JAMA 1976;236:361.

5. Read RC, Murphy ML, Hultgren HN, Takaro T. Survival of men treated for chronic stable angina pectoris. A cooperative randomized study. J Thorac Cardiovasc Surg 1978;75:1.

6. Reduto LA, Berger HJ, Geha A, Hammond G, Cohen LS, Gottschalk A, et al. Radionuclide assessment of ventricular performance during propranolol withdrawal prior to aortocoronary bypass surgery. Am Heart J 1978;96:714.

7. Roberts WC. Does thrombosis play a major role in the development of symptom-producing atherosclerotic plaques? Circulation 1973;48:1161.

8. Rogers WJ, Baim DS, Gore JM, Brown BG, Roberts R, Williams DO, et al. Comparison of immediate invasive, delayed invasive, and conservative strategies after tissue-type plasminogen activator. Results of the Thrombolysis in Myocardial Infarction (TIMI) Phase II-A Trial. Circulation 1990;81:1457.

9. Reichle FA, Stewart GJ, Essa N. A transmission and scanning electron microscopic study of luminal surfaces in Dacron and autogenous vein bypasses in man and dog. Surgery 1973;74:945.

10. Rogers WJ, Smith LR, Oberman A, Kouchoukos NT, Mantle JA, Russell RO Jr, et al. Surgical vs. nonsurgical management of patients after myocardial infarction. Circulation 1980;62:I67.

11. Rodriguez A, Boullon F, Perez-Balino N, Paviotti C, Liprandi MI, Palacios IF. Argentine randomized trial of percutaneous transluminal coronary angioplasty versus coronary artery bypass surgery in multi-vessel disease (ERACI): in-hospital results and 1-year follow-up. ERACI Group. J Am Coll Cardiol 1993;22:1060.

12. Rubenson DS, Tucker CR, London E, Miller DC, Stinson EB, Popp RL. Two-dimensional echocardiographic analysis of segmental left ventricular wall motion before and after coronary artery bypass surgery. Circulation 1982;66:1025.

13. Rogers WJ, Coggin CJ, Gersh BJ, Fisher LD, Myers WO, Oberman A, et al. Ten-year follow-up of quality of life in patients randomized to receive medicine therapy or coronary bypass graft surgery: the Coronary Artery Surgery Study (CASS). Circulation 1990;82:1647.

14. Reduto LA, Wickemeyer WJ, Young JB, Del Ventura LA, Reid JW, Glaeser DH, et al. Left ventricular diastolic performance at rest and during exercise in patients with coronary artery disease. Circulation 1981;63:1228.

15. Roffman JA, Fieldman A. Digoxin and propranolol in the prophylaxis of supraventricular tachydysrhythmias after coronary artery bypass surgery. Ann Thorac Surg 1981;31:496.

16. Rosengart TK, Lee LY, Patel SR, Sanborn TA, Parikh M, Bergman GW, et al. Angiogenesis gene therapy: phase I assessment of direct intramyocardial administration of an adenovirus vector expressing VEGF121 cDNA to individuals with clinically significant severe coronary artery disease. Circulation 1999;100:468.

17. Rentrop P, Blanke H, Wiegard V, Karsch KR. Acute myocardial infarction: intracoronary application of nitroglycerin and streptokinase. Clin Cardiol 1979;2:354.

18. Rentrop P, Blanke H, Karsch KR, Kaiser H, Kostering H, Leitz K. Selective intracoronary thrombolysis in acute myocardial infarction and unstable angina pectoris. Circulation 1981;63:307.

19. Rodewald G, Meffert HJ, Emskotter T, Gotze P, Lachenmayer L, Lamparter U, et al. "Head and Heart"—Neurological and psychological reactions to open heart surgery. Thorac Cardiovasc Surg 1988;36:254.

20. Rizzo RJ, Whittemore AD, Couper GS, Donaldson MC, Aranki SF, Collins JJ Jr, et al. Combined carotid and coronary revascularization: the preferred approach to the severe vasculopath. Ann Thorac Surg 1992;54:1099.

21. Richardson PD, Davies MJ, Born GV. Influence of plaque configuration and stress distribution on fissuring of coronary atherosclerotic plaques. Lancet 1989;2:941.

22. Ricci M, Karamanoukian HL, D'Ancona G, Bergsland J, Salerno TA. Exposure and mechanical stabilization in off-pump coronary artery bypass grafting via sternotomy. Ann Thorac Surg 2000;70:1736.

23. Roach GW, Kanchuger M, Mangano CM, Newman M, Nussmeier N, Wolman R, et al. Adverse cerebral outcomes after coronary bypass surgery. Multicenter Study of Perioperative Ischemia Research Group and the Ischemia Research and Education Foundation Investigators. N Engl J Med 1996;335:1857.

24. Royse AG, Royse CF, Tatoulis J, Grigg LE, Shah P, Hunt D, et al. Postoperative radial artery angiography for coronary artery bypass surgery. Eur J Cardiothorac Surg 2000;17:294.

S

1. Sones FM Jr, Shirey EK. Cine coronary arteriography. Mod Conc Cardiovasc Dis 1962;31:735.

2. Sewell WH. Improved coronary vein graft patency rates with side-to-side anastomosis. Ann Thorac Surg 1974;17:538.

3. See JR, Cohn PF, Holman BL, Roberts BH, Adams DF. Angiographic abnormalities associated with alterations in regional myocardial blood flow in coronary artery disease. Br Heart J 1976;38:1278.

4. Sharma B, Goodwin JF, Raphael MJ, Steiner RE, Rainbow RG, Taylor SH. Left ventricular angiography on exercise: a new method of assessing left ventricular function in ischaemic heart disease. Br Heart J 1976;38:59.

5. Sharma B, Taylor SH. Localization of left ventricular ischemia in angina pectoris by cineangiography during exercise. Br Heart J 1975; 37:963.

6. Symmes JC, Lenkei SC, Berman ND. Influence of aortocoronary bypass surgery on employment. Can Med Assoc J 1978;118:268.

7. Stratmann HG, Tamesis BR, Younis LT, Wittry MD, Amato M, Miller DD. Prognostic value of predischarge dipyridamole technetium 99m sestamibi myocardial tomography in medically treated patients with unstable angina. Am Heart J 1995;130:734.

8. Serruys PW, Rousseau MF, Cosyns J, Ponlot R, Brasseur LA, Detry JM. Hemodynamics during maximal exercise after coronary bypass surgery. Br Heart J 1978;40:1205.

9. Siegel W, Loop FD. Comparison of internal mammary artery and saphenous vein bypass grafts for myocardial revascularization: exercise test and angiographic correlations. Circulation 1976;54:III1.

10. Smith HC, Hammes LN, Gupta S, Vlietstra RE, Elveback L. Employment status after coronary artery bypass surgery. Circulation 1982;65:120.

11. Sergeant P, Lesaffre E, Flameng W, Suy R. Internal mammary artery: methods of use and their effect on survival after coronary bypass surgery. Eur J Cardiothorac Surg 1990;4:72.

12. Schaff HV, Gersh BJ, Fisher LD, Frye RL, Mock MB, Ryan TJ, et al. Detrimental effect of perioperative myocardial infarction on late survival after coronary artery bypass. Report from the Coronary Artery Surgery Study—CASS. J Thorac Cardiovasc Surg 1984; 88:972.

13. Sommers HM, Jennings RB. Experimental acute myocardial infarction. Lab Invest 1964;13:1491.

14. Solymoss BC, Nadeau P, Millette D, Campeau L. Late thrombosis of saphenous vein coronary bypass grafts related to risk factors. Circulation 1988;78:I140.

15. Sheldon WL, Sones FM Jr, Shirey EK, Fergusson DJ, Favaloro RG, Effler DB. Reconstructive coronary artery surgery: postoperative assessment. Circulation 1969;3940:I61.

16. Senning A. Strip grafting in coronary arteries: report of a case. J Thorac Cardiovasc Surg 1961;41:542.

17. Sesto M, Schwarz F. Regional myocardial function at rest and after rapid ventricular pacing in patients after myocardial revascularization by coronary bypass graft or by collateral vessels. Am J Cardiol 1979;43:920.

18. Slogoff S, Keats AS, Ott E. Preoperative propranolol therapy and aortocoronary bypass operation. JAMA 1978;240:1487.

19. Shelton ME, Forman MB, Virmani R, Bajaj A, Stoney WS, Atkinson JB. A comparison of morphologic and angiographic findings in long-term internal mammary artery and saphenous vein bypass grafts. J Am Coll Cardiol 1988;11:297.

20. Sergeant P, Blackstone E, Meyns B. Validation and interdependence with patient-variables of the influence of procedural variables on early and late survival after CABG. Leuven Coronary Surgery Program. Eur J Cardiothorac Surg 1997;12:1.

21. Sahn DJ, Barratt-Boyes BG, Graham K, Kerr A, Roche A, Hill D, et al. Ultrasonic imaging of coronary arteries in open-chest humans: evaluation of coronary atherosclerotic lesions during cardiac surgery. Circulation 1982;66:1034.

22. Sergeant P, Blackstone E, Meyns B. Is return of angina after coronary artery bypass grafting immutable, can it be delayed, and is it important? J Thorac Cardiovasc Surg 1998;116:440.

23. Stinson EB, Olinger GN, Glancy DL. Anatomical and physiological determinants of blood flow through aortocoronary vein bypass grafts. Surgery 1973;74:390.

24. Shaw PJ, Bates D, Cartlidge NE, Heaviside D, French JM, Julian DG, et al. Neurological complications of coronary artery bypass graft surgery: six month follow-up study. Br Med J 1986;293:165.

25. Suma H, Takeuchi A, Hirota Y. Myocardial revascularization with combined arterial grafts utilizing the internal mammary and the gastroepiploic arteries. Ann Thorac Surg 1989;47:712.

26. Schuster EH, Griffith LS, Bulkley BH. Preponderance of acute proximal left anterior descending coronary arterial lesions in fatal myocardial infarction: A clinicopathologic study. Am J Cardiol 1981; 47:1189.

27. Selinger SL, Berg R Jr, Leonard JL, Grunwald RP, O'Grady WP. Surgical treatment of acute evolving anterior myocardial infarction. Circulation 1981;64:II28.

28. Simon R, Amende I, Oelert H, Hetzer R, Borst HG, Lichtlen PR. Blood velocity, flow and dimensions of aortocoronary venous bypass grafts in the postoperative state. Circulation 1982;66:I34.

29. Smith SH, Geer JC. Morphology of saphenous vein-coronary artery bypass grafts: seven to 116 months after surgery. Arch Pathol Lab Med 1983;107:13.

30. Selzer A. On the limitation of therapeutic intervention trials in ischemic heart disease: a clinician's viewpoint. Am J Cardiol 1982;49:252.

31. Sigwart U, Grbic M, Essinger A, Bischof-Delaloye A, Sadeghi H, Rivier JL. Improvement of left ventricular function after percutaneous transluminal coronary angioplasty. Am J Cardiol 1982;49:651.

32. Swan HJ, Forrester JS, Diamond G, Chatterjee K, Parmley WW. Hemodynamic spectrum of myocardial infarction and cardiogenic shock: a conceptual model. Circulation 1972;45:1097.

33. Stanley JC, Sottiurai V, Fry RE, Fry WJ. Comparative evaluation of vein graft preparation media: electron and light microscopic studies. J Surg Res 1975;18:235.

34. Salomon NW, Page US, Bigelow JC, Krause AH, Okies JE, Metzdorff MT. Reoperative coronary surgery. Comparative analysis of 6591 patients undergoing primary bypass and 508 patients undergoing reoperative coronary artery bypass. J Thorac Cardiovasc Surg 1990;100:250.

35. Shub C, Vlietstra RE, Smith HC, Fulton RE, Elveback LR. The unpredictable progression of symptomatic coronary artery disease: a serial clinical-angiographic analysis. Mayo Clin Proc 1981;56:155.

36. Sergeant PT, Blackstone EH, Meyns BP. Does arterial revascularization decrease the risk of infarction after coronary artery bypass grafting? Ann Thorac Surg 1998;66:1.

37. Stewart WJ, Goormastic M, Healy BP, Lytle BW, Hoogwerf BJ, Cressman MD, et al. Clinical outcome ten years after coronary bypass: effects of cholesterol and triglycerides in 4,913 patients (abstract). J Am Coll Cardiol 1988;11:7.

38. Stewart WJ, Goormastic M, Lytle BW, Healy BP, Hoogwerf BJ, Cressman MD, et al. Saphenous vein graft patency after 2 years is related to preoperative serum cholesterol and triglyceride levels (abstract). J Am Coll Cardiol 1988;11:7.

39. Seyfer AE, Shriver CD, Miller TR, Graeber GM. Sternal blood flow after median sternotomy and mobilization of the internal mammary arteries. Surgery 1988;104:899.

40. Sabiston DC Jr, Ebert PA, Friesinger GC, Ross RS, Sinclair-Smith B. Proximal endarterectomy: arterial reconstruction for coronary occlusion at aortic origin. Arch Surg 1965;91:758.

41. Sergeant P, Blackstone E, Meyns B, Stockman B, Jashari R. First cardiological or cardiosurgical reintervention for ischemic heart disease after primary coronary artery bypass grafting. Eur J Cardiothorac Surg 1998;14:480.

42. Salomon NW, Page US, Bigelow JC, Krause AH, Okies JE, Metzdorff MT. Coronary artery bypass grafting in elderly patients. Comparative results in a consecutive series of 469 patients older than 75 years. J Thorac Cardiovasc Surg 1991;101:209.

43. Sergeant P, Lesaffre E, Flameng W, Suy R, Blackstone E. The return of clinically evident ischemia after coronary artery bypass grafting. Eur J Cardiothorac Surg 1991;5:447.

44. Sharma GV, Deupree RH, Khuri SF, Parisi AF, Luchi RJ, Scott SM, et al. Coronary bypass surgery improves survival in high-risk unstable angina. Results of a Veterans Administration cooperative study with an 8-year follow-up. Circulation 1991;84:III260.

45. Schmid C, Heublein B, Reichelt S, Borst HG. Steal phenomenon caused by a parallel branch of the internal mammary artery. Ann Thorac Surg 1990;50:463.

46. Schroeder E, Chenu P, Buche M, Marchandise B, Schoevaerdts JC, Chalant C, et al. Angiographic data of the epigastric artery. A new conduit for myocardial revascularization (abstract). J Am Coll Cardiol 1990;45:116.

47. Sani G, Mariani MA, Benetti F, Lisi G, Totaro P, Giomarelli PP, et al. Total arterial myocardial revascularization without cardiopulmonary bypass. Cardiovasc Surg 1996;4:825.

48. Schutz A, Mair H, Wildhirt SM, Gillrath G, Lamm P, Kilger E, et al. Re-OPCAB vs. Re-CABG for myocardial revascularization. Thorac Cardiovasc Surg 2001;49:144.

49. Stamou SC, Pfister AJ, Dullum MK, Boyce SW, Bafi AS, Lomax T, et al. Late outcome of reoperative coronary revascularization on the beating heart. Heart Surg Forum 2001;4:69.

50. Stamou SC, Bafi AS, Boyce SW, Pfister AJ, Dullum MK, Hill PC, et al. Coronary revascularization of the circumflex system: different approaches and long-term outcome. Ann Thorac Surg 2000;70:1371.

51. Suma H, Fukumoto H, Takeuchi A. Coronary artery bypass grafting by utilizing in situ right gastroepiploic artery: basic study and clinical application. Ann Thorac Surg 1987;44:394.

52. Suma H, Isomura T, Horii T, Sato T. Late angiographic result of using the right gastroepiploic artery as a graft. J Thorac Cardiovasc Surg 2000;120:496.

53. Savage MP, Douglas JS Jr, Fischman DL, Pepine CJ, King SB 3rd, Werner JA, et al. Stent placement compared with balloon angioplasty for obstructed coronary bypass grafts. Saphenous Vein De Novo Trial Investigators. N Engl J Med 1997;337:740.

54. Sim I, Gupta M, McDonald K, Bourassa MG, Hlatky MA. A meta-analysis of randomized trials comparing coronary artery bypass grafting with percutaneous transluminal coronary angioplasty in multivessel coronary artery disease. Am J Cardiol 1995;76:1025.

55. Sculpher MJ, Seed P, Henderson RA, Buxton MJ, Pocock SJ, Parker J, et al. Health service costs of coronary angioplasty and coronary artery bypass surgery: the Randomised Intervention Treatment of Angina (RITA) trial. Lancet 1994;344:927.

56. Sen PK, Daulatram J, Kinare SG, Udwadia TE, Parulkar GB. Further studies in multiple transmyocardial acupuncture as a method of myocardial revascularization. Surgery 1968;64:861.

57. Schofield PM, Sharples LD, Caine N, Burns S, Tait S, Wistow T, et al. Transmyocardial laser revascularisation in patients with refractory angina: a randomised controlled trial. Lancet 1999;353:519.

58. Schumacher B, Pecher P, von Specht BU, Stegmann T. Induction of neoangiogenesis in ischemic myocardium by human growth factors: first clinical results of a new treatment of coronary heart disease. Circulation 1998;97:645.

59. Sauve JS, Thorpe KE, Sackett DL, Taylor W, Barnett HJ, Haynes RB, et al. Can bruits distinguish high-grade from moderate symptomatic carotid stenosis? The North American Symptomatic Carotid Endarterectomy Trial. Ann Intern Med 1994;120:633.

60. Syed M, Lesch M. Coronary artery aneurysm: a review. Prog Cardiovasc Dis 1997;40:77.

61. Swaye PS, Fisher LD, Litwin P, Vignola PA, Judkins MP, Kemp HG, et al. Aneurysmal coronary artery disease. Circulation 1983;67:134.

62. Stratmann HG, Younis LT, Wittry MD, Amato M, Miller DD. Exercise technetium-99m myocardial tomography for the risk stratification of men with medically treated unstable angina pectoris. Am J Cardiol 1995;76:236.

63. Sergeant PT, Blackstone EH, Lesaffre E, Flameng W, Kirklin JW. Unpublished study; 1990.

64. Sergeant P, Blackstone E, Meyns B. Can the outcome of coronary bypass grafting be predicted reliably? Eur J Cardiothorac Surg 1997;11:2.

65. Sergeant P, Blackstone E, Meyns B. Validation and interdependence with patient-variables of the influence of procedural values on early and late survival after CABG. KU Leuven Coronary Surgery Program. Eur J Cardiothorac Surg 1997;12:1.

T

1. Tyras DH, Ahmad N, Kaiser GC, Barner HB, Codd JE, Willman VL. Ventricular function and the native coronary circulation five years after myocardial revascularization. Ann Thorac Surg 1979;27:547.

2. Trip MD, Cats VM, van Capelle FJ, Vreeken J. Platelet hyperreactivity and prognosis in survivors of myocardial infarction. N Engl J Med 1990;322:1549.

3. Theroux P, Ross J Jr, Franklin D, Kemper WS, Sasayama S. Coronary arterial reperfusion. III. Early and late effects on regional myocardial function and dimensions in conscious dogs. Am J Cardiol 1976;38:599.

4. Townes BD, Bashein G, Hornbein TF, Coppel DB, Goldstein DE, Davis KB, et al. Neurobehavioral outcomes in cardiac operations. A prospective controlled study. J Thorac Cardiovasc Surg 1989;98:774.

5. Topol EJ, Weiss JL, Guzman PA, Dorsey-Lima S, Blanck TJ, Humphrey LS, et al. Immediate improvement of dysfunctional myocardial segments after coronary revascularization: detection by intraoperative transesophageal echocardiography. J Am Coll Cardiol 1984;4:1123.

6. Tector AJ, McDonald ML, Kress DC, Downey FX, Schmahl TM. Purely internal thoracic artery grafts: outcomes. Ann Thorac Surg 2001;72:450.

7. Taylor HA, Deumite NJ, Chaitman BR, Davis KB, Killip T, Rogers WJ. Asymptomatic left main coronary artery disease in the Coronary Artery Surgery Study (CASS) Registry. Circulation 1989;79:1171.

8. Tector AJ, Schmahl TM, Janson B, Kallies JR, Johnson G. The internal mammary artery graft: its longevity after coronary bypass. JAMA 1981;246:2181.

9. Thistlethwaite PA, Tarazi RY, Giordano FJ, Jamieson SW. Surgical management of spontaneous left main coronary artery dissection. Ann Thorac Surg 1998;66:258.

U

1. Unni KK, Kottke BA, Titus JL, Frye RL, Wallace RB, Brown AL. Pathologic changes in aortocoronary saphenous vein grafts. Am J Cardiol 1974;34:526.

2. Ungerleider RM, Mills NL, Wechsler AS. Left thoracotomy for reoperative coronary artery bypass procedures. Ann Thorac Surg 1985;40:11.

3. Utley JR, Leyland SA. Coronary artery bypass grafting in the octogenarian. J Thorac Cardiovasc Surg 1991;101:866.

V

1. Vineberg A, Miller G. Internal mammary coronary anastomosis in the surgical treatment of coronary artery insufficiency. Can Med Assoc J 1951;64:204.

2. Varnauskas E, Olsson SB, Carlström E, Peterson LE. Prospective randomised study of coronary artery bypass surgery in stable angina pectoris: second interim report by the European Coronary Surgery Study Group. Lancet 1980;2:491.

3. Vlodaver Z, Edwards JE. Pathologic changes in aortic-coronary arterial saphenous vein grafts. Circulation 1971;44:719.

4. Varnauskas E. Survival, myocardial infarction, and employment status in a prospective randomized study of coronary bypass surgery. Circulation 1985;72:V90.

5. Vetrovec GW, Cowley MJ, Overton H, Richardson DW. Intracoronary thrombus in syndromes of unstable myocardial ischemia. Am Heart J 1981;102:1202.

6. Varnauskas E. Twelve-year follow-up of survival in the randomized European coronary surgery study. N Engl J Med 1988;319:332.

7. Vermeulen FE, Hamerlijnck RP, Defauw JJ, Ernst SM. Synchronous operation for ischemic cardiac and cerebrovascular disease: early results and long-term follow-up. Ann Thorac Surg 1992;53:381.

8. van Dijk D, Nierich AP, Jansen EW, Nathoe HM, Suyker WJ, Diephuis JC, et al. Early outcome after off-pump versus on-pump coronary bypass surgery: results from a randomized study. Circulation 2001;104:1761.

9. Voutilainen SM, Jarvinen AA, Verkkala KA, Keto PE, Heikkinen LO, Voutilainen PE, et al. Angiographic 20-year follow-up of 61 consecutive patients with internal thoracic artery grafts. Ann Surg 1999;229:154.

10. Vale PR, Losordo DW, Milliken CE, Maysky M, Esakof DD, Symes JF, et al. Left ventricular electromechanical mapping to assess efficacy of phVEGF$_{165}$ gene transfer for therapeutic angiogenesis in chronic myocardial ischemia. Circulation 2000;102:965.

11. Veterans Administration Coronary Artery Bypass Surgery Cooperative Study Group: eleven-year survival in the Veterans Administration randomized trial of coronary bypass surgery for stable angina. N Engl J Med 1984;311:1333.

W

1. Weisz D, Hamby RI, Aintablian A, Voleti C, Fogel R, Wisoff BG. Late coronary bypass graft flow: quantitative assessment by roentgendensitometry. Ann Thorac Surg 1979;28:429.

2. Webster MW, Chesebro JH, Smith HC, Frye RL, Holmes DR, Reeder GS, et al. Myocardial infarction and coronary artery occlusion: a prospective 5-year angiographic study (abstract). J Am Coll Cardiol 1990;15:218.

3. Webster JS, Moberg C, Rincon G. Natural history of severe proximal coronary artery disease as documented by coronary cineangiography. Am J Cardiol 1974;33:195.

4. Wainwright RJ, Brennand-Roper DA, Maisey MN, Sowton E. Exercise thallium-201 myocardial scintigraphy in the follow-up of aortocoronary bypass graft surgery. Br Heart J 1980;43:56.

5. Weiner DA, Ryan TJ, Parsons L, Fisher LD, Chaitman BR, Sheffield LT, et al. Long-term prognostic value of exercise testing in men and women from the Coronary Artery Surgery Study (CASS) Registry. Am J Cardiol 1995;75:865.

6. Wolf NM, Kreulen TH, Bove AA, McDonough MT, Kessler KM, Strong M, et al. Left ventricular function following coronary bypass surgery. Circulation 1978;58:63.

7. Whalen RE, Harrell FE Jr, Lee KL, Rosati RA. Survival of coronary artery disease patients with stable pain and normal left ventricular function treated medically or surgically at Duke University. Circulation 1982;65:49.

8. White LD, Lee TH, Cook EF, Weisberg MC, Rouan GW, Brand DA, et al. Comparison of the natural history of new onset and exacerbated chronic ischemic heart disease. J Am Coll Cardiol 1990;16:304.

9. Williams JB, Stephenson LW, Holford FD, Langer T, Dunkman WB, Josephson ME. Arrhythmia prophylaxis using propranolol after coronary artery surgery. Ann Thorac Surg 1982;34:435.

10. Wilson RF, Marcus ML, White CW. Effects of coronary bypass surgery and angioplasty on coronary blood flow and flow reserve. Prog Cardiovasc Dis 1988;31:95.

11. Wilson RF, White CW. Does coronary artery bypass surgery restore normal maximal coronary flow reserve? The effect of diffuse atherosclerosis and focal obstructive lesions. Circulation 1987;76:563.

12. Wechsler AS, Junod FL. Coronary bypass grafting in patients with chronic congestive heart failure. Circulation 1989;79:I92.

13. Wijnberg DS, Boeve WJ, Ebels T, van Gelder IC, van den Toren EW, Lie KI, et al. Patency of arm vein grafts used in aorto-coronary bypass surgery. Eur J Cardiothorac Surg 1990;4:510.

14. Watts GF, Lewis B, Brunt JN, Lewis ES, Coltart DJ, Smith LD, et al. Effects on coronary artery disease of lipid-lowering diet, or diet plus cholestyramine, in the St. Thomas' Atherosclerosis Regression Study (STARS). Lancet 1992;339:563.

15. Wareing TH, Davila-Roman VG, Barzilai B, Murphy SF, Kouchoukos NT. Management of the severely atherosclerotic ascending aorta during cardiac operations. A strategy for detection and treatment. J Thorac Cardiothorac Surg 1992;103:453.

16. Weinschelbaum EE, Macchia A, Caramutti VM, Machain HA, Raffaelli HA, Favaloro MR, et al. Myocardial revascularization with radial and mammary arteries: initial and mid-term results. Ann Thorac Surg 2000;70:1378.

17. Weintraub WS, Mauldin PD, Becker E, Kosinski AS, King SB 3rd. A comparison of the costs of and quality of life after coronary angioplasty or coronary surgery for multivessel coronary artery disease. Results from the Emory Angioplasty Versus Surgery Trial (EAST). Circulation 1995;92:2831.

18. Wennberg DE, Lucas FL, Birkmeyer JD, Bredenberg CE, Fisher ES. Variation in carotid endarterectomy mortality in the Medicare population: trial hospitals, volume, and patient characteristics. JAMA 1998;279:1278.

Y

1. Yeh TJ, Heidary D, Shelton L. Y-grafts and sequential grafts in coronary bypass surgery: a critical evaluation of patency rates. Ann Thorac Surg 1979;27:409.

2. Yeatman M, Caputo M, Ascione R, Ciulli F, Angelini GD. Off-pump coronary artery bypass surgery for critical left main stem disease: safety, efficacy and outcome. Eur J Cardiothorac Surg 2001;19:239.

3. Yeghiazarians Y, Braunstein JB, Askari A, Stone PH. Unstable angina pectoris. N Engl J Med 2000;342:101.

Z

1. Zeft HJ, Friedberg HD, King JF, Manley JC, Huston JH, Johnson WD. Reappearance of anterior QRS forces after coronary bypass surgery: an electrovectorcardiographic study. Am J Cardiol 1975;36:163.

2. Zir LM, Dinsmore R, Vexeridis M, Singh JB, Harthorne JW, Daggett WM. Effects of coronary bypass grafting on resting left ventricular contraction in patients studied 1 to 2 years after operation. Am J Cardiol 1979;44:601.

8 Left Ventricular Aneurysm

DEFINITION

A postinfarction left ventricular (LV) aneurysm is a well-delineated transmural fibrous scar, virtually devoid of muscle, in which the characteristic fine trabecular pattern of the inner surface of the wall has been replaced by smooth fibrous tissue. In such areas, the wall is usually thin, and both inner and outer surfaces bulge outward. During systole, the involved wall segments are akinetic (without movement) or dyskinetic (characterized by paradoxical movement).

Scars and infarcts are not considered aneurysms. Unlike aneurysms, they are not discrete, and the LV wall is not thin but rather predominantly muscle.

The definition of *aneurysm* and the criteria for separating an aneurysm from other types of LV scars are controversial, and some clinicians have adopted a broader, nonmorphologic definition rather than the one above. Johnson and colleagues defined aneurysm as "a large single area of infarction (scar) that causes the LV ejection fraction to be profoundly depressed (to approximately 0.35 or lower)."[J1] Although realistically the definition of LV aneurysm is less important to the surgeon than are criteria for and results of surgical excision of LV scars, lack of uniformity of definition complicates almost all discussions of this entity. For example, many reports indicate that most patients with LV aneurysms have single-system left anterior descending coronary artery (LAD) disease, whereas others find that nearly all patients have multiple-system disease.[A4] Many patients with multiple-system disease may have scars rather than true aneurysms.

HISTORICAL NOTE

Although John Hunter and others recognized very early that aneurysms of the LV occurred, it was not until the 1880s that the relationships among stenotic coronary artery disease, myocardial infarction, myocardial fibrosis, and LV aneurysm were recognized.[C1,L1,M1,T1,Z1] Until about 1950, few cases were diagnosed during life, but after that time, ability to diagnose LV aneurysms improved. In 1967, Gorlin and colleagues reported that a strong suspicion of aneurysm could be obtained in 75% of patients with this complication of myocardial infarction based on history, physical examination, and apex cardiographic, electrocardiographic, and radiologic studies.[G1] Many clinicians believe the prevalence of LV aneurysms has been decreasing since about 1980.

Surgical treatment of postinfarction LV aneurysm probably began in 1944, when Beck reinforced such a lesion with fascia lata in an effort to reduce expansile pulsation and prevent rupture. A closed ventriculoplasty, done with a special side-biting LV clamp, was reported in 1955 by Likoff and Bailey.[L2] A few years later, Bailey reported five survivors among six patients treated by this method. In 1959, Cooley and colleagues in Houston reported the first successful open excision of an LV aneurysm using cardiopulmonary bypass (CPB).[C2]

MORPHOLOGY
Gross Pathology

The wall of a mature aneurysm is a white fibrous scar, visible externally on the cut surface as well as endocardially. Characteristically, the aneurysmal portion of the LV wall is thin, the endocardial surface is smooth and nontrabeculated, and the area is clearly demarcated. In more than half the patients with classic LV aneurysms, varying amounts of mural thrombus are attached to the endocardial surface. The mural thrombus may calcify, as may the overlying pericardium, which is usually densely adherent to the epicardial surface of the aneurysm.[D1,P1]

Such classic LV aneurysms are at one end of the spectrum of postinfarction LV scars. At the other end are the diffuse, scattered, at times sparse punctate scars, frequently visible at operation in areas of previous myocardial infarction. These scars are usually not transmural, and the LV wall is not thinned. The endocardium beneath retains its trabeculations, and the area of scarring is not clearly demarcated from the rest of the wall. Mural thrombi are not commonly present, and the pericardium is not commonly adherent to the area.

Between these two extremes is a continuous spectrum of postinfarction LV scarring, because in an area of myocardial infarction, myocardial necrosis rarely involves an entire area homogeneously (see "Myocardial Infarction and Its Morphologic Sequelae" in Chapter 7).

Microscopic Pathology

A mature aneurysm consists almost entirely of hyalinized fibrous tissue. However, a small number of viable muscle cells are usually present.[G1] Fibrous tissue of the type present in aneurysms takes at least 1 month to form, although collagen is present within 10 days of infarction. Thus, when an aneurysm is said to be present (based on wall thinning and dilatation) within 1 week or so of a first infarction, the wall is composed largely of necrotic muscle and is not therefore by definition a true (mature) aneurysm.

Location

About 85% of LV aneurysms are located anterolaterally near the apex of the heart. Few are confined to the lateral (obtuse marginal) area, and only 5% to 10% are posterior, near the base of the heart.

Posterior, or inferior, aneurysms (i.e., those occurring in the diaphragmatic portion of the LV) are in some ways different from apical and anterolateral aneurysms. Nearly half of the posterior aneurysms are false aneurysms (see "False Left Ventricular Aneurysm" under Special Situations and Controversies), whereas nearly all anterolateral and apical aneurysms are true aneurysms.[B7] Virtually all lateral aneurysms are false aneurysms. True posterior wall postinfarction aneurysms are associated with a high prevalence of postinfarction mitral regurgitation secondary to ischemia of the papillary muscle[B7,V1] (see Chapter 10).

Coronary Arteries

Somewhat less than half the patients undergoing resection of classic LV aneurysms or scars have stenotic coronary artery disease confined to the LAD.[B1,B10,C7,D1-D3,D5,F1,K1, L3,R1,R2,S1,S11] More often, multiple-system disease is present. The discrepancy between the reported prevalence of single- and multiple-vessel disease may be related to differences in the definition of LV aneurysm; to different sources of the material (clinical, surgical, or postmortem); and, in the case of surgical material, to case selection. A patient with single-system disease is more apt to survive an acute infarction and appear in a surgical series than is a patient with multiple-system disease.

Left Ventricle

Postmortem studies indicate that most patients with classic LV aneurysms have increased cardiac volume and weight.[D1,G2,P1] The increase in volume is in part the result of simple thinning and bulging of the aneurysmal portion of the LV wall. However, nonaneurysmal portions of the LV also increase in volume and thickness secondary to hemodynamic stress placed on them by akinesia of the aneurysmal segment (remodeling) and by the LaPlace law. Inactivation (by akinesis or dyskinesis) of at least 20% of the LV wall area is required for LV enlargement to occur.[C4,K5] The larger the akinetic or dyskinetic area, the greater the enlargement of the rest of the ventricle. The time course of these events has not been clearly defined.

CLINICAL FEATURES AND DIAGNOSTIC CRITERIA

The morphologic diagnosis of postinfarction LV aneurysm can be made with assurance only at operation or autopsy. This is because the akinetic or dyskinetic segmental wall motion of an LV aneurysm can be mimicked by nontransmural scars or early infarcts that are not morphologic aneurysms. Thus, Froehlich and colleagues found no aneurysm at operation in 3 of 18 patients (17%; CL 7%-31%) with a preoperative diagnosis of aneurysm and only a questionable aneurysm, which was plicated, in an additional 4 patients (22%; CL 12%-37%).[F5]

Small and moderate-sized aneurysms are often associated with no specific symptoms, although the patient may experience angina because of stenoses in other portions of the coronary arterial tree. Patients with large LV aneurysms, however, usually present with dyspnea that often has persisted from the time of infarction. Heart failure requiring medication for control may have appeared by the time of presentation to the physician[B10,R1] (Table 8-1). In patients with LV aneurysms, 15% to 30% have symptoms related to ventricular tachycardia, which may become intractable to

medical treatment and cause death.[B10,G3] Although about half of aneurysms contain thrombus, thromboembolism occurs in only a small proportion of patients.[B10]

On physical examination, palpation over the heart often demonstrates a diffuse, sustained apical systolic thrust and a double impulse. On auscultation, usually a third heart sound and often a fourth (atrial) sound are present. There may be an apical pansystolic murmur if mitral regurgitation is present. Chest radiography and fluoroscopy may show an external bulge or convexity when the aneurysm is large enough and profiled.

Methods of LV imaging, namely, left ventriculography, two-dimensional echocardiography, transesophageal radionuclide cardiac blood pool imaging, computed tomography (CT), and magnetic resonance imaging (MRI), are all useful diagnostic techniques (Fig. 8-1).[B13,H8,L5] However, an incorrect preoperative or premortem diagnosis of aneurysm is still sometimes made. Ventriculography is probably the most sensitive imaging method. When there is akinesia or dyskinesia of the wall segment during systole, a permanent outward bulging or convexity,[G1,H3] thinning of the wall and lack of inner wall trabeculation, and clear demarcation of the area from the remaining ventricle, the diagnosis is probably correct. Wall thinning and even bulging of the contrast-medium-lined LV cavity may not be

■ **TABLE 8-1   Symptoms in Patients Operated on for Left Ventricular Aneurysm**

Symptoms	No.	% of 145
Severe angina[a] alone	45	31
CHF alone	30	21
CHF + severe angina	27	19
VT + other symptoms	22	15
CHF + mild angina	12	8
Mild angina[b] alone	8	5.5
Mild effort dyspnea	1	0.7
TOTAL	145	100

(Modified from Barratt-Boyes and colleagues.[B10])

Key: *CHF,* Congestive heart failure (severe dyspnea, orthopnea, paroxysmal nocturnal dyspnea, fluid retention, hepatomegaly); *VT,* ventricular tachycardia (two or more episodes of documented VT or ventricular fibrillation despite treatment with antiarrhythmic drugs).

[a] Severe = Canadian angina class 3 or 4.

[b] Mild = Canadian angina class 1 or 2.

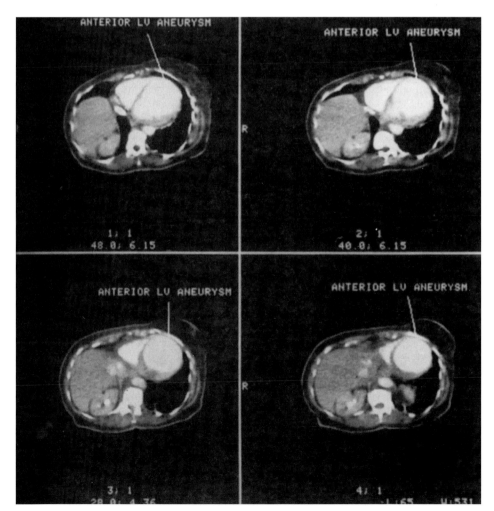

Figure 8-1   Cine (ultrafast) computed tomographic images at four adjacent anatomic levels (*upper left,* cranial to *lower right,* caudal) demonstrate an anterior left ventricular (LV) aneurysm. There is severe thinning of the anteroseptal and anterior walls and bulging of the LV anteriorly. (From Higgins.[H8])

detected when there is extensive smooth thrombus, and it is often difficult to define the margins of an area with akinesia. Identification of significant mural thrombus adds to the probability of aneurysm, as does presence of calcification in the wall. Right heart catheterization is useful because it enables measurement of pulmonary artery pressure and calculation of cardiac output. From the left heart study, LV end-diastolic pressure, ejection fraction, and end-diastolic volume are measured or calculated. Coronary angiography is always performed.

NATURAL HISTORY

Development of Left Ventricular Aneurysm

Historically, about 10% to 30% of patients who survived a major myocardial infarction developed an LV aneurysm.[A3,N1] Today, the prevalence appears to have lessened because of improved treatment of patients with acute myocardial infarction. The most important development may be widespread use of thrombolytic therapy and angioplasty, which have reduced the prevalence of permanently occluded LADs. Other improvements include better management of hypertension and avoidance of corticosteroids, both of which are risk factors for development of aneurysms.[B9,M5]

The mechanisms by which LV aneurysms form are not completely elucidated. Occurrence of a large transmural infarction is a prerequisite. It has been suggested that patients who develop LV aneurysms have few intercoronary collateral arteries.[B2,C3,H5] It is postulated that a rich collateral blood supply to an area of myocardial infarction tends to increase the number and size of the islands of viable myocardial cells in the area and to decrease the probability that the necrosis is extensive enough to result in a thin-walled transmural scar. This hypothesis is supported by Forman and colleagues, who studied 79 patients undergoing cardiac catheterization 6 months after a first myocardial infarction.[F8] They found total occlusion of the LAD and poorly developed collateral flow to be the determinants of LV aneurysm formation. Apparently, normal or supranormal systolic function in adjacent ventricular segments is necessary for generating sufficiently high intraventricular pressure and wall tension in the infarcted area to result in aneurysm formation.[A3]

Pathophysiologic Progression of Aneurysm

Whether large LV aneurysms are large from inception, or gradually enlarge once formed, is uncertain. However, they probably do not increase appreciably in size for more than 6 months after inception. The mechanism for increasing symptomatology that characterizes the life history of many patients with large LV aneurysms has not been clearly established.[C4,C7,H3] It may be due to a gradual increase in the size of the area of akinesia or dyskinesia and to a consequent gradual reduction in stroke volume and global ejection fraction.[A1,K5] The nonaneurysmal portion of the LV wall is subjected to increased systolic wall stress as ventricular size increases (as described by the LaPlace law) and may ultimately lose its systolic reserve and contribute to LV enlargement and failure.[K5] This process is aggravated by any myocardial ischemia that develops in the nonaneurysmal portion of the ventricular wall.

Left Ventricular Function

An aneurysm changes the curvature and thickness of the LV wall, and because these are determinants of LV afterload (wall stress), global LV performance can be expected to be altered.[D6,N5] Also, a large LV aneurysm leads to global cardiac remodeling with generalized dilatation.[W3] Variations in intrinsic properties of scar, muscle, and border zone tissue can affect both systolic and diastolic function.[K1] Finally, paradoxical movement in the aneurysmal portion of the wall reduces efficiency of the ventricle because systolic work is wasted on expansion of the aneurysm.[J3,S8]

Function in uninvolved segments of the LV per se (segmental ejection fraction) has been difficult to study because of the complexities of assessing ventricular function in this setting. However, when echocardiographically determined wall thickening is used as a measure of regional systolic function, it appears that systolic function is maintained in the remote nonaneurysmal portions of the ventricle.[N5] Early in systole, the aneurysm and border zones bulge outward (paradoxical movement) as systolic intraventricular pressure rises to a maximum.[N5] Later in systole, after the aortic valve has opened and wall stress is falling, some wall thickening occurs in the border zones, contributing to ejection.[N5]

Right Ventricular Function

Right ventricular (RV) function may be impaired in patients with LV aneurysm. This may result from akinesis or dyskinesis of the ventricular septum, impaired RV wall motion near the apex, increased pulmonary artery pressure, occlusive disease of the right coronary artery, and increased volume of the LV within the pericardial cavity.[B14,C13,G5]

Survival

The complexities of ischemic heart disease in general and the difficulties in identifying true LV aneurysms have mitigated against achieving a clear understanding of survival and risk factors for death of patients with LV aneurysms.

Patients with an LV akinetic area (not all of which are true aneurysms) are reported to have a 5-year survival without operation of 69%,[B3] perhaps only a little less than that dictated by their coexisting coronary artery disease. Patients with a dyskinetic area of LV wall (many of which are probably aneurysms) have a 54% 5-year survival, which is reduced to 36% when myocardial function in the remainder of the ventricle is reduced.[B3]

Size of the aneurysm is a risk factor for premature death in surgically untreated patients. In patients with small aneurysms (usually without symptoms of heart failure), the probability of survival is dictated primarily by the severity and extent of their coronary arterial stenoses and is greater in asymptomatic than in symptomatic patients (Fig. 8-2).[G3] Prognosis is adversely affected by *dyskinesia* rather than akinesia in the aneurysm; the former is usually associated

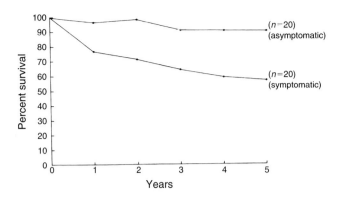

Figure 8-2   Five-year survival with left ventricular aneurysm but without operation for 20 patients with few or no symptoms and for 20 symptomatic patients. (Modified from Grondin and colleagues.[G3])

with a low global LV ejection fraction.[P2] The *functional characteristics* of the remainder of the ventricle are also major determinants of survival.

In addition, all the usual risk factors for premature death in patients with ischemic heart disease (see Table 7-2 in Chapter 7) pertain to patients with LV aneurysm.[F2]

TECHNIQUE OF OPERATION

Most patients who undergo resection of postinfarction LV aneurysms or other scars also require coronary artery bypass grafting (CABG). The following discussion augments the description of CABG in Chapter 7.

Preoperative and operating room preparations, removal or preparation of grafts, and median sternotomy are accomplished as described in Chapters 2 and 7. The pericardial adhesions over the LV are not disturbed at this point. If CABG is to be performed, and if the proximal anastomoses are to be placed first, this is done now. If the LAD is to be revascularized (and this is always done if possible), the left internal thoracic artery is prepared.

Moderately hypothermic CPB is established using double venous cannulation and caval taping or a single venous cannula. A left atrial or LV vent is not inserted. Dissection of adhesions between the LV and pericardium is deferred until the aorta is clamped, to avoid dislodging and embolizing mural thrombus.

Because patients with large LV aneurysms usually have heart failure and the operation may be a long one, warm induction of cardioplegia and controlled reperfusion with initially hyperkalemic, modified, and enriched blood may be used (see "Cold Cardioplegia, Controlled Aortic Root Reperfusion, and [When Needed] Warm Cardioplegic Induction" in Chapter 3). Retrograde cardioplegia (see "Technique of Retrograde Infusion" under Methods of Myocardial Management during Cardiac Surgery in Chapter 3) and a "no touch" technique may be particularly useful here.[G4]

When they are thin, adhesions can be mobilized over the entire aneurysm. If the classic method of repair is anticipated and the aneurysm is densely adherent to the pericardium, the LV can be separated from the aneurysm without

disturbing these adhesions. The aneurysm is incised at some convenient point. Loose thrombus is sought and removed. When the aneurysm contains considerable thrombus and debris, a sponge is placed deep inside the ventricle over the aortic and mitral valves to prevent debris from entering the aorta and left atrium. This sponge is removed after the dissection is completed. A small sump sucker is placed through the incision into the ventricle and is positioned so as to maintain a pool of blood within the open ventricle. This prevents air from entering the aorta and coronary ostia.

The incision is extended around the entire aneurysm, leaving a thin rim of scar tissue to facilitate closure. A classic aneurysm has a smooth endocardial surface. Thus, all of the LV free wall with a smooth endocardium should be removed. Additional endocardial tissue may be removed, and other procedures done, if the patient has a history of life-threatening ventricular arrhythmias (see Section 7, "Ventricular Tachycardia/Ventricular Fibrillation in Ischemic Heart Disease," in Chapter 45). When large amounts of thrombus are removed, the ventricular cavity is carefully inspected and irrigated to remove any debris. Otherwise, this is not done, to prevent air from entering the left atrium, aortic root, and coronary ostia. If the aneurysm is left adherent to the pericardium, thrombotic material is removed from it (this can be done later, during rewarming, after the ventricle is closed), and the avascular fibrous tissue is left attached to the pericardium.

Reconstruction of the Left Ventricle
Anterior Aneurysm

When reconstruction is performed with the classic technique (linear closure), a line of closure is selected that will least distort the LV. After opening the ventricle and excising the scar (Fig. 8-3, *A*), a stay suture is placed at each end of the line of closure (Fig. 8-3, *B*). If the aneurysm is small, closure of the LV can be accomplished with two rows of a simple continuous suture using No. 0 or 1 polypropylene on a large-curved needle. More often, closure is performed with heavy, double-armed sutures (No. 1 or 2 silk or polyester) that are placed horizontally immediately adjacent to one another, incorporating strips of PTFE (polytetrafluoroethylene) felt (see Fig. 8-3, *B*). These sutures are placed deep into the ventricular septum (see Fig. 8-3, *B* [inset]) to exclude as much septal scar as possible.[S3] As these sutures are tied, beginning at the basilar portion of the ventricle, volume from the pump-oxygenator is infused and the lungs are gently inflated to evacuate air from the pulmonary veins and left atrium. Saline can also be infused into the open LV. When this ventricular suture line is completed, it is reinforced with two continuous No. 0 or 1 polypropylene sutures that are positioned at each end of the incision, placed through the felt and through the edges of the myocardium superficial to the mattress sutures, and tied to each other (Fig. 8-3, *C*). Incorporation of the distal portion of the LAD into the suture lines should be avoided.

An alternative procedure is patch closure of the defect in the LV (Fig. 8-4).[C14,D4,F3] This technique has been termed "endoaneurysmorrhaphy" by Cooley[C14] and "endoventricular circular patch plasty repair" by Dor.[D4] The

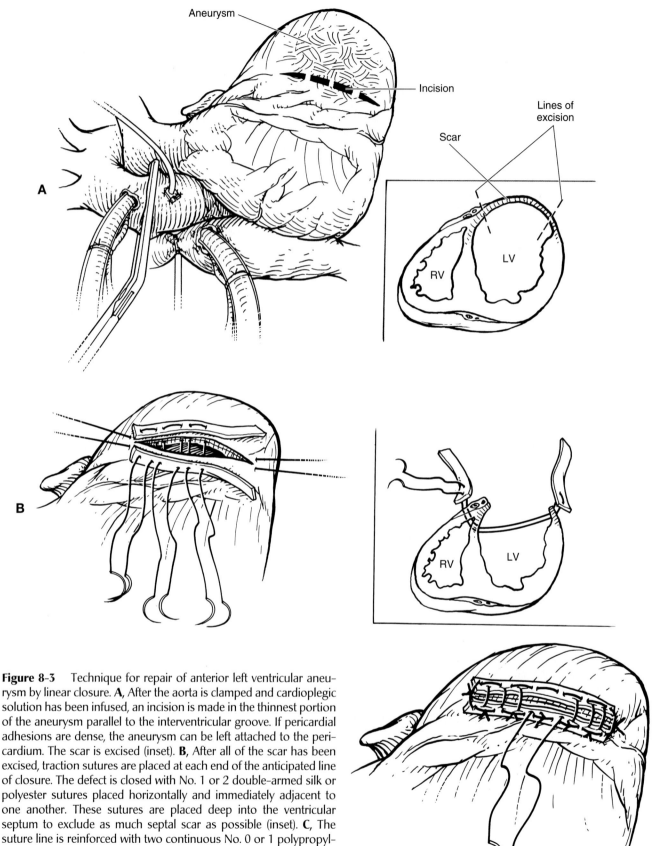

Figure 8-3   Technique for repair of anterior left ventricular aneurysm by linear closure. **A,** After the aorta is clamped and cardioplegic solution has been infused, an incision is made in the thinnest portion of the aneurysm parallel to the interventricular groove. If pericardial adhesions are dense, the aneurysm can be left attached to the pericardium. The scar is excised (inset). **B,** After all of the scar has been excised, traction sutures are placed at each end of the anticipated line of closure. The defect is closed with No. 1 or 2 double-armed silk or polyester sutures placed horizontally and immediately adjacent to one another. These sutures are placed deep into the ventricular septum to exclude as much septal scar as possible (inset). **C,** The suture line is reinforced with two continuous No. 0 or 1 polypropylene sutures positioned at each end of the incision, placed in the scar tissue superficially to the mattress sutures, and tied to each other.

Key: *LV,* Left ventricle; *RV,* right ventricle.

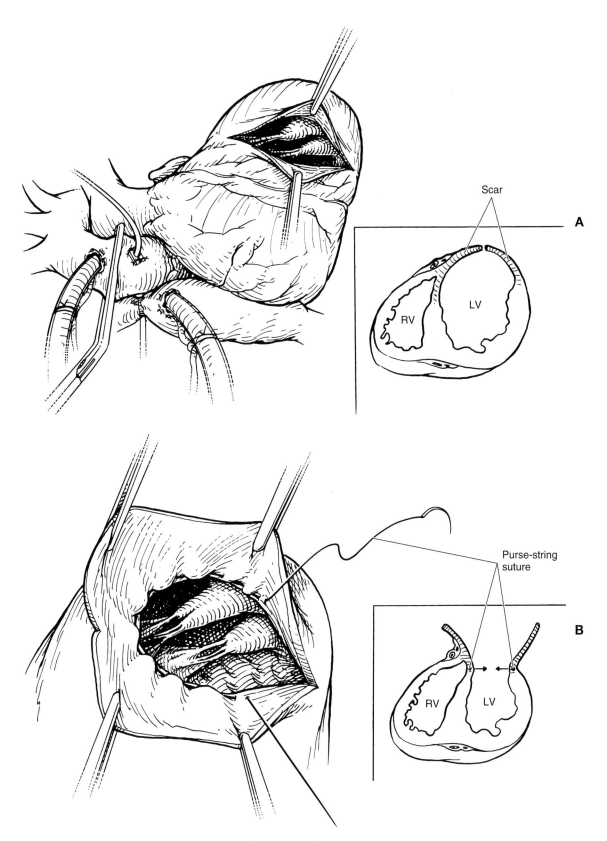

Figure 8-4   Technique for repair of anterior left ventricular aneurysm by patch closure. **A,** After the aorta is clamped and cardioplegic solution has been infused, an incision is made in the thinnest portion of the aneurysm parallel to the interventricular groove (inset). **B,** A purse-string suture of No. 2-0 polypropylene is placed at the line of demarcation between scar and contractile myocardium on the septum and free wall (inset). The longitudinal and transverse dimensions of the resulting defect are measured.

Key: *LV,* Left ventricle; *RV,* right ventricle.

Continued

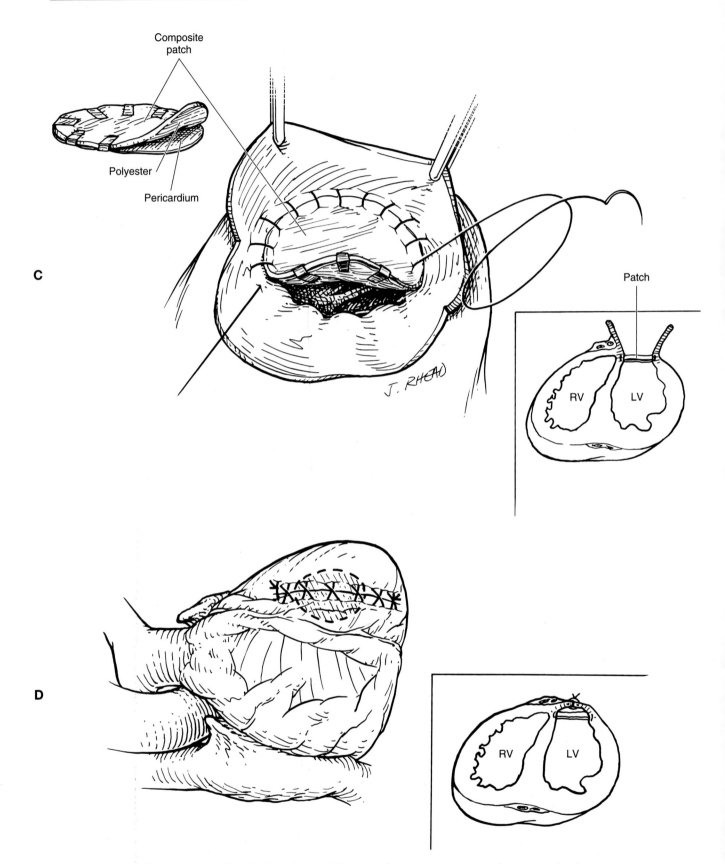

Figure 8-4, cont'd **C,** A patch of gelatin- or collagen-impregnated polyester or of polyester backed with pericardium (inset) is fashioned with slightly larger dimensions (0.5 cm) and is sutured into place, incorporating the purse-string suture, with a continuous No. 3-0 polypropylene suture. **D,** The remnant of the aneurysmal wall is trimmed and sutured securely over the patch with a continuous No. 2-0 polypropylene suture (inset).

Key: *LV,* Left ventricle; *RV,* right ventricle.

rationale for this technique is based in part on the fact that, coexisting with anterior LV aneurysm, scar tissue and akinesis or dyskinesis are present in the anterior portion of the LV septum. When a patch is used for closure, the area of septal scarring can be excluded from the reconstructed LV. This may result in improved LV function.[C14,D4,J4] Furthermore, curvature of the left anterior wall may be maintained.[H7]

Based on echocardiographic measurements in normal hearts, Fontan determined that the patch should be oval and should have a long diameter of 2 to 2.5 cm in situ. Thus, it should be made 2.5 to 3 cm in length to compensate for the space taken up by the suture line.[F3] A patch that is too large may result in too large an end-diastolic LV volume and thus a reduced global ejection fraction. A patch that is too small may reduce LV volume and compliance.[S13]

After opening the LV, the line of demarcation between scar and contractile LV myocardium is identified (Fig. 8-4, A [insert]). This may be facilitated by palpation if cardioplegia is not used during this portion of the operation.[A6] A purse-string suture of No. 2-0 polypropylene is placed at the junction of scar and contractile septal and free wall myocardium (Fig. 8-4, B). The longitudinal and transverse dimensions of the resulting defect are measured. A patch of gelatin or collagen-impregnated polyester (that can be lined with autologous pericardium) with slightly larger (0.5 cm) dimensions is fashioned and then sutured into place with a continuous No. 3-0 polypropylene suture (Fig. 8-4, C). Before completing the suture line, air is evacuated from the LV by infusion of volume from the pump-oxygenator, gentle inflation of the lungs, and injection of saline. This suture line must be watertight to avoid formation of a false aneurysm. The remnant of the aneurysm is trimmed, if necessary, and is closed securely over the patch with a continuous No. 2-0 polypropylene suture (Fig. 8-4, D).

A second alternative procedure in patients without a calcified aneurysm, and the rare patient with a small LV cavity, is direct LV reconstruction using multiple concentric purse-string sutures without a patch.[C16,M14]

Posterior Aneurysm

The techniques described for repair of anterior LV aneurysms are also applicable to posterior aneurysms. However, the defects remaining after excision of the scar or after circular reduction with a suture are generally smaller. Injury to the posterior papillary muscle at the lateral edge of the defect and to the posterior descending coronary artery on the medial edge of the defect must be avoided.

Associated Mitral Regurgitation

Some degree of mitral regurgitation is often present in patients with LV aneurysm. If repair of the valve is possible, it may be accomplished with standard techniques through a left atrial approach (see Technique of Operation in Chapter 11). Alternatively, the "edge to edge" repair technique proposed by Alfieri and colleagues can be performed through the ventriculotomy.[M10]

If replacement of the valve is indicated, it can be performed through the opened LV for posterior as well as anterior aneurysms (Fig. 8-5). The ventricle is opened as previously described, and the mitral valve is examined (Fig. 8-5, A). If replacement is indicated, the mitral valve leaflets are excised and all chordae tendineae are transected. A small remnant of anterior leaflet is left adjacent to the cusps of the aortic valve (Fig. 8-5, B). The valve holder apparatus is removed from the appropriately sized mechanical or bioprosthetic valve, and the valve is inverted and suspended by two hemostats. Interrupted, pledgeted mattress sutures of No. 2-0 polyester are placed through the mitral anulus, with the pledgets positioned on the atrial side (Fig. 8-5, C). These sutures are placed through the sewing ring of the prosthesis on the undersurface of the flanged portion (see Fig. 8-5, C). The valve is then lowered into the anulus and the sutures tied (Fig. 8-5, D). A soft rubber catheter is used to keep the leaflets of the prosthesis in the open position until air is evacuated from the pulmonary veins and left atrium. The LV is then reconstructed using one of the techniques previously described.

SPECIAL FEATURES OF POSTOPERATIVE CARE

Postoperative care is the same as that for other patients after intracardiac operations (see Chapter 5) and particularly after CABG. The detailed care late postoperatively required for patients undergoing CABG (see Special Features of Postoperative Care in Chapter 7) should also be applied to patients whose operation has included resection of a postinfarction LV aneurysm.

RESULTS

Survival

Early (Hospital) Death

Hospital mortality after LV aneurysm repair, with or without concomitant CABG, is about 5% to 7%,[E1,F3,J2,J4,K8,K9,M8,M9,M13,S12,V3] down from 10% to 20% in the earlier era (1958 to 1978) of cardiac surgery (Table 8-2).[B1,B10,C5,C7,L3,M2,M3,O1,R1,R2] The reduction in mortality over the past 10 to 20 years is related to improved surgical techniques, better myocardial management, greater efforts to perform concomitant CABG, better protection against embolization during operation, and use of adjunctive measures in patients with associated intractable ventricular tachycardia. No consistent difference in early mortality has been demonstrated between the classic (linear closure) and endoaneurysmorrhaphy (circular or patch closure) techniques.[J4,K8,K9,M13,S11,S12,V3]

Time-Related Survival

Overall time-related survival of heterogeneous groups of patients undergoing resection of LV aneurysms has varied, but in general, 30-day and 1-, 3-, and 5-year survival has been about 90%, 85%, 75%, and 65%, respectively[B1,B10,C2,E1,F4,F6,K8,S12] (Figs. 8-6 and 8-7). Several studies[M9,M13,V3] report higher 5-year survival (80% to 88%). This is generally better than survival after nonsurgical treatment.[C6,F4,G3] Not unexpectedly, the differences in outcome after surgical and nonsurgical treatment are particularly evident in patients with coexisting three-system disease.[F7]

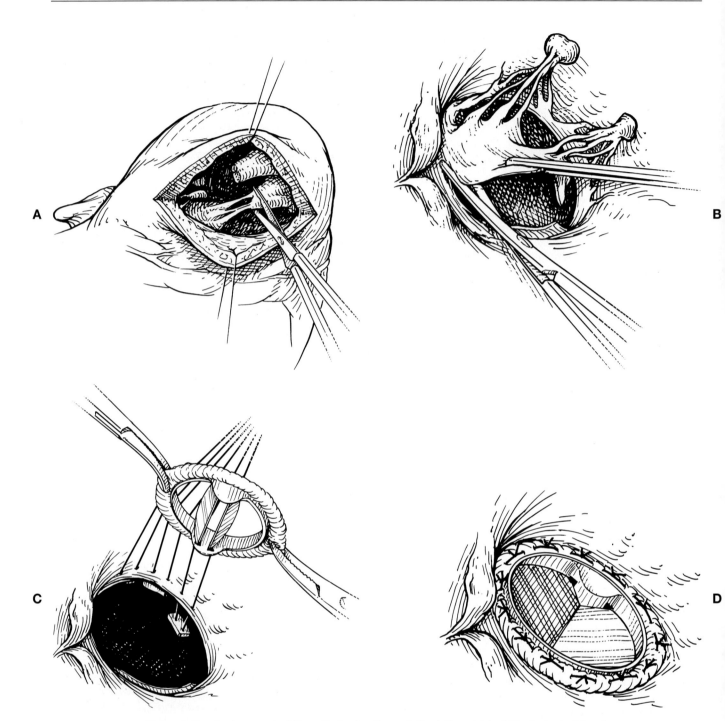

Figure 8-5 Replacement of the mitral valve through the left ventricle (LV). **A,** An incision is made in the thinnest portion of the aneurysm parallel to the interventricular groove, and the mitral valve is examined. The chordae tendineae are divided at the tips of the papillary muscles. **B,** The mitral valve leaflets are excised. A small rim of anterior leaflet is left adjacent to the cusps of the aortic valve. **C,** The valve holder apparatus is removed from the mechanical valve or bioprosthesis, and the valve is inverted and suspended by two hemostats. Interrupted, pledgeted mattress sutures of No. 2-0 polyester are placed through the mitral anulus, with the pledgets on the atrial side of the anulus. These sutures are then placed through the sewing ring of the prosthesis on the underside of the flanged portion. **D,** The valve is lowered into the anulus and the sutures tied. The LV is reconstructed using one of the techniques described in Figs. 8-3 and 8-4.

■ **TABLE 8-2   Early Results from Resection or Plication of Left Ventricular Aneurysms, Scars, and Infarcts (1969-1982)**

	n	No.	%	CL (%)
		Hospital Deaths		
True LVA	145	22	15	12-19
Scar or infarct	24	3	12	6-24
LVA + valve surgery	7	1	14	2-41
LVA or infarct + VSD surgery	3	0	0	0-47
False LVA	2	0	0	0-61
TOTAL	181	26	14	12-18

(Data from Barratt-Boyes and colleagues.[B10])

Key: *LVA,* Left ventricular aneurysm; *VSD,* ventricular septal defect.

Modes of Death

The most common mode of death early after operation is acute cardiac failure.[S12,V3,V4] In the late postoperative period, the mode of death is progressive chronic heart failure in about one third of patients and acute heart failure after another myocardial infarction in another third. Intractable ventricular tachycardia and sudden death have been the mode in about 15% of patients in the past, but the prevalence may be lower now as a result of more effective intraoperative management and medical and surgical treatment.

Incremental Risk Factors for Premature Death

In patients undergoing LV aneurysmectomy, risk factors for premature death and other unfavorable outcome events are generally the same as those in other patients with ischemic heart disease. The lower probability of time-related survival of patients undergoing LV aneurysmectomy (with or without concomitant CABG) is explained for the most part by their greater likelihood of having risk factors relating to myocardial scarring.[C12]

Severity and Extent of Coronary Arterial Stenoses

When complete revascularization is not accomplished in operations for ischemic heart disease, severity and extent of residual coronary arterial stenoses may appear as risk factors for most unfavorable outcome events. When severity and extent of coronary artery disease have not been identified as risk factors for death early or late after operation,[B5,C9,F1,K3,K8,R4,V3,W1] the presumption is that complete revascularization has been accomplished. In other groups of patients, preoperative severity and extent of coronary arterial stenoses have been risk factors.[B10] Presumably, they represent groups of patients in whom revascularization was necessarily incomplete.

Extent and Location of Myocardial Scar

By definition, patients with LV aneurysm have considerable myocardial scarring, and the scar is neither completely removed nor exteriorized by the operation. New scar formation occurs at the suture lines. Nonaneurysmal muscle may be scarred as well.

Risk factors for death both early and late after resection of LV aneurysms that are surrogates for myocardial scar include preoperative resting LV dysfunction and chronic heart failure[B1,K8,M6,M13,N4,R4,R5,W2] (Fig. 8-8). Other surrogates

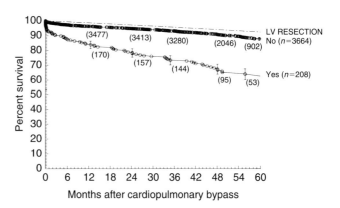

Figure 8-6   Survival of patients undergoing left ventricular (LV) resection for aneurysm and coronary artery bypass grafting compared with that of patients in whom no LV resection was done. Hospital deaths are included. The dash-dot-dash line represents survival of an age-sex-race–matched general population. (From UAB, 1977 to 1981.)

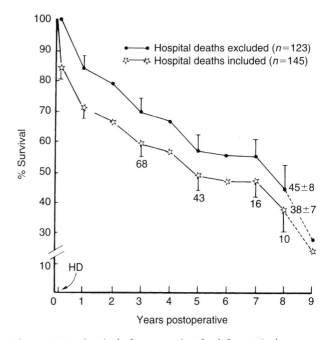

Figure 8-7   Survival after operation for left ventricular aneurysm, with and without hospital deaths included. The numbers of patients at risk are noted. (Data from Barratt-Boyes and colleagues.[B10])

identified as risk factors include preoperatively reduced cardiac output,[C7,K2,M2,S10] elevated LV end-diastolic pressure,[K6] impaired septal systolic function,[M3] higher New York Heart Association (NYHA) functional class (Fig. 8-9), poor segmental wall motion,[B1,B12,B14,R4] important mitral regurgitation,[M13] and ventricular tachycardia.[M13]

Also related to the extent and location of the myocardial scarring is the complication of *life-threatening ventricular tachycardia.* This is clearly a risk factor for death both early and late postoperatively[F6,M13] (see Section 7, "Ventricular Tachycardia/Ventricular Fibrillation in Ischemic Heart Disease," in Chapter 45).

Type of Operation

As in other cardiac operations, the risk of death after aneurysmectomy was higher in earlier eras.[B10]

Fontan and Dor and colleagues suggest that survival is improved by remodeling ventriculoplasty.[D4,F3] However, risk-adjusted comparisons, which are difficult to obtain, are required to be certain of long-term survival advantages. To date, no study has demonstrated a favorable effect of this procedure on late survival when compared with the linear closure technique.[J4,K9,S12,V3]

Other Risk Factors

Other risk factors for death and other unfavorable outcome events after CABG (see Tables 7-2, 7-7, and 7-8 in Chapter 7) also pertain to patients undergoing LV aneurysmectomy. For example, older age at operation is clearly a risk factor for death, both early and late after aneurysmectomy.[K8,R5]

Symptomatic Results

Most long-term survivors have substantial improvement in symptoms. The majority are in NYHA functional class I or II.[C10,D5,F4,K7,K8,M9,M13,S12] Improvement has also been demonstrated with exercise testing.[B8] Several[S12,V3,V4] but not all[K9] comparative studies have demonstrated greater symptomatic improvement among patients undergoing patch closure than among those who had linear closure of the ventriculotomy.

Late Postoperative Left Ventricular Function

Determining LV function late after resection of LV aneurysms presents the same problems and complexities as it

does in the case of the aneurysmal LV before operation (see "Left Ventricular Function" under Natural History earlier in this chapter). However, a reasonable amount of information is available.

The relationship between improvement in LV performance and symptomatic improvement is not entirely clear. Some patients with symptomatic improvement are without demonstrable improvement in LV function.[D3,F5] It is possible that current techniques of studying LV function may not identify the small increases in LV function that allow symptomatic improvement.

Although improvement is often noted in indices of LV function after aneurysmectomy without or with CABG,[C1,D5,D6,E1,K10,L5,M7,M13,S5,S12] it does not always occur. Possible mechanisms for failure to improve include:

- incomplete aneurysm resection (e.g., Froehlich and colleagues found in most of their patients that only 50% of the noncontractile area visualized by left ventriculography was resected[F5]);
- small size of the aneurysm, leading to small changes in function after resection (Fig. 8-10);
- large size of akinetic scar resulting from resection;[S5,S9] and
- intraoperative damage to nonaneurysmal portions of the ventricle.

Also, despite improved resting LV function, some patients show no improvement in exercise ejection frac-

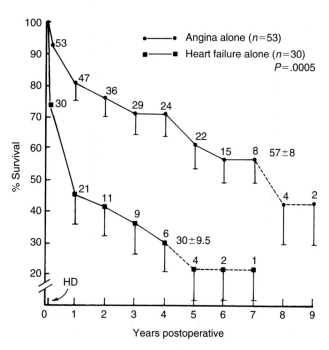

Figure 8-8   Survival after operation for isolated left ventricular aneurysm, comparing those with heart failure as the only symptom with those complaining only of angina. The numbers of patients at risk are noted. (Data from Barratt-Boyes and colleagues.[B10])

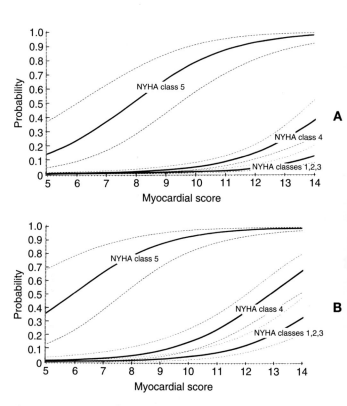

Figure 8-9   Nomogram of a multivariable logistic equation for probability of hospital death after left ventricular (LV) aneurysmectomy. Dashed lines enclose 70% confidence limits. The interacting incremental risks of a high myocardial score and poor functional status, related in part to poor LV function, are demonstrated. **A,** With ≤80 mg furosemide daily. **B,** With >80 mg furosemide daily. (Data from Barratt-Boyes and colleagues.[B10])

tion or stroke volume.[D6] Often, however, the improvement in global and regional ejection fraction during exercise is striking,[K10,M4,T2] and some experience suggests that the patch closure technique will produce even better results.[F3,K10]

Paradoxical movement in the segments in the border zone during isovolemic contraction is usually eliminated by aneurysmectomy.[N5] This effect may be the result of more favorable geometry in these segments, a reduction in wall stress related to decreased chamber size, or better coronary perfusion produced by CABG. Wall thickening increases in some but not all uninvolved (remote) segments; in some improved segments, operation fails to increase blood supply.[N5] The postoperative segmental wall function of these areas is well correlated ($r = .76$) with the patient's preoperative functional class, hence presumably with preoperative segmental wall motion. Thus, improvements in LV function are most evident in patients with heart failure preoperatively.[P5]

A reduction in end-diastolic pressure is well correlated with the clinical improvement in some patients.[S5] In three patients with single-system LAD disease and classic aneurysm, Harman and colleagues in 1969 demonstrated that simple resection, without CABG, increased LV ejection fraction, stroke volume, and stroke work, as well as cardiac index, and reduced LV end-diastolic pressure and volume.[H1] Two of the three patients were also relieved of angina pectoris. The data suggest that the resection and resultant decrease in LV volume decreased wall force according to the LaPlace law. The decreased tension (afterload) during systole probably increased the rate of fiber shortening, thereby increasing stroke volume, and decreased myocardial oxygen consumption, thereby decreasing angina pectoris (see "Ventricular Afterload" under Cardiac Output and Its Determinants in Section 1 of Chapter 5).

INDICATIONS FOR OPERATION

A large LV aneurysm in a symptomatic patient, particularly one with angina pectoris but also in one with heart failure, is an indication for operation. Appropriate CABG is indicated at the time of aneurysmectomy, as described in Chapter 7. Currently, the patch closure technique for remodeling ventriculoplasty appears to be preferable for the repair of anterolateral aneurysms.

In view of the high risk of operation in patients with advanced chronic heart failure, operation may not be indicated when the known risk factors are highly unfavorable to survival. It is apparent (see Fig. 8-9) that a patient with an LV aneurysm, NYHA class V, a myocardial score of 8 (two-system disease) or more, and severe heart failure has an 80% probability of hospital death (CL 55%-90%); if the myocardial score is 11 or greater, the risk approaches 100%. In both circumstances, operation may be contraindicated, although current methods of myocardial management may allow some such patients to survive operation and be clinically improved. The risk is lower when heart failure is less severe; under such circumstances, operation is clearly advisable. In borderline cases, akinesia or dyskinesia of the posterior-basal segment of the LV is recognized as an additional risk factor.

When the LV aneurysm is small or moderate in size, its presence is not an indication for operation per se. This conclusion is based in part on the fact that many preoperatively diagnosed aneurysms are not found to be aneurysms at operation or autopsy. Patients in such situations are advised about operation based on their coronary artery disease and LV function, as described in Chapter 7, rather than on their aneurysm. In this regard, it is noteworthy that an aneurysm that remains small 1 year after myocardial infarction is unlikely to enlarge progressively thereafter, and embolization from it is unlikely.

When indications for resection of an LV aneurysm are present, there is no reason to defer the operation for maturation of the aneurysm. Walker and colleagues, for example, report 1 hospital death among 20 patients (5%; CL 0.6%-16%) undergoing operation within 8 weeks of acute infarction.[W1] Six of the patients underwent early operation because of recurrent ventricular tachycardia. The long-term results were excellent, with 92% survival at 5 years.

LV scars encountered in the operating room during surgery for coronary artery disease may require excision if they clearly contain little muscle and are of important size. Di Donato, Dor, and colleagues have demonstrated comparable improvement in resting ejection fraction in patients with akinetic scars and those with dyskinetic scars (aneurysms) following endoventricular circular patch plasty repair.[D7,D8] They and others[A5,B15] have postulated that patients with heart failure, previous anterior myocardial infarction, and LV dilatation or akinesia may benefit from this type of repair as well. Preliminary results from a multicenter registry of 421 patients undergoing endoventricular patch plasty repair indicate a low operative mortality of 6.6% (CL 5.4%-8.1%) and survival of 95% at 1 month and 87% at 12 months.[A5] Among a cohort of the surviving patients, LV ejection fraction increased from 29%

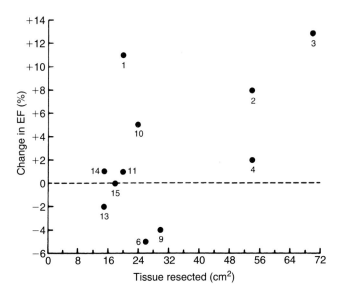

Figure 8-10 Relationship between size of resected left ventricular (LV) wall (aneurysm) and change in resting ejection fraction (EF) after LV aneurysmectomy with or without coronary artery bypass grafting. Although the number of patients is small, the data suggest that EF is increased postoperatively only when the aneurysm is large. (Data from Froehlich and colleagues.[F5])

to 39%, and LV end-systolic volume index decreased from 109 mL · m^{-2} to 69 mL · m^{-2}.

SPECIAL SITUATIONS AND CONTROVERSIES

Intractable Ventricular Tachyarrhythmias

Although intractable ventricular tachyarrhythmias occur in patients with ischemic heart disease in the absence of areas of LV scarring, they are more common in patients with LV aneurysms or extensive fibrosis. However, only a small proportion with LV aneurysms develop intractable ventricular tachycardia.[C11] Most patients in whom such an arrhythmia develops have poor global LV function,[A2] and it has been suggested that ventricular tachyarrhythmias are particularly likely to occur when the ventricular septum has been involved in the infarction. As a corollary, poor LV function and nonresponsiveness to drug therapy for ventricular tachycardia have been identified as risk factors for sudden cardiac death.[S7] Management of patients with the combination of LV aneurysm and intractable ventricular tachyarrhythmias is discussed in detail in Section 7, "Ventricular Tachycardia/Ventricular Fibrillation in Ischemic Heart Disease," in Chapter 45.

False Left Ventricular Aneurysm

The aneurysms discussed in this chapter, so-called true aneurysms, are formed by scarring, thinning, and stretching of an infarcted area of LV wall. This process produces a wide-mouthed aneurysm. By contrast, a *false aneurysm* develops after acute rupture of an infarcted area of LV. Such ruptures are usually fatal, but when the pericardium is sufficiently adherent to the epicardium, rupture may result only in a localized hemopericardium. Persistent communication of the hemopericardium with the LV cavity results in gradual expansion of the hemopericardium into a false aneurysm whose wall is composed of pericardium and adhesions[C8,R3] and occasionally of myocardium,[S14] and whose mouth is usually narrow.[V1] Such aneurysms have a strong tendency to rupture,[G6,V2] in contrast to so-called true aneurysms. False aneurysms are much more likely to occur posteriorly (on the diaphragmatic surface of the LV) or laterally than are true aneurysms.

Differentiation between true and false aneurysms can be difficult, because the imaging characteristics of the two entities are often similar.[B16] However, Doppler color flow imaging and transesophageal echocardiography are useful techniques for demonstrating the presence of a false aneurysm.[B17,R6]

Resection of an LV false aneurysm is clearly advisable.[G2,H2,S14,S15] The resection may pose formidable problems when the false sac extends anteriorly beneath the sternum. It is then necessary to begin CPB via cannulae introduced into the femoral artery and vein. If the false aneurysm is very large, the patient is cooled to 20°C before the sternum is opened. As soon as possible, the aorta is clamped, cardioplegia induced (see Chapter 3), and the operation begun. The false sac is entered, and blood from this sac is returned to the circuit using cardiotomy suckers. The aneurysmal wall is resected or left alone, and the LV is

reconstructed using techniques described earlier in this chapter (see Technique of Operation). When indicated, CABG is also performed.

Postinfarction Left Ventricular Free Wall Rupture

Acute rupture of the free wall of the LV may complicate acute myocardial infarction.[N2] It has been reported to occur in 4% to 24% of patients with acute infarction.[R7] It is the second most common cause of death following acute infarction (behind pump failure), accounting for up to 20% of early deaths.[R7,R8,S2] Rupture generally occurs between 1 and 7 days after the infarction.[R7,R8] Occasionally the rupture is massive, and death quickly results from exsanguination.[B4] Cardiac rupture is usually not a "blowout" phenomenon but a more gradual process that begins with small endocardial tears. These permit formation of a hematoma, which gradually dissects through the area of necrosis into the pericardium, resulting in sudden fatal pericardial tamponade.[K4,S2] Rupture occurs most commonly on the anterior or lateral wall of the LV, and more specifically at about the middle of the ventricle along the axis from the base to the apex.[S2,V5]

Myocardial free wall rupture should be suspected in patients with recent myocardial infarction who have recurrent or persistent chest pain, hemodynamic instability, syncope, pericardial tamponade, or transient electromechanical dissociation.[R8] The diagnosis can be made with echocardiography, which demonstrates a pericardial effusion or pericardial thrombus.[R8]

Operation is indicated unless the patient is moribund. If the patient is hemodynamically unstable with evidence of tamponade, rapid infusion of fluids and pericardiocentesis may permit stabilization. An intraaortic balloon should also be inserted.[P4] If the hemodynamic state does not improve, CPB can be established by peripheral cannulation (see "Cardiopulmonary Bypass Established by Peripheral Cannulation" under Special Situations and Controversies in Section 3 in Chapter 2). Preoperative coronary angiography is not advisable unless the hemodynamic state is very stable.

Several different approaches have been used for surgical treatment of ventricular free wall rupture. Padró and colleagues have reported success with a sutureless technique, applying a large PTFE felt patch over the myocardial tear and securing it to the surface of the LV with cyanoacrylate glue in 13 patients.[P6] The procedure was accomplished without the use of CPB in 12 of the 13. All survived the procedure and were alive during a mean follow-up interval of 26 months. Nunez and colleagues reported success in four of seven patients in whom a large PTFE patch was sutured to the normal myocardium surrounding the area of rupture.[N3] CPB was used for these procedures. Simple closure of the area of rupture on the anterior and lateral wall with pledgeted sutures has also been successfully employed.[S4] The more traditional approach involves the use of CPB, infarctectomy, and closure of the defect with a polyester patch.[D9,Y1] CABG can be added when appropriate. When surgical treatment is applied appropriately, long-term survival is possible.[B11,N3,P4,P6]

Congenital Left Ventricular Aneurysm

A congenital LV aneurysm is a rare malformation characterized by thinning of the myocardium, with complete layers intermingled with various amounts of fibrous tissue.[J5,M12] It is usually located at the apex of the LV and has a broad neck.[M12] This entity differs from a *congenital diverticulum* of the LV, which is a noncontractile bulging of the LV into the epigastrium.[H4] The latter is characterized by an elongated shape and a narrow connection with the LV cavity.[M12] It is also associated with midline thoracic and anterior abdominal defects.[E2] Both conditions are rare and have been treated surgically with good results.[H6,L4,S17]

Traumatic Left Ventricular Aneurysm

Rarely, violent nonpenetrating trauma to the chest produces such a severe contusion of the heart that a localized aneurysm forms.[G7,S6] Vascular injury and intramyocardial dissection resulting from blunt trauma may also lead to formation of an aneurysm.[C15,M11] The aneurysm, which is usually well localized and often thin walled, may be detected early after the trauma or not until several years later.[B6,P3,S16] Because of the thin wall and the propensity for rupture, a posttraumatic LV aneurysm should be resected whenever possible.

REFERENCES

A

1. Austen WG, Tsunekawa T, Bender HW, Ebert PA, Morrow AG. The acute hemodynamic effects of left ventricular aneurysm. J Surg Res 1962;2:161.
2. Arciniegas JG, Klein H, Karp RB, Kouchoukos NT, James TN, Kirklin JW, et al. Surgical treatment of life-threatening ventricular tachyarrhythmias (abstract). Circulation 1980;62:III42.
3. Arvan S, Badillo P. Contractile properties of the left ventricle with aneurysm. Am J Cardiol 1985;55:338.
4. Akins CW. Resection of left ventricular aneurysm during hypothermic fibrillatory arrest without aortic occlusion. J Thorac Cardiovasc Surg 1986;91:610.
5. Athanasuleas CL, Stanley AW Jr, Buckberg GD, Dor V, Di Donato M, Blackstone EH. Surgical anterior ventricular endocardial restoration (SAVER) in the dilated remodeled ventricle after anterior myocardial infarction. RESTORE group. Reconstructive endoventricular surgery: returning torsion original radius elliptical shape to the LV. J Am Coll Cardiol 2001;37:1199.
6. Athanasuleas CL, Stanley AW Jr, Buckberg GD. Restoration of contractile function in the enlarged left ventricle by exclusion of remodeled akinetic anterior segment: surgical strategy, myocardial protection, and angiographic results. J Card Surg 1998;13:418.

B

1. Burton NA, Stinson EB, Oyer PE, Shumway NE. Left ventricular aneurysm. Preoperative risk factors and long-term postoperative results. J Thorac Cardiovasc Surg 1979;77:65.
2. Banka VS, Bodenheimer MM, Helfant RH. Determinants of reversible asynergy. Effect of pathologic Q waves, coronary collaterals, and anatomic location. Circulation 1974;50:714.
3. Bruschke AV, Proudfit WL, Sones FM Jr. Progress study of 590 consecutive nonsurgical cases of coronary disease followed by 5-9 years. II. Ventriculographic and other correlations. Circulation 1973;47:1154.
4. Balakumaran K, Verbaan CJ, Essed CE, Nauta J, Bos E, Haalebos MM, et al. Ventricular free wall rupture: sudden, subacute, slow, sealed and stabilized varieties. Eur Heart J 1984;5:282.
5. Brawley RK, Schaff H, Stevens R, Ducci H, Gott VL, Donahoo JS. Influence of coronary artery anatomy on survival following resection of left ventricular aneurysms and chronic infarcts. J Thorac Cardiovasc Surg 1977;763:120.
6. Berkoff HA, Rowe GG, Crummy AB, Kahn DR. Asymptomatic left ventricular aneurysm: a sequela of blunt chest trauma. Circulation 1977;55:545.
7. Buehler DL, Stinson EB, Oyer PE, Shumway NE. Surgical treatment of aneurysms of the inferior left ventricular wall. J Thorac Cardiovasc Surg 1979;78:74.
8. Balu V, Hook N, Dean DC, Naughton J. Effect of left ventricular aneurysmectomy on exercise performance. Int J Cardiol 1984;5:210.

9. Bulkley BH, Roberts WC. Steroid therapy during acute myocardial infarction: a cause of delayed healing and of ventricular aneurysm. Am J Med 1974;56:244.
10. Barratt-Boyes BG, White HD, Agnew TM, Pemberton JR, Wild C. The results of surgical treatment of left ventricular aneurysms: an assessment of the risk factors affecting early and late mortality. J Thorac Cardiovasc Surg 1984;87:87.
11. Baudouy PY, Menashe P, Kural S, Wolff M, Piwnica A. Acute left ventricular rupture secondary to myocardial infarction. Report of long-term survival after early surgical repair. Thorac Cardiovasc Surg 1982;30:409.
12. Bogers AJ, Hermans J, Dubois SV, Huysmans HA. Incremental risk factors for hospital mortality after postinfarction left ventricular aneurysmectomy. Eur J Cardiothorac Surg 1988;2:160.
13. Buck T, Hunold P, Klaus U, Wentz KU, Tkalec W, Nesser HJ, et al. Tomographic three-dimensional echocardiographic determination of chamber size and systolic function in patients with left ventricular aneurysm. Circulation 1997;96:4286.
14. Banka VS, Agarwal JB, Bodenheimer MM, Helfant RH. Interventricular septal motion: biventricular angiographic assessment of its relative contribution to left and right ventricular contraction. Circulation 1981;64:992.
15. Buckberg GD. Defining the relationship between akinesia and dyskinesia and the cause of left ventricular failure after anterior infarction and reversal of remodeling to restoration. J Thorac Cardiovasc Surg 1998;116:47.
16. Brown SL, Gropler RJ, Harris KM. Distinguishing left ventricular aneurysm from pseudoaneurysm. Chest 1997;111:1403.
17. Burns CA, Paulsen W, Arrowood JA, Tolman DE, Rose B, Fabian JA, et al. Improved identification of posterior left ventricular pseudoaneurysms by transesophageal echocardiography. Am Heart J 1992;124:796.

C

1. Cohnheim J, Schulthess Rechberg AV. Uber die folgen der kranzarterienverschliessung für das Hertz. Virchows Arch [A] 1881;85:503.
2. Cooley DA, Henly WS, Amad KH, Chapman DW. Ventricular aneurysm following myocardial infarction: results of surgical treatment. Ann Surg 1959;150.
3. Cheng TO. Incidence of ventricular aneurysm in coronary artery disease: an angiographic appraisal. Am J Med 1971;50:340.
4. Cabin HS, Roberts WC. True left ventricular aneurysm and healed myocardial infarction: clinical and necropsy observations including quantification of degrees of coronary arterial narrowing. Am J Cardiol 1980;46:754.
5. Cooley DA, Hallman GL. Surgical treatment of left ventricular aneurysm: experience with excision of postinfarction lesions in 80 patients. Prog Cardiovasc Dis 1968;11:222.
6. Cullhed I, Delius W, Bjork I, Hallen A, Nordgren I. Resection of left ventricular aneurysm: late results. Acta Med Scand 1975;197:241.

7. Coopermann M, Stinson EB, Griepp RB, Shumway NF. Survival and function after left ventricular aneurysmectomy. J Thorac Cardiovasc Surg 1975;69:321.

8. Chesler E, Korns ME, Semba T, Edwards JF. False aneurysm of the left ventricle following myocardial infarction. Am J Cardiol 1969;23:76.

9. Cosgrove DM, Loop FD, Irarrazaval MG, Groves LK, Taylor PC, Golding LA. Determinants of long-term survival after ventricular aneurysmectomy. Ann Thorac Surg 1978;26:257.

10. Crosby IK, Wellons HA Jr, Martin RP, Schuch D, Muller WH Jr. Employability: a new indication for aneurysmectomy and coronary revascularization. Circulation 1980;62:I79.

11. Cohen M, Wienar I, Pichard A, Holt J, Smith H, Gorlin R. Determinants of ventricular tachycardia in patients with coronary artery disease and ventricular aneurysm: clinical, hemodynamic and angiographic factors. Am J Cardiol 1983;51:61.

12. Cohen DE, Vogel RA. Left ventricular aneurysm as a coronary risk factor independent of overall left ventricular function. Am Heart J 1986;111:23.

13. Cabin HS, Clubb KS, Wackers FJ, Zaret BL. Right ventricular myocardial infarction with anterior wall left ventricular infarction: an autopsy study. Am Heart J 1987;113:16.

14. Cooley DA. Ventricular endoaneurysmorrhaphy: a simplified repair for extensive postinfarction aneurysm. J Card Surg 1989;4:200.

15. Candell J, Valle V, Paya J, Cortadellas J, Esplugas E, Rius J. Post-traumatic coronary occlusion and early left ventricular aneurysm. Am Heart J 1979;97:509.

16. Calderia C, McCarthy PM. A simple method of left ventricular reconstruction without patch for ischemic cardiomyopathy. Ann Thorac Surg 2001;72:2148.

D

1. Dubnow MH, Burchell HB, Titus JL. Postinfarction ventricular aneurysm: a clinicomorphologic and electrocardiographic study of 80 cases. Am Heart J 1965;70:753.

2. Davis RW, Ebert PA. Ventricular aneurysm: a clinical-pathologic correlation. Am J Cardiol 1972;29:1.

3. Di Mattia DG, Di Biasi P, Salati M, Mangini A, Fundaró P, Santoli C. Surgical treatment of left ventricular post-infarction aneurysm with endoventriculoplasty: late clinical and functional results. Eur J Cardiothorac Surg 1999;15:413.

4. Dor V, Saab M, Coste P, Lornaszeweska M, Montiglio F. Left ventricular aneurysm: a new surgical approach. Thorac Cardiovasc Surg 1989;37:11.

5. Dor V, Sabatier M, Di Donato M, Maioli M, Toso A, Montiglio F. Late hemodynamic results after left ventricular patch repair associated with coronary grafting in patients with postinfarction akinetic or dyskinetic aneurysm of the left ventricle. J Thorac Cardiovasc Surg 1995;110:1291.

6. Dymond DS, Stephens JD, Stone DL, Elliott AT, Rees GM, Spurrell RA. Combined exercise radionuclide and hemodynamic evaluation of left ventricular aneurysmectomy. Am Heart J 1982;104:977.

7. Di Donato M, Sabatier M, Dor V, Toso A, Maioli M, Fantini F. Akinetic versus dyskinetic postinfarction scar: relation to surgical outcome in patients undergoing endoventricular circular patch plasty repair. J Am Coll Cardiol 1997;29:1569.

8. Dor V, Sabatier M, Di Donato M, Montiglio F, Toso A, Maioli M. Efficacy of endoventricular patch plasty in large postinfarction kinetic scar and severe left ventricular dysfunction: comparison with a series of large dyskinetic scars. J Thorac Cardiovasc Surg 1998;116:50.

9. Daggett WM, Buckley MJ, Akins CW, Leinbach RC, Gold HK, Block PC, et al. Improved results of surgical management of postinfarction ventricular septal rupture. Ann Surg 1982;196:269.

E

1. Elefteriades JA, Solomon LW, Salazar AM, Batsford WP, Baldwin JC, Kopf GS. Linear left ventricular aneurysmectomy: modern imaging studies reveal improved morphology and function. Ann Thorac Surg 1993;56:242.

2. Edgett JW Jr, Nelson WP, Hall RJ, Fishback ME, Jahnke EJ. Diverticulum of the heart. Part of the syndrome of congenital cardiac and midline thoracic and abdominal defects. Am J Cardiol 1969;24:580.

F

1. Fisher VJ, Alvarez AJ, Shah A, Dolgin M, Tice DA. Left ventricular scars: clinical and haemodynamic results of excision. Br Heart J 1974;36:132.

2. Faxon DP, Ryan TJ, Davis KB, McCabe CH, Myers W, Lesperance J, et al. Prognostic significance of angiographically documented left ventricular aneurysm from the Coronary Artery Surgery Study (CASS). Am J Cardiol 1982;50:157.

3. Fontan F. Transplantation of knowledge. J Thorac Cardiovasc Surg 1990;99:387.

4. Fontan F. The prognostic value of pre-operative left ventricular performance in left ventricular resection. Thorac Cardiovasc Surg 1979;27:281.

5. Froehlich RT, Falsetti HL, Doty DB, Marcus ML. Prospective study of surgery for left ventricular aneurysm. Am J Cardiol 1980;45:923.

6. Frank G, Klein H, Bednarska E, Gahl K, Flohr E, Trieb G, et al. Results after resection of postinfarction left ventricular aneurysms. Thorac Cardiovasc Surg 1980;28:423.

7. Faxon DP, Myers WO, McCabe CH, Davis KB, Schaff HV, Wilson JW, et al. The influence of surgery on the natural history of angiographically documented left ventricular aneurysm: the Coronary Artery Surgery Study. Circulation 1986;74:110.

8. Forman MB, Collins HW, Kopelman HA, Vaughn WK, Perry JM, Virmani R, et al. Determinants of left ventricular aneurysm formation after anterior myocardial infarction: a clinical and angiographic study. J Am Coll Cardiol 1986;8:1256.

G

1. Gorlin R, Klein MD, Sullivan JM. Prospective correlative study of ventricular aneurysm: mechanistic concept and clinical recognition. Am J Med 1967;42:512.

2. Gross H, Schwedel JB. The clinical course in ventricular aneurysm. N Y State J Med 1941;41:488.

3. Grondin P, Kretz JG, Bical O, Donzeau-Gouge P, Petitclerc R, Campeau L. Natural history of saccular aneurysms of the left ventricle. J Thorac Cardiovasc Surg 1979;77:57.

4. Gundry SR, Razzouk AJ, Vigesaa RE, Wang N, Bailey LL. Optimal delivery of cardioplegia for "redo" operations. J Thorac Cardiovasc Surg 1992;103:896.

5. Guez DH, Sideman S, Beyar R. Regional right ventricular endocardial motion in normal hearts and in hearts with left ventricular aneurysm: a three dimensional study. Int J Card Imaging 1997;13:281.

6. Gueron M, Wanderman KL, Hirsh M, Borman J. Pseudoaneurysm of the left ventricle after myocardial infarction: a curable form of myocardial rupture. J Thorac Cardiovasc Surg 1975;69:736.

7. Grieco JG, Montoya A, Sullivan HJ, Bakhos M, Foy BK, Blakeman B, et al. Ventricular aneurysm due to blunt chest injury. Ann Thorac Surg 1989;47:322.

H

1. Harman MA, Baxley WA, Jones WB, Dodge HT, Edwards S. Surgical intervention in chronic postinfarction cardiac failure. Circulation 1969;391:191.

2. Harper RW, Sloman G, Westlake G. Successful surgical resection of a chronic false aneurysm of the left ventricle. Chest 1975; 67:359.

3. Herman MV, Heinle RA, Klein MD, Gorlin R. Localized disorders in myocardial contraction: asynergy and its role in congestive heart disease. N Engl J Med 1967;277:222.

4. Hamaoka K, Onaka M, Tanaka T, Ohouchi Z. Congenital ventricular aneurysm and diverticulum in children. Pediatr Cardiol 1987; 8:169.

5. Hirai T, Fujita M, Nakajima H, Asanoi H, Yamanishi K, Ohno A, et al. Importance of collateral circulation for prevention of left ventricular aneurysm formation in acute myocardial infarction. Circulation 1989;79:791.

6. Hertzeanu H, Deutsch V, Yahini JH, Lieberman Y, Neufeld HN. Left ventricular aneurysm of unusual aetiology: report of two cases. Thorax 1976;31:220.

7. Hutchins GM, Brawley RK. The influence of cardiac geometry on the results of ventricular aneurysm repair. Am J Pathol 1980; 99:221.

8. Higgins CB. Newer cardiac imaging techniques: magnetic resonance imaging and computed tomography. In Braunwald E, ed. Heart disease. Philadelphia: WB Saunders, 1997, p. 336.

J

1. Johnson RA, Draggett WM Jr. Heart failure resulting from coronary artery disease. In Johnson RA, Haber E, Austen WG, eds. The practice of cardiology. Boston: Little, Brown, 1980, p. 345.

2. Jones EL, Craver JM, Hurst JW, Bradford JA, Bone DK, Robinson PH, et al. Influence of left ventricular aneurysm on survival following the coronary bypass operation. Ann Surg 1981;193:733.

3. Jan K. Distribution of myocardial stress and its influence on coronary blood flow. J Biomech 1985;18:815.

4. Jatene AD. Left ventricular aneurysmectomy: resection or reconstruction. J Thorac Cardiovasc Surg 1985;89:321.

5. Johansson L, Michaelsson M, Sjogren S. Congenital left ventricular apical aneurysm. Scand J Thorac Cardiovasc Surg 1976;10:135.

K

1. Kitamura S, Kay JH, Krohn BG, Magidson O, Dunne EF. Geometric and functional abnormalities of the left ventricle with a chronic localized noncontractile area. Am J Cardiol 1973;31:701.

2. Kiefer SK, Flaker GC, Martin RH, Curtis JJ. Clinical improvement after ventricular aneurysm repair: prediction by angiographic and hemodynamic variables. J Am Coll Cardiol 1983;2:30.

3. Kirklin JW, Blackstone EH, Rogers WJ. Bishop Lecture. The plights of the invasive treatment of ischemic heart disease. J Am Coll Cardiol 1985;5:158.

4. Kendall RW, DeWood MA. Postinfarction cardiac rupture: surgical success and review of the literature. Ann Thorac Surg 1978;25:311.

5. Klein MD, Herman MV, Gorlin R. A hemodynamic study of left ventricular aneurysm. Circulation 1967;35:614.

6. Kapelnaski DP, Al-Sadir J, Lambert JJ, Anagnostopoulos CE. Ventriculographic features predictive of surgical outcome for left ventricular aneurysm. Circulation 1978;58:1167.

7. Keenan DJ, Monro JL, Ross JK, Manners JM, Conway N, Johnson AM. Left ventricular aneurysm: the Wessex experience. Br Heart J 1985;54:269.

8. Komeda M, David TE, Malik A, Ivanov J, Sun Z. Operative risks and long-term results of operation for left ventricular aneurysm. Ann Thorac Surg 1992;53:22.

9. Kelser KA, Fiore AC, Naunheim KS, Sharp TG, Mahomed Y, Zollinger TW, et al. Anterior wall left ventricular aneurysm repair: a comparison of linear versus circular closure. J Thorac Cardiovasc Surg 1992;103:841.

10. Kawata T, Kitamura S, Kawachi K, Morita R, Yoshida Y, Hasegawa J. Systolic and diastolic function after patch reconstruction of left ventricular aneurysms. Ann Thorac Surg 1995;59:403.

L

1. Loeb J. Über partielle erweichende myocarditis (malacia cordis). Dissertation. University of Würzburg, Würzburg, West Germany, 1880.

2. Likoff W, Bailey CP. Ventriculoplasty: excision of myocardial aneurysm: report of a successful case. JAMA 1955;158:915.

3. Loop FD, Effler DB, Navia JA, Sheldon WC, Groves LK. Aneurysms of the left ventricle: survival and results of a ten-year surgical experience. Ann Surg 1973;178:399.

4. Lowe JB, Williams JC, Robb D, Cole D. Congenital diverticulum of the left ventricle. Br Heart J 1949;21:101.

5. Lu P, Liu X, Shi R, Mo L, Borer JS. Comparison of tomographic and planar radionuclide ventriculography in the assessment of regional left ventricular function in patients with left ventricular aneurysm before and after surgery. J Nucl Cardiol 1994;1:537.

M

1. Marie R. Anéyrisme de la pointe du coeur. Bull Soc Anat Paris 1896;11.

2. Moran JM, Scalon PJ, Nemickas R, Pifarre R. Surgical treatment of postinfarction ventricular aneurysm. Ann Thorac Surg 1976;21:107.

3. Mullen DC, Posey L, Gabriel R, Singh HM, Flemma RJ, Lepley D Jr. Prognostic considerations in the management of left ventricular aneurysms. Ann Thorac Surg 1977;23:455.

4. Mangschau A, Forfang K, Rootwelt K, Froysaker T. Improvement in cardiac performance and exercise tolerance after left ventricular aneurysm surgery: a prospective study. Thorac Cardiovasc Surg 1988;36:320.

5. Mourdjinis A, Olsen E, Raphael MJ. Clinical diagnosis and prognosis of ventricular aneurysm. Br Heart J 1968;30:497.

6. Marco JD, Kaiser GC, Barnes HE, Codd JE, Willman VL. Left ventricular aneurysmectomy. Arch Surg 1975;111:419.

7. Martin JL, Untereker WJ, Harken AH, Horowitz LN, Josephson ME. Aneurysmectomy and endocardial resection for ventricular tachycardia: favorable hemodynamic and antiarrhythmic results in patients with global left ventricular dysfunction. Am Heart J 1982;103:960.

8. Mills NL, Everson CT, Hockmuth DR. Technical advances in the treatment of left ventricular aneurysm. Ann Thorac Surg 1993;55:792.

9. Mickleborough LL, Maruyama H, Liu P, Mohamed S. Results of left ventricular aneurysmectomy with a tailored scar excision and primary closure technique. J Thorac Cardiovasc Surg 1994;107:690.

10. Maisano F, Torracca L, Oppizzi M, Stefano PL, D'Addario G, LaCanna G, et al. The edge-to-edge technique: a simplified method to correct mitral insufficiency. Eur J Cardiothorac Surg 1998;13:240.

11. Maselli D, Micalizzi E, Pizio R, Audo A, De Gasperis C. Posttraumatic left ventricular intramyocardial dissecting hematoma. Ann Thorac Surg 1997;64:830.

12. Matias A, Fredouille C, Nesmann C, Azancot A. Prenatal diagnosis of left ventricular aneurysm: a report of three cases and a review. Cardiol Young 1999;9:175.

13. Mickleborough LL, Carson S, Ivanov J. Repair of dyskinetic or akinetic left ventricular aneurysm: results obtained with a modified linear closure. J Thorac Cardiovasc Surg 2001;121:675.

14. Menicanti L, Dor V, Buckberg GC, Athanasuleas CL, Di Donato M, and the RESTORE group. Inferior wall restoration: anatomic and surgical considerations. Semin Thorac Cardiovasc Surg 2001;13:504.

N

1. Nagle RE, Williams DO. Natural history of ventricular aneurysm without surgical treatment (abstract). Br Heart J 1974;36:1037.

2. Norris RM, Sammel NL. Predictors of late hospital death in acute myocardial infarction. Prog Cardiovasc Dis 1980;23:129.

3. Nunez L, de la Llana R, Sendon JL, Coma J, Aguado MG, Larrea JL. Diagnosis and treatment of subacute free wall ventricular rupture after infarction. Ann Thorac Surg 1983;35:525.

4. Novick RJ, Stefanisyzn JH, Morin JE, Symes JF, Sniderman AD, Dobell AR. Surgery for postinfarction left ventricular aneurysm: prognosis and long-term follow-up. Can J Surg 1984;27:161.

5. Nicolosi AC, Spotnitz HM. Quantitative analysis of regional systolic function with left ventricular aneurysm. Circulation 1988;78:856.

O

1. Okies JE, Dietl C, Garrison HB, Starr A. Early and late results of resection of ventricular aneurysm. J Thorac Cardiovasc Surg 1978;75:255.

P

1. Phares WS, Edwards JE, Burchell HB. Cardiac aneurysms: clinico-pathologic studies. Proc Mayo Clin 1953;28:264.

2. Parmley WW, Chuck L, Kivowitz C, Matloff JM, Swan HJ. In vitro length–tension relations of human ventricular aneurysms: relation of stiffness to mechanical disadvantage. Am J Cardiol 1973;32:889.

3. Pupello DF, Daily PO, Stinson EB, Shumway NE. Successful repair of left ventricular aneurysm due to trauma. JAMA 1970;211:826.

4. Pifarre R, Sullivan JH, Grieco J, Montoya A, Bakhos M, Scanlon PF, et al. Management of left ventricular rupture complicating myocardial infarction. J Thorac Cardiovasc Surg 1983;86:441.

5. Palantianos GM, Craythorne CB, Schor JS, Bolooki H. Hemodynamic effects of radical left ventricular scar resection in patients with and without congestive heart failure. J Surg Res 1988;44:690.

6. Padró JM, Mesa JM, Silvestre J, Larrea JL, Caralps JM, Cerrón F, et al. Subacute cardiac rupture: repair with a sutureless technique. Ann Thorac Surg 1993;55:20.

R

1. Rogers WJ, Oberman A, Kouchoukos NT. Left ventricular aneurys-mectomy in patients with single vs. multivessel coronary artery disease. Circulation 1978;58:I50.

2. Rao G, Zikria EA, Miller WH, Samandani SR, Ford WB. Experience with sixty consecutive ventricular aneurysm resections. Circulation 1974;50:II149.

3. Roberts WC, Morrow AG. Pseudoaneurysm of the left ventricle: an unusual sequence of myocardial infarction and rupture of the heart. Am J Med 1967;43:639.

4. Rittenhouse EA, Sauvage LR, Mansfield PB, Smith JC, Davis CC, Hall DG, et al. Results of combined left ventricular aneurysmectomy and coronary artery bypass: 1974 to 1980. Am J Surg 1982;143:575.

5. Rizzoli G, Belloto F, Gallucci V, Gemelli M, Brumana T, Mazzucco A, et al. Early and late determinants of survival after surgery of left ventricular aneurysm. Eur J Cardiothorac Surg 1988;2:265.

6. Roelandt JR, Sutherland GR, Yoshida K, Yoshikawa J. Improved diagnosis and characterization of left ventricular pseudoaneurysm by Doppler color flow imaging. J Am Coll Cardiol 1988;12:807.

7. Reardon MJ, Carr CL, Diamond A, Letsou GV, Safi HJ, Espada R, et al. Ischemic left ventricular free wall rupture: prediction, diagnosis, and treatment. Ann Thorac Surg 1997;64:1509.

8. Raitt MH, Kraft CD, Gardner CJ, Pearlman AS, Otto CM. Subacute ventricular free wall rupture complicating myocardial infarction. Am Heart J 1993;126:946.

S

1. Sbokos CG, Monro JL, Ross JK. Elective operations for postinfarction left ventricular aneurysms. Thorax 1976;31:55.

2. Sutherland FW, Guell FJ, Pathi VL, Naik SK. Postinfarction ventricu-lar free wall rupture: strategies for diagnosis and treatment. Ann Thorac Surg 1996;61:1281.

3. Stoney WS, Alford WC Jr, Burrus GR, Thomas CS Jr. Repair of anteroseptal ventricular aneurysm. Ann Thorac Surg 1973;15:394.

4. Stryjer D, Friedensohn A, Hendler A. Myocardial rupture in acute myocardial infarction: urgent management. Br Heart J 1988;59:73.

5. Shaw RC, Connors JP, Hieb BR, Ludbrook PA, Krone R, Kleiger RE, et al. Postoperative investigation of left ventricular aneurysm resec-tion. Circulation 1977;56:II7.

6. Singh R, Molan SP, Schrank JP. Traumatic left ventricular aneurysm: two cases with normal coronary arteriograms. JAMA 1975;234:412.

7. Swerdlow CD, Winkle RA, Mason JW. Determinants of survival in patients with ventricular tachyarrhythmias. N Engl J Med 1983;308:1436.

8. Streeter D, Vaishnav R, Pater D, Spotnitz H, Ross J Jr, Sonnenblick E. Stress distribution in the canine left ventricle during diastole and systole. Biophys J 1970;10:345.

9. Sesto M, Schwartz F, Thiedemann KL, Flameng W, Schiepper M. Failure of aneurysmectomy to improve left ventricular function. Br Heart J 1979;41:79.

10. Swan HJ, Magnusson PT, Buchbinder NA, Mattoff JM, Gray RJ. Aneurysm of the cardiac ventricle: its management by medical and surgical intervention. West J Med 1978;129:26.

11. Sinatra R, Macrina F, Braccio M, Melina G, Luzi G, Ruvolo G, et al. Left ventricular aneurysmectomy; comparison between two tech-niques; early and late results. Eur J Cardiothorac Surg 1997;12:291.

12. Shapira OM, Davidoff R, Hilkert RJ, Aldea GS, Fitzgerald CA, Shemin RJ. Repair of left ventricular aneurysm: long-term results of linear repair versus endoaneurysmorrhaphy. Ann Thorac Surg 1997;63:701.

13. Salati M, Pajè A, Di Biasi P, Fundaró P, Cialfi A, Santoli C. Severe diastolic dysfunction after endoventriculoplasty. J Thorac Cardiovasc Surg 1995;109:694.

14. Stewart S, Huddle R, Stuard I, Schreiner BF, DeWeese JA. False aneurysm and pseudo-false aneurysm of the left ventricle: etiology, pathology, diagnosis, and operative management. Ann Thorac Surg 1981;31:259.

15. Shabbo FP, Dymond DS, Rees GM, Hill IM. Surgical treatment of false aneurysm of the left ventricle after myocardial infarction. Thorax 1983;38:25.

16. Stone DL, Fleming HA. Aneurysm of the left ventricular and left coronary artery after non-penetrating chest trauma. Br Heart J 1983;50:495.

17. Sherman SJ, Leenhouts KH, Utter GO, Litaker M, Lawson P. Prenatal diagnosis of left ventricular aneurysm in the late second trimester: a case report. Ultrasound Obstet Gynecol 1996;7:456.

T

1. Tantin LF. De quelques lésions des aretères coronaires comme causés d'altération du myocarde. Thèse, Paris, 1878.

2. Taylor NC, Barber R, Crossland P, Wraight EP, English TA, Petch MC. Does left ventricular aneurysmectomy improve ventricular func-tion in patients undergoing coronary bypass surgery? Br Heart J 1985;54:145.

V

1. Van Tassel RA, Edwards JE. Rupture of heart complicating myocar-dial infarction. Analysis of 40 cases including nine examples of left ventricular false aneurysm. Chest 1972;61:104.

2. Vlodaver Z, Coe JI, Edwards JE. True and false left ventricular aneurysms: propensity for the latter to rupture. Circulation 1975;51:567.

3. Vural KM, Sener E, Özatik MA, Tasdemir O, Bayazit K. Left ventricular aneurysm repair: an assessment of surgical treatment modalities. Eur J Cardiothorac Surg 1998;13:49.

4. Vicol C, Rupp G, Fischer S, Summer C, Bolte HD, Struck E. Linear repair versus ventricular reconstruction for treatment of left ventricu-lar aneurysm: a 10-year experience. J Cardiovasc Surg 1998;39:461.

5. Veinot JP, Walley VM, Wolfsohn AL, Chandra L, Russell D, Stinson WA, et al. Postinfarct cardiac free wall rupture: the relationship of rupture site to papillary muscle insertion. Mod Pathol 1995;8:609.

W

1. Walker WE, Stoney WS, Alford WC, Burrus GR, Glassford DM, Thomas CS. Results of surgical management of acute left ventricular aneurysm. Circulation 1980;62:II75.
2. Walker WE, Stoney WS, Alford WC, Burrus GR, Frist RA, Glassford DM, et al. Techniques and results of ventricular aneurysmectomy with emphasis on anteroseptal repair. J Thorac Cardiovasc Surg 1978; 76:824.
3. Weisman H, Bush D, Mannisi J, Bulkley B. Global cardiac remodeling after acute myocardial infarction: a study in the rat. J Am Coll Cardiol 1985;5:1355.

Y

1. Yamazaki Y, Eguchi S, Miyamura H, Hayashi J, Fukuda J, Ozeki H, et al. Replacement of myocardium with a Dacron prosthesis for complications of acute myocardial infarction (Torino). J Cardiovasc Surg 1989;30:277.

Z

1. Ziegler E. Über die Ursachen der Nierenschrumpfung nebst hemerkungen fiber die Unterschiedung Verschiedener Formen de Nephritis. Freiburg, West Germany, 1879, p. 586.

9 Postinfarction Ventricular Septal Defect

DEFINITION

Postinfarction ventricular septal defect (VSD) is a defect in the ventricular septum that results from rupture of acutely infarcted myocardium.

HISTORICAL NOTE

In 1847, Latham first described a postinfarction VSD at autopsy, but it was not until 1923 that Brunn made the diagnosis clinically.[B2] In 1957, Cooley and colleagues first reported the surgical repair of a postinfarction VSD, 11 weeks after myocardial infarction.[C1] The patient died 6 weeks later. The first long-term survivor of such repair was from the Mayo Clinic in 1963.[P1] Approach through the left ventricle was described in 1969 by Kay[K2] and Dubost[D3] and subsequently by Kitamura and colleagues,[K3] Javid and colleagues,[J1] and others.[D2,K1] The double-patch method was described by Iben and colleagues[I1] and subsequently modified by Gonzalez-Lavin and Zajtchuk[G4] and by Daggett and colleagues.[D1,M3] Repair of the ruptured septum through a right atrial approach was reported by Filgueira and colleagues in 1986.[F3] In 1987, David and colleagues introduced the concept of endocardial patch repair with infarct exclusion using autologous pericardium.[D8]

MORPHOLOGY

Postinfarction VSD is usually located in the anterior or apical portion of the ventricular septum (about 60% of cases)[S4] as a result of a transmural anterior myocardial infarction. About 20% to 40% of patients have a VSD in the posterior portion of the ventricular septum as a result of an inferior myocardial infarction.

Ventricular septal rupture usually occurs as a complication of a first acute myocardial infarction.[H2,M2,M4,P2] Also, a well-developed collateral coronary circulation is uncommon in hearts with a postinfarction VSD.[S5] The defect is generally associated with complete obstruction (rather than severe stenosis) of a coronary artery, usually the left anterior descending coronary artery.[S5] Important stenoses often coexist in the right coronary artery system.

The importance of concomitant right ventricular (RV) infarction in patients with postinfarction VSD has now become evident. For many years, evidence of RV dysfunction was thought simply to represent poor "adaptation" of the RV to the sudden increase in pulmonary blood flow imposed by the postinfarction VSD. Accumulated information now indicates that actual infarction of the inferior RV wall, or at least severe ischemia of that area, is responsible for the dysfunction.[C4,G5,H3,M4,R1]

VSDs may be multiple, and rather than simultaneously, they may develop separately several days apart.

A posterior VSD, in particular, may be accompanied by mitral valve regurgitation secondary to papillary muscle infarction or ischemia (see Chapter 10). In about 40% of patients who survive the early period of ventricular septal rupture, the remainder of the infarcted septum and ventricular wall may become aneurysmal.[J1,S2]

CLINICAL FEATURES AND DIAGNOSTIC CRITERIA

The first sign of ventricular septal rupture in a patient who has recently sustained a myocardial infarction is development of a *pansystolic murmur,* usually at the left lower sternal border, with or without radiation to the axilla, and of varying intensity. If the murmur is overlooked or its importance ignored, most patients with ventricular septal rupture die undiagnosed. The chest radiograph provides evidence of pulmonary venous hypertension and increased pulmonary blood flow.

A systolic murmur can result from acute mitral regurgitation secondary to myocardial infarction as well as from postinfarction VSD, and the two conditions may coexist. Thus, after detection of the murmur, an examination with two-dimensional echocardiography (either transthoracic or transesophageal) with Doppler color flow imaging is performed to define the site of the VSD, quantify the magnitude of the left-to-right shunt, and ascertain the presence or absence of mitral regurgitation. Echocardiography is highly sensitive and specific and provides safe and rapid diagnosis of a postinfarction VSD.[H1,R2] It also permits preoperative analysis of wall motion abnormalities in a high percentage of patients.[B4]

Magnitude of left-to-right shunt can also be quantified by the Fick principle (see "Whole Body Oxygen Consumption" under Cardiovascular Subsystem in Chapter 5). A pulmonary artery (Swan-Ganz) catheter is introduced at the bedside. Blood samples are obtained from the right atrium, pulmonary artery, and a peripheral artery. The left-to-right shunt is usually large, with a pulmonary-to-systemic blood flow ratio ($\dot{Q}p/\dot{Q}s$) of 2.0 or greater. Both pulmonary artery wedge pressure, reflecting left atrial and left ventricular (LV) end-diastolic pressures, and pulmonary artery pressure are usually elevated.

Once a left-to-right shunt is demonstrated and initial management implemented (see "Preoperative Preparation" under Technique of Operation), coronary angiography, cardiac catheterization, and left ventriculography may be performed if the patient is hemodynamically stable. Because evidence suggests that many patients with postinfarction VSD do well without the addition of invasive studies,[D9,S6] the role of preoperative coronary angiography remains controversial.[A1,C5,M5] The rationale for performing it is to identify important coronary artery stenoses or occlusions so that coronary artery bypass grafting (CABG) can be performed at the time of operation. Multiple-system coronary artery disease is present in more than 50% of patients with postinfarction VSD.[C6]

If echocardiographic studies have adequately identified the VSD, presence or absence of mitral regurgitation, and wall motion abnormalities, cardiac catheterization and left ventriculography are unnecessary.

NATURAL HISTORY

Oyamata and Queen[O1] and Jonas and colleagues[J2] have shown that postinfarction VSD complicates approximately 1% to 2% of cases of acute myocardial infarction. Septal rupture occurs an average of 2 to 3 days after infarction,[S3] but may occur any time in the first 2 weeks. Greatly reduced cardiac output follows, with all its sequelae.

Early death occurs frequently in patients with postinfarction VSD. Only about 75% survive the first 24 hours and only 50% the first week.[O1,S1] Less than 30% of patients survive 2 weeks and only 10% to 20% more than 4 weeks[C6] (Fig. 9-1). Risk of death is greatest immediately after a

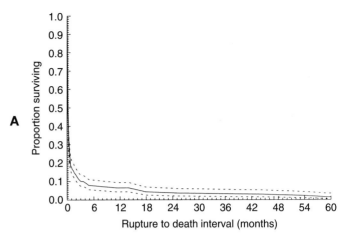

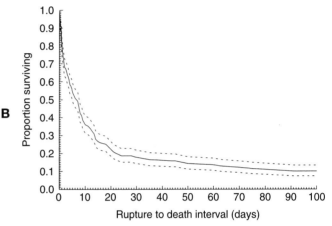

Figure 9-1 Survival without surgical treatment of patients with ventricular septal rupture after acute myocardial infarction, based on analysis of all proven cases ($n = 139$) reported in the literature until 1977. The solid line represents the proportion surviving, and the dashed lines enclose 70% confidence limits. **A,** Interval in months between rupture and death. **B,** Interval in days between rupture and death. Note that half the patients are dead within 7 days of rupture. (From Berger TJ, Blackstone EH, Kirklin JW: Unpublished observations; 1978.)

postinfarction ventricular septal rupture, then gradually declines thereafter.

TECHNIQUE OF OPERATION
Preoperative Preparation

Because most patients with postinfarction VSD are seriously ill and require operation early after septal rupture, their management before operation is of critical importance.

Once the diagnosis of acute postinfarction VSD has been confirmed by echocardiography and a pulmonary artery catheter has been inserted, additional diagnostic studies must be considered before proceeding with operation. (The only exception to this is the rare patient with essentially no systemic hemodynamic disturbance, as described in "Indications for Operation.") An intraaortic balloon catheter is inserted immediately, because these patients tend to deteriorate rapidly.[G1] If the patient is already critically ill, cardiopulmonary bypass (CPB) can be established by peripheral cannulation (see "Cardiopulmonary Bypass Established by Peripheral Cannulation" under Special Situations and Controversies in Section 3 of Chapter 2). If indicated, the patient is taken immediately to the cardiac catheterization laboratory for special studies (see "Clinical Features and Diagnostic Criteria" earlier in this chapter), with the intraaortic balloon or CPB in place and functioning. When the studies have been completed, or if they are not performed, operation is undertaken immediately, because permanent improvement is not achieved with support devices alone.[B3]

Initial Steps

After the usual initial preparations in the operating room (see "General Comments and Strategy" in Section 3 of Chapter 2), a median sternotomy incision is made. The heart is disturbed as little as possible before CPB is established, because of the patient's unstable hemodynamic state. While performing the median sternotomy, removal or preparation of grafts is accomplished in the usual manner (see Chapter 7). Because of the length and complexity of the operation, the surgical plan must be efficient so aortic clamp and CPB times are kept to a minimum.

CPB is promptly established using two venous cannulae and caval tapes. If CPB is established percutaneously before or immediately after the patient is brought to the operating room, surgical cannulations should be made and CPB established using a pump-oxygenator designed for operating room use. The femoral lines are clamped and removed, and the femoral artery and vein are repaired at the end of the procedure. The aorta is clamped.

Myocardial management may include warm induction of cardioplegia and controlled aortic root reperfusion (see "Cold Cardioplegia, Controlled Aortic Root Perfusion, and [When Needed] Warm Cardioplegic Induction" in Chapter 3). Because an acute coronary occlusion is typically present, the coronary sinus route of administration should be employed for part of the cardioplegic infusion (see "Technique of Retrograde Infusion" under Cold Cardioplegia [Multidose] in Chapter 3).

The caval tapes are snugged. A left atrial vent may be inserted, but usually is not necessary.

Repair of Defect

The VSD is usually approached through the LV. When located anteriorly, it is approached through the anterolateral infarction (or aneurysm) that is generally present (Fig. 9-2, A). The defect in the septum is typically found immediately beneath this area (Fig. 9-2, B). It is repaired using a collagen- or gelatin-impregnated polyester patch or a patch of autologous or bovine pericardium. The patch is made sufficiently large to cover the ventricular aspect of the intact but infarcted portion of the septum as well as the VSD. No part of the ventricular septum is resected. The patch is sewn into place on the LV side of the septum, with pledgeted mattress sutures placed away from the edge of the defect into noninfarcted myocardium. The sutures are placed close together and the pledgets placed on the RV

side of the defect (Fig. 9-2, C). Alternatively, the patch can be sutured into place with a continuous No. 3-0 or 4-0 polypropylene suture, securing the patch to noninfarcted myocardium on the ventricular septum (Fig. 9-2, D).[D6] Infarcted or aneurysmal myocardium on the anterolateral wall is excised, avoiding the anterolateral papillary muscle. If more than a small amount of tissue is removed from the anterolateral wall, it may be necessary to close the LV with a polyester or pericardial patch. If this is not necessary, the incision in the LV is closed with interrupted heavy (No. 0 or 2-0) silk or polyester sutures that are placed through strips of polytetrafluoroethylene (PTFE) felt and through the patch that has closed the VSD (Fig. 9-2, E). This suture line is reinforced with a continuous suture of No. 0 or 2-0 polypropylene, which is passed through both strips of PTFE felt, both edges of the myocardium, and the ventricular septal patch (Fig 9-2, F).

One technique involves suturing a pericardial patch to the endocardium of the LV adjacent to the area of the infarction.[D10] The LV is opened through an incision in the infarcted anterolateral wall. An oval patch (approximately 4×6 cm) of bovine pericardium is sutured to the endocardium of the inferior portion of the noninfarcted endocardium of the ventricular septum with a continuous No. 3-0 polypropylene suture (Fig. 9-3, A). The suture line is continued into the noninfarcted endocardium of the anterolateral ventricular wall (Fig. 9-3, B). When placing the continuous suture through the transition zones (superiorly and inferiorly) between the septum and the free wall of the LV, care must be taken to anchor the patch securely to the myocardium to prevent residual communications between the LV and RV.[P3] Separate interrupted sutures may be required. Once the patch is completely secured to the endocardium of the LV, the LV cavity is essentially excluded from the infarcted myocardium (Fig. 9-3, C). The ventriculotomy is closed using two strips of bovine pericardium or PTFE felt (Fig. 9-3, D).

When the VSD is in the apical portion of the septum and is associated with an apical myocardial infarction, the operation consists of amputation of the apex of the ventricle, including the involved portion of the ventricular septum (Fig. 9-4, A). The LV is opened through the infarcted myocardium and the septum examined. If the VSD is immediately adjacent to the area of apical infarction, the apex of the heart is excised, including the involved portion of the septum and adjacent RV (Fig. 9-4, B). Using strips of PTFE felt on each side of the septum and on the edges of the right and left ventricular myocardium, heavy mattress sutures of silk or polyester are placed through these four layers of felt as well as through the right and left ventricular myocardium and the ventricular septum (Fig. 9-4, C). These sutures are tied, thus closing the interventricular communication and the openings into both ventricles. The resulting suture line is reinforced with a continuous No. 0 or 2-0 polypropylene suture (Fig. 9-4, D).

VSDs located in the posterior septum are more difficult to expose and repair. The heart is lifted out of the pericardium with traction on the apex of the LV. The defect is approached through a vertical incision in the infarcted LV myocardium (Fig. 9-5, A). If the VSD is relatively small, the necrotic tissue can be excised, including the infarcted free wall of both the RV and LV, often with the overlying

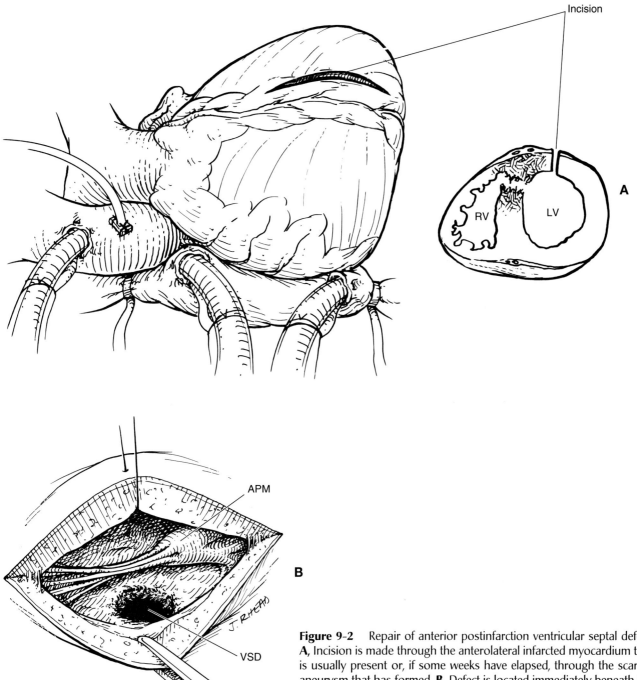

Figure 9-2   Repair of anterior postinfarction ventricular septal defect. **A,** Incision is made through the anterolateral infarcted myocardium that is usually present or, if some weeks have elapsed, through the scar or aneurysm that has formed. **B,** Defect is located immediately beneath the incision.

Key: *APM,* Anterior papillary muscle; *LV,* left ventricle; *RV,* right ventricle; *VSD,* ventricular septal defect.   *Continued*

occluded posterior descending coronary artery (Fig. 9-5, *B*). The VSD patch (collagen- or gelatin-impregnated polyester or bovine or autologous pericardium) is placed on the LV side of the septum and secured using mattress sutures of No. 2-0 polyester, with pledgets placed on the RV side of the septum (Fig. 9-5, *C*). If little or no free wall myocardium has been excised, LV and RV edges are approximated, incorporating the septal patch and two strips of PTFE felt. A large defect in the free wall requires a second patch.[D1] The free edge of the septal patch is sutured to the free wall

of the LV with interrupted mattress sutures of No. 2-0 polyester using pledgets on the patch and a strip of PTFE on the ventricular wall (Fig. 9-5, *D*). The patch for closure of the RV is attached to the septal patch already in position and to the free wall of the RV. Pledgets of felt are placed on the inner surface of the RV, and a strip of felt is placed on the outer surface (see Fig. 9-5, *D*).

Muehrcke and colleagues describe an alternative technique for closure of the free wall when there is extensive infarction.[M3] No infarcted muscle on the free walls of the

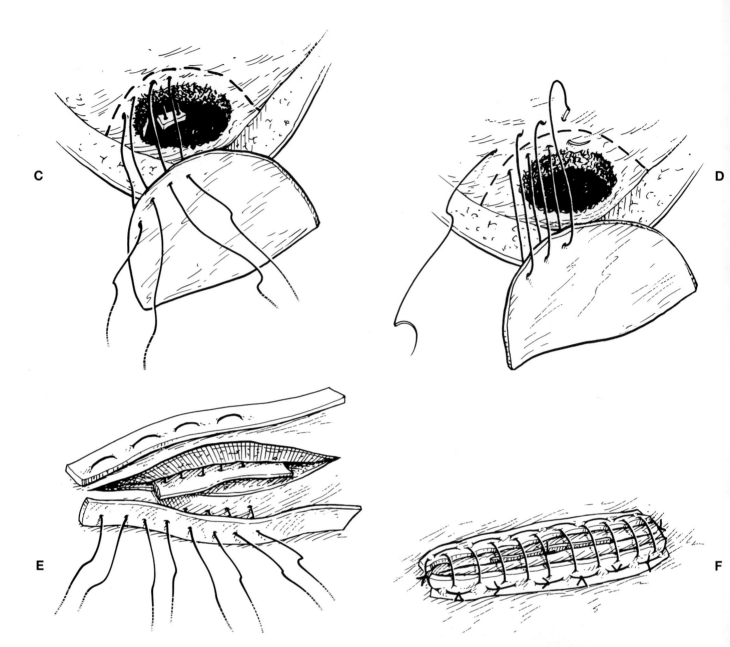

Figure 9-2, cont'd   **C,** If interrupted sutures are used, the patch is sewn into place on the left ventricular (LV) side of the septum, with pledgeted mattress sutures placed away from the edge of the defect into noninfarcted myocardium *(dashed line)*. The sutures are placed close together and the pledgets placed on the right ventricular side of the defect. **D,** If a continuous suture technique is used, the patch is sutured to noninfarcted myocardium on the ventricular septum adjacent to the area of infarction using a No. 3-0 or 4-0 polypropylene suture. **E,** If patch repair of the anterolateral wall is not required, the incision in the LV is closed with interrupted heavy silk or polyester sutures placed through strips of polytetrafluoroethylene (PTFE) felt, the edges of the myocardium, and the patch that has closed the ventricular septal defect. **F,** The suture line is reinforced with a continuous suture of No. 0 or 2-0 polypropylene, which is passed through both strips of PTFE felt, both edges of the myocardium, and the ventricular septal patch.

RV or LV is excised. The septal patch is sutured to the RV edge of the incision that was made to expose the septum. This suture line incorporates the infarcted free wall and a patch of polyester placed over the entire infarcted muscle of the free wall (Fig. 9-5, *E*). Pledgeted sutures are placed circumferentially around the area of infarcted muscle and

through the polyester patch, then tied over a strip of PTFE felt (Fig. 9-5, *F*).

The technique developed by David and colleagues involves an incision in the inferior wall of the LV parallel to the posterior descending coronary artery.[D10] Traction sutures are placed on the edges of the ventriculotomy to

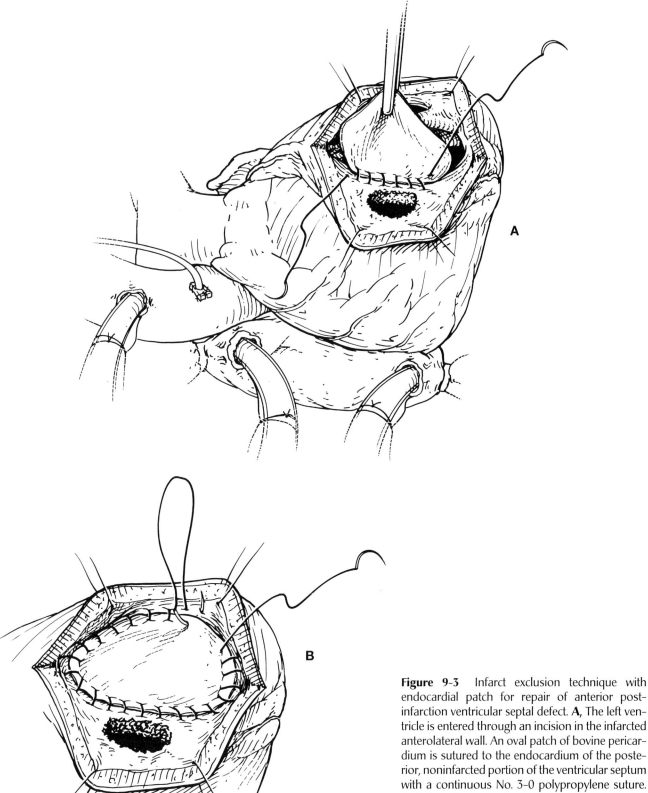

A

B

Figure 9-3 Infarct exclusion technique with endocardial patch for repair of anterior post-infarction ventricular septal defect. **A,** The left ventricle is entered through an incision in the infarcted anterolateral wall. An oval patch of bovine pericardium is sutured to the endocardium of the posterior, noninfarcted portion of the ventricular septum with a continuous No. 3-0 polypropylene suture. **B,** Suture line is continued into the noninfarcted endocardium of the anterolateral ventricular wall.

Continued

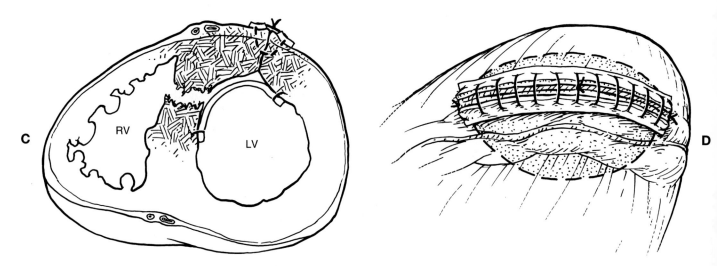

Figure 9-3, cont'd **C,** The left ventricular cavity is thus excluded from the infarcted myocardium. **D,** Ventriculotomy is closed using two strips of bovine pericardium or polytetrafluoroethylene (PTFE) felt and a continuous polypropylene suture.

Key: *LV,* Left ventricle; *RV,* right ventricle.

facilitate exposure (Fig. 9-6, *A*). The VSD is identified, and a triangular patch of bovine pericardium approximately 4×7 cm is sutured first to the fibrous anulus of the mitral valve using a continuous No. 3-0 polypropylene suture. The medial margin of the patch is sutured to noninfarcted muscle of the septum adjacent to the defect (Fig. 9-6, *B*). The lateral edge of the patch is then sutured to the endocardium of the LV free wall adjacent to the posterior papillary muscle (Fig. 9-6, *C*). This excludes all infarcted muscle from the LV cavity (Fig. 9-6, *D*). The ventriculotomy is closed with two layers of sutures buttressed with strips of bovine pericardium or PTFE felt (Fig. 9-6, *E*).

Associated Procedures

Occasionally, mitral regurgitation may be associated with acute septal rupture, particularly when the infarction is posterior. The mitral valve is replaced (or occasionally repaired) under such circumstances. Replacement is usually best performed through the left ventriculotomy using interrupted pledgeted mattress sutures, with the pledgets on the atrial side of the anulus (see Chapter 10).

When an LV aneurysm coexists with a postinfarction VSD, it is excised as the initial step in the operation.[F1] Then, after repair of the VSD, the aneurysm is generally repaired as usual (see Chapter 8). However, improvisation in the repair may be necessary.

Rarely, patients with postinfarction VSD are also found to have free wall rupture of the infarct. In surgical patients the rupture is usually small and can be repaired by excising the infarct. The possibility of such an associated lesion lends urgency to such situations.

In the case of important coronary artery stenosis, CABG should be performed. When feasible, the internal thoracic artery should be grafted to the left anterior descending coronary artery.

Completion

An essential part of the operation is controlled aortic root reperfusion (see "Cold Cardioplegia, Controlled Aortic Root Reperfusion, and [When Needed] Warm Cardioplegic Induction" in Chapter 3). During controlled aortic root reperfusion, all suture lines are examined. Additional measures are used, if necessary, to establish hemostasis.

The remainder of the operation is completed in the usual manner (see "Completing Operation" in Section 3 of Chapter 2). Particular care is taken to achieve hemostasis. Two right atrial and two right ventricular temporary pacing wires are placed so that atrioventricular sequential pacing is possible, if needed. Intraaortic balloon pumping (IABP) is resumed during the rewarming phase of CPB and usually is continued into the postoperative period. If CPB cannot be discontinued after about 30 minutes of normothermic partial CPB, temporary ventricular assistance may be required (see "Temporary Ventricular Assistance" in Chapter 5).

SPECIAL FEATURES OF POSTOPERATIVE CARE

Postoperative care is conducted as described in Chapter 5. IABP is continued in a one-to-one mode until cardiac output is adequate; it is then gradually discontinued and the balloon catheter removed. If ventricular assist devices are in place, flow through them is gradually decreased as ventricular function and cardiac output improve (see "Temporary Ventricular Assistance" in Chapter 5). Because patients are often critically ill during the early postoperative period, with low cardiac output and often with complicating arrhythmias, a full therapeutic regimen is usually required. This includes optimizing of preload with infusion (or removal) of volume, enhancing of contractility with inotropic agents, and reducing of afterload, if indicated. Attainment of a heart rate that results in optimal cardiac output by pacing or pharmacologic agents is also important.

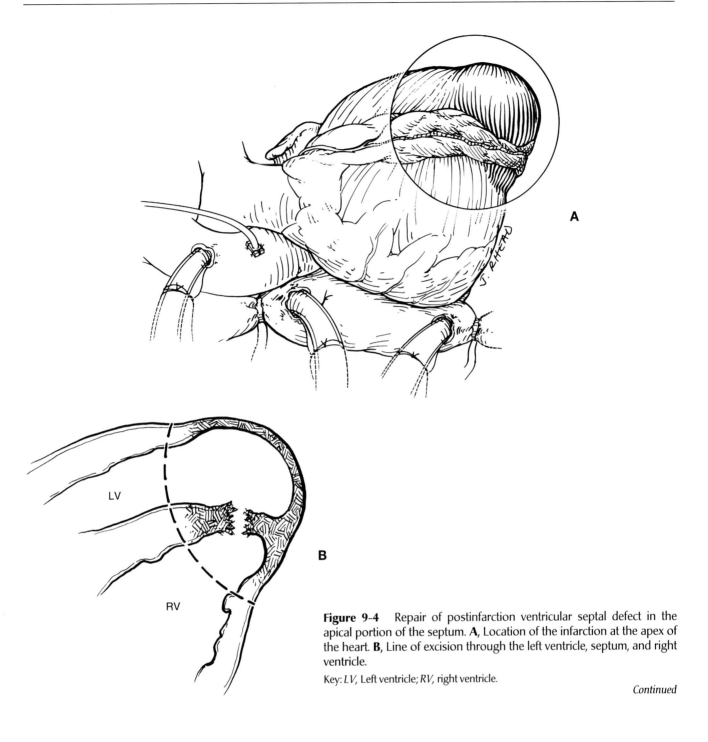

Figure 9-4   Repair of postinfarction ventricular septal defect in the apical portion of the septum. **A,** Location of the infarction at the apex of the heart. **B,** Line of excision through the left ventricle, septum, and right ventricle.

Key: *LV,* Left ventricle; *RV,* right ventricle.

Continued

Using the technique described earlier under "Clinical Features and Diagnostic Criteria," measurements are made to detect residual shunt, which can be present because of friability of the septum and relative insecurity of the repair. Transesophageal echocardiography is also useful for this purpose. If the Q̇p/Q̇s is 2.0 or greater and the hemodynamic state is poor, prompt reoperation should be considered.

Detailed care required late postoperatively by patients undergoing isolated CABG should be applied to those who have undergone repair of a postinfarction VSD (see "Special Features of Postoperative Care" in Chapter 7).

RESULTS

Early (Hospital) Death

Hospital mortality after VSD repair is approximately 30% to 40%.[A1,A3,D7,D9,D11,E1,M3] Death may be difficult to prevent because of the extent of myocardial necrosis associated with rupture of the ventricular septum. However, mortality might be reduced by prompt surgical repair, better methods of myocardial management, and more aggressive use of ventricular assistance in the postoperative period.

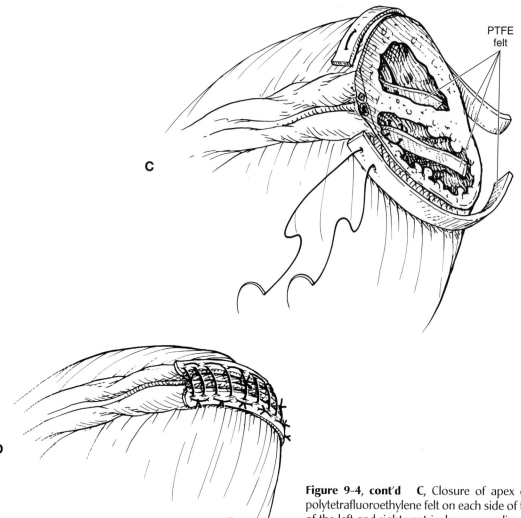

C

D

Figure 9-4, cont'd   C, Closure of apex of the heart using strips of polytetrafluoroethylene felt on each side of the septum and on the edges of the left and right ventricular myocardium. **D,** Suture line is reinforced with a continuous No. 0 or 2–0 polypropylene suture.

Key: *PTFE,* polytetrafluoroethylene.

Time-Related Survival

Time-related survival after repair of postinfarction VSD is less than optimal. In large series of patients with long-term follow-up, 5-year survival has ranged from 44% to 57% and 10-year survival from 29% to 36%[D7,D9,D11,M3] (Fig. 9-7, *A*). The hazard function for death after repair of postinfarction VSD has not only a high and rapidly declining early phase, but also an appreciable constant phase that is approximately five times greater than that after isolated CABG (Fig. 9-7, *B*).

Modes of Death

The mode of death in more than half and up to 90% of patients dying early after operation for postinfarction VSD is cardiac failure.[A1,A3,D7,E1,M3] This relatively high prevalence is related to extensive myocardial infarction, complexity of operation, and preoperative secondary subsystem failure. Bleeding, sepsis, stroke, gastrointestinal bleeding, and recurrent VSD are the other modes of early death. Cardiac failure is also the most common mode of late death. Other modes of late death include sudden death, stroke, sepsis, and myocardial infarction.[A1,D7,E1,M3]

Incremental Risk Factors for Death

Mortality is influenced by several factors that have been identified by a number of multivariable analyses.[D7,D9,D10,E1,M3,S6] From these and other studies in the literature,[A3,C1,C3] and from knowledge of the risk factors for death and other adverse outcomes in patients with ischemic heart disease (see "Results" in Chapter 7), some inferences can be made.

The most important risk factors for death in the early hazard phase are a poor hemodynamic state (cardiogenic shock) at the time of operation[D7,S6] and acute RV dysfunction (Fig. 9-8).[A1,A3,D7,D9,F2,G2,G3,L2,M1,M3,R1] The amount and distribution of myocardial necrosis and scar are responsible for both factors. A *poor hemodynamic state* becomes an even more severe risk factor when present for many hours before surgical intervention,[G3,L1,M1] as in the surgical treatment of acute myocardial infarction.[A2] Operation early

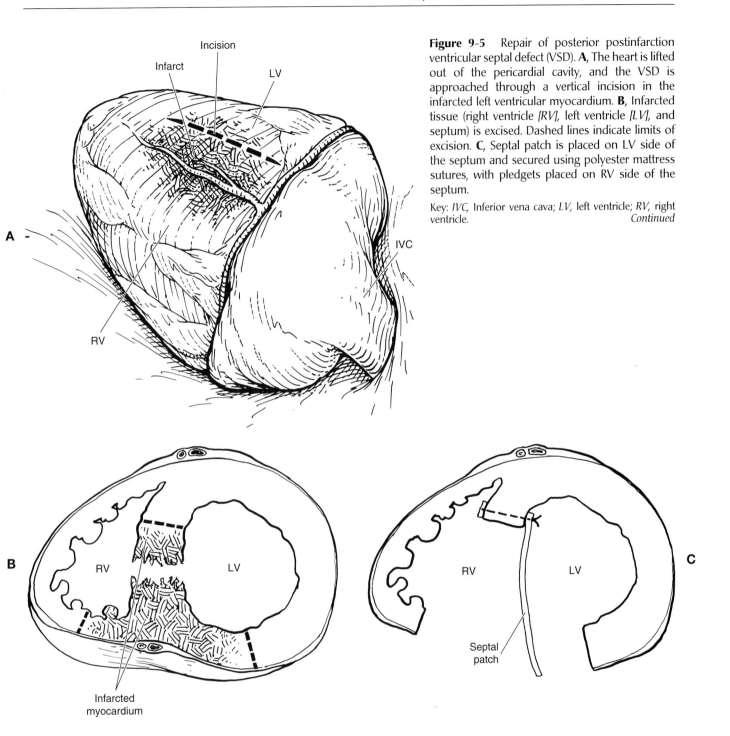

Figure 9-5   Repair of posterior postinfarction ventricular septal defect (VSD). **A,** The heart is lifted out of the pericardial cavity, and the VSD is approached through a vertical incision in the infarcted left ventricular myocardium. **B,** Infarcted tissue (right ventricle [RV], left ventricle [LV], and septum) is excised. Dashed lines indicate limits of excision. **C,** Septal patch is placed on LV side of the septum and secured using polyester mattress sutures, with pledgets placed on RV side of the septum.

Key: *IVC,* Inferior vena cava; *LV,* left ventricle; *RV,* right ventricle.   *Continued*

after rupture of the septum typically carries a higher risk than that undertaken many days or weeks later, probably because of the high prevalence of hemodynamic instability and extensive myocardial necrosis.[C2,D1,D5,G3,M3]

RV dysfunction results from ischemic damage or frank infarction of the RV and thus is more likely to be present when stenosis or occlusion in the right coronary artery system is located proximally.[A3,D7,J3] RV dysfunction may also occur after anterior myocardial infarction. The higher mortality associated with repair of defects located inferiorly in the septum probably relates to the higher prevalence of important right coronary stenosis and RV dysfunction in

this group.[A3,D1,D4,D9,G3,S6] Mortality may also be related to the greater complexity of posterior repairs and to more frequent involvement of the mitral valve.[A3]

Severity and distribution of the coronary artery disease are also risk factors, but are overshadowed by the patient's hemodynamic status at operation and amount of damaged myocardium.[R1]

Similarly, *comorbidities* such as older age at operation, diabetes, and preinfarction hypertension are likely risk factors for death in the early and constant hazard phases. The small number of patients in many series has made identification of these and other factors difficult.

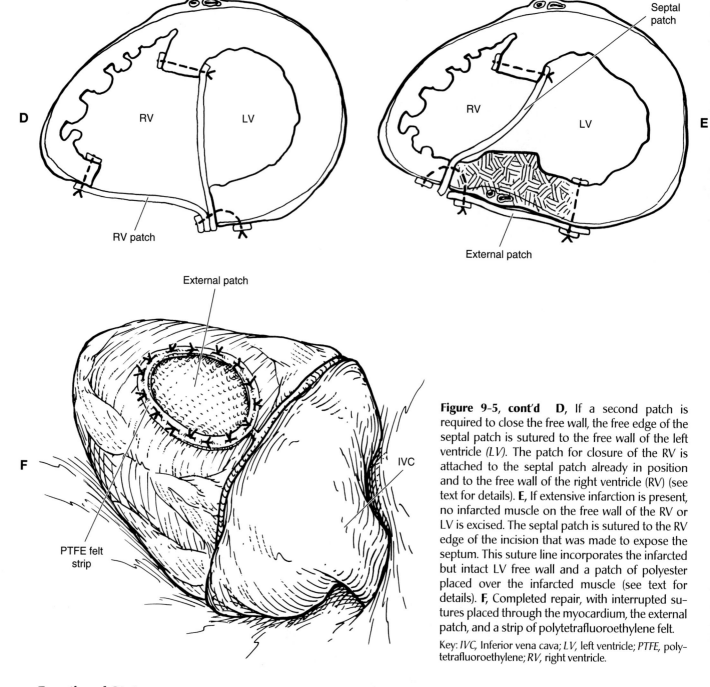

Figure 9-5, cont'd   D, If a second patch is required to close the free wall, the free edge of the septal patch is sutured to the free wall of the left ventricle *(LV)*. The patch for closure of the RV is attached to the septal patch already in position and to the free wall of the right ventricle (RV) (see text for details). **E,** If extensive infarction is present, no infarcted muscle on the free wall of the RV or LV is excised. The septal patch is sutured to the RV edge of the incision that was made to expose the septum. This suture line incorporates the infarcted but intact LV free wall and a patch of polyester placed over the infarcted muscle (see text for details). **F,** Completed repair, with interrupted sutures placed through the myocardium, the external patch, and a strip of polytetrafluoroethylene felt.

Key: *IVC,* Inferior vena cava; *LV,* left ventricle; *PTFE,* poly-tetrafluoroethylene; *RV,* right ventricle.

Functional Status

The functional status of most patients surviving the period of hospitalization is good. The majority of patients (70% to 95%) are in New York Heart Association (NYHA) functional class I or II.[A3,D5,D7,D9,D11,E1,M3]

Residual and Recurrent Defect

A residual VSD has been noted early or late postoperatively in 3% to 40% of patients.[B1,D7,D11,E1,S6] Residual VSD may be caused by (1) reopening of a closed defect, (2) presence of an overlooked VSD, or (3) development of a new VSD during the early postoperative period. Reoperation is required for closure of such residual defects when $\dot{Q}p/\dot{Q}s$

is greater than about 2.0 or with persistently low cardiac output, pulmonary edema, or other organ system dysfunction.

INDICATIONS FOR OPERATION

Postinfarction VSD is almost always an indication for operation, because it produces a large left-to-right shunt. The only question is the *timing* of operation.

Repair of postinfarction VSD 2 to 3 weeks or more after septal rupture is relatively safe. By then the edges of the defect have become tougher, and repair is more securely and safely accomplished. Therefore, when the patient presents with a stable hemodynamic state, repair can be

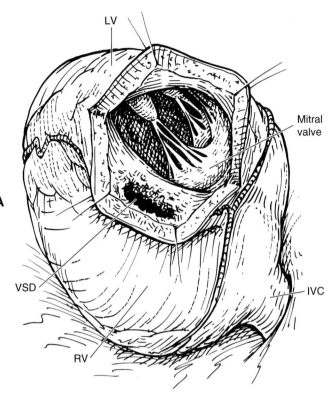

Figure 9-6   Infarct exclusion technique with endocardial patch for repair of posterior postinfarction ventricular septal defect. **A,** The left ventricle is entered posteriorly through an incision parallel and adjacent to the posterior descending coronary artery. Traction sutures are placed through the edges of the myocardium. **B,** Triangular-shaped patch of bovine pericardium is first sutured to the fibrous anulus of the mitral valve using a continuous No. 3-0 polypropylene suture. The medial edge of the patch is then sutured to the noninfarcted muscle of the septum adjacent to the defect.

Key: *IVC,* Inferior vena cava; *LV,* left ventricle; *RV,* right ventricle; *VSD,* ventricular septal defect.   *Continued*

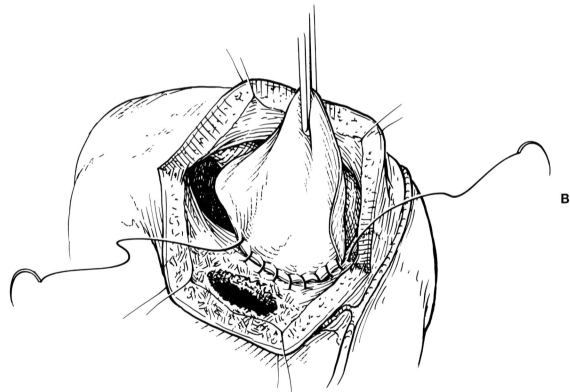

delayed, but there must be a high degree of certainty that the hemodynamic state is good. Otherwise, the patient's condition could suddenly deteriorate. The criteria for deferment include (1) adequate cardiac output, with no evidence of cardiogenic shock; (2) absence of symptoms of pulmonary venous hypertension, or easy control of initial symptoms with appropriate drug therapy; (3) absence of fluid retention,

or easy control by digitalis and diuretics; and (4) good renal function, with normal blood urea nitrogen (BUN) and creatinine levels. The natural history of postinfarction VSD suggests that such circumstances are uncommon.

In the vast majority of patients, septal rupture rapidly leads to a deteriorating hemodynamic state with cardiogenic shock, marked and intractable symptoms of pulmo-

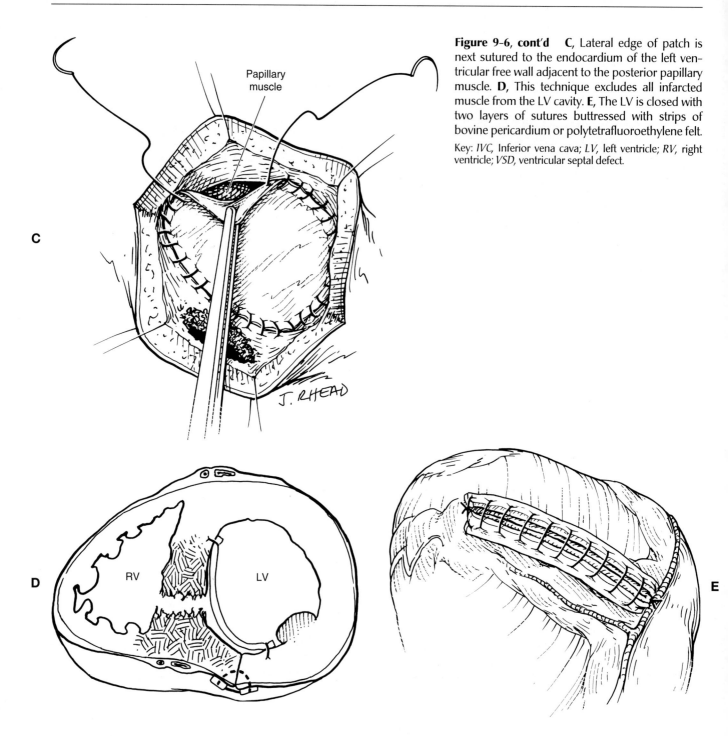

Figure 9-6, cont'd   C, Lateral edge of patch is next sutured to the endocardium of the left ventricular free wall adjacent to the posterior papillary muscle. **D,** This technique excludes all infarcted muscle from the LV cavity. **E,** The LV is closed with two layers of sutures buttressed with strips of bovine pericardium or polytetrafluoroethylene felt.

Key: *IVC,* Inferior vena cava; *LV,* left ventricle; *RV,* right ventricle; *VSD,* ventricular septal defect.

nary venous hypertension, and fluid retention. Immediate study and urgent operation are then indicated. Even if these signs and symptoms are absent and renal function deteriorates, as evidenced by rising BUN and creatinine levels, surgical intervention should be promptly undertaken. The increased risk of early repair is accepted because of the high risk without operation under such circumstances.

Delayed detection and referral for surgical treatment of seriously ill patients may make recovery so unlikely that it is appropriate to allow the natural history of the disease to unfold without surgical intervention. For example, the surgeon might see the patient only after profound cardiogenic shock has led to neurologic unresponsiveness, ischemic compromise of a limb or the bowel, or severe impair-

ment of renal function with anuria or greatly elevated BUN and creatinine levels.

SPECIAL SITUATIONS AND CONTROVERSIES

Repair of Defect Through a Right Atrial Approach

Repair of postinfarction VSD can be accomplished through a right atrial approach.[F3,M6] The potential advantage of this technique is that an incision in the LV myocardium is avoided. Experience with this procedure is limited. Massetti and colleagues have reported the largest series (12 patients).[M6] There were three early deaths (25%) and one late

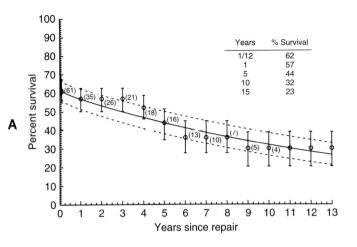

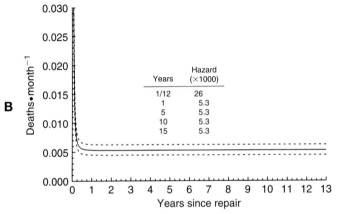

Figure 9-7   Survival after repair of postinfarction ventricular septal defect. **A**, Percent survival. **B**, Hazard function. The early, rapidly declining phase of hazard is followed by an appreciable constant phase about 3 months after operation. The constant-phase hazard is five times greater than after isolated coronary artery bypass grafting. (From Deville and colleagues.[D7])

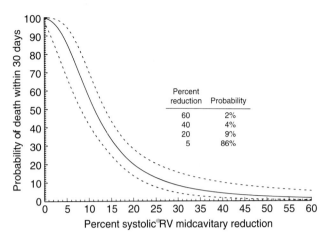

Figure 9-8   Association between right ventricular (RV) systolic dysfunction immediately before repair, as reflected in the percentage of systolic reduction of the midcavitary RV diastolic dimensions, and early mortality (probability of death within 30 days) after repair of postinfarction ventricular septal defect. (From Deville and colleagues.[D7])

Key: *RV,* Right ventricular.

Percutaneous Closure of Defect

Percutaneous techniques have been used successfully to close some congenital VSDs (see "Transcatheter Closure of Ventricular Septal Defects" under Special Situations and Controversies in Section 1 of Chapter 21). Lock and colleagues achieved successful percutaneous transcatheter closure of postinfarction VSDs in four patients with cardiogenic shock using the Rashkind double-umbrella device.[L2] The device embolized to the pulmonary artery in one patient, and the remaining three patients died with evidence of increased shunting across the defect over the ensuing several days. A Rashkind patent ductus arteriosus occluder system has also been used.[B5] Balloon catheters, which are inserted through the LV via the aorta or through the RV and then inflated, have been successful in temporarily reducing or eliminating the left-to-right shunt, thereby improving hemodynamic status and permitting a delay in surgical treatment.[A4,H4,K4,V1] Wider use of these or other minimally invasive techniques could substantially improve outcome.

death. One patient required reoperation for a residual defect 3 months postoperatively, and one had a small residual left-to-right shunt. Of the eight surviving patients who were followed for a mean of 5 years, three were NYHA functional class I, four were class II, and one was class III.

REFERENCES

A

1. Anderson DR, Adams S, Bhat A, Pepper JR. Post-infarction ventricular septal defect: the importance of site of infarction and cardiogenic shock on outcome. Eur J Cardiothorac Surg 1989;3:554.

2. Allen BS, Rosenkranz E, Buckberg GD, Davtyan H, Laks H, Tillisch J, et al. Studies on prolonged acute regional ischemia. VI. Myocardial infarction with left ventricular power failure: a medical/surgical emergency requiring urgent revascularization with maximal protection of remote muscle. J Thorac Cardiovasc Surg 1989;98:691.

3. Angelini GD, Penny WJ, Ruttley MS, Butchart EG, West RR, Henderson AH, et al. Post-infarction ventricular septal defect: the importance of right ventricular coronary perfusion in determining surgical outcome. Eur J Cardiothorac Surg 1989;3:156.

4. Abhyankar AD, Jagtap PM. Post-infarction ventricular septal defect: percutaneous transvenous temporary closure using a Swan-Ganz catheter. Catheter Cardiovasc Interv 1999;47:208.

B

1. Brandt B 3rd, Wright CB, Ehrenhaft JL. Ventricular septal defect following myocardial infarction. Ann Thorac Surg 1979;27:580.

2. Brunn F. Zur Diagnostic der erworbenen Ruptur der Kammerscheidowand des Horzons. Wien Arch Med 1923;6:533.

3. Buckley MJ, Mundth ED, Dagget WM, Gold HK, Leinbach RC, Austen WG. Surgical management of ventricular septal defects and mitral regurgitation complicating acute myocardial infarction. Ann Thorac Surg 1973;16:598.

4. Bishop HL, Gibson RS, Stamm RB, Beller GA, Martin RP. Role of two-dimensional echocardiography in the evaluation of patients with ventricular septal rupture postmyocardial infarction. Am Heart J 1981; 102:965.

5. Benton JP, Barker KS. Transcatheter closure of ventricular septal defect: a nonsurgical approach to the care of the patient with acute ventricular septal rupture. Heart Lung 1992;21:356.

C

1. Cooley DA, Belmonte BA, Zeis LB, Schnur S. Surgical repair of ruptured interventricular septum following acute myocardial infarction. Surgery 1957;41:930.

2. Campion BC, Harrison CE Jr, Giuliani ER, Schuttenberg TT, Ellis FH Jr. Ventricular septal defect after myocardial infarction. Ann Intern Med 1969;70:251.

3. Cummings RG, Califf R, Jones RN, Reimer KA, Kong YH, Lowe JE. Correlates of survival in patients with postinfarction ventricular septal defect. Ann Thorac Surg 1989;47:824.

4. Cummings RG, Reimer KA, Califf R, Hacket D, Boswick J, Lowe JE. Quantitative analysis of right and left ventricular infarction in the presence of postinfarction ventricular septal defect. Circulation 1988;77:33.

5. Cox FF, Plokker HW, Morshuis WJ, Kelder JC, Vermeulen FE. Importance of coronary revascularization for late survival after postinfarction ventricular septal rupture: a reason to perform coronary angiography prior to surgery. Eur Heart J 1996;17:1841.

6. Crenshaw BS, Granger CB, Birnbaum Y, Pieper KS, Morris DC, Kleiman NS, et al. Risk factors, angiographic patterns, and outcomes in patients with ventricular septal defect complicating acute myocardial infarction. Circulation 2000;101:27.

D

1. Daggett WM, Guyton RA, Mundth ED, Buckley MJ, McEnany MT, Gold HK, et al. Surgery for post-myocardial infarct ventricular septal defect. Ann Surg 1977;186:260.

2. Daggett WM, Burwell LR, Lawson DW, Austen WG. Resection of acute ventricular aneurysm and ruptured interventricular septum after myocardial infarction. N Engl J Med 1970;283:1507.

3. Dubost C. Discussion of paper by Iben AB et al.[11] Ann Thorac Surg 1969;8:252.

4. Donahoo JS, Brawley RK, Taylor D, Gott VL. Factors influencing survival following post-infarction ventricular septal defects. Ann Thorac Surg 1975;19:648.

5. Daggett WM, Buckley MJ, Akins CW, Leinbach RC, Gold HK, Block PC, et al. Improved results of surgical management of postinfarction ventricular septal rupture. Ann Surg 1982;196:269.

6. da Silva JP, Cascudo MM, Baumgratz JF, Vila JH, Macruz R. Postinfarction ventricular septal defect: an efficacious technique for early surgical repair. J Thorac Cardiovasc Surg 1989;987:86.

7. Deville C, Fontan F, Chevalier JM, Madonna F, Ebner A, Besse P. Surgery of post-infarction ventricular septal defect: risk factors for hospital death and long-term results. Eur J Cardiothorac Surg 1991;5:167.

8. David TE, Feindel CM, Ropchan GV. Reconstruction of the left ventricle with autologous pericardium. J Thorac Cardiovasc Surg 1987;94:710.

9. Dalrymple-Hay MJ, Langley SM, Sami SA, Haw M, Allen SM, Livesey SA, et al. Should coronary artery bypass grafting be performed at the same time as repair of a post-infarct ventricular septal defect? Eur J Cardiothorac Surg 1998;13:286.

10. David TE, Dale L, Sun Z. Postinfarction ventricular septal rupture: repair by endocardial patch with infarct exclusion. J Thorac Cardiovasc Surg 1995;110:1315.

11. Deja MA, Szostek J, Widenka K, Szafron B, Spyt TJ, Hickey MS, et al. Post infarction ventricular septal defect—can we do better? Eur J Cardiothorac Surg 2000;18:194.

E

1. Ellis CJ, Parkinson GF, Jaffe WM, Campbell MJ, Kerr AR. Good long-term outcome following surgical repair of post-infarction ventricular septal defect. Aust N Z J Med 1995;25:330.

F

1. Freeny PC, Schattenberg TT, Danielson GK, McGoon DC, Greenberg BH. Ventricular septal defect and ventricular aneurysm secondary to acute myocardial infarction. Circulation 1971;43:360.

2. Firt P, Hejnal J, Kramar R, Fabian J. Surgical treatment of post-infarction ventricular septal rupture. J Cardiovasc Surg 1984;25:25.

3. Filgueira JL, Battistessa SA, Hestable H, Lorenza A, Cassinelli M, Scola R. Delayed repair of an acquired posterior septal defect through a right atrial approach. Ann Thorac Surg 1986;42:208.

G

1. Gold HK, Leinbach RC, Sanders CA, Buckley MJ, Mundth ED, Austen WG. Intraaortic balloon pumping for ventricular septal defect or mitral regurgitation complicating acute myocardial infarction. Circulation 1973;47:1191.

2. Graham AF, Stinson EB, Daily PO, Harrison DC. Ventricular septal defects after myocardial infarction: early operative treatment. JAMA 1973;225:708.

3. Gaudiani VA, Miller DC, Stinson EB, Oyer PE, Reitz BA, Moreno-Cabral RJ, et al. Post-infarction ventricular septal defect: an argument for early operation. Surgery 1981;89:48.

4. Gonzalez-Lavin L, Zajtchuk R. Surgical considerations in the treatment of acute acquired ventricular septal defect. Thorax 1971;26:610.

5. Grose R, Spindola-Franco H. Right ventricular dysfunction in acute ventricular septal defect. Am Heart J 1981;101:67.

H

1. Harrison MR, MacPhail B, Gurley JC, Harlamert EA, Steinmetz JE, Smith MD, et al. Usefulness of color Doppler flow imaging to distinguish ventricular septal defect from acute mitral regurgitation complicating acute myocardial infarction. Am J Cardiol 1989;64:697.

2. Herlitz J, Samuelsson SO, Richter A, Hjalmarson A. Prediction of rupture in acute myocardial infarction. Clin Cardiol 1988;11:63.

3. Held AC, Cole PL, Lipton B, Gore JM, Antman EM, Hochman JS, et al. Rupture of the interventricular septum complicating acute myocardial infarction: a multicenter analysis of clinical findings and outcome. Am Heart J 1988;116:1330.

4. Hachida M, Nakano H, Hirai M, Shi CY. Percutaneous transaortic closure of postinfarctional ventricular septal rupture. Ann Thorac Surg 1991;51:655.

I

1. Iben AB, Pupello DF, Stinson EB, Shumway NE. Surgical treatment of postinfarction ventricular septal defects. Ann Thorac Surg 1969;8:252.

J

1. Javid H, Hunter JA, Najafi H, Dye WS, Julian OC. Left ventricular approach for the repair of ventricular septal perforation and infarctectomy. J Thorac Cardiovasc Surg 1972;63:14.

2. Jonas V, Hyncik V, Shlumsky J, Chlumska A. Eight-year survival after perforation of ventricular septum in myocardial infarction. Acta Univ Carol Med 1970;16:133.

3. Jones MT, Schofield PM, Dark JF, Moussalli H, Lawson RA, Ward C, et al. Surgical repair of acquired ventricular septal defect: determinants of early and late outcome. J Thorac Cardiovasc Surg 1987;93:680.

K

1. Kouchoukos NT. Infarction ventricular septal defect. In Cohn LH, ed. Modern techniques in surgery. Mount Kisco, N.Y.: Futura, 1979, p. 9.

2. Kay JH. Discussion of paper by Iben et al.[11] Ann Thorac Surg 1969;8:252.

3. Kitamura S, Mendez A, Kay JH. Ventricular septal defect following myocardial infarction. J Thorac Cardiovasc Surg 1971;61:186.

4. Kosuge M, Kimura K, Ishikawa T, Shimizu M, Himeno H, Ebina T, et al. Closure of ventricular septal rupture caused by acute myocardial infarction using a transaortic balloon catheter. Jpn Circ J 1993; 57:353.

L

1. Loisance DY, Cachera JP, Poulain H, Aubry PH, Juvin AM, Galey JJ. Ventricular septal defect after acute myocardial infarction: early repair. J Thorac Cardiovasc Surg 1980;80:61.

2. Lock JE, Block PC, McKay RG, Baim DS, Keane JF. Transcatheter closure of ventricular septal defects. Circulation 1988;78:361.

M

1. Matsui K, Kay JH, Mendez M, Pubiate P, Vanstrom N, Yokoyama T. Ventricular septal rupture secondary in myocardial infarction. JAMA 1981;245:1537.

2. Mann JM, Roberts WC. Cardiac morphologic observations after operative closure of acquired ventricular septal defect during acute myocardial infarction: analysis of 16 necropsy patients. Am J Cardiol 1987;60:981.

3. Muehrcke DD, Blank S, Daggett WM. Survival after repair of postinfarction ventricular septal defects in patients over the age of 70. J Card Surg 1992;7:290.

4. Moore CA, Nygaard TW, Kaiser DL, Cooper AA, Gibson RS. Postinfarction ventricular septal rupture: the importance of location of infarction and right ventricular function in determining survival. Circulation 1986;74:45.

5. Muehrcke DD, Daggett WM Jr, Buckley MJ, Akins CW, Hilgenberg AD, Austen WG. Postinfarct ventricular septal defect repair: effect of coronary artery bypass grafting. Ann Thorac Surg 1992;54:876.

6. Massetti M, Babatasi G, Le Page O, Bhoyroo S, Saloux E, Khayat A. Postinfarction ventricular septal rupture: early repair through the right atrial approach. J Thorac Cardiovasc Surg 2000;119:784.

O

1. Oyamada A, Queen FB. Spontaneous rupture of an interventricular septum following acute myocardial infarction with some clinicopathological observations of survival in five cases. Presented at the Pan-Pacific Pathology Congress, Tripler US Army Hospital, Honolulu, October 12, 1961.

P

1. Payne WS, Hunt JC, Kirklin JW. Surgical repair of ventricular septal defect due to myocardial infarction: report of a case. JAMA 1963;183:603.

2. Pohjola-Sintonen S, Muller JE, Stone PH, Willich SN, Antman EM, Davis VG, et al. Ventricular septal and free wall rupture complicating acute myocardial infarction: experience in the Multicenter Investigation of Limitation of Infarct Size. Am Heart J 1989;117:809.

3. Pett SB Jr, Follis F, Allen K, Temes T, Wernly JA. Posterior ventricular septal rupture: an anatomical reconstruction. J Card Surg 1998;13:445.

R

1. Radford MJ, Johnson RA, Daggett WM, Fallon JT, Buckley MJ, Gold HK, et al. Ventricular septal rupture: a review of clinical and physiologic features and an analysis of survival. Circulation 1981; 64:545.

2. Roelandt JR, Smyllie JH, Sutherland GR. The surgical complications of acute myocardial infarction: color Doppler evaluation. Int J Card Imaging 1989;4:45.

S

1. Sanders RJ, Kern WH, Blount SG Jr. Perforation of the interventricular septum complicating myocardial infarction: a report of eight cases, one with cardiac catheterization. Am Heart J 1956;51:736.

2. Schlichter J, Hellerstein HK, Katz LN. Aneurysm of the heart: a correlative study of one hundred and two proved cases. Medicine (Baltimore) 1954;33:43.

3. Selzer A, Gerbode F, Kerth WJ. Clinical, hemodynamic, and surgical considerations of rupture of the ventricular septum after myocardial infarction. Am Heart J 1969;78:598.

4. Swithinbank JM. Perforation of the interventricular septum in myocardial infarction. Br Heart J 1959;21:562.

5. Skehan JD, Carey C, Norrell MS, de Belder M, Balcon R, Mills PG. Patterns of coronary artery disease in post-infarction ventricular septal rupture. Br Heart J 1989;62:268.

6. Skillington PD, Davies RH, Luff AJ, Williams JD, Dawkins KD, Conway N, et al. Surgical treatment for infarct-related ventricular septal defects: improved early results combined with analysis of late functional status. J Thorac Cardiovasc Surg 1990;99:798.

V

1. Vajifdar B, Vora A, Narula D, Kulkarni H. Percutaneous balloon occlusion of post-infarction ventricular septal defect. Indian Heart J 1996;48:407.

DEFINITION

Mitral regurgitation from ischemic heart disease (ischemic mitral regurgitation) is mitral regurgitation *caused by* ischemic heart disease. This entity must not be confused with mitral regurgitation from other causes that *coexist* with ischemic heart disease.

HISTORICAL NOTE

Mitral regurgitation resulting from rupture of a papillary muscle has been long recognized as a rare and frequently catastrophic complication of acute myocardial infarction.[B3,S1] A case was identified at autopsy at The Johns Hopkins Hospital in 1935,[S2] but apparently the diagnosis was first made antemortem in 1948.[D1] Mitral regurgitation without papillary muscle rupture, occurring as an acute or chronic complication of ischemic heart disease with or without myocardial infarction, was described in 1963 by Burch and colleagues.[B2] These authors referred to this type of ischemic mitral regurgitation as "papillary muscle dysfunction," the presence of which was surmised rather than proved.

The first successful surgical correction of papillary muscle rupture was reported by Austen and colleagues at Massachusetts General Hospital in 1965.[A1]

MORPHOLOGY

Acute Mitral Regurgitation Complicating Myocardial Infarction

Rupture of Papillary Muscle

Rupture of a papillary muscle occurs as an acute complication of myocardial infarction, but its prevalence among patients with acute mitral regurgitation in the early stages of infarction is uncertain. About half of these patients have an actual rupture. About one third of patients with rupture may have a complete disruption of the papillary muscle, resulting in flailing of both the anterior and the posterior mitral leaflets.[B5,W1] About two thirds of patients have rupture of one or more heads of the papillary muscle rather than a complete rupture of the entire muscle.[B5]

The posteromedial papillary muscle is ruptured in about 75% of patients and the anterolateral muscle in about 25%.[B5,N1,W1] Correspondingly, most patients with acute mitral regurgitation during myocardial infarction have inferoposterior left ventricular (LV) infarction.[B5,E1] Also, at least in the study of Coma-Canella and colleagues, many have coexisting right ventricular infarction.[C1] Regardless, when the LV infarction is located inferoposteriorly rather than anterolaterally, the reason for more frequent rupture of the adjacent papillary muscle is not clear. The difference in collateral circulation to the two areas may play a role.[E2]

The size and nature of the coexisting acute LV infarction vary, perhaps because of the small number of cases in most series. Nishimura and colleagues reported that the infarction is often small,[N1] whereas Barbour and colleagues found infarction in more than 20% of the LV wall and septum in most patients.[B5] The infarction may be subendocardial rather than transmural.

Occasionally, papillary muscle rupture is associated with rupture of the ventricular septum[R1] as well as with rupture of the free wall of the left ventricle.[V1]

Papillary Muscle Necrosis without Rupture

About half the patients who develop severe mitral regurgitation during acute myocardial infarction do not have papillary muscle rupture, only papillary muscle necrosis. Papillary muscle dysfunction may contribute to resultant mitral regurgitation. However, contiguous myocardial infarction probably plays a more important role. The distribution of necrotic changes and extent of myocardial infarction are similar to those described for papillary muscle rupture.

Other Causes

Mitral regurgitation is a frequent complication of acute myocardial infarction. When Doppler echocardiography is used for diagnosis, mitral regurgitation has been detected in up to 39% of patients early after an infarction.[B7] Substantial (moderate or severe) mitral regurgitation is present in 3% to 19% of patients and is an important predictor of mortality.[L1,L2,T2,V3] Because papillary muscle rupture or necrosis occurs infrequently after acute infarction, other important causes of mitral regurgitation include (1) changes in configuration of the left ventricle, (2) global or segmental LV dysfunction, and (3) changes in function of the mitral valve resulting from leaflet prolapse, abnormal closure, or anular dilatation. Although papillary muscle dysfunction has been implicated as an important cause of ischemic mitral regurgitation,[B2] recent experimental and clinical studies employing two-dimensional echocardiography have demonstrated that it rarely is causative.[D2]

LV systolic dysfunction, increased LV chamber sphericity, and regional asynergy of the inferoposterolateral wall overlying the posterior papillary muscle may be the most important determinants of development of mitral regurgitation.[D2,V3] Van Dantzig and colleagues found that changes in the mitral valve anulus and leaflets were of limited importance in the pathogenesis of ischemic mitral regurgitation early after myocardial infarction.[V3] Thus, although there is usually no apparent structural abnormality of the mitral valve, changes in configuration and contractile function of the left ventricle after an acute infarction prevent adequate coaptation of the leaflets and result in mitral regurgitation.

Chronic Mitral Regurgitation from Ischemic Heart Disease

About half of the patients with ischemic heart disease and chronic mitral regurgitation have *coexisting* mitral regurgitation caused by rheumatic fever, myxomatous degeneration, or other conditions.[B6] In the other half, mitral regurgitation is likely the result of ischemic heart disease. At operation, distinction between mitral regurgitation coexisting with ischemic heart disease and that caused by ischemic heart disease can be difficult, because papillary muscle scarring or fibrosis is not always the result of earlier necrosis or adjacent myocardial infarction.[B4,C1,S3]

Nonetheless, chronic localized regurgitation through the mitral apparatus does follow an acute myocardial infarction in some patients.[I1,O1,T1] The regurgitation may be localized to the region of the posteromedial commissure or the anterolateral commissure or may occur at both commissures.[I1] Causes include underlying papillary muscle ischemic dysfunction, papillary muscle scarring and shortening, previous rupture of one head of the papillary muscle, adjacent asynergy of the adjacent LV wall, and LV remodeling, all of which may result from an earlier acute myocardial infarction.

Chronic mitral regurgitation secondary to ischemic heart disease may occur through the central part of the valve.[I1] This defect generally results from anular dilatation secondary to ischemic LV dysfunction. The severity and degree of the dysfunction may vary over time according to the remodeling (increased sphericity) that occurs in the individual patient after acute infarction.[D2,R2,V3]

CLINICAL FEATURES AND DIAGNOSTIC CRITERIA

Acute Mitral Regurgitation Complicating Myocardial Infarction

Papillary muscle rupture presents as an acute event within a few hours to 14 days after a myocardial infarction. The onset is usually characterized by pulmonary edema, hypotension, or both, typically 2 to 7 days after acute infarction.[N1,V1,W1] Rupture is signaled by worsening of the patient's clinical condition. Profound shock indicates gross mitral regurgitation from total rupture; less severe signs indicate less severe mitral regurgitation from partial rupture or LV dysfunction.[D2,V3] A new apical systolic murmur can be heard provided cardiac output is adequate and the regurgitation is not severe. The murmur is frequently absent in total rupture and usually present in partial rupture.[V1] An apical third heart sound is common, and pulmonary edema is often seen on chest radiography. The heart is usually normal in size or only slightly enlarged, and the left atrium is small.

A pulmonary artery (Swan-Ganz) catheter can provide important information, such as excluding the presence of left-to-right shunting and, when it is in the pulmonary artery wedge position, demonstrating a prominent *v* wave on the pressure tracing.

Echocardiography (two-dimensional or transesophageal) is a valuable diagnostic tool in mitral regurgitation associated with myocardial infarction.[N1] It is used to differentiate between papillary muscle rupture and LV dysfunction. In the latter the findings usually involve extensive wall motion abnormalities. With papillary muscle rupture the mitral leaflet becomes flail and extends into the left atrium during systole.[N1] The ruptured portion of the muscle may be directly visualized as a separate mass attached to the chordae.[E1,M2,N1]

Left ventriculography may be performed to confirm the diagnosis of mitral regurgitation (or ventricular septal defect or occasionally both) and to define areas of impaired LV contraction or aneurysm formation. In critically ill patients, however, left ventriculography is unnecessary when precatheterization studies have established the diagnosis, and only coronary angiography is performed.

When the patient is seriously ill, an intraaortic balloon pump should be used. If the patient's hemodynamic state remains unstable, cardiopulmonary bypass (CPB) can be established using a percutaneous technique (see "Cardiopulmonary Bypass Established by Peripheral Cannulation" under Special Situations and Controversies in Section 3 of Chapter 2). These devices can be left in place until cardiac catheterization is completed and the patient is taken to the operating room.

Chronic Mitral Regurgitation from Ischemic Heart Disease

Usually the patient presents with gradually increasing mitral regurgitation. When the murmur dates from a myocardial infarction, an ischemic etiology is assumed. There may be cardiac enlargement, including left atrial enlargement, hypokinesia, and akinesia at the infarction site. An LV aneurysm may coexist. Other diagnostic criteria are the same as for other types of chronic mitral regurgitation (see Chapter 11).

NATURAL HISTORY

Acute Mitral Regurgitation Complicating Myocardial Infarction

Rupture of a papillary muscle is an uncommon complication of acute myocardial infarction[W1] and probably even less common with current thrombolytic and percutaneous interventional therapy for acute infarction.[H1] Papillary muscle rupture is a life-threatening complication, with only about 25% of patients treated nonsurgically surviving more than 24 hours after total rupture.[S1,V1] Survival after partial papillary rupture is better; more than 70% of patients survive the first 24 hours, and about 50% survive more than 1 month. They are then considered to have *chronic* mitral regurgitation.

When the papillary muscle remains intact, the natural history of acute mitral regurgitation is less well defined. As previously noted, however, moderate or severe mitral regurgitation in the absence of papillary muscle rupture is present in 3% to 19% of patients early after an acute infarction and is an important predictor of mortality.[L1,L2,T2,V3] Using multivariable analysis, Lehmann and colleagues found that mitral regurgitation of any degree (as detected by left ventriculography) was a predictor of cardiovascular mortality at 1 year (relative risk 7.5; CL 2%-29%; $P = .0008$).[L1] In the study of Lamas and colleagues, cardiovascular mortality during 3½ years of follow-up was also higher in patients who developed mitral regurgitation early after acute infarction than in those who did not (29% versus 12%; $P < .001$).[L2] In the chronic phase after myocardial infarction, mitral regurgitation predicts mortality in excess of that anticipated

on the basis of patient characteristics and degree of LV dysfunction.[G5]

Chronic Mitral Regurgitation from Ischemic Heart Disease

Fortunately, severe chronic mitral regurgitation caused by ischemic heart disease is relatively uncommon, appearing in only about 3% of patients with chronic ischemic heart disease.[H1] Mild or moderate mitral regurgitation without papillary muscle rupture is episodic in some patients, presumably a result of changing prevalence and distribution of myocardial ischemia, loading characteristics of the LV, and variable LV function. Persistent and severe mitral regurgitation, often associated with moderate or severe LV dysfunction,[R1,V2] worsens the prognosis for patients with poor LV function. Furthermore, increasing severity of mitral regurgitation has an increasingly adverse effect on survival, regardless of type of treatment.[H1]

TECHNIQUE OF OPERATION

Acute Mitral Regurgitation Complicating Myocardial Infarction

In critically ill patients with this complication of acute myocardial infarction, intraaortic balloon pumping (IABP) is begun as soon as the condition is recognized,[B1] or CPB is established by percutaneous technique if indicated (see "Cardiopulmonary Bypass Established by Peripheral Cannulation" under Special Situations and Controversies in Section 3 of Chapter 2).

In the operating room the patient is prepared and draped for coronary artery bypass grafting (CABG); the sternotomy, graft preparation, and preparation for CPB are expeditiously accomplished. CPB is established using two venous cannulae. If CPB was established percutaneously before bringing the patient to the operating room, the cannulations just described should be made and CPB established by a pump-oxygenator designed for use in the operating room. The femoral lines are clamped but left in place. These cannulae are removed in the operating room at the end of the cardiac procedure, using an open technique and repair of the vessels.

Myocardial management may include warm induction of cardioplegia and controlled aortic root reperfusion (see "Cold Cardioplegia, Controlled Aortic Root Perfusion, and [When Needed] Warm Cardioplegic Induction" in Chapter 3). Because an acute coronary occlusion is typically present, the coronary sinus route of administration should be employed for part of the cardioplegic infusion (see "Technique of Retrograde Infusion" under Cold Cardioplegia [Multidose] in Chapter 3).

The distal anastomoses of the bypass grafts are performed before the mitral valve is repaired or replaced to avoid retracting the heart after a mitral prosthesis (valve or ring) has been inserted and thus prevent possible rupture of an area of infarcted LV.[H2] The proximal anastomoses of the grafts can be performed either immediately after completing the distal anastomoses and before opening the left atrium, or after closing the left atrium. If the left atrium has been closed, these anastomoses can be performed with the aorta still occluded or after removing the aortic clamp and placing a partially occluding clamp on the aorta while rewarming is completed.

The approach to the mitral valve is generally through the left atrium in the usual fashion, although an approach through the right atrium may be useful (see "Approach Across the Atrial Septum" under Special Situations and Controversies in Chapter 11). With acute total papillary muscle rupture, the mitral valve is replaced with a mechanical prosthesis or bioprosthesis. Because the mitral anular tissue is usually not thickened and may be more friable than normal, great care must be taken to (1) obtain adequate bites of tissue when placing the anular sutures and (2) avoid excessive traction on these sutures as the valve is lowered into position, to prevent them from pulling through the tissues. Pledgeted mattress or nonpledgeted simple interrupted sutures are preferred.

When the papillary muscle is not ruptured and the chordal mechanism is intact, or if only one head is ruptured and there is anular dilatation, reparative techniques and anuloplasty with or without use of an anuloplasty ring are preferable to valve replacement[H1,R2] (see "Mitral Regurgitation Repair" under Technique of Operation in Chapter 11). If inserting an anuloplasty ring or band, it is probably preferable to use one that is smaller than the sizer that fits the anulus. After CPB is discontinued and with cannulae still in place, competence of the valve is assessed, preferably by transesophageal echocardiography. Left atrial pressure should be at least 15 mmHg and systolic arterial pressure above 120 to 130 mmHg. Unless the valve is competent, CPB is reestablished, cardioplegia is reinfused, and the valve is either repaired again or replaced.

The remainder of the operation is completed as usual (see "Completing Cardiopulmonary Bypass" in Chapter 3). An IABP or temporary ventricular assistance may be needed (see "Treatment of Low Cardiac Output" under Cardiovascular Subsystem in Section 1 of Chapter 5).

Chronic Mitral Regurgitation from Ischemic Heart Disease

The techniques of repair and replacement of the chronically regurgitant mitral valve are described under "Technique of Operation" in Chapter 11. Difficulties in intraoperative decision making result from (1) time-related variability in the magnitude of regurgitation caused by ischemic heart disease, (2) uncertainty about the precise morphologic basis of the regurgitation, and (3) frequency with which regurgitation is associated with poor LV function. These considerations require careful evaluation of regurgitation and need for mitral repair or replacement preoperatively, in the operating room before CPB is established, after repair while CPB is still in place, and after CPB is discontinued. Evaluation includes visual examination of the morphology of the valve and identification of the location and magnitude of the regurgitation.

On direct visualization of the valve, diagnosis of an ischemic etiology for regurgitation is generally made by exclusion. The anulus appears normal or is only slightly dilated. The leaflets are usually normal in appearance, and the chordae tendineae are not shortened or elongated. The papillary muscles may be pale, scarred, or normal in appearance. In this setting, repair of the valve with some form of anuloplasty is usually possible (see Chapter 11).

Identifying the location and assessing the magnitude of regurgitation are accomplished by transesophageal echocardiography, recognizing that this technique can both overestimate and underestimate the degree of regurgitation. When the circulation is intact, echocardiographic assessments should be made with left atrial pressure at least 12 to 15 mmHg and systolic pressure above 120 to 130 mmHg.

When regurgitation is *severe* both preoperatively and intraoperatively and dominates the clinical picture, mitral repair or replacement is performed. When severity of regurgitation is *variable* preoperatively and variable and no more than moderate intraoperatively (particularly when severity lessens after the CABG portion of the operation is completed), and signs and symptoms of myocardial ischemia are dominant, the mitral valve may be left alone. However, this recommendation is controversial.[A2,A3,C2,D3,G2] *Intermediate situations* demand individual intraoperative decision making.

When a repair is performed, the functional status of the mitral valve is evaluated by transesophageal echocardiography after discontinuing CPB, with the cannulae still in place and with the systolic arterial pressure above 120 to 130 mmHg. If the hemodynamic situation or the repair is unsatisfactory, CPB can be reestablished and the mitral valve repaired again or replaced. If mitral replacement is necessary, every effort should be made to preserve the chordae tendineae to the posterior leaflet or to both leaflets.[G2,G3]

SPECIAL FEATURES OF POSTOPERATIVE CARE

The usual management protocols are followed (see Chapter 5). Because patients with mitral regurgitation from ischemic heart disease are apt to have low cardiac output postoperatively, catecholamine support and IABP are required more often than after other procedures.

RESULTS

Early (Hospital) Death

Acute Mitral Regurgitation Complicating Myocardial Infarction

For patients with rupture of a papillary muscle who undergo early operation, both excellent (no deaths among seven patients[N2]) and poor early survival (two deaths among five patients treated within 7 days of the infarction[B1]) have been reported. However, the small number of patients makes it unlikely that these experiences are similar (70%; CLs of early mortality were 0% to 24% in the first experience and 14% to 71% in the second). For patients without rupture of a papillary muscle who require operation for ischemic mitral regurgitation, hospital mortality is substantial (up to 67%), particularly for patients in cardiogenic shock.[D5,H3,R3,T3]

With use of appropriate myocardial management (see "Technique of Operation"), early mortality should depend primarily on extent of the myocardial infarction. This approach probably explains the favorable effect of early reperfusion after the infarction observed by Hickey and colleagues.[H1]

Chronic Mitral Regurgitation from Ischemic Heart Disease

Hospital mortality currently is about 9% to 15% for patients with chronic ischemic mitral regurgitation who undergo valve replacement or repair, usually in combination with CABG, and who are *not* in cardiogenic shock.[C4,D4,G4,H3,H4] Important predictors of increased hospital mortality include low ejection fraction (less than 30% to 35%), previous anterior infarction, extensive coronary artery disease, and advanced age.[G3,H1-H3,R1] Although mitral valve repair is clearly preferable to replacement, hospital mortality in several large series was not consistently lower among comparable patients who underwent repair.[C4,G4,H4] Concomitant procedures such as LV aneurysmectomy may be associated with increased hospital mortality.[G3,R1]

Time-Related Survival

When the operation is done acutely for rupture of a papillary muscle, late results are often good.[B1,C4,G4,N2]

Overall survival after CABG, including hospital mortality, is distinctly poorer in patients with ischemic mitral regurgitation than in those without it.[H1] Also, survival after CABG plus mitral valve replacement or repair is poorer when the regurgitation is ischemic in origin rather than rheumatic or degenerative.[G2,K1] These differences probably relate to impaired LV performance in patients with ischemic mitral regurgitation.[M1,R1]

Nonetheless, survival of patients with chronic ischemic mitral regurgitation who are treated surgically is better than that of those treated medically.[H1] Risk factors for poor outcomes in patients with ischemic heart disease in general apply to this group as well (see Chapter 7).

Addition of LV aneurysmectomy to the procedure adversely affects long-term survival. Miller and colleagues found poor late results in this group, with only 35% (CL 4% to 25%) of hospital survivors alive 3 years later.[M1] In a longer experience with valve replacement as an isolated or combined procedure, Karp and colleagues found that preoperative LV aneurysm was a significant incremental risk factor for premature late death.[K2]

In the study of Hickey and colleagues, mitral valve repair was associated with better long-term survival than mitral valve replacement.[H1] In a more recent nonrandomized study of surgery for ischemic mitral regurgitation, however, Hausmann and colleagues observed no difference in early or late survival among 197 patients treated by mitral valve replacement and 140 patients treated by mitral valve repair (Fig. 10-1).[H4] Seven-year survival was 67% and 62%, respectively, although it was better among patients who had no or minimal mitral regurgitation after the repair (77% at 7 years) than among those who had more extensive regurgitation or mitral valve replacement (Fig. 10-2).[H4] Gillinov and colleagues, using propensity analysis and multivariable hazard function regression, observed that in patients with ischemic mitral regurgitation who were not at high risk (younger age, lower New York Heart Association [NYHA] class, fewer

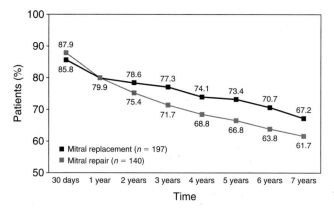

Figure 10-1   Survival after mitral valve replacement and mitral valve repair for patients with ischemic mitral regurgitation. (From Hausmann and colleagues.[H4])

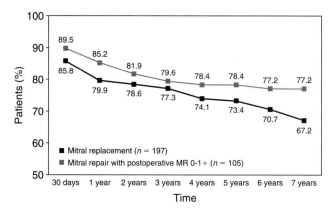

Figure 10-2   Survival after mitral valve replacement and mitral valve repair with either no or only grade 1+ mitral regurgitation postoperatively. (From Hausmann and colleagues[H4])

Key: *MR,* Mitral regurgitation.

wall motion abnormalities, no renal dysfunction), mitral valve repair was associated with higher survival at 5 years (58%) than was valve replacement (36%) ($P = .08$).[G4] There was no survival benefit for mitral valve repair among higher-risk patients.

Functional State

Symptomatic relief is generally good in survivors of mitral valve replacement and CABG for ischemic mitral regurgitation. Most patients experience considerable relief of their heart failure symptoms[R1] and are in NYHA class I or II between 3 to 5 years postoperatively (Fig. 10-3).[D4,R1] Less favorable results in such patients reported in 1973 by Glancy and colleagues may be related to the operation consisting of mitral valve replacement alone.[G1] Again, the less favorable outcomes in patients undergoing LV aneurysmectomy plus mitral replacement and coronary revascularization are evident in the data of Radford and colleagues; none of the three long-term survivors in this category had symptomatic improvement from that operation[R1] (see Fig. 10-3).

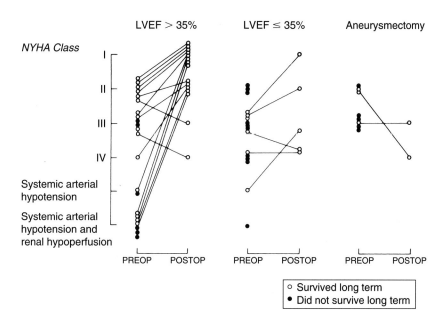

Figure 10-3   Functional status after valve replacement for ischemic mitral regurgitation: degree of heart failure (New York Heart Association [NYHA] functional class) before operation and during follow-up. The follow-up heart failure status is unknown for three long-term survivors; these patients are designated by preoperative symbols that are unconnected to postoperative symbols. Systemic arterial hypotension and renal hypoperfusion represent more advanced heart failure than implied by NYHA class IV. (From Radford and colleagues.[R1])

Key: *LVEF,* Left ventricular ejection fraction.

INDICATIONS FOR OPERATION

When a patient with an acute myocardial infarction suddenly develops acute mitral regurgitation, operation is advisable, recognizing that hospital mortality under such circumstances may be 30% or greater. As with acute rupture of the ventricular septum (see Chapter 9), operation should be done before severe hemodynamic deterioration occurs. When the hemodynamic state is reasonably good, one strategy has been to delay operation about 2 weeks to 2 months. However, Nishimura and colleagues reported sudden deterioration followed by death in five patients whose condition had initially stabilized with medical therapy.[N1] Therefore, all patients with papillary muscle rupture complicating acute myocardial infarction should have prompt investigation and operation. Operation should be avoided only when the patient is moribund.

When chronic mitral regurgitation results from ischemic heart disease, indications for operation are less well defined. Infrequently, and particularly when it develops acutely from partial rupture of a papillary muscle after myocardial infarction, mitral regurgitation dominates the clinical picture and causes the symptoms and disability.[R1] Then the decision for operation on the mitral valve is straightforward and based on the usual indications (see Chapter 11).

More often, however, patients with usual symptoms of ischemic heart disease have some signs of LV failure and clinical and angiographic evidence of mitral regurgitation. As already mentioned, the degree of regurgitation may fluctuate, but it may be constant and moderate or severe. In the latter circumstances, operation is indicated, including mitral valve replacement or repair. When the severity of regurgitation varies over time, it is more difficult to know when mitral valve surgery should be done at the time of CABG. The effect of CABG alone on this form of mitral regurgitation is not known with certainty. If mitral regurgitation is at least moderate (grade 3 or more on a scale of 1 to 6), however, as determined by intraoperative transesophageal echocardiography, mitral repair or replacement is indicated (see "Technique of Operation").

If mitral regurgitation is severe in patients with a low ejection fraction (10% to 20%), mitral valve replacement rather than repair may be indicated, because persistent mitral regurgitation after repair is associated with substantial early and late mortality.[H4] Patients with severe LV dysfunction and mitral regurgitation who are suitable surgical candidates should be considered for transplantation as an alternative to myocardial revascularization and mitral repair or replacement.[H3]

REFERENCES

A

1. Austen WG, Sanders CA, Averill JH, Friedlich AL. Ruptured papillary muscle: report of a case with successful mitral valve replacement. Circulation 1965;32:597.
2. Arcidi JM Jr, Hebeler RF, Craver JM, Jones EL, Hatcher CR Jr, Guyton RA. Treatment of moderate mitral regurgitation and coronary disease by coronary bypass alone. J Thorac Cardiovasc Surg 1988; 95:951.
3. Aklog L, Filsoufi F, Flores KQ, Chen RH, Cohn LH, Nathan NS, et al. Does coronary artery bypass grafting alone correct moderate ischemic mitral regurgitation? Circulation 2001;104:I68.

B

1. Buckley MJ, Mundth ED, Daggett WM, Gold HK, Leinbach RC, Austen WG. Surgical management of ventricular septal defects and mitral regurgitation complicating acute myocardial infarction. Ann Thorac Surg 1973;16:598.
2. Burch GE, DePasquale NP, Phillips JH. Clinical manifestations of papillary muscle dysfunction. Arch Intern Med 1963;112:158.
3. Breneman GM, Drake FH. Ruptured papillary muscle following myocardial infarction with long survival: report of two cases. Circulation 1962;25:862.
4. Brand FR, Brown JA, Berge KG. Histology of papillary muscle of the left ventricle in myocardial infarction. Am Heart J 1969;77:26.
5. Barbour DJ, Roberts WC. Rupture of a left ventricular papillary muscle during acute myocardial infarction: analysis of 22 necropsy patients. J Am Coll Cardiol 1986;8:558.
6. Bolling SF, Deeb GM, Bach DS. Mitral valve reconstruction in elderly, ischemic patients. Chest 1996;109:35.
7. Barzilai B, Gessler C Jr, Perez JE, Schaab C, Jaffe AS. Significance of Doppler-detected mitral regurgitation in acute myocardial infarction. Am J Cardiol 1988;61:220.

C

1. Coma-Canella I, Gamallo C, Onsurbe PM, Jadraque LM. Anatomic findings in acute papillary muscle necrosis. Am Heart J 1989;118:1188.
2. Christenson JT, Simonet F, Bloch A, Maurice J, Velebit V, Schmuziger M. Should a mild or moderate ischemic mitral valve regurgitation in patients with poor left ventricular function be repaired or not? J Heart Valve Dis 1995;4:484.
3. Czer LS, Maurer G, Bolger AF, DeRobertis M, Chaux A, Matloff JM. Revascularization alone or combined with suture annuloplasty for ischemic mitral regurgitation. Tex Heart Inst J 1996;23:270.
4. Cohn LH, Rizzo RJ, Adams DH, Couper GS, Sullivan TE, Collins JJ Jr, et al. The effect of pathophysiology on the surgical treatment of ischemic mitral regurgitation: operative and late risks of repair versus replacement. Eur J Cardiothorac Surg 1995;9:568.

D

1. Davidson S. Spontaneous rupture of a papillary muscle of the heart: a report of three cases and a review of the literature. Mt Sinai J Med 1948;14:941.
2. Dent JM, Spotnitz WD, Kaul S. Echocardiographic evaluation of the mechanisms of ischemic mitral regurgitation. Coron Artery Dis 1996;7:188.
3. Duarte IG, Shen Y, MacDonald MJ, Jones EL, Craver JM, Guyton RA. Treatment of moderate mitral regurgitation and coronary disease by coronary bypass alone: late results. Ann Thorac Surg 1999;68:426.
4. Dion R, Benetis R, Elias B, Guennaoui T, Raphael D, Van Dyck M, et al. Mitral valve procedures in ischemic regurgitation. J Heart Valve Dis 1995;4:S124.
5. Dion R. Ischemic mitral regurgitation: when and how should it be corrected? J Heart Valve Dis 1993;2:536.

E

1. Erbel R, Schweizer P, Bardos P, Meyer J. Two-dimensional echocardiographic diagnosis of papillary muscle rupture. Chest 1981;79:595.
2. Estes EH Jr, Dalton FM, Entman ML, Dixon HB II, Hackel DB. The anatomy and blood supply of the papillary muscles of the left ventricle. Am Heart J 1966;71:356.

G

1. Glancy DL, Stinson EB, Shepherd RL, Itscoitz SB, Roberts WC, Epstein SE, et al. Results of valve replacement for severe mitral regurgitation due to papillary muscle rupture or fibrosis. Am J Cardiol 1973;32:313.
2. Galloway AC, Grossi EA, Spencer FC, Colvin SB. Operative therapy for mitral insufficiency from coronary artery disease. Semin Thorac Cardiovasc Surg 1995;7:227.
3. Goor DA, Mohr R, Lavee J, Serraf A, Smolinsky A. Preservation of the posterior leaflet during mechanical valve replacement for ischemic mitral regurgitation and complete myocardial revascularization. J Thorac Cardiovasc Surg 1988;96:253.
4. Gillinov AM, Wierup PN, Blackstone EH, Bishay ES, Cosgrove DM, White J, et al. Is repair preferable to replacement for ischemic mitral regurgitation? J Thorac Cardiovasc Surg 2001;122:1125.
5. Grigioni F, Enriquez-Sarano M, Zehr KJ, Bailey KR, Tajik J. Ischemic mitral regurgitation: long-term outcome and prognostic implications with quantitative Doppler assessment. Circulation 2001;103:1759.

H

1. Hickey MS, Smith LR, Muhlbaier LH, Harrell FE, Reves JG, Hinohara T, et al. Current prognosis of ischemic mitral regurgitation: implications for future management. Circulation 1988;78:I51.
2. Harold JG, Bateman TM, Czer LS, Chaux A, Matloff JM, Gray RJ. Mitral valve replacement early after myocardial infarction: attendant high risk of left ventricular rupture. J Am Coll Cardiol 1987;9:277.
3. Hausmann H, Siniawski H, Hotz H, Hofmeister J, Chavez T, Schmidt G, et al. Mitral valve reconstruction and mitral replacement for ischemic mitral insufficiency. J Card Surg 1997;12:8.
4. Hausmann H, Siniawski H, Hetzer R. Mitral valve reconstruction and replacement for ischemic mitral insufficiency: seven years' follow up. J Heart Valve Dis 1999;8:536.

I

1. Izumi S, Miyatake K, Beppu S, Park YD, Nagata S, Kinoshita N, et al. Mechanism of mitral regurgitation in patients with myocardial infarction: a study using real-time two-dimensional Doppler flow imaging and echocardiography. Circulation 1987;76:777.

K

1. Kirklin JW, Blackstone EH, Rogers WJ. Bishop Lecture. The plights of the invasive treatment of ischemic heart disease. J Am Coll Cardiol 1985;5:158.
2. Karp RB, Cyrus RJ, Blackstone EH, Kirklin JW, Kouchoukos NT, Pacifico AD. The Bjork-Shiley valve. J Thorac Cardiovasc Surg 1981;81:602.

L

1. Lehmann KG, Francis CK, Dodge HT. Mitral regurgitation in early myocardial infarction. Incidence, clinical detection, and prognostic implications. TIMI Study Group. Ann Intern Med 1992;117:10.
2. Lamas GA, Mitchell GF, Flaker GC, Smith SC, Gersh BJ, Basta L, et al. Clinical significance of mitral regurgitation after acute myocardial infarction. Circulation 1997;96:827.

M

1. Miller DC, Stinson EB, Rossiter SJ, Oyer PE, Reitz BA, Shumway NE: Impact of simultaneous myocardial revascularization on operative risk, functional result, and survival following mitral valve replacement. Surgery 1978;84:848.
2. Mintz GS, Victor MF, Kotler MN, Parry WR, Segal BL. Two-dimensional echocardiographic identification of surgically correctable complications of acute myocardial infarction. Circulation 1981;64:91.

N

1. Nishimura RA, Schaff HV, Shub C, Gersh BJ, Edwards WE, Tajik AJ. Papillary muscle rupture complicating acute myocardial infarction: analysis of 17 patients. Am J Cardiol 1983;51:373.
2. Nishimura RA, Schaff HV, Gersh BJ, Holmes DR, Tajik AJ. Early repair of mechanical complications after acute myocardial infarction. JAMA 1986;256:47.

O

1. Ogawa S, Hubbard FE, Mardelli TJ, Dreifus LS. Cross-sectional echocardiographic spectrum of papillary muscle dysfunction. Am Heart J 1979;97:312.

R

1. Radford MJ, Johnson RA, Buckley MJ, Daggett WM, Leinbach RC, Godl HK. Survival following mitral valve replacement for mitral regurgitation due to coronary artery disease. Circulation 1979;60:I39.
2. Rankin JS, Hickey MS, Smith LR, Debruijn NP, Clements FM, Muhlbaier LH. Current management of mitral valve incompetence associated with coronary artery disease. J Card Surg 1989;4:25.
3. Rankin JS, Feneley MP, Hickey MS, Muhlbaier LH, Wechsler AS, Floyd D, et al. A clinical comparison of mitral valve repair versus valve replacement in ischemic mitral regurgitation. J Thorac Cardiovasc Surg 1988;95:165.

S

1. Sanders RJ, Neubuerger KT, Ravin A. Rupture of papillary muscles: occurrence of rupture of the posterior muscle in posterior myocardial infarction. Dis Chest 1957;36:316.

2. Stevenson RR, Turner WJ. Rupture of a papillary muscle in the heart as a cause of sudden death. Bull Johns Hopkins Hosp 1935;57:235.
3. Schwartz CJ, Mitchell JR. The relation between myocardial lesions and coronary artery disease. I. An unselected necropsy study. Br Heart J 1962;24:761.

T

1. Tallury VK, DePasquale NP, Burch GE. The echocardiogram in papillary muscle dysfunction. Am Heart J 1972;83:12.
2. Tcheng JE, Jackman JD Jr, Nelson CL, Gardner LH, Smith LR, Rankin JS, et al. Outcome of patients sustaining acute ischemic mitral regurgitation during myocardial infarction. Ann Intern Med 1992;117:18.
3. Tepe NA, Edmunds LH Jr. Operation for acute postinfarction mitral insufficiency and cardiogenic shock. J Thorac Cardiovasc Surg 1985; 89:525.

V

1. Vlodaver Z, Edwards JE. Rupture of ventricular septum or papillary muscle complicating myocardial infarction. Circulation 1977;55:815.
2. Vismara LA, Miller RR, DeMaria A, Mason DT, Amsterdam EA. Mitral regurgitation in patients with coronary artery disease: relation to extent of myocardial dysfunction (abstract). Am J Cardiol 1974; 33:175.
3. Van Dantzig JM, Delemarre BJ, Koster RW, Bot H, Visser CA. Pathogenesis of mitral regurgitation in acute myocardial infarction: importance of changes in left ventricular shape and regional function. Am Heart J 1996;131:865.

W

1. Wei JY, Hutchins GM, Bulkley BH. Papillary muscle rupture in fatal acute myocardial infarction: a potentially treatable form of cardiogenic shock. Ann Intern Med 1979;90:149.

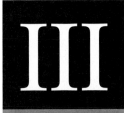

III Acquired Valvar Heart Disease

11 Mitral Valve Disease with or without Tricuspid Valve Disease

SECTION 1

Mitral Valve Disease

DEFINITION

This chapter describes the surgical aspects of acquired mitral valve disease, excluding ischemic mitral regurgitation (see Chapter 10). Associated or secondary tricuspid valve disease is also considered (see Section 2 of this chapter and Chapter 14), as is concomitant coronary artery surgery in patients with nonischemic mitral valve disease (see Section 3 of this chapter).

HISTORICAL NOTE

Mitral Stenosis

Sir Lauder Brunton was among the first surgeons to consider surgical treatment of mitral stenosis in his "preliminary note" in *The Lancet* in 1902.[B1] Cutler, then at Western Reserve University Medical School in Cleveland and later the Mosley Professor of Surgery at Harvard Medical School and Peter Bent Brigham Hospital in Boston, did experimental work on surgical approaches to mitral stenosis. In 1923, Cutler and Levine reported an operation via median sternotomy in which a special curved knife was inserted through the left ventricular apex to cut a stenotic mitral valve.[C1] In 1925, Souttar digitally opened a stenotic mitral valve through the left atrial appendage.[S1]

An effective closed surgical approach to mitral stenosis began with Harken and colleagues and Bailey in the United States and Brock and colleagues in London.[B2,B28,H1] Harken had been doing animal experiments involving mitral valve surgery at the Boston City Hospital in 1939 before serving with the United States Army in World War II, during which time he became well known for successful removal of missiles and shell fragments from the heart. After the war he continued his work on mitral valve surgery at the Boston City and Peter Bent Brigham Hospitals. Bailey was working primarily at Hahnemann Hospital in Philadelphia. Although their techniques and terminology were somewhat different, their approaches to opening the stenotic mitral valve through the left atrial appendage were similar. Technical modifications subsequently added to *closed commissurotomy* included Tubb's transventricular dilator, used with digital control by a finger inserted through the left atrial appendage.[A6]

In 1955, surgeons began to think of opening stenosed mitral valves by open techniques on cardiopulmonary bypass (CPB). However, closed operations produced such generally good results that the open technique did not come into wide use until after 1970.

Mitral Regurgitation

Although a few ingenious *closed* methods of surgically improving mitral regurgitation were reported during the 1950s, particularly by Bailey, Davila, Nichols, and their colleagues,[B29,D9,N3] an effective *open* approach using CPB was not made until 1957 by Lillehei and colleagues[L5] and Merendino and Bruce.[M4] McGoon described an effective repair for mitral regurgitation due to ruptured chordae in 1960.[M3] In subsequent years a number of surgeons have contributed technical advances in the repair of mitral regurgitation, particularly Carpentier, Duran, Frater, Reed, and their colleagues.[C35,D5,F7,R6]

Mitral Valve Replacement

A number of surgeons realized very early the need for replacement of at least some diseased mitral valves. However, it was Starr and Edwards from the University of Oregon Medical Center who, in 1961, first reported successful mitral valve replacement using a mechanical prosthesis.[S2]

MORPHOLOGY

Acquired mitral stenosis is usually a result of rheumatic heart disease, as is mixed stenosis and regurgitation. Pure mitral regurgitation may be rheumatic in origin, but is more frequently the result of another pathologic process.

Mitral Stenosis

Commissural fusion and *leaflet thickening* are the dominant features in clinically important mitral stenosis. The characteristic fusion of the edges of the mitral leaflets in commissural areas is a complex process, involving coapting edges of commissural, posterior (mural), and anterior (septal) leaflets at both the anterolateral and posteromedial commissures. Valve leaflets are thickened to varying degrees, particularly at their free edges and sites of fusion. Calcification often occurs in older patients, beginning at the commissures but at times extending posteriorly into the anulus.

Chordae tendineae are variably involved by the rheumatic process. Occasionally, in the presence of severe mitral stenosis, the chordae are nearly normal in appearance, and opening the valve commissures results in a wide orifice. More often, some degree of chordal thickening, fusion, and shortening is present in each commissural area. This process is extreme in some patients, particularly those in whom restenosis develops after an earlier commissurotomy, and results in an obstructing, tough, subcommissural mass on both sides of the narrow orifice. This advanced pathologic condition may be purely rheumatic in origin or may partly result from hemodynamic and (in the case of restenosis) surgical trauma. Subcommissural pathology may render the mitral apparatus severely stenotic, even after commissurotomy.

The *left atrium* is enlarged in pure mitral stenosis but usually not severely, and its wall is thickened. *Left ventricular* (LV) volume and mass are normal or slightly reduced.[K1] When fibrosis and particularly calcification involve the mitral anulus, regional wall motion at the base of the left ventricle (LV) is impaired, but overall LV systolic and diastolic function are often normal.[G6] Late in the disease, however, LV function may be impaired.

Pulmonary vascular resistance (Rp) may increase in patients with severe mitral stenosis. This increase may be the result of spasm in the pulmonary arterioles, presumably a reflex from left atrial hypertension. Organic pulmonary vascular disease may also increase Rp and is often found in young Polynesian and Asian patients, as well as in a small proportion of other patients with long-standing mitral stenosis. Rarely, the vascular disease may progress to obliteration of pulmonary arterioles.[P10] Increased Rp produces a rise in pulmonary artery and right ventricular pressure out of proportion to the valve stenosis and left atrial pressure increase, which leads to right ventricular hypertrophy and secondary tricuspid regurgitation.

Mitral Stenosis and Regurgitation

Mixed mitral stenosis and regurgitation is primarily rheumatic in origin. Stenosis is produced by varying degrees of commissural fusion and chordal thickening. Regurgitation results from fibrous retraction of the central unfused portion of the leaflets and either chordal shortening or chordal elongation. Shortening restricts leaflet motion and increases the gaping central orifice, whereas elongation permits cusp prolapse. Occasionally, chordae rupture as a result of the rheumatic process.

Endocarditis on a rheumatic stenotic valve adds regurgitation by eroding leaflet or chordal tissue.

Mitral Regurgitation

Regurgitation may be due to rheumatic valve disease, but has numerous other causes and morphologic patterns.

Rheumatic Mitral Regurgitation

Mitral regurgitation may occur as a severe lesion (sometimes combined with aortic regurgitation) during the acute rheumatic process in association with extensive myocarditis and sometimes pericarditis and pancarditis. Anular dilatation is the primary cause of regurgitation in this circumstance, with the valve leaflets frequently showing edema only and virtually normal chordae. After remission of the acute process, regurgitation may spontaneously regress, presumably because the myocarditis heals, the heart becomes smaller, and the anular dilatation regresses. In most cases, however, there is progressive leaflet thickening, particularly of the posterior leaflet, which becomes retracted and rolled with shortening of chordae. The anterior leaflet is less thickened, and major chordae are frequently elongated, allowing leaflet prolapse. The posterior chordae may also elongate, and occasionally one or more may rupture. Commissural leaflets are obliterated and fused, but the commissures remain more or less open. Calcification is uncommon. Anular dilatation is almost invariably progressive and produces increasing regurgitation.

Mitral Valve Prolapse

Prolapse of a mitral valve leaflet occurring as an isolated abnormality[1] is a relatively common and complex entity.[B6,D8,F9,J4] Infrequently, in its severe form, mitral prolapse results in important mitral regurgitation (10% of patients[M5]). Nonetheless, in the United States mitral valve prolapse has been reported as the most common cause of surgically treated isolated mitral regurgitation.[R14] The basic pathologic conditions are *mitral leaflet redundancy* and *myxomatous leaflet thickening,* resulting at least partly from acid mucopolysaccharide replacement of collagen in the leaflets. The redundant and elongated leaflets no longer meet properly to support each other during systole, and they begin to overshoot into the left atrium. Not only is the valve thereby rendered regurgitant, but abnormal strain is placed on the chordae as well. The chordae elongate, and ultimately some rupture, producing more regurgitation. Calcifications may occur in the mitral anulus, but do not appear to contribute to mitral valve dysfunction.[B34]

"Idiopathic" Chordal Rupture

"Idiopathic" and more or less localized chordal rupture is usually a variant of mitral valve prolapse syndrome,[J4] in which a considerable portion of leaflet tissue is uninvolved by the myxomatous process. In most cases the posteromedial portion of the posterior leaflet is involved; after chordal rupture, this becomes redundant and flail. More extensive posterior chordal rupture sometimes occurs. Localized chordal rupture may also occur in patients with Marfan syndrome.

Mitral Anular Calcification

Mitral anular calcification may occur in older patients without evident disease of the leaflets or chordae, but it may be more common in patients with myxomatous degeneration and prolapse of the mitral leaflets.[K11,N6,S16] Anular calcification is probably a degenerative disease, more common in elderly patients and apparently more common in women.[R14] It is seen also in patients with LV hypertrophy, particularly those with hypertrophic obstructive cardiomyopathy (HOCM; see Chapter 48). The process involves the posterior, or mural, portion of the anulus more often than other portions. Degenerative anular calcification often extends into the adjacent ventricular myocardium, and it may secondarily produce mitral regurgitation or stenosis. Anular calcification considerably complicates mitral repair or replacement.[C20,C37,M21]

Ischemic Papillary Muscle Dysfunction or Rupture

Papillary muscle dysfunction or rupture resulting from myocardial infarction or ischemic fibrosis can produce severe mitral regurgitation (see Chapter 10).

Infective Endocarditis

Endocarditis is a relatively uncommon cause of pure mitral regurgitation compared with its etiologic frequency in aortic regurgitation. When the aortic valve is infected and regurgitant, vegetations may drop down onto and infect the central portion of the anterior mitral leaflet, producing perforation and mitral regurgitation. In the absence of aortic valve disease, a normal or abnormal mitral valve may become infected,[B4] with destruction of cusps, chordae, or both (see Chapter 15).

Submitral Left Ventricular Aneurysms

Submitral LV aneurysms frequently result in mitral regurgitation. This unusual type of aneurysm is not ischemic in origin and occurs most often among the southern and western African black population.[A11,A12,C19] It may be multiloculated and have a well-defined neck situated immediately beneath the posterior mitral leaflet. Mitral regurgitation often coexists because of aneurysmal distortion of the posterior leaflet and leaflet prolapse. In rare instances the aneurysm bulges into the left atrium from behind, partly obstructing the mitral orifice.

CLINICAL FEATURES AND DIAGNOSTIC CRITERIA

Mitral Stenosis

Patients with moderate mitral stenosis are often asymptomatic at rest or with ordinary activities, particularly until the third or early part of the fourth decade of life. With severe exertion, typically sexual intercourse, pulmonary edema may develop suddenly.

Patients with severe mitral stenosis and *without* important elevation of Rp ("unprotected" mitral stenosis) have easy fatigability and effort dyspnea, orthopnea, and paroxysmal nocturnal dyspnea. When Rp rises, the alveolar bed is protected from sudden rises in capillary pressure with exertion, so that pulmonary edema does not occur and orthopnea and paroxysmal nocturnal dyspnea disappear.[W2] Hemoptysis is more common in this setting. The patient with advanced mitral stenosis who has low cardiac output and chronic heart failure secondary to high Rp is seldom seen today in developed countries. These patients tend to be women who have marked mitral facies, peripheral coldness, cyanosis, hepatic enlargement and pulsation, high jugular venous pressure with waves of tricuspid regurgitation, and sometimes ascites and peripheral edema.

In most patients, mitral stenosis can be diagnosed clinically based on history, physical examination, chest radiograph, and electrocardiogram. Auscultatory findings provide good evidence of mitral stenosis when they include a loud first sound, an opening snap, and the characteristic diastolic rumble with a presystolic crescendo when sinus rhythm is present. In severe stenosis the mid-diastolic murmur occupies more than half of diastole, and the opening snap is early.

In surgical candidates with important mitral stenosis, the chest radiograph typically shows some left atrial enlargement, although it is often only about grade 2 (on a scale of 1 to 6, with 6 being most severe). The left atrial appendage may or may not appear prominent along the left upper border of the cardiac silhouette. The LV is normal in size, but the right ventricle and pulmonary artery are usually somewhat enlarged. When Rp is elevated, the pulmonary trunk, branches, and hilar arteries are more enlarged; once tricuspid regurgitation occurs, there is considerable right

---

[1] Variously termed *myxomatous mitral valve prolapse, myxomatous mitral valve degeneration, floppy valve, "the symptom complex of midsystolic click and late systolic murmur,"* and *Barlow syndrome.*[B5]

atrial and right ventricular enlargement. The lung fields also show varying degrees of pulmonary venous hypertension on the plain chest radiograph (large pulmonary veins in upper lung fields, interstitial pulmonary edema, Kerley B lines, or alveolar pulmonary edema).

The electrocardiogram (ECG) is not diagnostic, but often shows P wave abnormalities characteristic of left atrial enlargement (P mitrale) or atrial fibrillation, and evidence of right ventricular hypertrophy when pulmonary hypertension is present.

Two-dimensional echocardiography is highly reliable for diagnosing and quantifying severity of mitral stenosis. It demonstrates degree of stenosis, leaflet mobility, thickening, and probable calcification, and any subvalvar obstruction. Doppler echocardiography, enhanced by color flow imaging to identify precise flow direction, is valuable for estimating severity of stenosis.[K10] Currently, these methods suffice for estimating mitral valve area as well as morphology and gradient across the valve.

Cardiac catheterization is usually unnecessary for diagnosing mitral stenosis and estimating its severity. Catheterization is necessary in patients over about age 35 to study the coronary arteries, however, because about 25% of patients over 40 with mitral stenosis and without angina have important coronary artery disease.[M14] When balloon valvotomy is used, prevalvotomy and postvalvotomy measurements are easily made by classic catheterization techniques or by echocardiography. *Pulmonary capillary wedge pressure* (PPCW) is measured to determine the severity of pulmonary venous hypertension. PPCW (which is similar to left atrial pressure) is compared with directly measured LV diastolic pressure to determine transmitral gradient; a resting end-diastolic gradient of 10 mmHg or more indicates important mitral stenosis. Mitral valve area is calculated from Gorlin's modified orifice equation[C2]; most symptomatic patients have a mitral valve area of 0.5 to 0.8 $cm^2 \cdot m^{-2}$, but occasionally the calculated area in patients with symptoms is as large as 1 $cm^2 \cdot m^{-2}$.

In a patient coming to treatment for mitral stenosis, the possibility of left atrial myxoma must always be considered. Echocardiography can detect a left atrial myxoma[N1] and is the type of screening performed when further information is needed (see Section 1, "Myxoma," in Chapter 47).

Mitral Regurgitation

Chronic

Patients with mitral regurgitation are often asymptomatic for many years, during which time LV size may steadily increase and LV contractility decrease. Eventually, effort intolerance develops, and symptoms of pulmonary venous hypertension evolve. Fluid retention and chronic heart failure, occasionally with cardiac cachexia, are characteristic of the late stage of the disease; by then, secondary tricuspid regurgitation is usually evident.

As with mitral stenosis, important mitral regurgitation can usually be diagnosed based on history, physical examination, chest radiograph, and ECG. The classic *apical systolic murmur* of mitral regurgitation is pansystolic, loudest at the apex, and radiates to the left axilla and left lung base. When regurgitation is the result primarily of ruptured chordae and prolapse of the posterior leaflet, however, the regur-

gitant jet is directed toward the roof (superior aspect) of the left atrium and is transmitted to the aortic root. Therefore, the murmur is maximal in the parasternal aortic area and may radiate into the carotid arteries. In contrast to the anterior radiation of posterior leaflet prolapse, the murmur of anterior prolapse radiates posteriorly to the infrascapular and posterior cervical area.[G14] As a result of large and rapid mitral valve flow during diastole, an LV filling sound (S_3) and a diastolic rumble may be present. Two important signs of the severity of regurgitation are an overactive LV impulse at the apex (from LV enlargement) and a precordial lift, the latter the result of systolic pulsation in the enlarged left atrium and right ventricle.

In severe chronic mitral regurgitation, the chest radiograph usually is highly characteristic. The left atrium generally is more enlarged than in patients with mitral stenosis, and the left atrial appendage is usually prominent. The LV may be enlarged, and there may be varying degrees of right atrial enlargement, depending on the amount of associated tricuspid regurgitation.

The ECG may remain normal even in the presence of severe mitral regurgitation. However, a pattern of LV hypertrophy is common.

As with mitral stenosis, two-dimensional echocardiography demonstrates the details of leaflet pathology. Both transthoracic (TTE) and transesophageal echocardiography (TEE) are useful. Prolapse of a specific leaflet can be visualized, and Doppler color flow imaging can identify the location and magnitude of the mitral regurgitant flow. Echocardiography may also be used to estimate both degree of LV enlargement and, by quantification of shortening fraction, ventricular contractility. Newer echocardiographic methods using three-dimensional techniques offer precise and accurate evaluation of leaflet physiology and specific areas of regurgitation within the valve apparatus.

Left ventriculography also demonstrates the regurgitant process at the mitral valve and can show leaflet prolapse. The degree of regurgitation can usually be estimated with reasonable accuracy, although if left atrial or LV enlargement is severe, the estimate is less valid. Fairly accurate calculations of regurgitant flow can be made from measurements of LV stroke volume by quantitative left ventriculography, and of forward flow by some measurement of cardiac output.[R11] LV ejection fraction can also be calculated by quantitative cineangiography or radioisotope techniques. Decisions about treatment of patients with mitral regurgitation may require additional studies from which inferences can be made about LV contractility (see "Mitral Regurgitation" under Natural History later in this section).

Acute

Mitral regurgitation may develop acutely as a result of chordal rupture or infective endocarditis or may complicate the course of acute myocardial infarction (see Chapter 10). Symptoms and signs of severe pulmonary venous hypertension suddenly appear. The left atrium and LV are normal in size or only slightly enlarged. The chest radiograph is dominated by signs of pulmonary venous hypertension, and left atrial pressure is high, as is the *v* wave. The mitral regurgitation murmur is often midsystolic and higher pitched compared with the pansystolic murmur of chronic mitral regurgitation.

NATURAL HISTORY

Mitral Stenosis

Rheumatic mitral stenosis develops slowly after the initial rheumatic involvement of the valve. In the New England area of the United States, the average age of the initial attack of rheumatic fever is 12 years, average age of onset of clinical signs of mitral stenosis 20 years, and age at onset of symptoms 31 years.[B3] Progression of valvar fibrosis and calcification is related in part to repeated episodes of rheumatic fever, but mechanical trauma and deposition of platelets and other blood substances resulting from stenosis-induced alterations of flow patterns also play a role.[S3] This progression is a major factor in increasing symptoms, ultimately causing death.

Most patients with mitral stenosis have normal LV wall thickness, volume, and systolic and diastolic function,[H13,S6] but do not increase cardiac output under stress, such as when LV afterload is acutely reduced by infusion of sodium nitroprusside.[B24] These findings suggest that the major cause of chronically reduced cardiac output in these patients is obstruction at the mitral valve.[B24,H3,H12] In some patients with long-standing mitral stenosis, however, minor posterobasal regional wall contraction abnormalities develop, perhaps from a rigid mitral valve complex.[H3]

In a small proportion of patients with apparently isolated mitral stenosis (usually older people), ejection fraction is substantially reduced.[B24,C11] Such patients have severe posterobasal segmental wall contraction abnormalities,[H3] sometimes anterolateral segmental contraction abnormalities, and occasionally diffuse hypokinesis.[B24,C11,H14] Anterolateral segmental contraction abnormalities may be caused by papillary muscle scarring and immobilization. Diffuse hypokinesia may result from scarring and decreased LV compliance secondary to chronic low cardiac output and low coronary blood flow.

Once symptoms develop after the so-called latent period, their progression to a state of total disability (New York Heart Association [NYHA] functional class IV) requires an estimated 7 to 10 years (Fig. 11-1).[R2,W2] The average age of death of patients with surgically untreated mitral stenosis is estimated to be 40 to 50 years.[R1,R2]

This general pattern of evolution is considerably shorter in some parts of the world and in some races. Polynesians in New Zealand, African-Americans in south central Alabama, Inuits in Alaska, and Asians experience a greatly accelerated evolution of signs, symptoms, and disability. Many reports suggest that, in addition to possible genetic factors, economic underdevelopment may play a role.[A4,A5,B25,C8,M6,R9]

Other events tend to occur during the lifetime of patients with surgically untreated mitral stenosis, and these in turn may alter the natural history of the disease. *Atrial fibrillation* usually develops, often occurring first in paroxysmal form. The first paroxysm, usually with tachycardia, may initiate symptoms because patients with mitral stenosis are particularly sensitive to loss of the atrial contribution to ventricular filling and to shortening of ventricular filling. Although originally incited by left atrial hypertension and hypertrophy, atrial fibrillation eventually becomes permanent because of disintegration of the architecture of atrial muscle.[B26] Because it reduces cardiac output and elevates

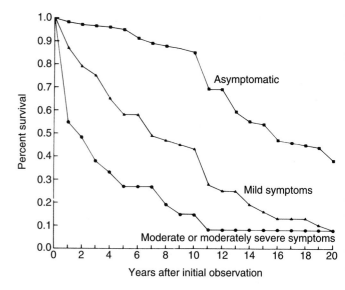

Figure 11-1 Survival of patients with nonsurgically treated mitral stenosis, according to symptomatic status at initial observation. (Modified from Rowe and colleagues.[R1])

left atrial pressure, atrial fibrillation accelerates the devolutionary course of patients with mitral stenosis and indicates a relatively advanced stage of the disease. It is an incremental risk factor for premature death of these patients. Olesen found that in patients with atrial fibrillation, 10- and 20-year survival was 25% and 10%, respectively, whereas in patients in sinus rhythm at initial observation, survival was 46% and 29%, respectively.[O1]

Systemic *arterial emboli,* most of which lodge in cerebral arteries, can suddenly complicate or kill patients with mitral stenosis. Most emboli originate in the left atrial appendage or left atrium, yet often no residual thrombus remains in the heart after embolization. Hoeksema and colleagues found that only 25% of patients with a history of arterial emboli had left atrial thrombi detected at closed commissurotomy.[H11] Also, some patients with large left atrial thrombi never have demonstrable embolization. Left atrial thrombosis and embolization are much more common when atrial fibrillation is present, but are not unknown in patients in sinus rhythm. At least 10% of surgically untreated patients develop arterial embolization during their lifetime, and a massive cerebral embolus may suddenly kill a mildly symptomatic patient.[S3]

Infectious endocarditis is unusual in patients with mitral stenosis.[R1]

Massive *pulmonary hemorrhage* may occasionally develop in patients otherwise mildly symptomatic from mitral stenosis. The association between mitral stenosis and hemorrhage is strongly suggested by its prompt and long-standing remission after surgical treatment of the stenosis.[R10]

In fact, the aforementioned features and criteria do not truly represent the "natural" (i.e., untreated) history of mitral stenosis, but rather the spectrum of mitral stenosis in *surgically untreated* patients receiving medical treatment available in the mid-twentieth century. The end stage of the disease in many patients is characterized by *cardiac cachexia,* a state infrequently seen before diuretic therapy became available. The true natural history of mitral stenosis in the first quarter of the twentieth century must have been different from that portrayed here, with the interval between onset of symptoms and death much shorter and with different patterns of death.

Likewise, evolution of the rheumatic disease complex is different in patients with mitral stenosis treated surgically versus medically. The course of the disease varies because the increased life span due to surgery now results in development of hemodynamically important rheumatic aortic valve disease and important tricuspid regurgitation in a considerably greater proportion of patients with mitral stenosis (Fig. 11-2).

Mitral Regurgitation

The natural history of mitral regurgitation is difficult to define because (1) etiology is variable; (2) age at onset is variable; (3) mitral regurgitation may be mild and nonprogressive for many years; and (4) LV function, an important determinant of symptoms and survival, deteriorates at different rates.

The effect of changes in global LV function in mitral regurgitation is modified by the fact that total LV load resisting shortening (afterload) is abnormally low in these patients (see "Ventricular Afterload" under Cardiac Output and Its Determinants in Chapter 5). Afterload is low as a result of ejection of part of the LV stroke volume into the low-pressure left atrium; because of this, the LV becomes small, and its wall thickens very early in systole.[B13,E1,U1] The more favorable relationships in Laplace's law that result reduce wall stress and afterload.[B36,H2] Because of this, LV contractility may gradually deteriorate while LV systolic function (*ejection fraction*) is maintained, the mechanism being reduction in afterload.[B36,C27,E1] The ejection fraction may even increase during exercise under these circumstances, while symptoms remain mild.[P2] Later, as mitral regurgitation becomes severe and LV contractility decreases, ejection fraction may diminish during exercise, even in asymptomatic patients.

These considerations have led to development of techniques for estimating LV function that are independent of preload and afterload.[C27] Foremost among these are those that use ventricular end-systolic pressure–volume relations. (see "Mitral Regurgitation" under Indications for Operation, Selection of Technique, and Choice of Device later in this section and "Cardiac Output and Its Determinants" in Section 1 of Chapter 5).[B39,B40,G7,M15,S17]

Patients with mitral regurgitation may develop tricuspid regurgitation, which also affects natural history (see Section 2).

Rheumatic Mitral Regurgitation

Patients with rheumatic mitral regurgitation are more likely to have had a previous severe attack of rheumatic fever than are those with mitral stenosis. The interval before the appearance of regurgitation also is shorter than for stenosis.

Patients with surgically untreated but hemodynamically important rheumatic mitral regurgitation have a survival curve surprisingly similar to those with mitral stenosis.[R2] Furthermore, the curve is different in different environmental and genetic situations, as it is in mitral stenosis. In

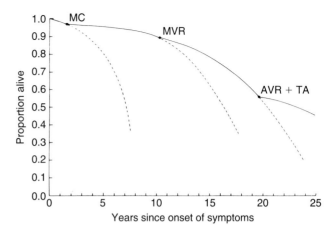

Figure 11-2   Schematic representation of life history and survival after initial development of symptoms in a large group of patients with mitral stenosis. Solid circles indicate a surgical procedure. Dashed lines represent estimated survival of patients not receiving the surgical procedure.

Key: *AVR*, Aortic valve replacement; *MC*, mitral commissurotomy; *MVR*, mitral valve replacement; *TA*, tricuspid anuloplasty.

San Francisco, for example, survival of such patients 5 years after initial evaluation was 80%, with 10-year survival of 60%, whereas in Venezuela 5-year survival was only 46%.[M1] Accelerated forms of rheumatic mitral regurgitation also occur in the same geographic areas where severe mitral stenosis appears in the pediatric population, with important symptoms by age 10 years.[S4]

Mitral Valve Prolapse

Mitral regurgitation associated with mitral valve prolapse has a complex natural history that entails more than leakage at the mitral valve. Mitral valve prolapse is believed to occur in about 2.5% to 5% of the adult population.[F9,H19,S20] The mitral leaflets not only prolapse in this condition, but are usually thickened as well.[M18] Mitral valve regurgitation is not the only event in patients with mitral prolapse. Serious but rarely fatal arrhythmias may occur in patients with only mild regurgitation,[P3] and psychiatric disturbances may develop. Symptoms may mimic thyrotoxicosis, hyperadrenergic states, or hypoglycemia.[B14,B15,C3,F2] Patients often have higher than normal catecholamine levels and other evidence of high adrenergic tone.[B14] As a further complication, patients with hyperthyroidism have an increased prevalence of mitral prolapse.[C12]

Patients with the classic form of mitral prolapse, which includes thickening of the leaflets as well as prolapse, have an increased prevalence of infective endocarditis[D13,M18]; those with normal leaflets do not. Both groups have a high prevalence of stroke.[M18]

Severe mitral regurgitation requiring valve repair or replacement rarely develops before age 50. Thereafter, the prevalence increases steeply, particularly in men.[W4] However, even men with mitral valve prolapse who have reached age 70 years have only about a 5% chance of requiring mitral valve repair or replacement. Once important mitral regurgitation appears, however, it tends to progress just as it does in patients with rheumatic mitral regurgitation. Presumably, as prolapse worsens, support in systole provided by closing of the two leaflets against each other ("stacked rifle effect") is lost. This puts an abnormally large load on the chordae, which elongate, become thick, and eventually rupture. This process worsens the regurgitation and accelerates the natural history of the disease.

Ruptured Chordae Tendineae

Patients with mitral regurgitation and ruptured chordae tendineae may have an insidious, slow development of symptoms. Ruptured chordae of the anterior or posterior leaflet, or both, are often found at operation, and the mitral valve leaflets have the appearance of myxomatous degeneration. These patients probably represent a subgroup of individuals with mitral valve prolapse. In fact, ruptured chordae may be present in patients with prolapse without important symptoms. Grenadier and colleagues found 11 (8%) of 134 patients with mitral valve prolapse to have ruptured chordae and few or no symptoms.[G5]

By contrast, important mitral regurgitation produced acutely by chordal rupture may occur in patients with no previous valve leakage. This happens predominantly in middle-age men.[S4] Often it is a complication in the life history of patients with midsystolic clicks and only trivial murmurs, but without previous evidence of mitral regurgitation. The anterior mitral leaflet and its chordae are frequently entirely normal, with the disease process limited to the medial aspect of the posterior mitral leaflet. In this group of patients with acute and severe symptoms, presumably initiated by sudden chordal rupture, the left atrium and LV are small, left atrial pressure is high, the v wave is greatly accentuated, and there is substantial clinical and radiologic evidence of pulmonary venous hypertension. TTE and TEE are diagnostic. The posteromedial segment of the valve (P_2, P_3) prolapses, and the ruptured chordae are flail or seen as thickened stubs on the affected portion of the leaflet. If the patient survives the acute event, the LV and left atrium enlarge moderately over time, and symptoms may lessen with appropriate medical management (as has been shown experimentally as well[T2]). The patient gradually regains a feeling of well-being. One year later, left atrial and ventricular enlargement may not have progressed, the LV and left atrium seemingly adapting to the volume overload. Years may pass before the self-aggravating tendency of mitral regurgitation results in increased regurgitation volume. After this, the classic natural history of important mitral regurgitation evolves.

In other patients with severe acute manifestations, symptoms improve only mildly with intense medical treatment. Although most patients survive, LV and left atrial enlargement progress steadily in the months after onset. Such patients have a large mitral regurgitant flow. When untreated surgically, they progress through the life history of severe mitral regurgitation more rapidly than do most patients, and without surgical intervention, they die within 2 to 5 years.

Infective Endocarditis

Infective endocarditis on a previously mildly abnormal mitral valve may produce acute mitral regurgitation. The natural history of that condition is similar to that described for acute chordal rupture, except that early mortality is higher. Infrequently, death is related to uncontrolled infection.

TECHNIQUE OF OPERATION

Tricuspid valve regurgitation may be associated with any type of mitral valve disease. Consequently, tricuspid anuloplasty or rarely replacement may need to be performed concomitantly with mitral valve surgery. Techniques for these operations are described in Chapter 14.

Closed Mitral Commissurotomy

After the usual preparations, including placing an arterial catheter in the right radial artery, the patient is positioned in the right lateral decubitus position. The hips are rotated to the patient's left. The left arm is placed at the patient's side and hanging slightly over the edge of a well-padded portion of the operating table, with the left hand beneath the hips. This position permits good access to the operative area.

After appropriate preparation of the skin and draping of the patient, an anterolateral incision is made over the interspace through which the impulse of the apex of the LV can be palpated. The incision in the interspace (typically the fifth or sixth) is carried posteriorly, but the latissimus dorsi usually does not require incision. At times the costal cartilage above or below the incision is transected.

The pericardium is opened anterior to the phrenic nerve. A purse-string suture is placed just off, and usually just lateral and superior to, the LV apex. The purse string is threaded into a Rummel tourniquet or similar device. A similar purse-string suture is placed around the tip of the left atrial appendage. With both the assistant and surgeon grasping their own side of the appendage with a sturdy thumb (tissue) forceps, an incision is made just off its tip. The incision must be of a size to accommodate the surgeon's right index finger snugly. While bleeding is controlled by opposing the thumb forceps, blood is allowed to escape for two or three brief periods so that small clots may emerge. The surgeon's right index finger is then insinuated through the appendage into the left atrium and passed directly to the mitral valve. After the valve is evaluated, pressure is applied with the exploring finger against the anterolateral commissure. Occasionally, this maneuver opens a pliable but severely stenotic valve widely and essentially completely, with no further action needed. In most cases, however, a Tubbs dilator is required and is inserted through a small stab wound in the center of the LV apical purse string (Fig. 11-3, *A*).

An assistant gently secures the Rummel tourniquet that has engaged the apical purse-string suture. Guided by the intraatrial finger and with the setscrew on the dilator positioned so that the maximal opening is 2.5 cm, the dilator is passed through the valve. The dilator blades are opened moderately for a few seconds to ensure that each dilating blade is against a leaflet and not a commissure (Fig. 11-3, *B*). This and each successive dilatation last only 5 to 6 seconds, and the heart is allowed to recover completely between dilatations. Successive dilatations are then performed, first with the maximum opening set at

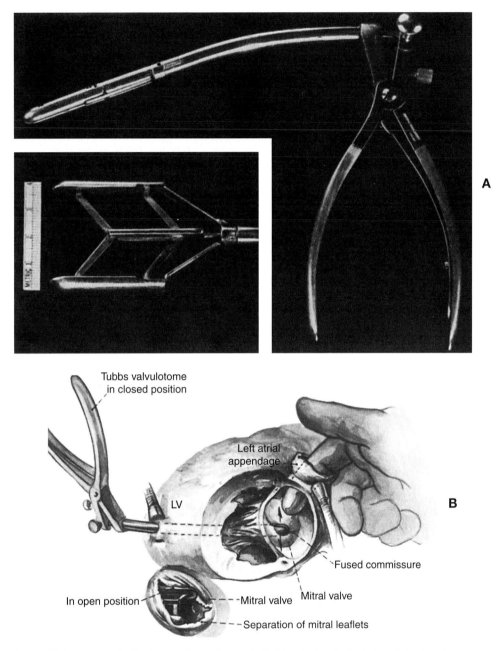

Figure 11-3 Closed mitral commissurotomy. **A**, Tubbs dilator (valvulotome). Note setscrew on handle and small size of closed tip. **B**, Dilator is advanced into mitral valve orifice against right index finger. The blades are opened against the leaflets, *not* against the commissures. (From Ellis.[E6])

Key: *LV*, Left ventricle.

2.5 cm and then at about 2.9, 3.3, 3.7, and finally 4.0 cm. In small patients the maximum dilator setting should be 3.3 to 3.5 cm. If important regurgitation develops after a dilatation, no larger settings should be attempted. Again, after the heart has recovered, the index finger is withdrawn as an assistant places a side-biting clamp across the lips of the incision in the appendage. At times, two Allis-Adair forceps close the incision well, and the clamp is not necessary. The purse string around the entrance of the Tubbs dilator is loosened slightly and then

secured as the dilator is removed. No effort is made to tighten the purse string so that *all* bleeding stops, lest the purse string cut through the ventricular muscle. Digital control suffices for residual bleeding. Several full-thickness interrupted stitches are placed in the stab wound, and the purse-string suture is removed from the tourniquet and tied snugly but not tightly. The incision in the atrial appendage is closed with a few interrupted stitches. Usually the purse string on the appendage is removed rather than tied because of the risk of dislodging a small thrombus that may have formed. A large (2-cm) window is made in the pericardium posteriorly, behind the phrenic nerve, for drainage into the left pleural space. The pericardium is then closed with widely spaced interrupted sutures. A catheter is placed posterolaterally in the left pleural space, hemostasis is secured, and the incision is closed in layers.

Open Mitral Commissurotomy

After the usual preparations and median sternotomy, pericardial stay sutures are placed and a left atrial catheter inserted (see "Preparation for Cardiopulmonary Bypass" in Section 3 of Chapter 2). Using intraoperative TEE chamber size is evaluated and mitral valve pathology confirmed, including degree of valve narrowing and any regurgitant jets. Often, subvalvar stenosis can be identified. Important tricuspid regurgitation or stenosis is noted.

The aortic cannula is inserted and venous cannulation accomplished with a single venous cannula, or bicaval cannulation may be used when the left atrium is small and exposure difficult. Cardiopulmonary bypass (CPB) is established, and the perfusate temperature is lowered to 18° to 20°C. A stab wound (part of the later left atriotomy) is made at the base of the right superior pulmonary vein for initial left atrial venting. A cardioplegic needle or aortic root catheter is placed in the ascending aorta, and a retrograde coronary sinus cardioplegic cannula may be introduced as well (see "Technique of Retrograde Infusion" in Chapter 3). The aorta is clamped, cold cardioplegic solution infused, and perfusate temperature stabilized at 28° to 32°C. The left atrium is opened vertically from the right side (Fig. 11-4, A). This may be done after developing the interatrial groove in cases of minimal left atrial enlargement, or the incision may be started medially on the right superior pulmonary vein without dissecting the groove. Superiorly, the incision is extended beneath the superior vena cava after the right pulmonary artery is dissected away from the superior aspect of the left atrium. Inferiorly, the incision may be extended by cutting behind the freed vena caval–right atrial junction. Rarely, when exposure remains poor because of the small size of the left atrium, the superior vena cava is transected on the atrial side of the cannulation site and the incision carried farther to the superior aspect of the left atrium.[B37] A Cooley left atrial retractor or a Deaver retractor is inserted (Fig. 11-4, B). An intracardiac sump sucker placed through the incision is positioned in the orifice of one of the left pulmonary veins to keep the operative field dry.

The mitral valve is examined to determine its suitability for commissurotomy, and judgment is made as to whether the leaflets will be sufficiently pliable after commissurotomy to open adequately at a low left atrial pressure. Determination is straightforward when the leaflets are pliable and noncalcified and there is little or no coalescence of chordae. However, mitral commissurotomy can often yield reasonably good results when the valve is less ideal and even when it is partially calcified.[E9,H23] Thus, if some reasonable degree of mobility remains in the central portion of the anterior leaflet, persistent attempts should be made to open the valve widely by commissurotomy.[H22]

If commissurotomy is chosen, one stay suture can be placed in the midportion of the free edge of the anterior leaflet and another placed similarly in the posterior leaflet. Retraction on these sutures puts tension on the leaflets and their commissures. With a sharp-pointed scalpel (#11 blade), a stab incision is made in the fused anterolateral commissure next to the anulus (see Fig. 11-4, B). The incision is extended with the scalpel toward the valve orifice, in the groove of the commissural fusion. A 3- to 4-mm incision reveals the fan of underlying chordae, making it easy to stay in the middle of the commissural tissue over the center of the fan.[R13] The incision is then carried into the valve orifice. Alternatively, a blunt-ended, long-handled hook is placed beneath each leaflet, and by trial and error these hooks are positioned exactly in the spot that provides the best exposure for division of each commissure. With the scalpel, an incision is made at the anterolateral commissure beginning at the valve orifice and extended toward the anulus. The surgeon takes care to follow the true line of the commissure, which extends more anteriorly than might be thought. With either method, when fused chordae are present beneath the commissure, they can usually be separated with the knife or scissors. When appropriate, the incision is carried down into the center of the papillary muscles, dividing them into anterior and posterior halves (Fig. 11-4, C).

The posteromedial commissure is usually less well defined and fused for a shorter distance than the anterolateral commissure. Using one of the techniques just described, this commissural leaflet tissue is incised. Chordae are often more fused beneath this commissure, and their separation by sharp dissection may be needed together with longitudinal division of the papillary muscle. If the chordae are fused together to form a fanlike fibrous sheet beneath either leaflet at one or both commissures, this sheet is fenestrated by removing a wedge of tissue from its center using a sharp-pointed scalpel. Localized but bulky calcium deposits are removed from the leaflets with bone-nibbling forceps.

A firm plastic catheter with multiple side holes (ideally a No. 24 French chest drainage tube) is placed through the valve into the LV and tied to the left atrial vent snare to secure it. Catheter placement frustrates the valve, and the side holes lying in the left atrium are an additional safeguard to prevent ejection by the LV into the aorta until de-airing is complete. The left atrium is closed with continuous No. 3-0 polypropylene suture, but with the loops left loose where the catheter exits through the left atrial incision. The left atrial vent is removed during this procedure to allow the left side of the heart to fill with blood. If return to the left atrium is inadequate, right atrial pressure is raised by returning blood to the patient (see "De-Airing the Heart" in Section 3 of Chapter 2). The LV apex is needled for air without dislocating the heart. With the patient's head down, the aortic clamp is released while suction is applied to the aortic vent needle. The heart is defibrillated if necessary, and the ventricle is allowed to eject into the left atrium and pericardium via the transmitral catheter until all air is clearly eliminated.

Alternatively, after completion of the commissurotomy, the left atrium is completely closed before beginning aortic root reperfusion and later removing the aortic clamp. Closure with No. 3-0 polypropylene suture is started at the superior angle, carried partway down, and held. With another suture, closure is begun at the inferior angle and

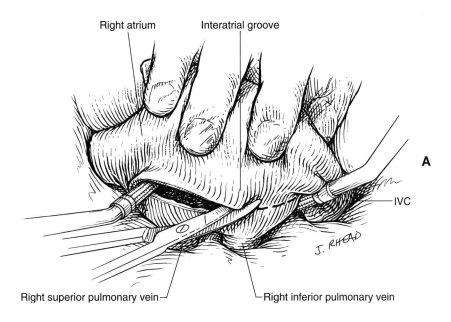

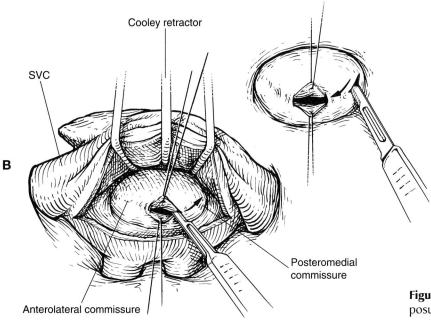

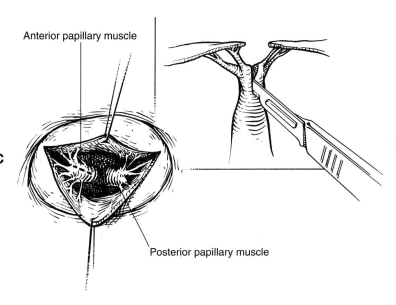

Figure 11-4 Open mitral commissurotomy. **A,** Exposure is through a median sternotomy. Left atrium is opened from the right side in front of right pulmonary veins. **B,** Cooley left atrial retractor is positioned. With traction on stay sutures in each leaflet, valve is well exposed for commissurotomy. An incision is made from valve orifice into posteromedial commissure; line to be incised is located by staying in leaflet tissue overlying center of underlying nest of chordae to posterior papillary muscle (see text for details). Note that correctly placed incision curves anteriorly. As incision is made, chordae beneath commissure are visualized and used as a guide for keeping the incision in leaflet tissue over micelles of chordal network. *Inset,* Alternatively, incision in the fused commissure is begun about 2 mm away from anulus and, as indicated by arrow, is carried centrally. A similar procedure is carried out at anterolateral commissure, where a longer commissural incision is usually possible. **C,** After opening valve at commissures, fused chordae beneath them can be separated. Incision is carried vertically down into the papillary muscles to attain a larger orifice.

Key: *IVC,* Inferior vena cava; *SVC,* superior vena cava.

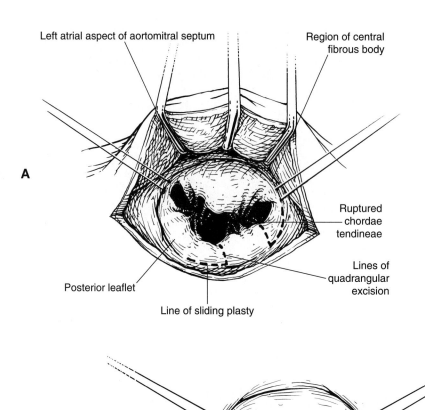

A

Left atrial aspect of aortomitral septum

Region of central fibrous body

Ruptured chordae tendineae

Lines of quadrangular excision

Posterior leaflet

Line of sliding plasty

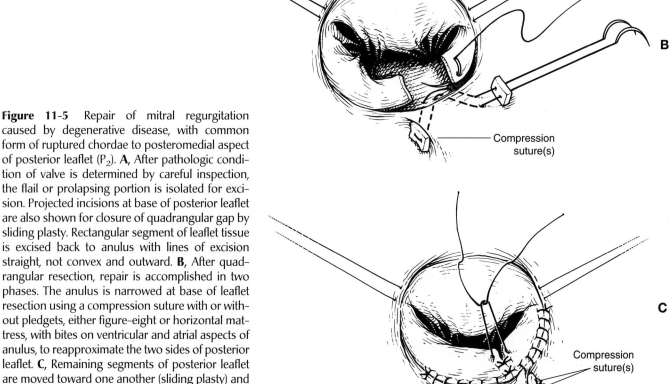

B

Compression suture(s)

C

Compression suture(s)

Figure 11-5   Repair of mitral regurgitation caused by degenerative disease, with common form of ruptured chordae to posteromedial aspect of posterior leaflet (P_2). **A,** After pathologic condition of valve is determined by careful inspection, the flail or prolapsing portion is isolated for excision. Projected incisions at base of posterior leaflet are also shown for closure of quadrangular gap by sliding plasty. Rectangular segment of leaflet tissue is excised back to anulus with lines of excision straight, not convex and outward. **B,** After quadrangular resection, repair is accomplished in two phases. The anulus is narrowed at base of leaflet resection using a compression suture with or without pledgets, either figure-eight or horizontal mattress, with bites on ventricular and atrial aspects of anulus, to reapproximate the two sides of posterior leaflet. **C,** Remaining segments of posterior leaflet are moved toward one another (sliding plasty) and reapproximated to base of leaflet. Leaflet repair is completed using fine interrupted, figure-eight, or continuous sutures.   *Continued on page 496*

carried superiorly until the other suture is reached. The closure must be done accurately, because it is difficult to see the angles later. The sump sucker is removed, and the left atrium is filled with saline solution just before the suture line is completed. The venous line is momentarily clamped, and while the lungs are inflated, a 13-gauge needle is inserted into the gently elevated apex of the LV to remove any air. Suction is placed on the aortic root catheter in the ascending aorta, the aortic clamp is released, and rewarming is begun (see "Completing Cardiopulmonary Bypass" in Section 3 of Chapter 2).

If the period of global myocardial ischemia has exceeded 30 minutes, the technique of controlled aortic root or retrograde perfusion may be used (see "Cold Cardioplegia, Controlled Aortic Root Reperfusion, and [When Needed] Warm Cardioplegic Induction" in Chapter 3). These maneuvers may aid in evacuating air from the coronary arteries. If careful observation reveals LV distention, a 13-gauge needle is inserted into the right ventricle and across the septum into the LV. After good cardiac action has returned, the usual de-airing procedures are followed (see "De-Airing the Heart" in Chapter 2).

As rewarming progresses, two right atrial and two right ventricular myocardial wires are placed. Before decannulation, examination by TEE should confirm no more than trivial or mild mitral regurgitation.

Repair of Mitral Regurgitation

Repair, rather than replacement, is the procedure of choice for treating mitral regurgitation,[C9,G12,S15] but not all cases are successfully managed in this fashion. Thus, at operation it must be determined whether repair will likely provide an acceptable result. This determination is aided appreciably by prebypass TEE. The magnitude and direction of the regurgitant jet can be assessed and the site of leaflet dysfunction accurately predicted. The abnormal valve physiology can often be characterized as restrictive, dilated, or prolapsing. These determinations allow informed decisions as to appropriate repair techniques. Repair can most confidently be performed when chordae are ruptured in a limited portion of the posterior leaflet and the anterior leaflet is essentially normal, or when there is simply prolapse of the posterior leaflet. Regurgitation from ruptured chordae to the anterior leaflet can be successfully repaired in some cases. Rheumatic mitral regurgitation can usually be repaired when distortion of the valve leaflets is minimal, as can certain cases of combined stenosis and regurgitation when commissurotomy precedes the repair. Nonrheumatic, noncalcific, almost pure mitral regurgitation in the adult, nearly always due to myxomatous degeneration, can usually be repaired. Regurgitation caused by infective endocarditis, with resultant chordal rupture or a perforated cusp, is reparable at times.[B32]

When regurgitation is associated with mitral valve prolapse, myxomatous degeneration, or chordal rupture, Carpentier's techniques have proven reproducible and durable. Carpentier and Kumar (of Duran's group) and their colleagues clarified the pathologic anatomy of the mitral valve.[C38,K17] Their observations are fundamental considerations for a repair. As observed by echocardiography or at operation, the disease process of the mitral apparatus can be classified as (1) restrictive, (2) normal with anular dilatation, or (3) degenerative (leaflet prolapse). The anterior leaflet is conveniently divided into two sectors, A_1 laterally and A_2 medially, and the posterior leaflet is divided into three sectors, P_1 laterally, P_3 medially, and P_2 centrally.[L14] (For an alternative [echocardiographic] classification, see Chapter 1.) When the cause of regurgitation is *prolapse of the posterior leaflet,* sectors P_2 and P_3 (Fig. 11-5) are usually involved. Additionally, there is some degree of anular dilatation.

Thus, with the mitral valve exposed as usual and using saline distention, areas of prolapse and regurgitation are identified. With forceps and blunt hooks (crochet hooks), each element of the valve apparatus (anulus, leaflets, chordae, papillary muscle) is examined for pathologic changes. In particular, the normal primary chordae are distinguished from the abnormal stretched or ruptured chordae to the offending prolapsed portion. A rectangular excision of the prolapsed sector of the posterior leaflet is done (see Fig. 11-5, *A*). This can involve 15% to 25% of the posterior leaflet. Further mobilization of the remaining leaflet may be accomplished by resecting some adjacent secondary and tertiary chordae. The resulting gap is bridged by a compacting (compression) suture at the base of the resected leaflet. Alternatively, with a sliding plasty, adjacent normal portions of the posterior leaflet are incised at their bases and moved centrally to obliterate the gap (see Fig. 11-5, *B* and *C*).[C38]

If a sliding plasty has been used, reconstruction is performed by suturing the mobilized leaflet to the posterior anulus and then reapproximating the cut edges of the leaflets with interrupted nonabsorbable sutures. Usually an anuloplasty ring is then sutured into place to both support the repair and narrow the anulus (see Fig. 11-5, *C* to *E*). Proper sizing of the anuloplasty ring (whether flexible or fixed) is essential to maintain competence and avoid postoperative LV outflow tract narrowing. If too large, the ring may produce or contribute to systolic anterior motion of the anterior leaflet and LV outflow tract obstruction. Basically, the ring must recreate the normal anteroposterior depth of the anulus, which typically is the anteroposterior length of the splayed anterior leaflet.

Anterior leaflet prolapse repair (sector A_2) is more difficult and less often successful than posterior leaflet repair. A triangular wedge of the involved leaflet is resected, the leaflet is reconstructed, and a ring is placed (Fig. 11-6). Often the repair involves other techniques described by Duran, Carpentier, Antunes, and Orszulak and their colleagues.[A10,C4,D28,O3] These maneuvers are technically demanding and not as reliable as those applied to the posterior leaflet. Techniques include chordal shortening, chordal transfer,[C4,C33] and occasionally reimplantation of partially ruptured papillary muscles.

Chordal transfer involves excising the leaflet insertion of a normal intact chord from the posterior leaflet, flipping it anteriorly, and attaching it to the flail anterior prolapsing sector (Fig. 11-7).[D17] *Chordal shortening* may also be used in such cases. The papillary muscle is split, and the chord is shortened by embedding it in the muscle.[D18,P12]

D

Sizer

Commissural markers

Anterior leaflet

Repaired posterior leaflet

Crochet hook

Sliding plasty

E

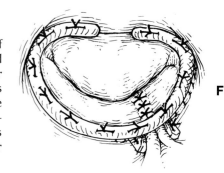

F

Figure 11-5, cont'd   **D,** Carpentier-Edwards or similar anuloplasty ring is inserted. Size of the ring is determined by height (depth) of anterior leaflet and by anterior intercommissural distance. Also, anterior leaflet is displayed using a crochet hook, and the two notches of sizer are approximated to anterolateral and posteromedial commissures. **E,** Anuloplasty ring is inserted using interrupted horizontal mattress sutures to create a purse-string effect at base of posterior leaflet, but using exactly matching intervals at base of anterior leaflet. Purse-string effect is attained both between the two arms of the suture and between each mattress suture. **F,** Completed ring insertion both narrows the anulus and bolsters the posterior repair. Only 10 to 12 double-armed mattress sutures are necessary to secure the ring.

Triangular resection of anterior leaflet

A

B

C

J. RHEAD

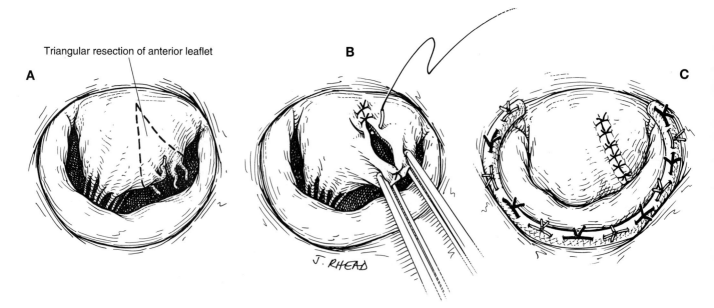

Figure 11-6   Repair of mitral regurgitation from the occasional isolated prolapse of anterior mitral leaflet or flail anterior leaflet from ruptured chordae. Valvuloplasty involves triangular resection, shown here for A_2, with repair of the leaflet using interrupted fine sutures (**B**), complemented by insertion of an anuloplasty ring (**C**). The triangular excision does not extend all the way to the base of the leaflet.

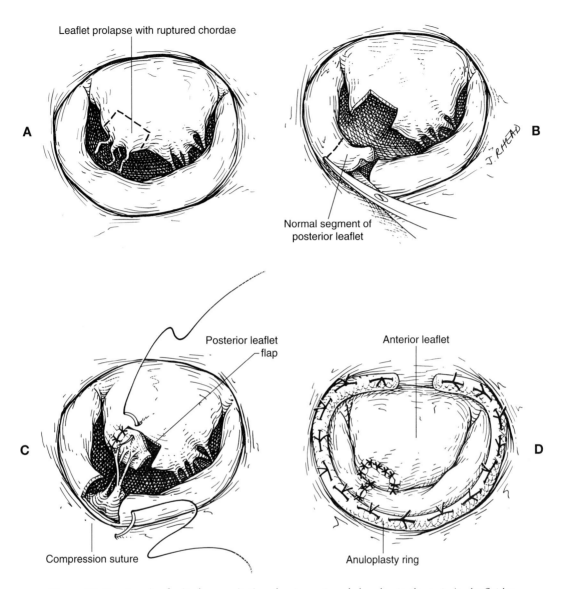

Figure 11-7   Repair of mitral regurgitation due to ruptured chordae to the anterior leaflet by chordal transfer. **A,** Area of anterior leaflet made flail secondary to ruptured chordae is resected. **B,** A small facing portion of normal posterior leaflet with its intact chordae is removed as a rectangular flap. **C,** Flap of posterior leaflet is flipped over to close defect in anterior leaflet, anchoring anterior leaflet with intact chordae. Base of flipped posterior leaflet segment is sutured to deepest aspect of anterior leaflet defect using fine polypropylene sutures. **D,** Quadrangular defect left in posterior leaflet is closed and the repair supported with an anuloplasty ring. (See Fig. 11-5, *B* and *C*.)

Alternatively, diseased chordae tendineae may simply be replaced by No. 5-0 expanded polytetrafluoroethylene (PTFE) sutures (Fig. 11-8).[D16,F7] A double-armed suture is passed twice through the usually fibrous tip of the papillary muscle and tied; each arm is then passed through the area of the leaflet where the native chordae are inserted, and then tied. Intermediate-term results with this technique have been good.[D16,Z2]

Alfieri and colleagues have described a simple technique that is especially useful for anterior leaflet prolapse (Fig. 11-9).[A19,A27] When the prolapse is near the commissure, the anterior and posterior leaflets are approximated "edge to edge" with one or two mattress sutures. When the

prolapse is in the central portion of the valve, one or two edge-to-edge leaflet-approximating sutures create a double-orifice mitral valve that functions adequately.[U2]

When there is *bileaflet prolapse* without anterior chordal pathology, often posterior leaflet resection and ring anuloplasty alone serve to correct the regurgitation, providing a durable repair without an additional procedure directed at the anterior leaflet.[G24]

When repair rather than replacement is done for *rheumatic mitral regurgitation* in adults, anuloplasty (generally using Carpentier's method, including an anuloplasty ring) has been the technique employed in most cases (see Fig. 11-5). When anuloplasty is necessary in young children

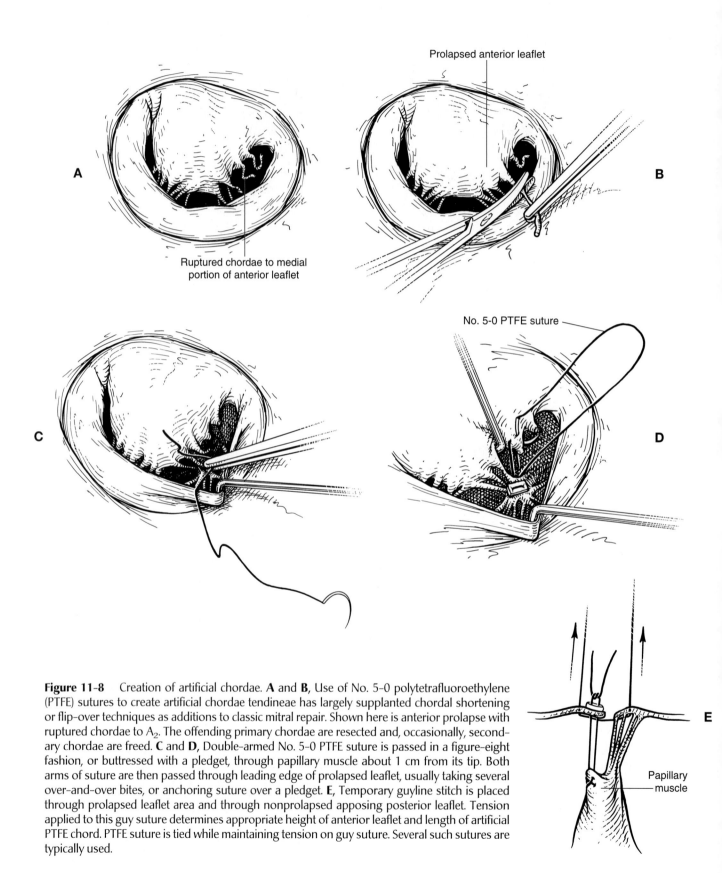

Prolapsed anterior leaflet

A

Ruptured chordae to medial portion of anterior leaflet

B

No. 5-0 PTFE suture

C

D

E

Papillary muscle

Figure 11-8   Creation of artificial chordae. **A** and **B**, Use of No. 5-0 polytetrafluoroethylene (PTFE) sutures to create artificial chordae tendineae has largely supplanted chordal shortening or flip-over techniques as additions to classic mitral repair. Shown here is anterior prolapse with ruptured chordae to A_2. The offending primary chordae are resected and, occasionally, secondary chordae are freed. **C** and **D**, Double-armed No. 5-0 PTFE suture is passed in a figure-eight fashion, or buttressed with a pledget, through papillary muscle about 1 cm from its tip. Both arms of suture are then passed through leading edge of prolapsed leaflet, usually taking several over-and-over bites, or anchoring suture over a pledget. **E**, Temporary guyline stitch is placed through prolapsed leaflet area and through nonprolapsed apposing posterior leaflet. Tension applied to this guy suture determines appropriate height of anterior leaflet and length of artificial PTFE chord. PTFE suture is tied while maintaining tension on guy suture. Several such sutures are typically used.

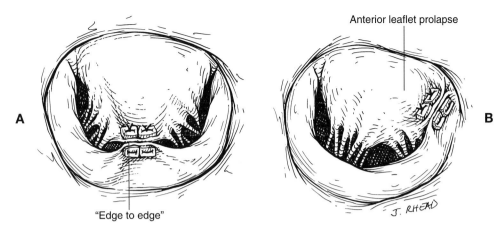

Figure 11-9   "Edge-to-edge" repair of ischemic mitral regurgitation. **A,** Pericardial buttressed horizontal mattress sutures of polypropylene are placed in leading edges of central portion of each leaflet and pulled together to create a double-orifice mitral valve. The resulting tethering effect, along with systolic leaflet apposition, prevents regurgitation. **B,** Edge-to-edge repair of prolapse of anterior leaflet involving its medial portion (A$_2$), bringing anterior and posterior leaflet tissue together to tether and shorten the prolapsed leaflet. (Modified from Alfieri and Maisano.[A27])

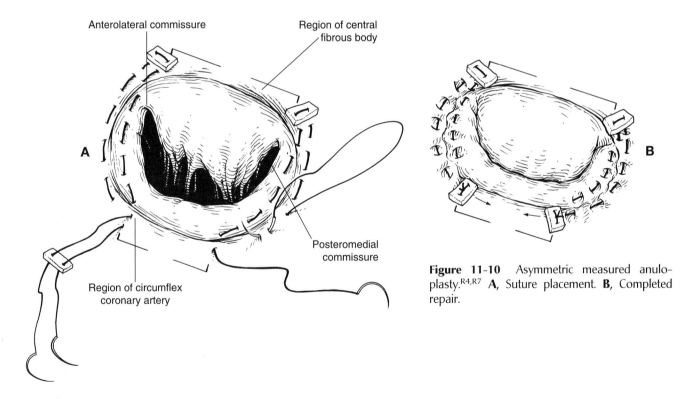

Figure 11-10   Asymmetric measured anuloplasty.[R4,R7] **A,** Suture placement. **B,** Completed repair.

with years of growth ahead, an anuloplasty ring is not employed. Instead, an asymmetric measured anuloplasty is done by the technique described by Reed and colleagues (Fig. 11-10).[R4,R7] This operation, as with most repairs of mitral regurgitation, is based on the fact that the central portion of the anterior mitral leaflet is usually pliable and of good quality. Its leading edge forms the line of closure for the repaired valve, both in the Reed repair and after insertion of a Carpentier ring.

Determination of competence of the repaired valve while the left atrium remains open is imprecise. Yacoub's maneu-

ver involves perfusing warm blood into the aortic root proximal to the clamp through the cardioplegic needle or aortic root catheter so that function of the repaired valve can be inspected with the heart beating.[Y1] A simpler method involves injecting saline under pressure through the valve into the LV. The distended leaflets and their opposing surfaces are examined, and areas of leakage, if present, are identified. The entire line of closure of the leaflets should be parallel to the mural part of the anulus, that is, to the hinge line of the posterior leaflet (or to this portion of the anuloplasty ring).[C33] If all this is satisfactory, the left atrium is closed,

Figure 11-11   *Mitral valve replacement: classic procedure. Approach is through a median sternotomy that opens left atrium from right side anterior to right pulmonary veins (see Fig. 11-4 legend). Two venous cannulae are illustrated, but a single venous cannula can be used. Cooley left atrial retractor is used. As described in text, incision in mitral leaflet is begun with knife anteriorly and about 2 mm from anulus, where leaflet usually is pliable and relatively free of disease. As incision is carried leftward with knife or scissors toward anterolateral commissure, underlying papillary muscle and fused chordae come into view and are incised. As incision is carried across anterolateral (illustrated here) and posteromedial commissural areas, care is taken to stay close to anulus so that valve is kept in one piece. This greatly facilitates completing the valve excision.*

Key: *Ao,* Ascending aorta; *SVC,* superior vena cava.

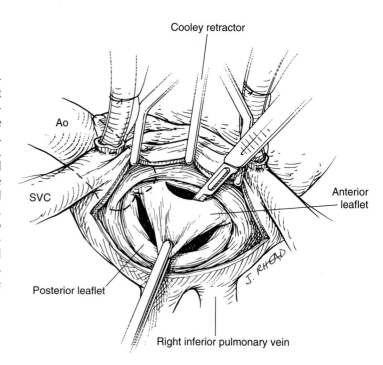

de-airing is performed as described under Open Mitral Commissurotomy, and CPB is discontinued. At this point, competence of the valve is assessed by TEE. If more than mild regurgitation is present, CPB is resumed and the mitral valve is either re-repaired or replaced. In one institution, intraoperative TEE identified 26 of 309 patients (8%) undergoing repair for mitral regurgitation who had immediate failure of the procedure and required further repair or replacement at the same operation. Used in this manner, intraoperative TEE can limit the number of those who require late reoperation for failed repair.[M22]

Repair of Mitral Regurgitation Associated with Submitral Left Ventricular Aneurysms

CPB and myocardial management are as described for other mitral valve operations. The left atrium is opened from the right side. The sac of the aneurysm is entered through an incision in the floor of the left atrium, parallel to and about 20 mm posterior to the hinge line of the posterior leaflet. The usually narrow pathway or "neck" between the LV and the aneurysm is then easily visualized.[A11] This pathway can be closed with interrupted pledgeted mattress sutures, bringing them anteriorly through the hinge line of the posterior leaflet. The opening from the left atrium into the aneurysm is then closed, draining the now-evacuated and exteriorized aneurysmal sac through its free wall into the pleural space if desired. Reparative operations can be performed for residual mitral regurgitation, if indicated.

Mitral Valve Replacement
Classic Procedure

Mitral valve replacement begins with exposure of the mitral valve as described for mitral commissurotomy, using one or two valve hooks to display the leaflets. To excise the valve,

an incision is begun with the knife in the center of the anterior mitral leaflet at approximately the 12-o'clock position, about 2 mm from the anulus, because at that point the leaflet tissue is typically pliable and free of disease (Fig. 11-11). The incision is carried from this point leftward and rightward, either with the knife or scissors, and on to the commissural leaflet tissue at the anterolateral and posteromedial commissures. The incisions through the commissural leaflet tissue are kept next to the anulus so that the anterior and posterior leaflets stay together. The underlying papillary muscle and fused chordae are cut just in front of the incision for better exposure.

Classically, the excision is continued to the posterior leaflet from both sides. Ordinarily the posterior leaflet and its chordae are left in place when they are thin and pliable.[G11] Thus, only the anterior leaflet is fully excised (but see "Chordal Sparing Procedure" later in this section). If this is not possible because of extensive disease, the secondary chordae that tether the posterior leaflet to the underlying ventricular myocardium are cut. When subanular calcification is present and can be excised without disturbing the anulus or the myocardium, it is removed. Otherwise, calcification is left in situ, because overzealous efforts may damage the circumflex coronary artery or precipitate postrepair ventricular rupture.

The mechanical prosthesis or bioprosthesis can be sewn into place with interrupted simple sutures, but preferably with horizontal mattress sutures using pledgets on the atrial side, or with a continuous No. 0 polypropylene suture (Figs. 11-12 and 11-13). All methods are associated with an extremely low prevalence of periprosthetic leakage (see "Periprosthetic Leakage" under Modes of Death later in this section).[D2] A technique employing interrupted pledgeted mattress sutures with the pledgets on the ventricular side may be chosen when heavy calcification remains in some areas of the anulus or, rarely, when exposure is particularly difficult. With this technique, all sutures are

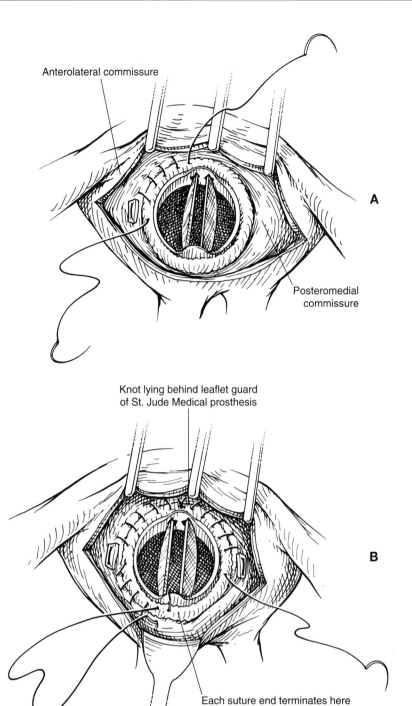

Figure 11-12 Mitral valve replacement: continuous suture technique. **A,** One end of a double-armed No. 0 polypropylene suture buttressed with a felt pledget is passed through mitral anulus just posterior to anterolateral commissure. Suture is then passed through prosthetic sewing ring, and valve without holder is lowered into place. Using about four throws, suture line is carried to the left, anteriorly passing stitches from anulus to sewing ring and taking deep bites, but avoiding noncoronary cusp of aortic valve. Suture is held midway across distance to posteromedial commissure. **B,** Other end of the suture, having been placed through mitral anulus as a mattress, is placed into prosthetic sewing ring and continued from anulus to sewing ring with four or five throws. It is helpful to move prosthesis in and out of anulus to accommodate needle passage. Suture is held. A second double-armed pledgeted suture is begun as a horizontal mattress just posterior to posteromedial commissure. Its ends are carried with four or five throws in each direction, first anteriorly and then posteriorly, to meet and tie with previously held ends. Knots then lie behind leaflet guards of the St. Jude Medical prosthesis depicted here.

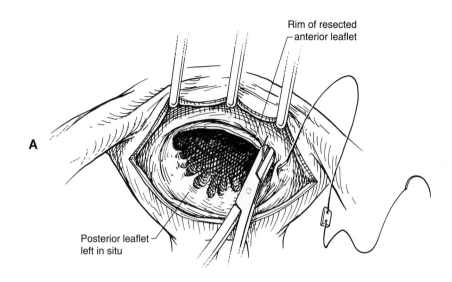

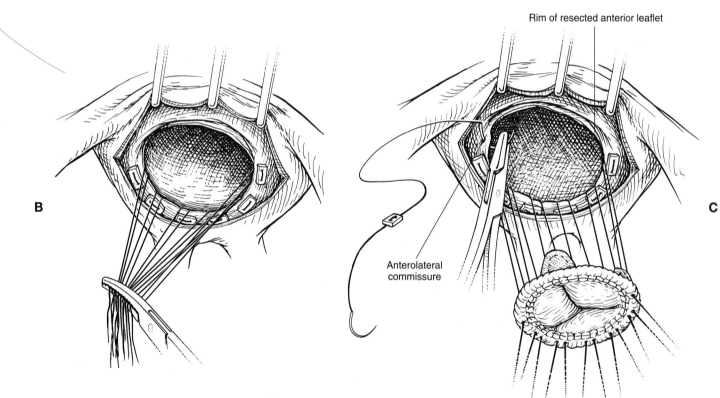

Figure 11-13   Mitral valve replacement: interrupted suture technique. **A,** Double-armed No. 0 polyester sutures are generally placed with pledgets on atrial aspect of anulus. It is convenient to place one arm of a mattress suture just behind posteromedial commissure, reserving other end for placement later and holding suture for exposure. **B,** Posterior suture line proceeds counterclockwise beginning at anterolateral commissure. Sutures are placed from atrial side to ventricular side of anulus and may either be held or placed in prosthetic sewing ring. **C,** Anterior suture line usually proceeds clockwise from anterolateral commissure to posteromedial commissure. Along whole circumference, suture bites encompass base of residual leaflet. Clockwise from anterolateral commissure are the aortic cusps, conduction system, atrioventricular septum, coronary sinus, and circumflex coronary artery, which are at risk when bites are taken too deeply. With all sutures in place and on tension, valve is lowered into place and sutures tied, with about 12 mattress sutures used. Before tying, device struts are inspected to ensure that no suture is looped around a strut or caught within the device.

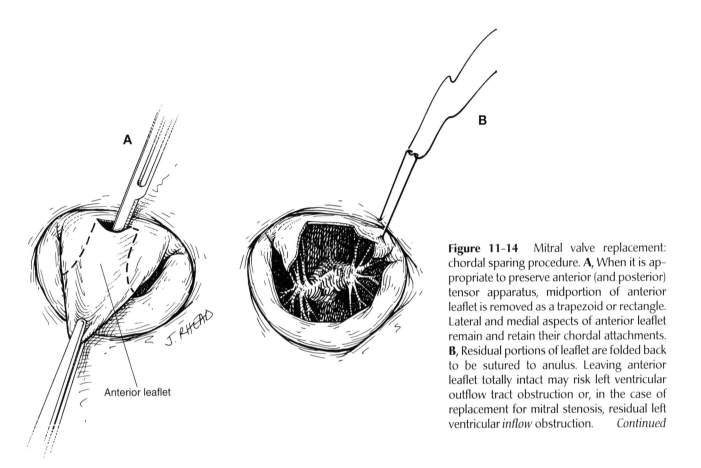

Figure 11-14   Mitral valve replacement: chordal sparing procedure. **A,** When it is appropriate to preserve anterior (and posterior) tensor apparatus, midportion of anterior leaflet is removed as a trapezoid or rectangle. Lateral and medial aspects of anterior leaflet remain and retain their chordal attachments. **B,** Residual portions of leaflet are folded back to be sutured to anulus. Leaving anterior leaflet totally intact may risk left ventricular outflow tract obstruction or, in the case of replacement for mitral stenosis, residual left ventricular *inflow* obstruction.   *Continued*

placed in the heart first and then passed through the valve sewing ring. The prosthesis can then be lowered into position and the sutures tied. Protruding suture ends can damage the leaflets of bioprostheses.

After completion of the valve insertion, a catheter is passed through the valve into the LV to act as a frustrator. The steps for exiting from the left side of the heart and de-airing are as described for mitral stenosis. However, because a rigid device is now sutured to the mitral anulus, the LV apex is elevated gently and air aspirated *before* commencing myocardial reperfusion.

Chordal Sparing Procedure

Information based on experimental observation and clinical experience indicates that retention (rather than resection) of the mitral tensor apparatus at mitral valve replacement results in better LV function postoperatively (see "Cardiac Performance" later in this section).[L17,M24,M28,M29,S29,Y4] To insert a prosthesis while retaining both the anterior and posterior chordal attachments, the anterior leaflet may be split centrally and folded laterally and the posterior leaflet left as is. Alternatively, both the intact anterior and intact posterior leaflets can be folded toward their bases, then a prosthesis inserted (Fig. 11-14). These maneuvers (including folding the anterior leaflet) do not result in LV outflow tract obstruction or prosthetic obstruction when done for mitral regurgitation.[E10]

SPECIAL FEATURES OF POSTOPERATIVE CARE

In both the operating room and intensive care unit, patients may display a large *v* wave in the left atrial pressure pulse. This is *not* a reliable indicator of mitral valve regurgitation because the height of the *v* wave is related primarily to the level of mean left atrial pressure,[B11] and in patients who have just undergone mitral valve repair or replacement, mean left atrial pressure is usually elevated. TEE can settle this issue.

Care of patients after mitral valve procedures is as described in Chapter 5. Ventricular unloading is an important aspect of the postoperative maintenance of optimal cardiac output in patients operated on for mitral regurgitation. Restoring mitral competence increases load-resisting shortening.[E11,M23] Thus, by removing a parallel low-resistance circuit, myocardial oxygen requirement increases along with impairment of myocardial contractile reserve. Nitroglycerin, nitroprusside, and phosphodiesterase inhibitors are useful for decreasing afterload and improving cardiac performance.

Patients undergoing mitral valve replacement, including those receiving bioprostheses and often those undergoing commissurotomy or repair of mitral regurgitation, are begun on anticoagulant therapy using warfarin the evening of postoperative day 1 or 2 (day of surgery is postoperative day 0). For adults with a normal prothrombin time (PT), the initial dose is generally 7.5 to 15 mg, followed by daily

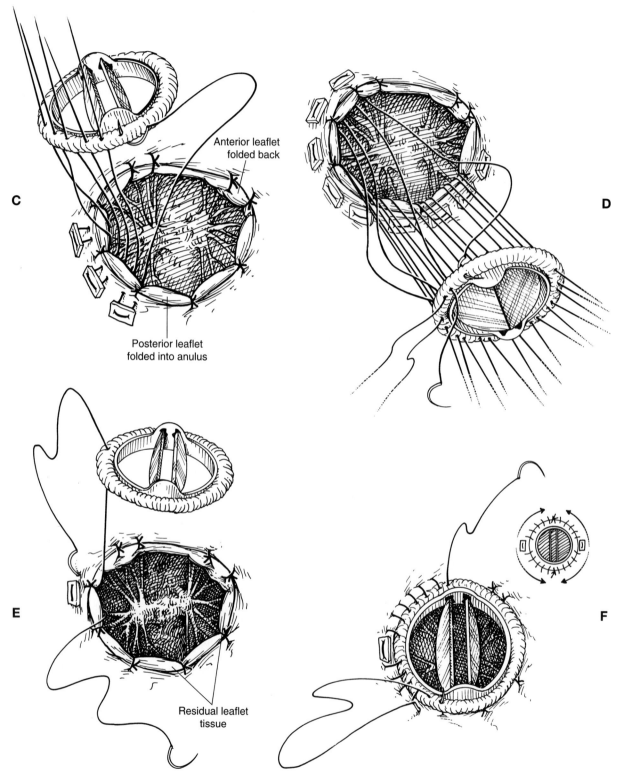

C

Anterior leaflet
folded back

Posterior leaflet
folded into anulus

D

E

Residual leaflet
tissue

F

Figure 11-14, cont'd Prosthesis is sutured into place using previously described interrupted (**C** and **D**) or continuous (**E** and **F**) suture technique. In either case, sutures surround retained leaflets, adding strength and purchase to the repair.

doses in the hospital guided by daily PT measurements. The goal is prothrombin activity 20% to 30% of normal or PT twice the control value. This is best monitored and regulated using the international normalized ratio (INR) terminology. The INR allows standardizing the determination of PTs by accounting for differences among commercial thromboplastin reagents.[R23] Optimal INR for patients after mitral valve replacement is 2.5 to 3.5.

When a mechanical valve has been inserted, this program is continued indefinitely, and the patient is educated about its extreme importance. Warfarin appears to be associated with a greater risk of excessive anticoagulation (hemorrhage) than reduced anticoagulation (thromboembolism and thrombosis). Thus, an appropriate recommendation is an INR of about 2.5 to 3.5.[C39,H25] Good results have been obtained, however, with warfarin regimens resulting in an INR of 1.5 to 2.0[C39] and also with a single dose of 2.5 mg · day.$^{-1}$[K19]

When a bioprosthesis is inserted or anuloplasty or valvotomy performed, anticoagulation is continued for 6 to 8 weeks. Lower INR values (1.5 to 2.0) are acceptable during this period.

RESULTS

Mitral Commissurotomy

Survival

In an earlier era, mortality after closed commissurotomy was high.[E3,G1,H11,H17] In the current era, *hospital mortality* after either closed or open commissurotomy approaches zero and late survival is similar in risk-adjusted comparisons.[H23,R21] A difference exists only in the prevalence of postcommissurotomy mitral regurgitation (see "Mitral Regurgitation" on p. 506).

In many institutions, percutaneous catheter valvotomy has almost completely replaced surgical commissurotomy

for isolated mitral stenosis. Procedure mortality approaches zero,[I2] and risk of complications (bleeding, severe regurgitation) requiring urgent operation is low. Intermediate-term survival is good in those with favorable immediate hemodynamic results (Fig. 11-15).

Mitral commissurotomy is not curative with either open or closed (or balloon) commissurotomy, with survival progressively diverging from that of the general population (Fig. 11-16).[C14,C23,E4,G1,N7,S10] However, few late deaths result directly from the effects of recurrent or residual mitral stenosis or regurgitation. Rather, they result from thromboembolism or early or later sequelae of reoperation and mitral valve replacement.

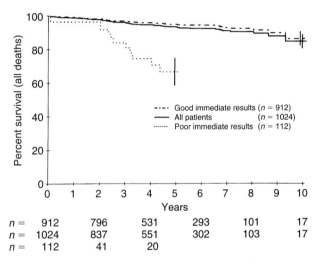

$n =$	912	796	531	293	101	17
$n =$	1024	837	551	302	103	17
$n =$	112	41	20			

Figure 11-15   Survival after percutaneous mitral commissurotomy. Of the 112 patients who had poor immediate results, only 19% ± 4% were free from surgery at 5 years. (From lung and colleagues.[I2])

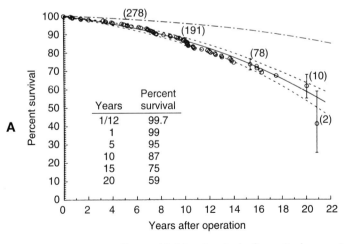

A

Years	Percent survival
1/12	99.7
1	99
5	95
10	87
15	75
20	59

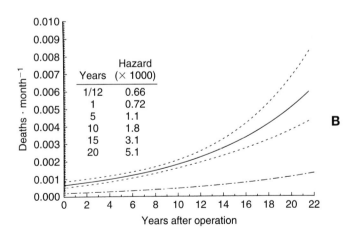

B

Years	Hazard (× 1000)
1/12	0.66
1	0.72
5	1.1
10	1.8
15	3.1
20	5.1

Figure 11-16   Survival after mitral commissurotomy by either closed or open technique. **A,** Survival. Each circle represents a death, positioned according to Kaplan–Meier estimator, vertical bars represent 70% confidence limits (CL), and numbers in parentheses are patients at risk. Solid line enclosed within dashed CLs is the parametric survival estimate. Dash-dot-dash curve is survival of an age-gender-ethnicity–matched general population. **B,** Hazard function for death. Note the steadily rising single hazard phase. Dashed lines are CLs. Dash-dot-dash line is hazard for an age-gender-ethnicity–matched general population. (From Hickey and colleagues.[H23])

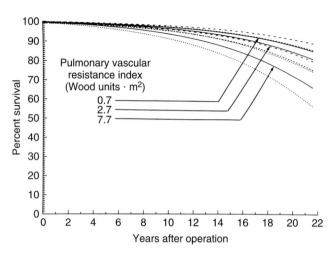

Figure 11-17 Nomogram of solution of multivariable equation (see Table 11-1), illustrating the effect of precommissurotomy pulmonary vascular resistance on risk-adjusted survival after commissurotomy. Dashed lines are 70% confidence limits. (See Hickey and colleagues[H23] for details of the equation.)

■ **TABLE 11-1   Incremental Risk Factors for Death after Mitral Commissurotomy** [a]

Risk Factor [b,c]	Hazard Phase	
	Early	**Late**
Demographic		
(Older) Age at commissurotomy		●
African–American	N	●
(Higher) Pulmonary vascular resistance index	O	●
Morphologic	N	
Leaflet calcification	E	●
(Greater) Left ventricular enlargement (grades 0–6)		●

(Data from Hickey and colleagues.[H23])

[a] UAB group, 1967 to 1988; $n = 339$; deaths = 65.

[b] Variables entered into the analysis, coefficients, and P values of the risk factors are provided in original article. Postcommissurotomy variables such as residual mitral regurgitation were excluded from this analysis.

[c] Type of commissurotomy (open or closed) was not a risk factor.

Incremental Risk Factors for Premature Death

Few deaths occur early after mitral commissurotomy,[H23,H24,S10] and no risk factors are associated with these. Risk factors associated with later deaths[H23,S10] include elevated Rp before commissurotomy, which directly affects survival rather than leading to reintervention, but its effect is moderate (Fig. 11-17 and Table 11-1). The aforementioned *morphologic* risk factors lead to recurrent symptoms and reintervention, usually valve replacement, and affect survival in this manner. Although not evident in a risk factor analysis using only preoperative variables, development of important mitral regurgitation after commissurotomy and occurrence of a thromboembolic event both adversely affect survival.

Mitral Regurgitation

Mitral regurgitation is a risk of mitral commissurotomy by any technique, but occurs in only 2% to 5% of patients who undergo open commissurotomy[S10] and in about 10% of patients who undergo closed commissurotomy.[H11,H17,H23] Rarely does the newly developed regurgitation require immediate operation, but it may lead to reoperation within a few months. Mild postcommissurotomy mitral regurgitation has little effect on survival or need for mitral valve replacement, but important postcommissurotomy regurgitation adversely affects both (Fig. 11-18).

Prevalence of new important mitral regurgitation is about 10% after percutaneous balloon mitral commissurotomy.[A16]

Cardiac Performance

Increase in calculated mitral valve area (or orifice size) produced by commissurotomy varies greatly and depends not only on the surgical opening but also on leaflet pliability and extent of subvalvar obstruction from fused chordae.[A3] Feigenbaum and colleagues found that closed mitral commissurotomy, usually with a transventricular

dilator, increased mitral valve area by an average of 1.3 to 2.6 cm², with postoperative mitral valve areas ranging from 0.7 to 5.8 cm².[F3] Younger patients tend to have a better functional result[C8] and to experience greater increases in calculated valve area than do older patients,[F3] perhaps because younger patients tend to have more pliable valves. The same general results are achieved by both open and closed commissurotomy and percutaneous balloon mitral valvotomy (Fig. 11-19). Enlargement after percutaneous balloon valvotomy results primarily from splitting of fused commissures.[M10]

Somewhat better orifices can be obtained by open than closed commissurotomy.[S10] Nakano and colleagues achieved valve areas of 2.52 ± 0.19 cm² in patients with pliable valves and minimal subvalvar disease, as well as good but smaller orifices in patients with extensive subvalvar diseases.[N7] Ben Farhat and colleagues reported an equivalent increase of mitral valve area (0.9 to 2.2 cm²) for open commissurotomy and percutaneous balloon valvotomy that was greater than for closed commissurotomy (0.9 to 1.6 cm²).[B48] The superior hemodynamic results continued over a 7-year follow-up period (see Fig. 11-19).

A secondary effect of increased orifice size is lowering of left atrial pressure, although it frequently remains above normal. On average, left atrial pressure at rest is about 12 mmHg after valvotomy, increasing to about 17 mmHg on exercise. LV end-diastolic pressure often is modestly higher after commissurotomy.[F3]

Cardiac output is usually increased by operation, and the amount of increase at rest and exercise correlates well with the increase in calculated valve area.[F3] Rp usually falls immediately, especially in young patients, as verified by Block and Palacios during percutaneous balloon commissurotomy.[B33] Pulmonary artery pressure usually falls, which correlates well with the decrease in left atrial pressure and Rp.

Thromboembolism

Successful mitral commissurotomy may reduce the likelihood of thromboembolism, although accurate comparisons are not available. About 90% of patients are free of a thromboembolic event 8 to 10 years after open commissurotomy.[C23,E4] The linearized rate of thrombo-

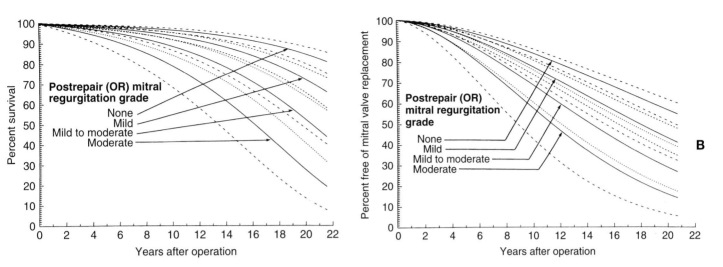

Figure 11-18   Nomograms representing solutions of multivariable equations, illustrating effect of postcommissurotomy mitral regurgitation on **A**, risk-adjusted survival, and **B**, freedom from mitral valve replacement. Dashed lines are 70% confidence limits. (See Hickey and colleagues[H23] for details of the equations.)

Key: *OR,* Operating room.

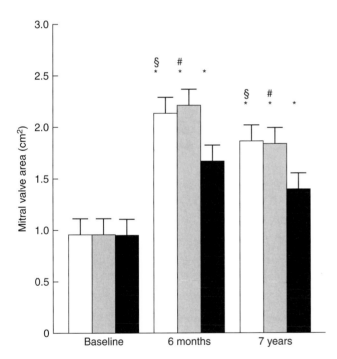

Figure 11-19   Mitral valve area determined by two-dimensional echocardiography at baseline and at follow-up in three groups of patients treated for mitral stenosis. *Open bar,* balloon mitral commissurotomy; *stippled bar,* open surgical commissurotomy; *solid bar,* closed surgical commissurotomy. (From Ben Farhat and colleagues.[B48])

*$P < .001$ for comparison of baseline value with its change at 6 months within each group.
§$P < .001$ for comparison of balloon commissurotomy with closed surgical commissurotomy.
#$P < .001$ for comparison of open versus closed surgical commissurotomy.

embolism has been reported at 1% to 2% per patient-year.[C23,E4,G1,H10,H23,S10] This statistic is not very useful, however, because the hazard function for a first or subsequent thromboembolic event is not constant (Fig. 11-20). Atrial fibrillation, older age, and a history of thromboembolism preoperatively are reported risk factors for postcommissurotomy thromboembolism.[E4,S10] Also, a postcommissurotomy thromboembolic event predisposes the patient to further events (Table 11-2). The type of surgical commissurotomy, open or closed, has not been shown to be a risk factor.[H23]

Functional Status

Successful open or closed mitral commissurotomy, in properly selected patients, results in dramatic relief of symptoms. More than 90% of patients are in NYHA functional class I or II during the first 1 or 2 postoperative years (Fig. 11-21).[G1,H5,H10,S10,V1] Lack of permanent favorable results from mitral commissurotomy is evident in the gradual decline in functional status. Redevelopment of symptoms results from gradual loss of leaflet pliability, as well as progression of subvalvar pathology and increase of valvar calcification. Although recurrence of rheumatic fever may

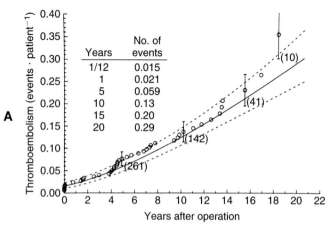
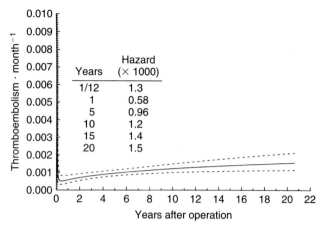

Figure 11-20 Depiction of all postcommissurotomy thromboembolic events, not only the first episode. Format is as in Fig. 11-16. **A,** Cumulative event function for all thromboembolism. **B,** Hazard function for any thromboembolic event after mitral commissurotomy. (From Hickey and colleagues.[H23])

■ **TABLE 11-2   Incremental Risk Factors for New Postcommissurotomy Thromboembolic Event after Mitral Commissurotomy** [a]

	Risk Factor	Hazard Phase	
		Early	Late
	Demographic		
(Older)	Age at commissurotomy (years)	●	
	History of thromboembolism before commissurotomy		●
(Greater)	Number of previous postcommissurotomy thromboembolic episodes (0, 1, 2)		●
	Morphologic		
(Greater)	Leaflet calcification (grade 0-5)		●
	Pliable leaflet		●

(Data from Hickey and colleagues.[H23] Database is same as in Table 11-1. Variables entered into the analysis, ordinal logistic coefficients, and *P* values are provided in the original article.)

[a] Thromboembolism was considered to be a modulated renewal process (event), and thus the first, second, or third events (total of 44) are included.

accelerate this pathology, progression seems to occur even without further rheumatic episodes. Thus, NYHA functional class correlates well with estimated area of the mitral orifice late postoperatively; the mean value is 2.0 cm² in class I patients, 1.7 in class II, and 1.6 in class III.[B38] Immobility of valve leaflets and obstructive subvalvar agglutination of chordae are the main risk factors for a poor early functional result.[H11] Calcification of a portion of the leaflet(s) does not preclude a satisfactory result.

Despite excellent early and intermediate results in the current era, durability of results is limited. Scarring from the rheumatic process in the valve seems to progress gradually. Eventually, although not until 20 years postoperatively in some patients, most patients lose their good functional status and return with restenosis or new-onset regurgitation (Fig. 11-22). Absence of leaflet pliability in the presence of valvar calcification is a risk factor for the rate of decline in functional status after all types of commissurotomy. Type of surgical commissurotomy

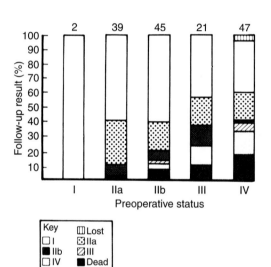

Figure 11-21 Comparison of preoperative and postoperative New York Heart Association functional status in 123 patients surviving an average of 48 months after open mitral valvotomy. (From Smith and colleagues.[S10])

Key: *Class IIa,* Breathlessness with unusually strenuous activity; *class IIb,* breathlessness with ordinary activity.

(open or closed) has not been shown to be a risk factor (Table 11-3).[H23]

Reintervention

Most patients undergoing mitral commissurotomy by any technique will require another procedure at some time, generally mitral valve replacement because of gradual loss of leaflet pliability, progression of subvalvar pathology, and increase of valvar calcification (Table 11-4; see Fig. 11-22).[C23,E4,E5,N7,N8] About 20% of patients undergoing surgical commissurotomy require valve replacement within 10 years, and about half require it by 20 years (Fig. 11-23).

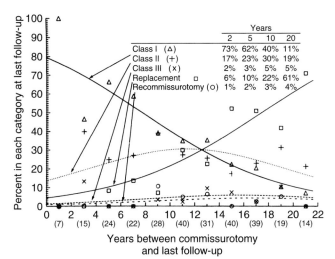

Figure 11-22 Declining percentage of patients in New York Heart Association functional class I after open or closed commissurotomy. Changes across time of functional classes II and III are also shown. The longer the time since commissurotomy, the greater is the percentage of patients undergoing mitral valve replacement. (From Hickey and colleagues.[H23])

■ **TABLE 11-3   Incremental Risk Factors for Poor Functional Status after Mitral Commissurotomy** [a]

	Risk Factor	Ordinal Logistic Coefficient	
		Estimate ± SD	P
(Older)	Age at commissurotomy	0.023 ± 0.0104	.03
(Higher)	Precommissurotomy NYHA class	0.74 ± 0.189	.0001
	Morphologic		
(Greater)	Valve calcification (grades 0-5)	1.02 ± 0.28	.0003
(Greater)	Leaflet immobility (grades 0-5)	0.36 ± 0.115	.002
(Longer)	Follow-up interval	0.0172 ± 0.0022	<.0001

(Data from Hickey and colleagues.[H23] Variables entered into the analysis, ordinal logistic coefficients, and P values are provided in the original article.)

Key: *NYHA*, New York Heart Association.

[a] UAB group; 1967 to 1988; *n* = 339; deaths = 65.

■ **TABLE 11-4   Cardiac Reinterventions and Mortality after Mitral Commissurotomy**

		All Deaths	
Type of Reintervention [a]	n	No.	%
Balloon mitral commissurotomy [b]	6	1	17
Closed mitral commissurotomy [c]	1	0	0
Open mitral commissurotomy [d]	4	1	25
MVR [e]	57	17	30
MVR + TVA	7	2	29
MVR + CABG	2	0	0
MVR + AVR	16	5	31
AVR	1	0	0
CABG	1	1	100
TOTAL	96	27	28

Key: *AVR*, Aortic valve replacement; *CABG*, coronary artery bypass grafting; *MVR*, mitral valve replacement; *TVA*, tricuspid valve anuloplasty.

(Data from Hickey and colleagues.[H23])

[a] Categories are not mutually exclusive.

[b] One patient, who lived, had subsequent MVR + CABG.

[c] One patient, who lived, had subsequent MVR.

[d] One patient, who died, had aortic valve replacement with concomitant open mitral commissurotomy and subsequently underwent aortobifemoral bypass.

A

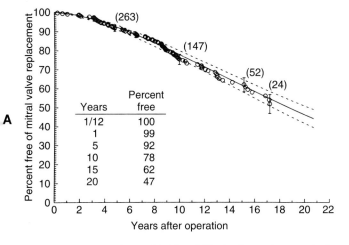

B

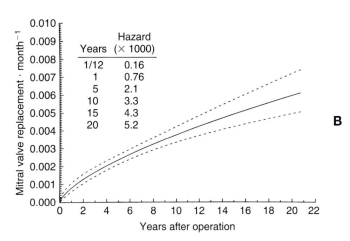

Figure 11-23 Mitral valve replacement after open or closed commissurotomy. Format is as in Fig. 11-16. **A**, Time-related freedom. **B**, Hazard function for mitral valve replacement after mitral commissurotomy. (From Hickey and colleagues.[H23])

The same variables that cause survival to vary probably cause prevalence of postcommissurotomy mitral valve replacement to vary (Table 11-5). Again, type of surgical commissurotomy (open or closed) has not been demonstrated to be a risk factor for subsequent mitral valve replacement.[H23] Morphology of the mitral valve powerfully affects the time-related prevalence of mitral valve replacement after surgical commissurotomy (Fig. 11-24) as well as after percutaneous balloon valvotomy. At 7 years, freedom from restenosis was 93% for the open and balloon procedures versus 63% after closed commissurotomy.

Percutaneous Balloon Valvotomy

Early hemodynamic, functional, and anatomic improvement after percutaneous mitral valvotomy is, as noted above, nearly equivalent to the results following open

■ **TABLE 11-5**   **Incremental Risk Factors for Mitral Valve Replacement after Mitral Commissurotomy**

	Risk Factor	Late Hazard Phase
	Morphologic	
(Smaller)	Preoperative mitral valve area	●
(Greater)	Leaflet immobility (grades 0-5)	●
	Leaflet calcification	●
(Greater)	Postrepair (OR) mitral valve regurgitation (grades 0-5)	●

Key: *OR,* Operating room.

(Data from Hickey and colleagues.[H23])

surgical commissurotomy. Long-term outcomes are not available. There is a progressive decrease in valve area that closely parallels that seen historically and in concurrent studies for surgical approaches. Degree of deterioration can be predicted by variables related to preoperative functional class and morphologic features of the mitral valve (Table 11-6 and Fig. 11-25).[E12] Thus, long-term survival and need for reintervention after the catheter approach should be similar to results after the open surgical approach.

Redo Mitral Commissurotomy

Survival after a second mitral commissurotomy is surprisingly good in view of the more advanced valvar pathology usually present at reoperation. Peper and colleagues report 5-, 10-, and 15-year survival of 96%, 83%, and 63%, respectively, after repeat open commissurotomy. Also, 16 (31%) of 52 hospital survivors underwent still another mitral operation, usually a replacement, an average of 8.25 years later.[P8]

Repair of Mitral Regurgitation

In general, early, intermediate, and long-term results of repair of mitral valve regurgitation have been good.[D15,S15]

Survival

Early (hospital) death. *Hospital mortality* after repair of isolated nonischemic mitral regurgitation approaches zero.[C4,D5,S15] Among 46 patients undergoing isolated mitral

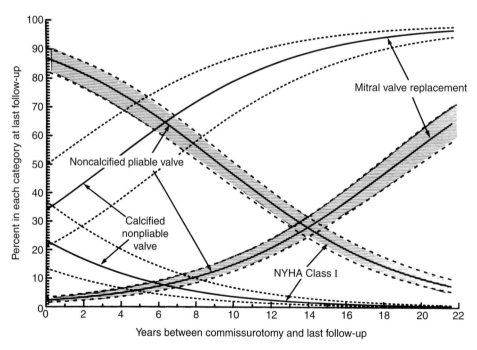

Figure 11-24   Nomogram of specific solution of a multivariate ordinal logistic risk factor equation, illustrating risk-adjusted effect of mitral calcification and absence of pliability on prevalence of mitral valve replacement after surgical commissurotomy. Also shown is the effect of valve morphology on rate of decline in percentage of patients in New York Heart Association functional class I after commissurotomy. Dashed lines enclose 70% confidence limits. (From Hickey and colleagues.[H23])

Key: *NYHA,* New York Heart Association.

valve repair at UAB (1975 to July 1983) and 43 patients at GLH (1972 to 1983), no deaths (0%; CL 0%-4%) occurred. More recently, Akins and colleagues reported 3.0% early mortality in 133 patients undergoing repair versus 11.5% in 130 patients undergoing replacement.[A21] The two groups of patients did not differ in any preoperative risk cate-

gory, including age, gender, prevalence of heart failure, or NYHA functional class.

Time-related survival. *Time-related survival,* including hospital deaths, of patients with mitral regurgitation undergoing repair with or without other cardiac procedures has been better than that of patients undergoing replacement (Fig. 11-26). Most groups have reported similar findings, with 4- or 5-year survival after repair varying from 74% to 94%.[A21,C40,D5,D20,E13,F12,N5,O3,P7,R8,S24,Y1] Ten-year survival of one group of patients undergoing repair with or without other procedures was 59%.[S15]

Variability in survival among reports and improved survival after repair compared with replacement are related in part to the differing prevalence of risk factors for death.[D19,G12] For example, in the UAB experience, patients undergoing repair were generally younger and less disabled than those undergoing replacement, which in part accounted for their improved survival.[S15] A more recent experience from the Mayo Clinic reported surgical mortality of 2.6% for repair and 10.3% for replacement (*P* = .002).[E13] Late survival (in surgical survivors) at 10 years was 69% ± 6% versus 58% ± 5% (*P* = .018), and

■ **TABLE 11-6   Predictors of Mitral Valve Restenosis after Balloon Mitral Valvotomy**

Predictor	P
Age at intervention	.12
Gender	.7
Cardiac rhythm	.09
Interval to follow-up	.03
Type of intervention	.2
Mitral valve morphology	
Thickening	.08
Mobility	.09
Calcification	.08
Subvalvar disease	.04
Composite valve score	.04

(From Essop and colleagues.[E12])

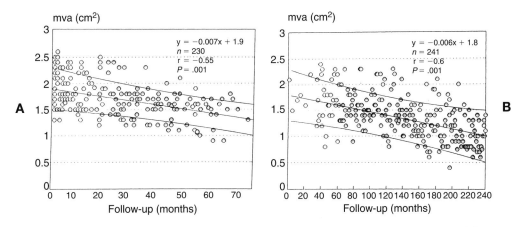

Figure 11-25   Relationship between Doppler mitral valve area and follow-up interval from intervention. **A,** Percutaneous balloon mitral valvotomy. **B,** Surgical mitral commissurotomy. Regression lines are shown with 95% confidence limits. Regression equation is shown at top right of each panel. Correlation coefficient is indicated by r. (From Essop and colleagues.[E12])

Key: *mva,* Mitral valve area.

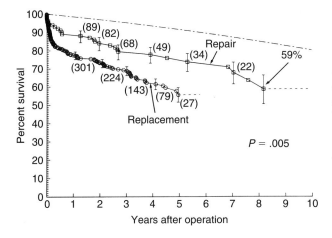

Figure 11-26   Survival after mitral valve repair and mitral valve replacement for mitral regurgitation, with or without associated cardiac procedures (UAB group, 1975 to July 1983; *n* = 490; total deaths = 158). Time zero is time of completion of the mitral valve operation. Each circle and square represents an individual death. Vertical bars enclose 70% confidence limits of the survival estimate. Numbers in parentheses describe the group at risk for each period. Dashed lines indicate patients traced beyond the last event. Risk factors for death likely differed between groups. Dash-dot-dash line represents survival of an age–gender–ethnicity–matched general population (U.S. life tables, 1977). (From Sand and colleagues.[S15])

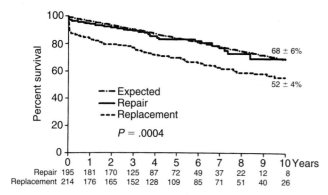

Figure 11-27 Overall survival comparison for mitral valve repair and replacement patients ($P = .0004$). Dash-dot-dash line represents expected survival. Numbers at the bottom indicate number of patients at risk for each interval. (From Enriquez-Sarano and colleagues.[E13])

late survival after valve repair did not differ from expected survival (Fig. 11-27). Again, the two groups differed mainly in degree of preoperative heart failure. To address comparison of repair versus replacement, Gillinov and colleagues used propensity score matching (see "Clinical Studies with Nonrandomly Assigned Treatment" in Chapter 6) and found that repair conferred a survival advantage in most (89%) patients that became evident after about 2 years.[G25]

Modes of Death

Modes of death early and late after mitral valve repair are similar to those after mitral valve replacement (Table 11-7).[S15] The most common mode is cardiac failure.

Incremental Risk Factors for Premature Death

Incremental risk factors for premature death after repair of mitral regurgitation are the same as those after replacement (Table 11-8). In the UAB experience, neither procedure was a risk factor vis-à-vis the other. More recent reports by Akins and Dujardin and their colleagues, however, indicate that mitral valve replacement is a risk factor for late mortality compared with mitral repair in a univariable analysis, but not by multivariable analysis.[A21,D20] In most studies, this reflects choice of replacement for those patients who are older or in a more advanced NYHA functional class. However, Gillinov and colleagues found by both multivariable analysis and propensity adjustment that replacement was a risk factor.[G25]

Residual or Recurrent Mitral Regurgitation

Many patients have no residual mitral regurgitation after repair.[S15,S18] Alvarez and colleagues reported that only 4.5% of 155 repair patients experienced repair failure within 6 months (Fig. 11-28).[A22] In Marwick's series, 26 of 309 patients (8%) had immediate (intraoperative) failure of repair (demonstrated by intraoperative TEE), necessitating a second run of CPB.[M22] Sixteen of these 26 patients had moderate or severe persistent regurgitation, and 10 had LV outflow tract obstruction. In a larger group of 1072 patients

■ **TABLE 11-7   Modes of Death at Any Time after Operation for Mitral Valve Regurgitation** [a]

Mode	Repair No.	Repair % of 27	Replacement No.	Replacement % of 131
Cardiac failure	13	48	59	45
Acute	3	11	16	12
Subacute	3	11	16	12
Chronic	7	26	27	21
Arrhythmic	1	4	7	5
Sudden	3	11	22	17
Neurologic	1	4	6	5
Hemorrhage	1	4	2	2
Cancer	3	11	3	2
Infection	0		4	3
Trauma	0		3	2
Miscellaneous	1	4	3	2
Acute pulmonary failure	0		1	1
Unrelated noncardiac operation	0		2	2
Sickle cell crisis	1	4	0	
After reoperation	3	11	12	9
Uncertain	1	4	10	8
TOTAL	27	100	131	100

[a] Data displayed are for patients undergoing repair or replacement, with or without associated cardiac procedures (UAB group, 1975 to July 1983; $n = 490$; deaths = 158).

■ **TABLE 11-8   Incremental Risk Factors for Premature Death after Valve Repair or Replacement for Mitral Regurgitation** [a]

	Risk Factor [b]	Hazard Phase Early and Decreasing	Hazard Phase Constant
	Demographic		
(Older)	Age	●	●
	African-American		●
	VA patient		●
	Morphologic		
	Papillary muscle ischemic disease	●	●
(Greater)	LV enlargement (grades 1-6)		●
	Clinical		
	Previous CABG		●
(Higher)	LVEDP		●
(Higher)	NYHA functional class (I-V)	●	
	Surgical		
	LV resection for aneurysm	●	

(Data from Sand and colleagues.[S15])

Key: *CABG,* Coronary artery bypass grafting; *LV,* left ventricular; *LVEDP,* left ventricular end-diastolic pressure; *NYHA,* New York Heart Association; *VA,* Veterans Administration.

[a] Patients with or without associated cardiac procedures are included in this study (UAB group, 1975 to July 1983; $n = 490$; deaths = 158). See original article for equations, P values, and coefficients.

[b] Mitral replacement as a risk factor has a P value of .14 (early phase only).

analyzed for late failure, only 30 repair patients needed late reoperation (freedom from reoperation at 10 years 93%; CL 91%-94%) valve.[G23] Recurrent regurgitation in these and other series is caused by either progression of disease or inadequate operation, including suture dehiscence.[G23] When studied by left ventriculography or Doppler echocardiography 1 to 3 years after repair, 9% to 20% of patients have important mitral regurgitation.[D5,K8,L6] This finding and other information[M13] suggest that in most patients,

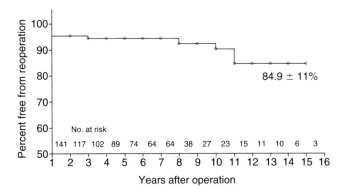

Figure 11-28   Freedom from reoperation for structural valve degeneration after mitral valve repair. (From Alvarez and colleagues.[A22])

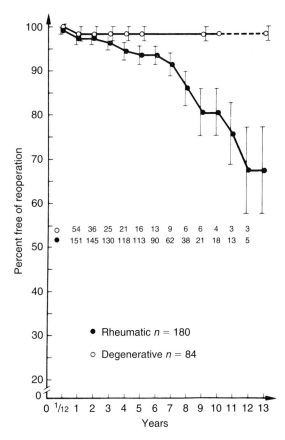

Figure 11-29   Freedom from reoperation after mitral valve repair in patients with rheumatic and degenerative etiologies for mitral regurgitation. A number of patients at risk in each group is shown below curves. Vertical bars indicate one standard deviation. (From Lessana and colleagues.[L15])

residual regurgitation is present immediately after repair rather than developing later. Although reoperation may underestimate the prevalence of late regurgitation, various groups report freedom from reoperation of 80% to 96% at 10- to 15-year follow-up, suggesting satisfactory durability of repair.[D15,D21,F10,L15,P11]

A clear relationship has not been established between technique of repair and prevalence of residual regurgitation. However, repair is clearly more effective for patients with *degenerative* (myxomatous) disease than for those with *restrictive* (rheumatic) disease (Fig. 11-29).[D21,L15] The best results may be in patients with ruptured chordae to the posterior leaflet,[S9] although Orszulak and colleagues have found almost equally good results when the ruptured chordae belong to the anterior leaflet.[M27,O3] For complex repairs and those involving the anterior leaflet, chordal replacement is superior to chordal shortening.[L15,P12]

Cardiac Performance

LV performance responds to mitral valve repair in the same general manner as it does to mitral valve replacement.[L6] Some regression of LV hypertrophy occurs, with decreased heart size, LV volume, and muscle mass.[D24,G16] Preoperative LV systolic function is more or less preserved, although ejection fraction is often moderately decreased.[C41] However, some studies document LV performance to be better after mitral valve repair than after replacement.[B27,C42] Corin and colleagues found that systolic and diastolic function returned to normal in mitral repair patients, but that global and regional systolic function as well as diastolic function were depressed in replacement patients.[C42] This difference is probably attributable to preservation of the tensor apparatus in the repaired valve, (Fig. 11-30)[T6,B27] but may also reflect earlier intervention in patients undergoing repair versus replacement.[E13,T7]

Thromboembolism

Patients undergoing mitral valve repair are generally free of late thromboembolic complications, even though they rarely receive anticoagulants. Duran and colleagues found 93% of patients free of thromboembolism within the first 4.5 years after repair, a prevalence similar to that for xenograft replacement in their experience.[D5]

Left Ventricular Outflow Obstruction

In about 5% to 10% of patients with mitral regurgitation associated with mitral valve prolapse, abnormal *systolic anterior motion* (SAM) of the mitral valve develops immediately after mitral anuloplasty with a Carpentier ring.[G8,K12,K13] Related to this, gradients of 60 mmHg across the LV outflow tract have been measured.[K12] This complication appears to be limited to patients with myxomatous degeneration[K13,M16,S19] and excessive redundancy of the anterior and posterior leaflets, although presence of a small hyperdynamic LV and excessive ventricular hypertrophy may also contribute. SAM is now believed to be the result of anterior displacement of leaflet coaptation.[L16] LV outflow tract obstruction has not been observed in patients undergoing suture (rather than ring) mitral anuloplasty.[D6] Cosgrove and colleagues have shown that simple removal of the rigid anuloplasty ring abolished the obstruction while retaining competence of the mitral valve.[C10] Substitution of a larger ring, flexible ring, or half-ring or addition of a posterior leaflet sliding plasty may also eliminate SAM. Grossi and colleagues noted a prevalence of 6.4% (28/438) in their series of valve repair. All patients were treated medically, with resolution of gradients in all patients and resolution of SAM in half of patients within a year.[G17]

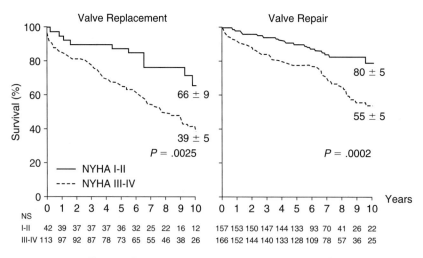

Figure 11-30 Overall survival comparison for patients in New York Heart Association functional class I-II and those in class III-IV who had mitral valve replacement *(left)* or repair *(right)*. (From Tribouilloy and colleagues.[T7])

Key: *NYHA,* New York Heart Association.

■ **TABLE 11-9** **Functional Status of Patients Alive and Without Reoperation after Surgery for Mitral Regurgitation** [a]

Postoperative NYHA Functional Class	Repair		Replacement	
	No.	% of 53	No.	% of 236
I	35	66%	142	60%
		} 49 (92%)		} 216 (92%)
II	14	26%	74	31%
III	3	6	18	8
IV	1	2	2	1
V	0	0	0	0
TOTAL	53	100	236	100
Unknown	6		9	

(Data from Sand and colleagues.[S15])

Key: *NYHA,* New York Heart Association.

[a] Study from UAB group, 1975 to July 1983.

Functional Status

Functional status of most patients is excellent after repair or replacement of a regurgitant mitral valve[E2,L10,S15] (Table 11-9).

Reoperation

Sand and colleagues reported that freedom from reoperation after mitral valve repair for mitral regurgitation was comparable to that for mitral valve replacement (Fig. 11-31).[S15] Others have reported freedom from reoperation late after mitral valve repair of 80% and 98%.[A7,A10,C10,P1,R6-R8,Y1]

Factors that may increase risk of reoperation late after repair include rheumatic disease (as opposed to degenerative disease), advanced degenerative changes involving the anterior leaflet, and residual regurgitation at completion of the initial procedure. When patients with 1+ or 2+ (of possible 4+) early postoperative regurgitation were compared with those with "echo-perfect" results (no regurgita-

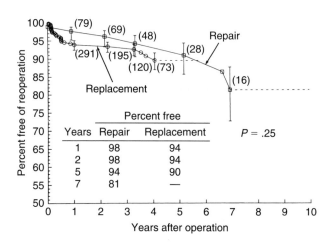

Figure 11-31 Freedom from mitral valve reoperation in patients with mitral regurgitation who have undergone repair or replacement (UAB group, 1975 to July 1983; *n* = 490). Format is as in Fig. 11-26. (From Sand and colleagues.[S15])

tion), Fix and colleagues found 83% freedom from reoperation in the former group versus 96% in the latter group at late follow-up (*P* = .07).[F14] Type of repair appears to have no effect on prevalence of reoperation.[S18] Reed, Chauvaud, and Ohno and their colleagues showed mitral repair to be as successful in children as in adults (Fig. 11-32).[C28,O5,R7]

The *hazard function* of reoperation after repair of mitral regurgitation is low, constant, and different from that of replacement (Fig. 11-33). Mitral valve repair does not have the peaking early hazard phase for reoperation, which in mitral replacement is related to periprosthetic leakage and prosthetic valve endocarditis. Furthermore, at least until now, no rising late hazard phase for reoperation after repair has been demonstrated, indicating the durability of this approach. In fact, in a 20-year experience reported by the

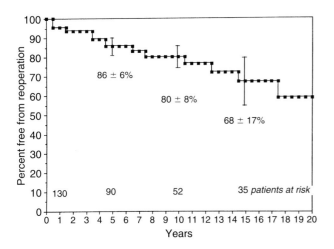

Figure 11-32 Freedom from reoperation after mitral valve repair in children younger than age 12 years. Vertical bars represent one standard error. (From Chauvaud and colleagues.[C44])

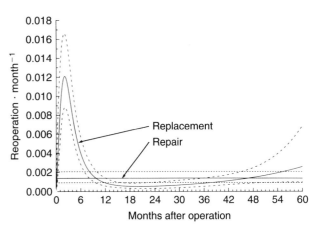

Figure 11-33 Separately determined hazards for mitral valve reoperation in patients with mitral regurgitation who have undergone repair or replacement (UAB group, 1975 to July 1983). (See original article for equations, *P* values, and coefficients.) (From Sand and colleagues.[S15])

■ **TABLE 11-10   Hospital and Total Mortality after Primary Mitral Valve Replacement** [a]

Procedure	*n*	Hospital Deaths			All Deaths	
		No.	%	CL (%)	No.	%
Isolated	415	10	2.4	1.6–3.5	85	20
Isolated repair after previous mitral repair	83	0	0	0–2.3	8	10
Isolated in HOC	8	2	25	9–50	3	38
+ CABG	138	12	9	6–12	43	31
Previous CABG	2	0	0	0–61	1	50
+ Tricuspid anuloplasty	64	8	12	8–18	25	39
+ TVR	4	2	50	18–82	2	50
+ ASD repair	9	1	11	1–33	2	22
SUBTOTAL (nonischemic MVD)	723	35	4.8	4.0–5.8	169	23
Isolated	1	0	0	6–85	1	100
+ CABG	89	17	19	1.5–24	46	52
Previous CABG	5	3	60	29–86	5	100
+ LV aneurysmectomy	1	0	0	0–85	1	100
SUBTOTAL (ischemic MVD)	96	20	21	16–26	53	55
TOTAL	819	55	6.7	5.8–7.7	222	27
$P(\chi^2)$		<.0001				

Key: *ASD,* Atrial septal defect; *CABG,* coronary artery bypass grafting; *CL,* 70% confidence limits; *HOC,* hypertrophic obstructive cardiomyopathy; *LV,* left ventricular; *MVD,* mitral valve disease; *TVR,* tricuspid valve replacement.

[a] Operations with concomitant procedures are included in this study (UAB group, 1975 to July 1983).

Mayo Clinic, the absolute prevalence of reoperation in the current era was 5% ± 2% for posterior leaflet repair and 10% ± 2% for anterior leaflet repair when assessed at the 10-year interval.[M27]

Infective Endocarditis

Infective endocarditis is rare after repair of mitral regurgitation.[G23] No cases were found in the UAB experience, with a follow-up of 21 to 120 months.[S15] This complication is more common when the affected valve is replaced rather than repaired.[S15]

Mitral Valve Replacement
Survival

Early (hospital) death. *Hospital mortality* after primary isolated mitral valve replacement for nonischemic valve disease is 2% to 7% (Table 11-10).[F5] Mortality after mitral valve replacement with tricuspid surgery is similar or slightly higher. As with all procedures, patient selection influences hospital mortality. For example, in 462 patients undergoing mitral repair (87%) or replacement (13%) through a ministernotomy, Gillinov and Cosgrove reported only a single death (0.2%).[G18] When mitral valve

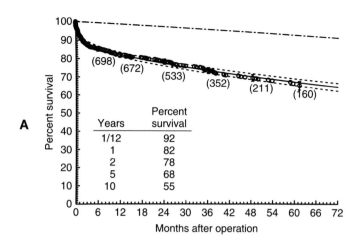

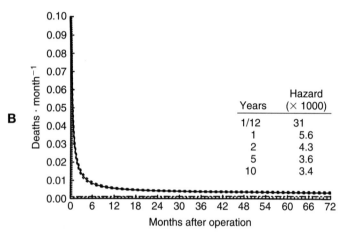

Figure 11-34   Patients undergoing primary isolated and combined mitral valve replacement. **A**, Survival. **B**, Hazard function for death (UAB group, 1975 to July 1983; $n = 819$; deaths = 222). Format is as in Fig. 11-16. (See Appendix 11A for details of the analysis.)

■ **TABLE 11-11**   **Hospital Mortality after Mitral Valve Surgery** [a]

		Hospital Deaths		
Previous Mitral Valve Surgery	**n**	**No.**	**%**	**CL (%)**
None	174	12	6.9	4.9–9.5
MV repair	38	5	13	7–21
MV replacement	50	2	4	1–9
Total	262	19	7.3	5.6–9.3
P(χ^2)			.2	

Key: *CL*, 70% confidence limits; *MV*, mitral valve.

[a] Patients undergoing primary or secondary mitral valve replacement with or without tricuspid surgery, with or without coronary artery bypass grafting, and with or without other cardiac surgery except aortic valve replacement are included in this study (GLH group, 1976 to 1980).

replacement has been preceded by mitral valve repair, hospital mortality is not affected appreciably (Table 11-11).

Time-related survival. Considering both isolated mitral valve replacement and replacement done concomitantly with other procedures, 1-, 5-, and 10-year survivals have been 82%, 68%, and 55%, respectively. The hazard function has a rapidly declining early phase but also a con-

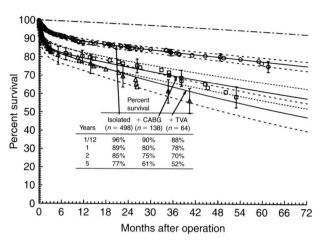

Figure 11-35   Nonparametric and parametric depictions of survival after mitral valve replacement for nonischemic mitral valve disease according to whether replacement was an isolated procedure (with or without previous mitral repair operation) or was performed with concomitant coronary artery bypass grafting or tricuspid valve anuloplasty. Depiction is as in Fig. 11-16. (UAB group, 1975 to July 1983; $n = 819$; same groups and data as in Table 11-10). (See Appendix 11B for coefficients and *P* values of parametric estimates.)

Key: *CABG*, Coronary artery bypass grafting; *TVA*, tricuspid valve anuloplasty.

stant phase extending as long as patients have been followed up (Fig. 11-34). *Time-related survival* has been higher in patients undergoing primary isolated mitral valve replacement than in those having replacement combined with other cardiac procedures (Fig. 11-35). Survivals similar to those reported here, including some 15-year survivals of 35% to 50%, have been reported by other groups.[B7,C21,K2,L1,L11,M12,T4,W1] Both early and late survival after primary mitral replacement are considerably improved over that obtained in earlier eras.[A1,B7,C5,H4,L3] Improvement is related to better myocardial management,[F5] reduction in technical problems such as atrioventricular rupture and air embolization, and improved mechanical and bioprosthetic valve replacement devices.

Survival both early and late after reoperation is less than that after original valve replacement (Fig. 11-36). This is related not only to technical aspects of reoperation, but also to the fact that prosthetic valve endocarditis is often the indication for reoperation, and reoperative patients as a group tend to have greater functional disability than those undergoing their first valve replacement.[B35]

Mitral valve replacement in children and adolescents has low early mortality, and time-related survival is probably equal to or superior to that of adults. However, mitral replacement in the first year of life may carry a higher risk; 9 of 25 patients died (36%; CL 25%-48%) in the experience of Kadoba and colleagues.[K20] Seven of the deaths were in patients with atrioventricular (AV) septal defects. Recent experience with improved repair of the left AV valve in AV septal defects, better myocardial management, and supraanular placement of the prosthesis have reduced early risk in infants considerably (see "Results" in Chapter 20). Time-related morbidity is attributable to reoperation

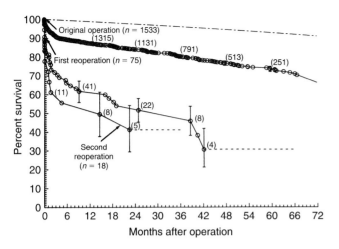

Figure 11-36   Survival after original and subsequent valve replacements. Depiction is as in Fig. 11-26. (Depiction is for *all* valve replacement operations, but is much the same as that for *only* mitral valve operations.) (From Blackstone and Kirklin.[B35])

■ **TABLE 11-13   Incremental Risk Factors for Death after Primary Mitral Valve Replacement** *a*

	Risk Factor	Hazard Phase	
		Early	Constant
	Demographic		
(Older)	Age at operation	●	●
	African-American		●
(Higher)	NYHA functional class	●	
	Valve disease		
	Nonischemic MV regurgitation *b*		●
	Ischemic MV regurgitation		●
(Greater)	LV enlargement (grades 0-6)	●	
	Important TV disease		●
	Surgical *c*		
	Previous CABG		●
	Concomitant LV resection in ischemic MVD	●	
(Longer)	Global myocardial ischemic time using cardioplegia	●	

Key: *CABG,* Coronary artery bypass grafting; *LV,* left ventricular; *MV,* mitral valve; *MVD,* mitral valve disease; *NYHA,* New York Heart Association; *TV,* tricuspid valve.

a Patients with or without concomitant procedures are included in this study (UAB group, 1975 to July 1983; *n* = 819; deaths = 222). See Appendix 11A for details of the analysis.

b P value for nonischemic mitral regurgitation = .098.

c Concomitant CABG was not a risk factor.

Modes of Death

■ **TABLE 11-12   Modes of Death Early and Late after Primary Mitral Valve Replacement** *a*

Mode *b*	No.	% of 179
Cardiac failure	96	54
Acute	31	17
Subacute	26	15
Chronic	39	22
Sudden	32	18
Neurologic	12	7
Cancer	12	7
Arrhythmia	8	4
Hemorrhage	6	3
Infection	6	3
Trauma	3	2
Miscellaneous	4	2
TOTAL	179	100

(Data from Ferrazzi and colleagues.[F5])

a Patients with or without concomitant cardiac procedures are included in this study (UAB group, 1975 to July 1983; *n* = 819; deaths = 222). A mode of death could not be identified in 16 patients.

b The 27 patients dying after reoperation are excluded.

associated with bioprosthetic tissue degeneration and acquired prosthetic stenosis associated with somatic growth.

Modes of Death

Most early deaths are attributable to cardiac failure, usually acute and within a few days of operation (Table 11-12). Subacute cardiac failure may be the mode of death in the hospital or within 1 to 2 months after hospital discharge. It is characterized by stable but low cardiac output and consequent widespread subsystem failure, often including cool (rarely frankly ischemic) extremities, abdominal distention, and occasionally ischemic bowel, gastrointestinal bleeding, jaundice, poor renal function, and mental confusion. Infection may occur as a terminal event.

Incremental Risk Factors for Premature Death

Some of the incremental risk factors for death that existed during the earliest eras of mitral valve replacement[B35] have

been neutralized by improvements in surgical technique, myocardial management (see Chapter 3), and perioperative care (see Chapters 4 and 5). Among specific improvements is sparing of the tensor apparatus, as demonstrated particularly by the Stanford group (see "Cardiac Performance" later in this section).[H26-28,M28,M29]

Older age.   Older age at operation continues to be an incremental risk factor in both the early and constant hazard phases (Table 11-13).[B35,C5,C34,F5,G2,P4,S8,W1] However, the increments are not great (Fig. 11-37) and appear to be related more to general risks of older age than to a specifically increased sensitivity to cardiac surgery; survival in the oldest group is predicted to be equivalent to or better than that in the general population (as is also the case after aortic valve replacement; see Chapter 12).

Nonischemic mitral regurgitation.   In contrast to mitral stenosis, nonischemic mitral regurgitation is probably a risk factor for death (see Table 11-13), but not to the extent that might be predicted from the sudden increase in LV afterload imposed when the regurgitant mitral valve is made competent. This is probably because a number of the other sudden hemodynamic changes (such as reduction in LV stroke work) are favorable.

Marked left ventricular enlargement.   LV enlargement is a risk factor for death early after repair (see Table 11-13). Presumably, marked LV enlargement connotes reduced ventricular contractility (see "Mitral Regurgitation" under Natural History earlier in this section), and this may actually be responsible for increased risk.

Left atrial enlargement.   Surprisingly, large size of the left atrium is a risk factor for poor outcome that approaches the risk imposed by LV enlargement.[R22]

Ischemic mitral regurgitation.   Ischemic etiology is a greater risk factor for death late after mitral valve replacement than is nonischemic etiology (Table 11-14).

Advanced functional disability.   Expressed as NYHA functional class, advanced disability is an important risk factor for death in the early phase of hazard[B7,B17,B35,C5,F5,G2,K2,L4,P4,S8,T7,W1] (see Table 11-13). In large part, this correlation is associated with the relation between functional status and left and right ventricular contractility.[C34,H18] The effect of preoperative functional class interacts with other incremental risk factors as well (Table 11-15; see also Tables 11-13 and 11-14). Neutralization of this risk factor depends on providing better intraop-

erative myocardial management for already damaged ventricles and preventing patients from reaching NYHA functional class IV or V before surgical intervention. Nonetheless, patients with mitral valve disease who have depressed left or right ventricular contractility appear to have better survival after surgical treatment than with continued medical treatment.[H18]

Global myocardial ischemic time. Global myocardial ischemic time has been an incremental risk factor for death in the early phase after operation.[B35,F5] Despite use of cold cardioplegia, this continues to be the case (see Table 11-13), although the magnitude of increase may be less in the current era. This can be seen from predicted 30-day mortality of 6% or less when global myocardial ischemic time is 120 minutes or shorter (Fig. 11-38). Almost all mitral valve operations, including those with concomitant coronary artery bypass grafting (CABG) and tricuspid anuloplasty, can be accomplished within that time.

Incremental risks of concomitant tricuspid anuloplasty and CABG are discussed separately under "Results" in Sections 2 and 3.

■ TABLE 11-14 **Percent Survival after Mitral Valve Replacement for Mitral Regurgitation According to Preoperative New York Heart Association Functional Class** [a]

	1-month Preoperative NYHA Class			5-year Preoperative NYHA Class		
Etiology	II	III	IV	II	III	IV
Nonischemic	98%	94%	80%	79%	72%	52%
Ischemic	97%	93%	80%	60%	55%	40%

Key: *NYHA*, New York Heart Association.

[a] Analysis from digital nomogram of a specific solution of multivariable risk-factor equation (see Table 11-13).

■ TABLE 11-15 **Hospital Mortality after Mitral Valve Replacement According to Symptoms and Lesion** [a]

NYHA Class	Mitral Stenosis				Mitral Regurgitation				Mixed Lesions				Total			
	n	No.	%	CL%	n	No.	%	CL%	n	No.	%	CL%	n	No.	%	CL%
I	1	0	0	0-85	6	0	0	0-27	2	0	0	0-61	9	0	0	0-19
II	9	0	0	0-19	28	0	0	0-7	5	1	20	3-53	42	1	2	0.3-7
III	13	1	8	1-24	64	3	5	2-9	22	2	9	3-20	99	6	6	4-10
IV	15	0	0	0-12	55	6	11	7-17	10	1	10	1-30	80	7	9	5-13
V	7	3	43	20-68	16	2	12	4-27					23	5	22	12-34
TOTAL	45	4	9	5-16	169	11	6.5	4.6-9.1	39	4	10	5-18	253	19	7.5	5.8-9.6
$P(\chi^2)$		.01				.25				.85				.05		

Key: *CL*, 70% confidence limits; *NYHA*, New York Heart Association.

[a] Patients undergoing primary or redo mitral valve replacement, with or without associated cardiac surgery but excluding nine patients (0 deaths) not coded for NYHA class, are represented in these data (GLH group, 1976 to 1980).

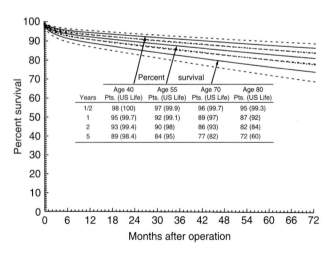

Figure 11-37 Nomogram depicting risk-adjusted survival of patients after isolated mitral valve replacement for mitral stenosis, with or without concomitant coronary artery bypass grafting, according to patient's age at operation. Solid lines represent parametric estimates and dashed lines 70% confidence limits. Age 80 has no line depiction. Percentages in parentheses are estimates of survival for an age-gender-ethnicity–matched general population (U.S. life tables, 1977). (See Appendix 11A for details.)

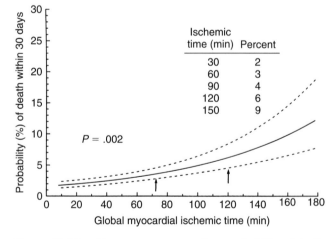

Figure 11-38 Nomogram representing probability of death within 30 days of mitral valve replacement, with or without concomitant cardiac procedures, in patients with mitral stenosis, according to length of global myocardial ischemic (aortic clamp) time when cold cardioplegia is used. (See Appendix 11A for details of constructing this nomogram.)

Devices. No device currently in use has been shown clearly to be a risk factor for premature death after mitral valve replacement.[B35,F8] Earlier, the "high profile" of caged-ball valves was alleged to be an incremental risk factor because of its supposed obstructive effect and detrimental effect on LV function. This may have been true, in view of the superior early results from 1970 to 1973 using a stent-mounted aortic allograft valve, suggesting that a nonobstructive device with a central orifice flow pattern is optimal. Also, at least in the experience of Cohn and colleagues, survival after mitral replacement with a bioprosthesis of any type was higher than after replacement with a prosthetic disc valve, perhaps related to fewer thromboembolic events and only infrequent anticoagulation in the former group[C29] (see "Mechanical Mitral Valve Replacement Devices" and "Bioprosthetic Mitral Valve Replacement Devices" later in this section).

Previous closed or open mitral valve repair or percutaneous balloon valvotomy cannot be considered incremental risk factors.

Cardiac Performance

Left AV valve function usually is greatly improved, but a transvalvar end-diastolic gradient is present in most patients.[G3,H6,J1] Magnitude of the gradient depends on patient size and physical activity (e.g., cardiac output at rest and during exercise), size of device inserted, and its type. Gradients are small when devices larger than 29 mm can be used, but they vary according to the device and are typically present with 29-mm, 27-mm, and 25-mm sizes (Table 11-16). Zero-pressure fixation techniques[B30] may improve the performance of porcine bioprostheses in the future by making the leaflets more pliable.

■ TABLE 11-16   **Hemodynamic Conditions after Insertion of Currently Available Mitral Valve Replacement Devices**

Devices and Standard Values	Mean Diastolic LA–LV Gradient (mmHg)		Effective Orifice Area (cm²)		Effective Orifice Area Index (cm² · m⁻²)		References
	Rest	Exercise	Rest	Exercise	Rest	Exercise	
25-mm Devices							
Starr-Edwards 6120			1.6	1.6			G9
St. Jude Medical	1.0-1.4	6	2.1	2.3	1.2	1.3	C15
Medtronic-Hall							
Omniscience	2						M19
Bjork-Shiley Monostrut	2.3-7.0		2.3				A15, A18
Carpentier-Edwards bioprosthesis							C16
Medtronic-Hancock bioprosthesis			2.2				K16, M8
CarboMedics							
27-mm Devices							
Starr-Edwards 6120	8	12	1.7	2.2			G3, H16, P5, S13
St. Jude Medical	1.9-3.0	3	2.3	3.6	1.4	2.3	C15, G9, G10, H15, N4
Medtronic-Hall	3.6		3.0				H8, M2
Omniscience	6.1						M19
Bjork-Shiley Monostrut	2.0-6.0		1.8				A15, A18
Carpentier-Edwards bioprosthesis							C16
Medtronic-Hancock bioprosthesis			1.0-1.2				K16, M8, S5
CarboMedics	3.5						B47
29-mm Devices							
Starr-Edwards 6120	7		1.7				G3, H16, P5, S13
St. Jude Medical	2-3	3.5-7.0	3.1-3.3	3.3	1.8		G10, H2, H9, M17, N4, S23, Y2
Medtronic-Hall	3		2.9				M2
Omniscience							M19
Bjork-Shiley Monostrut							
Carpentier-Edwards bioprosthesis							C16
Medtronic-Hancock bioprosthesis	5.0-12.1		1.4-2.5				K16, L9, S5
CarboMedics	3.4						B47
31-mm Devices							
Starr-Edwards 6120			1.9	1.9			F6, G9, W5
St. Jude Medical	1.6		3.9				M17, Y2
Medtronic-Hall	2		3.4				M2
Omniscience	5.4						M19
Bjork-Shiley Monostrut	2.3-4		2.5				A15, A18
Carpentier Edwards bioprosthesis							C16
Medtronic-Hancock bioprosthesis	2.3-10.4		1.8-2.1				K16, L2, L7, L8, S5
CarboMedics	3.5						B47
33-mm Devices							
CarboMedics							
Standard Values							
Normal	±0		4-6		3		
Severe stenosis	>12		<1		<0.6		
Desired Postoperative Value	<10	<15	>1.5		>0.9		

Key: *LA–LV,* Left atrium to left ventricle.

Response of LV performance to valve replacement in patients with mitral stenosis who have impaired function preoperatively has not been determined, but the abnormalities of compliance (which this type of impairment usually induces) probably remain.

Sudden ablation of mitral regurgitation by mitral valve replacement triggers a particularly complex LV response (see "Mitral Regurgitation" under Natural History earlier in this section).[K4,R5] If the LV is normal, as usually occurs in *acute* experimental or clinical regurgitation, sudden correction of regurgitation immediately increases forward flow (cardiac output) despite increased afterload.[S14] After valve replacement for *chronic* mitral regurgitation, however, ejection fraction (EF) is lower than preoperatively in most patients (Fig. 11-39).[B12,R5,S6] When preoperative LV enlargement is only mild or moderate (with an end-diastolic dimension of 7 cm or less and an end-systolic dimension of 5 cm or less, as determined by echocardiography[S6]), reduced EF after valve replacement generally remains within the normal range. Schuler and colleagues found that only

2 of 12 such patients (with values of 0.43 and 0.49) had an EF less than 0.5.[S6]

In patients with a more than moderately enlarged LV at operation (with an echocardiographically determined end-diastolic dimension greater than 7 cm or an end-systolic dimension greater than 5 cm[S6]), a condition accompanied by decreased LV contractility and increased myocardial degenerative changes,[F1] EF is greatly reduced 2 weeks after valve replacement and, at times, deteriorates still further during the later postoperative period. As noted later in this text or later in time, patients undergoing repair have better ejection indices postoperatively than similarly matched candidates after valve replacement. Tischler and colleagues reported reduction of rest and exercise EFs in 10 mitral replacement subjects, but no change in repair patients.[T6] Repair patients had a higher stroke volume and EF at rest and exercise (Fig. 11-40), associated with lower end-systolic wall stress (Fig. 11-41).

LV enlargement regresses after operation, with both end-diastolic (Fig. 11-42) and end-systolic dimensions re-

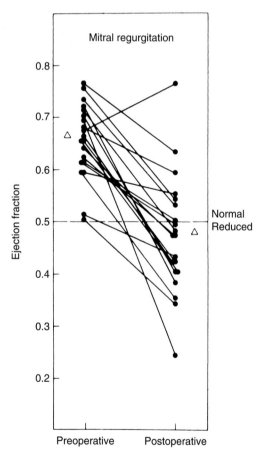

Figure 11-39   Ventricular systolic function (expressed along vertical axis as ejection fraction) before and early after mitral valve replacement for mitral regurgitation. Individual values are shown, and mean values are expressed by Δ. After operation, most patients with mitral regurgitation had an ejection fraction below normal. Broken line represents lower limit of normal (0.50). (From Boucher and colleagues.[B12])

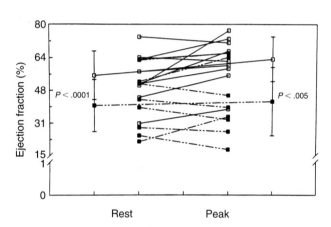

Figure 11-40   Plot of left ventricular ejection fraction at rest and peak exercise in patients with mitral valve repair (□) and mitral valve replacement (■). (From Tischler and colleagues.[T6])

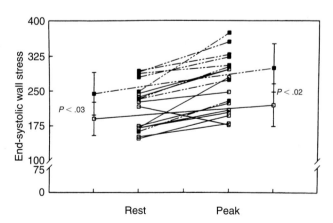

Figure 11-41   Plot of left ventricular end-systolic circumferential wall stress (kdyn · cm⁻²) at rest and peak exercise in patients with mitral valve repair (□) and mitral valve replacement (■). (From Tischler and colleagues.[T6])

turning toward normal.[B12,S6] LV contractility is probably normal or near normal preoperatively and remains so after operation.[K3,S6] In many patients, however, LV size is reduced early postoperatively (end-diastolic volume is less, and end-systolic volume is about the same), but increases late postoperatively (6 to 12 months after operation).[B12,S6] LV wall hypertrophy does not regress.[S6] In such patients the preoperative LV structural and contractile

abnormalities not only show *no regression* after valve replacement but in fact *progress* and account for many recurrences of symptoms 2 to 5 years postoperatively and for many deaths 2 to 10 years postoperatively.

These findings apply to conventional mitral valve replacement in which the tensor apparatus (chordae tendineae) of the native valve is excised or transected (see "Chordal Sparing" under Technique of Operation earlier in this section). Experiments done predominantly by Miller and colleagues have demonstrated that chordal division results in deterioration of LV systolic function in both isovolumic and ejecting heart preparations.[H26-H28] These observations were extended to animals with surgically induced mitral regurgitation.[Y3] Mitral valve replacement was performed with all chordae tendineae intact; LV systolic function was then assessed and subsequently remeasured after division of the chordae. End-systolic pressure volume (E_{es}) and end-systolic stress volume (M_s) relationships decreased by 46% and 36% when the chordae were divided ($P = .001$ and .0001), respectively, indicating deterioration in LV energetics and mechanical efficiency (Fig. 11-43).

Miller termed the effect of an intact tensor apparatus on optimal global ventricular function "valvular–ventricular interaction."[H26] Deterioration of function after division of the chordae resulted from an exacerbated mismatch of ventricular–arterial coupling with increased load resisting shortening. In fact, chordal sparing was first suggested by Lillehei in 1964,[L17] then later disputed by some.[R25] However, David and colleagues in 1983 and later Daenen, Miki, Goor, and Hennein and their colleagues produced clinical results suggesting that chordal sparing during mitral valve replacement improved hospital survival and global LV function.[D24,D25,G11,H29,M26] Carabello's group again documented preservation of systolic ejection performance in mitral valve replacement with intact tensor apparatus compared with otherwise similar mitral valve replacement patients without chordal preservation.[R26] Preservation resulted in postoperative decrease in diastolic

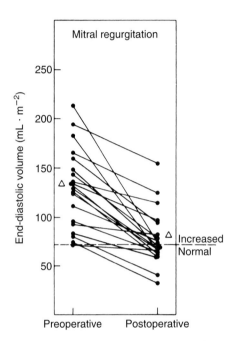

Figure 11-42   Representation as in Fig. 11-39, but with end-diastolic volume along the vertical axis. Preoperatively, end-diastolic volume was above the normal range in all but one patient. Postoperatively, volume decreased in all patients, becoming normal in 11. Broken line represents upper limit of normal (72 mL · m⁻²). (From Boucher and colleagues.[B12])

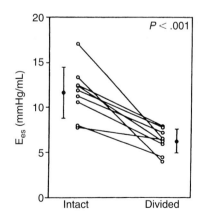
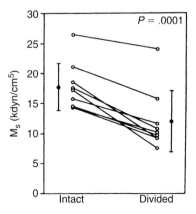

Figure 11-43   Effect of chordal division on left ventricular systolic performance in experimental animals, as reflected by the slope of end-systolic pressure volume and end-systolic stress volume relationships (open circles). Group mean values are also shown (closed circles). Vertical error bars indicate mean ± 1 standard deviation. (From Yun and colleagues.[Y3])

Key: E_{es}, End-systolic pressure volume; M_s, end-systolic stress volume.

volume, reduced end-systolic stress, and no reduction of ejection indices. In analogous experiments in dogs, these investigators found individual myocyte contractile function normal when global contractile indices returned to normal after chordal-sparing mitral valve replacement.[I3] Others have subsequently demonstrated a beneficial effect of chordal sparing on LV performance following mitral valve replacement for regurgitation.[D23,M24,O4,S25]

Although long-term survival and ventricular function are not yet known, it is apparent that some form of chordal continuity is desirable in mitral valve replacement for regurgitation.

Pulmonary Vascular Resistance

When severe pulmonary hypertension is present preoperatively, it is usually the combined result of simple back pressure from elevated left atrial pressure and of elevated Rp. Increased Rp may have both a *dynamic* element, which is immediately decreased by reducing left atrial pressure,[D4] and an *organic* element, which results from pulmonary vascular disease and may or may not regress after operation. Thus, even severe pulmonary hypertension will likely regress toward normal after mitral valve replacement. Kaul and colleagues reported on 30 patients with average preoperative pulmonary artery pressures of 110 mmHg systolic and 74 mmHg mean.[K5] Symptomatic improvement was striking. Restudy an average of 5.5 years after mitral valve replacement showed an average systolic pulmonary artery pressure of 48 mmHg and a mean of 31 mmHg. This drop often occurs soon after valve replacement and thus seems related largely to sudden reduction of left atrial pressure and reversal of severe spastic pulmonary vasoconstriction that accompanies left atrial hypertension in some patients.[B16] Although this initial reduction appears rapidly in most patients (Fig. 11-44),[B16,D4] Rp may continue to fall further in the months after operation. The changes are similar in operations performed for stenosis and for regurgitation.[B16]

Information derived from patients having balloon mitral valvotomy confirms these surgical observations. Immediately after valvotomy, pulmonary artery systolic pressure decreases, but no important change occurs in Rp. One year after the procedure, most patients experience a further decrease of pulmonary artery systolic pressure, and Rp decreases. In older patients and those with atrial fibrillation, normalization of Rp occurs less frequently.[F11,G19]

Thromboembolism

Table 11-17 shows the incidence of thromboembolism for currently available mechanical and bioprosthetic valves (Figs. 11-45 and 11-46). In general, the incidence is somewhat less with bioprostheses.[E7] The incidence and importance of thromboembolism and anticoagulant-related hemorrhage are sufficient to have unfavorable effects on the life expectancy of patients with mechanical valves.

Adequacy of warfarin therapy appears to be the most important determinant of the rate of thromboembolism in patients with mechanical valves in the mitral position. With

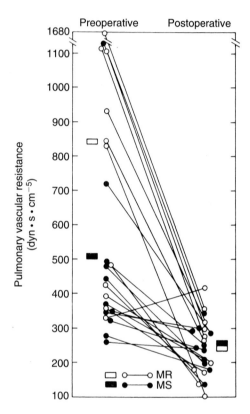

Figure 11-44 Comparison of preoperative and postoperative pulmonary vascular resistance in patients with predominant mitral regurgitation (MR) and mitral stenosis (MS). Horizontal bars represent mean values in each group. (From Braunwald and colleagues.[B16])

■ **TABLE 11-17**   **Thromboembolism after Mitral Valve Replacement According to Replacement Device**

	Freedom from First Event (%)			Linearized Rate of First	
Replacement Device	**5 Years**	**10 Years**	**15 Years**	**Event (%/patient-year)**	**References**
Starr-Edwards	73-78	60	54-57	4.5-5.7[a]	C21, H16, M7, S21
St. Jude Medical	88-96			1.5-1.75	A13, A17, B41, C17, C25, C31, D11, D12, H20, K14, K15, S22
Medtronic-Hall	89-95			1.3-3.1	A14, B42, B43, C24, H8
Omniscience	93			0.9-7.6	C24, D3, D14, E7, E8, M19, R18-R20
Bjork-Shiley Monostrut	95 (3 yr)			2.6-3.8	A15, B44, L12, T3
Carpentier-Edwards	78	80[b]			C18, M9
Medtronic-Hancock	92			1.5-2.0	B19, C6, C30, D1, H7
CarboMedics	94			1.0-2.5	A23, J6

[a] 9.5% when multiple events included.

[b] In patients 51 to 65 years of age at insertion.

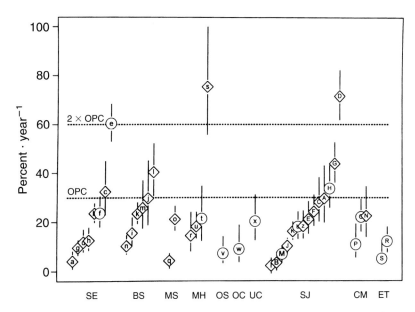

Figure 11-45   Summary of linearized rate of thromboembolism for mechanical mitral valve prostheses from reports published from 1989 to 2000, each containing at least 400 patient-years of follow-up. Vertical axis is linearized rate in units of percent per year (equivalent to events per 100 patient-years). Each symbol represents one series; height of symbol represents point estimate of event rate, and vertical bars show 95% confidence intervals. Series are grouped on the horizontal axis by valve model, shown below the axis by a two-letter abbreviation. Lower horizontal dashed line indicates the FDA's Objective Performance Criteria (OPC). For approval of a new valve, the upper confidence limit should be less than twice the OPC (upper dashed line). Circles indicate that only late events were used to calculate the rates; diamonds indicate that both early and late events were used. (From Grunkemeier and colleagues.[G15])

Key: *BS,* Bjork-Shiley; *CM,* CarboMedics; *ET,* Edwards Tekna; *MH,* Medtronic-Hall; *MS,* Monostrut; *OC,* Omnicarbon; *OPC,* Objective Performance Criteria; *OS,* Omniscience; *SE,* Starr-Edwards; *SJ,* St. Jude Medical; *UC,* Ultracor.

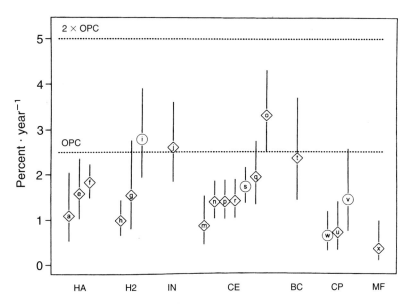

Figure 11-46   Summary of linearized rate of thromboembolism for mitral valve bioprostheses from reports published from 1989 to 2000, each containing at least 400 patient-years of follow-up. Format is as in Fig. 11-45. (From Grunkemeier and colleagues.[G15])

Key: *BC,* Biocor; *CE,* Carpentier-Edwards; *CP,* CE PERIMOUNT; *HA,* Hancock I; *H2,* Hancock II; *IN,* Medtronic Intact; *MF,* Mitroflow; *OPC,* objective performance criteria.

bioprostheses, warfarin therapy for 3 months, or aspirin indefinitely, appears to be as effective as long-term warfarin therapy.[E7]

Acute Thrombotic Occlusion

Acute thrombotic occlusion of a mitral prosthesis occurs more often with a mechanical device (3 per 100 patient-years) than with a bioprosthesis (1.9 per 100 patient-years)[E7] (see "Mechanical Mitral Valve Replacement Devices" later in this section).

The problem in using linearized rates is well exemplified in the case of acute thrombotic occlusion. Linearized rates assume a constant hazard function (see "General Comments" under Time-Related Events in Chapter 6). However, at least in the case of the Bjork-Shiley tilting-disc valve, the hazard function for this event had a single peaking phase that returned to a low level by 4 years after operation.[B35] This same shape was found by Lindblom.[L13] In addition to the scientific importance of this finding, the shape of the hazard function suggests the use of thrombectomy (through both the left atrium and aorta) rather than valve replacement. No recurrence has followed thrombectomy in three patients with thrombotic occlusion.[B35]

Acute thrombotic occlusion occurs primarily but not exclusively in patients receiving suboptimal anticoagulant therapy. A possible risk factor is female gender. Patients with this catastrophic complication usually become symptomatic only 1 to 3 days before admission to the hospital and present principally with extreme dyspnea and orthopnea. The patient may have noticed a decrease in intensity of prosthetic valve sounds at about the time symptoms began. Many experience chest pain, and signs of shock usually appear. Although regurgitation is often present, an apical systolic murmur is rarely heard. A fluoroscopic finding of limited disc movement supports the diagnosis, but an echocardiogram is diagnostic.[B18] Cardiac catheterization usually gives conclusive evidence of mitral obstruction, but such patients are usually too ill to withstand this procedure.[C7] Emergency operation is indicated. Surgical thrombectomy often achieves a good result.[M20] Thrombolysis has been used with mixed results (see previous text and "Thrombosis" under Results in Chapter 14).

Complications of Long-Term Anticoagulation

Complications of long-term anticoagulation with warfarin or warfarin-like compounds appear to be independent of type of prosthesis. Certainly the quality of the surveillance program for patients receiving long-term anticoagulation affects both freedom from anticoagulant-related hemorrhage and prevalence of thromboembolic complications. Percentage freedom from first anticoagulant-related hemorrhage at 5, 10, and 15 years is about 87%, 79%, and 71%, respectively. Linearized rate of important hemorrhage is generally estimated to average 2.3 to 3.4 per 100 patient-years in patients with mechanical prostheses who are taking warfarin,[A13,C24,C31,E7,H16,M7,S21,T4] although a recent meta-analysis suggests a lower rate of 1% to 2% per year.[G15] Many hemorrhagic episodes are relatively minor and do not require hospitalization and transfusion.[K2] Miller and colleagues found about one third of hemorrhagic events to be fatal.[M7]

There is no evidence that the hazard function for a bleeding event in a patient on warfarin therapy is anything other than a single constant phase, but this has not been rigorously studied.

Warfarin has a number of serious effects during pregnancy. It crosses the placenta and in about 10% of patients causes warfarin embryopathy if the fetus is exposed between the sixth and ninth weeks of gestation. If warfarin is taken during the second and third trimesters, optic atrophy and mental retardation occur in the fetus in about 3% of cases. Overall, miscarriage occurs in 70% to 75% of pregnancies when the mother has taken warfarin since conception.[E7]

Prosthetic Valve Endocarditis

Prosthetic valve endocarditis[2] is an uncommon but serious complication that results in the death of more than half of affected patients.[D2,I1] Endocarditis strongly predisposes the patient to periprosthetic leakage.[B35,D2] When it appears within 3 to 6 months of operation, prosthetic valve endocarditis is probably related to events in the operating room.[I1] When it develops later, it probably results from a new bacteremia (see Chapter 15).

When mitral prosthetic infection becomes evident within 6 months of implantation, prosthetic leakage is likely to occur and the risk of death is high. Intense antibiotic treatment, followed by early prosthetic replacement in most patients, is indicated. The organism and its antibiotic sensitivity should be identified and specific therapy used. In the unusual circumstance of excellent response to antibiotics, no evidence of peripheral embolization, and no evidence of periprosthetic leakage, reoperation may be deferred. The patient is followed closely under hospital conditions that permit immediate reoperation in the event any of these complications occur. When mitral prosthetic infection becomes apparent for the first time more than 6 months postoperatively, the same management protocols apply. More of these patients respond well to intense medical treatment alone than those with infections occurring in the first 6 months after operation.

Periprosthetic Leakage

At UAB, in an era when various suture techniques were used (1975 to July 1979), 13 of 452 (2.9%; CL 2.1%-3.9%) patients required reoperation for periprosthetic leakage. Currently, the incidence in uninfected patients approaches zero when suture techniques described in this chapter are used.[D2] Preoperative infectious endocarditis increases the risk of prosthesis dehiscence with periprosthetic leakage.[R15] Anular calcification also increases the risk.[D2]

Chronic Hemolysis

Well-functioning bioprosthetic and mechanical prostheses used in the current era rarely produce more than mild chronic hemolysis unless periprosthetic leakage is present.[A2] With periprosthetic leakage, hemolysis may be

---

[2] *Prosthetic valve endocarditis* and its abbreviation PVE are familiar, standard, and historical designations for infective endocarditis on any heart valve substitute. The rationale for a more appropriate term, *replacement device endocarditis,* is presented in Chapter 12.

■ **TABLE 11-18   New York Heart Association Functional Class after Primary Mitral Valve Replacement for Nonischemic Mitral Valve Disease** [a]

| | Postoperative NYHA Functional Class | | | | | | | | | | |
| | I | | II | | III | | IV | | | | |
Procedure	No.	% of 386	No.	% of 91	No.	% of 37	No.	% of 2	Total Alive	Dead	Unknown
Isolated [b]	288	59	132	34	22	6	4	1	386	93	19
+ CABG	50	55	33	36	7	8	1	1	91	43	4
+ TVA	20	54	9	24	6	16	2	5	37	25	2
+ TVR	0	0	2	100	0	0	0	0	2	2	0

[a] Data from UAB group, 1975 to July 1983. Information is from same database as for Table 11-10. *P* value (logistic) for difference in distribution of postoperative functional class between "with and without previous repair" and "+ CABG" is .40, and that between "with and without previous repair" and "+ TVA" is .05.

Key: *CABG,* Coronary artery bypass grafting; *MVR,* mitral valve replacement; *NYHA,* New York Heart Association; *TVA,* tricuspid valve anuloplasty; *TVR,* tricuspid valve replacement.

[b] With or without previous repair.

■ **TABLE 11-19   New York Heart Association Functional Class after Isolated Mitral Valve Replacement According to Preoperative Functional Class** [a]

| | | Postoperative NYHA Functional Class [c] | | | | | | | |
| | | I | | II | | III | | IV | |
Preoperative NYHA Functional Class [b]	*n* Alive and Known	No.	% of *n*	No.	% of *n*	No.	% of *n*	No.	% of *n*
I	7	6	86	1	14	0	0	0	0
II	42	32	76	9	21	1	2	0	0
III	306	175	57	111	36	17	6	3	1
IV	23	11	48	8	35	3	13	1	4
V	1	1	100	0	0	0	0	0	0

(Data from UAB group, 1975 to July 1983. *P* value [logistic] for difference in distribution of postoperative functional class between patients preoperatively in NYHA classes I and II and those in classes III and IV is .003, and the *P* value by linear regression for table as a whole is .001.)

Key: *NYHA,* New York Heart Association.

[a] Patients with or without previous mitral repair but without tricuspid valve surgery are represented. Information is from the same database as for Table 11-10.

[b] Unknown in seven patients.

severe with any device; red cell trauma and fragmentation may be extreme under these circumstances. A mechanical prosthesis of small size relative to body size and hemodynamics may result in severe hemolysis.[N2]

Functional Status

Symptoms are reduced and functional capacity increased in most patients (Table 11-18).[K2,W1] However, prevalence of an excellent functional status after replacement is related to preoperative functional class (Table 11-19). Only about half of patients with severe preoperative chronic functional disability return to NYHA functional class I. This finding suggests that many patients with mitral valve disease and advanced chronic disability have a secondary irreversible ventricular myopathy. Infrequently a patient may display striking symptomatic improvement for 2 to 5 years, after which important symptoms and disability gradually reappear despite good function of the prosthetic device. This sequence is believed to result from progression of a secondary cardiomyopathy that was present before operation or, occasionally, from progression of other valve lesions.

Reoperation

Reoperation, usually for periprosthetic leakage with or without infectious endocarditis or for bioprosthetic degeneration, has been required within 5 years of the original operation in about 5% of patients. Prevalence and particularly the hazard function for reoperation are different for mechanical and bioprosthetic devices; only bioprostheses exhibit degeneration and a late rising hazard function (Figs. 11-47 and 11-48). Risk of death after reoperation, both early and intermediate term (see Fig. 11-36), as well as the risk of reoperation (Fig. 11-49), subsequent prosthetic valve endocarditis (Fig. 11-50), and periprosthetic leakage (Fig. 11-51), increases with each succeeding reoperation.[B35,G2,K2]

Summary

Although not free of complications in all patients, mitral valve replacement provides a considerably better prognosis than could be expected according to natural history. About 70% of patients are alive and without complications for at least 5 years after valve replacement (Fig. 11-52).

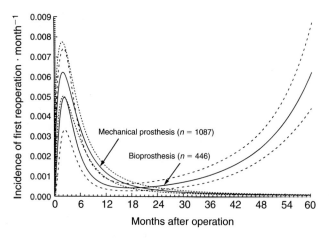

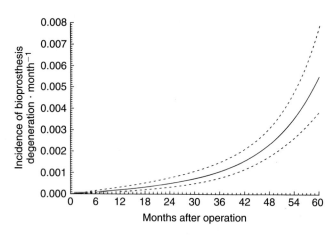

Figure 11-47 Hazard function for reoperation for mechanical prostheses and bioprostheses, determined by separate analyses. Hazard function for mechanical prostheses has an early peaking phase and a constant phase. Hazard function for bioprostheses has an early peaking phase and a second, late rising phase. (From Blackstone and Kirklin.[B35])

Figure 11-48 Hazard function for bioprosthetic degeneration after original valve replacement. There is a single, late rising hazard phase, which accounts for the unique shape of the hazard function for reoperation seen in Fig. 11-47. (From Blackstone and Kirklin.[B35])

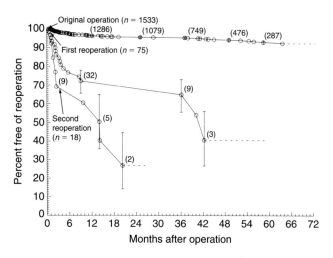

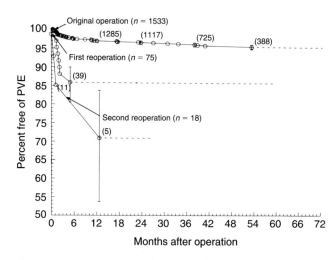

Figure 11-49 Freedom from reoperation after original and subsequent valve replacement procedures. (From Blackstone and Kirklin.[B35])

Figure 11-50 Freedom from prosthetic valve endocarditis after original and subsequent valve replacement procedures. (From Blackstone and Kirklin.[B35])

Key: *PVE,* Prosthetic valve endocarditis.

Figure 11-51 Freedom from periprosthetic leakage after original and subsequent valve replacement procedures. (From Blackstone and Kirklin.[B35])

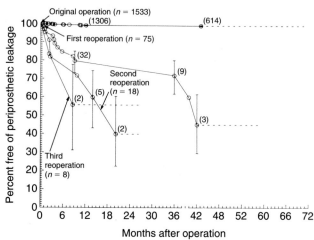

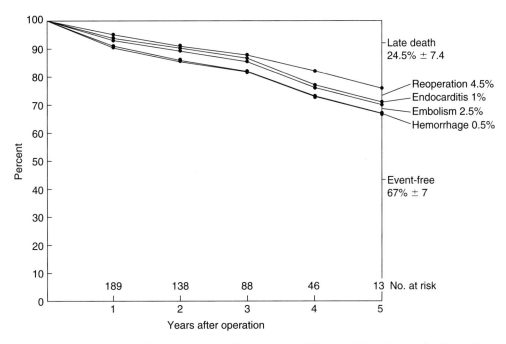

Figure 11-52   Cumulative complication-free events in 245 hospital survivors of mitral valve replacement with mechanical prostheses (45% of patients) and porcine bioprostheses (55% of patients) with or without tricuspid valve surgery. Only patients with mechanical valves received long-term anticoagulation therapy. Patients include those with first operations or reoperations and those with concomitant cardiac procedures, except procedures on the aortic valve, a left ventricular aneurysm, or an ascending aortic aneurysm. The ± indicates standard error (GLH group, 1976 to 1979).

INDICATIONS FOR OPERATION, SELECTION OF TECHNIQUE, AND CHOICE OF DEVICE

Mitral Stenosis

When an opening snap is prominent, when calcification cannot be demonstrated fluoroscopically, and when echocardiography demonstrates pliable leaflets and little or no subvalvar narrowing, good results from surgical mitral commissurotomy can usually be obtained. Under these circumstances, even mild symptoms (NYHA functional class II) in the presence of severe mitral stenosis are an indication for intervention. Percutaneous balloon mitral commissurotomy is often chosen, although surgical commissurotomy is a reasonable alternative. Particularly in young women, one acute episode of important paroxysmal nocturnal dyspnea or pulmonary edema in the presence of at least moderate mitral stenosis is an indication for intervention. It is particularly indicated before the onset of atrial fibrillation.[S10] Intervention is also advisable when there is an important increase in Rp, even in the absence of symptoms. Asymptomatic patients with multiple episodes of arterial emboli are advised to undergo intervention if commissurotomy is a strong possibility; in this setting and in the presence of demonstrated thrombi in the left atrium, open surgical commissurotomy is advisable.

In any event, commissurotomy rather than valve replacement is usually possible as the primary intervention for mitral stenosis. In the GLH experience between 1968 and 1976, only 16 patients among 154 having commissurot-omy required valve replacement (mean follow-up of 48 months).[S10] When a mitral valve replacement seems likely (because of absence of an opening snap, immobile leaflets, heavy mitral valve calcification, severe subvalvar disease,[A3] or associated mitral regurgitation), a more symptomatic state is demanded as the indication for operation because of the added long-term imponderables introduced by the device inserted. These would be more severe chronic symptoms (NYHA functional class III or higher) or several acute episodes of symptoms of pulmonary venous hypertension.

Advanced disability, associated tricuspid valve disease, and associated coronary artery disease are not contraindications to operation, nor is severe pulmonary hypertension.

Mitral Regurgitation

At operation, mitral valve repair rather than replacement is chosen whenever possible: in 50% to 70% of all patients and in up to 90% of patients with mitral valve prolapse (Fig. 11-53).[E14,S24] The decision to operate is more difficult in patients with mitral regurgitation than in those with mitral stenosis because of the following:

- Prediction of whether the valve can be repaired rather than replaced is more important and is made with less certainty.
- Conservation of LV contractility is the most important factor determining the ultimate effectiveness of repair or replacement.
- Determination of the preoperative contractile state is difficult.

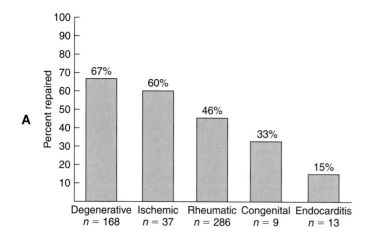

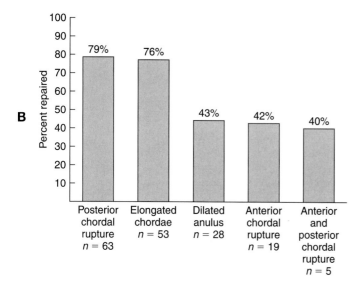

Figure 11-53 Prevalence of mitral valve repair. **A,** By etiology of mitral valve disease. **B,** By anatomy of degenerative mitral regurgitation. (From Chavez and colleagues.[C45])

Patients with mitral regurgitation may remain asymptomatic or may have only mild symptoms associated with long-standing disease and gradually deteriorating LV function because of the mitigating effect of regurgitant mitral flow on LV systolic function, EF, and cardiac output. Thus, whereas the diagnosis and symptoms of mitral stenosis generally provide sufficient evidence for decision making, special attention must also be paid to the status of the LV in mitral regurgitation.

In patients with chronic mitral regurgitation and in NYHA functional class I or II, any LV enlargement less than grade 3 (of grades 1 to 6, with 6 being extreme enlargement), as judged primarily by physical examination, chest radiograph, and echocardiogram, may support continued nonsurgical treatment. When LV enlargement is grade 3 or more in this clinical setting, secondary LV myopathy of mitral regurgitation usually has become prominent, portending its progression to an irreversible state. Operation is then advisable, even in the absence of disabling symptoms. Echocardiography, particularly TEE, can accurately predict specific mitral valve lesions and the functional anat-

omy of mitral regurgitation (88% to 99% overall accuracy in the Mayo Clinic experience).[E14] Moreover, echocardiographic anatomic and physiologic classification is a strong predictor of valve repairability, operative mortality, and long-term outcome. Therefore, patients with a floppy valve (prolapse, as opposed to ischemic or restrictive functional anatomy) who are asymptomatic are excellent candidates for early surgery because operative mortality is low (less than 2%), repairability is high (90%), and long-term survival is good.[E14,L18]

The role of left atrial enlargement in decision making is uncertain. More than moderate left atrial dilatation likely has a deleterious effect after valve repair or replacement and therefore favors operation.[R22]

Reference has been made to more sophisticated methods of assessing the functional state of the LV in patients with mitral regurgitation (see "Mitral Regurgitation" under Natural History earlier in this section). Zile, Schuler, and their colleagues identified groups of patients with elevated end-diastolic dimensions, elevated systolic dimensions, and low–normal LV EF in whom symptoms were not relieved, heart failure was persistent, or high mortality followed operation.[S27,Z3] If LV end-systolic dimension exceeded 26 mm · m^{-2} body surface area (BSA) and fractional shortening was less than 31%, consistent deterioration of LV function occurred postoperatively.[Z3] Based on these findings, Ross has suggested operation in patients with few or no symptoms if LV EF is less than 55%, fractional shortening is less than 30%, and end-systolic diameter approaches 50 mm (26 mm · m^{-2} BSA).[R27] These recommendations were recently reaffirmed in the ACC/AHA Procedure Guidelines for the Management of Patients with Valvular Heart Disease, which recommends operation for mitral regurgitation in patients with LV EF less than 60% and LV end-systolic dimension greater than 45 mm.[B45]

Diminished response of EF with exercise also has been found to be a predictor of postoperative LV dysfunction. Leung and colleagues found that patients with low postoperative EF (less than 0.50) had a preoperative change in exercise EF of –4% ± 9% versus +9% ± 10% (P = .005) for those with an adequate (greater than 0.50) postoperative EF.[L19]

Because these methods are not in general use for determining the time of elective surgery in patients with mitral regurgitation and in NYHA functional class I or II, a decline in LV contractility, assessed by end-systolic pressure–volume relationships or similar method, portends a state of irreversibility and may be used to advise operation in relatively asymptomatic patients. Additionally, operation in most of these asymptomatic patients is well advised if repair is probable, because it has been well documented that postoperative systolic and diastolic LV function are preserved after mitral valve reconstruction.[C42,S17]

When the patient with mitral regurgitation is in NYHA functional class III or IV, operation is clearly indicated. Currently, even advanced disability is not a contraindication to operation, although it is recognized that secondary LV myopathy associated with, and in part responsible for, this state has a deleterious effect on early and late results of operation. If a stage of irreversibility can be securely identified by preoperative studies, valve surgery may be ineffective and cardiac replacement indicated.

Nonischemic Chordal Rupture

The decision about operation is more difficult in patients with mitral regurgitation from nonischemic chordal rupture of recent onset. If the symptoms of pulmonary venous hypertension are brought promptly under control by medical management, as often occurs, operation may be deferred and the patient reevaluated at frequent intervals (see "Natural History" earlier in this section). Thereafter, the criteria used in chronic mitral regurgitation apply. If the pansystolic murmur radiates into the aortic area and neck, however, and if echocardiographic evidence shows that the ruptured chordae belong to the posterior leaflet, indications for operation should be liberalized because a durable reparative operation can be done at low risk.

Infective Endocarditis

Mitral regurgitation may develop acutely as a result of infective endocarditis. If symptoms are initially mild or moderate and are brought under good control, together with the infection, continuing in-hospital medical treatment is indicated. Surveillance must be close, however, because of possible rapid progression in severity of regurgitation. If this is suspected, operation is urgently indicated before hemodynamic deterioration occurs. Acute pulmonary edema, paroxysmal nocturnal dyspnea, or rising blood urea nitrogen or creatinine levels are indications for urgent operation. Systemic embolization during treatment or persistent active infection despite intense antibiotic treatment also indicate the need for operation (see Chapter 15).

Mixed Mitral Stenosis and Regurgitation

Patients with a mixture of important stenosis and mitral regurgitation usually have a clinical picture similar to that of patients with pure mitral stenosis. Valve replacement is usually required, and indications for operation are the same as in mitral stenosis.

Coexisting Mild Aortic Stenosis

A number of patients treated by percutaneous or surgical valvotomy for mitral stenosis have mild aortic involvement at the time of the procedure. Most do not progress to severe disease even after long follow-up, and aortic valve replacement is rarely needed. Thus, at initial mitral operation, prophylactic aortic valve replacement is not indicated.[V4]

Choice of Device for Valve Replacement

Some surgeons routinely use one device or another for mitral valve replacement, but the valve of choice varies widely. Rabago and Cooley and others have reviewed a number of factors involved in the choice of device.[G15,K18,R20,R24] Two of the most important considerations are durability and requirement for permanent anticoagulation.

Currently available xenograft bioprostheses degenerate more rapidly in young patients who would otherwise be good surgical candidates for tissue valves.[A8,A9] Advanced age and atrial fibrillation increase the probability of thromboembolism even in a patient with a bioprosthesis. Also,

Warnes and colleagues reported that bioprostheses degenerate more rapidly in the mitral position than in the aortic position.[W3] Bioprostheses are in a state of evolution; continuing improvements will probably lead to increased durability.[C13]

Prosthetic mechanical valves are also evolving, but there is no evidence that a device that does not require lifelong anticoagulation will soon be available. Hemodynamic characteristics and performance of the mitral valve prosthesis may also influence choices, particularly in very young patients.

For patients undergoing mitral valve replacement, the basic decision is whether to use a mechanical valve or a bioprosthesis. In patients older than about 60 years, survival may be better with a bioprosthesis because of thromboembolic and anticoagulant-related problems associated with mechanical valves. Also, reoperation 7 to 15 years later may be preferable to lifelong anticoagulant (warfarin) therapy. In patients younger than age 60, survival may be better with a mechanical valve because of the more rapid degeneration of bioprostheses in the young, despite need for lifelong anticoagulation. Infrequently, a bioprosthesis is used in young women, to be replaced electively after successful childbearing (see "Complication of Long-Term Anticoagulation" later in this section).

The newest approach to mitral valve substitute devices is use of a cryopreserved stentless allograft. Early reports suggest good hemodynamic performance and adequate freedom from thromboembolism (in the absence of anticoagulation).[A20] The important issue is durability. There are also scattered reports describing placement of a pulmonary valve autograft in the mitral position. The valve is implanted as a cylinder ("top hat") using two suture lines augmented with an atrial cuff.[G24,R24]

Mechanical Mitral Valve Replacement Devices

A discussion of modern mechanical valves is complicated by two factors: (1) changing availability of specific valves because of continuing introduction and withdrawal of new models and (2) variability in prevalence of use in different countries, in part because of regulatory agencies. In this section, only mechanical valves currently available and in use in at least several countries are discussed (see Table 11-16).

Starr-Edwards Silastic Ball Valve Prosthesis (Model 6120)

General considerations. The Starr-Edwards (S-E) mitral device (model 6120), available worldwide and approved for use in the United States by the Food and Drug Administration (FDA), is provided in sizes 5M (34 mm), 4M (32 mm), 3M (30 mm), 2M (28 mm), 1M (26 mm), 0M (22 mm), and 00M (20 mm). The ball is made of silicone rubber and contains barium sulfate for radiopacity. It has a flange-shaped sewing ring, with the flange overlapping the mitral anulus on the atrial side. The cage is made of stellite alloy. The sewing ring has a silicone rubber insert under the seamless PTFE or polyester cloth. Experience with currently available models covers more than 30 years; therefore, information is more secure than that for any other currently available mechanical valve. Anticoagulation with warfarin or similar drugs is recommended. Usual measures against prosthetic valve endocarditis are recommended for all patients.

Hemodynamics. Diastolic gradients across S-E prosthetic mitral valves in vivo are slightly greater, and effective orifice area slightly less, than for other available mechanical valves (see Table 11-16). No firm evidence indicates that the projection of the valve cage into the LV is functionally disadvantageous, except when the ventricle is unusually small.

Thromboembolism. Thromboembolism is probably more common with the S-E valve than with other valves and more common after mitral valve replacement than after aortic valve replacement. With the mitral device, 73% to 78% of patients are free of their first thromboembolic event for the first 5 years, but only 60% for the first 10 years and 54% to 57% for the first 15 years (see Table 11-17 and Fig. 11-45). About 4.5% of patients per year experience a first thromboembolic event, but the percentage is about twice this when each of multiple events in an individual patient is included.

Valve thrombosis. Linearized rate of valve thrombosis in the mitral position is very low, about 0.2% per patient-year.

Mechanical failure. Mechanical failures in the current S-E Silastic ball-valve prosthesis in the mitral position have not been reported.

St. Jude Medical Valve

General considerations. The St. Jude Medical (SJM) mitral device, available worldwide and approved for use in the United States by the FDA, is provided in the standard form (M-101) and in sizes 19, 21, 23, 25, 27, 29, 31, and 33 mm. The first implant of the SJM prosthetic valve was in October 1977. This device is bileaflet, and both the leaflets and orifice ring are fabricated from pyrolytic carbon. The leaflets are orifice oriented, and closing forces are supported by a pivot system. The pivot ears are raised above the housing, and leaflet motion is by rotation. Two relatively high-velocity regurgitant jets (seen on echocardiography) wash the pivot recess, producing approximately 10% regurgitation. The original SJM was not rotatable, but the newer Masters Series allows rotation to an "anatomical" or "anti-anatomical" position of the leaflets. The sewing cuff on the mitral prosthesis has a supraanular configuration and is provided in a standard (M-101) or expanded (MEC-102) polyester fiber cuff. It is also available with a PTFE fiber cuff (MT-103).

Anticoagulation with warfarin or similar drugs is recommended.[H21] Usual measures against prosthetic valve endocarditis are recommended.

Hemodynamics. Hemodynamic performance is excellent, as reflected in a relatively large effective orifice area (see Table 11-16). Regurgitant flow may be greater than optimal, particularly at low heart rates.[R17]

Thromboembolism. Performance is favorable in regard to thromboembolism (see Table 11-17). Between 88% and 96% of patients with device placement in the mitral position are free from their first thromboembolic event at 5 years after operation (see Table 11-17 and Fig. 11-54). Linearized rate of the first thromboembolic event is about 1.5% to 1.75% per patient-year.[B46,E7,J6,K15] Up to 75% of

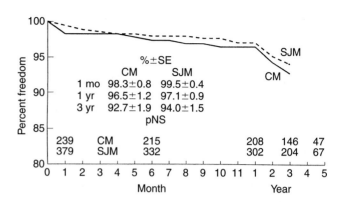

Figure 11-54   Freedom from major thromboembolism (including thrombosis and fatal) following mitral valve replacement with CarboMedics and St. Jude Medical prosthetic devices. (From Jamieson and colleagues.[J6])

Key: *CM,* CarboMedics; *pNS,* not statistically significant; *SE,* standard error; *SJM,* St. Jude Medical.

the thromboembolic episodes occur when anticoagulation is inadequate (INR < 2.5).[J6,K15]

Valve thrombosis. Thrombosis is uncommon. Incidence is approximately 0.1% per patient-year and is usually associated with inadequate anticoagulation.[I4]

Mechanical failure. Mechanical failure is uncommon.

Medtronic-Hall Valve

General considerations. The Medtronic-Hall (M-H) valve is a central pivoting-disc prosthesis and a descendant of the Lillehei-Kaster valve. The FDA-approved M-H valve was introduced in June 1977 and is available worldwide. The housing is one piece of machined titanium, and the valve has a rotatable knitted PTFE sewing ring. Model M7700 is supplied for mitral implantation in external diameter sizes 23, 25, 27, 29, 31, and 33 mm. Anticoagulation with warfarin or similar drugs is recommended. Usual measures against prosthetic valve endocarditis are recommended.

Hemodynamics. Hemodynamics are excellent and comparable to other wide-orifice mitral valve replacement prostheses[V2] (see Table 11-16).

Thromboembolism. Linearized rate of thromboembolic complications is low, about 2% per patient-year (see Table 11-17 and Fig. 11-45). Five-year freedom from a thromboembolic event is about 90%.

Valve thrombosis. Valve thrombosis appears to be rare. Linearized rate of thrombotic obstruction has been 0.2 to 1.2 per 100 patient-years.[B43,H8]

Mechanical failure. Mechanical failure has not been reported.

Omniscience Valve

General considerations. The Omniscience tilting-disc valve is provided in external diameter sizes of 19, 21, 23, 25, 27, 29, 31, and 33 mm for implantation in the mitral position. The FDA-approved valve, introduced in 1978 and distributed worldwide, is a pivoting occluder device consisting of a free-floating concave–convex disc of pyrolytic carbon within a one-piece titanium housing. Anticoagulation with warfarin or similar drugs is recommended. Usual measures against prosthetic valve endocarditis are recommended. The successor to the Omniscience valve is the Omnicarbon valve.

Hemodynamics. Hemodynamic performance is similar to that of other tilting-disc valves (see Table 11-16).

Thromboembolism. Thromboembolic complications have been the subject of considerable controversy. Several investigators have found linearized rates of thromboembolism to be considerably higher with the Omniscience valve than with other devices (see Table 11-17).[E8] However, DeWall and colleagues and others have found the rate of thromboembolism to be very low (see Fig. 11-45).[D3,D14] Although it provides interesting reading, this controversy is in essence a sad commentary on the variable quality of medical data collection and its reporting.[D14,E7,E8]

Valve thrombosis. Seven cases of valve thrombosis were observed among 65 patients.[C24] The linearized rate was 3.1% ± 1.1% per patient-year, higher ($P = .01$) than for Medtronic-Hall and Bjork-Shiley tilting-disc valves. Scotten and colleagues found a smaller regurgitant volume with the Omniscience valve than with some other devices.[S23] Thus, Cortina and colleagues have hypothesized a lesser degree of self-washing by this prosthesis as the explanation for the seemingly higher rate of valve thrombosis.[C24]

Mechanical failure. Few cases of mechanical failure have been encountered.

Bjork-Shiley Monostrut Valve

General considerations. The Bjork-Shiley (B-S) mitral replacement device, introduced in April 1982, is provided in odd-numbered external diameter sizes from 17 to 33 mm. It is available worldwide, is commonly used in Europe, but is not FDA approved for use in the United States. Earlier versions of the B-S valve are no longer available.[B8] The orifice ring and integral struts of the B-S Monostrut prosthesis are constructed from a cobalt–chromium alloy as a single piece. The pyrolytic carbon, concave–convex disc opens to 70 degrees. Anticoagulation with warfarin or similar drugs is recommended. Usual measures against prosthetic valve endocarditis are recommended for all patients.

Hemodynamics. Hemodynamics are good (see Table 11-16).[N9]

Thromboembolism. Available information suggests that in the mitral position, the valve has a relatively low rate of thromboembolism (see Table 11-17 and Fig. 11-45). Daenen and colleagues found that freedom from thromboembolism was 86% ± 4% at 6 years.[D25]

Valve thrombosis. No case of valve thrombosis has been reported.[D25]

Mechanical failure. No case of mechanical failure has been reported.

CarboMedics Valve

General considerations. The CarboMedics heart valve is a low-profile bileaflet prosthesis constructed of pyrolite carbon. The leaflet retention mechanism is within the pyrolyte housing and has no pivot ears, struts, or orifice projections. Leaflet motion is by rotation, with relatively

complete seating but allowing four small regurgitant jets (typically noted on echocardiography). The valve housing is rotatable within a carbon-coated polyester sewing ring. The mitral device is provided in sizes 19, 21, 23, 25, 27, and 29 mm. It has been in use since 1985 and was approved by the FDA in 1992 for use in the United States. Anticoagulation with warfarin or similar drugs is recommended. Usual measures against prosthetic valve endocarditis are recommended.

Thromboembolism. The valve has a favorable record for freedom from thromboembolism, with about 94% of patients event-free at 5 years (see Table 11-17 and Fig. 11-54).[J6] Linearized rate of thromboembolism is 1.0% to 2.5% per patient-year (see Fig. 11-45).[A23,J6]

Valve thrombosis. Thrombosis is uncommon. Prevalence is approximately 0.5 per 100 patient-years.[A24,F13]

Bioprosthetic Mitral Valve Replacement Devices

A number of stent-mounted bioprosthetic devices are in clinical use for mitral valve replacement, including those with leaflets made of allograft aortic valves, xenograft aortic valves, pericardium, fascia lata, and dura mater.

Carpentier-Edwards Glutaraldehyde-Preserved Porcine Xenograft

General considerations. The Carpentier-Edwards (C-E) bioprosthesis, FDA approved and distributed worldwide, is composed of porcine (xenograft) aortic valves preserved in buffered glutaraldehyde and mounted on a flexible lightweight frame made of a cobalt–chromium–nickel alloy (Elgiloy). Glutaraldehyde fixation reduces antigenicity and increases tissue stability.[C35,C36] The suture ring consists of a soft silicone rubber insert covered by porous, seamless PTFE. The valve is in a solution containing glutaraldehyde when purchased and must be thoroughly rinsed with saline and kept in saline until immediately before implantation. Anticoagulation of the patient for 2 months after insertion is recommended. For the mitral position (model 6625) the bioprosthesis is provided in sizes 27, 29, 31, 33, and 35 mm in the United States; elsewhere it is also available in a 25-mm size. The valve is also available with an extended sewing ring (model 6625-ESR).

The C-E valve, as well as the Medtronic-Hancock bioprosthesis, is subject to slow degeneration and at times calcification, particularly in young patients (see "Central Leakage" under Replacement Device Regurgitation under Results in Chapter 12).

Hemodynamics. Hemodynamic performance is good and comparable to that of other bioprostheses. In general, however, the effective orifice size in vivo is somewhat smaller than that of mechanical prostheses of the same external diameter. Thus, Carpentier suggested that the 31-mm or 33-mm valve be used in adults unless special circumstances demand a smaller valve.

Thromboembolism. Thromboembolism is sufficiently uncommon, as it is in other bioprostheses, that long-term anticoagulation is generally not recommended. However, thromboembolism does occur when the C-E device is in the mitral position, especially in elderly patients (see Table 11-17 and Fig. 11-46). The patient in atrial fibrillation presents a separate and definite indication for anticoagulation.

Valve thrombosis. Thrombosis has been reported but is uncommon.

Mechanical failure. Other than those from biologic deterioration, mechanical failures in bioprostheses such as the C-E are rare.

Medtronic-Hancock Glutaraldehyde-Preserved Porcine Xenograft (Standard Model). The original Hancock valve, introduced in 1970, consists of glutaraldehyde-preserved porcine aortic valves mounted on a polypropylene stent with polyester fabric and a molded silicone rubber sewing ring. The Medtronic-Hancock device is available for use in the mitral position worldwide and is FDA approved for use in sizes 25, 27, 29, 31, 33, and 35 mm.

Hemodynamic, thromboembolic, thrombotic, and tissue failure characteristics are similar to those of the Carpentier-Edwards prosthesis. Hemodynamic characteristics of the Hancock valve have been summarized by Khuri and colleagues, who emphasize the variability of the gradients, but noted their similarity to those of the Bjork-Shiley valve.[K16]

Medtronic Intact Glutaraldehyde-Preserved Porcine Xenograft. The Intact valve is a new-generation glutaraldehyde-treated porcine valve in which the fixation pressure is zero; toluidine blue is added in an attempt to inhibit calcium deposition. Although not FDA approved for use in the United States, the Intact valve is provided worldwide in odd-numbered sizes 25 to 35 mm for the mitral position. Because it is a relatively new device, its performance characteristics have been only partially evaluated,[J5,V3] but the information available indicates that its performance is good.[J5]

Carpentier-Edwards Pericardial Valve. This glutaraldehyde-fixed, stent-mounted pericardial valve for the mitral position has only recently become available in the United States, but has been used in Canada and Europe for a decade. It has a similar profile and configuration to the aortic C-E pericardial device (PERIMOUNT). Hemodynamic performance is comparable to other mitral bioprostheses. Ten-year freedom from thromboembolism was 93% ± 3% in the series reported by Poirer and colleagues.[P13] Freedom from structural deterioration at 10 years was 81% ± 7%, although no failures were noted in patients age 70 years or older.

SPECIAL SITUATIONS AND CONTROVERSIES

Alternative Surgical Approaches to Mitral Valve

Right Thoracotomy

Right thoracotomy was employed by Lillehei and colleagues in their first open operations for mitral valve disease and continues to be used by some surgeons.[L5] With this approach the incision is through the left atrium just behind the interatrial groove, as in the median sternotomy approach. The chief disadvantages of right thoracotomy are the limited field provided by the anterolateral interspace approach (with the patient positioned obliquely) and relative inaccessibility of the ascending aorta both for cannulation and for infusion of cardioplegic solution. The arterial cannula may need to be

positioned in the external iliac (or femoral) artery. A particular advantage of this approach may be in reoperations after median sternotomy when CABG was performed and when the patent venous or arterial grafts are at risk for injury during resternotomy. It may also be used in cases of previous sternotomy infection.

Left Thoracotomy

Left thoracotomy has been used in the past, but because venous cannulation is difficult, this approach cannot currently be recommended.

Approach through Superior Left Atrial Wall

Occasionally in large patients with small left atria, exposure is not optimal with the approach described earlier under "Technique of Operation." The "superior approach" through the most superior aspect of the left atrium, where it appears in the transverse sinus, is an attractive alternative (Fig. 11-55).[H24,R12,S7] The superior vena cava is mobilized and retracted laterally, and the aorta is retracted to the left (after clamping it and injecting cardioplegic solution, because retraction may make the aortic valve regurgitant). A transverse incision is made in the roof of the left atrium as far from the aortic root origin as possible (Fig. 11-55, C). The mitral valve is found to be very accessible; often, only stay sutures are required for retraction. Because of this, studying the competence of the valve after commissurotomy or repair is easier. Closure of this incision must be accurate, catching all layers (including the endocardium) with each stitch. Hemostasis should be secure before discontinuing CPB.

The superior approach is also useful when a short, limited upper sternotomy is used.[G20] A single-stage venous cannula is inserted through the right atrial appendage, and distal ascending aortic cannulation is used in combination with antegrade cardioplegia. Exposure is adequate.

Approach across Atrial Septum

Approach through the right atrium and across the atrial septum can be used, but may be unsatisfactory. Exposure is limited, and retraction is impeded by concern about injury to the AV node. Exposure can be improved by extending the incision onto the roof of the right atrium (see Fig. 11-55, B).[A19] A variation of this approach is that of Guiraudon and colleagues (Fig. 11-56).[G21] Incision is begun high on the right atrial free wall and is extended caudally on the interatrial septum. It is completed by extending the septal incision to the superior aspect (roof) of the left atrium. Exposure is excellent, although closure is somewhat tedious. It is useful for patients with deep chests and those with small left atria.

Mitral Valve Replacement with Allograft

Acar and colleagues revitalized interest in mitral valve replacement with a mitral allograft using new techniques for fixation of the papillary muscles (side-by-side, fine monofilament suture) and employing an anuloplasty ring in all cases (Fig. 11-57).[A25] Between 1992 and 1998, 98 cryopreserved allografts were implanted in the mitral position, 66 of which were total mitral valve replacements.

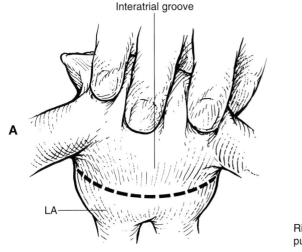

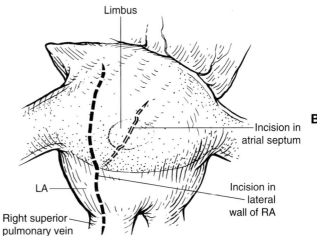

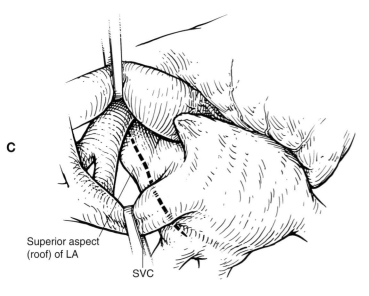

Figure 11-55   Three incisions for exposing mitral valve. **A,** Classic approach involves retracting lateral right atrial wall. Groove between posterior right atrium and left atrium is developed, and inferior aspect of left atrium is freed from pericardium behind inferior cavoatrial junction. Incision extends cephalad behind superior vena cava and caudad to the left under the inferior vena cava. **B,** Modification of DuBost transeptal approach. Vertical incision is made in lateral wall of right atrium. Interatrial septum is incised through the fossa ovalis, extending laterally to patient's right to meet the right atrial incision and continuing to ventral aspect of right superior pulmonary vein. Atrial septal component must not extend inferiorly or medially, which could put the tricuspid anulus, atrioventricular septum, or bundle of His at risk. **C,** "Superior approach" involves retracting superior vena cava laterally and the aorta to the left. Roof of left atrium is opened with the incision directed leftward and posteriorly, leaving an adequate rim of atrial tissue anteriorly so as not to infringe on the mitral anulus.

Key: *LA,* Left atrium; *RA,* right atrium; *SVC,* superior vena cava.

Perioperative mortality was 4.6%. Follow-up at 3 to 75 months showed trace or no mitral regurgitation in 87% of patients. Five valves were explanted (7.5%).

As of July 2002, there have been 168 cryopreserved mitral allografts implanted by 36 surgeons in the United States.[C43] Only 5 surgeons have implanted more than 10 grafts. Results show that this complex procedure is still in the early phase, even though implant techniques have been clearly described (see Fig. 11-57).[D27] Early explant of the valve during the first year after operation is the most important complication and is often caused by technical problems related to implantation. Twenty-two valves have been explanted early for a variety of causes (13%). Doty and colleagues implanted 24 valves in 20 patients; no patient died, and five valves were explanted (20%) during the first year after operation for papillary muscle dehiscence (1 patient), ruptured chordae tendineae (2), prolapse (1), and endocarditis (1).[D27]

When a technically adequate implant can be obtained, allograft valve function is good and appears to be stable.

Patients seem to favor the valve, with four of five patients requesting a second allograft when re-replacement was required. Methods for proper selection of valve size are being evaluated. Acar states that length of the anterior leaflet is the most reliable measurement because of correlation with papillary muscle length.[A26] Anatomic data from Sakai and colleagues, however, suggest that the anulopapillary muscle distance of the mitral valve correlates with mitral anular diameter.[S26] At present, valve size is chosen to match the diameter of the patient's anulus. Choice of type of anuloplasty ring has not been clarified, but a ring that remodels the anular shape seems to be desirable. Anticoagulation beyond the first 2 months after operation is not required. Long-term durability is unknown.

Surgical Plication of Giant Left Atrium

Massive enlargement of the left atrium can develop in patients with long-standing severe mitral regurgitation.[D10,O2,P6] Surgical reduction has been recommended

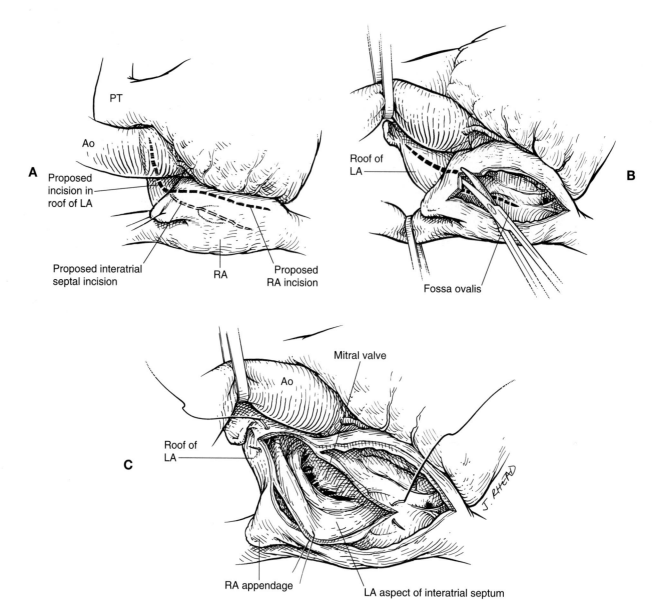

Figure 11-56   Biatrial approach of Guiraudon and colleagues, or "transplant" incision. **A** and **B**, Right atrium is opened transversely near atrioventricular groove. Atrial septum is incised vertically through fossa ovalis, and incision is extended superiorly to meet the right atrial incision. Where these two incisions meet, the incision is directed leftward through roof of left atrium toward left atrial appendage. Walls of atrial septum and left atrium are deflected by stay sutures. Mitral valve exposure is excellent. **C**, Atrial septum and roof of left atrium are closed with separate sutures, meeting superiorly. Right atrial portion is then closed.

Key: *Ao*, Ascending aorta; *LA*, left atrium; *PT*, pulmonary trunk; *RA*, right atrium.

since the early days of cardiac surgery, but has not been generally adopted.[J3] Kawazoe and colleagues have used a special plication procedure designed to reduce bronchial compression and improve LV performance; their experience suggests effective results.[K7] The procedure is probably indicated only when left atrial enlargement is causing severe compression of the left main bronchus.

Left Ventricular Rupture Complicating Mitral Valve Replacement

Massive intrapericardial hemorrhage may occur shortly after discontinuing CPB or in the intensive care unit a few

hours later. This complication is usually from LV rupture in or near the AV groove posteriorly. Nearly all patients die when the rupture occurs postoperatively, but some may be saved when it occurs while the chest is open.[B10] LV rupture with hemorrhage is more likely to occur in women and in patients with small left ventricles.

Several causes of LV rupture exist, but the surgeon must always assume that it is preventable. The most common contributing factors to LV rupture are (1) undue traction on the anulus during excision of the mitral valve or insertion of the prosthesis, (2) tearing of the anulus by sutures already placed when the heart is manually tilted up after the

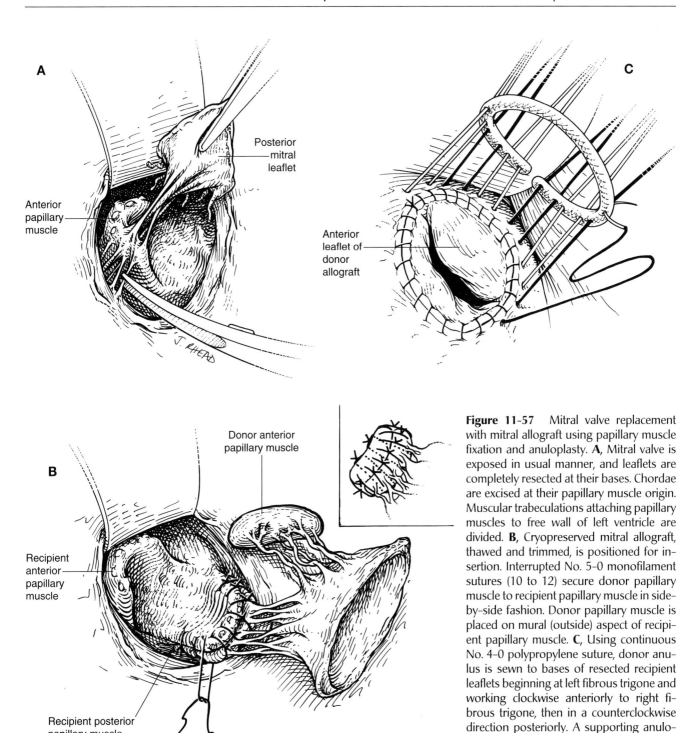

Figure 11-57   Mitral valve replacement with mitral allograft using papillary muscle fixation and anuloplasty. **A,** Mitral valve is exposed in usual manner, and leaflets are completely resected at their bases. Chordae are excised at their papillary muscle origin. Muscular trabeculations attaching papillary muscles to free wall of left ventricle are divided. **B,** Cryopreserved mitral allograft, thawed and trimmed, is positioned for insertion. Interrupted No. 5-0 monofilament sutures (10 to 12) secure donor papillary muscle to recipient papillary muscle in side-by-side fashion. Donor papillary muscle is placed on mural (outside) aspect of recipient papillary muscle. **C,** Using continuous No. 4-0 polypropylene suture, donor anulus is sewn to bases of resected recipient leaflets beginning at left fibrous trigone and working clockwise anteriorly to right fibrous trigone, then in a counterclockwise direction posteriorly. A supporting anuloplasty ring is added, and its anchoring sutures are placed before inserting the continuous leaflet suture.

mitral prosthesis is in place, and (3) penetration of stitches into the left AV groove posteriorly.[B9] These are particularly dangerous problems because the surgeon is usually unaware of producing them during the operation, which may otherwise have been a technically simple procedure. In the initial report on this problem, Roberts and Morrow indicated that LV rupture can also result from (1) perforation of the LV wall as papillary muscle is excised and (2) perforation of the AV groove as a calcific deposit is being removed.[R3]

Because of potential LV rupture, the surgeon must be very gentle in all maneuvers during mitral valve replacement. The heart should *not* be tipped up for air evacuation or ligation of the left atrial appendage or for routine inspection of the back of it after the prosthesis has been inserted. Excising only the chordae tendineae rather than the whole papillary muscle, and simply leaving in place deeply embedded calcific deposits in the anulus and placing sutures around them or only on their atrial side, should eliminate these causes of LV rupture. Alternatively, a chordal sparing mitral valve replacement can be performed.

LV rupture can occur in the midportion of the posterior wall rather than in the region of the AV valve anulus.[K6,R28] Whether the mechanism of this type of rupture is different is not certain, but LV trauma can be caused by penetration of a pillar of a stent-mounted valve.

Once massive hemorrhage has occurred, CPB must be reinitiated as quickly as possible while the hemorrhage is controlled digitally to the extent possible. A premature attempt to suture it will surely end in death, and even with proper management the risk of death is great. After establishing CPB, clamping the aorta, and administering cardioplegic solution, the left atrium is reopened and the valve removed. An appropriately shaped piece of pericardium is fashioned and positioned as an onlay patch on the inside of the heart, over the presumed or identified area of rupture, using multiple, large, felt-pledgeted sutures. Even though every attempt is made to avoid the proximal circumflex artery, it may be compromised by these sutures, so the area of the circumflex artery must be carefully inspected *before reinserting the valve*. If it is compromised, a saphenous vein bypass graft to a large marginal branch should be placed. The valve is then reinserted and the remainder of the procedure completed as usual. Great care must be taken with myocardial management throughout this procedure.

A small or moderate-sized hematoma is present in the left AV groove in 10% to 30% of all patients immediately after mitral valve replacement. If bleeding is not occurring, the patient's condition remains good, and the hematoma does not increase in size, it should be left untreated and uninspected with nothing further done. The hematoma rarely results in LV rupture, but false aneurysms occasionally develop in this area.

Treatment of Valve Thrombosis

Thrombosis of a mechanical mitral prosthesis is uncommon but devastating, usually affecting patients who are inadequately anticoagulated. Thrombosis may be subacute or may present as an urgent event characterized by low cardiac output and pulmonary venous hypertension and occasionally preceded by thromboembolism. Although auscultation and cardiac fluoroscopy were appropriate elements for diagnosis in the past, echocardiography is by far the most reliable diagnostic study.

Therapy remains controversial. Thrombolysis using streptokinase has been used by some groups (see "Thrombosis" under Results in Chapter 14). This approach is perhaps most effective for valves in the tricuspid position, but is also effective in some cases of acute mitral prosthetic thrombosis. Lysis may be incomplete, however, and consequently there can be associated systemic embolism. Hemorrhage, as well as allergic complications resulting from the lytic agents, can also occur. Late rethrombosis has been reported as well.

In general, surgical therapy is preferred for valve thrombosis. In some patients, simple thrombectomy is appropriate. In most patients, however, thrombotic material may be ad-

herent and often extends to the relatively inaccessible ventricular aspect of the prosthesis. Occasionally thrombotic material is indistinguishable from the vegetations of endocarditis. Thus, removal and replacement of the device is preferred. Mortality in these situations is 10% to 20%.[M25]

SECTION 2

Mitral Valve Surgery with Coexisting Tricuspid Valve Disease

MORPHOLOGY

Slightly under half of surgical patients exhibit some evidence of tricuspid regurgitation, which may be *organic* (rheumatic) in origin or, more frequently, *functional*.[C22] The importance of distinguishing between functional and organic tricuspid regurgitation in patients with mitral valve disease was illustrated by Duran and colleagues.[D7] When they ignored functional tricuspid regurgitation present at mitral valve surgery, tricuspid regurgitation was absent late postoperatively in all eight patients with low Rp postoperatively, but was present in all nine patients with high Rp late postoperatively ($P < .0001$). Untreated functional tricuspid regurgitation disappeared in eight (47%; CL 32%-62%) of 17 patients undergoing mitral valve surgery. In contrast, ignored organic tricuspid regurgitation disappeared in none (0%; CL 9%-13%) of 14 patients undergoing mitral valve surgery ($P = .003$). In 10% to 20% of patients undergoing mitral valve replacement, tricuspid anuloplasty is performed, but less than 1% of these patients require tricuspid valve replacement (see Table 11-10).[B31,F5,G4,S10]

CLINICAL FEATURES AND DIAGNOSTIC CRITERIA

Tricuspid regurgitation is apt to coexist when mitral regurgitation is rheumatic in origin and long-standing and when important symptoms have been present for more than about 6 years.[C22] This finding is probably related to low right ventricular EF (less than 30%) found in most patients with long-standing mitral regurgitation.[H18]

NATURAL HISTORY

Patients with functional tricuspid regurgitation secondary to mitral valve disease who do *not* undergo repair of regurgitation at mitral valve surgery have a variable course late postoperatively.[B23] Probably depending in part on the surgeon's indication for not repairing the tricuspid valve at the original mitral valve operation, 6% (CL 4%-9%)[S10] to 35%[S12] (CL 23%-49%) have moderate or severe regurgitation late postoperatively. In most patients, tricuspid regurgitation is a persistent form of the preoperative condition, but a few patients have a newly developed or worsening form of preoperative tricuspid regurgitation despite surgically improved mitral valve function.

Experimental work by Tsakiris and colleagues has shown that perfect tricuspid leaflet closure in systole depends on proper systolic shortening in circumference of the tricuspid anulus.[T1,T5] In support of this finding, Simon and colleagues have demonstrated a considerable increase in systolic shortening postoperatively in patients whose tricuspid regurgitation lessens after mitral valve surgery, and no change in those in whom it persists or worsens.[S12] In addition, an increased diastolic diameter of the tricuspid anulus results in tricuspid regurgitation; diastolic diameter is increased by pulmonary artery hypertension and by right ventricular myocardial failure and increased diastolic volume secondary to left-sided heart pathology.

Incremental risk factors for persisting or worsening tricuspid regurgitation after mitral valve repair or replacement without surgery to the tricuspid valve include the following:

- Persistent or recurrent mitral disease predisposes the patient to continuing or increasing tricuspid regurgitation.
- The more severe the unrepaired tricuspid regurgitation, the more likely it is to persist or increase late after mitral valve surgery. Thus, tricuspid regurgitation judged mild at operation rarely persists or progresses after adequate mitral valve surgery, whereas moderate or severe regurgitation may progress.[B22]
- Long-standing and perhaps irreversible right ventricular enlargement, secondary to mitral or pulmonary vascular disease, predisposes the patient to persistent tricuspid regurgitation. Such situations likely interfere with systolic shortening of the tricuspid anulus. Thus, tricuspid regurgitation that does not disappear promptly with intensive decongestive treatment preoperatively and is therefore fixed, rather than variable, is more likely to persist late postoperatively if not repaired.[C32]
- Organic tricuspid regurgitation, usually associated with some stenosis, is more likely to persist than is functional regurgitation.

TECHNIQUE OF OPERATION

Techniques of concomitant tricuspid valve surgery are discussed in detail under "Technique of Operation" in Chapter 14.

RESULTS

Assessing the results of repair of functional tricuspid regurgitation in patients undergoing mitral valve surgery is difficult because of insufficient information regarding the outcome had the patient's tricuspid regurgitation been left untreated. As a group, patients undergoing mitral valve replacement with concomitant tricuspid anuloplasty at UAB had higher hospital mortality (12%) than those undergoing isolated mitral valve replacement (2.4%), and the difference is unlikely to be due to chance alone ($P < .0001$) (see Table 11-10).[B20,B22,B31,J2,S11] This difference, however, was not as evident in the GLH experience ($P = .3$) (Table 11-20).

Intermediate-term survival is also lower in patients undergoing concomitant mitral valve replacement and tricuspid anuloplasty than in those undergoing isolated mitral valve replacement (see Fig. 11-35). When multivariable analysis accounts for other differences between patients undergoing mitral valve replacement alone and those undergoing concomitant tricuspid valve repair, important tricuspid regurgitation treated by anuloplasty is not a strong risk factor for death early after operation, but it is later after repair (see Table 11-13). These relationships are also reflected in the higher hazard function for death 3 or more months after operation for those undergoing mitral valve replacement plus tricuspid anuloplasty (Fig. 11-58). The inference is that, despite tricuspid valve repair, the right ventricular dysfunction usually associated with important preoperative tricuspid regurgitation persists in some patients and is a risk factor for death after mitral valve surgery. Nonetheless, survival is probably better than if the tricuspid regurgitation had been left untreated, although this has not been proved.

The functional result in patients surviving at least intermediate term after mitral valve replacement plus tricuspid valve repair is good. However, the prevalence of return to an excellent clinical status (NYHA functional class I or II) is less than when only mitral valve replacement is deemed necessary (see Table 11-18). This finding again suggests that, in general, patients requiring concomitant tricuspid anuloplasty have a more advanced cardiac condition than those requiring only mitral valve replacement.

■ TABLE 11-20   **Hospital Mortality after Mitral Valve Replacement and Tricuspid Valve Surgery According to New York Heart Association Functional Class** [a]

NYHA Class	Mitral Stenosis				Mitral Regurgitation + Mixed Lesions				Total			
	n	No.	%	CL (%)	n	No.	%	CL (%)	n	No.	%	CL (%)
I	–	–	–	–	2	0	0	0-61	2	0	0	0-61
II	1	0	0	0-85	5	0	0	0-32	6	0	0	0-27
III	3	0	0	0-47	13	1	8	1-24	16	1	6	0.8-20
IV	3	0	0	0-47	11	1	9	1-28	14	1	7	0.9-22
V	1	0	0	0-85	3	0	0	0-47	4	0	0	0-38
TOTAL	8	0	0	0-21	34	2	6	2-13	42	2	5	2-11

Key: *CL,* 70% confidence limits; *NYHA,* New York Heart Association.

[a] Patients with or without concomitant coronary artery bypass grafting, undergoing primary or redo operation, are included in these data (GLH group, 1976 to 1980). The table excludes one patient without NYHA class.

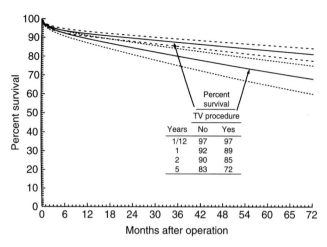

Figure 11-58 Nomogram depicting the effect (or absence) of tricuspid valve repair on risk-adjusted survival after mitral valve replacement, with or without concomitant cardiac procedures, in patients with mitral stenosis. (See Appendix 11B for details.)

INDICATIONS FOR OPERATION

Repair of tricuspid regurgitation often must be considered at operation for mitral valve disease. Decision for or against repair can be difficult. One reason is the uncertainty in estimating the presence and magnitude of tricuspid regurgitation both preoperatively and intraoperatively. Fournier, Carpentier, and Duran and their colleagues have emphasized that digital estimation at operation, with a finger through the right atrial appendage, is unreliable.[C32,D7,F4] However, information of some value can be obtained in this manner if (1) care is taken to ensure a good hemodynamic state when the observation is made, (2) the observer is experienced in detecting the relatively low-velocity and thus difficult-to-feel regurgitant stream of tricuspid regurgitation, and (3) it is recognized that the presence and degree of tricuspid regurgitation vary with time in a given patient. Availability of TEE in the operating room is helpful in this regard.

The patient should be transported to the operating room after a period of careful preoperative evaluation. Tricuspid anuloplasty is generally not indicated when (1) tricuspid regurgitation is variable preoperatively and is absent during periods of good medical control of heart failure, (2) organic tricuspid disease is excluded based on digital or echocardiographic examination of the valve at operation, (3) a good repair or replacement can be done for the mitral disease, and (4) Rp is low. If regurgitation is more severe under these circumstances, anuloplasty is indicated. When tricuspid regurgitation has been important and constant, surgical repair is usually indicated, as emphasized by Carpentier and colleagues.[C32] In these patients the surgeon usually finds tricuspid regurgitation greater than grade 3 by digital examination or by intraoperative TEE. Because the left-sided disease is long-standing and the possibility of irreversible left and right ventricular dysfunction high, a procedure directed at the tricuspid valve may decrease postoperative morbidity and avoid a second operation.

If tricuspid regurgitation has been left unrepaired, if right atrial pressure is the same or higher than left atrial

pressure immediately after CPB, and if tricuspid regurgitation is assessed digitally (or by TEE) as grade 3 or more, tricuspid anuloplasty is indicated, provided that temporary acute right ventricular dysfunction (usually from right coronary air embolization) can be excluded. This exclusion is made by resuming CPB; a vasoconstrictor is then given to ensure normal arterial blood pressure (see Chapter 4), the heart is "unloaded," and CPB is continued for 5 to 10 minutes.

Organic (rheumatic) tricuspid disease virtually always requires intervention, either repair or replacement.

SECTION 3

Mitral Valve Surgery with Coexisting Ischemic Heart Disease

MORPHOLOGY

In recent years, about 15% to 20% of patients undergoing mitral valve replacement for nonischemic mitral valve disease have undergone concomitant coronary artery bypass grafting (CABG).

NATURAL HISTORY

Reliable assessment of the results of isolated mitral valve surgery (without CABG) in patients with coexisting coronary artery disease is not available. Studies by Czer and Chaffin and their colleagues, however, suggest that survival is less satisfactory in these situations when operation is restricted to the mitral valve.[C5,C25]

TECHNIQUE OF OPERATION

Primary considerations in CABG accompanying mitral valve replacement or repair are (1) planning the operation to limit duration of CPB and global myocardial ischemia (aortic clamping) and (2) reducing the need to tilt the heart up *after* the valve is inserted or repaired (see "Left Ventricular Rupture Complicating Mitral Valve Replacement" in Section 1). Two methods can be recommended.

In one method, operation is begun by performing the distal anastomoses of vein grafts and in situ internal thoracic artery (see "Internal Thoracic Artery" under Technique of Operation in Chapter 7). After administering an additional dose of cardioplegia, the left atrium is opened from the right side and the mitral valve procedure performed. The left atrium is closed. After aspiration of air from the tip of the left ventricle (LV) and with strong suction on the aortic needle vent, the aortic clamp is removed and rewarming begun. Venous and arterial grafts are routed as usual, and the venous grafts are anastomosed to the openings in the exteriorized portion of the aorta. After the side-biting clamp is removed, the usual de-airing procedures are performed (see "De-Airing Heart" in Section 3 of Chapter 2). Operation is then completed in the usual manner. Unless urgently indicated the heart should not be tipped up for inspection of the posterior anastomoses, to avoid ventricular rupture. Alternatively, the proximal anastomoses are made with the aortic clamp still in

■ **TABLE 11-21   Hospital Mortality after Mitral Valve Replacement and Coronary Artery Bypass Grafting According to New York Heart Association Functional Class** [a]

NYHA Class	Mitral Stenosis				Mitral Regurgitation + Mixed Lesions				Total			
	n	No.	%	CL (%)	*n*	No.	%	CL (%)	*n*	No.	%	CL (%)
I	0				0				0			
II	2	0	0	0–61	3	1	33	4–76	5	1	20	3–53
III	1	0	0	0–85	13	1	8	1–24	14	1	7	0.9–22
IV	2	0	0	0–61	9	1	11	1–33	11	1	9	1–28
V	–	–	–	–	4	1	25	3–63	4	1	25	3–63
TOTAL	5	0	0	0–32	29	4 [b]	14	7–24	34	4	12	6–20

Key: *CL*, 70% confidence limits; *NYHA*, New York Heart Association.

[a] Patients with or without concomitant tricuspid valve surgery, undergoing primary or redo operation, are included in these data (GLH group, 1976 to 1980). The table excludes three patients without NYHA class.

[b] Two patients died with low cardiac output, one with cerebral air embolism, and one with left ventricular tear.

place. Operation proceeds as in isolated CABG, using the technique of initially hyperkalemic, controlled aortic root reperfusion (see "Cold Cardioplegia, Controlled Aortic Root Reperfusion, and [When Needed] Warm Cardioplegic Induction" in Chapter 3).

In the second method the proximal anastomoses are made directly after initiating CPB. Cardioplegic solution is then administered, and the distal anastomoses are performed as usual. Care is taken to ensure that the vein graft coursing to the right of the right atrium is slightly more redundant than usual to avoid damage from retraction during the mitral procedure. Particular care is taken to ensure the anastomoses are hemostatic, again to avoid the potentially dangerous maneuver of tilting up the heart *after* the mitral valve prosthesis is inserted. After infusing another dose of cardioplegic solution, small bulldog clamps are placed very proximally on each vein graft (they must be removed later, a minute or so after release of the aortic clamp) to prevent air that enters the aortic root during mitral replacement from entering the vein graft. Thereafter, the left atrium is opened and mitral valve repair or replacement carried out as usual. After the left atrium is closed, controlled aortic root reperfusion is begun, and the operation proceeds as in an isolated mitral valve procedure.

In both methods, TEE is useful to assess the adequacy of air removal from the cardiac chambers.

RESULTS

Early (Hospital) Death

Hospital mortality of patients undergoing mitral valve replacement and concomitant CABG is higher (9%) than that of patients undergoing isolated mitral valve replacement, with or without concomitant tricuspid valve anuloplasty (3.5%, $P = .008$) (Table 11-21; see also Table 11-10). Gillinov and colleagues compared survival in 447 patients undergoing mitral valve repair and 232 undergoing mitral valve replacement for degenerative disease, all with concomitant CABG, at the Cleveland Clinic from 1973 to 1999.[G25] Factors associated multivariably with greater likelihood of repair included isolated posterior chordal rupture ($P < .0001$), more recent date of operation ($P < .0001$), and younger age ($P = .0003$). Factors associated with a greater likelihood of replacement were bileaflet prolapse ($P < .0001$), retracted leaflet from abnormal chordal mesh

($P = .01$), and previous cardiac surgery ($P = .008$). Thirty patients died in the hospital (4.4%; CL 3.6%-5.4%), 16 after mitral valve repair (3.6%; CL 2.4%-4.7%) and 14 after mitral valve replacement (6.0%; CL 4.4%-8.1%, $P = .14$). Thirty-day mortality was 3.1% after mitral valve repair and 5.6% after replacement ($P = .12$), and operative mortality (hospital mortality and patients dying within 30 days) was 4.0% and 6.5% ($P = .16$), respectively.

Time-Related Survival

Intermediate-term survival is less satisfactory, and the hazard function for death in the constant phase is greater in patients undergoing mitral valve surgery and concomitant CABG than in those undergoing mitral surgery without concomitant CABG and thus presumably without coexisting ischemic heart disease (see Fig. 11-35). This finding is partly explained by coexistence of two diseases, but also partly by older age at operation of patients with the two existing diseases[3] and the longer global myocardial ischemic time when the two procedures are performed concomitantly. In the study by Gillinov and colleagues, for the mitral repair group, survival was 79% and 59% at 5 and 10 years, and for the mitral replacement group, it was 70% and 37%, respectively (Fig. 11-59, *A*).[G25] The unadjusted survival curves diverged at about 4 years because of earlier divergence (less than 2 years) of the late rising phase of hazard (Fig. 11-59, *B*), with patients undergoing mitral valve replacement having a marked increase in mortality risk compared with those undergoing repair.

Incremental Risk Factors for Death

Because patient characteristics differed between those undergoing mitral repair versus replacement, a propensity score was used to adjust the multivariable risk factor analysis for these differences (see "Clinical Studies with Nonrandomly Assigned Treatment" in Section 1 of Chapter 6). After using the propensity score to adjust for dissimilarities in patient characteristics between those undergoing mitral valve repair versus replacement in addition to other

---

[3] At UAB, age of patients undergoing isolated mitral valve replacement was 52 ± 13.7 [SD] years versus 61 ± 8.2 years in those with both diseases, $P < .0001$.

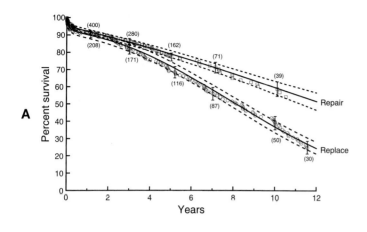

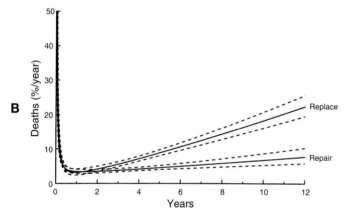

Figure 11-59   Time-related survival after coronary artery bypass grafting (CABG) and either mitral valve repair or replacement. **A,** Each symbol represents a death according to the Kaplan–Meier estimator. Vertical bars enclose asymmetric 68% confidence limits. Solid lines represent parametric survival estimates enclosed between dashed 68% confidence limits. Numbers in parentheses are numbers of patients traced beyond that point. **B,** Hazard functions (instantaneous risk) for death after CABG and mitral valve repair or replacement. (From Gillinov and colleagues.[G25])

variables for risk adjustment, replacement was identified as a risk factor for death in the late hazard phase, beginning about 2 years after surgery (Table 11-22). During the early hazard phase (surgery to 6 months), survival was similar after repair and replacement; in the constant hazard phase (6 months to 3.5 years), there was possibly improved survival in repair patients, but this varied with age.

Functional Status

Prevalence of good functional status (NYHA functional class I or II) among patients surviving at least the intermediate term after mitral valve replacement and concomitant CABG is as high as after isolated mitral valve replacement (see Table 11-18).[K9] This finding is probably related to coexisting coronary artery disease in this group of patients generally being moderate and well treated by CABG.

■ **TABLE 11-22   Incremental Risk Factors for Death after Mitral Valve Repair or Replacement for Degenerative Disease, with Concomitant Coronary Artery Bypass Grafting**

Risk Factor	Coefficient ± SE	P
Early Hazard Phase		
Mitral valve replacement	−0.005 ± 0.45	.9
Propensity adjustment [a]	−0.59 ± 0.70	.4
Older age [b]	1.03 ± 0.25	<.0001
Elongated chordae	1.00 ± 0.37	.007
Bilirubin	0.43 ± 0.17	.01
LITA graft	−1.12 ± 0.57	.05
Constant Hazard Phase		
Mitral valve replacement [c]	3.8 ± 2.5	.13
Propensity adjustment	−0.29 ± 1.01	.8
Older age [b]	0.49 ± 0.26	.06
Younger age in replacement patients [d]	−1.43 ± 0.65	.03
Higher NYHA functional class	0.69 ± 0.25	.006
Moderate or severe LV dysfunction	1.03 ± 0.33	.002
Preoperative atrial fibrillation	0.76 ± 0.33	.02
Preoperative BUN level	0.048 ± 0.011	<.0001
Late Hazard Phase		
Mitral valve replacement	1.24 ± 0.51	.01
Propensity adjustment	−0.71 ± 0.48	.13
Older age [b]	0.89 ± 0.19	<.0001
Diabetes	0.88 ± 0.30	.003
Smoking history	0.88 ± 0.24	.0002

(From Gillinov and colleagues.[G25])

Key: *BUN,* Blood urea nitrogen; *LITA,* left internal thoracic artery; *LV,* left ventricular; *NYHA,* New York Heart Association.

[a] Probability of receiving mitral valve repair.

[b] exp (age/50) exponential transformation.

[c] Represents increment to intercept for patients undergoing mitral valve repair.

[d] Interaction term.

INDICATIONS FOR OPERATION AND SELECTION OF TECHNIQUE

Chapter 10 discusses the special topic of ischemic mitral regurgitation.

Proper surgical procedure for patients with coronary artery disease who require mitral surgery for nonischemic mitral valve disease has been debated in the past. However, several studies have shown that ignoring coronary artery disease increases the risk of death.[C5,S8] In view of this finding and good results achieved in treating both diseases, important coronary artery disease should be treated surgically at the time of mitral repair or replacement.

Selection of Technique

Whether a patient should undergo repair or replacement of the mitral valve depends on the feasibility of repair and possible survival benefit if repair is done. The probability of valve calcification, for example, increases beyond about age 60 (Fig. 11-60). The probability of a survival benefit with repair rather than replacement is generally high (89%, Fig. 11-61); however, who benefits (and how much) and who does not is complicated. Therefore, Gillinov and colleagues devised an algorithm from which the 10-year survival difference can be calculated (Appendix 11C). To

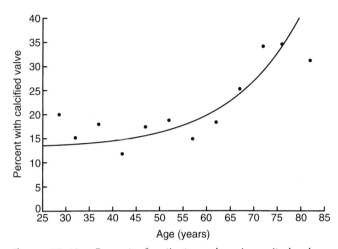

Figure 11-60   Percent of patients undergoing mitral valve repair or replacement for degenerative disease have either leaflet calcification or a calcified anulus (based on 1136 patients undergoing mitral valve repair or replacement for degenerative disease at the Cleveland Clinic).

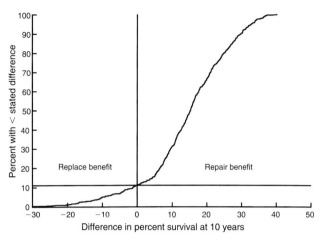

Figure 11-61   Cumulative distribution of differences in 10-year survival between mitral valve repair and replacement with concomitant coronary artery bypass grafting. Patients to the right of 0 difference are predicted to benefit from repair and those to the left from replacement. (From Gillinov and colleagues.[G25])

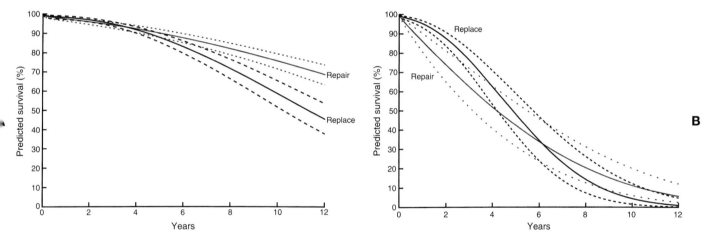

B

Figure 11-62   Nomograms representing solutions of the multivariable survival equation in Table 11-22 for specific patient characteristics in patients being considered for repair or replacement of the mitral valve for degenerative disease and concomitant coronary artery bypass grafting. The equation has been solved twice, once for mitral valve repair and again for replacement. Solid lines represent point estimates and dashed lines enclose 68% confidence limits. **A,** Predicted survival for a patient 70 years old, New York Heart Association (NYHA) class II, normal left ventricular function, chordal elongation = no, atrial fibrillation = no, diabetes = no, never smoked, blood urea nitrogen = 21 mg · dL^{-1}, left internal thoracic artery employed in bypass grafting. **B,** Predicted survival for a patient similar to the patient in A, except he is in NYHA class IV, has severe left ventricular dysfunction and diabetes, and is a smoker. (From Gillinov and colleagues.[G25])

illustrate, Fig. 11-62, *A,* shows predicted time-related survival for a 70-year-old patient coming to operation in NYHA class II with no other cardiac or noncardiac risk factors. Such a profile is typical of patients referred in the current era. Predicted survival after mitral valve repair and replacement with concomitant CABG diverges at about 4

years, with better survival after repair. In contrast, Fig. 11-62, *B,* shows predicted survival for a 70-year-old diabetic in NYHA class IV with severe LV dysfunction from previous myocardial infarcts. Survival is limited after mitral valve operation and concomitant CABG, with no advantage of either strategy for managing the mitral valve.

APPENDIX 11A

Parametric Time-Related Depictions, Including Multivariable Analysis, of Death after Mitral Valve Replacement[4]

Patients are depicted in Table 11-10, the multivariable equation is summarized in Table 11-13, and survivorship is displayed in Fig. 11-34. Follow-up data and other patient characteristics are described by Ferrazzi and colleagues.[F5] Parameter estimates for primary mitral valve replacement for the early hazard phase were $\mu_1 = 0.1420$, $\delta = 0$, $\rho = 2.928$, $v = 0$, $m = -2.150$, and for the constant hazard phase, $\mu_2 = 0.004276$.

Multivariable Analysis

Variables entered into the analysis included *demographic and socioeconomic* considerations, including age (years) at valve replacement; gender; African-American; patient at Birmingham Veterans Administration Hospital; *clinical state*, including New York Heart Association (NYHA) functional class I to V (class V is a patient with cardiogenic shock or hemodynamic instability); previous mitral valve repair; *concomitant ischemic heart disease,* including previous coronary artery bypass grafting (CABG); left ventricular (LV) aneurysmectomy; *ischemic mitral regurgitation; concomitant CABG with mitral valve replacement; mitral valve morphology and function,* including rheumatic pathology, degenerative pathology, ruptured chordae, ischemic mitral pathology (as noted above), native valve endocarditis, anular calcification, valve calcification, mitral regurgitation with no or mild stenosis, mitral stenosis with no or mild regurgitation, more than mild regurgitation, more than mild stenosis, mixed stenosis and regurgitation, and nonischemic regurgitation; *surgically assessed morphology,* including LV enlargement (grades 0 to 6) and left atrial enlargement (grades 0 to 6); and *surgical variables,* including date of operation, global myocardial ischemic time (minutes) when cardioplegia used, use of a mechanical or biologic prosthesis, number of distal CABG anastomoses, tricuspid anuloplasty, and tricuspid replacement.

The variables retained (see Table 11-13), their coefficients ±1 SD and *P* values, and shaping parameters for the *early hazard phase* were $\delta = 0$, $\rho = 3.508$, $v = 0$, $m = -2.108$, intercept $= -8.470$, age (years) at operation $= 0.02371 \pm 0.0101$ ($P = .02$), NYHA functional class (I to V) $= 1.172 \pm 0.1660$ ($P < .0001$), LV enlargement (grades 0 to 6) $= 0.2305 \pm 0.078$ ($P = .003$), LV resection $= 1.189 \pm 0.36$ ($P = .0009$), global myocardial ischemic time (using cardioplegia) $= 0.01242 \pm 0.0036$ ($P = .0006$). For the *constant hazard phase,* variables were intercept $= -7.739$, age (years) at operation $= 0.028922 \pm 0.0088$ ($P = .001$), African-American $= 0.8473$, previous CABG $= 1.727 \pm 0.48$ ($P = .0003$), ischemic mitral regurgitation $= 1.244 \pm 0.36$ ($P = .0005$), nonischemic mitral regurgitation $= 0.4776 \pm 0.28$ ($P = .09$), and tricuspid valve repair or replacement $= 0.7525 \pm 0.28$ ($P = .008$).

For the nomogram (see Fig. 11-37) portraying the effect of age on survival after mitral valve replacement for patients with mitral stenosis, with or without concomitant CABG, the mitral valve equation (see Table 11-13) was solved for African-American "no," NYHA class III, nonischemic and ischemic mitral valve regurgitation "no," tricuspid valve repair "no," LV enlargement absent, previous CABG "no," concomitant LV resection "no," and global myocardial ischemic time "42 minutes."

For the digital nomogram (see Table 11-14) portraying the effect of etiology of mitral regurgitation and preoperative NYHA functional class, the mitral valve equation (see Table 11-13) was solved for age at operation of 50 years, African-American "no," LV enlargement grade 3, important tricuspid valve disease "no," previous CABG "no," concomitant LV resection "no," and global myocardial ischemic time "42 minutes."

For the nomogram (see Fig. 11-38) portraying the relationship between global myocardial ischemic time during mitral valve replacement with or without concomitant procedures in patients with mitral stenosis, the mitral valve equation (see Table 11-13) was solved for age 57 years, African-American "no," NYHA class III, nonischemic and ischemic mitral regurgitation "no," LV enlargement "no," previous CABG "no," concomitant LV resection "no," and tricuspid valve repair "no."

For the nomogram (see Fig. 11-58) portraying the effect on survival of a tricuspid valve procedure (repair), the multivariable equation (see Table 11-13) was solved for age 57 years, African-American "no," NYHA class III, nonischemic and ischemic mitral regurgitation "no," LV enlargement "no," previous CABG "no," concomitant LV resection "no," and global myocardial ischemic time "42 minutes."

APPENDIX 11B

Parametric Coefficients and *P* Values for Three Separate Time-Related Depictions

Survival after isolated mitral valve replacement (MVR), after replacement plus tricuspid valve repair, and after replacement plus coronary artery bypass grafting (CABG)[5] is depicted in Fig. 11-35. Parameter estimates for isolated MVR for the early hazard phase were $\mu_1 = 0.09704$, $\delta = 0$, $\rho = 6.011$, $v = 0$, and $m = -1.875$, and for the constant hazard phase, $\mu_2 = 0.002653$. For MVR + CABG for the early hazard phase, estimates were $\mu_1 = 0.1645$, $\delta = 0$, $\rho = 1.921$, $v = 0$, and $m = -1.875$, and for the constant hazard phase, $\mu_2 = 0.005407$. For MVR + TVA for the early hazard phase, estimates were $\mu_1 = 0.1548$, $\delta = 0$, $\rho = 1.261$, $v = 0$, and $m = -2.093$, and for the constant hazard phase, $\mu_2 = 0.008277$.

APPENDIX 11C

Algorithm to Choose Mitral Valve Technique in Degenerative Mitral Valve Disease with Ischemic Heart Disease

Analysis of 10-year survival difference for mitral valve repair vs. replacement yields an algorithm that aids in deciding which strategy to pursue.[G25] Estimating the 10-year survival difference is a 4-step process. First, select one value for each of the three continuous variables from the columns below. Enter these values into the table on the following page.

---

[4] Data are from UAB group, 1975 to July 1983; $n = 819$; deaths = 222.

[5] Data are from UAB group, 1975 to July 1983.

Age	Value	BUN	Value	Bilirubin	Value
35	2.2	10	16.6	0.3	−0.43
40	2.9	12	16.1	0.4	−0.57
45	3.7	14	15.2	0.5	−0.71
50	4.5	16	14.2	0.6	−0.85
55	5.5	18	13.0	0.7	−0.99
60	6.5	20	11.9	0.8	−1.14
65	7.7	22	10.7	0.9	−1.28
70	8.9	24	9.6	1.0	−1.42
75	10.2	26	8.5	1.1	−1.56
80	11.6	28	7.5	1.2	−1.71
85	13.1	30	6.5	1.4	−1.99
		35	4.1	1.8	−2.55
		40	1.9	2.2	−3.12

Second, choose a value for each factor listed below. If the factor is not present, choose 0; otherwise, write in the value.

Variable	Value	Value Chosen
Age	See above	———
BUN	See above	———
Bilirubin	See above	———
NYHA class		
II	−3.7	———
III	−9.6	———
IV	−18.3	———
LV dysfunction [a]	−11.9	———
Atrial fibrillation	−8.5	———
Chordal rupture [b]	−1.2	———
Ever smoked	11.7	———
Diabetes [c]	9.7	———
Ventricular arrhythmias	1.7	———
TOTAL		———

[a] Grade 3 (moderately severe) or 4 (severe) left ventricular dysfunction.

[b] Only those of the posterior leaflet.

[c] Pharmacologically treated (real hypoglycemic agents or insulin).

Key: *BUN*, Blood urea nitrogen; *LV*, left ventricular; *NYHA*, New York Heart Association.

Third, sum all the numbers in the column marked "Value Chosen."

Fourth, interpret the total. The total is the estimated 10-year survival difference in percent. If the sum is positive, repair is favored; if negative, replacement is recommended. Approximate error of the survival difference is 5.5%.

Example: A 70-year-old (8.9) patient in sinus rhythm (0 for atrial fibrillation) without ventricular ectopy (0), with only posterior chordal rupture and leaflet prolapse (−1.2), in NYHA class III (−9.6) with 3-system coronary artery disease and well preserved left ventricular function (0), who has never smoked (0), has no history of diabetes (0), BUN of 18 (13.0), and bilirubin of 0.8 (−1.14). The total score is 9.96 ± 5.5, meaning mitral valve repair is recommended.

REFERENCES

A

1. Appelbaum A, Kouchoukos NT, Blackstone EH, Kirklin JW. Early risks of open heart surgery for mitral valve disease. Am J Cardiol 1976;37:201.

2. Ahmad R, Manohitharajah SM, Deverall PB, Watson DA. Chronic hemolysis following mitral valve replacement. A comparative study of the Bjork-Shiley, composite-seat Starr-Edwards, and frame-mounted aortic homograft valves. J Thorac Cardiovasc Surg 1976;71:212.

3. Akins CW, Kirklin JK, Block PC, Buckley MJ, Austen WG. Preoperative evaluation of subvalvular fibrosis in mitral stenosis: a predictive factor in conservative versus replacement surgical therapy. Circulation 1979;60:I71.

4. Angelino PF, Levi V, Brusca A, Actis-Dato A. Mitral commissurotomy in younger age group. Am Heart J 1956;51:916.

5. al-Bahrani IR, Thamer MA, al-Omeri MM, al-Naaman YD. Rheumatic heart disease in the young in Iraq. Br Heart J 1966;28:824.

6. Austen WG, Wooler GH. Surgical treatment of mitral stenosis by the transventricular approach with a mechanical dilator. N Engl J Med 1960;263:661.

7. Adebo OA, Ross JK. Conservative surgery for mitral valve disease: clinical and echocardiographic analysis of results. Thorax 1983; 38:565.

8. Antunes MJ, Santos LP. Performance of glutaraldehyde-preserved porcine bioprosthesis as a mitral valve substitute in a young population group. Ann Thorac Surg 1984;37:387.

9. Antunes MJ. Bioprosthetic valve replacement in children: long-term follow-up of 135 isolated mitral valve implantations. Eur Heart J 1984;5:913.

10. Antunes MJ, Magalhaes MP, Colsen PR, Kinsley RH. Valvuloplasty for rheumatic mitral valve disease: a surgical challenge. J Thorac Cardiovasc Surg 1987;94:44.

11. Antunes MJ. Submitral left ventricular aneurysms: correction by a new transatrial approach. J Thorac Cardiovasc Surg 1987;94:241.

12. Abrahams DG, Barton CJ, Cockshott WP, Edington GM, Weaver EJ. Annular subvalvular left ventricular aneurysm. Q J Med 1962;31:345.

13. Aron KV, Nicoloff DM, Kersten TE, Lindsay WG, Northrup WF 3rd. St. Jude Medical prosthesis: valve-related deaths and complications. Ann Thorac Surg 1987;43:591.

14. Antunes MJ, Wessels A, Sadowski RG, Schutz JG, Vanderdonck KM, Oliveira JM, et al. Medtronic-Hall valve replacement in a third-world population group. A review of the performance of 1000 prostheses. J Thorac Cardiovasc Surg 1988;95:980.

15. Aris A, Crexells C, Auge JM, Oriol A, Caralps JM. Hemodynamic evaluation of the integral Monostrut Bjork-Shiley prosthesis in the aortic position. Ann Thorac Surg 1985;40:234.

16. Abascal VM, Wilkins GT, Choong CY, Block PC, Palacios IF, Weyman AE. Mitral regurgitation after percutaneous balloon mitral valvuloplasty in adults: evaluation by pulsed Doppler echocardiography. J Am Coll Cardiol 1988;11:257.

17. Arom KV, Nicoloff DM, Kersten TE, Northrup WF 3rd, Lindsay WG, Emergy RW. Ten years' experience with the St. Jude Medical valve prosthesis. Ann Thorac Surg 1989;47:831.

18. Aris A, Padro JM, Camara ML, Crexells C, Auge JM, Caralps JM. Clinical and hemodynamic results of cardiac valve replacement with the Monostrut Bjork-Shiley prosthesis. J Thorac Cardiovasc Surg 1988;95:423.

19. Alfieri O, Sandrelli L, Pardini A, Fucci C, Zogno M, Ferrari M, et al. Optimal exposure of the mitral valve through an extended vertical transeptal approach. Eur J Cardiothorac Surg 1991;5:294.

20. Acar C, Gaer J, Chauvaud S, Carpentier A. Technique of homograft replacement of the mitral valve. J Heart Valve Dis 1995;4:31.

21. Akins CW, Hilgenberg AD, Buckley MJ, Vlahakes GJ, Torchiana DF, Daggett WM, et al. Mitral valve reconstruction versus replacement for degenerative or ischemic mitral regurgitation. Ann Thorac Surg 1994;58:668.

22. Alvarez JM, Deal CW, Lovebridge K, Brennan P, Eisenberg R, Ward M, et al. Repairing the degenerative mitral valve: ten- to fifteen-year follow-up. J Thorac Cardiovasc Surg 1996;112:238.

23. Aagaard J, Hansen CN, Tingleff J, Rygg I. Seven-and-a-half years clinical experience with the CarboMedics prosthetic heart valve. J Heart Valve Dis 1995;4:628.

24. Akins CW. Results with mechanical cardiac valvular prostheses. Ann Thorac Surg 1995;60:1836.

25. Acar C, Tolan M, Berrebi A, Caer J, Gouzeo R, Marchix T, et al. Homograft replacement of the mitral valve. Graft selection, technique of implantation, and results in forty-three patients. J Thorac Cardiovasc Surg 1996;111:367.

26. Acar C. The mitral homograft: an alternative to valve repair for the next millennium? Valvular Heart Disease Symposium, Mayo Clinic, 1999.

27. Alfieri O, Maisano F. An effective technique to correct anterior mitral leaflet prolapse. J Card Surg 1999;14:468.

B

1. Brunton L, Edin MD. Preliminary note on the possibility of treating mitral stenosis by surgical methods. Lancet 1902;1:352.

2. Bailey CP. The surgical treatment of mitral stenosis (mitral commissurotomy). Dis Chest 1949;15:377.

3. Bland EF, Jones TD. Rheumatic fever and rheumatic heart disease: a twenty-year report on 1000 patients followed since childhood. Circulation 1951;4:836.

4. Buchbinder NA, Roberts WC. Left-sided valvular active infective endocarditis. A study of forty-five necropsy patients. Am J Med 1972;53:20.

5. Barlow JB, Pocock WA, Marchand P, Denny M. The significance of late systolic murmurs. Am Heart J 1963;66:443.

6. Braunwald E. Heart disease: a textbook of cardiovascular medicine. 3rd Ed. Philadelphia: WB Saunders, 1980, p. 1045.

7. Barnhorst DA, Oxman HA, Connolly DC, Pluth JR, Danielson GK, Wallace RB, et al. Long-term follow-up of isolated replacement of the aortic or mitral valve with the Starr-Edwards prosthesis. Am J Cardiol 1975;35:228.

8. Bjork VO, Book K, Holmgren A. The Bjork-Shiley mitral valve prosthesis. A comparative study with different prosthesis orientations. Ann Thorac Surg 1974;18:379.

9. Bjork VO. Left ventricular rupture after mitral valve replacement (editorial). Ann Thorac Surg 1981;31:101.

10. Bjork VO, Henze A, Rodriguez L. Left ventricular rupture as a complication of mitral valve replacement. J Thorac Cardiovasc Surg 1977;73:14.

11. Book K, Holmgren A, Szamosi A. The left atrial V-wave after mitral valve replacement. Scand J Thorac Cardiovasc Surg 1975;9:9.

12. Boucher CA, Bingham JB, Osbakken MD, Okada RD, Strauss HW, Block PC, et al. Early changes in left ventricular size and function after correction of left ventricular volume overload. Am J Cardiol 1981;47:991.

13. Braunwald E. Mitral regurgitation: physiologic, clinical and surgical considerations. N Engl J Med 1969;281:425.

14. Boudoulas H, Reynolds JC, Mazzaferri E, Wooley CF. Metabolic studies in mitral valve prolapse syndrome: a neuroendocrine-cardiovascular process. Circulation 1980;61:1200.

15. Barlow JB, Pocock WA. The problem of nonejection clicks and associated mitral systolic murmurs: emphasis on the billowing mitral leaflet syndrome. Am Heart J 1975;90:636.

16. Braunwald E, Braunwald NS, Ross J Jr, Morrow AG. Effects of mitral valve replacement on the pulmonary vascular dynamics of patients with pulmonary hypertension. N Engl J Med 1965;273:509.

17. Barnhorst DA, Oxman HA, Connolly DC, Pluth JR, Danielson GK, Wallace RB, et al. Isolated replacement of the mitral valve with the Starr-Edwards prosthesis. J Thorac Cardiovasc Surg 1976;71:230.

18. Bernal-Ramirez JB, Phillips JH. Echocardiographic study of malfunction of the Bjork-Shiley prosthetic heart valve in the mitral position. Am J Cardiol 1977;40:449.

19. Borkon AM, McIntosh CL, Von Rueden TJ, Morrow AG. Mitral valve replacement with the Hancock bioprosthesis: five- to ten-year follow-up. Ann Thorac Surg 1981;32:127.

20. Baxter RH, Bain WH, Rankin RJ, Turner MA, Escarous AE, Thomson RM, et al. Tricuspid valve replacement: a five-year appraisal. Thorax 1975;30:158.

21. Babic UU, Pejcic P, Djurisic Z, Grujicic SM. Percutaneous transarterial balloon valvuloplasty for mitral valve stenosis. Am J Cardiol 1986;57:1101.

22. Breyer RH, McClenathan JH, Michaelis LL, McIntosh CL, Morrow AG. Tricuspid regurgitation. A comparison of nonoperative management, tricuspid annuloplasty, and tricuspid valve replacement. J Thorac Cardiovasc Surg 1976;72:867.

23. Braunwald NS, Ross J, Morrow AG. Conservative management of tricuspid regurgitation in patients undergoing mitral valve replacement. Circulation 1967;35:I63.

24. Bolen JL, Lopes MG, Harrison DC, Alderman EL. Analysis of left ventricular function in response to afterload changes in patients with mitral stenosis. Circulation 1975;52:894.

25. Borman JB, Stern S, Shapira T, Milvidsky H, Braun K. Mitral valvotomy in children. Am Heart J 1961;61:763.

26. Bailey GW, Braniff BA, Hancock EW, Cohn KE. Relation of left atrial pathology to atrial fibrillation in mitral valvular disease. Ann Intern Med 1968;69:13.

27. Bonchek LI, Olinger GN, Siegel R, Tresch DD, Keelan MH Jr. Left ventricular performance after mitral reconstruction for mitral regurgitation. J Thorac Cardiovasc Surg 1987;88:122.

28. Baker C, Brock RC, Campbell M. Valvulotomy for mitral stenosis: report of six successful cases. Br Med J 1950;1:1283.

29. Bailey CP, Bolton HE, Redondo-Ramirez HP. Surgery of the mitral valve. Surg Clin North Am 1952;32:1807.

30. Broom ND, Thomson FJ. Influence of fixation conditions on the performance of glutaraldehyde-treated porcine aortic valves: towards a more scientific basis. Thorax 1979;34:166.

31. Boyd AD, Engelman RM, Isom OW, Reed GE, Spencer FC. Tricuspid annuloplasty. Five and one-half years' experience with 78 patients. J Thorac Cardiovasc Surg 1974;68:344.

32. Barratt-Boyes BG. Surgical correction of mitral incompetence resulting from bacterial endocarditis. Br Heart J 1963;25:415.

33. Block PC, Palacios IF. Pulmonary vascular dynamics after percutaneous mitral valvotomy. J Thorac Cardiovasc Surg 1988;96:39.

34. Byram MT, Roberts WC. Frequency and extent of calcific deposits in purely regurgitant mitral valves: analysis of 108 operatively excised valves. Am J Cardiol 1983;52:1059.

35. Blackstone EH, Kirklin JW. Death and other time-related events after valve replacement. Circulation 1985;72:753.

36. Bove AA, Lazarow N, Kontos GJ, Owen RM, Mock MB. Temporal nonuniformity of left ventricular contraction in chronic mitral regurgitation (abstract). J Am Coll Cardiol 1985;5:486.

37. Barner HB. Combined superior and right lateral left atriotomy with division of the superior vena cava for exposure of the mitral valve. Ann Thorac Surg 1985;40:365.

38. Breyer RH, Mills SA, Hudspeth AS, Johnston FR, Watts LE, Nomeir AM, et al. Open mitral commissurotomy: long-term results with echocardiographic correlation. J Cardiovasc Surg 1985;26:46.

39. Borow KM, Green LH, Mann T, Sloss LJ, Braunwald E, Collins JJ, et al. End-systolic volume as a predictor of postoperative left ventricular performance in volume overload from valvular regurgitation. Am J Med 1980;68:655.

40. Braunwald E. Heart disease, 3rd Ed. Philadelphia: WB Saunders, 1988, p. 358.

41. Baudet EM, Oca CC, Roques XF, Laborde MN, Hafez AS, Collot MA, et al. A 5½ year experience with the St. Jude Medical cardiac valve prosthesis. Early and late results of 737 valve replacements in 671 patients. J Thorac Cardiovasc Surg 1985;90:137.

42. Butchart EG, Lewis PA, Kulatilake EN, Breckenridge IM. Anticoagulation variability between centres: implications for comparative prosthetic valve assessment. Eur J Cardiothorac Surg 1988;2:72.

43. Beaudet RL, Poirier NL, Doyle D, Nakhle G, Gauvin C. The Medtronic-Hall cardiac valve: 7½ years' clinical experience. Ann Thorac Surg 1986;42:644.

44. Bjork VO, Lindblom D. The Monostrut Bjork-Shiley heart valve. J Am Coll Cardiol 1985;6:1142.

45. Bonow RO, Carabello B, de Leon AC, Edmunds LH Jr, Fedderly BJ, Freed MD, et al. Practice guidelines for the management of patients with valvular heart disease: executive summary: a report of the American College of Cardiology/American Heart Association Task Force on Practice Guidelines (Committee on Management of Patients with Valvular Heart Disease). Circulation 1998;98:1949.

46. Baudet EM, Puel V, McBride JT, Grimaud JP, Roques F, Clerc F, et al. Long-term results of valve replacement with the St. Jude Medical prosthesis. J Thorac Cardiovasc Surg 1995;109:858.

47. Bjørnerheim R, Ihlen H, Simonsen S, Sire S, Svennevig J. Hemodynamic characterization of the CarboMedics mitral valve prosthesis. J Heart Valve Disease 1997;6:115.

48. Ben Farhat MB, Ayari F, Maatouk F, Betbout F, Gamra H, Jarrar M, et al. Percutaneous balloon versus surgical closed and open mitral commissurotomy: seven-year follow-up results of a randomized trial. Circulation 1998;97:245.

C

1. Cutler EC, Levine SA. Cardiotomy and valvulotomy for mitral stenosis: experimental observations and clinical notes concerning an operated case with recovery. Boston Med Surg J 1923;188:1023.

2. Cohen MV, Gorlin R. Modified orifice equation for the calculation of mitral valve area. Am Heart J 1972;84:839.

3. Criley JM, Lewis KB, Humphries JO, Ross PS. Prolapse of the mitral valve: clinical and cineangiographic findings. Br Heart J 1966;28:488.

4. Carpentier A, Relland J, Deloche A, Fabiani JN, D'Allaines C, Blondeau P, et al. Conservative management of the prolapsed mitral valve. Ann Thorac Surg 1978;26:294.

5. Chaffin JS, Daggett WM. Mitral valve replacement: a nine-year follow-up of risks and survivals. Ann Thorac Surg 1979;27:312.

6. Cohn LH, Sanders JH, Collins JJ Jr. Actuarial comparison of Hancock porcine and prosthetic disc valves for isolated mitral valve replacement. Circulation 1976;54:III60.

7. Copans H, Lakier JB, Kinsley RH, Colsen PR, Fritz VU, Barlow JB. Thrombosed Bjork-Shiley mitral prostheses. Circulation 1980;61:169.

8. Cherian G, Vytilingam KL, Sukumar JP, Gopinath N. Mitral valvotomy in young patients. Br Heart J 1964;26:157.

9. Carpentier A, Chauvaud S, Fabiani JN, Deloche A, Relland J, Lessana A, et al. Reconstructive surgery of mitral valve incompetence: ten-year appraisal. J Thorac Cardiovasc Surg 1980;79:338.

10. Cosgrove DM, Chavez AM, Lytle BW, Gill CC, Stewart RW, Taylor PC, et al. Results of mitral valve reconstruction. Circulation 1986;74:I82.

11. Curry GC, Elliott LP, Ramsey HW. Quantitative left ventricular angio-cardiographic findings in mitral stenosis. Detailed analysis of the anterolateral wall of the left ventricle. Am J Cardiol 1972;29:621.

12. Channick BJ, Adlin EV, Marks AD, Denenberg BS, McDonough MT, Chakko CS, et al. Hyperthyroidism and mitral valve prolapse. N Engl J Med 1981;305:497.

13. Carpentier A, Dubost C, Lane E, Nashef A, Carpentier S, Relland J, et al. Continuing improvements in valvular bioprostheses. J Thorac Cardiovasc Surg 1982;83:27.

14. Commerford PJ, Hastie T, Beck W. Closed mitral valvotomy: actuarial analysis of results in 654 patients over 12 years and analysis of preoperative predictors of long-term survival. Ann Thorac Surg 1982;33:473.

15. Chaux A, Gray RJ, Matloff JM, Feldman H, Sustaita H. An appreciation of the new St. Jude valvular prosthesis. J Thorac Cardiovasc Surg 1981;81:202.

16. Chaitman BR, Bonan R, Lepage G, Tubau JF, David PR, Dyrdra I, et al. Hemodynamic evaluation of the Carpentier-Edwards porcine xenograft. Circulation 1979;60:1170.

17. Chaux A, Czer LS, Matloff JM, DeRobertis MA, Stewart ME, Bateman TM, et al. The St. Jude Medical bileaflet valve prosthesis. A 5-year experience. J Thorac Cardiovasc Surg 1984;88:706.

18. Chesebro JH, Fuster V, Fisher LD, Danielson GK, Pluth JR, Orszulak TA, et al. Thromboembolism after biologic prosthetic heart valve replacement. J Am Coll Cardiol 1985;5:459.

19. Chesler E, Joffe N, Schamroth L, Meyers A. Annular subvalvular left ventricular aneurysms in the South African Bantu. Circulation 1965;32:43.

20. Cammack PL, Edie RN, Edmunds LH Jr. Bar calcification of the mitral anulus. J Thorac Cardiovasc Surg 1987;94,399.

21. Cobanoglu A, Grunkenmeier GL, Aru GM, McKinley CL, Starr A. Mitral replacement: clinical experience with a ball-valve prosthesis. Ann Surg 1985;202:376.

22. Cohen SR, Sell JE, McIntosh CL, Clark RE. Tricuspid regurgitation in patients with acquired, chronic, pure mitral regurgitation. I. Prevalence, diagnosis, and comparison of preoperative clinical and hemodynamic features in patients with and without tricuspid regurgitation. J Thorac Cardiovasc Surg 1987;94:481.

23. Cohn LH, Allred EN, Cohn LA, Disesa VJ, Shemin RJ, Collins JJ. Long-term results of open mitral valve reconstruction for mitral stenosis. Am J Cardiol 1985;55:731.

24. Cortina JM, Martinelli J, Artiz V, Fraile J, Rabago G. Comparative clinical results with Omniscience (STMI), Medtronic-Hall, and Bjork-Shiley convexo-concave (70 degrees) prostheses in mitral valve replacement. J Thorac Cardiovasc Surg 1986;91:174.

25. Czer LS, Matloff J, Chaux A, DeRobertis M, Yoganathan A, Gray RJ. A 6 year experience with the St. Jude Medical valve: hemodynamic performance, surgical results, biocompatibility and follow-up. J Am Coll Cardiol 1985;6:904.

26. Czer LS, Gray RJ, DeRobertis MA, Bateman TM, Stewart ME, Chaux A, et al. Mitral valve replacement: impact of coronary artery disease and determinants of prognosis following revascularization. Circulation 1984;70:I198.

27. Carabello BA, Nolan SP, McGuire LB. Assessment of preoperative left ventricular function in patients with mitral regurgitation: value of the end-systolic wall stress-end systolic volume ratio. Circulation 1981;64:1212.

28. Chauvaud S, Perier P, Touati G, Relland J, Kara SM, Benomar M, et al. Long-term results of valve repair in children with acquired mitral incompetence. Circulation 1986;74:I104.

29. Cohn LH, Allred EN, Cohn LA, Austin JC, Sabik J, DiSesa VJ, et al. Early and late risk of mitral valve replacement. A 12-year concomitant comparison of the porcine bioprosthetic disc mitral valves. J Thorac Cardiovasc Surg 1985;90:872.

30. Czer LS, Matloff JM, Chaux A, DeRobertis M, Gray RJ. Comparative clinical experience with porcine bioprosthetic and St. Jude valve replacement. Chest 1987;91:503.

31. Czer LS, Matloff JM, Chaux A, DeRobertis M, Stewart ME, Gray RJ. The St. Jude valve: analysis of thromboembolism, warfarin-related hemorrhage, and survival. Am Heart J 1987;114:389.

32. Carpentier A, Deloche A, Hanania G, Forman J, Sellier P, Piwnica A, et al. Surgical management of acquired tricuspid valve disease. J Thorac Cardiovasc Surg 1974;67:53.

33. Carpentier A. Cardiac valve surgery: the "French Correction." J Thorac Cardiovasc Surg 1983;86:323.

34. Christakis GT, Weisel RD, David TE, Salerno TA, Ivanov J. Predictors of operative survival after valve replacement. Circulation 1988;78:I25.

35. Carpentier A, Lemaigre G, Robert L, Carpentier S, Dubost C. Biological factors affecting long-term results of valvular heterografts. J Thorac Cardiovasc Surg 1969;58:467.

36. Carpentier A, Deloche A, Relland J, Fabiani JN, Forman J, Camilleri JP, et al. Six-year follow-up of glutaraldehyde-preserved heterografts. With particular reference to the treatment of congenital valve malformations. J Thorac Cardiovasc Surg 1974;68:771.

37. Carpentier AF, Pellerin M, Fuzellier JF, Relland JY. Extensive calcification of the mitral valve anulus: pathology and surgical management. J Thorac Cardiovasc Surg 1996;111:718.

38. Carpentier AF, Lessana A, Relland JY, Belli E, Mihaileanu S, Berrebi HS, et al. The "physio-ring": an advanced concept in mitral valve annuloplasty. Ann Thorac Surg 1995;60:1177.

39. Cannegieter SC, Rosendaal FR, Wintzen AR, van der Meer FJ, Vandenbroucke JP, Briet E. Optimal oral anticoagulation therapy in patients with mechanical heart valves. N Engl J Med 1995;333:11.

40. Cohn LH, Couper GS, Aranki SF, Rizzo RJ, Kinchla NM, Collins JJ Jr. Long-term results of mitral valve reconstruction for regurgitation of the myxomatous mitral valve. J Thorac Cardiovasc Surg 1994;107:143.

41. Corin WJ, Monrad ES, Murakami T, Nonogi H, Hess OM, Krayenbuehl HD. The relationship of afterload to ejection performance in chronic mitral regurgitation. Circulation 1987;76:59.

42. Corin WJ, Sutsch G, Murakami T, Krogmann ON, Turina M, Hess OM. Left ventricular function in chronic mitral regurgitation: preoperative and postoperative comparison. J Am Coll Cardiol 1995;25:113.

43. Capps S. CryoLife data, 1999.

44. Chauvaud S, Fuzellier JF, Houel R, Berrebi A, Mihaileanu S, Carpentier A. Reconstructive surgery in congenital mitral valve insufficiency (Carpentier's techniques): long-term results. J Thorac Cardiovasc Surg 1998;115:84.

45. Chavez AM, Cosgrove DM 3rd, Lytle BW, Gill CC, Loop FD, Stewart RW, et al. Applicability of mitral valvuloplasty techniques in a North American population. Am J Cardiol 1988;62:253.

D

1. Davila JC, Magilligan DJ Jr, Lewis JW Jr. Is the Hancock porcine valve the best cardiac valve substitute today? Ann Thorac Surg 1978;26:303.

2. Dhasmana JP, Blackstone EH, Kirklin JW, Kouchoukos NT. Factors associated with periprosthetic leakage following primary mitral valve replacement: with special consideration of the suture technique. Ann Thorac Surg 1983;35:170.

3. DeWall RA, Schuster B, Hicks G Jr, Pelletier C, Bonan R, Martineau JP, et al. Seventy-six month experience with the Omniscience cardiac valve. J Cardiovasc Surg 1987;28:328.

4. Dalen JF, Matloff JM, Evans GL, Hoppin FG Jr, Bhardwaj P, Harken DE, et al. Early reduction of pulmonary vascular resistance after mitral-valve replacement. N Engl J Med 1967;277:387.

5. Duran CG, Pomar JL, Revuelta JM, Gallo I, Poveda J, Ochoteco A, et al. Conservative operation for mitral insufficiency. Critical analysis supported by postoperative hemodynamic studies of 72 patients. J Thorac Cardiovasc Surg 1980;79:326.

6. Danilowicz D, Kronzon I, Doyle EF, Reed G. Echocardiographic patterns after mitral annuloplasty. Cardiology 1980;65:129.

7. Duran CM, Pomar JL, Colman T, Figueroa A, Revuelta JM, Ubago JL. Is tricuspid valve repair necessary? J Thorac Cardiovasc Surg 1980;80:849.

8. Devereux RB, Perloff JK, Reichek N, Josephson ME. Mitral valve prolapse. Circulation 1976;54:3.

9. Davila JC, Glover RP. Circumferential suture of the mitral valve for the correction of regurgitation. Am J Cardiol 1958;2:267.

10. DeSanctis RW, Dean DC, Bland FE. Extreme left atrial enlargement. Circulation 1964;29:14.

11. Douglas PS, Hirshfeld JW, Edie RN, Harken AH, Stephenson LW, Edmunds LH Jr. Clinical comparison of St. Jude and porcine aortic valve prostheses. Circulation 1985;72:II135.

12. Duncan JM, Cooley DA, Reul GJ, Ott DA, Hallman GL, Frazier OH, et al. Durability and low thrombogenicity of the St. Jude Medical valve at 5-year follow-up. Ann Thorac Surg 1986;42:500.

13. Danchin N, Voiriot P, Briancon S, Bairati I, Mathieu P, Deschamps JP, et al. Mitral valve prolapse as a risk factor for infective endocarditis. Lancet 1989;1:743.

14. DeWall RA. Thrombotic complications with the Omniscience valve: a current review (letter). J Thorac Cardiovasc Surg 1989;98:298.

15. Deloche A, Jebara VA, Relland JY, Chauvaud S, Fabiani JN, Perier P, et al. Valve repair with Carpentier techniques. The second decade. J Thorac Cardiovasc Surg 1990;99:990.

16. David TE, Bos J, Rakowski H. Mitral valve replacement of chordae tendineae with polytetrafluoroethylene sutures. J Thorac Cardiovasc Surg 1991;101:495.

17. Duran CG. Repair of anterior mitral leaflet chordae rupture or elongation (the flip-over technique). J Card Surg 1986;2:161.

18. Duran CG. Surgical management of elongated chordae of the mitral valve. J Card Surg 1989;4:253.

19. David TE, Armstrong S, Sun Z, Daniel L. Late results of mitral valve repair for mitral regurgitation due to degenerative disease. Ann Thorac Surg 1993;56:7.

20. Dujardin KS, Seward JB, Orszulak TA, Schaff HV, Bailey KR, Tajik AJ, et al. Outcome after surgery for mitral regurgitation. Determinants of postoperative morbidity and mortality. J Heart Valve Dis 1997;6:17.

21. David TE, Armstrong S, Sun Z. Replacement of chordae tendineae with Gore-Tex sutures: a ten-year experience. J Heart Valve Dis 1996;5:352.

22. Deutsch HJ, Curtius JM, Bongarth C, Behlke E, Borowski A, de Vivie ER, et al. Left ventricular geometry and function before and after mitral valve replacement. J Heart Valve Dis 1994;3:288.

23. David TE, Uden DE, Strauss HD. The importance of the mitral apparatus in left ventricular function after correction of mitral regurgitation. Circulation 1983;68:II76.

24. David TE, Burns RJ, Bacchus CM, Druck MN. Mitral valve replacement for mitral regurgitation with and without preservation of chordae tendineae. J Thorac Cardiovasc Surg 1984;88:718.

25. Daenen W, Van Kerrebroeck C, Stalpaert G, Mertens B, Lesaffre E. The Björk-Shiley Monostrut valve. Clinical experience in 647 patients. J Thorac Cardiovasc Surg 1993;106:918.

26. Doty DB, Acar C. Mitral valve replacement with homograft. Ann Thorac Surg 1998;66:2127.

27. Doty DB, Doty JR, Flores JH, Millar RC. Cardiac valve replacement with mitral homograft. Semin Thorac Cardiovasc Surg 2001;13:35.

28. Duran CM. Surgical techniques for the repair of anterior mitral leaflet prolapse. J Card Surg 1999;14:471.

E

1. Eckbert DL, Gault JH, Bouchard RL, Karliner JS, Ross J Jr. Mechanics of left ventricular contractions in chronic mitral regurgitation. Circulation 1973;47:1252.

2. Ellis FH Jr, Frye RL, McGoon DC. Results of reconstructive operations for mitral insufficiency due to ruptured chordae tendineae. Surgery 1966;59:165.

3. Ellis LB, Benson H, Harken DE. The effect of age and other factors on the early and late results following closed mitral valvuloplasty. Am Heart J 1968;75:743.

4. Eguaras MG, Luque I, Montero A, Moriones I, Granados J, Garcia MA, et al. Conservative operation for mitral stenosis. Independent determinants of late results. J Thorac Cardiovasc Surg 1988;95:1031.

5. Eguaras MG, Montero A, Moriones I, Granados J, Garcia MA, Luque I, et al. Conservative operation for mitral stenosis with densely fibrosed or partially calcified valves. J Thorac Cardiovasc Surg 1987;93:898.

6. Ellis FH. Surgery for acquired mitral valve disease. Philadelphia: WB Saunders, 1967.

7. Edmunds LH Jr. Thrombotic and bleeding complications of prosthetic heart valves (review). Ann Thorac Surg 1987;44:430.

8. Edmunds LH. Thrombotic complications with the Omniscience valve (letter). J Thorac Cardiovasc Surg 1989;98:300.

9. Eguaras MG, Luque I, Montero A, Garcia MA, Calleja F, Roman M, et al. A comparison of repair and replacement for mitral stenosis with partially calcified valve. J Thorac Cardiovasc Surg 1990;100:161.

10. Esper E, Ferdinand FD, Aronson S, Karp RB. Prosthetic mitral valve replacement: late complications after native valve preservation. Ann Thorac Surg 1997;63:541.

11. Eckberg DL, Gault JH, Bouchard RL, Karliner JS, Ross J Jr. Mechanics of left ventricular contraction in chronic severe mitral regurgitation. Circulation 1973;47:1252.

12. Essop R, Rothlisberger C, Dullabh A, Sareli P. Can the long-term outcomes of percutaneous balloon mitral valvotomy and surgical commissurotomy be expected to be similar? J Heart Valve Dis 1995;4:446.

13. Enriquez-Sarano M, Schaff HV, Orszulak TA, Tajik AJ, Bailey KR, Frye RL. Valve repair improves the outcome of surgery for mitral regurgitation. A multivariate analysis. Circulation 1995;91:1022.

14. Enriquez-Sarano M, Freeman WK, Tribouilloy CM, Orszulak TA, Khandheria BK, Seward JB, et al. Functional anatomy of mitral regurgitation: accuracy and outcome implications of transesophageal echocardiography. J Am Coll Cardiol 1999;34:1129.

F

1. Fuster V, Danielson MA, Robb RA, Broadbent JC, Brown AL Jr, Elveback LR. Quantitation of left ventricular myocardial fiber hypertrophy and interstitial tissue in human hearts with chronically increased volume and pressure overload. Circulation 1977;55:504.

2. Fontana ME, Pence HL, Leighton RF, Wooley CF. The varying clinical spectrum of the systolic click–late systolic murmur syndrome. Circulation 1970;41:807.

3. Feigenbaum H, Linback RE, Nasser WK. Hemodynamic studies before and after instrumental mitral commissurotomy. A reappraisal of the pathophysiology of mitral stenosis and the efficacy of mitral valvotomy. Circulation 1968;38:261.

4. Fournier C, Gay J, Gerbaux A. Long-term course of nonoperated tricuspid insufficiency following surgical correction of mitral and mitro-aortic valve disease. Arch Mal Coeur 1975;68:907.

5. Ferrazzi P, McGiffin DC, Kirklin JW, Blackstone EH, Bourge RC. Have the results of mitral valve replacement improved? J Thorac Cardiovasc Surg 1986;92:186.

6. Forrester JH, Wieting DW, Hall CW, DeBakey ME. A comparative study of the fluid flow resistance of prosthetic heart valves. Cardiovasc Res Cent Bull 1969;7:83.

7. Frater RW, Gabbay S, Shore D Factor S, Strom J. Reproducible replacement of elongated or ruptured mitral valve chordae. Ann Thorac Surg 1983;35:14.

8. Fiore AC, Naunheim KS, D'Orazio S, Kaiser GC, McBride LR, Pennington DG, et al. Mitral valve replacement: randomized trial of St. Jude and Medtronic-Hall prostheses. Ann Thorac Surg 1992;54:68.

9. Freed LA, Levy D, Levine RA, Larson MG, Evans JC, Fuller DL, et al. Prevalence and clinical outcome of mitral-valve prolapse. N Engl J Med 1999;341:1.

10. Fucci C, Sandrelli L, Pardini A, Toraracca L, Ferrari M, Alfieri O. Improved results with mitral valve repair using new surgical techniques. Eur J Cardiothorac Surg 1995;9:621.

11. Fawzy ME, Mimish L, Sivanandam V, Lingamanaicker J, Patel A, Khan B, et al. Immediate and long-term effect of mitral balloon valvotomy on severe pulmonary hypertension in patients with mitral stenosis. Am Heart J 1996;131:89.

12. Fernandez J, Joyce DH, Hirschfield KJ, Chen C, Yang SS, Laub GW, et al. Valve-related events and valve-related mortality in 340 mitral valve repairs: a late phase follow-up study. Eur J Cardiothorac Surg 1993;7:263.

13. Fiane AE, Gerian OR, Svennevig JL. Up to eight years' follow-up of 997 patients receiving the CarboMedics prosthetic heart valve. Ann Thorac Surg 1998;66:443.

14. Fix J, Isada L, Cosgrove D, Miller DP, Savage R, Blum K, et al. Do patients with less than "echo-perfect" results from mitral valve repair by intraoperative echocardiography have a different outcome? Circulation 1993;88:II39.

G

1. Gross RI, Cunningham JN Jr, Snively SL, Catinella FP, Nathan IM, Adams PX, et al. Long-term results of open radical mitral commissurotomy: ten-year follow-up study of 202 patients. Am J Cardiol 1981;47:821.

2. Grunkemeier GL, Macmanus Q, Thomas DR, Starr A. Regression analysis of late survival following mitral valve replacement. J Thorac Cardiovasc Surg 1978;75:131.

3. Glancy DL, O'Brien KP, Reis RL, Epstein SE, Morrow MG. Hemodynamic studies in patients with 2M and 3M Starr-Edwards prostheses: evidence of obstruction to left atrial emptying. Circulation 1969;39:I113.

4. Grondin P, Meere C, Limet R, Lopez-Bescos L, Delcan JL, Rivera R. Carpentier's annulus and De Vega's annuloplasty. J Thorac Cardiovasc Surg 1975;70:852.

5. Grenadier E, Alpan G, Keidar S, Palant A. The prevalence of ruptured chordae tendineae in the mitral valve prolapse syndrome. Am Heart J 1983;105:603.

6. Gash AK, Carabello BA, Cepin D, Spann JF. Left ventricular ejection performance and systolic muscle function in patients with mitral stenosis. Circulation 1983;67:148.

7. Grossman W, Braunwald E, Mann T, McLaurin LP, Green LH. Contractile state of the left ventricle in man as evaluated from end-systolic pressure-volume relations. Circulation 1977;56:845.

8. Galler M, Kronzon I, Slater J, Lighty GW Jr, Politzer F, Colvin S, et al. Long-term follow-up after mitral valve reconstruction: incidence of postoperative left ventricular outflow obstruction. Circulation 1986;74:I99.

9. Gabbay S, McQueen DM, Yellin EL, Becker RM, Frater RW. In vitro hydrodynamic comparison of mitral valve prostheses at high flow rates. J Thorac Cardiovac Surg 1978;76:771.

10. Gabbay S, Yellin EL, Frishman WH, Frater RW. In vitro hydrodynamic comparison of St. Jude, Bjork-Shiley and Hall-Kaster valves. Trans Am Soc Artif Intern Organs 1980;26:231.

11. Goor DA, Mohr R, Lavee J, Serraf A, Smolinsky A. Preservation of the posterior leaflet during mechanical valve replacement for ischemic mitral regurgitation and complete myocardial revascularization. J Thorac Cardiovasc Surg 1988;96:253.

12. Galloway AC, Colvin SB, Baumann FG, Grossi EA, Ribakove GH, Harty S, et al. A comparison of mitral valve reconstruction with mitral valve replacement: intermediate-term results. Ann Thorac Surg 1989;47:655.

13. Grossi EA, Galloway AC, Parish MA, Asai T, Gindea AJ, Harty S, et al. Experience with twenty-eight cases of systolic anterior motion after Carpentier mitral valve reconstruction. J Thorac Cardiovasc Surg 1992;103:466.

14. Giuliani ER. Mitral valve incompetence due to flail anterior leaflet: a new physical sign. Am J Cardiol 1967;20:784.

15. Grunkemeier GL, Li HH, Naftel DC, Starr A, Rahimtoola SH. Long-term performance of heart valve prosthesis. Curr Probl Cardiol 2000;25:73.

16. Gaasch WH, Zile MR. Left ventricular function after surgical correction of chronic mitral regurgitation. Eur Heart J 1991;12:B48.

17. Grossi EA, Galloway AC, Parish MA, Asai T, Gindea AJ, Harty S, et al. Experience with twenty-eight cases of systolic anterior motion after mitral valve reconstruction by the Carpentier technique. J Thorac Cardiovasc Surg 1992;103:466.

18. Gillinov AM, Cosgrove DM. Minimally invasive mitral valve surgery: ministernotomy with extended transseptal approach. Semin Thorac Cardiovasc Surg 1999;11:206.

19. Gamra H, Zhang HP, Allen JW, Lou FY, Ruiz CE. Factors determining normalization of pulmonary vascular resistance following successful balloon mitral valvotomy. Am J Cardiol 1999;83:392.

20. Gundry SR, Shattuck OH, Razzouk A Jr, del Rido MJ, Sardari FF, Bailey LL. Facile minimally invasive cardiac surgery via ministernotomy. Ann Thorac Surg 1998;65:1100.

21. Guiraudon GM, Ofiesh JG, Kaushik R. Extended vertical transatrial septal approach to the mitral valve. Ann Thorac Surg 1991;52:1058.

22. Gillinov AM, Cosgrove DM 3rd, Wahi S, Stewart WJ, Lytle BW, Smedira NG, et al. Is anterior leaflet repair always necessary in repair of bileaflet mitral valve prolapse? Ann Thorac Surg 1999;68:820.

23. Gillinov AM, Cosgrove DM, Blackstone EH, Diaz R, Arnold JH, Lytle BW, et al. Durability of mitral valve repair for degenerative disease. J Thorac Cardiovasc Surg 1998;116:734.

24. Gillinov AM, Blackstone EH, Alster JM, Craver JM, Baumgartner WA, Brewster SA, et al. The Carbomedics Top Hat supraanular aortic valve: a multicenter study. Ann Thorac Surg 2003;75:1175.

25. Gillinov AM, Faber C, Houghtaling PL, Blackstone EH, Lam BK, Diaz R, et al. Repair versus replacement for degenerative mitral valve disease with coexisting ischemic heart disease. J Thorac Cardiovasc Surg (in press).

H

1. Harken DW, Ellis LB, Ware PF, Norman LR. The surgical treatment of mitral stenosis. I. Valvuloplasty. N Engl J Med 1948;239:801.

2. Hood WP Jr, Rackley CE, Rolatt EL. Wall stress in the normal and hypertrophied human left ventricle. Am J Cardiol 1968;22:550.

3. Heller SJ, Carleton RA. Abnormal left ventricular contraction in patients with mitral stenosis. Circulation 1970;42:1099.

4. Hammermeister KE, Fisher L, Kennedy W, Samuels S, Dodge HT. Prediction of late survival in patients with mitral valve disease from clinical, hemodynamic, and quantitative angiographic variables. Circulation 1978;54:341.

5. Halseth WI, Elliott DP, Walker EL, Smith EA. Open mitral commissurotomy. J Thorac Cardiovasc Surg 1980;80:842.

6. Hawe A, Frye RL, Ellis FH Jr. Late hemodynamic studies after mitral valve surgery. J Thorac Cardiovasc Surg 1973;65:351.

7. Hetzer R, Hill JD, Kerth WJ, Ansbro J, Adappa MG, Rodvien R, et al. Thromboembolic complications after mitral valve replacement with Hancock xenograft. J Thorac Cardiovasc Surg 1978;75:651.

8. Hall KV, Nitter-Hauge S, Abdelnoor M. Seven and one-half years' experience with the Medtronic-Hall valve. J Am Coll Cardiol 1985;6:1417.

9. Horstkotte D, Haerten K, Herzen JA, Seipel L, Bircks W, Loogen F. Preliminary clinical and hemodynamic results after mitral valve replacement using St. Jude Medical prostheses in comparison with the Bjork-Shiley valve. Thorac Cardiovasc Surg 1981;29:93.

10. Housman LB, Bonchek L, Lambert L, Grunkemeier G, Starr A. Prognosis of patients after open mitral commissurotomy. Actuarial analysis of late results in 100 patients. J Thorac Cardiovasc Surg 1977;73:742.

11. Hoeksema TD, Wallace RB, Kirklin JW. Closed mitral commissurotomy: recent results in 291 cases. Am J Cardiol 1966;17:825.

12. Horwitz LD, Mullins CB, Payne RM, Curry GC. Left ventricular function in mitral stenosis. Chest 1973;64:609.

13. Halperin Z, Karasik A, Lewis BS, Geft IL, Gotsman MS. Echocardiographic left ventricular function in mitral stenosis. Isr J Med Sci 1978;14:841.

14. Holzer JA, Karliner JS, O'Rourke RA, Peterson KL. Quantitative angiographic analysis of the left ventricle in patients with isolated rheumatic mitral stenosis. Br Heart J 1973;35:497.

15. Horstkotte D, Haerten K, Herzer JA, Seipel L, Bircks W, Loogen F. Preliminary results in mitral valve replacement with the St. Jude Medical prosthesis: comparison with the Bjork-Shiley valve. Circulation 1981;64:II209.

16. Horstkotte D, Haerten K, Herzer JA, Loogen F, Scheibling R, Schulte HD. Five-year results after randomized mitral valve replacement with Bjork-Shiley, Lillehei-Kaster, and Starr-Edwards prostheses. Thorac Cardiovasc Surg 1983;31:106.

17. Holmes DR, Frye RL, Nishimura RA, Ilstrup DM, Hammes LN, Schaff HV, et al. Long-term follow-up of patients undergoing closed transventricular mitral valve commissurotomy (abstract). J Am Coll Cardiol 1989;13:A18.

18. Hochreiter C, Niles N, Devereux RB, Kligfield P, Borer JS. Mitral regurgitation: relationship of noninvasive descriptors of right and left ventricular performance to clinical and hemodynamic findings and to prognosis in medically and surgically treated patients. Circulation 1986;73:900.

19. Hickey AJ, Wolfers J, Wilcken DE. Mitral-valve prolapse: prevalence in an Australian population. Med J Aust 1981;1:31.

20. Horstkotte D, Haerten K, Seipel L, Korfer R, Budde T, Bircks W, et al. Central hemodynamics at rest and during exercise after mitral valve replacement with different prostheses. Circulation 1983;68:II161.

21. Hartz RS, LoCicero J 3rd, Kucich V, DeBoer A, O'Mara S, Meyers SN, et al. Comparative study of warfarin versus antiplatelet therapy in patients with a St. Jude Medical valve in the aortic position. J Thorac Cardiovasc Surg 1986;92:684.

22. Hvass U, Pansard Y, Himbert D, Touche T, Khoury W, Subayi JB, et al. Mitral stenosis with notable or important subvalvular changes. Complete open commissurotomies supported by chorda transfer. Arch Mal Coeur Vaiss 1986;79:1776.

23. Hickey MS, Blackstone EH, Kirklin JW, Dean LS. Outcome probabilities and life history after surgical mitral commissurotomy: implications for balloon commissurotomy. J Am Coll Cardiol 1991;17:29.

24. Hirt SW, Frimpong-Boateng K, Borst HG. The superior approach to the mitral valve—is it worthwhile? Eur J Cardiothorac Surg 1988;2:372.

25. Horstkotte D, Schulte H, Bircks W, Strauer B. Unexpected findings concerning thromboembolic complications and anticoagulation after complete 10 year follow-up of patients with St. Jude Medical prostheses. J Heart Valve Dis 1993; 2:291.

26. Hansen DE, Cahill PD, DeCampli WM, Harrison DC, Derby GC, Mitchell RS, et al. Valvular-ventricular interaction: importance of the mitral apparatus in canine left ventricular systolic performance. Circulation 1986;73:1310.

27. Hansen DE, Cahill PD, Derby GC, Miller DC. Relative contributions of the anterior and posterior mitral chordae tendineae to canine global left ventricular systolic function. J Thorac Cardiovasc Surg 1987;93:45.

28. Hansen DE, Sarris GE, Niczyporuk MA, Derby GC, Cahill PD, Miller DC. Physiologic role of the mitral apparatus in left ventricular regional mechanics, contraction synergy, and global systolic performance. J Thorac Cardiovasc Surg 1989;97:521.

29. Hennein HA, Swain JA, McIntosh CL, Bonow RO, Stone CD, Clark RE. Comparative assessment of chordal preservation versus chordal resection during mitral valve replacement. J Thorac Cardiovasc Surg 1990;99:828.

I

1. Ivert TS, Dismukes WE, Cobbs CG, Blackstone EH, Kirklin JW, Bergdahl LA. Prosthetic valve endocarditis. Circulation 1984;69:223.

2. Iung B, Garbarz E, Michaud P, Helou S, Farah B, Berdah P, et al. Late results of percutaneous mitral commissurotomy in a series of 1024 patients. Analysis of late clinical deterioration: frequency, anatomic findings, and predictive factors. Circulation 1999;99:3272.

3. Ishihara K, Zile MR, Kanazawa S, Tsutsui H, Urabe Y, DeFreyte G, et al. Left ventricular mechanics and myocyte function correction of experimental chronic mitral regurgitation by combined mitral valve replacement and preservation of the native mitral valve apparatus. Circulation 1992;86:II16.

4. Ibrahim M, O'Kane H, Cleland J, Gladstone D, Sarsam M, Patterson C. The St. Jude Medical prosthesis: a thirteen-year experience. J Thorac Cardiovasc Surg 1994;108:221.

J

1. Johnson AD, Daily PO, Peterson KL, LeWinter M, DiDonna GJ, Blair G, et al. Functional evaluation of the porcine heterograft in the mitral position. Circulation 1975;52:I40.

2. Jugdutt BI, Fraser RS, Lee SJ, Rossall RE, Callaghan JC. Long-term survival after tricuspid valve replacement. J Thorac Cardiovasc Surg 1977;74:20.

3. Johnson J, Danielson GK, MacVaugh H 3rd, Joyner CR. Plication of the giant left atrium at operation for severe mitral regurgitation. Surgery 1967;61:118.

4. Jeresaty RM, Edwards JE, Chawla SK. Mitral valve prolapse and ruptured chordae tendineae. Am J Cardiol 1985;55:138.

5. Jaffe WM, Barratt-Boyes BG, Sadri A, Gavin JB, Coverdale HA, Neutze JM. Early follow-up of patients with the Medtronic Intact porcine valve. A new cardiac bioprosthesis. J Thorac Cardiovasc Surg 1989;98:181.

6. Jamieson WR, Miyagishima RT, Tyers GF, Lichenstein SV, Munro AI, Burr LH. Bileaflet mechanical prostheses in mitral and multiple valve replacement surgery: influence of anticoagulant management on performance. Circulation 1997;96:II134.

K

1. Kennedy JW, Yarnall SR, Murray JA, Figley MM. Quantitative angiocardiography. IV. Relationships of left atrial and ventricular pressure and volume in mitral valve disease. Circulation 1970;41:817.

2. Karp RB, Cyrus RJ, Blackstone EH, Kirklin JW, Kouchoukos NT, Pacifico AD. The Bjork-Shiley valve: intermediate-term follow-up. J Thorac Cardiovasc Surg 1981;81:602.

3. Kennedy JW, Doces JG, Stewart DK. Left ventricular function before and following surgical treatment of mitral valve disease. Am Heart J 1979;97:592.

4. Kirklin JW. Replacement of the mitral valve for mitral incompetence. Surgery 1972;72:827.

5. Kaul TK, Bain WH, Jones JV, Lorimer AR, Thomson RM, Turner MA, et al. Mitral valve replacement in the presence of severe pulmonary hypertension. Thorax 1976;31:332.

6. Katske G, Golding LR, Tubbs RR, Loop FD. Posterior midventricular rupture after mitral valve replacement. Ann Thorac Surg 1979;27:130.

7. Kawazoe K, Beppu S, Takahara Y, Nakajima N, Tanaka K, Ichihashi K, et al. Surgical treatment of giant left atrium combined with mitral valvular disease. Plication procedure for reduction of compression to the left ventricle, bronchus, and pulmonary parenchyma. J Thorac Cardiovasc Surg 1983;85:885.

8. Kronzon I, Mercurio P, Winer HE, Colvin S. Echocardiographic evaluation of Carpentier mitral valvuloplasty. Am Heart J 1983; 106:362.

9. Kay PH, Nunley DL, Grunkemeier GL, Pinson CW, Starr A. Late results of combined mitral valve replacement and coronary bypass surgery. J Am Coll Cardiol 1985;5:29.

10. Khandheria BK, Tajik AJ, Reeder GS, Callahan MJ, Nishimura RA, Miller FA, et al. Doppler color flow imaging: a new technique for visualization and characterization of the blood flow jet in mitral stenosis. Mayo Clin Proc 1986;61:623.

11. Korn D, DeSanctis RW, Sell S. Massive calcification of the mitral annulus. N Engl J Med 1962;267:900.

12. Kronzon I, Cohen ML, Winer HE, Colvin SB. Left ventricular outflow obstruction: a complication of mitral valvuloplasty. J Am Coll Cardiol 1984;4:825.

13. Kreindel MS, Schiavone WA, Lever HM, Cosgrove D. Systolic anterior motion of the mitral valve after Carpentier ring valvuloplasty for mitral valve prolapse. Am J Cardiol 1986;57:408.

14. Kopf GS, Hammond GL, Geha AS, Elefteriades J, Hashim SW. Long-term performance of the St. Jude Medical valve: low incidence of thromboembolism and hemorrhagic complications with modest doses of warfarin. Circulation 1987;76:III132.

15. Kinsley RH, Antunes MJ, Colsen PR. St. Jude Medical valve replacement. An evaluation of valve performance. J Thorac Cardiovasc Surg 1986;92:349.

16. Khuri SF, Folland ED, Sethi GK, Souchek J, Oprian C, Wong M, et al. Six-month postoperative hemodynamics of the Hancock heterograft and the Bjork-Shiley prosthesis: results of a Veterans Administration cooperative prospective randomized trial. J Am Coll Cardiol 1988;12:8.

17. Kumar N, Kumar M, Duran CM. A revised terminology for describing surgical findings of the mitral valve. J Heart Valve Dis 1995;4:70.

18. Karp RB, Sand ME. Mechanical prostheses: old and new. Cardiovasc Clin 1993;23:235.

19. Katircioglu SF, Yamak B, Ulus AT, Tasdemir O, Bayazit K. Mitral valve replacement with St. Jude Medical prosthesis and low-dose anticoagulation in patients aged over 50 years. J Heart Valve Dis 1998;7:455.

20. Kadoba K, Jonas RA, Mayer JE, Castenada AR. Mitral valve replacement in the first year of life. J Thorac Cardiovasc Surg 1990;100:762.

L

1. Lefrak EA, Starr A. Cardiac valve prostheses. East Norwalk, Conn.: Appleton & Lange, 1979, p. 110.

2. Lakier JB, Khaja F, Magilligan DJ Jr, Goldstein S. Porcine xenograft valves. Long-term (60-89-month) follow-up. Circulation 1980;62:313.

3. Litwak RS, Silvay J, Gadboys HL, Lukban SB, Sakurai H, Castro-Blanco J. Factors associated with operative risk in mitral valve replacement. Am J Cardiol 1969;23:335.

4. Lepley D Jr, Flemma RJ, Mullen DC, Motl M, Anderson AJ, Weirauch E. Long-term follow-up of the Bjork-Shiley prosthetic valve used in the mitral position. Ann Thorac Surg 1980;30:164.

5. Lillehei CW, Gott VL, Dewall RA, Varco RL. Surgical correction of pure mitral insufficiency by annuloplasty under direct vision. Lancet 1957;1:446.

6. Lessana A, Herreman F, Boffety C, Cosma H, Guerin F, Kara M, et al. Hemodynamic and cineangiographic study before and after mitral valvuloplasty (Carpentier's technique). Circulation 1981;64:II195.

7. Lipson LC, Kent KM, Rosing DR, Bonow RO, McIntosh CL, Condit J, et al. Long-term hemodynamic assessment of the porcine heterograft in the mitral position. Late development of valvular stenosis. Circulation 1981;64:397.

8. Lurie AJ, Miller RR, Maxwell KS, Grehl TM, Vismara LA, Hurley AJ, et al. Hemodynamic assessment of the glutaraldehyde-preserved porcine heterograft in the aortic and mitral position. Circulation 1977;56:II104.

9. Levine FM, Carter JE, Buckley MJ, Daggett WM, Akins CW, Austen WG. Hemodynamic evaluation of Hancock and Carpentier-Edwards bioprostheses. Circulation 1981;64:II192.

10. Lessana A, Tran Viet T, Ades F, Kara SM, Ameur A, Ruffenach A, et al. Mitral reconstructive operations: a series of 130 consecutive cases. J Thorac Cardiovasc Surg 1983;86:553.

11. Lytle BW, Cosgrove DM, Gill CC, Stewart RW, Golding LA, Goormastic M, et al. Mitral valve replacement combined with myocardial revascularization: early and late results for 300 patients, 1970 to 1983. Circulation 1985;71:1179.

12. Lindblom D, Lindblom U, Henze A, Bjork VO, Semb BK. Three-year clinical results with the Monostrut Bjork-Shiley prosthesis. J Thorac Cardiovasc Surg 1987;94:34.

13. Lindblom D. Long-term clinical results after mitral valve replacement with the Bjork-Shiley prosthesis. J Thorac Cardiovasc Surg 1988;95:321.

14. Lambert AS, Miller JP, Merrick SH, Schiller NB, Foster E, Muhiudeen-Russell I, et al. Improved evaluation of the location and mechanism of mitral valve regurgitation with a systemic transesophageal echocardiography examination. Anesth Analg 1999;88:1197.

15. Lessana A, Carbone C, Romano A, Palsky E, Quan YH, Escorsin M, et al. Mitral valve repair: results and the decision-making process in reconstruction. Report of 275 cases. J Thorac Cardiovasc Surg 1990;99:622.

16. Lee KS, Stewart WJ, Lever HM, Underwood PL, Cosgrove DM. Mechanism of outflow tract obstruction causing failed mitral valve repair. Anterior displacement of leaflet coaptation. Circulation 1993;88:II24.

17. Lillehei CW, Levy MJ, Bannabeau RC. Mitral valve replacement with preservation of papillary muscles and chordae tendineae. J Thorac Cardiovasc Surg 1964;47:532.

18. Ling L, Enriquez-Sarano M, Seward J, Orszulak TA, Schaff HV, Bailey KR, et al. Early surgery in patients with mitral regurgitation due to flail leaflets: a long-term outcome study. Circulation 1997;96:1819.

19. Leung DY, Griffin BP, Stewart WJ, Cosgrove DM 3rd, Thomas JD, Marwick TH. Left ventricular function after valve repair for chronic mitral regurgitation: predictive value of preoperative assessment of contractile reserve by exercise echocardiography. J Am Coll Cardiol 1996;28:1198.

M

1. Munoz S, Gallardo J, Diaz-Gorrin JR, Medina O. Influence of surgery on the natural history of rheumatic mitral and aortic valve disease. Am J Cardiol 1975;35:234.

2. Medtronic Blood Systems. Medtronic-Hall prosthetic heart valve: 8 year experience. Minneapolis: Medtronic, 1985.

3. McGoon DC. Repair of mitral insufficiency due to ruptured chordae tendineae. J Thorac Cardiovasc Surg 1960;39:357.

4. Merendino KA, Bruce RA. One hundred seventeen surgically treated cases of valvular rheumatic heart disease: with a preliminary report of two cases of mitral regurgitation treated under direct vision with the aid of a pump-oxygenator. JAMA 1957;164:749.

5. Mills P, Rose J, Hollingsworth J, Amara I, Craige E. Long-term prognosis of mitral-valve prolapse. N Engl J Med 1977;297:13.

6. Manteuffel-Szoege L, Nowicki J, Wasniewska M, Sitkowski W, Turski C. Mitral commissurotomy: results of 1700 cases. J Cardiovasc Surg 1970;11:350.

7. Miller DC, Oyer PE, Stinson EB, Reitz BA, Jamieson SW, Baumgartner WA, et al. Ten to fifteen year reassessment of the performance characteristics of the Starr-Edwards Model 6120 mitral valve prosthesis. J Thorac Cardiovasc Surg 1983;85:1.

8. McIntosh CL, Michaelis LL, Morrow AG, Itscoitz SB, Redwood DR, Epstein SE. Atrioventricular valve replacement with the Hancock porcine xenograft: a 5-year clinical experience. Surgery 1975;78:768.

9. Marshall WG Jr, Kouchoukos NT, Karp RB, Williams JB. Late results after mitral valve replacement with the Bjork-Shiley and porcine prostheses. J Thorac Cardiovasc Surg 1983;85:902.

10. McKay RG, Lock JE, Safian RD, Come PC, Diver DJ, Baim DS, et al. Balloon dilation of mitral stenosis in adult patients: postmortem and percutaneous mitral valvuloplasty studies. J Am Coll Cardiol 1987;9:723.

11. Messmer FJ, Gattiker K, Rothlin M, Senning A. Reconstruction of the mitral valve. Ann Thorac Surg 1973;16:30.

12. Magovern JA, Pennock JL, Campbell DB, Pierce WS, Waldhausen JA. Risks of mitral valve replacement and mitral valve replacement with coronary artery bypass. Ann Thorac Surg 1985;39:346.

13. Maurer G, Czer LS, Chaux A, Bolger AF, DeRobertis M, Resser K, et al. Intraoperative Doppler color flow mapping for assessment of valve repair for mitral regurgitation. Am J Cardiol 1987;60:333.

14. Mattina CJ, Green SJ, Tortolani AJ, Padmanabham VT, Ong LY, Hall MH, et al. Frequency of angiographically significant coronary arterial narrowing in mitral stenosis. Am J Cardiol 1986;57:802.

15. Mehmel HC, Stockins B, Ruffman K, von Olshausen K, Schuler G, Kubler W. The linearity of the end-systolic pressure-volume relationship in man and its sensitivity for assessment of left ventricular function. Circulation 1981;63:1216.

16. Mihaileanu S, Marino JP, Chauvaud S, Perier P, Forman J, Vissoat J, et al. Left ventricular outflow obstruction after mitral valve repair (Carpentier's technique): proposed mechanisms of disease. Circulation 1988;78:I78.

17. McKay CR, Kawanishi DT, Kotlewski A, Parise K, Odom-Maryon T, Gonzalez A, et al. Improvement in exercise capacity and exercise hemodynamics 3 months after double-balloon, catheter balloon valvuloplasty treatment of patients with symptomatic mitral stenosis. Circulation 1988;77:1013.

18. Marks AR, Choong CY, Sanfilippo AJ, Ferre M, Weyman AE. Identification of high-risk and low-risk subgroups of patients with mitral valve prolapse. N Engl J Med 1989;320:1031.

19. Mikhail AA, Ellis R, Johnson S. Eighteen-year evolution from the Lillehei-Kaster valve to the Omni design. Ann Thorac Surg 1989;48:S61.

20. Montero CG, Mula N, Brugos R, Tellez G, Figuera D. Thrombectomy of the Bjork-Shiley prosthetic valve revisited: long-term results. Ann Thorac Surg 1989;49:824.

21. McEnany MT. Mitral valve replacement in the presence of severe valvular and annular calcification. J Card Surg 1993;8:117.

22. Marwick TH, Stewart WJ, Currie PJ, Cosgrove DM. Mechanisms of failure of mitral valve repair: an echocardiography study. Am Heart J 1991;122:149.

23. Mantle J, Hood W, Kouchoukos N, Karp RB, Zisserman P, Rackley C. Physiologic basis for afterload reduction following mitral valve replacement. Am J Cardiol 1978;41:420.

24. Moon MR, DeAnda A Jr, Daughters GT 2nd, Ingels NB Jr, Miller DC. Experimental evaluation of different chordal preservation methods during mitral valve replacement. Ann Thorac Surg 1994;58:931.

25. Martinall J, Jimenez A, Rábago G, Artiz V, Fraile J, Farre J. Mechanical cardiac valve thrombosis: is thrombectomy justified? Circulation 1991;84:III70.

26. Miki S, Kusuhara K, Ueda Y, Komeda M, Ohkita Y, Takahumi T. Mitral valve replacement with preservation of chordae tendineae and papillary muscles. Ann Thorac Surg 1988;45:28.

27. Mohty D, Orszulak TA, Schaff HV, Avierinos JF, Tajik JA, Enriquez-Sarano M. Very long-term survival and durability of mitral valve repair for mitral valve prolapse. Circulation 2001;104:I1.

28. Moon MR, DeAnda A Jr, Daughters GT 2nd, Ingels NB Jr, Miller DC. Effects of mitral valve replacement on regional left ventricular systolic strain. Ann Thorac Surg 1999;68:894.

29. Moon MR, DeAnda A Jr, Daughters GT 2nd, Ingels NB, Miller DC. Effects of chordal disruption on regional left ventricular torsional deformation. Circulation 1996;94:II143.

N

1. Nasser WK, Davis RH, Dillon JC, Tavel ME, Helmen CH, Feigenbaum H, et al. Atrial myxoma. I. Clinical and pathologic features in nine cases. Am Heart J 1972;83:694.

2. Nevaril CG, Lynch EC, Alfrey CP Jr, Hellums JD. Erythrocyte damage and destruction induced by shearing stress. J Lab Clin Med 1968;71:784.

3. Nichols HT. Mitral insufficiency: treatment by polar cross fusion of the mitral annulus fibrosis. J Thorac Cardiovasc Surg 1957;33:102.

4. Nicoloff DM, Emery RW, Arom KV, Northup WF 3rd, Jorgenson CR, Wang Y, et al. Clinical and hemodynamic results with the St. Jude Medical cardiac valve prosthesis. A three-year experience. J Thorac Cardiovasc Surg 1981;82:674.

5. Nunley DL, Starr A. The evolution of reparative techniques for the mitral valve. Ann Thorac Surg 1984;37:393.

6. Nestico PF, Depace NL, Morganrath J, Kotler MN, Ross J. Mitral annular calcification: clinical, pathophysiologic, and echocardiographic review. Am Heart J 1984;107:989.

7. Nakano S, Kawashima Y, Hirose H, Matsuda H, Shirakura R, Sato S, et al. Reconsiderations of indications for open mitral commissurotomy based on pathologic features of the stenosed mitral valve. J Thorac Cardiovasc Surg 1987;94:336.

8. Nakano S, Kawashima Y, Hirose H, Matsuda H, Sato S, Manabe H. Reoperation-free survival after closed mitral commissurotomy. A 28-year follow-up study in 469 patients. J Cardiovasc Surg 1986; 27:103.

9. Nakano S, Kawashima Y, Matsuda H, Sakai K, Taniguchi K, Kawamoto T, et al. A five-year appraisal and hemodynamic evaluation of the Bjork-Shiley Monostrut valve. J Thorac Cardiovasc Surg 1991;101:881.

O

1. Olesen KH. The natural history of 271 patients with mitral stenosis under medical treatment. Br Heart J 1962;24:349.

2. Owen I, Fenton WJ. A case of extreme dilatation of the left auricle of the heart. Trans Clin Soc Lond 1901;34:183.

3. Orszulak TA, Schaff HV, Danielson GK, Piehler JM, Pluth JR, Frye RL, et al. Mitral regurgitation due to ruptured chordae tendineae. Early and late results of valve repair. J Thorac Cardiovasc Surg 1985;89:491.

4. Okita Y, Miki S, Kusuhara K, Ueda Y, Tahata T, Yamanaka K, et al. Analysis of left ventricular motion after mitral valve replacement with a technique of preservation of all chordae tendineae. Comparison with conventional mitral valve replacement or mitral valve repair. J Thorac Cardiovasc Surg 1992;104:786.

5. Ohno H, Imai Y, Terada M, Hiramatsu T. The long-term results of commissure plication annuloplasty for congenital mitral insufficiency. Ann Thorac Surg 1999;68:537.

P

1. Pakrashi BC, Mary DA, Elmufti ME, Wooler GH, Ionescu MI. Clinical and haemodynamic results of mitral annuloplasty. Br Heart J 1974;36:768.

2. Peter CA, Austin EH, Jones RH. Effect of valve replacement from chronic mitral insufficiency on left ventricular function during rest and exercise. J Thorac Cardiovasc Surg 1981;82:127.

3. Pocock WA, Barlow JB. Postexercise arrhythmias in the billowing posterior mitral leaflet syndrome. Am Heart J 1970;80:740.

4. Phillips HR, Levine FH, Carter JE, Boucher CA, Osbakken MD, Okada RD, et al. Mitral valve replacement for isolated mitral regurgitation: analysis of clinical course and late postoperative left ventricular ejection fraction. Am J Cardiol 1981;48:647.

5. Pyle RB, Mayer JE Jr, Lindsay WG, Jorgensen CR, Wang Y, Nicoloff DM. Hemodynamic evaluation of Lillehei-Kaster and Starr-Edwards prostheses. Ann Thorac Surg 1978;26:336.

6. Parsonnet AE, Bernstein A, Martland HS. Massive left auricle with special reference to its etiology and mechanism: report of case. Am Heart J 1946;31:438.

7. Perier P, Deloche A, Chauvaud S, Fabiani JN, Rossant P, Bessou JP, et al. Comparative evaluation of mitral valve repair and replacement with Starr, Bjork, and porcine valve prostheses. Circulation 1984; 70:I187.

8. Peper WA, Lytle BW, Cosgrove DM, Goormastic M, Loop FD. Repeat mitral commissurotomy: long-term results. Circulation 1987; 76:III97.

9. Palacios I, Block PC. Percutaneous mitral balloon valvotomy (PMV): update of immediate results and follow-up (abstract). Circulation 1988;78:II490.

10. Parker F, Weiss S. The nature and significance of the structural changes in the lungs in mitral stenosis. Am J Pathol 1936;12:573.

11. Perier P, Clausnizer B, Mistarz K. Carpentier "sliding leaflet" technique for repair of the mitral valve: early results. Ann Thorac Surg 1994;57:383.

12. Phillips MR, Daly RC, Schaff HV, Dearani JA, Mullany CJ, Orszulak TA. Repair of anterior leaflet mitral valve prolapse: chordal replacement versus chordal shortening. Ann Thorac Surg 2000;69:25.

13. Poirer NC, Pelletier LC, Pellerin M, Carrier M. Fifteen-year experience with the Carpentier-Edwards pericardial bioprosthesis. Ann Thorac Surg 1998;66:S57.

R

1. Rowe JC, Bland EF, Sprague HB, White PD. The course of mitral stenosis without surgery: ten- and twenty-year perspectives. Ann Intern Med 1960;52:741.

2. Rapaport E. Natural history of aortic and mitral valve disease. Am J Cardiol 1975;35:221.

3. Roberts WC, Morrow AG. Causes of early postoperative death following cardiac valve replacement: clinicopathologic correlations in 64 patients studied at necropsy. J Thorac Cardiovasc Surg 1967; 54:422.

4. Reed GE, Tice DA, Clauss RH. Asymmetric exaggerated mitral annuloplasty: repair of mitral insufficiency with hemodynamic predictability. J Thorac Cardiovasc Surg 1965;49:752.

5. Rankin JS, Nicholas LM, Kouchoukos NT. Experimental mitral regurgitation: effects on left ventricular function before and after elimination of chronic regurgitation in the dog. J Thorac Cardiovasc Surg 1975;70:478.

6. Reed GE. Repair of mitral regurgitation: an 11-year experience. Am J Cardiol 1973;31:494.

7. Reed GE, Kloth HH, Kiely B, Danilowicz DA, Rader B, Doyle EF. Long-term results of mitral annuloplasty in children with rheumatic mitral regurgitation. Circulation 1974;50:II189.

8. Reed GE, Pooley RW, Moggio RA. Durability of measured mitral annuloplasty: seventeen-year study. J Thorac Cardiovasc Surg 1980; 79:321.

9. Roy SB, Gopinath N. Mitral stenosis. Circulation 1968;38:68.

10. Ramsey HW, De la Torre A, Bartley TD, Linhart JW. Intractable hemoptysis in mitral stenosis treated by emergency mitral commissurotomy. Ann Intern Med 1967;67:588.

11. Rackley CE, Hood WP Jr. Quantitative angiographic evaluation and pathophysiologic mechanisms in valvular heart disease. Prog Cardiovasc Dis 1973;15:427.

12. Richi AA, Sade RM, May MG, Hohn AR. Repair of left atrial abnormalities in children by the superior approach. Ann Thorac Surg 1981;31:433.

13. Rusted IE, Sheifley CH, Edwards JE, Kirklin JW. Guides to the commissures in operations upon the mitral valve. Mayo Clin Proc 1951;26:297.

14. Roberts WC. Morphologic features of the normal and abnormal mitral valve. Am J Cardiol 1983;51:1005.

15. Rizzoli G, Russo R, Resta M, Valfre C, Mazzucco A, Brumana T, et al. Mitral valve prosthesis dehiscence necessitating reoperation: an analysis of the risk factors involved. Thorac Cardiovasc Surg 1983;31:91.

16. Rediker DE, Block PC, Abascal VM, Palacios IF. Mitral balloon valvuloplasty for mitral restenosis after surgical commissurotomy. J Am Coll Cardiol 1988;11:252.

17. Rashtian MY, Stevenson DM, Allen DT, Yoganathan AP, Harrison EC, Edmiston WA, et al. Flow characteristics of four commonly used mechanical heart valves. Am J Cardiol 1986;58:743.

18. Rabago G, Martinell J, Fraile J. Results and complications with the Omniscience prosthesis. J Thorac Cardiovasc Surg 1984;87:136.

19. Rabago G, Fraile J, Martinell J. Omniscience thromboembolism rates (letter). J Thorac Cardiovasc Surg 1984;88:1040.

20. Rabago G, Cooley DA, eds. Heart valve replacement and future trends in cardiac surgery. New York: Futura, 1987.

21. Ravkilde JL, Hansen PS. Late results following closed mitral valvotomy in isolated mitral valve stenosis: analysis of thirty-five years of follow-up in 240 patients using Cox regression. Thorac Cardiovasc Surg 1991;39:133.

22. Reed D, Abbott RD, Smucker ML, Kaul S. Prediction of outcome after mitral valve replacement in patients with symptomatic chronic mitral regurgitation: the importance of left atrial size. Circulation 1991;84:23.

23. Rosendaal FR, Cannegieter SC, van de Meer FJ, Briet E. A method to determine the optimal intensity of oral anticoagulant therapy. Thromb Haemost 1993;69:236.

24. Ross DN, Kabbani S. Mitral valve replacement with a pulmonary autograft: the mitral top hat. J Heart Valve Dis 1997;6:542.

25. Rastelli GC, Kirklin JW. Hemodynamic state early after prosthetic replacement of mitral valve. Circulation 1966;34:448.

26. Rozich JD, Carabello BA, Usher BW, Kratz JM, Bell AE, Zile MR. Mitral valve replacement with and without chordal preservation in patients with chronic mitral regurgitation: mechanisms for differences in postoperative ejection performance. Circulation 1992;86:1718.

27. Ross J Jr. Afterload mismatch in aortic and mitral valve disease: implications for surgical therapy. J Am Coll Cardiol 1985;5:811.

28. Reardon MJ, Letsou GV, Reardon PR, Baldwin JC. Left ventricular rupture following mitral valve replacement. J Heart Valve Dis 1996;5:10.

S

1. Souttar HS. The surgical treatment of mitral stenosis. Br Med J 1925;2:603.

2. Starr A, Edwards ML. Mitral replacement: clinical experience with a ball valve prosthesis. Ann Surg 1961;154:726.

3. Selzer A, Cohn KE. Natural history of mitral stenosis: a review. Circulation 1972;45:878.

4. Selzer A, Katayama F. Mitral regurgitation: clinical patterns, pathophysiology and natural history. Medicine (Baltimore) 1972;51:337.

5. Sanders SP, Levy RJ, Freed MD, Norwood WI, Castaneda AR. Use of Hancock porcine xenografts in children and adolescents. Am J Cardiol 1980;46:429.

6. Schuler G, Peterson KL, Johnson A, Francis G, Dennish G, Utley J, et al. Temporal response of left ventricular performance to mitral valve surgery. Circulation 1979;59:1218.

7. Saksena DS, Tucker BI, Lindesmith GG, Nelson RM, Stiles QR, Meyer BW. The superior approach to the mitral valve. Ann Thorac Surg 1971;12:146.

8. Salomon NW, Stinson EB, Griepp RB, Shumway NE. Patient-related risk factors as predictors of results following isolated mitral valve replacement. Ann Thorac Surg 1977;24:519.

9. Selzer A, Kelly JJ Jr, Kerth WJ, Gerbode F. Immediate and long-range results of valvuloplasty for mitral regurgitation due to ruptured chordae tendineae. Circulation 1972;45,46:I52.

10. Smith WM, Neutze JM, Barratt-Boyes BG, Low JB. Open mitral valvotomy: effect of preoperative factors on result. J Thorac Cardiovasc Surg 1981;82:738.

11. Sanfelippo PM, Giuliani ER, Danielson GK, Wallace RB, Pluth JR, McGoon DC. Tricuspid valve prosthetic replacement. J Thorac Cardiovasc Surg 1976;71:441.

12. Simon R, Oelert H, Borst HG, Lichtlen PR. Influence of mitral valve surgery on tricuspid incompetence concomitant with mitral valve disease. Circulation 1980;62:I152.

13. Sala A, Schoevaerdts JC, Jaumin P, Ponlot R, Chalant CH. Review of 387 isolated mitral valve replacements by the model 6120 Starr-Edwards prosthesis. J Thorac Cardiovasc Surg 1982;84:744.

14. Spratt JA, Olsen CO, Tyson GS Jr, Glower DD Jr, Davis JW, Rankin JS. Experimental mitral regurgitation. Physiological effects of correction on left ventricular dynamics. J Thorac Cardiovasc Surg 1983;86:479.

15. Sand ME, Naftel DC, Blackstone EH, Kirklin JW, Karp RB. A comparison of repair and replacement for mitral valve incompetence. J Thorac Cardiovasc Surg 1987;94:208.

16. Savage DD, Garrison RJ, Castelli WP, McNamara PM, Anderson SJ, Kannel WB, et al. Prevalence of submitral (anular) calcium and its correlates in the general population-based sample (the Framingham Study). Am J Cardiol 1983;51:1375.

17. Sagawa K. The end-systolic pressure-volume relation of the ventricle: definition, modifications and clinical use (editorial). Circulation 1981;63:1223.

18. Spencer FC, Colvin SB, Culliford AT, Isom OW. Experiences with the Carpentier techniques of mitral valve reconstruction in 103 patients (1980-1985). J Thorac Cardiovasc Surg 1985;90:341.

19. Schiavone WA, Cosgrove DM, Lever HM, Stewart WJ, Salcedo EE. Long-term follow-up of patients with left ventricular outflow tract obstruction after Carpentier ring mitral valvuloplasty. Circulation 1988;78:I60.

20. Savage DD, Garrison RJ, Devereux RB, Castelli WP, Anderson SJ, Levy D, et al. Mitral valve prolapse in the general population. 1. Epidemiological features: the Framingham Study. Am Heart J 1983; 106:571.

21. Schoevaerdts JC, Buche M, el Gariani A, Lichtsteiner M, Jaumin P, Ponlot R, et al. Twenty years' experience with the Model 6120 Starr-Edwards valve in the mitral position. J Thorac Cardiovasc Surg 1987;94:375.

22. St. Jude Medical. Five-year multicenter experience. Minneapolis: St. Jude Medical, 1984.

23. Scotten LN, Racca RG, Nugent AH, Walker DK, Brownlee RT. New tilting disc cardiac prostheses: in vitro comparison of their hydrodynamic performance in the mitral position. J Thorac Cardiovasc Surg 1981;82:136.

24. Spencer FC, Galloway AC, Grossi EA, Ribakove GH, Delianides J, Baumann FG, et al. Recent development and evolving techniques of mitral valve reconstruction. Ann Thorac Surg 1998;65:307.

25. Straub UJ, Huwer H, Kalweit G, Volkmer I, Gams E. Improved regional left ventricular performance in mitral valve replacement with orthotopic refixation of the anterior mitral leaflet. J Heart Valve Dis 1997;6:395.

26. Sakai T, Okita Y, Ueda Y, Tahata T, Ogino H, Matsuyama K, et al. Distance between mitral anulus and papillary muscles: anatomic study in normal human hearts. J Thorac Cardiovasc Surg 1999;118:636.

27. Schuler G, Peterson KL, Johnson A, Francis G, Dennish G, Utley J, et al. Temporal response of left ventricular performance to mitral valve surgery. Circulation 1979;59:1218.

28. Shyu KG, Chen JJ, Lin FY, Tsai CH, Lin JL, Tseng YZ, et al. Regression of left ventricular mass after mitral valve repair of pure mitral regurgitation. Ann Thorac Surg 1994;58:1670.

29. Soga Y, Nishimura K, Ikeda T, Nishina T, Ueyama K, Nakamura T, et al. Chordal-sparing mitral valve replacement using artificial chordae tendineae for rheumatic mitral stenosis: experience of the "oblique" method. Artif Organs 2002;26:802.

T

1. Tsakiris AG, Mair DD, Seki S, Titus JL, Wood EH. Motion of the tricuspid valve annulus in anesthetized intact dogs. Circ Res 1975;36:43.

2. Taylor RR, Hopkins BE. Left ventricular response to experimentally induced chronic regurgitation. Cardiovasc Res 1972;6:404.

3. Thulin LI, Bain WH, Huysmans HH, van Ingen G, Prieto I, Basile F, et al. Heart valve replacement with the Bjork-Shiley Monostrut valve: early results of a multicenter clinical investigation. Ann Thorac Surg 1988;45:164.

4. Teply JF, Grunkemeier GL, Sutherland HD, Lambert LE, Johnson VA, Starr A. The ultimate prognosis after valve replacement: an assessment at twenty years. Ann Thorac Surg 1981;32:111.

5. Tsakiris AG, Sturm RE, Wood EH. Experimental studies on the mechanisms of closure of cardiac valves with use of roentgen videodensitometry. Am J Cardiol 1973;32:136.

6. Tischler MD, Cooper KA, Rowen M, LeWinter MM. Mitral valve replacement versus mitral valve repair. A Doppler and quantitative stress echocardiographic study. Circulation 1994;89:132.

7. Tribouilloy CM, Enriquez-Sarano M, Schaff HV, Orszulak TA, Bailey KR, Tajik AJ, et al. Impact of preoperative symptoms on survival after surgical correction of organic mitral regurgitation: rationale for optimizing surgical indications. Circulation 1999;99:400.

U

1. Urschel CW, Covell JW, Sonnenblick EH, Ross J Jr, Braunwald E. Myocardial mechanics in aortic and mitral valvular regurgitation: the concept of instantaneous impedance as a determinant of the performance of the intact heart. J Clin Invest 1968;47:867.
2. Umana JP, Salehizadeh B, DeRose JJ Jr, Nahar T, Lotvin A, Homma S, et al. "Bow-tie" mitral valve repair: an adjuvant technique for ischemic mitral regurgitation. Ann Thorac Surg 1998;66:1640.

V

1. Vega JL, Fleitas M, Martinez R, Gallo JI, Gutierrez JA, Colman T, et al. Open mitral commissurotomy. Ann Thorac Surg 1981;31:266.
2. Vallejo JL, Gonzalez-Santos JM, Albertos J, Riesgo MJ, Bastida ME, Rico MJ, et al. Eight years' experience with the Medtronic-Hall valve prosthesis. Ann Thorac Surg 1990;50:429.
3. Vesely I. Analysis of the Medtronic Intact bioprosthetic valve: effects of "zero pressure" fixation. J Thorac Cardiovasc Surg 1991;101:90.
4. Vaturi M, Porter A, Adler Y, Shapira Y, Sahar G, Vidne B, et al. The natural history of aortic valve disease after mitral valve surgery. J Am Coll Cardiol 1999;33:2003.

W

1. Williams JB, Karp RB, Kirklin JW, Kouchoukos NT, Pacifico AD, Zorn GL Jr, et al. Considerations in selection and management of patients undergoing valve replacement with glutaraldehyde-fixed porcine bioprostheses. Ann Thorac Surg 1980;30:247.
2. Wood P. An appreciation of mitral stenosis. Br Med J 1954;1:1051.
3. Warnes CA, Scott ML, Silver GM, Smith CW, Ferrans VJ, Roberts WC. Comparison of late degenerative changes in porcine bioprostheses in the mitral and aortic valve position in the same patient. Am J Cardiol 1983;51:965.
4. Wilcken DE, Hickey AJ. Lifetime risk for patients with mitral valve prolapse of developing severe valve regurgitation requiring surgery. Circulation 1988;78:10.

5. Walker DK, Scotten LN, Modi VJ, Brownlee RT. In vitro assessment of mitral valve prostheses. J Thorac Cardiovasc Surg 1980;79:680.

Y

1. Yacoub M, Halim M, Radley-Smith R, McKay R, Nijveld A, Towers M. Surgical treatment of mitral regurgitation caused by floppy valves: repair versus replacement. Circulation 1981;64:II210.
2. Yoganathan AP, Harrison EC, Corcoran WH. Prosthetic heart valves: Proceedings of the Fourteenth Annual Meeting of the Association for the Advancement of Medical Instrumentation. Pasadena, Calif.: Cal Tech Press, 1980, p. 181.
3. Yun KL, Rayhill SC, Niczyporuk MA, Fann JI, Zipkin RE, Derby GC, et al. Mitral valve replacement in dilated canine hearts with chronic mitral regurgitation: importance of the mitral subvalvular apparatus. Circulation 1991;84:III112.
4. Yun KL, Sintek CF, Miller DC, Pfeffer TA, Kochamba GS, Khonsari S, et al. Randomized trial comparing partial versus complete chordal-sparing mitral valve replacement: effects on left ventricular volume and function. J Thorac Cardiovasc Surg 2002;123:707.

Z

1. Zaretskii VV, Gromova GV, Kuznetsova LM, Dadabaev AD. Comparative evaluation of the dynamics of the echocardiographic parameters following open and closed mitral commissurotomy. Kardiologiia 1985;25:55.
2. Zussa C, Polesel E, Da Col U, Galloni M, Valfre C. Seven-year experience with chordal replacement with expanded polytetrafluoroethylene in floppy mitral valve. J Thorac Cardiovasc Surg 1994;108:37.
3. Zile M, Gaasch W, Carnall J, Levine HJ. Chronic mitral regurgitation: predictive value of preoperative echocardiographic indices, left ventricular function and wall stress. J Am Coll Cardiol 1984;3:235.

12 Aortic Valve Disease

DEFINITION

This chapter describes the surgical aspects of aortic valve disease, excluding congenital aortic stenosis in infants and children (see Chapter 33) and aortic regurgitation with either ventricular septal defect (see Chapter 21) or sinus of Valsalva aneurysm (see Chapter 22).

HISTORICAL NOTE

In 1947, Smithy and Parker at the University of South Carolina in Charleston first reported an experimental study of *aortic valvotomy.*[S2] During the early 1950s, Bailey and colleagues in Philadelphia used closed methods—either a dilator introduced transventricularly or a digital approach through a "poncho" sewn onto the ascending aorta—in clinical attempts to relieve severe aortic stenosis.[B2,B3] Modest success in some patients was obtained by them and by Ellis and Kirklin.[E3]

In 1951, Hufnagel in Washington, D.C., developed a *ball valve prosthesis* for rapid insertion into the descending thoracic aorta.[H1] (From his work with Gross in developing the coarctation operation, Hufnagel was well aware of the risk of paraplegia with aortic clamping and therefore emphasized the rapidity of insertion of his device; see Chapter 51.) The prosthesis could be inserted quickly because of two multi-point fixation rings, each placed around the aorta and over the end of the prosthesis lying within the aorta. Hufnagel and Harvey,[H2] Ellis and Kirklin,[E4] and others obtained fairly good palliation of severe aortic regurgitation in some patients with this device. However, upper body signs of aortic regurgitation became severe. During the early 1950s, Bailey and Likoff developed and used a number of ingenious but quite unsuccessful closed methods of overcoming aortic regurgitation.[B1]

A more effective approach to surgical treatment of aortic valve disease in adults began with the advent of clinical *cardiopulmonary bypass* in 1954 and 1955 (see Chapter 2). At first, aortic valvotomy and removal of calcific deposits were all that could be done.[H10,K11] Then Bahnson and colleagues and, independently, Hufnagel and Conrad developed a *single-leaflet prosthesis* that became commercially available.[B25,H8,M17] Generally, the leaflets were used to partially replace the aortic valve, but three leaflets could be used together for total aortic valve replacement. Probably the first *single-unit prosthesis* for total aortic valve replacement was the polytetrafluoroethylene sleeve prosthesis developed and first used by McGoon at the Mayo Clinic in 1961.[M6] Although this device was successful in terms of early results, competence was sometimes not achieved, leading to appreciable hospital mortality. Introduction of the ball valve prosthesis by Harken and colleagues and Starr and colleagues in 1960 (Starr and colleagues' report appeared in 1963) established aortic valve surgery on a firm basis.[H9,S16] Many types of prosthetic valves have subsequently appeared.

In 1956, Murray demonstrated that the aortic valve could be used as a valve transplant in the descending thoracic aorta in patients with aortic regurgitation,[M15] and a subsequent report by Kerwin and colleagues included 6-year follow-up.[K13] The first orthotopic insertions of an *allograft valve* using the double-suture-line technique were performed in 1962 by Barratt-Boyes and separately by Ross using a single-suture-line technique described by Duran and Gunning.[B27,D7,R10] At first, cadaveric valves were collected aseptically and implanted within a few days or weeks, but for logistic reasons this technique was soon replaced by unsterile collection and sterilization by beta-propiolactone, ethylene oxide, or irradiation.[H11,K12,P7] The allografts were then stored either in Hanks' balanced salt solution at 4°C or frozen and dried.[B26] In 1968, because of high occurrence of cusp rupture with these techniques, antibiotic sterilization was introduced.[B6] Cryopreservation, rather than wet preservation, was introduced in 1975 by O'Brien and colleagues.[O5] Yacoub and colleagues and Ross and colleagues expanded the use of allografts to include combined aortic valve and ascending aorta replacement.[D9,G9,R12]

In 1967, Ross and colleagues introduced the *pulmonary autograft* for aortic valve replacement,[G5,R3] after Lower and colleagues had shown the feasibility of the procedure experimentally in 1960.[L6] Subsequently, the pulmonary valve and artery were introduced as *autograft composite conduits* (cylinders) for replacing the aortic valve and ascending aorta.[R15]

Other biologic valves were introduced. Senning, in Zurich, replaced the aortic valve clinically with individual leaflets made of the patients' fascia lata.[S17] Because of high late postoperative occurrence of infective endocarditis, however, this method was abandoned. Use of autologous fascia lata mounted on a frame was described by Ionescu and Ross but abandoned because of late dehiscence.[I4] Allograft dura mater valves, stent-mounted and preserved in glycerol, were used for aortic valve replacement by Zerbini and colleagues in Brazil.[P5] Bovine pericardium, glutaraldehyde treated and frame mounted, was introduced by Ionescu and colleagues at Leeds, England, in 1971.[I5]

In 1965, Binet and colleagues in Paris implanted porcine aortic valves, sterilized and preserved in a special formaldehyde solution, directly into the aortic root.[B18] The valves degenerated rapidly, most likely because of suboptimal tissue preservation. This led to abandonment of direct xenograft valve implantation in favor of xenograft valves mounted on a stent-mounted frame. *Stent-mounted bioprostheses* are manufactured to provide a standard device that is easily implanted and provides reproducible results in the aortic position. Glutaraldehyde-preserved stent-mounted porcine valves were introduced by Carpentier and colleagues in Paris in 1967.[C3]

David and colleagues revived the concept of direct insertion of nonstented porcine xenografts into the aortic root.[D1] This valve was manufactured on a limited trial basis by Hancock Laboratory and by St. Jude Medical as the *Toronto SPV* (stentless porcine valve).

MORPHOLOGY

Aortic Valve Stenosis

Calcific Aortic Stenosis (Congenital)

Calcific aortic stenosis implies stenosis secondary to heavy dystrophic calcification of a congenitally abnormal valve (Fig. 12-1, *A* and *B*). Calcification is rarely present before age 20; thereafter it is slowly progressive and results in important stenosis, most often in the fifth and sixth decades of life, earlier in unicommissural than bicuspid valves, and earlier in men than women.[S19] The calcification presents as a bulky cauliflower-like mass within the leaflets, maximal at sites of commissural fusion or congenital buttress formation, often extending into the anulus (left ventricular–aortic junction) and adjacent aorta. Retrograde extension of calcification into the region beneath the right–noncoronary cusp commissure adjacent to the membranous septum may lead to complete heart block. The valvar orifice is slitlike, often eccentrically located and oriented in a sagittal (most often) or transverse plane, and fixed, which often results in trivial or mild aortic regurgitation. (For a detailed description of bicuspid, tricuspid, or unicommissural congenital aortic stenosis, see "Morphology" under Congenital Valvar Aortic Stenosis in Section 1 of Chapter 33.)

Rheumatic Aortic Stenosis

Rheumatic aortic stenosis is characterized primarily by diffuse, prominent fibrous leaflet thickening of a trileaflet valve (Fig. 12-1, *C*), with fusion to a variable extent of one or two commissures (rarely all three).[S19] The orifice is approximately central and is irregular in shape. Calcification other than a mild form is rarely present except in elderly patients, but is bulkiest at sites of commissural fusion. Rheumatic aortic stenosis is seldom if ever isolated, although at the

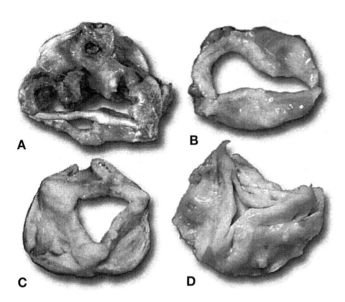

Figure 12-1   Morphology of aortic valve stenosis. **A,** Calcific aortic stenosis (congenital bicuspid valve). Valve is bicuspid due to fusion of one of the commissures. Calcification is bulky within the cusps. **B,** Calcific aortic stenosis (congenital unicuspid valve). Valve has only one open commissure. Calcification is not severe in this example. **C,** Rheumatic aortic stenosis. This morphology is characterized by diffuse fibrosis in leaflets of a tricuspid valve. Cusp edges are thick and rolled. Commissural fusion is variable, but is severe in this example. Calcification is mild. **D,** Degenerative aortic stenosis. Valve is tricuspid and without commissural fusion. Calcification occurs in diffuse nodular or eggshell deposits, which stiffen the valve and prevent opening. Calcification may involve the sinuses of Valsalva or ascending aorta. Degenerative aortic stenosis usually occurs in patients over age 65.

patient's first operation this may appear to be the case. In surgical series of apparently isolated aortic stenosis, prevalence of rheumatic etiology is low compared with that when patients with important mitral valve disease are included.

About half of patients with so-called rheumatic aortic stenosis fail to report a history of rheumatic fever, suggesting other unrecognized inflammatory processes as the cause.[P6] However, with the decline in known prevalence of rheumatic fever in the United States and other developed countries, rheumatic aortic stenosis decreased from a prevalence of 30% to 18% by the 1980s (and senile degenerative disease increased from 30% to 46%).[P3]

Degenerative Aortic Stenosis

Degenerative disease is often present in stenotic aortic valves of patients over age 65, and its prevalence increases with age. In a series of patients with mean age greater than 70, prevalence of degenerative aortic valve stenosis exceeded 70%.[K26] The valve is tricuspid, without commissural fusion; the leaflets are held in a closed position by deposits of diffuse nodular or eggshell calcification (Fig. 12-1, *D*). These deposits are not bulky and may also involve the sinuses of Valsalva and ascending aorta. Although degenerative (senile) aortic stenosis is presumed to be atheromatous,[W16] Hoagland and colleagues found no correlation between aortic stenosis in adults over age 50

and systemic hypertension, elevated serum cholesterol, smoking, or diabetes.[H12] A more recent study in 5201 subjects over age 65, however, found that clinical factors associated with aortic sclerosis and stenosis are similar to risk factors for atherosclerosis.[S26] Aortic valve sclerosis was present in 26% and aortic valve stenosis in 2% of the entire study cohort. In patients over age 75 the prevalence of aortic sclerosis was 37% and stenosis 2.6%. Smoking increased the risk by 35% and hypertension by 20%. Other factors associated with increased risk of aortic valve disease were high lipoproteins and low-density cholesterol levels. Age was directly associated with risk, with a twofold increase in risk for each 10-year increase in age.

Mitral anular calcification is common in elderly patients with calcific aortic stenosis.[N4] Presumably, both are degenerative in origin.

Aortic Valve Regurgitation

Morphologic characteristics of aortic regurgitation depend on etiology. These characteristics are not as easily categorized as in aortic stenosis. The terms *aortic regurgitation, aortic incompetence,* and *aortic insufficiency* are used interchangeably. *Regurgitation* is the preferred and most descriptive term.

Rheumatic Aortic Regurgitation

Rheumatic aortic regurgitation results from a different response of the valve to the rheumatic process than occurs when stenosis develops. Commissural fusion is minimal or absent, and the leaflets are only slightly thickened. Minor calcification is present in about 10% of affected valves. The major pathologic process is cicatricial shortening of the cusps between their free edge and their anular attachment, with rolling of the free edge. As time passes the aortic root widens in response to the regurgitation, increasing central valvar regurgitation further.

Anuloaortic Ectasia

Anuloaortic ectasia can produce valvar regurgitation of varying but sometimes severe degree, even though the cusps are normal. It is becoming a more common cause of regurgitation in surgical series.[O6] Anuloaortic ectasia is most often caused by cystic medial degeneration of the aorta and may be associated with *Marfan syndrome*. Even in the absence of Marfan syndrome, anuloaortic ectasia appears to be a genetic disease.[S18]

The process begins in the sinuses of Valsalva; at this stage, regurgitation is usually not present. With time the process extends to involve the proximal ascending aorta, producing a symmetric, pear-shaped aneurysmal enlargement. Regurgitation now appears and progresses because dilatation of the aortic wall at the sinotubular junction separates the commissures and tightens the free cusp edges, preventing coaptation during diastole. As dilatation of the aorta progresses, central aortic valve regurgitation increases. The left ventricular–aortic junction usually does not increase in size, even in patients with large aneurysms associated with anuloaortic ectasia. Size of the aortic valve prosthesis used in these patients (if indicated) is generally similar to that used for replacement in patients with rheumatic or other disease.[G15]

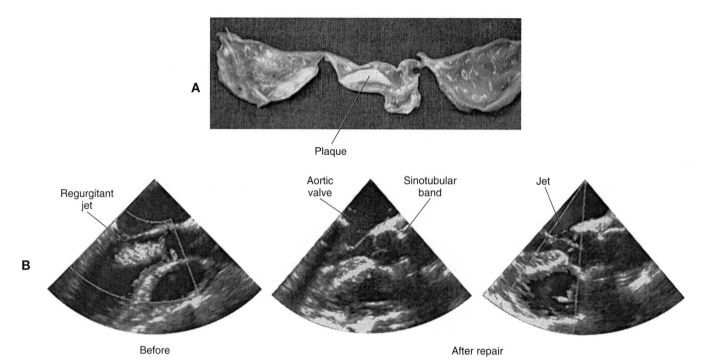

Figure 12-2   Iatrogenic aortic valve disease. Aortic valve regurgitation caused by physician intervention. **A,** Aortic valve affected by fenfluramine/phentermine (Fen/Phen). One cusp is contracted due to a fibrotic plaque. The other two cusps are normal. **B,** Echocardiogram of Fen/Phen iatrogenic aortic valve disease. A regurgitant jet indicates moderately severe aortic valve regurgitation before repair. Repair consisted of debridement of fibrotic plaques from the valve cusps and narrowing of the sinotubular junction by a prosthetic band. After repair, there is trivial aortic valve regurgitation.

The aneurysmal process eventually involves the entire ascending aorta, but usually stops just before the level at which the innominate artery originates, although the remainder of the arch may show cystic medial degeneration. The aneurysms are thin walled with a smooth lining. Dissection may begin within the aneurysms, extending proximally and distally or remaining localized (although most acute aortic dissections occur in the absence of an aortic root aneurysm). In patients with Marfan syndrome, about 30% of those operated on for anuloaortic ectasia and aneurysm of the ascending aorta have an aortic dissection. It is limited to the ascending aorta in about half the patients and extends into the transverse and descending aorta in the rest.[G6] Frequently, dissection is unexpectedly found at operation. With proximal extension of this dissection, the commissural attachment of the valve becomes separated from the outer aortic wall such that the valve prolapses centrally, and regurgitation may abruptly increase (see Chapter 52).

Native Valve Endocarditis

Native valve endocarditis, which may occur on a structurally normal valve or on congenitally or rheumatically deformed valves, is a common cause of aortic regurgitation. The regurgitation may result from a destroyed commissure and consequent cusp prolapse or from a perforation in the belly of the cusp. An infected pannus may appear below the cusps, or extensive destruction of the aortic root may occur, with a periaortic root abscess sometimes extending into the mitral anulus and anterior mitral leaflet. Mitral regurgita-

tion may also develop because of perforation of the anterior leaflet by a "drop lesion" caused by the infected regurgitant stream from the diseased aortic valve.

Congenital Aortic Valve Disease

A congenitally bicuspid or unicuspid valve can produce regurgitation from prolapse of the free edge of a redundant cusp.[R8] In such patients the regurgitation may be aggravated by infective endocarditis or an improper valvotomy (see Chapter 33). Lack of support of the aortic anulus in association with ventricular septal defect may result in aortic valve prolapse and regurgitation (see Chapter 21).

Floppy Aortic Valve

Occasionally, aortic regurgitation may be caused by prolapse of redundant aortic leaflets that are mildly thickened and myxomatous. The aortic root may be normal or dilated, usually with cystic medial necrosis, and mitral valve prolapse may also occur.[B36,W9]

Iatrogenic Aortic Valve Disease

Aortic valve regurgitation may be caused by a number of physician-related interventions. Perforation of the aortic valve cusps may result from diagnostic or balloon dilatation catheters. Even with newer methods and lower doses of mediastinal irradiation, occasional cases of mediastinal fibrosis occur, with injury to the pericardium, cardiac valves, coronary arteries, and myocardium. Cardiac valve disease has also been associated with migraine medications (ergotamine, methysergide) and appetite suppressants (fen-

■ TABLE 12-1   Time-Related Changes in Aortic Valve Morphology at Operation *ᵃ*

Morphology	AS (pure)		AS/AR (mixed)		AR (pure)	
	1965	1990	1965	1990	1965	1990
Bicuspid (congenital) (%)	49	36	20	17	17	14
Rheumatic (%)	33	9	61	17	47	14
Degenerative (%)	0	51	0	46	0	0
Dilatation ascending aorta (%)	0	0	0	0	19	50
Iatrogenic (%)	0	1	0	13	0	14
Infective endocarditis (%)	0	0	0	0	11	2
Other (%)	18	3	19	7	6	6
Patients (%)	32	65	39	10	29	25

(Data from William D. Edwards, MD, based on references D18, O6, P3, S19, and S25 and on surgical patients at the Mayo Clinic.)

Key: *AR,* Aortic regurgitation; *AS,* aortic stenosis; *AS/AR,* aortic stenosis and aortic regurgitation.

ᵃ Data presented as percent of the total number of patients in each category.

fluramine, with or without phentermine) (Fig. 12-2).[C40] Iatrogenic valve disease occurs unpredictably and depends on local availability and use of the causative agents.

Atherosclerotic and Syphilitic Ascending Aortic Aneurysms

Ascending aortic aneurysms also produce valvar regurgitation because of tightening of the free edges of the leaflets that results from aortic dilatation. In syphilitic ascending aortic aneurysm, aortic regurgitation is exacerbated by a valvulitis that produces thickening and retraction of the cusp edge. Neither condition, however, is generally associated with aortic dissection.

Aortitis

In some patients with rheumatoid arthritis, ankylosing spondylitis,[S4] or Reiter disease, an aortitis occurs that may lead to aneurysmal dilatation of the ascending aorta and aortic valvar regurgitation.[K10] The aortitis is characterized by dense adventitial inflammatory fibrosis involving the sinuses of Valsalva and proximal aorta, especially adjacent to the commissures.[B17] The process may extend below the base of the aortic valve to form a characteristic subvalvar ridge and may involve the base of the anterior mitral cusp or even the adjacent ventricular septum, causing conduction disturbances. Particularly in rheumatoid arthritis, the cusps may be thickened and shortened and may show rheumatoid nodules histologically.[R11]

Other Types of Aortic Regurgitation

Other causes of aortic valve regurgitation include spontaneous cusp rupture,[O2] rupture caused by severe closed-chest trauma,[M7,R13] and severe long-standing systemic hypertension with aortic root dilatation. In patients with long-standing hypertension, regurgitation may result from typical myxoid degeneration of the valve.[A5,L11,T6] Some instances of regurgitation are probably related to arthropathies with minimal joint involvement or to hypertension, psoriasis, giant cell aortitis,[G9] or Takayasu disease.

Occasionally the etiology of regurgitation may not be apparent.

Combined Aortic Stenosis and Regurgitation

The etiology and morphology of combined aortic stenosis and regurgitation are similar to those for aortic valve stenosis. In some cases an episode of endocarditis produces regurgitation in a previously stenotic valve.

Changing Etiology and Morphology

A time-related change in etiology and morphology has been observed at operation in patients with aortic valve disease. Although the overall prevalence of bicuspid aortic valves in the general population has not changed over the past 50 years,[S24] its relative frequency in the surgical population has decreased (Table 12-1). In surgical patients at the Mayo Clinic the relative frequency of bicuspid aortic valves fell from 49% in 1965 to 36% in 1990.[D18,S25] The relative frequency of patients with degenerative aortic valve disease increased greatly, however, and the prevalence of aortic stenosis doubled, from 32% to 65%. Mean age at operation increased from 49 years in 1965 to 66 years in 1990.[D18,O6,P3,S19,S25]

CLINICAL FEATURES AND DIAGNOSTIC CRITERIA

Aortic Stenosis

Patients with aortic stenosis are usually symptomatic when first seen. They may present without symptoms, however, having been referred because of a cardiac murmur. The classic triad of effort dyspnea, angina, and syncope is present in about one third of patients.[E5]

Angina pectoris is present as the only symptom or is combined with others in 50% to 70% of patients.[B7,E1] It is more common in patients with combined aortic stenosis and coronary artery disease than in those with isolated aortic stenosis.[L12] Angina in patients without coronary artery disease presumably results from an imbalance between coronary blood flow and oxygen demand in the hypertrophied left ventricle (LV). Angina appears to occur more frequently in patients with severe aortic stenosis than in those with less severe gradients across the aortic valve. Other morphologic and hemodynamic variables, such as LV wall thickness, wall stress, and wall tension, are similar in patients with aortic stenosis whether or not angina is present.[B7,B10]

From 30% to 50% of patients with important aortic stenosis have frank or incipient syncope. Among the many possible causes of syncope (and sudden death) in patients with aortic stenosis, the most likely is peripheral vasodilatation from a faulty baroreceptor mechanism.[J3] Symptoms of pulmonary venous hypertension (dyspnea, orthopnea, paroxysmal nocturnal dyspnea, or frank pulmonary edema) are present in 30% to 40% of patients, either alone or with other symptoms. These symptoms are associated with increased LV end-diastolic pressure and systolic wall stress and lower cardiac output and ejection fraction (EF).[D4]

A few patients (10%) survive typical symptoms long enough for secondary *right ventricular failure* to develop. These patients present with a clinical picture dominated by elevated right atrial and jugular venous pressure, hepatomegaly, cardiac cachexia, and rarely, tricuspid regurgitation. Patients often appear to have combined aortic stenosis and mitral regurgitation as well, even though this is not the case.

Diagnosis of important aortic stenosis can often be made by physical examination with reasonable certainty when, in addition to the presence of an aortic ejection murmur (usually best heard in the second right intercostal space beside the sternum and conducted to the carotids, but also often at the apex and in the second left intercostal space), the arterial pulse is of small volume with a slow upstroke. Support for the diagnosis may be obtained from expiratory splitting of the second heart sound and from evidence of LV hypertrophy provided by the character of the apex beat and electrocardiogram (ECG). Usually the ECG provides evidence of LV hypertrophy, with or without inverted T waves in lead V_6 (the so-called strain pattern). When chest radiography or fluoroscopy also shows calcification of the aortic valve and convexity along the upper part of the LV silhouette produced by LV hypertrophy, the diagnosis of calcific aortic stenosis becomes a near certainty.[E1]

At times, physical findings are less diagnostic. Systemic hypertension or, in older patients, inelasticity of aortic and arterial walls may alter the character of the arterial pulse wave and prevent development of a clinically recognizable slow upstroke or soft, weak pulse (pulsus parvus). Absence of the aortic component may prevent assessment of the respiratory behavior of the second heart sound, whereas in patients with right or left bundle branch block, splitting of this sound is of no value as a guide to the severity of aortic stenosis. In older patients especially, the character of the cardiac apex may be unreliable as a clinical guide to presence and degree of LV hypertrophy. The ECG also may fail to show the degree of LV hypertrophy associated with severe aortic stenosis and occasionally remains normal without showing evidence of LV involvement.

In these patients, judicious use of graded exercise testing may uncover a clinically silent state of LV dysfunction and functional aerobic impairment.[C30] Exercise has generally been considered dangerous in patients with severe aortic valve stenosis because of effort syncope. Experience has shown, however, that graded exercise testing is not a risky procedure in asymptomatic patients with aortic stenosis.[O10] Impaired exercise tolerance, occurrence of symptoms, inadequate blood pressure increase (10 mmHg · 30 watts^{-1} or less) or blood pressure drop (10 mmHg or greater), bradycardia, arrhythmia, conduction disturbance, and ST-segment depression (0.2 mV or more) indicate impaired aerobic or LV function. This information may be helpful in deciding on operative intervention or, if continued observation is advised, recommendations concerning vocational, recreational, or sports participation. Finally, in the terminal stages of low-output heart failure, the murmur may be so faint that aortic stenosis is not suspected, particularly in adult patients in whom the heart sounds are distant either because of chest wall thickness or inelastic and voluminous lungs.

When the clinical findings are classic, diagnosis of severe aortic stenosis can be made with a high degree of confidence, and special studies are not needed.[E1] *Doppler echocardiography* is a reliable means of establishing the presence of aortic stenosis and is usually performed in patients suspected of having aortic valve disease. In most patients with aortic stenosis, the degree of obstruction to outflow, aortic valve peak, mean gradient, and valve area can be reliably determined.[N8] Maximal instantaneous gradient is obtained by applying the modified Bernoulli equation to peak aortic velocity; this may be 30% to 40% higher than peak-to-peak gradient determined by cardiac catheterization. Mean gradient is more useful clinically and is obtained from the Doppler velocity curve at multiple intervals by converting instantaneous velocity to instantaneous pressure gradient. *Mean pressure gradient* is the arithmetic mean of the derived instantaneous gradients; it correlates well with mean pressure gradient obtained by cardiac catheterization. *Aortic valve area* may also be determined by echocardiography based on the continuity principle, which states that flow through a nonstenotic region of the heart should equal flow through a stenosis (assuming no regurgitation or shunt). Aortic valve area derived by cardiac catheterization is well correlated with this.[O9]

Hemodynamic data derived by Doppler echocardiography or cardiac catheterization can provide a grading of degree of stenosis. The aortic valve area must be reduced to one fourth its normal size before important changes occur in the circulation.[B46] The normal adult aortic valve area is 3.0 to 4.0 cm^2. Thus, an area 0.75 to 1.0 cm^2 may not be considered severely stenotic. Unless indexed to body size, these arbitrary limits may not provide a correct indication of stenosis severity. The American College of Cardiology/American Heart Association (ACC/AHA) Task Force on Practice Guidelines agrees that aortic valve stenosis is *mild* when aortic valve area is 1.5 cm^2 or greater, *moderate* when 1.0 to 1.5 cm^2, and *severe* when 1.0 cm^2 or less.[B46] Because pressure gradient is flow dependent, stenosis is considered severe when the gradient is 50 mmHg or higher and cardiac output is normal.[C6,W10] These hemodynamic criteria are helpful, but therapeutic decisions related to operative intervention are largely based on presence or absence of symptoms.

In patients over age 40, *coronary arteriography* is also performed when operation is being considered, because coronary artery disease coexists in many of these patients whether or not angina is present.[B10,G16,M3] At the time of coronary arteriography, systolic pressure gradient across the aortic valve is measured. Cardiac output can be measured and the valve area calculated by the Gorlin equation.

Aortic Regurgitation

Patients with aortic regurgitation present more frequently without symptoms than those with aortic stenosis, perhaps because of the more dramatic physical and radiographic findings and relatively long asymptomatic phase of regurgitation. In most patients the dominant symptoms reflect pulmonary venous hypertension (dyspnea, orthopnea, paroxysmal nocturnal dyspnea, pulmonary edema). Angina pectoris is often part of the presenting complaint, but is the chief complaint in less than one fourth of patients[B7,G2,S3] and is more common in older patients. Coronary artery disease is present in about 20% of patients with angina pectoris.[B7] Syncope is rare.

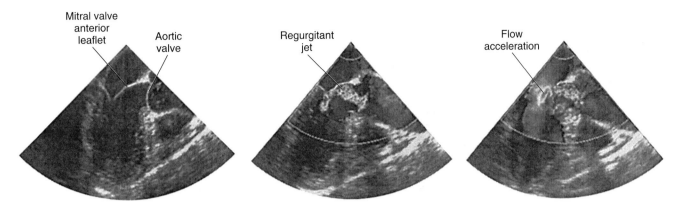

Figure 12-3   Echocardiogram of aortic valve regurgitation with Austin Flint murmur. Regurgitant jet through aortic valve is directed toward anterior leaflet of mitral valve, preventing complete opening during diastole. Thus, the mitral valve is held in semi-closed position during ventricular diastole (aortic valve is closed), causing partial obstruction of mitral valve orifice. Flow acceleration (and turbulence) through mitral valve orifice indicates obstruction to blood flow, resulting in the characteristic Austin Flint diastolic mitral valve murmur.

In severe aortic regurgitation, the LV apex is normally displaced and overactive in character. The carotid and other pulses are jerky to palpation in moderate regurgitation and collapsing or "water hammer" in severe regurgitation because of the wide pulse pressure and rapid rise and fall of the pulse wave. Blood pressure measured by Korotkoff sounds may reach 200 to 250 mmHg systolic and 50 to 0 mmHg diastolic. Normally brachial or radial pulse pressure measured by an arterial needle is less than that measured by Korotkoff sounds, and central aortic pulse pressure is even less. These phenomena, including systolic amplification between central aortic and radial artery blood pressures, are related to standing waves created by the pulsatile ejection of an unusually large LV stroke volume into the aorta and remainder of the arterial tree. If cardiac output is low because of severe cardiac failure, these phenomena are minimal.

Auscultation in the aortic area reveals an early diastolic murmur that radiates toward the apex of the heart. Intensity of the murmur has been shown to correlate with degree of aortic valve regurgitation.[D19] Murmur grade 3 or greater predicts severe aortic regurgitation in 71% of patients, whereas murmur grade 1 or less predicts that aortic regurgitation is not severe in 100% of patients. Often a systolic click or ejection murmur is present as well. At the apex a mid-diastolic murmur is frequently caused by fluttering of the anterior mitral leaflet from a prominent regurgitant jet *(Austin Flint murmur)*. This may be difficult to distinguish from the murmur of mitral stenosis, although in the latter an opening snap is often present. When mitral stenosis coexists, the ECG usually shows P mitrale and the left atrium is enlarged, although in severe and long-standing pure aortic regurgitation, the ECG may also show P mitrale. Two-dimensional echocardiography is useful in making the distinction between mitral stenosis and merely an Austin Flint murmur (Fig. 12-3). The chest radiograph confirms LV enlargement; the left atrium is usually normal or slightly enlarged. Radiographic evidence of pulmonary venous hypertension may or may not be present. Enlargement of the shadow of the ascending aorta to the right suggests an accompanying aneurysm of the ascending

aorta, but an aneurysm can be present without this sign. The ECG shows evidence of LV enlargement, often with the high-peaked T waves and prominent Q waves of LV volume overload. T wave inversion and ST-segment depression are seldom present until the LV is extremely large.

Diagnosis of aortic valve regurgitation can usually be made on the clinical findings, but other abnormalities in the aortic root allowing a rapid aortic runoff (such as ruptured sinus of Valsalva aneurysm and large patent ductus arteriosus with pulmonary valve regurgitation) cannot be entirely eliminated without special studies. Color flow Doppler echocardiography firmly establishes the diagnosis.

Doppler echocardiography can be used to quantify aortic valve regurgitation. Measurements are made of *regurgitant volume* (volume regurgitated per heartbeat) and of *regurgitant fraction* (proportion of total ejection of the LV). These measurements are highly dependent on technical experience, with overestimation the rule at first. Size of the jet visualized by color Doppler echocardiography may not represent the degree of aortic regurgitation. It is possible to measure the *vena contracta,* which is the size of the regurgitant jet within the regurgitant aortic valve orifice. This measurement correlates well with effective regurgitant orifice size. The width of the vena contracta just below the flow convergence is measured using the parasternal long axis view.[T8] Vena contracta of 7 mm or greater uniformly favor severe aortic valve regurgitation, whereas measurements of 5 mm or less correspond to less regurgitation. The degree of aortic regurgitation may also be quantified by cineangiography using an aortic root contrast injection in the right anterior oblique projection, but this method is difficult and often unreliable.

Coronary arteriography is indicated in patients over age 40.

Combined Aortic Stenosis and Regurgitation

Although many patients with severe aortic stenosis have mild regurgitation and a few patients with severe regurgitation have some stenosis, a small group of patients have virtually balanced lesions. Their symptoms are generally similar to those associated with aortic stenosis. This group may have a particularly unfavorable prognosis because there is both volume and pressure overload on the LV.

NATURAL HISTORY

Aortic Stenosis

The natural history of adults with aortic valve disease is incompletely known, although it is evident that severity of the stenosis gradually increases. Synthesis of four echocardiographic studies indicates that the average rate of decrease in aortic valve area is about 0.12 cm^2 per year.[B47,F9,O10,R20] Aortic stenosis appears to progress more rapidly in patients with degenerative disease than in those with congenital or rheumatic etiology.[B46] A complicating factor is that some degree of stenosis may have existed in childhood, often with associated regurgitation. The natural history in these patients may be more favorable than when the disease develops de novo and more rapidly later in life.

Survival

Grant reported that 35% of unoperated patients with usual symptoms of aortic stenosis are alive at 10 years.[G1] Wood stated that 46% of such patients were alive 1 to 7 years later.[W3] Frank and Ross reported that of 12 unoperated patients with severe aortic stenosis, only 18% were alive 5 years later.[F1] Based on their data, Ross and Braunwald concluded that average survival after onset of angina or syncope is 3 years and after onset of heart failure about 1½ years.[R1] ACC/AHA guidelines suggest that after onset of symptoms, average survival is less than 2 to 3 years.[B46] Thus, development of symptoms identifies a critical point in the natural history of aortic stenosis. O'Keefe and colleagues followed 50 symptomatic patients with severe aortic stenosis in whom operation was declined or deferred.[O7] Average age of these patients was 77 (60 to 89) years. Survival was 55%, 37%, and 25% at 1, 2, and 3 years, respectively, compared with a matched general population of 93%, 85%, and 77%. Death was from cardiac causes in all cases except one.

Although it is impossible to assemble such disparate data rigorously, a likely survival curve for adult patients with severe, unoperated aortic stenosis is estimated in Fig. 12-4. Deaths within the first 1 or 2 years are likely to be sudden, presumably associated with ventricular fibrillation (15% to 20% of all deaths in aortic stenosis are sudden[F1]) or, after a few hours or days of acute pulmonary edema, from sudden LV failure. Most unoperated patients die in the latter mode within about 5 years of diagnosis. Beyond 5 years of follow-up, some die of gradually worsening cardiac failure, with low cardiac output and gradually worsening symptoms of pulmonary venous hypertension. Moderate pulmonary artery hypertension develops in some patients who exhibit these findings; in a few, typical symptoms and signs of *right* ventricular failure become prominent.

Asymptomatic patients with severe aortic stenosis usually develop symptoms within a few years of diagnosis. Otto and colleagues showed that about one fourth of initially asymptomatic patients with aortic valve stenosis had developed symptoms,[O10] half by 3 years and three fourths by 4 years. When the Doppler outflow

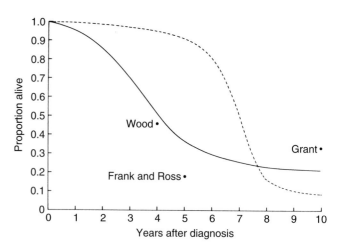

Figure 12-4   Nonrigorously derived survival curves for patients with surgically untreated severe aortic stenosis (*solid line*) and severe aortic regurgitation (*dashed line*). Time zero is the time of developing an important hemodynamic effect. Survival of patients with aortic stenosis reported by Wood,[W3] Frank and Ross,[F1] and Grant[G1] is shown by filled circles.

velocities were initially 4.0 m · s^{-1} or greater, progression was more rapid, with three fourths of patients symptomatic by 2 years. Thus, even in initially asymptomatic patients with aortic stenosis, progression to symptoms may be rapid, and patients should be monitored closely for progressive disease. Sudden death is uncommon in asymptomatic patients with aortic stenosis, occurring in less than 1% per year.[B46]

Left Ventricular Structure and Function

The LV hypertrophies progressively in the presence of important aortic stenosis. The resultant increase in LV mass that develops by the time of operation has complex interrelationships with systolic wall function.[K4] Schwartz and colleagues found good systolic function and only hypertrophic myocardial cells when the LV mass was less than 200 g · m^{-2}.[S7] When LV mass was 200 to 300 g · m^{-2}, degenerative changes were present, but mild. When LV mass was greater than 300 g · m^{-2}, systolic function was greatly depressed and multiple degenerative changes in ultrastructure were present (mitochondrial changes, disruption of sarcomeric units, nonoriented growth of fiber components, disappearance of organelles).[S7] Maron and colleagues also described these degenerative changes in detail.[M2] Krayenbuehl and colleagues found degenerative changes in the form of increased interstitial nonmuscular tissue in association with myocardial cellular hypertrophy.[K23] These changes are probably the morphologic basis for loss of inotropic (contractile) strength and irreversibility.

Myocardial hypertrophy in aortic valve stenosis is caused by new myofibrils added in parallel to myocytes. No new myocytes are added, but existing myocytes become thicker, not longer, compared with normal myocytes. The hypertrophy of myocardial cells (increased myocardial cell diameter) is a determinant of both increased systolic load stress and decreased LV diastolic function found in aortic stenosis,[S12] and is also related to reduction in EF.[K23] Myocardial fibrosis exerts little effect.

Thickening of the LV wall keeps LV afterload (systolic wall stress) more or less normal (see "Ventricular Afterload" under Cardiac Output and Its Determinants in Section 1 of Chapter 5), preserving LV systolic function. LV compliance and diastolic function are gradually impaired, to a degree primarily related to extent of LV hypertrophy.[F2] At a more advanced stage, hypertrophy and wall thickness may increase less than LV systolic pressure (afterload mismatch[R2]); the resulting increase in afterload impairs LV systolic function. However, the degree of LV hypertrophy and decrease in contractility that ultimately develop are more often the cause of declining cardiac function.[W5] Indices of systolic function (EF, end-systolic volume, LV fractional shortening, velocity of circumferential shortening) decline, cardiac output decreases gradually or acutely, and LV diastolic function decreases with a consequent increase in LV end-diastolic pressure.[G7,S12] By this time the condition is advanced, and chronic heart failure is present.

Occasionally, complete heart block develops in patients with extensive calcification of the stenotic aortic valve. It may be the result of gradually increasing pressure on the bundle of His by calcific deposits beneath the commissural area between the noncoronary and right coronary cusps.[W6] However, complete heart block sometimes occurs without calcific pressure on the bundle of His.[L5] Pressure in the LV is hypothesized to play a role. Rarely, relief of aortic stenosis relieves the heart block.[P4]

Aortic Regurgitation

Aortic regurgitation may develop acutely or more gradually as a chronic condition. Acute-onset of severe regurgitation imposes a sudden large regurgitant volume on the LV, which has been normal.[B46] There is little time to accommodate to the volume load, and LV end-diastolic and left atrial pressures increase rapidly. Tachycardia is the primary compensatory mechanism but may be insufficient, and the clinical situation may quickly deteriorate to pulmonary edema and circulatory shock.

Patients presenting with chronic aortic regurgitation have combined volume and pressure overload of the LV.[B46] Compensatory mechanisms are primarily recruitment of preload reserve and LV hypertrophy. Most patients remain asymptomatic through a long compensatory phase that may last for decades.[B46]

The natural history of patients with aortic regurgitation depends primarily on its severity.[H5] Mild or moderate aortic regurgitation appears to affect activity and life expectancy minimally. LV structure and function begin to be adversely affected, symptoms develop, and prognosis becomes more limited as severity of the aortic regurgitation increases.

Survival

Even when aortic regurgitation becomes severe, there may be a long latent period, 3 to 10 years, during which LV enlargement is only mild, symptoms are absent or mild,[S1] and the prognosis is good as long as the findings remain unchanged. Bonow and colleagues followed patients with chronic aortic regurgitation and normal EF.[B37] They found that 81% were alive and without need of aortic valve replacement 5 years later. Less than 6% per year required aortic valve replacement because of symptoms or LV dysfunction at rest, less than 3.5% per year developed asymptomatic LV systolic dysfunction, and less than 0.2% per year died suddenly. Vasodilator therapy using nifedipine may benefit such patients and delay surgical intervention.[S29] When important symptoms develop, however, prognosis becomes severely limited (see Fig. 12-4).

The probability of death increases with development of specific risk factors. Symptoms of cardiac failure, development of ventricular premature beats, marked cardiomegaly (cardiothoracic ratio greater than 0.6), and ECG evidence of severe LV hypertrophy all increased the risk of death in a group of 180 surgically untreated patients with isolated severe aortic regurgitation of rheumatic etiology.[S8]

When severe aortic regurgitation develops acutely, as from infective endocarditis, the natural history is much less favorable.[R16] Only 10% to 30% survive more than 1 year after onset.[D5,H5,T2]

Left Ventricular Structure and Function

Cardiac size gradually increases in the presence of important aortic regurgitation.[B14] Quantitative angiography has shown that increased LV end-diastolic volume is directly related to magnitude of aortic regurgitant flow.[M5]

Bonow and colleagues found a higher risk subgroup within patients who are asymptomatic and have normal LV systolic function.[B37] Progressive enlargement (dilatation) of the LV or reduction in resting EF identified by serial echocardiography heralds onset of symptoms. Patients at risk for sudden death are those with extreme LV dilatation or an LV cavity dimension of 80 mm or more at end-diastole and 55 mm or more at end-systole (normal values are ≤55 mm and ≤35 mm, respectively). As LV size and end-diastolic volume steadily increase, eventually there is a loss of LV reserve, and LV end-diastolic pressure then rises rapidly.

As the LV enlarges, LV hypertrophy begins to develop.[S8] In addition, the LV undergoes an increase in mass and wall thickness, and its shape and ultrastructure change.[P2] The myocardial cell hypertrophy and increase in interstitial nonmuscular tissue found in the pressure-overloaded LV of aortic stenosis are similar in the volume-overloaded LV of aortic regurgitation.[K23] Concomitant with hypertrophy, LV compliance decreases, compromising diastolic function. Finally, LV end-diastolic and left atrial pressures become elevated, with further increases during exercise.[K14]

At some point, LV stroke work fails to respond to increased wall stress (such as afterload increase by infusion of angiotensin). As LV systolic function decreases, LV end-systolic dimension steadily increases, and even in asymptomatic patients the rate of increase is about 7 mmHg per year.[H4]

Despite these changes and because of the complex interaction between aortic regurgitation and decreasing systemic vascular resistance, LV EF response to exercise is favorable for a considerable time. Eventually, however, it declines, and systolic function may even decrease during stress. Symptoms then worsen, and the decline in LV function accelerates.

TECHNIQUE OF OPERATION

Isolated Aortic Valve Replacement

Initial Steps

After the usual preparations and median sternotomy, cardiopulmonary bypass (CPB) is established at 34°C using a single two-stage venous cannula. A cardioplegia infusion catheter is positioned in the ascending aorta, and a coronary sinus perfusion catheter is passed through a purse-string stitch in the right atrium and positioned in the coronary sinus. The cardioplegic infusion catheter, on one arm of a Y assembly on the cardioplegic infusion tubing filled with cardioplegic solution, is positioned in the ascending aorta. The other arm of the Y assembly, now clamped, also has two arms. One is connected to a second Y assembly, on each arm of which is an O-ring cannula to be used for direct cardioplegic infusion into the coronary ostia. The other arm is attached to the coronary sinus retrograde perfusion catheter (see "Technique of Retrograde Infusion" in Chapter 3).

Perfusate temperature is lowered and adjusted to 25°C. Body temperature is brought to 28°C. The ascending aorta is occluded, promptly if ventricular fibrillation occurs to prevent distention of the LV. The operation may be performed without a vent; alternatively, a vent may be introduced into the left atrium from the right side through the right superior pulmonary vein and advanced into the LV. The vent catheter may be introduced before aortic occlusion if ventricular fibrillation occurs. Antegrade cold blood cardioplegia may then be infused into the aortic root provided there is no aortic regurgitation. Even the slightest leak at the aortic valve will cause ventricular filling, although a properly functioning LV vent may prevent ventricular distention. Subsequent to cardiac electromechanical arrest, cold cardioplegia may be infused into the coronary sinus. Cardioplegic arrest may be accomplished by exclusive perfusion of the coronary sinus in the presence of important aortic regurgitation. A small aortotomy should be made or the aortic root vented when coronary sinus perfusion is performed. Direct coronary artery orifice perfusion is reserved for the rare situation in which it is impossible to perfuse the coronary sinus.

An initial aortotomy is made about 15 mm downstream from the origin of the right coronary artery. Its precise location is very important not only for surgical exposure but also because of space for intraaortic positioning of an allograft, autograft, or xenograft valve, ease and security of closure, avoiding damage to the right coronary artery or its ostium, and facilitating aortic root enlargement if necessary. Exposure for this incision is facilitated by the first assistant's retraction of the fat pad along the right atrioventricular groove over the aortic root. The pulmonary artery may also need to be partially dissected from the aorta to avoid incising it. The initial incision is made directly anteriorly with the scissors, facilitated by the collapsed state of the aorta. Once this small incision is made, the inside of the aortic root is visualized, and a decision is made as to whether an allograft valve, a pulmonary autograft valve, or a prosthesis will be used or repair performed (see "Nonreplacement Aortic Valve Operations in Adults" under Special Situations and Controversies later in this chapter).

The incision is extended. The surgeon has a choice depending on the operation to be performed:

- Extend the incision transversely (Fig. 12-5, *A*). This is the most common approach and has the advantage of providing good exposure of the aortic root without distorting it. The sinotubular junction is not disturbed. Exposure at the level of the aortic valve and below into the LV outflow tract is usually very good.
- Extend the incision into the posterior commissure between the left and noncoronary cusps, should posterior enlargement of the aortic root be required.
- Extend the incision obliquely (Fig. 12-5, *B*) into the noncoronary sinus to a point near the aortic anulus, to provide maximal exposure at the level of the aortic valve and below into the LV outflow tract. This incision, which divides the sinotubular junction, can be extended for posterior aortic root enlargement into the anterior leaflet of the mitral valve.
- Extend the incision to divide the aorta (Fig. 12-5, *C*). This incision provides optimal exposure of the aortic root because the proximal aortic structures can be easily moved and displaced inferiorly and anteriorly so that the surgeon may visualize the intact aortic root and look directly into it. This incision is best for placing aortic allografts and stentless porcine bioprostheses inside the aortic root, as well as for aortic valve replacement with a pulmonary autograft or other procedures requiring replacement of the complete aortic root. The incision also provides excellent exposure for routine prosthetic valve implantation.

Traction stitches are placed just above the aortic valve commissures for optimal exposure of the aortic root structures, regardless of the type of incision.

The aortic valve is removed (Fig. 12-6, *A*). Unless the aortic valve disease is noncalcific, a short strip of narrow packing gauze is inserted through the valve orifice into the LV (and some foolproof system is used to ensure its removal) to trap all calcific fragments that may escape during valvectomy. Neat, complete removal of the valve, particularly when heavily calcified, without damage to the LV–aortic junction, ventricular septum, or aortic wall, is one of the critical aspects of the operation. Usually an area exists in about the midportion of the right coronary cusp where an initial scissors cut can be made from the free edge to the point of leaflet attachment. This incision allows entry of a knife blade to incise precisely along the attachment of the right coronary cusp toward the commissure between left and right coronary cusps. This commissure may also be calcified, but the incision can usually be carried between it and the aortic wall, often with scissors. The incision is then carried along the attachment of the left coronary cusp, stopping at a point about two thirds of the distance to the left coronary–noncoronary cusp commissure because beyond that point, there is a tendency to carry the incision *into* the aortic wall or LV–aortic junction.

Returning to the right coronary cusp, the incision is extended toward the right coronary–noncoronary cusp commissure. In this area and in this commissure the calcification is often especially abundant, sometimes extending onto the underlying ventricular septum or, especially at the commissure, onto the aortic wall or underlying membranous septum. Thus, in dissecting this area, great care must

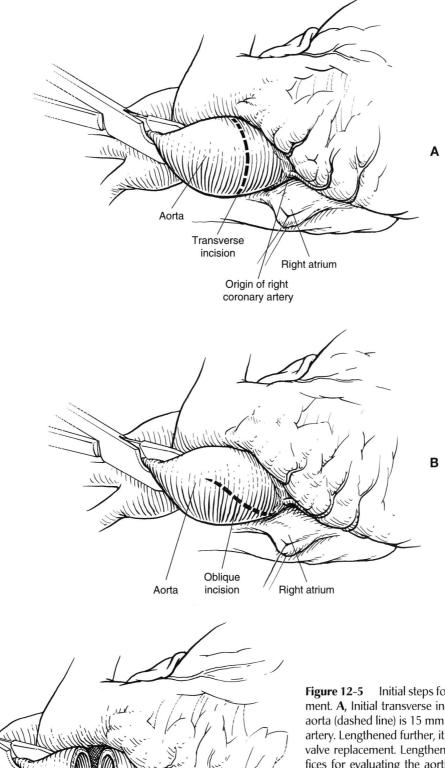

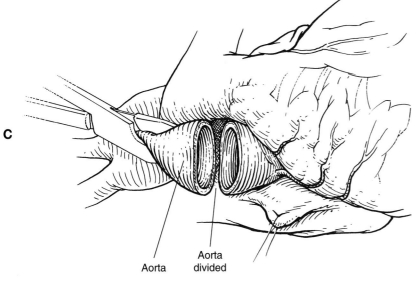

Figure 12-5   Initial steps for aortic valve replacement. **A,** Initial transverse incision into ascending aorta (dashed line) is 15 mm above right coronary artery. Lengthened further, it is sufficient for aortic valve replacement. Lengthened just a little, it suffices for evaluating the aortic valve and deciding on procedure to be used. **B,** Incision is extended into middle of noncoronary sinus of Valsalva, providing excellent exposure of aortic valve for its replacement with prosthetic device. **C,** Transverse incision may be extended to divide aorta above sinotubular junction. This permits working within the intact aortic root for correct positioning of aortic valve allografts or stentless xenografts below the coronary arteries (subcoronary technique).

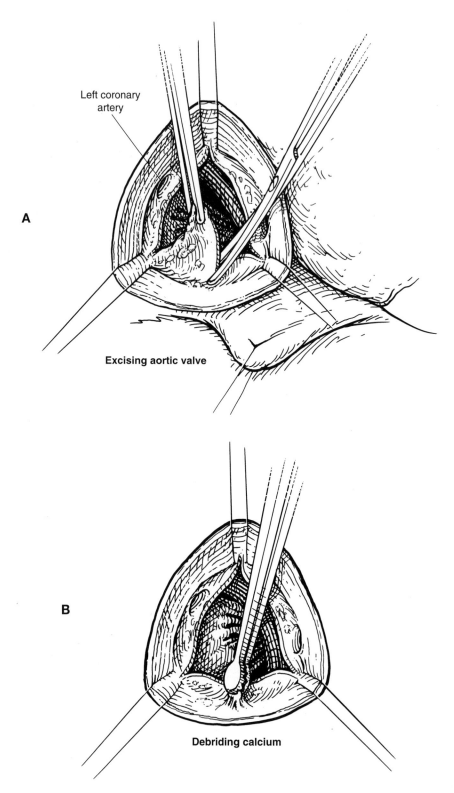

Figure 12-6   Excision of aortic valve and debridement. **A**, A scissors cut is made in aortic valve cusp, extending to, but *not into,* aortic wall. Valve excision is along hinge line of aortic valve cusp. Careful excision of valve usually includes removing most calcium deposits along with the valve. **B**, Residual calcium deposits are debrided from aortic anulus and sinus aorta. Sellman or other forceps and bone rongeurs are instruments commonly used to accomplish this.

be taken in deciding whether to cut through the calcific cusp attachment to the aortic wall or to go around some of the calcific material and leave it for later piece-by-piece removal. To the extent possible, one-piece removal is preferable, but perforation of the septum, LV–aortic junction, or aortic wall should not become a risk.

When the aortic valve is completely replaced by calcium deposits, or when the deposits extend into the sinus aorta or anterior leaflet of the mitral valve, it is useful to mobilize the calcified tissues by endarterectomy technique. Using a scalpel, a shallow incision is made in the aortic intima alongside the calcific deposit. This allows insertion of an endarterectomy spatula (Freer septum elevator) to lift the intact hard deposit away from the soft underlying aortic or mitral valve tissues without fragmenting the calcified material. The incision is carried down along the attachment of the noncoronary cusp, stopping about two thirds of the distance to the commissure between the noncoronary and left coronary cusps. The latter commissural area, which is at particular risk of junctional or aortic wall perforation during valvectomy, can then be approached with excellent visibility from both sides; the incision is carried through this area with firm upward traction on the valve.

After the valve is excised, the bed is examined and any loose calcific particles removed. Any remaining fragments are grasped with forceps or small rongeur and gently enucleated with a twisting motion (Fig. 12-6, *B*).

The downstream area of aorta is irrigated and examined for any loose calcific fragments, and the valve bed is wiped with gauze and irrigated with cold saline solution to remove any tiny fragments. The LV vent is turned off so that it will not suck fragments into the inaccessible depths of the ventricle, and the gauze strip is carefully removed from the LV cavity, most likely having trapped a few small calcific fragments. The LV cavity is then vigorously irrigated and aspirated with high-pressure suction and inspected for fragments. Generally, no fragments are found. With the precautionary measures against calcific embolization complete, the LV vent is again activated.

Prosthetic Aortic Valve

Insertion of a prosthetic aortic valve is the most common operation for replacing the aortic valve. The anulus is sized and an appropriate-size prosthesis selected. There is no advantage in choosing an oversized prosthesis that will erode the aortic anulus. Instead, if the aortic anulus is too small to accommodate a prosthesis that will provide adequate hemodynamic performance, a supraanular device may be chosen or the anulus enlarged (see "Managing the Small Aortic Root" under Special Situations and Controversies later in this chapter).

Interrupted suture technique. Synthetic suture material, with a compressed polytetrafluoroethylene (PTFE) pledget placed centrally and needles at each end, is used. Alternating suture colors (green, white) simplifies sorting so that sutures may be held together as a group for each aortic sinus. Mattress stitches are taken through the anulus of the aortic valve beginning at the commissure between the left and right coronary cusps. The suture is placed through the sewing ring of the prosthesis after completing each anular pass. Stitches are placed in the right coronary anulus working clockwise toward the commissure between

the right and noncoronary sinus (Fig. 12-7, *A*). Separate stitches are placed close to one another, and the space along the aortic anulus is taken beneath the pledget of the mattress stitch. The prosthesis is held away from the aortic anulus until all stitches have been placed.

The anulus of the left coronary sinus of Valsalva is then approximated to the sewing ring of the aortic valve prosthesis, working counterclockwise from the commissure between the left and right coronary cusps (Fig. 12-7, *B*). The anulus of the noncoronary sinus of Valsalva is then approximated to the valve prosthesis, working clockwise from the commissure between the right and noncoronary cusp toward the commissure between the left and noncoronary cusp (Fig 12-7, *C*). Needles are passed through the anulus in a "backhand" manner. The three groups of sutures are then strongly retracted so that the prosthesis may be slid over the suture loops into the aortic anulus. Position of the occluder mechanism may be adjusted before the valve holder is removed.

Sutures are sorted and tied down in order, working first in the noncoronary sinus in a counterclockwise approach. The first suture in the left coronary sinus closest to the commissure between the left and right coronary cusps is tied to secure seating of the prosthesis directly across the anulus from those sutures already tied in the noncoronary sinus. The sutures of the left coronary sinus are tied down counterclockwise. Sutures are tied in the right sinus, working clockwise to complete the procedure (Fig. 12-7, *D*). For valve prostheses that have any part of the device projecting below the sewing ring, so that it is positioned partially below the anulus in the LV outflow tract, the order of tying should be altered so that the prosthesis is first secured adjacent to the portions of the device below the anulus.

An alternative technique for placing the pledget stitches is used for the small aortic anulus (Fig. 12-7, *E*). Pledgets are placed below the anulus in the LV outflow tract by passing a double-needle suture with center pledget as a mattress stitch from below the anulus and up through the prosthesis. A larger prosthesis is thereby secured above the anulus as the anulus is compressed between the pledget and device.

Continuous suture technique. Continuous suture technique provides the advantage of tight approximation of the prosthesis to the aortic valve anulus, because the suture loops can slip through the tissues so that tension is equalized with heart motion.[D41] Inserting a slightly larger prosthesis may also be possible because an interrupted mattress suture technique may bunch tissues together.

The aortic anulus is divided into three segments by the commissures. During the valve replacement procedure the anulus is further subdivided into six subsegments at the midpoint on the anulus between the commissures. Polypropylene suture (No. 2-0) is used, with needles at each end and a compressed PTFE pledget in the center of the suture. An initial mattress stitch is placed at the center of the sinus of Valsalva through the anulus of the aortic valve and brought through the sewing ring of the prosthesis (Fig. 12-8, *A*). The prosthetic valve is held away from the anulus and positioned and retracted for added exposure. Exactly three stitches are placed between the initial pledgeted stitch and the commissure on each side of the sinus. The final stitch at each end is secured to the wound drapes by a hemostat. A loop of No. 0 suture is placed around the polypropylene suture as the first

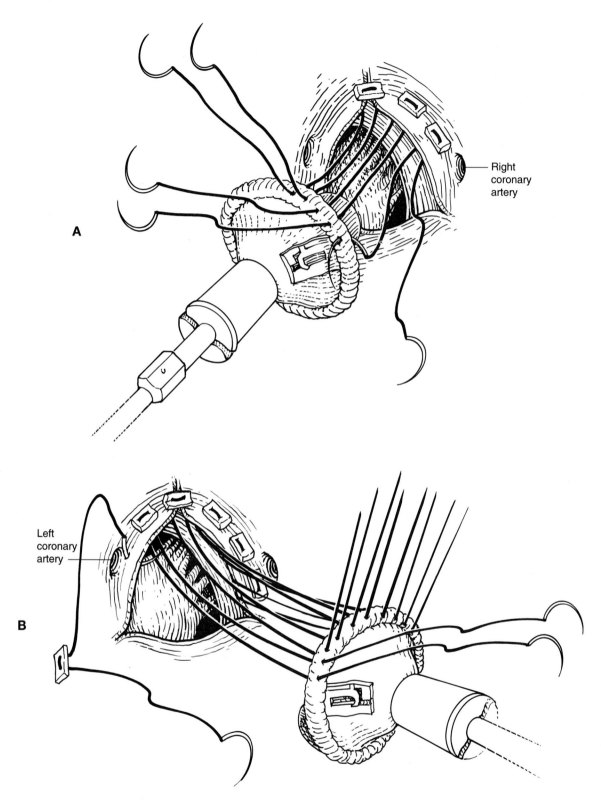

Right coronary artery

A

Left coronary artery

B

Figure 12-7   Aortic valve replacement with mechanical prosthesis or stent-mounted bioprosthesis, interrupted suture technique. **A,** Polytetrafluoroethylene felt pledget–reinforced No. 2-0
braided polyester suture is placed as interrupted horizontal mattress stitches passed from aortic
side through aortic anulus. Needles are then passed through sewing cuff of replacement device.
Suturing begins at commissure between left and right sinus of Valsalva and proceeds clockwise
in right coronary sinus to commissure between right and noncoronary sinus. Alternating color
of suture aids suture sorting. **B,** Suturing continues in left coronary sinus of Valsalva in a
counterclockwise fashion to commissure between left and noncoronary sinus.

Continued

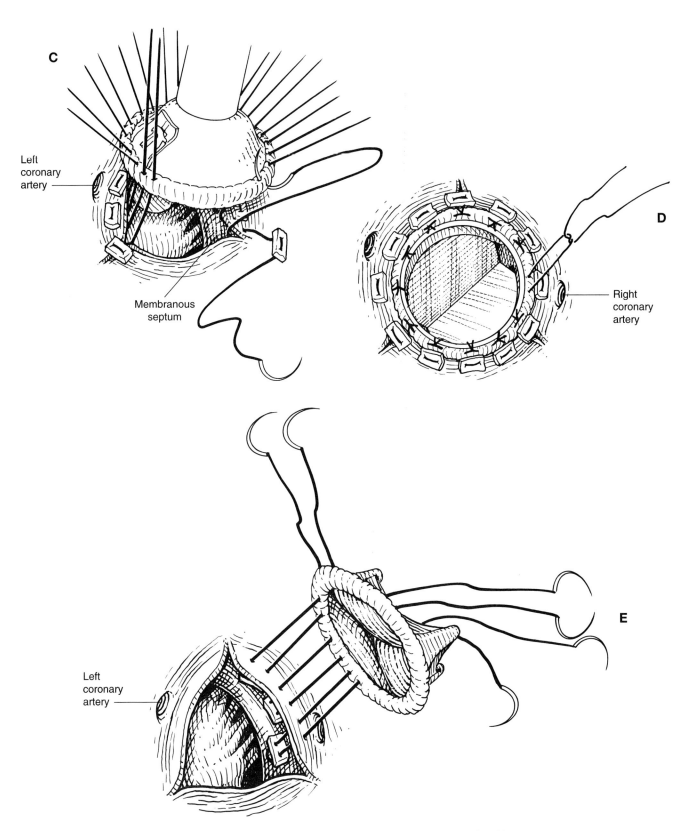

Figure 12-7, cont'd   C, Sutures surrounding anterior commissure should not penetrate tissues of membranous septum, to protect the His bundle from injury. Suturing is completed in noncoronary sinus of Valsalva. **D,** Prosthesis is passed over sutures into position on aortic anulus. Sutures are sorted and tied to fix prosthesis to aortic anulus. **E,** Some bioprostheses are designed to be implanted above aortic anulus (supraanular). When these devices are used, horizontal mattress stitches are passed from ventricular side of anulus to aortic surface and then through sewing cuff of bioprosthesis.

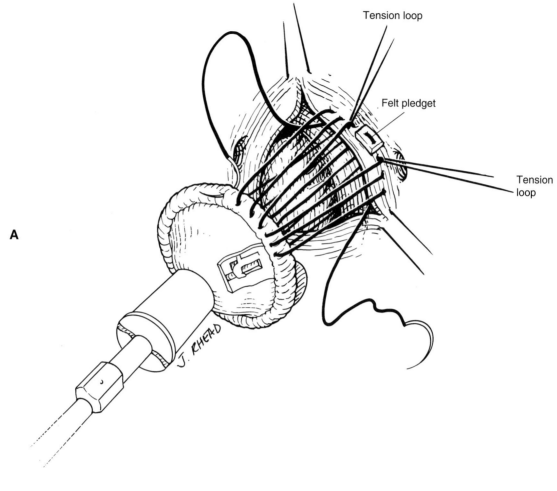

A

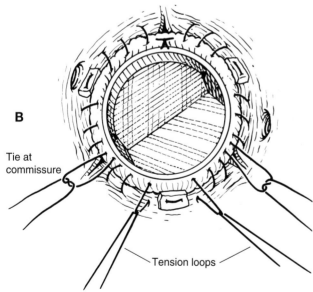

B

Tie at
commissure

Tension loops

Figure 12-8   Aortic valve replacement with mechanical prosthesis or stent-mounted bioprosthesis, continuous suture technique. **A,** Polytetrafluroethylene felt pledget–reinforced No. 2-0 polypropylene suture is placed through aortic anulus as a horizontal mattress stitch at midpoint of right coronary sinus. Stitch is brought through sewing cuff of prosthesis. Exactly three suture loops are placed through aortic anulus and sewing cuff between initial stitch and commissure. Tension loop is placed around first suture loop. After suturing right sinus, prosthesis is attached to left coronary sinus and finally to noncoronary sinus. **B,** Prosthesis is approximated to anulus of aortic valve by pulling up suture loops. Tension loops are pulled up to tightly approximate sewing cuff to deepest point in sinus of Valsalva. Suture ends at commissures are then pulled up to seat the valve in aortic root. Sutures are joined at commissures.

suture loop is completed through the prosthesis in each subsegment. This suture loop is held by a hemostat to be used to adjust tension on the suture line.

Sutures in the right coronary anulus are placed from the center toward the commissures in the first and second subsegments. The initial stitch in the left coronary sinus passes through the sewing ring of the prosthesis opposite

the last stitch of the second subsegment. Working from the center to the commissures in the left coronary sinus, the third and fourth subsegments are approximated to the prosthesis, and then the fifth and sixth subsegments are completed in the noncoronary sinus.

Traction is placed on the six No. 0 silk loop sutures to pull the prosthesis into the anulus of the aortic valve

(Fig. 12-8, *B*). The occluder of the prosthesis is opened, and the area below the prosthesis is checked to ensure that no loose suture loops exist in the LV outflow tract beneath the prosthesis.

The tension suture loops are removed sequentially and the ends of the polypropylene suture pulled up tightly to approximate the sewing ring of the prosthesis to the anulus. A final check of this approximation should be made with special attention to placement of the pledget, which should be above the anulus at the point of maximal stress deep in the center of the sinus of Valsalva. The suture ends are then joined by a knot at the three commissures (see Fig. 12-8, *B*).

Allograft Aortic Valve

Replacing the aortic valve with a transplanted human aortic valve became more feasible and available to surgeons because of improved cryopreservation techniques (Appendix 12A).

Subcoronary technique. Because with this technique the graft is to be sewn in "freehand" using the natural aorta for support, a clear understanding of the anatomy and spatial relationships of the aortic root is essential. Important deformity of the aortic sinuses should be appreciated and corrected or the procedure abandoned in favor of conventional valve replacement or aortic root replacement techniques.

A transverse aortotomy is made initially. After assessing aortic valve morphology and anatomy of the aortic root, the incision is extended to transect the aorta (see Fig. 12-5, *C*). The aortic valve is excised and anulus debrided by usual techniques. Diameter of the aortic root at the level of the ventriculoaortic junction (anulus) is determined using standard sizing devices. This dimension must be accurately measured and clearly visualized. The aortic valve allograft to be placed inside the aortic root will consume space simply because of the thickness of its wall. Therefore, it must be 1 to 2 mm smaller in internal diameter than the measured aortic anulus. This will allow some redundant aortic valve cusp to provide a larger than normal coaptation surface to accommodate the expected tissue shrinkage for several weeks after implantation.

The aortic allograft is removed from the liquid nitrogen freezer valve bank and thawed by protocol. The septal muscle is excised, with a finger placed inside the aorta to stabilize the graft, gauge the thickness of the trimmed graft, and remove endothelial cells that are antigenic.

Excess aorta is trimmed from the valve cusps, leaving a 3- to 4-mm rim of aorta beyond attachment of the cusps. Most of the sinus aorta is removed from the right and left coronary sinuses, leaving the noncoronary sinus intact (Fig. 12-9, *A*). This technique was described by Ross and colleagues in London and has been used successfully for many years.[K9,R18]

The graft is implanted in anatomic position. Three stitches are used to attach it to the outflow tract. The first suture is No. 3-0 polypropylene, placed using two small, strong needles (RB-1). This suture is chosen for high needle strength and low tissue drag. The suture is placed through the host aortic outflow tract below the medial commissure between the right and left coronary sinuses and through the septal myocardium below the corresponding commissure in

the graft. The stitch is placed below the anulus of the host aortic valve. The other two stitches are simply stay sutures placed to assist in aligning the allograft to the aortic root. These stitches are No. 4-0 polypropylene and will be removed because the primary suture line includes their position. They are placed beneath the appropriate commissure of the graft and directly below the anterior and posterior commissures of the host aorta.

The allograft valve is lowered into position in the aortic root. Commissures of the graft are inverted through its anulus into the LV of the host so as to expose the subvalvar edge of the graft. A knot is placed in the primary suture, and the stay sutures are tightened to align the graft with the LV outflow tract. Stitches are placed between the graft and the LV outflow tract at or below the level of the anulus, attempting to make a level suture line (Fig. 12-9, *B*). Because the aortic anulus is not circular but crescent shaped, the stitches are well below the fibrous anulus in the subcommissural region and through this fibrous tissue of the anulus at the midpoint of the aortic sinus (see "Cardiac Valves" in Chapter 1). The stitches below the left coronary sinus are placed first. The suture line is taken to a point below the posterior commissure. Using the opposite needle, the stitches between the graft and LV outflow tract are placed below the right coronary sinus and completed below the noncoronary sinus (Fig. 12-9, *B*).

The commissures of the aortic allograft are pulled out of the LV so that the allograft assumes its normal position and configuration. The commissures of the allograft are attached to the sinus aorta of the host using continuous No. 4-0 polypropylene sutures. Separate sutures are used for each aortic sinus. The first stitch is taken deep in the sinus aorta at midposition in the sinus slightly above the aortic anulus and then passed through the graft. Suturing proceeds along the sinus aorta toward the commissure, so as to place the graft flat against the host aortic wall. The final stitch is placed at the top of the commissure, leaving the suture to be secured later (Fig. 12-9, *C*). Suturing proceeds in each aortic sinus until the graft is completely attached. Generally, the right coronary sinus is completed first, sewing from the center point of the sinus to each of the commissures using opposite ends of the suture. The left sinus follows. The repair is completed in the noncoronary sinus by shortening the graft aorta to approximate the height of the intact noncoronary sinus of the host. The two edges of the aorta are simply oversewn by continuous suture so that the intact noncoronary sinus of the graft is completely enclosed within the aorta. The ends of the aorta are then reanastomosed by continuous suture.

Intraoperative echocardiography is used to confirm aortic valve competence.

Root-enlarging technique. An aortic allograft may be used for valve replacement as part of a root-enlarging operation.[M43] A transverse incision is made in the aorta. The incision is extended to the posterior aspect of the aorta and into the posterior commissure between the left and noncoronary sinuses. Incision into the triangular space of the commissure between the fibrous attachment of the native aortic valve opens the aortic root where there is little fibrous support so that the edges of the aortotomy will separate widely. The incision is taken to the upper edge of the anterior leaflet of the mitral valve, but it does not need

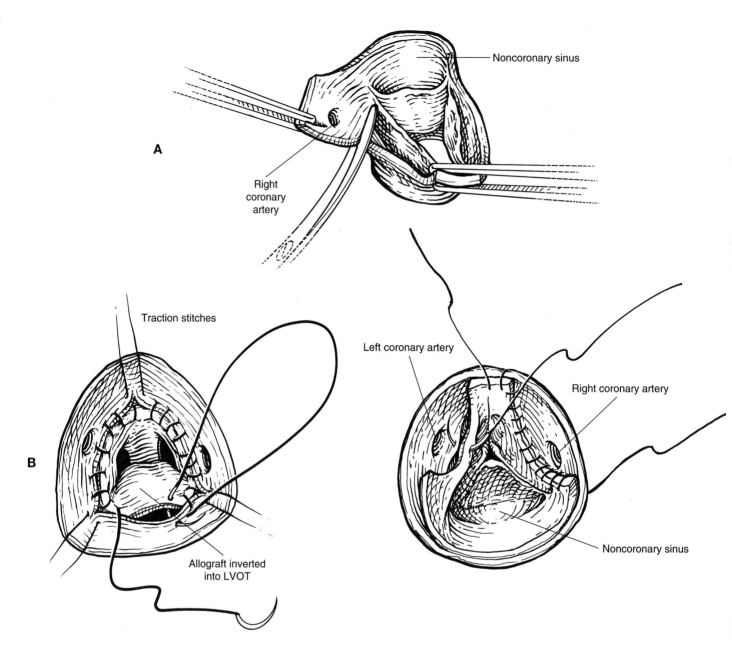

Figure 12-9 Aortic valve replacement with aortic valve allograft, subcoronary technique. **A,** Aortic allograft is chosen that is no more than 2 mm smaller in internal diameter than left ventricular (LV) outflow tract at aortic anulus. Cryopreserved aortic allograft is taken through the standard controlled thawing process. Septal myocardium is thinned out and anterior leaflet of mitral valve removed along with tissues below aortic valve to create a level plane. Aorta is removed from right and left coronary sinus of Valsalva leaving 3 to 4 mm of aorta beyond hinge point of valve. Noncoronary sinus remains intact, maintaining relationships of commissures on each side of sinus. **B,** Aorta is divided above sinotubular junction so that valve replacement may proceed within the intact aortic root. Traction stitches are placed above each commissure. Graft is inverted through its anulus into LV outflow tract. Graft is attached to aortic anulus and below commissures in a generally level plane using continuous stitches of No. 3-0 polypropylene suture. **C,** The allograft is pulled back into aorta. Sinus aorta of graft is attached to sinus aorta of patient below the coronary ostia. Sutures proceed progressively up commissures to accurately recreate relations of the aortic valve within aortic root. Suturing begins at lowest point of sinus of Valsalva and proceeds to top of each commissure. Separate sutures are used for each sinus and are joined at top of commissures. Intact noncoronary sinus of graft is sewn to patient's aorta by continuous suture.

Key: *LVOT,* Left ventricular outflow tract.

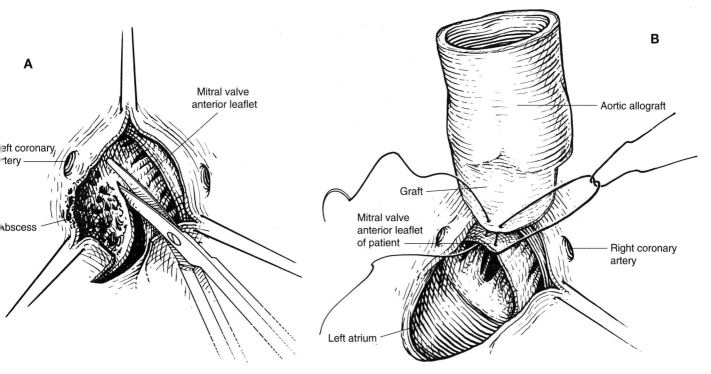

Figure 12-10   Aortic valve replacement with allograft, aortic root enlarging technique, or repair of anular abscess. **A,** Aortotomy is extended through posterior commissure into abscess of anterior leaflet of mitral valve. Abscess is debrided or simply incised if procedure is used to widen left ventricular (LV) outflow tract. **B,** Anterior leaflet of mitral valve is left attached to allograft and used to widen, LV outflow tract or repair defects caused by endocarditis. Anterior leaflet repair is done with interrupted stitches for greatest security. Defect in left atrium is closed with a patch of aorta from the graft.

to enter the leaflet tissue to provide the desired separation of the edges of the incision. The increased diameter of the aortic root is measured and an appropriate size aortic allograft chosen. The aortic allograft is trimmed, leaving the noncoronary sinus intact. The sinus aorta is removed from the left and right sinuses, leaving a few millimeters attached to the fibrous support of the cusps. The allograft is attached to the rim of the anterior leaflet of the mitral valve and superior aspect of the left atrium with interrupted No. 3-0 or 4-0 polypropylene sutures. The stitches are placed in the corresponding mitral valve and left atrium of the allograft's noncoronary sinus. A PTFE felt strip is fashioned to slightly more than the length of the unsupported area of the separated aortotomy. The sutures of the noncoronary sinus are then tied down over the felt strip so as to incorporate it and fill in any potential defects in the suture line. The commissures of the valve are inverted into the LV outflow tract, and the rest of the repair is completed according to the approach previously described under "Subcoronary Technique." The allograft's intact noncoronary sinus is used to close the aortotomy and widen the aortic root.

When greater enlargement of the LV outflow tract is required, or when there is infectious endocarditis with extension of anular abscess into the anterior leaflet of the mitral valve, the incision in the aorta is extended across the mitral valve anulus into the middle of the valve's anterior leaflet. Anular abscess may be thoroughly debrided

and much of the anterior leaflet of the mitral valve removed (Fig. 12-10, *A*). The anterior leaflet of the mitral valve is left attached to the aortic allograft and used to widen the LV outflow tract or repair defects in the patient's mitral valve (Fig. 12-10, *B*). The defect in the roof of the left atrium is closed with a patch taken from the aorta of the graft.

Aortic root replacement technique. An aortic allograft may be used to replace the aortic root completely when gross deformity is caused by infection or congenital anomaly or it may be used to enlarge the root.[D9] Many surgeons use this technique routinely because aortic valve competence is virtually assured due to retention of the valve relationships within the intact aortic root of the graft.

An initial transverse aortotomy is made (Fig. 12-11, *A*). After decision to proceed with aortic root replacement, the aorta is transected (Fig. 12-11, *B*). The sinus aorta is removed except for a rim surrounding the ostia of the coronary arteries. The aortic valve is removed and an appropriate size aortic allograft selected. The allograft is used intact and in natural anatomic orientation, with only the excess of septal myocardium and the anterior leaflet of the mitral valve removed. Size match is not nearly as important as it is for freehand subcoronary valve replacement, but if the aortic anulus is more than 3 mm larger in diameter than the largest available aortic allograft, the host aortic root should be narrowed to approximate the size of the graft. This can be done conveniently by placing a pledgeted mattress stitch through the aortic anulus along-

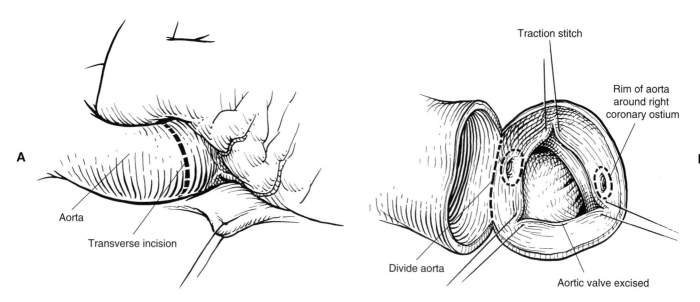

Figure 12-11 Aortic valve replacement, aortic root replacement technique. **A,** Transverse aortotomy is made. **B,** Traction stitches are placed in aorta above each commissure and aortic valve is excised. When the decision is made to proceed with complete replacement of aortic root, aortotomy is extended to divide aorta. Aorta is removed from sinuses of Valsalva except for generous buttons around coronary artery ostia. *Continued*

side the commissures so that when tied, the interleaflet triangle below the commissure is obliterated (see "Method for Reducing Diameter of Dilated Aortic Anulus" later in this chapter).

The allograft is attached to the LV outflow tract at the aortic anulus and below the commissures by simple interrupted stitches of No. 3-0 or 4-0 polypropylene (Fig. 12-11, *C*). The key to a hemostatic proximal suture line is use of a PTFE felt collar. The felt is approximately 5 mm wide and long enough to encircle the allograft. The allograft is slipped over the sutures into the desired position in the LV outflow tract. The sutures are then tied down, incorporating the felt strip within the suture loops (Fig. 12-11, *D*).

The coronary ostia on the allograft are removed to create openings 5 to 10 mm in diameter (Fig. 12-11, *E* and *F*). The coronary arteries are anastomosed to the allograft by continuous No. 5-0 or 4-0 polypropylene suture using a small needle (exact size depends on thickness of the tissues). The left coronary anastomosis is created first (Fig. 12-11, *E*), followed by the right coronary anastomosis (Fig. 12-11, *F*). Repair is completed by end-to-end anastomosis of the distal end of the allograft to the host aorta (Fig. 12-11, *G*). Continuous stitches of No. 3-0 or 4-0 polypropylene are used.

Cylinder technique. The aortic valve allograft may be inserted as a cylinder within the aortic root, using a technique described by O'Brien and colleagues.[O8]

Buttons of sinus aorta are excised, including the ostia of the left and right coronary arteries of the allograft.[O8] The resultant opening may need to be extended proximally because the allograft valve now lies a little downstream from its native position.[D11] This technique has the potential disadvantage of too much open space between the allograft and native aortic walls.

In a slight modification of the cylinder technique, the center of each sinus is removed before inserting the cylin-

der of allograft, leaving an intact strut of aortic wall over each sinus.[B34] This approach maintains the integrity and special relationships of the allograft until the majority of the second (downstream) suture line of each sinus is complete and the bar over that sinus excised.

Porcine Xenograft Stentless Bioprosthesis

Several manufacturers supply porcine xenograft stentless aortic valves. The devices most frequently used are manufactured by St. Jude Medical and Medtronic (Fig. 12-12, *A*). The St. Jude Medical device (Toronto SPV) is supplied for subcoronary valve replacement with the sinus aorta removed from all three sinuses of Valsalva.[D1] The device is covered with a thin polyester mesh. Proper insertion depends on near-normal diameter relationships of the aortic anulus and the sinotubular junction. The Medtronic device (Freestyle) is presented as the entire untrimmed aortic root and therefore may offer more flexibility and utility.

Subcoronary technique. The implant technique is similar to aortic valve replacement with aortic allografts.[D20] The aorta is divided about 1 cm above the sinotubular junction, or a transverse aortotomy is made in the same location. The proper size of graft is chosen using the sizing devices supplied by the manufacturer. The diameter of the aortic anulus is measured, and the same size graft is chosen for implantation. Some surgeons choose a graft 1 or 2 mm larger than the anulus because these flexible stentless bioprostheses fit easily into the aortic root. No advantage exists to greatly oversizing the prosthesis because oversized grafts increase the gradient across the valve.[N6] Downsizing is not required because the grafts are sized according to *outside* diameter of the device, in contrast to aortic allografts, which are sized according to *inside* orifice diameter.

The Medtronic Freestyle bioprosthesis requires trimming before implantation (see Fig. 12-12, *A*). The sinus

Figure 12-11, cont'd   **C**, Aortic allograft is minimally trimmed, removing anterior leaflet of mitral valve. Aortic allograft root is attached to anulus of native aortic valve with interrupted stitches of No. 3-0 or 4-0 polypropylene suture. Simple stitches are used. **D**, Suture loops are tied down over a narrow strip of polytetrafluroethylene felt or pericardium to support and fix diameter of aortic anulus and to seal spaces between stitches. **E**, Left coronary artery button is anastomosed to opening in allograft created by excising left coronary artery of graft. Continuous stitches of No. 4-0 or 5-0 polypropylene are used, depending on thickness of tissues.

Continued

aorta is removed from the right and left sinuses of Valsalva. The noncoronary sinus remains intact to fix the position of two of the three commissures of the valve. The lower edge of the aortic root of the graft is covered with polyester cloth to assist with implantation and to prevent shrinkage of the graft when graft septal myocardium is absorbed. This cloth limits how deeply the sinus aorta may be excised, especially in the right coronary sinus. Care should be taken not to disrupt the cloth covering.

The aortic valve is excised in the usual manner, and all calcific deposits are removed from the aortic anulus and sinus aorta. Exposure is enhanced by traction sutures placed at the sinus rim above each of the commissures. Markings on the cloth covering the lower edge of the graft correspond to each commissure. Continuous No. 3-0 polypropylene suture is used to attach the lower edge of the graft to the aortic anulus. A small needle with a taper-cut design is best to allow easier penetration of the polyester fabric. The suture line is started in the interleaflet triangle below the commissure between the left and right sinuses.

The valve is held away from the anulus as suture loops are placed (Fig. 12-12, *B*). A heavy suture (No. 0 or 2-0) is passed around every third suture loop to act as a tension-adjusting loop suture.[D41] These tension loops are secured by a small hemostat. Suturing proceeds below the right sinus to the commissure below the right and noncoronary

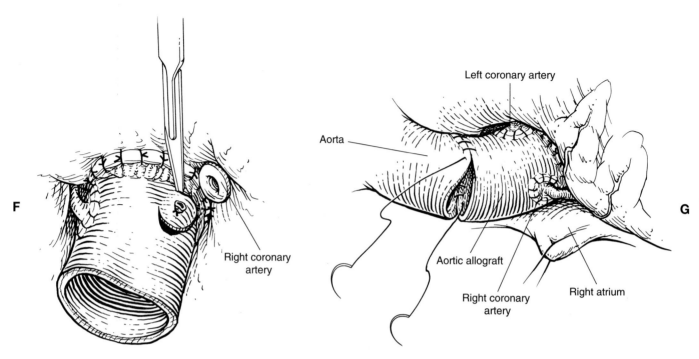

Figure 12-11, cont'd   **F,** Opening is made in allograft at position of right coronary artery unless aortic root of patient was greatly dilated. Dilatation of aortic root displaces right coronary artery; in this case, it is advisable to complete the aortic anastomosis so that aorta may be filled under pressure to properly locate position for anastomosis of right coronary artery. **G,** End-to-end anastomosis of graft to host aorta completes the repair.

sinuses. Stitches are placed mostly through the thick fibrous hinge of the aortic valve (anulus), attempting to level the plane of the suture line rather than strictly following the semilunar plane of the valve hinge (Fig. 12-12, *C*). From the midpoint of the right coronary sinus to the commissure between the right and noncoronary sinuses, the stitches must be through the anulus, not below and into the myocardium, to protect the conduction system from injury.

Suturing continues below the left sinus of Valsalva until below the commissure between the left and noncoronary sinuses. A separate suture is used for the noncoronary sinus repair. Tension loops are placed around every third stitch. The valve is seated in the aortic root by sequentially pulling up on the tension loops to approximate the fabric of the valve to the aortic anulus. Alternatively, the inflow suture line may be simple interrupted stitches placed with the graft held away from the anulus (see Fig. 12-12, *B*). Many surgeons prefer the interrupted stitch technique because it is similar to implanting prosthetic devices and avoids possibility of purse-string effect.

The sinus aorta of the graft is attached to the sinus aorta of the patient by continuous stitches of No. 4-0 polypropylene (Fig. 12-12, *D*). The initial stitch is placed in the host sinus aorta just below the right coronary ostia. The suture line comes very close to the coronary ostia to achieve proper fit of the xenograft tissues to the sinus aorta of the patient. This is especially true for the right coronary sinus of the graft, which is covered with cloth quite high on its external surface. The commissure between the right and left sinuses of the graft must be carefully located so as not to distort the graft. Suturing continues beneath the left coro-

nary artery to the top of each adjacent commissure (Fig. 12-12, *E*).

The noncoronary sinus repair is accomplished by trimming the graft to the same height as the patient's noncoronary sinus aorta. The two edges of tissue are approximated by direct suture (see Fig. 12-12, *E*). Sufficient space usually exists in the patient's noncoronary sinus of Valsalva to accommodate the graft without distortion. If the diameter (length) of the aorta at the sinotubular junction in the noncoronary sinus is greater than that of the sinotubular junction of the graft, the discrepancy can be compensated for by placing stitches more closely on graft side than patient aorta. The repair is completed by anastomosis of the aorta or closure of the transverse aortotomy.

Aortic root replacement technique. The Medtronic Freestyle device may be implanted as a complete aortic root replacement[D20,K26] (Fig. 12-12, *F*). This method is employed when the aortic root is distorted or when it is dilated enough that support for the graft as a subcoronary valve implant will be inadequate. The aorta is divided just above the sinotubular junction. The left and right coronary arteries are mobilized, retaining a generous rim of sinus aorta around the coronary ostia, and the noncoronary sinus aorta is excised. The device is implanted as a complete root. The inflow suture line is placed as for subcoronary implantation using continuous No. 2-0 polypropylene. The suture line is started in the intercusp triangle below the commissure between left and right sinuses. Suture loops are placed through the anulus of the aortic valve below the right sinus, then the left, then the noncoronary sinus. Tension loops are placed around the primary suture every third suture loop.

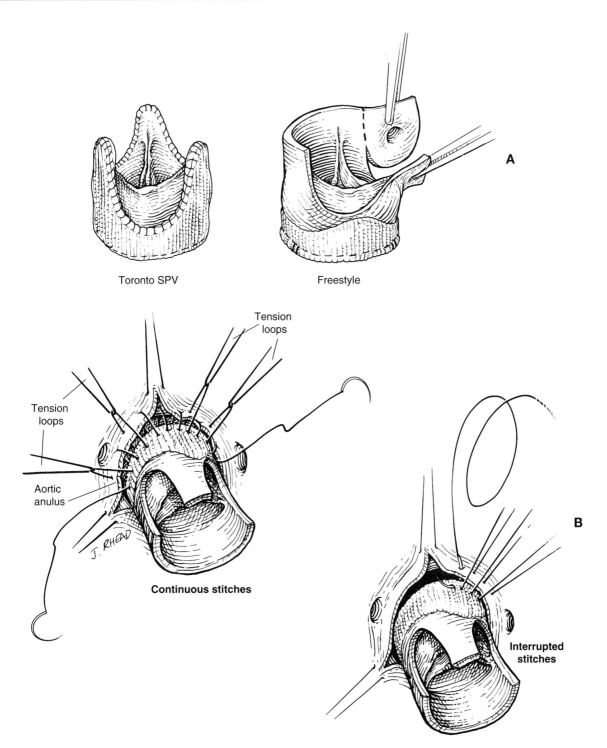

Figure 12-12   Aortic valve replacement, porcine xenograft stentless bioprosthesis. **A,** St. Jude Medical Toronto SPV bioprosthesis is presented with sinus aorta removed from all three sinuses of Valsalva. The device is covered with polyester fabric. Medtronic Freestyle porcine xenograft bioprosthesis is presented with intact aortic root with less fabric. There is an inflow sewing ring, and fabric covers portions of septal myocardium on aortic root. Aorta is removed by the surgeon from right and left coronary sinuses of Valsalva, leaving noncoronary sinus intact. **B,** Inflow sewing cuff of bioprosthesis (Freestyle) is attached to aortic valve anulus with continuous stitches of No. 3-0 polypropylene suture. Tension loops are placed around every third suture loop to make it easier to tighten suture and approximate bioprosthesis to aortic anulus. Alternatively, simple interrupted stitches of No. 2-0 or 3-0 braided polyester are used.

Key: *SPV,* Stentless porcine valve.   *Continued*

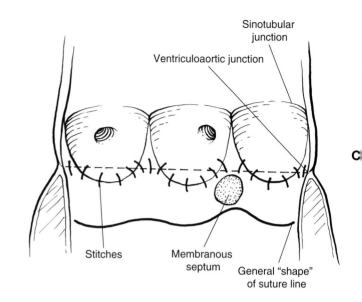

Figure 12-12, cont'd **C,** Placement of stitches to attach device to aortic anulus. A generally level plane is achieved by sewing through the anulus except in intercusp triangles, where stitches are placed below hinge point of aortic valve. Stitches should not be placed into membranous septum below anterior commissure, to protect conduction system from injury. **D,** Sinus aorta of graft is attached to sinus aorta of patient below right coronary artery. Continuous stitches of No. 4-0 polypropylene suture are used. Suturing continues around coronary ostium to smoothly attach graft to patient and to achieve correct positioning of commissures. Because it is fixed tissue, the graft will direct suture placement so as not to distort itself. That is, the patient's aorta is made to conform to the graft, rather than distorting the graft to conform to the shape of the patient's sinus of Valsalva. **E,** Suturing continues below left coronary artery and up edges of graft to attach adjacent commissures of graft to patient's aorta. Noncoronary sinus aorta of graft is trimmed to match height of noncoronary sinus aorta of patient so that the graft and host aorta may be attached by simple continuous suture.

Continued

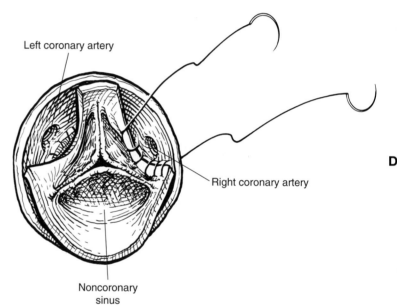

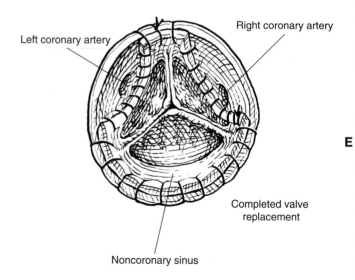

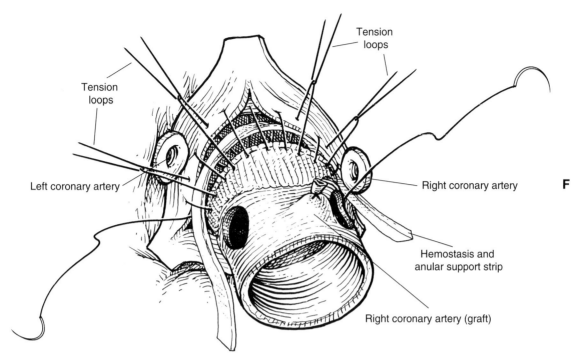

Figure 12-12, cont'd   F, Complete root replacement technique may be employed when Medtronic Freestyle device is used to repair aortic root disease. Inflow sewing cuff of graft is attached to aortic anulus by continuous or simple interrupted suture technique. A narrow strip of polytetrafluroethylene felt may be placed within suture loops for greater hemostasis. Left coronary artery of graft is removed and will always be the proper site for anastomosis of left coronary artery of the patient to the graft. Because porcine coronary arteries are closer together than 120 degrees, it is often necessary to position the opening for right coronary artery anastomosis further to the right than the location of the porcine right coronary artery.

Suture loops may be placed around a PTFE felt strip for added suture line hemostasis. Alternatively, simple interrupted sutures may be employed.

The device is firmly attached to the aortic valve anulus by tightening the suture loops. The ligature on the left coronary artery of the graft is cut away to create an opening into the graft. The left coronary artery is anastomosed using continuous No. 4-0 or 5-0 polypropylene suture. Although the left coronary artery always fits neatly to the position of the graft's left coronary artery, the right coronary artery may not fit properly to its counterpart because coronary arteries in the porcine aortic root are closer together than in humans. It is usually necessary to create another opening into the right coronary sinus of the graft at an appropriate location to prevent kinking of the right coronary artery. The position is usually to the right of the right coronary artery of the porcine root, although it may be placed on part of the base of the porcine right coronary artery. Proper location of the right coronary artery is facilitated by filling the right ventricle with blood from the pump-oxygenator. Any evidence of myocardial ischemia after aortic root replacement indicates need for revision of the location of the coronary anastomosis or for coronary artery bypass grafting.[L21]

Autograft Pulmonary Valve

The aortic valve may be replaced with the patient's own pulmonary valve (pulmonary autograft) and a pulmonary allograft used to replace the pulmonary valve. This opera-

tion was devised by Ross and appropriately carries his name.[R10] The operation has the advantage of placing autogenous tissue in the high-pressure aortic position that should last indefinitely, assuming the procedure is technically correct. The allograft tissue is placed in the low-pressure pulmonary position, where even if it should fail, valve regurgitation should be tolerated for a long time.

CPB is established using two cannulae for venous drainage. A right-angle cannula is placed directly into the superior vena cava at the pericardial reflection. The other is placed in the inferior vena cava through the right atrium at the diaphragm (see "Preparation for Cardiopulmonary Bypass" in Section 3 of Chapter 2). Alternatively, a single two-stage venous uptake cannula may be used, placing the second-stage opening low in the right atrium near the inferior vena cava orifice. Vacuum-assisted venous return provides more safety and reserve when the single-cannula technique is used, reducing the risk and consequences of air lock, which may occur in a gravity drainage system when the right ventricle is opened (see "Vacuum-Assisted Venous Return" in Section 1 of Chapter 2). Oxygenated blood is returned to the ascending aorta.

Pulmonary autograft technique. The aortic root is explored through the usual transverse incision. Once it is determined to proceed with the pulmonary autograft operation, the ascending aorta is divided, the aortic valve removed, and the entire sinus aorta excised except for a generous rim around the coronary ostia (Fig. 12-13, *A*).

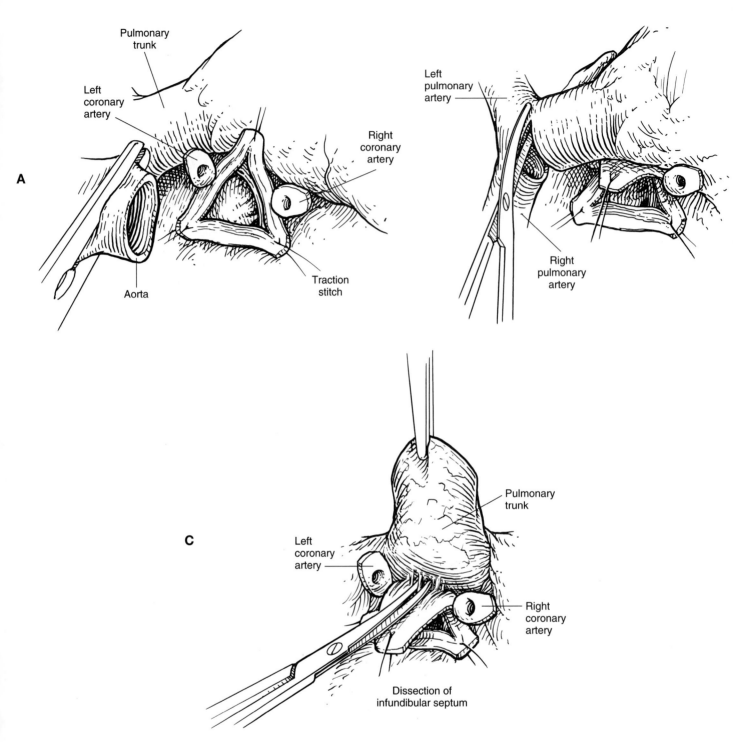

Figure 12-13   Aortic valve replacement with pulmonary autograft (Ross procedure), aortic root replacement technique. **A,** Ascending aorta is divided, aortic valve is removed, and all aorta from sinuses of Valsalva is excised except for generous buttons around coronary artery ostia. Traction stitches are placed above each commissure. **B,** Pulmonary trunk is divided at bifurcation. Pulmonary valve is inspected to assure normal morphology. **C,** Dissection between medial commissure of aortic valve and pulmonary trunk enters infundibular septum. Plane between infundibular septum and right ventricular outflow tract is identified and dissection carried as far behind pulmonary trunk as is convenient.   *Continued*

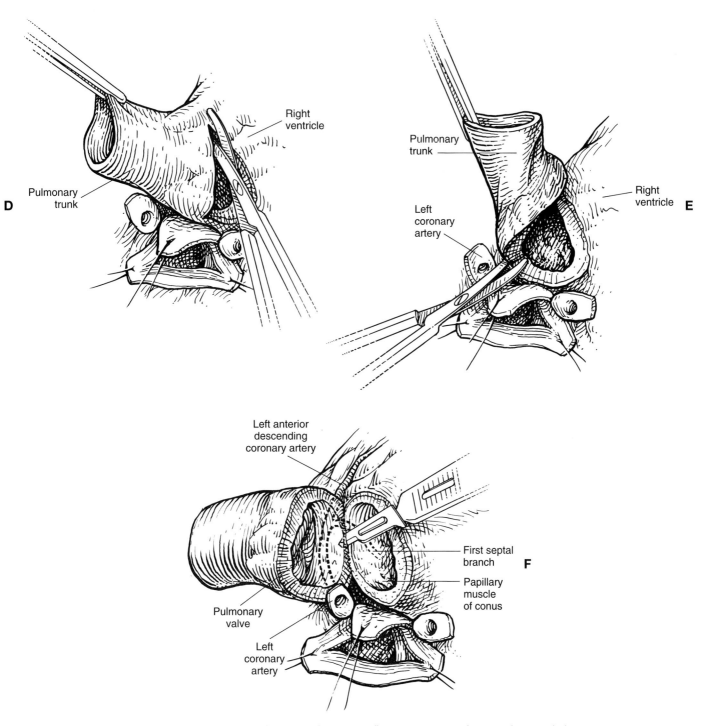

D

Pulmonary trunk

Right ventricle

Pulmonary trunk

Left coronary artery

Right ventricle

E

Left anterior descending coronary artery

First septal branch

F

Papillary muscle of conus

Pulmonary valve

Left coronary artery

Figure 12-13, cont'd   D, Right ventricular (RV) outflow tract is opened anteriorly 5 mm below pulmonary valve. **E,** Incision of the RV outflow tract is extended posteriorly to extent of previous dissection (**C**). **F,** Shallow incision is made below pulmonary valve posteriorly in the RV outflow tract joining extent of RV incisions. Angle of scalpel is changed so that ventricular myocardium may be shaved off infundibular septum without injuring underlying first septal branch of left anterior descending coronary artery.   *Continued*

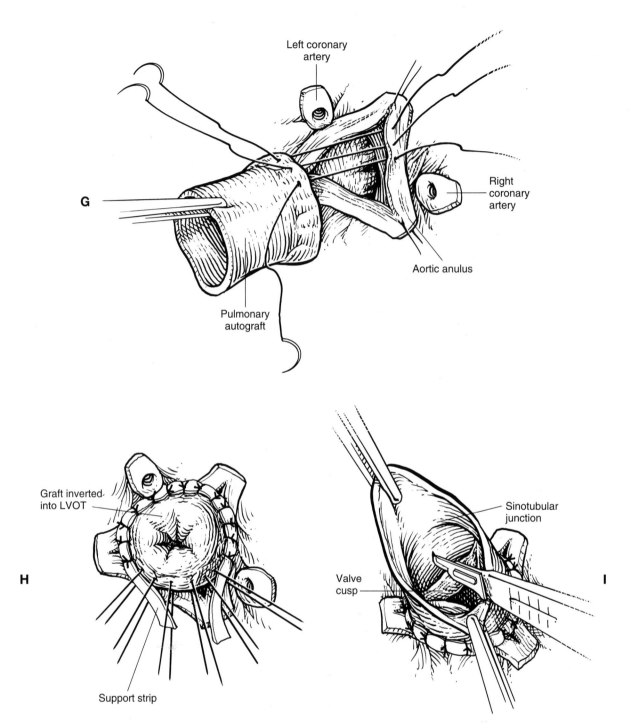

G

Left coronary
artery

Right
coronary
artery

Aortic anulus

Pulmonary
autograft

Graft inverted
into LVOT

H

Support strip

Sinotubular
junction

Valve
cusp

I

Figure 12-13, cont'd   G, Pulmonary autograft trunk is transferred to aortic position. Simple interrupted stitches of No. 3-0 polypropylene are used to attach pulmonary autograft to aortic anulus (see Fig. 12-11, *B*). **H,** Narrow strip of polytetrafluroethylene felt or pericardium is placed within suture loops. Pulmonary autograft is partially inverted into left ventricular outflow tract. Sutures are tied to secure pulmonary autograft to anulus of aortic valve, making sure that there is direct tissue approximation and keeping support strip to the outside. **I,** An opening is made in posterior sinus of Valsalva of pulmonary trunk and a narrow strip of tissue removed from one side to create a site for anastomosis of left coronary artery.

Key: *LVOT,* Left ventricular outflow tract.   *Continued*

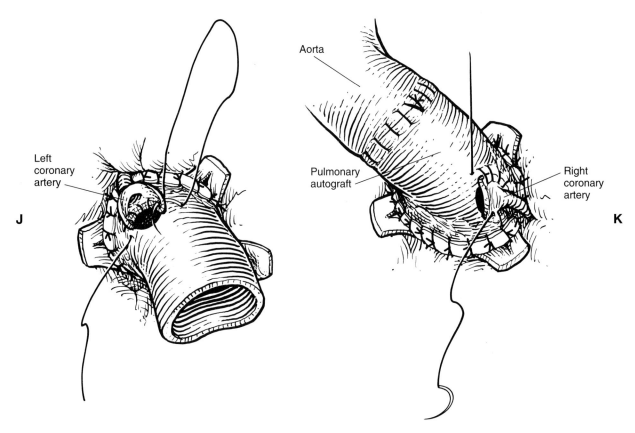

Figure 12-13, cont'd   **J**, Left coronary artery is anastomosed to pulmonary trunk using continuous stitches of No. 5-0 polypropylene. **K**, Pulmonary trunk is anastomosed in end-to-end fashion to ascending aorta. Aortic occlusion clamp is removed temporarily to fill pulmonary autograft under pressure so that proper position for right coronary artery anastomosis can be located. A small opening is made into graft, and right coronary artery is anastomosed to it.

Continued

Traction stitches on the aorta above the coronary arteries are helpful. Only the fibrous connection of the aortic cusps remains for attachment of the pulmonary autograft. Traction stitches are placed above each commissure. Diameter of aortic anulus is measured using Hegar dilator sizers.

The pulmonary trunk is separated from the aorta up to its bifurcation. It is divided at the bifurcation, taking care not to shorten the right pulmonary artery (Fig. 12-13, *B*). The pulmonary valve is inspected from above. If it is normal, operation may proceed. If it is abnormal, the pulmonary artery is reanastomosed and an aortic allograft used to replace the aortic root.

Dissection between the medial commissure of the aorta and the pulmonary trunk comes down onto the muscle of the right ventricular (RV) outflow tract (Fig. 12-13, *C*). Thorough dissection between the aorta and pulmonary trunk, especially low onto the RV in the plane between the RV outflow tract and the infundibular septum, makes removing the pulmonary trunk much easier.

The anterior interleaflet triangle below the anterior commissure is identified as a reference point for opening the RV outflow tract. A small right-angle clamp is placed precisely in the anterior interleaflet triangle and pushed through the anterior wall of the RV. The small opening is carefully enlarged. The pulmonary trunk is separated from the RV, looking inside frequently to maintain appropriate length of

the ventricle below the pulmonary valve (Fig. 12-13, *D*). Incision of the RV outflow tract continues on the right side and posterior to the extent of previous dissection (Fig. 12-13, *E*).

The critical and unique part of the Ross operation is separating the pulmonary trunk from the RV outflow tract above the infundibular septum. When done correctly, this part of the procedure makes the entire operation safe. Anatomy of the subpulmonary infundibulum is described in "Right Ventricle" under Cardiac Chambers and Major Vessels in Chapter 1.[M39] Injury to the underlying first septal branch of the left anterior descending coronary artery during dissection of the pulmonary trunk is a major source of morbidity in this operation. A shallow incision of the endocardial surface is made to join both ends of the partly excised pulmonary trunk (Fig. 12-13, *F*). The incision extends completely across the remaining undivided RV outflow tract. The angle of the scalpel is immediately changed to shave off the ventricular myocardium almost parallel to the endocardial surface. This shaves off the pulmonary trunk without injuring the underlying first septal branch. This part of the operation should be performed deliberately and under precise control. The septal excision eventually separates the pulmonary trunk completely, leaving the left main coronary artery and the first septal branch behind and

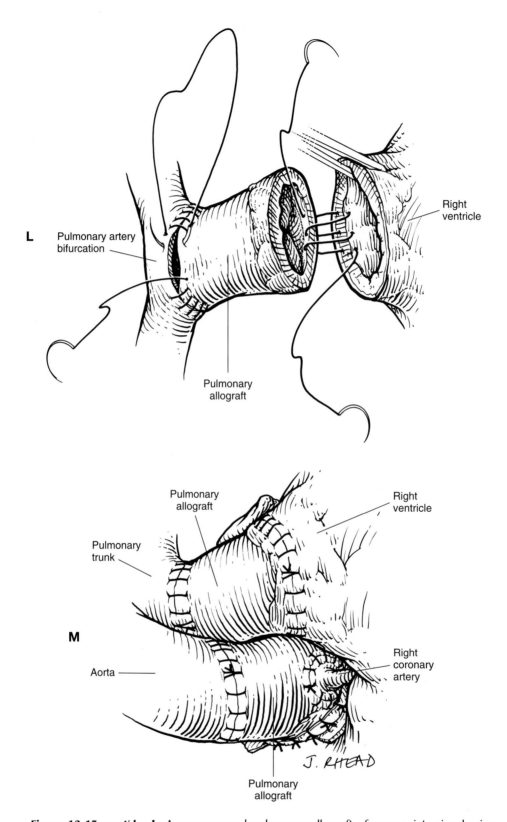

L   Pulmonary artery
     bifurcation

Right
ventricle

Pulmonary
allograft

Pulmonary
allograft

Right
ventricle

Pulmonary
trunk

M

Aorta

Right
coronary
artery

J. RHEAD

Pulmonary
allograft

Figure 12-13, cont'd   L, A cryopreserved pulmonary allograft of appropriate size, having previously been selected and thawed, is anastomosed in end-to-end fashion to pulmonary artery bifurcation. Exposure for this anastomosis is better if it is performed before the aortic anastomosis. Proximal end of pulmonary allograft is anastomosed to right ventricular outflow tract using continuous stitches of No. 3-0 polypropylene. Stitches are placed through only partial thickness of infundibular septum posteriorly over location of first septal branch of left anterior descending coronary artery. **M,** Completed repair: aortic valve replacement with pulmonary autograft, pulmonary trunk replacement with pulmonary allograft.

protected by a generous layer of tissue. The septal artery is occasionally seen in the myocardium.

The separated pulmonary trunk is placed in the pericardial sac for immediate use. The trunk is not removed from the operating field to prevent its misplacement or inadvertent mixture with the allograft. At this point it is convenient to measure the dimensions of the pulmonary anulus using standard prosthetic valve sizers and to choose a pulmonary allograft for preparation for later use.

The pulmonary autograft is attached to the unmodified LV outflow tract using interrupted stitches of No. 3-0 polypropylene (Fig. 12-13, *G*). Size discrepancy between the pulmonary autograft anulus and aortic anulus should not exceed 2 mm. A larger discrepancy indicates the need to adjust the anulus of the aorta to match that of the pulmonary autograft (see "Method for Reducing Diameter of Dilated Aortic Anulus" later in this chapter). The graft is marked below each of the commissures for orientation. The anterior commissure of the graft is oriented to approximate the commissure between the right and noncoronary sinuses. Suturing proceeds below each sinus, separating the stitches into three groups. Stitches are placed through the strong fibrous tissue of the aortic anulus, keeping the plane of repair as level as possible. A strip of PTFE felt about 5 mm wide is used to fix the diameter of the proximal suture line and to ensure hemostasis between the sutures (Fig. 12-13, *H*). A strip of autogenous pericardium may also be used. A "supported" repair is favored to prevent dilatation of the pulmonary autograft at the proximal suture line. Some surgeons prefer a continuous suture line using absorbable stitches without prosthetic material, especially for children in whom growth of the pulmonary autograft is desired. However, the accuracy of carefully spaced individual stitches and fixation support of the anulus seem best in adult patients. The felt or pericardial strip is placed within the suture loops so that it is incorporated as the sutures are tied down. The pulmonary autograft is partially inverted into the LV outflow tract as the sutures are tied to ensure that tissue approximation is accurate and that the support ring is to the outside rather than interposed between the tissues of the pulmonary autograft and the aortic anulus.

An opening is made into the left coronary sinus of the autograft using a scalpel (Fig. 12-13, *I*). Only minimal sinus tissue is excised because the delicate pulmonary artery dilates and separates readily. The sinotubular junction of the graft is preserved to maintain proper relationships of the commissures and cusps.

The left coronary anastomosis proceeds, working on the outside of the pulmonary graft (Fig. 12-13, *J*). Continuous stitches of No. 5-0 polypropylene are used. As a practical matter, it is best to perform the right coronary anastomosis after completing the aortic anastomosis so that the pulmonary trunk can be distended by temporarily removing the aortic clamp (Fig. 12-13, *K*). The right coronary anastomosis typically fits high in the right sinus or even above the sinotubular junction on the anterior wall of the pulmonary trunk. It may also be advisable to perform the anastomosis of the pulmonary allograft to the bifurcation of the pulmonary trunk before the aortic anastomosis if the medial aspect of the pulmonary anastomosis might be obscured by the overlying aorta (Fig. 12-13, *L*). Often the diameter of the aorta is larger than that of the pulmonary trunk, but the

pulmonary trunk is usually sufficiently long that a bevel can be created to take up any size discrepancy. With gross aortic enlargement or aneurysm, the entire ascending aorta may be removed and the pulmonary trunk extended with a prosthetic graft (see "Method for Extending Pulmonary Autograft" later in this chapter).

Pulmonary allograft technique. The cryopreserved pulmonary allograft is trimmed minimally. An end-to-end anastomosis of the pulmonary allograft to the pulmonary bifurcation is performed using continuous stitches of No. 4-0 polypropylene (see Fig. 12-13, *L*). Retracting the LV inferiorly and placing the graft in the space between the pulmonary bifurcation and the RV makes it easier to perform the anastomosis of the posterior wall of the pulmonary arteries. It is usually preferable to perform this anastomosis before constructing the aortic anastomosis. The proximal end of the pulmonary allograft trunk is anastomosed to the RV outflow tract (see Fig. 12-13, *L*). Continuous stitches of No. 3-0 polypropylene are used. Needle penetration must be through only part of the thickness in the infundibular septum to avoid injury to the underlying first septal branch of the left anterior descending coronary artery. A potentially weak point on the anastomosis at the transition from the infundibular septum to the medial aspect of the RV free wall may be reinforced with a PTFE pledget worked into the suture line. The completed repair produces a remarkably normal anatomic appearance (Fig. 12-13, *M*).

Method for lengthening pulmonary allograft. The pulmonary allograft may be tailored to achieve greater length, reducing the chance that the graft will be too tight between the RV outflow tract and pulmonary artery bifurcation. The entire left pulmonary artery may be retained on the graft. The right pulmonary artery is removed and closed by direct suture using No. 5-0 polypropylene to lengthen the graft (Fig. 12-14, *A*). The left pulmonary artery is cut back to the bifurcation to create a large circumference for anastomosis. Making the pulmonary allograft long or even slightly redundant may be important in maintaining proper graft length, because myocardium below the pulmonary allograft valve is resorbed and replaced with contracting scar.

Method for reducing diameter of dilated aortic anulus. When the patient's LV outflow tract at the level of the anulus is more than 2 mm in diameter greater than the pulmonary autograft, the patient's anulus may be narrowed to fit the autograft, taking up this variance in anular diameters. Interrupted mattress stitches of No. 2-0 braided suture reinforced with PTFE pledgets are placed through the fibrous tissue that supports the aortic leaflets alongside each of the commissures. The stitches are placed across the interleaflet triangle so that the triangle is obliterated on tying down the suture (Fig. 12-14, *B*).

Method for extending pulmonary autograft. When the ascending aorta is greatly dilated or aneurysmal, it is advisable to remove the affected aorta. A polyester tubular graft with the same diameter as the pulmonary autograft's distal end at the sinotubular junction is selected for replacement of the ascending aorta as an interposition graft (Fig. 12-14, *C*).

Method for fixing sinotubular junction. Evidence indicates that the pulmonary trunk may dilate up to 30% in diameter and length when exposed to systemic arterial

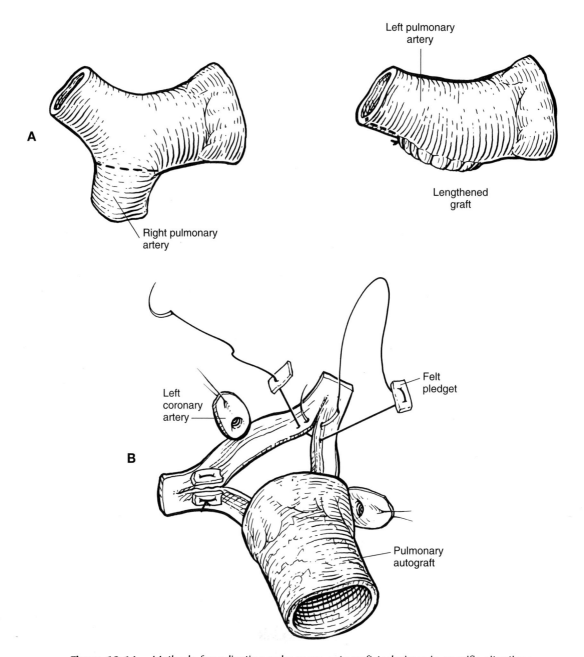

Figure 12-14 Methods for adjusting pulmonary autograft technique in specific situations. **A,** Method for lengthening pulmonary allograft to prevent tension on graft between right ventricular outflow tract and bifurcation of pulmonary artery as right ventricular myocardium on graft is reabsorbed and replaced with scar tissue. Left pulmonary artery is retained with pulmonary trunk; it may be cut back *(broken line)* to pulmonary bifurcation to create a large opening. Right pulmonary artery is removed and its origin closed by continuous suture. **B,** Method for reducing diameter of dilated aortic anulus for proper size match with pulmonary autograft. Pledget-reinforced horizontal mattress stitches are placed through the fibrous tissue adjacent to intercusp triangles posteriorly and medially to obliterate triangular space, thereby reducing anular diameter. *Continued*

pressure.[V3] Schmidtke and colleagues found the pulmonary trunk in the aortic position as a freestanding root assumed a diameter of 41 mm at the sinus level, compared with a 32-mm diameter when the autograft was placed within the natural aorta in patients undergoing the Ross procedure.[S27] The pulmonary trunk may also dilate in the clinical setting of bicuspid aortic valve with dilated ascending aorta.[D39]

Fixing the diameter of the sinotubular junction of the pulmonary autograft may be desirable and may prevent or correct pulmonary autograft regurgitation. A segment of a tubular polyester vascular prosthesis equal to or 1 to 2 mm greater than the diameter of the pulmonary autograft sinotubular junction (10% larger) is placed on the outside of the graft to fix the graft's diameter at its normal dimension. The

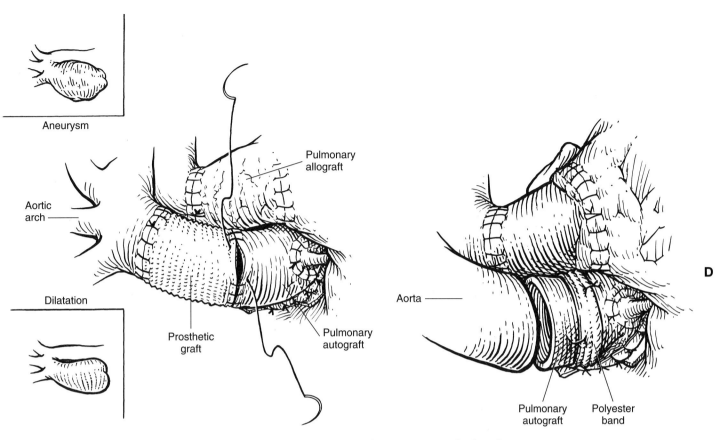

Labels in figure: Aneurysm; Aortic arch; Dilatation; Prosthetic graft; Pulmonary allograft; Pulmonary autograft; Aorta; Pulmonary autograft; Polyester band; **D**

Figure 12-14, cont'd   **C**, Method for extending pulmonary autograft when there is aneurysm or dilatation of ascending aorta. Aneurysmal aorta is removed. Pulmonary autograft is lengthened by attaching a tubular polyester graft of exactly the same diameter as the pulmonary artery just above valve commissures. **D**, Method of fixing sinotubular junction of pulmonary autograft to prevent dilatation. A segment of tubular polyester vascular prosthesis 10% smaller than measured diameter of pulmonary valve is placed around outside of autograft at level of sinotubular junction. A few interrupted stitches are placed to attach graft to pulmonary artery to prevent migration.

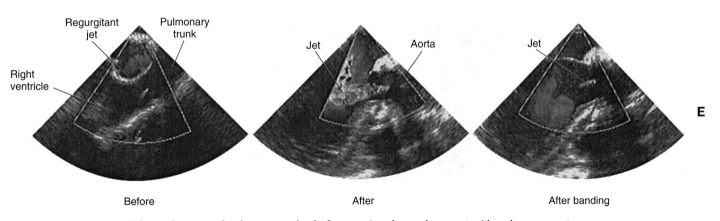

Labels in figure: Regurgitant jet; Pulmonary trunk; Right ventricle; Before; Jet; Aorta; After; Jet; After banding; **E**

E, Echocardiogram of pulmonary valve before aortic valve replacement with pulmonary autograft shows typical trivial central valve regurgitant jet. After pulmonary trunk is transferred to aortic position and subjected to systemic arterial pressure, there is moderate (2+) valve regurgitation. Narrowing the sinotubular junction with an external band restores valve to preoperative state of trivial regurgitation.

polyester segment is attached to the pulmonary autograft with a few simple stitches to prevent migration (Fig. 12-14, *D*). A PTFE felt strip works equally well, but the diameter of the finished band is more difficult to control. Surgeons not wanting to fix the diameter of the pulmonary autograft at the sinotubular junction may find that narrowing the graft with a felt strip may correct possibly important autograft regurgitation (Fig. 12-14, *E*).

Replacement of Aortic Valve and Ascending Aorta, En Bloc

Replacement of aortic valve and ascending aorta, en bloc, is most frequently performed for anuloaortic ectasia and ascending aortic aneurysm accompanied by aortic valve regurgitation. Occasionally, en bloc replacement is performed for infective endocarditis of the aortic root with extensive abscess formation and in the setting of acute or chronic aortic dissection with aortic valve regurgitation, where the technique of distal anastomosis may be somewhat different.

Initial Steps

The early steps of the en bloc operation differ somewhat from those of simple aortic valve replacement. The arterial cannula may need to be placed through the common femoral artery (see "Cardiopulmonary Bypass Established by Peripheral Cannulation" in Section 3 of Chapter 2). When the ascending aortic aneurysm stops short of the innominate artery origin, the distal ascending or proximal transverse arch can be cannulated in the usual manner.

A limited dissection is done, separating the right and contiguous portion of the pulmonary trunk from the back of the aorta and the aneurysm. This approach affords safe placement of the aortic occlusion clamp just proximal to the innominate artery. The procedure involves clean surgical separation of the right and contiguous portion of the pulmonary trunk from the back of the aorta and from the aneurysm, if possible.

CPB is established at 34°C using a single two-stage venous cannula and left atrial vent. The perfusate temperature is lowered to bring body temperature to 28°C. The aorta is occluded just proximal to the innominate artery. The ascending aorta is opened transversely in its midportion, stay sutures are applied, and cardioplegia is given.

The patient's aortic root is disconnected from the LV outflow tract and left atrium–mitral valve. The sinus aorta surrounding the coronary arteries is retained. The remaining sinus aorta is excised, leaving only fibrous aortic valve attachments, which are normal and uninvolved with the disease process being treated. The ascending aorta is divided by extension of the transverse aortotomy.

Allograft Aortic Valve Cylinder

When the ascending aorta is replaced along with the valve, sizing of the allograft valve is less critical than in the case of isolated aortic valve replacement. Aorta is usually sufficient on the graft to replace the ascending aorta. Length of the retained ascending aorta and arch are considered when choosing the graft (see Fig. 12-10). The distal aorta is tailored to fit the native aorta. The distal anastomosis is performed directly or under circulatory arrest with the patient's body temperature at 18°C.

Autograft Pulmonary Valve Cylinder

In young patients it may be desirable to use a pulmonary autograft as part of the en bloc operation. The pulmonary autograft is used as an intact pulmonary trunk to replace the aortic root as described earlier for isolated aortic valve replacement (see Fig. 12-14, *C*). The abnormal dilated or aneurysmal ascending aorta is excised. A crimped polyester tubular graft, collagen coated and of the same diameter as the distal end of the pulmonary autograft, is selected for replacement of the ascending aorta. This graft is anastomosed to the distal end of the pulmonary trunk. The graft is shortened and beveled appropriately for end-to-end anastomosis to the distal ascending aorta.

Composite Valve Conduit

Replacement of the aortic valve and ascending aorta as an en bloc procedure is most often done with a composite prosthesis containing a mechanical cardiac valve enclosed within a slightly larger tubular polyester graft. This operation is frequently referred to as the "Bentall" procedure.[B21] Previously these grafts required preclotting, but currently they have a collagen or gel coating that makes them impervious to blood.

The patient is placed on CPB using a single venous two-stage cannula, with oxygenated blood returned to the femoral artery in most cases. Occasionally, the amount of ascending aorta is sufficient to allow it or the transverse portion of the aortic arch to be perfused. The ascending aorta is occluded by a vascular clamp, and a vent catheter is placed through the right superior pulmonary vein to the left atrium and LV. A vertical incision is made in the aneurysm of the ascending aorta. Cold cardioplegic solution is administered to the coronary sinus by a retrograde coronary perfusion cannula. Traction stitches are placed above each aortic valve commissure to expose the aortic root (Fig. 12-15, *A*). The aortic valve is excised. The coronary arteries are mobilized, retaining a generous button of sinus aorta. A limited dissection of the coronary artery is sufficient to ensure that excision of the coronary artery is complete and that the coronary button will move easily up to the composite prosthesis without kinking or creating undue tension on the artery. The remaining sinus aorta is removed.

Diameter of the anulus is calibrated, and an appropriate size composite prosthesis, including the mechanical prosthetic aortic valve and attached crimped polyester tubular prosthesis, is selected. Stitches are placed through the anulus of the aortic valve and brought up through the sewing ring of the prosthesis using mattress stitches of No. 2-0 braided polyester with PTFE felt pledgets (Fig. 12-15, *B*). Suture placement is started in the right coronary sinus working clockwise, as for typical aortic valve replacement. Repair of the left coronary sinus follows, working counterclockwise. The repair is completed in the noncoronary sinus working clockwise.

Sutures are tied down to approximate the sewing ring of the prosthetic valve firmly to the aortic anulus (Fig. 12-15, *C*). A running suture technique is an acceptable method provided the anulus is strong and able to support the repair.

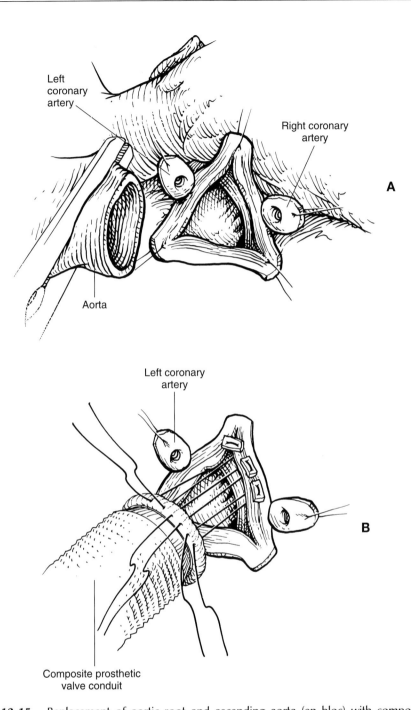

Figure 12-15   Replacement of aortic root and ascending aorta (en bloc) with composite prosthetic valve conduit. **A,** Aortic valve is excised. Aorta is removed from sinuses of Valsalva except for generous buttons around coronary ostia. Abnormal ascending aorta is removed. **B,** Composite prosthetic valve conduit is attached to anulus of aortic valve with pledget-reinforced horizontal mattress stitches of No. 2-0 braided polyester. Continuous suture technique may also be used.

Continued

A decision is then made regarding the method of reimplantating the coronary arteries to the graft. A direct anastomosis of the coronary ostia to the graft is usually made (Fig. 12-15, *D* and *E*). When aortic dissection involves the coronary ostia, it is necessary to repair the dissected aorta with biologic glue or reapproximate the dissected layers of aorta between PTFE felt "washers" (Fig. 12-15, *F*). In unusual circumstances

when the coronary ostia are displaced far laterally by a large-diameter aneurysm, it may be advisable to interpose a second graft between the coronary ostia and aortic graft to prevent tension on the coronary anastomosis, which is the most frequent point of hemorrhage after repair. Irreparable coronary ostial obstruction may require a bypass graft (saphenous vein) between the aortic graft and the affected coronary artery (Fig. 12-15, *G*). The

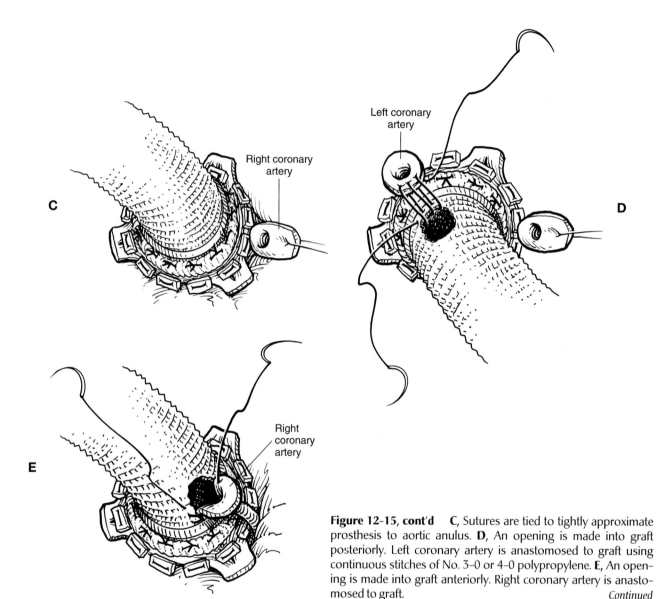

Figure 12-15, cont'd **C,** Sutures are tied to tightly approximate prosthesis to aortic anulus. **D,** An opening is made into graft posteriorly. Left coronary artery is anastomosed to graft using continuous stitches of No. 3-0 or 4-0 polypropylene. **E,** An opening is made into graft anteriorly. Right coronary artery is anastomosed to graft. *Continued*

primary ostium of the affected coronary artery is closed by suture.

The graft may be shortened appropriately to facilitate anastomosis of the coronary arteries to its side. Openings are made into the side of the graft exactly opposite the coronary artery ostia using scissors or battery-operated cautery.[B21,K15] Appropriately sized openings assist in creating the anastomosis. An adequate amount of graft should be left between the sewing ring of the prosthesis and the new coronary artery opening. The left coronary anastomosis is made first (see Fig. 12-15, *D*). The coronary ostium is approximated to the side of the graft by continuous stitches of No. 5-0, 4-0, or 3-0 polypropylene, depending on thickness of the aortic tissues. All the suture loops around the inferior rim of the coronary ostium are placed before pulling them up, so that this difficult area may be accurately approximated to the graft (see Fig. 12-15, *D*). Stitches are placed in "cartwheel" fashion around the coronary artery ostium, with deep bites into the aorta.

The right coronary anastomosis is performed after completing the left coronary anastomosis (see Fig. 12-15, *E*).

Both coronary ostia are approximated to the side of the graft in a similar manner.

The distal end of the graft is then shortened to approximate the distal end of the aorta. The aorta is completely divided to allow a direct end-to-end anastomosis. A short segment of graft is cut and placed as a collar over the main portion of the graft. The anastomosis is constructed using continuous stitches of No. 3-0 or 4-0 polypropylene, depending on the thickness and strength of the aorta. It is convenient to bring the first stitch from the outside of the aorta so that the stitching may continue from the inside surface of the graft. Several suture loops may be placed posteriorly before pulling the graft tightly against the aorta, to ensure accurate closure of the posterior wall of the anastomosis (Fig. 12-15, *H*).

The anastomosis is continued anteriorly and is completed by including all layers of the aorta in the graft. The graft collar is used to cover the completed anastomosis for hemostasis (Fig. 12-15, *I*).

Modifications are required when coronary artery ostia are either close to the anulus or widely separated laterally

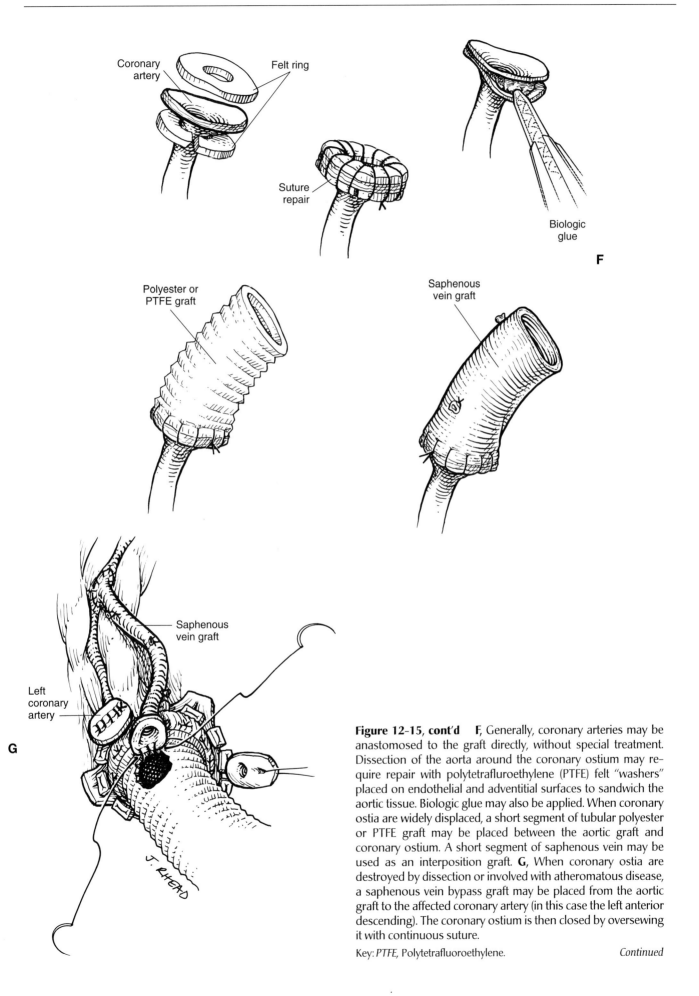

Figure 12-15, cont'd   F, Generally, coronary arteries may be anastomosed to the graft directly, without special treatment. Dissection of the aorta around the coronary ostium may require repair with polytetrafluoroethylene (PTFE) felt "washers" placed on endothelial and adventitial surfaces to sandwich the aortic tissue. Biologic glue may also be applied. When coronary ostia are widely displaced, a short segment of tubular polyester or PTFE graft may be placed between the aortic graft and coronary ostium. A short segment of saphenous vein may be used as an interposition graft. **G,** When coronary ostia are destroyed by dissection or involved with atheromatous disease, a saphenous vein bypass graft may be placed from the aortic graft to the affected coronary artery (in this case the left anterior descending). The coronary ostium is then closed by oversewing it with continuous suture.

Key: *PTFE,* Polytetrafluoroethylene.   *Continued*

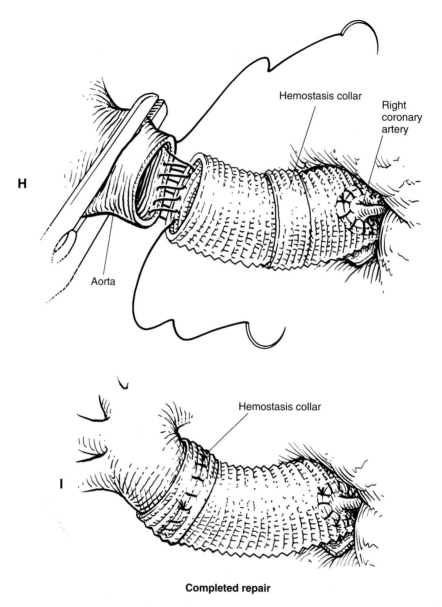

H

Hemostasis collar

Right
coronary
artery

Aorta

Hemostasis collar

I

Completed repair

Figure 12-15, cont'd **H,** End-to-end anastomosis of graft to aorta is constructed using continuous suture technique. A short segment of graft is cut and placed around the anastomosis to reinforce the suture line for hemostasis. **I,** Completed repair: replacement of aortic root and ascending aorta. Hemostasis collar is shown covering the graft to aorta anastomosis.

Continued

by an aortic aneurysm. When coronary artery ostia are bound tightly to the aortic anulus, usually by prior operation or valve replacement, it is impossible to create an accurate anastomosis to the tubular portion of a composite graft because the valve sewing ring may impinge on the coronary ostia. In this situation, a composite valve prosthesis is constructed by placing a prosthetic valve within a tubular polyester graft so that there is a short length of tubular graft extending below and a longer length of graft extending above the sewing ring of the valve (Fig. 12-15, *J*).[C22] The graft and sewing ring of the prosthetic valve are attached by continuous suture. The extension of the tubular graft below the prosthetic valve is attached to the aortic anulus, displacing the level of the prosthetic

valve cephalad above the bound down coronary ostia. Obstruction of the coronary ostia from contiguous placement of the thick sewing ring of the prosthetic valve is avoided. Ten-mm extension grafts from the aortic graft above the prosthetic valve to the coronary ostia complete the repair.

When the coronary artery ostia have been carried laterally and superiorly from the usual location relative to the aortic anulus by aneurysm or dilatation of the aortic root, it is necessary to create an extension from the composite prosthesis to the coronary arteries. Ten-mm tubular polyester grafts are attached to the coronary arteries and brought up to the anterior aspect of the composite prosthesis (Fig. 12-15, *K*).

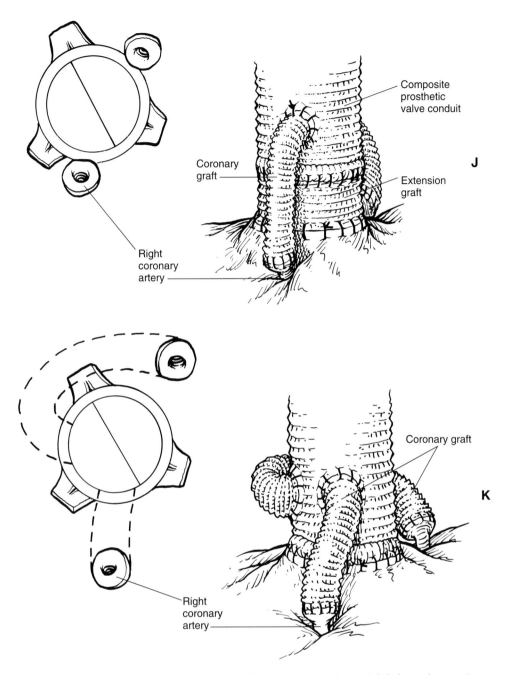

Figure 12-15, cont'd   **J,** Cabrol modification when coronary ostia are tightly bound to aortic anulus so that composite graft sewing cuff may impinge on the coronary ostia. A prosthetic valve is placed within a tubular polyester graft so that there is a short length of graft extending below the valve. The graft and the prosthetic valve are attached by continuous suture. The thin tubular graft is attached to the aortic anulus without obstructing the coronary arteries. Ten-mm tubular polyester grafts are used to extend the coronary arteries to the composite aortic graft above the location of the prosthetic valve. **K,** When the coronary arteries are carried laterally by aneurysm of the aortic root, extensions from the coronary arteries to the aortic graft are created following paths shown by broken lines. Ten-mm tubular polyester grafts are anastomosed to the coronary arteries and brought up to the aortic graft, where end-to-side anastomoses are created. The interposition graft prevents tension on the coronary artery anastomoses, thereby reducing chance of hemorrhage.

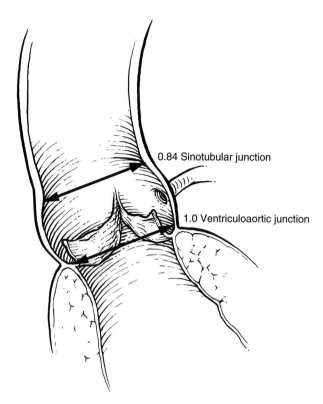

0.84 Sinotubular junction

1.0 Ventriculoaortic junction

Figure 12-16 Normal aortic root dimensions. Ratio of diameter of left ventricular outflow tract at ventriculoaortic junction (aortic anulus) to diameter at sinotubular junction is 0.84. (Based on data calculated at autopsy in normal young adults by Kunzelman and colleagues,[K27] recalculated by the author in 1997.)

Repair of Aortic Valve Regurgitation Caused by Aortic Dilatation or Aneurysm

Kunzelman and colleagues studied the relationships of the diameters at various levels in the aortic root, showing that the diameter at the sinotubular junction should be about 15% less than that at the base (anulus or ventriculoaortic junction) (Fig. 12-16).[K27] Grande and colleagues showed that minor dilatation of the aortic root (5% to 15%) caused increased stress on aortic valve cusps.[G18] In response to dilatation of the aortic root, strain on the valve cusps changes in order to maintain coaptation. This method of compensation fails at 30% to 50% dilatation of the aortic root, and cusp tissue is insufficient to maintain coaptation, resulting in aortic valve regurgitation. Frater demonstrated that simply adjusting the dimensions of the sinus rim or sinotubular junction can correct such regurgitation.[F3]

Beginning in 1979, Yacoub and colleagues[Y4] performed valve-preserving operations in patients with aneurysms of the ascending aorta and root (including those associated with Marfan syndrome.[B66]) and aortic dissection. The operation consists of removing all the sinus aorta except for a small rim of aortic tissue around the coronary ostia. Commissures are positioned to achieve good coaptation of the aortic valve cusps. The distance between the commissures is measured, and because this represents one third of the circumference at the sinotubular junction, a tubular graft three times that dimension is chosen. A 30-mm graft was used in 130 of 158 (82%) patients, fixing the sinotubular dimension at a diameter substantially larger than normal. Three slits are cut in the graft to about 1½ times the depth of the patient's sinuses. The graft is then attached to the aortic anulus, reconstructing the aortic sinuses with flaps of the graft that have been created. There is no circumferential fixation or reduction of diameter of the aortic anulus. Long-term results have been good, with 85% of patients free from reoperation at 15 years. Hvass described a similar technique, except that the polyester graft used to reconstruct the aortic root is placed as an inclusion cylinder within the intact aortic root.[H17] Improved flexibility of the prosthetic conduit may also improve dynamic features of the aortic valve cusps after valve–sparing operations.[D42]

David and Feindel described an aortic valve–sparing operation for patients with aortic regurgitation and aneurysm of the ascending aorta in which the aortic valve is reimplanted within a polyester tubular graft.[D15] The graft is secured to a level plane in the LV outflow tract just below the valve, except in the one sixth of the circumference occupied by the conduction system. Stitches are placed through the anulus, and a small wedge is removed from the graft to account for the higher level of suture placement. This fixes the diameter of the LV outflow tract, but one may reduce the diameter if necessary. The aortic valve is attached to the inside of the prosthetic graft (reimplanted). The graft determines the diameter of the sinotubular junction and is the same or slightly larger than the diameter of the anulus. This operation has been recommended for patients with Marfan syndrome who may have important dilatation of the ventriculoaortic junction and potential for further dilatation after repair. It could also be useful in aortic dissection by placing abnormal aortic tissues within the graft and thus reducing the risk of hemorrhage. Cochrane and colleagues modified the David operation to create pseudosinuses in the graft by removing three symmetric scallops from it, thereby lengthening the proximal suture line and restoring proper relationships at the sinotubular junction.[C31]

The pseudosinus method (Cochrane) and sinus-tailored method (Yacoub) result in simulated cusp stresses that are closer to normal than does the cylindrical technique (David).[G17] Again, the graft determines the diameter of the sinotubular junction, which in this operation should be smaller than the diameter of the anulus. The graft is usually 30 to 32 mm in diameter, although 28- or 34-mm grafts are occasionally used.

David recommended that when aortic root remodeling procedures, such as the Yacoub operation, are performed in patients with Marfan syndrome, or when the aortic anulus is dilated, an aortic anuloplasty should be performed.[D21,D22] A strip of prosthetic material is used on the outside of the LV outflow tract below the aortic valve to correct dilatation of the fibrous components of the LV outflow tract resulting from myxomatous changes in these tissues.

Identification of alterations of aortic root dimensions is the fundamental principle that allows accurate and reproducible aortic root reconstruction and restoration of aortic valve competence when the valve cusps are judged to be normal or near normal and morphology is thought to be related to abnormalities in the aorta. Intraoperative transesophageal echocardiography (TEE) identifies alterations of aortic root dimensions. The tubular graft used for reconstructing the aortic root then provides the unifying factor for accurately restorating aortic root dimensions for predictable aortic valve function. The graft is chosen after measuring the diameter of the LV outflow tract at the ventriculoaortic junction (aortic anulus). This dimension can be measured in all forms of aortic root abnormalities. Measuring the aortic anulus diameter is easier and more accurate than measuring the average length of the free edge of aortic valve leaflets, as proposed by David and colleagues, or the distance between commissures, as recommended by Morishita and colleagues.[D21,M31] The formulae for choice of proper graft diameter involve complicated mathematic and geometric relationships. Length of the free edge of the leaflet, however, must be directly related to the desired diameter of the aortic anulus.

Choo and Duran point out that the aortic root is dynamic, responding to pressure changes during the cardiac cycle that expand the aorta at the sinotubular junction by 35%, but the area at the base (anulus) by only 5%.[C32] Thus, they propose measuring the aortic root diameter at the base of the cusps as the most reliable method for appropriate graft sizing. The method proposed here is based on the measured diameter of the aortic anulus and simple arithmetic.[D2] When the diameter of the aortic anulus is normal, a graft is chosen that will narrow the sinotubular junction by 10% to 15%. When the diameter of the aortic anulus is enlarged, it is adjusted to normal diameter for body size using a graft diameter approximately 10% less than the desired aortic anular diameter. The geometry conveniently allows strips of the graft to support a reduction anuloplasty of five sixths the circumference of the anulus (avoiding the conduction system) while the graft adjusts the diameter of the sinotubular junction.

Intraoperative TEE is performed after induction of anesthesia and before incision. Aortic root dimensions are determined at the sinotubular junction and ventriculoaortic junction. Operations are performed on CPB using a single two-stage cannula for venous uptake, with oxygenated blood returned to a cannula placed high in the ascending aorta or arch or in the femoral artery. Deep hypothermia is used when the aneurysm extends beyond the ascending aorta.

The aorta is divided above the sinotubular junction and the aortic valve thoroughly examined. Normal aortic valve cusps suggest the possibility of a valve-sparing operation. Diameters of the sinotubular junction and ventriculoaortic junction are measured using Hegar dilators or accurate valve sizers. Alterations of aortic root dimensions are noted and will guide the steps taken to restore dimensions to normal.

Aortic Anulus Normal, Sinotubular Junction Enlarged

A normal aortic anulus with enlarged sinotubular junction is found in patients with aortic ectasia and aneurysm of the ascending aorta not involving the aortic sinuses.

A vascular graft the same diameter as the aortic anulus is selected. A 4- to 5-mm segment of the graft is prepared for placement on the outside of the aorta at the sinotubular junction (Fig. 12-17, A). The thickness of the aortic wall when compressed within the graft will reduce the inside diameter of the aorta to restore the normal dimension, which is 15% less than the diameter of the aortic anulus. Using this short segment of graft is easier and more accurate than attempting to attach a longer graft directly to the sinotubular junction.

Aortic Anulus Normal, Sinotubular Junction Normal

A normal aortic anulus with normal sinotubular junction is found in patients with aortic dissection.

A vascular graft 10% smaller than the diameter of the aortic anulus is selected, and three incisions are made into it at 120 degrees from each other (Fig. 12-17, B). The tips are removed from the flaps so created. The number of flaps depends on the sinuses involved in the dissection. The entire flap is removed corresponding to uninvolved sinuses. Dissected aortic sinus tissue is removed. The abnormal tissues should not cross the hinge point of the aortic valve leaflets (anulus). Flaps of the graft are used to reconstruct the sinuses, and if necessary, coronary arteries are reimplanted. Diameter at the sinotubular junction is restored to the diameter of the graft (see Fig. 12-17, E).

Aortic Anulus Enlarged, Sinotubular Junction Enlarged

An enlarged aortic anulus with enlarged sinotubular junction is found in patients with anuloaortic ectasia, some of whom have Marfan syndrome.

The sinus aorta is removed. The aortic anulus is reduced to a diameter appropriate for the patient's body size (Fig. 12-17, C), generally 25 mm for the average adult male, 27 mm for a large male, and 23 mm for an adult female. A vascular graft 10% to 15% smaller than that diameter is selected; thus, for a 25-mm anulus, a 22-mm graft is chosen. Two 4- to 5-mm segments (rings) of the graft are prepared to adjust the anulus diameter. The graft is tailored by making three incisions and trimming the flaps for sinus reconstruction and replacing the ascending aorta. To achieve an LV outflow tract 25 mm in diameter at the ventriculoaortic junction, the circumference of the aorta must be reduced to 78 mm ($25 \cdot \pi = 78$). This reduction is accomplished by "anuloplasty," using the short segments of graft to size the anulus accurately and to support the repair. Anuloplasty mattress stitches are placed in the LV outflow tract at a level plane just below the hinge point of the aortic valve. The stitches are placed beginning below the nadir or midpoint of the right coronary cusp of the aortic valve and working counterclockwise to the commissure between the noncoronary and right coronary cusps. This places the stitches on five sixths of the circumference, avoiding stitches in the one sixth of the ventricular septum that contains the conduction system. A strip of fabric to cover five sixths of the circumference and achieve a diameter of 25 mm is 65 mm in length ($78 \cdot \frac{5}{6} = 65$). It is convenient that a 22-mm crimped tubular polyester graft provides a strip of fabric 75 mm in length when the 4- to 5-mm segment is cut, opened, and stretched to length. From the strip of the graft, 10 mm of length is removed. The anuloplasty stitches are placed through the fabric strip and passed through the LV outflow tract to the outside as described. Thickness of tissue through which the needles pass is about 3 mm. Thus, the outside diameter to be

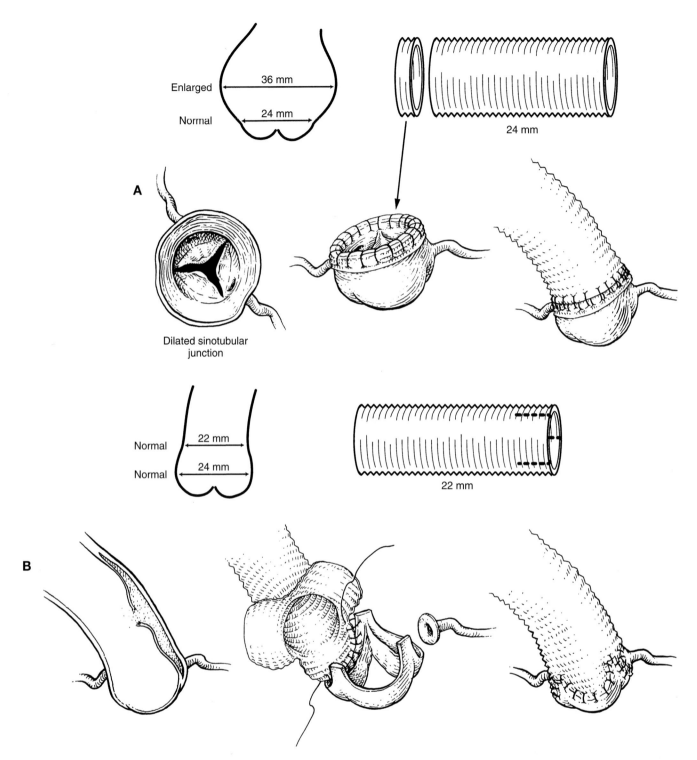

Figure 12-17   Repair of aortic valve regurgitation caused by dilatation or aneurysm of ascending aorta. **A,** Method for restoring aortic root dimensions in an aortic valve–sparing operation when aortic anulus is normal and sinotubular junction is enlarged. A 4- to 5- mm segment of graft the same diameter as the anulus is placed as a band on the outside of the aorta at the sinotubular junction to reduce the inside diameter 10%. **B,** Method for restoring aortic root dimensions in an aortic valve–sparing operation when aortic anulus and sinotubular junction are normal, as in aortic dissection. A vascular graft 10% smaller than the diameter of the aortic anulus is used to remodel the aortic root. Three slits are made into the graft at equal points on the circumference. The flaps created are rounded and attached to the aortic anulus from the lowest point to the top of the commissures. The "tailored" flaps recreate sinuses of Valsalva of the aortic root. Coronary arteries are reanastomosed to appropriate sinuses.

Continued

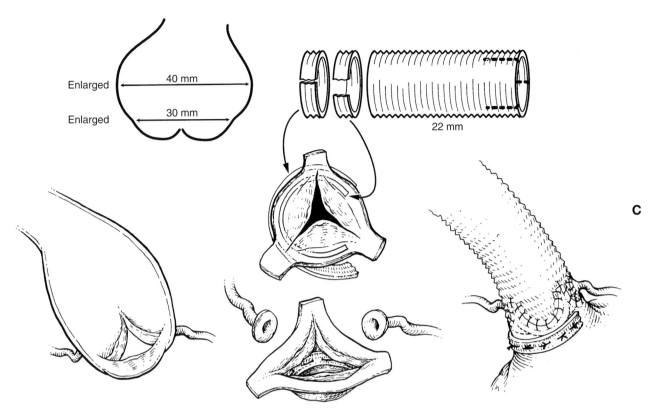

Figure 12-17, cont'd   C, Method for restoring aortic root dimensions in an aortic valve–sparing operation when the aortic anulus and sinotubular junction are enlarged, as in anuloaortic ectasia with Marfan syndrome. A vascular graft 10% to 15% smaller than the desired diameter of the aortic anulus is used to provide 4- to 5-mm strips of fabric that will support a reduction anuloplasty of ⅚ of the circumference of the left ventricular outflow tract (avoiding the conduction system) just below the aortic valve. Graft adjusts the diameter at sinotubular junction. Sinuses of Valsalva are reconstructed as in **B.**   *Continued*

supported will be about 28 mm in diameter. The length of fabric needed to support this diameter is, conveniently, about 75 mm $(28 \cdot \pi \cdot ⅚ = 74)$. The anuloplasty stitches are passed through the outside fabric strip. A 25-mm diameter Hegar dilator is placed in the LV outflow tract while the sutures are tied down. This narrows the LV outflow tract to a calculated diameter while distributing the tension equally over five sixths of its circumference.

The sinus aorta is reconstructed to the flap graft. Diameter of the sinotubular junction is accurately restored by the diameter of the graft chosen for the repair. Relationships just described should hold for the various graft sizes that might be chosen for reconstruction of the aortic root. Intraoperative TEE is performed with the heart contracting and ejecting at normal pressure to determine adequacy of the repair.

The Cochrane modification of the David operation has some advantages in patients with anuloaortic ectasia and Marfan syndrome in that the aortic valve is placed within the prosthetic aortic graft (Fig. 12-17, *D*).[C31,D15] This approach may provide more long-term strength to the repair of the aortic root. The aortic root is prepared by removing the entire aorta from the sinuses of Valsalva, retaining buttons of aorta around the coronary artery ostia. A 30- to 32-mm tubular polyester graft is selected. The graft is chosen by measuring the diameter of the aortic

anulus and adding 4 to 5 mm. The graft is scalloped to a depth of 4 to 5 mm at points 120 degrees on the circumference. Interrupted horizontal mattress stitches of No. 2-0 braided polyester are placed at a level plane just below the aortic valve from within the LV outflow tract and passed to the outside. The graft is attached using the sutures. It is then slid down to the outside of the LV outflow tract, placing the aortic valve entirely within the graft. The scalloped edge lengthens the circumference of the graft so that when sutures are tied down, pseudosinuses of Valsalva are created. Commissures of the aortic valve are positioned within the graft using a mattress stitch brought to the outside of the graft. The aortic valve is attached to the inside of the graft exactly as described for replacement of the aortic valve with an allograft (see Fig. 12-9, *C*).

Adequacy of aortic valve–sparing operations is confirmed by intraoperative TEE (Fig. 12-17, *E* and *F*).

The aortic root may be replaced with a stentless porcine bioprosthesis. Kon and colleagues replaced the aortic root with a stentless glutaraldehyde-processed porcine aortic root in 26 patients with 4% (CL 0.5%-12%) early mortality.[K26] In a multicenter trial (21 centers), 226 patients were implanted with a Medtronic Freestyle porcine aortic root bioprosthesis.[U1] Mean age was 70 ± 8.6 years. Two thirds of the patients were operated on for aortic valve regurgita-

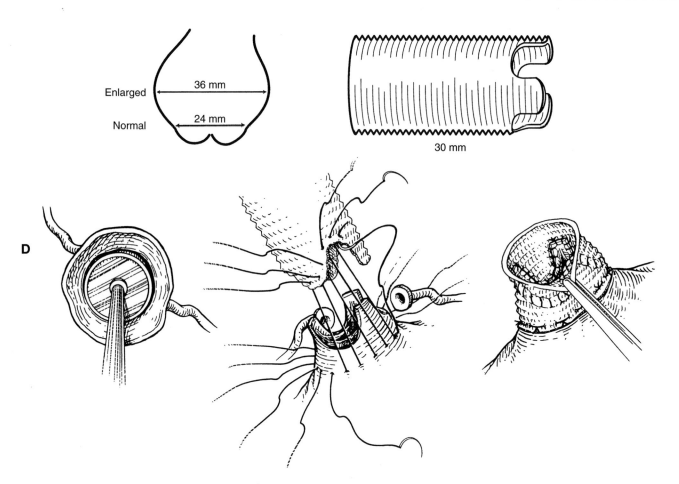

Figure 12-17, cont'd   **D,** Method for reconstructing aortic root using a graft with the aortic valve placed within it. A larger graft is used, usually about 30 mm in diameter. It is scalloped to a depth of 4 to 5 mm at three equidistant points on its circumference. These scallops lengthen the sewing circumference of graft so as to create "pseudo" sinuses of Valsalva. Graft is attached to aortic root by a series of interrupted horizontal mattress stitches placed below aortic valve from within left ventricular outflow tract. Aortic valve is attached to inside of graft in the manner described for aortic valve replacement with aortic allograft using the subcoronary technique. Coronary arteries are anastomosed to the appropriate pseudosinus (not shown).

tion or mixed stenosis–regurgitation, and 24% required ascending aorta replacement. Operative mortality was 11% in the older age group of patients with a high proportion of aortic pathology. Hemodynamic performance has been excellent, and the risk of thromboembolism leading to permanent deficit has been 1.0% per year over 6 years. The Freestyle bioprosthesis may be the device of choice for replacement of the aortic root in patients over age 70.

Aortic Valve Replacement and Coronary Artery Bypass Grafting

Preparation and draping of the patient and simultaneous removal and preparation of the saphenous vein are the same as in simple coronary artery bypass grafting (CABG) (see "Technique of Operation" in Chapter 7). Purse-string sutures for aortic cannulation are placed, with care taken that they are far enough distally (downstream) from the aortic valve to allow room for both the aortotomy and proximal venous graft anastomoses.

CPB is established. The operative procedure begins exactly as for isolated aortic valve replacement through excision of the aortic valve and selection of replacement device. The distal graft-to-coronary artery anastomoses are performed. Then the valve is replaced and the aortotomy closed. The vein grafts are routed and sized, and the proximal anastomoses to the aorta are performed. After de-airing the heart, CPB is discontinued and the operation completed as usual.

Redo Isolated Aortic Valve Replacement

Not all redo operations after primary aortic valve replacement involve a second replacement. Acute thrombosis may be treated by thrombectomy, and periprosthetic leakage of a mechanical valve or stent-mounted bioprosthesis may be successfully treated by simple resuture of the area of dehiscence. Prosthetic valve endocarditis, central leakages of all types, and extensive periprosthetic leakage typically require replacement.

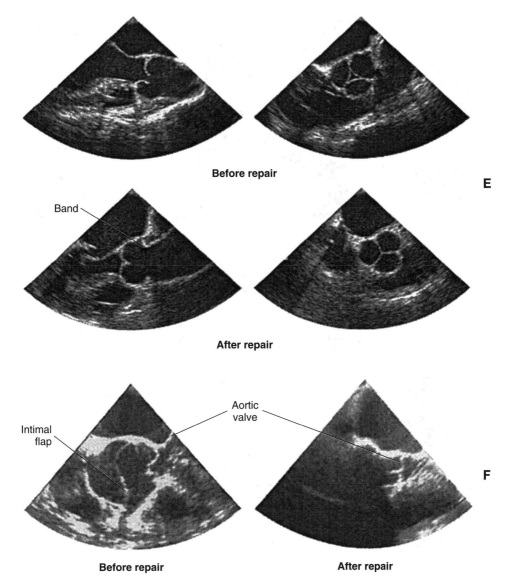

Before repair

E

Band

After repair

Intimal
flap

Aortic
valve

F

Before repair

After repair

Figure 12-17, cont'd   E, Two-dimensional echocardiograms before and after repair of aortic valve regurgitation caused by dilatation of ascending aorta. The sinotubular junction is narrowed by a band of appropriate size as described in **A. F,** Two-dimensional echocardiograms before and after aortic valve–sparing operation for aortic dissection using "tailored" flap method as in **B.** Aortic dissection resulted in dilatation of the aortic root, intima–media flap, and aortic valve regurgitation. After the repair using a tailored flap graft of appropriate size, the aortic valve is competent and aortic root dimensions are restored.

Technique of the operation embodies general principles of all redo cardiac operations (see "Secondary Median Sternotomy" under Incision in Section 3 of Chapter 2).

When a freehand-inserted allograft or xenograft requires rereplacement, the entire graft should be removed, including remnants of its aortic wall. The graft tissues are dissected from the sinus aorta and anulus using a Freer septum elevator, cutting suture material as required. This approach leaves an aortic root of good quality for insertion of either another allograft or other replacement device.

When a stent-mounted bioprosthesis or mechanical prosthesis has been used, the device is removed by pulling on the knots with a needle holder and using a No. 11 scalpel to cut individual sutures that were placed at the initial opera-

tion. Then using a Freer septum elevator, a dissection plane is established between the fabric of the prosthesis sewing ring and tissues of the aortic root. The prosthesis is thus removed intact and tissues of the aortic root remain in good condition to accept another prosthesis. Mechanical prostheses can also be removed by first separating the mechanical device from the sewing ring by sharply dividing the ring with a scalpel. The incision of the sewing ring is taken completely though the retaining thread that holds the ring to the mechanical device. Once these retaining threads are cut, the mechanical device comes away from the sewing ring. The fabric of the sewing ring is then more easily separated from the tissues by cutting the sutures placed at the initial operation.

Redo Aortic Valve and Ascending Aortic Replacement, En Bloc

The technique of reoperation needs to be modified from the standard approach because of an important risk of massive hemorrhage from the polyester tube graft at sternal reentry if the graft has adhered to the back of the sternum. Reentry is further complicated if aortic regurgitation is present. Under such circumstances, CPB is commenced through groin cannulation of the common femoral artery and vein using vacuum-assisted venous return (see "Vacuum-Assisted Venous Return" in Section 2 of Chapter 2). Core cooling is instituted to lower the nasopharyngeal temperature to about 20°C. When there is important aortic regurgitation, a limited left anterolateral thoracotomy may be made through the fifth intercostal space and a vent placed into the LV apex, monitoring LV end-diastolic pressure to maintain it at normal levels and prevent overdistention, even in the event of ventricular fibrillation. Alternatively, a large catheter (No. 12 French) is inserted percutaneously into the LV and its position confirmed by echocardiography. Adequate hypothermia permits the sternum to be opened with a vibrating saw without risk of exsanguinating hemorrhage. If the polyester tube is cut, CPB is stopped; blood escaping from the aorta is returned to the circuit by suction device, and control of the aorta distal to the tear is obtained before CPB is resumed. When infection is present, the prosthetic material should be removed entirely and replaced with an allograft. In the absence of infection, prosthetic material can be used again if desired.

SPECIAL FEATURES OF POSTOPERATIVE CARE

Postoperative care after adult aortic valve surgery is generally the same as after other types of cardiac surgery (see Chapter 5). Patients receiving a mechanical prosthesis are begun on lifelong sodium warfarin anticoagulant therapy on the evening of the second postoperative day. Intensity of anticoagulation should be specific for both prosthesis and patient.[B58] Modern mechanical prostheses are considered to have lower thrombogenicity than earlier devices. An international normalized ratio (INR) for prothrombin time of 2.5 is considered adequate to prevent valve thrombosis in the absence of abnormal intracardiac conditions. Atrial fibrillation alone does not raise the requirement for anticoagulation unless the left atrium is enlarged or LV function impaired. These additional risk factors dictate raising the intensity of anticoagulation to an INR of 3.0. Severe left atrial enlargement, greatly impaired LV function, or echocardiographic evidence of stasis in the left atrium require even higher levels of anticoagulation, with INR of 3.5 to 4.0. Some evidence indicates that adding aspirin (81 mg daily) further reduces risk of thromboembolism. Aspirin at higher levels (200 mg · day^{-1}) reduces total thromboembolic events, but morbidity associated with hemorrhage increases.[L16] Newer platelet antagonists have not been completely evaluated as adjuncts to warfarin therapy. Similarly, it is not known whether unfractionated heparin is necessary in a conservative anticoagulant protocol or if enoxaparin (Lovenox) should be started as soon as the first day after operation,

then continued for 5 days of combined therapy with warfarin until INR reaches a therapeutic level. Enoxaparin is usually administered as a fixed dose of 1 mg · kg^{-1} twice daily without any measure of its anticoagulant effect. This method of uncontrolled administration of a potent medication may expose the patient to excessive anticoagulation and added risk of postoperative hemorrhage. Patients are often autoanticoagulated early after operation with the prothrombin time and INR elevated above normal; this offers some protection against thrombus formation of the valve prosthesis.

Bioprostheses (human, porcine, bovine) in the aortic position of stent-mounted or stentless design do not require anticoagulation with warfarin. It is judicious to use aspirin therapy (81 mg daily) for 1 month, when risk of thromboembolism is greatest.

Patients in atrial fibrillation for more than 48 hours after operation are anticoagulated with warfarin until sinus rhythm is restored.

The thick-walled hypertrophied LV secondary to aortic valve disease requires a higher than usual filling pressure to distend it. Thus, a mean left atrial pressure of 8 to 10 mmHg, considered appropriate under many circumstances, may be inadequate to develop optimal LV *preload* early after operation in patients with important LV hypertrophy (see "Cardiac Output and Its Determinants" in Section 1 of Chapter 5). Reduction in myocardial compliance that occurs during cardiac surgery further increases the disparity between the usual mean left atrial pressure (LV filling pressure) and optimal preload.

For these reasons, unless cardiac performance is already optimal, left atrial pressure should be maintained at 15 to 18 mmHg by appropriate fluid infusion during the early hours after adult aortic valve surgery, particularly for severe aortic stenosis. This need is often less critical when operation has been done for aortic regurgitation, when the sudden reduction in LV stroke volume by the ablation of the aortic regurgitant flow improves left compared with right ventricular performance (see Chapter 5). Therefore, mean left atrial pressure may not be as elevated early postoperatively as when operation has been done for aortic stenosis.

Sinus tachycardia is frequently observed after operations on the aortic valve. When heart rate exceeds 100 beats · min^{-1} for several days and shows no signs of returning to normal, a beta-blocker should be administered to reduce the rate. It may be necessary to continue this therapy for 2 to 3 months until heart rate control mechanisms are restored.

RESULTS

Early (Hospital) Death

The Society of Thoracic Surgeons (STS) National Database reports a 3.4% (3.1% risk adjusted) hospital mortality for primary isolated aortic valve replacement[S35,S39] (Table 12-2). Risk is higher for women than men (3.9% versus 3.0%).[S39] When CABG is added to aortic valve replacement, the current risk of hospital death among STS National Database participants rises to 6.3%.[S35] These figures are similar to those reported in early experiences.[B29,C12,K8,M14,M18]

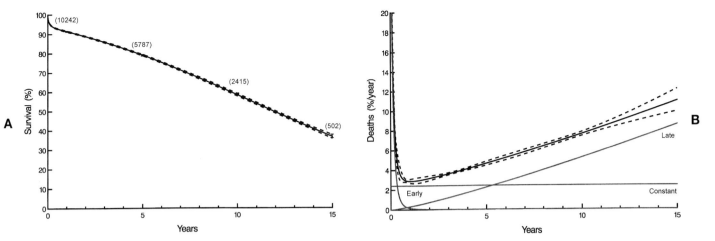

Figure 12-18   Survival after aortic valve replacement in a heterogeneous group of patients (see Appendix 12B for details). **A**, Survival. Parametric estimates *(solid line)* are enclosed within 68% confidence limits (CL). Numbers in parentheses represent number of patients still being followed at 1, 5, 10, and 15 years. Faintly visible at these same intervals are vertical bars representing CLs for the corresponding nonparametric Kaplan–Meier estimates. **B**, Hazard function (instantaneous risk of death). Solid curve enclosed within asymmetric 68% CLs represents parametric overall hazard estimates. Individual hazard components are labeled *early, constant,* and *late;* they sum to yield overall hazard. The rapidly falling early phase of risk lasted approximately 6 months (short-term survival), was dominated by operative mortality, and had the effective statistical power of 774 events. The constant hazard phase across all time dominated between 6 months and 5 years (intermediate-term survival) and had the statistical power of 1654 events. The late hazard phase, rising steadily from time zero, dominated beyond 5 years (late-term survival) and had the statistical power of 1470 events. Variables in multivariable analyses modulated the area beneath the early hazard phase, raised or lowered constant hazard, and tilted the late hazard component. (From Blackstone and colleagues.[B57])

■ TABLE 12-2   Hospital Mortality after Aortic Valve Replacement, 1962 through 2001

Year	n	Mortality (%)
GLH Experience		
1962-74	49	8.9
1974-80	95	9.5
1980-86	72	5.6
STS Database		
1995	7952	3.9
1996	9071	3.8
1997	9921	3.8
1998	9082	3.5
2001	3335	3.4

(Data from GLH experience [1962 to 1986] and Society of Thoracic Surgeons National Database Committee [1995 through 2001].[S35,S39])

Key: *STS,* Society of Thoracic Surgeons.

Time-Related Survival

Overall survival (including hospital deaths) after aortic valve replacement in heterogenous groups of patients is about 75% at 5 years, 60% at 10 years, and 40% at 15 years (Fig. 12-18, *A*).[B5,C4,H13,K1,M1,T1] These percentages are less than those in an age-gender-ethnicity–matched general population, except for elderly patients (Fig. 12-19). Many factors likely contribute to this, including the possible palliative nature of the operation, incomplete regression of LV remodeling after valve replacement, poor control of

chronic anticoagulation[B65] in patients receiving mechanical prostheses, reoperation for structural valve deterioration of bioprostheses, and other prostheses-related morbidity. Grunkemeier and colleagues report risk-unadjusted data suggesting that late survival is related to the type of device used to replace the aortic valve (Fig. 12-20)[G26]; patients with mechanical valve prostheses (mean age 57 years) had a survival advantage compared with those with bioprostheses (mean age 74 years). Adjusting for the age differences erased the apparent advantage of mechanical prostheses (see Fig. 12B-1 and Table 12B-2 in Appendix 12B).

The hazard function for death after aortic valve replacement is similar to that after other valve replacement operations in adults (Fig. 12-18, *B*). The early, rapidly declining hazard phase gives way to a late phase about 6 months after operation, which begins to rise as early as 5 years after operation.

Modes of Death

Of the few deaths early after aortic valve replacement, most are related to acute cardiac failure, neurologic complications, hemorrhage, and infection. Most late deaths are unrelated to the specific replacement device used. Cardiac failure and myocardial infarction are the most common modes of death, as after all valve replacement operations (Fig. 12-21). Sudden death occurs with surprising frequency, accounting for about 20% of late deaths. It may

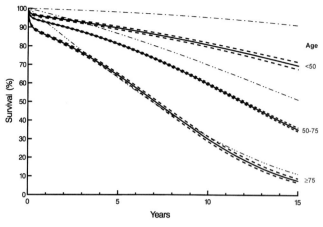

Figure 12-19 Survival after aortic valve replacement stratified by age group (see Appendix 12B for details). 1685 patients were age 50 years or younger; 1065 were alive and traced at 5 years, 539 at 10 years, and 160 at 15 years. 8224 were between age 50 and 75; 4010 were alive and traced at 5 years, 1725 at 10 years, and 303 at 15 years. 2636 were age 75 or older; 698 were alive and traced at 5 years, 140 at 10 years, and 10 at 15 years. For each age group, an age–gender–ethnicity–matched population life table curve is shown by the five dot–dash lines. Note that the younger the patient, the more marked is the departure from normal life expectancy. (From Blackstone and colleagues.[B57])

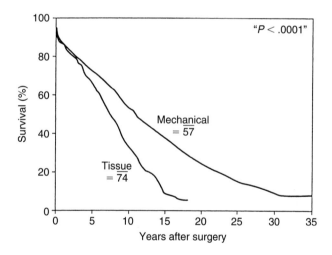

Figure 12-20 Long-term survival after aortic valve replacement comparing mechanical prostheses and bioprostheses (tissue). These data apparently strongly favor mechanical prostheses; however, mean age of patients in the mechanical group was 57 years, while it was 74 in the bioprosthesis (tissue) group. The "P" value is shown within quotation marks to indicate that when adjusted for differing age of patient populations, the survival curves are similar. (From Grunkemeier and colleagues.[G26])

result from thromboembolism in some patients, but its occurrence in patients with an allograft indicates other causes.

About 20% of deaths may be related to the device inserted, although the frequency may have decreased in recent years.[T4] Device-related deaths include thromboem-

■ **TABLE 12-3** **Average Remaining Lifetime** [a]

Age		Life Expectancy (Years)		
≤ years <		Total Population	Men	Women
20	25	56.7	53.5	59.8
25	30	52.0	48.9	55.0
30	35	47.3	44.3	50.1
35	40	42.7	39.8	45.4
40	45	38.1	35.4	40.6
45	50	33.6	31.0	35.9
50	55	29.2	26.7	31.4
55	60	24.9	22.6	27.0
60	65	20.9	18.8	22.8
65	70	17.3	15.3	18.9
70	75	14.0	12.2	15.3
75	80	10.9	9.5	11.9
80	85	8.3	7.1	8.9
85		6.0	5.2	6.4

(Data from National Center for Health Statistics, United States, 1993.)

[a] Survival curves for age-matched patient populations are generally presented as a gradually declining curve on a graph that plots percent survival versus time in years. Life tables are useful because they show the average number of remaining years of lifetime compared with age when considering choice of cardiac valve replacement valves.

bolism (and prosthetic thrombosis) and anticoagulation-induced hemorrhage (at least 10%), prosthetic valve endocarditis, and device failure, including bioprosthetic degeneration. When the aortic valve replacement device is an allograft, structural valve deterioration and endocarditis constitute the device-related modes of death.

Incremental Risk Factors for Premature Death

Table 12-4 summarizes incremental risk factors for premature death.

Older Age at Operation

Age of patients at operation has increased steadily since the beginning of aortic valve replacement and now approaches a mean of 70 years (Fig. 12-22).[G26] Overall survival curves are an artificial composite of patients of increasingly higher risk being served during increasingly safer years of calendar time. Older age at operation is a risk factor both early and late after aortic valve replacement, as after most cardiac operations.[B42,B65,C25,F7,K18,L14,M19,M24] However, elderly patients with any chronic illness are at increased risk of dying, and only death in the early phase is specific to the cardiac operation, as is evident in Fig. 12-19.

Strength of the risk factor of older age is less than might be expected.[C19,G21] Risk of death early after operation is about 1% at age 40 and about 8% in patients over 70 (Fig. 12-23).[B20,F7,M19] Risk of operative mortality for isolated aortic valve replacement among STS National Database participants is at least doubled when the operation is performed in patients over age 65 (4.9%) versus those under 65 (2.3%)[S35]; with associated coronary artery disease requiring CABG, the risk over age 65 increases to 7.6%, compared with 3.3% under 65. Levinson and colleagues reported that hospital mortality was 9.4% among 64 patients age 80 and older, 29 of whom underwent concomitant CABG.[L1] Five- and 10-year survival was 67% and

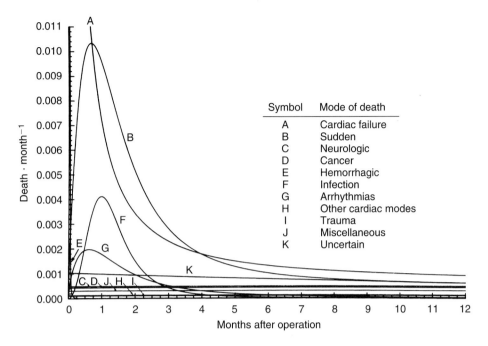

Figure 12-21   Hazard functions for each mode of death after primary aortic valve replacement in a group of 1533 patients. (An age-gender-ethnicity–matched general population has an incidence of deaths · month^{-1} of 0.001 across a 5-year period, similar to that for deaths in uncertain mode, marked K.) (From Blackstone and Kirklin.[B42])

49% among these elderly patients, and most enjoyed a satisfactory lifestyle. Similar results were obtained by Azariades and colleagues.[A10] Misbach and colleagues reported an even lower risk, with a hospital mortality of 3.4% (CL 2%-6%) in 101 patients over age 70, including 22 over age 80.[M19] Age is not so dominant a risk factor as to negate the effect of the other risk factors in elderly patients.[F7] Current risk of operation for aortic valve replacement combined with CABG in patients over age 80 is 10.1% (95%; CL 6.9%-13%), compared with 7.9% (95%; CL 6.6%-9.2%) in patients under age 80.[A18] Death early after operation in elderly patients tends to be related to excessive bleeding (in part attributable to the poor quality of the tissues), pulmonary dysfunction (in part related to generalized weakness and consequent delay in weaning from intubation and ventilation), and susceptibility to infection. Precise surgical techniques and acceleration of convalescence, with departure from the intensive care unit as quickly as possible, are helpful in neutralizing these risks.

Older age is also a risk factor for long-term mortality after aortic valve replacement. Grunkemeier and colleagues, analyzing data by decade of life, showed that probability of survival to 15 years in patients over age 70 is about 10%, compared with 65% in patients under 40 (Fig. 12-24).[G26]

Older patients may be more subject to important neurologic complications. Levinson and colleagues reported neurologic sequelae in 9% of 64 patients age 80 to 89 years undergoing isolated or combined aortic valve replacement.[L1] Alexander and colleagues reported associated neurologic events (15% versus 9.1%, $P < .05$) and renal failure (12% versus 6.8%, $P < .05$) were significantly higher in patients over 80 than in younger patients.[A18] These data

■ **TABLE 12-4   Incremental Risk Factors for Death Early and Late after Isolated and Combined Aortic Valve Replacement** [a]

	Risk Factors	Hazard Phase Early	Hazard Phase Late
	Demographic		
(Older)	Age	•	•
	African-American		•
	Clinical		
(Higher)	NYHA functional class (I-V)	•	•
(Greater)	Left ventricular enlargement (grades 0-4)	•	•
(More)	Aortic regurgitation (grades 0-5)	•	
	Angina	•	•
	Atrial fibrillation		•
	Morphologic (coexisting disease)		
(More)	Number of previous aortic valve replacement operations (grades 0-3)	•	•
	Coexisting coronary artery disease	•	•
	Coexisting aneurysm of ascending aorta	•	
	Prosthetic valve conduit		•
	Allograft aortic valve conduit	•	
	Autograft pulmonary valve conduit	•	
(More)	Left ventricular structural and functional abnormality (grades 0-4)	•	•
	Surgical		
(Earlier)	Era	•	
(Longer)	Global myocardial ischemic time	•	
	Type of replacement device		
	Mechanical prosthesis		•
	Bioprosthesis		•
	Allograft	•	
	Autograft	•	

Key: *NYHA*, New York Heart Association.

[a] Risk factors classified based on experience and published reports[B44,C25,C26] and not obtained by multivariable analysis.

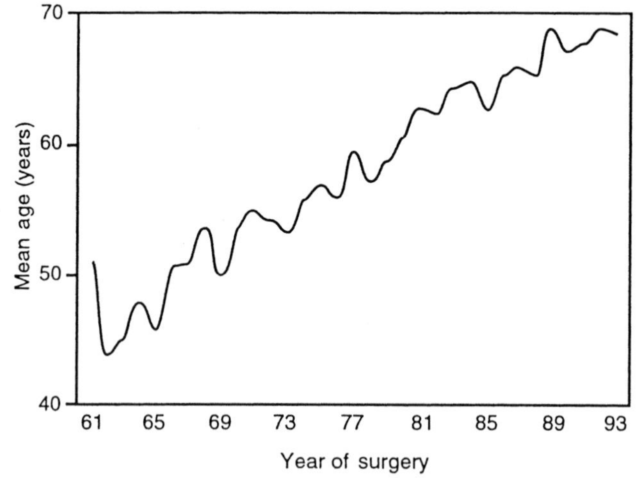

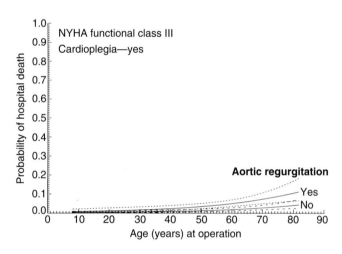

Figure 12-22   Age of patients at aortic valve replacement by year of operation. (From Grunkemeier and colleagues.[G26])

Figure 12-23   Relation of age at operation to probability of hospital death from all causes after primary isolated or combined aortic valve replacement. Nomogram of multivariable logistic equation. (From UAB group, 1975 to July 1979; $n = 842$.)

Key: *NYHA,* New York Heart Association.

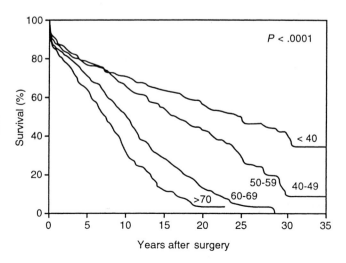

Figure 12-24   Survival after aortic valve replacement by age at operation (decades). Younger age at operation favors prolonged survival. (From Grunkemeier and colleagues.[G26])

■ **TABLE 12-5   Relationship of New York Heart Association Functional Class to Hospital Mortality after Aortic Valve Replacement** *ᵃ*

NYHA Class *ᵇ*	n	Hospital Deaths		
		No.	%	CL (%)
I	35	0	0	0-5
II	256	2	0.8	0.3-1.8
III	435	11	2.5	1.8-3.6
IV	97	7	7	5-11
V *ᶜ*	14	4	29	15-46
P		<.0001		

11/111
10% (CL 7%–14%)

Key: *CL*, 70% confidence limits; *NYHA*, New York Heart Association.

ᵃ Data from 842 patients undergoing primary aortic valve replacement with or without concomitant cardiac procedures at UAB, 1975 to July 1, 1979.

ᵇ Five patients could not be categorized.

ᶜ Class V indicates patients coming to the operating room in acute severe hemodynamic deterioration.

were compiled from results in 2035 patients having operations in 22 centers in the United States.

Ethnicity

African-Americans appear to be at increased risk of death late after aortic valve operations.[B42] The precise reasons for the ethnicity factor are unclear, but may include socioeconomic factors; compliance with therapy, such as anticoagulation; and genetic factors that predispose individuals to hypertension.

Functional Status

Poor functional status, as reflected in New York Heart Association (NYHA) functional class, is a risk factor for death, usually in cardiac failure, primarily early after isolated aortic valve replacement.[B4,B5,B42,C14,S14] The effect on the risk of premature death late postoperatively is less, probably because later survival is related preoperatively more to LV function, which is often not highly correlated with functional status.[K17] Risk of death is particularly increased when the disability is so advanced or acute that it is NYHA class V (Table 12-5), meaning hemodynamic instability or cardiogenic shock. However, risk of premature death late postoperatively is affected to some degree as well.[B5,K18,L10,L13]

Left Ventricular Morphology and Function

LV systolic and diastolic function are clearly important risk factors for premature death after aortic valve replacement,[B40] but other risk factors are surrogates. For example, LV enlargement, usually assessed easily based on physical examination, chest radiography, and echocardiography, is a risk factor for death both early and late after aortic valve replacement.[L14] However, LV enlargement may be a surrogate risk factor, because it is correlated with LV systolic and diastolic function as well as LV stroke volume associated with important aortic regurgitation. Increasing LV hypertrophy, reflected in mass index measured by echocardiography and normalized for gender (normally 107 ± 45 g · m^{-2} in men and 95 ± 41 g · m^{-2} in women), is a risk factor for early mortality.[M41]

Aortic Regurgitation

Aortic regurgitation is probably a risk factor for death early postoperatively under some circumstances. However, the interrelationship between aortic regurgitation and abnormalities of LV structure, size, and function indicates that these are likely the independent risk factors.

Gender

Gender is a risk factor for late mortality after operation for aortic valve regurgitation. Klodas and colleagues reported increased late mortality after aortic valve operations for women with aortic regurgitation in a multivariable analysis that considered patient size, LV dimension, and concomitant replacement of the ascending aorta for aneurysm.[K36] McDonald and colleagues found that this late mortality was influenced by coexisting aortic pathology and subsequent rupture of the aorta.[M40] Female gender (and body surface area less than 1.8 m^2) are risk factors for early mortality in patients over age 80.[B65]

Angina

Angina in patients with aortic valve disease increases the probability of coexisting coronary artery disease. Unless coronary artery disease is excluded or treated by concomitant CABG, angina becomes a risk factor for death after the operation.

Atrial Fibrillation

Using Cox regression analysis (univariable, multivariable, and age adjusted) to study 2359 patients with aortic valve replacement, Kvidal and colleagues found that atrial fibrillation was associated with a hazard ratio greater than 2 beyond 30 days of operation.[K35]

Coexisting Coronary Artery Disease

Coexisting coronary artery disease is a complex risk factor for premature death after operation.[K21,M19] Among STS National Database participants, aortic valve replacement with concomitant CABG carried a higher early mortality (6.3%) during the early phase after operation than either aortic valve replacement alone (3.9%) or CABG alone (2.8%).[S35] However, patients with both diseases are generally older at operation and have more functional disability, more angina, more previous myocardial infarctions, and a higher prevalence of hemodynamic instability than those with isolated aortic valve disease.[L12] These patients also usually require longer aortic occlusion time. Many of these factors have been found to increase risk of death after the combined operation.[K21] Some authors have not found concomitant CABG to be a risk factor for death during the early or intermediate period (up to 5 years) after aortic valve replacement operations,[B42,K18] but others have observed a somewhat lower 5- to 10-year survival than after isolated aortic valve replacement (Fig. 12-25).[A14,D25,L12]

Most important, despite the variability in comparisons of outcome after isolated aortic valve replacement with that after operation combined with CABG, patients who have combined aortic valve and coronary artery disease and who undergo *only* aortic valve replacement have a lower survival than patients who undergo concomitant CABG.[C9,K1,L12,M9,M25,W2] Also, Czer and colleagues found

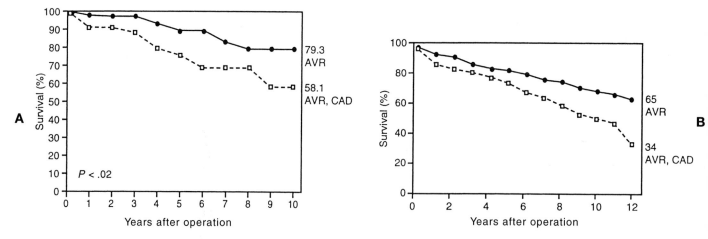

Figure 12-25 Survival after aortic valve replacement with and without coronary artery disease. The combination of aortic valve and coronary artery disease reduces survival after operation. Percent survival at 10 years indicated at right. **A**, Mechanical prosthesis (Medtronic-Hall). **B**, Stented bioprosthesis (Medtronic-Hancock II). (**A** from Akins[A14] and **B** from David and colleagues.[D25])

Key: *AVR*, Aortic valve replacement; *CAD*, coronary artery disease.

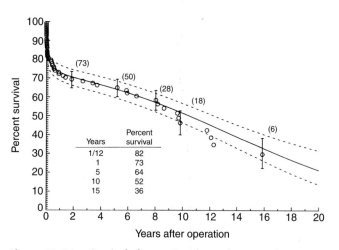

Figure 12-26 Survival after aortic valve replacement for acute native or prosthetic valve endocarditis. Depiction is as in Figure 12-18. (From Haydock and colleagues.[H15])

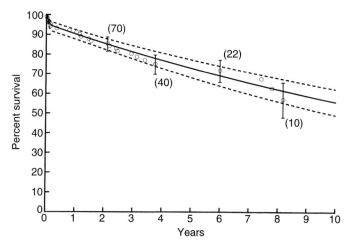

Figure 12-27 Survival after surgical treatment of aortic prosthetic valve endocarditis (PVE) by a strategy of radical debridement of infected tissue and aortic root replacement with cryopreserved aortic allografts. Each circle represents a death. Vertical bars are 68% confidence limits (CL) of Kaplan–Meier estimates. Solid line and its 68% CLs *(dashed lines)* are parametric estimates. Number of patients remaining at risk is depicted in parentheses. (From Sabik and colleagues.[S41])

sudden death late postoperatively to be more common in patients with combined aortic valve and coronary artery disease when concomitant CABG had *not* been performed than when it had.[C14]

Acute Aortic Valve Endocarditis

Surprisingly, *native valve endocarditis* at valve replacement is not a risk factor for long-term mortality (Fig. 12-26).[D16] For *replacement valve endocarditis*, radical debridement of infected tissue and aortic root replacement with cryopreserved aortic allografts can be accomplished with low early risk (Fig. 12-27).[S38]

Coexisting Ascending Aortic Aneurysm

Coexisting aneurysm of the ascending aorta has been associated with slightly decreased hospital and intermediate-term survival. However, coexisting aneurysm has not been

shown to be a risk factor overall,[B42] and the decreased survival may be attributable to other factors, including longer periods of global myocardial ischemia and CPB required for ascending aorta plus aortic valve replacement than for simple aortic valve replacement. Overall survival in patients with this combination who undergo only valve replacement probably is considerably lower.

Survival after combined replacement of the aortic valve and ascending aorta is partly determined by the replacement device. When a *composite valve conduit* has been used, 1-month and 1-, 5-, 10-, and 15-year survival, as reported by Kouchoukos and colleagues, has been 95%, 88%, 74%,

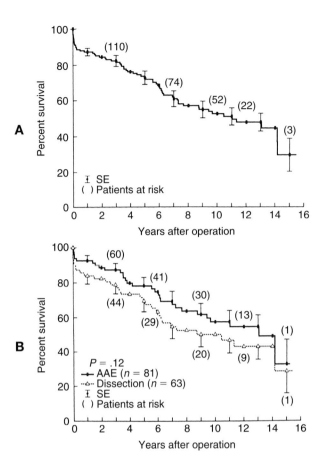

Figure 12-28   Survival among patients undergoing replacement of the aortic valve and ascending aorta with a prosthetic valve cylinder. **A,** Overall results in 168 patients. Vertical bars enclose 70% confidence limits (standard error). **B,** Survival according to whether the replacement was for anuloaortic ectasia or for acute or chronic dissection. (From Kouchoukos and colleagues.[K24])

Key: *AAE,* Anuloaortic ectasia; *SE,* standard error.

■ **TABLE 12-6   Hospital Mortality after Composite Prosthetic Valve-Graft Replacement of Aortic Valve and Ascending Aorta**

Aortic Disease	*n*	Hospital Deaths		
		No.	%	CL (%)
Anuloaortic ectasia	69	2	2.9	1.0–6.8
Chronic aortic dissection	39	1	2.6	0.3–8.5
Acute aortic dissection	12	2	17	6–11
Others [a]	7	1	14	2–41
TOTAL	127	6	4.7	2.8–7.5

(Data from Kouchoukos and colleagues.[K15])

Key: *CL,* 70% confidence limits.

[a] Includes syphilitic aortitis, replacement valve endocarditis, and extreme poststenotic aortic dilatation.

57%, and 32%, respectively (Fig. 12-28).[K15] Survival was somewhat better in patients with anuloaortic ectasia than in those operated on for ascending aortic dissection.[K24] Early (hospital) death was 4.7% (CL 2.8%-7.5%), although it was less in patients with anuloaortic ectasia or chronic aortic dissection (Table 12-6), as also reported by Gott and colleagues.[G6,G24] Most hospital deaths have been in acute cardiac failure.[K15] With methods of myocardial management now in use, early mortality may be even lower.

When an aortic valve-sparing operation is performed, survival is 88% at 5 years and 84% at 10 years.[B66,D43]

Need for emergency operation increases early risks, and overall survival may be somewhat less satisfactory in patients with Marfan syndrome. Using the inclusion technique in most patients (the interposition technique is now recommended; see "Replacement of Ascending Aorta" under Technique of Operation in Chapter 53), Kouchoukos and colleagues reported that 12% required reoperation early postoperatively for bleeding.[K15] The prevalence was half that when the interposition (open) technique was used.

Freedom from reoperation on the aortic valve or ascending aorta was 83% at 5 years after the original operation

and 78% at 10 years; most reoperations were performed on patients receiving the inclusion technique (Fig. 12-29). Patients with Marfan syndrome in particular tended to require subsequent operations on other portions of the aorta (Fig. 12-30).[K15]

Information on survival after replacement of the aortic valve and aortic root with an *allograft valve conduit* is limited. Results presented by Okita and colleagues from the experience of Ross suggest poorer overall survival with allograft replacement, but this is related primarily to higher hospital mortality than that reported by Kouchoukos and colleagues.[K15,O3] Also, the distribution of primary pathologies is quite different in the two series. However, Yacoub and colleagues reported 94% survival at 10 years in 74 patients having aortic root replacement with unprocessed viable ("homovital") aortic allografts.[Y1] They also reported a larger series of aortic root replacements with aortic allografts that included the homovital group plus a greater number of antibiotic-sterilized allografts.[L17] Survival at 20 years was 71%, excluding patients operated on for endocarditis or aneurysm of the ascending aorta or dissection, so this series does not provide the actual incremental risk for coexisting ascending aortic aneurysm.

Too few long-term follow-ups have been reported to define even tentatively the intermediate-term results after use of an *autograft pulmonary valve cylinder* for replacement of the aortic valve and ascending aorta. In one report, 3 patients (18%; CL 8%-32%) of 17 died early postoperatively from hemorrhage.[S21]

Era

Risk of hospital mortality has declined with each passing year since the beginning of operations to replace the aortic valve (see Table 12-2). Even in the current era, risk of early death after aortic valve replacement continues to decrease.

Global Myocardial Ischemic Time

Global myocardial ischemic time remains a risk factor for death early after isolated or combined aortic valve replacement. Although most aortic valve operations are performed using cold cardioplegia, it is difficult to document that mortality after aortic valve replacement has been improved by abandoning continuous coronary perfusion or hypothermic ischemic arrest as the method of myocardial management. The duration of relatively safe global myocardial ischemia has increased considerably with widespread use of

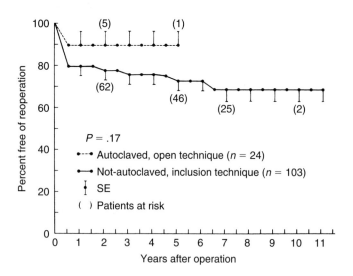

Figure 12-29 Freedom from reoperation among patients having undergone replacement of aortic valve and ascending aorta with a prosthetic valve cylinder, according to whether the interposition (open) or inclusion technique was used. (From Kouchoukos and colleagues.[K15])

Key: *SE*, Standard error.

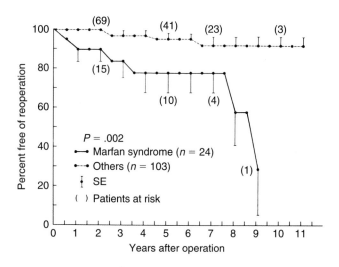

Figure 12-30 Freedom from reoperation on the remaining more distal aorta after prosthetic valve cylinder replacement of aortic valve and ascending aorta, according to whether Marfan syndrome was present. (From Kouchoukos and colleagues.[K15])

Key: *SE*, Standard error.

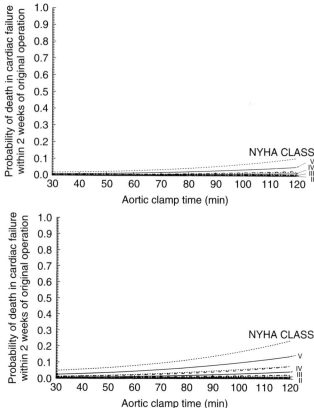

Figure 12-31 Nomogram illustrating risk–adjusted probability of cardiac death within 2 weeks of aortic valve replacement, according to aortic clamp time and preoperative New York Heart Association functional status (V represents patients with hemodynamic instability). **A,** Patients with aortic stenosis. **B,** Patients with aortic regurgitation. (From Blackstone and Kirklin.[B42] See original publication for equations.)

Key: *NYHA*, New York Heart Association.

When the hemodynamic state is unstable before CPB, the period of relatively safe global myocardial ischemia seems longer with current techniques of antegrade plus retrograde infusion of the cold cardioplegic solution, controlled aortic root reperfusion, and warm induction of cardioplegia and substrate enhancement of the cardioplegic solution (see "Cold Cardioplegia, Controlled Aortic Root Reperfusion, and [When Needed] Warm Cardioplegic Induction" in Chapter 3). These periods may be even longer with continuous warm cardioplegic infusion. These techniques should translate into increased survival.

Type of Replacement Device

Survival for at least 15 years is probably unrelated to the type of aortic valve replacement device used (see Appendix 12B).[B70,K38,M42] This inference has been supported by two randomized trials.[B8,B56,H7,H20] However, valve-related complications were more numerous in patients receiving mechanical valves, the result of considerably more nonfatal bleeding episodes in that group.[H7,K38] Grunkemeier and colleagues noted that these randomized trials were useful and important, but did little more than confirm information that was already known.[G28] Unfortunately, by the time the

cold cardioplegia (see "Cold Cardioplegia [Multidose]" under Methods of Myocardial Management during Cardiac Surgery in Chapter 3). As is always the case, the incremental risk of duration of global myocardial ischemic time is additive to, and at times interactive with, the effects of other risk factors. Thus, the risk of 120 minutes of global myocardial ischemia using cold cardioplegia is relatively low in patients with aortic stenosis. Risk is also low preoperatively in NYHA class II patients (Fig. 12-31, *A*) but higher in class V patients with aortic valve regurgitation and hemodynamic instability (Fig. 12-31, *B*).

trials were completed, some of the prosthetic devices studied were no longer in use.

The literature is replete with nonrandomized studies comparing various cardiac valve replacement devices and claims of survival superiority of one over the other. Grunkemeier and colleagues presented data that show a risk-unadjusted long-term advantage of using mechanical heart valves rather than tissue valves (see Fig. 12-20).[G26] However, the data also show that patients receiving each type of prosthesis are not comparable. For example, mean age of patients receiving mechanical valves was 57 years, whereas it was 74 years in patients receiving tissue valves. Correcting for age differences made the two groups comparable and showed no survival advantage for use of either type of heart valve. Grunkemeier and colleagues suggested that important clinical differences, such as structural failures or bleeding, do not require randomized trials to demonstrate statistical differences in properly controlled clinical evaluations.[G28]

Stentless valves. David and colleagues showed survival at 8 years of 91% ± 4% for patients receiving stentless porcine aortic valves and 69 ± 8% for those with a stent-mounted valve.[D33] They thought that superior hemodynamics of the stentless device conferred the better survival. Del Rizzo and colleagues also showed a survival advantage of stentless porcine aortic valves compared with stent-mounted valves.[D35] In patients under age 60 the probability of death was fivefold greater in the latter group. This advantage, however, diminished with advancing age. Age with persistent LV hypertrophy was an independent predictor of mortality, influencing survival after aortic valve replacement with a stentless bioprosthesis among 1173 patients. Mortality increased 8% for each year of age at surgery and by 1% for each $g \cdot m^{-2}$ increase in LV mass.

This association of mortality with LV mass is consistent with information from the Framingham study, which showed that LV hypertrophy has important prognostic implications even for patients free of clinically apparent cardiovascular disease. Levy and colleagues followed 3220 subjects older than 40 for 4 years, correcting for age, diastolic blood pressure, pulse pressure, treatment of hypertension, cigarette smoking, diabetes, obesity, and lipid ratios.[L22] They found that for each $50 \ g \cdot m^{-2}$ in LV mass corrected for height, the hazard ratio for death from all causes was 1.49 in men and 2.01 in women. However, inferences about the association of LV hypertrophy secondary to systemic hypertension may not be entirely transferable to that secondary to aortic valve disease. The former has complex systemic hemoral, cellular, and vascular aspects not generally present in the latter.

Studies comparing other stentless bioprostheses for aortic valve replacement are less conclusive for differences in survival.[D24] Yacoub and colleagues showed promising results with almost no decline in survival for the first 10 years after aortic valve replacement with homovital aortic allografts.[Y1] Cartier and colleagues compared stentless replacement devices for aortic valve replacement[C43]; survival at 5 years was 96% for pulmonary autografts (mean age 34 ± 16 years), 84% for aortic allografts (mean age 47 ± 19 years), and 84% for stentless porcine xenografts (mean age 68 ± 8 years). Knott-Craig and colleagues compared 10-year survival after aortic valve replacement with pulmonary

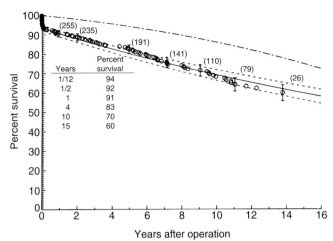

Figure 12-32   *Survival after replacement of the aortic valve with an allograft. Depiction as in Figure 12-18. (From O'Brien and colleagues.[O5])*

autografts and aortic allografts[K34]; survival was comparable (autograft 77%, allograft 67%), but valve degeneration and reoperation for valve-related causes appeared to favor the autograft group after 8 years. Aklog and Yacoub compared pulmonary autografts and aortic allografts (as an aortic root replacement) in a prospective randomized trial and found similar early risk and 5-year survival.[A15] Allograft aortic root replacement compares to aortic root replacement with that using a pulmonary autograft because of similarly exposed suture lines. After aortic valve replacement with a pulmonary autograft, death would be unusual, if not rare, as a result of bleeding from the pulmonary allograft used for RV outflow tract reconstruction. Serious hemorrhage more typically results from the aortic root reconstruction. Risk of infection or heart failure after either procedure is similar. Follow-up is insufficient, however, to determine durability of the repair. It will take 20 years to know if placing the allograft in the low-pressure, low-stress pulmonary circuit will allow the allograft tissue to last longer than placing it in the aortic position in adults.

Use of an allograft replacement device sewn freehand (subcoronary technique) into the aortic position has had no adverse effect on survival. This is evident from the previous discussions in this chapter, from the experience of O'Brien and colleagues (Fig. 12-32)[O5] and from the UAB experience (1981 to 1988) of no deaths (0%; CL 0%-2.5%) among 70 patients undergoing isolated aortic valve replacement and 7 undergoing concomitant CABG.

Stent-mounted porcine xenograft valves. These valves have not been shown to affect survival adversely when further replacements can be performed.[B7,M13] However, Lytle and colleagues found that the combination of a stent-mounted bioprosthesis and chronic anticoagulation decreased 10-year survival.[L7]

Mechanical valves. Mechanical replacement devices have not had an adverse effect on survival, but only because most bleeding complications from warfarin therapy are not fatal, although clinically important.[B39,C9,L10,L14] Zellner and colleagues followed patients having aortic valve replacement with the St. Jude Medical prosthesis and analyzed competing risks of outcomes (Fig. 12-33).[Z3] At 15

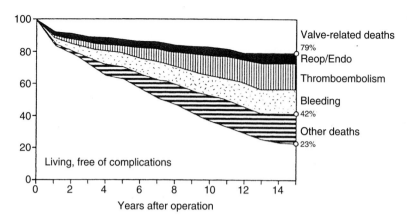

Figure 12-33 Competing risks of adverse events following aortic valve replacement with mechanical prosthesis (St. Jude Medical). Death related to the valve reduced survival to 79%. Complications related to reoperation, endocarditis, thromboembolism, and anticoagulant-related bleeding reduced complication-free survival to 42%. Other deaths reduced freedom from all complications in living patients to 23%. (From Zellner and colleagues.[Z3])

Key: *Reop/Endo,* Reoperation/endocarditis.

years, deaths related to the prosthesis reduced survival to 79%. Complications related to the valve (e.g., reoperation, endocarditis, thromboembolism, anticoagulant-related bleeding) that were not fatal occurred in 37% of patients, leaving only 42% free of death or complications related to the prosthetic valve. Non–valve-related deaths reduced the number of patients living and free of all complications to 23%.

Studies comparing mechanical prostheses usually do not show clinical advantages among different modern devices. A typical example is the study of Masters and colleagues comparing the St. Jude Medical device with the Medtronic-Hall device.[M37] Survival at 5 years appeared to be better with the St. Jude valve (86% ± 3% versus 68% ± 4% for the Medtronic-Hall, *P* = .0001). The authors were reluctant to conclude, however, that the prostheses differed significantly, noting that only 13 of the original 237 patients were at risk at 5 years in the St. Jude group and 64 of the original 272 patients in the Medtronic-Hall group. Instead, they concluded that both valves offered similar clinical performance. Antunes arrived at the same conclusion following a randomized trial in 182 patients.[A20] The CarboMedics bileaflet valve was compared to the Monostrut tilting-disc valve in a randomized study involving 200 patients[D38]; the authors concluded the two valves exhibited similar outcomes.

Pulmonary valve autograft. The potential for adverse effects from a pulmonary valve autograft as a replacement for the aortic valve has not been evaluated completely. Earlier information suggested no adverse effect,[G5,G19,G22,R6,R21] but current data suggest that 30-day mortality for this operation is 3.5% to 5.1% (Table 12-7).[E6,R21,S30]

Hospital Morbidity
Complete Heart Block

Infrequently, replacement of severely calcific aortic valves leads to complete heart block. It usually results from trauma to the bundle of His after removal of calcium from the region of the membranous septum and right

■ **TABLE 12-7 Morbidity and Survival after Aortic Valve Replacement: Pulmonary Autograft**

Events	Elkins[E6]	Stelzer[S30]	Registry[R21]
Mortality (< 30 days, %)	5.1	4.8	3.5
Survival (10 yr, %)	86	85 (7 yr)	88
Autograft explant (10 yr, % free)	96	89 (7 yr)	88
Allograft explant (10 yr, % free)	92	100	90

(Data from Elkins and colleagues,[E6] Ross Registry,[R21] and Stelzer and colleagues.[S30])

trigone beneath the noncoronary cusp–right coronary cusp commissure. Although this complication occasionally is unavoidable, care in removing calcium from these areas and rigorous avoidance of suture penetration of the membranous septum near its junction with the muscular septum should reduce its occurrence greatly. Heart block may be transient rather than permanent.

Neurologic Deficits

Neurologic complications after aortic valve replacement may mar an otherwise routine operation. The current risk of neurologic complications among STS National Database participants is 3.5%.[S35] With known atherosclerotic cardiovascular disease, the risk increases; when CABG is combined with aortic valve replacement, risk increases to 5.7%. Attention to the details of avoiding loss of calcific fragments during valve resection and to techniques for removing air from the heart after closing the aorta are the only methods available to reduce risk of neurologic complications associated with aortic valve replacement.

Symptomatic Improvement

The functional status of most surviving patients is good after aortic valve replacement. About 90% of patients traced 5 to 10 years (specifically, 8 years in the patients followed by Copeland and colleagues) are in NYHA functional class I or II.[C9] About 70% of patients preoperatively in NYHA class IV are in class I or II postoperatively, as are

80% of those preoperatively in class III and 90% of those preoperatively in class II. Hemodynamically efficient replacement devices appear to favor good functional results. After aortic valve replacement with aortic allografts in the subcoronary position, Prager and colleagues reported that at an average follow-up of 4.2 years, 100% and 97% of patients were in NYHA class I and II, respectively, when a root replacement technique was used.[P18] Doty and colleagues reported 94% of patients in functional class I and 4% in class II after aortic valve replacement with an allograft at an average follow-up of 4.6 years.[D31] The authors also reported 92% of a much older group of patients (mean age 71 ± 8.4 years) in class I or II after aortic valve replacement with stentless porcine aortic bioprostheses at an average follow-up of 2.3 years.[D32]

Exercise capacity tested objectively can approach normal after aortic valve replacement, as shown in patients with aortic stenosis, depressed preoperative exercise capacity, and near-normal resting LV end-diastolic pressure.[K5] In other situations, such as in many patients with aortic regurgitation and preoperatively increased LV end-diastolic pressure, exercise capacity is improved after operation but remains subnormal.[K5] Exercise capacity testing after aortic valve replacement with a pulmonary autograft has yielded impressive results. The Ross procedure provides excellent hemodynamic results at rest and exercise, with values indistinguishable from normal,[P19] including exercise capacity sufficient for athletic competition and ability to achieve extraordinarily high cardiac output with low pressure gradient across the LV outflow tract.[D34,O13]

Left Ventricular Structure and Function

The degree of improvement in LV structure and function, if any, after aortic valve replacement depends primarily on such factors as the type and extent of secondary cardiomyopathy at operation, coexisting disease, extent (if any) of permanent intraoperative LV damage, and energy loss and regurgitation across the valve replacement device.

Aortic Stenosis

Completeness of return of LV mass toward normal after normalization of LV systolic pressure by aortic valve replacement depends on extent of myocardial degenerative changes (and thus degree of LV hypertrophy) and related loss of LV reserve. When LV end-diastolic pressure is still low at operation, LV wall thickness and mass regress substantially, the latter from an average of $206 \text{ g} \cdot \text{m}^{-2}$ to $133 \text{ g} \cdot \text{m}^{-2}$ ($P < .05$) in a study by Kennedy and colleagues.[K5] The regression continues for more than a year postoperatively,[M27] but completely normal LV mass is rarely achieved.[K5,M10,P1]

In addition to reduction in mass, reversal of LV remodeling gradually returns the LV to a more spheroidal shape.[M27] When LV end-diastolic pressure has become importantly elevated before aortic valve replacement, either because of afterload mismatch (see "Natural History" earlier in this chapter) or reduced contractility, LV mass may be importantly reduced after operation.[C1,K5,S5] However, at this stage many patients fail to show a reduction in LV mass, presumably because of irreversible myocardial degenerative changes. Krayenbuehl and colleagues showed that the

preoperatively enlarged muscle fiber diameter shortens within 1 to 2 years after aortic valve replacement as part of this process, but with some increase in interstitial fibrosis.[K23] Interstitial fibrosis tended to decrease thereafter, but the myocardium did not return to normal, retaining some permanent fibrosis.

Rate and completeness of LV mass reduction after aortic valve replacement may be related to type of replacement device used and other factors at operation. LV function early after operation for aortic valve replacement with LV hypertrophy appears to be better when cold blood cardioplegia is employed versus other methods of myocardial management.[J10] Jin and colleagues showed more complete resolution of LV hypertrophy and greater improvement in LV function when an aortic allograft or stentless porcine bioprosthesis was used to replace the aortic valve than when a stent-mounted bioprosthesis or mechanical valve was employed.[J11] Walther and colleagues found regression of LV hypertrophy in all patients after aortic valve replacement in a randomized study comparing stentless and stent-mounted bioprostheses,[W14] but patients with stentless bioprostheses had greater regression at 6 months. Maselli and colleagues reported similar findings favoring aortic allografts and stentless bioprostheses, with the most rapid resolution of LV hypertrophy occurring when aortic allografts were used.[M33] Basarir and colleagues also found a greater decrease in LV hypertrophy with aortic allografts than with mechanical prostheses after aortic valve replacement.[B48]

Kleine and colleagues demonstrated that turbulence, and thus energy loss, caused by mechanical heart valves can be reduced simply by optimal orientation of the device relative to flow patterns created by LV ejection.[K32,K33] They state that turbulence may be an important factor in reversing ventricular remodeling after implantation of a prosthetic heart valve, as well as in relief or reduction of pressure gradient across the LV outflow tract. The premise is based on the observation that blood is ejected from the LV eccentrically at the level of the aortic valve. In humans (and pigs) the eccentric flow is toward the right posterior wall of the aorta, the location of the noncoronary sinus of Valsalva. Mechanical valves oriented to place the major flow orifice to take advantage of the eccentric flow pattern in the aorta have optimal performance in that orientation. Thus, a tilting-disc valve properly oriented can perform better than a bileaflet device, even though the latter is perceived as the better replacement device.

Functional response of the LV to sudden surgical normalization of systolic pressure can be anticipated from *morphologic* response.[K3,K23] LV end-diastolic and end-systolic volume indices decrease and EF increases within 6 months after aortic valve replacement.[H16] However, Hwang and colleagues found that 66% (CL 54%-76%) of patients with preoperative LV dysfunction still had abnormal values 6 months postoperatively.[H16] When LV wall stress is essentially normal at operation because of appropriate LV hypertrophy and increased wall thickness, indices of LV systolic function (including EF) remain normal or become supranormal postoperatively.[B23,K5,M10,S5] By the time of operation, when LV hypertrophy is insufficient to prevent afterload mismatch, the reduced EF and elevated end-diastolic pressure still may return to normal.[C1,K5] However, when these indices of LV function have deteriorated because of reduced contractility, usually associated with marked cardiomegaly, they often show little improvement after operation.

Hwang and colleagues developed a logistic risk factor equation for postoperative LV dysfunction after aortic valve replacement for aortic stenosis.[H16] The multivariably determined risk factors were lower preoperative EF, one or more myocardial infarctions preoperatively, low preoperative aortic valve gradient, and unrevascularized coronary artery disease.

Aortic Regurgitation

The increase in LV mass that develops in patients with important aortic regurgitation can occur insidiously and in the absence of symptoms. Also, LV mass can become much greater in these patients than in those with aortic stenosis.[J11,R9] At least experimentally, abolishing LV volume overload must be performed within 6 months of its inception to permit regression toward normal mass.[P2] This observation helps explain why reduction in LV mass after valve replacement for aortic regurgitation is often moderate in degree and unpredictable, even when indices of LV systolic and diastolic function improve after operation.[M5,O6] When these indices do not improve, the often massive increase in LV mass fails to regress and may even worsen several years after operation.

Regression of muscle fiber diameter after aortic valve replacement described for patients with aortic stenosis also occurs after operation for aortic regurgitation.[K23] Decrease in interstitial fibrous content is greater after valve replacement for aortic regurgitation, however.

Thus, it is not surprising that when LV contractility and EF are good and LV end-diastolic pressure is only mildly elevated, LV mass becomes almost normal late after replacing a regurgitant aortic valve.[D5,G3,M5,O6] When already severely diminished at valve replacement, LV systolic and diastolic function often remains compromised late postoperatively, and LV mass fails to regress.

When LV systolic function (estimated by resting and exercise EF, as well as end-systolic volume, LV fractional shortening, and velocity of circumferential shortening) is truly normal at aortic valve replacement (found in only about 10% of patients with symptomatic aortic regurgitation [B16]), LV diastolic function is usually normal and, with systolic function, remains normal postoperatively. When preoperative LV systolic and diastolic function is mildly or moderately depressed at rest or with stress testing, usually associated with only moderate cardiomegaly and increased LV mass, regression (but not normalization) of impaired resting function usually characterizes the postoperative period; however, the response of systolic function to stress usually remains abnormal.[B16,C5,K5] Impaired preoperative exercise capacity adversely affects the probability of important recovery of LV systolic function after valve replacement.[B15] Also, even with other factors equal, the longer the duration of preoperative limitation of LV systolic function, the less likely the possibility of appreciable return toward normal.[B38] When systolic function improves within 6 months of valve replacement, however, it usually improves still further over the next several years,[B33,F5,K23] although about one third of patients show no additional improve-

ment. Severe preoperative reduction of resting or stressed LV systolic function often indicates irreversible deterioration.[B15,G3,O1] Some patients may even show a progressive deterioration in LV systolic function and an increase in LV diastolic volumes, leading to death with heart failure a few months to a few years after operation.

Although LV diastolic function is often not improved by aortic valve replacement for aortic regurgitation,[G8,S12] the characteristically large LV end-diastolic volume is usually reduced toward normal within 10 days of ablation of regurgitation (and thus decrease in stroke volume).[G4,K5,S9] Further volume reduction occurs late postoperatively in many patients, with the greatest reduction in those with lesser degrees of abnormal LV structure and function preoperatively. Bonow and colleagues found that preoperative exercise capacity correlated well with postoperative reduction of LV end-diastolic dimensions. These fell strikingly and occasionally to near-normal values in patients with good preoperative exercise tolerance, whereas in patients with impaired exercise ability, some hearts were larger postoperatively, and few regressed in size late postoperatively (Fig. 12-34).[B15]

Failure of LV end-diastolic volume to regress toward normal indicates irreversible morphologic and functional LV damage and portends poor long-term results.[H4] By the time exercise ability has become impaired, the diastolic properties of the LV may have even become irreversibly impaired, and fixed cardiomegaly may be present (Fig. 12-35).[G3] These relationships are particularly important because exercise capacity becomes limited earlier in the course of aortic regurgitation than in aortic stenosis.[H3]

These same considerations apply to patients with periprosthetic leakage late postoperatively. The hemodynamic and functional variables after operation for aortic regurgitation appear to be very sensitive to the LV volume overload of periprosthetic leakage. Thus, Schwarz and colleagues found that such patients had importantly reduced LV systolic function late postoperatively compared with patients who had no periprosthetic leakage.[S10]

In summary, patients overall experience considerable reduction of LV diastolic volume, decrease in end-systolic volume, and increase in EF after aortic valve replacement for aortic regurgitation.[H16] However, about 60% of patients with preoperative dysfunction have dysfunction postoperatively. Some of the variability among reports of postoperative LV function may relate to the variable interval between operation and postoperative testing; LV systolic performance at rest and particularly during exercise improves still further after 1 year. Borer and colleagues reported improvement between the second and third postoperative years and observed no subsequent deterioration in patients who improved.[B44] LV systolic dysfunction preoperatively is the most predictive variable for postoperative LV dysfunction.[H16]

Left Ventricular–Aortic Energy Loss

All devices placed within the aortic root for replacement of the aortic valve are obstructive to some degree. This inherent obstruction may be minimized by complete replacement of the aortic root with an aortic allograft, stentless bioprosthesis, or pulmonary autograft. These oper-

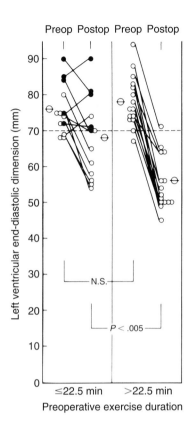

Figure 12-34 Changes in echocardiographic left ventricular end-diastolic dimension as a result of operation in symptomatic patients undergoing aortic valve replacement for regurgitation, according to preoperative exercise duration. Patients who completed stage 1 before operation (less than 22½ minutes) had a greater decrease in diastolic size than did patients who could not complete stage 1 (at least 22½ minutes). Dashed line at 70 mm indicates value of postoperative diastolic dimension above which patients have been shown to be at high risk of subsequent death from heart failure. (From Bonow and colleagues.[B15])

Key: *Open circle,* Alive; *closed circle,* Late death from operative heart failure; *Preop,* preoperative; *Postop,* postoperative.

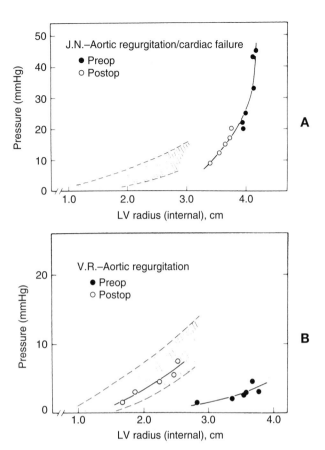

Figure 12-35 Relationship of left ventricular (LV) internal radius to corresponding LV pressure throughout the diastolic filling period in preoperative study *(closed circles)* and postoperative study approximately 1 year after aortic valve replacement for regurgitation *(open circles).* The dashed-line hatched areas define the range of pressure-radius values observed in a group of patients with normal LV function without aortic regurgitation. **A,** Patient (J.N.) with preoperatively depressed inotropic state. **B,** Patient (V.R.) with normal preoperative inotropic state. (From Gault and colleagues.[G3])

Key: *LV,* Left ventricular; *Preop,* preoperative; *Postop,* postoperative.

ations are more complex than replacement of the aortic valve with a mechanical or stent-mounted prosthesis.

Gradients are minimal after freehand insertion of an aortic allograft [B24,B30,J5,J6] or stentless aortic bioprosthesis,[D24] but are pronounced in patients receiving mechanical or stent-mounted prostheses.[S40] The magnitude of gradient varies greatly depending on characteristics of the prosthesis, size of the device relative to size of the patient, cardiac output (study done during rest, exercise, or pharmacologic stimulation), and abnormal conditions in or around the replacement device.

Fisher and colleagues evaluated mechanical and stent-mounted bioprosthetic valves in vitro with regard to pressure gradients generated at various flow rates (Fig. 12-36).[F10] In vivo measurement of pressure gradient over mechanical or bioprosthetic cardiac valves by Doppler ultrasound has been complicated by changes in blood flow

velocities associated with the prosthetic valve. [B50,Y5] Doppler ultrasound, although noninvasive, tends to overestimate energy loss resulting from pressure gradient over prosthetic valves. In addition, aortic curvature, arterial distensibility, arterial impedance, and unsteady flow appear to affect interpretation of pressure measurements.

Despite these limitations, reproducible estimates of pressure gradient are possible in vivo using Doppler ultrasound techniques. These values have been used to compare various prostheses and bioprostheses according to label size (Tables 12-8, *A,* and 12-8, *B*). Resting gradient under 10 mmHg is desirable. Comparative figures are subject to interpretation, recognizing that most values are obtained during rest, and even then, cardiac output (flow) may vary considerably from patient to patient. In addition, label size among different types of device is associated with widely variable valve orifice size. Comparing studies is also com-

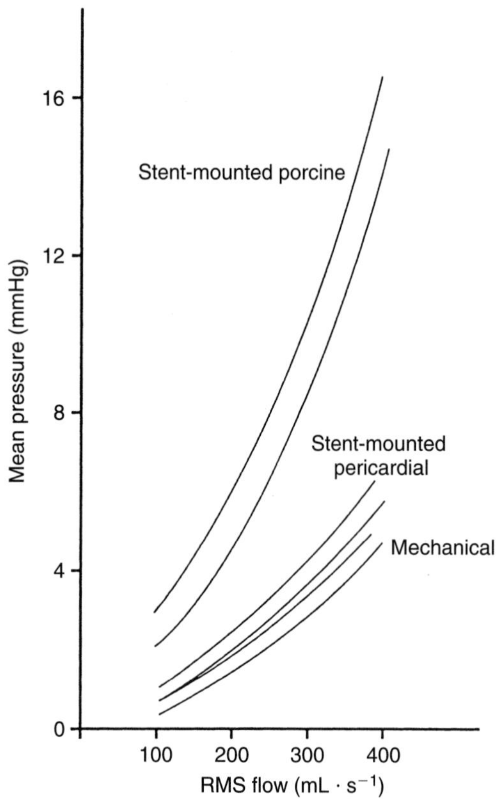

Figure 12-36 In vitro evaluation of mechanical and stent-mounted bioprosthetic valves. Bench testing of these devices for cardiac valve replacement compares root mean square forward flow through the device to the pressure gradient that is generated. Mechanical and stent-mounted pericardial prostheses show a performance advantage compared with first-generation stent-mounted porcine bioprostheses. (From Fisher and colleagues.[F10])

Key: *RMS*, Root mean square.

■ TABLE 12-8A   Systolic Left Ventricular to Aortic Pressure Gradient (mmHg): Mechanical Prostheses [a]

Prosthesis	Label Size (mm)			
	19	21	23	25
Starr-Edwards 1260	–	12	–	–
Medtronic-Hall	–	12-13	9	4
Monostrut	–	12	7-9	7
St. Jude	16-22	13-15	8-12	11-12
CarboMedics	17-19	12	9-10	8-9

[a] See Table 12-8, B.

■ TABLE 12-8B   Systolic Left Ventricular to Aortic Pressure Gradient (mmHg): Biologic Prostheses [a]

Prosthesis	Label Size (mm)				
	19	21	23	25	27
Carpentier-Edwards porcine	32	22	14	15	–
Hancock porcine	34	20	–	–	–
Hancock MO	17	15	9	11	–
Hancock II	–	12	12	11	8
Carpentier-Edwards pericardial	17-24	14-20	11-15	11-14	–
Medtronic Freestyle	13	11	9	6	5
St. Jude SPV	–	13	9	6	5

(Data from references A11, A12, C7, C15-C18, C34-C36, D25, J2, K28, L8, L9, L18, M4, N5, P8, P13, P14, R14, R19, T7, W7, W8, W13, and Z1.)

[a] Data represent in vivo mean pressure gradient measured by Doppler ultrasound.

plicated by what is reported: peak LV to aortic systolic gradient or mean systolic gradient, for example. After considering these confounding factors, however, hemodynamic performance characteristics clearly have improved with newer prosthetic valve designs. Also, most cardiac valve replacement devices function well at rest if greater than 23 mm in diameter. Some 21-mm devices are satisfactory, but 19-mm devices may have higher than desirable gradient even at rest.

Virtually all mechanical prostheses and bioprostheses larger than the 21-mm size can provide satisfactory performance in most adults. Some 21-mm mechanical prostheses and first-generation bioprostheses[C7] have high energy loss during periods of increased cardiac output. Among the 21-mm mechanical prostheses, the St. Jude Medical valve performs well in this regard.[W7] Other prostheses of either tilting-disc or bileaflet design also have good hemodynamic performance.

Because of the variability in the gradient usually present across the prostheses used for aortic valve replacement, unusual gradients may be difficult to identify. However, such abnormalities do develop from fibrous ingrowth below or above the device, dense clot around the valve (throm-

botic encasement), or leaflet calcification of a bioprosthesis.[B31] Gradients of 85 to 100 mmHg may be produced, but they can be much lower and more difficult to define as abnormal when cardiac output is reduced by these developments.

Effective Orifice Area

Acoustic anomalies caused by mechanical prosthetic valves after implantation make it difficult, if not impossible, to measure prosthetic valve area by ultrasound (echocardiography) using pressure half-time estimates.[Y5] These methods are most applicable to bioprosthetic heart valves. Mechanical prostheses cause changes in the flow velocity patterns across the aorta, and in vivo measurements are often subject to question as to sampling sites. A modified Bernoulli equation appears to be the most reproducible and accurate method for calculating prosthetic valve area by ultrasound. The mathematical constants of these equations are loaded into modern echocardiographic equipment so that estimation of valve area becomes a press of a button or a few key strokes for the echocardiographer.

Hemolysis

Patients with allograft valves sewn freehand into the aortic root do not have abnormal red blood cell hemolysis, even when there is periprosthetic or central leakage. Well-functioning stent-mounted xenografts generally do not produce hemolysis when central leakage develops, but they may do so with periprosthetic leakage. All well-functioning mechanical valves produce at least a small increase in hemolysis, with disc-type valves producing less than ball valves. Periprosthetic and intraprosthetic leakage produces increased amounts of hemolysis, the magnitude of which is related to the amount of regurgitation. Thrombotic narrowing of a prosthetic orifice also importantly increases hemolysis.

Replacement Device Regurgitation

Periprosthetic Leakage

Periprosthetic leakage may occur after replacement of the aortic valve with an allograft or stentless porcine bioprosthesis placed as a freehand subcoronary implant.[B42,D28] Elimination of the "dead space" between graft and host aorta by sutures is thought to reduce the occurrence of leakage, although these sutures may actually cause periprosthetic leak.[B32,B41,G10,O5,V2] Periprosthetic leakage in the presence of aortic allografts or freehand subcoronary-implanted bioprostheses is related to technical problems at the outflow or upper suture line. Buckling of the graft or dehiscence of sutures from the aortic wall results in dissection of blood along the native aortic wall into the space between the graft and aorta. Eventually, a passageway is created to the inflow or lower suture line. Although placing sutures between graft and aorta may reduce the space or may more securely approximate the graft and aorta at operation, it is virtually impossible to obliterate the space until healing has occurred. Sutures between the graft and aorta other than at the inflow and outflow suture line could actually open tracts to this space along the sutures and needle holes.

The best preventive measure against periprosthetic leakage is a secure outflow suture line, as confirmed by intraoperative echocardiography and a strict policy to repair any leakage found at operation.

With use of mechanical prostheses or bioprostheses, important periprosthetic leakage is uncommon in the absence of infection,[J1] although minor leakage may occur. Periprosthetic leakage usually becomes evident during the early months after operation.[B42,R17] Shean and colleagues reported a prevalence of minor periprosthetic leakage of 17% in the Massachusetts General Hospital series.[S23] In addition, 6% of patients (CL 5%-7%) had clinically recognizable hemolysis.

When periprosthetic leakage develops and no infection is present, the area of dehiscence is usually small and can be repaired with one or two pledgeted mattress sutures. The prosthesis does not have to be removed and replaced unless the area of dehiscence is large.

Central Leakage

Allograft aortic valves. Allograft valve central leakage has a variety of causes and a variable prevalence that relate to valve preparation, storage, and insertion techniques. For antibiotic-sterilized, wet-stored (at 4°C) valves, *degeneration* (cusp rupture with or without minor calcification) is the most common cause (Fig. 12-37), with a 10-year prevalence of up to 15% to 18%.[B41,O5,V2] The Stanford group reported a 30% 10-year prevalence of degenerative valve failure with antibiotic-treated valves.[M28] Differences in prevalence relate primarily to the definition of *degenerative failure*, which in the Stanford series[M28] was the appearance of a new regurgitant murmur, in the O'Brien series[O5] was

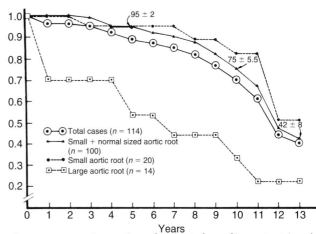

Figure 12-37   Proportion of patients free of important (moderate or severe) allograft valve regurgitation (antibiotic sterilization) after valve replacement. Ninety patients had isolated aortic valve disease, and 31 had multivalve disease, as detailed in an earlier publication.[B24] One hundred fourteen patients left the hospital alive. Two patients were lost to follow-up at 54 and 74 months. The other 48 survivors were followed for 132 to 162 months (average 12 years). Of the 29 instances of regurgitation occurring in the 100 patients with small or normal-sized roots, 24 were presumed or proven cusp rupture, 4 others were related to allograft valve endocarditis, and 1 was due to cusp malposition related to technical error at insertion. For small and normal-sized aortic roots compared with large aortic roots, $P = .0006$.

reoperation, and in the Barrett-Boyes series[B24] was moderate or severe regurgitation. Patients with mild or trivial regurgitation are not considered examples of valve failure because this may develop early after operation from imperfect cusp coaptation (Fig. 12-38).[B24] The instantaneous risk (hazard function) for reoperation for degenerative valve failure increases late postoperatively (Fig. 12-39).[O5]

A second, less common cause of important central leakage after freehand insertions is technical error, with leaflet distortion and prolapse or progressive host aortic root dilatation associated with bicuspid aortic valve or cystic medial necrosis of the aorta. The free edges of the cusps are overstretched and fail to meet centrally, but are otherwise intact. The latter mechanism can be prevented by avoiding freehand insertion in patients who have large aortic roots.

A third cause of central leakage is endocarditis (see "Replacement Device Endocarditis" later in this chapter).

Table 12-9 summarizes the incremental risk factors for central leakage caused by cusp degeneration. In *allograft preparation and storage,* integrity of cusp ground substance and fibroblasts is maintained either by short-duration, low-concentration antibiotic disinfection followed by cryopreservation[A7,O5,S20] and later insertion or by sterile collection, "wet" storage, and implantation within a few days (homovital).[C20,Y1] These techniques reduce cusp degeneration and central leakage to a prevalence of 2% to 10% by 10 years after insertion.[A8,C21,D31] Histologic findings in allograft cusps preserved by these techniques after implantation in animals[A3,A9,C20,K19] or retrieval after implantation in humans[G11,G12,O5] indicates better preservation of cusp

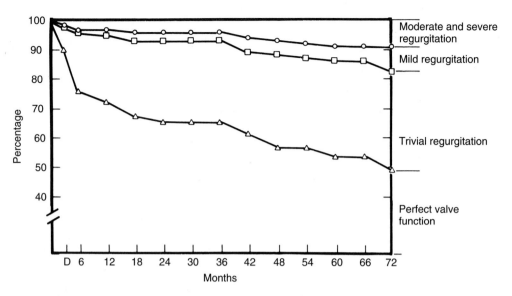

Figure 12-38 Prevalence of allograft aortic valve regurgitation in patients leaving the hospital. Both timing and severity of regurgitation are shown. Patients below the lowest line had no diastolic aortic murmur. (From Barratt-Boyes and colleagues.[B24])

Key: *D*, Discharge from hospital.

■ **TABLE 12-9 Incremental Risk Factors for Central Leakage from Cusp Degeneration of Allograft Aortic Valves Used for Aortic Valve Replacement** *a*

	Risk Factor	
	Allograft preparation and storage	
	Chemical sterilization (beta-propiolactone)	•
	Sterilization by irradiation	•
(Greater)	Donor age	•
(Larger)	Aortic root diameter	•
(Younger)	Recipient age	•
	Native valve regurgitation	•
	Technique of insertion	•
	Stent mounting	•
	Faulty freehand insertion	•

a Risk factors assembled based on experience and published reports[B6,B43,C21,O5,V2] and not obtained by multivariable analysis.

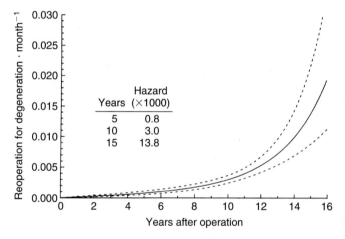

Figure 12-39 Hazard function for reoperation for degeneration (cusp rupture) after allograft aortic valve replacement with antibiotic-sterilized "nonviable" valves. Depiction as in Fig. 12-18. (From O'Brien and colleagues.[O5])

architecture and fibroblasts than when other methods are used. The allograft valve is antigenic,[H14] however, and both endothelial cells and fibroblasts are probably destroyed by an immunologic process. Antibiotic sterilization and cryopreservation are thought to reduce antigenicity of allograft valves,[Y2,Y3] but low-grade rejection still may occur and promote graft degeneration. Tissue matching and immunosuppressive therapy fail to reduce degeneration.[Y2]

Donor age appears to be a continuous variable that affects the rate of cusp degeneration, but its effect is weak until after about 50 years. The effect is probably produced by age-related structural changes in the cusp. Cusp calcification is also more common in valves from older donors, which presumably explains why most allograft valves that develop stenosis come from donors over age 60.[A6,K20,L15] The age effect is such that prevalence of valve degeneration by 10 years after insertion is 8%, 25%, and 40% when donor age is under 20 years, 20 to 50 years, and over 50 years, respectively (Fig. 12-40).[B41]

Although *aortic root diameter* is also a continuously variable risk factor, its effect becomes strong only when it is greater than 30 mm (corresponding to an allograft inner diameter of greater than 28 mm). Thus, central leakage within 10 years is approximately 40% when the aortic root diameter is at least 30 mm and 10% when it is less than 30 mm (Fig. 12-41).[B24,B42]

The incremental risk of *young age* on cusp degeneration and central leakage is much weaker than with stent-mounted xenograft valves. With freehand-inserted allograft valves the degeneration does not seem to be accompanied by cusp calcification.

Although difficult to examine, *imperfect freehand insertion* of an allograft results in altered stress and strain on the cusps, which in turn predispose to rupture in the cusp belly or

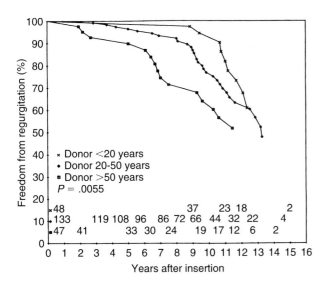

Figure 12-40   Freedom from important allograft aortic valve regurgitation according to age of donor providing "nonviable" valves. Only regurgitation from valve wear (degeneration) is included. Numbers at risk are noted. (From Barratt-Boyes and colleagues.[B41])

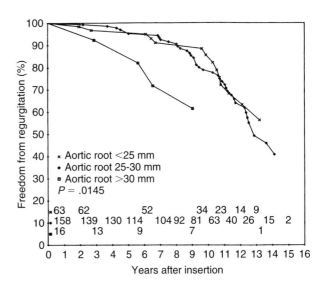

Figure 12-41   Freedom from important regurgitation according to aortic root diameter after allograft aortic valve insertion. Data set and format is as in Fig. 12-40. (From Barratt-Boyes and colleagues.[B41])

even at the commissures where stresses are minimal in the native valve. Asymmetric location of the graft valve commissures at implantation or distortion of the commissural location during closure of an oblique aortotomy that extends into the noncoronary sinus of Valsalva may be an important cause of altered stress on the graft cusp tissues. Fig. 12-42 shows how commissural positional abnormality results in lengthening and stretching of the right and left coronary cusps, compared with redundancy of the noncoronary cusp. Calcium deposits are greatest in the anulus and sinus of the redundant cusp, whereas the stretched cusps are subject to cusp tear or disruption. Septal myocardium left on the allograft is broken down and absorbed, because no myocardium is seen on the graft at explantation. This may explain why an aortic valve allograft inserted by the subcoronary freehand technique may show perfect function at operation but become regurgitant within a few weeks or months. In support of this, the prevalence of aortic regurgitation several months after operation is considerably greater with freehand aortic allografts than with aortic valve allografts or pulmonary autografts inserted as part of an aortic root replacement or "mini" aortic root replacement.[D14]

Stent mounting of allograft aortic valves used as aortic valve replacements has resulted in a higher prevalence of cusp degeneration and valve regurgitation than has freehand insertion.[A1]

Risk factors are incremental. Therefore, results appear to be best with cryopreserved or homovital valves when donor age is restricted to less than 50 years, to recipient age greater than 15 years, and to aortic root diameter less than 30 mm. Even with antibiotic-preserved valves stored at 4°C, these restrictions can reduce central leakage to 6% at 9 years, although the prevalence rises sharply thereafter (Fig. 12-43).

Pulmonary autograft. Cusp degeneration or central regurgitation of a pulmonary autograft implanted freehand

into the aortic valve position (Ross procedure) may result from technical factors similar to those associated with freehand-inserted aortic valve allografts.[C47] It is important to note, however, that 84% of pulmonary autografts are now inserted by the full aortic root replacement technique.[R21] When regurgitation occurs in this situation, it is likely caused by technical problems with insertion, cusp shrinkage (which should be minimal or absent), and progressive changes of connective tissue related to genetic factors either in the native aortic root tissues that support the pulmonary autograft or in the autograft itself. Technical problems at operation relate primarily to matching diameter of the pulmonary autograft to the LV outflow tract at the position of attachment. The LV outflow tract should be sized up or down to a diameter within 2 or 3 mm of that of the autograft. The autograft should not be stretched over a larger LV outflow tract, and the size of the autograft should not be "taken up" during implantation to an importantly smaller aortic anulus. Use of an interrupted suture technique probably provides the most accurate method of suture placement for implanting the autograft and may result in more perfect valve function later. Addition of a support or reinforcement ring to the LV outflow tract suture line is associated with greater freedom from important regurgitation of the pulmonary autograft (Fig. 12-44).[D30]

Connective tissue abnormalities, such as fibrillin deficiency associated with Marfan syndrome, are considered contraindications to aortic valve replacement with pulmonary autograft because the pulmonary artery will likely have the same tendency for dilatation as the aorta. Elkins and colleagues noted fibrillin or elastin abnormalities in the resected aorta in a high proportion of patients undergoing the Ross procedure for aneurysm or dilatation of the ascending aorta.[E8] Changes in pulmonary autograft dimensions did not correlate with the observed changes in fibrillin or elastin. Concern about potential dilatation of the pulmo-

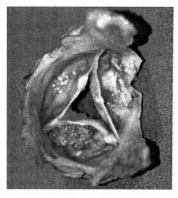 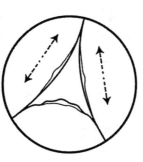

A

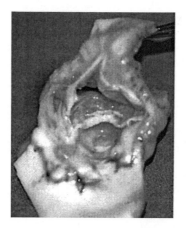 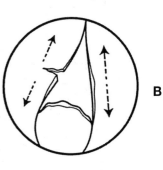

B

Figure 12-42   Effect of commissural position error in aortic valve replacement with an aortic allograft. **A,** Minor position error. An explanted aortic allograft is shown in surgeon's view with diagram of the major findings alongside. Distance (length of aorta) between the commissures bordering the noncoronary sinus of Valsalva is shorter than that between the commissures bordering the left coronary sinus and the commissures bordering the right coronary sinus. Presumably this is the result of closing an oblique incision in the noncoronary sinus with some aortic tissue loss. This commissural positional abnormality places stress on the right and left coronary cusps. Calcium deposits appear greatest in the noncoronary cusp. **B,** Major position error. An explanted aortic allograft is shown in surgeon's view with diagram alongside. The commissure between the left and noncoronary sinuses is drawn far to the right above the noncoronary sinus rather than following the natural position posteriorly. The commissure between the right and noncoronary sinuses is drawn far to the right, producing a similar deformity so that the commissures nearly touch in the noncoronary sinus. This is the result of closure of an oblique incision in the noncoronary sinus of Valsalva with large tissue bites, which draws the adjacent commissures toward each other, as well as simply not following the anatomic contours of the aortic valve. Stress on the left and right coronary cusps resulted in leaflet tear, and the noncoronary cusp is redundant, prolapsed, and contains calcium deposits.

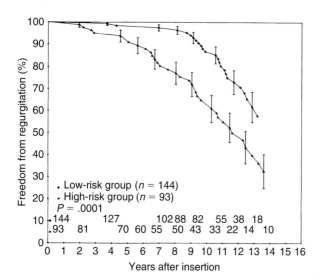

Figure 12-43   Freedom from important allograft regurgitation in patients in a low-risk group (>15 years of age + donor valve <50 years + aortic root size <30 mm) versus high-risk group not meeting these characteristics. Bars represent 1 standard error (70% CL). Data set is as in Fig. 12-40. (From Barratt-Boyes and colleagues.[B41])

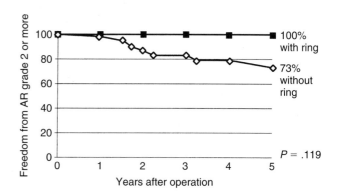

Figure 12-44   Freedom from regurgitation grade 2 or more after aortic valve replacement with pulmonary autograft. Effect of anular support (with ring). Fixing diameter of pulmonary autograft at the anastomosis to the aortic anulus during implantation virtually eliminated autograft regurgitation. (From Dossche and colleagues.[D30])

Key: *AR,* Aortic regurgitation.

nary autograft, resulting in aortic valve regurgitation in a bicuspid aortic valve and dilatation of the aortic root and ascending aorta, appears to be overstated. Long-term series do not report this complication when the aortic anulus is supported and its diameter fixed.[E6,E8,S30]

Although aortic root dilatation is common late after autograft root replacement, it is probably not related to bicuspid aortic valve disease or preexisting degenerative changes in the pulmonary trunk. Histologic abnormalities of the pulmonary trunk are rare and equally prevalent in patients with bicuspid and tricuspid aortic valves.[L23] As noted in "Autograft Pulmonary Valve" under Isolated Aortic Valve Replacement earlier in this chapter, the pulmonary trunk may dilate up to 30% when subjected to systemic arterial pressure.[V3]

Stent-mounted xenograft (porcine) and pericardial (bovine) glutaraldehyde-treated aortic valves. These valves, mounted on a cloth-covered stent, may develop central leakage because of cusp rupture either in the commissural region or in the cusp belly.[S6,T2] Rupture is often associated with cusp calcification, in contrast to the situation with allograft valves inserted freehand. Also, the calcification may produce stenosis rather than rupture.[M26] Although most ruptures in this type of bioprosthesis are precipitated by collagen fatigue and fracture and subsequent invasion of the cusp by macrophages,[B19,F6] some may be caused by abrasion of the cusp against a poorly designed stent. A few cases have resulted from cusp perforation by the long, cut ends of rigid suture material projecting inward from the sewing ring toward the cusp base. Detachment of the valve's aortic remnant from the stent pillar, in contrast to stent-mounted allograft valves and previously used formaldehyde-treated stent-mounted xenografts, is rare and associated with failure of host tissue overgrowth across the polyester bias strip onto the graft.[M21] Presumably the collagen cross-linkage that results from glutaraldehyde preservation of porcine aortic and bovine pericardial valves strengthens the aortic tissue sufficiently to prevent tearing and detachment.

Risk factors for central leakage from degeneration (structural valvar deterioration, SVD) of the cusps of a stent-mounted glutaraldehyde-fixed xenograft include gender and age of the recipient (Fig. 12-45). Xenograft valves in the aortic position degenerate more rapidly in young patients, but this accelerated rate of degeneration rapidly declines with advancing age. In patients older than about 65 years, the failure rate at 10 years is less than 5%.[B42] Jamieson and colleagues showed that degeneration of first-generation porcine xenograft valves was related to age, with risk being higher for younger decades of life. Degeneration decreased after age 60 and was almost imperceptible in patients over 70.[J8,J12] A similar age-related effect on durability of bovine pericardial bioprostheses has been observed (Fig. 12-46); chance of valve explant for struc-

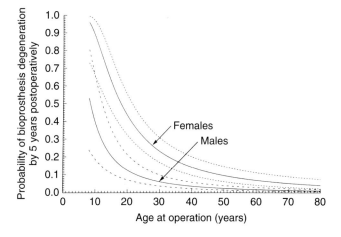

Figure 12-45 Nomogram of estimated risk-adjusted probability of bioprosthetic degeneration within 5 years of inserting first-generation stent-mounted porcine xenografts, according to patient's gender and age at insertion. (From Blackstone and Kirklin.[B42])

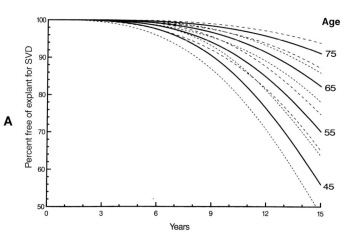
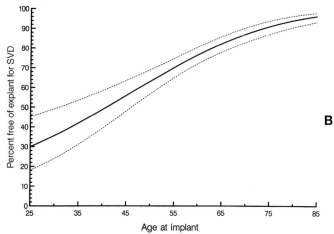

Figure 12-46 Age-related explant for structural valve deterioration (SVD) of bovine pericardial aortic valve prostheses. Dashed lines enclose 68% confidence limits of estimates. **A,** Freedom from explant for SVD for a patient whose valve was implanted at age 45, 55, 65, and 75. **B,** Fifteen-year freedom from explant for SVD across a spectrum of ages. (From Banbury and colleagues.[B68])

Key: *SVD,* Structural valve deterioration.

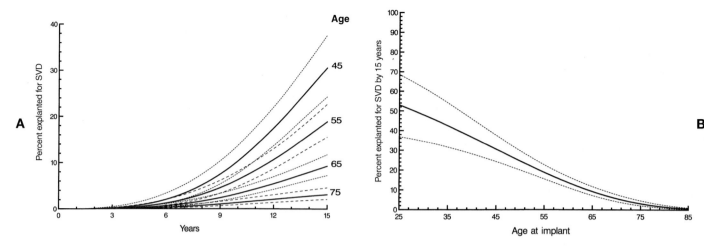

Figure 12-47   Risk-adjusted estimates of age-related explant for structural valve deterioration (SVD) of bovine pericardial aortic valve prostheses. Depiction is from a competing risks analysis that accounts for death before valve explant (see "Competing Risks" under Analyses in Section 4 of Chapter 6); vertical axis is cumulative incidence. For this figure, the patient was assumed to be a male in New York Heart Association functional class III, undergoing first valve replacement, and not undergoing concomitant coronary artery bypass grafting or ascending aorta replacement. Dashed lines enclose 68% confidence limits of estimates. **A,** Evolution of SVD across time for a patient age 45, 55, 65, and 75 at implant. **B,** Fifteen-year freedom from explant for SVD in a similar patient, but across a continuous spectrum of ages. (From Banbury and colleagues.[B68])

Key: *SVD,* Structural valve deterioration.

tural deterioration was less than 10% at 15 years in patients over age 65 years (Fig. 12-47).[B68] Statistical methodology also affects interpretation of the apparent frequency of degeneration[G29] (see "Computing Risks" in Section 4 of Chapter 6). Kaplan–Meier analysis estimates accurately the biologic frequency of SVD among living patients as an isolated event; competing risks analysis places SVD into the context of mortality before SVD occurs. Thus, in older patients, not only does the biologic behavior of the xenograft contribute to a lower incidence of SVD, but mortality decreases the probability that the patient will survive long enough to experience the event (Table 12-10).

Method of valve preservation is also probably a risk factor, because glutaraldehyde fixation at pressures above zero abolishes the normal collagen crimp and importantly diminishes cusp pliability (distensibility). As a result, the cusp kinks rather than stretches on opening, leading to compression fracture of the collagen at the sites of kinking.[B12,B19,B28] In contrast, zero-pressure fixation retains collagen crimp and produces a more pliable cusp with mechanical properties that closely approach those of fresh cusp tissue.[M29] Second-generation zero-pressure–fixed bioprostheses (Medtronic Intact) and third-generation bioprostheses (Medtronic Mosaic and Freestyle) may perform better over time than first-generation pressure-fixed valves.[J7] Also, substances introduced into the fixation protocol may reduce risk of cusp calcification.

Accumulating data demonstrate that second- and third-generation bioprostheses last longer than first-generation devices (Fig. 12-48).[F11,U1-U3] The Hancock II porcine aortic xenograft with improved stent and anticalcification treatment (T6) and the Edwards Lifesciences bovine pericardial valve with flexible stent and anticalcification treat-

■ TABLE 12-10   Freedom from Structural Valve Deterioration at 15 Years after Aortic Valve Replacement According to Age and Statistical Method [a]

Age Group		AVR (%)		MVR (%)	
≤ Years <		% Free	Cumulative Incidence (%) [b]	% Free	Cumulative Incidence (%) [b]
20	40	31	50	18	61
40	50	50	35	20	52
50	60	68	21	30	37
60	70	76	14	30	32
70		89	2	91	4

(Data from Jamieson and colleagues.[J13])

Key: *AVR,* Aortic valve replacement; *MVR,* mitral valve replacement.

[a] Kaplan–Meier estimates.

[b] Competing risks analysis (see "Competing Risks Analysis" in Chapter 6) expressed as cumulative incidence. Patients with Carpentier-Edwards standard porcine bioprosthesis.

ment (Tween 80) are showing less degeneration at 10 years than first-generation devices.[B12,D25,L20] Cryopreserved and homovital aortic allografts appear on the same curve as second-generation xenografts. Data are limited beyond 5 years with third-generation stentless porcine valves treated with alpha-amino oleic acid (Freestyle), but structural integrity appears good.

Stentless xenograft (porcine) aortic valves. Absence of a stent has the theoretic advantages of making the device less stenotic and decreasing perivalvar leakage. Also, by analogy with allografts, degeneration may occur more slowly in stentless than in first-generation stent-mounted xenografts. Experimental and short-term clinical results in a small number of patients are compatible with this

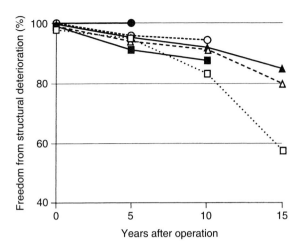

Third-generation stentless porcine (FreeStyle)

Second-generation stentless porcine (Hancock II)

Stent-mounted bovine pericardial (Edwards Life sciences)

Allograft (cryopreserved)

Allograft (homovital)

First-generation stent-mounted porcine
(Carpentier-Edwards & Hancock)

Figure 12-48   Comparison of freedom from structural deterioration of bioprostheses after aortic valve replacement among first-, second-, and third-generation devices. (From Fann and colleagues[F11] and U.S. IDE Centers.[U1–U3])

hypothesis.[D1,D3,D4] Midterm data show that the prevalence of primary periprosthetic leak at 4 years is 2.2% and that virtually no central aortic valve regurgitation of 1+ or greater occurs with the Medtronic Freestyle.[D32] These data exclude five valves explanted earlier for periprosthetic leakage and one valve explanted for central regurgitation, as well as two patients who died from causes related to periprosthetic leakage. Changes in the aorta, however, independent of degeneration of the valve may affect performance of the Toronto SPV bioprosthesis[D23]; dilatation of the sinotubular junction may result in aortic valve regurgitation and may be prevented by restricting the aorta above the valve with a circumferential band.[D44]

Mechanical valve replacement devices. Mechanical replacements develop important central leakage only with mechanical failure (such as poppet escape) or entrapment of a suture. Also, tissue or thrombosis may encroach into the seating area of the device, although the occurrence appears low.

Replacement Device Endocarditis

Endocarditis on the device used for aortic valve replacement is an uncommon but serious complication; overall, only about 30% of patients are long-term survivors.[I3]

Prevalence and Incidence

The prevalence of endocarditis on an aortic valve replacement device is low, with 95% to 97% of patients free of this complication 5 years postoperatively (Fig. 12-49). Risk of

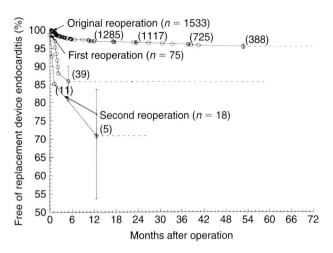

Figure 12-49   Freedom from replacement device endocarditis, after an original valve replacement operation, first reoperation, and second reoperation. Note expanded vertical axis. Each symbol represents an infection; dashed lines indicate patients traced and free of endocarditis, numbers in parentheses are patients at risk, and vertical bars are 70% confidence limits. (From Blackstone and Kirklin.[B42])

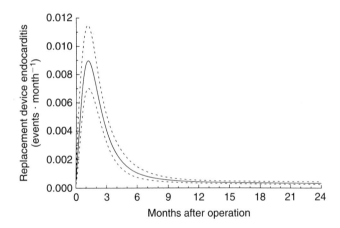

Figure 12-50   Hazard function for replacement device endocarditis after primary valve replacement. Graph is applicable to patients undergoing aortic valve replacement. Initial peaking phase of hazard merges with a constant phase about 6 months after operation. Depiction as in Figure 12-11. (From Ivert and colleagues.[I3])

endocarditis (incidence) generally is greatest about 6 weeks after insertion of the replacement device, then gradually declines to a low constant hazard function by about 9 months (Fig. 12-50). The general shape of the hazard function has been confirmed by others.[B13,B42,H15,L4]

Etiology

Endocarditis early after valve replacement (within 3 months) is usually caused by organisms already present in the operative field or introduced at operation or within the next few days. The organisms are usually staphylococci, gram-negative cocci, or mixed organisms.[I3] The rare fungal infection is typically fatal. Replacement device endocarditis occurring late after operation is the result of a transient bacteremia, most often with streptococcal organisms.

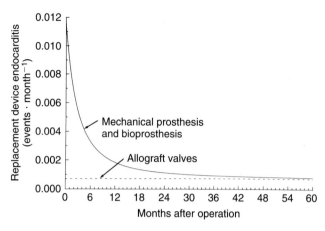

Figure 12-51   Hazard function for replacement device endocarditis. Patients are stratified into those receiving allograft aortic valves versus those receiving mechanical prostheses and bioprostheses. (From GLH: prostheses 1976 to 1980, *n* = 147, 11 events; allografts 1968 to 1981, *n* = 71, 4 events.)

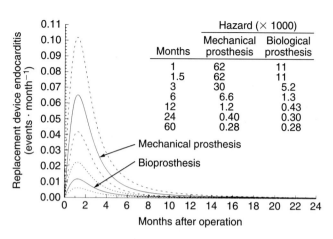

Figure 12-52   Hazard function for replacement device endocarditis after valve replacement for native valve endocarditis, according to whether the device was a mechanical prosthesis or bioprosthesis. Depiction is as in Fig. 12-11. In both cases the early peaking hazard phase merges at 3 to 12 months, with a low constant of hazard. (From Ivert and colleagues.[13])

■ **TABLE 12-11   Incremental Risk Factors for Replacement Device Endocarditis after Primary Operation**

	Hazard Phase	
Risk Factor	**Early**	**Constant**
Demographic variables		
Male gender	•	
African-American	•	•
Endocarditis	•	
Surgical variables		
Mechanical prosthesis	•	

(Data from Blackstone and Kirklin.[B42])

■ **TABLE 12-12   Incremental Risk Factors for Replacement Device Endocarditis after Reoperations on Valve**

Risk Factor	**Single Hazard Phase**
Male gender	•
Mitral replacement at original operation	•

(Data from Blackstone and Kirklin.[B42])

Incremental Risk Factors

Incremental risk factors for developing endocarditis after primary aortic valve replacement (the same as after primary mitral valve replacement) (Table 12-11) are different from those after reoperation (Table 12-12). When the valve replacement operation is performed for endocarditis on either the native valve or a previously inserted replacement device, no risk factors for subsequent endocarditis other than the endocarditis have been identified, probably because of the dominant risk of infection already present.

Of particular therapeutic importance is the finding that a mechanical prosthesis is a risk factor for replacement device infection because of the high early phase of hazard associated with its use (Figs. 12-51 to 12-53). The allograft aortic valve, inserted freehand into the aortic position, is unique in having no early hazard phase (Fig. 12-54), even when the operations are performed on already infected native valves or replacement devices (see Fig. 12-53).

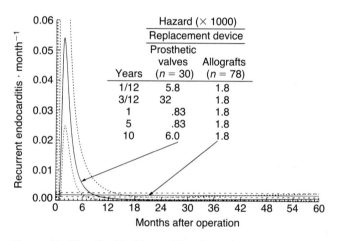

Figure 12-53   Stratified hazard function of recurrent postoperative endocarditis in patients with acute native or prosthetic aortic valve endocarditis undergoing aortic valve replacement. The hazard, when allograft valves were used, was predicted to be higher with localized endocarditis than with extensive endocarditis (*P* for difference = .07). (From Haydock and colleagues.[H15])

Bioprostheses seem less likely to develop "prosthetic valve endocarditis" than mechanical prostheses.

Presence of native valve endocarditis has some adverse effects on subsequent freedom from replacement device endocarditis (Fig. 12-55). Replacement device endocarditis tends to develop after a redo operation more often than after an original valve operation (Fig. 12-56).

Early (Hospital) Death and Time-Related Survival

Replacement device endocarditis is a serious complication; in one study, 50% of patients were dead within 6 months of its identification (Fig. 12-57). Mortality was less with allograft aortic valves inserted freehand; even though the operation was performed on already infected valves, only about 20% of patients died within 6 months. This result,

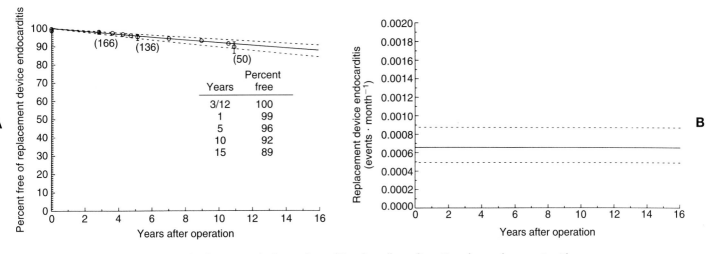

Figure 12-54   Replacement device endocarditis after allograft aortic valve replacement, with or without concomitant coronary artery bypass grafting. Depiction is as in Fig. 12-11. **A,** Freedom from endocarditis. **B,** Hazard function for allograft valve endocarditis. (From O'Brien and colleagues.[O5])

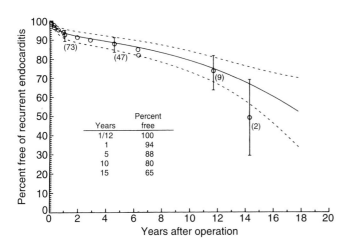

Figure 12-55   Freedom from replacement valve endocarditis after aortic valve replacement for acute native or prosthetic valve endocarditis in 108 patients. Depiction is as in Fig. 12-18. (From Haydock and colleagues.[H15])

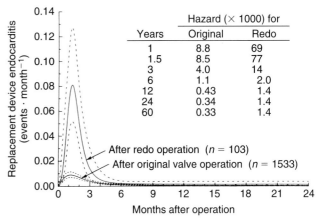

Figure 12-56   Hazard function for replacement device endocarditis after original valve operation and after redo valve operation. Depiction is as in Fig. 12-18. (From Blackstone and Kirklin.[B42])

however, may reflect operations performed in patients with less extensive infections than those requiring aortic root replacement techniques for aortic root abscess, as well as infectious processes extending beyond the aortic valve cusp tissues. In contrast, Sabik and colleagues reported that radical debridement and aortic root replacement with a cryopreserved aortic allograft resulted in 5- and 10-year survival of 73% and 56%, respectively.[S38]

Table 12-13 lists the risk factors for death after valve replacement for native valve or prosthetic endocarditis.

Treatment

When endocarditis develops early or late after an aortic valve replacement operation, the causative organism is identified so that specific treatment with appropriate antibiotics can be started. Endocarditis on aortic valve replacement devices is often destructive of the entire aortic anular

support mechanism and may be associated with anular abscess. Infection may extend to contiguous cardiac structures beyond the aortic root. Reconstruction of the aortic root destroyed by infection may be best accomplished by use of aortic allograft.

Thromboembolism

Risk (hazard) of thromboembolism is approximately constant beyond the first month after operation. The authoritative report by Edmunds indicates that the overall linearized rate of thromboembolism in patients with mechanical device replacement of the aortic valve is 2 ± 1 per 100 patient-years and about half that value in patients with stent-mounted xenograft valves.[E2] The comprehensive study of Grunkemeier and colleagues showed considerable variance in rate of thromboembolism among

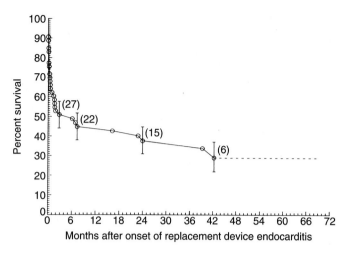

Figure 12-57 Survival after onset of replacement device endocarditis. Depiction is as in Fig. 12-18. (From Ivert and colleagues.[13])

■ **TABLE 12-13 Incremental Risk Factors for Death after Aortic Valve Replacement for Acute Infectious Endocarditis**

		Hazard Phase	
	Risk Factors[a]	Early	Constant[b]
(Older)	Age at operation	•	
(Higher)	NYHA class (I-V)	•	
(Larger)	Number of previous aortic valve procedures[c]	•	

(Data from Haydock and colleagues.[H15])

Key: *NYHA*, New York Heart Association.

[a] Nonuse of an allograft aortic valve inserted by freehand technique did not remain in the final model (equation); *P* was .3 in early hazard phase and .9 in constant hazard phase.

[b] No risk factors in constant phase.

[c] When number of previous aortic valve procedure was 0, endocarditis was on the native valve.

published series of patients.[G28] Thromboembolism rate is about the same for the various mechanical devices; median rate for the St. Jude valve is $1.33\% \cdot year^{-1}$, for the Medtronic-Hall $1.20\% \cdot year^{-1}$, and for the CarboMedics valve $1.16\% \cdot year^{-1}$. Rates for stent-mounted bioprostheses are also similar; median rate for the Hancock porcine is $0.78\% \cdot year^{-1}$, for the Carpentier-Edwards porcine $0.87\% \cdot year^{-1}$, and for the Carpentier-Edwards bovine $1.22\% \cdot year^{-1}$. The rate is lower for allografts, with a median of $0.23\% \cdot year^{-1}$. All these rates fall below the objective performance criteria required for U.S. Food and Drug Administration (FDA) approval of $3.0\% \cdot year^{-1}$ for mechanical valves and $2.5\% \cdot year^{-1}$ for bioprostheses. Adequacy of warfarin therapy is the key determinant of the rate in patients with mechanical aortic valves. Thromboembolism is unusual in patients receiving pulmonary autografts in the aortic position.

Thrombosis of the replacement device itself is uncommon. The linearized rate for mechanical prostheses is about $0.1\% \cdot year^{-1}$. Thrombosis occurs even less often in patients with stent-mounted xenograft valves.

Complications of Anticoagulation

Complications of chronic warfarin therapy in patients who have undergone aortic valve replacement are the same as in other patients (see "Complications of Long-Term Anticoagulation" under Results in Section 1 of Chapter 11). Excessive anticoagulation is accompanied by threat of bleeding. Anticoagulant levels above therapeutic values but with INR less than 5 indicate need to withhold warfarin until INR returns to therapeutic range, then restarting the medication at a lower dose. Warfarin is withheld in patients with INR of 5 to 9, and oral vitamin K (1.25 to 2.5 mg) is considered if the patient is at increased risk of bleeding. Vitamin K (2.5 to 5 mg) is given orally to patients with INR greater than 9, and if the patient has serious bleeding, it is given intravenously (10 mg) accompanied by transfusion of fresh frozen plasma.

Frequent questions arise about managing potential bleeding in patients with mechanical heart valves taking warfarin who require cardiac catheterization, percutaneous catheter intervention, noncardiac surgery, or a dental procedure. Most dental procedures can be managed without interrupting anticoagulation. For patients with minimal risk of thromboembolism, warfarin should be stopped about 3 days before elective operation so that the procedure may be performed when INR is 1.5 or less. Warfarin is restarted as soon as risk for bleeding has ceased, usually 24 to 48 hours after completing the procedure. Where there is increased risk (atrial fibrillation with large atria, enlarged or poorly contractile LV), unfractionated heparin (enoxaparin) is administered when INR is less than 2. The short-acting anticoagulant is discontinued for the procedure, restarted along with warfarin after risk of bleeding has ceased, and continued for a 3- to 5-day overlap until INR is again therapeutic. Enoxaparin administered to patients prior to cardiac operations, however, increases risk of postoperative bleeding requiring re-entry.[J14] When emergency operation is required, operation proceeds immediately as indicated, with reversal of warfarin's effect by transfusion of fresh frozen plasma as required to achieve adequate clotting.

More accurate control of level of anticoagulation by self-testing of prothrombin time has been associated with a reduction in major bleeding events.[B43,B59] In a randomized trial of 325 patients, Byeth and Landefeld reported reduction of major bleeding events in the first 6 months of therapy with warfarin.[B60] Providing appropriate devices to allow patients to measure prothrombin time themselves and teaching them how to adjust the warfarin dose early after operation is effective in reducing complications related to anticoagulant therapy.[A16,A17,K37]

Aortic Root Complications
Aneurysms

Three unsuspected small aneurysms were found among 100 patients studied by aortography 6 to 9 months after aortic valve replacement by Bjork and colleagues.[B11] One was at the aortotomy suture line, and two seemed to originate from the left coronary sinus. Thus, at operation, a secure full-thickness closure must always be obtained to prevent not only acute postoperative bleeding but also late aneurysm formation.

After composite graft reconstruction using the inclusion technique,[B21] there has been an important occurrence of aneurysm, most often arising from partial dehiscence of the anastomosis to the graft of the aorta around the coronary ostia [K6,K15] and less often from the distal graft to aorta suture line. To overcome dehiscence, Cabrol and colleagues recommend routine use of a separate 8-mm polyester tube graft, the extremities of which are anastomosed to the aorta around the right and left coronary orifices. A large side-to-side anastomosis is then made between the center of this graft and the front of the 30-mm polyester tube.[C22] Alternatively, and probably preferably, an aortic button containing the coronary ostium is anastomosed directly to a window in the polyester graft (see "Technique of Operation" earlier in this chapter). Dehiscence at the distal graft suture line is avoided by using a prosthetic collar (cut from the primary graft) to cover the distal suture line.

False aneurysm at the proximal suture line has been observed when the full root replacement technique is employed for implanting an aortic allograft or pulmonary autograft (Ross procedure).[O15] This rare complication may be eliminated by routine use of a support collar at the proximal suture line and partial inversion of the graft while it is tied to the aortic anulus to ensure direct tissue approximation during implantation.

Infection

Infection in the aortotomy is rare in the absence of infection in the valve replacement device, even when ascending aortic root replacement has been part of the operation.

Cessation of Gastrointestinal Bleeding

In patients with aortic stenosis who have a history of gastrointestinal bleeding, an unusual but characteristic syndrome, nearly all (93% of 91 patients in one study[K7]) are free of bleeding after aortic valve replacement. In contrast, abdominal procedures for gastrointestinal bleeding are successful only occasionally.[K7]

Reoperation

Reoperation may be necessary early or late after aortic valve replacement. The nature of the reoperation varies with its indication. When performed for acute thrombosis, thrombectomy can be an effective procedure, although valve replacement is often required. When performed for periprosthetic leakage, simple suture repair is often possible and effective. Valve replacement is required in a few patients when dehiscence of the valve from aortic root tissues is extensive. When the reoperation is for endocarditis, re-replacement is indicated when there is active infection. In unusual circumstances, when infection has been controlled and arrested for weeks or months and there is residual periprosthetic leakage, it may be possible to repair the leak and retain the valve.

Although hospital mortality can be low for a first-time aortic valve re-replacement (3.9%; CL 2.4%-6.0% in one study[W1]), replacement of an already replaced aortic valve has serious implications.

Jones and colleagues[J15] have shown that operative mortality for repeat heart valve surgery has declined with each

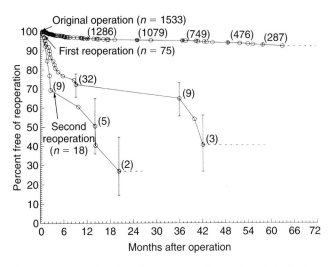

Figure 12-58   Freedom from reoperation after original valve replacement operation, after first reoperation, and after second reoperation. Depiction is similar to format of Fig. 12-49. (From Blackstone and Kirklin.[B42])

decade of experience. Mortality for aortic valve re-replacement was 6.4%. Risk increased with increasing age of the patient, presence of coronary artery bypass grafts, and indication for operation (particularly for valve thrombosis or endocarditis). Replacing a dysfunctional mechanical valve had 2.25 times the risk of replacing a bioprosthetic valve. Hasnat and colleagues report an early mortality of 3.4% (CL 1.9%-5.8%) for replacing an aortic valve allograft with a second one.[H25] In their experience a second aortic valve allograft was associated with good long-term survival; accelerated degeneration did not occur. Byrne and colleagues[B67] reported 11% hospital mortality for aortic valve allograft re-replacement in 18 patients, 14 of whom (67%) received mechanical prostheses at reoperation. At least in the case of prosthetic and bioprosthetic valves, after each reoperation there is an increasing prevalence of still another reoperation (Fig. 12-58), of periprosthetic leakage (Fig. 12-59), and of prosthetic valve endocarditis (see Fig. 12-49). In addition, each reoperation increases the risk of early death.[B42] Many factors contribute to the increasing prevalence of unfavorable outcome events as the reoperations accumulate, including increased fibrosis and decreasing local vascularity in the interior of the aortic root. This emphasizes the importance of making the first valve replacement operation the only one whenever possible.

The prevalence and incidence of a first reoperation vary to some extent with the circumstances. Thus, the shape of the hazard function for reoperation for mechanical devices differs from that for stent-mounted xenografts (Fig. 12-60). Mechanical replacement devices have an early phase of hazard for reoperation that peaks at about 3 months and is usually caused by prosthetic valve endocarditis and periprosthetic leakage. This phase of hazard steadily declines thereafter, and a constant phase cannot be identified. By contrast, stent-mounted xenograft valves not only have the early peaking hazard phase for reoperation like mechanical devices, but also a second late-rising hazard phase related to the increasing incidence of bioprosthesis degeneration as time passes. In the case of freehand allografts, provided the

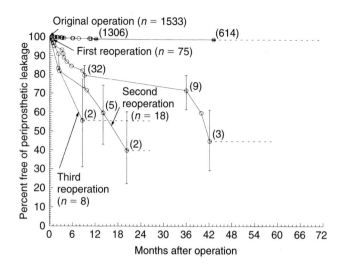

Figure 12-59 Freedom from periprosthetic leakage without evident infection after original valve replacement operation and after first, second, and third reoperation. Depiction is similar to format of Fig. 12-49. (From Blackstone and Kirklin.[B42])

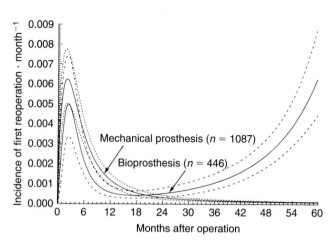

Figure 12-60 Hazard function for reoperation for mechanical prostheses and bioprostheses, determined by separate analyses. In the hazard function for mechanical prostheses, there is an early peaking hazard phase and a constant hazard phase; in that for bioprostheses, there is an early peaking phase and a second rising late hazard phase. (From Blackstone and Kirklin.[B42])

device is properly inserted, without the prevalence of early regurgitation attributable to technical error, there is no early hazard phase of reoperation, but rather a gradually increasing late postoperative phase (see Fig. 12-39).[B41,O5]

Late reoperation may be required after composite prosthetic graft reconstruction for graft or prosthetic valve infection, for prosthetic valve thrombosis or perivalvar leak, and for pseudoaneurysm. Freedom from reoperation was 81% at 7 years in one series.[K15]

INDICATIONS FOR OPERATION, SELECTION OF TECHNIQUE, AND CHOICE OF DEVICE

Advances in diagnostic techniques, understanding of natural history, and operative procedures for aortic valve disease have resulted in enhanced diagnosis, more scientific selection of patients for surgery, and increased survival of patients with aortic valve disorders. The extensive literature on valvar heart disease, however, consists mostly of single-institution experiences in relatively small numbers of patients. ACC/AHA charged the Committee on Management of Patients with Valvular Heart Disease with the task of compiling an information base and making recommendations for diagnosis and treatment. The task force's report, Guidelines for Management of Patients with Valvular Heart Disease, represents the most definitive treatise on this subject. The document is available as an abbreviated executive summary[B46] with a few key references or as full text[B52] with references to 737 published articles on the subject.

Box 12-1 summarizes the indications for operation in patients with aortic valve disease.

Aortic Stenosis

Symptomatic Patients

Patients with symptoms of angina pectoris, dyspnea, or syncope caused by aortic valve stenosis have symptomatic

improvement and increased survival after aortic valve replacement, even with LV dysfunction.[C29,K30,L19,M34,S36,S37] Therefore, aortic valve replacement is indicated in virtually all symptomatic patients. Patients with severe, symptomatic aortic valve stenosis associated with low transvalvar pressure gradient also have hemodynamic improvement and better functional results.[B53] Elderly patients over age 85 with severe heart failure and associated coronary artery disease may be exceptions. Even severe concomitant noncardiac disease rarely contraindicates aortic valve replacement, although advanced chronic obstructive pulmonary disease, widespread arteriosclerosis, and advanced neurologic disease may greatly increase the risk of operation or render it inadvisable.

The urgency of operation in patients with important aortic stenosis and syncope (or near-syncope) as the only complaint has been debated. This presentation generally does not make operation urgent but does make it advisable.

Asymptomatic Patients

Controversy surrounds the approach to patients with absent or trivial symptoms. When stenosis is clearly severe (peak systolic gradient 50 mmHg or higher, aortic valve area 1.0 cm^2 or less), operation is usually advisable even though some patients may have no symptoms. Some clinicians, however, may be reluctant to proceed.[C41] Even though the perioperative risk of operation is low, long-term morbidity and mortality related to the replacement device may be appreciable. The combined risk of operation and late complications of the replacement device may exceed the 1% per year risk of sudden death in asymptomatic patients. Some asymptomatic patients may be at higher risk for sudden death without surgery, although supporting data are limited. These patients may have LV systolic dysfunction, abnormal response to exercise (hypotension), ventricular tachycardia, marked LV hypertrophy (15 mm or greater), or valve area

BOX 12-1   Indications for Operation for Aortic Valve Disease

Aortic Stenosis
1. Symptomatic patients with severe stenosis
2. Patients with moderate or severe stenosis having operation for coronary artery disease, other heart valve disease, or aortic disease
3. Asymptomatic patients with severe aortic stenosis
   a. LV systolic dysfunction
   b. Abnormal response to exercise (hypotension)
   c. Ventricular tachycardia
   d. Marked LV hypertrophy (≥15 mm)
   e. Aortic valve area (<0.6 cm²)

Aortic Regurgitation
1. Symptomatic patients with severe chronic regurgitation
   a. Preserved LV systolic function (EF >0.5)
   b. Advanced LV dysfunction (EF <0.25, end-systolic dimension >60 mm), risk increased
   c. Progressive LV dilatation, declining EF, or positive exercise test performance
   d. Angina without coronary artery disease
2. Symptomatic or asymptomatic patients
   a. Mild to moderate LV dysfunction (EF 0.25-0.49)
   b. Having operation for coronary artery disease, other heart valve disease, or aortic disease
3. Asymptomatic patients
   a. Normal systolic function (EF >0.5) with dilated left ventricle (end-systolic dimension >55 mm, end-diastolic dimension >75 mm)
   b. Normal systolic function (EF >0.5) with decline in EF during exercise
   c. Severe systolic dysfunction (EF <0.25)
4. Acute and severe aortic regurgitation

Modified from Bonow and colleagues.[B52]
Key: *EF*, Ejection fraction; *LV*, left ventricular.

less than 0.6 cm². Such high-risk patients are usually symptomatic but if not will become so in a short time.[B52]

Patients with Ischemic Heart Disease

Patients with severe aortic valve stenosis and important ischemic heart disease should have aortic valve replacement at the time of CABG. The approach is less clear if aortic valve stenosis is moderate or even mild, because it is difficult to predict when these patients will develop severe aortic stenosis after coronary revascularization. Some patients manifest rapid progression of aortic valve stenosis of up to 0.3 cm² · year⁻¹ and an increase in pressure gradient of up to 15 to 19 mmHg · year⁻¹. Most patients, however, show little or no change. The average rate of reduction in valve area seems to be about 0.12 cm² · year⁻¹.[O10] Mean time to reoperation for aortic valve replacement after CABG is 5 to 8 years.[C42,F11,H19,O14] Experienced surgeons tend to be more aggressive in treating mild and moderate aortic valve stenosis in conjunction with coronary artery disease because of the unpredictable progression of the aortic valve disease.[K25,P10] Patients over age 45, those over 35 with angina as a part of their symptomatology (which makes coexisting coronary artery disease more likely[L12]), and those with a strong family history of arteriosclerotic disease require coronary angiography before operation.

Patients with Other Heart Valve or Thoracic Aorta Disease

Patients with moderate (gradient 30 mmHg or greater) or severe aortic valve stenosis should have aortic valve replacement in conjunction with operations on the aorta or other heart valves.

Aortic Regurgitation

Patients with pure, chronic aortic regurgitation should have aortic valve replacement only if the regurgitation is severe.[B52] Patients with symptoms and only mild or moderate aortic regurgitation may have other conditions, such as coronary artery disease, hypertension, or cardiomyopathy.

Symptomatic Patients

Aortic valve replacement is recommend for patients with normal systolic function (EF 0.5 or greater at rest) and symptoms in NYHA functional class III or IV or angina pectoris in Canadian Heart Association class 2 to 4.[B52] Patients with new onset of mild symptoms require special attention and are usually considered for operation, even without reaching threshold values for LV size and function.

Symptomatic Patients with Left Ventricular Dysfunction

Patients having symptoms of heart failure or angina pectoris and mild to moderate LV dysfunction (EF 0.25 to 0.49) should have aortic valve replacement. Postoperative survival and recovery of systolic function are reduced, however, compared with less symptomatic patients.[B33,B40] Symptomatic patients with advanced LV dysfunction (EF less than 0.25, end-systolic dimension greater than 60 mm) present more difficult management problems; some recover LV function after aortic valve replacement, but many do not because of irreversible myocardial changes. Operative mortality in these patients approaches 10%.[B52] Chance of good results is better in patients with recent onset of symptoms in NYHA functional class II or III. Operation is usually recommended for patients with class II symptoms and normal EF who show evidence of progressive LV dilatation or declining EF at rest on serial echocardiographic or radionuclide studies. Even in the high-risk group with NYHA class IV symptoms, aortic valve replacement is usually a better alternative than the higher risks of long-term medical management.

Asymptomatic Patients

Aortic valve replacement in asymptomatic patients with aortic regurgitation is controversial, but most agree that operation is indicated in patients with LV systolic dysfunction.[B54] Aortic valve replacement is generally recommended for asymptomatic patients when EF is less than 0.50. Severe LV dilatation (end-diastolic dimension greater than 75 mm, end-systolic dimension greater than 55 mm) is also an indication for operation, even if EF remains normal, because these patients have an increased risk of sudden death and postoperative results are good.[B55,K31,T9] Patients with systemic hypertension, coronary artery disease, concomitant mitral valve stenosis, or who are women deserve special attention and may be recommended for aortic valve replacement at reduced LV dimension thresholds.[B52] Reduced EF during exercise, progressive decline in EF, or minor increases in LV dimensions less than those just detailed are not usually indications for operation in asymptomatic patients with aortic regurgitation.[B52,H6,H18] Improving methods of aortic valve replacement, however, may reduce objective thresholds for recommending operation.

Patients with Ischemic Heart Disease, Other Heart Valve Disease, or Aortic Disease

Coronary artery disease coexists with aortic regurgitation less frequently than with aortic stenosis. Patients having CABG or other heart valve replacement usually have aortic valve replacement for moderate or severe aortic regurgitation. Mild aortic valve regurgitation has a long natural history and is usually not an indication for aortic valve replacement in association with other cardiac operations. Operations for primary disease of the aorta with associated aortic regurgitation require special attention. Indications for operation are usually based on severity and degree of the aortic pathology rather than on the condition of the aortic valve. Surgical intervention is indicated when the aortic diameter reaches or exceeds 50 mm (but see McDonald and colleagues for indications based on aortic dimensions normalized to body size[M40]).[B52] These dimensions should be lowered to 45 mm for patients with Marfan syndrome to prevent progression of aortic valve regurgitation and aortic dissection. Aortic valve–sparing operations are often possible when operation is performed before the aortic root is greatly enlarged.[G24,S18]

Native Aortic Valve Endocarditis

Native aortic valve endocarditis in a hemodynamically stable patient should be treated in the hospital with appropriate antimicrobial therapy and serial echocardiographic examination of the aortic valve and root. If aortic regurgitation develops and progresses, if evidence of aortic root or mitral anular abscess appears, or if septic embolization or vegetation is observed, operation must be undertaken promptly, before hemodynamic deterioration increases the risks associated with operation.

An allograft valve is clearly the aortic replacement device of choice in these patients and may be used even when an aortic root abscess is present.[K22] A pulmonary autograft may also be used in patients with active endocarditis on aortic valve cusps, limited anular involvement with no associated medical comorbidity, and a life expectancy exceeding 20 years.[N9,O17] Extensive aortic root destruction indicates aortic root replacement with an allograft aortic root.[G23] Rarely, the infected valve may be repaired rather than replaced.[D17]

Selection of Technique and Choice of Device

After 50 years of experience with heart valve devices,[D40] it would seem reasonable that a single type of device should have emerged that is ideal for all circumstances when replacement of the aortic valve is necessary. Unfortunately, this is not the case. The surgeon must choose from an ever-increasing number of replacement devices; new devices are constantly being designed, tested, and added to the market after short-term clinical trials. By the time

■ **TABLE 12-14   Types of Aortic Valve Replacement Devices Used (%), 1995 through 2001**

Device	1995	1996	1997	1998	1999	2000	2001
Mechanical	57	53	50	44	41	40	36
Bioprosthetic	36	40	43	47	50	54	60
Allograft	1.9	2.1	2.3	2.2	2.7	2.2	2.6
Not known	4.7	4.0	4.2	4.4	4.7	2.9	1.5

(Data from Society of Thoracic Surgeons National Database Committee.[S35,S39])

midterm or long-term performance data are known, an equal number of valves are discarded in favor of new and unproven devices.

Type of Replacement Device

The type of operation performed on the aortic valve has changed over time as replacement devices have changed and improved. Current practice indicates a trend toward less frequent use of mechanical prostheses and more use of bioprosthetic devices (Table 12-14).[S35,S39] Allograft aortic valve procedures are limited by donor availability to about 2% of aortic valve replacements.

Comparative information concerning performance specifications of the various valves is confusing. The body of literature on valve performance and outcome statistics is enormous; an individual surgeon cannot assimilate sufficient data to make informed recommendations. DeWall and colleagues reviewed the evolution of mechanical heart valves from the introduction of the ball-in-tube design of Hufnagel to contemporary devices.[D40,H1] Grunkemeier and colleagues evaluated the long-term performance of heart valve prostheses using statistics extracted from published articles on results.[G28] Their database is the most extensive information available.

Marketing ploys by device manufacturers further confound the issue. Actual sizer dimensions supplied by manufacturers and dimensions of prostheses vary considerably from labeled diameters.[B61,B62,W17] However, a few constants are of some value in interpreting performance characteristics of the various cardiac valve replacement devices. The manufacturer's label size (mm) expresses only approximately the size (diameter) of the prosthesis. For stent-mounted bioprosthesis the label size correlates with the outside diameter of the stent, not the outer diameter including the sewing ring as it does for mechanical devices. Label size is always larger than the primary orifice or inside diameter of the device (Fig. 12-61 and Box 12-2).

The primary orifice is often referred to as the *internal orifice area* or the *measured geometric orifice* (cm²). The internal orifice area is always larger than functional *in vitro orifice area,* which is calculated by testing the valve in the laboratory in vitro with either steady flow or pulsatile flow. The in vitro orifice area is generally larger than the area measured in vivo by Doppler ultrasound after the valve is implanted (the exception is bioprostheses tested at low steady flow rates). The orifice area calculated either in vitro or in vivo is also called the *effective orifice area* (EOA, cm²), which may be indexed to body size by dividing by body surface area (indexed EOA = EOA ÷ BSA). Body surface area is calculated from both height and weight, however, so obesity may distort this figure.

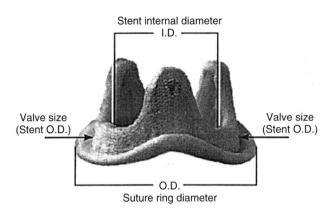

Figure 12-61 Manufacturer's specifications and definition of dimensions for stent-mounted porcine bioprosthesis (Medtronic-Hancock II). Valve label size correlates with outside diameter of stent. Primary orifice refers to internal diameter of stent and does not reflect the actual orifice once the bioprosthetic valve is mounted within the confines of the stent. Outer diameter of the device is called the *suture ring diameter* and is the dimension that must be fitted within the aortic root. (Courtesy Medtronic, Inc.)

Key: *I.D.,* Internal diameter; *O.D.,* outer diameter.

BOX 12-2   Size Relationships of Aortic Valve Prostheses

- Manufacturer's *label size* (mm) expresses prosthesis size (diameter) and is larger than the *primary (geometric) orifice diameter.*

- *Internal orifice area* (measured geometric orifice in cm²) is larger than *in vitro orifice area* (measured in pulse duplicator).

- In vitro orifice area is larger than *in vivo orifice area* (measured after implant by Doppler).

Devices for replacement of the aortic valve are divided into two groups: mechanical prostheses and bioprostheses, the latter commonly referred to as "tissue valves." A complete listing of all available devices would serve little useful purpose. The focus here is on the devices that have been most widely used throughout the world, recognizing their high-volume use in the United States. Generally, valves within a grouping have similar performance characteristics, and choice is usually based on surgeon preference, handling characteristics of the device, availability, technical and service support, and cost.

Mechanical Aortic Valve Replacement Devices

Ball-in-cage devices

Starr-Edwards Silastic Ball Valve Prosthesis (Model 1260). The Starr-Edwards valve is a first-generation device of great historical importance. The first device in this line was used in the first successful human valve replacement operation. Only model 1260 has been available in recent years. In small sizes in the aortic position, the valve has somewhat more energy loss across it than other devices.

Tilting-disc devices

Medtronic-Hall. The model A7700 Medtronic-Hall valve for aortic valve replacement has improved hemodynamic performance compared with ball-in-cage devices.[A14] The design is a tilting carbon-coated disc with a small central hole. The disc is retained and guided during opening and closing by a strut that protrudes through this central hole. The housing and retaining strut are machined from a single piece of titanium. Thromboembolism occurs less often with this second-generation device in the aortic position (92% freedom for at least 5 years) than with ball-in-cage devices. The tilting disc can be rotated inside the sewing ring.

Omniscience, Omnicarbon. The Omniscience valve (Medical Incorporated) is an evolution of the discontinued Lillehei-Kaster pivoting disc valve. The Omnicarbon valve is an all–pyrolytic carbon design of the Omniscience valve. Pyrolytic carbon is a ceramic material that is extraordinarily hard.

Ultracor. The Ultracor valve is manufactured by Aortech (Scotland). It incorporates features of the Lillehei-Kaster, Omniscience, and Omnicarbon valves.

Monostrut (Bjork-Shiley, Sorin, Alliance Medical Technologies). The Bjork-Shiley Monostrut valve for aortic valve replacement (model ABMS) also has improved hemodynamic performance. Two struts retain a grooved, pyrolytic carbon–coated disc. The housing and struts are machined from a single block of titanium for strength. Freedom from a thromboembolic event for at least 5 years in the aortic position is 93%.[N7] This valve is not available presently.

Bileaflet devices

St. Jude. The St. Jude Medical bileaflet valve was introduced in 1977. The valve mechanism, unchanged since its first clinical use, consists of two semicircular leaflets with small ears that pivot in a butterfly-shaped recess in the housing of the device. It is manufactured from pyrolytic carbon and is durable, with leaflet fracture virtually nonexistent.[L3]

The St. Jude valve is available in a variety of models, all based on variations of the sewing ring; the basic mechanical device is the same in all models. It is available in rotatable and nonrotatable, standard, expanded, or reduced sewing rings and with silver impregnation (Silzone) to prevent infection (see "Silver-Coated Sewing Rings" under Special Situations and Controversies later in this chapter). Hemodynamic performance of even the 19-mm device is adequate, and sizes 21 mm and larger show good performance. Freedom from thromboembolism is good.[A4,C24,D12]

CarboMedics. The CarboMedics valve is available in various designs of sewing cuff, but the basic mechanical valve is the same in all models. The bileaflet design has flat, pyrolytic carbon–coated leaflets in a pyrolytic carbon housing strengthened by a radiopaque titanium ring.

Edwards Tekna. The Edwards Tekna device was originally called the Duromedics valve. Its unique design features are curved leaflets and a hinge mechanism below the inflow edge of the housing. After initial mechanical failures, minor modifications have apparently corrected the problems.

Sorin Bicarbon. The Bicarbon device was introduced in 1990. It has a solid titanium housing and a bileaflet carbon mechanism. The sewing ring is carbon coated.

■ **TABLE 12-15** **Primary Orifice Area (cm²): Manufacturers' Specifications for Mechanical Prostheses**

	Label Size (mm)				
Prosthesis	**19**	**21**	**23**	**25**	**27**
Starr-Edwards 1260	–	1.41	1.67	–	2.16
Medtronic-Hall	–	2.01	2.54	3.14	3.80
Monostrut	1.5	2.0	2.0	3.1	3.8
St. Jude	1.63	2.06	2.55	3.09	3.67
CarboMedics	1.59	2.07	2.56	3.16	3.84

(Data from Walker and Scotten.[W11])

■ **TABLE 12-16** **Effective Orifice Area (cm²) from In Vitro Studies on Mechanical Prostheses**

	Label Size (mm)				
Prosthesis	**19**	**21**	**23**	**25**	**27**
Starr-Edwards 1260	–	1.23	–	1.62	1.75
Medtronic-Hall	–	1.74	2.26	3.07	3.64
Monostrut	1.07	1.45	2.00	2.62	3.34
St. Jude	1.21	1.81	2.24	3.23	4.09
CarboMedics	1.12	1.66	2.28	3.14	3.75

(Data from Yoganathan and colleagues.[Y5])

ATS (Advancing the Standard) Open Pivot. The ATS valve is unique in that the hinge socket is on the cusp, whereas the protrusion of the hinge mechanism is on the housing. The purpose is to reduce thromboembolism by better washing of the pivot mechanism. It was introduced in 1995.

MCRI (Medical Carbon Research Institute) On-X. The On-X device is manufactured from an improved and more pure form of pyrolytic carbon for greater strength. It has an elongated housing and flared inlet to provide hemodynamic advantages.

Specifications for mechanical prostheses. Table 12-15 lists manufacturers' reported primary orifice area for the common mechanical cardiac valve prostheses.[W11] Compared with in vitro pulse duplicator studies, the effective orifice is smaller than measured geometric orifice (Table 12-16).[Y5] In vivo performance studies of mechanical heart valves are often subject to error artifacts caused by turbulence and alterations of blood flow patterns by the prosthetic material in the LV outflow tract. Also, some manufacturers' labeled-size valves are mechanically equivalent, meaning that the same housing is used but the sewing rings are different, enabling the manufacturer to label the device differently. For example, Medtronic-Hall label sizes 20 and 21 mm share the same housing, as do sizes 22 and 23 and sizes 29 and 31. For the St. Jude prostheses, HP valves have label size 2 mm less than the standard valve sharing the same size housing.

Mechanical cardiac valve prostheses produce sounds that are audible to patients. Occasionally the sound is disturbing. Sezai and colleagues interviewed patients 1 month and 1 year after aortic valve replacement with the St. Jude Medical or ATS prosthesis.[S28] Many patients (52% St. Jude Medical, 8.3% ATS) reported that the valve was audible 1 year after implantation. The sound was sometimes disturbing in 9% of patients with the St. Jude Medical valve (0% ATS) and resulted in sleep disturbances in 9% and a desire for a less noisy valve in 9%. Reported loudness of the valve sound is the best measurement of a patient's adverse reaction to the sound; this may be modified by hearing loss in patients.[B45] Erickson and colleagues studied mechanical heart valve sound loudness in vitro and found that the quietest valves were the St. Jude Medical and the CarboMedics.[E9] The Sorin Bicarbon valve was 10% louder. Loudness was doubled with the Edwards Tekna and Monostrut valves. The loudest of all was the Medtronic-Hall valve. The St. Jude Medical valve was confirmed as quiet in another study.[B45] Sezai and colleagues' data, how-

ever, indicate there may be some advantage in quietness of the ATS valve.[S28]

Bioprosthetic Aortic Valve Replacement Devices

Stent-mounted devices. The many stent-mounted bioprosthetic devices in clinical use include those with valve cusps made of xenograft aortic valves, pericardium, fascia lata, and dura mater. Theoretically, according to the physical characteristics of biologic materials, only cusp tissue should be considered appropriate for this purpose, but pericardium has proved to be remarkably durable.

Carpentier-Edwards Glutaraldehyde-Preserved Porcine Xenograft (Edwards Lifesciences). The Carpentier-Edwards bioprosthesis model 2625 is used for aortic valve replacement. The effective orifice in smaller sizes of this device may be slightly smaller than that of equivalent mechanical prostheses; however, EOA in bioprostheses, unlike mechanical prostheses, is flow dependent. Incidence of thromboembolism is low, so the device may be implanted without anticoagulating the patient. Durability is better in the aortic position than in the mitral position and is related to patient age. The device is more durable in patients over age 60 (see Table 12-10).[J13]

Hancock Glutaraldehyde-Preserved Porcine Xenograft (Medtronic). The original Hancock I valve (standard model) has an appreciable gradient across it in all sizes in the aortic position. This bioprosthesis is also available with a modified orifice. In the modified version, the right coronary cusp, with its muscular bar at the base, is replaced by a muscle-free noncoronary cusp from a second valve. This modification has not reduced the device's long-term durability.[D13] The Hancock Modified Orifice bioprosthesis has been free of structural deterioration in 78% of patients over age 65 (7% cumulative incidence of SVD) and 84% of patients over 70 (3% cumulative incidence of SVD) at 19 years.[M35] It differs from the Hancock I in having a lower gradient across the valve.

Hancock II Glutaraldehyde-Preserved Porcine Xenograft (Medtronic). The Hancock II porcine xenograft is a second-generation device with a porcine aortic valve fixed at low pressure. The anticalcification agent sodium dodecyl sulfate surfactant (T6) is added to the fixative. A flexible, high-strength stent is made of acetyl homopolymer (Delrin) with reduced implant height. Flow area is maximized. The stent is covered with polyester and is less bulky so that a larger valve can be implanted. The inflow edge and sewing ring are scalloped to allow supraanular implantation of a larger valve. Hemodynamic performance, reduced thromboembolic complications, and durability are improved compared with first-generation devices.[D25,L20] Anticoagulation is not required.

Intact Glutaraldehyde-Preserved Porcine Xenograft (Medtronic). The Intact xenograft is a newer generation glutaraldehyde-treated porcine valve in which the fixation pressure is zero and toluidine blue is added to inhibit calcium deposition. Zero-pressure fixation preserves the collagen crimp of the porcine aortic valve so that it is more flexible and presumably more durable.[C33] This device has been used in large series of patients in New Zealand, Canada, and South Africa. Explantation of the valve has not been done in any patients over age 60 at 8½ years.[B49]

Biocor (St. Jude Medical). The Biocor stent-mounted aortic valve bioprosthesis was developed in Brazil. This porcine aortic valve is fixed at zero pressure, and the stent has a supraanular configuration.

Mosaic Glutaraldehyde-Preserved Porcine Xenograft (Medtronic). The Mosaic xenograft is a third-generation stent-mounted bioprothesis in which the porcine valve is subjected to physiologic aortic root fixation. Glutaraldehyde at 40 mmHg pressure is applied in the LV outflow tract below the valve and also to the aorta above the valve. The effect is to apply zero net pressure to the valve leaflets to preserve collagen crimp and flexibility while applying sufficient pressure to the aorta and sinuses of Valsalva to fix the aorta in anatomic relationships. Mechanical properties are such that they can withstand stress equivalent to normal valve leaflets.[C44] Alpha-amino oleic acid, an anticalcification agent, is chemically bound to glutaraldehyde for permanence in the tissues. Wong and colleagues reported no structural failures occurring during 3-year follow-up of 98 patients.[W15]

PERIMOUNT Glutaraldehyde-Preserved Bovine Pericardial Xenograft (Edwards Lifesciences). The PERIMOUNT pericardial xenograft is a second-generation bioprosthesis. Bovine pericardium is fixed in glutaraldehyde at low pressure and applied to a flexible stent with distensible struts by infrastent tissue mounting. The anticalcification agent polysorbate (Tween 80) is added. The prosthesis has proved to be remarkably durable, with 80% freedom from structural deterioration at 14 years in the aortic position.[B68,P12] The postapproval IDE study showed 84% freedom from structural valve deterioration.[U2] The stent and method of tissue mounting provide for a very good EOA, perhaps the best of all stent-mounted bioprostheses.[C49]

Mitroflow. The Mitroflow bioprosthesis is constructed from bovine pericardium mounted on a stent. It was introduced to clinical practice and received the CE mark of the European Community for the international market in 1997.

Stentless devices

Freestyle Glutaraldehyde-Preserved Porcine Aortic Root Bioprosthesis (Medtronic). The Freestyle porcine bioprosthesis is a third-generation device presented as the complete porcine aortic root with a thin polyester covering of the septal myocardium. It has no support stent. The tissue is fixed in glutaraldehyde using the physiologic root pressure technique described for the Mosaic valve: there is zero net pressure applied to the valve leaflets to preserve collagen crimp while the aorta is distended to normal configuration. The graft may be implanted as a valve replacement in the subcoronary position, as an inclusion root cylinder, or as a full aortic root replacement. Thus, as the name Freestyle implies, the surgeon may choose the method of implantation. Hemodynamic performance of the device is excellent because without a stent, a large EOA valve may be implanted. Short-term durability has been excellent, with 99.7% freedom from SVD at 5 years.[U1]

Alpha-amino oleic acid is added to prevent or retard calcification. Effectiveness of anticalcification treatment is not known, but evidence suggests that it is beneficial. Electron beam computed tomography showed a low amount of calcification in the aortic wall of the Freestyle bioprosthesis compared with homovital aortic allografts at 18 months.[M16] Calcium deposits have been noted in the aortic wall of the graft, but the cusps remain free of calcification up to 4 years.[F12] A Freestyle bioprosthesis removed at autopsy 68 months after implantation showed minimal calcification in the aortic tissue at the commissures and no calcium deposits in cusp tissue.

Toronto SPV Glutaraldehyde-Preserved Porcine Xenograft (St. Jude Medical). The Toronto SPV (stentless porcine valve) is a low-pressure glutaraldehyde-fixed aortic valve. The aortic tissue is removed from all three sinuses, and the graft is covered with a thin coat of polyester. It can only be implanted as a subcoronary valve replacement. With no support stent, a large valve can be implanted with greater effective orifice area compared with stented devices. Hemodynamic performance has been excellent and equivalent to the Medtronic Freestyle device. Durability has been good, with freedom from structural deterioration of 85% at 9 years.[D23]

Edwards Prima. The Prima device is a low-pressure glutaraldehyde-fixed porcine aortic root similar to the Freestyle device. Markings on the outside of the aortic root guide the trimming of the aorta for subcoronary valve implantation.

CryoLife-O'Brien. The CryoLife-O'Brien stentless porcine aortic valve is a manufactured composite of the noncoronary sinus and cusp from three porcine aortic roots. It is designed to be implanted below the coronary arteries in a supraanular position in the sinuses of Valsalva by a single suture line. Experience is limited to a few centers, and the technical aspects of implantation may be more difficult than with other stentless bioprostheses.

Cryopreserved Aortic Allograft. Human donor aortic valve allografts are presented as the complete aortic root, ascending aorta, and some or all of the aortic arch. The anterior cusp of the mitral valve usually remains attached unless it has been removed for a mitral valve graft. The tissue is harvested under sterile conditions, the internal diameter at the ventriculoaortic junction measured, quality of the valve assured, and the graft packaged. The tissue is frozen using liquid nitrogen with the temperature drop controlled at 1°C per minute between +5°C and –40°C, in a tissue culture media containing 10% dimethyl sulfoxide (DMSO) to facilitate water transfer across cell membranes during the freezing process. The tissue is placed in liquid nitrogen for storage at –180°C. (See Appendix 12A for details.) Cryopreserved aortic allografts are free of structural deterioration in 80% of patients at 15 years.[O12]

■ **TABLE 12-17**   **Primary Orifice Diameter (mm): Manufacturer's Specifications for Biologic Prostheses**

| | Label Size (mm) | | | | | | | | | |
| | 19 | | 21 | | 23 | | 25 | | 27 | |
Prosthesis	I.D.	O.D.	I.D.	O.D.	I.D.	O.D.	I.D.	O.D.	I.D.	O.D.
Carpentier-Edwards porcine	17	24	19	27	21	29	23	31	25	34
Hancock porcine	16	25	18	28	20	29	22	32	23	34
Hancock MO	16	25	18	28	20	31	22	35	–	–
Hancock II	–	–	18.5	27	20.5	30	22.5	33	24	36
Carpentier-Edwards pericardial	18	28	20	31	22	33	24	35	26	38

(Data from manufacturers' package inserts.)

Key: *I.D.*, Internal (stent) diameter; *O.D.*, outer (suture ring) diameter.

Pulmonary autograft and cryopreserved pulmonary allograft. The patient's own pulmonary trunk, including the pulmonary valve, may be used to replace the aortic valve, usually as a full aortic root replacement. The pulmonary trunk is then replaced with a cryopreserved pulmonary allograft, as described earlier in this chapter. This operation (Ross procedure) is hemodynamically superior to other procedures for replacing the aortic valve because the patient's own pulmonary valve is properly sized to accept cardiac output with little or no pressure gradient, even during the high cardiac output state of extreme exercise.[O13] In fact, the pulmonary valve is usually slightly larger than the aortic valve (see "Dimensions of Normal Cardiac and Great Artery Pathways" in Chapter 1). The pulmonary valve in the aortic position appears to function well over time.

Mechanical differences are minimal between aortic and pulmonary valve tissues, and the tensile strength of pulmonary valve cusps equals or exceeds that of aortic valve cusp tissues.[G20,V3] Goffin and colleagues studied tissues removed at autopsy 17 months after the Ross procedure.[G27] Pulmonary autograft valve cusp tissues showed essentially normal histology, with preserved fibroblasts and some endothelial cells on the surfaces. Schoof and colleagues showed in growing pigs that developing pulmonary autograft wall in the aortic position becomes normally revascularized, remains viable without major degenerative phenomena, and retains morphologic features typical for pulmonary artery rather than remodeling to thickness similar to aorta.[S22] Smooth muscle rearrangement and increased collagen were observed in response to increased pressure on the vascular matrix, strengthening the vascular wall without increasing wall thickness. A meta-analysis based on current evidence calculated average reoperation-free life expectancy of the pulmonary autograft as 16 years after implantation.[T11]

The cryopreserved pulmonary allograft is extensively devitalized, with valve cusps devoid of endothelial cells and few fibroblasts present.[G27] This phenomenon is likely immunologically mediated as measured by presence of classes I and II anti-HLA antibodies after implanting cryopreserved allograft material in patients.[H21,H22] Degree of histocompatability, however, does not appear to be related to humoral response.[B69] Implanting decellularized human valve allografts does not provoke a panel reactive antibody response nor encourage host recellularization.[E10] Stenosis of the pulmonary allograft, manifest by pressure gradients across the graft of 30 mmHg or more, occurs in 17% of patients after the Ross procedure with a mean follow-up of 48 months; only 3% of the patients, however, require reoperation.[C48] Cause of stenosis appears to be an inflam-

■ **TABLE 12-18**   **Effective Orifice Area (cm²) from In Vitro Studies on Biologic Prostheses**

| | Label Size (mm) | | | | |
Prosthesis	19	21	23	25	27
Carpentier-Edwards porcine	1.17	1.38	–	2.36	2.74
Hancock porcine	1.15	1.31	1.73	1.93	2.14
Hancock MO	1.22	1.43	1.94	2.16	–
Hancock II	–	1.48	1.81	2.10	2.36
Carpentier-Edwards pericardial	1.56	1.88	–	3.25	3.70
Medtronic Freestyle	1.84	2.17	2.69	3.41	3.75

(Data from Yoganathan and colleagues.[Y5])

matory reaction to the pulmonary allograft leading to extrinsic compression or shrinkage. The reaction may be immunologically mediated, but could also be related to other as yet unexplained mechanisms.

Specifications for bioprostheses. Manufacturer specifications for bioprostheses are more complicated than they are for mechanical cardiac valve prostheses. It is not practical to measure true internal orifice area because of the irregular shape presented by the biologic tissues mounted within the stent. Therefore the manufacturers' specifications refer to the *inner diameter* or the *outside diameter* of the mounting stent. The actual outside diameter including the sewing ring is always considerably larger than the diameter of the mounting stent, *which is used for the label size* (actually from midpoint to midpoint of the mounting stent).

Table 12-17 presents comparison data of widely used first- and second-generation stent-mounted bioprostheses. Stentless bioprostheses are labeled as the outside diameter of the device. In this respect, Medtronic Freestyle and St. Jude Medical Toronto SPV devices are equivalent. In vitro studies allow benchmarking of the EOA (cm²) of the various devices (Table 12-18). Second-generation stent-mounted bioprostheses (Hancock II, Carpentier-Edwards pericardial) have improved EOA compared with first-generation devices because of improved mounting stents. Third-generation stentless bioprostheses (Medtronic Freestyle, St. Jude Toronto SPV) are even better because the mounting stent has been eliminated, and generally a graft with a larger label size can be implanted.

Selection of Technique and Choice of Device for Isolated Aortic Valve Replacement

Mechanical prostheses. Mechanical prostheses are useful because of their durability under all circumstances and because of their good performance, even in relatively small aortic roots.[B22] Although these prostheses carry the disadvantages of thrombogenicity requiring lifelong antico- agulation with its complications of thromboembolism and bleeding, they are rarely contraindicated; exceptions in- clude premenopausal women (because of risk to fetus and mother) and those with unusual risk of hemorrhage, such as from severe peptic ulcer disease, ulcerative colitis, and hazardous occupation. Mechanical valves are particularly indicated for patients at any age who are willing to avoid undue physical hazards, who can follow a regimented medical protocol,[B71] and who prefer the low risks of chronic warfarin therapy to the lower potential risk, but greater anxiety and discomfort, of a second valve replace- ment operation.

Stent-mounted glutaraldehyde-preserved porcine xeno- graft valve. This type of valve is appropriate in patients over age 70, particularly those in sinus rhythm, because of ease of insertion and long-term durability in this age group, with no need for warfarin anticoagulation (although long- term treatment with aspirin, 80 to 375 mg · day^{-1}, is prudent).[J9] This type of valve should be used only under unusual circumstances in persons under age 45 (because of more rapid structural valve deterioration in this age group) or when a size smaller than 23 mm is needed; a larger size can be used by surgically enlarging the aortic root. Chronic renal failure, with high calcium turnover, is a contraindica- tion to the xenograft valve. If rate of degeneration proves slower in newer xenograft valves, such as those in which zero-pressure fixation is used,[J7,M29] indications for xeno- graft valves may broaden.

Stent-mounted glutaraldehyde-preserved bovine pericardial valve. Second-generation stent-mounted bo- vine pericardial bioprostheses have proved to be durable and are a good choice for patients over age 70, and possibly younger, particularly those in sinus rhythm. They are easy to insert, and anticoagulation with warfarin is not required.

Stentless glutaraldehyde-preserved porcine xenograft valve. This type of bioprosthesis is appropriate for patients over age 70 and for select younger patients because of its excellent hemodynamic performance and no requirement for anticoagulation with warfarin. Long-term outcomes are unknown, but at midterm (5 to 10 years) performance and durability are good.

Cryopreserved aortic allograft valve. Inserted free- hand inside the aorta, the allograft valve has been chosen for aortic valve replacement because of excellent hemody- namic performance, lack of thromboembolism, no need for anticoagulation with warfarin, and resistance to infection in patients requiring valve replacement for infective endocar- ditis of either native or prosthetic aortic valves. Allograft aortic valve replacement is primarily indicated in patients under age 55 and in select older patients, generally for endocarditis. The primary contraindications include an aor- tic root with a left ventricular–aortic junction or aorta at the level of the leaflet commissures that is 30 mm or more in diameter or an aortic root with dimensions that are 2 mm larger than those of the largest available allograft. Under these circumstances the aortic root may be reduced in diameter (tailored), and aortic root replacement may be used. The allograft aortic valve is less desirable than mechanical or biologic prostheses when the ascending aorta is diffusely enlarged and thin walled and when severe and poorly controlled systemic hypertension is present.

Pulmonary valve autograft. A pulmonary valve auto- graft is considered by Ross and colleagues to be "an almost ideal means of aortic valve replacement in appropriate patients."[R6] Hemodynamic performance of the pulmonary autograft in the aortic position is superior to any other replacement device. It is therefore indicated in younger patients, usually under age 50, when an active lifestyle or athletic performance requires superior hemodynamics. An- ticoagulation with warfarin is not required. The pulmonary autograft procedure may be used in select patients with endocarditis. This two-valve procedure is substantially more complex than isolated aortic valve replacement and carries more risk.

Because of the added complexity and length of the operation, patients with associated medical problems should not have a pulmonary autograft, especially those with chronic renal or pulmonary disease or with coronary artery disease that requires revascularization of more than one artery.[D37] Patients with connective tissue diseases, such as systemic lupus erythematosus and rheumatoid arthritis, particularly those taking corticosteroids, should probably not have a pulmonary autograft. Marfan syndrome is usually considered a contraindication for the operation. Active rheumatic fever or rheumatic disease with associ- ated mitral valve disease requires special caution.[C46]

Choice of Device for Replacing Aortic Valve and Ascending Aorta, En Bloc

The optimal device to replace the aortic valve and ascend- ing aorta en bloc is controversial. Use of a *composite* prosthetic valve within a polyester cylinder probably offers the lowest early mortality (4.7%; CL 2.8%-7.5%) and the least risk of late postoperative complications, but it requires lifelong anticoagulation with warfarin and carries the usual risks of prosthetic valve thromboembolism.

Kouchoukos and colleagues reported early mortality of only 0.9% in patients with anuloaortic ectasia undergoing replacement of aortic root and ascending aorta.[K15] This se- ries was folded into a large multi-institutional study, and the results were reported by Gott and colleagues.[G24] Of the 675 patients studied, 604 had composite graft replacement, indi- cating that this was the treatment of choice from 1968 to 1996. Early mortality in this group was 1.5% (CL 1.0%- 2.4%) among 455 patients having elective repair and 2.6% (CL 1.1%-5.1%) among 117 patients having operation per- formed urgently. Risk climbed to 11.7% (CL 8.3%-16%) among 103 patients having emergency operation.

Composite graft replacement is currently the procedure of choice in patients age 55 to 70 years because of demonstrated durability of the prosthetic valve. Operations that preserve the aortic valve are gaining more favor for these patients. Yacoub and colleagues had excellent results with an operation to preserve the aortic valve while replac- ing the aortic root and ascending aorta with a prosthetic graft.[Y4] None of the 68 patients died after operation, and 85% remained free of reoperation at 15 years.

Use of an *autograft* pulmonary valve cylinder could be considered the ideal replacement device when the aortic valve and aortic root or ascending aorta are replaced en bloc, because the autograft is the patient's own tissue. Even when the surgeon has specialized knowledge of the proce- dure, however, early mortality is 3.5% to 5.1% for this complex two-valve operation.[E6,R21,S30] Even with this initial risk, the operation could be the procedure of choice in patients under 55 to 60 years of age. It may be particularly advantageous in children because the transferred pulmonary valve and trunk may grow.[E7]

Use of an *allograft* valve and ascending aortic cylinder is another option. The operation is less complex than when an autograft is used, but the replacement device is less durable, with a useful life of about 15 to 20 years. Early risk of the operation is low. O'Brien reported 30-day hospital mortality of $1.13\% \pm 1\%$.[O11] Of 67 patients of Yacoub who had complete aortic root replacement with an aortic allograft, 56% were free of tissue failure and 90% free of reoperation for valve replacement at 15 years, as reported by Lind and colleagues.[L17] O'Brien reported only seven valves removed for structural deterioration over almost 15 years after full aortic root replacement in 350 patients using a cryopreserved allograft.[O11] The allograft is preferred when there is active native valve endocarditis with root abscess or infection from a previously placed prosthetic valve.[L11,P11,Z2]

SPECIAL SITUATIONS AND CONTROVERSIES

Small Aortic Root and Small Prosthesis: Prosthesis–Patient Mismatch

Controversy surrounds whether a device used for aortic valve replacement can be too small for a patient and affect immediate- and long-term outcomes. Foster and colleagues showed that prostheses as small as 17 mm in diameter can provide acceptable clinical results.[F4] Adams and colleagues, on the other hand, showed that the combination of a 19-mm prosthesis and male gender increased the risk of operative death; however, the number of patients was only 9.[A21] Data from a multi-institutional meta-analysis of 13,258 patients having aortic valve replacement showed that small valve size increased operative mortality by less than 1% in the 10% of patients receiving a small valve relative to body size, but did not reduce midterm (6 months to 5 years) and late (5 to 15 years) survival (see Appendix 12B).[B57] Similarly, Medalion and colleagues did not find that small aortic valve prostheses affected incidence of early or late mortality or cardiac events in patients, even when the prosthesis diameter was as much as four standard deviations below normal predicted for body size.[M36,M38]

Superior hemodynamics with a valve prosthesis, generally associated with a large orifice size and valve efficiency, should translate to a survival advantage. Such logic does not apply in this case, however, which may indicate that a marker other than survival should be analyzed when considering replacement of the aortic valve with a small aortic root. Izzat and colleagues argue that prosthesis–patient mismatch is not a problem of clinical significance.[I2] Pibarot and Dumesnil countered with a strong argument that when valve size and body size are used to calculate an indexed effective valve area, a strong relationship exists between small prosthetic valve size (19 or 21 mm) and pressure gradient across the valve during rest and exercise.[P20] This held for bileaflet mechanical and stent-mounted bioprosthetic valves. Del Rizzo and colleagues showed that indexed EOA less than $0.8 \ cm^2 \cdot m^{-2}$ affected the extent of

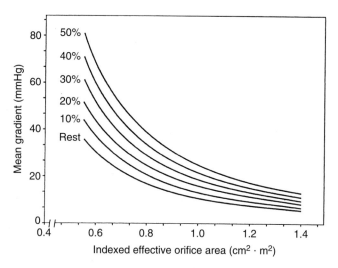

Figure 12-62 Hemodynamic performance of prosthetic heart valves during rest and exercise. Indexed effective orifice area is compared with mean pressure gradient across the prosthesis at rest and during increasing levels of exercise. Prosthetic heart valves show steep rise in pressure gradient when indexed effective orifice is less than $0.85 \ cm^2 \cdot m^{-2}$. (From Dumesnil and Yoganathan.[D29])

LV mass regression after aortic valve replacement with stentless bioprostheses.[D36] Dumesnil and Yoganathan showed that indexed EOA predicts performance of prosthetic valves during exercise (Fig. 12-62).[D29] Indexed EOA greater than $0.85 \ cm^2 \cdot m^{-2}$ will keep pressure gradient from rising during exercise on the steep part of performance curves; indexed EOA less than that is considered to represent prosthesis–patient mismatch because of the rapid rise in mean pressure gradient observed during exercise. This is especially important when choosing a mechanical prosthesis or stented bioprosthesis, because these devices tend to be on the ascending portion of performance curves more frequently than stentless bioprostheses, allografts, or autografts (Fig. 12-63).[P17]

In vitro valve performance data from Yoganathan can be compared with patient body surface area for an estimate of minimum prosthetic valve size that will perform adequately.[Y5] The surgeon can then seek optimal device performance for the patient rather than being caught up in the unresolved argument of whether or not the size of the prosthesis will affect midterm or long-term survival.

Managing the Small Aortic Root

Some adult patients have a smaller than usual LV–aortic junction or a narrow aortic aortic waist at the level of the commissural attachment of the cusps (see discussion of true congenital subvalvar or supravalvar aortic narrowing in Sections 2 and 3 of Chapter 33).

The simplest technique in patients with a small aortic anulus is placing the device partly in a supraanular position (Fig 12-64, *A*). This takes advantage of the bulging of the noncoronary sinus of Valsalva. A replacement device one size larger than the aortic anulus can be used by suturing it to the anulus along the left and right sinuses and in the supraanular position along the noncoronary sinus. In that

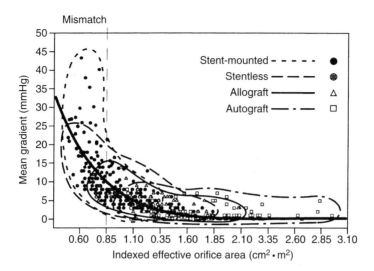

Figure 12-63   Hemodynamic performance of bioprosthetic heart valves in vivo. Indexed effective orifice area plotted against mean pressure gradient across the aortic bioprosthesis. Pulmonary autografts and aortic allografts are on the flat part of the curve. Stentless porcine aortic bioprostheses may show an increase in pressure gradient when indexed effective orifice area is less than 0.85. Stent-mounted porcine aortic xenografts often have indexed effective orifice area less than 0.85 accompanied by high pressure gradient across the device. (From Pibarot and colleagues[P17] and unpublished composite data provided by J.G. Dumesnil.)

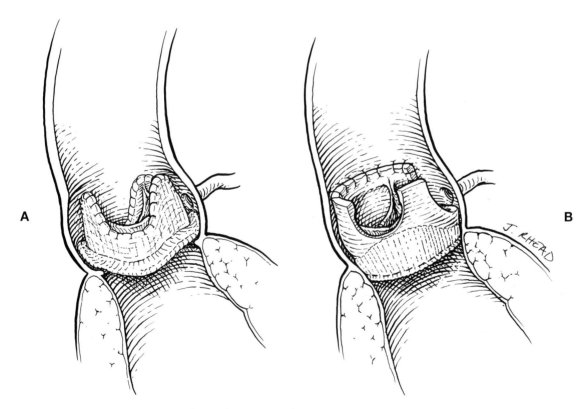

Figure 12-64   Aortic valve replacement in the small aortic root. **A,** Supraanular implant of stent-mounted xenograft. Contoured design of second-generation xenografts allows implantation of device above anulus of the aortic valve, taking advantage of space in the sinuses of Valsalva. A larger bioprosthesis may be implanted without obstructing the coronary arteries for better hemodynamic function. **B,** Intraanular subcoronary implant of stentless porcine bioprosthesis. Improved hemodynamic performance provided by absence of the support stent allows mounting of a stentless porcine xenograft even in the small aortic root.

area, pledgeted mattress sutures are placed from outside in or on the ventricular side of the aortic anulus.[D8,G14,O4]

The freehand (subcoronary) aortic allograft is the best device in the small aortic root. Appropriate-sized allografts are available in graft banks and can be inserted within the aortic root, resulting in minimal gradient.[J5,J6] Subcoronary valve replacement using a stentless porcine bioprosthesis is also effective for the small aortic root. These devices are designed to be implanted in the intraanular position in the LV outflow tract (Fig. 12-64, *B*). Absence of a supporting stent allows insertion of a valve with an effective orifice large enough to provide good hemodynamic function even in the small aortic root. Sintek and colleagues implanted 19- and 21-mm Freestyle bioprostheses and found the average LV–aortic gradient was 13 mmHg for 19-mm valves and 8 mmHg for 21-mm devices.[S31] Doty and colleagues noted similar results, concluding that this stentless bioprosthesis could be used in patients with a small aortic root.[D20]

When a mechanical prosthesis is used, a size smaller than 23 mm often results in considerable obstruction, depending on the device and the patient's body surface area. Replacement device mismatch is a serious iatrogenic disease that produces persistent or increasing LV dysfunction, hemolysis, and a very difficult reoperation.[J2,S11] Reoperation is difficult because, at the initial operation, the largest possible prosthesis has been inserted in a small passageway, which often results in erosion of anular support. Coronary ostia are usually drawn close to the sewing ring, increasing the possibility of coronary obstruction. Reoperation often requires full root reconstruction. All these increase difficulty and risk.

A 19-mm device may be obstructive, but could be used cautiously, thoughtfully, and infrequently in some circumstances in small and sedentary patients. Modern bileaflet or tilting-disc mechanical prostheses may be less obstructive than stent-mounted bioprostheses of the same label size. Second- and third-generation bioprostheses and mechanical prostheses may provide adequate hemodynamic performance in small and sedentary patients provided a 21-mm device can be implanted. Otherwise, enlargement of the aortic root by one of several methods to allow use of a larger prosthesis will provide better hemodynamics and reduce the chance of residual LV outflow tract obstruction. A stentless bioprosthesis (autograft, allograft, or xenograft) implanted in the subcoronary position or as a full-root replacement may also accomplish the desired hemodynamic performance.

When the narrowing is only at the supraanular level at the top of the sinuses of Valsalva, *supraanular enlargement* with a patch graft into the noncoronary sinus of Valsalva is used.[N1] A patch of pericardium has the advantage of ease of handling and insertion, and the suture line is easily made hemostatic (Fig. 12-65, *A* and *B*). Piehler and colleagues followed patients nearly 20 years and showed that a pericardial patch in this position does not become aneurysmal.[P9] Alternatively, a knitted or woven polyester velour or felt patch with pericardium on the inner surface may be used. Patches of either knitted or woven polyester sealed with collagen or other gel are the most hemostatic and easiest to use of the available materials.

Another method when the anulus is also involved is *supraanular and anular enlargement* by patch graft en-largement that is carried across the anulus and into the aortic–mitral anulus below it (Fig. 12-65, *C* to *E*). Nicks and colleagues described this method, with a slight modification by Blank and colleagues.[B13,N2]

Enlargement of both supraanular and anular areas can also be achieved by extending the aortotomy through the left coronary–noncoronary commissural area and into the underlying aortic–mitral anulus.[M11,M12,R7,S13] The valve is excised and need for aortic root enlargement determined. The aortotomy is extended posteroinferiorly directly through the left coronary–noncoronary commissural area (see Fig. 12-65, *A*), across the anulus, and into the base of the aortic–mitral anulus where it adheres to the left atrial wall. The incision does not reach the hinge point of the mitral cusp. The left atrium is first dissected away and may or may not be opened as the incision is made. A broad, teardrop-shaped patch, generally about 4 cm wide, is created. Beginning at the midpoint of the bottom of the incision, interrupted felt pledget–supported horizontal mattress sutures of No. 3-0 polyester are placed through the aorta and patch. Special care is used because it is difficult to see this area again after the stitches are tied and the aortic clamp removed. The valve is sewn into place using interrupted horizontal mattress sutures in the region of the patch, bringing these in from the outside to secure the valve against the patch (see Fig. 12-65, *B*). The remainder of the circumference of the prosthetic valve is attached to the anulus of the aortic valve as usual with continuous or interrupted mattress stitches. The valve is seated in the LV outflow tract in the intraanular position. The prosthetic patch is used to close all or part of the aortotomy using continuous stitches of No. 4-0 or 3-0 polypropylene.

The aortic incision is extended across the anulus of the mitral valve and into the midportion of its anterior cusp when more diameter enlargement is required. Degree of enlargement is related to depth of incision into the anterior cusp. Diameter increase of up to 4 to 5 mm may be possible with aggressive incision to the free edge of the mitral valve. The roof of the left atrium is entered as the incision crosses the mitral anulus, creating a defect in the atrium. The defect in the anterior leaflet of the mitral valve is repaired with a prosthetic patch, which is extended across the aortic–mitral anulus into the aorta. Interrupted stitches of No. 3-0 braided suture are used to attach the patch to the mitral cusp tissues. Continuous stitches are probably less desirable than simple interrupted ones in terms of strength and accuracy of repair. Interrupted mattress stitches of No. 2-0 braided suture with PTFE felt pledgets are used to approximate an appropriate size prosthetic valve to the prosthetic patch. These stitches may be started in the rim of the left atrial defect if the atrial tissues are sufficiently flexible to allow approximation to the prosthetic patch without tension. Otherwise, the atrial defect is filled in with a separate patch of autologous pericardium. The prosthetic patch is tailored to a point and used to close all or part of the aortotomy.

An alternative to all these methods is *replacing* the aortic root and first part of the ascending aorta with a porcine aortic root bioprosthesis, an *allograft* aortic valve cylinder, or an *autograft* pulmonary valve cylinder. Excision of almost all the aortic root except for buttons of sinus aorta around the coronary arteries often opens up the narrow aortic anulus. Excision of the residual commissures

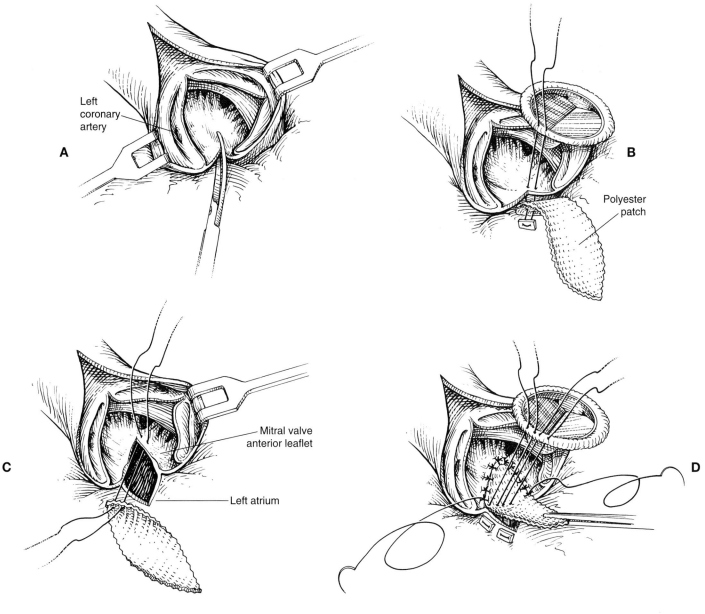

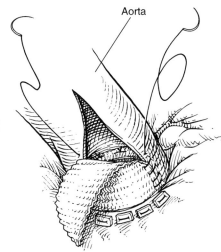

Figure 12-65 Aortic root enlargement. **A**, Incision is made through commissure between left and noncoronary sinuses. It is extended into intercusp triangle to the level of mitral valve anulus. Loose connective tissues in triangle allow edges of aorta to separate. **B**, Teardrop-shaped patch of collagen-coated polyester is placed into defect in aortic wall. Pledget-reinforced mattress sutures placed from outside of patch, through aorta and through sewing ring of a prosthesis, create tight closure of widened left ventricular (LV) outflow tract. **C**, Extending incision across mitral valve anulus into its anterior leaflet provides even greater separation of edges of the aorta and widens further the LV outflow tract. The left atrium is also entered. A collagen-coated polyester patch is inserted to close defect in mitral valve and aorta. Interrupted stitches are used to attach patch to mitral valve leaflet tissues up to level of aortic valve anulus. **D**, Pledget-reinforced horizontal mattress sutures are placed through edge of defect in left atrium (if the tissue is flexible and mobile), brought through the polyester patch, then through sewing ring of the prosthesis. A separate patch is used to close the left atrium if there is any tension on the closure. **E**, Patch is trimmed appropriately and used to fill defect in aorta.

to open into the intercusp triangles allows the more flexible tissues in the triangle to expand and enlarge the aortic root. The aortic root is then replaced with an appropriate size porcine bioprosthesis aortic allograft or the patient's own pulmonary trunk (autograft). In this technique the conduit will represent an important "size up" compared with the original diameter of the aortic anulus and aortic root.

Associated subvalvar LV outflow tract narrowing may be anatomic hypoplasia or acquired from excessive compensatory LV hypertrophy. In former practice this was an indication for aortoventriculoplasty (Konno-Rastan operation).[K2,R4,R5] Clarke described a modification of this operation using an aortic allograft with its attached anterior mitral leaflet.[C23,M30] These complex operations have largely been replaced by a modification of the pulmonary autograft procedure in which the Konno-Rastan type incision is less deep into the LV septum. The shallower incision virtually eliminates injury to the first septal branch of the left anterior descending coronary artery and resultant septal myocardial infarction and injury to the conduction system. The pulmonary autograft is implanted deeper into the LV outflow tract below the aortic anulus for complete relief of the outflow tract obstruction.

Use of an *LV apicoabdominal aortic valve conduit*[C8,N3] has nearly been abandoned. It should not be considered the primary approach to the problem of a small anulus or aortic root in patients requiring valve replacement. When the patient is facing a second or third replacement, however, and has no periprosthetic leakage, such a conduit might be considered as an alternative to aortic root enlargement.

Managing the Large Aortic Root

When the aortic root is large, it may be tailored to a size that will accommodate an allograft, pulmonary autograft, or stentless xenograft. Tailoring is accomplished by extending an incision in the noncoronary sinus across the base of the noncoronary cusp into the aortic–mitral anulus. The left atrium is dissected away as deeply as possible first, but whether this chamber is entered at the lowest point of the incision is not important. A second parallel incision is made posteriorly and tapered to remove an ellipse of aortic root with its widest point at "anulus" level. The amount of aortic wall to be removed to reduce the diameter appropriately can be calculated but can also be judged visually, remembering that further reduction in circumference occurs when the sutures are placed several millimeters from the edge and tied down. The lowest part of the defect so created is closed using interrupted figure-of-eight or simple sutures through strong tissue, including the adjacent left atrial wall if it has been opened.

This technique was used frequently in the past. Residual aortic valve regurgitation after this procedure was common. Current practice is full aortic root replacement in the presence of large, dilated aortic root pathology. It may be necessary to reduce the diameter at the ventriculoaortic junction (anulus) so that an aortic root allograft or stentless porcine xenograft may fit perfectly into the LV outflow tract. These methods are described earlier under "Repair of Aortic Valve Regurgitation Caused by Aortic Dilatation or Aneurysm."

Percutaneous Balloon Aortic Valvotomy

Percutaneous balloon aortic valvotomy (euphemistically termed "valvuloplasty") suddenly burst into the therapeutic world in 1987.[C2,M22] This procedure was enthusiastically endorsed by some interventional cardiologists as the treatment of choice for elderly patients with "critical aortic stenosis" (an emotion-laden phrase virtually never used previously by surgeons seeing this same condition). In fact, some centers developed the practice of bringing terminally ill, elderly patients with extensive coexisting disease from nursing homes or home care to undergo balloon aortic valvotomy; large numbers of patients underwent this procedure.[C2,C10,D10,I1,J4,M20]

In some patients the valve orifice is initially enlarged by the procedure, probably from fracture of calcific nodules, partial separation of fused commissures (although commissural fusion is uncommon in senile calcific aortic stenosis), and leaflet fracture.[C10,M2,S15] Increased valvar regurgitation and embolization can be complications of the procedure.

Hospital death in 125 patients (80% over age 70) was 10% (CL 7%-13%) in the experience of Lewin and colleagues.[L2] In terms of functional improvement in seriously ill patients and enhanced survival for at least 12 months, overall effectiveness of the procedure remains to be determined. Earlier experiences with surgical valvotomy and valvar debridement[H10,K11] predict that balloon aortic valvotomy for calcific aortic stenosis in elderly patients will be relatively ineffective and will be used infrequently. The few remaining indications will probably be in younger patients with fused commissures or noncalcified rheumatic valves.[B9]

Despite the associated morbidity and mortality and limited long-term results, balloon valvotomy may have a role in temporarily managing patients at high risk for aortic valve replacement.[R22] Patients with refractory pulmonary edema or circulatory shock might be sufficiently improved and in stable condition for later operation to replace the aortic valve. Patients requiring urgent noncardiac surgery may also be considered candidates for balloon valvotomy, but they are usually successfully treated by other measures.[O16,T10] In summary, balloon aortic valvotomy has an important role in treating adolescents and young adults with aortic stenosis but a limited role in older adults.[B52]

Nonreplacement Aortic Valve Operations in Adults

Nonreplacement operations for aortic stenosis are probably quite different from procedures accomplished with the balloon and have given reasonably good results in selected patients.[K16,M23] At a few centers the procedure has been augmented by using ultrasonic decalcification. However, the prevalence of immediate and delayed cusp rupture is sufficient to make the technique of doubtful value.[C28,F8] In most patients, valve replacement operations yield better and more predictable overall results.

A few groups have performed reparative operations for adults with aortic regurgitation.[C11,C27,D6,F3] Generally these procedures involve plicating the commissures or pursestring narrowing of the LV–aortic junction, as well as excising a portion of one or more cusps and suture reconstruction. Casselman and colleagues report repair of bicuspid aortic valve with aortic regurgitation in 94 patients.[C45] Repair was by triangular resection of the prolapsing cusp in 66 patients. Freedom from reoperation was 84% at 7 years. The major risk factor for reoperation was presence of residual aortic regurgitation at operation. Late aortic regurgitation did not progress over time. The indications for and results of these procedures are not well defined.

Silver-Coated Sewing Rings

Silver salts and colloidals have a long history as antimicrobials. Silver has a broad spectrum of action against bacteria. Silver toxicity can be a problem if serum level is greater than 300 parts per billion (ppb).[W12] Ion beam–assisted deposition of silver as a coating on polyethylene terephthalate (polyester) fabric appears to be safe and is probably effective as an antimicrobial agent for use in the sewing cuffs of mechanical heart valves.[T3] Healing at the sewing rings in animal studies was not impaired, but pannus formation was thinner on the silver fabric.[T5]

Silver coating (Silzone) was introduced onto the sewing rings of mechanical cardiac valves by St. Jude Medical to reduce infection on the device. More than 30,000 St. Jude Medical Silzone valves have been implanted. Some questions have been raised regarding reduced healing and increased thromboembolism. Ionescu and colleagues showed higher incidence of ischemic stroke and peripheral embolism when the Silzone sewing cuff was used ($17.1\% \cdot$ patient-year^{-1}) compared with the standard sewing cuff ($0.85\% \cdot$ patient-year^{-1}).[I6] The study groups were not randomized or even concurrent, but patient characteristics were similar.

A large randomized study comparing standard and silver-coated sewing rings (AVERT) enrolled patients to determine effectiveness of prevention of infective endocarditis. Enrollment in the study was suspended in January 2000 when audit of the data revealed 11 of 398 (2.8%) patients in the Silzone group had periprosthetic leakage, with eight (2.01%) requiring reoperation for explant. Four of 394 (1.02%) patients in the conventional sewing cuff group had periprosthetic leakage, with one requiring explant (0.25%). The company voluntarily recalled all products with silver coating. Subsequent analysis of the data confirmed that the risk of explant for periprosthetic leakage was greater in the Silzone group ($P < 0.02$).[G13] Other studies, independent of the AVERT study, however, subsequently demonstrated no differences in the prevalence of periprosthetic leakage between the silver-coated and standard St. Jude Medical prostheses.[A23,H23,H24] No differences were found in the incidence of thromboembolism or endocarditis. Continued follow-up of the patients may determine if there is any antimicrobial advantage of silver coating on the sewing ring of prosthetic cardiac valves.

Aortic Valve Replacement through Smaller Incisions

A number of reports have described a variety of incisions that are smaller than the standard median sternotomy for cardiac valve operations. Initial interest in performing cardiac valve operations through a minimal incision was stimulated by port access technology applied experimentally.[P15]

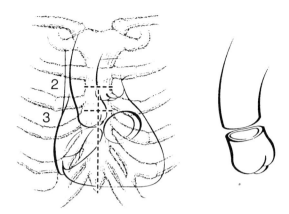

Figure 12-66   Aortic valve replacement through smaller incision, lower partial sternotomy. This incision is favored for all cardiac valve operations when an incision smaller than standard midline sternotomy is desired. The sternum is divided transversely at level of second or third intercostal space and vertically from that point through lower portion of sternum. Cardiopulmonary bypass is established using small cannulae passed through primary incision. Active venous uptake using vacuum-assisted venous return is employed (see "Vacuum-Assisted Venous Return" in Chapter 2). Aorta is transected for optimum exposure of aortic valve.

The Society of Thoracic Surgeons National Adult Cardiac Surgery Database has shown steady growth in the percentage of minimally invasive cardiac valve procedures, but they still represent a small fraction of all approaches.[S35] For isolated aortic valve replacement, 8.0% of operations were attempted by a minimally invasive approach. In the 2002 Cleveland Clinic experience, minimally invasive isolated aortic valve replacement reached 65%.

The most popular incision for aortic valve procedures has evolved to a *limited partial sternotomy*. Reardon and colleagues studied the anatomy of partial sternotomy.[R23] Usually the incision is made vertically through the upper half or two thirds of the sternum for aortic valve operations, with a number of variations for the transverse section of the sternum, including T-, J-, C-, or even Z-shaped incisions.[D26,G25,K29,S32,S33] Parasternal and transverse sternal incisions have been tried and mostly abandoned because of limited exposure, injury to the internal thoracic arteries, and lung hernia.[C37-C39] A lower-half sternotomy, however, provides a small incision that is so versatile that most, if not all, cardiac operations can be performed through this standard incision.[D27,M32]

To perform the partial lower half or lower two-thirds sternotomy, a body habitus is studied after the patient is placed in supine position for operation. The angle of Louis (second rib) and the second and third intercostal spaces are located (Fig. 12-66). Length of the sternum is evaluated and shape of the thorax observed. It is desirable to make an incision over the location of the cardiac valves large enough to accommodate the surgeon's hand should direct palpation of the heart be required. When the sternum is long and the patient's habitus slender, dividing the sternum in the third intercostal space is sufficient for most cardiac valve operations. When the patient's sternum is short or body habitus stocky or obese, a second intercostal transverse sternal incision will provide better access. Complex valve operations such as the Ross procedure are easier to perform through a second interspace incision. Third interspace incisions are shorter and cosmetically more appealing. The skin incision is made in the midline over the sternum, extending from the interspace selected to near the end of the sternum. The pectoralis major and intercostal muscles are dissected away from the sternum in the second or third intercostal space on each side of the sternum to free the internal thoracic vascular pedicle. The sternum is divided transversely at the second or third intercostal space and vertically from that point through the xiphoid process using an oscillating saw. The upper one third or half of the sternum, including the manubrium, remains intact.

CPB is established using a small (29/37 French) two-stage or three-stage (29/29 French) cannula for venous uptake, with oxygenated blood returned to a small (24 French) cannula placed in the ascending aorta. Active venous uptake is used in all patients through a vacuum-assisted venous return system (see "Vacuum-Assisted Venous Return" in Section 2 of Chapter 2). The cannulae are brought through the primary incision. The aortic occlusion clamp is brought through a stab incision on the right side below the clavicle and passed through the open right pleural space into the pericardial sac to occlude the aorta. A small (12 French) vent cannula is introduced through the right superior pulmonary vein. Cold blood cardioplegic solution is perfused into the coronary sinus through the usual cannula designed for this purpose. The aortic valve is exposed by dividing the aorta above the sinotubular junction. Retraction stitches are placed just above each of the commissures, which rotates the aortic root anteriorly and elevates it for optimum exposure.

Several reports suggest that smaller incisions lessen surgical morbidity as well as the cost of the procedure.[C37,C39,D26,G25,M8,P16] Aris and colleagues, however, found that reduced pulmonary function associated with aortic valve replacement was not prevented by a smaller incision.[A19,A22] Szwerc and colleagues compared partial upper sternotomy with median sternotomy for aortic valve replacement and found similar results.[S34] They showed that partial sternotomy offered a cosmetic benefit but did not reduce pain, length of stay, or cost. They also noted that upper sternotomy does not provide access to the heart other than at the aorta and the base. This cardiac access problem is overcome by lower partial sternotomy, which centers the incision over the heart.

Arom and colleagues have compared port access to less invasive procedures in which a small incision is made but the aorta and atria are cannulated directly.[A13] They found that port access procedures required more operating room time, longer operative and aortic clamp time, and more cost than the less invasive procedures. Their experience concurs with that of other surgeons. Therefore the trend in cardiac valve operations is toward direct cannulation of the aorta and heart when small incisions are used. Byrne and colleagues have reported use of a partial upper hemisternotomy for reoperative aortic valve replacement.[B51] They found operative bleeding was reduced as well as operating time compared with standard full sternotomy during reoperations.

In a diverse patient population, it seems that the approach at operation, age of the patient, and other comorbid factors are the major influences on outcomes, frequency of complications, and costs.

Functional Mitral Regurgitation Associated with Aortic Valve Disease

Important organic mitral regurgitation may coexist with severe aortic valve disease, and repair or replacement of both valves is the proper surgical procedure (see Chapter 13). However, mitral regurgitation of grade 1 or 2 (based on grades 1 to 4) may occur in the presence of aortic valve disease even when the mitral leaflets are normal, presumably because of anular dilatation. The mitral regurgitation is usually abolished or considerably reduced by aortic valve replacement.[A2]

When encountering this situation, the surgeon should evaluate the mitral valve by intraoperative TEE. If it seems structurally normal and regurgitation is no more than grade 2, the valve should not be repaired or replaced. In borderline cases, it is best to discontinue CPB after repair or replacement of the aortic valve and to reassess mitral valve function using TEE with the heart beating and ejecting. If mitral regurgitation continues to be important, CPB is recommended, and the mitral valve is repaired with an anuloplasty band or ring.

APPENDIXES

APPENDIX 12A
Method of Allograft Valve Preparation

Collection Technique
The aortic valve, ascending and transverse aorta, proximal portion of its branches, and pulmonary valve and pulmonary artery trunk with right and left pulmonary arteries, along with the heart, are removed through a median sternotomy from a subject who is serving as a tissue donor. The procedure is done aseptically and in an operating room.

The heart, ascending aorta transverse arch, and pulmonary arteries are removed in exactly the same manner as for cardiac transplantation. Gentle rinsing with saline solution removes blood from the cardiac chambers and aorta. The heart and 200 mL of saline solution are placed sequentially in a plastic bag, a second bag, a lid-sealed plastic container, another bag, and an ice-filled chest. The temperature is thus maintained at 4°C during transfer to the tissue-processing laboratory.

Blood is collected from the donor heart at postmortem and tested for hepatitis B antigen and human immunodeficiency virus (HIV) antibodies by appropriate tests. Valves from antigen positive donors are discarded.

Valves are acceptable from donors up to age 55 whose body has been refrigerated after death for up to 24 hours. Exceptions are death from endocarditis, septicemia, and hepatitis. Carcinoma is not a contraindication. The valve cusps must be free of important atheroma and any calcification, normally formed and tricuspid, and free of major fenestrations that might weaken the commissural cusp attachment.

Dissection

Prompt dissection of the allograft from the fresh heart in an aseptic environment with normal surgical discipline is important. The dissection is done under a laminar flow cabinet. The epicardium is raised and dissected from the aorta down to the aortic root, or, if thin, it may be retained. The coronary arteries are identified and cut about 3 mm from the ostia, and the aorta is dissected from the pulmonary trunk. Once the septal myocardium is identified, cutting in a downward direction may be done more decisively. Continuing with dissection toward the left atria will expose the mitral valve leaflet; this should be dissected from the atrial wall as closely as possible. The same procedure is followed for the right atrium and tricuspid valve leaflets.

Great care is required not to cut through the membranous septum. Another hazard is accidentally cutting the sinus of Valsalva when it is large.

The aortic valve may now be cut clear of the cardiac mass. The aorta is left long distally so that the allograft may be used as a valved extracardiac conduit, and the aortic root is trimmed proximally at a level 1 cm below the lower point of the aortic cusp attachment. Trimming away excess myocardium reduces the aortic root; the moist gloved finger is gently placed through the valve from below. The myocardium rests against the finger and can be trimmed with scissors. The thickness of the myocardium should be reduced to about 5 mm. The valve is then vigorously rinsed in modified Hanks' solution.

Valve Inspection and Sizing

A pair of dissecting forceps is passed carefully through the valve, the cut aortic wall is grasped, and the valve is turned inside out. The cusps are then carefully examined. Fenestrations are usually acceptable unless severe, but any congenital variation, unless mild, is unacceptable. Unfortunately, many variations are not seen until this stage is reached. In cases of death by trauma, damage to the cusps and myocardium should be sought. Any cusp atheroma is also unacceptable. After examination of the cusps, the allograft is uninverted.

The valve ring is rinsed again in Hanks' solution, and a moist obturator is passed into the anulus. Sizing is most easily done before trimming the aortic root, because the mitral cusp remnant can be grasped with forceps and the anulus lifted as the obturator is passed inside. The anulus must not be stretched. The aorta is sized in a similar manner. These details are recorded, together with the valve number, date and time after death of dissection, cause of donor death, and brief comment concerning any defects in the graft. A strip of tissue is cut from the aorta and divided into nine pieces. The valve is again rinsed in Hanks' solution. When the valve is moved up and down in the solution, the movement of the cusps can be observed. The valve is placed in a jar of sterile antibiotic Hanks' solution, and six pieces of aortic tissue are added. The remaining three pieces are put into another sterile jar, and about 10 mL of the final rinse is added. The two jars are immediately transferred to the microbiology department for further processing.

Antibiotic Solution

Suitable dilutions[1] of the appropriate antibiotics[S20] are prepared freshly in sterile distilled water and added aseptically to 1 L of modified Hanks' solution.[2] The prepared solution is dispensed into suitable jars for allograft storage, for example, wide-mouthed 200-mL jars fitted with lids that provide an airtight seal. This solution is stable for 1 week when stored at 4°C; the pH should be 6.8 to 7.0.

Processing

The valve is stored at 4°C and transferred to fresh antibiotic solution after 24 hours. The valve is prepared for freezing as soon as possible, under sterile conditions, by first placing it in tissue culture medium containing 10% dimethyl sulfoxide (DMSO) and transferring it to a plastic bag.[3] The bag is sealed and placed in two institutional plastic bags of increasing size. The bags are packed in a layer of cotton wool, sealed in a fourth plastic bag, and then frozen immediately.

Microbiologic Culture

The pieces of tissue not exposed to antibiotics and the samples of fluid in which each allograft was rinsed are placed in thioglycollate broth[4] and Sabouraud dextrose broth with antibiotics.[5] Broth cultures are incubated at 37°C, except for one Sabouraud dextrose broth, which is kept at 27°C for 6 weeks. Broths showing visible growth of microorganisms are subcultured at 3 days onto appropriate solid media and incubated aerobically, anaerobically, and in 7% carbon dioxide. Those samples not showing growth are subcultured at 7 days and kept for a further 5 weeks. When each allograft is transferred to fresh antibiotic solution at 24 hours, two of the pieces treated with it are placed in two thioglycollate broths. At 48 hours, when each allograft is frozen, two pieces are again placed in thioglycollate broths and one piece in Sabouraud dextrose broth without antibiotics. Thioglycollate broths are incubated at 37°C for 1 week and, if the results are negative, a further 5 weeks. The Sabouraud dextrose broth is incubated at 27°C for 6 weeks.

All microorganisms isolated are identified according to the method of Cowan and Steel[C13] and tested for sensitivity to the antibiotics used in the disinfecting solution by standard techniques.[S19]

Cold Storage

Allografts are frozen in a freezing chamber (CRFC-1-Linde).[6] Freezing is controlled at 1°C · min^{-1} to –40°C, the temperature at which the allograft is transferred to its permanent storage in liquid nitrogen. Valves are packed in polystyrene containers and suspended in the vapor phase of a liquid nitrogen refrigerator (about –180°C). Allografts may be stored indefinitely. This is the method developed and used at the Department of Cardiac Surgery, Prince Charles Hospital, Brisbane, by O'Brien and colleagues.[O5,W4] If the cultured aortic wall fragments taken immediately before freezing prove to be contaminated, the valve is discarded.

Preparation for Insertion

When needed, the frozen allograft in its container is removed from its storage position in the liquid nitrogen and placed in a container containing 2 L of saline solution at 42°C. The allograft is gently removed from its container and placed in 42°C tissue culture fluid with 10% DMSO. It is then passed through three successive gentle rinses and warming, each for 1 minute, and each with decreasing concentrations of DSMO. A final warm rinse in pure tissue culture medium is done. Trimmings from the aorta and the solution in which the valve was thawed are cultured for microorganisms.

The valve is now ready for final trimming and use as a replacement for the aortic valve or aortic root. The valve or a similarly prepared pulmonary valve and artery can also serve as a replacement for a pulmonary pathway if a pulmonary autograft was used or as a valved extracardiac conduit (see "Technique of Operation" in Section 1 of Chapter 24).

---

[1] Antibiotic solution (CLPVA) ($\mu g \cdot L^{-1}$ Hanks' balanced salt solution): cefoxitin, 240; lincomycin, 120; polymyxin B, 100; vancomycin hydrochloride, 50; amphotericin B, 25.

[2] Hanks' balanced salt solution: sodium chloride (NaCl), 8.0 g; potassium chloride (KCl), 0.4 g; magnesium sulfate ($MgSO_4 \cdot 7H_2O$), 0.1 g; magnesium chloride ($MgCl_2$ $6H_2O$), 0.1 g; Na_2HPO_4 $12H_2O$, 0.12 g; KH_2PO_4, 0.06 g; dextrose, 1.0 g; sodium bicarbonate ($NaHCO_3$), 0.35 g; water for injection, 1.0 L.

[3] Cryovac B620 barrier bags: Grand Island Biological Company (GIBCO), Grand Island, NY.

[4] Thioglycollate broth (as for cerebrospinal and blood culture): Baltimore Biological Laboratories (BBL). Thioglycollate without indicator, 30 g; distilled water, 1 L; normal saline solution, 5 mL; liquid Roche, 0.5 g. This is dispensed in 20-mL volumes into 25-mL McCarney bottles.

[5] Sabouraud dextrose broth: GIBCO animal tissue polypeptone, 10 g; dextrose, 40 g; distilled water, 1 L. Sabouraud dextrose broth with antibiotics is prepared in the same way but with the following antibiotics added: chloramphenicol, 100 mg · L^{-1} gentamicin, 40 mg · L^{-1}.

[6] Made by a Division of Union Carbide, Danbury, CT 06817.

■ TABLE 12B-1   Sources of Individual Patient Data for Multi-Institutional Study of Aortic Valve Replacement

Source	Location	Inclusive Dates [a]	n
Cleveland Clinic Foundation	Cleveland, Ohio, United States	5/1975 to 6/1999	4768
University of British Columbia	Vancouver, British Columbia, Canada	3/1976 to 7/1996	2046
Northern New England Cardiovascular Disease Study Group	Lebanon, New Hampshire, United States [b]	9/1989 to 1/1997	1928
Northwest Surgical Associates	Portland, Oregon, United States [c]	3/1976 to 12/1998	1164
Stanford University	Stanford, California, United States	8/1971 to 3/1990	1153
University Hospital	Cardiff, Wales, United Kindom	2/1980 to 4/1994	729
Instituto Chirurgia Cardiovascolore, University of Padova	Padova, Italy	3/1970 to 12/1997	692
Harefield Hospital	London, United Kingdom	9/1969 to 1/1993	518
Edwards Lifesciences Corporation	Irvine, California, United States	9/1981 to 1/1984	260
TOTAL			13,258

(Data from Blackstone and colleagues.[B57])

[a] Rounded to nearest month.

[b] A multi-institutional collaboration.

[c] A multi-institutional collaboration of Health Data Research, Inc., Portland, Oregon, United States.

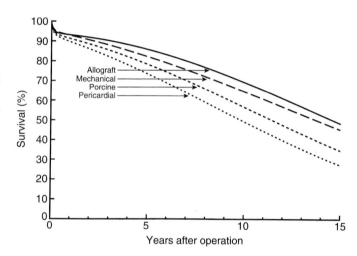

Figure 12B-1   Non–risk-adjusted survival after aortic valve replacement according to variety of prosthesis inserted: allograft, mechanical, stent-mounted bovine pericardial (pericardial), or stent-mounted porcine xenograft (porcine). (From Blackstone and colleagues.[B57])

Key: *Pericardial,* Stent-mounted bovine pericardial prosthesis; *porcine,* stent-mounted porcine xenograft.

APPENDIX 12B

Multi-Institutional Study of Survival after Aortic Valve Replacement

Patients

Individual patient data were assembled on 13,258 aortic valve replacements from nine sources (Table 12B-1). *Included* were adults ≥18 years for whom prosthesis type, model, and label size were recorded. *Excluded* were patients (1) having a preexisting valve prosthesis in a location other than aortic, (2) undergoing a multiple valve operation, (3) having native or prosthetic valve endocarditis, (4) undergoing emergent aortic valve replacement, or (5) having concomitant procedures other than coronary artery bypass grafting (CABG). Patients undergoing aortic root enlargement were not excluded. Half the operations were performed before 1990.

Deidentified data were assembled from existing registries and clinical research databases. This combination of individual patient data from multiple sources has been termed a *meta-analysis of individual patient data* (IPD).[B64]

Prostheses

Prostheses were of four varieties: stented porcine xenografts (n = 5757, designated *porcine),* stented bovine pericardial xenografts

(n = 3198, designated *pericardial),* mechanical devices (n = 3583, of which 2125 were bileaflet and 1458 monoleaflet), and allografts (n = 720).

Survival

Study end point was all-cause mortality, including hospital mortality.[L24] 69,780 patient-years of follow-up were available for analysis (mean 5.3 ± 4.7 years); 2427 patients (18%) were followed 10 or more years and 498 (4%) more than 15 years (up to 27 years).

Survival overall was 95.8% at 30 days, and 91%, 79%, 58%, and 37% at 1, 5, 10, and 15 years (see Fig. 12-18, *A).* Instantaneous risk of death peaked immediately after operation, fell rapidly during the first 6 postoperative months, and then rose steadily (see Fig. 12-18, *B).* These represent three additive hazard phases, labeled early, constant, and late. To determine the independent influence of prosthesis–patient size on long-, intermediate-, and short-term survival, a multiphase hazard decomposition method was employed (see "Parametric Survival Estimation" under Time-Related Events in Section 4 of Chapter 6). Each hazard phase incorporates an independent set of risk factors, permitting quantification of the effects of various risk factors within each time frame determined by the data themselves, not arbitrarily, without assuming proportional hazards.[B63]

■ **TABLE 12B–2   Variables Associated with Use of 19-mm or Smaller Prosthesis for Aortic Valve Replacement**

Variable	Logistic Coefficient ± SD	P
Demography		
Older age [a]	1.00 ± 0.34	.003
Younger age [b]	–1.15 ± 0.48	.02
Smaller BSA in women [c]	4.7 ± 0.60	< .0001
Smaller BSA in men [c]	9.6 ± 1.37	< .0001
Clinical Status		
NYHA functional class I or II	0.39 ± 0.079	< .0001
Pathophysiology		
Pure aortic stenosis	0.93 ± 0.124	< .0001
Mixed lesion	0.78 ± 0.142	< .0001
Procedures		
Previous AVR	0.74 ± 0.114	< .0001
Concomitant CABG	0.52 ± 0.076	< .0001
Experience		
More recent date of operation [d]	1.07 ± 0.136	< .0001
Intercept for women	–6.4	
Intercept for men	–11.7	

(Data from Blackstone and colleagues.[B57])

Key: *AVR*, Aortic valve replacement; *BSA*, body surface area; *CABG*, coronary artery bypass grafting; *NYHA*, New York Heart Association; *SD*, standard deviation.

[a] $(age/50)^3$ cubic transformation.

[b] $exp(age/50)$ exponential transformation.

[c] $1/[BSA (m^2)]$ inverse transformation.

[d] Ln(years since 1/1/1969) natural logarithmic transformation.

Systematic survival decrements were identified according to *variety of prosthesis* (Fig. 12B-1). However, these differences were largely accounted for by differing patient characteristics, in particular age (see Fig. 12-19). This is because selection of device has favored allografts (age 51 ± 14.0 years) and mechanical (age 60 ± 12.1 years) devices in younger patients and porcine (age 65 ± 12.9 years) and pericardial (age 72 ± 8.9 years) bioprostheses in the elderly.

Selection factors are also apparent in label size of prosthesis. Compared with other patients, the 1109 who received a prosthesis size 19 mm or less were older, smaller, and more likely to have aortic stenosis, previous aortic valve replacement, and concomitant CABG (Table 12B-2).

Incremental Risk Factors for Death
Statistical significance and direction of the association of factors associated with time-related survival after aortic valve replacement are shown in Table 12B-3. Associations include the strong effect of patient factors such as advanced age, advanced symptoms, aortic regurgitation, previous aortic valve replacement, and ischemic heart disease. Mortality in the early hazard phase decreased throughout the experience. Small and generally statistically nonsignificant differences in mortality were observed among models of aortic prosthesis, with the exception of higher early risk in patients receiving allografts, and across data sources.

■ **TABLE 12B–3   Incremental Risk Factors for Death after Aortic Valve Replacement (direction of association with mortality [+, increased; –, decreased] indicated in parentheses)**

Factor	Hazard Phase Early	Hazard Phase Constant	Hazard Phase Late
Demography			
Women	.03 (+)	< .0001 (–)	.5 (+)
Older age	< .0001	< .0001	< .0001
Smaller size (BSA)	.001	.01	.03
Larger size (BSA)	–	–	.01
Clinical Status			
Previous aortic valve replacement	< .0001 (+)	.0003 (+)	.4 (+)
NYHA functional class II [a]	.7 (–)	.4 (+)	.5 (+)
NYHA functional class III [a]	.04 (+)	.002 (+)	.2 (+)
NYHA functional class IV [a]	< .0001 (+)	.001 (+)	.17 (+)
Pathophysiology [b]			
Pure aortic stenosis	.5 (–)	.7 (+)	.2 (–)
Pure aortic regurgitation	.4 (+)	.001 (+)	.96 (–)
Procedures			
Previous aortic valve replacement	< .0001 (+)	.0003 (+)	.4 (+)
Concomitant CABG	< .0001 (+)	.3 (–)	< .0001 (+)
Experience			
Date of operation (earlier)	< .0001	< .0001	–[c]
Data Source [d]			
A	.11 (+)	.11 (+)	.03 (–)
B	.2 (+)	.11 (–)	.08 (–)
C	.2 (+)	.97 (–)	.17 (–)
D	.11 (–)	.2 (–)	–[e]
E	.6 (+)	.7 (+)	.6 (–)
F	.7 (–)	.11 (–)	.6 (–)
G	.9 (–)	.9 (–)	.8 (–)
H	.12 (–)	.02 (–)	.16 (+)
Prosthesis [f]			
Stented xenograft			
Hancock Model 242	.2 (+)	.5 (–)	.14 (+)
Hancock Model 250	.8 (+)	.97 (–)	.7 (+)
Carpentier-Edwards Model 2625	.4 (–)	.9 (–)	.4 (–)
Carpentier-Edwards SAV Model 2650	.18 (+)	.9 (+)	.11 (–)
Mechanical			
St. Jude Medical Model A-101	.9 (–)	.2 (–)	.8 (–)
St. Jude Medical Model AHP-105	.7 (–)	.4 (+)	–[g]
Medtronic-Hall Model A7700	.4 (+)	.18 (–)	.4 (ı)
Sorin	.8 (+)	.6 (–)	.9 (+)
Allograft			
Cryopreserved	.04 (+)	.5 (–)	.13 (+)

(Data from Blackstone and colleagues.[B57])

Key: *BSA*, Body surface area; *CABG*, coronary artery bypass grafting; *NYHA*, New York Heart Association.

[a] Versus NYHA functional class I.

[b] Versus mixed aortic stenosis and aortic regurgitation.

[c] Confounded with length of follow-up.

[d] Versus Center I.

[e] Confounded with prosthesis model.

[f] Versus Carpentier-Edwards PERIMOUNT RSR Model 2700.

[g] Insufficient follow-up of this prosthesis for late-phase estimation.

REFERENCES

A

1. Angell WW, Oury JH, Lamberti JJ, Koziol J. Durability of the viable aortic allograft. J Thorac Cardiovasc Surg 1989;98:48.

2. Austen WG, Kastor JA, Sanders CA. Resolution of functional mitral regurgitation following surgical correction of aortic valvular disease. J Thorac Cardiovasc Surg 1967;53:255.

3. Armiger LC, Gavin JB, Barratt-Boyes BG. Histological assessment of orthotopic aortic valve leaflet allografts: its role in selecting graft pretreatment. Pathology 1983;15:67.

4. Arom KV, Nicoloff DM, Kersten TE, Northrup WF 3rd, Lindsay WG, Emery RW. Ten years' experience with the St. Jude Medical valve prosthesis. Ann Thorac Surg 1989;47:831.

5. Allen WM, Matloff JM, Fishbein MC. Myxoid degeneration of the aortic valve and isolated severe aortic regurgitation. Am J Cardiol 1985;55:439.

6. Anderson ET, Hancock EW. Long-term follow-up of aortic valve replacement with the fresh aortic homograft. J Thorac Cardiovasc Surg 1976;72:150.

7. Angell JD, Hawtrey CO, Angell WM. A fresh viable homograft valve bank: sterilization, sterility testing and cryogenic preservation. Transplant Proc 1976;8:139.

8. Angell WW, Angell JD, Oury JH, Lamberti JJ, Grehl TM. Long-term follow-up of viable frozen aortic homografts. A viable homograft valve bank. J Thorac Cardiovasc Surg 1987;93:815.

9. Angell WW, Pillsbury RC, Shumway NE. Storage and function of the canine aortic valve homograft. Arch Surg 1969;99:92.

10. Azariades M, Fessler CL, Ahmad A, Starr A. Aortic valve replacement in patients over 80 years of age: a comparative standard for balloon valvuloplasty. Eur J Cardiothorac Surg 1991;5:373.

11. Aris A, Ramirez I, Camara ML, Carreras F, Borras X, Pons-Llado G. The 20 mm Medtronic-Hall prosthesis in the small aortic root. J Heart Valve Dis 1996;5:459.

12. Aupart M, Neville P, Dreyfus X, Meurisse Y, Sirinelli A, Marchand M. The Carpentier-Edwards pericardial aortic valve: intermediate results in 420 patients. Eur J Cardiothorac Surg 1994;8:277.

13. Arom KV, Emery RW, Kshettry VR, Janey PA. Comparison between port-access and less invasive valve surgery. Ann Thorac Surg 1999; 68:1525.

14. Akins CW. Long-term results with the Medtronic-Hall valvular prosthesis. Ann Thorac Surg 1996;61:806.

15. Aklog L, Carr-White GS, Birks EJ, Yacoub M. Pulmonary autograft versus aortic homograft for aortic valve replacement: interim results from a prospective randomized trial. J Heart Valve Dis 2000;9:176.

16. Anderson DR, Harrison L, Hirsh J. Evaluation of a portable prothrombin time monitor for home use by patients requiring long-term oral anticoagulant therapy. Arch Intern Med 1993;153:1441.

17. Ansell JE. Empowering patients to monitor and manage oral anticoagulation therapy. JAMA 1999;281:182.

18. Alexander KP, Anstrom KJ, Muhlbaier LH, Grosswald RD, Smith PK, Jones RH, et al. Outcomes of cardiac surgery in patients age 80 years: results from the National Cardiovascular Network. J Am Coll Cardiol 2000;35:731.

19. Aris A, Camara ML, Casan P, Litvan H. Pulmonary function following aortic valve replacement: a comparison between ministernotomy and median sternotomy. J Heart Valve Dis 1999;8:605.

20. Antunes MJ. Clinical performance of St. Jude and Medtronic-Hall prostheses: a randomized comparative study. Ann Thorac Surg 1990; 50:743.

21. Adams DH, Chen RH, Kadner A, Aranki SF, Allred EN, Cohn LH. Impact of small prosthetic valve size on operative mortality in elderly patients after aortic valve replacement for aortic stenosis: does gender matter? J Thorac Cardiovasc Surg 1999;118:815.

22. Aris A, Camara ML, Montiel J, Delgado LJ, Galan J, Litvan H. Ministernotomy versus median sternotomy for aortic valve replacement: a prospective randomized study. Ann Thorac Surg 1999; 67:1583.

23. Auer J, Berent R, Ng CK, Punzengruber C, Mayer H, Lassnig E, et al. Early investigation of silver-coated Silzone™ heart valves prosthesis in 126 patients. J Heart Valve Dis 2001;10:717.

B

1. Bailey CP, Likoff W. The surgical treatment of aortic insufficiency. Ann Intern Med 1955;42:388.

2. Bailey CP, Glover RP, O'Neill TJ, Redondo-Ramirez HP. Experience with the experimental surgical relief of aortic stenosis: a preliminary report. J Thorac Surg 1950;20:516.

3. Bailey CP, Redondo-Ramirez HP, Larzelere HB. Surgical treatment of aortic stenosis. JAMA 1952;150:1647.

4. Barnhorst DA, Oxman HA, Connolly DC, Pluth JR, Danielson GK, Wallace RB, et al. Long-term follow-up of isolated replacement of the aortic or mitral valve with the Starr-Edwards prosthesis. Am J Cardiol 1975;35:228.

5. Barnhorst DA, Oxman HA, Connolly DC, Pluth JR, Danielson GK, Wallace RB, et al. Isolated replacement of the aortic valve with the Starr-Edwards prosthesis: a 9 year review. J Thorac Cardiovasc Surg 1975;70:113.

6. Barratt-Boyes BG. Long-term follow-up of aortic valvar grafts. Br Heart J 1971;33:60.

7. Basta LL, Raines D, Najjar S, Kioschos JM. Clinical, haemodynamic, and coronary angiographic correlates of angina pectoris in patients with severe aortic valve disease. Br Heart J 1975;37:150.

8. Bloomfield P, Kitchin AH, Wheatley DJ, Walbaum PR, Lutz W, Miller HC. A prospective evaluation of the Bjork-Shiley, Hancock, and Carpentier-Edwards heart valve prostheses. Circulation 1986;73:1213.

9. Bulle TM, Dean LS. Double-valve percutaneous balloon dilatation. J Thorac Cardiovasc Surg 1989;98:633.

10. Baxter RH, Reid JM, McGuiness JB, Stevenson JG. Relation of angina to coronary artery disease in mitral and in aortic valve disease. Br Heart J 1978;40:918.

11. Bjork VO, Henze A, Jereb M. Aortographic follow-up in patients with the Bjork-Shiley aortic disc valve prosthesis. Scand J Thorac Cardiovasc Surg 1973;7:1.

12. Butany J, Yu W, Silver MD, David TE. Morphologic findings in explanted Hancock II porcine bioprostheses. J Heart Valve Dis 1999;8:4.

13. Blank RH, Pupello DF, Bessone LN, Harrison EE, Sbar S. Method of managing the small aortic anulus during valve replacement. Ann Thorac Surg 1976;22:356.

14. Bolen JL, Holloway EL, Zener JC, Harrison DC, Alderman EL. Evaluation of left ventricular function in patients with aortic regurgitation using afterload stress. Circulation 1976;53:132.

15. Bonow RO, Borer JS, Rosing DR, Henry WL, Pearlman AS, McIntosh CL, et al. Preoperative exercise capacity in symptomatic patients with aortic regurgitation as a predictor of postoperative left ventricular function and long-term prognosis. Circulation 1980; 62:1280.

16. Borer JS, Rosing DR, Kent KM, Bacharach SL, Green MV, McIntosh CJ, et al. Left ventricular function at rest and during exercise after aortic valve replacement in patients with aortic regurgitation. Am J Cardiol 1979;44:1297.

17. Bulkley BH, Roberts WC. Ankylosing spondylitis and aortic regurgitation: description of the characteristic cardiovascular lesion from study of eight necropsy patients. Circulation 1973;48:1014.

18. Binet JP, Duran CG, Carpenter A, Langlois J. Heterologous aortic valve transplantation. Lancet 1965;2:1275.

19. Broom ND. Fatigue induced damage in glutaraldehyde-preserved heart valve tissue. J Thorac Cardiovasc Surg 1978;76:202.

20. Bessone LN, Pupello DF, Hiro SP, Lopez-Cuenca E, Glatterer MS Jr, Ebra G. Surgical management of aortic valve disease in the elderly: a longitudinal analysis. Ann Thorac Surg 1988;46:264.

21. Bentall H, De Bono A. A technique for complete replacement of the ascending aorta. Thorax 1968;23:338.

22. Bjork VO, Henze A, Holmgren A, Szamosi A. Evaluation of the 21 mm Bjork-Shiley tilting disc valve in patients with narrow aortic roots. Scand J Thorac Cardiovasc Surg 1973;7:203.

23. Borow K, Green LH, Mann T, Sloss LJ, Collins JJ Jr, Cohn L, et al. End systolic volume as a predictor of postoperative left ventricular function in volume overload from valvular regurgitation (abstract). Circulation 1977;55/56:III40.

24. Barratt-Boyes BG, Roche AH, Whitlock RM. Six-year review of the results of freehand aortic valve replacement using an antibiotic sterilized homograft valve. Circulation 1977;55:353.

25. Bahnson HT, Spencer FC, Busse EF, Davis FW Jr. Cusp replacement and coronary artery perfusion in open operations on the aortic valve. Ann Surg 1960;152:494.

26. Barratt-Boyes BG. A method for preparing and inserting a homograft aortic valve. Br J Surg 1965;52:847.

27. Barratt-Boyes BG. Homograft aortic valve replacement in aortic incompetence and stenosis. Thorax 1964;19:131.

28. Broom ND, Thomson FJ. Influence of fixation conditions on the performance of glutaraldehyde-treated porcine aortic valves: towards a more scientific basis. Thorax 1979;34:166.

29. Barratt-Boyes BG, Lowe JB, Cole DS, Kelly DT. Homograft valve replacement for aortic valve disease. Thorax 1965;20:495.

30. Barratt-Boyes BG. Cardiothoracic surgery in the Antipodes. J Thorac Cardiovasc Surg 1979;78:804.

31. Barratt-Boyes BG, Roche AH, Brandt PW, Smith JC, Lowe JB. Aortic homograft valve replacement: a long-term follow-up of an initial series of 101 patients. Circulation 1969;40:763.

32. Barratt-Boyes BG, Roche AH. A review of aortic valve homografts over a six and one-half year period. Ann Surg 1969;170:483.

33. Bonow RO, Dodd JT, Maron BJ, O'Gara PT, White GG, McIntosh CL, et al. Long-term serial changes in left ventricular function and reversal of ventricular dilatation after valve replacement for chronic aortic regurgitation. Circulation 1988;78:1108.

34. Bailey WW. A modified freehand technique for homograft aortic valve replacement. J Cardiac Surg 1987;2:193.

35. Borkon AM, McIntosh CL, Jones M, Lipson LC, Kent KM, Morrow AG. Hemodynamic function of the Hancock standard orifice aortic valve bioprosthesis. J Thorac Cardiovasc Surg 1981;82:601.

36. Bellitti R, Caruso A, Festa M, Mazzei V, Icsu S, Falco A, et al. Prolapse of the "floppy" aortic valve as a cause of aortic regurgitation: a clinico-morphologic study. Int J Cardiol 1985;9:399.

37. Bonow RO, Rosing DR, McIntosh CL, Jones M, Maron BJ, Lan KK, et al. The natural history of asymptomatic patients with aortic regurgitation and normal left ventricular function. Circulation 1983;68:509.

38. Bonow RO, Rosing DR, Maron BJ, McIntosh CL, Jones M, Bacharach SL, et al. Reversal of left ventricular dysfunction after aortic valve replacement for chronic aortic regurgitation: influence of duration of preoperative left ventricular dysfunction. Circulation 1984;70:570.

39. Borkon AM, Soule LM, Baughman KL, Aoun H, Baumgartner WA, Gardner TJ, et al. Comparative analysis of mechanical and bioprosthetic valves after aortic valve replacement. J Thorac Cardiovasc Surg 1987;94:20.

40. Bonow RO, Picone AL, McIntosh CL, Jones M, Rosing DR, Maron BJ, et al. Survival and functional results after valve replacement for aortic regurgitation from 1976 to 1983: impact of preoperative left ventricular function. Circulation 1985;72:1244.

41. Barratt-Boyes BG, Roche AH, Subramanyan R, Pemberton JR, Whitlock RM. Long-term follow-up of patients with the antibiotic-sterilized aortic homograft valve inserted freehand in the aortic position. Circulation 1987;75:768.

42. Blackstone EH, Kirklin JW. Death and other time-related events after valve replacement. Circulation 1985;72:753.

43. Butchart EG, Lewis PA, Grunkemeier GL, Kulatilake N, Breckenridge IM. Low risk of thrombosis and serious emboli events despite low-intensity anticoagulation: experience with 1,004 Medtronic-Hall valves. Circulation 1988;78:166.

44. Borer JS, Herrold EM, Hochreiter C, Romain M, Supino P, Devereux RB, et al. Natural history of left ventricular performance at rest and during exercise after aortic valve replacement for aortic regurgitation. Circulation 1991;84:III133.

45. Blome-Eberwein SA, Mrowinski D, Hofmeister J, Hetzer R. Impact of mechanical heart valve prosthesis sound on patients' quality of life. Ann Thorac Surg 1996;61:594.

46. Bonow RO, Carabello B, de Leon AC Jr, Edmunds LH Jr, Fedderly BJ, Freed MD, et al. ACC/AHA Guidelines for the Management of Patients with Valvular Heart Disease: Executive Summary; a report of the American College of Cardiology/American Heart Association Task Force on Practice Guidelines (Committee on Management of Patients with Valvular Heart Disease). Circulation 1998;98:1949.

47. Brener SJ, Duffy CI, Thomas JD, Stewart WJ. Progression of aortic stenosis in 394 patients: relation to changes in myocardial and mitral valve dysfunction. J Am Coll Cardiol 1995;25:305.

48. Basarir S, Islamoglu F, Ozkisacik E, Atay Y, Boga M, Bakalim T, et al. Comparative analysis of left ventricular hemodynamics and hypertrophy after aortic valve replacement with homografts or mechanical valves. J Heart Valve Dis 2000;9:45.

49. Barratt-Boyes BG, Jaffee WM, Ko PH, Whitlock RM. The zero pressure fixed Medtronic Intact porcine valve: an 8.5 year review. J Heart Valve Dis 1993;2:604.

50. Baumgartner H, Khan S, DeRobertis M, Czer L, Maurer G. Effect of prosthetic aortic valve design on the Doppler-catheter gradient correlation: an in vitro study of normal St. Jude, Medtronic-Hall, Starr-Edwards, and Hancock valves. J Am Coll Cardiol 1992;19:324.

51. Byrne JG, Aranki SF, Couper GS, Adams DH, Allred EN, Cohn LH. Reoperative aortic valve replacement: partial upper hemisternotomy versus conventional sternotomy. J Thorac Cardiovasc Surg 1999;118:991.

52. Bonow RO, Carabello B, de Leon AC Jr, Edmunds LH Jr, Fedderly BJ, Freed MD, et al. ACC/AHA Guidelines for the Management of Patients with Valvular Heart Disease: a report of the American College of Cardiology/American Heart Association Task Force on Practice Guidelines (Committee on Management of Patients with Valvular Heart Disease). J Am Coll Cardiol 1998;32:1486.

53. Brogan WC 3rd, Grayburn PA, Lange RA, Hillis LD. Prognosis after valve replacement in patients with severe aortic stenosis and a low transvalvular pressure gradient. J Am Coll Cardiol 1993;21:1657.

54. Bonow RO. Asymptomatic aortic regurgitation: indications for operation. J Card Surg 1994;9:170.

55. Bonow RO, Lakatos E, Maron BJ, Epstein SE. Serial long-term assessment of the natural history of asymptomatic patients with chronic aortic regurgitation and normal left ventricular systolic function. Circulation 1991;84:1625.

56. Bloomfield P, Wheatley DJ, Prescott RJ, Miller HC. Twelve-year comparison of a Bjork-Shiley mechanical heart valve with porcine bioprostheses. N Engl J Med 1991;324:573.

57. Blackstone EH, Cosgrove DM 3rd, Jamieson WR, Birkmeyer NJ, Lemmer JH Jr, Miller DC, et al. Prosthesis size and long-term survival after aortic valve replacement. J Thorac Cardiovasc Surg 2003 (in press).

58. Butchart EG. Prosthetic heart valves. In Verstraete M, Fuster V, Topol EF, eds. Cardiovascular thrombosis: thrombocardiology and thromboneurology, 2nd Ed. Philadelphia: Lippincott-Raven, 1998, p. 395.

59. Bussey HI, Chiquette E, Bianco TM, Lowder-Bender K, Kraynak MA, Linn WD. A statistical and clinical evaluation of fingerstick and routine laboratory prothrombin time measurements. Pharmacotherapy 1997;17:861.

60. Byeth RJ, Landefeld CS. Prevention of major bleeding in older patients treated with warfarin: results of a randomized trial (abstract). J Gen Intern Med 1997;12:66.

61. Bonchek LI, Burlingame MW, Vazales BE. Accuracy of sizers for aortic valve prostheses. J Thorac Cardiovasc Surg 1987;94:632.

62. Bartels C, Leyh RG, Matthias, Bechtel JF, Joubert-Hubner E, Sievers HH. Discrepancies between sizer and valve dimensions: implications for small aortic root. Ann Thorac Surg 1998;65:1631.

63. Blackstone EH, Naftel DC, Turner ME Jr. The decomposition of time-varying hazard into phases, each incorporating a separate stream of concomitant information. J Am Stat Assoc 1986;81:615.

64. Berry DA, Stangl DK. Meta-analysis in medicine and health policy. New York: Marcel Dekker; 2000.

65. Bloomstein LZ, Gielchinsky I, Bernstein AD, Parsonnet V, Saunders C, Karanam R, et al. Aortic valve replacement in geriatric patients: determinants of in-hospital mortality. Ann Thorac Surg 2001;71:597.

66. Birks EJ, Webb C, Child A, Radley-Smith R, Yacoub MH. Early and long-term results of a valve-sparing operation for Marfan Syndrome. Circulation 1999;100:II29.

67. Byrne JG, Karavas AN, Aklog L, Adams DH, Cheung AC, Cohn LH, et al. Aortic valve reoperation after homograft or autograft replacement. J Heart Valve Dis 2001;10:451.

68. Banbury MK, Cosgrove DM 3rd, White JA, Blackstone EH, Frater RW, Okies JE. Age and valve size effect on the long-term durability of the Carpentier-Edwards aortic pericardial bioprosthesis. Ann Thorac Surg 2001;72:753.

69. Bechtel JF, Bartels C, Schmidtke C, Skibba W, Muller-Steinhardt M, Kluter H, et al. Does histocompatibility affect homograft valve function after the Ross procedure? Circulation 2001;104:I25.

70. Birkmeyer NJ, Birkmeyer JD, Tosteson AN, Grunkemeier GL, Marrin CA, O'Connor GT. Prosthetic valve type for patients undergoing aortic valve replacement: a decision analysis. Ann Thorac Surg 2000; 70:1946.

71. Butchart EG, Payne N, Li HH, Buchan K, Mandana K, Grunkemeier GL. Better anticoagulation control improves survival after valve replacement. J Thorac Cardiovasc Surg 2002;123:715.

C

1. Carabello BA, Green LH, Grossman W, Cohn LH, Koster JK, Collins JJ Jr. Hemodynamic determinants of prognosis of aortic valve replacement in critical aortic stenosis and advanced congestive heart failure. Circulation 1980;62:42.

2. Cribier A, Savin T, Berland J, Rocha P, Mechmeche R, Saoudi N, et al. Percutaneous transluminal balloon valvuloplasty of adult aortic stenosis: report of 92 cases. J Am Coll Cardiol 1987;9:381.

3. Carpentier A, Lemaigre G, Robert L, Carpentier S, Dubost C. Biological factors affecting long-term results of valvular heterografts. J Thorac Cardiovasc Surg 1969;58:467.

4. Cheung D, Flemma RJ, Mullen DC, Lepley D Jr, Anderson AJ, Weirauch E. Ten-year follow-up in aortic valve replacement using the Bjork-Shiley prosthesis. Ann Thorac Surg 1981;32:138.

5. Clark DG, McAnulty JH, Rahimtoola SH. Valve replacement in aortic insufficiency with left ventricular dysfunction. Circulation 1980; 61:411.

6. Currie PJ, Seward JB, Reeder GS, Vlietstra RE, Bresnahan DR, Bresnahan JF, et al. Continuous-wave Doppler echocardiographic assessment of severity of calcific aortic stenosis: a simultaneous Doppler-catheter correlative study in 100 adult patients. Circulation 1985;71:1162.

7. Cohn LH, Sanders JH Jr, Collins JJ Jr. Aortic valve replacement with the Hancock porcine xenograft. Ann Thorac Surg 1976;22:221.

8. Cooley DA, Norman JC. Severe intravascular hemolysis after aortic valve replacement. J Thorac Cardiovasc Surg 1977;74:322.

9. Copeland JG, Griepp RB, Stinson EB, Shumway NE. Long-term follow-up after isolated aortic valve replacement. J Thorac Cardiovasc Surg 1977;74:875.

10. Commeau P, Grollier G, Lamy E, Foucault JP, Durand C, Maffei G, et al. Percutaneous balloon dilatation of calcific aortic valve stenosis: anatomical and haemodynamic evaluation. Br Heart J 1988;59:227.

11. Carpentier A. Cardiac valve surgery: the "French correction." J Thorac Cardiovasc Surg 1983;86:323.

12. Christakis GT, Weisel RD, Fremes SE, Teoh KH, Skalenda JP, Tong CP, et al. Can the results of contemporary aortic valve replacement be improved? J Thorac Cardiovasc Surg 1986;92:37.

13. Cowan ST, Steel KJ. Manual for the identification of medical bacteria, 2nd Ed. New York: Cambridge University Press, 1974.

14. Czer LS, Gray RJ, Stewart ME, De Robertis M, Chaux A, Matloff JM. Reduction in sudden late death by concomitant revascularization with aortic valve replacement. J Thorac Cardiovasc Surg 1988;95:390.

15. Craver JM, King SB 3rd, Douglas JS, Franch RH, Jones EL, Morris DC, et al. Late hemodynamic evaluation of Hancock modified orifice aortic bioprosthesis. Circulation 1979;60:I93.

16. Chaitman BR, Bonan R, Lepage G, Tubau JF, David PR, Dyrda I, et al. Hemodynamic evaluation of the Carpentier-Edwards porcine xenograft. Circulation 1979;60:1170.

17. Cohn LH, Koster JK, Mee RB, Collins JJ Jr. Long-term follow-up of the Hancock bioprosthetic heart valve: a 6-year review. Circulation 1979;60:I87.

18. Chaux A, Gray RJ, Matloff JM, Feldman H, Sustaita H. An appreciation of the new St. Jude valvular prosthesis. J Thorac Cardiovasc Surg 1981;81:202.

19. Craver JM, Goldstein J, Jones EL, Knapp WA, Hatcher CR Jr. Clinical, hemodynamic, and operative descriptors affecting outcome of aortic valve replacement in elderly versus young patients. Ann Surg 1984;199:733.

20. Cleveland RJ, Madge GE, Lower RR. Homovital graft replacement of the aortic valve. Surg Forum 1967;18:124.

21. Cohen DJ, Myerowitz PD, Young WP, Chopra PS, Berkoff HA, Kroncke GM, et al. The fate of aortic valve homografts 12 to 17 years after implantation. Chest 1988;93:482.

22. Cabrol C, Pavie A, Mesnildrey P, Gandjbakhch I, Laughlin L, Bors V, et al. Long-term results with total replacement of the ascending aorta and reimplantation of the coronary arteries. J Thorac Cardiovasc Surg 1986;91:17.

23. Clarke DR. Extended aortic root replacement in 12 patients with complex left ventricular outflow tract obstruction. In Yankah AC, Hetzer R, Miller DL, Ross DN, Somerville J, Yacoub MH, eds. Cardiac valve allografts. 1962-1987. New York: Springer-Verlag, 1988, p. 157.

24. Czer LS, Matloff JM, Chaux A, De Robertis M, Stewart ME, Gray RJ. The St. Jude valve: analysis of thromboembolism, warfarin-related hemorrhage, and survival. Am Heart J 1987;114:389.

25. Christakis GT, Weisel RD, David TE, Salerno TA, Ivanov J. Predictors of operative survival after valve replacement. Circulation 1988; 78:I25.

26. Craver JM, Weintraub WS, Jones EL, Guyton RA, Hatcher CR Jr. Predictors of mortality, complications, and length of stay in aortic valve replacement for aortic stenosis. Circulation 1988;78:I85.

27. Cosgrove DM 3rd, Rosenkranz ER, Hendren WG, Bartlett JC, Stewart WJ. Valvuloplasty for aortic insufficiency. J Thorac Cardiovasc Surg 1991;102:571.

28. Cosgrove DM 3rd, Ratliff NB, Schaff HV, Edwards WD. Aortic valve decalcification: history repeated with a new result. Ann Thorac Surg 1990;49:689.

29. Connolly HM, Oh JK, Orszulak TA, Osborn SL, Roger VL, Hodge DO. Aortic valve replacement for aortic stenosis with severe left ventricular dysfunction: prognostic indicators. Circulation 1997; 95:2395.

30. Clyne CA, Arrighi JA, Maron BJ, Dilsizian V, Bonow RO, Cannon RO 3rd. Systemic and left ventricular responses to exercise stress of asymptomatic patients with valvular aortic stenosis. Am J Cardiol 1991;68:1469.

31. Cochrane RP, Kunzelman KS, Eddy AC, Hofer BO, Verrier ED. Modified conduit preparation creates a pseudosinus in an aortic valve-sparing procedure for aneurysm of the ascending aorta. J Thorac Cardiovasc Surg 1995;109:1049.

32. Choo SJ, Duran CM. A surgical method for selecting appropriate size of graft in aortic root remodeling (letter). Ann Thorac Surg 1999; 67:599.

33. Christie GW. Anatomy of aortic heart valve leaflets: the influence of glutaraldehyde fixation on function. Eur J Cardiothorac Surg 1992;6:S25.

34. Carrel T, Zingg U, Jenni R, Aeschbacher B, Turina MI. Early in vivo experience with the Hemodynamic Plus St. Jude Medical heart valves in patients with narrowed aortic annulus. Ann Thorac Surg 1996; 61:48.

35. Chambers J, Cross J, Deverall P, Sowton E. Echocardiographic description of the CarboMedics bileaflet prosthetic heart valve. J Am Coll Cardiol 1993;21:398.

36. Cartier PC, Dumesnil JG, Metras J, Desaulniers D, Doyle DP, Lemieux MD, et al. Clinical and hemodynamic performance of Freestyle aortic root bioprosthesis. Ann Thorac Surg 1999;67:345.

37. Cohn LH, Adams DH, Couper GS, Bichell DP, Rosborough DM, Sears SP. Minimally invasive cardiac valve surgery improves patient satisfaction while reducing costs of cardiac valve replacement and repair. Ann Surg 1997;226:421.

38. Cosgrove DM 3rd, Sabik JF. Minimally invasive approach for aortic valve operations. Ann Thorac Surg 1996;62:596.

39. Cosgrove DM 3rd, Sabik JF, Navia JL. Minimally invasive valve operations. Ann Thorac Surg 1998;65:1535.

40. Connolly HM, Crary JL, McGoon MD, Hensrud DD, Edwards BS, Edwards WD, et al. Valvular heart disease associated with fenfluramine-phentermine. N Engl J Med 1997;337:581.

41. Carabello BA. Timing of valve replacement in aortic stenosis: moving closer to perfection. Circulation 1997;95:2241.

42. Collins JJ Jr, Aranki SF. Management of mild aortic stenosis during coronary artery bypass graft surgery. J Card Surg 1994;9:145.

43. Cartier PC, Metras J, Dumesnil JG, Pibarot P, Lemieux M. Midterm follow-up of unstented biological valves. Semin Thorac Cardiovasc Surg 1999;2:22.

44. Christie GW, Gross JF, Eberhardt CE. Fatigue-induced changes to the biaxial mechanical properties of glutaraldehyde-fixed aortic valve leaflets. Semin Thorac Cardiovasc Surg 1999;11:201.

45. Casselman FP, Gillinov AM, Akhrass R, Kasirajan V, Blackstone EH, Cosgrove DM 3rd. Intermediate-term durability of bicuspid aortic valve repair for prolapsing leaflet. Eur J Cardio Thorac Surg 1999; 15:302.

46. Choudhary SK, Mathur A, Sharma R, Saxena A, Chopra P, Roy R, et al. Pulmonary autograft: should it be used in young patients with rheumatic disease? J Thorac Cardiovasc Surg 1999;118:483.

47. Chambers JC, Somerville J, Stone S, Ross DN. Pulmonary autograft procedure for aortic valve disease: long-term results of the pioneer series. Circulation 1997;96:2206.

48. Carr-White GS, Kilner PJ, Hon JK, Rutledge T, Edwards S, Burman ED, et al. Incidence, location, pathology, and significance of pulmonary homograft stenosis after the Ross operation. Circulation 2001;104:116.

49. Cosgrove DM. Carpentier pericardial valve. Semin Thorac Cardiovasc Surg 1996;8:269.

D

1. David TE, Pollick C, Bos J. Aortic valve replacement with stentless porcine aortic bioprosthesis. J Thorac Cardiovasc Surg 1990;99:113.

2. Doty DB, Arcidi JM Jr. Methods for graft size selection in aortic valve-sparing operations. Ann Thorac Surg 2000;69:648.

3. David TE, Ropchan GC, Butany JW. Aortic valve replacement with stentless porcine bioprostheses. J Card Surg 1988;3:501.

4. Dineen E, Brent BN. Aortic valve stenosis: comparison of patients with to those without chronic congestive heart failure. Am J Cardiol 1986;57:419.

5. Degeorges M, Delzant JF. Elements de pronostic de l'insuffisance aortique isolee recueillis chez 206 malades agés de moins de 50 ans. Sem Hop Paris 1966;42:1171.

6. Duran CG. Reconstructive techniques for rheumatic aortic valve disease. J Card Surg 1988;3:23.

7. Duran CG, Gunning AJ. A method for placing a total homologous aortic valve in the subcoronary position. Lancet 1962;2:488.

8. David TE, Uden DE. Aortic valve replacement in adult patients with small aortic annuli. Ann Thorac Surg 1983;36:577.

9. Donaldson RM, Ross DM. Homograft aortic root replacement for complicated prosthetic valve endocarditis. Circulation 1984;70:I178.

10. DiMario C, Beatt KJ, de Feyter P, van den Brand M, Essed CE, Serruys PW. Percutaneous aortic balloon dilatation for calcific aortic stenosis in elderly patients: immediate hemodynamic results and short term follow-up. Br Heart J 1987;58:644.

11. Dziatkowiak AJ, Pfitsner R, Andres J, Podolec P, Marek Z, Sarska M. Modified techniques for subcoronary insertion of allografts. In Yankah AC, Hetzer R, Miller DC, Ross DN, Somerville J, Yacoub MH, eds. Cardiac valve allografts. 1962-1987. New York: Springer-Verlag, 1988, p. 141.

12. Duncan JM, Cooley DA, Reul GJ, Ott DA, Hallman GL, Frazier OH, et al. Durability and low thrombogenicity of the St. Jude Medical valve at 5-year follow-up. Ann Thorac Surg 1986;42:500.

13. DiSesa VJ, Allred EN, Kowalker W, Shemin RJ, Collins JJ Jr, Cohn LH. Performance of a fabricated trileaflet porcine bioprosthesis. J Thorac Cardiovasc Surg 1987;94:220.

14. Davila-Roman VG, Barzilai B, Murphy S, Brown P, Kouchoukos NT. Doppler echocardiography of aortic valve allografts and pulmonary autografts: a comparison of free-hand valve and aortic root replacement (abstract). J Am Coll Cardiol 1991;17:40.

15. David TE, Feindel CM. An aortic valve-sparing operation for patients with aortic incompetence and aneurysm of the ascending aorta. J Thorac Cardiovasc Surg 1992;103:617.

16. David TE, Bos J, Christakis GT, Brofman PR, Wong D, Feindel CM. Heart valve operations in patients with active infective endocarditis. Ann Thorac Surg 1990;49:701.

17. Dreyfus G, Serraf A, Jebara VA, Deloche A, Chauvaud S, Couetil JP, et al. Valve repair in acute endocarditis. Ann Thorac Surg 1990; 49:706.

18. Dare AJ, Veinot JP, Edwards WD, Tazelaar HD, Schaff HV. New observations on the etiology of aortic valve disease: a surgical pathologic study of 236 cases from 1990. Hum Pathol 1993;24:1330.

19. Desjardins VA, Enriquez-Sarano M, Tajiik AJ, Bailey KR, Seward JB. Intensity of murmurs correlates with severity of valvular regurgitation. Am J Med 1996;100:149.

20. Doty JR, Flores JH, Millar RC, Doty DB. Aortic valve replacement with Medtronic Freestyle bioprosthesis: operative technique and results. J Card Surg 1998;13:208.

21. David TE, Feindel CM, Bos J. Repair of the aortic valve in patients with aortic insufficiency and aortic root aneurysm. J Thorac Cardiovasc Surg 1995;109:345.

22. David TE. Current practice in Marfan's aortic root surgery: reconstruction with aortic valve preservation or replacement? What to do with the mitral valve. J Card Surg 1997;12:147.

23. David TE, Feindel CM, Scully HE, Bos J, Rakowski H. Aortic valve replacement with stentless porcine aortic valves: a ten-year experience. J Heart Valve Dis 1998;7:250.

24. Del Rizzo DF, Abdoh A. Clinical and hemodynamic comparison of the Medtronic Freestyle and Toronto SPV stentless valves. J Card Surg 1998;13:398.

25. David TE, Armstrong S, Sun Z. The Hancock II bioprosthesis at 12 years. Ann Thorac Surg 1998;66:S95.

26. De Amicis V, Ascione R, Innelli G, Di Tommaso L, Monaco M, Spampinato N. Aortic valve replacement through minimally invasive approach. Texas Heart Inst J 1997;24:353.

27. Doty DB, DiRusso GB, Doty JR. Full-spectrum cardiac surgery through a minimal incision: mini-sternotomy (lower half) technique. Ann Thorac Surg 1998;65:573.

28. Doty DB, Cafferty A, Kon ND, Huysmans HA, Krause AH Jr, Westaby S. Medtronic Freestyle aortic root bioprosthesis: implant techniques. J Card Surg 1998;13:369.

29. Dumesnil JG, Yoganathan AP. Valve prosthesis hemodynamics and the problem of high transprosthetic pressure gradients. Eur J Cardiothorac Surg 1992;6:S34.

30. Dossche KM, de la Riviere AB, Morshuis WJ, Schepens MA, Ernst SM, van den Brand JJ. Aortic root replacement with the pulmonary autograft: an invariably competent aortic valve? Ann Thorac Surg 1999;68:1302.

31. Doty JR, Salazar JD, Liddicoat JR, Flores JH, Doty DB. Aortic valve replacement with cryopreserved aortic allograft: ten-year experience. J Thorac Cardiovasc Surg 1998;115:371.

32. Doty DB, Cafferty A, Cartier P, Huysmans HA, Kon ND, Krause AH, et al. Aortic valve replacement with Medtronic Freestyle bioprosthesis: 5-year results. Semin Thorac Cardiovasc Surg 1992;2:35.

33. David TE, Puschmann R, Ivanov J, Bos J, Armstrong S, Feindel CM. Aortic valve replacement with stentless and stented porcine valves: a case-match study. J Thorac Cardiovasc Surg 1998;116:236.

34. Doty DB, Flores JH, Yanowitz FG, Oury JH. Maximum exercise after aortic valve replacement with pulmonary autograft. Asian Ann Cardiovasc Thorac Surg 1999;7:37.

35. Del Rizzo DF, Abdoh A, Cartier P, Doty D, Westaby S. The effect of prosthetic valve type on survival after aortic valve surgery. Semin Thorac Cardiovasc Surg 1999;2:1.

36. Del Rizzo DF, Abdoh A, Cartier P, Doty D, Westaby S. Factors affecting left ventricular mass regression after aortic valve replacement with stentless valves. Semin Thorac Cardiovasc Surg 1999; 2:114.

37. Doty DB. Aortic valve replacement with homograft and autograft. Semin Thorac Cardiovasc Surg 1996;8:249.

38. De la Fuente A, Sanchez R, Romero J, Berjon J, Imizcoz MA, Fernandez JL, et al. CarboMedics and Monostrut valves: clinical and hemodynamic outcomes in a randomized study. J Heart Valve Dis 2000;9:303.

39. David TE, Omran A, Ivanov J, Armstrong S, de Sa MP, Sonnenberg B, et al. Dilation of the pulmonary autograft after the Ross procedure. J Thorac Cardiovasc Surg 2000;119:210.

40. DeWall RA, Qasim N, Carr L. Evolution of mechanical heart valves. Ann Thorac Surg 2000;69:1612.

41. Doty DB, Nelson RM. Aortic valve replacement: continuous-suture technique. J Card Surg 1986;1:379.

42. De Paulis R, De Matteis GM, Nardi P, Scaffa R, Buratta MM, Chiariello L. Opening and closing characteristics of the aortic valve after valve-sparing procedures using a new aortic root conduit. Ann Thorac Surg 2001;72:487.

43. David TE, Armstrong S, Ivanov J, Feindel CM, Omran A, Webb G. Results of aortic valve-sparing operations. J Thorac Cardiovasc Surg 2001;122:39.

44. David TE, Ivanov J, Eriksson MJ, Bos J, Feindel CM, Rakowski H. Dilation of the sinotubular junction causes aortic insufficiency after aortic valve replacement with the Toronto SPV bioprosthesis. J Thorac Cardiovasc Surg 2001;122:929.

E

1. Eddleman EE Jr, Frommeyer WB Jr, Lyle DP, Turner ME Jr, Bancroft WH Jr. Critical analysis of clinical factors in estimating severity of aortic valve disease. Am J Cardiol 1973;31:687.

2. Edmunds LH Jr. Thrombotic and bleeding complications of prosthetic heart valves. Ann Thorac Surg 1987;44:430.

3. Ellis FH Jr, Kirklin JW. Aortic stenosis. Surg Clin North Am 1955;35:1029.

4. Ellis FH Jr, Kirklin JW. Aortic insufficiency. Surg Clin North Am 1955;35:1035.

5. Emery RW, Arom KV, eds. The aortic valve. Philadelphia: Hanley & Belfus, 1991.

6. Elkins RC, Lane MM, McCue C, Ward KE. Pulmonary autograft root replacement: mid-term results. J Heart Valve Dis 1999;8:499.

7. Elkins RC, Knott-Craig CJ, Ward KE, McCue C, Lane MM. Pulmonary autograft in children: realized growth potential. Ann Thorac Surg 1994;57:1387.

8. Elkins RC, Lane MM, McCue C, Chandrasekaran K. Ross operation and aneurysm or dilation of the ascending aorta. Semin Thorac Cardiovasc Surg 1999;2:50.

9. Erickson RL, Thulin LI, Richard GJ. An in vitro study of mechanical heart valve sound loudness. J Heart Valve Dis 1994;3:330.

10. Elkins RC, Dawson PE, Goldstein S, Walsh SP, Black KS. Decellularized human valve allografts. Ann Thorac Surg 2001;71:S428.

F

1. Frank S, Ross J Jr. The natural history of severe, acquired valvular aortic stenosis. Am J Cardiol 1967;19:128.

2. Fifer MA, Borow KM, Colan SD, Lorell BH. Early diastolic left ventricular function in children and adults with aortic stenosis. J Am Coll Cardiol 1985;5:1147.

3. Frater RW. Aortic valve insufficiency due to aortic dilatation: correction by sinus rim adjustment. Circulation 1986;47:I136.

4. Foster AH, Tracy CM, Greenberg GJ, McIntosh CL, Clark RE. Valve replacement in narrow aortic roots: serial hemodynamics and long-term clinical outcome. Ann Thorac Surg 1986;42:506.

5. Fioretti P, Roelandt J, Sclavo M, Domenicucci S, Haalebos M, Bos E, et al. Postoperative regression of left ventricular dimensions in aortic insufficiency: a long-term echocardiographic study. J Am Coll Cardiol 1985;5:856.

6. Ferrans VJ, Spray TL, Billingham ME, Roberts WC. Structural changes in glutaraldehyde-treated porcine heterografts used as substitute cardiac valves. Am J Cardiol 1978;41:1159.

7. Fremes SE, Goldman BS, Ivanov J, Weisel RD, David TE, Salerno T. Valvular surgery in the elderly. Circulation 1989;80:1.

8. Freeman WK, Schaff HV, Orszulak TA, Tajik AJ. Ultrasonic aortic valve decalcification: serial Doppler echocardiographic follow-up. J Am Coll Cardiol 1990;16:623.

9. Faggiano P, Ghizzoni G, Sorgato A, Sabatini T, Simoncelli U, Gardini A, et al. Rate of progression of valvular aortic stenosis in adults. Am J Cardiol 1992;70:229.

10. Fisher J, Reece IJ, Wheatley DJ. In vitro evaluation of six mechanical and six bioprosthetic valves. Thorac Cardiovasc Surg 1986;34:157.

11. Fann JI, Miller DC, Moore KA, Mitchell RS, Oyer PE, Stinson EB, et al. Twenty-year clinical experience with porcine bioprostheses. Ann Thorac Surg 1996;62:1301.

12. Fyfe BS, Schoen FJ. Pathological analysis of nonstented Freestyle aortic root bioprostheses treated with amino oleic acid. Semin Thorac Cardiovasc Surg 1999;2:151.

G

1. Grant RT. After histories for ten years of a thousand men suffering from heart disease: a study in prognosis. Heart 1933;16:275.

2. Goldschlager N, Pfeifer J, Cohn K, Popper R, Selzer A. The natural history of aortic regurgitation. Am J Med 1973;54:577.

3. Gault JH, Covell JW, Braunwald E, Ross J Jr. Left ventricular performance following correction of free aortic regurgitation. Circulation 1970;42:773.

4. Gaasch WH, Andrias CW, Levine HJ. Chronic aortic regurgitation: the effect of aortic valve replacement on left ventricular volume, mass and function. Circulation 1978;58:825.

5. Gula G, Wain WH, Ross DN. Ten years' experience with pulmonary autograft replacements for aortic valve disease. Ann Thorac Surg 1979;28:392.

6. Gott VL, Pyeritz RE, Magovern GJ Jr, Cameron DE, McKusick VA. Surgical treatment of aneurysms of the ascending aorta in the Marfan syndrome. N Engl J Med 1986;314:1070.

7. Gaasch WH, Levine JH, Quinones MA, Alexander JK. Left ventricular compliance: mechanisms and clinical implications. Am J Cardiol 1976;38:645.

8. Grossman W, McLaurin LP, Moos SP, Stefadouros M, Young DT. Wall thickness and diastolic properties of the left ventricle. Circulation 1974;49:129.

9. Gula G, Pomerance A, Bennet M, Yacoub MH. Homograft replacement of aortic valve and ascending aorta in a patient with non-specific giant cell aortitis. Br Heart J 1977;39:581.

10. Gonzalez-Lavin L, Barratt-Boyes BG. Surgical considerations in the treatment of ventricular septal defect associated with aortic valvular incompetence. J Thorac Cardiovasc Surg 1969;57:422.

11. Gavin JB, Herdson PB, Monro JL, Barratt-Boyes BG. Pathology of antibiotic treated human heart valve allografts. Thorax 1973;28:473.

12. Gavin JB, Barratt-Boyes BG, Hitchcock GC, Herdson PB. Histopathology of "fresh" human aortic valve allografts. Thorax 1973;28:482.

13. Grunkemeier GL, Kennard E, Holubkov R. Ex tempore analysis of the AVERT study data. St. Paul, Minn.: St. Jude Medical, 2000.

14. Girardet RW, Wheat MW Jr. Technique of aortic valve replacement. J Thorac Cardiovasc Surg 1976;71:446.

15. Guiney TE, Davies MJ, Parker DJ, Leech GJ, Leatham A. The aetiology and course of isolated severe aortic regurgitation: a clinical, pathological, and echocardiographic study. Br Heart J 1987;58:358.

16. Green SJ, Pizzarello RA, Padmanabhan VT, Ong LY, Hall MH, Tortolani AJ. Relation of angina pectoris to coronary artery disease in aortic valve stenosis. Am J Cardiol 1985;55:1063.

17. Grande-Allen KJ, Cochran RP, Reinhall PG, Kunzelman KS. Re-creation of sinuses is important for sparing the aortic valve: a finite element study. J Thorac Cardiovasc Surg 2000;119:753.

18. Grande-Allen KJ, Cochran RP, Reinhall PG, Kunzelman KS. Mechanisms of aortic valve incompetence: finite element modeling of Marfan syndrome. J Thorac Cardiovasc Surg 2001;122:946.

19. Gonzalez-Lavin L, Robles A, Graf D. The Ross operation: the autologous pulmonary valve in the aortic position. J Card Surg 1988;3:29.

20. Gorczynski A, Trenkner M, Anisimowicz L, Gutkowoski R, Drapella A, Kwiatkowska E, et al. Biomechanics of the pulmonary autograft in the aortic position. Thorax 1982;37:535.

21. Galloway AC, Colvin SB, Grossi EA, Baumann FG, Sabban YP, Esposito R, et al. Ten-year experience with aortic valve replacement in 482 patients 70 years of age or older: operative risk and long-term results. Ann Thorac Surg 1990;49:84.

22. Gerosa G, McKay R, Ross DN. Replacement of the aortic valve or root with a pulmonary autograft in children. Ann Thorac Surg 1991;51:424.

23. Glazier JJ, Verwilghen J, Donaldson RM, Ross DN. Treatment of complicated prosthetic aortic valve endocarditis with annular abscess formation by homograft aortic root replacement. J Am Coll Cardiol 1991;17:1177.

24. Gott VL, Greene PS, Alejo DE, Cameron DE, Naftel DC, Miller DC, et al. Replacement of the aortic root in patients with Marfan's syndrome. N Engl J Med 1999;340:1307.

25. Gundry SR. Aortic valve surgery via limited incisions. In Oz MC, Goldstein DJ, eds. Contemporary cardiology: minimally invasive cardiac surgery. Totowa, N.J.: Humana, 1999, p. 205.

26. Grunkemeier GL, Li HH, Starr A. Heart valve replacement: a statistical review of 35 years' results. J Heart Valve Dis 1999;8:466.

27. Goffin YA, Narine KR, Alexander JP, Van Goethem J, Daenen WJ. Histopathologic comparison of a pulmonary autograft and pulmonary homograft in a patient 17 months after a Ross procedure: an autopsy study. J Heart Valve Dis 1998;7:327.

28. Grunkemeier GL, Li HH, Naftel DC, Starr A, Rahimtoola SH. Long-term performance of heart valve prostheses. Curr Probl Cardiol 2000;25:73.

29. Grunkemeier GL, Wu YX. Mean time to 'actual' failure for porcine heart valves. J Heart Valve Dis 2001;10:449.

H

1. Hufnagel CA. Aortic plastic valvular prosthesis. Bull Georgetown Univ Med Ctr 1951;4:128.

2. Hufnagel CA, Harvey WP. The surgical correction of aortic regurgitation. Bull Georgetown Univ Med Ctr 1953;6:60.

3. Hirshfeld JW Jr, Epstein SE, Roberts AJ, Glancy DL, Morrow AG. Indices predicting long-term survival after valve replacement in patients with aortic regurgitation and patients with aortic stenosis. Circulation 1974;50:1190.

4. Henry WL, Bonow RO, Borer JS, Ware JH, Kent KM, Redwood DR, et al. Observations on the optimum time for operative intervention for aortic regurgitation. I. Evaluation of the results of aortic valve replacement in symptomatic patients. Circulation 1980;61:471.

5. Hegglin R, Scheu H, Rothlin M. Aortic insufficiency. Circulation 1968;38:77.

6. Henry WL, Bonow RO, Rosing DR, Epstein SE. Observations on the optimum time for operative intervention for aortic regurgitation. II. Serial echocardiographic evaluation of asymptomatic patients. Circulation 1980;61:484.

7. Hammermeister KE, Henderson WG, Burchfiel CM, Sethi GK, Souchek J, Oprian C, et al. Comparison of outcome after valve replacement with a bioprosthesis versus a mechanical prosthesis: initial 5 year results of a randomized trial. J Am Coll Cardiol 1987;10:719.

8. Hufnagel CA, Conrad PW. The direct approach for the correction of aortic insufficiency. JAMA 1961;178:275.

9. Harken DE, Soroff HS, Taylor WJ, Lefemine AA, Gupta SK, Lunzer S. Partial and complete prostheses in aortic insufficiency. J Thorac Cardiovasc Surg 1960;40:744.

10. Hurley PJ, Lowe JB, Barratt-Boyes BG. Debridement-valvotomy for aortic stenosis in adults: a follow-up of 76 patients. Thorax 1967;22:314.

11. Hoeksima TD, Titus JL, Giuliani ER, Kirklin JW. Early results of use of homografts for replacement of the aortic valve in man. Circulation 1967;35/36:I9.

12. Hoagland PM, Cook EF, Flatley M, Walker C, Goldman L. Case-control analysis of risk factors for presence of aortic stenosis in adults (age 50 years or older). Am J Cardiol 1985;55:744.

13. Hackett D, Fessatidis I, Sapsford R, Oakley C. Ten year clinical evaluation of Starr-Edwards 2400 and 1260 aortic valve prostheses. Br Heart J 1987;57:356.

14. Heslop BF, Wilson SE, Hardy BE. Antigenicity of aortic valve allografts. Ann Surg 1973;177:301.

15. Haydock D, Barratt-Boyes B, Macedo T, Kirklin JW, Blackstone E. Aortic valve replacement for acute infectious endocarditis in 108 patients. J Thorac Cardiovasc Surg 1992;103:130.

16. Hwang MH, Hammermeister KE, Oprian C, Henderson W, Bousvaros G, Wong M, et al. Preoperative identification of patients likely to have left ventricular dysfunction after aortic valve replacement. Circulation 1989;80:I65.

17. Hvass U. A new technique for sparing the aortic valve in patients with aneurysm of the ascending aorta and root. J Thorac Cardiovasc Surg 2000;119:1048.

18. Herreman F, Ameur A, de Vernejoul F, Bourgin JH, Gueret P, Guerin F, et al. Pre-and postoperative hemodynamic and cineangiocardiographic assessment of left ventricular function in patients with aortic regurgitation. Am Heart J 1979;98:63.

19. Hoff SJ, Merrill WH, Stewart JR, Bender HW Jr. Safety of remote aortic valve replacement after prior coronary artery bypass grafting. Ann Thorac Surg 1996;61:1689.

20. Hammermeister KE, Sethi GK, Henderson WG, Oprian C, Kim T, Rahimtoola S. A comparison of outcomes in men 11 years after heart-valve replacement with a mechanical valve or bioprosthesis: Veterans Affairs Cooperative Study on Valvular Heart Disease. N Engl J Med 1993;328:1289.

21. Hawkins JA, Breinholt JP, Lambert LM, Fuller TC, Profaizer T, McGough EC, et al. Class I and class II anti-HLA antibodies after implantation of cryopreserved allograft material in pediatric patients. J Thorac Cardiovasc Surg 2000;119:324.

22. Hoekstra FM, Witvliet M, Knoop CY, Wassenaar C, Bogers AJ, Weimar W, et al. Immunogenic human leukocyte antigen class II antigens on human cardiac valves induce specific alloantibodies. Ann Thorac Surg 1998;66:2022.

23. Herijgers P, Herregods MC, Vandeplas A, Meyns B, Flammeng W. Silzone™ coating and paravalvular leak: an independent, randomized study. J Heart Valve Dis 2001;10:712.

24. Houel R, Kirsch M, Hillion ML, Loisance D. Silzone™-coated St. Jude Medical valve: a safe valve. J Heart Valve Dis 2001;10:724.

25. Hasnat K, Birks EJ, Liddicoat J, Hon JK, Edwards S, Glennon S, et al. Patient outcome and valve performance following a second aortic valve homograft replacement. Circulation 1999;100:II42.

I

1. Isner JM, Salem DN, Desnoyers MR, Hougen TJ, Mackey WC, Pandian NG, et al. Treatment of calcific aortic stenosis by balloon valvuloplasty. Am J Cardiol 1987;59:313.

2. Izzat MB, Kadir I, Reeves B, Wilde P, Bryan AJ, Angelini GD. Patient-prosthesis mismatch is negligible with modern small-size aortic valve prostheses. Ann Thorac Surg 1999;68:1657.

3. Ivert TS, Dismukes WE, Cobbs GC, Blackstone EH, Kirklin JW, Bergdahl LA. Prosthetic valve endocarditis. Circulation 1984;69:223.

4. Ionescu MI, Ross DN. Heart-valve replacement with autologous fascia lata. Lancet 1969;2:1.

5. Ionescu MI, Pakrashi BC, Holden MP, Mary DA, Wooler GH. Results of aortic valve replacement with frame-supported fascia lata and pericardial grafts. J Thorac Cardiovasc Surg 1972;64:340.

6. Ionescu AA, Fraser AG, Butchart EG. High incidence of embolism after St. Jude Silzone prosthetic valve implantation (abstract). Circulation 1999;100:I524.

J

1. Jacobs ML, Fowler BN, Vezeridis MP, Jones N, Daggett WM. Aortic valve replacement: a 9-year experience. Ann Thorac Surg 1980;30:439.

2. Jones EL, Craver JM, Morris DC, King SB 3rd, Douglas JS Jr, Franch RH, et al. Hemodynamic and clinical evaluation of the Hancock xenograft bioprosthesis of aortic valve replacement (with emphasis on management of the small aortic root). J Thorac Cardiovasc Surg 1978;75:300.

3. Johnston AM. Aortic stenosis, sudden death, and the left ventricular baroreceptors. Br Heart J 1971;33:1.

4. Jackson G, Thomas S, Monaghan M, Forsyth A, Jewitt D. Inoperable aortic stenosis in the elderly: benefit from percutaneous transluminal valvuloplasty. Br Med J 1987;294:83.

5. Jaffe WM, Coverdale HA, Roche AH, Brandt PW, Ormiston JA, Barratt-Boyes BG. Doppler echocardiography in the assessment of the homograft aortic valve. Am J Cardiol 1989;63:1466.

6. Jaffe WM, Coverdale HA, Roche AH, Whitlock RM, Neutze JM, Barratt-Boyes BG. Rest and exercise hemodynamics of 20 to 23 mm allograft, Medtronic Intact (porcine), and St. Jude Medical valves in the aortic position. J Thorac Cardiovasc Surg 1990;100:167.

7. Jaffe WM, Barratt-Boyes BG, Sadri A, Gavin JB, Coverdale HA, Neutze JM. Early follow-up of patients with the Medtronic Intact porcine valve: a new cardiac bioprosthesis. J Thorac Cardiovasc Surg 1989;98:942.

8. Jamieson WR, Burr LH, Miyagishima RT, Germann E, Anderson WN. Actuarial versus actual freedom from structural valve deterioration with the Carpentier-Edwards porcine bioprostheses. Can J Cardiol 1999;15:973.

9. Jones EL, Weintraub WS, Craver JM, Guyton RA, Cohen CL, Corrigan VE, et al. Ten-year experience with the porcine bioprosthetic valve: interrelationship of valve survival and patient survival in 1,050 valve replacements. Ann Thorac Surg 1990;49:370.

10. Jin XY, Gibson DG, Pepper JR. Early changes in regional and global left ventricular function after aortic valve replacement: comparison of crystalloid, cold blood, and warm blood cardioplegias. Circulation 1995;92:II155.

11. Jin XY, Zhang ZM, Gibson DG, Yacoub MH, Pepper JR. Effects of valve substitute on changes in left ventricular function and hypertrophy after aortic valve replacement. Ann Thorac Surg 1996;62:683.

12. Jamieson WR, Munro AI, Miyagishima RT, Allen P, Burr LH, Tyers GF. Carpentier-Edwards standard porcine bioprosthesis: clinical performance to seventeen years. Ann Thorac Surg 1995;60:999.

13. Jamieson WR, Burr LH, Janusz MT, Munro AI, Hayden RI, Miyagishima RT, et al. Carpentier-Edwards standard and supraannular porcine bioprostheses: comparison of technology. Ann Thorac Surg 1999;67:10.

14. Jones HU, Muhlestein JB, Jones KW, Bair TL, Lavasani F, Schrevardi M, et al. Preoperative use of enoxaparin compared with unfractionated heparin increases the incidence of re-exploration for post operative bleeding after open-heart surgery in patients who present with an acute coronary syndrome: clinical investigation and reports. Circulation 2002;106:I19.

15. Jones JM, O'Kane H, Gladstone DJ, Sarsam MA, Campalani G, MacGowan SW, et al. Repeat heart valve surgery: risk factors for operative mortality. J Thorac Cardiovasc Surg 2001;122:913.

K

1. Karp RB, Cyrus RJ, Blackstone EH, Kirklin JW, Kouchoukos NT, Pacifico AD. The Bjork-Shiley valve: intermediate-term follow-up. J Thorac Cardiovasc Surg 1981;81:602.

2. Konno S, Imai Y, Iida Y, Nakajima M, Tatsuno K. A new method for prosthetic valve replacement in congenital aortic stenosis associated with hypoplasia of the aortic valve ring. J Thorac Cardiovasc Surg 1975;70:909.

3. Krayenbuehl HP, Turina M, Hess OM, Rothlin M, Senning A. Pre- and postoperative left ventricular contractile function in patients with aortic valve disease. Br Heart J 1979;41:204.

4. Kennedy JW, Twiss RD, Blackmon JR, Dodge HT. Quantitative angiocardiography. 3. Relationships of left ventricular pressure, volume, and mass in aortic valve disease. Circulation 1968;38:838.

5. Kennedy JW, Doces J, Stewart DK. Left ventricular function before and following aortic valve replacement. Circulation 1977;56:944.

6. Kouchoukos NT, Karp RB, Blackstone EH, Kirklin JW, Pacifico AD, Zorn GL. Replacement of the ascending aorta and aortic valve with a composite graft. Results in 86 patients. Ann Surg 1980;192:403.

7. King RM, Pluth JR, Giuliani ER. The association of unexplained gastrointestinal bleeding with calcific aortic stenosis. Ann Thorac Surg 1987;44:514.

8. Karp RB, Lell W. Evaluating techniques of myocardial preservation for aortic valve replacement: operative risk. J Thorac Cardiovasc Surg 1976;72:206.

9. Khanna SK, Ross JK, Monro JL. Homograft aortic valve replacement: seven years' experience with antibiotic-treated valves. Thorax 1981;36:330.

10. Kawasuji M, Hetzer R, Oelert H, Stauch G, Borst HG. Aortic valve replacement and ascending aorta replacement in ankylosing spondylitis: report of three surgical cases and review of the literature. Thorac Cardiovasc Surg 1982;30:310.

11. Kirklin JW, Mankin HT. Open operation in the treatment of calcific aortic stenosis. Circulation 1960;21:578.

12. Karp RB, Kirklin JW. Replacement of diseased aortic valves with homografts. Ann Surg 1969;169:921.

13. Kerwin AJ, Lenkei SC, Wilson DR. Aortic valve homograft in the treatment of aortic insufficiency: report of nine cases with one followed for six years. N Engl J Med 1962;266:852.

14. Kawanishi DT, McKay CR, Chandraratna PA, Nanna M, Reid CL, Elkayam U, et al. Cardiovascular response to dynamic exercise in patients with chronic symptomatic mild-to-moderate and severe aortic regurgitation. Circulation 1986;73:62.

15. Kouchoukos NT, Marshall WG Jr, Wedige-Stecher TA. Eleven-year experience with composite graft replacement of the ascending aorta and aortic valve. J Thorac Cardiovasc Surg 1986;92:691.

16. King RM, Pluth JR, Giuliani ER, Piehler JM. Mechanical decalcification of the aortic valve. Ann Thorac Surg 1986;42:269.

17. Karaian CH, Greenberg BH, Rahimtoola SH. The relationship between functional class and cardiac performance in patients with chronic aortic insufficiency. Chest 1985;88:553.

18. Kay PH, Nunley D, Grunkemeier GL, Carcia C, McKinley CL, Starr A. Ten-year survival following aortic valve replacement: a multivariate analysis of coronary artery bypass as a risk factor. J Cardiovasc Surg 1986;27:494.

19. Kosek JC, Iben AB, Shumway NE, Angell WW. Morphology of fresh heart valve homografts. Surgery 1969;66:269.

20. Kosinki EJ, Cohn PF, Grossman W, Cohn LH. Severe stenosis occurring in antibiotic sterilized homograft valves. Br Heart J 1978;40:194.

21. Kirklin JK, Naftel DC, Blackstone EH, Kirklin JW, Brown RC. Risk factors for mortality after primary combined valvular and coronary artery surgery. Circulation 1989;79:I185.

22. Kirklin JK, Kirklin JW, Pacifico AD. Aortic valve endocarditis with aortic root abscess cavity: surgical treatment with aortic valve homograft. Ann Thorac Surg 1988;45:674.

23. Krayenbuehl HP, Hess OM, Monrad ES, Schneider J, Mall G, Turina M. Left ventricular myocardial structure in aortic valve disease before, intermediate, and later after aortic valve replacement. Circulation 1989;79:744.

24. Kouchoukos NT, Wareing TH, Murphy SF, Perrillo JB. Sixteen-year experience with aortic root replacement. Results of 172 operations. Ann Surg 1991;214:308.

25. Kennedy KD, Nishimura RA, Holmes DR Jr, Bailey KR. Natural history of moderate aortic stenosis. J Am Coll Cardiol 1991;17:313.

26. Kon ND, Westaby S, Amarasena N, Pillai R, Cordell AR. Comparison of implantation techniques using freestyle stentless porcine aortic valve. Ann Thorac Surg 1995;59:857.

27. Kunzelman KS, Grande KJ, David TE, Cochran RP, Verrier ED. Aortic root and valve relationships: impact on surgical repair. J Thorac Cardiovasc Surg 1994;107:162.

28. Khan SS, Mitchell RS, Derby GC, Oyer PE, Miller DC. Differences in Hancock and Carpentier-Edwards porcine xenograft aortic valve hemodynamics: effect of valve size. Circulation 1990;82:IV117.

29. Kasegawa H, Shimokawa T, Matsushita Y, Kamata S, Ida T, Kawase M. Right-sided partial sternotomy for minimally invasive valve operation: "open door method." Ann Thorac Surg 1998;65:569.

30. Kouchoukos NT, Davila-Roman VG, Spray TL, Murphy SF, Perrillo JB. Replacement of the aortic root with a pulmonary autograft in children and young adults with aortic-valve disease. N Engl J Med 1994;330:1.

31. Klodas E, Enriquez-Sarano M, Tajik AJ, Mullany CJ, Bailey KR, Seward JB. Aortic regurgitation complicated by extreme left ventricular dilation: long-term outcome after surgical correction. J Am Coll Cardiol 1996;27:670.

32. Kleine P, Perthel M, Nygaard H, Hansen SB, Paulsen PK, Riis C, et al. Medtronic-Hall versus St. Jude Medical mechanical aortic valve: downstream turbulences with respect to rotation in pigs. J Heart Valve Dis 1998;7:548.

33. Kleine P, Hasenkam MJ, Nygaard H, Perthel M, Wesemeyer D, Laas J. Tilting disc versus bileaflet aortic valve substitutes: intraoperative and postoperative hemodynamic performance in humans. J Heart Valve Dis 2000;9:308.

34. Knott-Craig DJ, Elkins RC, Santangelo K, McCue C, Lane MM. Aortic valve replacement: comparison of late survival between autografts and homografts. Ann Thorac Surg 2000;69:1327.

35. Kvidal P, Bergstrom R, Horte LG, Stahle E. Observed and relative survival after aortic valve replacement. J Am Coll Cardiol 2000;35:747.

36. Klodas E, Enriquez-Sarano M, Tajik AJ, Mullany CJ, Bailey KR, Seward JB. Surgery for aortic regurgitation in women: contrasting indications and outcomes compared with men. Circulation 1996;94:2472.

37. Kortke H, Korfer R. International normalized ratio self-management after mechanical heart valve replacement: is an early start advantageous? Ann Thorac Surg 2001;72:44.

38. Kahn SS, Trento A, DeRobertis M, Kass RM, Sandhu M, Czer LS, et al. Twenty-year comparison of tissue and mechanical valve replacement. J Thorac Cardiovasc Surg 2001;122:257.

L

1. Levinson JR, Akins CW, Buckley MJ, Newell JB, Palacios IF, Block PC, et al. Octogenarians with aortic stenosis: outcome after aortic valve replacement. Circulation 1989;80:I49.

2. Lewin RF, Dorros G, King JF, Mathiak L. Percutaneous transluminal aortic valvuloplasty: acute outcome and follow-up of 125 patients. J Am Coll Cardiol 1989;14:1210.

3. Lund O, Nielsen SL, Arildsen H, Ilkjaer LB, Pilegaard HK. Standard aortic St. Jude valve at 18 years: performance profile and determinants of outcome. Ann Thorac Surg 2000;69:1459.

4. Lindblom D. Long-term clinical results after aortic valve replacement with the Bjork-Shiley prosthesis. J Thorac Cardiovasc Surg 1988;95:658.

5. Lev M. The normal anatomy of conduction system in man and its pathology in A-V block. Ann NY Acad Sci 1964;III817.

6. Lower RR, Stofer RC, Shumway NE. Autotransplantation of the pulmonic valve into the aorta. J Thorac Cardiovasc Surg 1960;39:680.

7. Lytle BW, Cosgrove DM 3rd, Taylor PC, Goormastic M, Stewart RW, Golding LA, et al. Primary isolated aortic valve replacement: early and late results. J Thorac Cardiovasc Surg 1989;97:675.

8. Lee G, Grehl TM, Jaye JA, Kaku RF, Harter W, DeMaria AN, et al. Hemodynamic assessment of the new aortic Carpentier-Edwards bioprosthesis. Catheter Cardiovasc Diagn 1978;4:373.

9. Levine FH, Buckley MJ, Austen WG. Hemodynamic evaluation of the Hancock-modified orifice bioprosthesis in the aortic position. Circulation 1978;58:I33.

10. Lytle BW, Cosgrove DM 3rd, Loop FD, Taylor PC, Gill CC, Golding LA, et al. Replacement of aortic valve combined with myocardial revascularization: determinants of early and late risk for 500 patients, 1967-1981. Circulation 1983;68:1149.

11. Lakier JB, Copans H, Rosman HS, Lam R, Fine G, Khaja F, et al. Idiopathic degeneration of the aortic valve: a common cause of isolated aortic regurgitation. J Am Coll Cardiol 1985;5:347.

12. Lund O, Nielsen TT, Pilegaard HK, Magnussen K, Knudsen MA. The influence of coronary artery disease and bypass grafting on early and late survival after valve replacement for aortic stenosis. J Thorac Cardiovasc Surg 1990;100:327.

13. Lund O, Voeth M. Prediction of late results following valve replacement in aortic valve stenosis: seventeen years of follow-up examined with the Cox regression analysis. J Thorac Cardiovasc Surg 1987;35:295.

14. Lytle BW, Cosgrove DM 3rd, Gill CC, Taylor PC, Stewart RW, Golding LA, et al. Aortic valve replacement combined with myocardial revascularization. J Thorac Cardiovasc Surg 1988;95:402.

15. Lorch G, Kennedy JW, Gould KL. Severe stenosis of a viable homograft aortic valve. J Thorac Cardiovasc Surg 1976;71:932.

16. Laffort P, Roudaut R, Roques X, Lafitte S, Deville C, Bonnet J, et al. Early and long-term (one-year) effects of the association of aspirin and oral anticoagulant on thrombi and morbidity after replacement of the mitral valve with the St. Jude Medical prosthesis. J Am Coll Cardiol 2000;35:739.

17. Lund O, Chandrasekaran V, Grocott-Mason R, Elwidaa H, Mazhar R, Khaghani A, et al. Primary aortic valve replacement with allografts over twenty-five years: valve-related and procedure-related determinants of outcome. J Thorac Cardiovasc Surg 1999;117:77.

18. Laske A, Jenni R, Maloigne M, Vassalli G, Bertel O, Turina MI. Pressure gradients across bileaflet aortic valves by direct measurement and echocardiography. Ann Thorac Surg 1996;61:1418.

19. Lund O. Preoperative risk evaluation and stratification of long-term survival after valve replacement for aortic stenosis: reasons for earlier operative intervention. Circulation 1990;82:124.

20. Legarra JJ, Llorens R, Catalan M, Segura I, Trenor AM, de Buruaga JS, et al. Eighteen-year follow-up after Hancock II bioprosthesis insertion. J Heart Valve Dis 1999;8:16.

21. Luciani GB, Casali G, Mazzucco A. Risk factors for coronary complications after stentless aortic root replacement. Semin Thorac Cardiovasc Surg 1999;2:126.

22. Levy D, Garrison RJ, Savage DD, Kannel WB, Castelli WP. Prognostic implications of echocardiographically determined left ventricular mass in the Framingham Heart Study. N Engl J Med 1990;322:1561.

23. Luciani GB, Barozzi L, Tomezzoli A, Casali G, Mazzucco A. Bicuspid aortic valve disease and pulmonary autograft root dilatation after the Ross procedure: a clinicopathologic study. J Thorac Cardiovasc Surg 2001;122:74.

24. Lauer MS, Blackstone EH, Young JB, Topol EJ. Cause of death in clinical research: time for a reassessment? J Am Coll Cardiol 1999;34:618.

M

1. MacManus Q, Grunkemeier GL, Lambert LE, Starr A. Non-cloth-covered caged-ball prostheses: the second decade. J Thorac Cardiovasc Surg 1978;76:788.

2. Maron BJ, Ferrans VJ, Roberts WC. Myocardial ultrastructure in patients with chronic aortic valve disease. Am J Cardiol 1975;35:725.

3. Moraskl RE, Russell RO Jr, Mantle JA, Rackley CE. Aortic stenosis, angina pectoris, coronary artery disease. Catheter Cardiovasc Diagn 1976;2:157.

4. Morris DC, King SB 3rd, Douglas JS Jr, Wickliffe CW, Jones EL. Hemodynamic results of aortic valvular replacement with the porcine xenograft valve. Circulation 1977;56:841.

5. Miller GA, Kirklin JW, Swan HJ. Myocardial function and left ventricular volumes in acquired valvular insufficiency. Circulation 1965;31:374.

6. McGoon DC. Prosthetic reconstruction of the aortic valve. Mayo Clin Proc 1961;36:88.

7. McIlduff JB, Foster ED. Disruption of a normal aortic valve as a result of blunt chest trauma. J Trauma 1978;18:373.

8. Machler HE, Bergmann P, Anelli-Monti M, Dacar D, Rehak P, Kenz I, et al. Minimally invasive versus conventional aortic valve operations: a prospective study in 120 patients. Ann Thorac Surg 1999;67:1001.

9. Miller DC, Stinson EB, Oyer PE, Rossiter SJ, Reitz BA, Shumway NE. Surgical implications and results of combined aortic valve replacement and myocardial revascularization. Am J Cardiol 1979;43:494.

10. Mirsky I, Henschke C, Hess OM, Krayenbuehl HP. Prediction of postoperative performance in aortic valve disease. Am J Cardiol 1981;48:195.

11. Manouguian S, Seybold-Epting W. Patch enlargement of the aortic valve ring by extending the aortic incision into the anterior mitral leaflet: new operative technique. J Thorac Cardiovasc Surg 1979;78:402.

12. Mori T, Kawashima Y, Kitamura S, Nakano S, Kawachi K, Nakata T. Results of aortic valve replacement in patients with a narrow aortic annulus: effects of enlargement of the aortic annulus. Ann Thorac Surg 1981;31:111.

13. Milano AD, Bortolotti U, Mazzucco A, Guerra F, Magni A, Gallucci V. Aortic valve replacement with the Hancock standard, Bjork-Shiley, and Lillehei-Kaster prostheses. J Thorac Cardiovasc Surg 1989;98:37.

14. McGoon DC, Moffett EA. Total prosthetic reconstruction of the aortic valve. J Thorac Cardiovasc Surg 1963;45:162.

15. Murray G. Homologous aortic valve segment transplant as surgical treatment for aortic and mitral insufficiency. Angiology 1956;7:466.

16. Melina G, Rubens MB, Birks EJ, Bizzarri F, Khaghani A, Yacoub MH. A quantitative study of calcium deposition in the aortic wall following Medtronic Freestyle compared with homograft aortic root replacement: a prospective randomized trial. J Heart Valve Dis 2000;9:97.

17. McGoon DC, Mankin HT, Kirklin JW. Results of open heart operation for acquired aortic valve disease. J Thorac Cardiovasc Surg 1963;45:47.

18. McGoon DC, Ellis FH Jr, Kirklin JW. Late results of operation for acquired aortic valvular disease. Circulation 1965;31/32:I108.

19. Misbach GA, Allen MD, Stewart DK, Kruse AP, Ivey TD. Aortic valve replacement in the elderly: a standard for percutaneous valvuloplasty. J Thorac Cardiovasc Surg (in press).

20. McKay RG, Safian RD, Lock JE, Diver DJ, Berman AD, Warren SE, et al. Assessment of left ventricular and aortic valve function after aortic balloon valvuloplasty in adult patients with critical aortic stenosis. Circulation 1987;75:192.

21. Maxwell L, Gavin JB, Barratt-Boyes BG. Uneven host tissue on-growth and tissue detachment in stent mounted heart valve allografts and xenografts. Cardiovasc Res 1989;23:709.

22. McKay RG, Safian RD, Lock JE, Mandell VS, Thurer RL, Schnitt SJ, et al. Balloon dilatation of calcific aortic stenosis in elderly patients: postmortem, intraoperative, and percutaneous valvuloplasty studies. Circulation 1986;74:119.

23. Mindich BP, Guarino T, Goldman ME. Aortic valvuloplasty for acquired aortic stenosis. Circulation 1986;74:I130.

24. Magovern JA, Pennock JL, Campbell DB, Pae WE, Bartholomew M, Pierce WS, et al. Aortic valve replacement and combined aortic valve replacement and coronary artery bypass grafting: predicting high risk groups. J Am Coll Cardiol 1987;9:38.

25. Mullaney CJ, Elveback LR, Frye RL, Pluth JR, Edwards WD, Orszulak TA, et al. Coronary artery disease and its management: influence on survival in patients undergoing aortic valve replacement. J Am Coll Cardiol 1987;10:66.

26. Maxwell L, Gavin JB, Barratt-Boyes BG. Differences between heart valve allografts and xenografts in the incidence and initiation of dystrophic calcification. Pathology 1989;21:5.

27. Monrad ES, Hess OM, Murakami T, Nonogi H, Corin WJ, Krayenbuehl HP. Time course of regression of left ventricular hypertrophy after aortic valve replacement. Circulation 1988;77:1345.

28. Miller DC, Shumway NE: "Fresh" aortic allografts. long-term results with free-hand aortic valve replacement. J Card Surg 1987;185.

29. Mayne AS, Christie GW, Smaill BH, Hunter PJ, Barratt-Boyes BG. An assessment of the mechanical properties of leaflets from four second-generation porcine bioprostheses with biaxial testing techniques. J Thorac Cardiovasc Surg 1989;98:170.

30. McKowen RL, Campbell DN, Woelfel GF, Wiggins JW Jr, Clarke DR. Extended aortic root replacement with aortic allografts. J Thorac Cardiovasc Surg 1987;93:366.

31. Morishita K, Abe T, Fukada J, Sato H, Shiiku C. A surgical method for selecting appropriate size of graft in aortic root remodeling. Ann Thorac Surg 1998;65:1795.

32. Moreno-Cabrol RJ. Mini-T sternotomy for cardiac operations (letter). J Thorac Cardiovasc Surg 1997;113:810.

33. Maselli D, Pizi R, Bruno LP, Di Bella I, De Gasperis C. Left ventricular mass reduction after aortic valve replacement: homografts, stentless and stented valves. Ann Thorac Surg 1999;67:966.

34. Murphy ES, Lawson RM, Starr A, Rahimtoola SH. Severe aortic stenosis in patients 60 years of age or older: left ventricular function and 10-year survival after valve replacement. Circulation 1981;64:II184.

35. Mahoney CB, Miller CD, Kahn SS, Hill JD, Cohn LH. Twenty-three year, three-institution evaluation of the Hancock modified orifice aortic valve durability: comparison of actual and actuarial results. Circulation 1998;98:II88.

36. Medalion B, Lytle BW, McCarthy PM, Stewart RW, Arheart KL, Arnold JH, et al. Aortic valve replacement for octogenarians: are small valves bad? Ann Thorac Surg 1998;66:699.

37. Masters RG, Pipe AL, Walley VM, Keon WJ. Comparative results with the St. Jude Medical and Medtronic-Hall mechanical valves. J Thorac Cardiovasc Surg 1995;110:663.

38. Medalion B, Blackstone EH, Lytle BW, White J, Arnold JH, Cosgrove DM 3rd. Aortic valve replacement: is valve size important? J Thorac Cardiovasc Surg 2000;119:963.

39. Merick AF, Yacoub MH, Ho SY, Anderson RH. Anatomy of the muscular subpulmonary infundibulum with regard to the Ross procedure. Ann Thorac Surg 2000;69:556.

40. McDonald ML, Smedira NG, Blackstone EH, Grimm RA, Lytle BW, Cosgrove DM 3rd. Reduced survival in women after valve surgery for aortic regurgitation: impact of aortic enlargement and late aortic rupture. J Thorac Cardiovasc Surg 2000;119:1205.

41. Mehta RH, Bruckman D, Das S, Tsai T, Russman P, Karavite D, et al. Implications of increased left ventricular mass index on in-hospital outcomes in patients undergoing aortic valve surgery. J Thorac Cardiovasc Surg 2001;122:919.

42. McGiffin DC, O'Brien MF, Galbraith AJ, McLachlan GJ, Stafford EG, Gardner MA, et al. An analysis of risk factors for death and mode-specific death after aortic valve replacement with allograft, xenograft, and mechanical valves. J Thorac Cardiovasc Surg 1993; 106:895.

43. Milsom FP, Doty DB. Aortic valve replacement and mitral valve repair with allograft. J Card Surg 1993;8:350.

N

1. Najafi H, Ostermiller WE Jr, Javid H, Dye WS, Hunter JA, Julian OC. Narrow aortic root complicating aortic valve replacement. Arch Surg 1969;99:690.

2. Nicks R, Cartmill T, Bernstein L. Hypoplasia of the aortic root. Thorax 1970;25:339.

3. Norman JC, Nihill MR, Cooley DA. Valved apico-aortic composite conduits for left ventricular outflow tract obstructions. Am J Cardiol 1980;45:1265.

4. Nair CK, Sketch MH, Ahmed I, Thomson W, Ryschon K, Woodruff MP, et al. Calcific valvular aortic stenosis with and without mitral anular calcium. Am J Cardiol 1987;60:865.

5. Nicoloff DM, Emery RW, Arom KV, Northup WF 3rd, Jorgensen CR, Wang Y, et al. Clinical and hemodynamic results with the St. Jude Medical cardiac valve prosthesis. J Thorac Cardiovasc Surg 1981; 82:674.

6. Nagy ZL, Fisher J, Walker PG, Watterson KG. The effect of sizing on the hydrodynamic parameters of the Medtronic freestyle valve in vitro. Ann Thorac Surg 2000;69:1408.

7. Nakano S, Kawashima Y, Matsuda H, Sakai K, Taniguchi K, Kawamoto T, et al. A five-year appraisal and hemodynamic evaluation of the Bjork-Shiley Monostrut valve. J Thorac Cardiovasc Surg 1991; 101:881.

8. Nishimura RA, Tajik AJ. Quantitative hemodynamics by Doppler echocardiography: a noninvasive alternative to cardiac catheterization. Prog Cardiovasc Dis 1994;36:309.

9. Niwaya K, Knott-Craig CJ, Santangelo K, Lane MM, Chandrasekaran K, Elkins RC. Advantage of autograft and homograft valve replacement for complex aortic valve endocarditis. Ann Thorac Surg 1999;67:1603.

O

1. O'Toole JD, Geiser EA, Reddy PS, Curtiss EI, Landfair RM. Effect of preoperative ejection fraction on survival and hemodynamic improvement following aortic valve replacement. Circulation 1978;58:1175.

2. O'Brien KP, Hitchcock GC, Barratt-Boyes BG, Lowe JB. Spontaneous aortic cusp rupture associated with valvular myxomatous transformation. Circulation 1968;37:273.

3. Okita Y, Franciosi G, Matsuki O, Robles A, Ross DN. Early and late results of aortic root replacement with antibiotic-sterilized aortic homograft. J Thorac Cardiovasc Surg 1988;95:696.

4. Olin CL, Bomfim V, Halvazulis V, Holmgren AG, Lamke BJ. Optimal insertion technique for the Bjork-Shiley valve in the narrow aortic ostium. Ann Thorac Surg 1983;36:567.

5. O'Brien MF, Stafford EG, Gardner MA, Pohlner PG, McGiffin DC. A comparison of aortic valve replacement with viable cryopreserved and fresh allograft valves, with a note on chromosomal studies. J Thorac Cardiovasc Surg 1987;94:812.

6. Olson LJ, Subramanian R, Edwards WD. Surgical pathology of pure aortic insufficiency: a study of 225 cases. Mayo Clin Proc 1984; 59:835.

7. O'Keefe JH Jr, Vlietstra RE, Bailey KR, Holmes DR Jr. Natural history of candidates for balloon aortic valvuloplasty. Mayo Clin Proc 1987;62:986.

8. O'Brien MF, McGiffin DC, Stafford EG. Allograft aortic valve implantation: techniques for all types of aortic valve and root pathology. Ann Thorac Surg 1989;48:600.

9. Oh JK, Hatle LK, Seward JB, Danielson GK, Schaff HV, Reeder GS, et al. Diagnostic role of Doppler echocardiography in constrictive pericarditis. J Am Coll Cardiol 1994;23:154.

10. Otto CM, Burwash IG, Legget ME, Munt BI, Fujioka M, Healy NL, et al. Prospective study of asymptomatic valvular aortic stenosis: clinical, echocardiographic, and exercise predictors of outcome. Circulation 1997;95:2262.

11. O'Brien MF. The 28-year, 99.3% follow-up of 1022 homograft aortic valve replacement patients (abstract). Presented at World Symposium on Heart Valve Disease, London, 1999.

12. O'Brien MF, Stafford EG, Gardner MA, Pohlner PG, Tesar PJ, Cochrane AD, et al. Allograft aortic valve replacement: long-term follow-up. Ann Thorac Surg 1995;60:S65.

13. Oury JH, Doty DB, Oswalt JD, Knapp JF, Mackey SK, Duran CM. Cardiopulmonary response to maximal exercise in young athletes following the Ross procedure. Ann Thorac Surg 1998;66:S153.

14. Odell JA, Mullany CJ, Schaff HV, Orszulak TA, Daly RC, Morris JJ. Aortic valve replacement after previous coronary artery bypass grafting. Ann Thorac Surg 1996;62:1424.

15. Oury JH, Mackey SK, Duran CM. Critical analysis of the Ross procedure: do its problems justify wider application? Semin Thorac Cardiovasc Surg 1999;2:55.

16. O'Keefe JH Jr, Shub C, Rettke SR. Risk of noncardiac surgical procedures in patients with aortic stenosis. Mayo Clin Proc 1989; 64:400.

17. Oswalt J. Management of aortic infective endocarditis by autograft valve replacement. J Heart Valve Dis 1994;3:377.

P

1. Pantely G, Morton M, Rahimtoola SH. Effects of successful, uncomplicated valve replacement on ventricular hypertrophy, volume, and performance in aortic stenosis and in aortic incompetence. J Thorac Cardiovasc Surg 1978;75:383.

2. Papadimitriou JM, Hopkins BE, Taylor RR. Regression of left ventricular dilation and hypertrophy after removal of volume overload. Circ Res 1974;35:127.

3. Passik CS, Ackermann DM, Pluth JR, Edwards WD. Temporal changes in the causes of aortic stenosis: a surgical pathologic study of 646 cases. Mayo Clin Proc 1987;62:119.

4. Pakrashi BC, Mary DA, Garcia JB, Ionescu MI. Recovery from complete heart block following aortic valve replacement. Arch Surg 1974;108:373.

5. Puig LB, Verginelli G, Belotti G, Kawabe L, Frack CC, Pileggi F, et al. Homologous dura mater cardiac valve: preliminary study of 30 cases. J Thorac Cardiovasc Surg 1972;64:154.

6. Pomerance A. Isolated aortic stenosis. In Pomerance A, Davies MI, eds. The pathology of the heart. London: Blackwell, 1975, p. 327.

7. Pacifico AD, Karp RB, Kirklin JW. Homografts for replacement of the aortic valve. Circulation 1972;45/46:I36.

8. Pyle RB, Mayer JE Jr, Lindsay WG, Jorgensen CR, Wang Y, Nicoloff DM. Hemodynamic evaluation of Lillehei-Kaster and Starr-Edwards prostheses. Ann Thorac Surg 1978;26:336.

9. Piehler JM, Danielson GK, Pluth JR, Orszulak TA, Puga FJ, Schaff HV, et al. Enlargement of the aortic root or anulus with autogenous pericardial patch during aortic valve replacement. J Thorac Cardiovasc Surg 1983;86:350.

10. Pellikka PA, Nishimura RA, Bailey KR, Tajik AJ. The natural history of adults with asymptomatic, hemodynamically significant aortic stenosis. J Am Coll Cardiol 1990;15:1012.

11. Petrou M, Wong K, Albertucci M, Brecker SJ, Yacoub MH. Evaluation of unstented aortic homografts for the treatment of prosthetic aortic valve endocarditis. Circulation 1994;90:II198.

12. Poirier NC, Pelletier C, Pellerin M, Carrier M. 15-year experience with the Carpentier-Edwards pericardial bioprosthesis. Ann Thorac Surg 1998;66:S57.

13. Perin EC, Jin BS, de Castro CM, Ferguson JJ, Hall RJ. Doppler echocardiography in 180 normally functioning St. Jude Medical aortic valve prostheses. Chest 1991;100:988.

14. Pelletier LC, LeClerc Y, Bonan R, Crepeau J, Dyrda I. Aortic valve replacement with the Carpentier-Edwards pericardial bioprosthesis: clinical and hemodynamic results. J Card Surg 1988;3:405.

15. Pompili MF, Stevens JH, Burdon TA, Siegel LC, Peters WS, Ribakove GH, et al. Port-access mitral valve replacement in dogs. J Thorac Surg 1996;112:1268.

16. Pau KK, Yakub A, Awang Y. Minimally invasive aortic valve surgery: pocket AVR. J Thorac Cardiovasc Surg 1998;115:255.

17. Pibarot P, Dumesnil JG, Jobin J, Cartier P, Honos G, Durand LG. Hemodynamic and physical performance during maximal exercise in patients with an aortic bioprosthetic valve. J Am Coll Cardiol 1999;34:1609.

18. Prager RL, Fischer CR, Kong B, Byrne JP, Jones DJ, Hance ML, et al. The aortic homograft: evolution of indications, techniques, and results in 107 patients. Ann Thorac Surg 1997;64:659.

19. Porter GF, Skillington PD, Bjorksten AR, Morgan JG, Yapanis AG, Grigg LE. Exercise hemodynamic performance of the pulmonary autograft following the Ross procedure. J Heart Valve Dis 1999;8:516.

20. Pibarot P, Dumesnil JG. Patient-prosthesis mismatch is not negligible. Ann Thorac Surg 2000;69:1983.

21. Pibarot P, Dumesnil JG, Cartier PC, Metras J, Lemieux MD. Patient-prosthesis mismatch can be predicted at the time of operation. Ann Thorac Surg 2001;71:S265.

R

1. Ross J Jr, Braunwald E. Aortic stenosis. Circulation 1968;38:V61.

2. Ross J Jr. Afterload mismatch and preload reserve: a conceptual framework for the analysis of ventricular function. Prog Cardiovasc Dis 1976;18:255.

3. Ross DN. Replacement of aortic and mitral valves with a pulmonary autograft. Lancet 1967;2:956.

4. Rastan H, Koncz J. Plastische Erweiterung der linken Ausflussbahn: eine neue Operationsmethode. Thorax Chir 1975;23:169.

5. Rastan H, Abu-Aishah N, Rastan D, Heisig B, Koncz J, Bjornstad PG, et al. Results of aortoventriculoplasty in 21 consecutive patients with left ventricular outflow tract obstruction. J Thorac Cardiovasc Surg 1978;75:659.

6. Robles A, Vaughan M, Lau JK, Bodnar E, Ross DN. Long-term assessment of aortic valve replacement with autologous pulmonary valve. Ann Thorac Surg 1985;39:238.

7. Rittenhouse EA, Sauvage LR, Stamm SJ, Mansfield PB, Hall DG, Herndon PS. Radical enlargement of the aortic root and outflow tract to allow valve replacement. Ann Thorac Surg 1979;27:367.

8. Roberts WC, Morrow AG, McIntosh CL, Jones M, Epstein SE. Congenitally bicuspid aortic valve causing severe, pure aortic regurgitation without superimposed infective endocarditis. Am J Cardiol 1981;47:206.

9. Richardson JV, Karp RB, Kirklin JW, Dismukes WE. Treatment of infective endocarditis: a 10-year comparative analysis. Circulation 1978;58:589.

10. Ross DN. Homograft replacement of the aortic valve. Lancet 1962;2:487.

11. Roberts WC, Kehoe JA, Carpenter DF, Golden A. Cardiac valvular lesions in rheumatoid arthritis. Arch Intern Med 1980;122:141.

12. Ross DN, Martelli V, Wain WH. Allograft and autograft valves used for aortic valve replacement. In Ionescu MI, ed. Tissue heart valves. London: Butterworth, 1979.

13. Rehr RB, Mack M, Firth BG. Aortic regurgitation and sinus of Valsalva–right atrial fistula after blunt thoracic trauma. Br Heart J 1982;48:420.

14. Rossiter SJ, Miller DC, Stinson EB, Oyer PE, Reitz BA, Moreno-Cabral RJ, et al. Hemodynamic and clinical comparisons of the Hancock modified orifice and standard orifice bioprostheses in the aortic position. J Thorac Cardiovasc Surg 1980;80:54.

15. Randolph JD, Toal K, Stelzer P, Elkins RC. Aortic valve and left ventricular outflow tract replacement using allograft and autograft valves: a preliminary report. Ann Thorac Surg 1989;48:345.

16. Rapaport E. Natural history of aortic and mitral valve disease. Am J Cardiol 1975;35:221.

17. Rizzoli G, Russo R, Valente S, Mazzucco A, Valfre C, Brumana T, et al. Dehiscence of aortic valve prostheses: analysis of a ten-year experience. Int J Cardiol 1984;6:207.

18. Ross DN. Applications of homografts in clinical surgery. J Card Surg 1987;2:175.

19. Rothkopf M, Davidson T, Lipscomb K, Narahara K, Hillis LD, Willerson JT, et al. Hemodynamic evaluation of the Carpentier-Edwards bioprosthesis in the aortic position. Am J Cardiol 1979;44:209.

20. Roger VL, Tajik AJ, Bailey KR, Oh JK, Taylor CL, Seward JB. Progression of aortic stenosis in adults: new appraisal using Doppler echocardiography. Am Heart J 1990;119:331.

21. Ross Registry International Summary Report, 1999, Missoula, Montana.

22. Rahimtoola SH. Catheter balloon valvuloplasty for severe calcific aortic stenosis: a limited role. J Am Coll Cardiol 1994;23:1076.

23. Reardon MJ, Conklin LD, Philo R, Letsou GV, Safi HJ, Espada R. The anatomical aspects of minimally invasive cardiac valve operations. Ann Thorac Surg 1999;67:266.

S

1. Spagnuolo M, Kloth H, Taranta A, Doyle E, Pasternack B. Natural history of rheumatic aortic regurgitation: criteria predictive of death, congestive heart failure, and angina in young patients. Circulation 1971;44:368.

2. Smithy HG, Parker EF. Experimental aortic valvulotomy: preliminary report. Surg Gynecol Obstet 1947;34:625.

3. Segal J, Harvery WP, Hufnagel C. A clinical study of one hundred cases of severe aortic insufficiency. Am J Med 1956;21:200.

4. Spangler RD, McCallister BD, McGoon DC. Aortic valve replacement in patients with severe aortic valve incompetence associated with rheumatoid spondylitis. Am J Cardiol 1970;26:130.

5. Schwarz F, Flameng W, Thormann J, Sesto M, Langebartels F, Hehrlein F, et al. Recovery from myocardial failure after aortic valve replacement. J Thorac Cardiovasc Surg 1978;75:854.

6. Spray TL, Roberts WC. Structural changes in porcine xenografts used as substitute cardiac valves. Am J Cardiol 1977;40:319.

7. Schwarz F, Schaper J, Flameng W, Hehrlein FW. Correlation between left ventricular function and myocardial ultrastructure in patients with aortic valve disease (abstract). Circulation 1976;53/54:II67.

8. Smith HJ, Neutze JM, Roche AH, Agnew TM, Barratt-Boyes BG. The natural history of rheumatic aortic regurgitation and the indications for surgery. Br Heart J 1976;38:147.

9. Schuler G, Peterson KL, Johnson AD, Francis G, Ashburn W, Dennish G, et al. Serial noninvasive assessment of left ventricular hypertrophy and function after surgical correction of aortic regurgitation. Am J Cardiol 1979;44:585.

10. Schwarz F, Flameng W, Langebartels F, Sesto M, Walter P, Schlepper M. Impaired left ventricular function in chronic aortic valve disease: survival and function after replacement by Bjork-Shiley prosthesis. Circulation 1979;60:48.

11. Schaff HV, Borkon AM, Hughes C, Achuff S, Donahoo JS, Gardner TJ, et al. Clinical and hemodynamic evaluation of the 19 mm Bjork-Shiley aortic valve prosthesis. Ann Thorac Surg 1981;32:50.

12. Schwarz F, Flameng W, Schaper J, Hehrlein F. Correlation between myocardial structure and diastolic properties of the heart in chronic aortic valve disease: effects of corrective surgery. Am J Cardiol 1978;42:895.

13. Seybold-Epting W, Hoffmeister HE. Clinical experience with enlargement of the aortic anulus by extension of the aortic incision into the anterior mitral leaflet. Thorac Cardiovasc Surg 1980;28:420.

14. Scott WC, Miller DC, Haverich A, Dawkins K, Mitchell RS, Jamieson SW, et al. Determinants of operative mortality for patients undergoing aortic valve replacement. J Thorac Cardiovasc Surg 1985;89:400.

15. Safian RD, Mandell VS, Thurer RE, Hutchins GM, Schnitt SJ, Grossman W, et al. Postmortem and intraoperative balloon valvuloplasty of calcific aortic stenosis in elderly patients: mechanisms of successful dilation. J Am Coll Cardiol 1987;9:655.

16. Starr A, Edwards ML, McCord CW, Griswold HE. Aortic replacement: clinical experience with a semirigid ball-valve prosthesis. Circulation 1963;27:779.

17. Senning A. Fascia lata replacement of aortic valves. J Thorac Cardiovasc Surg 1967;54:465.

18. Savunen T. Cardiovascular abnormalities in the relatives of patients operated upon for annulo-aortic ectasia. Eur J Cardiothorac Surg 1987;1:3.

19. Subramanian R, Olson LJ, Edwards WD. Surgical pathology of pure aortic stenosis: a study of 374 cases. Mayo Clin Proc 1984;59:683.

20. Strickett MG, Barratt-Boyes BG, MacCulloch D. Disinfection of human heart valve allografts with antibiotics in low concentration. Pathology 1983;15:457.

21. Stelzer P, Jones DJ, Elkins RC. Aortic root replacement with pulmonary autograft. Circulation 1989;80:III209.

22. Schoof PH, Gittenberger-De Groot AC, De Heer E, Bruijn JA, Hazekamp MG, Huysmans HA. Remodeling of the porcine pulmonary autograft wall in the aortic position. J Thorac Cardiovasc Surg 2000;120:55.

23. Shean FC, Austen WG, Buckley MJ, Mundth ED, Scannell JG, Daggett WM. Survival after Starr-Edwards aortic valve replacement. Circulation 1971;44:1.

24. Sabet HY, Edwards WD, Tazelaar HD, Daly RC. Congenitally bicuspid aortic valves: a surgical pathology study of 542 cases (1991 through 1996) and a literature review of 2,715 additional cases. Mayo Clin Proc 1999;74:14.

25. Subramanian R, Olson LJ, Edwards WD. Surgical pathology of combined aortic stenosis and insufficiency: a study of 213 cases. Mayo Clin Proc 1985;60:247.

26. Stewart BF, Siscovick D, Lind BK, Gardin JM, Gottdiener JS, Smith VE, et al. Clinical factors associated with calcific aortic valve disease. J Am Coll Cardiol 1997;29:630.

27. Schmidtke C, Bechtel JF, Hueppe M, Noetzold A, Sievers HH. Size and distensibility of the aortic root and aortic valve function after different techniques of the Ross procedure. J Thorac Cardiovasc Surg 2000;119:990.

28. Sezai A, Shiono M, Orime Y, Hata H, Yagi S, Negishi N, et al. Evaluation of valve sound and its effects on ATS prosthetic valves in patients' quality of life. Ann Thorac Surg 2000;69:507.

29. Scognamiglio R, Rahimtoola SH, Fasoli G, Nistri S, Dalla Volta S. Nifedipine in asymptomatic patients with severe aortic regurgitation and normal left ventricular function. N Engl J Med 1994;331:689.

30. Stelzer P, Weinrauch S, Tranbaugh RF. Ten years of experience with the modified Ross procedure. J Thorac Cardiovasc Surg 1998; 115:1091.

31. Sintek CF, Fletcher AD, Khonsari S. Small aortic root in the elderly: use of stentless bioprosthesis. J Heart Valve Dis 1996;5:S308.

32. Svensson LG. Minimal-access "J" or "j" sternotomy for valvular aortic and coronary operations or reoperations. Ann Thorac Surg 1997;64:1501.

33. Svensson LG, D'Agostino RS. "J" incision minimal-access valve operations. Ann Thorac Surg 1998;66:1110.

34. Szwerc MF, Benckart DH, Weichmann RJ, Savage EB, Szydlowski GW, Magovern GJ Jr, et al. Partial versus full sternotomy for aortic valve replacement. Ann Thorac Surg 1999;68:2209.

35. Society of Thoracic Surgeons National Database Committee. Annual Report 1999. Durham, N.C.: STS, 2000, p. 52.

36. Schwarz F, Bauman P, Manthey J, Hoffman M, Schuler G, Mehmel HC, et al. The effect of aortic valve replacement on survival. Circulation 1982;66:1105.

37. Smith N, McAnulty JH, Rahimtoola SH. Severe aortic stenosis with impaired left ventricular function and clinical heart failure: results of valve replacement. Circulation 1978;58:255.

38. Sabik JF, Lytle BW, Blackstone EH, Marullo AG, Pettersson GB, Cosgrove DM. Aortic root replacement with cryopreserved allograft for prosthetic valve endocarditis. Ann Thorac Surg 2002;74:650.

39. Society of Thoracic Surgeons National Database Committee. Grover FL, Chairman, Peterson ED, Principal Investigator. Annual Report 2001, Durham N.C., p. 46.

40. Silberman S, Shaheen J, Merin O, Fink D, Shapira N, Liviatan-Strauss N, et al. Exercise hemodynamics of aortic prostheses: comparison between stentless bioprostheses and mechanical valves. Ann Thorac Surg 2001;72:1217.

T

1. Thompson R, Yacoub M, Ahmed M, Seabra-Gomes R, Rickards A, Towers M. Influence of preoperative left ventricular function on results of homograft replacement of the aortic valve for aortic stenosis. Am J Cardiol 1979;43:929.

2. Tompsett R, Lubash GD. Aortic valve perforation in bacterial endocarditis. Circulation 1961;23:662.

3. Tweden KS, Cameron JD, Razzouk AF, Holmberg WR, Kelly SJ. Biocompatibility of silver-modified polyester for antimicrobial protection of prosthetic valves: J Heart Valve Dis 1997;6:553.

4. Tepley JF, Grunkemeier GJ, Sutherland HD, Lambert LE, Johnson VA, Starr A. The ultimate prognosis after valve replacement: an assessment at twenty years. Ann Thorac Surg 1981;32:111.

5. Tweden KS, Cameron JD, Razzouk AJ, Bianco RW, Holmberg WR, Bricault RJ, et al. Silver modification of polyethylene terephthalate textiles for antimicrobial protection. ASΛIO J 1997;43:M475.

6. Tonnemacher D. Myxomatous degeneration of the aortic valve is a common cause of severe pure aortic regurgitation (abstract). J Am Coll Cardiol 1985;5:505.

7. Tatineni S, Barner HB, Pearson AC, Halbe D, Woodruff R, Labovitz AJ. Rest and exercise evaluation of St. Jude Medical and Medtronic-Hall prostheses: influence of primary lesion, valvular type, valvular size, and left ventricular function. Circulation 1989;80:I16.

8. Tribouilloy CM, Enriquez-Sarano M, Bailey KR, Tajik AJ, Seward JB, Tajik AJ. Assessment of severity of aortic regurgitation using the width of the vena contracta: a clinical color Doppler imaging study. Circulation 2000;102:558.

9. Turina J, Turina M, Rothlin M, Krayenbuehl HP. Improved late survival in patients with chronic aortic regurgitation by earlier operation. Circulation 1984;70:I147.

10. Torsher LC, Shub C, Rettke SR, Brown DL. Risk of patients with severe aortic stenosis undergoing noncardiac surgery. Am J Cardiol 1998;81:448.

11. Takkenberg JJ, Eikemans MJ, van Herwerden LA, Steyerberg EW, Grunkemeier GL, Habbema JD, et al. Estimated event-free life expectancy after autograft aortic root replacement in adults. Ann Thorac Surg 2001;71:S344.

U

1. U.S. IDE Centers, Medtronic. 1999 Post Approval Report, Freestyle.
2. U.S. IDE Centers, Medtronic. 1999 Post Approval Report, Hancock II.
3. U.S. IDE Centers, Baxter Healthcare. 1997 Post Approval Report, PERIMOUNT 2700.

V

1. Verheul HA, van den Brink RB, Bouma BJ, Hoedemaker G, Moulijn AC, Dekker E, et al. Analysis of risk factors for excess mortality after aortic valve replacement. J Am Coll Cardiol 1995;26:1280.
2. Virdi IS, Monro JL, Ross JK. Eleven year experience of aortic valve replacement with antibiotic sterilized homograft valves in Southampton. Thorac Cardiovasc Surg 1986;34:277.
3. Vesely I, Casarotto DC, Gerosa G. Mechanics of cryopreserved aortic and pulmonary homografts. J Heart Valve Dis 2000;9:27.

W

1. Wideman FE, Blackstone EH, Kirklin JW, Karp RB, Kouchoukos NT, Pacifico AD. The hospital mortality of rereplacement of the aortic valve: incremental risk factors. J Thorac Cardiovasc Surg 1981;82:870.
2. Williams JB, Karp RB, Kirklin JW, Kouchoukos NT, Pacifico AD, Zorn GL Jr, et al. Considerations in selection and management of patients undergoing valve replacement with glutaraldehyde-fixed porcine bioprostheses. Ann Thorac Surg 1980;30:247.
3. Wood P. Aortic stenosis. Am J Cardiol 1958;1:553.
4. Watts LK, Duffy P, Field RB, Stafford EG, O'Brien MF. Establishment of a viable homograft cardiac valve bank: a rapid method of determining homograft viability. Ann Thorac Surg 1976;21:230.
5. Wisenbaugh T, Booth D, DeMaria A, Nissen S, Waters J. Relationship of contractile state to ejection performance in patients with chronic aortic valve disease. Circulation 1986;73:47.
6. Warshawsky H, Abramson W. Complete heart block in calcareous aortic stenosis. Ann Intern Med 1947;27:1040.
7. Wortham DC, Tri TB, Bowen TE. Hemodynamic evaluation of the St. Jude Medical valve prosthesis in the small aortic anulus. J Thorac Cardiovasc Surg 1981;81:615.
8. Winter TQ, Reis RL, Glancy L, Roberts WC, Epstein SE, Morrow AG. Current status of the Starr-Edwards cloth-covered prosthetic cardiac valves. Circulation 1972;45/46:I1.
9. Woldow AB, Parameswaran R, Hartman J, Kotler MN. Aortic regurgitation due to aortic valve prolapse. Am J Cardiol 1985;55:1435.
10. William GA, Labovitz AJ, Nelson JG, Kennedy HL. Value of multiple echocardiographic views in the evaluation of aortic stenosis in adults by continuous-wave Doppler. Am J Cardiol 1985;55:445.
11. Walker DK, Scotten LN. A database obtained from in vitro function testing of mechanical heart valves. J Heart Valve Dis 1994;3:561.

12. Wan AT, Conyers RA, Coombs CJ, Masterton JP. Determination of silver in blood, urine, and tissues of volunteers and burn patients. Clin Chem 1991;37:1683.
13. Wiseth R, Levang OW, Sande E, Tangen G, Skjaerpe T, Hatle L. Hemodynamic evaluation by Doppler echocardiography of small (less than or equal to 21 mm) prostheses and bioprostheses in the aortic valve position. Am J Cardiol 1992; 70:240.
14. Walther T, Falk V, Langebartels G, Kruger M, Schilling L, Kiegeler A, et al. Regression of left ventricular hypertrophy after stentless versus conventional aortic valve replacement. Semin Thorac Cardiovasc Surg 1999;11:I8.
15. Wong SP, Legget ME, Greaves SC, Barratt-Boyes BG, Milsom FP, Raudkivi PJ. Early experience with the Mosaic bioprosthesis: a new generation porcine valve. Ann Thorac Surg 2000;69:1846.
16. Westaby S, Horton M, Jin XY, Katsumata T, Ahmed O, Pillai R, et al. Survival difference between stentless and stented bioprosthesis patients. Presented at the Society of Thoracic Surgeons 36th Annual Meeting, Ft. Lauderdale, Florida, 2000.
17. Walther T, Falk V, Weigl C, Diegeler A, Rauch T, Autschbach R, et al. Discrepancy of sizers for conventional and stentless aortic valve implants. J Heart Valve Dis 1997;6:145.

Y

1. Yacoub M, Rasmi NR, Sundt TM, Lund O, Boyland E, Radley-Smith R, et al. Fourteen-year experience with homovital homografts for aortic valve replacement. J Thorac Cardiovasc Surg 1995;110:186.
2. Yacoub MH. Applications and limitations of histocompatibility in clinical cardiac valve allograft surgery. In Yankah AC, Hetzer R, Miller DC, Ross DN, Somerville J, Yacoub MH, eds. Cardiac valve allografts 1962-1987. New York: Springer-Verlag, 1988, p. 95.
3. Yandah AC, Wottge HU, Muller-Ruchholtz W. Antigenicity and fate of cellular components of heart valve allografts. In Yankah AC, Hetzer R, Miller DC, Ross DN, Somerville J, Yacoub MH, eds. Cardiac valve allografts 1962-1987. New York: Springer-Verlag, 1988, p. 77.
4. Yacoub MH, Gehle P, Chandrasekaran V, Birks EJ, Child A, Radley-Smith R. Late results of a valve-preserving operation in patients with aneurysms of the ascending aorta and root. J Thorac Cardiovasc Surg 1998;115:1080.
5. Yoganathan AP, Heinrich RS, Fontaine AA. Fluid dynamics of prosthetic valves. In Otto CM, ed. The practice of clinical echocardiography. Philadelphia: WB Saunders, 1997.

Z

1. Zusman DR, Levine FH, Carter JE, Buckley MJ. Hemodynamic and clinical evaluation of the Hancock modified-orifice aortic bioprosthesis. Circulation 1981;64:II189.
2. Zwischenberger JB, Shalaby TZ, Conti VR. Viable cryopreserved aortic homograft for aortic valve endocarditis and annular abscesses. Ann Thorac Surg 1989;48:365.
3. Zellner JL, Kratz JM, Crumbley AJ 3rd, Stroud MR, Bradley SM, Sade RM, et al. Long-term experience with the St. Jude Medical valve prosthesis. Ann Thorac Surg 1999;68:1210.

13 Combined Aortic and Mitral Valve Disease with or without Tricuspid Valve Disease

DEFINITION

Acquired diseases of both the aortic and mitral valves severe enough to require simultaneous surgery (replacement, repair, or valvotomy) are considered in this chapter. Because tricuspid valve disease may form part of this spectrum and require simultaneous surgery, it is also considered, although discussed in more detail in Chapter 14.

HISTORICAL NOTE

Surgical treatment of combined aortic and mitral valve disease began during the early 1950s by closed methods. In 1955, Likoff and colleagues reported 74 patients who had undergone simultaneous closed repair of aortic and mitral stenosis by Bailey and Glover in Philadelphia.[L1] In 1958, Lillehei and colleagues were the first to report simultaneous repairs of both valves by open techniques using cardiopulmonary bypass (CPB).[L2] In 1963, soon after introduction of durable mechanical prostheses, Cartwright and colleagues first reported simultaneous aortic and mitral valve replacement.[C1] In 1964, Starr and colleagues reported 13 patients who had undergone multiple valve replacements, including one who received mechanical aortic, mitral, and tricuspid prostheses.[S1]

MORPHOLOGY

Morphology of diseases involving mitral, aortic, and tricuspid valves is described in Chapters 11, 12, and 14. In most patients, multivalvar disease is rheumatic in origin, but each valve may manifest a separate pathologic condition, for example, rheumatic aortic valve disease and mitral regurgitation from infective endocarditis, idiopathic chordal rupture, or ischemic papillary muscle dysfunction.

The effect of combined disease on morphology of the left ventricle (LV) is of great importance. Thus, at the extremes, combined aortic and mitral regurgitation imposes a large volume overload on the LV, and LV volume and wall thickness increase severely; combined aortic and mitral stenosis results in a small, thick-walled, noncompliant LV.

CLINICAL FEATURES AND DIAGNOSTIC CRITERIA

In general, clinical criteria and noninvasive diagnostic tests are the same for mitral and aortic valve disease whether they are combined or isolated, but additional cardiac catheterization and angiography data are more frequently needed when they are combined. In patients older than 40 years of age, coronary angiography is indicated routinely, and the valve lesions are assessed at that time.

One lesion is usually dominant and may modify the clinical signs of the less dominant one. A frequent problem is assessing severity of the less dominant lesion, because if it is mild, or even mild to moderate, it may not require simultaneous correction. Historically, it was sometimes possible to obtain reliable information on the second lesion during operation by palpating an atrial chamber to detect systolic pulsation, by feeling the valve directly with the finger before beginning cardiopulmonary bypass (CPB), or by exposing the valve. Today, with two-dimensional and color Doppler echocardiography, the status of the aortic, mitral, and tricuspid valves is usually known before the patient enters the operating room. Intraoperative use of transesophageal echocardiography (TEE) verifies this status, if necessary.

Dominant Aortic Stenosis

Dominant aortic stenosis is diagnosed by the same techniques used in isolated aortic stenosis (see Chapter 12). Dominant aortic stenosis may complicate diagnosing coexisting mitral stenosis by simple methods. The auscultatory signs of moderate mitral stenosis may be masked, and transmission of the aortic systolic murmur to the apex may confuse the assessment of mitral regurgitation. However, Doppler echocardiography can render as precise a diagnosis as in isolated mitral stenosis. Severity of pure mitral stenosis associated with aortic stenosis can be verified by pressure measurements (left atrium to LV) on the operating table, although varying cardiac output sometimes makes interpretation difficult. In questionable cases, the valve may be palpated on CPB or examined directly by opening the left atrium through the superior approach (see Chapter 11).

The most convincing sign of important mitral regurgitation associated with aortic stenosis is a right parasternal systolic lift, especially if associated with an apical third heart sound when the venous and hepatic pulses do not indicate important tricuspid regurgitation. More than modest left atrial enlargement on the posteroanterior chest radiograph and also P mitrale in the electrocardiogram strongly suggest important associated mitral valve disease. Two-dimensional echocardiography with Doppler color flow interrogation is helpful in identifying mitral regurgitation both preoperatively and intraoperatively.

Dominant Aortic Regurgitation

As noted in Chapter 12, an Austin Flint murmur can mimic that of mitral stenosis, the absence of which can be confirmed by two-dimensional echocardiography with Doppler color flow interrogation. If in addition to a mid-diastolic murmur there is an opening snap, left atrial enlargement

above grade 2, and P mitrale, then important mitral stenosis is usually present.

With dominant aortic stenosis, severity of associated mitral regurgitation requires careful assessment by two-dimensional echocardiography, particularly because it is frequently secondary to LV enlargement or dysfunction. If it is less than grade 2 in severity, it usually regresses after the aortic regurgitation is corrected. When the LV is severely enlarged, it is likely that both aortic and mitral regurgitation are severe.

Dominant Mitral Stenosis

Dominant mitral stenosis may minimize the usual signs and symptoms of coexisting aortic regurgitation. When aortic regurgitant flow is moderate or large, its presence and severity are readily assessed clinically by the character of the arterial pulse and blood pressure. At times, however, what seems to be less than grade 2 regurgitation becomes clearly moderate or severe after surgical relief of the mitral stenosis. Magnitude of aortic regurgitation cannot be assessed reliably at operation. Visual inspection of the aortic valve may provide information about extent of the rheumatic condition but not about magnitude of the leakage. Thus, evaluating the aortic valve preoperatively with two-dimensional echocardiography Doppler color flow interrogation is important before undertaking mitral valve surgery. Intraoperative TEE can be of value as well. The size of the jet visualized by color Doppler echocardiography may not represent the degree of aortic regurgitation. It is possible to measure the *vena contracta,* which is the size of the regurgitant jet within the regurgitant aortic valve orifice. This measurement correlates well with effective regurgitant orifice. Width of the vena contracta is measured from the parasternal view long axis, just below the flow convergence. Vena contracta greater than or equal to 7 mm uniformly indicates severe aortic valve regurgitation, whereas measurements of 5 mm or less correspond to regurgitation that is moderate or less.

Moderate (grade 2) associated aortic stenosis can usually be identified clinically by characteristic physical findings (see Chapter 12), and LV–aortic gradient can be measured at operation, but flow may not be known. Therefore, an estimate of aortic valve orifice size by two-dimensional echocardiography or cardiac catheterization (see Chapter 12) should be available when mitral valve surgery is undertaken.

Dominant Mitral Regurgitation

The same considerations discussed for dominant mitral stenosis apply to aortic valve disease associated with dominant mitral regurgitation.

Dominant Tricuspid Valve Disease

In uncommon cases of dominant tricuspid stenosis or regurgitation, accurate clinical assessment of downstream lesions in the mitral and aortic valves is seldom possible. Preoperative two-dimensional echocardiographic study is required, and occasionally cardiac catheterization as well.

NATURAL HISTORY

The natural history of combined aortic and mitral valve disease is complicated by the same variability in dominance of one lesion over the other that makes diagnosis and decision making difficult. For example, in rheumatic aortic valve disease, the mitral valve is involved almost universally, although the lesions—either stenosis or regurgitation—may be so mild that operation is not required until many years after replacement of the aortic valve. Double valve surgery in such patients is sequential. Patients with rheumatic mitral valve disease often have only mild rheumatic aortic valve disease at the time of their original mitral operation. The longer these patients survive, the more likely it is that a mild rheumatic aortic lesion will become important and require operation. Choudhary and colleagues followed 284 patients with rheumatic heart disease who had mild aortic valve involvement at the time of mitral valve surgery.[C4] After a mean interval of about 5 years, 35% of those with mild aortic valve stenosis had progressed to moderate or severe stenosis. Freedom from development of moderate or severe aortic valve stenosis was 75% ± 6%, 62% ± 9%, and 46% ± 11% at 5, 10, and 15 years, respectively. Mild aortic valve regurgitation at the time of mitral valve intervention, on the other hand, progressed slowly, with only 5% of patients developing moderate or severe aortic valve regurgitation after a mean interval of 12 years. Freedom from development of moderate or severe aortic valve regurgitation was 100%, 97% ± 2%, and 87% ± 5% at 5, 10, and 15 years.

Simultaneous development of important aortic and mitral valve disease usually results from a particularly severe and prolonged attack of rheumatic fever or from recurrent attacks, and there may be a florid myocarditis and pericarditis as well. Regurgitant combined valve lesions may mature particularly rapidly, requiring operation by the second decade of life.

When dominant aortic stenosis coexists with mitral stenosis, prognosis may be worse than that of isolated aortic stenosis. When dominant mitral stenosis coexists with important aortic stenosis, survival is shorter than for isolated mitral stenosis, with sudden death being a particular risk. When severe aortic and mitral regurgitation coexist, reduction of LV afterload by mitral regurgitation provides a protective effect (see Chapter 11), and patients with aortic regurgitation tend to remain asymptomatic, despite advanced left ventricular dysfunction (see Chapter 12). Consequently, it is likely that patients with this combination will remain asymptomatic well beyond the stage when left ventricular dysfunction becomes irreversible.

TECHNIQUE OF OPERATION

After induction of general inhalation anesthesia and during appropriate preparation of the skin and draping of a sterile field, an echocardiography probe is inserted into the esophagus (see Chapter 4). Two-dimensional ultrasound imaging is used to evaluate valve morphology and color Doppler ultrasound to evaluate valvar hemodynamics. The plan for operation is then refined. The aortic valve is replaced in most circumstances, but it may be repaired if there is aortic valve regurgitation that is judged to be secondary to dilatation of the aortic root or to dilatation or aneurysm of the ascending aorta. The mitral valve may be repaired or replaced. The tricuspid valve may not need intervention or may be repaired. The crux of the operation usually involves the intervention that is judged necessary for the mitral valve, because there are more options available for the aortic valve, and the tricuspid valve is usually reparable.

A median sternotomy is performed. The cardiac valves lie in close proximity to each other so that an extensive incision is unnecessary. The pericardium is opened and suspended to provide optimal exposure of the heart. A systematic evaluation is made by assessing cardiac chamber size and palpating for thrills caused by turbulent blood flow. CPB is established using a single venous uptake cannula or two venous cannulae if the left atrium is small. Two venous cannulae and caval tapes with tourniquets are required for operations involving the tricuspid valve (see Chapter 2). Oxygenated blood is returned through a cannula placed in the ascending aorta. Multiple valve operations are enhanced by using small cannulae and vacuum-assisted venous return (see "Vacuum-Assisted Venous Return" in Chapter 2). The perfusate may be cooled to lower the body temperature to 28°C.

Operations involving more than one cardiac valve are most conveniently performed using intermittent retrograde administration of cardioplegic solution via the coronary sinus (see "Technique of Retrograde Infusion" in Chapter 3). A perfusion cannula is inserted into the coronary sinus through the right atrial wall for aortic and mitral valve operations, or directly after opening the right atrium for operations involving the tricuspid valve.

A vascular clamp occludes the ascending aorta. A vent catheter is inserted through the right superior pulmonary vein and advanced across the mitral valve into the LV. A transverse aortotomy is made and cold cardioplegia administered. For tricuspid valve operations, the right atrium is opened parallel to the atrioventricular groove, the coronary sinus cannula is inserted, and cold cardioplegia is administered.

The aortotomy is extended into the noncoronary sinus of Valsalva or extended to divide the aorta above the sinotubular junction. The aortic valve is inspected for the possibility of repair. If it is not reparable, it is excised. Calcareous deposits are removed from the aortic anulus. Diameter of the LV outflow tract at the aortoventricular junction (aortic anulus) is measured.

The operation then focuses on the mitral valve. The left atrium is opened on the right side posterior to the interatrial groove at the junction of the right pulmonary vein, and the incision is extended superiorly behind the superior vena cava and inferiorly behind the inferior vena cava. Alternatively, the superior aspect of the left atrium is opened medial to the superior vena cava and behind the aortic anulus. This superior approach is particularly useful when the aorta has been divided. When operation on the tricuspid valve is required, a transseptal approach is employed, extending the right atrial incision superiorly medial to the superior vena cava and onto the superior aspect of the left atrium. The atrial septum is cut back inferiorly through the fossa ovalis to the inferior wall of the left atrium. A self-retaining retractor maintains exposure of the mitral valve.

The mitral valve is inspected for the possibility of repair. If repair is feasible, the valve is usually replaced with a mechanical prosthesis, although second- or third-generation stent-mounted bioprostheses may be used in patients over about 70 years of age. This influences the choice of replacement device for the aortic valve, because it is usually replaced with the same type of valve as the mitral valve (see "Choice of Device" in Chapter 12). The only exception to mixing rather than matching the type of prosthesis is in the case of a very small aortic root, when a stentless bioprosthesis (allograft or xenograft) may be chosen (see "Small Aortic Root and Small Prosthesis: Prosthesis–Patient Mismatch" in Chapter 12). If the mitral valve is reparable, more selection options are available for the aortic valve, with weight given to a bioprosthesis to avoid anticoagulation if the cardiac rhythm is likely to be normal sinus after operation. The tricuspid valve is usually repaired regardless of choices made for the aortic and mitral positions. Occasionally the tricuspid valve is involved by rheumatic disease and requires replacement.

Coronary artery bypass grafting (CABG) may be required in combination with multiple valve procedures. It is usually performed after the valves are excised but before the prostheses are inserted, to reduce risk of atrioventricular groove disruption during cardiac retraction to expose the posterior wall of the LV. Proximal vein graft anastomoses to the aorta for left-sided grafts may be performed after completing distal anastomoses to the coronary arteries. For right-sided grafts, the proximal anastomosis is deferred until the atria and aorta are closed.

SPECIAL FEATURES OF POSTOPERATIVE CARE

Postoperative care of patients who have undergone combined aortic and mitral valve surgery is the same as that for other patients undergoing cardiac surgery with the aid of CPB (see Chapter 5). Anticoagulants are indicated in patients with atrial fibrillation.

RESULTS

Survival

Early (Hospital) Death

Simultaneous aortic and mitral valve replacement is often accompanied by other procedures. In the UAB group's early experience (1967 to 1981), 22% of patients underwent concomitant procedures. The complexity of the operation explains, in part, hospital mortality of 9.7% after double valve replacement (Table 13-1). Others reported hospital mortality up to 20% in this early era.[A4,L3] Early mortality for combined aortic and mitral valve replacement in contemporary collected series has changed little over time. In the Society of Thoracic Surgeons National Adult Cardiac Surgery Database, operative mortality during the 1990s ranged from 6.9% to 9.9%.[S2] Hannan and colleagues reported hospital mortality of 9.6% in 1418 multiple valvuloplasty or replacement operations from 1995 to 1997 in the state of New York.[H1] John and colleagues reported 9.2% hospital mortality among 456 patients having aortic and mitral valve replacements,[J1] whereas Mueller and colleagues reported 5%.[M4] When

■ **TABLE 13-1   Hospital Mortality after Primary Combined Aortic and Mitral Valve Procedures** [a]

Procedure	n	Hospital Deaths		
		No.	%	CL (%)
AVR + MVR	442	43	9.7 [b]	8.3–11.4
AVR + MVR + CABG	42	7	17	11–25
AVR + MVR + tricuspid annuloplasty	34	4	12	6–20
AVR + MVR + tricuspid replacement	46	12	26	19–34
AVR, MVR, tricuspid surgery, + CABG	5	0	0	0–32
Total	569	66	11.6	10.2–13.2

Key: *AVR,* Aortic valve replacement; *CABG,* coronary artery bypass grafting; *CL,* 70% confidence limits; *MVR,* mitral valve replacement.

[a] The data set of 569 patients undergoing primary combined aortic and mitral valve replacements, with or without concomitant procedures, is from the UAB experience 1967 to 1981. Patients who had undergone a previous valve replacement are excluded, but 73 patients had previously undergone one or more closed or open valve repairs.

[b] Hospital mortality was 5.9% (CL 4.3%–8.1%) among the 219 patients who underwent operation from 1975 to 1981 (13 hospital deaths).

CABG was added to the multiple valve operation, operative mortality doubled to 19% in the state of New York experience.[H1]

Time-Related Survival

Time-related survival of heterogeneous groups of patients undergoing simultaneous combined aortic and mitral valve replacement, including those undergoing concomitant tricuspid valve surgery and CABG, is lower than after single valve replacement.[A2-A4,G1,L3,M3,T1] In the UAB group's experience, it was 88%, 77%, 63%, 47%, and 23% at 1 month and 1, 5, 10, and 20 years after operation, respectively (Fig. 13-1). The hazard function for death has a rapidly declining early phase of risk, giving way to a second, slowly increasing hazard phase about 3 months postoperatively (Fig. 13-2). The increasing phase of hazard may reflect an imperfect postoperative hemodynamic state dating from the time of operation.

Modes of Death

Most deaths early after primary combined aortic and mitral valve replacement are from acute or subacute cardiac failure. However, an unusually high prevalence of death with hemorrhage has occurred in this group of patients in the past (Table 13-2). This is because of the ease with which left atrioventricular rupture can be produced at the time of double valve replacement. Currently, greater attention to this detail has considerably lessened the prevalence of this early postoperative complication.

Mode of death occurring after hospitalization discharge is most commonly due to chronic heart failure. Even when tricuspid valve regurgitation and right ventricular dysfunction have seemed to be absent before operation, a number of patients present late postoperatively with increasing evidence of tricuspid regurgitation, right atrial enlargement, and progressing hepatomegaly. The reason for the unusually high prevalence is not apparent. However, the primary feature appears to be right ventricular dysfunction, and tricuspid valve replacement at this stage generally does not improve the patient's condition.

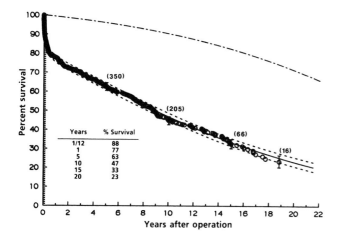

Figure 13-1 Survival after primary combined aortic and mitral valve replacement, with or without tricuspid valve surgery and coronary artery bypass grafting, in 569 patients (UAB group, 1967 to 1981). Dash-dot-dash line represents survival of an age-gender-ethnicity–matched general population. Circles represent deaths, vertical bars 70% confidence limits of Kaplan–Meier estimate, and numbers in parentheses patients traced beyond that interval. Solid line enclosed within 70% confidence limits represents parametric survival estimates.

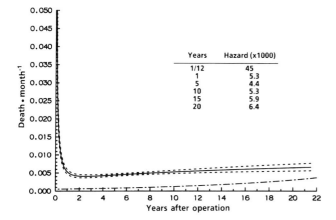

Figure 13-2 Hazard function for death after primary combined aortic and mitral valve replacement, enclosed within 70% confidence limits. Data are as in Fig. 13-1.

Incremental Risk Factors for Death
Double Valve Replacement

Double valve replacement itself is an incremental risk factor for death (9.4%) compared with isolated replacement of the mitral (5.7%) or aortic valve (3.5%).[S2] This is evident early after operation, and particularly in intermediate and long-term follow-up, when many deaths occur because of increasing tricuspid regurgitation progressing to right atrial enlargement, hepatomegaly, and finally cardiac cachexia. These types of death occur much less frequently after isolated mitral valve replacement and rarely after isolated aortic valve replacement. The relative roles of decreasing LV performance, increasing pulmonary vascular resistance, and decreasing right ventricular performance in

■ TABLE 13-2 Modes of Death after Primary Combined Aortic and Mitral Valve Replacement [a]

Mode of Death	Early (30 days)		Intermediate and Late	
	n	% of 84	n	% of 267
Cardiac failure	54	64	109	41
Acute	28	33	19	7
Subacute	26	31	12	5
Chronic	0	0	73	27
Not specified	0	0	5	2
Hemorrhage	9	11	5	2
Sudden	3	4	37	14
Neurologic	0	0	28	10
Acute			13	5
Subacute			1	0.4
Chronic			2	0.7
Not specified			12	4
Arrhythmia	2	2	5	2
Cancer	0	0	12	4
Pulmonary failure	0	0	3	1.1
Acute			1	0.4
Subacute			1	0.4
Chronic			1	0.4
Trauma	0	0	4	1
Heat stroke	0	0	2	0.7
Polymyositis	0	0	1	1
Acute abdominal event [b]	0	0	1	0.4
Uncertain	0	0	35	13
Death after valve reoperation or rereplacement	16	19	25	9
Total	84	100	267	100

[a] Data are from 569 patients (UAB group, 1967 to 1981).

[b] Rupture of undiagnosed splenic artery aneurysm.

this late deterioration after double valve replacement are uncertain.

Mitral Valve Replacement Rather than Repair

One-stage mitral and aortic valve operations may not involve replacement of both valves. When they do not, the early risks have generally been less, even when concomitant tricuspid valve surgery is performed, and the intermediate and long-term results are better.[A2,G3,T1,T2] Gillinov and colleagues reported hospital mortality of 5.4% when the mitral valve was repaired and 7.0% when it was replaced.[G3] They also reported 15-year survival of 46% when the mitral valve was repaired compared with 34% when it was replaced (*P* = .01; Fig. 13-3). The instantaneous risk of death was highest immediately postoperatively, decreased to its lowest level at 1 year, and increased slowly thereafter (Fig. 13-4). The late phase of hazard was consistently higher after mitral valve replacement than after repair.

Previous Operations

Approximately 15% of patients undergoing first-time simultaneous replacement of the aortic and mitral valves have had a previous valve operation. This has not, however, increased the risks of the double valve replacement.

Choice of Replacement Device

Choice of replacement device does not affect long-term survival. Caus and colleagues compared a matched population age 60 ± 3 years having aortic and mitral valve

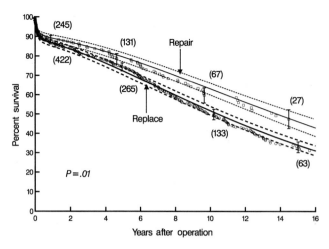

Figure 13-3 Survival after combined aortic and mitral valve operation. Open squares represent patients having aortic valve replacement and mitral valve repair; open circles are those having replacement both valves. Format is as in Fig. 13-1. (From Gillinov and colleagues.[G3])

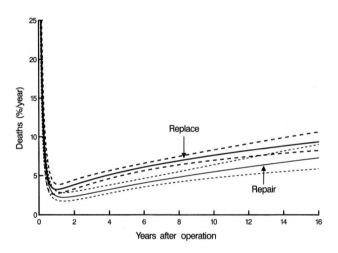

Figure 13-4 Risk of death after combined aortic and mitral valve operation (hazard function) according to mitral valve replacement or repair. (From Gillinov and colleagues.[G3])

replacement with either mechanical prostheses or bioprostheses.[C5] Survival at 5, 10, and 15 years was similar, although reoperation was more common in the bioprostheses group and thromboembolic complications were more common in the mechanical valve group.

Age at Operation

Historically, age at operation has not been identified as an incremental risk factor for death during the first 30 days after operation (Table 13-3). However, more patients are now being operated on in their eighth and ninth decades of life, so older age is probably a risk factor for early postoperative death in the current era. It clearly is a risk factor for death late postoperatively, especially for patients older than 70 years at the time of operation

■ **TABLE 13-3** Synthesis of Incremental Risk Factors for Death after Primary Aortic and Mitral Valve Repair or Replacement [a]

	Risk Factor	Early	Late
	Demographic		
(Older)	Age (years)		●
(Larger)	Body surface area (m²)	●	
	African-Americans		●
	Clinical and Hemodynamic Status		
(Higher)	NYHA class (I–V)	●	●
	Moderate or severe LV dysfunction		●
(Higher)	Pulmonary vascular resistance (units · m²)		●
	Morphologic		
	Nonrheumatic etiology	●	●
	Important aortic and mitral regurgitation	●	
(Greater)	LV enlargement (grades 1–6)		●
	Cardiac Comorbidity		
	Atrial fibrillation		●
	Coronary artery disease, left main stenosis	●	
	Noncardiac Comorbidity		
	Renal disease		●
(Higher)	BUN	●	

Key: *BUN*, Blood urea nitrogen; *LV*, left ventricular; *NYHA*, New York Heart Association.
[a] Based on analysis of 569 patients, including those with concomitant procedures, from UAB group, 1967 to 1981, and of 813 patients having aortic valve replacement and mitral valve repair or replacement at the Cleveland Clinic, 1975 to 1998.[G3]

(Fig. 13-5).[G3,H1,M4] Gillinov and colleagues demonstrated a 20% survival advantage for patients having operation at age 50 years versus those having operation at age 65.

Left Ventricular Function and Preoperative Functional Status

The more advanced the heart failure, and thus the functional disability, the greater the early and late risks of death (Fig. 13-6). Patients whose condition necessitates an emergency operation can be expected to be particularly at risk early postoperatively.[M4] Even patients in New York Heart Association (NYHA) functional class II have reduced late survival.

LV ejection fraction below 30% increased hospital mortality in multiple valve replacement in the New York State study to 13%, compared with 9.3% when it was higher.[H1] Mueller and colleagues found that LV ejection fraction below 50% increased risk of all deaths ($P < .001$).[M4] Moderate or severe LV dysfunction was a risk factor for death in the late hazard phase.[G3,T2]

Left Ventricular Enlargement

Greater LV enlargement is a powerful risk factor for death late postoperatively. Because of the large volume overload, combined severe aortic and mitral regurgitation has a strong tendency to produce marked LV enlargement; the outcome after operation for patients with severe LV enlargement and this combination of valve lesions is particularly poor, with 5-, 10-, and 20-year survival of 64%, 37%, and 9%, respectively (Fig. 13-7).

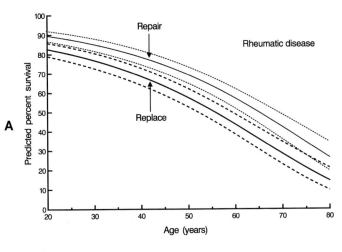

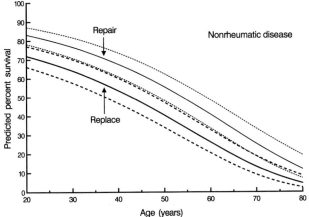

Figure 13-5   Age and 16-year survival after combined aortic and mitral valve operation. **A,** Mitral valve repair versus replacement in rheumatic valve disease. The depiction is a nomogram from the multivariable analysis in which patient characteristics were New York Heart Association functional class II, left ventricular dysfunction grade <3, no important coronary artery disease, normal sinus rhythm, blood urea nitrogen 20 mg·dL^{-1}, and no renal disease. **B,** Mitral repair versus replacement in nonrheumatic valve disease. Depiction is as in **A.** (From Gillinov and colleagues.[G3])

Valve Pathology

Imperfect outcome after double valve replacement is well illustrated by survival of patients with the most favorable valve pathology, namely, important stenosis at one or both valves with only grade 2 LV enlargement (see Fig. 13-7). The combination of severe mitral regurgitation and severe aortic regurgitation has mildly increased the risk of death early after operation (see Fig. 13-7). Mueller and colleagues also found that aortic valve stenosis is a risk factor in the early hazard phase.[M5]

Patients having multiple valve operations for rheumatic valvar heart disease have greater survival benefit than those having operations for nonrheumatic disease. John and colleagues reported survival of 85% at 15 years and 82% at 24 years in patients with a mean age of 33 years having aortic and mitral valve replacement for rheumatic valve

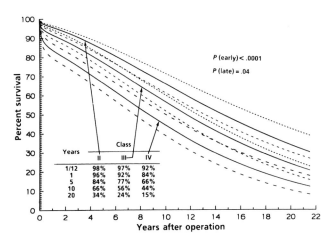

Figure 13-6   Risk-adjusted probability of survival after primary combined aortic and mitral valve replacement as it is affected by the preoperative functional status of the patient. The plot is a nomogram of a specific solution of the multivariable equation. (See Appendix 13A for details.)

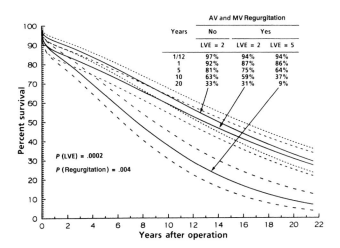

Figure 13-7   Effect of important regurgitation at both valves and left ventricular enlargement on risk-adjusted survival after primary combined aortic and mitral valve replacement. The plot is a nomogram of a specific solution of the multivariable equation. (See Appendix 13A for details.)

Key: *AV,* Aortic valve; *LVE,* left ventricular enlargement; *MV,* mitral valve.

disease.[J1] Mueller and colleagues reported survival of 56% at 15 years and a linearized death rate of 2.3% per patient-year in a group of older patients (mean age 56 years) in whom 55% underwent operation for rheumatic disease.[M4] Gillinov and colleagues also reported that patients with rheumatic disease had greater predicted survival benefit than patients with nonrheumatic disease and that repair of the mitral valve further improved survival[G3] (Fig. 13-8). Nonrheumatic disease reduced survival in even the lowest-risk patients, and age at operation further reduced the chance of surviving for 16 years after aortic valve replacement and mitral valve repair or replacement (see Fig. 13-5, *B*).

Cardiac Comorbidity

Early mortality is increased by the presence of important tricuspid regurgitation, necessitating associated annuloplasty or, particularly, valve replacement, although this is not evident in all analyses.[G1,G2,M3,T1] It is also increased by presence of ischemic heart disease requiring concomitant CABG, especially left main coronary artery stenosis.[A3,G3,M4] Pulmonary vascular resistance that is elevated before operation affects late survival. Mueller and colleagues also found that pulmonary systolic pressure of 60 mmHg or more is a risk factor for early death.[M5] Atrial fibrillation is a risk factor for death in the late hazard phase, presumably because of the added risk of embolism and late heart failure related to the atrial dysrhythmia.[G3] Tricuspid valve operations in combination with aortic and mitral valve procedures reduce early and late survival.[M2,T2]

Noncardiac Comorbidity

Renal disease increases risk of death in the late hazard phase, and elevated blood urea nitrogen adds risk in the early phase after operation.[G3] Dialysis at the time of operation increases early relative risk ninefold.[H2] Diabetes mellitus also increments risk.[H1,M4] Hepatic failure increased early risk of operation from 9.2% to 26% in the New York State series.[H1]

Functional Status

Most surviving patients are considerably improved by double valve replacement.[A2] However, by 10 years after operation, only 51% are in NYHA functional class I and 34% are in class II (Fig. 13-9). The proportion of surviving patients who are in NYHA functional class I gradually declines as follow-up becomes longer, reaching only 35% by 20 years (Fig. 13-9). Because only 47% of patients undergoing aortic and mitral valve replacement with or without concomitant procedures are alive 10 years after operation (see Fig. 13-1), only one fourth of patients operated on are alive and in NYHA functional class I 10 years after operation; at 20 years after operation, the percentage is only 8%. John and colleagues reported 72% in functional class I, 25% in class II, and 3.1% in class III at median 8.5 years of follow-up after aortic and mitral valve replacement for rheumatic disease.[J1] As noted earlier, this patient group was also young (mean age 33 years).

Freedom from Thromboembolism

Freedom from thromboembolism after primary combined aortic and mitral valve replacement (Fig. 13-10) is similar to that after isolated mitral valve replacement.[A1,K1] The use

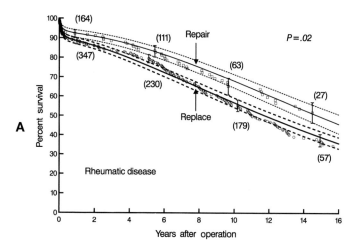

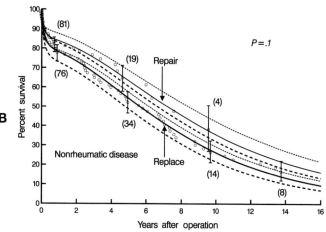

Figure 13-8   Survival after combined aortic and mitral valve operation, according to etiology. Format is as in Fig. 13-3. **A,** Survival in patients with rheumatic valve disease etiology stratified according to mitral valve replacement or repair. **B,** Survival in patients with nonrheumatic valve disease etiology stratified according to mitral valve replacement or repair. (From Gillinov and colleagues.[G3])

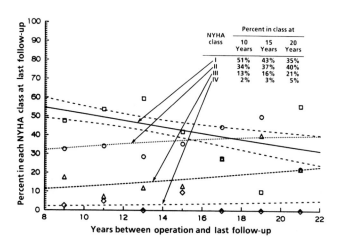

Figure 13-9   Time-related prevalence of New York Heart Association (NYHA) functional classes among patients surviving after primary combined aortic and mitral valve replacement with or without other procedures. The longest follow-up is 22 years. Lines to which arrows point are parametric estimates; dashed lines enclose 70% confidence limits for class I. Symbols represent prevalences at 2-year intervals of NYHA classes. Squares represent class I, circles class II, triangles class III, and diamonds class IV. (See Appendix 13B for details.) (Data from UAB group, 1970 to 1981.)

of bioprostheses in both positions has not eliminated late postoperative thromboembolic episodes.[W1] Mueller and colleagues found similar results in a group of patients in which 82% had double valve replacement with bileaflet mechanical valves.[M4] Freedom from thromboembolism was 89% at 5 years, 74% at 10 years, and 66% at 15 years. Mitral valve repair did not reduce the risk compared with double valve replacement.

Just as after mitral valve replacement mitral commissurotomy, risk of a subsequent thromboembolic event is increased by more postoperative thromboembolic events (see Fig. 13-10) as well as those occurring prior to operation.

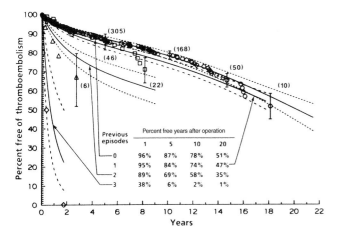

Figure 13-10   Freedom from thromboembolism after primary simultaneous aortic and mitral valve replacement, with or without other procedures, according to number of previous postoperative thromboembolic events. The graph was constructed by reentering patients at a new time zero at the time of each thromboembolic event (see "Repeated Events" in Chapter 6). (Data from UAB group, 1967 to 1981; $n = 569$.)

Complications of Anticoagulant Therapy

Prevalence of hemorrhage related to anticoagulant therapy is no different after double valve replacement than after single valve replacement (see "Complications of Long-Term Anticoagulation" under Mitral Valve Replacement in Chapter 11). In patients in whom mechanical prostheses were used (bileaflet in 82%), freedom from bleeding events was 89% at 5 years, 81% at 10 years, and 73% at 15 years. Linearized rates of valve-related thromboembolism and bleeding with bileaflet prostheses are listed in Table 13-4.

Hemolysis and Valve Thrombosis

With two mechanical prostheses, hemolysis and valve thrombosis are greater than with one. Both complications are rare.

Reoperation

As has been the experience with reoperations after valve replacement in general, the risk of yet another reoperation becomes greater after each (Fig. 13-11).

Need to reoperate is usually determined by the durability of the repair or replacement device applied in the mitral position (Fig. 13-12). Reoperation is done least frequently when mechanical prostheses are used. More than 90% of patients are free of reoperation at 15 years when a mechanical valve is used to replace the mitral valve in double valve operations; in contrast, that figure drops to 25% when a stented bioprosthesis is used.

The choice of replacement or repair of the mitral valve affects the procedure chosen for the aortic position. Patients requiring anticoagulant therapy for atrial fibrillation or recurrent deep vein thrombosis, for example, derive greatest benefit from the durability of mechanical prostheses. Extensive calcification of the mitral valve is usually best treated by mitral valve replacement. Severe mitral stenosis with thickening of the valve and subvalvar apparatus is usually treated by mitral valve replacement.

■ **TABLE 13-4   Linearized Rate of Thromboembolism and Bleeding after Double Valve Replacement with Bileaflet Prostheses**

Author and Year	Valve Type	Number of Patients	Embolism ($\% \cdot$ patient-year^{-1})	Bleeding ($\% \cdot$ patient-year^{-1})
Kinsley et al., 1986[K2]	SJM	126	1.7	–
Armenti et al., 1987[A2]	SJM	92	4.6	1.2
Burckhardt et al., 1988[B1]	SJM	81	1.1	–
Arom et al., 1989[A4]	SJM	100	1.3	0
Czer et al., 1990[C2]	SJM	74	2.0	3.1
Smith et al., 1993[S3]	SJM	64	0.3	0.3
de Luca et al., 1993[D1]	CM	76	0.3	0.6
Nakano et al., 1994[N1]	SJM	223	0.8	0.1
Ibrahim et al., 1994[I1]	SJM	70	5.0	2.1
Baudet et al., 1995[B2]	SJM	132	1.6	1.0
Copeland, 1995[C3]	CM	144	3.1	1.2
Mueller et al., 1998[M4]	SJM, CM, ATS	163	2.6	2.6
Range		0.3–5.0	0.0–3.1	
Median		1.6	1.1	
Interquartile range		1.1–2.6	0.2–2.4	

(Modified from Mueller and colleagues.[M4])

Key: *ATS*, Advancing the Standard; *CM*, CarboMedics; *SJM*, St. Jude Medical.

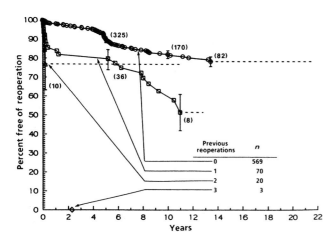

Figure 13-11   Freedom from reoperation after primary combined aortic and mitral valve replacement, according to the number of previous reoperations. Construction of the graph is as in Fig. 13-10. (Data are from UAB group, 1967 to 1981; *n* = 569.)

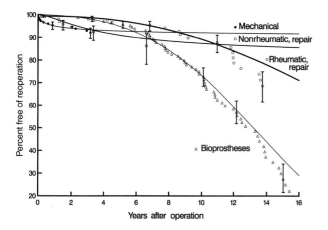

Figure 13-12   Freedom from reoperation after mitral valve repair or replacement in combined aortic and mitral valve operations. Filled circles represent reoperation after replacement of the mitral valve with a mechanical prosthesis; triangles represent mitral valve replacement with a bioprosthesis; squares represent mitral valve repair in nonrheumatic etiologies; and circles represent mitral valve repair in rheumatic valve etiology. Parametric estimates are represented by solid lines; their confidence limits are suppressed for clarity. (From Gillinov and colleagues.[G3])

Repair of both the mitral and aortic valves can be accomplished with acceptable early and late mortality and valve-related morbidity.[G4] Unfortunately, the durability of both mitral and aortic valve repairs is limited. Freedom from reoperation for valve dysfunction was 94%, 82%, and 65% at 1, 5, and 10 years, respectively.[G4] However, results of repair of rheumatic-type mitral valves decrease between 10 and 15 years.

INDICATIONS FOR OPERATION

Remarkably few data exist to guide management of multiple valve disease objectively. Each case must be considered individually, and management must be based on hemodynamics and ventricular function as well as on the probable benefit of medical versus surgical intervention.[A5] The most logical approach is to operate when valvar disease produces more than mild symptoms, or, in the case of dominant aortic valve stenosis, when patients have only mild symptoms.[A5] In regurgitant dominant lesions, surgery can be delayed until symptoms of LV dysfunction develop in asymptomatic patients. Use of vasodilators to delay surgery in mixed valve disease is untested.

Aortic and mitral valve operation is required when the patient's symptoms are important (NYHA functional class III or greater) despite an appropriate and intense medical regimen. Such an approach, which is more conservative than that with isolated mitral or aortic valve replacement, is indicated by the higher early and late risks of double valve replacement and the probably increased late morbidity when there are two, rather than one, artificial devices in situ. Despite these early and late risks, outcome after double valve replacement is surely superior to that which can be accomplished with nonsurgical means. Because of the markedly increased risks with advanced heart disease, it is unwise to insist on severe limitation (NYHA class IV) before recommending double or triple valve surgery. It is particularly unwise to keep deferring operation until it suddenly becomes necessary to perform an emergency operation on a class V patient, because then the early and late risks become high.

Exceptions to these general indications are cases of combined aortic and mitral regurgitation. These patients are advised to undergo operation when LV enlargement is grade 2 or higher (based on grades 1 to 6), *even though symptoms are absent or mild.* Otherwise, there is a strong tendency to develop extreme LV enlargement *before* symptoms become important, considerably lowering long-term survival and increasing the probability of developing ventricular arrhythmias and sudden death.

Patients with active rheumatic carditis, severe aortic and mitral regurgitation, and critical heart failure must be operated on when it is clear that the acute episode is not subsiding. Patients with severe aortic and mitral regurgitation and active bacterial endocarditis, in whom neither infection nor heart failure can be controlled medically, must also undergo operation without delay.

SPECIAL SITUATIONS AND CONTROVERSIES

Multiple Valve Replacement through Small Incisions

It has become possible to perform almost all cardiac valve operations through incisions smaller than standard median sternotomy. Experience and familiarity with smaller incisions have shown that exposure of cardiac valves is not compromised, and even though the smaller incision provides more confined dimensions within which the surgeon must work, results have been equivalent. The frequency with which the minimally invasive approach to cardiac valves is used has increased, but it is still a small fraction of the total.

A lower half partial sternotomy approach may be considered for any cardiac valve operation.[D2] This approach allows the minimally invasive operation not only in isolated single valve replacement but also in complex cardiac valve operations. The incision is centered over the location of the cardiac valves. Cadaveric dissections performed by Reardon and colleagues affirm the lower half sternotomy exposure.[R1] They found the pulmonary valve behind the third left costal cartilage, the aortic valve behind the sternum opposite the third intercostal space, and the mitral and tricuspid valves related to the fourth costal cartilage and fourth interspace.

Operations on the aortic valve are facilitated by dividing the ascending aorta above the sinotubular junction. The aortic root may then be positioned for direct visualization, allowing precise examination. The mitral valve approach through standard left atriotomy posterior to the intraatrial groove on the right side is comfortable and familiar to the surgeon. When aortic and mitral valve operations are combined, the mitral valve is easily accessible through the superior aspect of the left atrium, especially with the aorta divided and aortic root retracted inferiorly. A transatrial septal approach is used (1) when the mitral valve is repaired or replaced in conjunction with operations on the tricuspid valve, or (2) for triple valve operations.

Complex operations are easier when the transverse section of the sternum is through the second intercostal space. The longer the sternal incision, the less the incision qualifies as "minimally invasive." Nevertheless, it is not wise to compromise exposure or needlessly confine the incision to the point that the operation becomes tedious and prolonged. When either the third or second interspace is used, the entire manubrium remains intact, along with the

clavicular attachment. This should be of substantial benefit to the patient in terms of chest wall stability after operation and should eliminate the possibility of dehiscence of the sternal repair at the manubrium.

Small-diameter cannulae as used in vacuum-assisted venous return considerably aid placement of aortic and venous cannulae through the primary incision. Vacuum-assisted venous return has also been helpful in providing more reserve and safety in the venous drainage system to the reservoir of the oxygenator (see "Vacuum-Assisted Venous Return" in Chapter 2). The right heart remains empty and collapsed more consistently than with gravity drainage, and air entrainment with air lock, frequently seen with gravity drainage, is eliminated. This and other advances in cardiopulmonary technology have made operating through a small incision easier, and the technology is transferable to full sternotomy operations.

Doty and colleagues studied the partial sternotomy (lower half) approach in 16 patients undergoing double valve operations.[D2] One patient died (6.3%). Triple valve operations were performed in five patients, none of whom died. They concluded that this approach provides a smaller, less invasive incision through which essentially all cardiac valve operations may be performed. It provides standard exposure to the cardiac valves, and standard instruments and retraction devices are employed. Maintaining the integrity of the manubrium and upper sternum should be beneficial for patient mobilization and rehabilitation after operation, and the smaller incision is appreciated by patients of all ages. Data are not available, however, to justify the approach based on cost, length of hospital stay, or decreased pain.

APPENDIXES

APPENDIX 13A

Survival and Related Matters

This appendix discusses survival and related matters in patients undergoing simultaneous combined aortic and mitral valve replacement, with or without concomitant cardiac procedures, and excluding only those patients with a previous aortic or mitral valve replacement operation (UAB group, 1967 to 1981, $n = 569$). Follow-up extended to 22 years.

Parameter Estimates

Shaping parameter estimates, the risk factors retained in the analysis, their coefficients, standard deviations, and (in parentheses) P values were as follows:

Early phase: $\delta = 0$, $\rho = 7.989$, $\nu = 1$, $m = -2.519$, intercept 7.134, body surface area 0.9023 ± 0.41 ($P = .03$), preoperative NYHA functional class 0.8177 ± 0.139 ($P < .0001$), aortic and mitral regurgitation 0.6092 ± 0.21 ($P = .004$), use of cardioplegia -1.054 ± 0.28 ($P = .0002$), global myocardial ischemic time (using cardioplegia) 0.02138 ± 0.0080 ($P = .007$), surgeon X 0.9934 ± 0.46 ($P = .03$)

Late phase: $\tau = 1$, $\gamma = 1$, $\alpha = 1$, $\eta = 1.458$, intercept -10.64, age at operation 0.02698 ± 0.0060 ($P < .0001$), African-American 0.7758 ± 0.20 ($P = .0001$), preoperative NYHA functional class 0.2528 ± 0.124 ($P = .04$), pulmonary resistance index 0.04011 ± 0.020 ($P = .05$), left ventricular (LV) enlargement grade 0.2654 ± 0.072 ($P = .0002$), concomitant coronary artery bypass grafting (CABG) 0.7388 ± 0.26

($P = .005$), Bjork–Shiley prostheses used in aortic and mitral position -0.6490 ± 0.156 ($P < .0001$)

Specific Solutions of the Multivariable Equation

Figure 13-6: Age was entered as 65 years, African-American 15%, body surface area as 1.7 m², pulmonary vascular resistance as 4.3 μ · m², important aortic and mitral regurgitation = no, LV enlargement grade 3, CABG = no, and global myocardial ischemic time as 80 minutes, with cardioplegia.

Figure 13-7: The entries were similar, and NYHA was entered as class III.

APPENDIX 13B

Ordinal Logistic Equation for NYHA Functional Class

The NYHA functional class on the date of latest follow-up (November to December 1988) in living patients was analyzed using the ordinal logistic model for an ordered categorical response variable. The intercepts and regression coefficient, its standard deviation, and P value are as follows: intercept 1, -0.7283; intercept 2, -2.417; intercept 3, -4.389; interval (months) from operation to last follow-up 0.005665 ± 0.0030 ($P = .06$).

REFERENCES

A

1. Aberg B. Surgical treatment of combined aortic and mitral valvular disease. A clinical, haemodynamic and experimental evaluation of the standard and convexo-concave models of Bjork-Shiley tilting disc valve prosthesis. Scand J Thorac Cardiovasc Surg 1980;14:1.
2. Armenti F, Stephenson LW, Edmunds LH Jr. Simultaneous implantation of St. Jude Medical aortic and mitral prostheses. J Thorac Cardiovasc Surg 1987;94:733.
3. Akins CW, Buckley MJ, Daggett WM, Hilgenberg AD, Austen WG. Myocardial revascularization with combined aortic and mitral valve replacements. J Thorac Cardiovasc Surg 1985;90:272.
4. Arom KV, Nicoloff DM, Kersten TE, Northrup WF III, Lindsay WG, Emery RW. Ten-year follow-up study of patients who had double valve replacement with the St. Jude Medical prosthesis. J Thorac Cardiovasc Surg 1989;98:1008.
5. ACC/AHA guidelines for the management of patients with valvular heart disease. A report of the American College of Cardiology/American Heart Association. Task Force on Practice Guidelines. J Am Coll Cardiol 1998;32:1486.

B

1. Burckhardt D, Striebel D, Vogt S, Hoffmann A, Roth J, Weiss P, et al. Heart valve replacement with St. Jude Medical valve prosthesis: long-term experience in 743 patients in Switzerland. Circulation 1988;78:118.
2. Baudet EM, Puel V, McBride JT, Grimaud JP, Roques F, Clerc F, et al. Long-term results of valve replacement with the St. Jude Medical prosthesis. J Thorac Cardiovasc Surg 1995;109:858.

C

1. Cartwright RS, Giacobine JW, Ratan RS, Ford WB, Palich WE. Combined aortic and mitral valve replacement. J Thorac Cardiovasc Surg 1963;45:35.
2. Czer LS, Chaux A, Matloff J, DeRobertis MA, Nessim SA, Scarlata D, et al. Ten year experience with the St. Jude Medical valve for primary valve replacement. J Thorac Cardiovasc Surg 1990;100:44.
3. Copeland JG III. An international experience with the CarboMedics prosthetic heart valve. J Heart Valve Dis 1995;4:56.
4. Choudhary SK, Talwar S, Juneja R, Kumar AS. Fate of mild aortic valve disease after mitral valve intervention. J Thorac Cardiovasc Surg 2001;122:583.
5. Caus T, Rouviere P, Collart F, Mouly-Bandini A, Monties JR, Mesana T. Late results of double-valve replacement with biologic or mechanical prostheses. Ann Thorac Surg 2001;71:S261.

D

1. de Luca L, Vitale N, Giannolo B, Cafarella G, Piazza L, Cortrufo M. Mid-term follow-up after heart valve replacement with CarboMedics bileaflet prosthesis. J Thorac Cardiovasc Surg 1993;106:1158.
2. Doty DB, Flores JH, Doty JR. Cardiac valve operations using a partial sternotomy (lower half) technique. J Card Surg 2000;15:35.

G

1. Gersh BJ, Schaff HV, Vatterott PJ, Danielson GK, Orszulak TA, Piehler JM, et al. Results of triple valve replacement in 91 patients: perioperative mortality and long-term follow-up. Circulation 1985;72:130.
2. Galloway AC, Grossi EA, Baumann FG, LaMendola CL, Croake GA, Harris LJ, et al. Multiple valve operation for advanced valvular heart disease: results and risk factors in 513 patients. J Am Coll Cardiol 1992;19:725.
3. Gillinov AM, Blackstone EH, Cosgrove DM 3rd, White JW, Kerr P, Marullo A, et al. Mitral valve repair and aortic valve replacement is superior to double valve replacement. J Thorac Cardiovasc Surg (in press).

4. Gillinov AM, Blackstone EH, White J, Howard M, Ahkrass R, Marullo A, Cosgrove DM. Durability of combined aortic and mitral valve repair. Ann Thorac Surg 2001;72:20.

H

1. Hannan EL, Racz MJ, Jones RH, Gold JP, Ryan TJ, Hafner JP, et al. Predictors of mortality for patients undergoing cardiac valve replacements in New York State. Ann Thorac Surg 2000;70:1212.

I

1. Ibrahim M, O'Kane H, Cleland J, Gladstone D, Sarsam M, Patterson C. The St. Jude medical prosthesis: a thirteen-year experience. J Thorac Cardiovasc Surg 1994;108:221.

J

1. John S, Ravikumar E, John CN, Bashi VV. 25-year experience with 456 combined mitral and aortic valve replacement for rheumatic heart disease. Ann Thorac Surg 2000;69:1167.

K

1. Karp RB, Cyrus RJ, Blackstone EH, Kirklin JW, Kouchoukos NT, Pacifico AD. The Bjork-Shiley valve: intermediate-term follow up. J Thorac Cardiovasc Surg 1981;81:602.
2. Kinsley RH, Antunes MJ, Colsen PR. St. Jude Medical valve replacement: an evaluation of valve performance. J Thorac Cardiovasc Surg 1986;92:349.

L

1. Likoff W, Berkowitz D, Denton C, Goldberg H. A clinical evaluation of the surgical management of combined mitral and aortic stenosis. Am Heart J 1955;49:394.
2. Lillehei CW, Gott VL, DeWall RA, Varco RL. The surgical treatment of stenotic and regurgitant lesions of the mitral and aortic valves by direct vision utilizing a pump-oxygenator. J Thorac Surg 1958;35:154.
3. Lindblom D, Lindblom U, Aberg B. Long-term clinical results after combined aortic and mitral valve replacement. Eur J Cardiothorac Surg 1988;2:347.

M

1. Melvin DB, Tecklenberg PL, Hollingsworth JF, Levine FH, Glancy DL, Epstein SE, et al. Computer-based analysis of preoperative and postoperative prognostic factors in 100 patients with combined aortic and mitral valve replacement. Circulation 1973;48:III56.
2. Midell AL, DeBoer A. Multiple valve replacement: an analysis of early and late results. Arch Surg 1972;104:471.
3. Mullany CJ, Gersh BJ, Orszulak TA, Schaff HV, Puga FJ, Ilstrup DM, et al. Repair of tricuspid valve insufficiency in patients undergoing double (aortic and mitral) valve replacement. J Thorac Cardiovasc Surg 1987;94:780.
4. Mueller XM, Tevaearai HT, Stumpe F, Fischer AP, Hurni M, Ruchat P, et al. Long-term results of mitral-aortic valve operations. J Thorac Cardiovasc Surg 1998;115:1298.
5. Mueller XM, Tevaearai HT, Ruchat P, Hurni M, Fischer AP, Stumpe F, et al. Perioperative morbidity and mortality in combined aortic and mitral valve surgery. J Heart Valve Dis 1997;6:387.

N

1. Nakano K, Koyanagi H, Hashimoto A, Kitamura M, Endo M, Nagashima M, et al. Twelve years' experience with the St. Jude Medical valve prosthesis. Ann Thorac Surg 1994;57:697.

R

1. Reardon MJ, Conklin LD, Philo R, Letsou GV, Safi HJ, Espada R. The anatomical aspects of minimally invasive cardiac valve operations. Ann Thorac Surg 1999;67:266.

S

1. Starr A, Edwards M, McCord CW, Wood J, Herr R, Griswold HE. Multiple-valve replacement. Circulation 1964;29:30.
2. STS National Database Committee, Grover FL, Chair. Annual report 1999, p. 137.
3. Smith JA, Westlake GW, Mullerworth MH, Skillington PD, Tatoulis J. Excellent long-term results of cardiac valve replacement with the St. Jude Medical valve prosthesis. Circulation 1993;88:49.

T

1. Teoh KH, Christakis GT, Weisel RD, Tong CP, Mickleborough LL, Scully HE, et al. The determinants of mortality and morbidity after multiple-valve operations. Ann Thorac Surg 1987;43:353.
2. Turina J, Stark T, Seifert B, Turina M. Predictors of long-term outcome after combined aortic and mitral valve surgery. Circulation 1999; 100:II48.

W

1. Williams JB, Karp RB, Kirklin JW, Kouchoukos NT, Pacifico AD, Zorn GL Jr, et al. Considerations in selection and management of patients undergoing valve replacement with glutaraldehyde-fixed porcine bio-prostheses. Ann Thorac Surg 1980;30:247.

14 Tricuspid Valve Disease

DEFINITION

This chapter discusses regurgitation and stenosis of the tricuspid valve in those uncommon situations in which it occurs as an isolated lesion, as well as tricuspid valve disease associated with mitral or combined mitral and aortic valve disease.

Tricuspid valve abnormalities or disease may be associated with various conditions discussed in other chapters, including atrioventricular septal defect in Chapter 20, ventricular septal defect (straddling tricuspid valve) in Chapter 21, pulmonary atresia and intact ventricular septum in Chapter 26, Ebstein anomaly in Chapter 28, and right atrial myxoma in Chapter 47. Rarely, isolated tricuspid valve disease is secondary to chronic cor pulmonale,[K2,K3] inferior myocardial infarction,[C2,M3,Z1] administration of methysergide,[B7,M7] scleroderma,[S3] lupus erythematosus,[G1] primary phospholipid syndrome,[H3] and hypereosinophilic syndrome.[C3,S4,V1]

MORPHOLOGY

Functional (Secondary) Tricuspid Regurgitation

The tricuspid anulus shortens during systole when the tricuspid valve is competent.[T1,T2] When right ventricular (RV) dilatation develops, usually as a consequence of important disease of the left-sided heart valves in association with pulmonary arterial hypertension, the tricuspid anulus also dilates (lengthens) and fails to shorten during systole.[U1] The leaflets and chordae remain normal in appearance.[W2] The septal leaflet portion of the anulus lengthens least in this process, because it is fixed between the right and left trigones and the atrial and ventricular septa. The remaining two thirds of the anulus lengthens greatly, particularly that part giving origin to the posterior leaflet.[B6,C5,T2] The anular dilatation results in failure of leaflet coaptation, contributed to in some patients by chordal shortening secondary to the RV dilatation.

It is these mechanisms that may produce tricuspid regurgitation late after isolated mitral valve operations or after combined aortic and mitral valve operations (see Chapters 11 and 13).

Rheumatic Tricuspid Stenosis and Regurgitation

Rheumatic tricuspid valve disease occurs in association with rheumatic involvement of the mitral valve, the mitral and aortic valves combined, or rarely, the aortic valve alone. It is not seen as an isolated lesion.

Rheumatic tricuspid disease usually results in a regurgitant valve with variable amounts of stenosis, but in rare cases there may be pure stenosis.[Y1] In tricuspid stenosis, the orifice is larger than in mitral stenosis, even when hemodynamically there is severe obstruction. This is because the vis à tergo of blood reaching the right atrium is less than that reaching the left atrium; therefore, the hemodynamic effects of anatomically moderate tricuspid stenosis are the equivalent of tight mitral stenosis. Borders of the stenotic tricuspid orifice are usually fibrous and thickened, although peripheral portions of the leaflets remain thin.[C4]

The hallmark of organic tricuspid stenosis is commissural fusion. All commissures are usually equally fused, but occasionally fusion is limited to the anteroseptal commissure. Chordal thickening and fusion are usually mild, and calcification is usually absent.

Tricuspid Valve Endocarditis

Acute tricuspid valve endocarditis is rare and usually associated with habitual intravenous self-administration of drugs.[A1] The most common etiologic organism is *Pseudomonas aeruginosa,* followed by *Staphylococcus aureus.*[S9] A variety of gram-negative bacilli may be involved. Rarely, *Candida albicans* is the infective organism. The organisms may form masses on the valve leaflets, or simply erode and destroy large portions of leaflets and chordae (see Chapter 15).

Traumatic Rupture of Tricuspid Valve

Tricuspid regurgitation is an uncommon result of severe, nonpenetrating chest injury, and in this setting is due to rupture of one or more papillary muscles or chordae (see "Atrioventricular Valve Rupture" in Section 2 of Chapter 46).[K6] Usually it is the anterior tricuspid leaflet that becomes flailed. Rarely, the ventricular septum may rupture.[S2] Occasionally a transvenous ventricular pacing lead is associated with important tricuspid regurgitation. This may be due to perforation, laceration, or scarring.[P4] Apical electric activation may also contribute.

Carcinoid Tricuspid Valve Disease

Carcinoid tumors originate from Kulchitsky cells in the gastrointestinal tract, which produce serotonin (5-hydroxytryptamine), a substance inactivated in the liver. However, carcinoid tumors that metastasize to the liver produce serotonin there, and this powerful substance passes into the pulmonary and, to a lesser extent, systemic circulation (because a good deal of it is inactivated in the lungs). Thereby, the carcinoid syndrome may be produced, with bronchospasm, diarrhea, nausea, malabsorption, flushing, and telangiectasia. In some of these patients, cicatricial deformity of the tricuspid and pulmonary valves also develops (see "Carcinoid Heart Disease" in Chapter 47).

Typical carcinoid symptoms are considerably more common in carcinoid patients with valvar involvement than in noncardiac carcinoid patients.[R2] Tricuspid commissures are fused, chordae tendineae thickened and fused, and leaflets thickened and shortened,[C1] resulting in combined stenosis and regurgitation. Microscopically, a deposition of loose or compact fibrous tissue is present on both surfaces of the tricuspid leaflets. Tricuspid regurgitation is the most common cardiac manifestation of the carcinoid syndrome. Tricuspid valve replacement may be required, but operative mortality is high (due to comorbidity), particularly in patients above the age of 60.[H1,H2,R3]

CLINICAL FEATURES AND DIAGNOSTIC CRITERIA

Tricuspid Stenosis

Moderate degrees of tricuspid stenosis may be overlooked, particularly if the patient is in atrial fibrillation. If sinus rhythm is present, there is a dominant *a* wave in the jugular venous pulse (immediately preceding the carotid pulse). Other signs include a mid-diastolic, often high-pitched murmur maximal over the lower left sternal edge, which increases on inspiration; there may be a tricuspid opening snap. The murmur can be confused with an aortic early diastolic murmur (because its timing may be relatively early) or with a conducted mitral diastolic murmur. The liver is enlarged but not pulsatile (unless from forceful atrial contraction that produces a presystolic pulse).

The chest radiograph shows right atrial enlargement, and the electrocardiogram shows a prominent P wave unless atrial fibrillation is present. Two-dimensional echocardiography is helpful in establishing the presence of leaflet thickening. Cardiac catheterization with simultaneous measurement of right atrial and RV pressures identifies a diastolic gradient (greater than 4 mm) across the valve.

Tricuspid Regurgitation

History and physical signs are sufficient to suggest diagnosis of important tricuspid regurgitation. The jugular venous pulse shows a dominant fused *c* and *v* wave, followed by a sharp, deep *y* descent. The murmur, maximal over the lower left sternal edge, is pansystolic, often high pitched, and increases on inspiration. The enlarged liver shows systolic pulsation. However, when tricuspid regurgitation is severe (such as after excision of the tricuspid valve), a murmur may be absent.[F1] In advanced cases, there are other signs of right heart failure, including peripheral edema and ascites. Mitral or aortic valve disease signs can dominate the findings, and severe right heart failure may occur under such conditions without tricuspid valve regurgitation.

Quantification of the degree of tricuspid regurgitation is important when surgical treatment of valvar heart disease is being considered, but preoperative assessment is often difficult because of the confounding effect of severe cardiac failure. In this regard, two-dimensional echocardiography is particularly useful, because presence of the cardiac catheter across the tricuspid valve interferes with angiographic assessment. Both contrast and Doppler echocardiography have been useful, but the increasing precision of color flow mapping and Doppler color flow map-guided interrogation have made them the favored methods for estimating tricuspid regurgitant flow.[C6,C7] Echocardiography can also detect reversal of flow in the inferior vena cava, as well as paradoxical ventricular septal motion and shift of the atrial septum toward the left atrium in isolated tricuspid regurgitation. Maximum circumference of the tricuspid anulus is larger in patients with tricuspid regurgitation than in normal adults (14 ± 0.7 cm and 11.9 ± 0.9 cm, respectively), and its reduction during systole is less ($10\% \pm 2\%$ versus $19\% \pm 4\%$).[C7,T2]

Despite these refinements in diagnosis, the presence and severity of tricuspid regurgitation need to be assessed in the operating room. The patient's hemodynamic state must be optimized by the anesthesiologist for any form of assessment to have validity. The surgeon's finger, inserted through the right atrial appendage, can appreciate a tricuspid regurgitant jet. Severe tricuspid regurgitation correlates reasonably well with a jet of greater intensity, greater width, and increased propagation from the valve orifice. If regurgitation is severe, however, there may not be a jet with sufficient velocity to be identified in this manner. Fortunately, intraoperative echocardiography, either with contrast Doppler or color mapping, and use of a handheld epicardial or intraesophageally positioned transducer add precision to the pre- and post-repair evaluation of tricuspid regurgitation and tricuspid anular circumference.[C7,C8,G2,G3]

In the special setting of tricuspid valve *endocarditis in drug addicts,* the valve is usually rapidly destroyed, and classic signs and symptoms of severe regurgitation develop. The illness is usually only 1 to 3 weeks in duration before the patient presents for medical care. Frequently, pulmonary symptoms and signs secondary to septic pulmonary emboli are marked.[R1] The diagnosis can be strongly suspected from a history of drug abuse, evidence of pulmonary infection, elevated jugular venous pressure, pulsatile neck veins, and pulsatile liver. These features, combined with positive blood cultures (in samples withdrawn from the RV or pulmonary artery) and echocardiography, are usually sufficient to establish the diagnosis.[K1]

Diagnosis of *traumatic* tricuspid regurgitation is usually easily established by signs of severe regurgitation and a history of a blow to the chest. Occasionally, however, the relationship of these signs to a history of injury is not obvious. In patients with traumatic tricuspid regurgitation, right-to-left shunting may occur across a patent foramen ovale, which can lead to the mistaken diagnosis of Ebstein anomaly.

NATURAL HISTORY

The natural history of patients with dominantly *stenotic* tricuspid valve disease is usually determined primarily by the associated rheumatic mitral or aortic valve disease. No doubt, however, the increased systemic venous pressure, hepatomegaly, and peripheral edema accelerate deterioration of patients with rheumatic tricuspid stenosis.

Tricuspid regurgitation has an inherent tendency to progress, just as do other types of valvar regurgitation.

However, the deleterious effects of ventricular volume overload on the right side of the heart are slower to develop than on the left. For example, in patients with traumatic tricuspid regurgitation who survive the initial trauma, regurgitation may be well tolerated for many months or years.[B1,M2] Ultimately, however, symptoms develop as regurgitation increases; by 5 to 10 years after trauma, they are usually severe and incapacitating. In patients with acute tricuspid endocarditis caused by *S. aureus,* tricuspid vegetations greater than 1 cm in diameter (visualized by two-dimensional echocardiography) worsen the natural history of tricuspid regurgitation.[B3]

Functional (secondary) tricuspid valve regurgitation also tends to progress occasionally, even after adequate treatment of the left-sided valvar lesion. King and colleagues reported that 66% of patients returning for tricuspid valve procedures late after mitral valve replacement had only mild tricuspid regurgitation at the time of the initial valve operation.[K4] In this regard, preoperative echocardiography at initial operation may be helpful. If the tricuspid anular diameter is greater than 30 mm with or without important regurgitation, reduction to a diameter of 24 mm or so may be adequate to prevent residual tricuspid regurgitation in the long term.[T3] When there is no remaining left-sided stenosis or regurgitation, progression is most frequently related to persistent pulmonary hypertension or progressing secondary RV dysfunction (see "Mitral Valve Surgery with Coexisting Tricuspid Valve Disease" in Chapter 11).

TECHNIQUE OF OPERATION

Tricuspid Valve Anuloplasty

Anuloplasty Ring Technique

Because isolated tricuspid valve disease is rare, the technique of operation is given for tricuspid valve regurgitation accompanying left-sided valve disease. When evaluation before cardiopulmonary bypass (CPB) indicates important tricuspid regurgitation, two venous cannulae are used. The tricuspid procedure may be done in the beating, perfused heart during rewarming of the patient, with suction on the aortic vent needle after the left heart has been carefully de-aired, or during continuing antegrade/retrograde cold cardioplegia with addition of external cardiac cooling.

After the mitral procedure is completed, the right atrium is opened with the usual oblique incision (Fig. 14-1). When an anuloplasty is performed using a ring, length of the base of the tricuspid septal leaflet is measured with calipers, or area of the anterior leaflet with a sizer, and on this basis the proper-sized ring is selected.[C4] The Carpentier-Edwards anuloplasty ring, for example, is a modified oval corresponding to the configuration of the tricuspid anulus, with a gap in the portion designed to overlie the atrioventricular (AV) node so that the conduction tissue is not compromised.[B4] Rings correct regurgitation by returning the anulus to slightly less than its normal size by plicating that portion at the base of the posterior (posteroinferior) leaflet and at the commissure between that and the anterior leaflet. Thus, the ring effectively "bicuspidizes" the tricuspid valve. The anulus is not plicated at either the attachment of the septal leaflet or along the major part of the attachment of the large

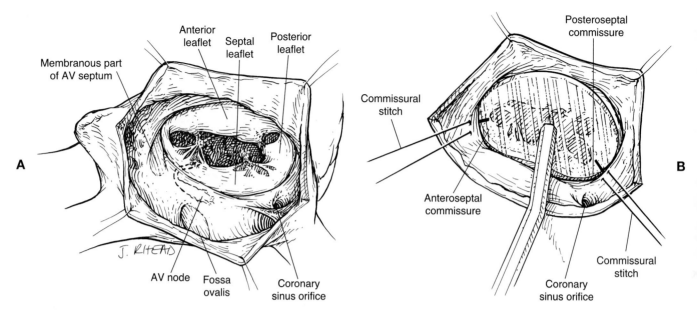

Figure 14-1 Tricuspid ring anuloplasty. **A,** Exposure is through the usual oblique right atriotomy. Venous cannulae are inserted directly into the superior and inferior venae cavae (for alternatives, see Chapter 2). **B,** Stay sutures provide excellent exposure (alternatively, a Cooley retractor may be used). The surgeon identifies the anteroseptal tricuspid valve commissure, membranous part of the atrioventricular septum, and coronary sinus orifice, and can then mentally visualize the location of the AV node and penetrating portion of the bundle of His. Using appropriate sizers, notched at points corresponding to the anteroseptal and posteroseptal commissures at both ends of the septal tricuspid leaflet, a proper-sized tricuspid anuloplasty ring is selected.

Key: *AV,* Atrioventricular.

anterior leaflet. A flexible "half ring" (Cosgrove) accomplishes a similar function, leaving the base of the septal leaflet untouched but plicating the anulus at the attachment of the anterior and posterior leaflets.[M5] It is unwise to select too small a ring in the belief that it will be more effective, because it distorts and narrows the orifice and may subsequently detach. Because tissues around the tricuspid valve are usually tenuous, sutures must take adequate bites, beginning in the atrial wall and passing into the deeper part of the anulus itself, carefully avoiding leaflet tissue.

An alternative technique is to shorten the circumference of the tricuspid anulus by simply excluding that part to which the posterior leaflet is attached.[B5,K5,K7,N1] To accomplish this, a No. 2-0 or 3-0 polyester suture is passed through the anulus at the anteroposterior commissure, then at the center of the posterior leaflet, and then through the anulus at the posteroseptal commissure. The suture is tied snugly, and a second one is placed for reinforcement. Pledgeted mattress sutures also may be used. A further modification that incorporates a flexible strip into the posterior leaflet anuloplasty has been reported to be useful.[B6] The repaired tricuspid valve should have about a normal diameter (see "Dimensions of Normal Cardiac and Great Artery Pathways" in Chapter 1.)

De Vega Technique

The De Vega technique is used in patients with no more than moderate regurgitation from ring dilatation, where it is

anticipated that good long-term function is not dependent on integrity of the repair.[D2] This technique has the advantages of simplicity and low cost. A No. 2-0 polyester suture (not monofilament polypropylene) is passed in a counterclockwise direction as a circular stitch deeply into the junction of the anulus and right ventricular wall from 1 or 2 cm medial to the posteroseptal commissure to the base of the anterior leaflet 2 to 4 cm medial to the anteroseptal commissure (Fig. 14-2). The same suture is then reversed and passed in clockwise direction slightly peripherally to the first stitch back to the starting point. Separate pledgets of polyester felt are incorporated in the suture at each end to prevent its pulling through the tissues. The suture is tightened until the orifice will admit an appropriate sizer (24 to 30 mm) and is then tied.

After discontinuing CPB and before decannulation, competence of the valve is assessed by two-dimensional echocardiography, using either a handheld or esophageal probe. Presence of moderate or severe regurgitation is an indication for valve replacement. If the heart is beating and normothermic, a reasonable assessment of competence of the repair is possible as soon as it is completed. With the atrium still open, the RV is allowed to fill with blood and the tricuspid leaflet apposition is assessed. If apposition is obviously inadequate, the valve is replaced. If it appears adequate, the right atrium is closed, air is aspirated from the RV and pulmonary artery, and the operation is completed in the usual manner (see "Completing Operation" in Section 3 of Chapter 2).

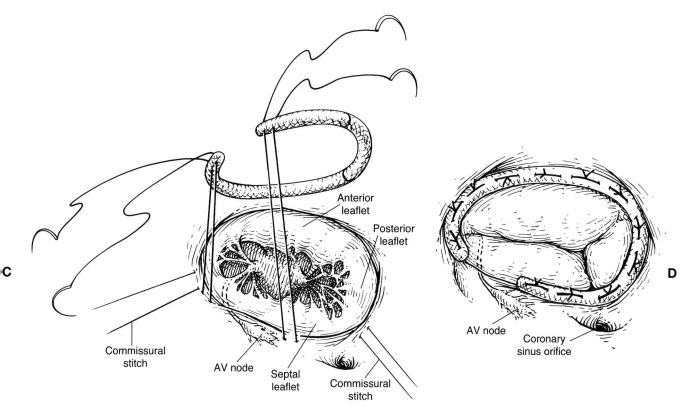

Figure 14-1, cont'd   C, The first stitch, of No. 2-0 or 3-0 polyester, is positioned exactly at the midpoint of the septal leaflet anulus, and only two further mattress stitches are needed for the septal portion of the ring. Small pledgets may be used on these mattress sutures. These and all other sutures are passed first through host tissue and then through the cloth of the undersurface of the ring, just as in suturing the ring for mitral anuloplasty (see Chapter 11). **D,** Five or six mattress stitches are needed in the portion of the anulus to be plicated, which is adjacent to the posterior leaflet, and these are passed through the cloth of the ring close together (marking stitches are present on the ring cloth to guide the surgeon). The remainder of the ring, corresponding to about half its circumference, is attached to the anulus at the base of the anterior cusp with, at most, four fairly widely spaced mattress sutures. The ring is lowered into position along the sutures and the sutures tied, with great care taken not to pull upward strongly on them, lest they tear out. In some cases the anuloplasty ring can be secured in place with three or four interrupted mattress sutures along the septal leaflet and then with continuous sutures for the remainder.

Key: *AV,* Atrioventricular.

Tricuspid Valve Replacement

When tricuspid valve replacement is elected, the leaflets are excised, and a 2- to 3-mm fringe of leaflet tissue is left on the anulus (Fig. 14-3). Interrupted pledgeted mattress sutures are placed in the fringe of leaflet tissue along the area occupied by the septal leaflet, to avoid damaging the AV node and bundle of His. Either a continuous polypropylene suture or interrupted pledgeted mattress sutures may be used for the remainder of the insertion. Alternatively, simple interrupted sutures may be used throughout. Infrequently, to avoid heart block, the suture line for valve insertion can be placed on the atrial aspect above the coronary sinus and base of the septal defect.

Tricuspid Valve Excision

In drug addicts with active tricuspid valve endocarditis, the three leaflets and their chordae tendineae can simply be excised, using the general techniques described earlier.[A2,A3,M1,S1,W1] However, postoperative convalescence and late cardiac performance are compromised by the resulting severe tricuspid regurgitation. In addition, later valve replacement is more difficult.

Stern and colleagues suggest that primary bioprosthetic valve replacement is preferable to valve excision and is not followed by recurrent endocarditis unless intravenous drug abuse continues.[S9]

SPECIAL FEATURES OF POSTOPERATIVE CARE

Long-term anticoagulation is needed when a mechanical valve has been used or if there is an additional mechanical prosthesis in either the mitral or aortic position. Warfarin administration is begun on the evening of postoperative day 2 (see "Special Features of Postoperative Care" in

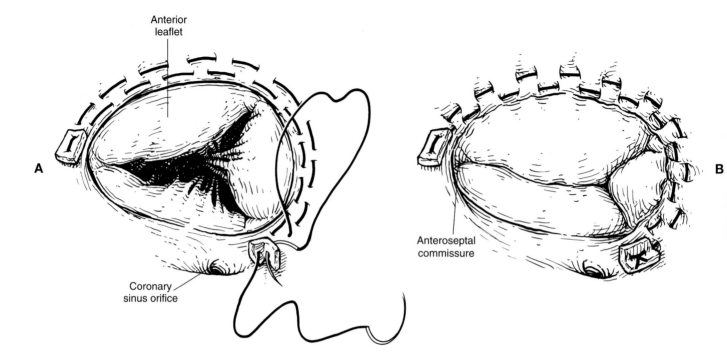

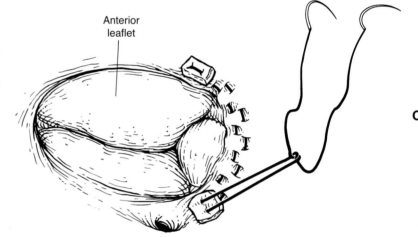

Figure 14-2   De Vega anuloplasty. **A,** The classic De Vega anuloplasty is accomplished using a double-armed No. 2-0 braided polyester suture. It is designed to narrow the tricuspid anulus at the base of the anterior and posterior leaflets, avoiding the area of the penetrating bundle of His and atrioventricular membranous septum. One arm and then the other arm of the suture pass into the tricuspid anulus, taking 8 to 10 fairly deep bites. **B,** Suture is tied over a felt pledget, producing a purse-string effect and narrowing the orifice to admit a 24- to 30-mm sizer. **C,** Often a sufficient repair can be done by narrowing the anulus only in the lateral half of the anterior leaflet and the base of the posterior leaflet.

Chapter 11). If a bioprosthesis is used and has also been used for all other valve replacement, long-term anticoagulation is controversial.

Because of the risk of complete heart block in the latter part of the hospital stay, electrocardiographic monitoring should be continued until a stable rhythm is established at an adequate heart rate.

Fluid retention is prominent among patients with tricuspid valve disease. Characteristically, their postoperative care requires aggressive use of diuretic agents.

RESULTS

Results of tricuspid valve operations have probably changed little since data were assembled by Barratt-Boyes and colleagues at GLH and Kirklin and colleagues at UAB; therefore, they have been retained and designated in the text as GLH, UAB, or combined GLH–UAB.

Tricuspid Valve Anuloplasty
Survival

Because tricuspid anuloplasty is rarely performed as an isolated procedure, its effect on early and intermediate-term survival is difficult to assess directly. However, in combined operations including tricuspid annuloplasty, early mortality can be similar to that in operations in which tricuspid anuloplasty was not required[B8] (Table 14-1). Intermediate-term survival (Fig. 14-4) may be compromised by persistence of important RV dysfunction that often accompanies tricuspid regurgitation (see "Mitral Valve Surgery with Coexisting Tricuspid Valve Disease" in Chapter 11).

Tricuspid Valve Competence

Anuloplasty of the tricuspid valve results in valvar competence in most patients (Table 14-2). Freedom from

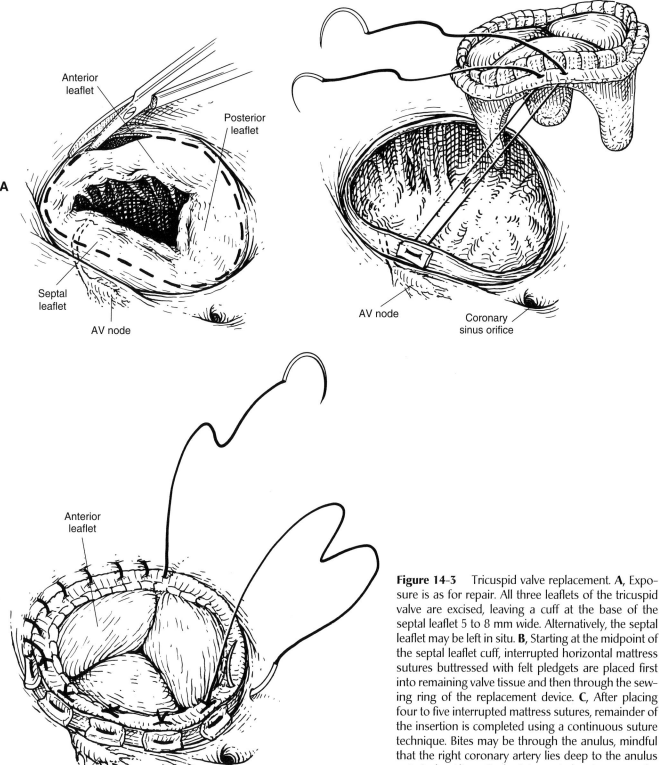

Figure 14-3   Tricuspid valve replacement. **A**, Exposure is as for repair. All three leaflets of the tricuspid valve are excised, leaving a cuff at the base of the septal leaflet 5 to 8 mm wide. Alternatively, the septal leaflet may be left in situ. **B**, Starting at the midpoint of the septal leaflet cuff, interrupted horizontal mattress sutures buttressed with felt pledgets are placed first into remaining valve tissue and then through the sewing ring of the replacement device. **C**, After placing four to five interrupted mattress sutures, remainder of the insertion is completed using a continuous suture technique. Bites may be through the anulus, mindful that the right coronary artery lies deep to the anulus anteriorly. Alternatively, interrupted sutures can be used circumferentially.

Key: *AV*, Atrioventricular.

■ TABLE 14-1   Hospital Death after Tricuspid Valve Surgery for Acquired Tricuspid Valve Disease[a]

	1965 to 1973				1973 to 1982												Total			
	TV Replacement				TV Replacement				TV Anuloplasty				Total							
	Hospital Deaths					Hospital Deaths					Hospital Deaths					Hospital Deaths					Hospital Deaths		
Procedure	n	No.	%	CL	n	No.	%	CL	n	No.	%	CL	n	No.	%	CL	n	No.	%	CL
TVS alone	3	0	0	0-47	5	0	0	0-32	1	0	0	0-85	6	0	0	0-27	9	0	0	0-19
TVS+MVS	30	10	33	24-44	39	2	5	2-12	80	4	5	3-9	119	6	5	3-8	149	16	11	8-14
TVS+MVS+AVS	12	5	42	25-60	17	1	6	0.8-19	32	2	6	2-14	49	3	6	3-12	61	8	13	9-19
TVS+AVS	1	0	0	0-85	1	1	100	85-100	2	1	50	7-93	3	2	67	24-96	4	2	50	18-82
TVS+excision AAA[b]	0				0				2	1	50	7-93	2	1	50	7-93	2	1	50	7-93
TVS+MVS+CABG	0				0				5	1	20	3-53	5	1	20	3-53	5	1	20	3-53
TOTAL	46	15	33	25-41	62	4	6	3-11	122	9	7	5-11	184	13	7.1	5.1-9.6	230	28	12	10-15
P(x²)		.5				.002				.03				.0002				.08		

Key: *AAA*, Ascending aortic aneurysm; *AVS*, aortic valve surgery; *CABG*, coronary artery bypass grafting; *CL*, 70% confidence limits; *MVS*, mitral valve surgery; *TV*, tricuspid valve; *TVS*, tricuspid valve surgery.

[a] Data are from 246 operations in 230 patients (GLH group, 1965 to 1982). Replacement device was a stent-mounted allograft semilunar valve in 91 operations, a stent-mounted porcine xenograft in 20, and a mechanical prosthesis in 9. Tricuspid anuloplasty (not done before 1973) was by the De Vega method in 18 operations and by a Carpentier ring in 108.

[b] One also had aortic valve replacement and one also had aortic and mitral valve replacement.

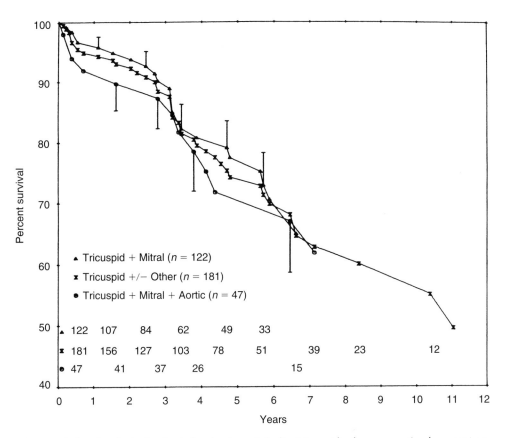

Figure 14-4   Survival of patients leaving hospital after tricuspid valve surgery (replacement or repair) with or without other valve surgery (n = 193 operations in 181 traced patients). Bars represent 1 standard error. (From Barratt-Boyes and colleagues.[B8])

moderate or severe recurrent tricuspid regurgitation in 98 anuloplasty patients (mostly Carpentier rings) was 85% at 6 years (GLH).[B8] Carpentier and colleagues found that with use of the Carpentier ring, no tricuspid regurgitation was present late postoperatively in 17 (68%; CL 56%-79%) of 25 patients with preoperatively moderate or severe regurgitation, and mild regurgitation was present in 7 (28%; CL 18%-40%). Only one patient had moderate regurgitation late postoperatively; that patient had severe regurgitation preoperatively.[C4] Long-term relief of tricuspid regurgitation by use of the Carpentier ring has been confirmed by postoperative two-dimensional echocardiography with Doppler color flow mapping.[C8]

Kay and colleagues have also reported satisfactory results in a sizable group of patients after suture bicuspidization anuloplasty.[K7,N1]

A small experience with the De Vega anuloplasty (GLH, 18 patients) has also provided good results (see Table 14-2), confirmed in larger series by echocardiography.[A5,K8,P2]

However, there are risk factors for persisting tricuspid regurgitation after repair. Recurrence is more likely when mitral disease progresses or severe pulmonary hypertension persists[B8] (see Table 14-2; see also "Mitral Valve Surgery with Coexisting Tricuspid Valve Disease" in Chapter 11). Duran and colleagues found that when functional tricuspid regurgitation was repaired, 31 (89%; CL 80%-94%) of 35 patients with low late postoperative pulmonary vascular resistance (less than 6 units · m^2) had no regurgita-

tion, whereas this was true of only 6 (43%; CL 27%-60%) of 14 patients with high pulmonary vascular resistance (P = .001).[D1]

Reoperation

Reoperation for tricuspid valve dysfunction is infrequent following Carpentier ring anuloplasty, with 97% of this group being free of reoperation 3 years postoperatively.[B8] Nakano and colleagues reported that after suture anuloplasty for important functional tricuspid regurgitation, 94% of patients were free of reoperation 10 years later, as were 70% 17 years later.[N1] Usually, redeveloped tricuspid regurgitation is associated with persisting or developed pulmonary hypertension.

Functional Status

Functional status as assessed by the New York Heart Association (NYHA) functional class is usually improved by tricuspid anuloplasty.[B8]

Tricuspid Valve Replacement
Survival

Early mortality for tricuspid valve replacement with or without double or triple valve surgery is currently 6% (CL 3%-11%) (see Table 14-1), less than in earlier years (see "Risk Factors for Premature Death after Tricuspid Valve Surgery" later in this chapter). Scully and Armstrong,[S8]

■ TABLE 14-2 Tricuspid Valve Dysfunction at Late Follow-up after Tricuspid Valve Surgery [a]

Device Used and Type of Dysfunction	n	Recurrent Tricuspid Dysfunction — Severe No.	Severe %	Severe CL	Moderate No.	Moderate %	Moderate CL	Total No.	Total %	Total CL	Tricuspid Reoperation No.	Reop %	Reop CL	Associated Lesions [b] — MVD No.	MVD %	MVD CL	AVD No.	AVD %	AVD CL	PH No.	PH %	PH CL
Allograft [c]	75	15	20	15-26	3	4	2-8	18	24	19-30	12	16	12-22	10	13	9-19	2	2.7	0.9-6.2	5	7	4-11
Regurgitation		14	19	14-24	3	4	2-8	17	23	17-29	11	15	10-20	10	13	9-19	2	2.7	0.9-6.2	5	7	4-11
Stenosis		1	1.3	0.2-4.5	0	0	0-2.6	1	1.3	0.2-4.5	1	1.3	0.2-4.5	0	0	0-2.6	0	0	0-2.6	0	1.2	0.2-4.0
Carpentier Ring, regurgitation [d]	84	5	6	3-10	5	6	3-10	10	12	8-17	3	6	3-10	3	6	3-10	0	0	0-2.3	1		
De Vega repair, regurgitation [e]	14	0	0	0-13	0	0	0-13	0	0	0-13	0	0	0-13	0	0	0-13	0	0	0-13	0	0	0-13
Stent-mounted porcine xenograft, stenosis [f]	15	1	7	0.9-21	0	0	0-12	1	7	0.9-21	1	7	0.9-21	1	7	0.9-21	0	0	0-12	0	0	0-12
Bjork–Shiley, stenosis [g]	3	1	33	4-76	0	0	0-47	1	33	4-76	0	0	0-47	0	0	0-47	0	0	0-47	0	0	0-47
Braunwald-Cutter, stenosis	1	0	0	0-85	1	100	15-100	1	100	15-100	0	0	0-85	0	0	0-85	0	0	0-85	0	0	0-85
Starr-Edwards, stenosis	1	0	0	0-85	0	0	0-85	0	0	0-85	0	0	0-85	0	0	0-85	0	0	0-85	0	0	0-85
TOTAL	193	22	11	9-14	9	4.7	3.1-6.8	31	16	13-19	16	8.3	6.2-10.9	14	7.3	5.3-9.7	2	1.0	0.3-2.4	7	3.6	2.3-5.6
$P(\chi^2)$															.3			.8			.06	

Key: AVD, Aortic valve disease; CL, 70% confidence limits; MVD, mitral valve disease; PH, pulmonary hypertension.

[a] Database is the same as for Table 14-1.

[b] An associated lesion is one present when the tricuspid valve dysfunction was identified late postoperatively. This was either native aortic or mitral valve disease not evident or mild at the time of tricuspid valve surgery or malfunction or failure of the repair or replacement of one of those valves performed at the time of tricuspid valve surgery. Late postoperatively, the mitral valve disease was severe in two patients, moderate in six, and mild in six. Aortic valve disease was severe regurgitation in both. In three of the seven patients with residual severe pulmonary hypertension, it was not associated with residual left-sided valve disease.

[c] Duration of follow-up 67 ± 41.5 months.

[d] Duration of follow-up 35 ± 24.2 months.

[e] Duration of follow-up 20 ± 11.8 months.

[f] Duration of follow-up 31 ± 18.1 months.

[g] Duration of follow-up 34 ± 27.7 months.

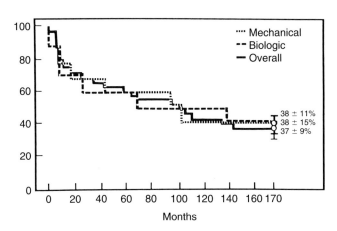

Figure 14-5 Survival (including hospital deaths) of 60 patients undergoing tricuspid valve replacement (1978 to 1993). Isolated tricuspid replacement was done in five patients; the remainder had another valve procedure or an associated repair of a congenital malformation. A bioprosthesis was used in 28 patients and a mechanical device in 32 patients. (From Scully and Armstrong.[S8])

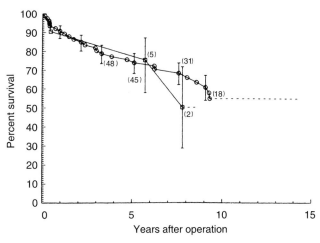

Figure 14-6 Survival of patients leaving the hospital alive after tricuspid valve replacement. Squares represent patients having only tricuspid valve replacement (n = 21). Circles represent patients having tricuspid and mitral valve replacement with or without aortic valve replacement (UAB group, 1967 to 1981; n = 77).

■ **TABLE 14-3   Late Results of Tricuspid Valve Replacement** [a]

Procedure	Hospital Survivors (n)	Late Death			Reoperation for TV Problem			Late Pacemaker Insertion [b]		
		No.	%	CL	No.	%	CL	No. (n)	% of n	CL
TVR alone	21	4	19	10–32	2	10	3–21	0 (20)	0	0–9
TVR + MVR	34	11	32	23–44	1	3	0.4–10	3 (32)	9	4–18
TVR + MVR + AVR	43	15	35	27–44	1	2	0.3–8	3 (40)	8	3–15
TVR + other [c]	5	2	40	14–71	1	20	3–53	0 (5)	0	0–32
TOTAL	103	32	31	26–36	5	5	3–8	6 (97)	6	4–10

Key: *AVR,* Aortic valve replacement; *CL,* 70% confidence limits; *MVR,* mitral valve replacement; *TV,* tricuspid valve; *TVR,* tricuspid valve replacement.

[a] Data are from 106 operations in 103 patients (UAB group, 1967 to 1981). Median follow-up was 7.0 years (6.6 months to 14.4 years); median age at operation was 43 years (5.7 to 76 years).

[b] n = 97 for hospital survivors without pacemakers. In addition, two patients had pacemakers preoperatively, and four had pacemakers implanted during initial hospitalization (three were TVR + MVR + AVR; one was TVR + MVR).

[c] Two patients had TVR + AVR, two had TVR + orthotopic or heterotopic PVR, and one had TVR + AVR + PVR.

however, reported a 27% operative mortality in 60 patients, with all deaths occurring in patients in NYHA class III or IV, those having repeat operations, or those with complex congenital heart disease (Fig. 14-5).

Survival at 10 years is approximately 55%, including hospital deaths (Fig. 14-6; see also Fig. 14-4). Most of these patients have multivalvar disease, and tricuspid valve failure is seldom the dominant factor in late death.[B8]

Mode of Premature Late Death

Following tricuspid valve surgery, most late deaths are related to advanced RV dysfunction or arrhythmias. Endocarditis and cerebrovascular accidents are uncommon modes of death, as are recurrent moderate or severe tricuspid stenosis or regurgitation resulting from malfunction of the replacement devices or failed anuloplasty. Thus, among 284 patients followed over nearly 10 years (combined GLH–UAB), prevalence of these complications was similar

after either tricuspid valve repair or replacement and accounted for 9 (11%; CL 8%-16%) of the late deaths, or 3.2% of the entire group (CL 2%-5%).

Complete Heart Block

Complete heart block occasionally develops late after tricuspid valve replacement, occurring in 6 (6%; CL 3%-9%) of 108 patients (GLH). Five of the 6 had associated mitral valve replacement,[B8] as did all those developing complete heart block in the UAB experience (Table 14-3). This association is undoubtedly related to the position of the AV node between the two replacement devices. In all, approximately 10% of patients undergoing both tricuspid and mitral replacement required insertion of a pacemaker late postoperatively because of heart block, and up to 10 years postoperatively the prevalence is 25% (Fig. 14-7). None of the patients undergoing tricuspid replacement as an isolated procedure (UAB) had this complication (*P* for

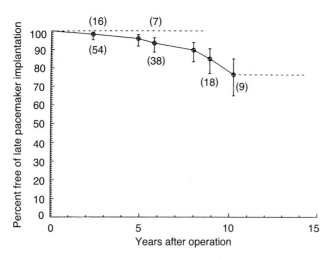

Figure 14-7 Freedom from pacemaker implantation late postoperatively. Circles represent patients undergoing tricuspid and mitral valve replacement with or without aortic valve replacement who left the hospital alive without a pacemaker (n = 73 traced patients). Dashed lines represent those undergoing only tricuspid valve replacement (n = 20 traced patients) (UAB group, 1967 to 1981).

difference = .16). Late development of complete heart block is uncommon after tricuspid anuloplasty, occurring in only 1 (1.6%; CL 0.5%-4%) of 113 survivors (GLH).[B8]

Thromboembolism

Pulmonary embolization is a rare complication of tricuspid valve surgery. Only 1 of 103 patients had probable large pulmonary emboli on follow-up (UAB). Because that patient also had deep vein thrombophlebitis in one leg, it is not certain that the emboli originated from the tricuspid replacement device.

Thrombosis

After tricuspid valve replacement, thrombosis may occur, more often of mechanical devices than of bioprostheses. The older types of mechanical prostheses (Smelloff-Cutter, Bjork-Shiley) apparently had a greater risk than present bileaflet valves. The linearized thrombosis rate in Van Nooten's series of 146 tricuspid replacements was approximately 1% per patient-year.[V2] Initial thrombolytic treatment using streptokinase may relieve obstruction in many cases. Hurrell and colleagues have reviewed the efficacy of thrombolytic therapy for all valve positions, and this approach seems particularly effective for prostheses in the tricuspid position (Table 14-4).[H4]

Streptokinase is administered as in treatment of acute myocardial infarction: 1 million units over 45 to 60 minutes optionally followed by 150,000 units · h^{-1} for 4 to 6 hours. Alternatively, urokinase may be infused intravenously at 50,000 to 150,000 units · h^{-1} for up to 24 hours.

Allergy to streptokinase is manifested by hypotension and fever. An unusual reaction to urokinase is severe rigor, which can be treated with meperidine hydrochloride.

■ **TABLE 14-4 Efficacy of Thrombolytic Therapy and Recurrence of Valve Obstruction, Stratified by Valve Position**

Position	n	Therapeutic Success		Recurrence of Obstruction	
		No.	%	No. (n) [a]	% of n
Mitral	122	99	81	21 (114)	18
Aortic	51	44	86	8 (49)	16
Tricuspid	28	24	86	5 (26)	19
Pulmonary	6	6	100	1 (6)	17
TOTAL	207	173	84	35 (195)	18
P (x^2)			.6		.99

Overall success of thrombolytic therapy was 84%. Success for right-sided valves (88%) was similar to that for left-sided valves (83%; P = .4). (From Hurrell and colleagues.[H45])

[a] Based on patients (n) with reported follow-up.

Functional Status

Late functional status of patients undergoing tricuspid valve surgery is influenced more by the multivalvar nature of most of the procedures than by the tricuspid repair or replacement itself. Nonetheless, most patients are considerably improved by the surgical procedure. Thus, in the GLH–UAB follow-up group, 42% of 103 patients were in NYHA class I late postoperatively. This is more impressive when it is realized that of these, 34 were preoperatively in class V,[1] 62 in class IV, and 6 in class III. In both series, less than 15% were in class IV late postoperatively.

Symptoms of Systemic Venous Hypertension

Most patients remain free of systemic venous hypertension late postoperatively. However, peripheral edema and hepatomegaly, with or without ascites, were present at follow-up in 28 (29%) of 97 patients after tricuspid replacement with mechanical prostheses or bioprostheses in whom these features were assessed (UAB). These symptoms could be the result of functional or organic obstruction of the tricuspid replacement device, residual left-sided cardiac failure with or without left-sided valvar disease, or important residual pulmonary hypertension (high pulmonary vascular resistance) or residual RV dysfunction. In this regard, Silver and colleagues reported higher right atrial pressures after tricuspid valve replacement than before in patients with Ebstein anomaly, but they also noted marked symptomatic improvement in cardiac function.[S6]

Performance of Replacement Devices

Small gradients of 4 to 10 mmHg exist across *stent-mounted xenografts* in the tricuspid position (Table 14-5). These bioprostheses seem to degenerate at about the same rate and with the same age-related occurrence in the tricuspid position as they do in the mitral and aortic

---

[1] Class V is cardiogenic shock or hemodynamic instability requiring emergency operation. This class augments the usual NYHA class IV, based on the observation of the UAB group that this subgroup of class IV was generally at higher risk than patients simply confined to bed.

■ **TABLE 14-5**   **Doppler Echocardiographic Data for Various Valve Prostheses**

Prosthesis	n	Early Velocity (m · s^{-1}) Mean ± SD	Mean Gradient (mmHg) Mean ± SD	Pressure Half-Time (ms) Mean ± SD (n [a])	Regurgitation % [b]
Stent-mounted porcine xenograft	41	1.3 ± 0.2	3.2 ± 1.1	146 ± 39 (29)	22
Caged ball	33	1.3 ± 0.2	3.1 ± 0.8	144 ± 46 (29)	9
St. Jude Medical	7	1.2 ± 0.3	2.7 ± 1.1	108 ± 32 (6)	29
Bjork-Shiley	1	1.3	2.2	144	0
Total	82	1.3 ± 0.2	3.1 ± 1.0	142 ± 42 (65)	17

Hemodynamic performance of various tricuspid valve replacement prostheses obtained by Doppler echocardiographic interrogation. (Modified from Connolly and colleagues.[C9])

Key: *SD*, Standard deviation.

[a] Pressure half-time not measured in patients with fusion of early and atrial velocities.

[b] Percentage of tricuspid prostheses with mild regurgitation or less.

■ **TABLE 14-6**   **Reoperations on Tricuspid Replacement Device** [a]

Original Replacement Device	n [b]	Age of Patient [c]	Interval [d] (years)	Indication
Starr-Edwards	46	43	9.3	Prosthetic valve endocarditis
Bjork-Shiley	23	39	6.1	Thrombotic encapsulation
Braunwald-Cutter	8	15	7.8	Thrombotic encapsulation
Stent-mounted porcine xenograft	29	9	3.7	Structural valve degeneration
Stent-mounted porcine xenograft	29	18	2.6	Structural valve degeneration

[a] Database is the same as in Table 14-3. At reoperation, two of the five patients died.

[b] The variable n refers to the total number of patients receiving that device in the tricuspid position.

[c] Age (years) at initial valve replacement operation.

[d] Years between initial replacement and re-replacement.

positions (see "Reoperation" under Mitral Valve Replacement and Results in Section 1 of Chapter 11; see also "Central Leakage" under Replacement Device Regurgitation in Chapter 12). In the combined GLH–UAB experience with 33 bioprostheses in the tricuspid position, three patients underwent reoperation, two of whom were younger than 20 years of age and required reoperation at 2.6 and 3.7 years after insertion (Table 14-6).

The Starr-Edwards ball valve *mechanical prosthesis* has performed well in the tricuspid position. Only 1 of 46 patients (UAB) required reoperation over a median follow-up of 7 years (see Table 14-6). No instances of acute or recurrent occlusion or encapsulation were seen. The Bjork-Shiley mechanical prosthesis also performed well in the tricuspid position, although no doubt it has a gradient in virtually all cases, as do all mechanical prostheses.[W3] One Bjork-Shiley valve required reoperation for thrombotic encapsulation. P'eterffy and Bjork reported this complication in two of five patients undergoing tricuspid valve replacement with this device.[P1] The St. Jude Medical valve appears also to exhibit good hemodynamic performance in the tricuspid position; Singh and colleagues reported no diastolic gradient in six patients with this device and a gradient of 2 mm in a seventh patient.[S5]

Reoperation

Most patients who have undergone tricuspid valve replacement are free of the need for reoperation up to 10 years later. Of those receiving mechanical or xenograft valves at UAB, 96% were free from tricuspid reoperation at 5 years, and 89% at 9 years. In McGrath's series of 530 patients having a procedure involving the tricuspid valve, freedom from reoperation was 26% at 15 years.[M4] However, be-

cause of the competing risk of 81 late deaths, cumulative incidence of reoperation was 59% at 15 years (see "Competing Risks under Time-Related Events" in Chapter 6).[M4]

Tricuspid Valve Excision

Survival

Early death occurs in 12% of drug addicts after excision without replacement of the tricuspid valve.[A1,A4] Late survival in such patients is 63% at 15 years, with death due to return to drug addiction and not to right-sided endocarditis.[A4]

Hemodynamic Status

After excision of the tricuspid valve, the expected hemodynamic state develops. Cardiac murmurs are usually absent, but hepatomegaly with systolic pulsation is often present.[F1] Jugular venous pulsations, with prominent v waves, are universal as a result of the dramatic increase in right atrial pressure during systole.

The volumes of the right atrium and RV are considerably increased within a few months of tricuspid valve removal. The atrial septum shifts to the left with each ventricular systole, and the left atrium is compressed.

Functional Status

Most young patients are in NYHA functional class II for at least several years. Ankle edema and mild exercise intolerance are noted in about half the patients. Hemodynamic and functional states begin to deteriorate progressively after about 5 years, often in association with troublesome substernal fullness, which is worse in the recumbent position.[S7]

Risk Factors for Premature Death after Tricuspid Valve Surgery

A general understanding of the results of tricuspid valve surgery per se, especially of the risk factors for surgical failure, is difficult to obtain because of the relative infrequency of these operations, variety of operations, numerous concomitant procedures, and heterogeneity of the patient population. It is possible to have low hospital mortality across all components of this heterogeneity (see Table 14-1), but this has not been the experience universally.

Tricuspid valve excision without replacement is clearly a risk factor for a poor early and long-term result.[A1] The need for tricuspid anuloplasty and replacement, particularly the latter, has been associated with an increased risk of early death in multivalvar disease (see "Mitral Valve Surgery with Coexisting Tricuspid Valve Disease" under Results in Chapter 11).[M4] However, early mortality after these combined procedures need not necessarily be determined by the tricuspid procedure[B8] (Table 14-7). Multivariable analysis of risk factors for both early and late deaths indicates that neither repair nor replacement is associated with a greater risk than the other; the type of replacement device (allograft, mechanical, bioprosthetic) was not a risk factor.[M4]

Earlier date of operation was a risk factor for death early after operation (Table 14-8).

Older age has been a risk factor for death early and late after operation[B8] (Table 14-9), as has preoperative functional disability, as reflected in NYHA class, particularly when the disability was severe and associated with cardiomegaly.[B2,B3] Prior valve surgery was also a risk factor for premature late death.

INDICATIONS FOR OPERATION

When isolated severe tricuspid regurgitation is present, operation is indicated. This should be annuloplasty rather than replacement, unless competence cannot be achieved. In intravenous drug users with endocarditis, simple valve excision may suffice, but tricuspid valve replacement is preferred over total excision; partial valve excision and reconstruction can be considered for less extreme valvar destruction.[A6] (Indications for operation in functional tricuspid regurgitation associated with mitral valve disease are discussed in detail under "Mitral Valve Surgery with Coexisting Tricuspid Valve Disease" in Chapter 11.) Because most tricuspid procedures are done to accompany left-sided valve operations, the left-sided hemodynamics usually determines indications for operation. However, because NYHA class IV, severe heart failure, high mean pulmonary artery pressure, and icterus are incremental risks for mortality when a tricuspid procedure is done, intervention early rather than late in multiple valve disease is prudent.[P3,V2]

When important tricuspid valve regurgitation occurs late after mitral valve replacement, 5-year survival after subsequent operation is only 44%, and most patients who fail to survive have little or no symptomatic improvement from the tricuspid valve procedure.[K4] This suggests the frequent presence of severe and irreversible RV failure in such patients. Thus, tricuspid regurgitation after previously adequate mitral valve operation is an uncommon indication for tricuspid valve operation.

Choice of Replacement Device

In no other valve position is the choice between durability of a mechanical prosthesis and lack of thrombogenicity of a xenograft more apparent. It can be argued that younger

■ **TABLE 14-7   Tricuspid Valve Surgery as Part of a Multivalve Operation**

Type of Operation	n	Hospital Deaths		
		No	%	CL
Triple valve replacement	13	1	8	1–24
Double valve replacement + repair of third valve	31	1	3	0.4–11
Single valve replacement + repair of two other valves	6	1	17	2–46
Double valve replacement	44	3	7	3–13
Single valve replacement + repair of one other valve	78	7	9	6–14
Double valve repair	18	0	0	0–10
TOTAL	190	13	6.8	4.9–9.3
$P (x^2)$			.6	

(From GLH group, 1973 to 1982.)

Key: *CL*, 70% confidence limits.

■ **TABLE 14-8   Relationship between NYHA Functional Class and Hospital Mortality after Isolated or Multivalve Tricuspid Valve Surgery in Two Eras** [a]

NYHA Class	1965 to 1973				1973 to 1982				Total			
		Hospital Deaths				Hospital Deaths				Hospital Deaths		
	n	No.	%	CL	n	No.	%	CL	n	No.	%	CL
I	0				0				0			
II	0				1	0	0	0–85	1	0	0	0–85
III	1	0	0	0–85	18	1	6	0.7–18	19	1	5	0.7–17
IV	30	5	17	9–27	109	2	1.8	0.6–4.3	139	7	5	3.1–7.7
V	17	10	59	43–73	70	10	14	10–20	87	20	23	18–29
TOTAL	48	15	31	24–40	198	13	6.6	4.7–8.9	246	28	11	9–14
$P(\text{logistic})$ [b]		.004				.01				.003		

Key: *CL*, 70% confidence limits; *NYHA*, New York Heart Association.

[a] From GLH group, 1965 to 1982; includes patients requiring hospitalization and intense decongestive therapy for up to 4 weeks preoperatively because of heart failure.

[b] Multivariable logistic test for era and NYHA class: $P(\text{era}) = .0001$; $P(\text{NYHA}) = .0002$.

■ TABLE 14–9 Relationship between Age at Operation and Hospital Death after Tricuspid Valve Surgery[a]

Age (Years)	TVS Alone				TVS + MVS				TVS + MVS + AVS				TVS + AVS				Total			
		Hospital Deaths				Hospital Deaths				Hospital Deaths				Hospital Deaths				Hospital Deaths		
	n	No.	%	CL	n	No.	%	CL	n	No.	%	CL	n	No.	%	CL	n	No.	%	CL
< 10	0	0			1	0	0	0-85	1	0	0	0-85	0				2	0	0	0-61
10–20	0	0			21	1	5	0.6-15	11	1	9	1-28	0				32	2	6	2-14
20–30	2	0	0	0-61	32	1	3	0.4-10	12	1	8	1-26	1	0	0	0-85	47	2	4	1-10
30–40	1	0	0	0-85	30	0	0	0-6	11	1	9	1-28	2	0	0	0-61	44	1	2	0.3-8
40–50	3	0	0	0-47	19	1	5	0.7-17	5	1	20	2.6-53	0				27	2	7	2-17
50–60	0	0			14	1	7	0.9-22	6	0	0	0-27	0				20	1	5	0.6-16
60–70	1	0	0	0-85	16	3	19	8-34	5	0	0	0-32	1	1	100	85-100	23	4	17	9-29
70–80	0	0			2	0	0	0-61	0				1	1	100	85-100	3	1	33	4-76
TOTAL	7	0	0	0-24	135	7	5.2	3.2-8.0	51	4	8	4-14	5	2	40	14-71	198	13	6.6	4.7-8.0
$P(\chi^2)$							.3				.9				.17				.09 (logistic)	

Key: AVS, Aortic valve surgery; CL, 70% confidence limits; MVS, mitral valve surgery; TVS, tricuspid valve surgery.

[a] Database includes 198 operations in 184 patients (GLH group, 1973 to 1982).

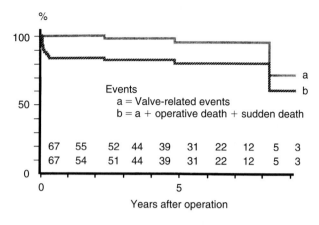

Figure 14-8 Freedom from valve-related events *(a)* and valve-related events plus operative and sudden deaths *(b)* in tricuspid valve replacements using an inverted bovine pericardial bioprosthesis. (Carpentier-Edwards model 2700 aortic xenograft). (From Nakano and colleagues.[N2])

patients with a better prognosis should receive a low-profile mechanical device, and older patients a xenograft.[V2] Nakano and colleagues report satisfactory valve performance using an inverted Carpentier-Edwards pericardial valve.[N2] (Fig. 14-8). Others prefer porcine xenografts for all patients despite a 10% to 40% prevalence of structural deterioration within 7 to 10 years.[K9,M6] In all cases a large device should be implanted. There is no evidence favoring use of a xenograft in the tricuspid area when mechanical prostheses are implanted on the left side, and vice versa.

REFERENCES

A

1. Arbulu A, Asfaw I. Tricuspid valvulectomy without prosthetic replacement. J Thorac Cardiovasc Surg 1981;82:684.

2. Arbulu A, Thomas NW, Wilson RF. Valvulectomy without prosthetic replacement: a lifesaving operation for tricuspid pseudomonas endocarditis. J Thorac Cardiovasc Surg 1972;64:103.

3. Arneborn P, Bjork VO, Rodriguez L, Svanbom M. Two-stage replacement of tricuspid valve in active endocarditis. Br Heart J 1977;39:1276.

4. Arbulu A. Discussion (Stern JH, Sisto DA, Strom JA, Soeiro R, Jones SF, Frater RW. Immediate tricuspid valve replacement for endocarditis. J Thorac Cardiovasc Surg 1986;91:163). J Thorac Cardiovasc Surg 1986;91:167.

5. Abe T, Tukamoto M, Yanagiya M, Morikawa M, Watanabe N, Komatsu S. De Vega's annuloplasty for acquired tricuspid disease: early and late results in 110 patients. Ann Thorac Surg 1989;48:670.

6. Allen MD, Slachman F, Eddy AC, Cohen D, Otto CM, Pearlman AS. Tricuspid valve repair for tricuspid valve endocarditis: tricuspid valve "recycling." Ann Thorac Surg 1991;51:593.

B

1. Beasley K. Traumatic tricuspid insufficiency. Tex Med 1973;69:71.

2. Baughman KL, Kallman CH, Yurchak PM, Daggett WM, Buckley MJ. Predictors of survival after tricuspid valve surgery. Am J Cardiol 1984;54:137.

3. Bayer AS, Blomquist IK, Bello E, Chiu CY, Ward JI, Ginzton LE. Tricuspid valve endocarditis due to *Staphylococcus aureus*. Chest 1988;93:247.

4. Bharati S, Lev M, Kirklin JW. Cardiac surgery and the conduction system, 2nd ed. Mount Kisco, NY: Futura, 1992.

5. Boyd AD, Engelman RM, Isom OW, Reed GE, Spencer FC. Tricuspid annuloplasty. Five and one-half years' experience with 78 patients. J Thorac Cardiovasc Surg 1974;68:344.

6. Bex JP, Lecompte Y. Tricuspid valve repair using a flexible linear reducer. J Card Surg 1986;1:151.

7. Barrillon A, Baragan J. Methysergide and tricuspid valve lesions (letter). Circulation 1978;58:578.

8. Barratt-Boyes BG, Rutherford JD, Whitlock RM, Pemberton JR. A review of surgery for acquired tricuspid valve disease, including an assessment of the stented semilunar homograft valve, and the results of operation for multivalvular heart disease. Aust N Z J Surg 1988;58:23.

C

1. Carpena C, Kay JH, Mendez AM, Redington JV, Zubiate P, Zucker R. Carcinoid heart disease: surgery for tricuspid and pulmonary valve lesions. Am J Cardiol 1973;32:229.

2. Collins P, Daly JJ. Tricuspid incompetence complicating acute myocardial infarction. Postgrad Med J 1977;53:51.

3. Chusid MJ, Dale DC, West BC, Wolffe SM. The hypereosinophilic syndrome: analysis of fourteen cases with review of the literature. Medicine (Baltimore) 1975;54:1.

4. Carpentier A, Deloche A, Hanania G, Forman J, Sellier P, Piwnica A, et al. Surgical management of acquired tricuspid valve disease. J Thorac Cardiovasc Surg 1974;67:53.

5. Come PC, Riley MF. Tricuspid annular dilatation and failure of tricuspid leaflet coaptation in tricuspid regurgitation. Am J Cardiol 1985;55:599.

6. Curtius JM, Thyssen M, Breuer HW, Loogen F. Doppler versus contrast echocardiography for diagnosis of tricuspid regurgitation. Am J Cardiol 1985;56:333.

7. Chopra HK, Nanda NC, Fan P, Kapur KK, Goyal R, Daruwalla D, et al. Can two-dimensional echocardiography and Doppler color flow mapping identify the need for tricuspid valve repair? J Am Coll Cardiol 1989;14:1266.

8. Czer LS, Maurer G, Bolger A, DeRobertis M, Kleinman J, Gray RJ, et al. Tricuspid valve repair: operative and follow-up evaluation by Doppler color flow mapping. J Thorac Cardiovasc Surg 1989;98:101.

9. Connolly HM, Miller FA Jr, Taylor CL, Naessens JM, Seward JB, Tajik AJ. Doppler hemodynamic profiles of 82 clinically and echocardiographically normal tricuspid valve prostheses. Circulation 1993;88:2722.

D

1. Duran CM, Pomar JL, Colman T, Figueroa A, Revuelta JM, Ubago JL. Is tricuspid valve repair necessary? J Thorac Cardiovasc Surg 1980;80:849.

2. De Vega NG. La anuloplastia selectiva, regulable permanente. Rev Esp Cardiol 1972;25:555.

F

1. Friedman G, Kronzon I, Nobile J, Cohen ML, Winer HE. Echocardiographic findings after tricuspid valvectomy. Chest 1985;87:668.

G

1. Gibson R, Wood P. The diagnosis of tricuspid stenosis. Br Heart J 1955;17:552.
2. Goldman M, Mindich B, Guarino T, Fuster V. Intraoperative contrast echo: a new method to evaluate tricuspid regurgitation (abstract). J Am Coll Cardiol 1985;54:459.
3. Goldman ME, Guarino T, Fuster V, Mindich B. The necessity for tricuspid valve repair can be determined intraoperatively by two dimensional echocardiography. J Thorac Cardiovasc Surg 1987; 94:542.

H

1. Honey M, Paneth M. Carcinoid heart disease: successful tricuspid valve replacement. Thorax 1975;30:464.
2. Hendel N, Leckie B, Richards J. Carcinoid heart disease: eight-year survival following tricuspid valve replacement and pulmonary valvotomy. Ann Thorac Surg 1980;30:391.
3. Hojnik M, George J, Ziporen L, Shoenfield Y. Heart valve involvement (Libman-Sacks endocarditis) in the antiphospholipid syndrome (review). Circulation 1996;93:1579.
4. Hurrell DG, Schaff HV, Tajik AJ. Thrombolytic therapy for obstruction of mechanical prosthetic valves (review). Mayo Clin Proc 1996; 71:605.

K

1. Kisslo J, Von Ramm OT, Haney R, Jones R, Juk SS, Behar VS. Echocardiographic evaluation of tricuspid valve endocarditis: an M-mode and two-dimensional study. Am J Cardiol 1976;38:502.
2. Keller BD, Boal BH, Lewin A, Kaltman AJ. Development of tricuspid valvular regurgitation during the course of chronic cor pulmonale. Chest 1970;57:196.
3. Khosla SN, Arora BS. Tricuspid incompetence in chronic cor pulmonale. J Assoc Physicians India 1972;20:571.
4. King RM, Schaff HV, Danielson GK, Gersh BJ, Phil D, Orszulak TA, et al. Surgery for tricuspid regurgitation late after mitral valve replacement. Circulation 1984;70:I193.
5. Kay JH, Maselli-Campagna G, Tsuji KK. Surgical treatment of tricuspid insufficiency. Ann Surg 1965;162:53.
6. Katz NM, Pallas RS. Traumatic rupture of the tricuspid valve: Repair by chordal replacements and annuloplasty. J Thorac Cardiovasc Surg 1986;91:310.
7. Kay JH, Mendez AM, Zubiate P. A further look at tricuspid annuloplasty. Ann Thorac Surg 1976;22:498.
8. Kulshrestha P, Das B, Iyer KS, Sampathkumar A, Sharma ML, Rao IM, et al. Surgical experience with diseases of the tricuspid valve. Cross-sectional and Doppler echocardiographic evaluation following De Vega's repair. Int J Cardiol 1989;23:19.
9. Kuwaki K, Komatsu K, Morishita K, Tsukamoto M, Abe T. Long-term results of porcine bioprostheses in the tricuspid position. Jpn J Surg 1998;28:599.

M

1. Michl L, Shumacker HB Jr. Tricuspid valvulectomy. Surg Gynecol Obstet 1973;137:590.
2. Marvin RF, Schrank JP, Nolan SP. Traumatic tricuspid insufficiency. Am J Cardiol 1973;32:723.
3. McAllister RG Jr, Friesinger GC, Sinclair-Smith BC. Tricuspid regurgitation following inferior myocardial infarction. Arch Intern Med 1976;136:95.
4. McGrath LB, Gonzalez-Lavin L, Bailey BM, Grunkemeier GL, Fernandez J, Laub GW. Tricuspid valve operations in 530 patients: twenty-five year assessment of early and late phase events. J Thorac Cardiovasc Surg 1990;99:124.
5. McCarthy JF, Cosgrove DM III. Tricuspid valve repair with the Cosgrove-Edwards annuloplasty system. Ann Thorac Surg 1997; 64:267.
6. McGrath LB, Chen C, Bailey BM, Fernandez J, Laub GW, Adkins MS. Early and late phase events following bioprosthetic tricuspid valve replacement. J Card Surg 1992;7:245.

N

1. Nakano S, Kawashima Y, Hirose H, Matsuda H, Shimazaki Y, Taniguchi K, et al. Evaluation of long-term results of bicuspidalization annuloplasty for functional tricuspid regurgitation. J Thorac Cardiovasc Surg 1988;95:340.
2. Nakano K, Eishi K, Kosakai Y, Isobe F, Sasako Y, Nagata S, et al. Ten-year experience with the Carpentier-Edwards pericardial xenograft in the tricuspid position. J Thorac Cardiovasc Surg 1996;111:605.

P

1. P'eterffy A, Bjork VO. Surgical treatment of Ebstein's anomaly. Scand J Thorac Cardiovasc Surg 1979;13:1.
2. Pasaoglu I, Demiricin M, Dogan R, Hatipglu A, Gunay I, Ersoy U, et al. De Vega's tricuspid annuloplasty: analysis of 195 patients. Thorac Cardiovasc Surg 1990;38:365.
3. Poveda JJ, Bernal JM, Matorras P, Hernando JP, Oliva MJ, Ochoteco A, et al. Tricuspid valve replacement in rheumatic disease: preoperative predictors of hospital mortality. J Heart Valve Dis 1996;5:26.
4. Paniagua D, Aldrich H, Liberman E, Lamas G, Agaston A. Increased prevalence of significant tricuspid regurgitation in patients with transvenous pacemaker leads. Am J Cardiol 1998;82:430.

R

1. Reisberg BE. Infective endocarditis in the narcotic addict. Prog Cardiovasc Dis 1979;22:193.
2. Robiolio PA, Rigolin VH, Wilson JS, Harrison JK, Sanders LL, Bashoire TM, et al. Carcinoid heart disease: correlation of high serotonin levels with valvular abnormalities detected by cardiac catheterization and echocardiography. Circulation 1995;92:790.
3. Robiolio PA, Rigolin VH, Harrison JK, Lowe JE, Moore JO, Bashore TM, et al. Predictors of outcome of tricuspid valve replacement in carcinoid heart disease. Am J Cardiol 1995;75:485.

S

1. Sethia B, Williams BT. Tricuspid valve excision without replacement in a case of endocarditis secondary to drug abuse. Br Heart J 1978; 40:579.
2. Stephenson LW, MacVaugh H 3rd, Kastor JA. Tricuspid valvular incompetence and rupture of the ventricular septum caused by nonpenetrating trauma. J Thorac Cardiovasc Surg 1979;77:768.
3. Sackner MA, Heinz ER, Steinberg AJ. The heart in scleroderma. Am J Cardiol 1966;17:542.
4. Solley GO, Maldonado JE, Gleich GJ, Giuliani ER, Hoagland HC, Pierre RV, et al. Endomyocardiopathy with eosinophilia. Mayo Clin Proc 1976;51:697.
5. Singh AK, Christian FD, Williams DO, Georas CS, Riley RR, Nanian KB, et al. Follow-up assessment of St. Jude Medical prosthetic valve in the tricuspid position: clinical and hemodynamic results. Ann Thorac Surg 1984;37:324.
6. Silver MA, Cohen SR, McIntosh CL, Cannon RO III, Roberts WC. Late (5 to 132 months) clinical and hemodynamic results after either tricuspid valve replacement or annuloplasty for Ebstein's anomaly of the tricuspid valve. Am J Cardiol 1984;54:627.
7. Slone RM, Hill JA, Akins EW, Conti CR. Magnetic resonance imaging late after tricuspid valvectomy. Am J Cardiol 1987;59:1426.
8. Scully HE, Armstrong CS. Tricuspid valve replacement. Fifteen years of experience with mechanical prostheses and bioprostheses. J Thorac Cardiovasc Surg 1995;109:1035.
9. Stern HJ, Sisto DA, Strom JA, Soeiro R, Jones SR, Frater RW. Immediate tricuspid valve replacement for endocarditis. Indications and results. J Thorac Cardiovasc Surg 1986;91:163.

T

1. Tsakiris AG, Mair DD, Seki S, Titus JL, Wood EH. Motion of the tricuspid valve annulus in anesthetized intact dogs. Circ Res 1975; 36:43.

7. Misch KA. Development of heart valve lesions during methysergide therapy. Br Med J 1974;2:365.

2. Tei C, Pilgrim JP, Shah PM, Ormiston JA, Wong M. The tricuspid valve annulus: study of size and motion in normal subjects and in patients with tricuspid regurgitation. Circulation 1982;66:665.

3. Tager R, Skudicky D, Mueller U, Essop R, Hammond G, Sareli P. Long-term follow-up of rheumatic patients undergoing left-sided valve replacement with tricuspid annuloplasty: validity of preoperative echocardiographic criteria in the decision to perform tricuspid annuloplasty. Am J Cardiol 1998;81:1013.

U

1. Ubago JL, Figueroa A, Ochoteco A, Colman T, Duran RM, Duran CG. Analysis of the amount of tricuspid valve anular dilatation required to produce functional tricuspid regurgitation. Am J Cardiol 1983;52:155.

V

1. Van Slyck EJ, Adamson TC III. Acute hypereosinophilic syndrome: successful treatment with vincristine, cytarabine, and prednisone. JAMA 1979;242:175.

2. Van Nooten GJ, Caes F, Taeymans Y, Van Belleghem Y, Francois K, De Bacquer D, et al. Tricuspid valve replacement: postoperative and long-term results. J Thorac Cardiovasc Surg 1995;110:672.

W

1. Wright JS, Glennie JS. Excision of tricuspid valve with later replacement in endocarditis of drug addiction. Thorax 1978;33:518.

2. Waller BJ, Moriarty AT, Ebie JN, Davey DM, Hawley DA, Pless JE. Etiology of pure tricuspid regurgitation based on anular circumference and leaflet area: analysis of 45 necropsy patients with clinical and morphologic evidence of pure tricuspid regurgitation. J Am Coll Cardiol 1986;7:1063.

3. Weerasena N, Spyt TJ, Pye M, Bain WH. Clinical evaluation of the Bjork-Shiley disc valve in the tricuspid position: long-term results. Eur J Cardiothorac Surg 1990;4:19.

Y

1. Yousef AM, Shafer MZ, Endrys G, Khan N, Simo M, Cherian G. Tricuspid stenosis and regurgitation in rheumatic heart disease: a prospective cardiac catheterization study in 525 patients. Am Heart J 1985;110:60.

Z

1. Zone DD, Botti RE. Right ventricular infarction with tricuspid insufficiency and chronic right heart failure. Am J Cardiol 1976;37:445.

15 Infective Endocarditis

BOX 15-1   Glossary

Endocarditis: Exudative and proliferative inflammatory alterations of the endocardium, characterized by vegetations on the endocardial surface or within the endocardium. It may occur as a primary disorder *(infective endocarditis)* or as a complication of or in association with another disease (e.g., lupus erythematosus, rheumatic heart disease).

Infective endocarditis: Invasion and multiplication of microorganisms on the endocardial surface, within the endocardium, or on prosthetic materials within and around cardiac structures. It includes conditions in which structures of the heart, most frequently the valves, harbor an infective process that leads to valvar dysfunction, localized or generalized sepsis, or sites for embolism. The term covers:
- Acute, subacute, and chronic processes
- Infection of bacterial, viral, rickettsial, or fungal etiology
- Involvement of either native or prosthetic valves (or other prosthetic material)

Acute endocarditis: A severe form of infective endocarditis caused by virulent pyogenic microorganisms such as hemolytic streptococci or staphylococci. It can become life threatening within days.

Subacute endocarditis: A form of infective endocarditis that develops subtly over a period of weeks to several months. It may produce symptoms for months before heart valve damage or emboli make the diagnosis clear. It is usually caused by *Streptococcus viridans* or *S. fecalis.*

Active endocarditis: A surgical term indicating an operation carried out in the presence of obvious local cardiac infection manifested by inflammation, active vegetations, abscesses, burrowing sinuses, or fistulae. If such an operation is carried out while a patient is being treated with antibiotics for active infection, or has been treated within 2 weeks of operation, the disease is considered active.

Healed endocarditis: A surgical term indicating an operation carried out in the absence of obvious local cardiac infection and inflammation, generally following treatment and supposed eradication of microorganisms. It is characterized by lack of local inflammation; vegetations may be present but are generally endothelialized, and abscesses have resulted in well-defined and stable cavities, including sinuses and fistulae.

Native valve endocarditis: Infectious endocarditis involving a patient's own (native) heart valve.

Prosthetic valve endocarditis: Infectious endocarditis involving a surgically implanted prosthetic heart valve. *Prosthetic valve endocarditis* and its abbreviation PVE are familiar, standard, and historical designations for infective endocarditis on any heart valve substitute. However, "prosthetic" is at times a misnomer (e.g., infection of a pulmonary autograft). The rationale for a more appropriate term, *replacement device endocarditis,* is presented in Chapter 12. In this chapter the historical term is maintained for sake of familiarity.

DEFINITION

Infective endocarditis includes conditions in which structures of the heart, most frequently the valves, harbor an infective process that leads to valvar dysfunction, localized or generalized sepsis, or sites for embolism (Box 15-1). The term *infective endocarditis* includes acute, subacute, and chronic processes; infection of bacterial, viral, rickettsial, or fungal etiology; and involvement of either native or prosthetic valves. As such, the term has no implication as to duration of the processes, infecting agent, or site of infection, and thus supplants previously used terms such as "subacute bacterial endocarditis."

HISTORICAL NOTE

In 1806, Corvisart described mitral valve vegetations found at autopsy in a 39-year-old man.[C1] In their book on heart disease, Bertin and Bouillaud discuss induration and vegetations on the valves of patients dying with endocarditis.[B1] The term *endocarditis* was introduced by Bouillard in 1841, when he described clinical and pathologic features of the disease.[B2] Earlier, Morgagni, Lancisi, and Sandifort had described hearts with probable endocardial vegetations.[M1,L1,S1]

Weinstein and Brusch report that in 1886, Wyssokowitch and Orth designed an experimental model for endocarditis in which aortic valve leaflets of animals were traumatized and the animals subsequently injected with bacterial suspensions from patients with endocarditis.[O1,W1,W2] The animals developed murmurs, embolic complications, and valve lesions at autopsy.

At the 1885 Gulstonian Lecture, Osler described the classic features of endocarditis.[O2] By 1909, he had refined his understanding of the pathologic anatomy ("proliferative vegetations") and introduced the clinical finding of changing murmurs.[O3] Along with Horder, Osler emphasized the role of blood cultures for diagnosis.[H1,O2,O3]

Successful treatment of endocarditis lagged behind pathologic and clinical descriptions. In the 1940s, the era of sulfa drugs, cure was achieved in about 5% of patients.[W1] By 1950, however, principles of antibiotic therapy had been established, including high-dose penicillin, long duration of treatment, and antibiotic suppression.[C2,G1,L2] It was also recognized at that time that delay in treatment, congestive heart failure, advanced age, and preexisting rheumatic valvulitis were adverse prognostic factors.[C2]

Direct surgical treatment of infective endocarditis (IE) began in 1961, when Kay and colleagues reported successful treatment of *Candida* endocarditis of the tricuspid valve. The native valve was debrided and an accompanying ventricular septal defect closed.[K1] In 1940, Tauroff and Vessell successfully ligated a patent ductus arteriosus in treating a 2-year-old female with endocarditis.[T1]

In 1957, Bahnson and colleagues reported occurrence of staphylococcal infection on silk sutures used for great vessel and intracardiac repairs.[B3] The first report of replacement of a cardiac valve for native IE was published in 1965 by Wallace and colleagues.[W3] Their patient was a 45-year-old man who had severe aortic regurgitation with heavy *Klebsiella* vegetations on each cusp. Although treated intensively with antibiotics over 3 weeks, there was resistant active infection and heart failure. Valve replacement was successful, eradicating the infection and restoring satisfactory hemodynamics.

In 1972, Merendino's group from the University of Washington reported the collective results of cardiac operations for endocarditis in 139 patients, 24 of whom were treated by mitral valve repair, mechanical prosthetic mitral replacement, and replacement of the aortic valve with beta-propriolactone–sterilized allografts. Seventeen of 24 patients survived.[M2] The report emphasized continuing sepsis and heart failure as indications for operation, compared native ("primary") to prosthetic ("secondary") valve endocarditis, and differentiated between active and healed lesions.

Most of the modern concepts of surgical treatment of IE were articulated by the late 1970s and reviewed in publications by Stinson and by Richardson and colleagues.[R1,S2]

PATHOGENESIS AND MORPHOLOGY
Pathogenesis

Several predisposing factors have been identified that may contribute to or be responsible for development of IE. Despite Osler's initial observations, valvulitis of rheumatic fever was often confused histologically with IE.[O2] However, as opposed to rheumatic valvulitis, IE is not characterized in its early stages by global neovascularization or global inflammation of valve leaflets. In most cases the *valvar endocardial surface must be altered* to allow deposition of fibrin and platelets and subsequent attachment of bacteria. This injury may result from preexisting valvar lesions, such as rheumatic valvulitis, anular or valvar calcification, or catheter trauma. Hemodynamic factors may contribute, such as the jet effect of blood flow through a patent ductus arteriosus or restrictive ventricular septal defect, mitral valve prolapse, or bicuspid aortic valve. Bacteremia must occur in IE. Frequent, transient bacteremias are found in 60% to 80% of normal individuals, but the number of organisms is small, and without the presence of one or more of the above factors, infection and vegetations do not result.[W1]

Several lines of evidence have demonstrated the importance of a *compromised or altered immune system* in the pathogenesis of IE. Histopathologic analysis of kidney tissue in patients with IE may reveal diffuse proliferative glomerulonephritis, with evidence of deposition of immunoglobulin G (IgG) and IgM.[B6] Circulating immune complexes (CICs) may be found in the glomerular basement membrane and in the retina and peripheral lesions (Roth spots and Janeway lesions).[B7,G3] Various manifestations of complement activation have been found in IE.[O5] Hooper and colleagues identified CICs in patients with prosthetic valve endocarditis[1] (PVE).[H2] Kauffmann and colleagues found a positive correlation between CIC levels and duration of illness,[K2] and several investigators have noted a decline in CIC levels with successful treatment.[B7,C3]

Staphylococcus aureus binds to porcine valvar endothelial cells by a mechanism that is specific and receptor mediated.[J2] This characteristic most likely represents a specific *physiochemical interaction* between microbial adhesins and a host cell receptor that involves fibronectin lipoteichoic acid.[G4,R2,V1] IE involving a previously normal valve is often caused by *S. aureus*.

In several studies, one quarter of IE cases occurred on normal valves.[M4,W5] Common factors were presence of overwhelming sepsis, resuscitation from shock, use of long-term indwelling catheters, intravenous (IV) drug abuse, and fungemia associated with prolonged antibiotic therapy. Only about 5% of patients with catheter sepsis are found to have IE, and this is generally due to staphylococcal organisms. *Iatrogenic* IE most frequently occurs in patients undergoing chronic hemodialysis who have frequent staphylococcal bacteremias and also may have sclerotic aortic or mitral valves. A few patients develop endocarditis of normal valves. Likely organisms are those that have increased adhesion molecules noted on dextran polymerization, namely, *Staphylococcus, Streptococcus viridans,* and *Enterococcus.*

---

[1] *Prosthetic valve endocarditis* and its abbreviation PVE are familiar, standard, and historical designations for infective endocarditis on any heart valve substitute. However, "prosthetic" is surely at times a misnomer (e.g., infection of a pulmonary autograft). The rationale for a more appropriate term, *replacement device endocarditis,* is presented in Chapter 12. In this chapter the historical term is maintained for sake of familiarity.

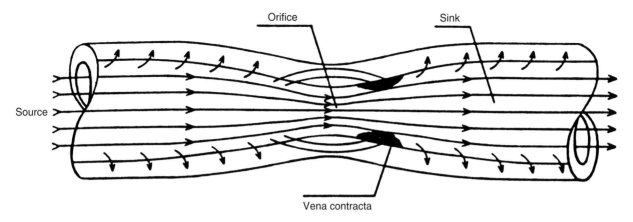

Figure 15-1   Flow through a permeable tube. High-pressure source drives fluid through an orifice into a low-pressure sink. Curved arrows leaving the stream entering the wall in the upstream segment represent normal perfusion of lining layer. Velocity is maximal and perfusing pressure is low immediately beyond the orifice, where momentum of stream converges stream-lines to form a vena contracta. Low pressure in this segment results in reduced perfusion and may cause retrograde flow from deeper layers of the vessel into the flowing stream. It is at the vena contracta that bacteria and other formed elements in the blood accumulate. (From Rodbard.[R3])

It has long been acknowledged that usual bacterial vegetation of IE can result from seeding of a platelet–thrombin nidus after mechanical trauma. Garrison and Freedman produced endocarditis in rabbits by inserting a catheter into the endocardium and injecting bacterial isolates from humans with endocarditis.[G5] This model remains the principal experimental paradigm for the mechanical basis of IE.

Perhaps the most persuasive hypothesis for the pathogenesis of IE has been put forward by Rodbard.[R3] Basically, high-velocity jets of blood from a high-pressure source occur at an orifice and enter a low-pressure sink. Venturi currents deposit bacteria immediately beyond the orifice to form vena contracta and result in mechanical erosion and deposition of platelets and thrombin (Fig. 15-1). These mechanical conditions exist beyond stenotic valves, on the pulmonary artery opposite a patent ductus arteriosus (Fig. 15-2) and on the left atrial aspect of a regurgitant mitral valve. Because most IE lesions of the aortic valve begin on the ventricular aspect, however, this suggests a role for valvar regurgitation in the pathogenesis of these lesions, and the Venturi effect would also apply (Table 15-1).

Morphology

Usual sites for IE found at operation in patients with NVE not related to IV drug use are shown in Fig. 15-3. Vegetations and erosive cavities are on the ventricular aspect of the aortic valve cusps and at the base of the atrial aspect of the mitral valve leaflets, often resulting in separation or discontinuity at the ventriculoarterial or atrioventricular junction. Less often, discrete perforations caused by isolated vegetations are located on the aortic cusps themselves. Occasionally, "drop lesions" from the aortic valve occur on the anterior mitral leaflet or the tensor apparatus of the mitral valve.

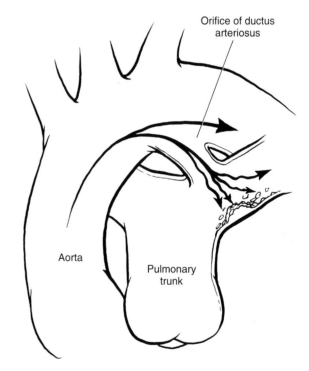

Figure 15-2   Representation of infective endocarditis at a patent ductus arteriosus. Vegetations are deposited on the pulmonary artery wall opposite a high-velocity jet through an open ductus.

In the vast majority of non–drug-related cases of native valve endocarditis (NVE), valve deposits are left sided. In IV-drug–related IE, the tricuspid valve is involved in about half the cases and aortic or mitral valves in the remainder.[M5] Perianular pseudoaneurysms (abscesses) are more frequently associated with aortic than with mitral

■ **TABLE 15-1** **Loci of Infective Endocarditic Lesions**

Condition	High-Pressure Source	Orifice	Low-Pressure Sink	Location of Lesions [a]	Satellite Lesions
Coarctation of aorta	Central aorta	Coarctation	Distal aorta	Downstream wall of aorta	Lateral wall peripheral to stenotic lesion
Patent ductus arteriosus	Aorta	Ductus	Pulmonary artery	Pulmonary artery	Pulmonary artery Tricuspid valve
Arteriovenous fistula	Artery	Fistula	Vein	Communications and veins	
Ventricular septal defect	Left ventricle	Defect	Right ventricle	Right ventricular surface of defect	Pulmonary artery
Aortic regurgitation	Aorta	Closed aortic valves	Left ventricle	Ventricular surface of aortic valves	Mitral chordae
Mitral regurgitation	Left ventricle	Closed mitral valves	Left atrium	Atrial surface of mitral valves	Atrium
Pulmonary regurgitation	Pulmonary artery	Closed pulmonary valves	Right ventricle	Ventricular surface Pulmonary valves	
Tricuspid regurgitation	Right ventricle	Closed tricuspid valves	Right atrium	Atrial surface Tricuspid valves	

(Modified from Rodbard[R3]; in Weinstein and Schlesinger.[W5])

[a] Add adjacent downstream surfaces.

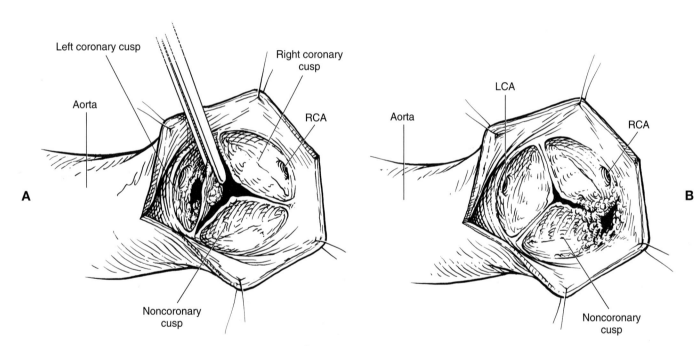

Figure 15-3 Usual sites of native valve infective endocarditis. **A,** Aortic valve with vegetation on noncoronary cusp and partial destruction of left coronary cusp. **B,** Aortic valve with vegetation between noncoronary and right coronary cusps extending as an anular abscess.

Key: *RCA,* right coronary artery; *LCA,* left coronary artery. *Continued*

endocarditis and occur in about one third of cases studied by transesophageal echocardiography (TEE). *S. aureus* is the predominant organism.[T3] Clinically, presence of pericarditis, rapid progression of symptoms, and a high degree of atrioventricular block are associated with perianular abscess.[A2]

In PVE, all or most of the vegetations are on the ventricular aspect of the prosthesis. Only a small area of "sewing ring" detachment may be apparent and may appear "sterile." At operation, therefore, a thorough search must be made beneath the prosthesis for the bulk of the pathologic process. As noted in some series, there may be important detachment without apparent vegetations; this may occur in either the presence or absence of positive blood cultures.[I1] This represents PVE and requires replacement of the prosthesis.

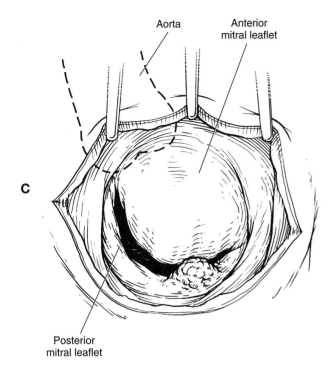

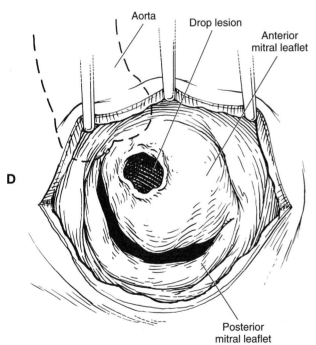

Figure 15-3, cont'd   C, Leaflet vegetation and ring abscess of posterior medial aspect of mitral valve. **D,** Mitral valve with drop lesion of anterior leaflet.

CLINICAL FEATURES AND DIAGNOSTIC CRITERIA

Infective endocarditis is present when defined in accordance with New York Heart Association (NYHA) criteria[N1]: positive blood cultures associated with either new or changing murmurs or with embolic phenomena; or new or changing murmurs in a patient with a congenital cardiac

---

BOX 15-2   Diagnostic Criteria for Infective Endocarditis (IE)

Major Criteria
- Positive blood culture for IE
  Typical microorganisms for IE from two separate blood cultures
  Viridans streptococci, [a] *Streptococcus bovis,* HACEK group, or community-acquired *Staphylococcus aureus* or enterococci, in absence of a primary focus, *or*
  Persistently positive blood culture, defined as recovery of a microorganism consistent with IE from:
  (i) Blood cultures drawn more than 12 hours apart, *or*
  (ii) All of three or majority of four or more separate blood cultures, with first and last drawn at least 1 hour apart
- Evidence of endocardial involvement:
  Positive echocardiogram for IE
  (i) Oscillating intracardiac mass, on valve or supporting structures, *or* in path of regurgitant jets, *or* on implanted material, in absence of an alternative anatomic explanation, *or*
  (ii) Abscess, *or*
  (iii) New partial dehiscence of prosthetic valve, *or* New valvar regurgitation (increase or change in preexisting murmur not sufficient)

Minor Criteria
  Predisposition: predisposing heart condition *or* IV drug use
  Fever: ≥38°C
  Vascular phenomena: major arterial emboli, septic pulmonary infarcts, mycotic aneurysm, intracranial hemorrhage, conjunctival hemorrhages, Janeway lesions
  Immunologic phenomena: glomerulonephritis, Osler nodes, Roth spots, rheumatoid factor
  Microbiologic evidence: positive blood culture but not meeting major criterion [b] *or* serologic evidence of active infection with organism consistent with IE
  Echocardiogram: consistent with IE but not meeting major criterion

Key: *HACEK, Haemophilus* spp., *Actinobacillus actinomycetemcomitans, Cardiobacterium hominis, Eikenella* spp., and *Kingella kingae.*
[a] Including nutritional variant strains.
[b] Excluding single positive cultures for coagulase-negative staphylococci and organisms that do not cause endocarditis.

---

anomaly or with prior valve damage, associated with either embolic phenomena or sustained fever, anemia, and splenomegaly. Most authorities accept a modification of that definition to include progressive heart failure in the presence of positive blood cultures. In an effort to improve specificity and sensitivity for diagnosis IE, investigators at Duke University have proposed criteria modeled after the Jones criteria for diagnosing rheumatic fever[D1] (Box 15-2). These criteria include major and minor signs and symptoms, echocardiographic findings, possible iatrogenic and nosocomial factors (e.g., indwelling catheters), and history of intravenous (IV) drug abuse.[B4]

The most common clinical manifestation of IE is *fever,* which is present in 95% to 100% of patients. This applies to both *NVE* and *PVE.* The fever may be low grade or spiking and generally follows peaks of bacteremia by about 2 hours.

Positive blood cultures are obtained in about 95% of patients even when right-sided endocarditis, endocarditis caused by fungus, endocarditis in addicts, and endocarditis caused by fastidious organisms are included.

A heart murmur is found in about 85% to 95% of IE patients. Changing murmurs occur much less frequently (about 15% to 20%). Although the concept of changing murmurs has been classically associated with IE since Osler's Gulstonian Lecture in 1885, clinically changing murmurs are not often appreciated.[O2] Ten percent of IE patients lack murmurs, particularly those with tricuspid involvement. Infection involving the aortic valve and root is often characterized by a relatively short diastolic murmur. There may be a murmur only in early systole or midsystole, although murmurs are often obscured by tachycardia. The murmur of mitral regurgitation caused by IE is similar to that of other mitral regurgitation murmurs and may exhibit a typical radiation posteriorly when anterior leaflet perforation is present. There also may be signs of mitral stenosis secondary to obstruction by large vegetations, in which the murmur may be diastolic.

Pulse pressure may be normal or even narrowed in aortic regurgitation if IE is acute or important heart failure exists. Narrowed pulse pressure is caused by high left ventricular end-diastolic pressure with low cardiac output. There is frequently a gallop rhythm.

Infection of the mitral valve and its supporting structures is less frequent than aortic valve endocarditis, but may be more indolent in its course. *Right-sided endocarditis* is almost uniquely related to the tricuspid valve. Right-sided lesions are associated with fever, but often a cardiac murmur is initially absent.

Anemia frequently occurs in IE patients and has multifactorial causes, but primarily it results from marrow suppression secondary to chronic disease. Arthritis and arthralgias are infrequently seen today, generally because endocarditis is diagnosed earlier. Myalgias are common and may be associated with bacteremia or occasionally may result from muscle microabscesses, generally occurring in staphylococcal bacteremia.

Severity of heart failure in a hospitalized IE patient is not appropriately quantified by NYHA functional class. In general, heart failure can be termed *mild* when only small doses of diuretic or digitalis are necessary; *moderate* when large doses of diuretic, afterload-reducing medications, and bed rest are necessary; and *severe* when cardiogenic shock is present and inotropic agents are needed.

Embolization is the presenting manifestation in about 10% to 15% of patients with left-sided IE. These emboli seem about evenly distributed between cerebral and peripheral sites. Classic peripheral signs of endocarditis—Osler nodes, Janeway lesions, Roth spots, petechiae, and clubbing—are late manifestations and are infrequently seen in a surgical practice. The one exception may be Janeway lesions, and when noted, the infecting organism is almost always *Staphylococcus.*

Diagnosis of IE is made most often by the *presence of positive blood cultures* and a cardiac lesion characterized by new stenosis, new regurgitation, or echocardiographic evidence for a vegetation. There are many more individuals with sepsis and positive blood cultures, but without cardiac manifestations, and they are not considered to have IE.

An excellent microbiology laboratory is essential for accurate and prompt diagnosis. With current techniques, ability to culture fastidious organisms (e.g., Q fever, *Mycoplasma*) is high. Thus, diagnosis of IE involving cardiac valves or congenital malformations is made on a constellation of findings, usually fever, positive blood cultures, and hemodynamic derangement within the cardiac structures that is best assessed and followed by echocardiography.

Echocardiography has become a standard modality for diagnosis and continuing observation of patients with IE.[M3] In all situations, *transesophageal echocardiography* has greater sensitivity and specificity than does *transthoracic echocardiography* (TTE).[S3] Specificity for TEE is approximately 90% and sensitivity 95%.[B5,D2] For TTE, accuracy ranges from 40% to 80%. These figures apply equally to NVE and PVE. Perivalvar or perianular cavities associated with prosthetic valves are more easily delineated with TEE, and in the view of some authorities, these represent pseudoaneurysms rather than abscess cavities in most patients.[T3]

An algorithm for diagnosis of IE begins with fever, requires positive blood cultures, includes some sign or symptom referable to the heart, and receives anatomic corroboration with TEE. From TEE, vegetation size, mobility, and position can be documented; degree of stenosis and regurgitation associated with the valve lesion can be assessed; and in PVE the presence of prosthetic leakage or perianular cavities can be determined.

The decision to use *cardiac catheterization and angiography* has varied over the years and continues to be a case-by-case decision. In few cases have vegetations been disturbed by intraarterial or venous catheters, and a reasonable policy is that if coronary artery disease or coronary embolization is suspected, coronary angiography should be undertaken before operation.

Neurologic abnormalities may occur in as many as 25% to 30% of IE patients. They are protean in nature and include cerebrovascular accident (stroke), transient ischemic attack, toxic encephalopathy, meningitis, brain abscess, loss of vision, seizures, headache, backache, and acute mononeuropathy.[J1] Funduscopic examination (Roth spots or flame hemorrhages), cerebrospinal fluid examination, and computed tomography (CT) scanning or magnetic resonance imaging (MRI) of the brain are performed as indicated, and results may alter timing of surgical therapy (see following discussion). Gillinov and colleagues identified 34 patients among 247 individuals with NVE who presented with preoperative neurologic deficits.[G2] Most had an embolic cerebrovascular accident, and CT demonstrated a cerebral lesion in 29 of 32 patients studied. Embolic events are reported frequently in IE patients (24% to 67%). Prevalence is probably higher in IV drug–related endocarditis and perhaps slightly lower in PVE. The brain is the most frequently identified site of emboli.[S4]

Involvement of *abdominal viscera* varies. Ting and colleagues reported that 19% of patients with IE secondary to IV drug abuse developed splenic abscesses.[T2] A more reasonable figure is 5% in the usual type of left-sided NVE. Metastatic infection of viscera is typically caused by *Staphylococcus.*

NATURAL HISTORY

Crude incidence of NVE in a Swedish population study was 6.2 per 100,000 inhabitants per year, and highest in the oldest age group.[H3] Older age is also implicated in occur-

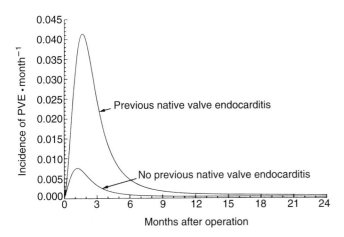

Figure 15-4   Hazard function for prosthetic valve endocarditis in patients with and without previous native valve endocarditis. (From Ivert and colleagues.[I1])

Key: *PVE,* Prosthetic valve endocarditis.

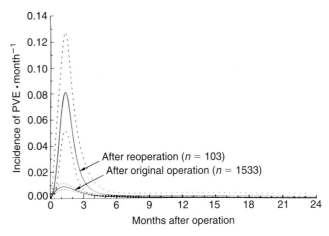

Figure 15-5   Hazard functions for prosthetic valve endocarditis after original valve replacement and after reoperation. Both have early peaking and constant phases. (From Blackstone and Kirklin.[B8])

Key: *PVE,* Prosthetic valve endocarditis.

rence of nosocomial IE. Terpenning and colleagues found that indwelling catheters were implicated as the source of bacteremia in half the cases of nosocomial IE.[T4]

In a large study of adult patients, occurrence of PVE was 4.1% at 48 months after valve replacement in 1465 consecutive hospital survivors, and 64% of these patients died.[I1] Other studies report an annual incidence of PVE ranging from 0.12% to 0.4% per patient-year.[D3] In contrast, indwelling pacemaker leads are infrequently disposed to IE.[R4]

It is difficult to identify a precise causative factor for PVE. However, intraoperative surface contamination, introduction of contaminated blood or blood substitute, bacterial colonization of a member of the surgical team, bacterial aerosolization in ventilators, nasal colonization of the patient, and preexisting urosepsis have all been implicated. The hazard for developing PVE is greater in patients operated on for NVE than in patients with valve replacement for other reasons (Fig. 15-4).[B8,I1] In addition to NVE as a risk factor for PVE, placement of a mechanical prosthesis (versus a tissue valve), black race, male gender, and longer cardiopulmonary bypass time are incremental risk factors for subsequent development of PVE. Finally, prosthetic valve reoperation is a greater hazard for development of PVE than primary valve replacement (Fig. 15-5).

Among the pediatric population, IE most often occurs in patients with ventricular septal defects (VSD) and valvar aortic stenosis. Incidence is low (14.5 per 10,000 person-years), but 35 times that of the normal population.[G6] Incidence of IE in patients with VSD is reduced by about 50% after surgical closure. Postoperative endocarditis in children most often occurs after aortic valvotomy, valve replacement, or use of a right ventricular–pulmonary trunk conduit.[A1] In both pediatric and adult populations, mitral valve prolapse has emerged as a frequent preexisting malformation in the spectrum of IE (29% of patients in McKinsey and colleagues' series[M4]).

S. aureus predominates as the infecting organism in the majority of hospital-acquired and drug-related cases of

■ **TABLE 15-2   Comparison of Infecting Organisms Recovered in Children with Infective Endocarditis during Two Eras at Columbia Presbyterian Hospital**

Type	1953 to 1972		1970 to 1990	
	No. (%)	CL (%)	No. (%)	CL (%)
Streptococcus	44 (41)	36–41	14 (29)	22–37
Staphylococcus aureus	33 (30)	26–30	13 (27)	20–30
Uncommon organisms[a]	16 (15)	11–19	16 (33)	26–42
No organisms recovered	15 (14)	10–18	5 (11)	6–17
TOTAL	108 (100)		48 (100)	

(Modified from Awadallah and colleagues.[A1])

Key: *CL,* 70% confidence limits.

[a] Includes three patients with fungal endocarditis in second era; no cases of fungal endocarditis occurred in first era.

IE. Distribution of infecting organisms in the usual NVE population, however, may vary among institutions and temporally[A1,R1,S4,W4] (Tables 15-2 and 15-3).

In IE cases confirmed by echocardiography, autopsy, or operation, positive blood cultures are obtained in 95% of cases with two blood specimens and in 98% with four specimens.[W5] However, occurrence of negative-culture endocarditis rises to about 10% in most surgical series,[S4] and PVE predominates in this group of patients.[H4] A history of antibiotic therapy or serologic evidence of *Mycoplasma* or *Chlamydia* species are likely responsible for negative-culture IE.

Complications

The most frequent cardiac complication of NVE is *heart failure,* primarily caused by valvar regurgitation. However, NVE occasionally results in mitral or tricuspid valve stenosis and infrequently in aortic valve stenosis. Perianular leakage and abscess and occasionally stenosis are the major causes of heart failure in PVE. Myocardial abscess, conduction abnormalities, and myocardial perforation may

■ **TABLE 15-3   Spectrum of Infecting Organisms Recovered in Adults with Infective Endocarditis** [a]

			PVE	
	NVE	IVDA	Early	Late
Microorganism	n = 80 (%)	n = 15 (%)	n = 7 (%)	n = 35 (%)
Staphylococcus aureus	24 (30)	6 (40)	0	6 (18)
Streptococci	34 (43)	1 (7)	0	9 (27)
Enterococci	4 (5)	1 (7)	0	3 (9)
Coagulase-negative staphylococci	1 (1.3)	0	4 (57)	8 (24)
Corynebacterium jeikeium	0	0	0	1 (3)
Escherichia coli	1 (1.3)	0	0	1 (3)
Pseudomonas aeruginosa	0	2 (13)	0	0
HACEK group	4 (5)	0	0	0
Others	3 (4)	0	0	1 (3)
Culture negative	7 (9)	1 (7)	3 (43)	3 (9)

(Modified from Sandre and Shafran.[S4])

Key: *HACEK, Haemophilus* spp., *Actinobacillus actinomycetemcomitans, Cardiobacterium hominis, Eikenella* spp., and *Kingella kingae. IVDA,* intravenous drug abuser; *NVE,* native valve endocarditis; *PVE,* prosthetic valve endocarditis.

[a] 135 cases, 1985 to 1993, University of Alberta.

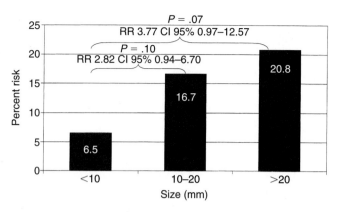

Figure 15-6   Risk of embolic events according to vegetation size in patients followed 1 to 942 days (mean 151 days) after initiation of antibiotic treatment for left-sided infective endocarditis (217 episodes in 211 patients). (Multicenter study from Vilacosta and colleagues[V2]; April 1996 to June 2000.)

Key: *CI,* Confidence interval; *RR,* relative risk.

complicate IE. Pericarditis typically occurs in association with anular abscess or myocardial perforation. Multiple coronary emboli may result in myocardial infarction and ventricular dysfunction.

Renal complications of IE take at least four forms: prerenal failure secondary to low cardiac output, microabscesses caused by septic emboli, glomerular dysfunction resulting from circulating immune complexes, and renal failure caused by antibiotic toxicity.

Embolic events are common in IE patients, with a reported prevalence of 43% in NVE, 67% in IV-drug–associated IE, and 25% in PVE.[S4] Ting and colleagues report a 19% occurrence of splenic emboli in their series of patients with IV-drug–related endocarditis.[T2] Other classic peripheral manifestations of IE (e.g., petechiae, Osler nodes, splinter hemorrhages) are infrequently seen now, probably because of earlier intervention in the disease process.

About half the embolic complications of IE are associated with neurologic manifestations, and about a third of patients with NVE or PVE at some time have neurologic complications.[S5] Presence of *S. aureus* increases the risk of neurologic complications,[D4,V2] but neurologic manifestations do not increase overall mortality in IE. *Stroke* (cerebrovascular accident) is the most common neurologic event. Vegetations were seen on echocardiography in 38% of patients with neurologic complications and in 28% of patients without neurologic sequelae (*P* = .26).[S5] Some characteristics of vegetations visualized on TTE or TEE, such as density or mobility, may not be helpful in defining emboli risk.[D4] After instituting antibiotic therapy, however, both absolute vegetation size and observed increase in vegetation size are associated with increased embolic risk (Fig. 15-6).[V2]

Medical treatment alone (versus operative) increases risk of embolism.[L4] However, delaying repair of the cardiac lesion is usually advised in the presence of central nervous system (CNS) complications.[G2] Morbidity is less when repair is done in the presence of cerebral infarction versus cerebral hemorrhage.[E1] Evidence indicates that cerebral mycotic emboli will regress after extirpation of the valvar septic lesion, so early cardiac operation in patients with mycotic aneurysm and cerebral abscess may be advisable.[M6]

TECHNIQUE OF OPERATION

Goals of operative therapy are to (1) remove infected tissue and drain abscesses, (2) restore or reconstruct atrioventricular or ventriculoarterial continuity, and (3) reverse the hemodynamic abnormality. Drainage of abscesses, debridement of areas of necrosis, and improvement of mechanical function by repair or replacement of infected valves are done as required. Operation is also aimed at closing acquired defects (e.g., VSD, ring abscess, fistula, aneurysm) and in children may include repairing the underlying malformation.

All operations for IE are done through a partial or total median sternotomy. Presence of adhesive or suppurative pericarditis is strong evidence of previous perforation at the aortic or mitral ring or ring abscess.[F1,U1] It is prudent to use bicaval cannulation to allow flexibility in the presence of burrowing abscesses, acquired septal perforation, unexpected right-sided valve involvement, and complex aortic root reconstruction. Intraoperative TEE is extremely useful to diagnose and plan treatment of the various manifestations of the infectious process. In left-sided IE, minimal manipulation of the heart should be the rule to avoid dislodging infected thrombotic material or vegetations. As in other valvar procedures, myocardial management is accomplished with antegrade and retrograde cardioplegia supplemented with moderate systemic hypothermia. Thorough excision of infected tissue is performed with drainage of abscesses and closure of defects.

Operation for aortic endocarditis should involve examining the anterior leaflet of the mitral valve and its chordae for drop lesions. It is sometimes necessary to open the left atrium to examine the posterior leaflet apparatus. Similarly, when mitral endocarditis is present, the possibility of concomitant aortic vegetations should be considered. However, absence of a murmur or thrill, presence of a competent aortic valve, and no echocardiographic evidence of vegetations at the aortic area argue against aortic involvement and preclude the need for inspection of the valve.

Reparative procedures may be done on the mitral valve when the vegetation is healed, small, or discrete and does not involve a major portion of the tensor apparatus. It may include closing small perforations of the posterior or anterior leaflet using autologous or bovine pericardium or direct suturing (Fig. 15-7). Small vegetations may be stripped from chordae tendineae. When minor lesions are causing minor regurgitation, reconstruction can be performed. Major regurgitation in the presence of all but the tiniest vegetations dictates valve replacement. In the absence of active endocarditis, as defined by positive blood cultures and overt inflammation at the site of vegetation, mitral repair of the classic type can be accomplished. Triangular resection of a portion of the anterior leaflet or quadrangular resection of a portion of the posterior leaflet may be performed, supplemented by inserting a partial or complete anular ring. Partial leaflet resection and anuloplasty procedures for tricuspid valve endocarditis can be applied on a more liberal basis (Fig. 15-8).

At the time of mitral valve resection, the posteroinferior portion of the mitral anulus should be inspected because the usual myocardial ring abscess occurs in this location. In resection of the aortic valve, the abscess is usually found just posterior to the membranous portion of the ventricular septum or at the posterior portion of the septum just anterior to the orifice of the left coronary artery. When found, abscesses should be totally evacuated and surrounding tissue debrided. The concept of atrioventricular or ventriculoarterial discontinuity must be kept in mind. The infecting process often erodes those junctions, with potential or actual separation. In mitral valve IE with left atrioventricular discontinuity, the defect can be handled in several ways. Often a simple variation of the usual valve replacement technique is appropriate; interrupted horizontal mattress sutures anchored with felt or pericardial pledgets are placed on the ventricular aspect of the mitral anulus, brought up through the left atrial aspect, and then through the prosthetic sewing ring. Deep bites are necessary. This can be done only after thorough debridement of the infected tissue within the mitral ring (Fig. 15-9).

In more extensive ring abscess or often in PVE with abscess, a different type of reconstruction is necessary. The atrioventricular discontinuity is bridged by a patch fashioned from a sheet of autologous or bovine pericardium. The ventricular aspect is anchored to the endocardium and myocardium using deep bites of continuous No. 3-0 or 4-0 polypropylene suture. The superior aspect of this tissue reconstruction is anchored to the atrial endocardium with a similar suture. The new prosthesis is anchored to the composite suture line on the ventricular aspect of the suture line using interrupted horizontal mattress sutures buttressed with felt pledgets.[D5]

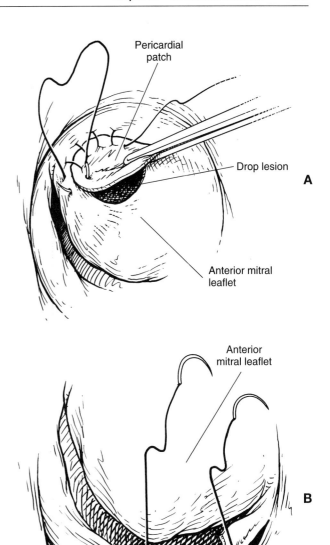

Figure 15-7 Repair of infective endocarditis involving the mitral valve. **A,** Closure of a drop lesion defect of mitral valve using a pericardial patch. **B,** Step in repair of a lesion (see Fig. 15-3, *C*) using a limited quadrangular resection and sliding plasty.

Various maneuvers have been suggested for seating valves in the aortic position in the presence of frank abscesses of the aortic root. The advantage of tissue valves over mechanical valves in terms of preventing reinfection has not been conclusively demonstrated. In the aortic area, however, stentless tissue valves, either allografts or xenografts, have some advantage in that their pliability allows some flexibility in reconstructing continuity between the ventricle and aorta. When stent-mounted valves, either mechanical or tissue, are used, a technique using felt-buttressed horizontal mattress sutures is advised. The mattress is placed on the ventricular aspect of the aortic anulus

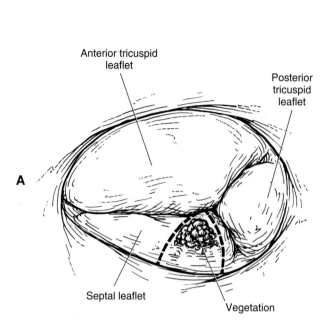

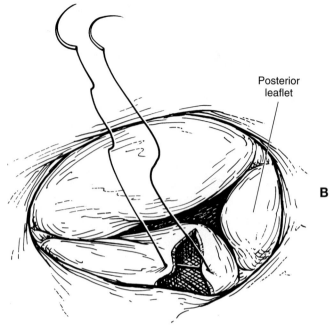

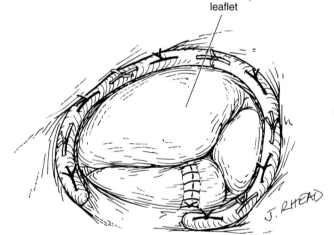

Figure 15-8   Repair of tricuspid valve infective endocarditis in which vegetation is localized to a portion of septal leaflet. **A**, Line of leaflet resection. **B**, Repair of defect using fine interrupted sutures. **C**, Completed repair supported by an anuloplasty ring.

or from outside the aortic wall, dissecting the aortic root upstream in its noncoronary and posterior left coronary aspects and occasionally opening the right ventricular outflow tract to place pledgeted sutures from the infundibular septum through the aortic anulus.

When a simple small abscess lies under the left coronary ostium, evacuation, debridement, and patch closure of the defect can be accomplished. The stent-mounted or stentless tissue prosthesis is then placed in its usual orthotopic position using techniques similar to those required in noninfected cases (see Chapter 12). In many patients with important aortic valve IE, full root replacement offers the most satisfactory solution (Fig. 15-10). Infected tissue is first debrided, and formal root replacement is done in the usual way, with particular emphasis on locating the upstream (proximal) suture line within the left ventricular outflow tract, thus appropriately bridging the left ventricular–aortic discontinuity. All infected tissue is thus exteriorized.

Ancillary procedures during valve replacement may be helpful. Some authorities suggest soaking the prosthetic device in an appropriate antibiotic, and others have irrigated or swabbed the local area with antiseptic solution such as povidone-iodine (Betadine). In fungal endocarditis, irrigation of the local area with amphotericin or other antifungal agents is thought to be efficacious.[H6,M13,N3]

When both the aortic and mitral valves are involved, but the infection is limited to the leaflets, usual sequencing of operation is followed: aortotomy, then aortic valve resection, followed by left atriotomy and mitral valve resection. The mitral anulus is then sized and an appropriate mechanical device or bioprosthesis inserted. The aortic anulus is then sized and an appropriate mechanical or tissue prosthesis inserted. When the infection is not limited to the leaflets, there may be destruction of aortomitral continuity with absence of the aortomitral curtain. In this case, seating of the mitral prosthesis is modified because much of the

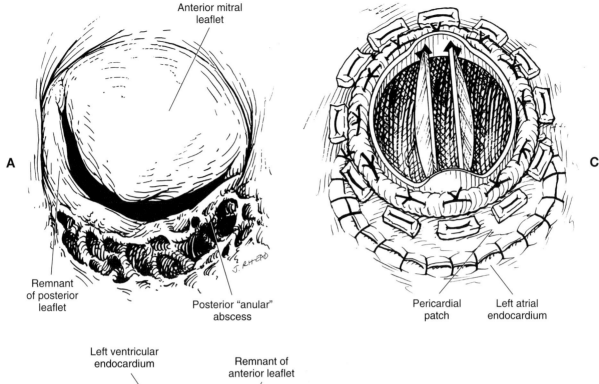

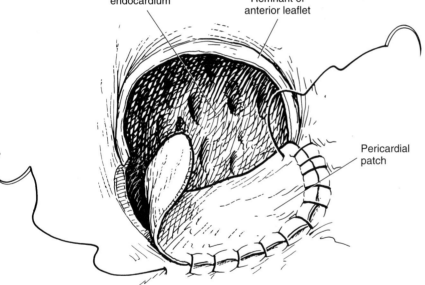

Figure 15-9   Infective endocarditis producing a ring abscess involving base of posterior leaflet of mitral valve. **A,** Abscess is evacuated and debrided. **B,** Defect is covered by a pericardial patch anchored within the left ventricle and extending up across the base of the portion of the posterior leaflet, then sewn to the left atrial wall. **C,** Prosthesis is sutured into place, siting the posterior suture line either on the patch (in this case) or, occasionally, below the patch on the ventricular wall.

anterior lateral suture attachment of the sewing ring will be absent. As much of the mitral prosthesis as possible is inserted in the usual way. Attention is then redirected to the aortic exposure, and a new synthetic aortomitral curtain is formed with polyester or pericardium. Upstream or proximal anchoring is done with sutures to the sewing ring of the mitral prosthesis, and downstream aortoventricular continuity is established by suturing this curtain to the root of the aorta. Thereafter, the aortic prosthesis is inserted as usual, attaching the prosthesis in its right lateral aspect (noncoronary sinus aspect) to the reconstructed mitral curtain. Alternatively, the sewing ring of the aortic prosthesis can

be attached where it interfaces directly to the sewing ring of the mitral prosthesis.[D7]

Treatment of associated infection, particularly peripheral mycotic aneurysm; brain, spleen, or liver abscess; and renal parenchymal infection, usually takes second priority to the intracardiac operation. Use of cardiopulmonary bypass does not generally exacerbate associated neurologic deficits, except in the specific case of cerebral hemorrhage. Persisting infection after valve replacement should alert the surgeon to splenic and liver abscesses. Similarly, continued renal decompensation suggests the presence of renal parenchymal disease.

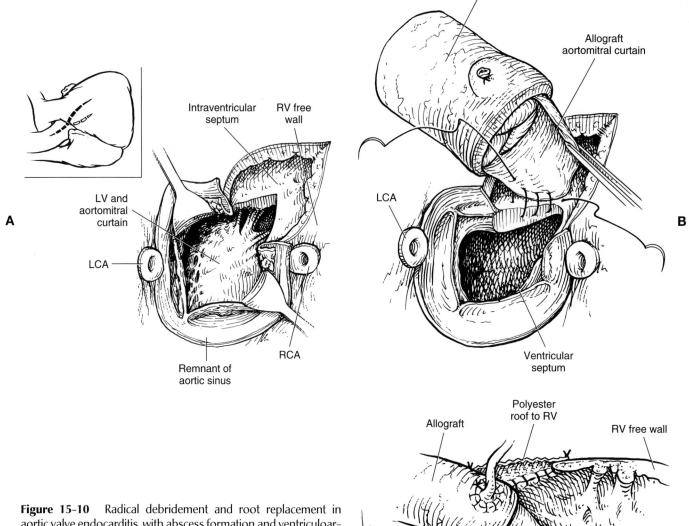

Figure 15-10   Radical debridement and root replacement in aortic valve endocarditis, with abscess formation and ventriculoarterial discontinuity. **A,** Aortic valve has been resected and burrowing septal abscess debrided using a Konno approach (see Chapter 12). *Inset,* Initially a vertical aortotomy is used and extended across right ventricular outflow tract to the left of the right coronary artery. Later, after resection of the aortic sinuses, the aorta is transected at the sinotubular junction. **B,** Using a cryopreserved allograft with its attached aortomitral curtain, the septal defect is reconstructed and allograft root replacement performed as usual. Allograft anulus is placed within left ventricular outflow tract. **C,** If involved, mitral valve is replaced, anchoring it anterior to residual native aortomitral curtain.

Key: *LA,* Left atrium; *LCA,* left coronary artery; *LV,* left ventricle; *RCA,* right coronary artery; *RV,* right ventricle.

SPECIAL FEATURES OF POSTOPERATIVE CARE

In general, patients undergoing operations for complications of IE are subject to the same early postoperative monitoring and intervention algorithms as non–IE patients undergoing similar operations for valve replacement or repair (see Chapter 5). Hemodynamic state is assessed by measuring or estimating cardiac output and measuring left atrial, right atrial, or pulmonary artery pressures, combined with assessing blood pressure and peripheral perfusion.

Occasionally, patients with an acute septic syndrome manifest decreased peripheral resistance with low, normal, or high cardiac output early postoperatively. Appropriate treatment may include use of phenylephrine, levarterenol,

■ **TABLE 15-4   Results of Treatment for Native Valve Infective Endocarditis (1967 to 1977) According to Degree of Heart Failure**

Degree of heart failure	Nonsurgical Treatment				Surgical Treatment				P
		Hospital Deaths				Hospital Deaths			
	n	No.	%	CL (%)	n	No.	%	CL (%)	
Absent, mild	22	3	14	6-26	49	3	6	3-12	0.2
Moderate	30	19 66%	63	52-73	20	4 25%	20	10-33	< .003
Severe	2	2 (55%-75%)	100	39-100	12	4 (17%-35%)	33	18-52	.08
TOTAL	54	24	44	37-52	81	11	14	10-19	.0001

(Data from Richardson and colleagues.[R1])

Key: *CL*, 70% confidence limits.

---

or less often arginine vasopressin to increase peripheral resistance. Mobilizing extravascular lung water may be important to facilitate extubation. Adequate diuretic therapy and positive end-expiratory pressure ventilation early postoperatively are then indicated.

In all patients, tissue should be obtained for Gram stain and subsequent culture and histologic analysis. Results of these studies are integrated into the postoperative care plan with initiation of or changes in antibiotic regimen. Because renal function often is compromised, antibiotic levels are followed at intervals, initially every 2 days.

Patients with compromised renal function often have increased blood urea nitrogen (BUN) and creatinine levels early postoperatively, followed by a decline to near-normal levels over the next 3 to 7 days. Monitoring of renal function is therefore important, and pharmacologic therapy with large doses of diuretics is often indicated. In some patients, temporary renal dialysis is necessary. Some surgeons may want to follow white blood counts or phase reactants over the postoperative period to monitor resolution of sepsis. If a septic picture continues, possible involvement of peripheral sites should be investigated.

Protocols for anticoagulation are the same in IE patients as in those having similar devices who have not undergone surgical intervention for IE.

Antibiotic treatment, most often administered intravenously, is continued for 4 to 6 weeks based on the type of organism and its sensitivity to antimicrobials. In the case of fungal endocarditis, oral treatment with ketoconazole or fluconazole may be appropriate for 3 to 6 months.

RESULTS

Early (Hospital) Death

Native Valve Endocarditis

Hospital mortality for valve operations (and associated procedures) in patients with IE varies between 4% and 30%.[B9,D5,D6,G7,H5,J3,L5,M7,M10] The variation can be ascribed to several factors, most notably, the difference in risk between operation in the acute versus healed stages of endocarditis. Surgery for *acute* IE is defined as an operation undertaken during antibiotic treatment in the presence of obvious local cardiac inflammation, including active vegetations, abscesses, burrowing sinuses, or fistulae. By contrast, *healed* IE is characterized by lack of local inflammation; vegetations may be present but are generally endothelialized; abscesses have resulted in well-defined and stable cavities, including sinuses and fistulae. In general,

■ **TABLE 15-5   Native Valve Infective Endocarditis According to Operative Category** [a]

Operative Category	n	Hospital Deaths			
		No.	%	CL (%)	
Elective	38	2	5	2-12	
Urgent	31	5	16	9-26	P = .14
Emergency	12	4	33	18-52	
TOTAL	81	11	14	10-19	

(Data from Richardson and colleagues.[R1])

Key: *CL*, 70% confidence limits.

[a] UAB experience, 1967 to 1977.

operations for healed IE are performed after a full course of antibiotic therapy.

Other factors affecting the variation in reported hospital mortality reflect the incremental risks for an operation, as discussed later.

Operative treatment of IE is in reality a combined medical–surgical treatment, and *timing* of the operation is an important factor in patient survival. However, it is convenient to compare strictly medical (nonoperative) treatment of IE with results of operative treatment. In general, the more urgent the surgical indication and the more severe the heart failure, the better are the surgical results compared with medical therapy. However, no prospective or randomized studies have been done, and thus patients in the nonoperative medical group may not be strictly comparable to those in the surgical group. Richardson and colleagues reported that operative treatment in 81 patients with NVE resulted in 11 deaths (14%; CL 10%-19%), compared with 24 deaths (44%; CL 37%-52%) in 54 patients treated medically (Table 15-4).[R1] Operative mortality was affected by urgency of operation (Table 15-5). For elective operations (next convenient operative date), mortality was 5%, for urgent operations (next day) 16%, and for emergency operations in patients with severe heart failure and low cardiac output (immediate operation) 33%.

Operations in IE patients often demand complex procedures, which may affect hospital mortality after valve repair or replacement.[D6,L5] Complexity of the procedure is often dictated by duration of the illness and particularly by the infecting organism. Tissue destruction is characteristic of staphylococcal and some gram-negative organisms and is much less likely to occur in streptococcal or pneumococcal endocarditis. In reports from Bauernschmitt and Middlemost and their colleagues, however, early results of valve

■ **TABLE 15-6** Results of Surgical Treatment of Left-Sided Native Valve Endocarditis in the Present Era (203 Patients)

Variables	AV No. (%)	MV No. (%)	DV No. (%)
Prevalence	110 (54)[a]	50 (25)	43 (21)
Preoperative Findings			
Urgent surgery	62 (56)	18 (36)	28 (65)
Mean interval to surgery (days)	12	13	8
Embolism	11 (10)	7 (14)	7 (16)
Surgical Findings			
Extensive infection	45 (41)[a]	7 (14)	12 (28)
Abscess	38 (35)[b]	1 (2)	7 (16)
Fistula	5 (5)	–	–
Pericardial involvement	19 (17)	7 (14)	5 (12)
Aortic clamp time (min)	57[b]	38	67[c]
Early Postoperative Events			
Ring leaks	5 (5)	1 (2)	1 (2)
Early prosthetic infection	4 (4)	–	1 (2)
Embolism	–	3 (6)	3 (7)
In-hospital death	6 (5)	1 (2)	1 (2)

(Data from Middlemost and colleagues.[M7])

Key: *AV,* Aortic valve; *MV,* mitral valve; *DV,* double valve.

[a] *P* < .005 versus mitral infection.

[b] *P* < .001 versus mitral infection.

[c] *P* < .01 versus mitral infection.

■ **TABLE 15-7** Risk Factors by Multivariable Analysis for Operative Death and Late Death in Patients with Infective Endocarditis

Risk Factor	Operative Death Odds Ratio (± 95% CL)	P	Freedom from Late Death Hazards Ratio (± 95% CL)	P
Heart failure	1.76 (0.49, 6.28)	.4	1.49 (0.71, 3.17)	.3
Emboli	0.56 (0.14, 2.32)	.4	0.39 (0.17, 0.92)	.03
Sepsis	4.56 (0.87, 24.00)	.07	1.83 (0.89, 3.80)	.10
ARF	[a]	[a]	0.35 (0.05, 2.72)	.3
Vegetations	1.21 (0.27, 5.37)	.8	1.65 (0.74, 3.69)	.2
Age >60 yr	2.47 (0.78, 7.87)	.13	1.40 (0.73, 2.73)	.3
PVE	3.50 (1.05, 11.68)	.04	2.20 (1.13, 4.31)	.02
AVR	1.33 (0.27, 6.46)	.7	1.39 (0.57, 3.34)	.5
MVR	1.07 (0.25, 4.6)	.9	1.49 (0.67, 3.30)	.3

(Data from Larbalestier and colleagues.[L5])

Key: *ARF,* Acute renal failure; *AVR,* aortic valve replacement; *MVR,* mitral valve replacement; *PVE,* prosthetic valve endocarditis.

[a] No operative deaths.

replacement did not seem to be adversely affected by excessive complexity of the procedure (Table 15-6).[B9,M7] Rather, preoperative complications and severity indices had a more profound influence on mortality (Table 15-7).

Often, IE can be successfully treated in children without operative intervention. Nomura and colleagues reported on 98 patients seen over 13 years, 30 of whom were treated operatively, with a hospital mortality of 6.7%.[N2] The remaining patients were treated medically, with a 10% hospital mortality. Tolan and colleagues reviewed 132 published reports in which children underwent operative intervention during active endocarditis.[T5] Hospital survival was 77%. Only 67% of patients had preoperative conditions thought to predispose them to IE, and about one quarter of

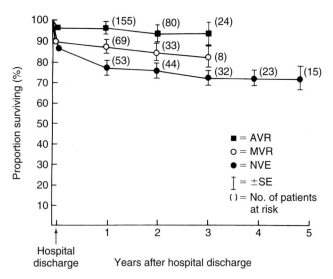

Figure 15-11 Comparison of survival in patients operated on for native valve endocarditis with patients having isolated aortic or mitral valve replacement without infective endocarditis during the same era (*P* > .1 at 3 years). (From Richardson and colleagues.[R1])

Key: *AVR,* Aortic valve replacement; *MVR,* mitral valve replacement; *NVE,* native valve endocarditis; *SE,* standard error.

those were operated on for infection associated with patent ductus ateriosus.

Prosthetic Valve Endocarditis

PVE is an incremental risk factor for operative mortality in the domain of all IE.[R1] Again, overall survival for patients with PVE is improved in those treated operatively compared with those treated medically. Although results may not be strictly comparable, most series report a difference in outcome when operative treatment of NVE is compared with PVE. In the Brigham and Women's Hospital experience, mortality was 22% in 49 PVE patients versus 6% in 109 NVE patients.[L5] Several factors more prevalent in the PVE group are likely responsible for this difference, including reoperation, prevalence of abscess, anular erosion and perianular aneurysm, insidious onset of infection, and fastidious or fungal organisms. However, Sabik and colleagues at the Cleveland Clinic report a 3.9% (CL 2%-7%) hospital mortality among 103 patients managed with radical debridement of infected tissue and aortic root replacement with a cryopreserved allograft.[S7]

Time-Related Survival

Late survival after valve replacement for NVE is good, but not as good as with similar operations done in the absence of endocarditis (Fig. 15-11). Death and other events late after operation often are not related to IE or recurrent IE but rather to other conditions associated with heart disease, such as the valve replacement device and associated complications, myocardial dysfunction, and coronary artery disease. Using mechanical valves exclusively, Bauernschmitt and colleagues reported 81.1% survival among 138 patients after 8 years (Fig. 15-12).[B9]

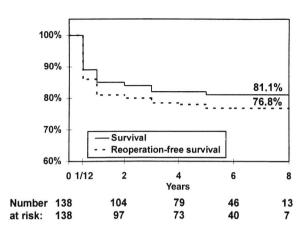

Figure 15-12   Survival and reoperation-free survival in 138 patients receiving mechanical prostheses for infective endocarditis between 1988 and 1996. (From Bauernschmitt and colleagues.[B9])

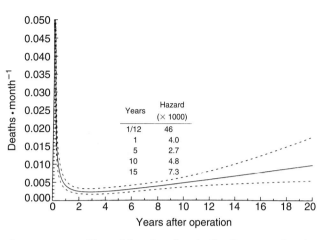

Figure 15-13   Hazard function for death after operation in 108 patients undergoing aortic valve replacement for infective endocarditis. (From Haydock and colleagues.[H5])

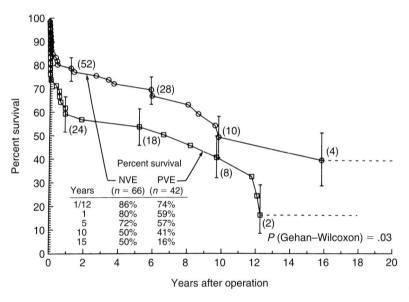

Figure 15-14   Survival according to initial native valve endocarditis or prosthetic valve endocarditis in 108 patients undergoing aortic valve replacement (*P* = .03). (From Haydock and colleagues.[H5])

Key: *NVE,* Native valve endocarditis; *PVE,* prosthetic valve endocarditis.

In the GLH group's series of 108 IE patients who underwent aortic valve replacement for IE, 1-, 5-, and 15-year survival was 73%, 64%, and 36%, respectively.[H5] There was an early, high peaking hazard for death and then a constant later phase (Fig. 15-13). Survival was lower in those patients who had PVE than in those with NVE (Fig. 15-14). In this group of patients, recurrent IE, nonstreptococcal organisms, and heart failure were statistically associated with late death after valve replacement.

Data for long-term survival after heart valve replacement in IE patients are typified by those reported by d'Udekem and colleagues[D6] from Toronto. Survival at 10 years was 61% ± 6%.[D6] Aranki and colleagues, in two separate publications from Brigham and Women's Hospital, reported 81% to 83% 5-year survival and 61% to 63% 10-year survival for both mitral and aortic valve replacement.[A3,A4]

Incremental Risk Factors

Several factors portend higher mortality with operative treatment for IE. A strong risk is hemodynamic deterioration,[B9,D5,H5] characterized as preoperative shock, advanced heart failure, or advanced NYHA functional class. Some have also found a relationship with low preoperative cardiac index.[L5] A second important risk factor is the infecting organism. Nonstreptococcal organisms, primarily staphylococci, increase operative risk. Staphylococcal infection is generally associated with abscesses, and abscesses independently may also increase risk.[B9,H5,L5] Likewise, most studies report that PVE is associated with a lower early postoperative survival than NVE.[B9,L5,M9] Additional incremental risk factors are older age, renal dysfunction, longer CPB time, acute versus healed IE, insidious onset of infection, and associated procedures (Fig. 15-15).

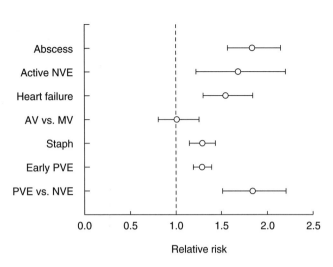

Figure 15-15 Factors influencing operative mortality after surgical treatment of patients with infective endocarditis. Data are presented as relative risk (see Chapter 6 for definition) for each factor plus 95% confidence limits, as determined by meta-analysis of 30 major studies. (From Moon and colleagues.[M10])

Key: *AV,* Aortic valve; *MV,* mitral valve; *NVE,* native valve endocarditis; *PVE,* prosthetic valve endocarditis; *Staph, Staphylococcus aureus* or *S. epidermidis.*

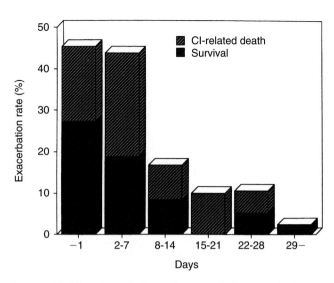

Figure 15-16 Exacerbation of cerebral damage, including death related to cerebral injury, according to interval from onset of cerebral infarction until cardiac operation. (From Eishi and colleagues.[E1])

Key: *CI,* Cerebral infarction.

In-hospital Morbidity

A few IE patients have continuing episodes of sepsis despite an apparently adequate cardiac operation. Almost uniformly the source of this sepsis is not the heart; however, an overlooked valvar lesion must be sought, generally by repeat TEE. There is a high prevalence of splenic and other visceral infarcts, emboli, or abscesses,[M11] but usually these do not cause continuing sepsis and are amenable to continued antibiotic therapy. Renal parenchymatous disease as a cause of sepsis is rare, as are cerebral mycotic aneurysms. Peripheral mycotic aneurysms may ultimately be found to be the cause of continuing sepsis.

New or evolving conduction abnormalities preoperatively reflect evolution of the cardiac sepsis or may result from coronary emboli. Postoperatively, heart block occurs more often than in patients without endocarditis. In most situations, this is a predictable occurrence resulting from the radical debridement necessary to eradicate infections around the aortic root, mitral valve apparatus, and ventricular septum.

Most observers have noticed increased postoperative bleeding. Inflamed tissue, inflammatory pericarditis, complex reconstructions, renal dysfunction, and platelet dysfunction may play a role in excessive bleeding. Use of aprotinin intraoperatively may diminish bleeding without increased complications.[T7]

A devastating complication is a new or deepening neurologic deficit after valve replacement. Even with meticulous surgical technique, friable vegetations may dislodge to cause new CNS deficits. More frequently, however, an existing CNS finding is aggravated by operation. Ting and colleagues found evidence of cerebral septic emboli in 45 (42%) of 106 patients who underwent valve replacement for IE.[T6] Neurologic complications after valve

replacement included postoperative strokes in 6%, cerebral abscesses in 2%, and seizures in 1%. Presence of a hemorrhagic infarct preoperatively predisposed patients to perioperative stroke. Eishi and colleagues collected 2523 surgical cases of IE and found that 10% of patients had associated cerebral complications.[E1] In-hospital mortality of those patients was 11%; cerebral infarction occurred in 65%, cerebral bleeding in 32%, and abscess in 3%. Exacerbation of cerebral complications (including death), according to interval from onset of cerebral infarction to cardiac operation, occurred in 46% of patients operated on within 24 hours and 44% of those operated on days 2 through 7, 17% of those operated on days 8 through 14, 10% of those operated on days 15 through 28, and just 2% of those operated on after 4 weeks. Thus, an important correlation existed between the interval from onset of cerebral complications to operation and exacerbation of cerebral complications (*P* = .008). Preoperative risk factors affecting exacerbation of cerebral complications were severity of cerebral complication, interval between complication and surgery, and uncontrolled heart failure. Postoperative exacerbation of cerebral complications is more likely in those patients with more severe preoperative manifestation of brain infarction. In the Eishi study of 51 patients without exacerbation of their cerebral complication, operation occurred an average of 15 days after diagnosis, compared with 8 days among 17 patients having exacerbation[E1] (*P* = .01). Thus, exacerbation is inversely related to interval between diagnosis and operation (Fig. 15-16). If cerebral infarction is not associated with hemorrhage, however, earlier operation is better tolerated.

Recurrent Infection

Some institutions report few cases of subsequent reinfection even when operation is done early in the course of

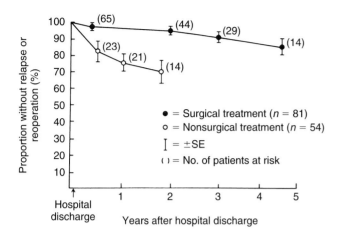

Figure 15-17   Probability of event-free survival in patients with native valve endocarditis, comparing surgical and non-surgical patients (*P* < .0001 at 2 years). (From Richardson and colleagues.[R1])

Key: *SE,* Standard error.

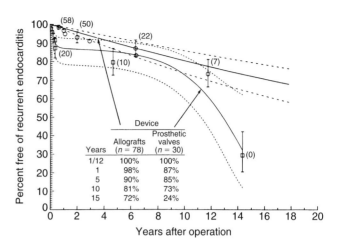

Figure 15-18   Recurrent endocarditis according to whether the replacement device was a freehand (subcoronary technique, see "Allograft Aortic Valve" in Chapter 12) allograft *(circles)* or a prosthetic valve *(squares)*. (From Haydock and colleagues.[H5])

NVE. Despite 20% of patients requiring valve replacement in the UAB series having uncontrolled infection at operation, no cases of subsequent PVE occurred[R1] (Fig. 15-17). This finding is similar to the experience of Utley and Mills and of Okies and colleagues, who reported that reinfections were rare in such patients and emphasized the importance of adequate debridement of infected areas.[O4,U2] In each of the studies, however, follow-up was relatively short. Indeed, recurrent infection after valve replacement (or repair) does occur. In Larbalestier and colleagues' report, 18 of 109 patients surviving surgery for NVE underwent reoperation.[L5] Eight had developed recurrent endocarditis. Recurrent IE is more common when the initial organism is nonstreptococcal and when there has been major destruction of the anulus or surrounding valve structures. This finding is reflected in Aranki's report, in which freedom from recurrent endocarditis in *acute* aortic IE surgical patients was 89% ± 3% at 5 years and 83% ± 4% at 10 years, versus 96% ± 3% at 5 years and 86% + 6% at 10 years in patients with *healed* aortic valve IE.[A3] Freedom from reoperation is higher when the mitral valve is involved (compared with the aortic valve), reflecting less anular destruction. In a series reporting results of operation for mitral valve IE at Brigham and Women's Hospital, freedom from reoperation at 5 and 10 years was 92% ± 4% and 62% ± 13% for acute endocarditis and 94% ± 4% and 84% ± 10% for healed endocarditis (*P* = .7), respectively.[A4] The Brigham and Women's Hospital group of 158 patients operated on in the acute phase underwent 49 operations for PVE. There was little difference in recurrent IE at 10 years for those patients operated on for NVE (85%) versus PVE (82%), although long-term survival was better for those with NVE. Reinfection with the same or different organism is common in drug abusers, and late mortality is greater in that group. In Hiraztka's experience, late mortality was 39% in drug abusers versus 7% for non–drug users.[H2]

There is some controversy as to whether a tissue valve, particularly a cryopreserved allograft, is preferable for use in aortic NVE. In 108 patients, Haydock and colleagues reported a small but statistically significant difference in incidence of recurrent IE in patients having allografts versus prosthetic valves (Fig. 15-18).[H5] Hazard functions were qualitatively different for allografts; there was a constant phase of hazard when an allograft was used, but an early peaking hazard phase and late rising phase when a prosthetic device was used (Fig. 15-19). In a similar study from the same institution, McGiffin and colleagues noted that allografts in the aortic position had a higher freedom from *recurrent endocarditis* than mechanical or xenograft valves (Fig. 15-20).[M9] Thus, if there is an advantage among valve substitutes, it is conferred uniquely by allografts. In both Haydock's and McGiffin's series, where aortic valve replacement was done with allograft valves, freedom from recurrent endocarditis was about 80%. Not all institutional experience supports this view, however.[H5,M10,M14] In 138 patients who received only mechanical valves, *reoperation-free survival* was similar (77%), suggesting that mechanical prostheses may perform as well as allografts when operation is done for aortic NVE.[B9] However, reoperation-free survival does not comparably address differences in early hazard for recurrent infection.

Lytle and colleagues reoperated on 146 patients with PVE. There were 19 (13%) in-hospital deaths.[L3] Subsequent reoperation was performed in 15% of hospital survivors, and in those who had aortic valve replacement, *reoperation-free survival* was similar among those who received biologic, mechanical, or allograft valves (Fig. 15-21).

Thus, for aortic NVE, some evidence suggests that an allograft is the preferable replacement device. For all aortic PVE, mitral NVE, or mitral PVE operations, there is no evidence indicating the superiority of xenografts over mechanical devices.

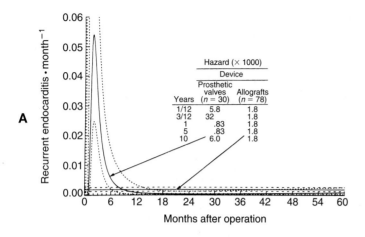

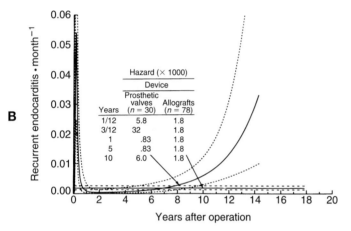

Figure 15-19 Hazard function for recurrent endocarditis in patients with freehand (subcoronary technique, see "Allograft Aortic Valve" in Chapter 12) allografts compared with those receiving prosthetic mechanical or bioprosthetic valves. **A,** Patients with originally localized endocarditis had a constant rate of 3.1 events per 1000 patients per month, and those with originally extensive endocarditis had a constant rate of 0.45 events per 1000 patients per month. **B,** Same depiction extending 20 years. (From Haydock and colleagues.[H5])

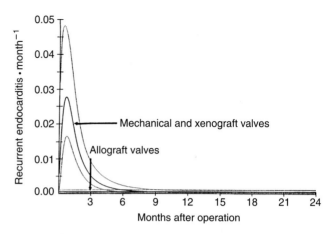

Figure 15-20 Aortic valve replacement for infective endocarditis. Hazard function *(solid lines)* for recurrent endocarditis repaired using 141 mechanical and xenograft valves (18 events) and 53 allograft valves (2 events). Dotted lines enclose 70% confidence limits. (From McGiffin and colleagues.[M9])

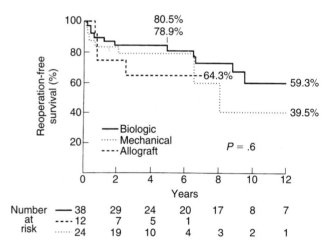

Figure 15-21 Reoperation-free survival in a group of patients with aortic prosthetic valve endocarditis. Results are equivalent regardless of type of device used. (*P* = .6). (From Lytle and colleagues.[L3])

INDICATIONS FOR OPERATION

In *healed* NVE, indications for operation are related primarily to hemodynamic severity of the valvar lesion or defect. It follows that, in general, results of operation in healed endocarditis are identical to those in patients without endocarditis having the same hemodynamic disturbance. For *active* NVE, principal indications for operation are presence of moderate or severe heart failure, major embolic episodes, important arrhythmias, progressive renal failure, and staphylococcal endocarditis (except right-sided cases). Fungal endocarditis and uncontrolled sepsis are also indications.[H7]

For *early* PVE, presence of mild heart failure with evidence of valvar obstruction caused by vegetations or of a regurgitant murmur and staphylococcal endocarditis with any degree of heart failure are indications for valve replacement. The clinical presentation and natural history of *late*

PVE (more than 2 months after initial operation) are similar to those of active NVE. Therefore, indications for valve replacement in *late* PVE—advanced degree of heart failure, emboli, continuing sepsis, and staphylococcal organism—are similar to those for NVE. Timing of operation for either NVE or PVE should be based on clinical considerations, not on duration of antibiotic treatment.

Echocardiography has become an integral part of the algorithm for diagnosing and treating endocarditis. Presence of mobile vegetations, vegetations larger than 10 mm, and obstructing vegetations warrant consideration for operative therapy. In left-sided NVE, Sanfilippo and colleagues found that vegetation size, extent, mobility, and consistency were univariate predictors of complications (Fig. 15-22).[S6] Patients with a vegetation greater than 10 mm in diameter on echocardiography have a significantly higher risk of embolic phenomena than those with

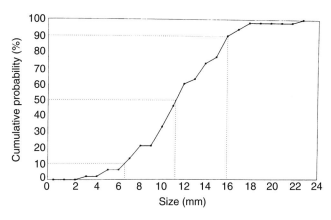

Figure 15-22 Nomogram of cumulative probability of complications relative to increasing size of vegetations, as measured by echocardiography. (From Sanfilippo and colleagues.[S6])

BOX 15-3 Echocardiographic Features Suggesting Potential Need for Surgical Intervention in Patients with Infective Endocarditis

Vegetation

Persistent vegetation after systemic embolization
  Anterior mitral valve leaflet vegetation, particularly with size 10 mm
  One or more embolic events during first 2 weeks of antimicrobial therapy[a]
  Two or more embolic events during or after antimicrobial therapy[a]
  Increase in vegetation size after 4 weeks of antimicrobial therapy[b]

Valvar Dysfunction

Acute aortic or mitral regurgitation with signs of ventricular dilatation[b]
Heart failure unresponsive to medical therapy[b]
Valve perforation or rupture[b]

Perivalvar Extension

Valvar dehiscence, rupture, or fistula[b]
New heart block[b]
Large abscess, or extension of abscess despite appropriate antimicrobial therapy[b]

[a] Surgery may be required because of risk of embolization.
[b] Surgery may be required because of heart failure or failure of medical therapy.

---

small or no vegetations (47% versus 19%).[M8] It must be stressed that vegetation size is only one of several criteria recognized as indications for surgical intervention (Box 15-3). In several studies, vegetation size was no different in patients with and without severe heart failure or in patients surviving or dying during acute IE.[B10]

Right-sided endocarditis in IV drug abusers is caused by *S. aureus* in 80% of patients. Tricuspid valve replacement has been advocated in IE patients who have large vegetations and fever that persist for more than 3 weeks despite appropriate antibiotic therapy. Bayer and colleagues, however, correlating echocardiographic findings with clinical outcome in 53 patients with tricuspid NVE secondary to *S. aureus,* found that 50 patients were cured with antibiotics,

while only 3 required surgery. Of 38 vegetations detected, 21 were 10 mm or greater in diameter. Similarly, recurrent pulmonary emboli were not correlated with demonstrable vegetations or with size of the vegetation.[B11]

Indications for surgical intervention in *children* are much the same as those in adults: heart failure, continuing sepsis, and embolization. In children, however, large masses associated with chronic right-sided indwelling catheters are often indications for surgical extirpation. Small right-sided masses associated with indwelling catheters in both children and adults can be treated with antibiotics, heparinization, and nonsurgical removal of the catheter.

SPECIAL SITUATIONS AND CONTROVERSIES

Three situations in patients with endocarditis present special problems. The first is timing of operation in patients with preoperative CNS events. The data lean heavily in favor of delay if possible in patients with stroke secondary to endocarditis. Risk of deepening stroke or death resulting from a neurologic problem is particularly serious in patients with demonstrable cerebral hemorrhage (as opposed to infarction), as diagnosed with brain CT or MRI. On the other hand, a number of studies have shown that cardiopulmonary bypass is not particularly dangerous in patients with cerebral infarction without hemorrhage or in those with cerebral mycotic aneurysm. In fact, mycotic aneurysms have been shown to regress in the presence of an adequate cardiac operation and continued antibiotic therapy.[M6]

Early surgical treatment of staphylococcal NVE, regardless of hemodynamic compromise, is usually advocated. However, there are isolated reports of successful medical treatment for staphylococcal NVE. Likewise, surgical intervention in early PVE usually is recommended, particularly when the offending organism is *Staphylococcus* or a fastidious organism. In the absence of heart failure, emboli, or a large vegetation, however, nonsurgical treatment may suffice.

Because recidivism is common in drug abusers, surgical treatment of right-sided endocarditis may occasionally be appropriately delayed or abandoned in favor of nonsurgical treatment. This approach may be particularly appropriate when replacement is more likely to be done than repair, because reinfection often follows tricuspid valve replacement. Tricuspid valve resection without replacement is also an option, although hemodynamic sequelae are important limitations to this approach (see Chapter 14).[D8]

Preferred Device for Operation

Choice of valve replacement device depends on several factors, including durability, need for anticoagulation, availability, and ease of insertion. However, factors such as adequate eradication of foci of infection and "best fit" also apply. For that reason, a number of choices may be available for patients with aortic IE. When small abscesses can be excluded by a pliable allograft, this device may be preferable. On the other hand, when root replacement is necessary, insufficient evidence exists to indicate that a tissue valve is superior to a mechanical valved conduit.

Because tricuspid valve endocarditis frequently accompanies IV drug abuse, repair is preferred over replacement. If replacement is necessary, choice of device depends on the usual factors associated with tricuspid valve replacement (see Chapter 14).

Repair is occasionally successful in mitral valve endocarditis, but the preponderance of repairs is done when IE is healed rather than acute.[M12] In the acute stage a mechanical valve is preferable.[M14]

APPENDIX

APPENDIX A
Antibiotic Prophylaxis for Infective Endocarditis

Prophylaxis Recommended
High-risk category
- Prosthetic cardiac valves, including bioprosthetic and allograft valves
- Previous infective endocarditis
- Complex cyanotic congenital heart disease (e.g., single-ventricle states, transposition of great arteries, tetralogy of Fallot)

Moderate-risk category
- Most other congenital cardiac malformations (other than those for high-risk and negligible-risk categories)
- Acquired valve dysfunction (e.g., rheumatic heart disease)
- Hypertrophic cardiomyopathy
- Mitral valve prolapse with valvar regurgitation/thickened leaflets

Prophylaxis Not Recommended
Negligible-risk category (no greater risk than in general population)
- Isolated secundum atrial septal defect
- Surgical repair of atrial septal defect, ventricular septal defect, or patent ductus arteriosus (without residua beyond 6 months)
- Previous coronary artery bypass graft surgery
- Mitral valve prolapse without valvar dysfunction
- Physiologic, functional, or innocent heart murmurs
- Previous Kawasaki disease without valvar dysfunction
- Cardiac pacemakers (intravascular, epicardial) and implanted defibrillators

(Modified from Dajani and colleagues.[D8])

REFERENCES

A
1. Awadallah SM, Kavey RE, Byrum CJ, Smith FC, Kveselis DA, Blackman MS. The changing pattern of infective endocarditis in childhood. Am J Cardiol 1991;68:90.
2. Arnett EN, Roberts WC. Valve ring abscess in active infective endocarditis. Frequency, location, and clues to clinical diagnosis from the study of 95 necropsy patients. Circulation 1976;54:140.
3. Aranki SF, Santini F, Adams DH, Rizzo RJ, Couper GS, Kinchla NM, et al. Aortic valve endocarditis. Determinants of early survival and late morbidity. Circulation 1994;90:1175.
4. Aranki SF, Adams DH, Rizzo RJ, Couper GS, Sullivan TE, Collins JJ Jr, et al. Determinants of early mortality and late survival in mitral valve endocarditis. Circulation 1995;92:143.

B
1. Bertin RJ, Bouillaud J. Traits des maladies du coeur. Paris: Bailliere, 1824, p. 169.
2. Bouillaud J. Traits clinique des maladies du coeur, Vol. 2. Paris: Bailliere, 1841, p. 1.

3. Bahnson HT, Spencer FC, Bennett IL Jr. Staphylococcal infections of the heart and great vessels due to silk sutures. Ann Surg 1957;146:399.
4. Bayer AS, Ward JI, Ginzton LE, Shapiro SM. Evaluation of new clinical criteria for the diagnosis of infective endocarditis. Am J Med 1994;96:211.
5. Birmingham GD, Rahko PS, Ballantyne F 3rd. Improved detection of infective endocarditis with transesophageal echocardiography. Am Heart J 1992;123:774.
6. Bayer AS, Theofilopoulos AN. Immune complexes in infective endocarditis. Springer Semin Immunopathol 1989;11:457.
7. Bayer AS, Theofilopoulos AN, Eisenberg R, Dixon FJ, Guze LB. Circulating immune complexes in infective endocarditis. N Engl J Med 1976;295:1500.
8. Blackstone EH, Kirklin JW. Death and other time-related events after valve replacement. Circulation 1985;72:753.
9. Bauernschmitt R, Jakob HG, Vahl CF, Lange R, Hagl S. Operation for infective endocarditis: results after implantation of mechanical valves. Ann Thorac Surg 1998;65:359.

10. Bayer AS, Bolger AF, Taubert KA, Wilson W, Steckelberg J, Karchmer AW, et al. Diagnosis and management of infective endocarditis and its complications. Circulation 1998;98:2936.

11. Bayer AS, Blomquist IK, Bello E, Chiu CY, Ward JI, Ginzton LE. Tricuspid valve endocarditis due to Staphylococcus aureus. Correlation of two-dimensional echocardiography with clinical outcome. Chest 1998;93:247.

C

1. Corvisart dM, Nicolas J. Essai sur les maladies et les lesions organiques du coeur et des gros vaisseaux. Paris: Migneret, 1806, p. 220.

2. Cates JR, Christie RV. Subacute bacterial endocarditis. Q J Med 1951;20:93.

3. Cabane J, Godeau P, Herreman G, Acar J, Digeon M, Bach JF. Fate of circulating immune complexes in infective endocarditis. Am J Med 1979;66:277

D

1. Durack DT, Lukes AS, Bright DK. New criteria for diagnosis of infective endocarditis: utilization of specific echocardiographic findings. Duke Endocarditis Service. Am J Med 1994;96:200.

2. Daniel WG, Mugge A, Grote J, Hausmann D, Nikutta P, Laas J, et al. Comparison of transthoracic and transesophageal echocardiography for detection of abnormalities of prosthetic and bioprosthetic valves in the mitral and aortic positions. Am J Cardiol 1993;71:210.

3. De Gevigney G, Pop C, Delahaye JP. The risk of infective endocarditis after cardiac surgical and interventional procedures. Eur Heart J 1995;16:7.

4. De Castro S, Magni G, Beni S, Cartoni D, Fiorelli M, Venditti M, et al. Role of transthoracic and transesophageal echocardiography in predicting embolic events in patients with active infective endocarditis involving native cardiac valves. Am J Cardiol 1997;80:1030.

5. David TE, Bos J, Christakis GT, Brofman PR, Wong D, Feindel CM. Heart valve operations in patients with infective endocarditis. Ann Thorac Surg 1990;49:701.

6. d'Udekem Y, David TE, Feindel CM, Armstrong S, Sun Z. Long-term results of surgery for active infective endocarditis. Eur J Cardiothorac Surg 1997;11:46.

7. David TE, Kuo J, Armstrong S. Aortic and mitral valve replacement with reconstruction of the intervalvular fibrous body. J Thorac Cardiovasc Surg 1997;114:766.

8. Dajani AS, Taubert KA, Wilson W, Bolger AF, Bayer A, Ferrieri P, et al. Prevention of bacterial endocarditis. Recommendations by the American Heart Association. Circulation 1997;96:358.

E

1. Eishi K, Kawazoe K, Kuriyama Y, Kitoh Y, Kawashima Y, Omae T. Surgical management of infective endocarditis associated with cerebral complications. Multi-center retrospective study in Japan. J Thorac Cardiovasc Surg 1995;110:1745.

F

1. Frantz PT, Murray GF, Wilcox BR. Surgical management of left ventricular-aortic discontinuity complicating bacterial endocarditis. Ann Thorac Surg 1980;29:1.

G

1. Geraci J, Martin W. Antibiotic therapy of bacterial endocarditis. IV. Successful short term (2 weeks) combined pencillin dihydrostreptomycin therapy in subacute bacterial endocarditis caused by pencillin sensitive streptococci. Circulation 1953;8:494.

2. Gillinov AM, Shah RV, Curtis WE, Stuart RS, Cameron DE, Baumgartner WA, et al. Valve replacement in patients with endocarditis and acute neurologic deficit. Ann Thorac Surg 1996;61:1125.

3. Gutman RA, Striker GE, Gilliland BC, Cutler RE. The immune complex glomerulonephritis of bacterial endocarditis. Medicine 1972;51:1.

4. Gould K, Ramirez-Ronda CH, Holmes RK, Sanford JP. Adherence of bacteria to heart valves in vitro. J Clin Invest 1975;56:1364.

5. Garrison PK, Freedman LR. Experimental endocarditis. I. Staphylococcal endocarditis in rabbits resulting from placement of a polyethylene catheter in the right side of the heart. Yale J Biol Med 1970;42:394.

6. Gersony WM, Hayes CJ, Driscoll DJ, Keane JF, Kidd L, O'Fallon WM, et al. Bacterial endocarditis in patients with aortic stenosis, pulmonary stenosis, or ventricular septal defect. Circulation 1993;87:I121.

7. Glazier JJ, Verwilghen J, Donaldson RM, Ross DN. Treatment of complicated prosthetic aortic valve endocarditis with annular abscess formation by homograft aortic root replacement. J Am Coll Cardiol 1991;17:1177.

H

1. Horder RJ. Infective endocarditis with an analysis of 150 cases with special reference to the chronic form of the disease. Q J Med 1909;2:289.

2. Hooper DC, Bayer AS, Karchmer AW, Theofilopoulos AN, Swartz MN. Circulating immune complexes in prosthetic valve endocarditis. Arch Intern Med 1983;143:2081.

3. Hogevik H, Olaison L, Andersson R, Lindberg J, Alestig K. Epidemiologic aspects of infective endocarditis in an urban population. A 5-year prospective study (review). Medicine 1995;74:324.

4. Hoen B, Selton-Suty C, Lacassin F, Etienne J, Briancon S, Leport C, et al. Infective endocarditis in patients with negative blood cultures: analysis of 88 cases from a one-year nationwide survey in France. Clin Infect Dis 1995;20:501.

5. Haydock D, Barratt-Boyes B, Macedo T, Kirklin JW, Blackstone E. Aortic valve replacement for active infectious endocarditis in 108 patients. J Thorac Cardiovasc Surg 1992;103:130.

6. Hiratzka LF, Nelson RJ, Oliver CB, Jengo JA. Operative experience with infective endocarditis. Drug users compared with non-drug users. J Thorac Cardiovasc Surg 1979;77:355.

7. Hogevik H, Alestig K. Fungal endocarditis: a report on seven cases and a brief review. Infection 1996;24:17.

I

1. Ivert TS, Dismukes WE, Cobbs CG, Blackstone EH, Kirklin JW, Bergdahl LA. Prosthetic valve endocarditis. Circulation 1984;69:223.

J

1. Jones HR Jr, Siekert RG. Neurological manifestations of infective endocarditis. Review of clinical and therapeutic challenges. Brain 1989;112:1295.

2. Johnson CM, Hancock GA, Goulin GD. Specific binding of Staphylococcus aureus to cultured porcine cardiac valvular endothelial cells. J Lab Clin Med 1988;112:16.

3. Jault F, Gandjbakhch I, Rama A, Nectoux M, Bors V, Vaissier E, et al. Active native valve endocarditis: determinants of operative death and late mortality. Ann Thorac Surg 1997;63:1737.

K

1. Kay JH, Bernstein S, Feinstein D, Biddle M. Surgical cure of Candida albicans endocarditis with open heart surgery. N Engl J Med 1961;264:907.

2. Kauffmann RH, Thompson J, Valentijn RM, Daha MR, Van Es LA. The clinical implications and the pathogenetic significance of circulating immune complexes in infective endocarditis. Am J Med 1981;71:17.

L

1. Lancisi GM. De subitaneis mortibus. Venice, Poleti, 1708, p. 225.
2. Loewe L, Rosenblatt P, Green HJ, et al. Combined pencillin and heparin therapy of subacute bacterial endocarditis. Report of seven consecutive successfully treated patients. JAMA 1944;124:14.
3. Lytle BW, Priest BP, Taylor PC, Loop FD, Sapp SK, Stewart RW, et al. Surgical treatment of prosthetic valve endocarditis. J Thorac Cardiovasc Surg 1996;111:198.
4. Lancellotti P, Galiuto L, Albert A, Soyeur D, Pierard LA. Relative value of clinical and transesophageal echocardiographic variables for risk stratification in patients with infective endocarditis. Clin Cardiol 1998;21:572.
5. Larbalestier RI, Kinchla NM, Aranki SF, Couper GS, Collins JJ Jr, Cohn LH. Acute bacterial endocarditis. Optimizing surgical results. Circulation 1992;86:II68.

M

1. Morgagni JB. The seats and causes of diseases, Vol 1, tr Benjamin Alexander. London, Millar and Candell, 1769, Book II, Letter XXIV, Article 18, p. 730.
2. Manhas DR, Mohri H, Hessel EA 2nd, Merendino KA. Experience with surgical management of primary infective endocarditis: a collected review of 139 patients. Am Heart J 1972;84:738.
3. Mugge A. Echocardiographic detection of cardiac valve vegetations and prognostic implications. Infect Dis Clin North Am 1993;7:877.
4. McKinsey DS, Ratts TE, Bisno AL. Underlying cardiac lesions in adults with infective endocarditis: the changing spectrum. Am J Med 1987;82:681.
5. Mathew J, Addai T, Anand A, Morrobel A, Maheshwari P, Freels S. Clinical features, site of involvement, bacteriologic findings, and outcome of infective endocarditis in intravenous drug users. Arch Intern Med 1995;155:1641.
6. Morawetz RB, Karp RB. Evolution and resolution of intracranial bacterial (mycotic) aneurysms. Neurosurgery 1984;15:43.
7. Middlemost S, Wisenbaugh T, Meyerowitz C, Teeger S, Essop R, Skoularigis J, et al. A case for early surgery in native left-sided endocarditis complicated by heart failure: results in 203 patients. J Am Coll Cardiol 1991;18:663.
8. Mugge A, Daniel WG, Frank G, Lichtlen PR. Echocardiography in infective endocarditis: Reassessment of prognostic implications of vegetation size determined by the transthoracic and the transesophageal approach, J Am Coll Cardiol 1989;14:631.
9. McGiffin DC, Galbraith AJ, McLachlan GJ, Stower RE, Wong ML, Stafford EG, et al. Aortic valve infection. Risk factors for death and recurrent endocarditis after aortic valve replacement. J Thorac Cardiovasc Surg 1992;104:511.
10. Moon MR, Stinson EB, Miller DC. Surgical treatment of endocarditis. Prog Cardiovasc Dis 1997;40:239.
11. Mansur AJ, Grinberg M, da Luz PL, Bellotti G. The complications of infective endocarditis. A reappraisal in the 1980s. Arch Intern Med 1992;152:2428.
12. Muehrcke DD, Cosgrove DM 3rd, Lytle BW, Taylor PC, Burgar AM, Durnwald CP, et al. Is there an advantage to repairing infected mitral valves? Ann Thorac Surg 1997;63:1718.
13. Muehrcke DD, Lytle BW, Cosgrove DM. Surgical and long-term antifungal therapy for fungal prosthetic valve endocarditis. Ann Thorac Surg 1995;60:538.
14. Moon MR, Miller DC, Moore KA, Oyer PE, Mitchell RS, Robbins RC, et al. Treatment of endocarditis with valve replacement: the question of tissue versus mechanical prosthesis. Ann Thorac Surg 2001;71:1164.

N

1. Nomenclature and criteria for diagnosis of disease of the heart and great vessels, 8th Ed. The Criteria Committee of the New York Heart Association. Boston: Little Brown, 1979, p. 61.
2. Nomura F, Penny DJ, Menahem S, Pawade A, Karl TR. Surgical intervention for infective endocarditis in infancy and childhood. Ann Thorac Surg 1995;60:90.
3. Nasser RM, Melgar GR, Longworth DL, Gordon SM. Incidence and risk of developing fungal prosthetic valve endocarditis after nosocomial candidemia. Am J Med 1997;103:25.

O

1. Orth J. Ueber die aetiologie der esperimentellen Myocotischem endocarditis. Arch Pathol Anat 1886;103:23.
2. Osler W. The Gulstonian Lectures on malignant endocarditis. Br J Med 1885;1:467.
3. Osler W. Chronic infective endocarditis. Q J Med 1909;2:219.
4. Okies JE, Bradshaw MW, Williams TW Jr. Valve replacement in bacterial endocarditis. Chest 1973;63:898.
5. O'Connor DT, Weisman MH, Fierer J. Activation of the alternate complement pathway in Staphylococcus aureus infective endocarditis and its relationship to thrombocytopenia, coagulation abnormalities and acute glomerulonephritis. Clin Exp Immunol 1978;34:179.

R

1. Richardson JV, Karp RB, Kirklin JW, Dismukes WE. Treatment of infective endocarditis: a 10-year comparative analysis. Circulation 1978;58:589.
2. Ramirez-Ronda CH, Guiterrez-Nunez JJ, Bernude RH. Effects of teichoic acid on adherence of staphylococci to heart valves in vitro. Clin Res 1980;28:377A.
3. Rodbard S. Blood velocity and endocarditis. Circulation 1963,27:18.
4. Rubio-Alvarez J, Duran-Munoz D, Sierra-Quiroga J, Garcia-Bengochea JB. Right heart endocarditis and endocardial pacemakers. Ann Thorac Surg 1989;48:147.

S

1. Sandifort E. Observations anatomico-pathologicae. Leyden, v.d. Eyk and Vygh, 1777.
2. Stinson EB. Surgical treatment of infective endocarditis. Prog Cardiovasc Dis 1979;22:145.
3. Shapiro SM, Young E, De Guzman S, Ward J, Chiu CY, Ginzton LE, et al. Transesophageal echocardiography in diagnosis of infective endocarditis. Chest 1994;105:377.
4. Sandre RM, Shafran SD. Infective endocarditis: review of 135 cases over 9 years. Clin Infect Dis 1996;22:276.
5. Salgado AV, Furlan AJ, Keys TF, Nichols TR, Beck GJ. Neurologic complications of endocarditis: a 12-year experience. Neurology 1989;39:173.
6. Sanfilippo AJ, Picard MH, Newell JB, Rosas E, Davidoff R, Thomas JD, et al. Echocardiographic assessment of patients with infectious endocarditis: prediction of risk for complications. J Am Coll Cardiol 1991;18:1191.
7. Sabik JF, Lytle BW, Blackstone EH, Marullo AG, Pettersson GB, Cosgrove DM. Aortic root replacement with cryopreserved allograft for prosthetic valve endocarditis. Ann Thorac Surg 2002;74:650.

T

1. Tauroff AS, Vessell H. Subacute Streptococcus viridians endocarditis complicating patent ductus arteriosus. JAMA 1940;115:1270.
2. Ting W, Silverman NA, Arzouman DA, Levitsky S. Splenic septic emboli in endocarditis. Circulation 1990;82:105.
3. Tingleff J, Egeblad H, Gotzsche CO, Baandrup U, Kristensen BO, Pilegaard H, et al. Perivalvular cavities in endocarditis: abscesses versus pseudoaneurysms? A transesophageal Doppler echocardiographic study in 118 patients with endocarditis. Am Heart J 1995;130:93.
4. Terpenning MS, Buggy BP, Kauffman CA. Hospital-acquired infective endocarditis. Arch Intern Med 1988;148:1601.
5. Tolan RW Jr, Kleiman MB, Frank M, King H, Brown JW. Operative intervention in active endocarditis in children: report of a series of cases and review. Clin Infect Dis 1992;14:852.

6. Ting W, Silverman N, Levitsky S. Valve replacement in patients with endocarditis and cerebral septic emboli. Ann Thorac Surg 1991;51:18.
7. Taylor KM. Improved outcome for seriously ill open heart surgery patients: focus on reoperation and endocarditis. J Heart Lung Transplant 1993;12:S14.

U

1. Utley JR, Mills J, Hutchinson JC, Edmunds LH Jr, Sanderson RG, Roe BB. Valve replacement for bacterial and fungal endocarditis. A comparative study. Circulation 1973;48:III42.
2. Utley JR, Mills J. Annular erosion and pericarditis: complications of endocarditis of the aortic root. J Thorac Cardiovasc Surg 1972;64:76.

V

1. Vaudaux P, Suzuki R, Waldvogel FA, Morgenthaler JJ, Nydegger UE. Foreign body infection: role of fibronectin as a ligand for the adherence of Staphylococcus aureus. J Infect Dis 1984;150:546.
2. Vilacosta I, Graupner C, San Roman JA, Sarria C, Ronderos R, Fernandez C, et al. Risk of embolization after institution of antibiotic therapy for infective endocarditis. J Am Coll Cardiol 2002;39:1489.

W

1. Weinstein L, Brusch JL. Infective endocarditis. New York: Oxford University Press, 1996, p. 5.
2. Wyssokowitch W. Beatrage zur lehre von der endocarditis. Arch Pathol Anat 1886;103:21.
3. Wallace AG, Young WO Jr, Osterhout J. Treatment of acute bacterial endocarditis by valve excision and replacement. Circulation 1965;31:450.
4. Watanakunakorn C. Infective endocarditis as a result of medical progress. Am J Med 1978;64:917.
5. Weinstein L, Schlesinger JJ. Pathoanatomic, pathophysiologic and clinical correlations in endocarditis. N Engl J Med 1974;291:832.

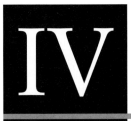

IV Congenital Heart Disease

Atrial Septal Defect and Partial Anomalous Pulmonary Venous Connection

DEFINITION

An *atrial septal defect* (ASD) is a hole of variable size in the atrial septum. A patent foramen ovale that is functionally closed by overlapping of limbic tissue superiorly and the valve of the fossa ovalis inferiorly (in response to the normal left-to-right atrial pressure gradient) is excluded. ASDs generally permit left-to-right shunting at the atrial level. *Partial anomalous pulmonary venous connection* (PAPVC) is a condition in which some, but not all, of the pulmonary veins connect to the right atrium or its tributaries, rather than to the left atrium. The term *connection* is preferred to the term "return" because connection is anatomic and return is governed by hemodynamic factors. PAPVCs may occur as isolated anomalies or may be combined with ASDs.

These two groups of anomalies are considered together in this chapter because they manifest similar physiology and result in similar clinical findings. *Total* anomalous pulmonary venous connection is considered in Chapter 17. ASDs typically occur in association with other cardiac anomalies, and these are considered in chapters dealing with those anomalies.

HISTORICAL NOTE

Clinical recognition of an ASD has been possible only in about the past 60 years. Thus, among the 62 recorded autopsy cases of ASD analyzed by Roesler in 1934, only one had been correctly diagnosed during life.[R1] By 1941, Bedford and colleagues were able to make the diagnosis clinically in a number of patients.[B4] When cardiac catheterization came into general use during the late 1940s and early 1950s, a secure diagnosis became possible. The first description of PAPVC is said to be that by Winslow in 1739[B7] or by Wilson in 1798.[M6] The first diagnosis of PAPVC during life appears to have been made by Dotter and colleagues in 1949.[D6]

A number of ingenious closed methods for repair of ASDs and related conditions were proposed and studied experimentally in the productive and expansive surgical era following the end of World War II in 1945. Probably the first clinical trial was Murray's closure of an ASD in a child by external suturing in Toronto in 1948.[M3] Several other closed methods had clinical trials, including Bailey and colleagues' "atrioseptopexy" and Søndergard's purse-string suture closure.[B3,S2] However, limited applicability of these methods was always apparent, and they were soon discarded.

The technique of hypothermia induced by surface cooling and inflow stasis for repair of ASDs was introduced during the early 1950s (see "Historical Note" in Section 1 of Chapter 2). Lewis and Taufic reported the first successful open repair of an ASD with this method in 1953.[L1] At about the same time, Gross invented the ingenious atrial well technique, a semi-open approach in which a rubber, open-bottomed well or cone was sutured to an incision in a clamp-exteriorized portion of the right atrial wall.[G3,K2] When the clamp was released, the blood rose into the well, and through this pool of blood the surgeon could place sutures under digital control for direct or patch closure of the defect. Gibbon started the era of open heart surgery in 1953, when he successfully repaired an ASD in a young woman using a pump-oxygenator.[G1] Although these three methods—hypothermia and inflow stasis, atrial well, and cardiopulmonary bypass (CPB)—were all used during the late 1950s and provided similar early results, by the late 1960s almost all surgeons used CPB exclusively for these repairs. Percutaneous catheter techniques for closing a fossa ovalis ASD using a polyester double umbrella device were introduced by King and Mills in 1974.[K11]

The first reported treatment for a type of PAPVC was lobectomy in 1950.[D5] In 1953, Neptune and colleagues reported repair using a closed technique in 17 patients with PAPVC of the right lung to the right atrium associated with ASD.[N3] It is not certain who first repaired the sinus venosus syndrome, but the malformation was clearly illustrated by Bedford and colleagues in 1957.[B1] Repair of PAPVC to the inferior vena cava was performed by Kirklin and colleagues at the Mayo Clinic in 1960 and was also subsequently reported by Zubiate and Kay in 1962 and by the UAB group in 1971.[M8,Z1] Correction of anomalous connection of the left pulmonary veins to the left innominate vein and other forms of PAPVC was reported from the Mayo Clinic in 1953[G5,K3] and later in 1956.[K5]

BOX 16-1   Types of Atrial Septal Defect [a]

- Fossa ovalis defect [b]
- Posterior defect
- Coronary sinus defect
- Sinus venosus defect (superior caval ASD)
- Confluent defect
- Ostium primum defect (absence of atrioventricular septum)

[a] Fossa ovalis, posterior, and most confluent defects can be classified as *secundum* type.
[b] Varies in size from small, valvar incompetent foramen ovale ASD to complete absence of septum primum tissue with resultant ASD extending to inferior vena cava.
Key: *ASD*, Atrial septal defect.

MORPHOLOGY

Types of Atrial Septal Defect

As viewed from the right atrial side (see Fig. 1-2), the normal atrial septum may have defects in almost any location (Box 16-1). Although the morphology of these defects has been known since the early descriptions by Robitansky in 1875,[R2] the advent of open heart surgery emphasized their surgically important aspects. The papers by Lewis and colleagues in 1955 and Bedford and colleagues in 1957 are excellent examples of this surgical focus (Fig. 16-1).[B1,L4]

Fossa Ovalis Defect

The most common ASD is the fossa ovalis type, also called *foramen ovale type* or *ostium secundum defect*. This defect lies within the perimeter inscribed by the limbus anteriorly, superiorly, and posteriorly (Fig. 16-2). The smallest defects are essentially valvar incompetent foramina ovale, which occur beneath the superior limbus, between it and the valve (floor) of the fossa ovalis. The floor of the fossa ovalis (remnant of septum primum) may in this situation have multiple fenestrations of various sizes (Fig. 16-3). When

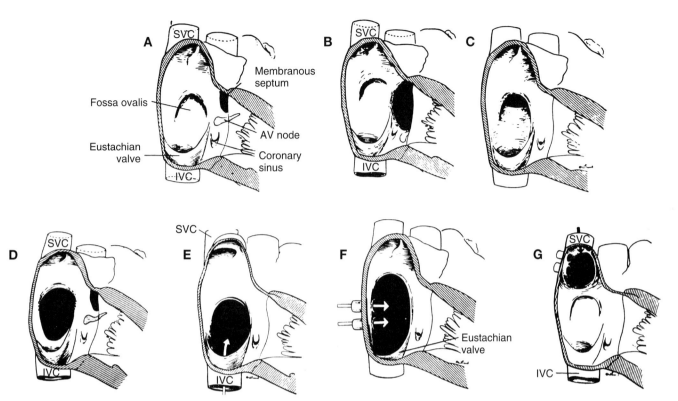

Figure 16-1   Anatomy of atrial septal defect (ASD), viewed from the right atrium, as accurately depicted and described by Bedford and colleagues in 1957.[B1] Original terminology is modified to reflect current usage. **A,** Normal atrial septum. **B,** Atrioventricular (primum) type of atrial septal defect. **C,** Widely patent foramen ovale. **D,** Fossa ovalis defect with complete septal rim (secundum). **E,** Low fossa ovalis ASD astride inferior caval orifice with large eustachian valve. **F,** Large fossa ovalis ASD without posterior rim, with pseudoanomalous right pulmonary veins. **G,** Superior caval type of ASD, or sinus venosus defect. (From Bedford and colleagues.[B1])

Key: *AV,* Atrioventricular; *IVC,* inferior vena cava; *SVC,* superior vena cava.

more of the floor of the fossa ovalis is absent, a larger fossa ovalis defect is present. When all fossa ovalis tissue is absent, the ASD is confluent with the orifice of the inferior vena cava (IVC). The eustachian valve of the IVC then overhangs the ASD and must not be mistaken for its inferior edge at operation. Size of this type of ASD is also affected by any hypoplasia of the limbus that may be present. When the limbus is quite hypoplastic anteriorly, there is only a thin rim of tissue above the atrioventricular (AV) valves (formerly this was called an *intermediate defect* and was sometimes confused with an ostium primum defect). The limbus may also be hypoplastic superiorly or posteriorly.

Normally the IVC–right atrial junction is partly to the left of the plane of the limbus, so that when the floor of the fossa ovalis is absent and an ASD of fossa ovalis type extends to the IVC, the caval ostium overrides (or straddles) the defect onto the left atrium.[V1] This defect results in some right-to-left shunting of IVC blood to the left atrium in virtually all patients with a large fossa ovalis type of ASD (as documented in experimental studies[K8,M5,S11]) and severe shunting with cyanosis in a few patients.[W5] Also, the position of the normally connected right pulmonary veins next to the atrial septal remnant results in preferential left-to-right shunting of their venous drainage.[B10,S11]

Posterior Defect

A defect in the most posterior and inferior part of the atrial septum, with absence, hypoplasia, or anterior displacement of the posterior limbus, is termed a *posterior ASD*. The orifices of the right pulmonary veins usually open directly into the area of the defect, but true anomalous pulmonary venous connection (APVC) of the right lung frequently coexists. In the pure form of this type of ASD, the tissue of the fossa ovalis (including the posterior limbus) is present, and the ASD is an oval defect posterior to this tissue (Fig. 16-4).

Sinus Venosus Defect

The ASD that occurs in sinus venosus syndrome (subcaval defect, superior vena caval defect) is located immediately beneath the orifice of the superior vena cava (SVC), superior to the limbic tissue, and is usually associated with APVC of the right superior pulmonary vein to the SVC near or at the SVC–right atrial junction. The lower margin of the defect is a sharply defined crescentic edge of atrial septum, whereas its upper margin is devoid of septum, being continuous with the posterior SVC wall, which in turn is continuous with the upper edge of the left atrium. The SVC usually overrides the atrial septum onto the left atrium to some extent (see "Sinus Venosus Malformation [Syndrome]" later in this chapter).

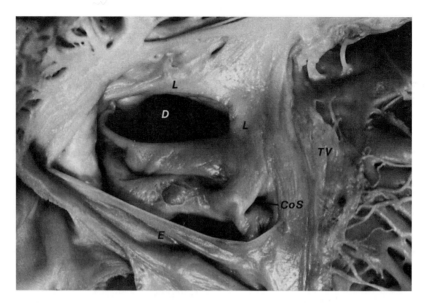

Figure 16-2 Specimen with fossa ovalis atrial septal defect, viewed in anatomic orientation with superior vena cava above and inferior vena cava and its eustachian valve below. The limbus forms the anterior, superior, and posterior rim of the defect, and remnants of the floor (valve) of fossa ovalis form the inferior rim.

Key: *CoS,* Coronary sinus; *D,* atrial septal defect; *E,* eustachian valve; *L,* limbus; *TV,* septal leaflet of tricuspid valve.

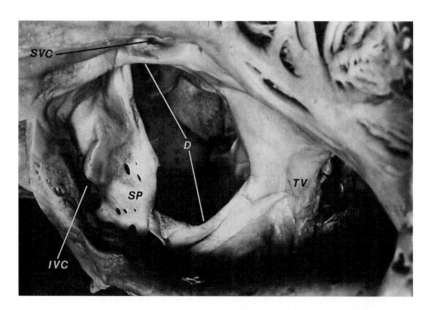

Figure 16-3 Specimen with large fossa ovalis atrial septal defect, viewed from opened right atrium in same orientation as Fig. 16-2. The thin remnant of septum primum (floor of the fossa ovalis) shows numerous perforations.

Key: *D,* Atrial septal defect; *IVC,* inferior vena cava; *SP,* septum primum; *SVC,* superior vena cava; *TV,* tricuspid valve.

Coronary Sinus Defect

Coronary sinus ASDs are part of *unroofed coronary sinus syndrome*. When the sinus is completely unroofed and no partition is present to separate it from the left atrium, the ostium of the coronary sinus is a hole in the atrial septum that permits free communication between left and right atria (see Chapter 19). Occasionally a fenestration may exist in this partition in the midportion of the coronary sinus, particularly in hearts with tricuspid atresia, or rarely the fenestration may be almost at the ostium of the coronary sinus (Fig. 16-5).[R6]

Confluent Defect

Large ASDs may represent a confluence of two of the defects already described. Thus, a fossa ovalis defect coexisting with absence of the posterior limbus can present

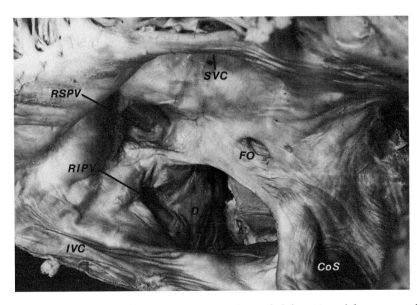

Figure 16-4   Specimen with large posterior atrial septal defect, viewed from opened right atrium. Orientation is as in the previous anatomic figures. The fossa ovalis is intact, but there is a patent foramen ovale. The right inferior pulmonary vein certainly drains anomalously but is probably normally connected. The right superior pulmonary vein is anomalously connected to the right atrium.

Key: *CoS,* Coronary sinus; *D,* atrial septal defect; *FO,* fossa ovalis; *IVC,* inferior vena cava; *RIPV,* right inferior pulmonary vein; *RSPV,* right superior pulmonary vein; *SVC,* superior vena cava.

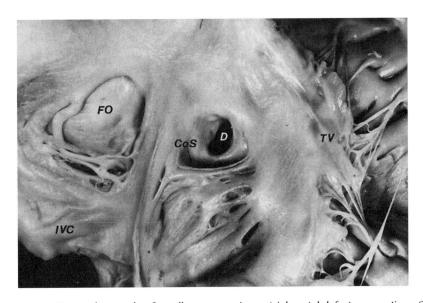

Figure 16-5   Unusual example of small coronary sinus atrial septal defect near ostium. Other anomalies include patent foramen ovale, ventricular septal defect, mild aortic regurgitation, and possible mitral regurgitation.

Key: *CoS,* Coronary sinus; *D,* atrial septal defect; *FO,* fossa ovalis; *IVC,* inferior vena cava; *TV,* tricuspid valve.

as a very large ASD with no septal remnant posteriorly. Another confluent defect occasionally seen is a combination of coronary sinus and fossa ovalis ASDs.

Ostium Primum Defect

An ASD occurs anterior to the fossa ovalis (and the anterior limbus) when the AV septum is *absent.* Such defects are called *AV canal defects, atrioventricular septal defects,* or *ostium primum atrial septal defects,* and are considered in Chapter 20. When essentially the entire atrial septum is absent (common atrium), the defect includes absence of the AV septum (see "Atrial Septal Deficiency and Interatrial Communications" under Morphology in Chapter 20).

Types of Partial Anomalous Pulmonary Venous Connection

Sinus Venosus Malformation (Syndrome)

The most common type of PAPVC is the defect present in sinus venosus syndrome, in which the anomaly coexists with a superior caval ASD. In sinus venosus syndrome the right upper and middle lobe pulmonary veins (right superior pulmonary vein) attach to the low SVC or the SVC–right atrial junction, an arrangement that is present in about 95% of patients with a superior caval ASD.[C3,L7,S10] Most often the APVC is through two anomalous veins from upper and middle lobes, one superior to the other, but there

may be three or rarely four veins, with the uppermost entering the SVC near the azygos vein entry. Infrequently, only part of the right superior vein connects anomalously, with the inferior (right middle lobe) portion of that vein connecting to the left atrium. Rarely, both the right superior and right inferior pulmonary veins connect anomalously to the low SVC or the SVC–right atrial junction (Fig. 16-6).

The lowermost part of the SVC that receives the anomalous veins is usually wider than normal, although it may be relatively small, particularly when there is also a well-formed left SVC, which is not uncommon.[T5] The SVC typically overrides the atrial septum to some extent and

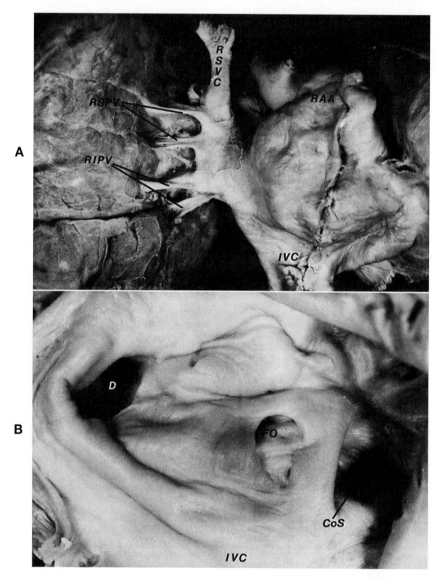

Figure 16-6   Unusual example of sinus venosus malformation (syndrome). **A,** Specimen with typical subcaval atrial septal defect (ASD), but with both right superior and right inferior pulmonary veins entering superior vena caval–right atrial junction. In addition, the left pulmonary veins form a common channel connected to the left atrium and right superior vena cava. Left superior vena cava and mitral atresia were also present. **B,** Interior of right atrium showing the subcaval ASD high in the septum and the enlarged coronary sinus ostium to which is connected the left superior vena cava.

Key: *CoS,* Coronary sinus; *D,* atrial septal defect; *FO,* fossa ovalis; *IVC,* inferior vena cava; *RAA,* right atrial appendage; *RIPV,* right inferior pulmonary vein; *RSPV,* right superior pulmonary vein; *RSVC,* right superior vena cava.

enters partly into the left atrium, resulting in a right-to-left shunt of some SVC blood to the left atrium.

In a few patients SVC overriding is severe enough to produce a large right-to-left shunt and marked cyanosis.[S7] The overriding may also be complete, so that the SVC drains directly and completely into the left atrium.[B14,P6,T6] The relationship between anomalous connection of the SVC to the left atrium without an ASD and sinus venosus syndrome is indicated by connection of pulmonary veins from the right upper lobe to the cardiac end of the SVC in some patients with PAPVC.[B15,E1,K8,P6] This relationship also occurs in patients with no ASD, but in whom the pulmonary veins from the right upper lobe are connected to the cardiac end of the SVC, with the SVC connected to the left atrium by a large opening and to the right atrium by a small opening.[B14,S7]

Rarely a typical high, superior caval ASD is present without APVC; right pulmonary veins connect to the left atrium, but more superiorly than normal.

Right Superior Pulmonary Vein to Superior Vena Cava

Occasionally the entire right superior pulmonary vein connects to the SVC without an associated superior caval ASD. The connection is then usually well above (superior to) the SVC–right atrial junction, and the lower part of the SVC is not dilated. Rarely, even when no superior caval ASD is present, the connection may be in the typical low position of sinus venosus syndrome. Occasionally, only a *portion* of the right superior pulmonary vein draining one or two segments of the right upper lobe connects directly to the SVC. The PAPVC may be isolated or associated with a fossa ovalis ASD.

Right Pulmonary Veins to Right Atrium

Right pulmonary veins may connect directly to the right atrium, either in toto, where they may connect as two or three separate veins, or only through the superior (or rarely inferior) right pulmonary vein. This anomaly may exist as an isolated defect, without an ASD or with only a patent foramen ovale, with the plane of the atrial septum altered from coronal to near-sagittal because of leftward displacement of its lateral attachment. The plane of the right pulmonary vein is actually altered minimally from normal. Because the posterior limbus is present in such defects, the veins are clearly anomalously connected to the right atrium. In ASDs with absence of posterior limbus (posterior ASD) and at times in large fossa ovalis ASDs, the plane of division between right and left atria posteriorly can be questionable, and thus the atrial connection of the right pulmonary veins in this area is debatable. In such defects, however, true anomalous connection of the right pulmonary veins may be present (see Fig. 16-4).[M7,S6]

Right Pulmonary Veins to Inferior Vena Cava (Scimitar Syndrome)

An anomalous right pulmonary vein, generally draining the entire right lung but occasionally only the middle and lower lobes, may descend in a cephalad-to-caudad direction toward the diaphragm, more or less parallel to the pericardial border but with a crescentic (scimitar) shape, and then curve sharply to the left just above or below the IVC–right

■ **TABLE 16-1   Scimitar Syndrome: Presentation and Outcome**

Presentation and Outcome	Infant [a] (n = 19)		Adult (n = 13)	
	No.	%	No.	%
Symptomatic	19	100	9	69
Outcome				
No Repair	13	68	2	15
Deaths	5	38	0	0
Right lung blood flow [b]	3	25	0	0
Repair [c]	6	32	11	85
Deaths	0	0	0	0
Right lung blood flow [b]	1	19	3	27

(Modified from Najm and colleagues.[N5])

[a] Age less than 12 months.

[b] By perfusion scan as percentage of total lung flow.

[c] Complete repair; there were 12 palliative operations, including occlusion of arterial collaterals, pneumonectomy, and dilatation of pulmonary artery stenosis.

atrial junction.[K4] The anomalous pulmonary venous trunk usually passes anterior to the hilum of the right lung, but occasionally is posterior to it. Entrance into the IVC is just superior to the hepatic vein orifices. The atrial septum may be intact, or a fossa ovalis ASD may be present. Occasionally the anomalous vein also connects to *left* atrium,[G6,M9] and rarely scimitar syndrome can exist with connection of the anomalous vein *only* to left atrium.[M10] Pulmonary venous *drainage* is then normal. (Rarely, the left lung may connect via a scimitar-shaped vein to the IVC.[D7,M11])

Right-sided scimitar syndrome occurs as an isolated malformation in a minority of cases. In most patients, anomalies of the right lung are also present.[N5] The most common anomaly is *right lung hypoplasia,* which is associated with a marked mediastinal shift and dextroposition of the heart, and in its severe form with the entire heart lying in the right side of the chest. Blood supply to the hypoplastic right lung comes mainly from a branch of the abdominal aorta in the region of the celiac axis, which ascends through the inferior pulmonary ligament to supply the lower lobe or more often the entire right lung. A small pulmonary artery may be present, but often the central and hilar portions of the right pulmonary artery are absent (Table 16-1). Occasionally a true right lower lobe bronchopulmonary sequestration may exist, with secondary intrapulmonary cyst formation.

Associated cardiac anomalies are often present in scimitar syndrome. In one study, for example, 11 of 13 infants had associated malformations, seven of whom had left-sided hypoplastic conditions.[G11] Diaphragmatic anomalies occurred in about 20% of the cases reviewed by Kiely and colleagues.[K4] These defects included herniation of the right lung through the foramen of Bochdalek and abnormal attachments of the diaphragm.

Rare Connections of Right Pulmonary Veins

Rarely, right pulmonary veins may connect anomalously to the azygos vein or coronary sinus with or without a fossa ovalis ASD.

Left Pulmonary Venous Connections

Left pulmonary veins may connect to the left innominate vein by way of an anomalous vertical vein.[S8] Anomalous drainage is usually from the entire left lung, but may be only from the left upper lobe.[B7] A fossa ovalis ASD coexists in some patients, and in others the atrial septum is intact.[H7]

Rarely, left pulmonary veins connect anomalously to the coronary sinus, a right-sided SVC, or the right atrium.

Bilateral Partial Pulmonary Venous Connection

Partial but bilateral APVC is rare. The most common variant is probably the defect in which the atrial septum is intact, the left superior pulmonary vein attaches to the left innominate vein by way of an anomalous vertical vein, and the right superior pulmonary vein attaches to the SVC–right atrial junction. In another form, a common pulmonary venous chamber is present (see "Pulmonary Venous Anatomy" under Morphology in Chapter 17 for definition), and some veins from both lungs connect to it. All but one lobe or only one lobe from each side may connect to the sinus. The common venous sinus may connect to the right atrium or innominate vein.

Cardiac Chambers in Atrial Septal Defect and Related Conditions

Typically in ASD and related conditions, the right atrium is greatly enlarged (at least grade 3 or 4, on a scale of 1 to 6) and thick walled. The left atrium is not enlarged. This discrepancy occurs in the absence of any flow or pressure restriction between the two, speculatively because the right atrial wall is more distensible than the left.

RV diastolic size is increased, often greatly, because of volume overload imposed by the left-to-right shunt. Whereas normal RV diastolic dimensions are between 0.6 and 1.4 cm · m^{-2}, in patients with large left-to-right shunts at atrial level they average 2.66 cm · m^{-2} and may be as large as 4 cm · m^{-2}.[P2] Consequently, the cardiac apex is often formed by the RV.

Morphologically, the LV is normal or slightly decreased in size. However, important left ventricular dynamic abnormalities are present in most patients (see "Mitral Prolapse" in the text that follows).

Mitral Valve and Atrial Septal Defects

Mitral Prolapse

Mitral valve prolapse occurs in association with fossa ovalis ASD, sinus venosus syndrome,[T5] and probably other types of ASDs and related conditions that result in left-to-right shunts at the atrial level. Prevalence of true prolapse is about 20%,[L3] increasing with age and with magnitude of the pulmonary-to-systemic blood flow ratio ($\dot{Q}p/\dot{Q}s$).[L3,S4]

Schreiber and colleagues have clarified a previously confused subject by relating mitral valve prolapse to abnormalities of LV shape[S4] in patients with ASD.[L2,L8,W2] Alteration in LV configuration results from leftward shift of the ventricular septum, a process that begins as a slight decrease in the normal rightward convexity and progresses with time to flattening and then reversal, with a resultant central bulge into the LV. This process is a response to RV enlargement, which is secondary to volume overload. This etiologic basis of mitral valve prolapse is supported by its decreased degree or elimination in most cases by ASD closure, with return of LV geometry to normal.[A2,S4]

Mitral Regurgitation

Mitral prolapse in ASD can lead to mitral regurgitation, as does ordinary mitral prolapse. True prevalence of regurgitation in unselected patients varies, because older patients and those with larger pulmonary blood flows have a higher prevalence of this abnormality and prolapse. Prevalence of mitral regurgitation severe enough to require correction at the time of ASD repair may be as low as 2% or as high as 10%, occurring in 6% of operated patients at the Mayo Clinic. The data of Leachman and colleagues strongly suggest that this type of mitral prolapse can also precipitate chordal rupture, as it can in Barlow syndrome.[L3]

Cleft Mitral Leaflets

Cleft anterior or posterior mitral leaflets that cause mitral regurgitation are reported to occur occasionally in patients with ASD.[D1,G4,H4] However, judging from some of the illustrations of such "clefts," they may simply be *spaces* between commissural and main leaflets in prolapsed valves.

Lungs and Pulmonary Vasculature

Pulmonary arteries are considerably dilated and elongated when pulmonary blood flow is increased. This dilatation involves even the smallest branches, which tend to compress the smaller airways, with resultant retention of secretions and bronchiolitis.

Hypertensive pulmonary vascular disease develops infrequently in patients with ASD, and then usually not until the third or fourth decade of life (see "Pulmonary Vascular Disease" under Morphology in Chapter 21). This contrasts sharply with ventricular septal defects, complete AV septal defects, and patent ductus arteriosus, in which pulmonary vascular disease may be present early in life. In ASD, pulmonary vascular disease is caused mainly by secondary thrombosis in the dilated pulmonary artery branches, with changes in the intima and media of vessels usually playing a minor role. Haworth has suggested, however, that an increase in pulmonary arterial smooth muscle may be the only finding.[H9]

Associated Cardiac Conditions

ASDs and related conditions may coexist with almost all varieties of congenital heart disease, but such cases are not considered here unless the left-to-right shunt at atrial level is the dominant hemodynamic lesion. A wide spectrum of cardiac anomalies coexist with ASD as the dominant lesion (Table 16-2).

Valvar heart disease may coexist with hemodynamically important ASDs. Six cases with moderate or severe rheumatic mitral stenosis and a hemodynamically significant ASD (Lutembacher syndrome) were included among 443 patients with an ASD at GLH (1957 to 1983). Eleven cases of moderate or severe mitral regurgitation were included, in three of which regurgitation was rheumatic in origin. Both mitral stenosis and regurgitation increase left-to-right shunting.

Tricuspid regurgitation of variable severity frequently complicates ASDs in older patients with heart failure, the

■ **TABLE 16-2   Associated Cardiac Anomalies in Patients with Atrial Septal Defect or Partial Anomalous Pulmonary Venous Connection** [a]

Anomaly	No.	% of 443
Left superior vena cava	24	5
Mild or moderate pulmonary artery stenosis	16	4
Peripheral pulmonary artery stenosis	4	1
Azygos extension of inferior vena cava	4	1
Small ventricular septal defect	2	0.01
Small patent ductus arteriosus	2	0.01
Mild coarctation of aorta	2	0.01
Small coronary artery–pulmonary trunk fistula	2	0.01
Anomalous right subclavian artery	2	0.01
Dextrocardia (isolated)	1	0.005

[a] Data from 443 patients undergoing repair at GLH from 1957 to 1983. Some patients had more than one anomaly, so the figures are not cumulative.

Key: *ASD,* Atrial septal defect; *PAPVC,* partial anomalous pulmonary venous connection.

mechanism generally being right ventricular and tricuspid anular dilatation. In 10 of 443 patients undergoing repair of ASD at GLH, tricuspid regurgitation required surgical treatment.

Related Conditions

Rarely, ASD may occur in patients with Marfan, Turner, Noonan, or Holt-Oram syndromes.

CLINICAL FEATURES AND DIAGNOSTIC CRITERIA

The symptoms, clinical features, and signs in ASD and related conditions producing left-to-right shunting at atrial level are related largely to size of the left-to-right shunt.[1] Thus, in general, when $\dot{Q}p/\dot{Q}s$ is less than 1.5, there are neither signs nor symptoms of the shunt, and this is often true with a $\dot{Q}p/\dot{Q}s$ up to 1.8. When $\dot{Q}p/\dot{Q}s$ is larger than this, usually signs of the shunt are present and symptoms appear eventually (see "Changes in Pulmonary/Systemic Blood Flow over Time" in Natural History later in the chapter). Infants present an exception to these generalizations. Their clinical features are often atypical; for example, splitting of the second heart sound is unrelated to $\dot{Q}p/\dot{Q}s$.[H11]

---

[1] Left-to-right shunting across a nonrestrictive (>2 cm in an adult) ASD under ordinary circumstances is a function of the relative compliance (reflected in the diastolic pressures) of right and left ventricles (RV and LV). RV compliance in particular is unpredictable and is one factor causing variability in $\dot{Q}p/\dot{Q}s$ from one patient to another. A compliant distensible RV (in association with a normal pulmonary vascular bed) will permit a large shunt; a less compliant one (such as may result from pulmonary hypertension or from morphologic RV changes that occur later in life[J1,P5]) permits a more modest shunt. LV compliance tends to decrease with age, which tends to increase $\dot{Q}p/\dot{Q}s$ as patients become older. Shunting is increased by systemic hypertension when this results in decreased LV compliance. Mitral regurgitation or stenosis increases $\dot{Q}p/\dot{Q}s$. When the ASD is small and flow is restrictive, left-to-right shunting is limited. Even then, mitral stenosis may elevate left atrial pressure sufficiently that a large left-to-right shunt through all phases of the cardiac cycle results, leading to a soft continuous murmur.

Symptoms

Symptoms may be absent for several decades, but consist of effort breathlessness when they occur and a tendency toward recurrent respiratory tract infections. Palpitation from paroxysmal atrial tachycardia or atrial fibrillation may occur later in life. Older adults may present with chronic heart failure with fluid retention, hepatomegaly, and severe cardiac cachexia. Occasionally an infant with ASD and a large left-to-right shunt, often in association with PAPVC, may have heart failure with tachypnea, but this is uncommon. In such infants, other associated malformations may contribute to the heart failure.

Atypical presentations occur. An unequivocal history of cyanosis may bring a patient with an uncomplicated ASD to medical attention,[J1,M13,M14] as in one of the 340 patients in the UAB surgical series. He was a 12-year-old child with normal pulmonary artery pressure, a large fossa ovalis ASD extending to the IVC, and considerable right-to-left shunting from the IVC to the left atrium. This coincides with occasional bidirectional shunting in patients with otherwise uncomplicated ASDs,[G8] usually older patients.[G8] For the same anatomic reasons (see "Morphology" earlier in this chapter), patients may present with paradoxical emboli or cerebral infarctions; two patients (1%) in the UAB series presented in this way, one 33 and the other 38 years old. Both had normal pulmonary artery pressures. This presentation occurred in nine (2%) of the Mayo Clinic series of 546 patients.[R4] Infrequently the presentation may be modified by presence of severe pulmonary hypertension, in which case cyanosis, effort intolerance, and hemoptysis may be present.

Signs

Clinical signs diagnostic of a large ($\dot{Q}p/\dot{Q}s$ greater than 1.8 to 2.0) shunt at atrial level are as follows:
- Overactive left parasternal systolic lift
- Fixed splitting of the second heart sound throughout the respiratory cycle (absent when large $\dot{Q}p/\dot{Q}s$ is from PAPVC with an intact atrial septum)
- A soft pulmonary midsystolic flow murmur (in second and third left intercostal spaces)
- A mid-diastolic tricuspid flow murmur (in fourth and fifth left intercostal spaces) present in borderline situations only on inspiration

This last sign is occasionally absent, however, particularly in older patients and in those with a larger shunt. In addition, an extremely large shunt produces a more marked left-sided precordial right ventricular lift, occasionally some prominence of the left anterior chest wall, and leftward displacement of the cardiac apex. Many such patients are short and thin.

When heart failure is present, jugular venous pressure is elevated, the liver is enlarged, and there is gross cardiomegaly. Tricuspid regurgitation produces systolic liver pulsation and a greater tendency to ascites and peripheral edema.

Important pulmonary hypertension is evident clinically by accentuation of the second heart sound and a more marked right ventricular and pulmonary artery lift. A pulmonary regurgitation murmur may be heard, as well as a murmur of tricuspid regurgitation.

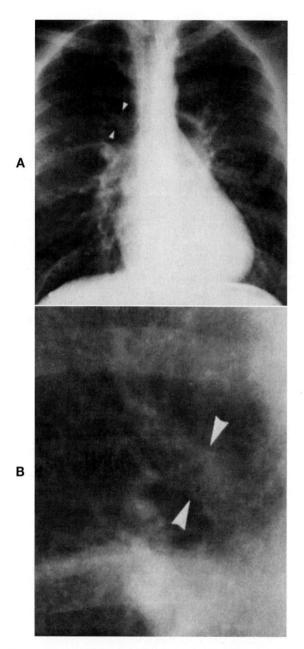

Figure 16-7 Chest radiograph of sinus venosus malformation. **A**, Usual view. **B**, Magnification copy. Arrowheads indicate right superior pulmonary vein.

Chest Radiography

Chest radiography reflects the large $\dot{Q}p/\dot{Q}s$. The right atrium and right ventricle are large. The pulmonary trunk shadow in the upper left portion of the cardiac silhouette is enlarged, and the right and left pulmonary arteries are enlarged to the periphery of the lung field. In general, pulmonary vascular markings are increased, or plethoric. The shadow of the transverse aortic arch is abnormally small. Patients with heart failure may have interstitial pulmonary edema and areas of pulmonary consolidation and atelectasis. These signs are probably secondary to compression of smaller airways by enormously enlarged small pulmonary vessels.

The chest radiograph may suggest the specific anatomic diagnosis. Occasionally the right superior pulmonary vein can be identified lying more superiorly than normal (Fig.

16-7), leading to suspicion of sinus venosus syndrome. A crescentic shadow more or less parallel to the right-sided heart border (Fig. 16-8) suggests the diagnosis of APVC of right pulmonary veins to IVC (scimitar syndrome).

Electrocardiography

Electrocardiogram (ECG) almost always shows the pattern of incomplete right bundle branch block and a clockwise frontal loop. Left axis deviation and a counterclockwise loop strongly suggest an AV septal defect, although this pattern occurs in about 10% of patients with fossa ovalis ASDs.

Echocardiography

Clinical diagnosis of ASD, particularly of the foramen ovale type, can be confirmed by visualizing the defect directly using two-dimensional echocardiography[F3,L2,S12] (Fig. 16-9). Echocardiography also gives indirect evidence of ASD in demonstrating right ventricular volume overload, which includes increased right ventricular diastolic size and abnormal (flat or paradoxical) septal motion.[M4,T4] However, two-dimensional echocardiography has been unreliable (less than 75% sensitivity) in detecting anomalous connection of right pulmonary veins to SVC. More often these sinus venosus defects can be detected by *transesophageal echocardiography* (TEE). TEE also can localize fossa ovalis defects to the high, low, or posterior septum. AV septal defects can be separated from secundum defects, and localization of subcaval defects and APVC is usually possible. The addition of Doppler color flow interrogation allows a reasonable estimate of $\dot{Q}p/\dot{Q}s$.

Cardiac Catheterization and Cineangiography

When diagnosis of a typical and apparently uncomplicated ASD has been made by noninvasive methods in children, adolescents, and young adults, cardiac catheterization is not required.[S14] The surgeon then becomes responsible for confirming the type of ASD at operation and presence or absence of any APVCs. Cardiac catheterization and appropriate cineangiography are indicated in infants (because of possible associated anomalies), in many adults (for assessing possible pulmonary hypertension and status of mitral valve), and in any patient in whom noninvasive tests suggest PAPVC. Coronary angiography is performed in patients older than 35 to 40 years.

Assessment of operability in patients with pulmonary hypertension is a particular problem. Even in Eisenmenger syndrome with shunt reversal at atrial level, pulmonary artery pressure (PpA) is rarely more than two thirds that of systemic pressure. (There is no transmission of systemic pressure across the defect, as is the case with large defects at ventricular or ductus levels; see "Cardiac Catheterization" under Clinical Features and Diagnostic Criteria in Chapter 21.)

The most reliable criterion of inoperability is the absolute level of pulmonary vascular resistance normalized to body surface area (RpI) and calculated when possible using measured, rather than assumed, oxygen uptake.[N4] Pulmonary to systemic flow ratios or resistance ratios are much less discriminating. In fact, precise criteria have not been established as accurately for ASD as for ventricular septal defect (VSD). Using VSD criteria (with no reason to

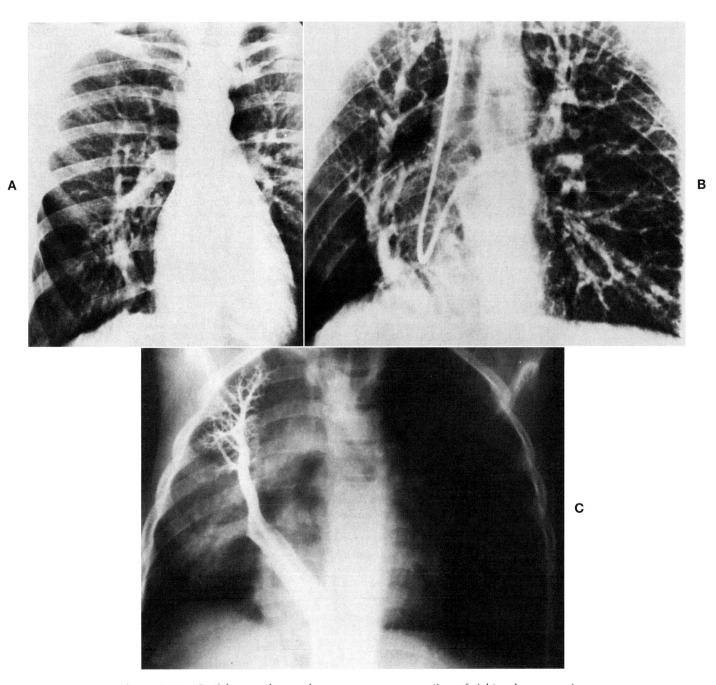

Figure 16-8   Partial anomalous pulmonary venous connection of right pulmonary veins to inferior vena cava in patient with scimitar syndrome. **A**, Plain chest radiograph, frontal view, showing crescentic shadow of anomalous pulmonary vein. **B**, Levophase of pulmonary angiogram showing anomalous pulmonary vein draining into inferior vena cava. **C**, Selective angiogram into anomalous pulmonary vein.

believe these are not equally applicable to ASD), a resting RpI of 8 U · m² or more may preclude complete operative closure. In this event, RpI must also be calculated while using a pulmonary vasodilator (isoproterenol,[N4] tolazoline,[M16] or 100% oxygen[M17]). If arterial desaturation (less than 97%) exists when measured by the usual finger sensor, cardiac catheterization is indicated in both adults and children. Interventions such as 100% O_2, exercise, and perhaps nitric oxide (NO) are appropriate to gauge pulmonary vascular reactivity, response of pulmonary vascular resistance, and reversion to a strictly left-to-right shunt

condition. If arterial oxygen saturation (SaO_2) increases to normal levels and pulmonary vascular resistance falls, operation can be done even in the presence of intermittent arterial desaturation (right-to-left shunt). The vasodilator must produce a fall in RpI to below 7 U · m² before the patient can be considered operable,[L10,M16,N4] because only then can the pulmonary vascular disease be expected to regress. Otherwise, disease is likely to progress despite closure of the ASD. Progressive pulmonary vascular disease is less well tolerated when the atrial septum is intact, because the right side of the heart is then unable to

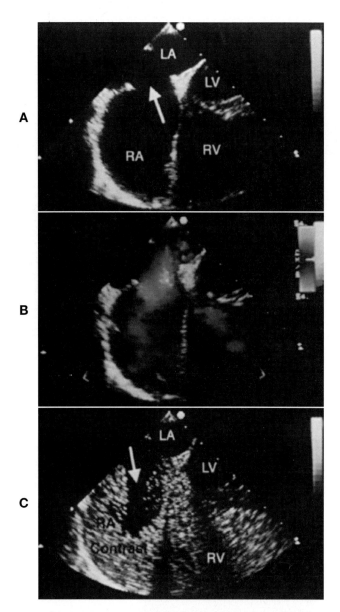

Figure 16-9   Transesophageal echocardiogram of fossa ovalis atrial septal defect. **A,** Arrow indicates dropout of atrial septum with clear evidence of tissue superiorly and inferiorly (above atrioventricular valves), diagnostic of fossa ovalis (secundum) defect. **B,** Blood flow is directed through the defect left to right from left to right atrium. **C,** Negative image of left-to-right flow during injection of saline (as contrast). (From Lang and Marcus.[L12])

Key: *LA,* left atrium; *LV,* left ventricle; *RA,* right atrium; *RV,* right ventricle.

decompress through a right-to-left shunt at atrial level; thus, ASD closure under such circumstances usually decreases life expectancy.

Cardiac catheterization and angiography are also useful in defining anatomic details of related conditions that can cause shunting at the atrial level. Increased SaO_2 in the low SVC provides presumptive evidence of sinus venosus syndrome, and this becomes virtually certain if the catheter can be passed through a subcaval ASD into the left atrium. An indicator dilution curve obtained after injecting dye into the SVC may show some right-to-left shunting, which is

generally completely absent in patients with a fossa ovalis ASD (who may have right-to-left shunting from the IVC). In addition, curves obtained after injection into the right pulmonary artery generally show a much larger left-to-right shunt, a result of the anomalously draining right pulmonary veins, than curves obtained after injection into the left pulmonary artery. Identification of the specific anatomic details of sinus venosus syndrome is best accomplished by angiography after right pulmonary artery injection because the typical location and drainage of the right superior pulmonary vein can then be seen. Pulmonary artery injection may confirm anomalous connection of the right pulmonary veins to the right atrium or IVC (see Fig. 16-8), of left veins to innominate or other veins, or of bilateral APVCs.

When anomalous connection of the right pulmonary veins to the IVC is demonstrated, *aortography* should also be done to identify any anomalous systemic arteries from the abdominal or thoracic aorta to the right lower lobe. If the right lung is small, if the right lower lobe is contracted or seems otherwise abnormal on chest radiography, or if the patient gives a history of hemoptysis or recurrent pulmonary infections, *bronchoscopy* or *bronchography* is also indicated.

Calculations of Q̇p/Q̇s are of particular importance in patients with isolated PAPVC of only a part of one lung. An operation is not indicated when the ratio is less than 1.8. This approach is especially relevant with isolated connection of some of the right upper lobe veins to the high SVC, because diversion or transfer to the left atrium is quite difficult (and probably needless). Even when only the right superior pulmonary vein is involved and the atrial septum is intact, the shunt may be greater than this, presumably because right atrial and caval pressures are distinctly lower than left atrial pressures, producing a larger-than-usual pulmonary venous gradient.[H2]

NATURAL HISTORY

The natural history of persons born with ASDs and related conditions producing left-to-right shunts at atrial level is not known precisely, but its general characteristics have been described.[C4,C5]

Survival

In 1970, Campbell published the most detailed study available on survival of patients with ASD treated nonsurgically.[C5] Transformation of these findings into conventional survival format and comparison with life expectancy of the general population provide good insight into the life expectancy of patients with ASD (Fig. 16-10).

Campbell's data support the idea that only 0.1% of individuals born with a large ASD and no other important cardiac anomaly die in infancy and that few who are unrepaired die in the first or second decade. About 5% to 15% die in the third decade, usually with pulmonary hypertension and Eisenmenger syndrome.[C4] Premature late death with heart failure occurs in an increasing proportion after the fifth decade. Even so, probably no more than 25% of persons born with a large ASD die from the defect, because lethal manifestations of the disease tend to occur so late in life that other unrelated conditions cause death first.

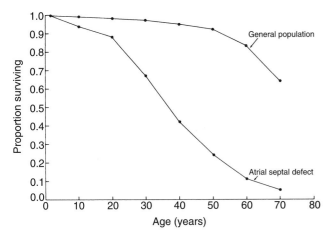

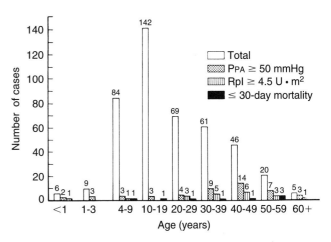

Figure 16-10   Plot of Campbell's survival computations of life expectancy for surgically untreated patients with atrial septal defects (ASD) who reach age 1 year, based on three sets of collected data. Spread among the data sets indicates confidence limits of modest width around point estimates (confidence limits cannot be calculated from data). Life expectancy of the general population at age 1 year is also from Campbell and is close to that computed from U.S. life tables. The data suggest that 99.9% of patients born with ASD reach the first year of life unless unrelated conditions cause their death. (From Campbell.[C5])

Figure 16-11   Histogram showing frequency of pulmonary hypertension and increased pulmonary vascular resistance in a series of surgically treated patients with atrial septal defects (data set is same as in Table 16-2). Of these patients, 372 were catheterized, and in the remaining 71, pulmonary artery systolic pressure was assumed to be less than 50 mmHg and RpI less than 4.5 U · m[2].

Key: P_{PA}, Pulmonary artery systolic pressure, RpI, pulmonary vascular resistance index.

The natural history of patients with sinus venosus syndrome[H7] and most other types of PAPVC and ASD[B8,S9] is similar to that of patients with large fossa ovalis ASD. Patients with sinus venosus syndrome in the fourth to sixth decades present with heart failure or with severe pulmonary hypertension from pulmonary vascular disease.

The natural history of scimitar syndrome is not clear. Presumably, patients without important anomalies of the right lung and with a large left-to-right shunt have a life history similar to that of patients with a large fossa ovalis ASD. Those with right lung hypoplasia, however, often have a life history dominated by their pulmonary pathology, including hemoptysis and recurrent pulmonary infections.

When there is isolated PAPVC of part of one lung and Qp/Qs is less than 1.8, life expectancy may be normal. Rarely, paradoxical emboli occur in patients with sinus venosus syndrome (from SVC) as well as in those with fossa ovalis ASDs (from IVC).

Pulmonary Hypertension

In the UAB surgical series, 14% of patients catheterized had pulmonary hypertension with a mean pulmonary artery pressure (P_{PA}) greater than 25 mmHg. In the GLH surgical series, systolic P_{PA} was greater than 50 mmHg in 13% of catheterized patients and 11% of the total series (Fig. 16-11). Prevalence of elevated RpI (4 U · m[2] or greater) was 4.5% and rare (1%) in patients less than 20 years of age. In a few locations where individuals reside at high altitude, however, prevalence of pulmonary hypertension is greater. Cherian and colleagues report that in their region of India, pulmonary hypertension was present in 13% of patients under age 10 years.[C6]

■ **TABLE 16-3   Relationship between New York Heart Association Functional Class and Age at Operation** [a]

Preoperative NYHA Class	Age (years)		
	Mean	**Median**	**Range**
I	16	12	3.3-63
II	32	30	4.2-72
III	50	54	0.9-68
IV	51	57	2.2-66

[a] Data from 340 patients undergoing repair of atrial septal defect at UAB, 1967 to 1979.

Key: NYHA, New York Heart Association.

Pulmonary hypertension is particularly prevalent in patients with scimitar syndrome partly caused by increased pulmonary blood flow but also by stenosis of the anomalous vein, presence of systemic arterial collaterals to the right lung, or reduction of the pulmonary vascular bed on the right side.[N5]

Functional Status

Probably only about 1% of patients born with a large ASD have symptoms during the first year.[A1,D2,H5,N1,S5] Most are asymptomatic through the first and second decades, although many are short and thin. Effort intolerance and easy fatigability may develop in the second or third decade or as late as the fifth or sixth decade. These symptoms progress gradually to fluid retention, hepatomegaly, and elevated jugular venous pressure, leading to gradually increasing disability. These phenomena are well exemplified in the surgical experience, in which preoperative New York Heart Association (NYHA) functional class and age at operation are moderately well correlated ($r = .61$, $P < .05$) (Table 16-3). When heart failure becomes advanced, both mitral and tricuspid regurgitation are likely to have developed.

Spontaneous Closure

Spontaneous closure of a hemodynamically significant isolated ASD occasionally occurs in the first year.[M3] Cockerham and colleagues found closure in 22% of 87 patients[C7] and Ghisla and colleagues in 14%.[G9] Smaller left-to-right shunts were present in patients whose defects spontaneously closed than in those whose did not.[C7] Spontaneous closure is uncommon after the first year,[C1,G2,H1,H7,M1,M2] although Ghisla and colleagues found that closure occasionally occurred in the second year.[G9]

Changes in Pulmonary/Systemic Blood Flow over Time

As already noted, decreasing LV compliance increases $\dot{Q}p/\dot{Q}s$ in patients with ASD, and this may develop during the fifth and sixth decades. Systemic arterial hypertension accelerates this process and may unmask an ASD that was not an important shunt before onset of decreased LV compliance.

It is also likely that most ASDs increase in size as time passes; this has been clearly demonstrated in the case of patent foramen ovale.[H10] The direct relationship between $\dot{Q}p/\dot{Q}s$ and the tendency toward mitral valve prolapse also supports the concept that the shunt increases with age.[S4] These increases in $\dot{Q}p/\dot{Q}s$ with time do not occur when the shunt is from APVC without ASD. $\dot{Q}p/\dot{Q}s$ decreases when pulmonary hypertension develops, a result of decreased RV compliance that accompanies RV hypertrophy (see footnote 1 on p. 723).

Right Ventricular Function

Right ventricular (RV) volume overload and consequent increased RV diastolic dimensions are characteristic of patients with a hemodynamically significant ASD or PAPVC. The ventricular septum is displaced posteriorly and leftward under such circumstances.[W2] However, systolic anterior motion of the septum occurs.[H3,P1] These features are well tolerated by the RV for many years, much longer than for the volume-overloaded *left* ventricle and probably longer than for volume overload produced by acute tricuspid or pulmonary valve regurgitation. RV failure eventually occurs, however, with decreased RV ejection fraction and hypokinesia. Doty and colleagues demonstrated loss of coronary reserve in patients with ASD and volume-induced RV hypertrophy,[D8] which contributes further to development of RV failure. Associated signs and symptoms of elevated systemic venous pressure then develop (peripheral edema, elevated jugular venous pressure, hepatomegaly, and finally ascites), often with tricuspid regurgitation.

These RV phenomena have been documented by several studies. Liberthson and colleagues found increased RV volume but normal (64%) ejection fraction in 9 asymptomatic patients with a mean age of 25 years. However, 11 symptomatic patients with a mean age of 52 years had diffuse RV hypokinesia and ejection fraction averaging 36%, in addition to increased RV volume.[L5] In a possibly related finding, adult patients with ASD but without pulmonary hypertension occasionally have marked pulmo-

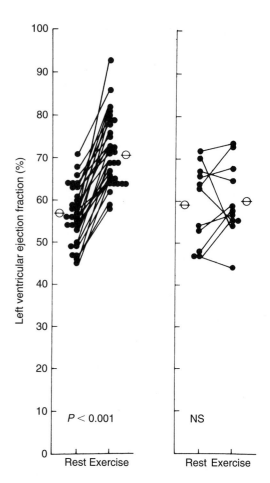

Figure 16-12 *Left,* Normal response of increased left ventricular ejection fraction with maximal exercise. *Right,* In contrast, adult patients with atrial septal defects generally do not increase ejection fraction with maximal exercise. (From Bonow and colleagues.[B6])

Key: *NS,* Not significant.

nary valve regurgitation,[L6] which disappears after repair of the ASD.

Left Ventricular Function

Most adult patients with hemodynamically significant ASD or PAPVC have normal left ventricular (LV) systolic dimensions but subnormal diastolic dimensions.[B6,P1,T3] Some loss of LV functional reserve is present in most adult patients and in some children with ASD. Thus, in contrast to normal persons, such individuals do not increase LV ejection fraction during maximal exercise[B6] (Fig. 16-12), although resting ejection fraction is usually within normal limits.[B6,P1] Popio and colleagues also reported abnormal sequences of LV contraction.[P1]

These preoperative LV abnormalities are convincingly ascribed by Bonow and colleagues to the effects of the volume-overloaded *right* ventricle.[B6] Other studies have established that, even in the absence of symptoms of systemic venous hypertension from RV failure, LV structure and function in patients with ASDs are influenced by the increased RV volume rather than changes in LV compliance.[K1,L8,W2]

Atrioventricular Valvar Dysfunction

As discussed earlier, important mitral regurgitation is present in 2.5% to 10% of adults with large ASDs,[H8] and both mitral and tricuspid regurgitation may become prominent in older patients who develop heart failure. When viewed at operation, the tricuspid valve does not appear to be intrinsically abnormal. Presumably, regurgitation develops because of anular dilatation and lack of proper shortening of the tricuspid anulus during systole secondary to RV enlargement resulting from long-standing volume overload.[T1,T2]

Supraventricular Arrhythmias

After the third decade, supraventricular arrhythmias complicate the natural history of patients with large ASDs and related conditions in increasing numbers over time. Most often this begins with paroxysmal atrial fibrillation, which gradually becomes permanent. Atrial fibrillation was present in 15 (20%; CL 15%-26%) of 75 patients over age 40 operated on by Magilligan and colleagues.[M6] Of 19 patients preoperatively in NYHA class III or IV, 47% (CL 34%-64%) had this arrhythmia, compared with 11% (CL 6%-17%) of 56 patients in class I or II. St. John Sutton and colleagues found that 56% of their patients over age 60 had atrial fibrillation at operation.[S1]

In addition to evident supraventricular arrhythmias, more subtle abnormalities of conduction system function develop. Benedini and colleagues found concealed sinus node dysfunction in 17 (65%; CL 53%-76%) of 26 adult patients with fossa ovalis ASD, which became evident only with electrophysiologic testing.[B11] Such abnormalities are less common in children with ASDs.[R5]

Systemic Arterial Hypertension

Adult patients with hemodynamically important ASDs are likely to have systemic arterial hypertension. At the Mayo Clinic, St. John Sutton and colleagues found that 25 (38%) of their 66 patients had systemic arterial blood pressure above 150/90, a higher proportion ($P < .01$) than in an age-matched general population.[S1] As noted, this relationship may result partly from the effect of hypertension on shunt size.

TECHNIQUE OF OPERATION
Fossa Ovalis Atrial Septal Defect

Anesthetic management, positioning and preparation of the patient, median sternotomy, and preparations for CPB are discussed in detail in Section 3 of Chapter 2 and in Chapter 4. An alternative to the midline skin incision may be used for cosmetic reasons; in this approach, a bilateral fourth interspace submammary skin incision is made and a skin flap raised superiorly and inferiorly before the sternum is incised vertically in the usual way. However, some surgeons have expressed concern regarding breast development and symmetry late following right submam-mary incisions in females. Alternatively, a right anterolateral fifth intercostal space incision may be used if the patient expresses concern about the cosmetic effects of a midline scar. Repair of ASD may also be accomplished using the small lower sternotomy approach and also a small vertical right parasternal incision. Each requires modification of the setup for caval cannulation (see Section 3 in Chapter 2).

In children and young adults with uncomplicated ASDs, a routinely placed left atrial pressure monitoring catheter is considered unnecessary by some authorities, but such monitoring should be done routinely in older patients, whose left atrial pressure may be considerably higher than right atrial pressure after repair. Routine use of a left atrial catheter also may be advisable in very young patients.

After the incision is made and the pericardial stay sutures placed, intrapericardial anatomy is assessed. The characteristically large right atrium and RV of ASD are noted, as well as the normal-sized left atrium and LV. A left SVC in the fold of Marshall is sought. The external position and connections of the right and left superior and inferior pulmonary veins are noted. Often the ASD can be palpated through the atrial wall. Optimally, TEE is available to establish the position of the ASD, relationship of the pulmonary veins, and function of the mitral and tricuspid valves.

The patient is heparinized and arterial cannula inserted. Two venous cannulae are used, one inserted through the right atrial appendage and the other through the low right atrial wall. Alternatively, direct caval cannulation with angled cannulae is employed.

CPB is established with the perfusate temperature at 34°C. The cardioplegic needle or aortic root catheter is now placed in the ascending aorta, the aorta is clamped, and cold cardioplegic solution is injected. Rewarming of the patient with the perfusate is begun once the heart is cold and isolated. The caval tapes are "snugged," and the right atrium is opened obliquely (Fig. 16-13). A left atrial suction catheter is *not* inserted through the left atrial wall in fossa ovalis ASD because it is unnecessary and imposes a remote risk of cerebral air embolism.

A few fine stay sutures are placed on the edges of the atriotomy incision. Blood in the left atrium is suctioned only enough to expose clearly the edges of the ASD, because evacuation of more blood than this from the left side of the heart needlessly exposes the patient to risk of air entrapment and subsequent air embolization. An exception to this policy is presence of mitral valve pathology.

The entire right atrial internal anatomy is examined, particularly identifying the limbus and defining any rim of the ASD. The relationship of the defect to the ostium of the coronary sinus, membranous portion of the AV septum, and commissural area between the septal and anterior tricuspid leaflets is studied because these features serve as guides to the location of the AV node and penetrating portion of the bundle of His (see Fig. 16-13). Possible fenestrations in the valve (floor) of the fossa ovalis are sought; these are usually between the fossa ovalis and limbus anteriorly or near the IVC inferiorly. When present in thin tissue, fenestrations may be joined to the main defect by excising

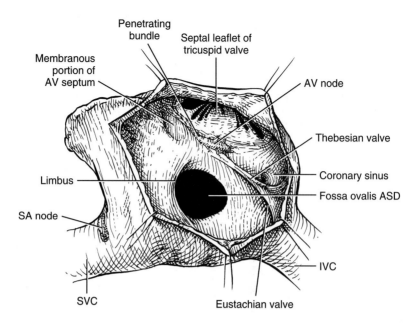

Figure 16-13 Internal anatomy of a fossa ovalis (secundum) atrial septal defect as seen through usual atrial incision. The sinus node is lateral at the cavoatrial junction at the superior aspect of the crista terminalis. The anterior inferior rim of the defect lies near the atrioventricular (AV) node, which lies in the muscular portion and just inferior to the membranous portion of the AV septum.

Key: *ASD*, Atrial septal defect; *AV*, atrioventricular; *IVC*, inferior vena cava; *SA*, sinoatrial; *SVC*, superior vena cava.

sufficient tissue to create an edge strong enough to hold sutures well, or the fenestrated tissue simply may be imbricated into the suture line.

Usually the fossa ovalis ASD is closed directly (see "Direct Suture versus Patch Repair" under Special Situations and Controversies later in this chapter). The suturing is begun at the inferior angle by placing a half purse-string stitch. Care is taken to catch good, substantial anterior and posterior limbic tissue with the first and last bites of this stitch (Fig. 16-14), which must be inferior to any remaining fenestrations. Great care is taken to avoid confusing the eustachian valve of the IVC with the remnant of the floor of the fossa ovalis. Such an error results in connecting the IVC to the *left* atrium, which can occur when the operation is done under circulatory arrest and there is no IVC cannula, or when direct caval cannulation is used. After this half purse-string stitch is tied, the ASD assumes a slitlike appearance. The suture line is now carried superiorly, catching tough limbic tissue anteriorly and posteriorly. The sutures must not be placed too far from the edge anteriorly to avoid damage to the AV node. Before the last few stitches are pulled up, a clamp or tissue forceps is placed in the aperture, and the anesthesiologist inflates the lung to expel any air from the left atrium. The suture line is snugged while lung inflation is maintained, and an additional bite is taken with the stitch, which is then tied. After the right atrium is sucked dry, once again the lungs are inflated to drive through left atrial blood and thus identify any defects in the suture line. If seen, defects are closed with interrupted sutures.

The right atrium is then closed. The caval tapes are released, the apex of the upturned LV is aspirated for air, strong suction is placed on the aortic needle vent or catheter, and the aortic clamp is released. Generally the clamp has been in place about 10 minutes for this procedure.

After good cardiac action has developed, usual de-airing procedures are carried out (see "De-Airing Heart" in Section 3 of Chapter 2). Atrial wires are placed routinely or may be omitted in young patients. CPB is now discontinued, with care taken not to overdistend the left side of the heart in the process. Even when a left atrial catheter is not left for the postoperative period, left atrial pressure is measured at this time (or estimated by palpation of the pulmonary artery) and noted to be 5 to 15 mmHg higher than right atrial pressure. This increase is related to small size and decreased compliance of the LV compared with that of the RV (see footnote 1 on p. 723 and "Relative Performance of Left and Right Ventricles" under Cardiac Output and Its Determinants in Section 1 of Chapter 5). The remainder of operation is completed as usual.

Posterior Atrial Septal Defect

If the anomaly is a pure posterior ASD, closure by direct suture is possible in a manner similar to that described in the previous text. If the posterior ASD is confluent with a fossa ovalis ASD, the defect may be too large for direct closure. Then a patch of pericardium, knitted polyester velour, or polytetrafluoroethylene (PTFE) is used.

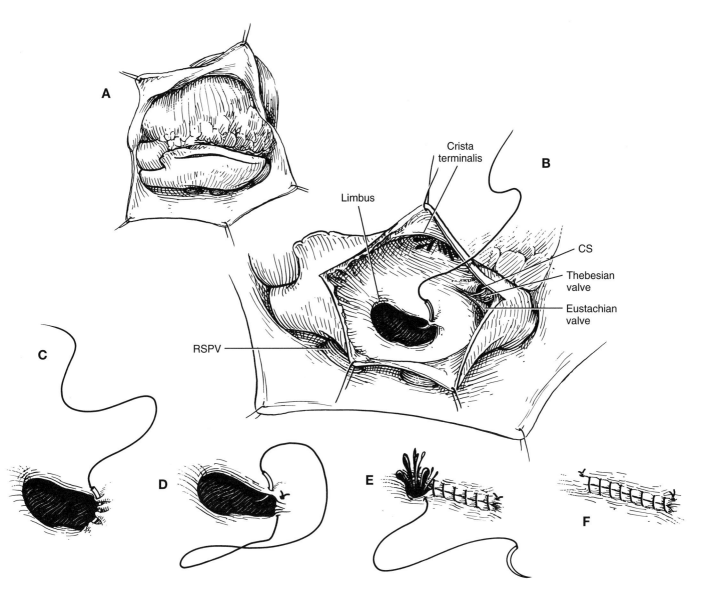

Figure 16-14   Repair of fossa ovalis atrial septal defect (ASD). **A,** Usual oblique right atriotomy is made and retracting sutures placed. **B** and **C,** After exposure is arranged and all structures examined (orifices of pulmonary veins, valve of inferior vena cava [eustachian] coronary sinus), the first sutures are taken as a half purse–string stitch. If ASD extends to the inferior vena cava (IVC), initial sutures are placed in floor of the IVC; eustachian valve of the IVC must be noted so that it is not erroneously included. **D,** After first set of stitches is tied, ASD becomes slitlike. **E,** Before last stitch is tied, anesthesiologist places positive pressure on lung to express air from left atrium. **F,** Completed repair.

Key: *CS,* Coronary sinus; *RSPV,* right superior pulmonary vein.

Coronary Sinus Atrial Septal Defect

Because coronary sinus ASDs are close to the AV node (Fig. 16-15), stitches must be placed close to the edge of the defect superiorly, in tissue that may not be strong. For these reasons, patch closure is generally advisable. Additionally, when a coronary sinus ASD is identified, presence of a completely or partially unroofed coronary sinus must be ruled out (see Chapter 19). These defects are often associated with a left SVC. Inappropriate simple closure of the defect may result in a right-to-left shunt.

Sinus Venosus Malformation

Preparation and positioning of the patient are as usual. After sternotomy, the pericardium is cleared of pleural reflections bilaterally, and a large pericardial piece is removed and set aside between moist towels or in 0.6%

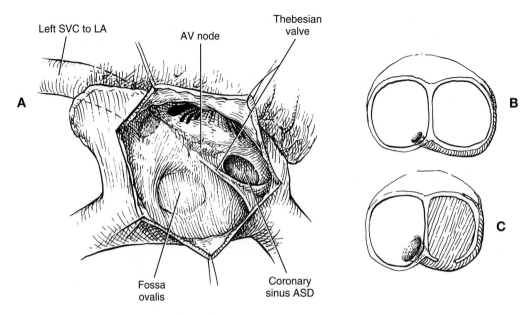

Left SVC to LA

AV node

Thebesian valve

A

B

C

Fossa ovalis

Coronary sinus ASD

Figure 16-15   Repair of coronary sinus atrial septal defect *(ASD)*. **A,** Anatomy of coronary sinus ASD showing its proximity to atrioventricular *(AV)* node. ASD is closed with a patch sutured to edges of the defect to avoid AV node, but only after the surgeon is assured that there is no unroofing of coronary sinus. If the sinus is unroofed, a different type of repair is done by opening the atrial septum for better access (see "Technique of Operation" in Chapter 19). **B,** Normal coronary sinus without ASD, diagrammed in transverse section. **C,** Coronary sinus ASD associated with unroofed coronary sinus allowing left-to-right (and obligatory right-to-left) shunt. A large coronary sinus defect suggests an unroofed coronary sinus, whereas a small defect indicates an ASD.

Key: *ASD,* Atrial septal defect; *AV,* atrioventricular; *LA,* left atrium; *SVC,* superior vena cava.

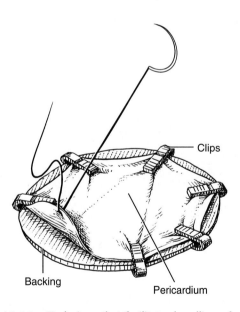

Clips

Backing

Pericardium

Figure 16-16   Technique that facilitates handling of pericardial patch and avoids need for stay sutures. The piece of excised pericardium is flattened onto a piece of wet toweling or cardboard with its shiny serosa uppermost. Pericardium and backing are both cut to appropriate shape. A suture can be positioned without distorting the pericardium. Pericardium and backing are both lowered into the heart, and the backing is not withdrawn until the pericardial patch is appropriately positioned.

glutaraldehyde.[2] After the remaining pericardium is widely opened, stay sutures are placed and the anatomy is examined. The right superior pulmonary vein is easily seen, attached to the low SVC or SVC–right atrial junction. At this point the pulmonary vein (or veins) should be differentiated from the azygos vein, which is slightly more cephalad and directed more medially. Size of the SVC is noted, as is the possible presence of a left SVC, in which case the right-sided SVC is likely to be small. The right atrium and RV are usually considerably enlarged.

Purse-string sutures are inserted, including those for direct caval cannulation. Sutures for SVC cannulation are placed on the anterior aspect of the SVC cephalad to the area of abnormal connection of the right superior pulmonary vein. Alternatively, the innominate vein can be cannulated with a right-angle cannula directed toward the left and small enough to allow flow around it.

CPB is then established, the aorta clamped, and cold cardioplegia infused (see "Cold Cardioplegia, Controlled Aortic Root Reperfusion, and [When Needed] Warm

[2] A special technique for using a pericardial patch was developed many years ago and has had long use in our centers (Fig. 16-16). The pericardium is spread on a thin sheet of cardboard, excess cardboard is trimmed, edges of the pericardium are attached firmly to the cardboard with a few clips, and the resulting patch assembly is immersed in 0.6% glutaraldehyde for 5 to 30 minutes. The technique improves handling characteristics of the pericardium and greatly facilitates trimming the patch and beginning its insertion.

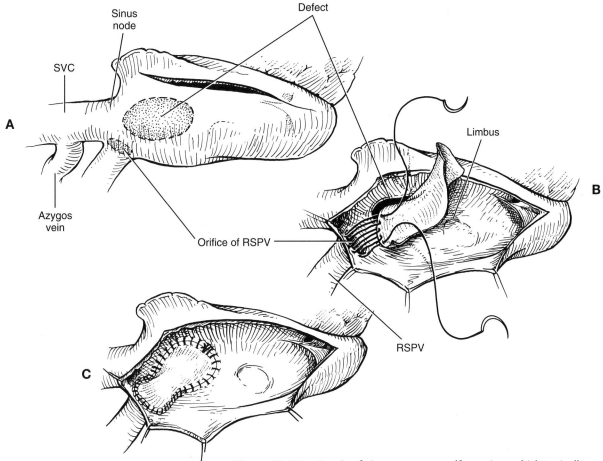

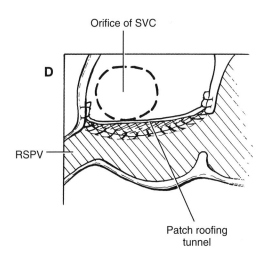

Figure 16-17   Repair of sinus venosus malformation, which typically consists of subcaval atrial septal defect (ASD) associated with partial anomalous pulmonary venous connection of right superior pulmonary vein *(RSPV)* to low superior vena cava *(SVC)*. **A,** Usual atriotomy is away from sinus node. **B,** Incision can be extended superiorly and medially to sinoatrial node. Subcaval ASD is superior to limbus. At times the SVC overrides the defect to drain in part directly into the left atrium. ASD is far removed from tricuspid valve and atrioventricular node. First stitches for inserting pericardial patch are shown at right lateral edge of SVC orifice at its junction with laterally placed orifice of RSPV. Patch is sewn into place with continuous No. 4-0 or 5-0 polypropylene suture. Suture line continues medially in an anterior and posterior direction to form a tunnel or roof leading the anomalous RSPV through the ASD. **C,** Convex roof of the tunnel has been completed, and blood from anomalously connected RSPV drains beneath this roof into left atrium. Pathway from SVC to right atrium is unobstructed. When SVC is cannulated directly, exposure is good through this incision, and augmentation of the atrial closure is not necessary. **D,** Transverse section through repair seen from below.

Key: *SVC,* superior vena cava; *RSPV,* right superior pulmonary vein.

Cardioplegic Induction" in Chapter 3). The caval tapes are secured. In infants, repair may be done with a single venous cannula and hypothermic circulatory arrest. When the aorta is clamped, the perfusate temperature is stabilized at 25° to 32°C.

When configuration of the superior pulmonary vein is usual and the SVC–right atrial junction is wide, the right atrium is opened through the usual oblique incision beginning at the base of the right atrial appendage and extending down toward the IVC cannula (Fig. 16-17). This does not damage the sinoatrial node or its artery. Stay sutures are placed. A pump sump-sucker is placed across the foramen ovale into the left atrium (or through a stab wound), or no left atrial vent may be used. When the cardiac end of the SVC is small, as with a large left SVC, or the anomalous pulmonary veins are three or four in number and some enter the SVC more superiorly than usual, a vertical atriotomy is made posteriorly and extended into the SVC posterior to the sinus node and just in front of the anomalous veins (Fig. 16-18), in preparation for a V-Y–plasty enlargement of the SVC.

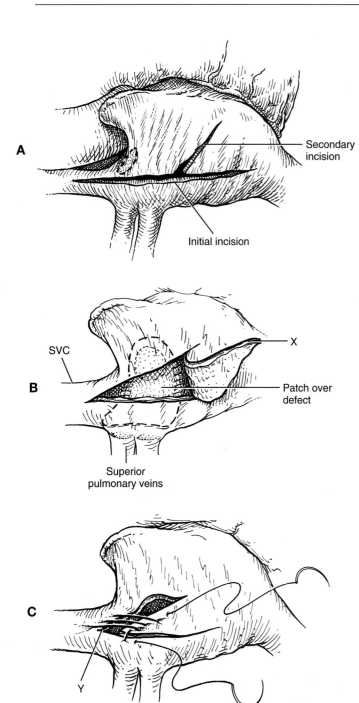

The repair directs pulmonary venous drainage through the ASD into the left atrium while closing the interatrial communication (see Fig. 16-17). A pericardial baffle forms approximately the anterior half of this internal conduit. Width of the pericardial patch should be about 1.5 times the diameter of the ASD, and length about 1.25 times the estimated length of the distances from the superior edge of the anomalous vein to the inferior edge of the ASD. This ensures an adequate pulmonary venous pathway and does not obstruct the SVC.

After the ASD repair is repaired, the sump (if used) is removed and the created defect closed. Rewarming is begun, and with suction on the needle vent in the ascending aorta, the aortic clamp is released. The right atriotomy is closed, and the operation is completed as usual (see "Completing Cardiopulmonary Bypass" in Section 3 of Chapter 2).

Anomalous Connection of Right Pulmonary Veins to Right Atrium

The operation begins exactly as described for sinus venosus malformation, including opening the right atrium through the usual oblique incision. The interior of the right atrium is examined, anomalous connections of the right pulmonary veins and normal connections of the left pulmonary veins to the left atrium are confirmed, and any defects in the atrial septum are identified.

When the atrial septum is intact, repair can often be accomplished by making a longitudinal incision in it next to the atrial wall posteriorly and resuturing it to the lateral right atrial wall in front of the right pulmonary vein orifices. Alternatively, and particularly when geometry in the right atrium does not lend itself to this simple repair, the fossa ovalis and posterior limbic tissue may be excised and a pericardial, PTFE, or knitted polyester patch used for baffle reconstruction (Fig. 16-19).

When an ASD is present, repair is similar. When the defect is large and of the fossa ovalis or confluent type, a patch similar to the one shown in Fig. 16-19 is used. Occasionally, and particularly when the associated ASD is posterior, repair by direct suture is possible.

Anomalous Connection of Right Pulmonary Veins to Inferior Vena Cava (Scimitar Syndrome)

Initial stages of the operation for scimitar syndrome proceed as described for sinus venosus malformation. An internal conduit is then constructed within the right atrium to conduct the right pulmonary venous blood from its entrance into the IVC across the atrial septum into the left atrium.

In small infants the entire repair may be done during hypothermic circulatory arrest. In older patients, part of the repair can be performed during hypothermic circulatory arrest; alternatively, the entire repair can be performed during conventional CPB at 20° to 28°C. In the latter approach, the IVC tape may be passed inferior (caudad) to the entrance of the anomalous pulmonary vein

Figure 16-18   V-Y atrioplasty technique for enlarging superior vena cava *(SVC)*. **A,** Initial incision is longitudinal and does not cross the SVC–right atrial junction unless it is thought that SVC enlargement will be required. In such cases, secondary incision is then added to create a V flap of right atrial wall. **B,** SVC is enlarged by advancing the tip of the V flap to the apex of the SVC incision. **C,** Augmentation is completed with a continuous suture line (X in **B** is brought to Y in **C**).

Key: *SVC,* superior vena cava.

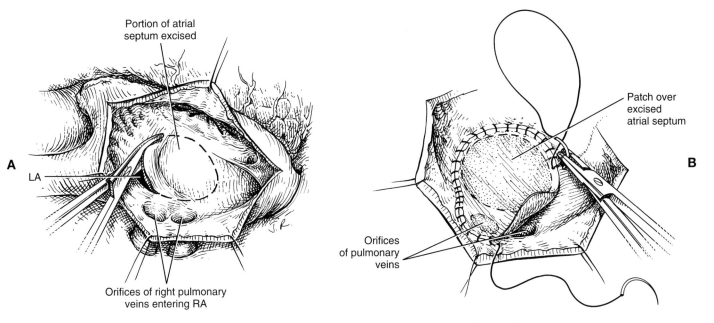

Figure 16-19   Repair of anomalous connection of right superior and inferior pulmonary veins to right atrium without atrial septal defect. **A,** Right atrial incision is the usual oblique transverse one, and fossa ovalis and posterior limbus are excised. **B,** Repair is made by replacing excised portion of atrial septum with a patch, sewn to right of (anterior to) the right pulmonary vein orifices.

Key: *LA,* Left atrium; *RA,* right atrium.

into the IVC, and a right-angled metal cannula can be used to cannulate the IVC inferior to this point. This possibility depends on whether the anomalous vein enters at the IVC–right atrial junction. If it does, the common femoral or external iliac vein can be cannulated for IVC return.

In any case, CPB is established with two venous cannulae, and if part of the repair is to be made with circulatory arrest, the IVC tape is placed on the cardiac side of the IVC entrance of the anomalous vein. The aorta is clamped and cold cardioplegic solution infused. After caval tapes have been tightened, the right atrium is opened with the usual oblique incision and carried right down to the IVC. If present, the valve of the fossa ovalis is completely excised to create a large ASD (Fig. 16-20). The pericardial patch is trimmed according to the measurements made, and stay sutures are applied at the four corners.

Circulatory arrest is established with the patient's nasopharyngeal temperature at 18°C when this modality is used, and the IVC cannula is removed. Otherwise, repair proceeds during CPB. The pericardial patch is sewn into place so as to form the anterior wall of a conduit between the entrance of the anomalous vein and the defect created in the atrial septum (see Fig. 16-20). If repair has been done during circulatory arrest, the IVC cannula is reinserted, caval tape retightened, CPB reestablished, and rewarming of the patient with the perfusate begun. The anomalous vein is observed from time to time to ensure pressure in it is not elevated, because its drainage is now

temporarily obstructed by the IVC tape. The right atrium is closed and the caval tapes promptly released. The apex of the LV is aspirated for air, and with suction on the aortic needle vent, the aortic clamp is released.

Alternatively, the anomalous pulmonary vein can be disconnected from its low insertion at the cavoatrial junction and reimplanted higher on the right atrial wall with connection via a baffle to the left atrium.[T7] As a third option, after disconnection, the anomalous vein can be implanted directly onto the left atrial wall at its rightmost aspect because this area is "bare" (having no natural entrance of right pulmonary veins).[H11]

Usually, repair of the anomalous venous connection should be complemented by interrupting the aberrant systemic subphrenic arterial collateral supply to the right lower lobe. This can be accomplished by surgical ligation or catheter intervention. In neonates, it may be sufficient simply to interrupt the aberrant arterial supply and leave the anomalous venous connection intact.

Anomalous Connection of Left Pulmonary Veins to Innominate Vein

When the atrial septum is intact or there is only a valve-competent foramen ovale, operation is performed using a closed technique. The left chest is entered through a posterolateral incision (Fig. 16-21). The anomalous left vertical vein is dissected up to the innominate vein. Left superior and inferior veins are dissected and mobilized as much as possible. A tape is placed around the left pulmo-

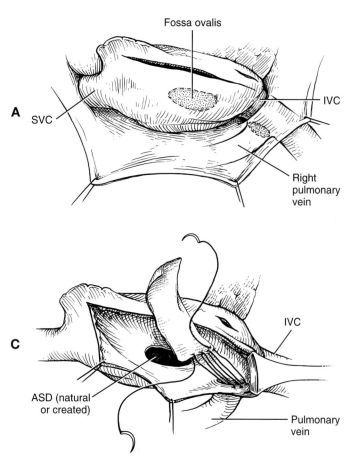

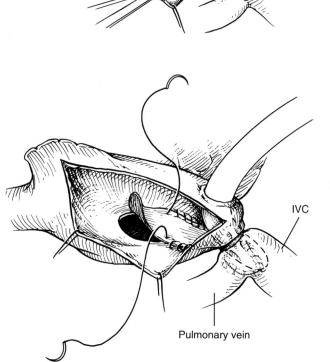

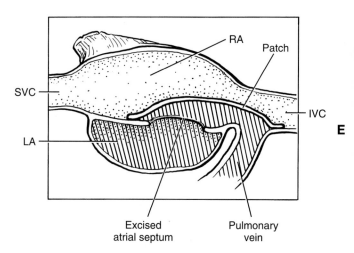

Figure 16-20 Repair of partial anomalous pulmonary venous connection, right pulmonary veins to inferior vena cava (scimitar syndrome). **A,** Usual oblique right atriotomy is made, extending it to inferior vena cava *(IVC)*. **B,** Valve (floor) of fossa ovalis (septum primum) is excised, creating an atrial septal defect that extends almost to IVC. **C,** During a short period of circulatory arrest or with sucker trickle flow, IVC cannula is removed. Distance between inferior aspect of orifice of the anomalous vein entrance into the IVC and superior limbus is measured, as is width of the fossa ovalis. Pericardial patch is trimmed in a rectangular shape with length about 1.25 times the measured length and width about 1.5 times the width of the fossa ovalis. Using a continuous polypropylene suture, patch insertion is begun at inferior aspect of orifice of anomalous pulmonary vein in IVC, after this orifice and that of the hepatic vein are positively identified. Suture line between patch and floor of IVC is carried to patient's left and then up toward and onto anterior limbus, where it is held. With the other arm of original suture, patch is attached above orifice of anomalous vein as suture line is carried superiorly. IVC cannula is reinserted, and cardiopulmonary bypass is resumed at usual flow. **D,** Patch is then attached successively to posterior limbus, superior limbus, and anterior limbus, and tied there to other end of suture. **E,** Patch now forms approximately half of an intraatrial internal conduit conducting right pulmonary vein blood across defect created in the fossa ovalis into the left atrium. This is drawn in parasagittal section.

Key: *ASD,* Atrial septal defect; *IVC,* inferior vena cava; *LA,* left atrium; *RA,* right atrium; *SVC,* superior vena cava.

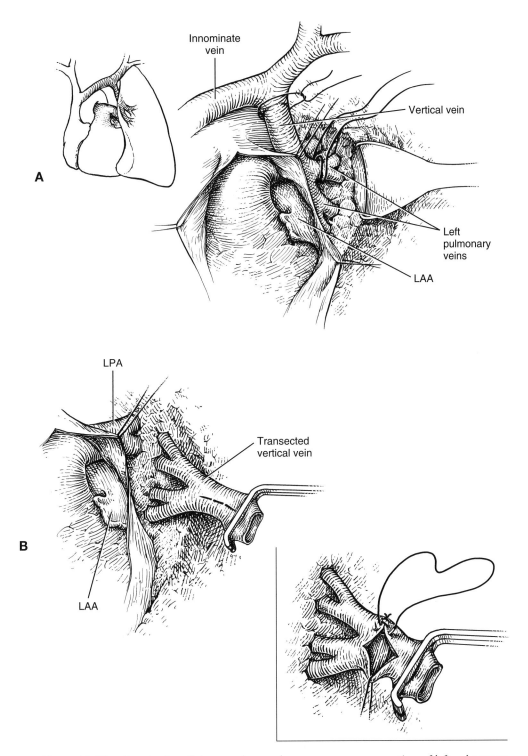

Figure 16-21   Repair of partial anomalous pulmonary venous connection of left pulmonary veins to innominate vein. **A,** Often, veins of the left lung drain anomalously through a vertical vein into the innominate vein. Through a left thoracotomy and without cardiopulmonary bypass, the vertical vein is connected to the left atrial appendage. **B,** Left pulmonary artery and left pulmonary veins are temporarily occluded, and vertical vein is divided near its insertion into the innominate vein. *Inset,* Occasionally a counterincision is made in the vertical vein to widen it.

Key: *LAA,* Left atrial appendage; *LPA,* left pulmonary artery.   *Continued*

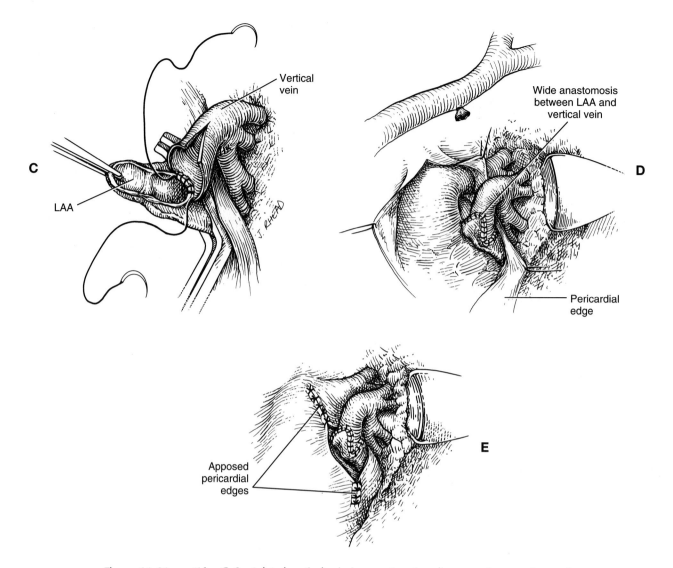

Figure 16-21, cont'd   **C,** Spatulated vertical vein is sewn to a trapdoor opening near base of left atrial appendage. **D,** Wide opening at this anastomosis must result. **E,** Pericardium is closed loosely to prevent herniation.

Key: *LAA*, Left atrial appendage.

nary artery. The pericardium is opened, usually behind the phrenic nerve, and a large window is made. A clamp is placed across the very base of the left atrial appendage, and most of the appendage is amputated. The left pulmonary artery is temporarily occluded, the left vertical vein is ligated flush with the innominate vein, a clamp is placed across its proximal portion, and it is divided as near the ligature as safety allows. The vein is positioned with great care to avoid any rotation and is anastomosed to the base of the left atrial appendage. At least part of the anastomosis is made with interrupted sutures to avoid any possible purse-string effect. Before releasing the clamps, care is taken that no air is in the vein.

When there is an associated fossa ovalis ASD, both the left APVC and ASD should be repaired. (The first patient undergoing repair of this type of APVC, reported from the Mayo Clinic in 1953, required later closure of the ASD, at which time the previously made anastomosis was function-

ing well.[K3]) This repair can all be accomplished through a median sternotomy with CPB.

The anastomosis between the vertical vein and left atrial appendage can be modified when CPB is used. Ports and colleagues make a long incision in the lateral aspect of the left atrial appendage, carrying it down onto the left atrium.[P4] The anomalous vein is cut transversely, then a T extension is made posteriorly. The end-to-side anastomosis is thus extremely wide. Alternatively, a side-to-side vertical vein–left atrial anastomosis is made, ligating the vertical vein at its junction with innominate vein.

Other Anomalous Pulmonary Venous Connections

Bilateral PAPVCs and rare right or left anomalous connections require individual techniques using principles described for standard repairs.

Treatment of Associated Mitral or Tricuspid Valve Disease

Mitral stenosis is treated by valvotomy. Mitral and tricuspid regurgitation are treated by anuloplasty when possible (see "Repair of Mitral Regurgitation" under Technique of Operation in Chapter 11). If mitral valve replacement is necessary, great care is required because the anulus tends to be friable.

SPECIAL FEATURES OF POSTOPERATIVE CARE

Convalescence of most children and adolescents who have had repair of an uncomplicated ASD, as well as most adults operated on before they have reached NYHA functional class IV, is uneventful. They are extubated in the operating room or within a few hours of leaving it. Arterial blood pressure is monitored until the next morning via an arterial catheter and the atrial pressures via the polyvinyl catheters placed at operation.

Occasionally, older patients have unusually high left atrial pressures (20 to 25 mmHg) in the early hours after repair, presumably because systolic and diastolic LV functions are more impaired than usual by the aging process or by coexisting coronary artery disease, systolic arterial hypertension, or residual important mitral regurgitation that has been underestimated preoperatively. In contrast to a few examples reported in the literature,[B2,B5] in which urgent reoperation was performed and the ASD reopened because of severe left-sided heart failure with pulmonary edema, in 35 years of experience with this malformation at GLH, the Mayo Clinic, and UAB, no ASD has been reopened. A partial explanation for this may be that ASD closure has not been recommended when the *primary* problem was LV cardiomyopathy. However, because of these considerations, left atrial pressure is routinely monitored intraoperatively and for about 24 hours postoperatively in older patients. Occasionally, when mitral regurgitation has been underestimated preoperatively and there are signs of severe pulmonary venous hypertension postoperatively, an urgent echocardiographic study or LV angiogram may be required. If these show important residual mitral regurgitation, reoperation may be necessary to repair or replace the mitral valve.

All patients over age 35 years at operation receive sodium warfarin prophylactically, beginning on the evening of the second postoperative day and continuing for 8 to 12 weeks after repair. The rationale is that both pulmonary and systemic arterial embolization occur after repair in patients over about age 35.[H2] Occurrence is particularly high in elderly patients in atrial fibrillation (see "Results" in the text that follows), in whom permanent anticoagulation is usually warranted.

RESULTS

Early (Hospital) Death

Hospital mortality for repair of ASDs and related conditions has approached zero for many years in most cardiac surgical centers throughout the world. Even during the early years of cardiac surgery, mortality was low. Among 696 patients undergoing repair at the Mayo Clinic between 1954 and 1965, some of whom had pulmonary vascular disease,[S16] only 22 (3.2%) died in hospital.[R4]

■ **TABLE 16-4   Hospital Mortality after Repair of Isolated Atrial Septal Defect** [a]

Location (Type) of ASD	n	Hospital Deaths No.	Hospital Deaths %
Fossa ovalis	317	3	0.9
Posterior (absence of posterior limbus)	12	0	
Confluent (fossa ovalis plus absence of posterior limbus)	7	0	
Not classified	4	0	
TOTAL	340	3	0.9 (CL 0.4-1.8)

Key: *ASD,* Atrial septal defect; *CL,* 70% confidence limits.

[a] Data from 340 patients operated on at UAB, 1967 to 1979. Ages ranged from 11 months to 72 years; 236 females and 104 males. Isolated sinus venosus atrial septal defects (ASD) are in Table 16-6. All patients with coronary sinus ASDs had major associated cardiac anomalies (see "Morphology" in Chapter 19). Excluded are patients with ASD and partial or total anomalous pulmonary venous connection, atrioventricular septal defect, major associated cardiac anomalies, associated coronary artery bypass grafting (13 patients, no deaths), or valve replacement for unrelated mitral valve disease (10 patients, no deaths).

■ **TABLE 16-5   Hospital Mortality after Repair of Partial Anomalous Pulmonary Venous Connection According to Morphologic Category** [a]

Category	n	Hospital Deaths No.	Hospital Deaths %
Sinus venosus syndrome	101	3	3
Part or all of right superior pulmonary veins to SVC without subcaval ASD	12	0	0
Right superior and inferior pulmonary veins to right atrium	28	1	4
Posterior ASD (absent posterior limbus) and anomalous connection of right pulmonary veins to right atrium	14	0	0
Right pulmonary veins to IVC (scimitar syndrome)	12	0	0
Right pulmonary veins to coronary sinus	1	0	0
Left pulmonary veins to left innominate vein	5	0	0
Bilateral but subtotal anomalous pulmonary venous connection	6	0	0
TOTAL	179	4	2.2 (CL 1.1-4)
$P(\chi^2)$			.98

Key: *ASD,* Atrial septal defect; *CL,* 70% confidence limits; *IVC,* inferior vena cava; *SVC,* superior vena cava.

[a] Data from UAB (1967 to 1981) and GLH (1957 to 1983). Only three patients in the GLH series had no ASD. Three of the deaths were before 1966.

In the combined UAB–GLH experience (1967 to 1979), five deaths (1.0%; CL 0.5%-1.6%) occurred among 518 patients undergoing repair of ASD alone, and one death (0.7%; CL 0.1%-2.5%) occurred among patients undergoing repair of PAPVC with or without ASD (Tables 16-4 to 16-6).

Time-Related Survival

Time-related survival of patients with ASD or PAPVC repaired during the first few years of life is that of the matched general population. When operation is performed later in childhood or in early adult life, survival is nearly as good. In older patients, repair of ASD improves life expectancy, but survival is lower than in the matched population.[M15]

■ TABLE 16-6 Hospital Mortality after Repair of Sinus Venosus Syndrome [a]

		Hospital Deaths	
Malformation	n	No.	%
Typical	52	1	2
Subcaval ASD only	2	0	0
Upper portion of right superior PV anomalously connected and inferior part to LA	1	0	0
Right superior and inferior PV to low SVC	1	0	0
TOTAL	56	1	1.8 (CL 2-6)

Key: *ASD,* Atrial septal defect; *CL,* 70% confidence limits; *LA,* left atrium; *PV,* pulmonary vein; *SVC,* superior vena cava.

[a] Data from UAB, 1967 to 1981. The one death was in a 69-year-old man, New York Heart Association class IV with associated tricuspid regurgitation, from sepsis and multiple subsystem failure.

■ TABLE 16-7 Preoperative Status and Hospital Mortality after Repair of Atrial Septal Defect [a]

		Hospital Deaths	
Preoperative NYHA Class (Mean Age in Years)	n	No.	% [b]
I (16)	171	1	0.6
II (32)	112	1	0.9
III (50)	41	0	0
IV (51)	13	1	8 (CL 1-24) [b]
Unknown	3	0	0
TOTAL	340	3	0.9 (CL 0.4-1.8)
P (logistic)			.2

Key: *CL,* 70% confidence limits; *NYHA,* New York Heart Association.

[a] Data from UAB, 1967 to 1979, as in Table 16-4.

[b] For NYHA classes I, II, and III, two deaths in 324 patients: 0.6% (CL 0.2%–1.5%).

[c] P for difference (Fisher) = .11 comparing 1 death in 13 to 2 deaths in 324.

In an observational study, Konstantinides and colleagues compared surgical closure of ASD to medical treatment in 179 patients over age 40 (mean age 56 ± 9 years). Ten-year survival of the surgically treated patients was 95% versus 84% for those treated medically.[K10]

Modes of Death

The rare patient who dies in hospital after repair of an ASD or PAPVC usually has a serious coexisting condition, such as pulmonary vascular disease or old age. The exception is the rare occurrence of death from air embolization, about the only risk in repair of ASDs, and the reason for using the particular surgical techniques described (see "Technique of Operation" earlier in this chapter).

Premature late death likewise occurs infrequently and almost exclusively in the types of patients just described. Horvath and colleagues found that premature late death occurred more often in patients undergoing surgery in adulthood when preoperative systolic P_{PA} was 30 mmHg or greater than when it was less (survival 85% ± 1% versus 99% ± 6% at 10 years; $P < .0002$).[H6] Neurologic failure from cerebral embolization or hemorrhage is the most common mode of late death in elderly patients, most of whom have hypertension. Heart failure is the next most common cause of death, again in elderly patients.[S1] In rare

■ TABLE 16-8 Age and Hospital Mortality after Repair of Atrial Septal Defect [a]

Age			Hospital Deaths	
≤ years <		n	No.	%
	2	1 [b]	0	0
2	5	19	0	0
5	10	71	1	1.4
10	20	82	1	1.2
20	30	40	0	0
30	40	27	0	0
40	50	39	0	0
50	60	34	1	2.9
60	70	26	0	0
70		1	0	0
TOTAL		340	3	0.9 (CL 0.4-1.8)
P (logistic)				.9

Key: *CL,* 70% confidence limits.

[a] Data from UAB, 1967 to 1979, as in Table 16-4.

[b] 11 months old.

instances, late death results from severe supraventricular arrhythmias.

Incremental Risk Factors for Death

In contrast to most types of congenital heart disease, patients with ASD or PAPVC rarely have serious important coexisting cardiac anomalies. Therefore, this incremental risk factor is absent. Likewise, neither morphology of the ASD (see Tables 16-5 and 16-6) nor morphology of most types of PAPVC (see Table 16-6) is a risk factor for death. Again, in contrast to most types of congenital and acquired heart disease, preoperative functional class is not a confirmed risk factor for death, probably because the operation is relatively atraumatic and requires only a short duration of CPB and global myocardial ischemia (Table 16-7).

Pulmonary Vascular Disease

Preoperative pulmonary hypertension severe enough to indicate important pulmonary vascular disease is a risk factor for death, and if severe enough, death may be early after operation.[F4,S16] This risk factor appears in various forms in different analyses; in the study by Murphy and colleagues, for example, pulmonary vascular disease appears as the level of systolic P_{PA}.[M15] Elevation of RpI becomes a major risk factor when greater than 6 U · m² and may be an irreversible risk when RpI reaches about 12 U · m² (see "Special Situations and Controversies" later in this chapter).

Older Age at Operation

Neither older age at operation nor young age at operation is a risk factor for hospital death (Tables 16-8 and 16-9). Older age is a risk factor for premature late death, identifiable after the first decade and becoming progressively more powerful as age increases.[M15] Patients in the first decade have about a 98% chance of surviving at least 25 years after repair, those in the third decade a 93% chance, and those in the fourth decade an 84% chance; patients older than about 40 years have even less

■ **TABLE 16-9   Repair of Atrial Septal Defect in Patients under Age 2 at Operation** [a]

Age (Months)	Type of Defect	Associated Anomalies
2	FO, APVC all R lung to RA	Moderate or severe PS
2	FO, APVC all R lung to RA	Mild coarctation of aorta, mild aortic stenosis, anomalous R subclavian artery, LSVC
3	FO	Small PDA
5	FO	Large Morgagni hernia, small VSD, LSVC, isolated dextrocardia
6	FO, APVC all R lung to RA	
8	FO, APVC all R lung to IVC	Severe bronchiolitis
15	FO	
22	FO, APVC all R lung to RA	

Key: *APVC,* Anomalous pulmonary venous connection; *FO,* fossa ovalis (see Box 16-1); *IVC,* inferior vena cava; *LSVC,* left superior vena cava; *PDA,* patent ductus arteriosus; *PS,* pulmonary stenosis; *R,* right; *RA,* right atrium; *VSD,* ventricular septal defect.

[a] Data from GLH, 1957 to 1983. Heart failure, recurrent respiratory infections, and growth retardation were present in all patients. Hypothermic circulatory arrest was used in those under 12 months of age. All patients survived.

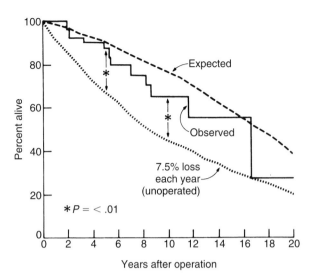

Figure 16-22   Late survival of patients over age 60 years after undergoing repair of atrial septal defect (hospital survivors only) compared with survival of an age–gender–matched general population ("Expected") and with that of patients of the same age treated nonsurgically ("Unoperated"). (From St. John Sutton and colleagues.[S1])

probability of long-term survival.[G7] St. John Sutton and colleagues found that 10-year survival was 64% after repair of ASD in patients older than age 60, importantly better than that of similar patients treated nonsurgically but not as good as that of a matched general population (Fig. 16-22).[S1]

It remains uncertain whether age at operation in the first decade has an effect on long-term outcome. Cardiomegaly before repair in a 5-year-old patient often remains late postoperatively, suggesting that repair ideally should be performed in the first few years of life.

Anatomic Type of Interatrial Communication

The anatomic type of interatrial communication or PAPVC does not appear to affect survival.[D3,H2,K6,S1,T5] An exception may be scimitar syndrome, with the right pulmonary veins connecting anomalously to the IVC. Increased risk is caused primarily by abnormalities in the right lung rather than by PAPVC itself.

Functional Status

Asymptomatic children have no symptoms after operation, but symptomatic infants undergoing repair of ASD may also experience complete relief of symptoms.[P3] Older symptomatic patients typically show improvement.[D4,R3,S3] Forfang and colleagues found that ASD closure in patients over age 40 improved symptomatic state by one NYHA functional class in every patient.[F1]

Both Konstantinides and Gatzoulis and their colleagues reported improved functional status in their surgically treated groups that were over age 40.[G10,K10] Even patients undergoing surgery after age 60 showed striking functional and symptomatic improvement[N2,P7]: 87% improved at least one NYHA functional class. Among the 31 patients preoperatively in NYHA class III or IV in the study by St. John Sutton and colleagues, only two (6%) remained severely disabled.[S1]

This striking symptomatic improvement, even in older patients whose cardiomegaly does not always regress, has been documented by Pearlman and colleagues.[P2] Excellent treadmill exercise performance and normal maximal oxy-

gen consumption were found in all 14 consecutive patients studied late after repair of ASD, despite 9 with persistently large RV diastolic dimensions.

Hemodynamic Results

Important hemodynamic changes occur immediately after closure of an uncomplicated ASD. Mean pressure in the ascending aorta increases, as does mean aortic blood flow.[S13] There is an immediate reduction in pulmonary blood flow.[L9] Right atrial pressure decreases and left atrial pressure increases; Søndergard and Paulsen found an average immediate rise of 8 mmHg.[S13]

The small amount of available information indicates that in older patients, RpI drops negligibly late after operation.

Ventricular Function

RV diastolic dimensions are strikingly decreased after operation,[B6] but are still above normal in many patients (Fig. 16-23).[L5,M12,S4] This finding is consistent with Young's early observation that some children had important residual cardiomegaly years after complete repair of their ASD, which he correctly ascribed to the secondary cardiomyopathy resulting from chronic RV volume overload.[Y1] Pearlman and colleagues showed an effect of age at operation in this regard; 7 (64%; CL 44%-81%) of 11 patients age 10 years or less at operation had normal or near-normal RV diastolic volumes late postoperatively, whereas only 3 (21%; CL 10%-38%) of 14 patients over age 25 displayed this finding (*P* [Fisher] for difference = .04).[P2]

In adult patients with preoperatively decreased RV wall motion and ejection fraction, most of whom have elevated right atrial pressure and are importantly symptomatic, reduction in RV size after surgical repair is less, and

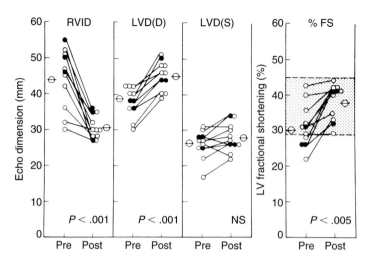

Figure 16-23 Effect of atrial septal defect repair on echocardiographic right ventricular internal dimension at end-diastole, left ventricular dimension at end-diastole and end-systole, and left ventricular fractional shortening. *Stippled area,* normal range of fractional shortening (29% to 45%); *open circles with bars,* mean values; *solid symbols,* three symptomatic patients with marked drop in ejection fraction during exercise. (From Bonow and colleagues.[B6])

Key: *D,* End-diastole; *FS,* fractional shortening; *LV,* left ventricular; *LVD,* left ventricular dimension; *NS,* not significant; *Pre,* preoperative; *Post,* postoperative; *RVID,* right ventricular internal dimension; *S,* end-systole.

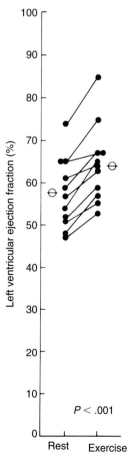

Figure 16-24 Left ventricular ejection fraction at rest and during exercise after repair of atrial septal defect. *Open circles with bars,* mean values. (From Bonow and colleagues.[B6])

ejection fraction, although higher than preoperatively, remains abnormally low (47% in the experience of Liberthson and colleagues[L5]). These patients are improved by operation but do not become asymptomatic. Analogies between this and response to surgery of the volume-overloaded LV are apparent (see "Left Ventricular Structure and Function" under Results in Chapter 12).

Postoperatively, in contrast to the preoperative condition, LV ejection fraction increases normally with maximal exercise (Fig. 16-24). Even in patients who have undergone repair in adult life, exercise ejection fraction is normal. This favorable change is the result of ablation of the RV volume overload by closure of the ASD. Also, LV diastolic dimensions, when abnormally small preoperatively, increase to normal within 6 months of operation.[B6,W1] The abnormalities of LV geometry present preoperatively are also corrected by repair of the ASD.

Arrhythmic Events

Closure of ASDs in children has been shown to improve AV conduction, decrease AV nodal refractory periods, and improve sinus node function in most patients early postoperatively.[B13,K9] Presumably this improvement results from reduction in RV and right atrial volume after ablation of the left-to-right shunt at the atrial level. However, Bolens and Friedli found loss of sinus node function after operation and an atrial ectopic rhythm.[B13] Although possibly the result of direct surgical damage to the sinus node, these effects may represent the unmasking of preoperatively concealed sinus node dysfunction.[B11]

Little specific information is available on arrhythmias late after repair of ASDs in infants and children, but presumably these are uncommon. Forfang and colleagues, as well as other groups, found that arrhythmic symptoms regress less frequently than other symptoms.[F1] Thus, most adult patients with atrial fibrillation preoperatively continue to experience it late postoperatively.[B12] Shah and colleagues, however, as well as Konstantinides, noted a persistent occurrence of new arrhythmias and thromboembolic events in adults followed long term after surgical repair.[K10,S17] Furthermore, at least in patients over about age 40 years, almost half of those not in atrial fibrillation preoperatively develop it late postoperatively.[H2,M6] This tendency to atrial fibrillation or flutter late postoperatively may be less when venous cannulation is directly into the venae cavae rather than through the right atrial appendage.[B9]

Essentially these same findings apply after repair of PAPVC, particularly of sinus venosus malformation, so the pessimistic view expressed by Clark and colleagues is not justified.[C2] Twenty-three (79%; CL 69%-87%) of the 29 patients followed by Trusler and colleagues after repair of sinus venosus malformation were in sinus rhythm late postoperatively, and 6 were in junctional rhythm (one of whom had it preoperatively).[T5] Also, prevalence of changed heart rhythms after repair is similar in patients with fossa ovalis ASDs and those with sinus venosus syndrome. Twenty-six (84%; CL 74%-91%) of 31 patients undergoing repair of sinus venosus malformation had no change in their preoperative rhythm during the first 7 days after operation, compared with 190 (92%; CL 89%-94%) of 207 such patients undergoing repair of fossa ovalis defects ($P[\chi^2] = .16$) (Rouse RG, MacLean WH, Kirklin JW; unpublished study 1979). Trusler and colleagues reported similar findings; 4 of 29 children had sick sinus syndrome or junctional rhythm late postoperatively, and all 4 had an atriotomy across the cavoatrial junction.[T5]

Thromboembolism

Both systemic and pulmonary emboli tend to occur in patients with ASDs. Among 587 hospital survivors of ASD repair at the Mayo Clinic between 1953 and 1963, Hawe and colleagues found postoperative embolization as late as 11 years after repair.[H2] A higher incidence was found in patients over age 40, especially those with atrial fibrillation (Fig. 16-25).

Reintervention

Recurrent ASD has required reoperation in about 2% of patients. Recurrence of ASD is particularly likely in older patients with heart failure preoperatively. In one infant repaired under circulatory arrest, reoperation was required because the IVC was misdirected to the left atrium.

Reoperation is likewise rarely necessary after repair of PAPVC. In the UAB experience, 1 of 56 hospital survivors required reoperation for partial patch dehiscence resulting in partial SVC obstruction and diversion of the SVC largely to the left atrium. At reoperation an entirely new patch was placed with a good result. Two of 12 patients required reoperation after repair of scimitar syndrome because of stenosis of the surgically created channel. Both had right lung hypoplasia with a $\dot{Q}p/\dot{Q}s$ of 1.6.

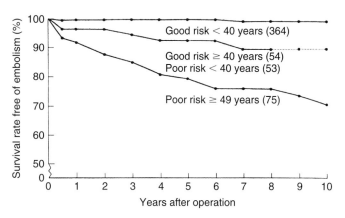

Figure 16-25 Estimates of survival in hospital patients who were free of embolization after repair of atrial septal defect. "Good-risk" patients did not have preoperative embolization, preoperative pulmonary hypertension, or postoperative atrial fibrillation. "Poor-risk" patients had one or more of these conditions. Good-risk patients age 40 or older and poor-risk patients younger than age 40 are combined in a single line because their curves were similar. Numbers in parentheses represent number of patients in the group initially. (From Hawe and colleagues.[H2])

Reoperation carries negligible low risk; no deaths occurred in the UAB experience. When occurring beneath a pericardial or polyester tunnel, however, stenosis may be difficult to relieve.

INDICATIONS FOR OPERATION

Presence of an uncomplicated ASD or of PAPVC with evidence of RV volume overload is an indication for operation. The indication can be restated as a $\dot{Q}p/\dot{Q}s$ of 2.0 or more and at times, if the anomaly is uncomplicated, of greater than 1.5. An exception is patients with scimitar syndrome who have severe hypoplasia of the right lung and a $\dot{Q}p/\dot{Q}s$ of less than 2.0. Operation, usually lobectomy or pneumonectomy with ligation of the anomalous arterial supply, may be required in these patients because of complications of bronchopulmonary sequestration. Isolated PAPVC of a part of one lung without an ASD is not an indication for operation when the $\dot{Q}p/\dot{Q}s$ is less than 1.8, particularly because the shunt under such circumstances does not increase with age. Isolated PAPVC of a whole lung is an indication for repair; whenever an entire lung drains anomalously and the atrial septum is intact, only the opposite, correctly draining lung can return oxygenated blood to the systemic circuit. If this normal lung is importantly compromised (e.g., by pneumonia, pneumothorax, or atelectasis from inhaled foreign body or tumor), potentially fatal hypoxia occurs.

Optimal age for operation is 1 to 2 years because of the deleterious effects of longer periods of RV volume overload. However, the opportunity to intervene surgically as early as age 1 year is not always present because diagnosis is often made later in life. Very young or very old age is not a contraindication to operation. Mainwaring and colleagues, however, caution that infants presenting with major symptoms and large fossa ovalis defects may not benefit from ASD closure.[M18] The inference is that these young patients' failure to thrive is not related to presence of the defect.

Pulmonary vascular disease of sufficient severity to raise RpI to 8 to 12 U · m² at rest and to prevent its decrease to less than 7 units with a pulmonary vasodilator is a contraindication to operation (see "Cardiac Catheterization and Cineangiography" earlier in this chapter). Such conditions are usually present with a resting Q̇p/Q̇s of less than 1.5 in patients with elevated PₚA, but may be present with a Q̇p/Q̇s of 2.0. These ideas are inferential and based on postoperative studies in patients with VSDs and elevated RpI.[N4]

Associated tricuspid or mitral regurgitation, which occurs especially in older patients, is not a contraindication to operation. If important, such conditions are repaired at closure of the ASD. Grading of mitral regurgitation by angiography and echocardiography may be misleading when major runoff occurs from the left to the right atrium through the ASD, and the regurgitation becomes more important when the ASD is closed. For these reasons, moderate mitral regurgitation is usually an indication for mitral valve repair.

SPECIAL SITUATIONS AND CONTROVERSIES

Closure of Atrial Septal Defects by Percutaneous Techniques

At least some ASDs can be closed with a device known as the "clam shell," introduced and manipulated percutaneously.[R7] The procedure has been successfully performed on an outpatient basis. Currently, 60% to 70% of patients with a fossa ovalis ASD are treated by percutaneous techniques at the few institutions worldwide with the necessary devices and experienced operators. The technique must be considered investigational and not suitable for all types of ASDs.

Transcatheter closure is an inferior technique for routine closure of fossa ovalis defects. The procedure is limited to "central" defects with well-defined margins and size of 5 to 20 mm. The procedure is associated with initial failure up to 10%, device migration, embolization requiring urgent operation, and residual shunts.[L11,R8] Simple foramen ovale defects permitting right-to-left shunting and a paradoxical embolus in elderly patients are ideally managed by transcatheter closure.[E2]

Need for Cold Cardioplegic Myocardial Protection

Repair of uncomplicated ASDs was done safely before the advent of cold cardioplegic myocardial protection and requires only a brief time inside the heart. These facts support performing the operation with the patient under simple ischemic arrest. When using this approach, however, even this simple operation can result in some myocardial necrosis (see "Profoundly Hypothermic Global Myocardial Ischemia" in Chapter 3). Furthermore, risk of air embolism can be reduced to an absolute minimum with cold cardioplegia, and operation can be performed more perfectly and elegantly and thus more safely with this technique. More-

over, cold cardioplegia adds no more than a few minutes to the operative procedure and may minimize risk of RV functional damage. For these reasons its use is advocated. The period of global myocardial ischemia is usually less than 30 minutes, so controlled aortic root reperfusion is usually unnecessary.

Direct Suture versus Patch Repair

Cardiac surgeons vary as to the frequency with which they use a patch (usually pericardium, PTFE, or knitted polyester velour) to close ASDs. For example, this approach was used in 17% of patients in the Mayo Clinic experience,[H2] approximately 30% of those in the GLH experience, and 3% of those at UAB. Provided a patch is used when the defect is particularly large or the tissues are unduly friable, there appears to be no difference in end results, including early or late thromboembolic complications.[H2] Under such circumstances the ease and simplicity of direct suturing support its use in most patients.

Patch Material in Atrial Septum

Pericardium is the material of choice for interatrial patches (1) when a regurgitant jet may strike the patch, such as after repair of AV septal defects (prosthetic patches may produce severe hemolysis under these circumstances); (2) when pericardium forms part of the wall of an intracardiac conduit, the precise contour (position) of which is primarily determined by pressures on the two sides; and (3) when the patch is sewn to a very delicate area. In other situations, knitted polyester and PTFE patches are suitable alternatives.

Complications after Repair of Sinus Venosus Malformation

Late postoperative narrowing of the SVC is rare after repair of sinus venosus malformation by the techniques described.[S15] For this reason, minimal information is available to recommend the more complex repairs that are the subject of reports by numerous groups,[W3,W4] particularly when long-term results are not yet known.

In those rare cases in which the SVC compartment is found at operation to be too small following placement of the ASD patch in front of the ostia of the anomalous pulmonary veins, the SVC needs to be enlarged. Inserting a pericardial patch for this purpose is undesirable because it may lead to postoperative SVC stenosis. Stenosis occurred in one of four such patients in Trusler's series who were recatheterized late postoperatively and in 6 of 14 patients reported by Friedlo and colleagues in whom the repair had produced a much smaller SVC before patching compared with Trusler's patients.[F2,T5] Moreover, late retraction and thickening of a pericardial patch could compromise the sinus node because the suture line inevitably lies close to this structure. Fortunately, the lateral right atrial wall employing a V-Y atrioplasty may be used as an alternative (see Figure 16-20 and "Technique of Operation" earlier in this chapter).

An alternative point of view is that any incision across the SVC–right atrial junction risks early or late develop-

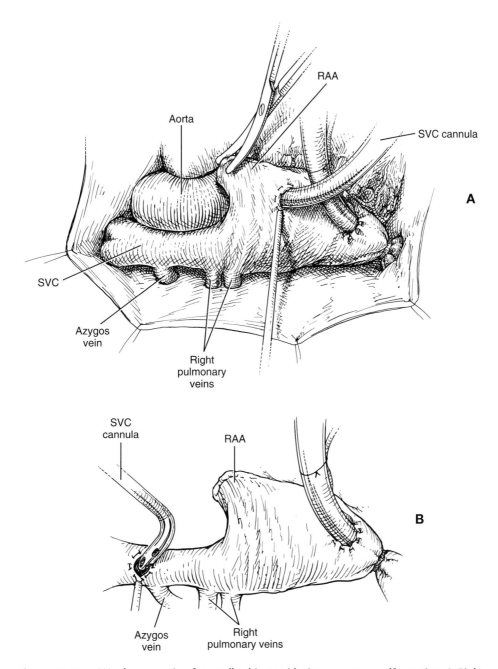

Figure 16-26   Warden operation for small subjects with sinus venosus malformation. **A,** Right pulmonary veins entering right atrium. Right atrial appendage is amputated. **B,** Cephalad end of transected superior vena cava is anastomosed to amputated right atrial appendage. For mobilization, azygos vein is divided.

Key: *RAA,* Right atrial appendage; *SVC,* superior vena cava.   *Continued*

ment of a junctional rhythm with all its potentially serious complications. For this reason the *Warden operation* may be used (Fig. 16-26).^W4 The SVC is divided cephalad to the anomalously connected right pulmonary veins. The central end is closed, and as a final step in operation, the distal end is anastomosed to the right atrial appendage.

From within the right atrium the inferior lip of the subcaval ASD is joined to the right atrial wall anterior and lateral to the caval orifice. This closes the interatrial communication and diverts pulmonary venous drainage from the anomalously connected right pulmonary veins to the left atrium.

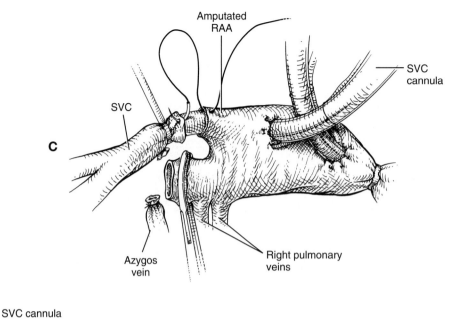

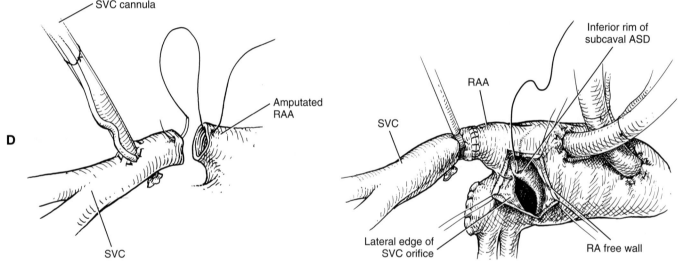

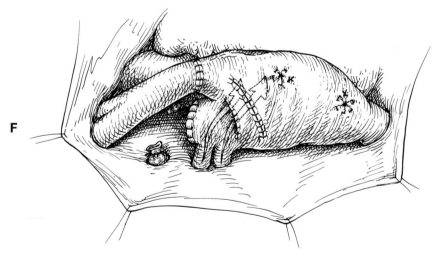

Figure 16-26, cont'd   **C** and **D,** Alternatively, the superior vena cava *(SVC)* can be cannulated directly. **E,** Small incision is made in right atrial wall. Lateral edge of SVC orifice is sutured to lower rim of subcaval atrial septal defect *(ASD).* Cardiac end of transected SVC is closed. **F,** Right pulmonary vein blood now flows *(arrows)* across the roofed ASD into left atrium. (From Warden and colleagues.[W4])

Key: *RA,* Right atrium; *RAA,* right atrial appendage; *SVC,* superior vena cava.

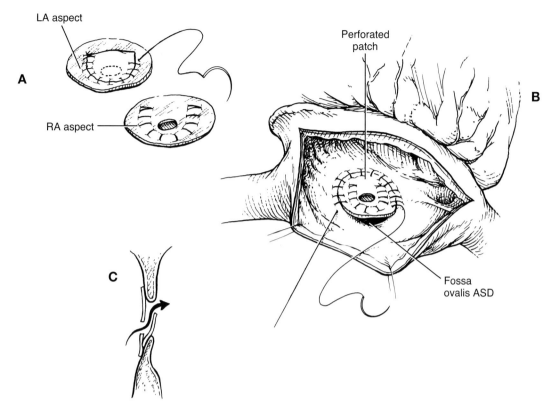

Figure 16-27   Operation for patients with atrial septal defect and high pulmonary vascular resistance. **A,** Suggested operation using perforated flap-valve patch. **B,** Complex patch is created such that higher right atrial pressure opens flap leftward. Thus, flap is placed on left atrial side of patch. **C,** Coronal section through repaired atrial septum.

Key: *ASD,* Atrial septal defect; *LA,* left atrial; *RA,* right atrial.

Repair in Presence of Increased Pulmonary Vascular Resistance

Some information indicates that a few patients with high RpI (greater than 6 U · m^2) may benefit from closure of the ASD using a flap-valve patch (Fig. 16-27).[A3-A5,Z2] The flap opens right to left, such that if right atrial pressure exceeds left atrial pressure in severe pulmonary hypertension, the right atrium will decompress to the left atrium, supporting systemic cardiac output (see "Lateral Tunnel Fontan with Deliberately Incomplete Atrial Partitioning" in Section 4 of Chapter 27). It is inferred that as P$_{PA}$ and RpI decrease late postoperatively, the flap valve will close by cicatrix.

REFERENCES

A

1. Adams CW. A reappraisal of life expectancy with atrial shunts of the secundum type. Dis Chest 1965;48:357.
2. Angel J, Soler-Soler J, Garcia del Castillo H, Anivarro I, Batlle-Diaz J. The role of reduced left ventricular end diastolic volume in the apparently high prevalence of mitral valve prolapse in atrial septal defect. Eur J Cardiol 1980;11:341.
3. Ad N, Barak J, Birk E, Snir E, Vidne BA. Unidirectional valve patch. Ann Thorac Surg 1996;62:626.
4. Ad N, Birk E, Barak J, Diamant S, Snir E, Vidne BA. A one-way valved atrial septal patch: a new surgical technique and its clinical application. J Thorac Cardiovasc Surg 1996;111:841.
5. Ad N, Barak J, Birk E, Diamant S, Vidne BA. A one-way, valved, atrial septal patch in the management of postoperative right heart failure: an animal study. J Thorac Cardiovasc Surg 1994;108:134.

B

1. Bedford DE, Sellors TH, Somerville W, Belcher JR, Besterman EM. Atrial septal defect and its surgical treatment. Lancet 1957;272:1255.
2. Beyer J. Atrial septal defect: acute left heart failure after surgical closure. Ann Thorac Surg 1978;25:36.
3. Bailey CP, Nichols HT, Bolton HE, Jamison WL, Gomez-Almedia M. Surgical treatment of forty-six interatrial septal defects by atrioseptopexy. Ann Surg 1954;140:805.
4. Bedford DE, Papp C, Parkinson J. Atrial septal defect. Br Heart J 1941;3:37.
5. Beyer J, Brunner L, Hugel W, Kreuzer E, Reichart B, Sunder-Plassmann L, et al. Acute left heart failure following repair of atrial septal defects. Thoraxchir Vask Chir 1975;23:346.

6. Bonow RO, Borer JS, Rosing DR, Bacharach SL, Green MV, Kent KM. Left ventricular functional reserve in adult patients with atrial septal defect: Pre- and postoperative studies. Circulation 1981; 63:1315.

7. Brody H. Drainage of the pulmonary veins into the right side of the heart. Arch Pathol 1942;33:221.

8. Babb JD, McGlynn TJ, Pierce WS, Kirkman PM. Isolated partial anomalous venous connection: a congenital defect with late and serious complications. Ann Thorac Surg 1981;31:540.

9. Bink-Boelkens MT, Meuzelaar KJ, Eygelaar A. Arrhythmias after repair of secundum atrial septal defect: the influence of surgical modification. Am Heart J 1988;115:629.

10. Bowes DE, Kirklin JW, Swan HJ. Effect of large atrial septal defects in dogs. Am J Physiol 1954;179:620.

11. Benedini G, Affatato A, Bellandi M, Cuccia C, Niccoli L, Renaldini E, et al. Pre-operative sinus node function in adult patients with atrial septal defect (ostium secundum type). Eur Heart J 1985;6:261.

12. Brandenburg RO Jr, Holmes DR Jr, Brandenburg RO, McGoon DC. Clinical follow-up study of paroxysmal supraventricular tachyarrhythmias after operative repair of a secundum type atrial septal defect in adults. Am J Cardiol 1983;51:273.

13. Bolens M, Friedli B. Sinus node function and conduction system before and after surgery for secundum atrial septal defect: an electrophysiologic study. Am J Cardiol 1984;53:1415.

14. Bharati S, Lev M. Direct entry of the right superior vena cava into the left atrium with aneurysmal dilatation and stenosis at its entry into the right atrium with stenosis of the pulmonary veins: a rare case. Pediatr Cardiol 1984;5:123.

15. Braudo M, Beanlands DS, Trusler G. Anomalous drainage of the right superior vena cava into the left atrium. Can Med Assoc J 1968;99:715.

C

1. Cayler GG. Spontaneous functional closure of symptomatic atrial septal defects. N Engl J Med 1967;276:65.

2. Clark EB, Rolad JM, Varghese PJ, Neill CA, Haller JA. Should the sinus venosus type ASD be closed? A review of the atrial conduction defects and surgical results in twenty-eight children (abstract). Am J Cardiol 1975;35:127.

3. Cooley DA, Ellis PR, Bellizi ME. Atrial septal defects of the sinus venosus type: surgical considerations. Dis Chest 1961;39:158.

4. Craig RJ, Selzer A. Natural history and prognosis of atrial septal defect. Circulation 1968;37:805.

5. Campbell M. Natural history of atrial septal defect. Br Heart J 1970; 32:820.

6. Cherian G, Uthaman CB, Durairaj M, Sukumar IP, Krishnaswami S, Jairaj PS, et al. Pulmonary hypertension in isolated secundum atrial septal defect: high frequency in young patients. Am Heart J 1983; 105:952.

7. Cockerham JT, Martin TC, Gutierrez FR, Hartmann AF Jr, Goldring D, Strauss AW. Spontaneous closure of secundum atrial septal defect in infants and young children. Am J Cardiol 1983;52:1267.

D

1. Davies RS, Green DC, Brott WH. Secundum atrial septal defect and cleft mitral valve. Ann Thorac Surg 1977;24:28.

2. Dimich I, Steinfeld L, Park SC. Symptomatic atrial septal defect in infants. Am Heart J 1973;85:601.

3. Daicoff GR, Brandenburg RO, Kirklin JW. Results of operation for atrial septal defect in patients forty-five years of age and older. Circulation 1967;35:I143.

4. Dave KS, Pakrashi BC, Wooler GH, Ionescu MI. Atrial septal defect in adults. Am J Cardiol 1973;31:7.

5. Drake EH, Lynch JP. Bronchiectasis associated with anomaly of the right pulmonary vein and right diaphragm. J Thorac Surg 1950;19:433.

6. Dotter CT, Hardisty NM, Steinberg I. Anomalous right pulmonary vein entering the inferior vena cava: two cases diagnosed during life by angiocardiography and cardiac catheterization. Am J Med Sci 1949;218:31.

7. D'Cruz IA, Arcilla RA. Anomalous venous drainage of the left lung into the inferior vena cava: a case report. Am Heart J 1964;67:539.

8. Doty DB, Wright CB, Hiratzka LF, Eastham CL, Marcus ML. Coronary reserve in volume-induced right ventricular hypertrophy from atrial septal defect. Am J Cardiol 1984;54:1059.

E

1. Ezekowitz MD, Alderson PO, Bulkley BH, Dwyer PN, Watkins L, Lappe DL, et al. Isolated drainage of the superior vena cava into the left atrium in a 52-year-old man. Circulation 1978;58:751.

2. Ende DJ, Chopra PS, Rao PS. Transcatheter closure of atrial septal defect or patent foramen ovale with the buttoned device for prevention of recurrence of paradoxic embolism. Am J Cardiol 1996;78:233.

F

1. Forfang K, Simonsen S, Andersen A, Efskind L. Atrial septal defect of secundum type in the middle-aged. Am Heart J 1977;94:44.

2. Friedli B, Guerin R, Davignon A, Fouron JC, Stanley P. Surgical treatment of partial anomalous pulmonary venous drainage: a long-term follow-up study. Circulation 1972;45:159.

3. Forfar JC, Godman MJ. Functional and anatomical correlates in atrial septal defect. An echocardiographic analysis. Br Heart J 1985;54:193.

4. Fiore AC, Naunheim KS, Kessler KA, Pennington DG, McBride LR, Barner HB, et al. Surgical closure of atrial septal defect in patients older than 50 years of age. Arch Surg 1988;123:965.

G

1. Gibbon JH. Application of a mechanical heart-lung apparatus to cardiac surgery. Minn Med 1954;37:171.

2. Giardina AC, Raptoulis AS, Engle MA, Levin AR. Spontaneous closure of atrial septal defect with cardiac failure in infancy. Chest 1979;75:395.

3. Gross RE, Pomeranz AA, Watkins E Jr, Goldsmith EI. Surgical closure of defects of the interauricular septum by use of an atrial well. N Engl J Med 1952;247:455.

4. Goodman DJ, Hancock EW. Secundum atrial septal defect associated with a cleft mitral valve. Br Heart J 1973;35:1315.

5. Geraci JE, Kirklin JW. Transplantation of left anomalous pulmonary vein to left atrium: report of case. Mayo Clin Proc 1953;28:472.

6. Gazzaniga AB, Matloff JM, Harken DE. Anomalous right pulmonary venous drainage into the inferior vena cava and left atrium. J Thorac Cardiovasc Surg 1969;57:251.

7. Gault JH, Morrow AG, Gay WA Jr, Ross J Jr. Atrial septal defect in patients over the age of 40 years: clinical and hemodynamic studies and the effects of operation. Circulation 1968;37:261.

8. Galve E, Angel J, Evangelista A, Anivarro I, Permanyer-Miralda G, Soler-Soler J. Bidirectional shunt in uncomplicated atrial septal defect. Br Heart J 1984;51:480.

9. Ghisla RP, Hannon DW, Meyer RA, Kaplan S. Spontaneous closure of isolated secundum atrial septal defects in infants: an echocardiographic study. Am Heart J 1985;109:1327.

10. Gatzoulis MA, Redington AN, Somerville J, Shore DF. Should atrial septal defects in adults be closed? Ann Thorac Surg 1996;61:657.

11. Gao YA, Burrows PE, Benson LN, Rabinovitch M, Freedom RM. Scimitar syndrome in infancy. J Am Coll Cardiol 1993;22:873.

H

1. Hoffman JI, Rudolph AM, Danilowicz D. Left-to-right atrial shunts in infants. Am J Cardiol 1972;30:868.

2. Hawe A, Rastelli GC, Brandenburg RO, McGoon DC. Embolic complications following repair of atrial septal defects. Circulation 1969;39:I185.

3. Hagan AD, Francis GS, Sahn DJ, Karliner JS, Friedman WF, O'Rourke RA. Ultrasound evaluation of systolic anterior septal motion in patients with and without right ventricular volume overload. Circulation 1974;50:248.

4. Hara M, Char F. Partial cleft of septal mitral leaflet associated with atrial septal defect of the secundum type. Am J Cardiol 1966;17:282.

5. Hastreiter AR, Wennemark JR, Miller RA, Paul MH. Secundum atrial septal defects with congestive heart failure during infancy and early childhood. Am Heart J 1962;64:467.

6. Horvath KA, Burke RP, Collins JJ Jr, Cohn LH. Surgical treatment of adult atrial septal defect: early and long-term results. J Am Coll Cardiol 1992;20:1156.

7. Hickie JB, Gimlette TM, Bacon AP. Anomalous pulmonary venous drainage. Br Heart J 1956;18:365.

8. Hynes KM, Frye RL, Brandenburg RO, McGoon DC, Titus JL, Giuliani ER. Atrial septal defect (secundum) associated with mitral regurgitation. Am J Cardiol 1974;34:333.

9. Haworth SG. Pulmonary vascular disease in secundum atrial septal defect in childhood. Am J Cardiol 1983;51:265.

10. Hagen PT, Scholz DG, Edwards WD. Incidence and size of patent foramen ovale during the first 10 decades of life: an autopsy study of 965 normal hearts. Mayo Clin Proc 1984;59:17.

11. Honey M. Anomalous pulmonary venous drainage of right lung to inferior vena cava (scimitar syndrome): clinical spectrum in older patients and role of surgery. Q J Med 1977;46:463.

J

1. Joffe HS. Effect of age on pressure flow dynamics in secundum atrial septal defect. Br Heart J 1984;51:469.

K

1. Kelly DT, Spotnitz HM, Beiser GD, Pierce JE, Epstein SE. Effects of chronic right ventricular volume and pressure loading on left ventricular performance. Circulation 1971;44:403.

2. Kirklin JW, Ellis FH Jr, Barratt-Boyes BG. Technique for repair of atrial septal defect using the atrial well. Surg Gyn Obst 1956;103:646.

3. Kirklin JW. Surgical treatment of anomalous pulmonary venous connection (partial anomalous pulmonary venous drainage). Mayo Clin Proc 1953;28:476.

4. Kiely B, Filler J, Stone S, Doyle EF. Syndrome of anomalous venous drainage of the right lung to the inferior vena cava. Am J Cardiol 1967;20:102.

5. Kirklin JW, Ellis FH Jr, Wood ED. Treatment of anomalous pulmonary venous connections in associations with interatrial communications. Surgery 1956;39:389.

6. Kyger ER 3rd, Frazier OH, Cooley DA, Gillette PC, Reul GJ Jr, Sandiford FM, et al. Sinus venosus atrial septal defect: early and late results following closure in 109 patients. Ann Thorac Surg 1978;25:44.

7. Kirklin JW, Swan HJ, Wood EH, Burchell HB, Edwards JE. Anatomic, physiologic, and surgical considerations in repair of interatrial communications in man. J Thorac Surg 1955;29:37.

8. Kirsch WM, Carlsson E, Hartmann AF Jr. A case of anomalous drainage of the superior vena cava into the left atrium. J Thorac Cardiovasc Surg 1961;41:550.

9. Karpawich PP, Antillon JR, Cappola PR, Agarwal KC. Pre- and postoperative electrophysiologic assessment of children with secundum atrial septal defect. Am J Cardiol 1985;55:519.

10. Konstantinides S, Geibel A, Olschewski M, Görnandt L, Roskamm H, Spillner G, et al. A comparison of surgical and medical therapy for atrial septal defect in adults. N Eng J Med 1995;333:469.

11. King TD, Mills NL. Nonoperative closure of atrial septal defects. Surgery 1974;75:383.

L

1. Lewis FJ, Taufic M. Closure of atrial septal defects with the aid of hypothermia: experimental accomplishments and the report of the one successful case. Surgery 1953;33:52.

2. Lieppe W, Scallion R, Behar VS, Kisslo JA. Two-dimensional echocardiographic findings in atrial septal defect. Circulation 1977;56:447.

3. Leachman RD, Cokkinos DV, Cooley DA. Association of ostium secundum atrial septal defects with mitral valve prolapse. Am J Cardiol 1976;38:167.

4. Lewis FJ, Taufic M, Varco RL, Niazi S. The surgical anatomy of atrial septal defects: experiences with repair under direct vision. Ann Surg 1955;142:401.

5. Liberthson RR, Boucher CA, Strauss HW, Dinsmore RE, McKusick KA, Pohost GM. Right ventricular function in adult atrial septal defect. Am J Cardiol 1981;47:56.

6. Liberthson RR, Buckley MJ, Boucher CA. Pulmonary regurgitation in large atrial shunts without pulmonary hypertension. Circulation 1976;54:966.

7. Lewis FJ. High defects of the atrial septum. J Thorac Cardiovasc Surg 1958;36:1.

8. Levin AR, Liebson PR, Ehlers KH, Diamant B. Assessment of left ventricular function in secundum atrial septal defect: evaluation by determination of volume, pressure and external systolic time indices. Pediatr Res 1975;9:894.

9. Lucas CL, Wilcox BR, Coulter NA. Pulmonary vascular response to atrial septal defect closure in children. J Surg Res 1975;18:571.

10. Lupi-Herrera E, Sandoval J, Seoane M, Bialostozky D, Attie F. The role of isoproterenol in the preoperative evaluation of high pressure high resistance ventricular septal defects. Chest 1982;81:42.

11. Lloyd TR, Rao PS, Beekham RH 3rd, Mendelsohn AM, Sideris EB. Atrial septal defect occlusion with the buttoned device (a multi-institutional U.S. trial). Am J Cardiol 1994;73:286.

12. Lang RM, Marcus RH. Images in clinical medicine. Ostium secundum atrial septal defect. N Engl J Med 1995;332:1337.

M

1. Menon VA, Wagner HR. Spontaneous closure of secundum atrial septal defect. N Y State J Med 1975;75:1068.

2. Mody MR. Serial hemodynamic observations in secundum atrial septal defect with special reference to spontaneous closure. Am J Cardiol 1973;32:978.

3. Murray G. Closure of defects in cardiac septa. Ann Surg 1948;128:843.

4. Meyer RA, Schwartz DC, Benzing G 3rd, Kaplan S. Ventricular septum in right ventricular volume overload: an echocardiographic study. Am J Cardiol 1972;30:349.

5. Marshall HW, Helmholz HF, Wood EH. Physiologic consequences of congenital heart disease. In Hamilton WF, ed. Handbook of physiology: circulation, Vol. 1. Washington, DC: American Physiologic Society, 1962, p. 417.

6. Magilligan DJ Jr, Lam CR, Lewis JW Jr, Davila JC. Late results of atrial septal defect repair in adults. Arch Surg 1978;113:1245.

7. McCormack RJ, Pickering D. A rare type of atrial septal defect. Thorax 1968;23:350.

8. Murphy JW, Kerr AR, Kirklin JW. Intracardiac repair for anomalous pulmonary venous connection of right lung to inferior vena cava. Ann Thorac Surg 1971;11:38.

9. Mohiuddin SM, Levin HS, Runco V, Booth RW. Anomalous pulmonary venous drainage: a common trunk emptying into the left atrium and inferior vena cava. Circulation 1966;34:46.

10. Morgan JR, Forker AD. Syndrome of hypoplasia of the right lung and dextroposition of the heart: "scimitar sign" with normal pulmonary venous drainage. Circulation 1971;43:27.

11. Mardini MK, Sakati NA, Nyhan WL. Anomalous left pulmonary venous drainage to the inferior vena cava and through the pericardiophrenic vein to the innominate vein: left-sided scimitar syndrome. Am Heart J 1981;101:860.

12. Meyer RA, Korfhagen JC, Covitz W, Kaplan S. Long-term follow-up study after closure of secundum atrial septal defect in children: an echocardiographic study. Am J Cardiol 1982;50:143.

13. Morishita Y, Yamashita M, Yamada K, Arikawa K, Taira A. Cyanosis in atrial septal defect due to persistent eustachian valve. Ann Thorac Surg 1985;40:614.

14. Morrison JG, Merrill WH, Friesinger GC, Bender HW Jr. Cyanosis, interatrial communication, and normal pulmonary vascular resistance in adults. Am J Cardiol 1986;58:1128.

15. Murphy JG, Gersh BJ, McGoon MD, Mair DD, Porter CJ, Ilstrup DM, et al. Long-term outcome after surgical repair of isolated atrial septal defect. Follow-up at 27 to 32 years. N Engl J Med 1990;323:1645.

16. Momma K, Takao A, Ando M, Nakazawa M, Takamizawa K. Natural and postoperative history of pulmonary vascular obstruction associated with ventricular septal defect. Jpn Circ J 1981;45:230.

17. Marshall HW, Swan HJ, Burchell HB, Wood EH. Effect of breathing oxygen on pulmonary artery pressure and pulmonary vascular resistance in patients with ventricular septal defect. Circulation 1961;23:241.

18. Mainwaring RD, Mirali-Akbar H, Lamberti JJ, Moore JW. Secundum-type atrial septal defects with failure to thrive in the first year of life. J Card Surg 1996;11:116.

N

1. Nakamura FF, Hauck AJ, Nadas AS. Atrial septal defect in infants. Pediatrics 1964;34:101.

2. Nasrallah AT, Hall RJ, Garcia E, Leachman RD, Cooley DA. Surgical repair of atrial septal defect in patients over 60 years of age. Long-term results. Circulation 1976;53:329.

3. Neptune WB, Bailey CP, Goldberg H. The surgical correction of atrial septal defects associated with transposition of the pulmonary veins. J Thorac Cardiovasc Surg 1953;25:623.

4. Neutze JM, Ishikawa T, Clarkson PM, Calder AL, Barratt-Boyes BG, Kerr AR. Assessment and follow-up of patients with ventricular septal defect and elevated pulmonary vascular resistance. Am J Cardiol 1989;63:327.

5. Najm HK, Williams WG, Coles JG, Rebeyka IM, Freedom RM. Scimitar syndrome: twenty years' experience and results of repair. J Thorac Cardiovasc Surg 1996;112:1161.

P

1. Popio KA, Gorlin R, Teichholz LE, Cohn PF, Bechtel D, Herman MV. Abnormalities of left ventricular function and geometry in adults with an atrial septal defect. Am J Cardiol 1975;36:302.

2. Pearlman AS, Borer JS, Clark CE, Henry WL, Redwood DR, Morrow AG, et al. Abnormal right ventricular size and ventricular septal motion after atrial septal defect closure. Am J Cardiol 1978;41:295.

3. Phillips SJ, Okies JE, Henken D, Sunderland CO, Starr A. Complex of secundum atrial septal defect and congestive heart failure in infants. J Thorac Cardiovasc Surg 1975;70:696.

4. Ports TA, Turley K, Brundage BH, Ebert PA. Operative correction of total left anomalous pulmonary venous return. Ann Thorac Surg 1979;27:246.

5. Perloff JK. Ostium secundum atrial septal defect: survival for 87 and 94 years. Am J Cardiol 1984;53:388.

6. Park HM, Summerer MH, Preuss K, Armstrong WF, Mahomed Y, Hamilton DJ. Anomalous drainage of the right superior vena cava into the left atrium. J Am Coll Cardiol 1983;2:358.

7. Paolillo V, Dawkins KD, Miller GA. Atrial septal defect in patients over the age of 50. Int J Cardiol 1985;9:139.

R

1. Roesler H. Interatrial septal defect. Arch Intern Med 1934;54:339.

2. Robitansky CF. Die Defect der Scheidewande des Herzens. Vienna: Wilhelm Braumuller, 1875, p. 153.

3. Richmond DE, Lowe JB, Barratt-Boyes BG. Results of surgical repair of atrial septal defects in the middle-aged and elderly. Thorax 1969;24:536.

4. Rahimtoola SH, Kirklin JW, Burchell HB. Atrial septal defect. Circulation 1968;38:V2.

5. Ruschhaupt DG, Khoury L, Thilenius OG, Replogle RL, Arcilla RA. Electrophysiologic abnormalities of children with ostium secundum atrial septal defect. Am J Cardiol 1984;53:1643.

6. Russell GA, Stovin PG. Coronary sinus type atrial septal defect in a child with pulmonary atresia and Ebstein's anomaly. Br Heart J 1985; 53:465.

7. Rome JJ, Keane JF, Perry SB, Spevak PJ, Lock JE. Double umbrella closure of atrial defects. Circulation 1990;82:751.

8. Rao PS, Sideris EB, Hausdorf G, Rey C, Lloyd TR, Beekman RH, et al. International experience with secundum atrial septal defect occlusion by the buttoned device. Am Heart J 1994;128:1022.

S

1. St. John Sutton MG, Tajik AJ, McGoon DC. Atrial septal defect in patients ages 60 years or older: operative results and long-term postoperative follow-up. Circulation 1981;64:402.

2. Søndergard T. Closure of atrial septal defects: report of three cases. Acta Chir Scand 1954;107:492.

3. Saksena FB, Aldridge HE. Atrial septal defect in the older patient. Circulation 1970;42:1009.

4. Schreiber TL, Feigenbaum H, Weyman AE. Effect of atrial septal defect repair on left ventricular geometry and degree of mitral valve prolapse. Circulation 1980;61:888.

5. Spangler JG, Feldt RH, Danielson GK. Secundum atrial septal defect encountered in infancy. J Thorac Cardiovasc Surg 1976;71:398.

6. Sturm JT, Ankeney JL. Surgical repair of inferior sinus venosus atrial septal defect. J Thorac Cardiovasc Surg 1979;78:570.

7. Shapiro EP, Al-Sadir J, Campbell NP, Thilenius OG, Anagnostopoulos CE, Hays P. Drainage of right superior vena cava into both atria. Circulation 1981;63:712.

8. Snellen HA, Van Ingen HC, Hoefsmit EC. Patterns of anomalous pulmonary venous drainage. Circulation 1968;38:45.

9. Saalouke MG, Shapiro SR, Perry LW, Scott LP 3rd. Isolated partial anomalous pulmonary venous drainage associated with pulmonary vascular obstructive disease. Am J Cardiol 1977;39:439.

10. Swan HJ, Kirklin JW, Becu LM, Wood EH. Anomalous connection of right pulmonary veins to superior vena cava with interatrial communications: hemodynamic data in eight cases. Circulation 1957;16:54.

11. Silver AW, Kirklin JW, Wood EH. Demonstration of preferential flow of blood from inferior vena cava and from right pulmonary veins through experimental atrial septal defects in dogs. Circ Res 1956;14:413.

12. Shub C, Dimopoulos IN, Seward JB, Callahan JA, Tancredi RG, Schattenberg TT, et al. Sensitivity of two-dimensional echocardiography in the direct visualization of atrial septal defect utilizing the subcostal approach: experience with 154 patients. J Am Coll Cardiol 1983;2:127.

13. Søndergard T, Paulsen PK. Some immediate hemodynamic consequences of closure of atrial septal defects of the secundum type. Circulation 1984;69:905.

14. Shub C, Tajik AJ, Seward JB, Hagler DJ, Danielson GK. Surgical repair of uncomplicated atrial septal defect without "routine" preoperative cardiac catheterization. J Am Coll Cardiol 1985;6:49.

15. Stewart S, Alexson C, Manning J. Early and late results of repair of partial anomalous pulmonary venous connection to the superior vena cava with a pericardial baffle. Ann Thorac Surg 1986;41:498.

16. Steele PM, Fuster V, Cohen M, Ritter DG, McGoon DC. Isolated atrial septal defect with pulmonary vascular obstructive disease—long-term follow-up and prediction of outcome after surgical correction. Circulation 1987;76:1037.
17. Shah D, Azhar M, Oakley CM, Cleland JG, Nihoyannopoulos P. Natural history of secundum atrial septal defect in adults after medical or surgical treatment: a historical prospective study. Br Heart J 1994; 71:224.

T

1. Tsakiris AG, Mair DD, Seki S, Titus JL, Wood EH. Motion of the tricuspid valve annulus in anesthetized intact dogs. Circ Res 1975;36:43.
2. Tsakiris AG, Sturm RE, Wood EH. Experimental studies on the mechanisms of closure of cardiac valves with use of roentgen videodensitometry. Am J Cardiol 1973;32:136.
3. Tikoff G, Schmidt AM, Kuida H, Hecht HH. Heart failure in atrial septal defect. Am J Med 1965;39:533.
4. Tajik AJ, Gau GT, Ritter DG, Schattenberg TT. Echocardiographic pattern of right ventricular diastolic volume overload in children. Circulation 1972;46:36.
5. Trusler GA, Kazenelson G, Freedom RM, Williams WG, Rowe RD. Late results following repair of partial anomalous pulmonary venous connection with sinus venosus atrial septal defect. J Thorac Cardiovasc Surg 1980;79:776.
6. Tuchman H, Brown JF, Huston JH, Weinstein AB, Rowe GG, Crumpton CW. Superior vena cava draining into left atrium. Am J Med 1956;21:481.
7. Torres AR, Dietl CA. Surgical management of the scimitar syndrome: an age-dependent spectrum. Cardiovasc Surg 1993;1:432.

V

1. Van Praagh R, Van Praagh S. Does connection of the IVC with the LA exist? (letter.) Pediatr Cardiol 1987;8:151.

W

1. Wanderman KL, Ovsyshcher I, Gueron M. Left ventricular performance in patients with atrial septal defect: evaluation with noninvasive methods. Am J Cardiol 1978;41:487.
2. Weyman AE, Wann S, Feigenbaum H, Dillon JC. Mechanism of abnormal septal motion in patients with right ventricular volume overload: a cross-sectional echocardiographic study. Circulation 1976;54:179.
3. Williams WH, Zorn-Chelton S, Raviele AA, Michalik RE, Guyton RA, Dooley KJ, et al. Extracardiac atrial pedicle conduit repair of partial anomalous pulmonary venous connection to the superior vena cava in children. Ann Thorac Surg 1984;38:345.
4. Warden HE, Gustafson RA, Tarnay TJ, Neal WA. An alternative method for repair of partial anomalous pulmonary venous connection to the superior vena cava. Ann Thorac Surg 1984;38:601.
5. Winters WL Jr, Cortes F, McDonough M, Tyson RR, Baier H, Gimenez J, et al. Venoarterial shunting from inferior vena cava to left atrium in atrial septal defects with normal right heart pressures. Am J Cardiol 1967;19:293.

Y

1. Young D. Later results of closure of secundum atrial septal defect in children. Am J Cardiol 1973;31:14.

Z

1. Zubiate P, Kay JH. Surgical correction of anomalous pulmonary venous connection. Ann Surg 1962;156:234.
2. Zhou Q, Lai Y, Wei H, Song R, Wu Y, Zhang H. Unidirectional valve patch for repair of cardiac septal defects with pulmonary hypertension. Ann Thorac Surg 1995;60:1245.

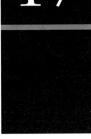

17 Total Anomalous Pulmonary Venous Connection

DEFINITION

Total anomalous pulmonary venous connection (TAPVC) is a cardiac malformation in which there is no direct connection between any pulmonary vein and the left atrium; rather, all the pulmonary veins connect to the right atrium or one of its tributaries. Although not part of the malformation, a patent foramen ovale or atrial septal defect is present in essentially all persons with TAPVC and is necessary for survival after birth.

This chapter concerns TAPVC in hearts with concordant atrioventricular and ventriculoarterial connections without other major cardiac anomalies except patent ductus arteriosus. TAPVC in hearts with atrial isomerism is considered in Chapter 44.

HISTORICAL NOTE

TAPVC was apparently first described by Wilson in 1798.[W1] In 1951, Muller, while at the University of California Medical Center in Los Angeles, reported the first successful surgical approach.[M1] His correction was partial, achieved by anastomosing the common pulmonary venous sinus to the left atrial appendage using a closed technique. In 1956, Lewis, Varco, and colleagues[L1] at the University of Minnesota reported successful open repair of this malformation using moderate hypothermia induced by surface cooling and temporary occlusion of venous inflow to the heart. The same year, Burroughs and Kirklin reported successful repair of TAPVC using cardiopulmonary bypass (CPB).[B1] Their report also described a successful operation several years earlier using the atrial well technique of Gross and colleagues.[G1]

Subsequently, it became apparent that mortality for repair of TAPVC in infants using CPB was strikingly higher than that for older patients, but attempts to improve the results by staged operation or palliative measures were generally unsuccessful.[B2,C1,M2,M3,S1] Successes were reported from time to time, however, even for critically ill infants with infracardiac connection.[W2]

Improvement in intraoperative techniques eventually substantially improved results in infants. In 1967, Dillard and colleagues achieved good results using hypothermic circulatory arrest without CPB,[D1] and in 1971, Malm, Gersony, and colleagues reported success in a small group of young infants using standard, normothermic CPB.[G2] Hypothermic circulatory arrest and limited CPB were used in 1969 with strikingly improved results.[B3,B4]

MORPHOLOGY

Pulmonary Venous Anatomy

TAPVC is supracardiac in about 45% of cases, cardiac in about 25%, infracardiac in about 25%, and mixed in about 5% (Fig. 17-1).[B5,B6,D2,D3] The connection in *supracardiac TAPVC* is usually to a left vertical vein draining into the left innominate vein, less often to the superior vena cava, usually at its junction with the right atrium, and rarely to the azygos vein. In *cardiac TAPVC,* the connection is usually to the coronary sinus and less often to the right atrium directly. The most common sites of connection in patients with *infracardiac (infradiaphragmatic) TAPVC* are the portal vein (65% of cases, according to Duff and colleagues[D4]) and ductus venosus; less common are the gastric vein, right or left hepatic vein, and inferior vena cava. Uncommonly, the pulmonary venous drainage may be through two connections.[A4] Also, part of the pulmonary venous drainage may be to one site and part to another in what is termed *mixed TAPVC.* In the most common connections in mixed TAPVC, the left lung (usually the upper lobe) drains to a left vertical vein and the remainder of both lungs drains to the coronary sinus.

No matter what the final connection or termination may be, the individual right and left pulmonary veins usually converge to form a *common pulmonary venous sinus,* which in turn connects to the systemic venous system in one of the ways noted earlier. It is usually posterior to the pericardium. Its long axis is usually oriented transversely, with the pulmonary veins of the left lung converging to form its left extremity and those from the right lung to form its right extremity. When the drainage is infracardiac, the right and left pulmonary veins slope downward to converge into a vertical sinus, with the entire arrangement having a Y, T, or tree shape.[C2,K2,T1] Rarely, there are two vertical veins that are not confluent until below the diaphragm.[W9]

A common pulmonary venous sinus may be absent in some cases with cardiac or mixed connections. Its apparent absence in some patients may be an illusion attributable to a defect in the anterior wall of the sinus. That defect is the orifice connecting it to the coronary sinus or right atrium.

Pulmonary venous obstruction is a severe associated condition usually resulting from a stenosis involving the vein connecting the common pulmonary venous sinus to the systemic venous system. A localized stenosis may occur at the junction of the left vertical vein with either the left innominate vein or the common pulmonary venous sinus, or at the junction of a connecting vein that joins the superior vena cava.

A severe obstruction may be due to the so-called *vascular vice,* in which the left vertical vein passes posterior rather than anterior to the left pulmonary artery and is compressed between it and the left main bronchus.[S17] When TAPVC is to the coronary sinus, a stenosis may occur where the common pulmonary venous sinus joins the coronary sinus or, rarely, at the coronary sinus ostium.[A3,J2] In infracardiac connection, the connecting vein may be similarly narrowed at its junction with the portal vein or ductus venosus, or it may be compressed where it penetrates the diaphragm. In those varieties of infracardiac connection in which the ductus venosus is not available to bypass the liver, the portal sinusoids offer additional important obstruction to venous return. Finally, pulmonary venous obstruction may result simply from the length of a comparatively narrow connecting vein.

Important pulmonary venous obstruction of these various types exists in nearly all patients with infracardiac connection and in almost all with connections to the azygos vein, in 65% of those with connections to the superior vena cava, in 40% of those with connections to the left innominate vein, and in 40% with connections of the mixed type (see Table 17-3).[D3] It is less common in patients with a cardiac connection, although it has been found in 20% of patients in whom the connection is to the coronary sinus.[J2] Rarely, pulmonary venous obstruction is the result of stenoses of individual pulmonary veins at or close to their connections to the common pulmonary venous sinus.[G3]

Functional pulmonary venous obstruction arguably occurs in patients having a patent foramen ovale rather than an atrial septal defect, although this occurrence may be limited to those with a small orifice at the foramen ovale.

Cardiac Chamber and Septal Anatomy

For survival after birth, a communication between systemic and pulmonary circulations must exist. Nearly always, an atrial septal defect or patent foramen ovale is present. However, in the review of Delisle and colleagues, one of 93 autopsy cases was an 11-year-old with an intact atrial septum and multiple ventricular septal defects, and Hastreiter and colleagues reported a 6-week-old patient with TAPVC to the ductus venosus, a patent ductus, and a closed foramen ovale.[D3,H1] Atrial communication in TAPVC is usually of adequate size and not obstructive,[B2,G3] although the GLH group reported that the defect was small in about half the infants operated on.[W3] There is frequently no pressure gradient between the two atria even when the defect is small.[E1,W3]

The right atrium is enlarged and thick walled in patients with TAPVC, and the left atrium is abnormally small.[B5,B7] Cineangiographic studies by Mathew and colleagues have shown left atrial volume to be 53% of predicted normal.[M4] These investigators noted that the left atrial appendage was normal in size and believed that left atrial smallness could be explained by absence of the pulmonary vein component. In addition, in patients with TAPVC to the right atrium, the posterior attachment of the atrial septum is shifted to the left, so the septum lies nearer to the sagittal than the usual coronal plane.

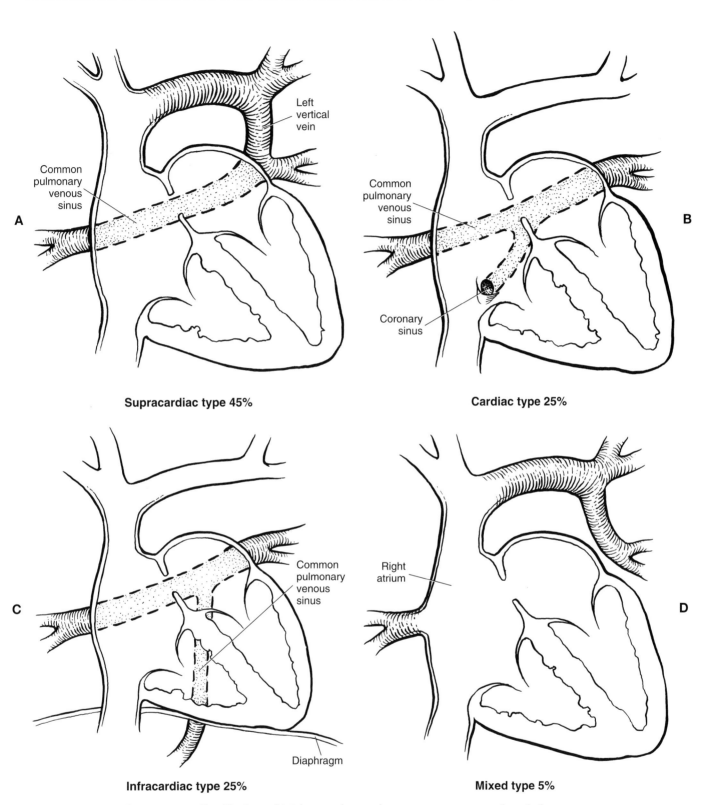

Supracardiac type 45%

Cardiac type 25%

Infracardiac type 25%

Mixed type 5%

Figure 17-1   Classification of total anomalous pulmonary venous connection. **A,** Supracardiac type (45% of cases), in which the common pulmonary venous sinus connects by a vertical vein on the left side to the left innominate vein. **B,** Cardiac type (25% of cases), in which the common pulmonary venous sinus connects to the coronary sinus in the right atrium. **C,** Infracardiac type (25% of cases), in which the common pulmonary venous sinus connects to the portal vein or ductus venosus below the diaphragm. **D,** Mixed type (5% of cases), in which there is no common pulmonary venous sinus and pulmonary veins connect randomly to the heart.

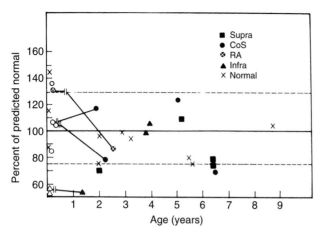

Figure 17-2 Preoperative left ventricular end-diastolic volume, expressed along the vertical axis as percent of predicted normal, according to age and cardiac morphology. Dashed horizontal lines enclose ±2 SD from the mean normal value. Open symbols represent preoperative values in seven patients, and closed symbols represent postoperative values. When both values were measured in the same patient, symbols are connected by solid lines, with two short, vertical parallel lines indicating time of repair. X represents values in normal patients. (From Whight and colleagues.[W3])

Key: *CoS*, Coronary sinus TAPVC; *Infra*, infracardiac TAPVC; *RA*, right atrial cardiac TAPVC; *Supra*, supracardiac TAPVC.

Anatomic studies have shown that the left ventricle (LV) is usually normal in size.[B5,R5] Haworth and Reid's quantitative study showed that inflow measurements of the LV were normal in eight of nine dying infants with TAPVC.[H2] In one infant, however, LV inflow measurements were abnormally small, and weight of the free LV wall plus the septum was less than that of a normal fetus at full term. In all nine infants, LV free wall thickness was normal. In a quantitative autopsy study of infants with TAPVC, Bove and colleagues found LV mass to be normal as well.[B8] However, they found the LV cavity small because of leftward displacement of the septum secondary to right ventricular (RV) pressure–volume overload (see "Mitral Prolapse" under Morphology in Chapter 16). Correspondingly, Nakazawa and colleagues reported that angiographically determined LV end-diastolic volume (LVEDV) was 79% less than normal (*P* = .009) in a group of infants with TAPVC and severe pulmonary hypertension.[N1] Hammon and colleagues also reported small LVEDV in infants with TAPVC.[H3] These findings are all compatible with those of Whight and colleagues[W3] (Fig. 17-2).

The RV varies in size, depending on the magnitude of pulmonary blood flow, presence or absence of pulmonary venous stenosis, and the point at which anomalous pulmonary veins connect. When connection was infracardiac, Haworth and Reid found that the RV was neither dilated nor hypertrophied.[H2] In cases in which venous connection was supradiaphragmatic, the septum and RV were hypertrophied and the RV dilated.

Pulmonary Vasculature

Because most infants with TAPVC have marked pulmonary hypertension, structural changes are usually found in the lungs of even the youngest infants dying with the malformation.[N2] Haworth and Reid demonstrated increased pulmonary arterial muscularity in all infants dying with TAPVC, including an 8-day-old neonate, as shown by increased arterial wall thickness and extension of muscle into smaller and more peripheral arteries than normal.[H2] Vein wall thickness was increased in all but the youngest child.

Associated Conditions

Except for an atrial communication, most infants presenting with severe symptoms from TAPVC have either no associated condition or a small or large patent ductus arteriosus. Patent ductus arteriosus is present in nearly all infants coming to operation in the first few weeks of life with pulmonary venous obstruction and, overall, in about 15% of cases. Ventricular septal defects occasionally occur.

However, more than one third of cases coming to autopsy, few of which are infants, have other major associated cardiac anomalies.[D3] These include tetralogy of Fallot, double-outlet right ventricle, interrupted aortic arch,[B9] and other lesions.[D9] The combination of TAPVC with other major cardiac anomalies is especially likely to occur when there is atrial isomerism[B5,D3,S2] (see Chapter 44).

CLINICAL FEATURES AND DIAGNOSTIC CRITERIA

Presentation

Usually, patients with TAPVC present as seriously and often critically ill neonates.[C3] The diagnosis frequently has been missed because of lack of florid signs and symptoms. TAPVC must be suspected in any neonate who has unexplained tachypnea, the cardinal symptom of this anomaly. During the first 2 weeks of life, there are other causes of tachypnea that may be impossible to distinguish clinically from TAPVC, particularly a diffuse pneumonic process and retention of fetal lung fluid.[S3] Meconium aspiration and myocarditis may also confound the diagnosis. Respiratory distress syndrome should not be difficult to differentiate, because of its classic radiologic features: prematurity and intercostal and sternal indrawing. Cyanosis is usually unimpressive in TAPVC unless there is marked pulmonary venous obstruction or a widely open ductus arteriosus that permits right-to-left shunting.

Both LV and RV functions are depressed compared with normal (*P* < .001 in both instances) in infants presenting when seriously ill with TAPVC and marked pulmonary hypertension.[H3,N1] Severe metabolic acidosis develops soon after birth, when pulmonary venous obstruction is severe, rapidly leading to myocardial necrosis. Some neonates are so critically ill that they require intubation immediately upon hospital admission and before evaluation is begun.

Examination

In infants, the heart is not particularly overactive on examination. There may be an unimpressive precordial systolic murmur and gallop sound (the latter often proves to be a tricuspid flow murmur). The second heart sound is usually single or narrowly split. In older children, the signs are those of a large atrial septal defect unless there is increased pulmonary vascular resistance.

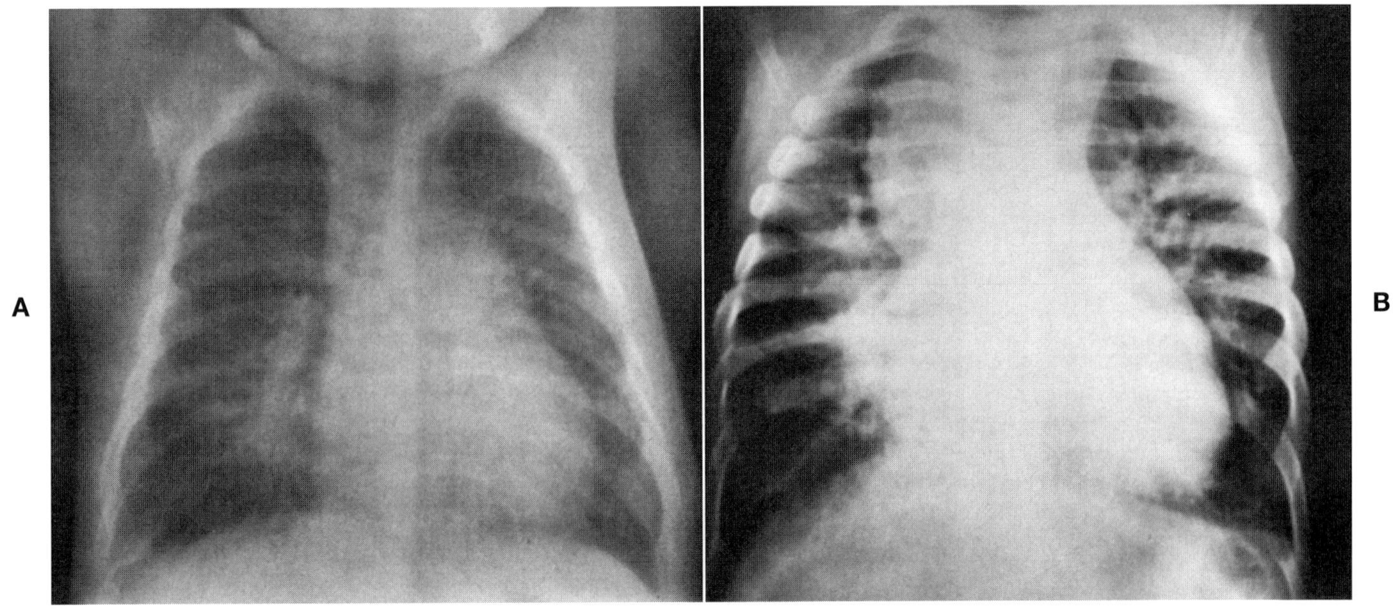

Figure 17-3   Chest radiographs of patients with total anomalous pulmonary venous connection (TAPVC). **A**, A 2.5-month-old infant with infracardiac TAPVC. Note the mild cardiac enlargement and evidence of pulmonary venous hypertension. Even less radiologic change is seen in neonates. **B**, "Snowman" or "figure-of-eight" configuration in a 1-year-old patient with TAPVC to the left innominate vein. Shadow on the left above the heart is the large left vertical vein. Shadow on the right is cast by the large superior vena cava.

Chest Radiography

On chest radiography, heart size is usually near normal if there is pulmonary venous obstruction, but it may be large when there is increased pulmonary blood flow. The latter is associated with plethora (Fig. 17-3, *A*), but the more common pulmonary venous obstruction is evident as a diffuse haziness or, in its severe forms, a ground glass appearance. This sign is reduced when the pulmonary circuit can decompress via a patent ductus arteriosus. Older infants with TAPVC to the left innominate vein have a characteristic "figure-of-eight" or "snowman" configuration on the chest radiograph[S3] (Fig. 17-3, *B*).

Echocardiography

Two-dimensional echocardiography is remarkably accurate in assessing the morphology of TAPVC (Fig. 17-4).[S9] Along with Doppler color flow interrogation, it is diagnostic in almost all infants with this condition.[C4,G7,H5] Echocardiographic features of TAPVC include criteria for RV diastolic overload and an echo-free space posterior to the left atrium.[P2] However, a second drainage site might be overlooked.[C4]

Echocardiography is accepted as the definitive diagnostic procedure in neonates with important pulmonary venous obstruction, because contrast medium is not required.[S16,W8] Cardiac catheterization delays operation and exacerbates myocardial failure and pulmonary edema. Magnetic resonance imaging correlates well with echocardiography, but offers no advantages and is time consuming and difficult to perform.[C6]

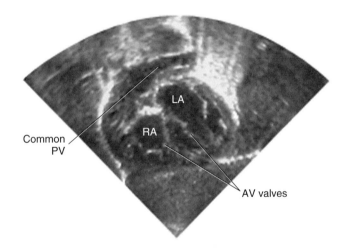

Figure 17-4   Two-dimensional echocardiograph of an infant with total anomalous pulmonary venous connection. There is no connection of the common pulmonary vein to the left atrium.

Key: *AV*, Atrioventricular; *LA*, left atrium; *PV*, pulmonary venous sinus; *RA*, right atrium.

Cardiac Catheterization and Cineangiography

Angiograms obtained by pulmonary artery or pulmonary vein injections define the malformation, identify the site of drainage, and often localize the site of pulmonary venous obstruction. This procedure is diagnostic in nearly all patients.[G3] However, it should not be used in seriously ill neonates (see previous discussion).

When the connection is to a left vertical vein, the common pulmonary venous sinus and vertical vein can usually be demonstrated (Fig. 17-5, *A*). When the anomalous connection is to the coronary sinus, it appears as an ovoid opacification over the left side of the spine within the right atrial contour.[R1] When it is infracardiac, the descending vein can usually be demonstrated, although its precise infradiaphragmatic connection may not be seen (Fig. 17-5, *B*). Tynan and colleagues have pointed out that in neonates, umbilical vein catheterization permits direct injection of contrast medium into the anomalously connecting infradiaphragmatic vein and an accurate diagnosis of its connections.[T1] Where injections of contrast medium are made into the pulmonary trunk and there is a patent ductus arteriosus, virtually all the contrast medium passes down the descending aorta; hence, the injection must be repeated more distally in the left pulmonary artery.

The site of pulmonary venous obstruction may be identified as a discrete narrowing on the angiogram, or by slow clearing of dye from the lungs or slow filling of the area to which the connection is made. Presence of pulmonary venous obstruction is established by demonstrating a gradient between left atrial and pulmonary artery wedge pressures. In the common left vertical vein connection, it is usually possible to pass a catheter retrogradely from the innominate vein into the common pulmonary venous chamber and to localize the site of obstruction on catheter withdrawal. Greene and colleagues employ superimposition digital subtraction angiography to define pulmonary venous anatomy, relationship of common pulmonary vein to left atrium, and size of left atrium.[G8]

Physiology of Common Mixing Chamber

In TAPVC, the right atrium is theoretically a common mixing chamber.[B10] This situation is reflected in the frequent finding of close similarity of oxygen content and saturations from the right atrium, left atrium, pulmonary artery, and systemic artery.[F1] There is considerable deviation from this pattern, however, because of streaming of systemic venous return in the right atrium, directing inferior vena caval blood through the foramen ovale to the mitral valve and superior vena caval blood through the tricuspid valve. Thus, in infracardiac TAPVC, systemic arterial saturation is typically higher than pulmonary artery saturation.

Because TAPVC has this common mixing chamber, in most patients who live beyond infancy, a direct relationship exists between the magnitude of pulmonary blood flow and arterial oxygen saturation, assuming a constant oxygen consumption and blood hemoglobin level. This relationship was formulated into a nomogram by Burchell[B10] (Fig. 17-6). Because the pulmonary–systemic blood flow ratio ($\dot{Q}p/\dot{Q}s$) in such patients is determined primarily by magnitude of the pulmonary blood flow, and because their pulmonary vascular resistance is inversely related to pulmonary blood flow, arterial oxygen saturation in children (not in seriously ill neonates and young infants) is a rough guide to the patient's operability vis-à-vis pulmonary vascular disease. When in children and adults the arterial oxygen saturation is less than about 80%, the $\dot{Q}p/\dot{Q}s$ is likely to be less than 1.4 and pulmonary vascular resistance greater than 10 U · m².

NATURAL HISTORY

TAPVC is relatively uncommon, accounting for only about 1.5% to 3% of cases of congenital heart disease.[B5,K1] Infants born with TAPVC have a generally unfavorable prognosis, with only about 20% surviving the first year of life.[B7,B11,K3] Only about 50% survive beyond 3 months, with death occurring during the first few weeks or months of life in most neonates in whom tachypnea, cyanosis, and clinical evidence of low cardiac output develop. Such infants usually have pulmonary venous obstruction, long

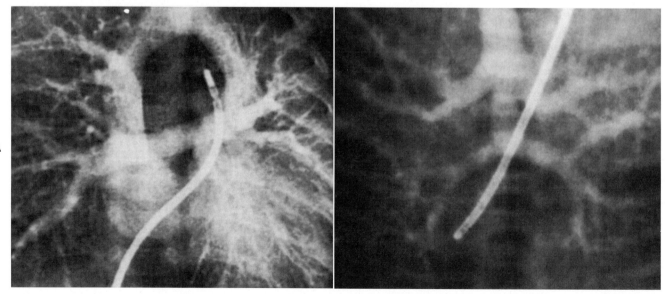

Figure 17-5 Angiograms of infants with total anomalous pulmonary venous connection (TAPVC). **A**, TAPVC to left innominate vein. **B**, TAPVC draining infradiaphragmatically.

pulmonary venous pathways, and a small patent foramen ovale.[B7] Survival past the critical first few weeks and months does not portend a favorable prognosis, because only about half the patients surviving to age 3 months survive to 1 year.

Infants who survive the first few weeks of life usually have cardiomegaly and a large pulmonary blood flow, with mild cyanosis. Most have some degree of pulmonary artery hypertension.[G3] Their clinical syndrome includes tachypnea, recurrent episodes of severe pulmonary congestion, failure to thrive, fluid retention, and hepatomegaly.

Those with TAPVC who survive the first year of life without surgical treatment usually have a large atrial septal defect. Characteristically, they exhibit important physical underdevelopment similar to that of patients with other kinds of large left-to-right shunts, mild cyanosis, and mild exercise intolerance (see "Survival" under Natural History in Chapter 16). Like patients with isolated large atrial septal defects, they tend to have a stable hemodynamic state for 10 to 20 years, with little change in pulmonary vascular resistance and thus little change in pulmonary artery pressure, blood flow, and arterial oxygen levels.[G3] In the second decade of life, pulmonary vascular disease develops in some patients, and there is increasing cyanosis as pulmonary blood flow diminishes (Eisenmenger complex).[S13]

To quantify the natural history, Hazelrig and colleagues analyzed data from 183 autopsied cases of surgically untreated TAPVC reported in the literature.[H8] Median survival was 2 months, with the shortest survival being 1 day and the longest 49 years. Ninety percent of deaths occurred in the first year of life. Obstruction of the pulmonary venous pathway importantly reduced median survival ($P < .0001$) (Fig. 17-7), from 2.5 months in the nonobstructed group to 3 weeks in the obstructed group. Patients with supracardiac and cardiac connections had a similar history, with median survival of 2.5 and 3 months, respectively, whereas those with infracardiac connections had a worse prognosis, with median survival of 3 weeks (Fig. 17-8). Only three patients had mixed connections; two died at 5 months and one at 3.3 months. Presence of an atrial septal defect (rather than a patent foramen ovale) was associated with increased survival, particularly when the connection was not infracardiac (Fig. 17-8).

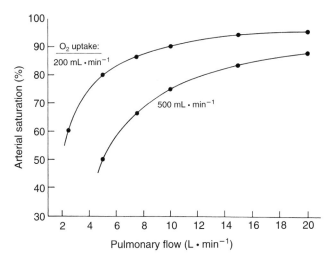

Figure 17-6   Relation between percent arterial oxygen saturation and pulmonary blood flow in persons with common mixing chambers, formulated on theoretical grounds by Burchell.[B10] The upper curve is at rest; the lower is at moderate exercise. Systemic blood flow is assumed to be 25 L · min⁻¹. (From Burchell.[B10])

TECHNIQUE OF OPERATION

Operation should be undertaken as an emergency, immediately after diagnosis by two-dimensional echocardiography, in neonates and infants who enter the hospital critically ill. Preoperative preparation and stabilization should be brief.

Hypothermic circulatory arrest with limited CPB may be used routinely in neonates and infants. Alternatively, in patients weighing more than about 2.5 kg, hypothermic CPB may be used and the repair performed during reduced

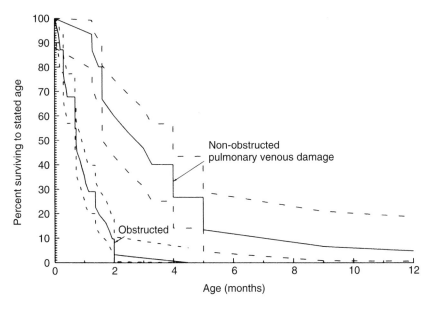

Figure 17-7   Survival of surgically untreated persons with total anomalous pulmonary venous connection, according to clearly present or clearly absent obstruction to pulmonary venous drainage; based on 31 cases among 183 in which the autopsy protocol was clear in this regard. Dashed lines represent 70% confidence limits (*P* for difference < .0001). (From Hazelrig and colleagues.[H8])

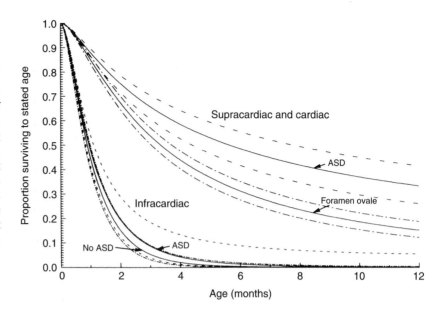

Figure 17-8 Nomogram of multivariable equation relating survival of surgically untreated persons with total anomalous pulmonary venous connection ($n = 183$) to type of connection and presence or absence of an atrial septal defect. Survival was not different for supracardiac and cardiac types. Solid lines represent probabilities; dashed lines represent 70% confidence limits. The separation into atrial septal defect and foramen ovale groups was based simply on the words used in the autopsy protocol, under the presumption that atrial septal defect denoted larger holes. (From Hazelrig and colleagues.[H8])

Key: *ASD*, Atrial septal defect.

flows and short periods of circulatory arrest. The ductus arteriosus must be dissected and closed routinely in infants (see Chapter 20, Fig. 20-29, in 2nd edition of this book), even if not visualized in preoperative studies.[B16,F3] This is usually accomplished just after CPB is established and before cooling is begun. Although no longer generally used, preliminary surface cooling to low temperature has the advantage of ease of exposure of the aorta for cannulation permitted by low intravascular pressures. In the tiny infant with TAPVC, the aorta is very small and hidden by the large and hypertrophied RV outflow tract. Retraction of this tract for exposure and aortic cannulation at normothermia can precipitate severe persistent hypotension.

The stringent technical demands of surgical correction of TAPVC in neonates and young infants require, for at least part of the repair, the perfect operating conditions of hypothermic circulatory arrest. With induction of hypothermia by CPB in preparation for circulatory arrest, in a few instances it has been noted that the heart has become very hard and fibrillates soon after the start of cooling.[R2,W7] This type of damage has not been observed by other experienced groups.[J3] Nonetheless, a thick ventricular wall and small LV volume (due to the smallness of the infant and occasionally to a small normalized LV volume) may increase wall tension markedly, severely limit perfusion of inner layers of both the RV and LV, and predispose the heart to such an occurrence.[A2,B15] An alternative explanation for this unfavorable response of the ventricles is that severe preoperative acidosis may be present, and possibly myocardial ischemia from obstruction to retrograde aortic (and thus coronary) flow by the arterial cannula (Jonas RA: personal communication; 1992). Avoiding addition of calcium to the perfusate (because it is citrated blood) or using warm induction of cardioplegia before reducing the temperature of the perfusate may be important in minimizing this problem (see "Cold Cardioplegia, Controlled Aortic Root Perfusion, and [When Needed] Warm Cardioplegic Induction" in Chapter 3).

Total Anomalous Pulmonary Venous Connection to Left Innominate Vein

After establishing CPB and cardioplegia and while core cooling is under way, posterior pericardial attachments of the heart are cut[K6] (Fig. 17-9, *A*). The common pulmonary venous sinus, lying behind the pericardium, is identified after lifting up the apex of the heart for a moment to visualize the retrocardiac portion of the pericardium. The right pulmonary artery, running parallel and just cephalad to the sinus, is also identified to avoid confusing it with the common pulmonary venous sinus. The vertical vein connecting the common pulmonary venous sinus to the left innominate vein can sometimes be seen inside the pericardium, but in most cases the pericardium on the left must be retracted toward the patient's right and the persistent left vertical vein identified beneath the mediastinal pleura. The vein is isolated after carefully freeing the left phrenic nerve. A ligature is tied to the tip of the left atrial appendage for leftward retraction.

When circulatory arrest is used, the baby's body temperature reaches 18° to 20°C about the time these preparations have been completed; thus, the aorta may simply be clamped and circulatory arrest established. Alternatively, cold cardioplegia, after warm induction, has already been established. When the repair is to be done in part during CPB, perfusate temperature is stabilized at 18° to 20°C and flow reduced to 0.5 to 1.0 L · min^{-1} · m^{-2}, with circulatory arrest used to improve exposure whenever needed. The persistent vertical vein is doubly ligated. The common pulmonary venous sinus is mobilized and opened (Fig. 17-9, *B* and *C*), and the posterior left atrial wall is opened. Anastomosis is then made between the common pulmonary venous sinus and left atrium (see Fig. 17-9, *D*, *E*, and *F*). Sutures must be placed precisely and rather close together to avoid postoperative bleeding. The continuous portion of the suture line must not be pulled up so tightly as to pursestring the anastomosis and narrow it.

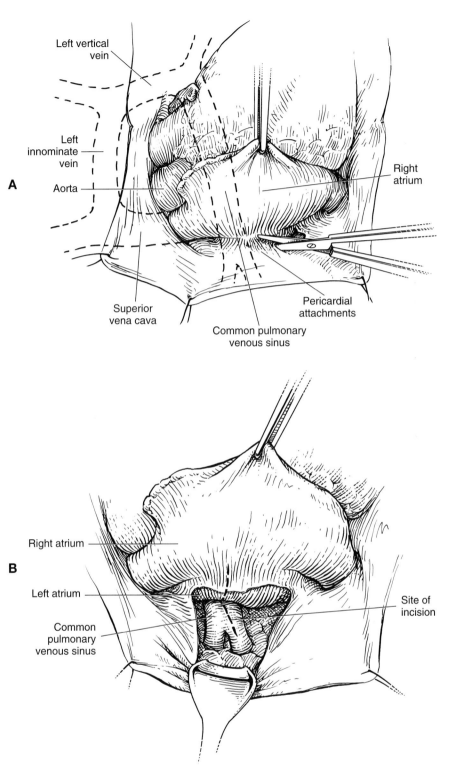

A

Left vertical vein

Left innominate vein

Aorta

Superior vena cava

Common pulmonary venous sinus

Pericardial attachments

Right atrium

B

Right atrium

Left atrium

Common pulmonary venous sinus

Site of incision

Figure 17-9   Repair of total anomalous pulmonary venous connection (TAPVC) to left innominate vein, right lateral approach. **A,** Posterior pericardial attachments of heart are cut, allowing cavae and atria to be lifted completely free of common pulmonary venous sinus, which is behind the pericardium. Left vertical vein is exposed, preferably from within the pericardium. If extrapericardial exposure is required, the phrenic nerve is elevated off the pericardium and vein. This dissection must be done sharply and with perfect exposure and visibility, because damage to this vein might necessitate its premature ligation. In this case, the common pulmonary venous sinus would have to be opened immediately to prevent severe pulmonary venous hypertension. Also, the dissection must identify the site of connection of the uppermost left pulmonary vein, so that the vertical vein may be ligated *superior* to that point. **B,** With ventricles in their normal position in the pericardium, exposure for repair (and for repair of other types of TAPVC) is obtained by elevating the atria up and to the left.[K6] Posterior pericardium over the common pulmonary venous sinus and anterior wall of the sinus are opened parallel to the long axis of the sinus.   *Continued*

The right atrium is opened (if this has not already been done) and the foramen ovale closed. Then the atrium is closed. If a single venous cannula has been used, it is reinserted and CPB is reestablished. Rewarming is begun and the aortic clamp is removed with strong suction on the needle vent, or controlled aortic root reperfusion is begun (see "Cold Cardioplegia, Controlled Aortic Root Reperfusion, and [When Needed] Warm Cardioplegic

Induction" in Chapter 3). The remainder of the operation is completed in the usual manner, including the de-airing procedure (see "Completing Cardiopulmonary Bypass" in Section 3 of Chapter 2).

An alternative method of repairing TAPVC to the left innominate vein is via a right atrial approach.[D10] This method has the advantage of allowing the anastomosis of the common pulmonary venous sinus to the left atrium to

Figure 17-9, cont'd **C,** Incision should be made over full length of sinus. Orifices of left and right pulmonary veins are located and inspected, and care is taken to avoid damaging them. A corresponding incision is made more or less transversely in the back wall of the left atrium. The incision may need to be carried onto the base of the left atrial appendage to gain sufficient length. It is carried to the atrial septum on the right, but care is taken not to enter the septum itself. When in doubt about initial placement of the left atrial incision, it is helpful to pass a small, curved clamp through an incision in the right atrial wall and through the foramen ovale, so that its tip tents the back wall of the left atrium outward. **D,** Traction sutures of No. 5-0 polypropylene are placed on inferior and superior lips of the incision into the common pulmonary venous sinus; both the sinus wall and posterior pericardium are caught with these sutures and with the suture line. Anastomosis is begun at the point shown, with the first stitch placed from outside to inside in the atrial wall, allowing suture line to be made from inside the vessels. **E,** Suture line is carried toward and around the left-sided angle of the incisions and along most of the superior side. The previously held other end of the double-armed No. 6-0 or 7-0 polypropylene or polydioxanone stitch is then used to approximate, in similar fashion, the inferior edge. Here the stitches are placed from outside to inside on the sinus and from inside to outside on the atrial wall. Suture line is carried nearly to the right–sided angle. **F,** Suture line is then completed, either with a few interrupted stitches or as a continuous stitch.

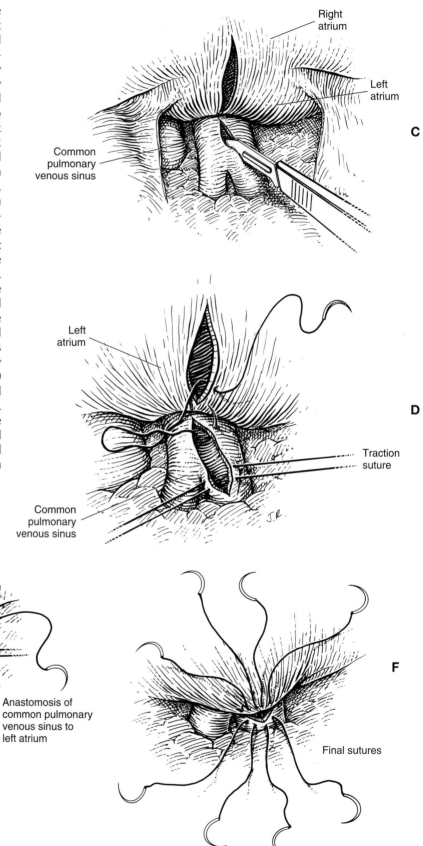

be performed in precise anatomic relationships, because there is no retraction or displacement of critical structures to gain exposure. The right atrium is incised parallel to the atrioventricular groove (Fig. 17-10, *A*), exposing the atrial septum. The membrane of the foramen ovale is excised to gain entry to the left atrium. The posterior wall of the left atrium is incised transversely (Fig. 17-10, *B*) into the free pericardial space behind the atrium. The common pulmonary venous sinus is identified lying beneath the pericardium directly behind the incision in the left atrium. An incision is made in the pulmonary venous sinus, which extends from the bifurcation on the left side to the bifurcation on the right side (see Fig. 17-10, *C*). A large anastomosis is constructed between the common pulmonary venous sinus and left atrium using fine polypropylene or polydioxanone suture (Fig. 17-10, *D*). This anastomosis has little chance for distortion because it is performed without displacing anatomically adjacent structures. Repair is completed by closing the foramen ovale with a pericardial patch (Fig. 17-10, *E*). The patch serves both to repair the atrial septum and to enlarge the left atrial filling capacity.

Fine polyvinyl catheters are left in the right atrium, inserted through the left atrial appendage into the left atrium, and inserted through the free wall of the RV and advanced into the pulmonary trunk; these are essential for appropriate postoperative monitoring.

Total Anomalous Pulmonary Venous Connection to Superior Vena Cava

A common pulmonary venous sinus is usually present in the rare anomaly of TAPVC to the superior vena cava, providing free communication between right and left pulmonary veins. When the presence of this sinus is confirmed during cooling (see "Total Anomalous Pulmonary Venous Connection to Left Innominate Vein" earlier in this chapter), the operation proceeds in the same manner as described for patients with TAPVC to the left innominate vein. The usual right atrial incision is made. The connection into the lower part of the superior vena cava is identified, and palpation is performed with a right-angled clamp to confirm the anatomic details. The sinus is disconnected from the superior vena cava by cutting across the connection. The resultant opening in the sinus is extended in both directions and the sinus–to–left atrial anastomosis made. The site of connection into the superior vena cava is then easily closed from within the right atrium, using a pericardial patch. The right atrium is then closed, rewarming begun, and the remainder of the operation completed as described for patients with connection to the left innominate vein.

Total Anomalous Pulmonary Venous Connection to Coronary Sinus

The operation proceeds as already described. The right atrium is opened by the usual oblique incision, and stay sutures are applied to the edges of the incision. The repair most commonly used includes excision of both the roof of the coronary sinus, so that it communicates freely with the left atrium, and the fossa ovalis (Fig. 17-11, *A* and *B*). The resulting large defect is then closed with a pericardial patch (Fig. 17-11, *C*).

However, occurrence of stenosis at the repair site late after operation has prompted use of the technique described by Van Praagh and colleagues.[V1] The foramen ovale is enlarged to obtain an adequate exposure within the left atrium (Fig. 17-12, *A*). The wall between the coronary sinus and left atrium is incised (Fig. 17-12, *B*), and the incision is enlarged as much as possible in both directions. The foramen ovale and coronary sinus ostium are closed separately (Fig. 17-12, *C*). The pulmonary veins then drain into the left atrium through the surgically unroofed coronary sinus (see Fig. 17-12, *D*). The remainder of the operation is completed as described for other types of TAPVC.

Obstructed pulmonary venous drainage occurs in patients with TAPVC to the coronary sinus. Thus, the surgeon must be prepared to abandon usual approaches if a stenosis is proximal to the coronary sinus itself, and proceed to anastomose the common pulmonary venous sinus, which is actually the junction of the right and left pulmonary veins, to the back of the left atrium.[J2]

Total Anomalous Pulmonary Venous Connection to Right Atrium

The repair most used in the past has been an intraatrial one in which the fossa ovalis is excised and a baffle of pericardium (or polytetrafluoroethylene [PTFE]) is placed to divert the pulmonary venous blood across the resulting defect into the left atrium. Because of occasional occurrence of late stenosis when this technique is used, whenever possible the common pulmonary venous sinus is anastomosed to the back of the left atrium directly, in a manner similar to the repair employed for TAPVC to the left innominate vein. Because the heart cannot be rotated up off the common sinus, repair is made from within the left atrium, or the anomalous connection is severed so that the anastomosis can be made from behind the heart.[B1]

Initial stages of the operation are as described for other types of TAPVC. The right atrium is opened obliquely and stay sutures applied. The anomalous connection is explored with an instrument to verify the presence of a confluent pulmonary venous sinus. The foramen ovale is then enlarged, and, working through it, an incision is made in the posterior left atrial wall. The heart is rotated up and to the right, and the point at which the opening is to be made in the common pulmonary venous sinus is marked with a suture. Working again from within the heart and through the left atrial posterior wall incision, the anterior wall of the common sinus is incised. This opening is enlarged and anastomosed to the left atrial incision, still working from within the atria. The enlarged foramen ovale is closed by direct suture. The original connection of the common pulmonary venous sinus to the right atrium is closed with a relatively small pericardial patch; it must be remembered that the pulmonary venous pathway from the right lung is beneath the patch. Alternatively, as described for the repair of TAPVC to the superior vena cava, the common pulmonary venous sinus can be detached from the right atrium, the opening in the common pulmonary venous sinus enlarged and used for anastomosis to the left atrium, and the resulting defect in the posterior atrial wall

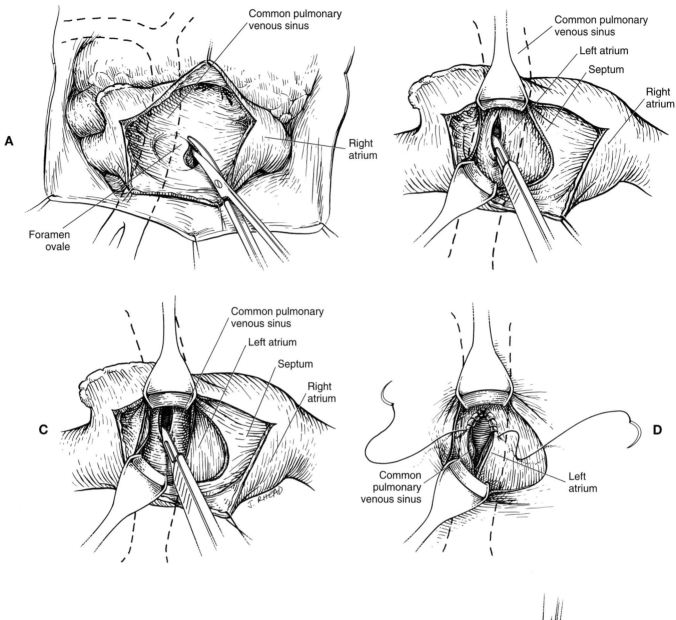

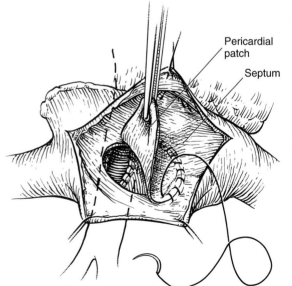

Figure 17-10   Repair of total anomalous pulmonary venous connection to left innominate vein, right atrial approach. **A**, Right atrium is incised parallel to atrioventricular groove. Membrane of foramen ovale is excised. **B**, Posterior wall of left atrium is incised transversely into the pericardial space behind it. **C**, A long incision is made in the common pulmonary venous sinus, which extends from the pulmonary vein bifurcation on the left side to the right side. **D**, Common pulmonary venous sinus is anastomosed to left atrium using continuous stitches of No. 7-0 polypropylene or polydioxanone suture. Suture line is started at apex of pulmonary venous sinus incision on the left side, placing stitches from inside the pulmonary vein. **E**, Foramen ovale is closed with pericardial patch to increase capacity of left atrium.

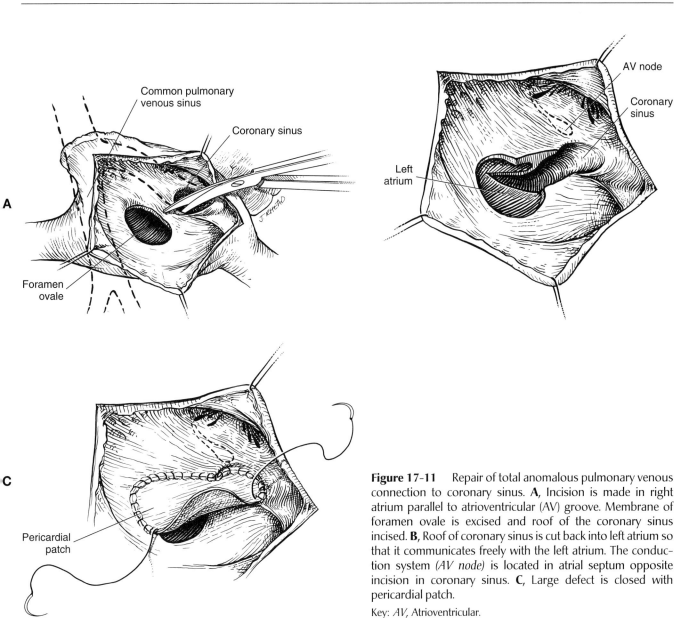

Figure 17-11   Repair of total anomalous pulmonary venous connection to coronary sinus. **A,** Incision is made in right atrium parallel to atrioventricular (AV) groove. Membrane of foramen ovale is excised and roof of the coronary sinus incised. **B,** Roof of coronary sinus is cut back into left atrium so that it communicates freely with the left atrium. The conduction system (AV node) is located in atrial septum opposite incision in coronary sinus. **C,** Large defect is closed with pericardial patch.

Key: *AV,* Atrioventricular.

closed. The remainder of the operation is completed as usual.

Total Anomalous Pulmonary Venous Connection to Infradiaphragmatic Vein

In TAPVC to an infradiaphragmatic vein, the distal (inferior) portion of the common pulmonary venous sinus is vertical, and proximally (superiorly) it forms a Y or T connection with the left and right pulmonary veins. Therefore, after initial stages of the operation have been performed as described for other types of TAPVC, a decision is made about the approach, which may be similar to that for other types, through the opened right atrium, or through the back of the left atrium directly after tilting the apex of the heart up and to the right (Fig. 17-13, *A*). Good results have been obtained by all approaches. The methods have in common (1) ligating the vertical vein at the diaphragm

(after making sure that the point of ligature is *below* the entrance of the right and left pulmonary veins into the common pulmonary venous sinus), (2) dividing the common pulmonary venous sinus above the ligature, (3) incising the anterior wall of the sinus from the transection upward and usually out onto the left pulmonary vein and sometimes the right, and (4) opening the posterior wall of the left atrium more vertically than usual and into the left atrial appendage[P3,T2] (see Fig. 17-13, *A*). The foramen ovale is closed after making the repair by whatever approach is used.

The heart is freed from its posterior attachments and the back of the left atrium is exposed (see Fig. 17-13, *A*). The common pulmonary venous sinus and left atrium are incised (Fig. 17-13, *B*). The common pulmonary venous sinus is anastomosed to the back of the left atrium (Fig. 17-13, *C*) and is ligated, and may be divided to allow the anastomosis to conform better. Alternatively, the right atrium is opened,

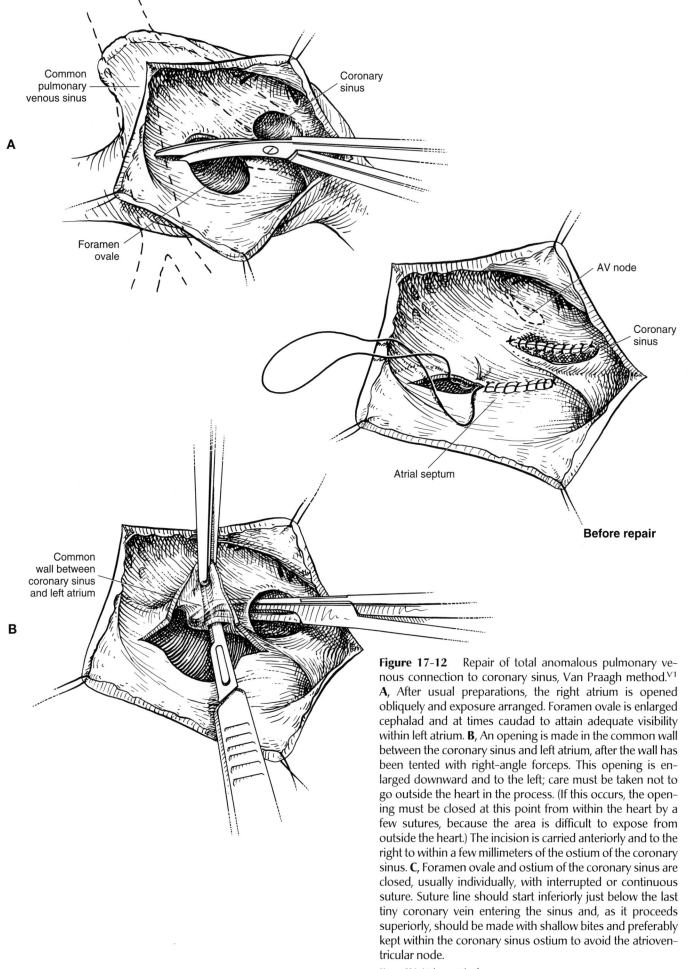

A Common pulmonary venous sinus

Coronary sinus

Foramen ovale

B Common wall between coronary sinus and left atrium

AV node

Coronary sinus

Atrial septum

C

Before repair

Figure 17-12 Repair of total anomalous pulmonary venous connection to coronary sinus, Van Praagh method.[V1] **A,** After usual preparations, the right atrium is opened obliquely and exposure arranged. Foramen ovale is enlarged cephalad and at times caudad to attain adequate visibility within left atrium. **B,** An opening is made in the common wall between the coronary sinus and left atrium, after the wall has been tented with right-angle forceps. This opening is enlarged downward and to the left; care must be taken not to go outside the heart in the process. (If this occurs, the opening must be closed at this point from within the heart by a few sutures, because the area is difficult to expose from outside the heart.) The incision is carried anteriorly and to the right to within a few millimeters of the ostium of the coronary sinus. **C,** Foramen ovale and ostium of the coronary sinus are closed, usually individually, with interrupted or continuous suture. Suture line should start inferiorly just below the last tiny coronary vein entering the sinus and, as it proceeds superiorly, should be made with shallow bites and preferably kept within the coronary sinus ostium to avoid the atrioventricular node.

Key: *AV,* Atrioventricular.

Before repair

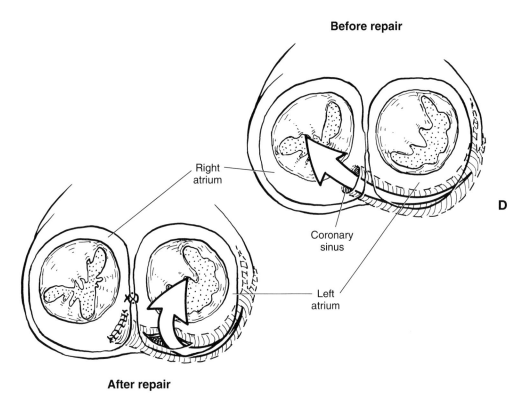

Right
atrium

Coronary
sinus

Left
atrium

D

After repair

Figure 17-12, cont'd   D, Arrow indicates the path of blood flow through the coronary sinus to the right atrium before repair. After repair, blood flow from the coronary sinus is to the left atrium above the mitral valve through the unroofed coronary sinus.

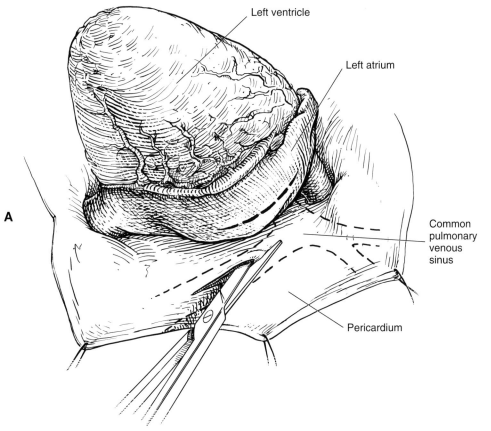

Left ventricle

Left atrium

Common
pulmonary
venous
sinus

Pericardium

A

Figure 17-13 Repair of total anomalous pulmonary venous connection draining infradiaphragmatically. **A**, Exposure of common pulmonary venous sinus and posterior wall of the left atrium is obtained by tilting the heart superiorly and to the right. The pulmonary venous sinus is identified behind the pericardium posteriorly.   *Continued*

Figure 17-13, cont'd   B, Posterior wall of left atrium is incised beginning at base of the appendage and somewhat more vertically than for other types of repair of TAPVC. A long incision is made in the common pulmonary venous sinus. Alternatively, the common pulmonary venous sinus may be ligated and divided *(inset)*. **C,** Anastomosis of common pulmonary venous sinus to left atrium is constructed using No. 6-0 or 7-0 polypropylene or polydioxanone suture. Anastomosis is started at the apex superiorly, working from within the left atrium and pulmonary venous sinus. The technique with the venous sinus divided is also shown *(inset)*.

Left atrial appendage

Common pulmonary venous sinus

B

Division of venous sinus

Anastomosis of common pulmonary venous sinus to left atrium

C

Venous sinus divided

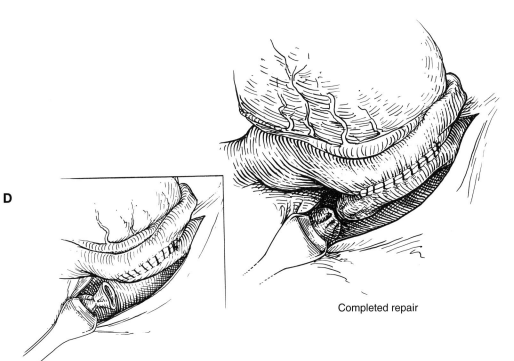

D

Completed repair

Figure 17-13, cont'd   D, Common pulmonary venous sinus is ligated below anastomosis, with care taken to place ligature below any pulmonary vein branch. The sinus may be divided to allow the anastomosis to conform better *(inset).*

foramen ovale enlarged, back of the left atrium opened, and anastomosis made as described, but from within the left atrium.

Miscellaneous Types of Total Anomalous Pulmonary Venous Connection

Some rare types of TAPVC occur, such as connection to the azygos vein. When at operation the connection cannot readily be found or dissected out, the common pulmonary venous sinus is opened and the connection identified from within it. After the connection is closed, the usual anastomosis is made between the common pulmonary venous sinus and left atrium.

Mixed Total Anomalous Pulmonary Venous Connection

Patients with mixed TAPVCs present a diagnostic as well as surgical challenge. Management of each patient must be individualized, based on analysis of the mixture presented. Techniques used for correction of some forms of partial anomalous pulmonary venous connection apply to repair of mixed type TAPVC (see Chapter 16). In some small babies in whom an extensive operation would be required for complete one-stage repair, subtotal repair can be successful, leaving unrepaired, for example, anomalous connection of the left upper lobe to the left innominate vein.

SPECIAL FEATURES OF POSTOPERATIVE CARE

The overall management of patients after correction of TAPVC is accomplished in the usual way (see Chapter 5). The relationship between left and right atrial pressures is of

particular importance. Left atrial pressure may be considerably higher than right when the pulmonary artery pressure decreases immediately after repair, particularly when a small and noncompliant left atrium acts more like a conduit than a reservoir.[P1] The left atrial pressure pulse after operation is then characterized by a steep *y* descent (Fig. 17-14). A small or borderline-sized LV contributes to this situation.

In infants and particularly neonates who present for operation in critical condition with pulmonary venous obstruction, pulmonary artery pressure and resistance may remain high in the early postoperative period, which in part may reflect the damaging effects of CPB (see Chapter 2) and postoperative acidemia. Because of this, continuous monitoring of pulmonary artery pressure for at least 48 hours after repair is essential.[S14] When pulmonary artery systolic pressure remains elevated to two thirds or more of systemic arterial systolic pressure, right atrial and RV end-diastolic pressures are usually higher than left atrial pressure, and RV stroke volume is likely to be reduced. When this situation is present, acidemia must be vigorously treated; in addition, $PaCO_2$ should be kept low (25 to 30 mmHg) by hyperventilation.[D7] Fentanyl should be continued for at least 36 hours postoperatively, and all features of the regimen to minimize the occurrence of paroxysmal pulmonary hypertension should be employed (see "Pulmonary Hypertensive Crises" under Pulmonary Subsystem in Section 1 of Chapter 5). Drugs that dilate the pulmonary vascular bed, such as tolazoline hydrochloride, prostacyclin (PGI_2), and possibly dobutamine and milrinone, may be beneficial, because vasospasm probably plays an important role in the pulmonary artery hypertension. Tolazoline hydrochloride is given initially as a bolus of $2 \text{ mg} \cdot \text{kg}^{-1}$, followed by a continuous infusion (1 to 2 $\text{mg} \cdot \text{kg}^{-1} \cdot \text{h}^{-1}$),[S10] but the precise dose of prostacyclin remains uncertain. The dose of both drugs may need to be lowered if blood pressure declines unduly.

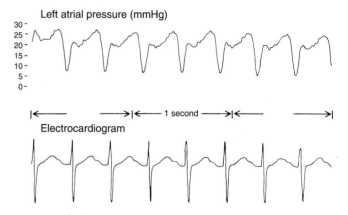

Right atrial pressure (mmHg)

Left atrial pressure (mmHg)

|← →|← 1 second →|← →|

Electrocardiogram

Figure 17-14 Left and right atrial pulses and electrocardiogram in an infant a few hours after repair of TAPVC. The left atrial pressure pulse is characterized by a rapid *y* descent, probably because of low left atrial compliance. The right atrial pressure pulse has an essentially normal contour, because of its large size and normal compliance. The electrocardiogram shows that the *y* descent coincides with the opening of the mitral valve. (From Parr and colleagues.[P1])

RESULTS

Results of operation for TAPVC can be excellent, but two types of complication still occur and can be fatal: (1) a strong tendency to early postoperative paroxysms of pulmonary hypertension and (2) delayed development and progression of pulmonary vein stenosis.

The results of repair of TAPVC at UAB from 1967 to 1991 are still relevant and form the basis for much of the discussion below. This was an unpublished study of 112 patients with concordant atrioventricular and ventriculoarterial connections (see "UAB Study," Appendix 16A in Chapter 16 of the 2nd edition of this book). The type of TAPVC in these patients is shown in Table 17-1. Thirty-seven patients had associated atrial septal defects (rather than a patent foramen ovale), and two had a ventricular septal defect. Follow-up ranged from 7.2 months to 24 years, median 11.9 years, mean 11.8 ± 6.05 (SD) years. Ten percent of patients were followed longer than 19 years, 25% longer than 16 years, 50% longer than 11 years, and 75% longer than 7 years.

Survival

Early (Hospital) Death

Although hospital mortality for repair of TAPVC in infants was high before the 1970s,[D4] for those few patients who survived beyond the first year of life without severe pulmonary vascular disease, it has been relatively low since the early days of cardiac surgery.[B1,C1,G4] This is not of much practical importance, however, because virtually all operations for this condition are done early in life. Thus, the remainder of the discussion primarily concerns this group.

Hospital mortality for repair of TAPVC in the first year of life does not approach zero, but as demonstrated by Sano and colleagues, it can be low even in patients with ob-

■ **TABLE 17-1** **Type of Connection in Patients with Total Anomalous Pulmonary Venous Connection** [a]

Type of Connection	No.	Percent of 112
Infracardiac	23	21
Cardiac	30	27
To coronary sinus	19	
To right atrium	10	
To right atrium and coronary sinus	1	
Supracardiac	53	47
To innominate vein	43	
To left superior vena cava	1	
To superior vena cava	4 [b]	
To azygos vein	2	
To multiple supracardiac sites	3	
Mixed	6	5
TOTAL	112	100%

[a] Data are from 112 patients undergoing repair (UAB group, 1967 to 1991).

[b] In three patients, there was a common pulmonary venous sinus.

structed pulmonary venous drainage.[S11] Hospital mortality in the current era in institutions with special competence in surgical treatment of congenital heart disease varies between 2% and 20%.[B12,G6,J2,L2,O1,R6,S11,T2,Y1]

Theoretically, hospital mortality should approach zero in this completely corrective operation in which the ventricles are not opened. However, the severity of the condition in most neonates and young infants presenting for treatment, combined with the small size of most patients, general inability to stabilize seriously ill neonates before operation, and relative rarity of the condition (and thus infrequency of the operation in any one center), makes this situation sensitive to even small errors. Thus, Bove and colleagues found severe acidosis on admission to be the most impor-

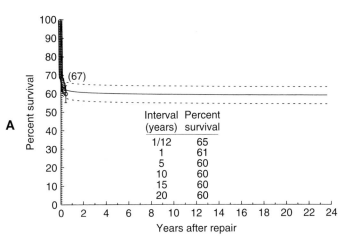

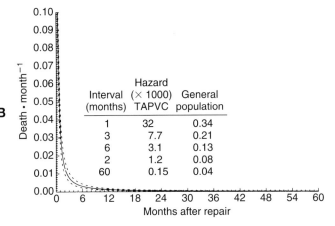

Figure 17-15   Survival and hazard function of a heterogeneous group of 112 patients after repair of total anomalous pulmonary venous connection (UAB group, 1967 to 1991). **A,** Survival. Each circle represents a death (Kaplan–Meier estimator), and solid line enclosed within 70% confidence limits is the parametric estimate. **B,** Hazard function.

Key: *TAPVC,* Total anomalous pulmonary venous connection.

tant risk factor for hospital death after repair of infracardiac TAPVC.[B16]

Time-Related Survival

Long-term survival is determined by early mortality, because death after the first few postoperative months is rare[G4,L2] (Fig. 17-15). Thus, the hazard function for death becomes similar to that of the general population by about 24 months after operation.

Modes of Death

The most common modes of death in hospital after repair are acute and subacute cardiac failure and, less often, hypertensive pulmonary artery crises (Table 17-2). In the UAB study, all deaths after hospital discharge following repair were associated with pulmonary vein stenosis except two; these occurred in patients dying 3.0 months and 3.6 months after operation for whom insufficient information was available to assign a mode of death. This has been the experience of Sano and colleagues as well.[S11]

■ **TABLE 17-2   Modes of Death after Repair of Total Anomalous Pulmonary Venous Connection** [a]

Mode of Death	Patients Dying in Hospital after Repair	Patients Dying after Hospital Discharge
Acute cardiac failure	25	0
Subacute cardiac failure	3	0
Acute pulmonary failure	1	0
Acute cardiac and pulmonary failure	2	0
Unexpected after tracheal suctioning	1 [b]	0
Catastrophic surgical event	1	0
Hemorrhage	1	0
Sudden	1 [b]	0
Uncertain	0	2
Pulmonary vein stenosis	0	8 [c]
TOTAL	35	10

[a] Data are from 112 patients undergoing repair at UAB (1967 to 1991).

[b] Probably represents hypertensive pulmonary artery crisis after repairs in 1973 and 1981.

[c] Four died in hospital with acute cardiac failure after reoperation for pulmonary vein stenosis; one died in hospital with subacute cardiac failure after reoperation for pulmonary vein stenosis; one died after hospital discharge but 1.7 months after reoperation for pulmonary vein stenosis; two died without reoperation but with certain diagnosis and awaiting reoperation.

■ **TABLE 17-3   Incremental Risk Factors for Death after Repair of Total Anomalous Pulmonary Venous Connection** [a]

	Risk Factor	Single Hazard Phase *P*
(Younger)	Age at repair	.006
	Cardiac, infracardiac, or mixed type of connection	.08
(Higher)	NYHA class I-V[K8]	.01
(Higher)	PA systolic pressure	.01
(Lower)	LV systolic pressure	.02
	Previous balloon atrial septostomy	.0006

Key: *LV,* Left ventricular; *NYHA,* New York Heart Association; *PA,* pulmonary arterial.

[a] Data are from 112 patients undergoing repair at UAB (1967 to 1991).

Incremental Risk Factors for Death

Because all deaths, except those surely or probably related to development of pulmonary vein stenosis, occurred in hospital after repair, the risk factors are essentially those for death early after repair (Table 17-3). Because of the confounding effect of the many correlated variables, interpreting the multivariable analysis is difficult, although its predictive performance is exemplary (Fig. 17-16).

Taking into account this incremental risk factor equation, interrelationships between variables, work of others, and other multivariable equations, it is clear that *infracardiac connection* (Fig. 17-17), *pulmonary venous obstruction* (see Fig. 17-16), and a *poor preoperative state* are the basic risk factors for death.[B16,B17,H3,K8,M7,T2] In some patients without a true atrial septal defect, the patent foramen ovale appears to be sufficiently small that pulmonary venous obstruction results, even though there is no anatomic narrowing of the pulmonary veins or common sinus; such a small foramen ovale probably contributes to a poor hemodynamic state in a few neonates and thus is a risk factor for death. The finding in the multivariable analysis

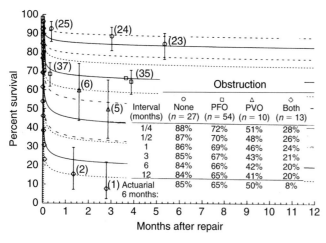

Figure 17-16 Relationship between pulmonary venous obstruction and survival among 112 patients operated on at UAB, 1967 to 1991. Format is similar to Fig. 17-15, *A*, except the solid lines, with their 70% confidence intervals enclosed by the dashed lines, were obtained by solving the multivariable equation (see Table 17-3) for each patient in the group and averaging (a method of validation).[F4]

Key: *PFO*, Patent foramen ovale; *PVO*, pulmonary venous obstruction.

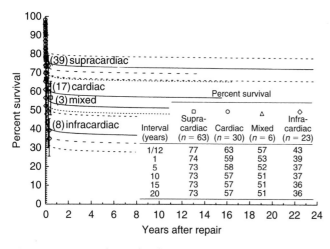

Figure 17-17 Relationship between type of connection and time-related survival among 112 patients operated on at UAB, 1967 to 1991. Format is similar to Fig. 17-15, *A*.

that a balloon atrial septostomy performed before repair is a risk factor for death, not an ameliorating factor, suggests that obstruction at the patent foramen ovale is infrequent and that cardiac catheterization and ballooning have an unfavorable effect in the critically ill neonate. On the other hand, catheter balloon dilatation of the left vertical vein in supracardiac TAPVC may provide important clinical improvement and short-term hemodynamic stability before operation.[B18]

Possibly, preoperatively small pulmonary veins predispose patients to develop the lethal postoperative complication of pulmonary vein stenosis.[J1] Therefore, this finding is also a risk factor for death after repair. Further study may

show that in rare circumstances, the pulmonary veins are so small that the probability of this complication developing is high, necessitating something other than the usual repair of TAPVC. Small size of the coronary sinus in cardiac TAPVC may also be a risk factor for death after repair.[B19]

Severe pulmonary artery hypertension in neonates is a risk factor for death (see Table 17-3), but it is highly correlated with, and secondary to, pulmonary venous obstruction and, in turn, the type of connections and clinical state preoperatively. In older patients, a mild or moderate increase in pulmonary vascular resistance increases the risk of operation,[G4,L3] and severe elevation makes older patients inoperable. The situation in these older patients is analogous to that in patients with atrial septal defect (see "Indications for Operation" in Chapter 16).

There may be a few patients with TAPVC in which the LV is so small that it per se represents an incremental risk factor. However, this is rare. Fortunately, major associated cardiac anomalies in this condition are rare as well.

Functional Status

The functional result in most surviving patients who undergo repair in infancy is excellent. At follow-up evaluation in one UAB study, 64 patients (96% of living patients) were in New York Heart Association (NYHA) functional class I, two (3%) were in class II, and one surviving patient's functional status was unknown. Surviving patients are usually asymptomatic and grow normally.

Hemodynamic Result

Pulmonary artery pressure is normal in patients recatheterized after repair unless there is abnormal cardiac rhythm.[W3] Cardiac index is normal and ranged from 2.9 to 5.2 $L \cdot min \cdot m^{-2}$ (average 3.7 $L \cdot min^{-1} \cdot m^{-2}$) in the study of Whight, Barratt-Boyes, and colleagues.[W3]

Postoperative cineangiographic studies of infants have shown that left atrial volumes are mostly within normal range, with the exceptions more often large than small. Incorporation of the pulmonary venous sinus, and the coronary sinus in some types of TAPVC, probably increases left atrial size (which was small before repair) to normal for age postoperatively. Some functional left atrial abnormality is present early and late postoperatively, perhaps based on abnormally low compliance of part of the atrium, because left atrial pressure tracings are often abnormal both early[P1] and late postoperatively.[W3]

RV volume, variable but often increased preoperatively, is normal or only mildly enlarged late postoperatively.[H3] LV end-diastolic volume, normal or abnormally small preoperatively, increases to normal late postoperatively.[H3] LV systolic function, often markedly depressed before operation, returns to normal late postoperatively[H3] (Fig. 17-18). Part of the explanation for this may be the improved LV geometry resulting from reduction in RV size (see "Ventricular Function" under Results in Chapter 16).

Cardiac Rhythm

Normal sinus rhythm is present in nearly all patients, unless there is rhythm abnormality preoperatively. However, at

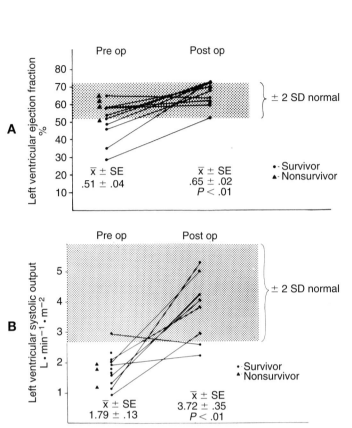

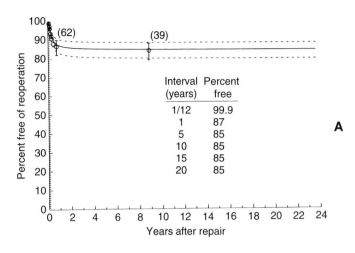

A

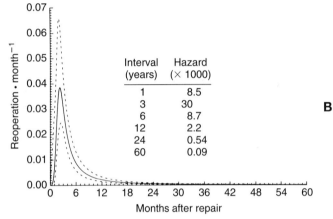

B

Figure 17-18 Depressed preoperative left ventricular (LV) systolic function returning to normal late after repair of total anomalous pulmonary venous connection (TAPVC) in infancy. **A,** Changes in LV ejection fraction. **B,** Changes in LV systolic output. (From Hammon and colleagues.[H3])

Key: *SD,* standard deviation; *SE,* standard error.

Figure 17-19 Freedom from reoperation after repair of total anomalous pulmonary venous connection in 112 patients at UAB, 1967 to 1991. **A,** Freedom from reoperation. Format is similar to Fig. 17-15, *A.* **B,** Hazard function for reoperation. Note that hazard function for reoperation peaks within 6 months of repair and declines rapidly thereafter.

least some of the preferential pathways of conduction from the sinus node to the atrioventricular node (see "Internodal Pathways" under Conduction System in Chapter 1) could be damaged by the repair.[D8] Thus, Holter monitoring after repair demonstrates that asymptomatic ectopic atrial pacemaker activity and other abnormalities are present in most patients.[B8,S15] To date, these conditions appear not to have handicapped patients.

Reoperation and Development of Postoperative Pulmonary Venous Obstruction

Reoperations are performed for two reasons: *severe anastomotic stenosis* and *pulmonary vein stenosis.* They have been necessary in every experience and are directed against pulmonary venous obstruction.[A1,G6,J2,K4,L2,O1,R4,S12,W3,Y1] With rare exceptions, they are required within the first 6 to 12 months of repair (Fig. 17-19). Patients usually become symptomatic with development of recurrent dyspnea and signs of pulmonary venous congestion, but ideally the diagnosis should be made before that stage.

Two-dimensional pulsed Doppler echocardiography is a powerful tool for evaluating patients with respect to pulmonary venous obstruction *before* hospital discharge after repair.[S6] Ideally, it should be repeated on several occasions during the first postoperative year. High-velocity turbulent flow at either the anastomosis or the pulmonary vein orifices suggests stenosis. Prompt angiographic restudy may further clarify the anatomic point of stenosis. The pulmonary veins are entered retrogradely from the left atrium to make a direct pulmonary vein angiogram and to determine pressure gradient across the site of the anastomosis.

Anastomotic Stenosis

In 5% to 10% of patients, strictures appear to develop at the anastomosis (Table 17-4 and Fig. 17-20). They usually occur within a few months of repair. However, results of reoperation are occasionally disappointing, with an important chance of a subsequent restenosis, as reported by Breckenridge and colleagues.[B13]

Despite theoretical considerations favoring use of interrupted sutures,[S4] there is no correlation between

■ **TABLE 17-4   Prevalence of Anastomotic Strictures after Repair of Total Anomalous Pulmonary Venous Connection** [a]

| | | Anastomotic Stricture | | |
Source	*n*	No.	%	CL (%)
GLH, 1969 to 1977[W3]	8	0	0	0-21
UAB, 1967 to July 1977[A1,K4]	32	3	9	4-18
GOS, 1963 to January 1970[B2]	11	1	9	1-33
GOS, May 1971 to February 1973[B13]	11	2	18	6-38
Cooley et al., 1995 to 1964[C1]	16 [b]	1	6	1-20
Hawkins et al., 1982 to 1988[H6]	23 [c]	4	17	9-29
Hawkins et al., 1989 to 1994[H6]	32 [d]	1	3	0.4-10
TOTAL	133	12	9	6-12
$P(\chi^2)$			.4	

Key: *CL*, 70% confidence limits; *GLH*, Green Lane Hospital, Auckland; *GOS*, Great Ormond Street Hospital, London; *UAB*, University of Alabama at Birmingham.

[a] The variable *n* refers to number of hospital survivors. Except in the GLH patients, in whom routine postoperative cardiac catheterization was performed, the data concern patients dying or requiring reoperation for stricture formation. The 70% confidence limits of the individual proportions all overlap; this overlap and the *P* value make institutional differences in prevalence unlikely.

[b] This may include some infants with a cardiac connection.

[c] These patients had anastomosis with polypropylene suture.

[d] These patients had anastomosis with polydioxanone suture.

stricture formation and method of suturing. It is likely, however, that the open technique of anastomosis is preferable to use of clamps.[B13,D5] Suture material may influence formation of anastomotic stricture. Absorbable polydioxanone suture as a continuous stitch has been recommended by Hawkins and colleagues for constructing the left atrium to common pulmonary venous sinus anastomosis.[H6] Late anastomotic stricture occurred in 1 (3.2%; CL 0.4%-10%) of 32 survivors having anastomosis with polydioxanone compared with 4 (17%; CL 9%-29%) of 23 patients having anastomosis with nonabsorbable suture. However, groups compared in this series were not concurrent. Based on complete absence of this complication late postoperatively, it is likely that anastomoses grow appropriately as patients grow.

Pulmonary Vein Stenosis

Unlike anastomotic stenosis, pulmonary vein stenosis may occur months to years after repair (see Table 17-2). In most instances the stenosis is due to diffuse fibrosis and thickening of the vein wall, and often to localized narrowing at the vein–left atrial junction.[F2,F3,G3,L4,T2] Pulmonary vein stenosis may be accompanied by anastomotic stenosis.

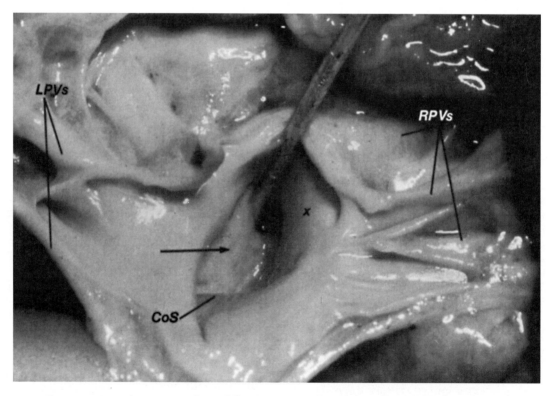

Figure 17-20   Autopsy specimen following repair of total anomalous pulmonary venous connection to coronary sinus using conventional operation with a pericardial patch. Operation was performed in a 3-month-old patient, and death occurred 6 weeks later from stenosis at repair site. Specimen has been opened from behind. The probe lies in stenotic surgically created ostium (3.5-mm diameter) between coronary sinus and pericardial patch (x). Arrow indicates a still intact portion of the roof of the coronary sinus that forms one boundary of the stenosis.

Key: *CoS*, Coronary sinus; *LPVs*, left pulmonary veins; *RPVs*, right pulmonary veins.

Pulmonary vein stenosis is usually lethal, even with reoperation and extensive attempts at revision or repair.

Lacour-Gayet and colleagues reported that of 178 patients having correction of TAPVC, progressive pulmonary vein stenosis developed in 16 (9%) within a median interval of 4 months after operation.[L5] The obstruction was bilateral in seven patients. Fifteen underwent reoperation, and four (27%) died afterward. Those authors recommended using in situ pericardial patch technique to relieve the stenosis.

Development of pulmonary vein stenosis many years after repair is exceedingly rare, but it has been reported. Kveselis and colleagues reported successful repair of infracardiac TAPVC in a 17-day-old infant who had a demonstrated absence of pulmonary vein obstruction when recatheterized 3.7 years after surgery. This patient continued to be healthy without limitations until 12 years of age, at which time he became symptomatic and important obstruction was demonstrated at the anastomosis.[K9] Reoperation successfully corrected the problem.

The only risk factor that has been identified with near certainty is preoperative size of the individual pulmonary veins.

INDICATIONS FOR OPERATION

Investigation must be undertaken promptly in any neonate or infant, no matter how young, who develops signs and symptoms suggestive of TAPVC. Procrastination leads to death in babies with obstructive TAPVC (and in some without it) or to admission to hospital in a semi-moribund state, which importantly increases operative mortality.

Once the diagnosis is made, operation should be undertaken immediately in any neonate or infant importantly ill with TAPVC. This policy should lead to surgical intervention during the first few days or week of life, frequently in the first month of life, and usually before 6 months of age.

In infants in whom the diagnosis is made between 6 and 12 months of age, operation should be undertaken promptly, because risk of operation is low, and even infants who appear to be doing well are at risk of dying before age 1 year.[B11,K3]

Rarely, individuals survive into childhood or early adult life with TAPVC and are first seen for surgical consideration at that time. Operation is advisable if severe pulmonary vascular disease has not developed; the criteria for operability are the same as for patients with atrial and ventricular septal defects (see "Indications for Operation" in Chapters 16 and 21). In TAPVC, degree of cyanosis is not helpful, because of the common mixing chamber, nor is height of mean pulmonary artery pressure relative to systemic pressure, because the shunt is not at systemic level. When pulmonary vascular disease is suspected clinically, measurement of pulmonary vascular resistance is required at preoperative cardiac catheterization. Using the Fick principle, the patient's response to a continuous isoproterenol infusion is assessed. When resistance is greater than $8 \ U \cdot m^2$, operation is indicated only when the resistance declines to $7 \ U \cdot m^2$ or less during isoproterenol infusion.[N3]

SPECIAL SITUATIONS AND CONTROVERSIES

Pulmonary Vein Stenosis

Pulmonary vein stenosis may be either a postoperative complication (as discussed previously) or a primary congenital anomaly.[H7] Congenital lesions are classified as (1) diffuse hypoplasia, (2) long segment (tubular) focal stenosis, and (3) ostial (discrete) stenosis. Diffusely hypoplastic pulmonary veins extending into the lung parenchyma usually require heart–lung or lung transplantation, and prognosis is poor. Long segment tubular stenoses of pulmonary veins with normal caliber intraparenchymal pulmonary veins may be treated, but prognosis is also poor. Treatment includes operative patch venoplasty, catheter dilatation and stent placement, or a combination of therapies. Short segment discrete stenoses located at or near the left atrial ostium of the pulmonary vein have the best chance for success with operation (patch venoplasty) or catheter dilatation and stent placement. Stent placement at operation with the left atrium open is another option. In general, congenital pulmonary vein stenosis has a poor prognosis because of development of pulmonary venous hypertension, followed by pulmonary arterial hypertension.

Mixed Total Anomalous Pulmonary Venous Connection

Repair of mixed TAPVC has been associated with high mortality, but there are several reports of successful corrections.[B13,D6,G4,K5,W4] Better outcomes are being obtained as a result of more precise preoperative study and more precise surgical correction. Occasionally in infants with mixed TAPVC, as noted earlier, subtotal correction may be appropriate at the first operation.

Delayed Operation

Opinions differ regarding the policy of immediate emergency operation described earlier. Some have advised initial balloon atrial septostomy and delay of operation for several months in critically ill neonates and small infants who are without anastomotic pulmonary venous obstruction.[M5,M6,S5,W6] In critically ill neonates and young infants whose obstruction is primarily at the atrial level (an unusual situation), balloon atrial septostomy (with a blade if necessary) and delay of operation *for 1 to 2 days* are reasonable approaches.

Preoperative preparation of the critially ill neonate by infusion of prostaglandin E_1 combined with low-dose dopamine for a few hours has been advised by Serraf and colleagues.[S14] However, such treatment may shunt blood away from the lungs and increase cyanosis in neonates with severe pulmonary venous obstruction and pulmonary venous hypertension.

Operative Exposure

Correction of TAPVC by anastomosis of the common pulmonary venous sinus to the left atrium has been carried out from a variety of exposures. From 1955 to 1956 at the Mayo Clinic, the right atrium and then the atrial septum were opened, and an incision for the anastomosis was made in the back of the left atrium. The common pulmonary venous sinus was visualized through this incision and incised, and the anastomosis was performed between it and the left atrium. This anastomosis was carried across the septum and onto the back of the right atrium when necessary, and a new septum was inserted to the right of the anastomosis. Cooley and Ochsner later described this same approach,[C5] and it continues to be used by some surgeons.[D10,H4]

A left posterolateral thoracotomy was employed in Muller's first partial correction.[M1] Roe then recommended this exposure in repair of supracardiac TAPVC using CPB.[R3] Most surgeons have, however, adopted exposure through a median sternotomy for all types of TAPVC.

Shumacker and King described carrying a transverse right atriotomy onto the lateral left atrial wall.[S7] This procedure permitted the left atrial–pulmonary venous trunk anastomosis to be accomplished essentially from outside the heart. Williams and colleagues described elevation of the apex of the heart to gain exposure for construction of the left atrial–pulmonary venous sinus anastomosis from outside the heart.[W5] Successful use of this technique was reported by Sano, Brawn, and Mee.[S11] Tucker and colleagues described exposing the structures for anastomosis of the common pulmonary venous sinus to the left atrium through the transverse sinus between the aorta and the superior vena cava.[T3]

Kirklin described incision of the posterior pericardial attachments, so that the heart and cavae are easily elevated and retracted to the left to bring the posterior left atrium and pulmonary venous sinus into good view.[K6] With this method there is virtually no risk of kinking or twisting of the anastomosis, which is the essential factor in successful repair of TAPVC.

Surgical Enlargement of Left Atrium

Trusler and colleagues found in dogs that a decrease in atrial volume of more than 50% resulted in an important reduction in cardiac output.[T4] Brighton and colleagues, using a mechanical model, obtained substantial improvement in cardiac output by adding a flexible atrium to the inlet of their artificial heart.[B14] In studying the effect of atrial compliance on cardiac performance with a mathematical electrical analog, Suga found that cardiac performance was markedly improved by increasing atrial compliance while maintaining constant ventricular contractility.[S8] Analysis suggested that increased atrial compliance facilitated the reservoir function of the atrium and maintenance of a relatively high mean atrial pressure during ventricular filling. These facts, combined with the preoperatively observed small left atrium in patients with TAPVC, have made its enlargement by shifting the atrial septum to the right attractive.[D10,G5,K7]

Katz and colleagues, on the other hand, found similar survival with and without left atrial enlargement.[K4] This may be because surgical efforts to improve left atrial size are not effective, or because adequate left atrial enlargement may result from incorporating the common pulmonary venous sinus into the left atrium.[M4,W3] Also, lack of left atrial reservoir function may rarely be critical early or late postoperatively if other aspects of the situation favor survival. Nonetheless, the repair must be done in a manner that does *not decrease* the size of the left atrium.

REFERENCES

A

1. Applebaum A, Kirklin JW, Pacifico AD, Bargeron LM Jr. The surgical treatment of total anomalous pulmonary venous connection. Israel J Med 1975;11:89.
2. Archie JP Jr. Determinants of regional intramyocardial pressure. J Surg Res 1973;14:338.
3. Arciniegas E, Henry JG, Green EW. Stenosis of the coronary sinus ostium. J Thorac Cardiovasc Surg 1980;79:303.
4. Arciprete P, McKay R, Watson GH, Hamilton DI, Wilkinson JL, Arnold RM. Double connections in total anomalous pulmonary venous connection. J Thorac Cardiovasc Surg 1986;92:146.

B

1. Burroughs JT, Kirklin JW. Complete surgical correction of total anomalous pulmonary venous connection: report of three cases. Mayo Clin Proc 1956;31:182.
2. Behrendt DM, Aberdeen E, Waterston DJ, Bonham-Carter RE. Total anomalous pulmonary venous drainage in infants. I. Clinical and hemodynamic findings, methods, and results of operation in 37 cases. Circulation 1972;46:347.
3. Barratt-Boyes BG, Simpson M, Neutze JM. Intracardiac surgery in neonates and infants using deep hypothermia with surface cooling and limited cardiopulmonary bypass. Circulation 1971;43:I25.

4. Barratt-Boyes BG. Primary definitive intracardiac operations in infants: total anomalous pulmonary venous connection. In Kirklin JW, ed. Advances in cardiovascular surgery. Orlando, Fla.: Grune & Stratton, 1973, p. 127.
5. Bharati S, Lev M. Congenital anomalies of the pulmonary veins. Cardiovasc Clin 1973;5:23.
6. Brody H. Drainage of the pulmonary veins into the right side of the heart. Arch Pathol Lab Med 1942;33:221.
7. Burroughs JT, Edwards JE. Total anomalous venous connection. Am Heart J 1960;59:913.
8. Bove KE, Geiser EA, Meyer RA. The left ventricle in anomalous pulmonary venous return. Arch Pathol Lab Med 1975;99:522.
9. Barratt-Boyes BG, Nicholls TT, Brandt PW, Neutze JM. Aortic arch interruption associated with patent ductus arteriosus, ventricular septal defect and total anomalous pulmonary venous connection: total correction in an eight day old infant using profound hypothermia and limited cardiopulmonary bypass. J Thorac Cardiovasc Surg 1972;63:367.
10. Burchell HB. Total anomalous pulmonary venous drainage: clinical and physiologic patterns. Mayo Clin Proc 1956;31:161.
11. Bonham-Carter RE, Capriles M, Noe Y. Total anomalous pulmonary venous drainage. Br Heart J 1969;31:45.

12. Buckley MJ, Behrendt DM, Goldblatt A, Laver MB, Austin WS. Correction of total anomalous pulmonary venous drainage in the first month of life. J Thorac Cardiovasc Surg 1972;63:269.

13. Breckenridge IM, de Leval M, Stark J, Waterston DJ. Correction of total anomalous pulmonary venous drainage in infancy. J Thorac Cardiovasc Surg 1973;66:447.

14. Brighton JA, Wade ZA, Pierce WS, Phillips WM, O'Bannon W. Effect of atrial volume on the performance of a sac-type artificial heart. Trans Am Soc Artif Intern Organs 1973;19:567.

15. Barnard RJ, Buckberg GD, Manganaro AJ. Ventricular volume a major determinant of minimum subendocardial vascular resistance (abstract). Circulation 1978;58:87.

16. Bove EL, de Leval MR, Taylor JF, Macartney FJ, Szarnicki RJ, Stark J. Infradiaphragmatic total anomalous pulmonary venous drainage: surgical treatment and long-term results. Ann Thorac Surg 1981;31:544.

17. Barratt-Boyes BG. Corrective surgery for congenital heart disease in infants with the use of profound hypothermia and circulatory arrest techniques. Aust N Z J Surg 1979;47:737.

18. Bu'Lock FA, Jordan SC, Martin RP. Successful balloon dilatation of ascending vein stenosis in obstructed supracardiac total anomalous pulmonary venous connection. Pediatr Cardiol 1994;15:78.

19. Bhan A, Saxena A, Sharma R, Venugopal P. Coronary sinus size a determinant of outcome in cardiac TAPVC (letter). Ann Thorac Surg 1996;62:940.

C

1. Cooley DA, Hallman GL, Leachman RD. Total anomalous pulmonary venous drainage: correction with the use of cardiopulmonary bypass in 62 cases. J Thorac Cardiovasc Surg 1966;51:88.

2. Cooley DA, Balas PE. Total anomalous pulmonary venous drainage into the inferior vena cava: report of successful surgical correction. Surgery 1962;51:798.

3. Carter RE, Capriles M, Noe Y. Total anomalous pulmonary venous drainage: a clinical and anatomical study of 75 children. Br Heart J 1969;31:45.

4. Chin AJ, Sanders SP, Sherman F, Lang P, Norwood WI, Castaneda AR. Accuracy of subcostal two-dimensional echocardiography in prospective diagnosis of total anomalous pulmonary venous connection. Am Heart J 1987;113:1153.

5. Cooley DA, Ochsner A Jr. Correction of total anomalous pulmonary venous drainage: technical considerations. Surgery 1957;42:1014.

6. Choe YH, Lee HJ, Kim HS, Ko JK, Kim JE, Han JJ. MRI of total anomalous pulmonary venous connections. J Comput Assist Tomogr 1994;18:243.

D

1. Dillard DH, Mohri H, Hessel EA II, Anderson HN, Nelson RJ, Crawford EW, et al. Correction of total anomalous pulmonary venous drainage in infancy utilizing deep hypothermia with total circulatory arrest. Circulation 1967;35:I105.

2. Darling RC, Rothney WB, Craig JM. Total pulmonary venous drainage into the right side of the heart. Lab Invest 1957;6:44.

3. Delisle G, Ando M, Calder AL, Zuberbuhler JR, Rochenmacher S, Alday LE, et al. Total anomalous pulmonary venous connection: report of 93 autopsied cases with emphasis on diagnostic and surgical considerations. Am Heart J 1976;91:99.

4. Duff DF, Nihill MR, McNamara DG. Infradiaphragmatic total anomalous pulmonary venous return: review of clinical and pathological findings and results of operation in 28 cases. Br Heart J 1977;39:619.

5. Davignon A. Cure du retour veineux anormal total du nourisson: pont de vue de médicin. Journées de Cardiologie Pediatrique. Château de Feillac. October 7, 1972.

6. de Leval M, Stark J, Waterston DJ. Mixed type of total anomalous pulmonary venous drainage: surgical correction in 3 infants. Ann Thorac Surg 1973;16:464.

7. Drummond WH, Gregory GA, Heymann MA, Phibbs RA. The independent effects of hyperventilation, tolazoline and dopamine on infants with persistent pulmonary hypertension. J Pediatr 1981;98:603.

8. Davis JT, Ehrlich R, Hennessey JR, Levine M, Morgan RJ, Bharati S, et al. Long-term follow-up of cardiac rhythm in repaired total anomalous pulmonary venous drainage. Thorac Cardiovasc Surg 1986;34:172.

9. DeLeon SY, Gidding SS, Ilbawi MN, Idriss FS, Muster AJ, Cole RB, et al. Surgical management of infants with complex cardiac anomalies associated with reduced pulmonary blood flow and total anomalous pulmonary venous drainage. Ann Thorac Surg 1987;43:207.

10. Doty DB. Cardiac surgery: operative technique. St Louis: Mosby-Yearbook Inc, 1997, p. 74.

E

1. el-Said GM, Mullins CE, McNamara DG. Management of total anomalous pulmonary venous return. Circulation 1972;45:1240.

F

1. Friedlich A, Bing RJ, Blount SG Jr. Physiological studies in congenital heart disease. IX. Circulatory dynamics in the anomalies of venous return to the heart including pulmonary arteriovenous fistula. Bull Johns Hopkins Hosp 1950;86:20.

2. Friedli B, Davignon A, Stanley P. Infradiaphragmatic anomalous pulmonary venous return: surgical correction in a newborn infant. J Thorac Cardiovasc Surg 1971;62:301.

3. Fleming WH, Clark EB, Dooley KJ, Hofschire PJ, Ruckman RN, Hopeman AR, et al. Late complications following surgical repair of total anomalous pulmonary venous return below the diaphragm. Ann Thorac Surg 1979;27:435.

4. Ferrazzi P, McGiffin DC, Kirklin JW, Blackstone EH, Bourge RC. Have the results of mitral valve replacement improved? J Thorac Cardiovasc Surg 1986;92:186.

G

1. Gross RE, Watkins E Jr, Pomeranz AA, Goldsmith EI. A method for surgical closure of interauricular septal defects. Surg Gynecol Obstet 1953;96:1.

2. Gersony WM, Bowman FO Jr, Steeg CN, Hayes CJ, Jesse MJ, Malm JR. Management of total anomalous pulmonary venous drainage in early infancy. Circulation 1971;43:I19.

3. Gathman GE, Nadas AS. Total anomalous pulmonary venous connection: clinical and physiologic observations of 75 pediatric patients. Circulation 1970;42:143.

4. Gomes MM, Feldt RH, McGoon DC, Danielson GK. Total anomalous pulmonary venous connection: surgical considerations and results of operation. J Thorac Cardiovasc Surg 1970;60:116.

5. Goor DA, Yellin A, Frand M, Smolinsky A, Neufeld N. The operative problem of small left atrium in total anomalous pulmonary venous connection: report of 5 patients. Ann Thorac Surg 1976;72:245.

6. Galloway AC, Campbell DN, Clarke DR. The value of early repair for total anomalous pulmonary venous drainage. Pediatr Cardiol 1985;6:77.

7. Goswami KC, Shrivastava S, Saxena A, Dev V. Echocardiographic diagnosis of total anomalous pulmonary venous connection. Am Heart J 1993;126:433.

8. Greene CA, Case CL, Oslizlok P, Gillette PC. "Superimposition" digital subtraction angiography: evaluation of total anomalous pulmonary venous connection. Pediatr Cardiol 1993;14:47.

H

1. Hastreiter AR, Paul MH, Molthan ME, Miller RA. Total anomalous pulmonary venous connection with severe pulmonary venous obstruction. Circulation 1962;25:916.

2. Haworth SG, Reid L. Structural study of pulmonary circulation and of heart in total anomalous pulmonary venous return in early infancy. Br Heart J 1977;39:80.

3. Hammon JW Jr, Bender HW Jr, Graham TP Jr, Boucek RJ Jr, Smith CW, Erath HG Jr. Total anomalous pulmonary venous connection in infancy: ten years' experience including studies of postoperative ventricular function. J Thorac Cardiovasc Surg 1980;80:544.

4. Hawkins JA, Clark EB, Doty DB. Total anomalous pulmonary venous connection. Ann Thorac Surg 1983;36:548.

5. Huhta JC, Gutgesell HP, Nihill MR. Cross sectional echocardiographic diagnosis of total anomalous pulmonary venous connection. Br Heart J 1985;53:525.

6. Hawkins JA, Minich LL, Tani LY, Ruttenberg HD, Sturtevant JE, McGough EC. Absorbable polydioxanone suture and results in total anomalous pulmonary venous connection. Ann Thorac Surg 1995;60:55.

7. Herlong JR, Jaggers JJ, Ungerleider RM. Congenital heart surgery nomenclature and database project: pulmonary venous anomalies. Ann Thorac Surg 2000;69:S56.

8. Hazelrig JB, Turner ME Jr, Blackstone EH. Parametric survival analysis combining longitudinal and cross-sectional-censored and interval-censored data with concomitant information. Biometrics 1982;38:1.

J

1. Jenkins KJ, Sanders SP, Coleman L, Mayer JE Jr, Colan SD. Individual pulmonary vein size and survival in infants with totally anomalous pulmonary venous connection. J Am Coll Cardiol 1993;22:201.

2. Jonas RA, Smolinsky A, Mayer JE, Castaneda AR. Obstructed pulmonary venous drainage with total anomalous pulmonary venous connection to the coronary sinus. Am J Cardiol 1987;59:431.

3. Jonas RA, Krasna M, Sell JE, Wessel D, Mayer JE, Castaneda AR. Myocardial failure is a rare cause of death after pediatric cardiac surgery (abstract). J Am Coll Cardiol 1991;17:110A.

K

1. Keith JD, Rowe RD, Vlad P, eds. Heart disease in infancy and childhood, 2nd Ed. New York: Macmillan, 1967, p. 493.

2. Kawashima Y, Matsuda H, Nakano S, Miyamoto IC, Fujino M, Kozaka T, et al. Tree-shaped pulmonary veins in intracardiac total anomalous pulmonary venous drainage. Ann Thorac Surg 1977;23:436.

3. Keith JD, Rowe RD, Vlad P, O'Hanley JH. Complete anomalous pulmonary venous drainage. Am J Med 1954;16:23.

4. Katz NM, Kirklin JW, Pacifico AD. Concepts and practices in surgery for total anomalous pulmonary venous connection. Ann Thorac Surg 1978;25:479.

5. Klint R, Weldon C, Hartmann A Jr, Schad N, Hernandez A, Goldring D. Mixed-type total anomalous pulmonary venous drainage. J Thorac Cardiovasc Surg 1972;63:164.

6. Kirklin JW. Surgical treatment of total anomalous pulmonary venous connection in infancy. In Barratt-Boyes BG, Neutze JM, Harris EA, eds. Heart disease in infancy: diagnosis and surgical treatment. Edinburgh: Churchill Livingstone, 1973, p. 89.

7. Kirklin JW. Corrective surgical treatment of cyanotic congenital heart disease. In Bass AD, Moe GK, eds. Congenital heart disease. Washington, DC: American Association for the Advancement of Science, 1960, p. 329.

8. Kirklin JK, Blackstone EH, Kirklin JW, McKay R, Pacifico AD, Bargeron LM Jr. Intracardiac surgery in infants under age 3 months: incremental risk factors for hospital mortality. Am J Cardiol 1981;48:500.

9. Kveselis DA, Chameides L, Diana DJ, Ellison L, Rowland T. Late pulmonary venous obstruction after surgical repair of infradiaphragmatic total anomalous pulmonary venous return. Pediatr Cardiol 1988;9:175.

L

1. Lewis FJ, Varco RL, Taufic M, Niazi SA. Direct vision repair of triatrial heart and total anomalous pulmonary venous drainage. Surg Gynecol Obstet 1956;102:713.

2. Lamb RK, Qureshi SA, Wilkinson JL, Arnold R, West CR, Hamilton DI. Total anomalous pulmonary venous drainage. J Thorac Cardiovasc Surg 1988;96:368.

3. Leachman RD, Cooley DA, Hallman G, Simpson JW, Dear WE. Total anomalous pulmonary venous return: correlation of hemodynamic observations and surgical mortality in 58 cases. Ann Thorac Surg 1969;7:5.

4. Lucas RV, Anderson RC, Amplatz K, Adamas P Jr, Edwards JE. Congenital causes of pulmonary venous obstruction. Pediatr Clin North Am 1963;10:781.

5. Lacour-Gayet F, Zoghbi J, Serraf AE, Belli E, Piot D, Rey C, et al. Surgical management of progressive pulmonary venous obstruction after repair of total anomalous pulmonary venous connection. J Thorac Cardiovasc Surg 1999;117:679.

M

1. Muller WH. The surgical treatment of transposition of the pulmonary veins. Ann Surg 1951;134:683.

2. Mustard WT, Keon WJ, Trusler GA. Transposition of the lesser veins (total anomalous pulmonary venous drainage). Prog Cardiovasc Dis 1968;11:145.

3. Mustard WT, Keith JD, Trusler GA. Two-stage correction for total anomalous pulmonary venous drainage in childhood. J Thorac Cardiovasc Surg 1962;44:477.

4. Mathew R, Thilenius OG, Replogle RL, Arcilla RA. Cardiac function in total anomalous pulmonary venous return before and after surgery. Circulation 1977;55:361.

5. Miller WW, Rashkind WJ, Miller RA, Hastreiter AR, Green EW, Golinko RJ, et al. Total anomalous pulmonary venous return: effective palliation of critically ill infants by balloon atrial septostomy (abstract). Circulation 1967;35:II11.

6. Mullins CE, el-Said GM, Neches WH, Williams RL, Vargo TA, Nihill MR, et al. Balloon atrial septostomy for total anomalous pulmonary venous return. Br Heart J 1973;35:752.

7. Mazzucco A, Rizzoli G, Fracasso A, Stellin G, Valfre C, Pellegrino P, et al. Experience with operation for total anomalous pulmonary venous connection in infancy. J Thorac Cardiovasc Surg 1983;85:686.

N

1. Nakazawa M, Jarmakini JM, Gyepes MT, Prochazka JV, Yabek SM, Marks RA. Pre- and postoperative ventricular function in infants and children with right ventricular volume overload. Circulation 1977;55:479.

2. Newfeld EA, Wilson A, Paul MH, Reisch JS. Pulmonary vascular disease in total anomalous pulmonary venous drainage. Circulation 1980;61:103.

3. Neutze JM, Ishikawa T, Clarkson PM, Calder AL, Barratt-Boyes BG, Kerr AR. Assessment and follow-up of patients with ventricular septal defect and elevated pulmonary vascular resistance. Am J Cardiol 1989;63:327.

O

1. Oelert H, Schafers HJ, Stegmann T, Kallfelz HC, Borst HG. Complete correction of total anomalous pulmonary venous drainage: experience with 53 patients. Ann Thorac Surg 1986;41:392.

P

1. Parr GV, Kirklin JW, Pacifico AD, Blackstone EH, Lauridsen P. Cardiac performance in infants after repair of total anomalous pulmonary venous connection. Ann Thorac Surg 1974;17:561.

2. Paquet M, Gutgesell H. Electrocardiographic features of total anomalous pulmonary venous connection. Circulation 1975;51:599.

3. Phillips SJ, Kongtahworn C, Zeff RH, Skinner JR, Chandramouli B, Gay JH. Correction of total anomalous pulmonary venous connection below the diaphragm. Ann Thorac Surg 1990;49:738.

R

1. Rowe RD, Glass IH, Keith JD. Total anomalous pulmonary venous drainage at cardiac level: angiocardiographic differentiation. Circulation 1961;23:77.

2. Rebeyka IM, Hanan SA, Borges MR, Lee KF, Yeh T Jr, Tuchy GE, et al. Rapid cooling contracture of the myocardium. The adverse effect of prearrest cardiac hypothermia. J Thorac Cardiovasc Surg 1990; 100:240.

3. Roe BB. Posterior approach to correction of total anomalous pulmonary venous return. J Thorac Cardiovasc Surg 1970;59:748.

4. Reardon MJ, Cooley DA, Kubrusly L, Ott DA, Johnson W, Kay GL, et al. Total anomalous pulmonary venous return: report of 201 patients treated surgically. Tex Heart Inst J 1985;12:131.

5. Rosenquist GC, Kelly JL, Chandra R, Ruckman RN, Galioto FM Jr, Midgley FM, et al. Small left atrium and change in contour of the ventricular septum in total anomalous pulmonary venous connection: a morphometric analysis of 22 infant hearts. Am J Cardiol 1985;55:777.

6. Raisher BD, Grant JW, Martin TC, Strauss AW, Spray TL. Complete repair of total anomalous pulmonary venous connection in infancy. J Thorac Cardiovasc Surg 1992;104:443.

S

1. Sloan H, Mackenzie J, Morris JD, Stern A, Sigmann J. Open heart surgery in infancy. J Thorac Cardiovasc Surg 1962;44:459.

2. Stanger P, Rudolph AM, Edwards JE. Cardiac malpositions. Circulation 1977;56:159.

3. Swischuk LE, ed. Radiology of the newborn and young infant. Baltimore: Williams & Wilkins, 1973, p. 40.

4. Sauvage LR, Harkins HN. Growth of vascular anastomoses: an experimental study of the influence of suture type and suture method with a note on certain mechanical factors involved. Bull Johns Hopkins Hosp 1952;91:276.

5. Serratto M, Bucheleres HG, Bicoff P, Miller RA, Hastreiter AR. Palliative balloon atrial septostomy for total anomalous pulmonary venous connection in infancy. J Pediatr 1968;73:734.

6. Smallhorn JF, Burrows P, Wilson G, Coles J, Gilday DL, Freedom RM. Two-dimensional and pulsed Doppler echocardiography in the postoperative evaluation of total anomalous pulmonary venous connection. Circulation 1987;76:298.

7. Shumacker HB Jr, King H. A modified procedure for complete repair of total anomalous pulmonary venous drainage. Surg Gynecol Obstet 1961;112:763.

8. Suga H. Importance of atrial compliance in cardiac performance. Circ Res 1974;35:39.

9. Smallhorn JF, Sutherland GR, Tommasini G, Hunter S, Anderson RH, Macartney FJ. Assessment of total anomalous pulmonary venous connection by two-dimensional echocardiography. Br Heart J 1981; 46:613.

10. Shinebourne EA, Del Torso S, Miller GA, Jones OD, Capuani A, Lincoln C. Total anomalous pulmonary venous drainage (TAPVD): medical aspects and surgical indications. In Parenzan L, Crupi G, Graham G, eds. Congenital heart disease in the first three months of life. Bologna: Patron Editore, 1981, p. 447.

11. Sano S, Brawn WJ, Mee RB. Total anomalous pulmonary venous drainage. J Thorac Cardiovasc Surg 1989;97:886.

12. Schafers HJ, Luhmer I, Oelert H. Pulmonary venous obstruction following repair of total anomalous pulmonary venous drainage. Ann Thorac Surg 1987;43:432.

13. Schamroth CL, Sareli P, Klein HO, Davidoff R, Barlow JB. Total anomalous pulmonary venous connection with pulmonary venous obstruction: survival into adulthood. Am Heart J 1985;109:1112.

14. Serraf A, Bruniaux J, Lacour-Gayet F, Chambran P, Binet JP, Lecronier G, et al. Obstructed total anomalous pulmonary venous return. Towards neutralization of a major risk factor. J Thorac Cardiovasc Surg 1991;101:601.

15. Saxena A, Fong LV, Lamb RK, Monro JL, Shore DF, Keeton BR. Cardiac arrhythmias after surgical correction of total anomalous pulmonary venous connection: late follow-up. Pediatr Cardiol 1991;12:89.

16. Sreeram N, Walsh K. Diagnosis of total anomalous pulmonary venous drainage by Doppler color flow imaging. J Am Coll Cardiol 1992;19:1577.

17. Seo JW, Lee HJ, Choi JY, Choi YH, Lee JR. Pulmonary veins in total anomalous pulmonary venous connection with obstruction: demonstration using silicone rubber casts. Pediatr Pathol 1991;11:711.

T

1. Tynan M, Behrendt D, Urquhart W. Portal vein catheterization and selective angiography in diagnosis of total anomalous pulmonary venous connection. Br Heart J 1974;36:115.

2. Turley K, Tucker WY, Ullyot DJ, Ebert PA. Total anomalous pulmonary venous connection in infancy: influence of age and type of lesion. Am J Cardiol 1980;45:92.

3. Tucker BL, Lindesmith GG, Stiles QR, Meyer BW. The superior approach for correction of the supracardiac type of total anomalous pulmonary venous return. Ann Thorac Surg 1976;22:374.

4. Trusler GA, Bull RC, Hoeskema T, Mustard WT. The effect on cardiac output of a reduction in atrial volume. J Thorac Cardiovasc Surg 1963;46:109.

V

1. Van Praagh R, Harken AH, Delisle G, Ando M, Gross RE. Total anomalous pulmonary venous drainage to the coronary sinus: a revised procedure for its correction. J Thorac Cardiovasc Surg 1972;64:132.

W

1. Wilson J. A description of a very unusual formation of the human heart. Philos Trans R Soc Lond 1798;88:346.

2. Woodwark GM, Vince DJ, Ashmore PG. Total anomalous pulmonary venous return to the portal vein: report of a case of successful surgical treatment. J Thorac Cardiovasc Surg 1963;45:662.

3. Whight CH, Barratt-Boyes BG, Calder L, Neutze JM, Brandt PW. Total anomalous pulmonary venous connection: long-term results following repair in infancy. J Thorac Cardiovasc Surg 1978;75:52.

4. Wukasch DC, Deutsch M, Reul GJ, Hallman GL, Cooley DA. Total anomalous pulmonary venous return: review of 125 patients treated surgically. Ann Thorac Surg 1975;19:622.

5. Williams GR, Richardson WR, Campbell GS. Repair of total anomalous pulmonary venous drainage in infancy. J Thorac Cardiovasc Surg 1964;47:199.

6. Ward KE, Mullins CE, Huhta JC, Nihill MR, McNamara DG, Cooley DA. Restrictive interatrial communication in total anomalous pulmonary venous connection. Am J Cardiol 1986;57:1131.

7. Williams WG, Rebeyka IM, Tibshirani RJ, Coles JG, Lightfoot NE, Mehra A, et al. Warm induction blood cardioplegia in the infant: a technique to avoid rapid cooling myocardial contracture. J Thorac Cardiovasc Surg 1990;100:896.

8. Wang JK, Lue HC, Wu MH, Young ML, Wu FF, Wu JM. Obstructed total anomalous pulmonary venous connection. Pediatr Cardiol 1993;14:28.

9. Wyttenbach M, Carrel T, Schupbach P, Tschappeler H, Triller J. Total anomalous pulmonary venous connection to the portal vein. Cardiovasc Intervent Radiol 1996;19:113.

Y

1. Yee ES, Turley K, Hsieh WR, Ebert PA. Infant total anomalous pulmonary venous connection: factors influencing timing of presentation and operative outcome. Circulation 1987;76:III83.

18 Cor Triatriatum

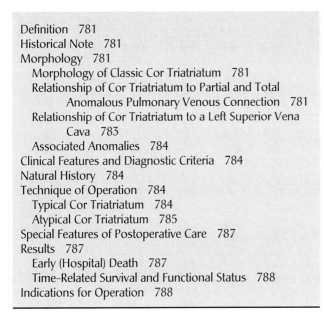
DEFINITION

Classic (or typical) cor triatriatum, or cor triatriatum sinister, is a rare congenital cardiac anomaly in which the pulmonary veins typically enter a "proximal" left atrial chamber separated from the "distal" left atrial chamber by a diaphragm in which there are one or more restrictive ostia.[1]

HISTORICAL NOTE

Cor triatriatum was apparently first described in 1868 by Church.[C1] The name *cor triatriatum* was applied to the malformation by Borst in 1905.[B1] The angiographic diagnosis seems first to have been made at the Mayo Clinic and described by Miller and colleagues in 1964.[M1] The echocardiographic diagnosis of this cardiac anomaly was described by Ostman-Smith and colleagues in 1984 and by Wolf in 1986.[O2,W2] The first surgical correction is believed to

have been performed by Vineberg and Gialloreto in 1956; the second, by Lewis and colleagues, followed shortly thereafter.[L1,V3]

MORPHOLOGY

It is unfortunate that cor triatriatum was first defined as "an abnormal septum in the left atrium,"[C1] because the description obscures the surgically important concepts about cor triatriatum, as does the phrase *subdivided left atrium*.[R1,T1]

Morphology of Classic Cor Triatriatum

Typically, the common pulmonary venous chamber (proximal chamber) is somewhat larger than the left atrium (distal chamber). The common wall between them, which may have one or more openings in it, is usually thick and fibromuscular (Fig. 18-1). Occasionally, rather than an aperture in the common wall or diaphragm, the connection is tubular.[M2,R1]

The proximal chamber is usually thick-walled, whereas the distal left atrium containing the mitral valve and left atrial appendage is thin-walled (Fig. 18-2). Despite high pressure in the proximal chamber, the pulmonary veins are not dilated. Entry of the right pulmonary veins into the proximal chamber usually bears the same relationship to the right atrium and superior vena cava as in the normal heart (Fig. 18-3).

The right ventricle is usually enlarged, but this enlargement depends on the presence and degree of left-to-right shunting at the atrial level. The left ventricle is usually normal in size or small.

The fossa ovalis may be in the septum between the common pulmonary venous chamber and right atrium, but occasionally is in the septum between the left and right atria.[N1] The foramen ovale is usually patent and stretched.

Relationship of Cor Triatriatum to Partial and Total Anomalous Pulmonary Venous Connection

In normal hearts with atrioventricular (AV) concordant connection and normally positioned ventricles (D-loop in situs solitus; see Appendix 1A in Chapter 1), the left atrium contains the left atrial appendage and empties into the left ventricle through the mitral valve. An atrial septum, with or without a foramen ovale, separates the left atrium from the

---

[1] *Cor triatriatum dexter* is a term used to describe the partially divided right atrium present in some cardiac malformations. This condition is considered later in the chapter on tricuspid atresia (see "Morphology" in Chapter 27) and is unrelated to cor triatriatum sinister.

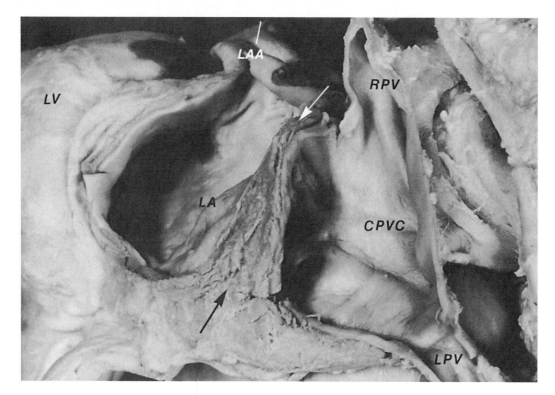

Figure 18-1 Autopsy specimen of cor triatriatum showing opened common pulmonary venous chamber (proximal chamber) separated by thick diaphragm (between arrows) from opened left atrium (distal chamber). The diaphragm has a restrictive orifice (not illustrated here) in its center. The relationship of this anomaly to total anomalous pulmonary venous connection is evident from this specimen.

Key: *CPVC,* Common pulmonary venous chamber; *LA,* left atrium; *LAA,* left atrial appendage; *LPV,* left pulmonary veins; *LV,* left ventricle; *RPV,* right pulmonary veins.

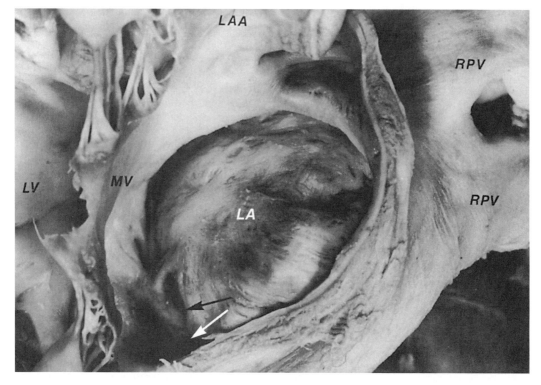

Figure 18-2 Autopsy specimen in which only the left atrium and left ventricle have been opened. Arrows indicate two small openings in the diaphragm that communicate with the common pulmonary venous chamber, to which all pulmonary veins are attached.

Key: *LA,* Left atrium; *LAA,* left atrial appendage; *LV,* left ventricle; *MV,* mitral valve; *RPV,* right pulmonary veins.

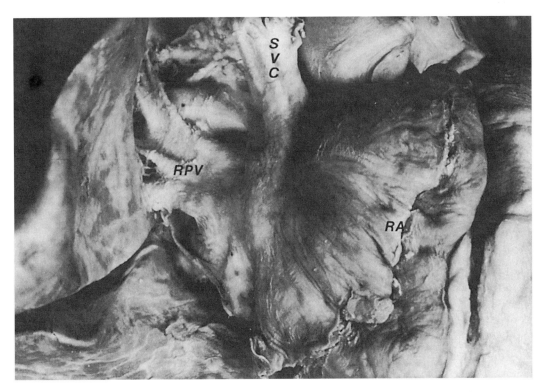

Figure 18-3   Same specimen as in Fig. 18-2, oriented anatomically with the great vessels at the top. Specimen is viewed from in front, and an incision made in the right atrium has been closed. Note normal relationship between right pulmonary veins and superior vena cava and right atrium.

Key: *RA,* Right atrium; *RPV,* right pulmonary veins; *SVC,* superior vena cava.

right atrium. In cor triatriatum, the right and left pulmonary veins can be considered as not joining the left atrium but rather as entering a chamber generally posterior and a little superior or medial to the left atrium that is analogous to the common pulmonary venous sinus found in many patients with total anomalous pulmonary venous connection (see Chapter 17). Indeed, Van Praagh and Corsini did not use the term *proximal left atrial chamber* but called it the *common pulmonary vein chamber* of cor triatriatum.[V1] Marin-Garcia and colleagues used similar terminology.[M2]

Consistent with cor triatriatum being, in essence, total anomalous pulmonary venous *connection* to rudimentary left atrium (and usually normal *drainage* to the left atrium) are details of morphology in patients in whom *partial anomalous pulmonary venous connection* coexists with cor triatriatum. When partial anomalous right pulmonary connection coexists, these veins alone may connect to the proximal chamber, with the left pulmonary veins connecting to the left atrium.[T1] Partial anomalous left pulmonary venous connection (from left upper lobe only or from the entire left lung) may connect to a left vertical vein that connects to the left innominate vein, with all other pulmonary veins entering into the proximal chamber (that is, into the common pulmonary venous chamber).[R1,S1,V1] Partial anomalous venous connection may consist of all the left pulmonary veins connecting to the coronary sinus, with the proximal chamber receiving only the right pulmonary veins and connecting through the usual small orifice into the distal left atrial chamber.[G2]

The proximal chamber, receiving all pulmonary veins, may have an imperforate portion between it and a typical distal chamber and instead connect to the *right* atrium, whereas the right and left atria are in communication through a coronary sinus atrial septal defect, with the coronary sinus itself being completely unroofed (see Chapter 19). All pulmonary veins may fail to join an otherwise typical proximal chamber separated from the distal left atrial chamber by a perforated membrane, and instead connect to a common pulmonary venous sinus behind the heart that may connect to the coronary sinus, superior vena cava, or infradiaphragmatically.[K1,V4] Thus, cor triatriatum is similar to total anomalous pulmonary venous connection, but the pulmonary veins in cor triatriatum are incorporated into the structure of the left atrium, whereas in total anomalous pulmonary venous connection, the pulmonary veins connect to sites separate from the left atrium.

Relationship of Cor Triatriatum to a Left Superior Vena Cava

A left superior vena cava coexists with cor triatriatum considerably more frequently than with other types of congenital heart disease.[A1,G2,O3] One proposed pathogenesis of cor triatriatum is impingement of a left superior vena cava on the developing left atrium.[G3] Ascuitto and colleagues reported cases in which a persistent left superior vena cava joining a dilated coronary sinus impinged on the posterior wall of the left atrium and divided it into two chambers, both of which had defects that communicated with the right atrium.[A2] It seems clear that a relationship exists between these two anomalies, at least in some patients.

Associated Anomalies

In addition to partial anomalous pulmonary venous connection and unroofed coronary sinus with a left superior vena cava joining the left atrium, other associated anomalies include ventricular septal defect, coarctation of the aorta, atrioventricular septal defect, tetralogy of Fallot, and, rarely, asplenia and polysplenia.[M2]

CLINICAL FEATURES AND DIAGNOSTIC CRITERIA

Infants with classic cor triatriatum, with a small opening between the common pulmonary venous chamber and left atrium, usually present with evidence of low cardiac output, including pallor, tachypnea, poor peripheral pulses, and growth failure.[W1] When there is associated left-to-right shunting because of an opening of the proximal chamber into the right atrium or because of associated partial anomalous pulmonary venous connection, evidence of pulmonary overcirculation and venous obstruction may be present in the chest radiograph, and right ventricular enlargement is prominent.

In children and young adults, the classic presentation is with signs and symptoms of pulmonary venous hypertension. However, like mitral stenosis, cor triatriatum may present with less classic symptoms.[S1]

Diagnosis is made by echocardiography. Originally, M-mode echocardiography provided strong clues to the diagnosis[G1,N2]; now, two-dimensional echocardiography is the standard[M3,S3] (Fig. 18-4). Cardiac catheterization and cineangiographic studies are no longer considered necessary unless major associated cardiac anomalies are suspected. However, further evidence may be obtained from selective cineangiographic studies and pressure measurements in the common pulmonary venous chamber and left atrium. If the catheter cannot be manipulated into the proximal and distal chambers from the right atrium, sometimes an arterial catheter can be advanced into the left ventricle and retro-

gradely across the mitral valve and into the distal and then proximal chamber.[V2] Gradients of 20 to 25 mmHg have been demonstrated between the two chambers.[V2]

NATURAL HISTORY

Natural history depends on the effective size of the hole in the partition (diaphragm) between the common pulmonary venous chamber and left atrium. When the hole is small, the infant becomes critically ill during the early months of life with signs of pulmonary venous obstruction (Fig. 18-5, A). Without surgical treatment, such patients die at that young age.[J1,O1,P1,W1] If the hole is larger, the patient presents in childhood or young adulthood with the signs, symptoms, and prognosis of mitral stenosis.[B2]

In most patients, the hole is severely restrictive, and approximately 75% of persons born with classic cor triatriatum die in infancy. However, when the common pulmonary venous chamber communicates with the right atrium through a fossa ovalis atrial septal defect, prognosis is better, because the proximal chamber decompresses into the right atrium (Fig. 18-5, B). These patients present with signs of a large left-to-right shunt and generally do better than those with an obstructive diaphragm.

Rarely, cor triatriatum may be discovered in an adult.[A3,M4] Delay in diagnosis may be accounted for by a lesser degree of obstruction by the membrane or by a unilateral pulmonary venous obstruction.[K2]

TECHNIQUE OF OPERATION
Typical Cor Triatriatum

Treatment of cor triatriatum is primarily by operation. However, percutaneous balloon dilatation using a double balloon technique similar to that proposed for mitral valve stenosis is possible.[K3] Relief of symptoms is good, but follow-up is too short (3 months) to establish confidence in this method of treatment.

Enlargement of the proximal (common pulmonary venous) chamber in typical cor triatriatum unassociated with other cardiac anomalies makes the surgical approach through an incision in the right side of this chamber attractive; under such circumstances, this approach is recommended. The common pulmonary venous chamber may not be enlarged to the right, and the right atrium may be enlarged because of a large left-to-right shunt from the proximal chamber directly into the right atrium. In such a situation and in small infants, an approach through the right atrium is preferable.

After usual preparations, moderately hypothermic cardiopulmonary bypass (CPB) using two venous cannulae is established (see Section 3 of Chapter 2). If the patient is an infant, hypothermic circulatory arrest may be employed. Cold cardioplegia is established as usual after clamping the aorta (see "Cold Cardioplegia, Controlled Aortic Root Reperfusion, and [When Needed] Warm Cardioplegic Induction" in Chapter 3). The common pulmonary venous chamber is opened through a vertical incision anterior to the right pulmonary veins (Fig. 18-6, A) exactly as for mitral valve surgery (see "Technique of Operation" in Chapter 11). After insertion of an appropriately sized Richardson retractor or similar instrument, the diaphragm is

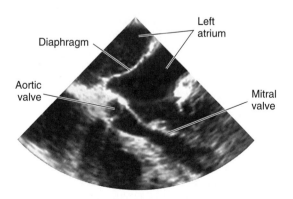

Figure 18-4 Two-dimensional echocardiogram of cor triatriatum. Computer-enhanced image shows diaphragm subdividing the left atrium.

exposed and holes in it identified. A preliminary incision out from the holes improves exposure for the definitive excision (Fig. 18-6, *B*). Orifices of the pulmonary veins on both sides are located. Position of the atrial septum is also identified, if necessary by opening the right atrium and inserting a curved clamp to displace the atrial septum into either the left atrium or common pulmonary venous chamber. Most of the common wall between the proximal and distal chambers is then excised to make as large an opening as possible (see Fig. 18-6, *C*). This procedure is usually easily and quickly done.

When an approach through the right atrium is indicated because of an atrial septal defect (which may be a foramen ovale) situated between the common pulmonary venous chamber and right atrium, this opening is enlarged (Fig. 18-7, *A*) to provide good exposure within the common pulmonary venous chamber. The diaphragm is easy to identify and expose by this approach (Fig. 18-7, *B*). The procedure described for the left-side approach is carried out and the opening in the atrial septum closed with a pericardial patch (Fig. 18-7, *C*).

The cardiotomy is closed, the heart having been filled with blood or saline solution before the last few sutures were placed. The remainder of the operation is completed in the usual fashion (see "Completing Cardiopulmonary Bypass" in Section 3 of Chapter 2).

Atypical Cor Triatriatum

As noted under "Morphology" earlier in this chapter, occasionally, patients become importantly symptomatic and present for treatment early in life with congenital cardiac anomalies that resemble cor triatriatum, but they could have total anomalous pulmonary venous connection. Others may have partial anomalous pulmonary venous connection coexisting with an anomaly that resembles cor triatriatum. Other important cardiac anomalies may coexist. A persistent left superior vena cava may be present, connecting to the coronary sinus or directly to the upper left atrium, with "unroofing" of the coronary sinus.[V5] Because almost any number of specific combinations may be encountered, the general surgical approach is described rather than a detailed description of each possible combination.

Before operation, the surgeon must determine with reasonable certainty the connections and drainage of all pulmonary and systemic veins, including the possible presence and connection of a left superior vena cava. The possible presence of both a confluence of all (or some of) the pulmonary veins behind the heart *and* a proximal left atrial chamber should be investigated. The possible connections, through apertures in the wall, of the proximal chambers with both the distal left atrial chamber *and* right atrium are determined.

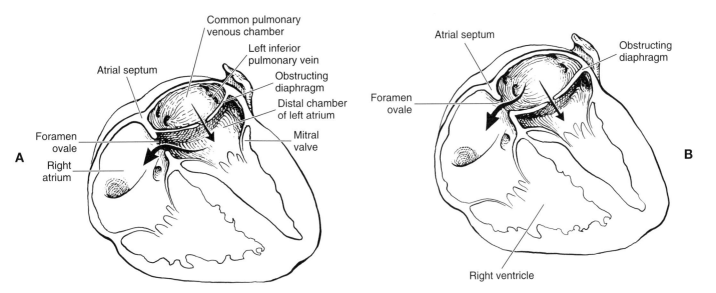

Figure 18-5   Morphology of cor triatriatum. **A**, Cor triatriatum with patent foramen ovale below obstructing diaphragm. The common pulmonary venous chamber is separated from distal chamber of left atrium by an obstructing diaphragm. The diaphragm is attached to the atrial septum medially and immediately below the left inferior pulmonary vein laterally. The lateral attachment is also closely related to the mitral valve. The left atrial appendage is in the distal chamber. Clinical presentation is that of pulmonary venous obstruction (like mitral valve stenosis) when the hole in the diaphragm is small. Distal chamber communicates with right atrium through foramen ovale, but left-to-right shunt is small. **B**, Cor triatriatum with patent foramen ovale above obstructing diaphragm, through which the common pulmonary venous chamber may communicate with the right atrium. Clinical presentation in this situation is that of a large left-to-right shunt or may mimic total anomalous pulmonary venous connection. Right ventricle may be enlarged.

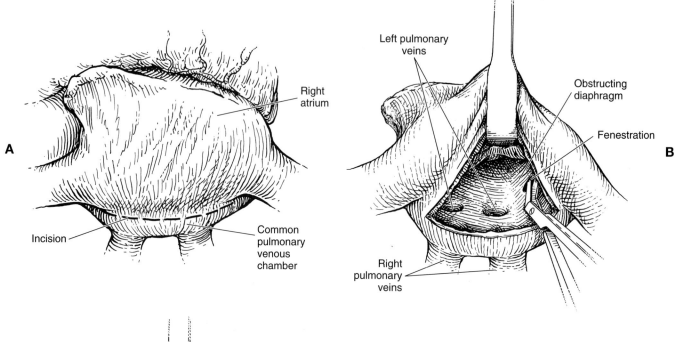

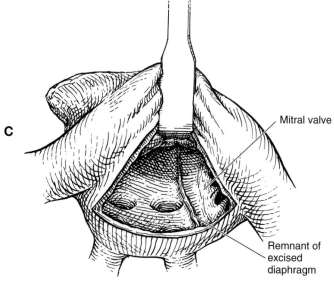

Figure 18-6   Technique of operation, left side approach. **A,** When the common pulmonary venous chamber is enlarged in older children and adults, incision is made into the chamber on the right side behind the interatrial groove, as for mitral valve operations. **B,** Anterior retraction of atrial septum exposes obstructing diaphragm with its central fenestration. Positions of the four pulmonary veins are located, noting the proximity of left inferior pulmonary vein to lateral attachment of diaphragm. Structures in distal left atrial chamber are not visible. Excision of obstructing diaphragm is started by opening the fenestration. Structures below obstructing diaphragm are identified as opening is enlarged. **C,** Excision of obstructing diaphragm proceeds to the left once its position relative to left inferior pulmonary vein and mitral valve is clarified. Diaphragm is completely excised, taking care not to penetrate free wall of left atrium. Foramen ovale and left atriotomy are closed to complete the repair.

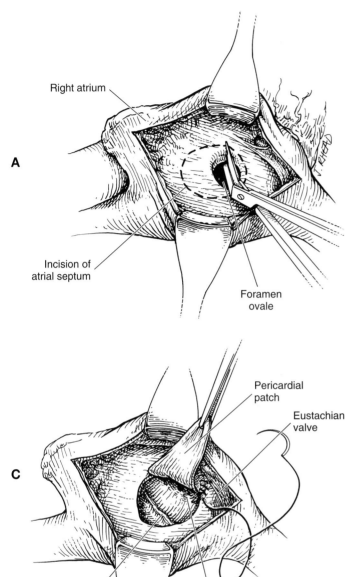

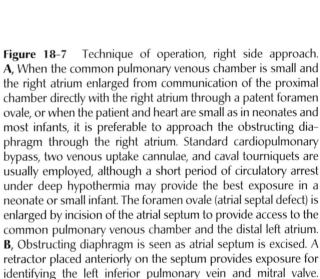

Figure 18-7 Technique of operation, right side approach. **A,** When the common pulmonary venous chamber is small and the right atrium enlarged from communication of the proximal chamber directly with the right atrium through a patent foramen ovale, or when the patient and heart are small as in neonates and most infants, it is preferable to approach the obstructing diaphragm through the right atrium. Standard cardiopulmonary bypass, two venous uptake cannulae, and caval tourniquets are usually employed, although a short period of circulatory arrest under deep hypothermia may provide the best exposure in a neonate or small infant. The foramen ovale (atrial septal defect) is enlarged by incision of the atrial septum to provide access to the common pulmonary venous chamber and the distal left atrium. **B,** Obstructing diaphragm is seen as atrial septum is excised. A retractor placed anteriorly on the septum provides exposure for identifying the left inferior pulmonary vein and mitral valve. **C,** Obstructing diaphragm is completely excised. Atrial septum is repaired using a pericardial patch.

The largest "atrial" chamber appearing on the right side of the heart should be opened initially at operation. If this is not the right atrium, the right atrium often should be opened subsequently to complete a thorough examination of the morphologic details, all of which must be verified at operation.

The repair itself is usually some combination of the repair of typical cor triatriatum, partial and total anomalous pulmonary venous connections (see "Technique of Operation" in Chapters 16 and 17), and unroofed coronary sinus syndrome (see Chapter 19).

SPECIAL FEATURES OF POSTOPERATIVE CARE

Postoperative care is as usual (see Chapter 5), with special attention given to support of the respiratory subsystem, which may be compromised by pulmonary venous obstruction existing before operation.

RESULTS

Early (Hospital) Death

Hospital deaths are uncommon after repair of *classic cor triatriatum*. Those that occur are in critically ill infants and must be considered to be related to inadequate myocardial management.[R2] Thus, between 1955 and 1967 at the Mayo Clinic[M1] and from 1967 to 1991 at UAB, 10 patients, 6 of whom were seriously ill infants, underwent repair of classic cor triatriatum, with one (10%; CL 1%-30%) hospital death. Other experiences are similar.[C2,S2]

Atypical cor triatriatum can also be successfully repaired. In the UAB experience, one critically ill young infant presented with signs of low cardiac output; the common pulmonary venous chamber drained to the left atrium through a 3-mm perforation and opened into the right atrium through a large aperture in the region of the posterior limbus, and the right atrium opened into the left atrium through a patent foramen ovale that was 3 mm in diameter. Repair was successful. This patient's malformation was the same as that described in several patients by Niwayama.[N1] Another patient, age 3 years, had a large and nonrestrictive orifice between the superiorly placed common pulmonary venous chamber and distal left atrium, a large left superior vena cava attached to the upper left corner of the left atrium, absence of the coronary sinus, a large coronary sinus atrial septal defect (unroofed coronary sinus syndrome) and tetralogy of Fallot. This patient also survived repair. Mortality after repair of atypical complex cor triatriatum is difficult to ascertain because patients are categorized according to coexisting cardiac anomalies, of which atypical cor triatriatum is a part.

Time-Related Survival and Functional Status

Life expectancy after repair of classic cor triatriatum approaches that of the general population, especially when the operation is done in infancy.[S2] Richardson and colleagues reported one late death attributed to pulmonary vein stenosis in their group of eight hospital survivors.[R1] The association of pulmonary vein stenosis with cor triatriatum reinforces the interrelationship between cor triatriatum and total anomalous pulmonary venous connection (see "Pulmonary Vein Stenosis" under Reoperation and the Development of Pulmonary Venous Obstruction in Chapter 17).

Another unfavorable late event is restenosis of the orifice between the common pulmonary venous chamber and left atrium.[J1] This may be the result of an inadequate original operation in which the common wall between the two chambers was incompletely resected.

INDICATIONS FOR OPERATION

Classic cor triatriatum, with a restrictive aperture in the partition between the proximal common pulmonary venous sinus (or chamber) and the distal left atrium, is an urgent indication for operation because 75% of patients with such malformations die in infancy. When older patients present with chronic symptoms, operation is also urgently indicated.

In atypical cor triatriatum, when the common pulmonary venous chamber opens into the right atrium, a restrictive opening or no opening is present between the common pulmonary venous chamber and left atrium, and only a small patent foramen ovale exists between the right atrium and left atrium, a large left-to-right shunt, combined with restricted left atrial and left ventricular inflow, produces severe symptoms during the early months of life, and operation is urgently indicated.

REFERENCES

A

1. Arciniegas E, Farooki ZQ, Hakimi M, Perry BL, Green EW. Surgical treatment of cor triatriatum. Ann Thorac Surg 1981;32:571.
2. Ascuitto RJ, Ross-Ascuitto NT, Kopf GS, Fahey J, Kleinman CS, Hellenbrand WE, et al. Persistent left superior vena cava causing subdivided left atrium: diagnosis, embryological implications, and surgical management. Ann Thorac Surg 1987;44:546.
3. al-Abdulla HM, Demany MA, Zimmerman HA. Cor triatriatum: preoperative diagnosis in an adult patient. Am J Cardiol 1970;26:310.

B

1. Borst H. Ein Cor triatriatum. Zentralbl Allg Pathol 1905;16:812.
2. Belcher JR, Somerville W. Cor triatriatum (stenosis of the common pulmonary vein): successful treatment of a case. Br Med J 1959;1:1280.

C

1. Church WS. Congenital malformation of the heart: abnormal septum in left auricle. Trans Pathol Soc Lond 1867/1868;19:188.
2. Carpena C, Colokathis B, Subramanian S. Cor triatriatum. Ann Thorac Surg 1974;17:325.

G

1. Gibson DG, Honey M, Lennox SC. Cor triatriatum: diagnosis by echocardiography. Br Heart J 1974;36:835.
2. Geggel RL, Fulton DR, Chernoff HL, Cleveland R, Hougen TJ. Cor triatriatum associated with partial anomalous pulmonary venous connection to the coronary sinus: echocardiographic and angiocardiographic features. Pediatr Cardiol 1987;8:279.
3. Gharagozloo F, Bulkley BH, Hutchings GM. A proposed pathogenesis of cor triatriatum: impingement of the left superior vena cava on the developing left atrium. Am Heart J 1977;94:618.

J

1. Jorgensen CR, Ferlic RM, Varco RL, Lillehei CW, Eliot RS. Cor triatriatum: Review of the surgical aspects with a follow-up report on the first patient successfully treated with surgery. Circulation 1967;36:101.

K

1. Kirk AJ, Pollock JC. Concomitant cor triatriatum and coronary sinus total anomalous pulmonary venous connection. Ann Thorac Surg 1987;44:203.
2. Kerensky RA, Bertolet BD, Epstein M. Late discovery of cor triatriatum as a result of unilateral pulmonary venous obstruction. Am Heart J 1995;130:624.
3. Kerkar P, Vora A, Kulkarni H, Narula D, Goyal V, Dalvi B. Percutaneous balloon dilatation of cor triatriatum sinister. Am Heart J 1996;132:888.

L

1. Lewis FJ, Varco RL, Taufic M, Niazi SA. Direct vision repair of triatrial heart and total anomalous pulmonary venous drainage. Surg Gynecol Obstet 1956;102:713.

M

1. Miller GA, Ongley PA, Anderson MW, Kincaid OW, Swan HJ. Cor triatriatum: hemodynamic and angiocardiographic diagnosis. Am Heart J 1964;68:298.
2. Marin-Garcia J, Tandon R, Lucas RV Jr, Edwards JE. Cor triatriatum: study of 20 cases. Am J Cardiol 1975;35:59.
3. Muhiudeen-Russell IA, Silverman NH. Images in cardiovascular medicine. Cor triatriatum in an infant. Circulation 1997;95:2700.
4. McGuire LB, Nolan TB, Reeve R, Dammann JF. Cor triatriatum as a problem of adult heart disease. Circulation 1965;30:263.

N

1. Niwayama G. Cor triatriatum. Am Heart J 1960;59:291.
2. Nimura Y, Matsumoto M, Beppu S, Matsuo H, Sakakibara H. Noninvasive preoperative diagnosis of cor triatriatum with ultrasonocardiotomogram and conventional echocardiogram. Am Heart J 1974;88:240.

O

1. Oelert H, Breckenridge IM, Rosland G, Stark J. Surgical treatment of cor triatriatum in a 4½-month-old infant. Thorax 1973;28:242.
2. Ostman-Smith I, Silverman NH, Oldershaw P, Lincoln C, Shinebourne EA. Cor triatriatum sinistrum: diagnostic features on cross sectional echocardiography. Br Heart J 1984;51:211.
3. Oglietti J, Cooley DA, Izquierdo JP, Ventemiglia R, Muasher I, Hallman GL, et al. Cor triatriatum: operative results in 25 patients. Ann Thorac Surg 1983;35:415.

P

1. Perry LW, Scott LD, McClenathan JE. Cor triatriatum: preoperative diagnosis and successful repair in a small infant. J Pediatr 1967;71:840.

R

1. Richardson JV, Doty DB, Siewers RD, Zuberbuhler JR. Cor triatriatum (subdivided left atrium). J Thorac Cardiovasc Surg 1981;81:232.
2. Rodefeld MD, Brown JW, Heimansohn DA, King H, Girod DA, Hurwitz RA, et al. Cor triatriatum: clinical presentation and surgical results in 12 patients. Ann Thorac Surg 1990;50:562.

S

1. Somerville J. Masked cor triatriatum. Br Heart J 1966;28:55.
2. Salomone G, Tiraboschi R, Crippa M, Ferri F, Bianchi T, Parenzan L. Cor triatriatum. Clinical presentation and operative results. J Thorac Cardiovasc Surg 1991;101:1088.
3. Shuler CO, Fyfe DA, Sade R, Crawford FA. Transesophageal echocardiographic evaluation of cor triatriatum in children. Am Heart J 1995;129:507.

T

1. Thilenius OG, Bharati S, Lev M. Subdivided left atrium: an expanded concept of cor triatriatum sinistrum. Am J Cardiol 1976;37:743.

V

1. Van Praagh R, Corsini I. Cor triatriatum: pathologic anatomy and a consideration of morphogenesis based on 13 postmortem cases and a study of normal development of the pulmonary vein and atrial septum in 83 human embryos. Am Heart J 1969;78:379.
2. van der Horst RL, Gotsman MS. Cor triatriatum: angiographic diagnosis by retrograde catheterization of the dorsal accessory chamber. Br J Radiol 1971;44:273.
3. Vineberg A, Gialloreto O. Report of a successful operation for stenosis of common pulmonary vein (cor triatriatum). Can Med Assoc J 1956;74:719.
4. Vouhe PR, Baillot-Vernant F, Fermont L, Bical O, Leca F, Neveus JY. Cor triatriatum and total anomalous pulmonary venous connection: a rare, surgically correctable anomaly. J Thorac Cardiovasc Surg 1985;90:443.
5. van Son JA, Autschbach R, Mohr FW. Repair of cor triatriatum associated with partially unroofed coronary sinus. Ann Thorac Surg 1999;68:1414.

W

1. Wolf RR, Ruttenberg HD, Desilets DT, Mulder DE. Cor triatriatum. J Thorac Cardiovasc Surg 1968;56:114.
2. Wolf WJ. Diagnostic features and pitfalls in the two-dimensional echocardiographic evaluation of a child with cor triatriatum. Pediatr Cardiol 1986;6:211.

in this chapter, despite the controversy concerning proper classification of such anomalies (see "Atrial Isomerism" under Morphology later in this chapter; see also Chapter 44).

HISTORICAL NOTE

Unroofed coronary sinus syndrome was unknown to cardiac pathologists before the era of cardiac catheterization and cardiac surgery. In 1954, Campbell and Deuchar referred to instances of LSVC attached to the left atrium.[C1] Although they did not have such an example in their own series of LSVC, they appreciated that in such cases there was no true coronary sinus. That same year, Winter, a radiologist at Hahnemann Hospital in Philadelphia, published a report that identified persistent LSVC attached to the left atrium, and 2 years later, Friedlich and colleagues identified LSVC entering the left atrium by cardiac catheterization in four patients.[F1,W1] An isolated case was also reported by Tuchman and colleagues in 1956.[T1] However, true understanding of the morphology of the syndrome awaited the classic paper by Raghib, Edwards, and colleagues in 1965.[R2] The descriptive phrase "unroofed coronary sinus" was first used by Helseth and Peterson in 1974.[H2]

In cyanotic patients with a communication between the left and right SVC, the LSVC was first ligated (appropriately) by Hurwitt and colleagues in 1955 and then by Davis and colleagues in 1959.[D1,H1] In 1965, Taybi and colleagues reported a ligation and mentioned "transferring the left SVC to the right atrium," but presumably this was unsuccessful, because no further details were given.[T2] The first report of successful repair was from the Mayo Clinic in 1963.[R1] In this case, a tunnel was constructed from the posterior wall of the left atrium. In a second case, a large pericardial atrial baffle was constructed that corrected the anomalous connection of both the SVC and the inferior vena cava (IVC) to a left-sided atrium.[M2] This procedure was also described by Helseth and Peterson in 1974.[H2]

MORPHOLOGY

Completely Unroofed Coronary Sinus with Persistent Left Superior Vena Cava

In one form of unroofed coronary sinus syndrome, the coronary sinus does not exist, because the common wall between it and the left atrium is absent. A persistent LSVC, which usually becomes continuous with the coronary

DEFINITION

Unroofed coronary sinus syndrome is a spectrum of cardiac anomalies in which part or all of the common wall between the coronary sinus and the left atrium is absent.

Hearts with atrial isomerism and a left-sided superior vena cava (LSVC) entering a left-sided atrium are included

sinus, connects to the left upper corner of the left atrium.[S1] The site of connection of the LSVC to the left atrium appears to be constant and lies between the opening of the left atrial appendage anteriorly and slightly superiorly and the opening of the left pulmonary veins posteriorly and inferiorly. The pulmonary veins may enter the left atrium more superiorly than usual in this form of the syndrome. A coronary sinus atrial septal defect (ASD) is present in the posteroinferior region of the atrial septum, in the usual position of the ostium of the coronary sinus (see Chapter 16, Fig. 16-5). The ASD is separated from the atrioventricular (AV) valve ring by a remnant of atrial septum (in contrast to an ostium primum ASD), and its posterior margin is formed by the atrial wall where it joins the IVC. There may be a separate foramen ovale ASD or a single large ASD formed by the confluence of both defects. The coronary sinus ASD may be confluent with an ostium primum ASD, or there may be a common atrium.

Because the coronary sinus does not exist, individual coronary veins connect separately to the inferior aspect of the left atrium. Some also connect to the right atrium.

Of considerable surgical importance is the fact that the left innominate vein is absent in 80% to 90% of cases of unroofed coronary sinus syndrome and LSVC.[Q1,R1] The right SVC is frequently small and may be absent. The IVC not infrequently crosses to the left side below the diaphragm to enter the left hemiazygos vein, which joins the LSVC. The hepatic veins usually enter the inferior aspect of the right atrium, but they too may enter the inferior wall of the left atrium. When all the systemic veins enter a morphologically left atrium, total anomalous systemic venous connection is present.

Completely Unroofed Coronary Sinus without Persistent Left Superior Vena Cava

In some cases, the syndrome is characterized by a completely unroofed coronary sinus without a persistent LSVC. Such cases consist of a coronary sinus type of ASD and total absence of the coronary sinus because of absence of the partition between it and the left atrium.

Partially Unroofed Midportion of Coronary Sinus

Another form of the syndrome is characterized by a partially unroofed midportion of the coronary sinus (also called biatrial opening of coronary sinus, or coronary sinus-to-left atrial window or fenestration). In this anomaly, an aperture is present in the midportion of the wall between the coronary sinus and left atrium. Through this aperture, a left-to-right or right-to-left shunt occurs, depending on whether obstruction is present to left atrial or right atrial outflow.[F2]

When this rare form of unroofed coronary sinus syndrome occurs as an isolated lesion, there may be a large left-to-right shunt.[A1,M1] It has also been reported as a major cardiac anomaly associated with tricuspid atresia, recognized only after the Fontan repair has elevated the right atrial pressure and produced a right-to-left shunt.[F2,R3,R4]

When midportion unroofing occurs in the presence of LSVC, there is a right-to-left shunt into the left atrium.

Partially Unroofed Terminal Portion of Coronary Sinus

Particularly in the presence of an atrioventricular septal defect (see "Complete Unroofed Coronary Sinus with Left Superior Vena Cava" under Morphology in Chapter 20), the coronary sinus ostium may open into the left atrium rather than the right. Also, a localized unroofing of the sinus may occur just before it enters the ostium of the coronary sinus, resulting in a coronary sinus ASD with preservation of the coronary sinus (see "Coronary Sinus Defect" under Morphology in Chapter 15). Such anomalies can be considered to be unroofing (or absence) of the terminal portion of the coronary sinus.

Relationship of Unroofed Coronary Sinus Syndrome to Cor Triatriatum and Atrioventricular Septal Defect

As indicated, when a completely unroofed coronary sinus with persistent LSVC is present, both the left and right pulmonary veins may enter the left atrium more superiorly than usual. Sometimes this condition is accompanied by a mild or moderate narrowing between the portion of the left atrium to which the pulmonary veins are attached (the common pulmonary venous chamber) and that to which the LSVC, left atrial appendage, and mitral valve are attached (see "Relationship of Cor Triatriatum to a Left Superior Vena Cava" under Morphology in Chapter 18).

Unroofed coronary sinus syndrome has as its most common major associated cardiac anomaly an atrioventricular septal defect, not infrequently with a common atrium (see Chapter 20). Interestingly, atrioventricular septal defects are more commonly associated with persistent LSVC than are other types of ASD.

Atrial Isomerism

Many patients with an LSVC connecting to a left-sided atrium have atrial isomerism (see Chapter 44), and the majority of such patients have an atrioventricular septal defect. Thus, in an unpublished autopsy series from GLH of 26 hearts with the LSVC connecting to the left-sided atrium, only three were examples of classic unroofed coronary sinus syndrome. Twenty-three hearts had atrial isomerism, 17 with bilateral morphologically right atria (most with asplenia) and six with bilateral morphologically left atria (most with polysplenia). Of the 23, 20 had an atrioventricular septal defect in addition to numerous other cardiac anomalies. When bilateral morphologically right atria are present, the LSVC enters the left-sided right atrium behind a typical crista terminalis and is not therefore an example of unroofed coronary sinus, even though the coronary sinus is usually absent. When bilateral morphologically left atria are present, the LSVC may or may not be part of an unroofed coronary sinus syndrome. In such cases, however, the coronary sinus is frequently absent.

CLINICAL FEATURES AND DIAGNOSTIC CRITERIA

In most cases, diagnosis of unroofed coronary sinus syndrome is made by two-dimensional echocardiography and confirmed at operation. Demonstration of an LSVC by catheter passage into the vein or by cineangiography suggests the diagnosis, which is confirmed at operation if the LSVC can also be shown to drain into the left atrium. Diagnosis of a partially unroofed midportion of the coronary sinus can be made by cineangiography after injection into the right atrium, when right atrial pressure is higher than left (such as after the Fontan operation). Konstam and colleagues have pointed out that radionuclide angiography can be diagnostic, because intravenous injections into the left arm show much larger right-to-left shunting than those into the right arm.[K1] Diagnosis sometimes can be made by cross-sectional and contrast echocardiography.[S3]

Generally, however, diagnosis is made by the surgeon viewing external and internal morphology of the heart at operation.

NATURAL HISTORY

Cyanosis from right-to-left shunting dominates the clinical picture of isolated completely unroofed coronary sinus with persistent LSVC and determines its natural history. In the series of Quaegebeur and colleagues, cyanosis was mild (all patients were younger than age 17), but it was severe in some older patients in other series.[Q1]

Cerebral embolization manifested by transient ischemic attacks or stroke and brain abscess complicate the life history in 10% to 25% of patients[Q1,R2] (Table 19-1). This situation is similar to that in other types of right-to-left shunting. Presumably, life expectancy is considerably reduced by these complications and by other problems associated with increasing cyanosis and polycythemia.

TECHNIQUE OF OPERATION

Isolated Completely Unroofed Coronary Sinus with Persistent Left Superior Vena Cava

Anesthesia and preparation of the patient for repair of isolated completely unroofed coronary sinus with persistent LSVC are as described in Section 3 of Chapter 2. When the diagnosis is known preoperatively, the anesthesiologist inserts a pressure-monitoring line into the *left* external or, preferably, internal jugular vein.

Operation may be done with cardiopulmonary bypass (CPB) at 25°C and the usual direct caval cannulation (see "Clinical Methodology of Cardiopulmonary Bypass" in Section 3 of Chapter 2); venous blood from the LSVC is collected with a sump sucker connected to the pump-oxygenator. Alternatively, in infants, a single venous cannula and repair during hypothermic circulatory arrest may be used. Myocardial management is conducted as for other cardiac operations (see "Methods of Myocardial Management during Cardiac Surgery" in Chapter 3).

Intracardiac Repair

After sternotomy a large piece of pericardium is excised and set aside (see Chapter 16). After aortic clamping and infusion of cardioplegic solution, the right atrium is opened through

■ **TABLE 19-1   Some Details of Eight Patients with Isolated Completely Unroofed Coronary Sinus with Left Superior Vena Cava**

Data	No. of Patients [a]
Age	
1-11 years	8
History	
Brain abscess or TIA	2
Mild arterial desaturation	8
Anatomy	
LSVC to upper corner of left atrium	8
LSVC to innominate vein	1
Coronary sinus type ASD	4
Isolated	2
With foramen ovale	2
Confluent ASD (coronary sinus plus fossa ovalis type)	4
Management	
Ligation of LSVC and closure of ASD	1
Roofing of coronary sinus	
With posterior wall of left atrium	4
With pericardium	2
With opened polyester tube	1

(Data from Quaegebeur and colleagues.[Q1])

Key: *ASD,* Atrial septal defect; *LSVC,* left superior vena cava; *TIA,* transient ischemic attack.

[a] Numbers are not cumulative.

the usual oblique incision. Orifices of the three cavae are identified with certainty. Repair can be accomplished satisfactorily using one of two methods (the original method of "reroofing the coronary sinus"[Q1,R1,S2] is no longer used because of its technical difficulty and because the left pulmonary veins are at risk of obstruction by the baffle). One method consists of excising the entire atrial septum except for the anterior limbus, which is preserved as a protection for the AV node and bundle of His.[C2,M2] A pericardial patch is sutured into place as a repositioned atrial septum, and all three caval orifices are positioned on the right side of this septum (Figs. 19-1 and 19-2). This method is particularly useful when a common atrium is part of the cardiac anomaly.

A second method, described by Sand and colleagues, consists of "rerouting the coronary sinus" to the roof of the left atrium (Fig. 19-3) and then reconstructing the atrial septum.[S4]

After the right atriotomy is closed, the caval tapes are released and the aortic clamp is removed. Usual de-airing maneuvers are performed (see "De-airing the Heart" in Section 3 of Chapter 2), and the operation is completed.

Extracardiac Repair

A third method involves extracardiac correction of the unroofed coronary sinus in combination with the associated intracardiac repair. If the innominate vein is absent, the LSVC is divided at its junction with the left atrium, and the opening in the left atrium is oversewn. The divided end of the LSVC is anastomosed to the side of the right SVC either anterior or posterior to the aorta.[R5,V1] Alternatively, the LSVC can be anastomosed to the right atrial appendage or to the left pulmonary artery as a bidirectional superior cavopulmonary shunt.[F3,R5,S1,T2] A continuous No. 6-0 or 7-0 absorbable monofilament suture is used for these anastomoses.

If the innominate vein is present but restrictive, it can be enlarged with a patch of autologous pericardium.[V2] The LSVC is then divided at its junction with the left atrium, and both ends are oversewn.

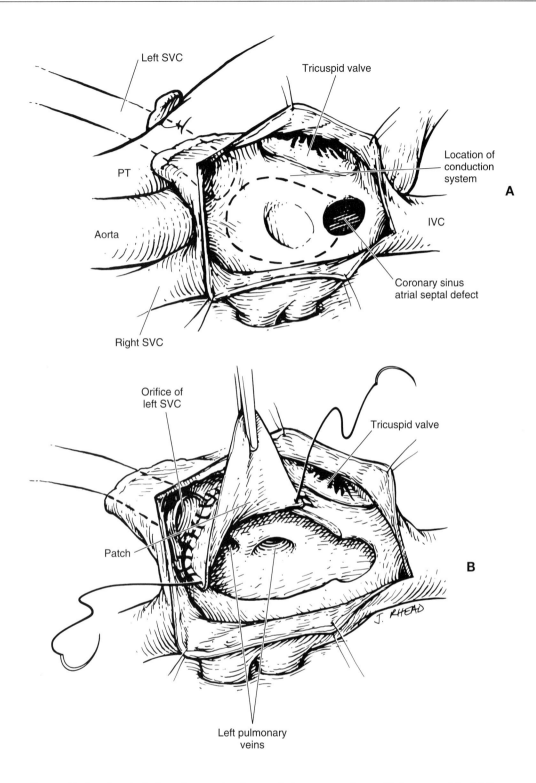

Figure 19-1   One technique for repair of unroofed coronary sinus with large persistent left superior vena cava (LSVC) entering the upper left corner of the left atrium. **A,** Exposure is through an oblique right atriotomy. Dashed circle represents line of incision in atrial septum. **B,** Atrial septum has been excised, with care taken to preserve anterior limbus as protection for atrioventricular node and bundle of His. Orifices of left pulmonary veins are visible. Anterosuperior to these orifices is the orifice of the LSVC, and just anterior to that is the left atrial appendage. A pericardial patch is sutured to the posterior rim of the LSVC using a continuous No. 4-0 or 5-0 polypropylene suture.

Key: *IVC,* Inferior vena cava; *PT,* pulmonary trunk; *SVC,* superior vena cava.   *Continued*

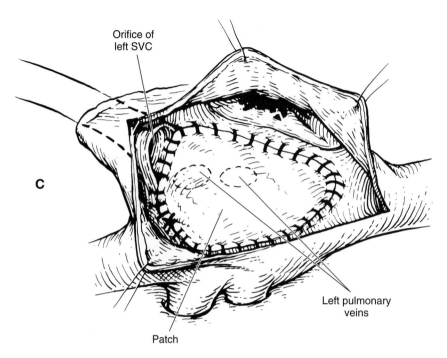

Orifice of
left SVC

C

Left pulmonary
veins

Patch

Figure 19-1, cont'd **C,** The suture line is continued along the rim of the atrial septum and the rim of the coronary sinus atrial septal defect.

Key: *SVC,* Superior vena cava.

These extracardiac techniques eliminate the need for constructing an intraatrial baffle or tunnel. They can be performed during the period of rewarming after correction of associated intracardiac anomalies, thus reducing the durations of myocardial ischemia and CPB. They also eliminate the potential for creation of a small left atrium with reduced compliance and reduce the potential for development of pulmonary venous obstruction.

Partially Unroofed Midportion of Coronary Sinus

Repair of a partially unroofed midportion of the coronary sinus is made through a right atrial approach. The important step is defining the aperture, which is accomplished by passing a small forceps or clamp into the coronary sinus, through the defect, and into the left atrium, verifying that the tip has, in fact, entered the left atrium. Closure can usually be made from within the coronary sinus, whether there is an LSVC or not. Alternatively, repair can be made from the left atrial side, approaching the defect through an opening in the atrial septum.

Partially Unroofed Terminal Portion of Coronary Sinus

A partially unroofed terminal portion of the coronary sinus occurs primarily in association with atrioventricular septal

defects. The coronary sinus ostium is simply left to drain into the left atrium by the repair (see Chapter 20).

Unroofed Coronary Sinus Syndrome with Left Superior Vena Cava and Atrioventricular Septal Defect

For unroofed coronary sinus syndrome with LSVC and atrioventricular septal defect, repair is made exactly as described for uncomplicated cases except that, rather than being attached to the limbus, the pericardial baffle is attached to the crest of the ventricular septum and AV valves (partial atrioventricular septal defect) or to the top of the polyester patch that is used to close the interventricular communication (complete atrioventricular septal defect) (see Fig. 19-2; see also Chapter 44 and Fig. 44-4).

Completely Unroofed Coronary Sinus Associated with Other Complex Cardiac Anomalies

No simple description can be given of repairing complex anomalies in which unroofed coronary sinus syndrome is but a part. Such cases are often unique, and the surgeon must study the malformation in detail and plan the repair according to the findings. General comments concerning atypical cor triatriatum may be applicable (see Chapter 18).

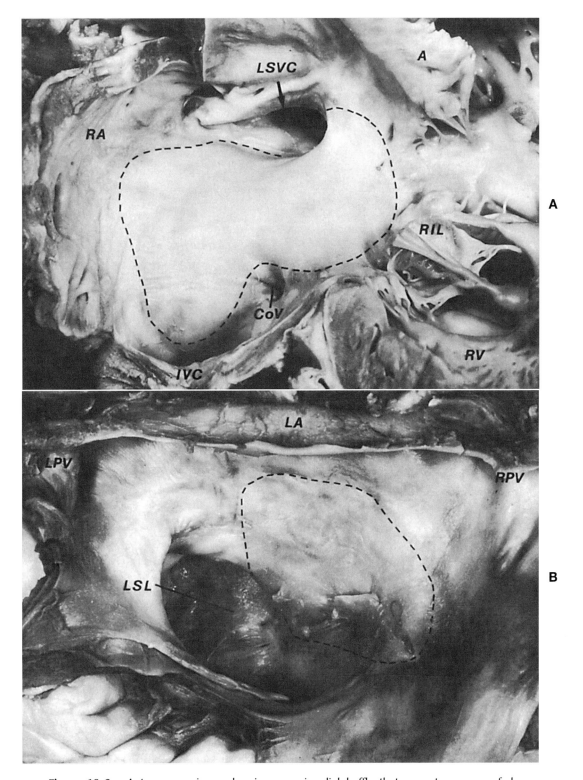

Figure 19-2 Autopsy specimen showing a pericardial baffle that corrects an unroofed coronary sinus syndrome (left superior vena cava [*LSVC*] to left atrium) in association with a common atrium and partial atrioventricular septal defect. Operation was performed on a patient 20 months of age; the child died at 13 years of age, probably from arrhythmia. In both views, the pericardial baffle suture line is identified by a dashed line. **A,** Exposure from opened right atrium and right ventricle. Baffle suture line passes behind the LSVC ostium to reach the ventricular septal crest between right and left atrioventricular valves and then behind inferior vena caval ostium. There is no right superior vena cava in this heart. **B,** Viewed from the opened left atrium.

Key: *A,* Anterior leaflet right atrioventricular valve; *CoV,* opening of large coronary vein into atrium; *IVC,* inferior vena cava; *LA,* left atrium; *LPV,* left pulmonary veins; *LSL,* left superior atrioventricular valve leaflet; *RA,* right atrium; *RIL,* right inferior atrioventricular valve leaflet; *RPV,* right pulmonary veins; *RV,* right ventricle.

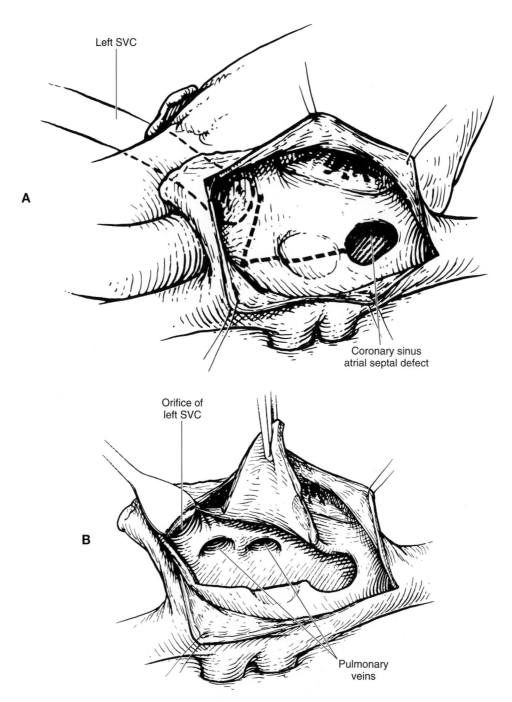

Figure 19-3 Repair of left superior vena cava (LSVC) entering left atrium. **A,** In a patient with only a small coronary sinus atrial septal defect (completely unroofed coronary sinus), an incision is made in the atrial septum as shown by the angled dashed lines. **B,** The atrial septal incision has been made and the flap retracted. The orifice of the entrance of the LSVC into the left atrium is shown in its usual position just anterior and superior to the orifices of the pulmonary veins.

Key: *SVC,* Superior vena cava.

Continued

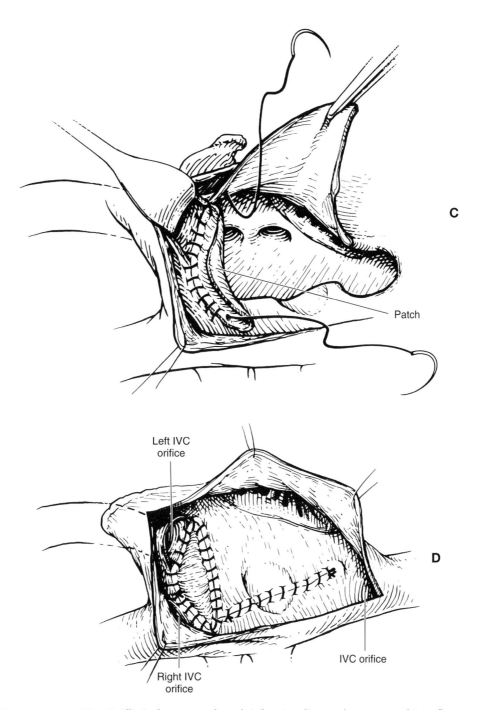

Figure 19-3, cont'd   **C**, Elliptical, contoured patch (of pericardium, polyester, or polytetrafluo-roethylene is sutured into place posteriorly to begin creation of a pathway for diverting blood from LSVC to right atrium. Care is taken to avoid encroachment of suture line or patch on orifice of the left superior pulmonary vein. **D**, Atrial flap has been laid back into position. Posteriorly and inferiorly, it is resutured to remnant of atrial septum to close the coronary sinus atrial septal defect. Superiorly, the flap is sewn to the other edge of contoured patch; before this, the patch is trimmed to be as narrow as possible to avoid any encroachment on pulmonary veins. Note free access of all three caval orifices to the right atrium.

Key: *IVC,* Inferior vena cava.

■ **TABLE 19-2**   **Repair of Unroofed Coronary Sinus Syndrome**

Category	n	No. of Hospital Deaths
Pure, with LSVC	8	0
With simple cardiac malformations	10	0
With LSVC	5	
Common atrium with partial AVSD		4
Tetralogy of Fallot		1
Without LSVC	5	
Partial AVSD (partially unroofed)		3
Complete AVSD (partially unroofed)		1
Tetralogy of Fallot		1
With complex cardiac malformations [a]	6	3
Common atrium, complete AVSD, DORV, polysplenia	2	
Common atrium, complete AVSD, DORV, PS, TASVC, hypoplastic LV, asplenia	1 [b]	
TAPVC, polysplenia	1 [b]	
Dextroversion, iolated ventricular inversion, polysplenia	1 [b]	
Situs inversus totalis, complete AVSD, DORV, PS	1 [b]	
TOTAL	24	3

(Data from Quaegebeur and colleagues.[Q1])

Key: *AVSD*, Atrioventricular septal defect; *DORV*, double outlet right ventricle; *LSVC*, left superior vena cava; *LV*, left ventricle; *PS*, pulmonary stenosis; *TAPVC*, total anomalous pulmonary venous connection; *TASVC*, total anomalous systemic venous connection.

[a] Atrial situs ambiguous or inversus.

[b] Patient died.

RESULTS

Early (Hospital) Death

Risk of repairing simple unroofed coronary sinus syndrome is low. No deaths occurred among 18 patients (0%; CL 0%-10%) reported by Quaegebeur and colleagues[Q1] (Table 19-2).

When the syndrome is part of a complex anomaly associated with atrial isomerism, risk has been much higher. Three of six patients (50%; CL 24%-76%) in the same series died[Q1] (see Table 19-2). A similar experience was reported by Cherian and Rao.[C3] Better understanding of morphology and improved operative methods, including avoidance of intracardiac repair, should result in improved outcomes (for further details, see Chapter 44).

Time-Related Survival and Functional Status

No late deaths occurred after repair of simple unroofed coronary sinus syndrome in the series of Quaegebeur and col-

leagues, but one of the patients required reoperation after 8 years because of tunnel obstruction.[Q1] In the series of Cherian and Rao, one of eight hospital survivors required reoperation for closure of a coronary sinus ASD.[C3] At the time of the reports, surviving patients in both series were without symptoms, including the ones who required reoperation.

INDICATIONS FOR OPERATION

When diagnosis of isolated completely unroofed coronary sinus with persistent LSVC is made, operation is advisable because of arterial desaturation, risk of cerebral emboli, and satisfactory results of operation. Indications for repair of the rare, isolated completely unroofed coronary sinus without persistent LSVC (coronary sinus ASD) are the same as for other types of ASD[L1] (see Chapter 16). When unroofed coronary sinus is associated with complex cardiac anomalies, the associated anomaly usually presents a clear indication for operation.

SPECIAL SITUATIONS AND CONTROVERSIES

Ligation of Left Superior Vena Cava

When the innominate vein is absent or restrictive, some surgeons ligate the LSVC in this and other conditions even when the jugular venous pressure goes as high as 30 mmHg after temporary occlusion of the LSVC. No ill effects have been reported late postoperatively, although venous engorgement, facial edema, and chylothorax may be early complications.[D2]

We do not recommend ligation in this circumstance, because the other methods described are safe and widely applicable. An alternative practice, when correction of unroofed coronary sinus may complicate intracardiac repair of a coexisting condition and extracardiac repair is not possible, involves temporarily occluding the LSVC and ligating if the increase in left jugular venous pressure does not exceed 15 to 20 mmHg. Even in this setting, however, creating an LSVC to left pulmonary artery anastomosis (bidirectional Glenn) would seem preferable to ligating the LSVC. This procedure is technically simple and is feasible in essentially all circumstances except in the presence of pulmonary hypertension. Increasing experience with the bidirectional pulmonary stent as part of a two-ventricle repair (the "one and a half ventricle repair") has shown that this physiologic arrangement is well tolerated when applied to a variety of morphologic conditions (see Chapters 20, 26, 27, and 41).[H3,R6,V3]

REFERENCES

A

1. Allmendinger P, Dear WE, Cooley DA. Atrial septal defect with communication through the coronary sinus. Ann Thorac Surg 1974;17:193.

C

1. Campbell M, Deuchar DC. The left-sided superior vena cava. Br Heart J 1954;16:423.
2. Chiu IS, Hegerty A, Anderson RH, de Leval M. The landmarks to the atrioventricular conduction system in hearts with absence or unroofing of the coronary sinus. J Thorac Cardiovasc Surg 1985;90:297.
3. Cherian KM, Rao SG. Surgical correction of the unroofed coronary sinus syndrome. Indian Heart J 1994;46:91.

D

1. Davis WH, Jordaan FR, Snyman HW. Persistent left superior vena cava draining into the left atrium, as an isolated anomaly. Am Heart J 1959;57:616.
2. de Leval MR, Ritter DG, McGoon DC, Danielson GK. Anomalous systemic venous connection. Surgical considerations. Mayo Clin Proc 1975;50:599.

F

1. Friedlich A, Bing RJ, Blount SG Jr. Circulatory dynamics in the anomalies of venous return to the heart including pulmonary arteriovenous fistula. Bull Johns Hopkins Hosp 1956;86:20.
2. Freedom RM, Culham JA, Rowe RD. Left atrial to coronary sinus fenestration (partially unroofed coronary sinus). Morphological and angiocardiographic observations. Br Heart J 1981;46:63.
3. Foster ED, Baeza OR, Farina MF, Shafer RM. Atrial septal defect associated with drainage of the left superior vena cava to left atrium and absence of the coronary sinus. J Thorac Cardiovasc Surg 1978;76:718.

H

1. Hurwitt ES, Escher DJ, Citrin LI. Surgical correction of cyanosis due to entrance of left superior vena cava into left auricle. Surgery 1955;38:903.
2. Helseth HK, Peterson CR. Atrial septal defect with termination of left superior vena cava in the left atrium and absence of the coronary sinus. Recognition and correction. Ann Thorac Surg 1974;17:186.
3. Hanley FL. The one and a half ventricular repair—we can do it, but should we do it? J Thorac Cardiovasc Surg 1999;117:659.

K

1. Konstam MA, Levine BW, Strauss HW, McKusick KA. Left superior vena cava to left atrial communication diagnosed with radionuclide angiocardiography and with differential right to left shunting. Am J Cardiol 1979;43:149.

L

1. Lee ME, Sade RM. Coronary sinus septal defect. Surgical considerations. J Thorac Cardiovasc Surg 1979;78:563.

M

1. Mantini E, Grondin CM, Lillehei CW, Edwards JE. Congenital anomalies involving the coronary sinus. Circulation 1966;33:317.
2. Miller GA, Ongley P, Rastelli GC, Kirklin JW. Surgical correction of total anomalous systemic venous connection: report of a case. Mayo Clin Proc 1965;40:532.

Q

1. Quaegebeur J, Kirklin JW, Pacifico AD, Bargeron LM Jr. Surgical experience with unroofed coronary sinus. Ann Thorac Surg 1979;27:418.

R

1. Rastelli GC, Ongley PA, Kirklin JW. Surgical correction of common atrium with anomalously connected persistent left superior vena cava: report of a case. Mayo Clin Proc 1965;40:528.
2. Raghib G, Ruttenberg HD, Anderson RC, Amplatz K, Adams P Jr, Edwards JE. Termination of left superior vena cava in left atrium, atrial septal defect, and absence of coronary sinus. Circulation 1965;31:906.
3. Rose AG, Beckman CB, Edwards JE. Communication between coronary sinus and left atrium. Br Heart J 1974;36:182.
4. Rumisek JD, Pigott JD, Weinberg PM, Norwood WI. Coronary sinus septal defect associated with tricuspid atresia. J Thorac Cardiovasc Surg 1986;92:142.
5. Reddy VM, McElhinney DB, Hanley FL. Correction of left superior vena cava draining to the left atrium using extracardiac techniques. Ann Thorac Surg 1997;63:1800.
6. Reddy VM, McElhinney DB, Silverman NH, Marianeschi SM, Hanley FL. Partial biventricular repair for complex congenital heart defects: an intermediate option for complicated anatomy or functionally borderline right complex heart. J Thorac Cardiovasc Surg 1998;116:21.

S

1. Shumacker HB Jr, King H, Waldhausen JA. The persistent left superior vena cava. Surgical implications, with special reference to caval drainage into the left atrium. Ann Surg 1967;165:797.
2. Sherafat M, Friedman S, Waldhausen JA. Persistent left superior vena cava draining into the left atrium with absent right superior vena cava. Ann Thorac Surg 1971;11:160.
3. Schmidt KG, Silverman NH. Cross-sectional and contrast echocardiography in the diagnosis of interatrial communications through the coronary sinus. Int J Cardiol 1987;16:193.
4. Sand ME, McGrath LB, Pacifico AD, Mandke NV. Repair of left superior vena cava entering the left atrium. Ann Thorac Surg 1986;42:560.

T

1. Tuchman H, Brown JF, Huston JH, Weinstein AB, Rowe GC, Crumpton CW. Superior vena cava draining into left atrium. Am J Med 1956;21:481.
2. Taybi H, Kurlander GJ, Lurie PR, Campbell JA. Anomalous systemic venous connection to the left atrium or to a pulmonary vein. Am J Roentgenol Radium Ther Nucl Med 1965;94:62.

V

1. van Son JA, Hambsch J, Mohr FW. Repair of complex unroofed coronary sinus by anastomosis of left to right superior vena cava. Ann Thorac Surg 1998;65:280.
2. van Son JA, Falk V, Mohr FW. Pericardial patch augmentation of restrictive innominate vein and division of left superior vena cava in unroofed coronary sinus syndrome. J Thorac Cardiovasc Surg 1997;114:132.
3. Van Arsdell GS, Williams WG, Maser CM, Streitenberger KS, Rebeyka IM, Coles JG, et al. Superior vena cava to pulmonary artery anastomosis: an adjunct to biventricular repair. J Thorac Cardiovasc Surg 1996;112:1143.

W

1. Winter FS. Persistent left superior vena cava. Angiology 1954;5:90.

20 Atrioventricular Septal Defect

DEFINITION

Atrioventricular (AV) septal defects are characterized by a deficiency or absence of septal tissue immediately above and below the normal level of the AV valves, including the region normally occupied by the AV septum, in hearts with two ventricles. The AV valves are abnormal to a varying degree.

These defects have also been called AV canal defects, AV defects, endocardial cushion defects, ostium primum atrial septal defects (ASDs) (when there is no interventricular communication), and common AV orifice (when there is only a single AV valve orifice).[B21]

HISTORICAL NOTE

Morphology

Abbott apparently recognized ostium primum ASD and common AV "canal" defect, but it was Rogers and Edwards who in 1948 recognized their morphologic similarity.[A2,R4] This concept was further elaborated by Wakai and Edwards in 1956 and 1958.[W1,W2] The terms *partial* and *complete atrioventricular canal defects* were introduced by these investigators, who realized nonetheless that not all cases fit their definitions. During this period, Lev was formulating his concepts of ostium primum ASD (or partial AV canal) and common AV orifice (or complete AV canal), and he described the position of the AV node and bundle of His in these malformations.[L4] Wakai and Edwards and later Bharati and Lev became dissatisfied with trying to compress all cases into two categories and added the terms *intermediate* and *transitional*.[B5,W1,W2] During this period, Van Mierop's scholarly studies added a great deal of knowledge to the overall anatomic features of AV septal defects.[V3,V6]

By the early 1960s, surgical treatment of these defects provided a stimulus to further morphologic studies. In 1966, Rastelli and colleagues at the Mayo Clinic described in more detail the morphology of AV valve leaflets in cases with common AV orifice.[R3] The error made in this study was to compress into the designation *common anterior leaflet* a leaflet that was in fact divided in two by a commissure (that is, the divided common anterior leaflet of type A). The description of AV valve leaflets by Rastelli and colleagues was accepted for some years, but in 1976 a publication by Ugarte and colleagues emphasized the idea of leaflets *bridging* the ventricular septum, a concept also held by Lev.[U1] Meanwhile, based on anatomic and cineangiographic studies and in accordance with the description of Baron and colleagues and Van Mierop and colleagues, it was recognized in the late 1960s that the basic defect in these malformations was *absence of the AV septum*.[B4,B10,V3] This concept is particularly important, because the AV septum can be imaged by echocardiography and in the left ventriculogram in the right anterior oblique projection. These concepts were further expanded by Piccoli and colleagues, under the direction of R.H. Anderson, who further emphasized that all the variations of the defect were part of a spectrum (Fig. 20-1).[P5,P6]

Surgical Treatment

In 1952 at the University of Minnesota Hospitals in Minneapolis, after a long period of laboratory investigation, Dennis and Varco attempted for the first time a cardiac operation in a human using a pump-oxygenator. The preoperative diagnosis was ASD, and at operation the defect was thought to be closed. The patient died, and autopsy showed the true diagnosis to be partial AV septal defect (Edwards JE: personal communication; 1980). The first successful repair of a complete AV septal defect was performed by Lillehei and colleagues in 1954, using cross-circulation and direct suture of the atrial rim of the septal defect to the crest of the ventricular septum.[L1] In 1954, Kirklin and colleagues successfully repaired a partial AV septal defect through the atrial well of Watkins and Gross and in 1955 began repairing AV septal defects by open cardiotomy and use of the pump-oxygenator.[K6,K10,R2,W3]

Early experiences with complete AV septal defects were all associated with a high hospital mortality, often related to complete heart block, postrepair left AV valve regurgitation, or creation of subaortic stenosis.[C1,E1,L2,S4] Interestingly, in many of these early operations a two-patch technique was used (see "Two-Patch Technique" under Technique of Operation later in this chapter). In 1958, Lev's description of the location of the bundle of His provided the basis for techniques of repair that avoid heart block.[L4] In 1959, Dubost and Blondeau reported their early experience and emphasized that the "cleft" in the "mitral leaflet" need not be sutured in repairing partial AV septal defects, a concept currently challenged.[D2] In 1962, Maloney and colleagues described two cases in which a single patch was used to close both defects and with the valve tissue suspended from the patch.[M1] This technique was again described by Gerbode in 1962 and led to a decrease in hospital

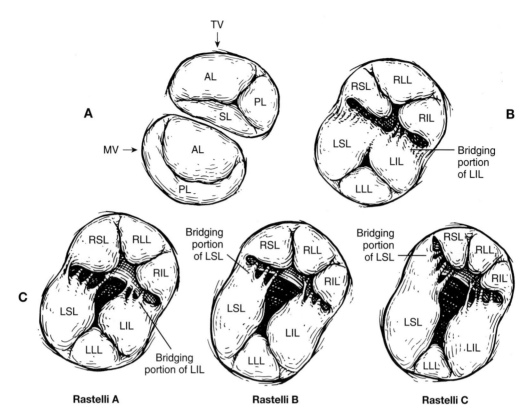

Figure 20-1 Diagrammatic representation of atrioventricular (AV) valves viewed from atrial side (surgical orientation). **A,** Normal, with anterior and posterior mitral valve leaflets and septal, anterior, and posterior tricuspid valve leaflets. **B,** Leaflets in partial AV septal defects. Left superior, left inferior, and left lateral leaflets form the left AV valve; right superior, right inferior, and right lateral leaflets form the right AV valve. **C,** Leaflets in complete AV septal defects, or common AV orifice, are similar to those in **B.** However, left superior and left inferior leaflets are not connected. The left inferior leaflet usually bridges a little (grade 1 or 2, based on 1 to 5) across crest of ventricular septum. The left superior leaflet may bridge slightly or not at all (grade 0 or 1, Rastelli type A), moderately (grade 2 or 3, Rastelli type B), or markedly (grade 4 or 5, Rastelli type C).

Key: *AL,* Anterior leaflet; *LIL,* left inferior leaflet; *LLL,* left lateral leaflet; *LSL,* left superior leaflet; *MV,* mitral valve; *PL,* posterior leaflet; *RIL,* right inferior leaflet; *RLL,* right lateral leaflet; *RSL,* right superior leaflet; *SL,* septal leaflet; *TV,* tricuspid valve.

mortality.[G2,R1] McGoon recognized the importance of "taking from the tricuspid valve" to leave sufficient tissue from which to create an adequate left AV valve. These technical advances allowed repair of even the more complex variants of the defect.[P1,R5,Z1] Subsequently, good results were obtained in patients older than about 2 years of age, but results in infants remained relatively poor.[B1,B2,G1,H1,K1,M2,M4,R1,V1] Between 1968 and 1971, Barratt-Boyes successfully repaired this anomaly in four severely ill infants[B12]; subsequently, improved results in infants were reported by many others.[A1,B2,B3,C3,C5,M3,M5,N3]

In 1978, Carpentier again emphasized (as did Dubost and Blondeau[D2]) that generally, the left AV valve functions best when repaired as a three-leaflet valve.[C6] As a result of these advances, risks of operation for nearly all types of AV septal defect are now low.[B1,C2,S2]

MORPHOLOGY
General Morphologic Characteristics

AV septal defects have as defining characteristics a deficiency or absence of the AV septum, resulting in an ostium primum defect immediately above the AV valves and a deficiency (or scooped-out area) in the inlet (basal) portion of the ventricular septum immediately below the AV valves.

Patients with partial AV septal defects have a normal length of atrial septum, and the ostium primum ASD is the result of absence of the relatively small AV septum plus some deficiency in the inlet portion of the ventricular septum.[G9] The deficiency in the inlet portion of the ventricular septum is variable, but on average is greater in patients with complete AV septal defects than in those with partial defects.[G9,P9]

■ **TABLE 20-1   Size of Interatrial Communication in Atrioventricular Septal Defects** [a]

	Prevalence	
Size	No.	% of 310
0 [b]	2	0.6
1	2	0.6
2	27	8.7
3	35	11.3
4	223	71.9
5 [c]	21	6.8

(Data from Studer and colleagues.[S2])

[a] Study is based on data from 310 surgical patients.

[b] Condition in which the characteristic atrioventricular (AV) septal deficiency is present but the AV valves are adherent on their atrial side to the edge of the defect, resulting in no interatrial communication.

[c] Common atrium.

■ **TABLE 20-2   Size of Interventricular Communication in Atrioventricular Septal Defects**

	Beneath Left Superior Leaflet		Beneath Left Inferior Leaflet	
Size	No.	% of 310	No.	% of 309 [a]
0 [b]	158	51	176	57
1	3	1.0	3	1.0
2	9	2.9	9	2.9
3	4	1.3	16	5.2
4	9	2.9	22	7.1
5 [c]	127	41	82	27

(Data from Studer and colleagues.[S2])

[a] Data not available for one patient.

[b] Condition in which the characteristic atrioventricular (AV) septal deficiency is present but the AV valves are adherent on their ventricular side to the crest of the ventricular septum, resulting in no interventricular communication (if this occurs under both left AV valve leaflets, it is commonly called "partial AV septal defect". If size greater than 1 occurs under both AV valve leaflets, the condition is commonly called "complete AV septal defect").

[c] Very large communication but not common ventricle.

These septal deficiencies may or may not result in interatrial or interventricular communications, depending on configuration and attachments of the AV valves (Tables 20-1 and 20-2). Whereas the basic defect in these malformations is absence of the AV septum, whether the ventricular septal or atrial septal deficiency or the AV valve abnormality is the result only of AV septal absence is still debated. [B4,B10,V3]

Five or more AV valve leaflets of variable size are usually present (see Fig. 20-1), but there is often variability in completeness of commissures and prominent crenations in the leaflets (Fig. 20-2). For example, among the 43 hearts with all types of AV septal defects and two ventricles in the GLH autopsy series in which the number of leaflets could be accurately assessed, 10 (23%) had four leaflets, 18 (42%) had five leaflets, 14 (33%) had six leaflets, and one (2%) had seven leaflets. When a large interventricular communication was present (complete AV septal defect), the most common number of leaflets was five (16 of 28, or 57%).

The left superior leaflet (LSL) and left inferior leaflet (LIL) are particularly variable in size, connections one to another (Table 20-3), and degree of bridging across the

■ **TABLE 20-3   Left Superior and Left Inferior Leaflet Connections in Atrioventricular Septal Defects**

Degree of LSL-LIL Connection [a]	No Interventricular Communication (n = 154)		Interventricular Communication (n = 156)	
	No.	% of 154	No.	% of 156
0	2	1.3	139	89
1	55	36	11 [b]	7
2	82	53	5 [b]	3
3	9	6	0	—
4	5	3	0	—
5	1	0.6	0	—
Connected, unknown degree	0	0	1 [b]	0.6

(Data from Studer and colleagues.[S2])

Key: *LIL*, Left inferior leaflet; *LSL*, left superior leaflet.

[a] 0, separate LSL and LIL, such as in common AV orifice; 1 and 2, narrow connections (deep cleft in "anterior mitral leaflet"); 3 and 4, broad connection (shallow cleft or notch); 5, no cleft, anterior mitral leaflet.

[b] Among these 17, in four the LSL and LIL were connected but free-floating, with large interventricular communications beneath them and their connections (Bharati type C[B9]). In 11, very small interventricular communications were present beneath the LSL and/or LIL. In two, no interatrial communication was present.

■ **TABLE 20-4   Left Superior Leaflet Bridging in Atrioventricular Septal Defects**

Degree of LSL Bridging	Without Interventricular Communication (n = 154)		With Interventricular Communication (n = 156)		
	No.	% of 153 [a]	No.	% of 154 [b]	
0	150	98	65	42	} Rastelli type A
1	3	2.0	23	15	
2			5	3.2	} Rastelli type B
3			10	6.5	
4			8	5.2	} Rastelli type C
5			43	28	

(Data from Studer and colleagues.[S2])

Key: *LSL*, Left superior leaflet.

[a] Data not available for one patient.

[b] Data not available for two patients.

■ **TABLE 20-5   Type of Atrioventricular Valve Orifices in Atrioventricular Septal Defects** [a]

Type	No.	% of 310
Two AV valves	171 [b]	55
Common AV valve	139	45

(Data from Studer and colleagues.[S2])

Key: *AV*, Atrioventricular.

[a] Database is same as in Table 20-1.

[b] Includes the 154 patients without interventricular communications; 11 with small interventricular communications beneath the left superior (LSL) and/or inferior leaflets (LIL); four with connected but free-floating and connected LSL and LIL (see Table 20-3); and two with no interatrial communication but large interventricular communication (not inlet atrioventricular septal-type ventricular septal defects).

crest of the ventricular septum (Table 20-4; see Figs. 20-1 and 20-2). There may be one or two AV valve orifices (Table 20-5).

Hearts with AV septal defects are also characterized by absence of the usual wedged position of the aortic valve

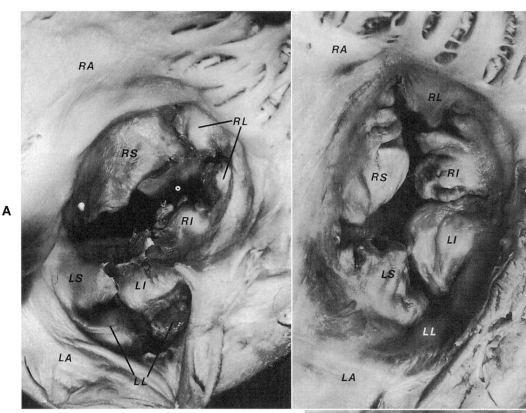

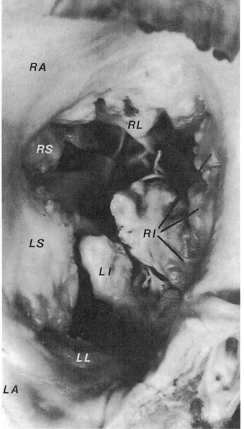

Figure 20-2   Atrioventricular (AV) valves in AV septal defects viewed from atrial aspect in a series of fixed specimens. **A,** Specimen with partial AV septal defect in which left superior and left inferior leaflets are adherent to crest of ventricular septum and there is no interventricular communication. Arrow marks line of closure between left superior and left inferior leaflets, formerly called the *cleft in the anterior mitral leaflet.* Note that, as usual, left superior leaflet does not bridge septum (there is no leaflet tissue in the position of the superior portion of the normal tricuspid septal leaflet). In this heart, as is not uncommon, there are two left lateral and two right lateral leaflets. **B,** Specimen with complete AV septal defect in which there are interventricular communications beneath left superior and left inferior leaflets. Left superior leaflet does not bridge crest of septum. Right superior leaflet is characteristically large. Left inferior leaflet is bridging (grade 2) and very distinct from right inferior leaflet. **C,** Specimen of a complete AV septal defect in which left superior leaflet markedly bridges crest of septum. Correspondingly, right superior leaflet is small. Left superior leaflet is characteristically larger than left inferior leaflet.

Key: *LA,* Left atrium; *LI,* left inferior leaflet; *LL,* left lateral leaflet; *LS,* left superior leaflet; *RA,* right atrium; *RI,* right inferior leaflet; *RL,* right lateral leaflet; *RS,* right superior leaflet.

above the AV valves. Instead, it is elevated and deviated anteriorly.[G6,P5,V3,V5,V6] Details of the aortic–mitral fibrous continuity often differ from those in the normal heart. Thus, continuity was abnormal in more than half of 21 specimens with normally related great arteries in the GLH autopsy series; continuity was to the base of the noncoronary cusp in only five (24%) and to both the noncoronary and right coronary cusps in seven (33%). In addition, the left ventricular (LV) inflow tract is shortened in relationship to length of the outflow portion, and there is a related reduction in length of the diaphragmatic wall of the LV.[G3,G7,P5,V3,V5] The LV outflow tract is also narrowed, although rarely is the narrowing sufficient to be of hemodynamic importance in the unrepaired heart.[P7]

AV septal defects include a spectrum of malformations. At one end is the simplest type, in which there is an interatrial communication but no interventricular communication and a connection of variable width between the left superior and left inferior leaflets; this is called a *partial AV septal defect* or *ostium primum defect*. At the other end of the spectrum is the most extreme form, with large deficiencies in the atrial and ventricular septa, a common AV valve orifice, and large interatrial and interventricular communications; this is called a *complete AV septal defect*. Because a continuous spectrum of gradations lies between these extremes, some anomalies have been grouped as *intermediate AV septal defects*. Added complexity is provided by occurrence of a large variety of major and minor associated cardiac anomalies (Tables 20-6 through 20-8). In addition, Down syndrome is common, particularly in patients with an interventricular communication.

Because it is virtually impossible to subdivide the spectrum of AV septal defects into satisfactory noncontroversial subgroups, this chapter describes cases based on morphologic and functional variables rather than categorizing them into subgroups. Problems in diagnosis, surgical treatment, and results can then be analyzed in a clearer and more meaningful way.[S2] The older, imprecise terms continue to be useful as shorthand, and in this chapter, *partial*

AV septal defect refers to a malformation with two AV valve orifices and no interventricular communication, whereas *complete AV* septal defect refers to a defect with a common AV valve orifice and large (grade 2 or more) interventricular communication.

Atrial Septal Deficiency and Interatrial Communications

Partial Atrioventricular Septal Defect

Usually there is an interatrial communication related to *deficiency of the AV septum,* the so-called ostium primum ASD (Fig. 20-3). The defect is bounded below by the inferiorly displaced AV valve leaflets and above by a crescentic ridge of atrial septum that fuses with the AV valve anulus only at its extremities.

Generally, there is little atrial septal tissue at the superior point of fusion of the atrial septum with the valve anulus

■ **TABLE 20-6 Major Associated Cardiac Anomalies in Atrioventricular Septal Defects**

Anomaly	No.	% of 310
None	237	76
Patent ductus arteriosus	31	10.0
Tetralogy of Fallot	20	6.5
Completely unroofed coronary sinus with left SVC	9	2.9
Situs ambiguus	7	2.3
DORV without PS	6	1.9
Additional VSDs	5	1.6
DORV + PS	3	1.0
Situs inversus totalis	3	1.0
TAPVC	2	0.6
Left ventricular outflow obstruction	2	0.6
Transposition of the great arteries	1	0.3
PS, supravalvar mitral stenosis, Ebstein malformation, coarctation, isolated dextrocardia	1 each	0.3

(Data from Studer and colleagues.[S2])

Key: *DORV*, Double outlet right ventricle; *PS*, pulmonary stenosis; *SVC*, superior vena cava; *TAPVC*, total anomalous pulmonary venous connection; *VSD*, ventricular septal defect.

■ **TABLE 20-7 Minor Associated Cardiac Anomalies in Atrioventricular Septal Defects**

	Without Interventricular Communication (n = 154)			With Interventricular Communication (n = 156)		
Anomaly	No.	% of 154	CL (%)	No.	% of 156	CL (%)
(Sizable) ASD[a]	17	11	8–14	32	21	17–24
Left SVC without unroofed coronary sinus	10	6	4–9	7	4	3–7
Partially unroofed coronary sinus	5	3	1–5	2	1	0.4–3
Azygos extension of IVC	4	3	1–5	3	1	0.6–3
IVC to lower left common atrium				1	1	0.1–2
Bilateral IVCs	1	1	0.1–2			
TASVC to common atrium				1	1	0.1–2
Right PVs to RA	1	1	0.1–2			
Anomalous origin LAD from RCA (TF)				1	1	0.1–2
Origin stenosis LPA (not TF)	1	1	0.1–2			
Wolff–Parkinson–White syndrome	1	1	0.1–2			
Spontaneous heart block	1	1	0.1–2			
Coronary artery disease requiring CABG	1	1	0.1–2			

(Data from Studer and colleagues.[S2])

Key: *ASD*, Atrial septal defect; *CABG*, coronary artery bypass grafting; *CL*, 70% confidence limits; *IVC*, inferior vena cava; *LAD*, left anterior descending coronary artery; *LPA*, left pulmonary artery; *PV*, pulmonary vein; *RA*, right atrium; *RCA*, right coronary artery; *SVC*, superior vena cava; *TASVC*, total anomalous systemic venous connection; *TF*, tetralogy of Fallot.

[a] Does not include patent foramen ovale.

adjacent to the aorta, but more tissue is usually present inferiorly adjacent to the coronary sinus (Fig. 20-4). The distance between the crescentic atrial margin of the defect and the AV valves (and thus the size of the interatrial communication) is variable. In most cases the fossa ovalis is normally formed, and there is a patent foramen ovale or an associated fossa ovalis ASD. Usually, the interatrial communication through the ostium primum defect is mod-

■ TABLE 20-8   Conditions Associated with Atrioventricular Septal Defects in Autopsied Hearts with Two Ventricles [a]

Associated Condition	No.	% of 69
Down syndrome	9	13
Trisomy E	3	4
Asplenia[b]	19	28
Polysplenia[b]	4	6
Other complex congenital heart disease	18	26

[a] Data from GLH autopsy series of nonsurgical and surgical cases; number with Down syndrome may not be representative, in view of case selection.

[b] In the rest of this chapter, including other tables, cases with atrial isomerism are not included (they are discussed in Chapter 44).

erate in size. When the interatrial communication is small, the atrial septal deficiency is restricted to the area normally occupied by the AV septum.[V7] The communication may be still smaller because of fusion of the base of the left superior or inferior leaflets to the edge of the adjacent portion of the atrial septum. Rarely, there may be an accessory "parachute" of fibrous tissue narrowing or obstructing the defect. Under such circumstances a pressure difference exists between the two atria.

Common Atrium

Deficiencies in the anterior limbus or fossa ovalis may be associated with AV septal defects, resulting in a larger interatrial communication. Occasionally the entire limbus and fossa ovalis are absent, along with the AV septum. The condition is then termed *common atrium* (see Table 20-1).[E3,G5,R6,R7]

Absence of Interatrial Communication

Rarely, AV valve tissue is attached completely to the edge of the atrial septum, and no interatrial communication

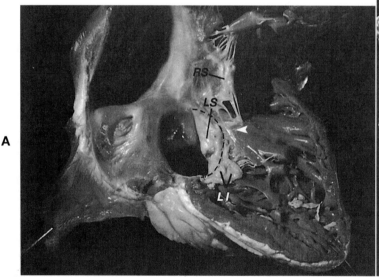
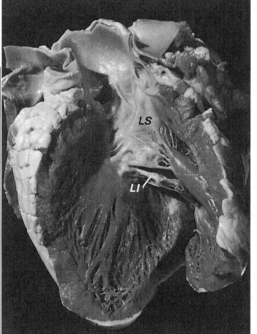

Figure 20-3   Partial atrioventricular (AV) septal defect. **A,** View from right atrium and right ventricle. Large ostium primum atrial septal defect is seen above AV valve leaflets. No interventricular communication is present beneath the leaflets. However, deficiency of basal (inlet) portion of the ventricular septum is apparent. Left superior leaflet is attached firmly by fibrous tissue to crest of septum *(dashed line)* and does not bridge onto right ventricular side. There is thus a bare area on right side of the superior aspect of the ventricular septum *(arrow).* Left inferior leaflet bridges on right ventricular side. Right superior leaflet is clearly visible, but right lateral and inferior leaflets are not in photograph. **B,** Left ventricular outflow view. Left superior and left inferior leaflets are firmly attached to crest of ventricular septum. Narrowing and elongation of left ventricular outflow tract are apparent. This figure makes clear why, in describing the position of the two leaflets attached to the ventricular crest, the terms *superior* and *inferior* are preferable to *anterior* and *posterior,* terms that lead to confusion with normal mitral leaflets. (Courtesy Dr. Maurice Lev.)

Key: *LI,* Left inferior leaflet; *LS,* left superior leaflet; *RS,* right superior leaflet.

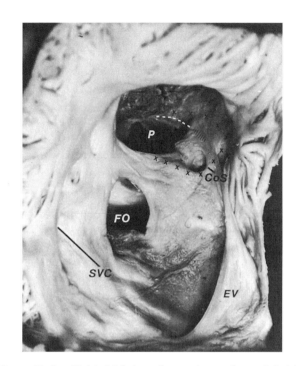

Figure 20-4 Right atrial view of a specimen of a partial atrioventricular (AV) septal defect. Coronary sinus ostium is seen inferior and posterior to ostium primum defect in atrial septum. Approximate position of AV node and His bundle is shown as a dashed line. Placement of inferior part of patch suture line is shown by the line of x's.

Key: *CoS*, Coronary sinus ostium; *EV*, eustachian valve of inferior vena cava; *FO*, fossa ovalis; *P*, ostium primum; *SVC*, superior vena cava.

exists despite the deficiency in the septum (see Table 20-1).[P5,S2] In this unusual variant, the characteristic deficiency of the inlet (basal) portion of the ventricular septum is also present and is associated with a large interventricular communication beneath the leaflets. The functionally left AV valve, consisting only of those portions of the left superior and left inferior leaflets on the *left* side of their attachment to the atrial septum, tends to be competent. As seen from a right atrial approach, part of the right AV valve may have chordal attachments across the ventricular defect to the left side of the septum, that is, it is straddling. When viewed from the ventricular side, the appearance is typical of a complete AV septal defect. It is distinct from an inlet type of perimembranous VSD that is sometimes called inlet septal, AV septal, or AV canal type of VSD, which is unrelated to deficiency of the AV septum (see "Inlet Septal Type of Ventricular Septal Defect" under Morphology in Chapter 21).

Ventricular Septal Deficiency and Interventricular Communications

Partial Atrioventricular Septal Defect

Some degree of deficiency of the inlet portion of the ventricular septum immediately beneath the AV valves is a constant finding. Thus, the inlet portion of the ventricular septum is shortened. There is usually no interventricular communication when left superior and inferior leaflets are connected and attached to the downwardly displaced crest

of the septum throughout its length (Fig. 20-5; see also Fig. 20-3), the situation described as a partial AV septal defect. Occasionally, one or several small interventricular communications are present beneath the attachment of the AV valve to the septum (see Fig. 20-5, *B*).

Complete Atrioventricular Septal Defect

With ventricular septal deficiency generally greater than that in a partial AV septal defect, a moderate or large interventricular communication may be present, and usually, left superior and inferior leaflets are separate. This anomaly is described as a *complete AV septal defect* (see Fig. 20-5, *C*). Deficiency of the inlet portion of the ventricular septum (the "scoop") is generally deeper in hearts with complete AV septal defects than in those with partial AV septal defects.[A4,E9,F5] Often the communication is particularly large beneath the LSL and smaller beneath the LIL (see Table 20-2), whereas in about 5% of cases there is a larger interventricular communication beneath the LSL and none beneath the LIL. Rarely, there is no VSD beneath the LSL and a large one beneath the LIL.

A remnant of the membranous ventricular septum may be present (see Fig. 20-5, *B*). This was the case in 8 of 27 (30%) GLH autopsy specimens of AV septal defect with normally related great arteries. In 19 specimens the membranous septum could not be identified.

Atrioventricular Valves

Attachments of the AV valves to the crest of the ventricular septum in partial AV septal defects, as well as their chordal attachments in complete AV septal defects, are displaced toward the apex of the heart because of deficiency of the inlet (basal) portion of the septum. This alters orientation of the AV orifices relative to the aortic orifice (that is, the aortic valve is no longer wedged between the AV valves) and provides an important diagnostic imaging criterion of this malformation.[A9,B6,B7,B10]

Two Atrioventricular Valve Orifices

Typically, when two AV valve orifices are present, as in partial AV septal defects, the LSL and LIL are joined together to a variable extent anteriorly, near the crest of the ventricular septum, by leaflet tissue (see Figs. 20-1 and 20-3). Thus, together they resemble an anterior (septal) mitral leaflet with a cleft, but in fact the left AV valve is tricuspid and oriented differently from the normal valve (see Figs. 20-1 and 20-2). The connection between the LSL and LIL may be only a thin strand of tissue (complete cleft), but more commonly it is 2 to 4 mm or more deep (see Table 20-3). This connection, too, is usually fused to the crest of the ventricular septum in partial AV septal defects. Occasionally, chordae pass from opposing edges of the LSL and LIL to the muscular ventricular septum beneath.[E2] Yilmaz and colleagues identify a difference in this area of separation and distinguish between a commissure that is supported by chordal apparatus on either side of the gap and a cleft that is relatively unsupported and bereft of chordae at its edges.[Y2] In addition, the chordae that originate from the central edges of the LSL and LIL attach to different papillary muscles, which can cause a distracting force on the leaflets during closure. This contrasts with the

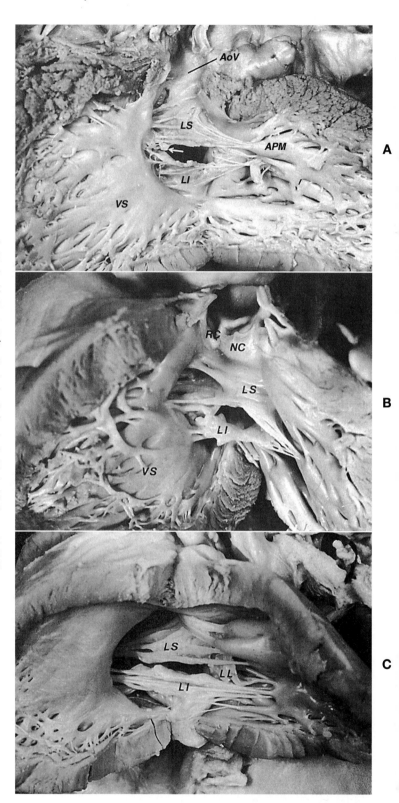

Figure 20-5   Left ventricular aspect of atrioventricular (AV) septal defects. **A,** Partial AV septal defect viewed from opened left ventricle. Left superior and left inferior leaflets are completely attached to crest of a deficient ventricular septum. Area of contact or closure between left superior and left inferior leaflets is indicated by arrow. In this specimen, only the anterior papillary muscle is present (parachute mitral valve). **B,** Intermediate type of AV septal defect from left ventricular view. Numerous small interventricular communications are present between thick, short chordae that tether both left superior and left inferior leaflets to ventricular crest. Fibrous tissue extending from superior leaflet to below right coronary aortic cusp represents a remnant of membranous septum. **C,** Complete AV septal defect viewed from left ventricular aspect. Left superior and left inferior bridging leaflets are free floating, and there is a large interventricular communication between them and the underlying crest of the ventricular septum. This specimen also has double outlet right ventricle.

Key: *AoV,* Aortic valve; *APM,* anterior papillary muscle; *LI,* left inferior leaflet; *LL,* left lateral leaflet; *LS,* left superior leaflet; *NC,* noncoronary aortic cusp; *RC,* right coronary aortic cusp; *VS,* septal surface of left ventricle.

normal commissure in which the chordae from adjacent leaflet edges attach to a single papillary muscle, encouraging coaptation. Rarely, separation into LSL and LIL is represented only by a notch in the center of the free edge of a nearly normal "anterior mitral leaflet." The left lateral leaflet (LLL) is usually smaller than the other two leaflets and is triangular.

In aggregate, these left AV valve leaflet anomalies may make the valve regurgitant to a variable degree, sometimes severely (Table 20-9). When LSL and LIL are nearly completely separated (connection grades 1 and 2; see Table 20-3), an appreciable gap may occur during systole, producing regurgitation. When there is failure of valve coaptation at this site, leaflet tissue forming the margin usually

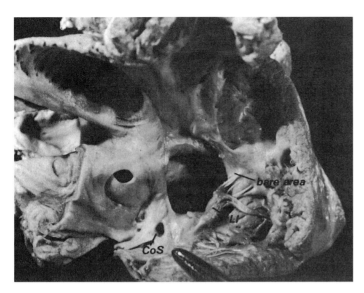

Figure 20-6   Complete atrioventricular septal defect viewed from right ventricular side in a specimen in which left inferior leaflet bridges over crest of septum onto right ventricular side. Left superior leaflet (poorly seen) does not bridge, resulting in a bare area of crest of ventricular septum on right ventricular side, where in a normal heart the superior aspect of the septal leaflet touches the septum. A small fossa ovalis atrial septal defect is also present.

Key: *CoS,* Coronary sinus; *LI,* left inferior leaflet.

■ **TABLE 20-9   Preoperative Atrioventricular Valve Regurgitation in Patients with Atrioventricular Septal Defect without Major Associated Cardiac Anomalies**

Magnitude of AV Valve Regurgitation	Total		Without Interventricular Communication			With Interventricular Communication		
	No.	% of 305 [a]	No.		% of 154	No.		% of 151 [a]
0	29	10	15		10	14		9
1	39	13	26		17	13		9
2	85	28	48		31	37		25
3	98	32	41	}	27	57	}	38
4	43	14	16	65/154 (42%) [b]	10	27	87/151 (58%) [b]	18
5	11	4	8		5	3		2
TOTAL	305		154		151			

(Data from Studer and colleagues.[S2])

[a] No information on five patients.

[b] $P(\chi^2)$ for difference = .007.

becomes thickened and rolled. In other cases, regurgitation appears to be due to deficiency of leaflet tissue, particularly in the LIL.[B9,M15] The mechanism of severe left AV valve regurgitation is, however, not evident in some cases. The jet of regurgitation is usually directed into the right atrium. Rarely, the left AV valve is stenotic, but this usually is associated with hypoplasia of the LV.[B16]

The right AV valve is also abnormal when there are two AV orifices, although less attention has been paid to it. It may consist of three leaflets—right superior leaflet (RSL), right lateral leaflet (RLL), and right inferior leaflet (RIL)—or of two or four leaflets (see Figs. 20-1 and 20-2). Leaflet tissue attached directly or by chordae to the crest or right side of the crest of the septum, and thus contributing to closure of the right AV valves, is considered to represent bridging of the LSL or LIL (see Fig. 20-1).

Usually, in cases without an interventricular communication, the LSL does not bridge at all (previously, this finding was interpreted as absence or hypoplasia of the superior part of the tricuspid septal leaflet) and the LIL bridges moderately (see Fig. 20-2, *A*). Even with abnormalities of the right AV valve, regurgitation is rare (unless right heart failure develops).

Common Atrioventricular Orifice

When the AV valve orifice is a common one and the interventricular communication is large (complete AV septal defect), LSL and LIL are separate, and a bare area is exposed on the crest of the ventricular septum (Fig. 20-6; see Figs. 20-1 and 20-5, *C*). The LSL may be entirely on the LV side of the septum or may, to a variable degree, bridge the septum and extend onto the right ventricular side (see Fig. 20-2, *B, C* and Table 20-4). This variability formed the basis for the classification by Rastelli and colleagues into types A, B, and C.[R3] Chordal attachments of the right ventricular extremity of the LSL vary according to degree of bridging (Fig. 20-7).[P6] When there is no bridging, chordal attachments are to the ventricular crest (see Fig. 20-7, *A*). With mild bridging, they are to the medial papillary muscle in the right ventricle; with moderate bridging, to an accessory (often large) apical papillary muscle (see Fig. 20-7, *B*); and with marked bridging, to the normally positioned (although often bifid) anterolateral papillary muscle of the right ventricle (see Fig. 20-7, *C*). When the LSL bridges the septum moderately or markedly and extends into the right ventricle, it is usually unattached to the underlying ventricular crest (free-floating), but it may

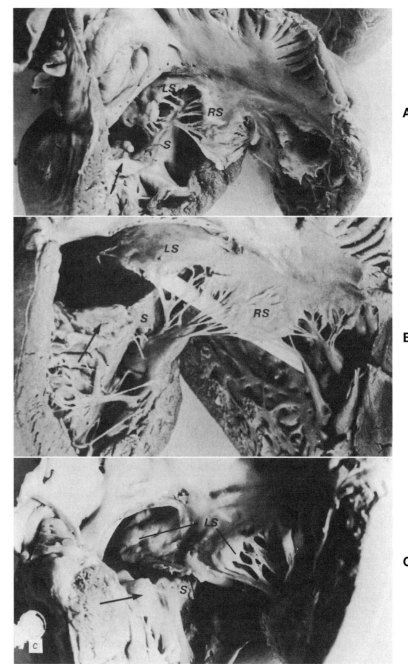

Figure 20-7 Complete atrioventricular septal defects with varying degrees of bridging of left superior leaflet. **A,** Nonbridging (bridging grade 0) left superior leaflet (Rastelli type A). This surgical specimen (the patch having been removed) is viewed from right atrium. Arrow marks mildly bridging left inferior leaflet. **B,** Moderate (grade 2 or 3) bridging of left superior leaflet. Chordae from its right ventricular extremity go to a papillary muscle in right ventricle. Arrow indicates bridging portion of left inferior leaflet. (Rastelli and colleagues termed this *type B,* but it is just part of the spectrum of bridging.) **C,** Marked (grade 5) bridging of left superior leaflet (Rastelli type C). Arrow marks bridging part of left inferior leaflet. (From Rastelli and colleagues.[R3])

Key: *LS,* Left superior leaflet; *RS,* right superior leaflet; *S,* ventricular septal crest.

occasionally be attached by chordae (tethered). Length of the chordal or fibrous attachments to the right side or crest of the ventricular septum varies according to the size of the interventricular communication or the position of the leaflet.

The LIL typically bridges moderately, but it too varies in this respect. It is not uncommon for a bridging left inferior leaflet to be attached to the underlying ventricular crest either completely or by short, thick chordae with interchordal spaces.

Chordal attachments of the leftward components of the common AV valve in the LV are usually relatively normal, although the posterior papillary muscle is displaced more laterally than normal and a third papillary muscle may be

present.[C6] There may be only one papillary muscle, producing a "parachute" type valve that is difficult to repair.[C6] This was the case in 7 of 53 (13%) cases in the GLH autopsy series, in 14% of the specimens described by David and colleagues, and in 4% of 155 surgical cases reported by Ilbawi and colleagues.[D5,I1]

The right ventricular portion of the common AV valve has superior, lateral, and inferior leaflets, but, as in partial AV septal defects, they vary considerably in number and size (see Fig. 20-2). When bridging of the LSL is absent or mild, the RSL is large, whereas with more extensive bridging, it is smaller.[P6]

When leaflets of the common AV valve close appropriately during ventricular systole, AV valve regurgitation is

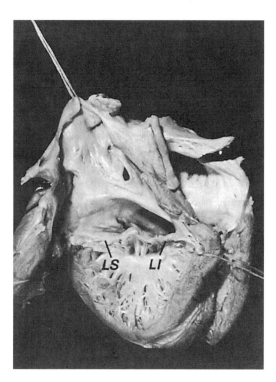

Figure 20-8   Intermediate type of atrioventricular (AV) septal defect viewed from left ventricular aspect. Left superior leaflet is connected to left inferior leaflet by leaflet tissue, resulting in two AV valve orifices; yet there are interventricular communications between short, thick chordae connecting the leaflets and their connection to the scooped-out underlying ventricular septum. Left superior and inferior leaflets, particularly the latter, are deficient. (From Bharati and colleagues.[B9])

Key: *LI,* Left inferior leaflet; *LS,* left superior leaflet.

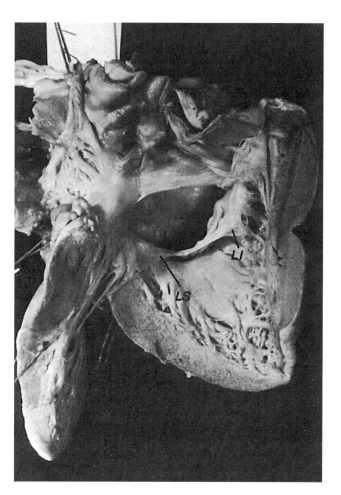

Figure 20-9   Intermediate type of atrioventricular septal defect viewed from left ventricular aspect. Left superior and left inferior leaflets are connected by leaflet tissue, and thus two AV valve orifices are present. However, the interventricular communication is large, and neither the connection nor leaflets are attached to the scooped-out underlying ventricular septum. (From Bharati and colleagues.[B9])

Key: *LI,* Left inferior leaflet; *LS,* left superior leaflet.

absent or mild. However, important left AV valve regurgitation may be present (see Table 20-9). The mechanism of the regurgitation is often not clearly understood.

Unusual Atrioventricular Combinations

Other unusual combinations of size, connections, attachments, and degree of bridging of AV valve leaflets in the spectrum of AV septal defects prompted Wakai and Edwards, Bharati and colleagues, and others to use a transitional or intermediate category.[B9,W1,W4] Rarely, in patients with two AV valve orifices with no interventricular communication beneath the LSL and LIL, these leaflets are connected only by a fibrous strand adherent to the ventricular septal crest (see Tables 20-3 and 20-5), forming what Bharati and colleagues have called a *"pseudomitral" leaflet,* rather than an *"anterior mitral leaflet with a complete cleft."*[B9]

In such patients, deficiency of LIL tissue and severe left AV valve regurgitation are common. Occasionally, when LSL and LIL are connected and thus two AV valve orifices are present, one or multiple small interchordal interventricular communications are present beneath the leaflets (see Tables 20-2 and 20-5), and occasionally one or two larger holes may be present (Fig. 20-8; see Fig. 20-5, *B*). In about 1% of cases, the connected LSL and LIL have large interventricular communications beneath them; in these patients, the connection is a thin strand of valve tissue,

beneath which there is also a large interventricular communication (Fig. 20-9), but two AV valve orifices can be said to be present (see Table 20-5). Bharati and colleagues have referred to this also as *intermediate type C.*[B9]

Accessory Orifice

An accessory orifice (double left AV valve orifice) is present in the commissure on one side, usually the inferior side, of the LLL in about 5% of cases[11,L10,M15,W2] (Table 20-10). A ring of chordae surrounds the orifice, and a very small papillary muscle is usually beneath it.[B20,E8] The accessory orifice may be conceptualized as an incomplete commissure, and the fibrous tissue "bridge" between the accessory orifice and main orifice consists of valvar tissue and chordae.[B20] This emphasizes the danger of producing regurgitation by cutting the bridge. The LLL is often underdeveloped when an accessory orifice is present.[D1] Accessory orifices predispose patients to stenosis after repair.

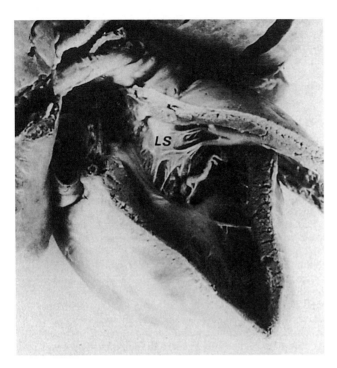

Figure 20-10 Left ventricular aspect of a complete atrioventricular septal defect with no bridging of left superior leaflet and connection of leaflet to underlying ventricular septum by long chordae. Narrowness of left ventricular outflow tract is apparent. (From Rastelli and colleagues.[R3])

Key: *LS,* Left superior leaflet.

■ **TABLE 20-10   Left Atrioventricular Valve Orifice in Atrioventricular Septal Defect**

	Without Interventricular Communication (*n* = 154)		With Interventricular Communication (*n* = 156)	
Left AV Valve Orifice	**No.**	**% of 154**	**No.**	**% of 156**
Single	149	97	147	94
Double	5	3[a]	9	6[a]

(Data from Studer and colleagues.[S2])

[a] $P(\chi^2)$ for difference = .3.

Single Papillary Muscle

A single papillary muscle in the LV uncommonly (about 5% of cases) complicates AV septal defects, most commonly the complete type.[D5,T8] All chordae of the left AV valve leaflets insert into this single papillary muscle, which is usually situated anteriorly in the LV. In complete AV septal defect with a free-floating and bridging LSL, no LV inflow obstruction results. Otherwise, or after repair, the situation is entirely analogous to a true "parachute mitral valve" (see "Papillary Muscle Anomalies" under Morphology in Chapter 36), and inflow obstruction can complicate intracardiac repair.[D1,D5,I1,T8]

Ventricles

The LV outflow tract is characteristically elongated and narrowed (Fig. 20-10) in all types of AV septal defect (see

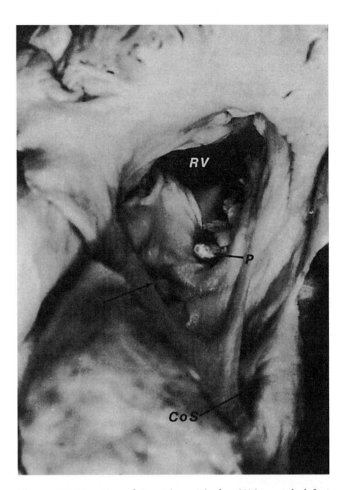

Figure 20-11 Complete atrioventricular (AV) septal defect with hypoplasia of left ventricle and a dominant right ventricle. Specimen is viewed from its right atrial aspect, and a probe passes into left ventricular cavity. The common AV valves open almost entirely into right ventricle. Arrow indicates superior margin of the ostium primum atrial septal defect.

Key: *CoS,* Coronary sinus; *P,* probe; *RV,* right ventricle.

"General Morphologic Characteristics" under Morphology earlier in this chapter).

In AV septal defect with large interventricular communications, the LV may be abnormally large. However, its size is variable, both absolutely and in relation to the right ventricle.[B5] In the severely right dominant type of AV septal defect, the LV is severely hypoplastic (Fig. 20-11).[S2] In such cases the atrial septum may be displaced leftward in relation to the plane of the ventricular septum, in which case it overrides the left AV valve to a varying degree and may be associated with hypoplasia of the left atrium.[T2,U1] This variant is therefore sometimes included in "hypoplastic left heart physiology."

The right ventricle has no specific anomalies but is usually enlarged secondary to the left-to-right shunt. Its size is also variable, and occasionally it is importantly hypoplastic (Thanopoulos and colleagues: personal communication; 1981).

The left or right ventricle is severely hypoplastic in about 7% of patients born with complete AV septal defect.[C7] Prevalence of the two types is similar. Presence of severe ventricular hypoplasia can increase risk of surgical correction and may demand a Fontan-type repair, alone or with a technique for correcting of the hypoplastic left heart physiology (see Chapter 35).[C7,F4,S2]

Septal Malalignment

Usually the two AV valves or common AV valve orifice lies in proper proportion over the two ventricles. When one ventricle is hypoplastic, the ventricular septum is malaligned and lies more to the side of the hypoplastic ventricle (see Fig. 20-11).

Less commonly, the atrial septal remnant is malaligned, and then usually leftward. When this is severe, both AV valves (or common AV valve orifice) are accessible only from the right atrium, and blood exists from the left atrium only through the ostium primum defect (so-called double outlet right atrium).[A3,C8,W8]

Left Ventricular Outflow or Inflow Obstruction

Important LV outflow tract obstruction occurs rarely in unoperated hearts (about 1% of cases) in all types of AV septal defect.[C7,P7,S2,S4,T2] It more often becomes apparent as a postoperative complication. It is surprising that it is not more frequent, in view of the elongation and narrowing of this area in affected hearts.[D7,E6]

Part of the elongation and narrowing is due to the more extensive area of direct fibrous continuity between the aortic valve and the LSL than is present normally between the aortic and mitral valves.[E7] This is formed in part by the short, thick chordae that often anchor the LSL to the crest of the ventricular septum.[C9,V2] Also, the anterolateral muscle bundle of the LV (muscle of Moulaert) bulges more into the LV outflow tract in hearts with AV septal defects than in normal hearts, contributing to the tendency to outflow obstruction after repair.[D7] In addition to these basic arrangements tending to narrow the LV outflow tract, LV obstruction may be contributed to by morphologically discrete subaortic stenosis or by excrescences of AV valve tissue heaped up in the LV outflow tract.[B14,P7,S3,T5] It may also result from abnormally positioned papillary muscles.[P7] Occasionally, its presence is overlooked preoperatively, and it becomes apparent or develops only after operation.

Important LV inflow obstruction may occur rarely.[P7] This may be from simple narrowing of the AV valve entrance into the LV, usually associated with marked right ventricular dominance. It may be related to presence of an accessory AV valve orifice on the left side, or it may result from cor triatriatum (see Chapter 18) or a supravalvar fibrous ring.[T7] These associated cardiac anomalies appear to be more prevalent in patients without Down syndrome than in those with it.[D6,V8]

Conduction System

The defect in the AV septum often displaces the coronary sinus ostium inferiorly. (It may appear to lie in the left atrium, especially when the ostium primum atrial defect is particularly large.) The AV node is also displaced inferiorly (caudally) and lies in the posterior right atrial wall between the orifice of the coronary sinus and ventricular crest[L4]

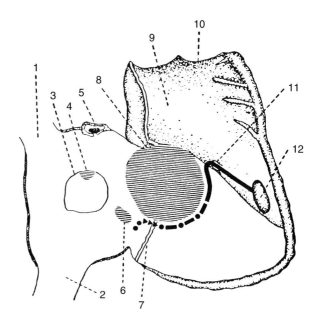

Figure 20-12   Diagrammatic sketch of the course of atrioventricular (AV) node, His bundle, and right bundle branch in common AV septal defect, right atrial and ventricular view. (Sinoatrial node is normal.) (From Lev.[L4])

Key: •, Atrioventricular node; ▲, penetrating portion of the atrioventricular bundle; • ■■, branching portion of the atrioventricular bundle; ■■■, right bundle branch; 1, superior vena cava; 2, inferior vena cava; 3, limbus; 4, patent foramen ovale; 5, cut edge of atrial appendage; 6, entry of coronary sinus; 7, base of atrioventricular valve; 8, atrioventricular septal communication; 9, infundibulum; 10, base of pulmonary valve; 11, muscle of Lancisi; 12, cut edge of moderator band.

(Fig. 20-12), in what has been termed the *nodal triangle*.[T6] The bundle of His passes forward and superiorly from the node to the ventricular crest, reaching it where the crest fuses posteriorly with the AV valve anulus.[B18] It then courses along the top of the ventricular septum, beneath the bridging portion of the LIL, giving off the left bundle branches. As it reaches the midpoint of the crest of the ventricular septum, it becomes the right bundle branch, which continues along the crest a little farther before it descends toward the muscle of Lancisi and moderator band. These anatomic findings have been supported by electrophysiologic studies at operation.[K3-K5] This morphology of the conduction system is a determinant of the electrocardiographic pattern usually seen in AV septal defects and is of obvious surgical importance.[F2,T6]

Major Associated Cardiac Anomalies

Table 20-6 presents the prevalence of the major cardiac anomalies associated with AV septal defects.

Patent Ductus Arteriosus

A *patent ductus arteriosus* is present in about 10% of patients with AV septal defects. It is particularly common in those with an interventricular communication.

Tetralogy of Fallot

Typical tetralogy of Fallot is present in about 5% of patients with complete AV septal defects, and about 1% of patients with tetralogy of Fallot have associated complete AV septal defects.[B13,K11,N3] The LSL bridges markedly and is free-floating over the crest of the ventricular septum, and the interventricular communication beneath it is large and juxtaaortic.[D4,F3,L8,T3] An interventricular communication beneath the LIL is present in only about half of cases.[V9] Rarely, the LSL and LIL are connected by a fibrous (or valvar) band, beneath which also is a large interventricular communication. The right ventricular outflow tract has typical tetralogy morphology (see Chapter 24) that may be so severe that pulmonary atresia is present. Localized narrowing occasionally occurring in that portion of the LV outflow tract just upstream from the recess formed by the subaortic deficiency of the ventricular septum further complicates the situation in rare cases.

Double Outlet Right Ventricle

Double outlet right ventricle without pulmonary stenosis complicates complete AV septal defect in about 2% of cases.[B11,B13,R3,S2,S7,T3] As in tetralogy of Fallot, usually deficiency of the ventricular septum is large and juxtaaortic beneath the extensively bridging and free-floating LSL. However, occasionally the interventricular communication is far from the aortic and pulmonary valves and is "noncommitted."[B11] Rarely, Taussig-Bing type of double outlet right ventricle is present.[B13,S7] Double outlet right ventricle combined with severe pulmonary stenosis coexists with complete AV septal defects in about 1% of cases.[S2] These combinations of double outlet right ventricle and AV septal defect with large interventricular communication frequently also have situs ambiguus or situs inversus, common atrium, completely unroofed coronary sinus with left superior vena cava, azygos extension of the inferior vena cava, or total anomalous pulmonary venous connection.[P3,S7]

Transposition of the Great Arteries

Very rarely, *transposition of the great arteries* (discordant ventriculoarterial connection) is associated[B13] (see Table 20-6).

Completely Unroofed Coronary Sinus with Left Superior Vena Cava

Completely unroofed coronary sinus with persistent left superior vena cava (see Chapter 19) attached to left atrium occurs in about 3% of patients with an interventricular communication and in about 3% without, and is more frequent when common atrium is present.[Q1] A *partially unroofed* distal end of the coronary sinus, resulting in drainage of the coronary sinus into the left atrium, occasionally occurs, but is a minor and unimportant associated anomaly.[Y1] When complete AV septal defect is associated with persistent left superior vena cava and unroofed coronary sinus, atrial isomerism is also frequent.[A7]

Minor Associated Cardiac Anomalies

Table 20-7 lists minor cardiac anomalies associated with AV septal defects.

Pulmonary Vascular Disease

In partial AV septal defects, as in other types of ASDs, pulmonary vascular disease is uncommon, whereas in complete AV septal defects, as with large VSDs, pulmonary vascular disease usually appears early in life and progresses.[H3]

Morphologically, pulmonary vascular disease associated with complete AV septal defects is similar to that associated with large VSDs (see "Pulmonary Vascular Disease" under Morphology in Section 1 of Chapter 21). However, it tends to progress more rapidly in patients with complete AV septal defects. Correlation between histologic findings and pulmonary vascular resistance is similar in the two conditions.[F6] The pulmonary vascular changes probably are more frequent and occur at an earlier age in patients with Down syndrome with complete AV septal defects compared with patients without Down syndrome.[C11,Y3]

Down Syndrome

Down syndrome is rare in patients with partial AV septal defects but common (about 75%) in those with complete AV septal defects.[W6] Left-sided obstructive lesions are 10 times less common in Down syndrome patients[D6,V8]; other associated anomalies are probably also less common.[P9] As noted earlier, advanced pulmonary vascular disease may be more frequent.[F6]

Inlet Septal Type of Ventricular Septal Defect

It is important to note that an isolated inlet (AV septal) type of VSD (see "Morphology" in Section 1 of Chapter 21) occurs without any of the features of an AV septal defect as defined in this chapter, except that it involves the inflow portion of the ventricular septum beneath the septal tricuspid valve leaflet and usually also the area of the membranous ventricular septum. The AV septum is, however, intact, and the mitral and tricuspid anuli and aortic orifice lie in normal positions. This feature allows these VSDs to be readily differentiated echocardiographically and angiographically from AV septal defects. Interestingly, in isolated inlet VSD, the anterior mitral leaflet is occasionally cleft.

CLINICAL FEATURES AND DIAGNOSTIC CRITERIA

Pathophysiology

Left-to-right shunting is present in AV septal defects unless severe pulmonary vascular disease has developed or important pulmonary stenosis coexists. When there is no interventricular communication, the shunt is at atrial level and usually large. It may, however, be small or moderate, and in such cases a pressure gradient can be demonstrated between left and right atria. When the shunt is large and left AV valve regurgitation is mild or absent, the hemodynamic state of the patient is identical to that in isolated ASD (see "Clinical Features and Diagnostic Criteria" in Chapter 16); only right ventricular stroke volume is increased. When important left AV valve regurgitation is present, the left-to-right shunt becomes much larger; in fact, the regurgitation jet usually goes directly from LV to right atrium. Left as well as right ventricular stroke volume is increased, and marked cardiomegaly and heart failure develop early in life.

When a large interventricular communication is also present (complete AV septal defect), the left-to-right shunt is large, and right ventricular and pulmonary artery pres-

■ **TABLE 20-11   Preoperative Pulmonary Artery–Aortic Pressure Ratios in Patients without Major Associated Cardiac Anomalies**

P~PA~/P~AO~		Without Interventricular Communication (n = 140)		With Interventricular Communication (n = 97)	
≤ ratio <		No.	% of 97 [a]	No.	% of 74 [b]
	.03	65	67 ⎫ 85/97	5	7 ⎫ 12/74
.03	.05	20	21 ⎬ (88%)	7	9 ⎬ (16%)
.05	.07	5	5	10	14
.07	.09	6	6 ⎫ 7/97	29	39 ⎫ 52/74
.09		1	1 ⎬ (7%)	23	31 ⎬ (70%)

(Data from Studer and colleagues.[S2])

Key: *AO*, Aortic; *PA*, pulmonary artery.

[a] Data not available for 43 patients.

[b] Data not available for 23 patients.

sures approach or equal systemic pressures (Table 20-11). Pulmonary vascular resistance rises rapidly and is usually importantly elevated after age 6 to 12 months and sometimes before.[N1] When present, AV valve regurgitation adds greatly to the ventricular volume overload. For some reason, however, the overload usually seems to enlarge the right ventricle more than the left.

Atrioventricular Valve Regurgitation

Prevalence of regurgitation at the left AV valve or common AV valve is now considered to be less than before echocardiographic studies were available. Probably 10% to 15% of patients with partial AV septal defect have important regurgitation, not 40% as was estimated earlier (see Table 20-9). Moderate AV valve regurgitation is present in about 20% of infants with complete AV septal defects and severe regurgitation in only about 15%.[A5,B1,C2,W7] AV valve regurgitation may be considerably more prevalent in older patients with complete AV septal defects.

A not uncommon site of regurgitation is through the gap between the LSL and LIL, particularly near the leaflet hinge or base; partly for this reason, regurgitant flow frequently goes directly into the right atrium. Under such circumstances the left atrium remains small and the right becomes large; but, when the interatrial communication is smaller or the regurgitation is sited elsewhere, regurgitation may enter the left atrium, which enlarges.

Although the precise mechanism of AV valve regurgitation is often unclear, it apparently varies considerably, as would be expected from variations in the number, size, and configuration of the leaflets and their chordal attachments. In patients with partial AV septal defects and important left AV valve regurgitation, the LIL is commonly severely hypoplastic.

Symptoms and Physical Findings

Patients without an interventricular communication (partial AV septal defect) and with absent or mild left AV valve regurgitation often present in the first decade of life, but they may remain asymptomatic well beyond that age. Their clinical presentation is virtually identical to that of patients with the more common fossa ovalis ASD (see "Fossa

Ovalis Defect" under Morphology in Chapter 16), except that they may have an apical systolic murmur when mild left AV valve regurgitation is present, and left axis deviation and a counterclockwise frontal plane loop.[O1,T1]

Moderate or severe (grade 3, 4, or 5) left AV valve regurgitation in patients with partial AV septal defects may produce symptoms earlier, and progressive severe heart failure may require treatment in infancy.[B12] In addition to the usual signs of ASD, the heart is more active in association with a loud apical pansystolic murmur, and the apex of the LV may be palpable. Tachypnea and hepatomegaly are often evident.

In patients with complete AV septal defect, presentation is usually in the first year of life, and frequently during the first months, as a result of progressive severe heart failure, which may not be controllable medically. There is associated tachypnea, poor peripheral perfusion, and failure to thrive. Occasionally, heart failure is minimal early in life, and presentation may be delayed until some years later, by which time there is almost always severe hypertensive pulmonary vascular disease and Eisenmenger complex (see "Clinical Findings" under Clinical Features and Diagnostic Criteria in Section 1 of Chapter 21). On physical examination, cardiomegaly with increased ventricular activity is apparent. The second heart sound at the base is split and usually fixed, with accentuation of the second component caused by elevated pulmonary artery pressure. A systolic murmur is audible over the left precordium from the shunt at ventricular level and is increased in intensity and nearer the apex when there is important AV valve regurgitation. A mid-diastolic flow murmur is characteristically widely heard both over the lower left precordium and at the apex secondary to the large diastolic flow across the malformed AV valve leaflets (depending on both the left-to-right shunt and any AV valve regurgitation).

In those patients with morphology intermediate between the partial and complete AV septal defects, clinical features depend on size of the interventricular communication and severity of left AV valve regurgitation.

Chest Radiograph

In patients without an interventricular communication or important left AV valve regurgitation, the chest radiograph is the same as in other large ASDs. When moderate or severe left AV valve regurgitation is present, the radiograph usually shows marked cardiomegaly, with evidence of LV, right ventricular, and right atrial enlargement and marked pulmonary plethora. Left atrial enlargement is not apparent unless the ostium primum defect is restrictive.

In complete AV septal defect, cardiomegaly and pulmonary plethora are evident in infants and young children presenting with heart failure. In patients who survive beyond this age, severely increased pulmonary vascular resistance usually dominates, and the heart is less enlarged, central pulmonary arteries are large, and lung fields are clear.

Electrocardiogram

Electrocardiographic findings are rather specific.[D3] They usually indicate marked right ventricular hypertrophy and may show LV hypertrophy as well. The PR interval is

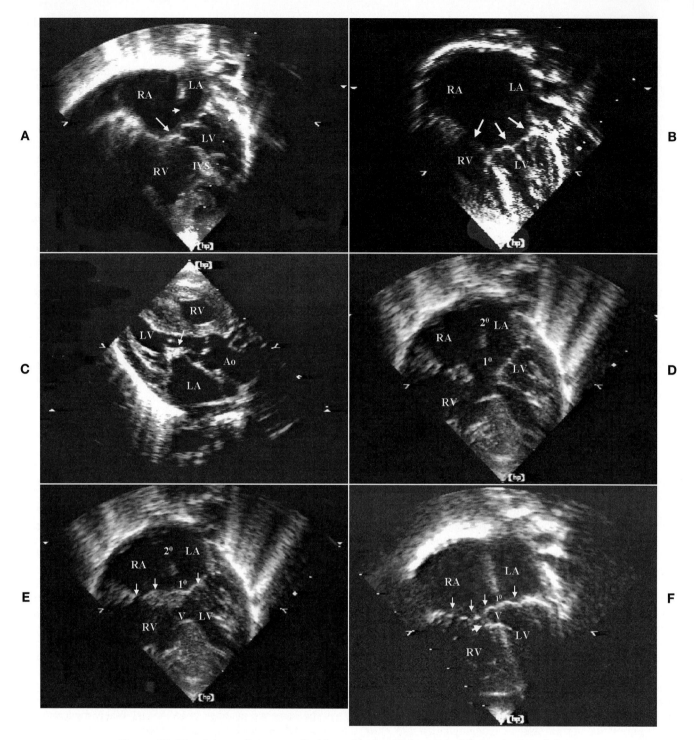

Figure 20-13 Echocardiograms of atrioventricular (AV) septal defects. **A,** Apical four-chamber view of a heart with an unbalanced AV septal defect. In this figure, the common AV valve *(arrow)* is positioned such that there is malalignment between interatrial septum and interventricular septum and a disproportionate size of the ventricles. Smaller arrow shows primum atrial septal defect. **B,** Apical four-chamber view showing common AV valve *(arrows)* with virtual absence of interatrial septum. **C,** Parasternal long axis view showing a "gooseneck" appearance of left ventricular outflow tract caused by displacement of left-sided portion of a common AV valve *(arrow)*. **D,** Coronal image of heart as viewed from apex (apical four-chamber view). This heart has a complete AV septal defect. There are both primum and secundum atrial septal defects. **E,** Coronal image of a heart with a complete AV septal defect as viewed from the apex (apical four-chamber view). Arrows point to the common AV valve. There are both primum and secundum atrial septal defects. **F,** Coronal image of a heart with a partial AV septal defect as viewed from the apex (apical four-chamber view). Thin arrows point to common AV valve. Thick arrow points to tissue occluding the inlet ventricular septal defect right AV valve pouch formation.

Key: *Ao,* Aorta; *IVS,* interventricular septum; *LA,* left atrium; *LV,* left ventricle; *RA,* right atrium, *RV,* right ventricle; *V,* inlet ventricular septal defect; *1°,* primum; *2°,* secundum.

frequently prolonged. Of considerable diagnostic importance is the vectorcardiogram.[T1] Ongley and colleagues conclude that a counterclockwise frontal plane loop anterior and to the right strongly suggests, but does not prove, the diagnosis.[O1]

Two-Dimensional Echocardiogram

In AV septal defects without an interventricular communication or important left AV valve regurgitation, two-dimensional echocardiography, together with clinical presentation, chest radiograph, and electrocardiogram, is diagnostic, and cardiac catheterization with cineangiography is not necessary.[L5,S9] Two-dimensional echocardiography, particularly with Doppler color flow imaging and, when possible, with a transthoracic window, can also provide full information for complete AV septal defects.[C10,S12]

The common AV orifice is easily seen in the four-chamber view (Fig. 20-13). Characteristically, left and right AV valves (separated or common) exist at the same level, in contrast to the cephalad displacement of the normal mitral valve. The elongated outflow septum and unwedged position of the aortic valve are also identifiable. Chordal attachment and degree of leaflet bridging can also be assessed. Finally, the degree of AV valve regurgitation is assessed with color flow.

Limitations of echocardiography include lack of sensitivity for double orifice left AV valve and inability to assess quantitatively pulmonary vascular resistance and reactivity.

Cardiac Catheterization and Cineangiogram

Direction and magnitude of shunting; pulmonary and systemic pressures, resistances, and flows; and right and left ventricular pressures can be measured and calculated from data obtained at cardiac catheterization (see "Cardiac Catheterization" under Clinical Features and Diagnostic Criteria in Section 1 of Chapter 21).[F1,P2] However, these studies are now required only when major cardiac anomalies coexist and when operability is questioned because of evidence of pulmonary vascular disease.

Angiocardiographic features of AV septal defects were well described by Baron and colleagues in 1964 and further refined by the work of Brandt and colleagues, Bargeron and colleagues, and Macartney and colleagues.[B4,B6,B7,B10,M12,S8] Both oblique and axial views are used.[B7,B10] They demonstrate absence of the AV septum and deficiency of the inlet portion of the ventricular septum, elongation of the LV outflow tract in relationship to the inflow tract, elevation and anterior displacement of the aortic valve vis-à-vis the AV valves, and the anomalous relationship of anterior components of the left AV valve to the aorta. These are well portrayed by the line drawings of Baron and colleagues and representative cineangiograms (Figs. 20-14 through 20-16).[B4] The anomalous left AV valve's relationship to the aorta results in change in direction of left AV valve movement. Interatrial and interventricular shunting can also be demonstrated, as can presence of one or two AV valve orifices. With high-quality studies, leaflets of the left AV valve often can be visualized in motion to delineate the degree, location, and mechanism of valvar regurgitation.

The relative size of the two ventricles and of AV orifices must be determined by whatever technique, echocardiography or angiography, is preferred. Severe hypoplasia of one or the other ventricle must be identified preoperatively, because such hypoplasia makes it unlikely that anatomic correction will be successful.[C7]

Special Situations and Associated Defects

Presence of *common atrium* generally can be identified preoperatively by echocardiography or a cineangiogram, which show nearly complete absence of both atrial and AV septum (see Fig. 20-13). Finding mild arterial desaturation in a patient with clinical findings of an AV septal defect, but without an interventricular communication or pulmonary artery hypertension, suggests presence of common atrium.[D3,F1,M8,R6,R7] Presence of a left superior vena cava in such a setting suggests both unroofed coronary sinus syndrome and common atrium, because they frequently coexist.[Q1,R7] In patients with common atrium and atrial isomerism, even more complex associations occur, including double outlet right ventricle, partial or total anomalous pulmonary venous connection, and azygos extension of the inferior vena cava (see "Morphology" in Chapter 44).[D1,K7,P3,S5,T4]

A patent ductus arteriosus can be identified on aortography. Likewise, associated malformations, such as tetralogy of Fallot, double outlet right ventricle, transposition of the great arteries, and additional VSDs, are identified by a combination of echocardiography and cineangiography.

It is essential to recognize functionally important LV outflow tract obstruction. Narrowing of this tract is inherent in AV septal defects, but rarely results in a systolic pressure gradient. Distortion results from the shortened inflow axis of the LV and anterior displacement of the left AV valve complex (Fig. 20-17).[V10] Thus, LV outflow obstruction is most prevalent in patients with Rastelli type A valve morphology.[P4,S14] This distortion is rarely evident preoperatively as LV outflow obstruction. More frequently, important obstruction becomes evident postoperatively, both early and later. Usually it takes the form of subaortic "discrete membranous" stenosis, but the process may be relatively diffuse along the outflow tract. Infrequently, it occurs as a result of the ventricular patch component pulling the left AV valve apically and anteriorly such that the new "mitral" valve apparatus narrows the outflow tract. Thus, the initial AV septal repair must place the left AV valve at the appropriate level: caudad toward the apex may result in LV outflow tract obstruction; cephalad toward the atria may result in left AV valve regurgitation.

NATURAL HISTORY

The life history of patients with surgically untreated AV septal defects depends on morphologic and functional details of their malformation. When there is a *partial AV septal defect, only mild left AV valve regurgitation,* and *no major associated cardiac anomaly,* life history without surgical treatment is similar to that of patients with large fossa ovalis ASDs (see "Natural History" in Chapter 16). Important pulmonary vascular disease develops in a small number of patients in their twenties, thirties, and forties.[P2]

Text continued on p. 823

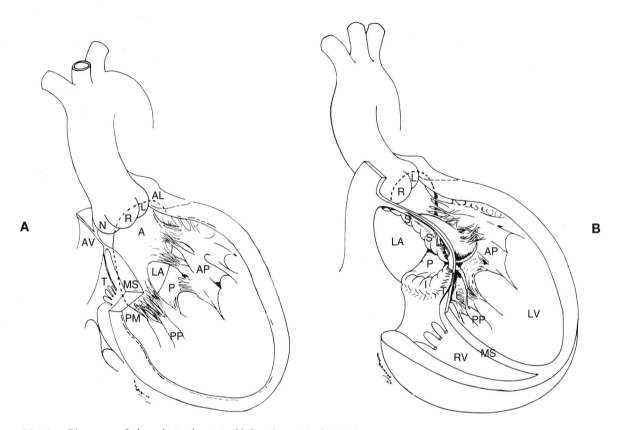

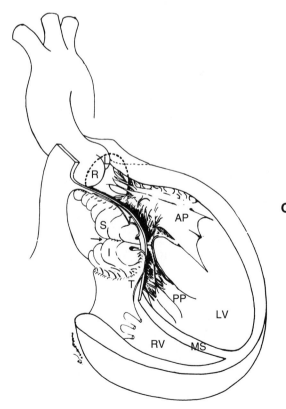

Figure 20-14   Diagrams of altered attachment of left atrioventricular *(AV)* valve leaflets in AV septal defect compared with normal heart. Heart is shown in its in vivo position as seen in a frontal angiogram. Right ventricle and most of the ventricular septum and right atrium have been removed. Dashed line indicates portion of line of attachment of left AV valve that is hidden by other structures. **A,** Normal heart. Attachment of anterior mitral leaflet begins at anterolateral commissure and runs anteriorly for a short distance along free wall of left ventricle. It is then continuous with the root of the aorta in relation to adjacent portion of left coronary and noncoronary aortic cusps. Line of attachment proceeds downward along AV septum to posteromedial commissure. Attachment of mitral valve to AV septum is profiled in right anterior oblique view (see Fig. 20-15). **B, C,** Partial AV septal defect shown in diastole (**B**) and systole (**C**). Scooped-out crest of basal portion of ventricular septum is shown considerably thinner than it actually is. Right AV valve leaflets are shown only at their sites of attachment. Diastolic figure (**B**) depicts left superior and left inferior leaflets as open; their line of attachment to aortic root is nearly normal, but it then passes along the superior rim of the scooped-out ventricular septal crest. Left superior leaflet is displaced upward into the left ventricular outflow tract, narrowing it. Left inferior leaflet is folded back against left ventricular aspect of sinus septum. In systolic figure (**C**), left superior and inferior leaflets are closed. Increased left ventricular pressure balloons them toward the atria. Arrow marks their point of coaptation. (From Baron and colleagues.[B4])

Key: *A,* Anterior mitral leaflet; *AL,* anterolateral commissure of mitral valve; *AP,* anterior papillary muscle; *AV,* atrioventricular septum; *I,* left inferior leaflet of atrioventricular valve; *L,* left coronary aortic cusp; *LA,* left atrium; *LV,* left ventricle; *MS,* muscular ventricular septum; *N,* noncoronary aortic cusp; *P,* posterior mitral leaflet; *PM,* posteromedial commissure of mitral valve; *PP,* posterior papillary muscle; *R,* right aortic cusp; *RV,* right ventricle; *S,* left superior leaflet of atrioventricular valve; *T,* tricuspid valve.

A

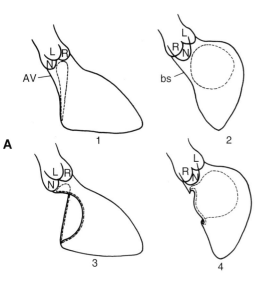

Figure 20-15   Diagrammatic representations of cineangiograms of a normal heart and hearts with atrioventricular *(AV)* septal defects, in oblique and axial views. **A,** Mitral valve orifice and leaflet attachments *(interrupted line)* in right anterior oblique (RAO) and left anterior oblique (LAO) projections. *(1)* Normal mitral orifice is approximately profiled in 40° RAO projection, but is overlapped by left ventricular (LV) outflow tract. Rightward posterior border of normal LV outflow tract is formed by AV septal tissue, not mitral valve. *(2)* In 50° LAO projections, the rightward anterior margin of the normal outflow tract consists of the basal ventricular sinus (inlet) septum: membranous above, muscular below. Mitral valve attachments do not reach the septal margin. *(3, 4)* In AV septal defects, absence of AV septum and adjacent deficiency of basal (inlet) ventricular septum modify left AV valve attachments and position and shape of left AV orifice and LV outflow tract. **B,** LV cineangiograms in 40° RAO projections. *(1, 2)* Normal features can be compared with those of typical partial *(3, 4)* and complete *(5, 6)* AV septal defect in systole and diastole. In the normal heart, mitral (left AV valve) leaflets contribute only to the lowest portion of the rightward posterior LV outflow margin in systole, the relatively immobile AV septum forming the remainder of this margin throughout the cardiac cycle in diastole. Line of attachment *(m)* of mural (posterior) leaflet of mitral valve can be identified, because contrast is trapped between the leaflet and adjacent LV wall. In AV septal defects, rightward posterior margin of LV outflow tract consists of mobile leaflet tissue: left superior leaflet *(s)* above and left inferior leaflet *(i)* below. AV septum is absent. Mural leaflet attachment lies in relatively normal position. When there is complete attachment of left superior and inferior leaflets to septal crest *(dashed line),* the LV outflow tract deformity is well marked in systole, and position of septal crest can be identified in diastole, with contrast being trapped between the open leaflets and septum. When there is a large interventricular communication with superior and inferior leaflets that are free-floating or attached to the septal crest by thin chordae only *(5, 6),* the systolic deformity may be less marked and septal crest may be invisible, because contrast is washed away by nonradio–opaque inflow. RAO view separates an AV regurgitant stream *(AVR)* from an interventricular shunt *(VS).*

Key: *AV,* Atrioventricular septum; *AVR,* atrioventricular regurgitant stream; *bs,* basal (inlet) portion of ventricular septum; *i,* left inferior leaflet; *L,* left coronary sinus of aortic root, *m,* line of attachment of posterior mitral leaflet; *N,* noncoronary sinus of aortic root; *R,* right coronary sinus of aortic root; *s,* left superior leaflet; *VS,* ventricular shunt.

Continued

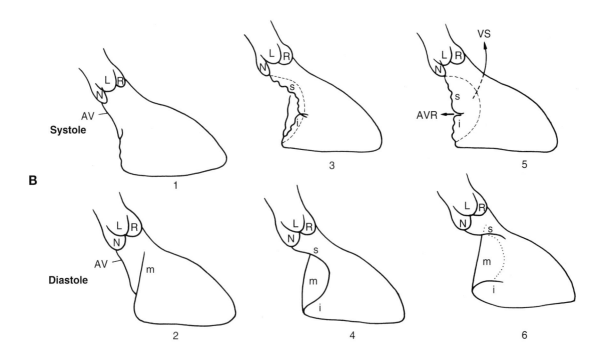

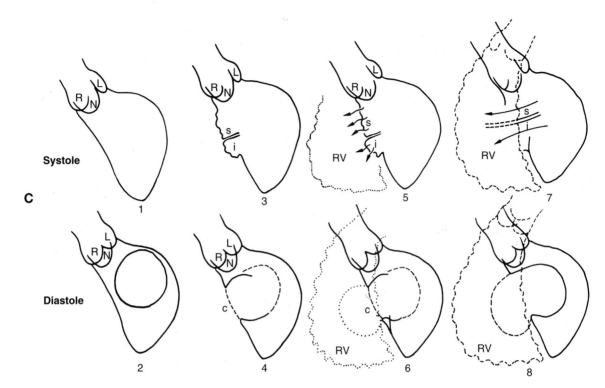

C

Systole

Diastole

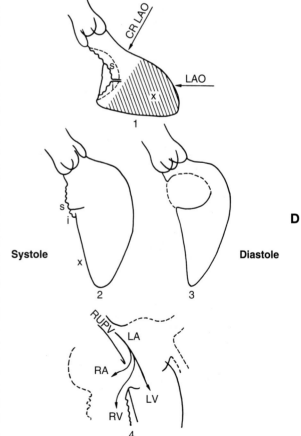

D

Systole

Diastole

Figure 20-15, cont'd **C,** Left ventricular *(LV)* cineangiograms in 50° left anterior oblique *(LAO)* projection. *(1, 2)* In the normal heart, septal margin of the LV outflow tract is uninterrupted in systole and diastole. In AV septal defect *(3 to 8)*, septal margin is interrupted by defect in basal (inlet) ventricular septum, the defect being continuous with left AV orifice. *(3, 4)* When left superior and inferior leaflets are completely attached to septal crest, as in partial AV septal defect, leaflet tissue bulges into defect in systole, and position of septal crest *(c)* can be identified in diastole. *(7, 8)* When there is a large interventricular communication, systolic flow into right ventricle can be observed passing beneath left superior *(upper arrow)* or left inferior *(lower arrow)* leaflets. In diastole, a common AV orifice is identified. *(5, 6)* In some cases, attachments to septal crest are present but leave smaller interventricular communications. AV valve regurgitation tends to obscure valve detail as overlying atria opacify. **D,** LV or left atrial cineangiograms of AV septal defect in 50° LAO with cranial angulation (axial, hepatoclavicular, or four-chamber view). *(1)* Arrows in 40° RAO view illustrate why conventional LAO (part **C**) shows full height of the AV orifice, providing the best separation of left superior from left inferior leaflets. Cranially tilted version of LAO *(CR LAO)* foreshortens AV orifice and tends to superimpose these leaflets. *(2, 3)* However, the characteristic deformity of septal and AV orifice anatomy seen in conventional LAO view can be appreciated in axial LAO views, which are shown in both systole and diastole. In addition, midmuscular and apical parts of the sinus septum are better separated from basal defect so that additional muscular defects in cross-hatched area (for example, at *x)* may be identified. AV valve regurgitation obscures detail, but partial separation of atria from ventricles improves differentiation of regurgitation from interventricular shunting. With a left atrial or right upper pulmonary venous injection in 50° LAO with cranial angulation *(4)*, contrast flow *(arrows)* early in the sequence shows position of atrial septal defect adjacent to AV valves. Contrast enters right atrium, right ventricle, and left ventricle. Cranial angulation rarely achieves a perfect profile of AV anulus, and ventricular opacification obscures detail later in the sequence.

Key: *c,* Septal crest; *CR LAO,* cranial left anterior oblique; *i,* left inferior leaflet; *L,* left coronary sinus of aortic root; *LA,* left atrium; *LAO,* left anterior oblique; *LV,* left ventricle; *N,* noncoronary sinus of aortic root; *R,* right coronary sinus of aortic root; *RA,* right atrium; *RUPV,* right upper pulmonary venous injection; *RV,* right ventricle; *s,* left superior leaflet.

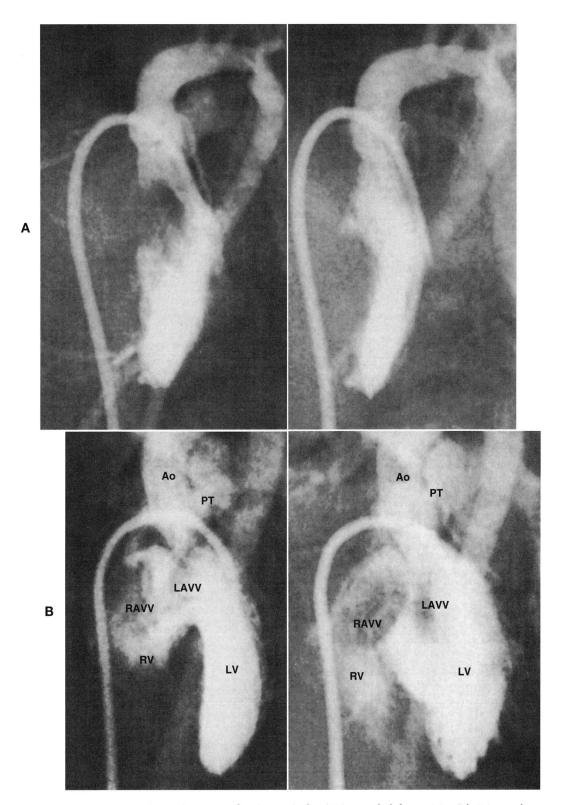

Figure 20-16   Cineangiograms of atrioventricular (AV) septal defects. **A,** Partial AV septal defect shown by left ventriculogram in four-chamber position: diastolic frame (left) and systolic frame (right). Loss of straight line contour from aortic valve to crux cordis indicates absence of major part of AV septum. **B,** AV septal defect with two AV valve orifices and an interventricular communication.

Key: *Ao,* Aorta; *LAVV,* left atrioventricular valve; *LV,* left ventricle; *PT,* pulmonary trunk; *RAVV,* right atrioventricular valve; *RV,* right ventricle.   *Continued*

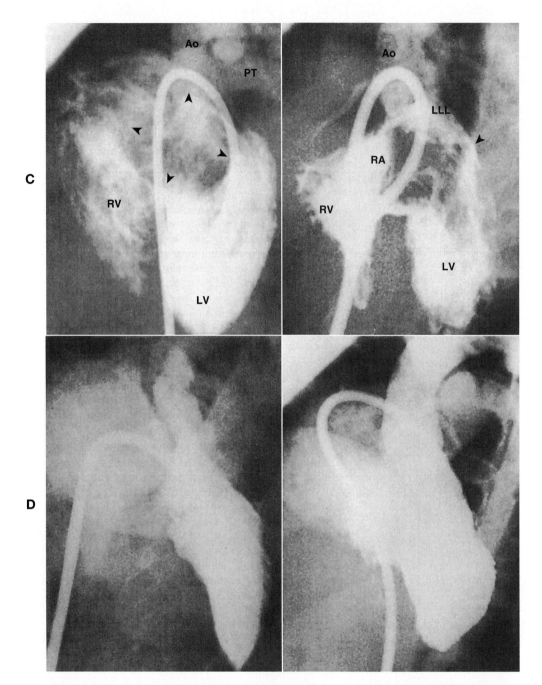

Figure 20-16, cont'd   C, Complete atrioventricular (AV) septal defect shown by left ventriculo-gram in four-chamber view. On the left, anulus of valve is seen as a negative shadow formed by accumulation of contrast medium between the leaflets and ventricular free wall *(arrows)*. The anulus includes right and left ventricles in almost equal proportions. On the right, contrast medium outlines left lateral leaflet, which is related to the aorta and separated from left superior leaflet by a commissure *(arrow)* marking position of papillary muscle of conus. Outline of left superior leaflet is separated from left lateral leaflet by a commissure marking position of anterior papillary muscle of left ventricle. This represents an example of Rastelli type A defect. **D,** Partial AV septal defects with moderate (left) and severe (right) regurgitation of left AV valve. Contrast medium has passed from left ventricle into right atrium through regurgitant valve.

Key: *Ao,* Aorta; *LLL,* left lateral leaflet; *LV,* left ventricle; *PT,* pulmonary trunk; *RA,* right atrium; *RV,* right ventricle.

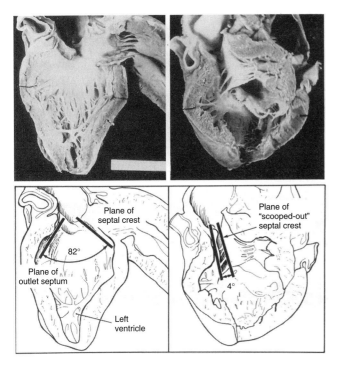

Figure 20-17   Anatomic specimens (above) and drawings of them (below) contrasting outflow angle in a normal heart compared to that in atrioventricular (AV) septal defect. *Left,* wide angle between plane of outlet septum and plane of septal crest (outflow angle) in a normal heart. *Right,* Narrow angle in a heart with AV septal defect. Septal crest is scooped out, shortened, and anteriorly displaced; outflow axis is elongated. (From Van Arsdell and colleagues.[V12])

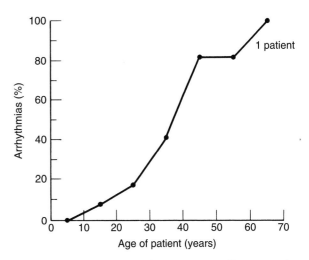

Figure 20-18   Cardiac arrhythmias in surgically untreated patients with a partial atrioventricular septal defect according to age. Increased prevalence in older patients is striking. (From Somerville.[S6])

As in other types of large ASD, symptomatic deterioration of patients in adult life often coincides with development of atrial fibrillation (Fig. 20-18).[S6]

Patients with a *partial AV septal defect* and *moderate or severe left AV valve regurgitation* have a different natural history. Because of a nonrestrictive interatrial communication, severe left atrial and pulmonary venous hypertension are absent, but the left-to-right shunt is large and pulmonary artery pressure usually at least moderately elevated. Probably at least 20% of such individuals are severely symptomatic in infancy, and without surgical treatment, many would die in the first decade of life.

Patients with a *complete AV septal defect* have a still more unfavorable natural history. Because no group of infants known to have this malformation has been followed from birth without surgical intervention, the ideal database for delineation of their natural history does not exist. The closest approach is the prospective study of 56,109 live births by Mitchell and colleagues that included 10 infants judged to have isolated complete AV septal defect (excluding four stillbirths with the malformation), four of whom died within the first 3 years of life.[M11] This information is inconclusive, however, because of the small number of patients involved; failure to obtain a positive diagnosis by surgery, autopsy, or cardiac catheterization in all patients in

the study; use of surgical intervention in some cases; and nonreporting of specific ages of the six survivors.

An important event in the natural history is development of severe pulmonary vascular disease. This complication becomes apparent at 7 to 12 months of age in up to 30% of patients with complete AV septal defect and is probably present in 90% of such patients by age 3 to 5 years.[F6,N1] Thus, its prevalence in early life is higher in patients with complete AV septal defect than in those with large VSD.

In the absence of a definitive prospective study, approximation of natural history of complete AV septal defect has been constructed from 39 patients in two reports of autopsies.[B8] This analysis indicates that about 80% of patients who do not undergo operation die by age 2 years (Fig. 20-19). A child surviving to age 1 year has only about a 15% chance of living to age 5. Those who die in the first 1 to 2 years of life usually do so with heart failure, with or without recurrent pulmonary infections, as a result of the large left-to-right shunt and moderate-to-severe AV valve regurgitation present in 60%.[S2] The high incidence of death in the first year of life has been confirmed by Samánek.[S11] Thereafter, valve regurgitation and increasing pulmonary vascular disease become dominant factors in the natural history. Newfeld and colleagues showed histologically that advanced pulmonary vascular disease (Heath-Edwards grade 3 and 4; see "Pulmonary Vascular Disease" under Morphology in Section 1 of Chapter 21) is occasionally present in such infants, even in the first year of life.[N1] However, it is present in nearly 90% of patients older than age 1 year (7 of their 8 specimens).

Bull and colleagues dispute these inferences and deduce a more favorable prognosis for infants with complete AV septal defects based on a study of patients with Down syndrome and this anomaly.[B19] Careful study of their report generates uncertainty as to the appropriateness of analyses underlying their inferences, however.[K14,W6]

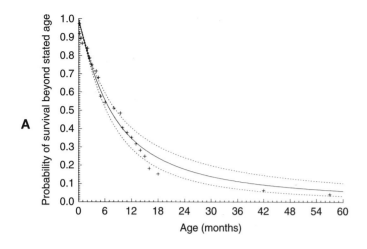

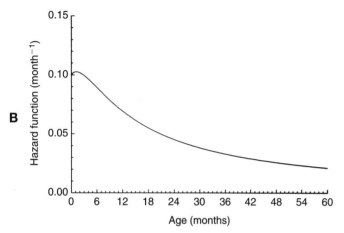

Figure 20-19   Life expectancy without surgery of patients with complete atrioventricular septal defects. **A**, Plus signs represent nonparametric survival estimates; solid line, with its 70% confidence limits *(dotted lines)*, represents parametric survival estimates. Note that probability of surviving beyond 6 months is 50%, and beyond a year is only 30%. **B**, Hazard function according to age. Note that risk of dying is highest in the first few months of life. (From Berger and colleagues.[B8])

Another aspect of the natural history of patients with AV septal defects is the tendency of their offspring to have similar defects or other congenital cardiac malformations. Emanuel and colleagues found that 14% of children of mothers with AV septal defects have congenital heart disease[E5]; half have tetralogy of Fallot, and half have AV septal defects. This prevalence is much higher than the 2% to 4% among children of parents with other types of congenital heart disease.[N2]

TECHNIQUE OF OPERATION

Surgical treatment of AV septal defects is directed toward (1) closing the interatrial communication, which is virtually always present; (2) closing the interventricular communication, if one is present; (3) avoiding damage to the AV node and bundle of His; and (4) maintaining or creating two competent, nonstenotic AV valves.

Repair techniques vary considerably, but when used properly, all appear to provide good results.[E9,L9,L11] For example:

- One or two patches may be used to repair the malformation when there is large interventricular communication.[R1]
- A markedly bridging LSL may be divided to facilitate the repair, or it may be left intact.[B15,R5,S2]
- The AV node and bundle of His may be avoided by staying on the LV and left atrial side (McGoon DC: personal communication; 1978) or by staying on the right side of the septum.[S2]
- Contiguous surfaces of the LSL and LIL may be sutured together, or the left AV valve may be left as a tricuspid structure.[C6,R2]
- The patch may be attached to leaflet tissue by simple sutures or by pledgeted mattress sutures with some sort of sandwich method,[S2] with assortment of techniques employed to establish AV valve competence.[C6]

Methods described in this chapter are the product of experiences in several centers and have improved surgical results. They avoid functionally important damage to the conduction system, provide complete and permanent closure of interatrial and interventricular communications, and are suitable for the many variations across the spectrum of AV septal defects. They are well adapted to cases with major associated cardiac anomalies. They retain AV valve competence when it is present, minimize occurrence of valve repair dehiscence, and generally abolish or lessen AV valve regurgitation, although in this regard the results are imperfect, particularly in patients without interventricular communications.[K8,S2] The same improvements have been obtained while retaining the single patch technique. Addition of intraoperative transesophageal echocardiography to assess completeness of repair provides a further safeguard against an imperfect anatomic and functional result.[R9]

Repair of Complete Atrioventricular Septal Defect with Little or No Bridging of Left Superior and Left Inferior Leaflets: Rastelli Type A

Two-Patch Technique

After the usual preparations a median sternotomy is made, a large piece of pericardium is removed and set aside (see footnote 2, "Pericardial Patch Preparation," under Technique of Operation in Chapter 16), and pericardial stay sutures are applied. External cardiac anatomy is evaluated and a left superior vena cava sought. If one is present, there is a 50% chance of associated unroofed coronary sinus syndrome. Purse-string sutures are placed.

In patients weighing less than 8 kg, repair may be performed with limited cardiopulmonary bypass (CPB) with a single venous cannula and hypothermic circulatory arrest; in larger patients, standard CPB is used. Alternatively, in both infants and older children, hypothermic CPB at 20°C and cold cardioplegia may be used. In this method, the cavae are cannulated directly with thin-walled, right-angled metal cannulae (see "Venous Cannulation" in Section 3 of Chapter 2). CPB flow is reduced to about

$1.2 \; L \cdot min^{-1} \cdot m^{-2}$ when the patient's temperature reaches 20°C. Short periods of circulatory arrest are occasionally used if visibility is not excellent. As cooling proceeds, the right atrium is opened widely, and a pump sump sucker is passed through the foramen ovale into the left atrium. Stay sutures are applied, the aorta is clamped, and cold cardioplegic solution is injected.

The malformation is examined and each morphologic detail noted (Fig. 20-20). Morphology of the LSL and LIL is noted carefully with the leaflets in both the closed and open positions. Cold saline solution is injected once or twice through the valve and the closure pattern and any regurgitant leaks studied (Fig. 20-21, *A-C*). The most anterior point of LSL–LIL opposing edges is found, and a double-armed No. 6-0 or 7-0 polypropylene suture is placed through it. Leaflet stay and marking sutures are placed, measurements are made, and the polyester interventricular patch is trimmed.

The patch is sutured to the right side of the crest of the ventricular septum with continuous polypropylene suture (Fig. 20-21, *D* and *E*). Chordae of RSL and RIL stay on the right ventricular side of the patch; those of LSL and LIL stay on the LV side, and some may be cut if they interfere with the suturing, because the anterior edges of these leaflets will be sutured to the polyester patch.

When this phase is completed, the marking suture on anterior edges of the coapting surfaces of the LSL–LIL complex is passed through the appropriate point of the edge of the polyester ventricular defect patch. The pericardial interatrial patch is then trimmed to appropriate shape and size, and the first part of its insertion is accomplished (Fig. 20-21, *F*). For this, interrupted mattress sutures of No. 6-0 polyester are placed to enclose anterior edges of LSL and LIL between the polyester patch below and pericardial patch above. Alternatively, left-sided leaflet tissue is anchored as a separate maneuver to the polyester patch; the pericardial atrial septal patch is then sewn to the leaflet-patch line of attachment. Great care is taken to ensure alignment of left AV valve leaflets is perfect and without distortion during this process.

Saline solution is again injected through the left-sided portion of the AV valves (two orifices are present once the interventricular patch is in place) to study its closure pattern and competence. A few additional "tailoring sutures" are placed without tension along the coapting surfaces of LSL and LIL near the patch, if needed, to prevent systolic eversion or prolapse; usually they are not required. If a central leak (at the point of junction of LSL, LIL, and LLL) persists, an anuloplasty stitch is placed in the region of the commissure between LSL and LLL. If necessary and if the orifice is large enough, a similar stitch can be placed at the LLL–LIL commissure, the surgeon being certain not to approach the AV node. This part of the operation is critically important and requires patience and ingenuity.

Assessment of both left and right AV valves at this point includes consideration of their size. The diameter of each is estimated with Hegar dilators and considered acceptable if within 2 SD of normal for the size of the patient (*Z* value is −2 or greater; see Chapter 1, Appendix 1D, Table 1D-2).

Repair is completed by suturing the rest of the pericardial interatrial patch in place, with the suture line passing *around* the AV node and bundle of His and not across them

(Fig. 20-21, *G* and *H*). The right-sided leaflets are usually not sutured to the patch because they close competently without this. If any commissural tissue between LSL and RSL or LIL and RIL is cut, the right side of this (as well as the left side) is sutured to the patch.

Rewarming of the patient is begun (see "Completing Cardiopulmonary Bypass" in Section 3 of Chapter 2). A few sutures are placed, but not pulled up or tied, for closure of the foramen ovale, leaving the pump sump-sucker in place. The first stitch for closure of the right atriotomy is placed at its inferior angle.

Closure of the right atriotomy is continued up to the midportion. Usually cardiac action has begun by then, so the pump sump-sucker is removed and sutures closing the foramen ovale are tied, with care taken to avoid trapping air in the left atrium. The remainder of the right atrium is closed and caval tapes released. Assessment at this stage of the morphologic and functional result by transesophageal two-dimensional color flow Doppler echocardiography is useful.[S12] If important abnormalities are present, CPB and cardioplegia are reestablished and corrections made. Otherwise, the remainder of the operation is completed in the usual manner (see "Completing Cardiopulmonary Bypass" in Section 3 of Chapter 2 and "Cold Cardioplegia, Controlled Aortic Root Reperfusion, and [When Needed] Warm Cardioplegic Induction" in Chapter 3). Left and right atrial and pulmonary artery pressure-monitoring catheters are placed.

Alternatively, when hypothermic circulatory arrest is used in infants, circulatory arrest is continued until the right atrium is closed, provided the procedure can be completed within 45 minutes (which is usually possible). The single venous cannula is then reinserted, the heart is de-aired, CPB for rewarming is begun, and the remainder of the procedure continues as usual. (For repair that requires more than 45 minutes, the sequence described in Chapter 2, Section 4, is adopted.)

Repair of Complete Atrioventricular Septal Defect with Bridging of Left Superior Leaflet: Rastelli Type B or C

Repair is similar to that just described, but special consideration is given to the LSL. Whether bridging is moderate (Rastelli type B) or marked (Rastelli type C), the commissure between it and the RSL is generally only slightly on the right ventricular side of the intersection of the atrial (and ventricular) septum with the anulus. This location is critically important, because, again, suturing for insertion of the interventricular polyester patch usually begins in the anulus at the level of this commissural tissue. If suturing in the anulus is too far anterior, that is, too far on the right ventricular side of the junction of anulus with atrial septum, either by error or because the LSL–RSL commissure is far anterior, the right AV valve orifice will be too narrow. Narrowing of its orifice can also be produced by attaching the interventricular polyester patch too far to the right of the crest of the septum with the first few superior (cephalad) stitches. Compensation too far leftward narrows the LV outflow tract.

The interventricular patch is slid beneath the chordae going from the right extremity of the LSL to right ventricu-

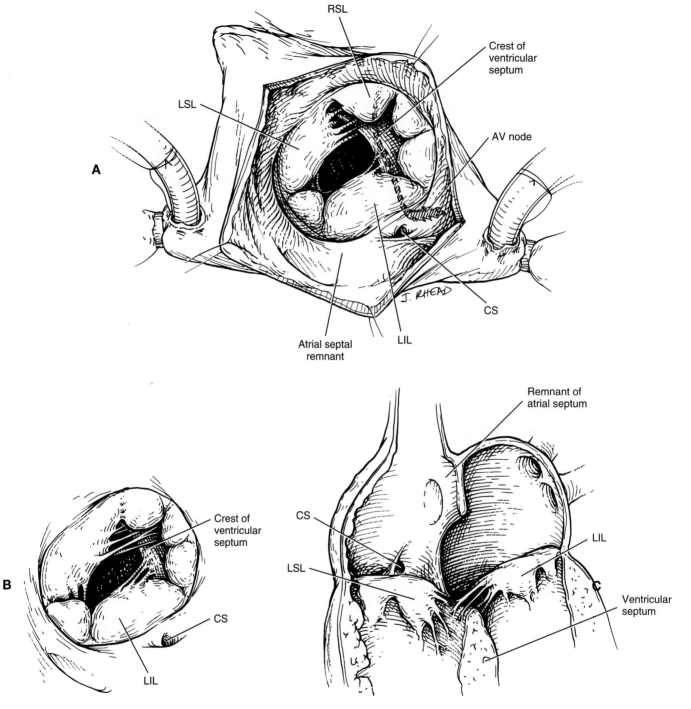

Figure 20-20   Repair of complete atrioventricular (AV) septal defect; right atrial view, showing two variations of bridging. **A**, Bridging grade 1. **B**, Bridging grade 4. In both there is a common AV orifice and interventricular communication. AV node lies on right side of inferior (caudad) atrial septal remnant at its junction with floor of the right atrium over the crux cordis. The node pierces the abnormally formed central fibrous body to become the short penetrating portion of His bundle. This structure immediately becomes the branching bundle, which gives off left bundle branches earlier than normal as it travels along the crest of the ventricular septum. **C**, A cross-section through AV septal defect with common AV valve orifice showing mild bridging of left inferior leaflet and the scooped-out crest of ventricular septum. View is anterior to posterior.

Key: *AV*, Atrioventricular; *CS*, Coronary sinus; *LIL*, left inferior leaflet; *LSL*, left superior leaflet; *RSL*, right superior leaflet.

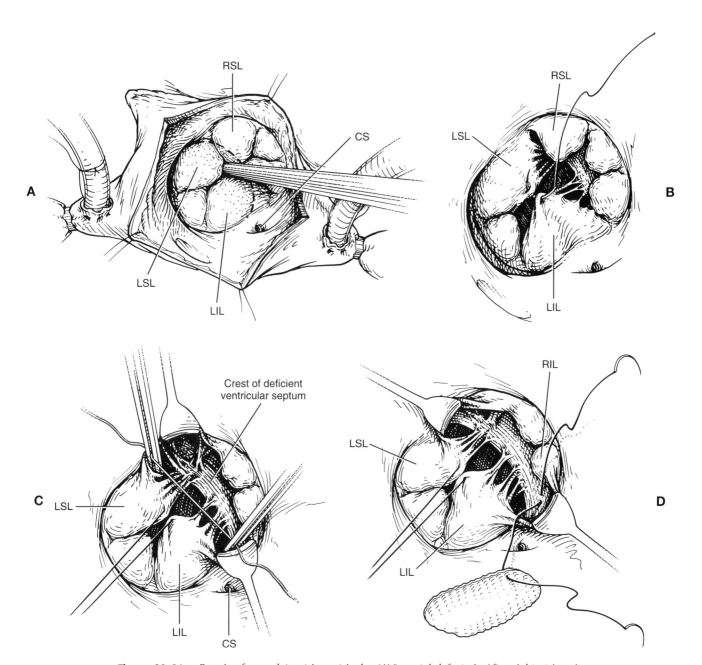

Figure 20-21 Repair of complete atrioventricular (AV) septal defect. **A**, After right atrium is opened, valve leaflets are often closed exactly as they are in systole. If, instead, they are open, saline is injected into left ventricle to close them. At this point, morphology of the leaflets, particularly their closure pattern, is studied and information obtained is used to plan repair of any regurgitation present or to accommodate any lack of left AV valve tissue. **B**, A fine polypropylene suture is placed between left superior leaflet *(LSL)* and left inferior leaflet *(LIL)* in position shown (anterior aspect) and left loose. **C**, The leaflets are allowed to open and details of atrial and ventricular septal deficiencies and of interatrial and interventricular communications are studied. Position of coronary sinus is noted, and the course of the unseen AV node and bundle of His is conceptualized by the surgeon from knowledge of the anatomy. The leaflets are retracted as much as possible and projected width (shown here) and depth of AV patch estimated. The planned suture line of the interventricular patch to the ventricular septum and free wall is thus visualized by the surgeon. **D**, Polyester ventricular patch is trimmed to a flat, rectangular–pyramidal shape. Suture line may begin anywhere along ventricular septum, but it must be on the right ventricular side of all chordae from left-sided leaflets, including those from any bridging components of the LIL. Retractor in right inferior aspect of the common valve marks the position in which base of RIL is sandwiched between ventricular and atrial patches. Suture line here stays well back from crest of interventricular septum and catches some of the base of the RIL to avoid the bundle of His.

Key: *CS,* Coronary sinus; *LIL,* left inferior leaflet; *LSL,* left superior leaflet; *RIL,* right inferior leaflet; *RSL,* right superior leaflet.
Continued

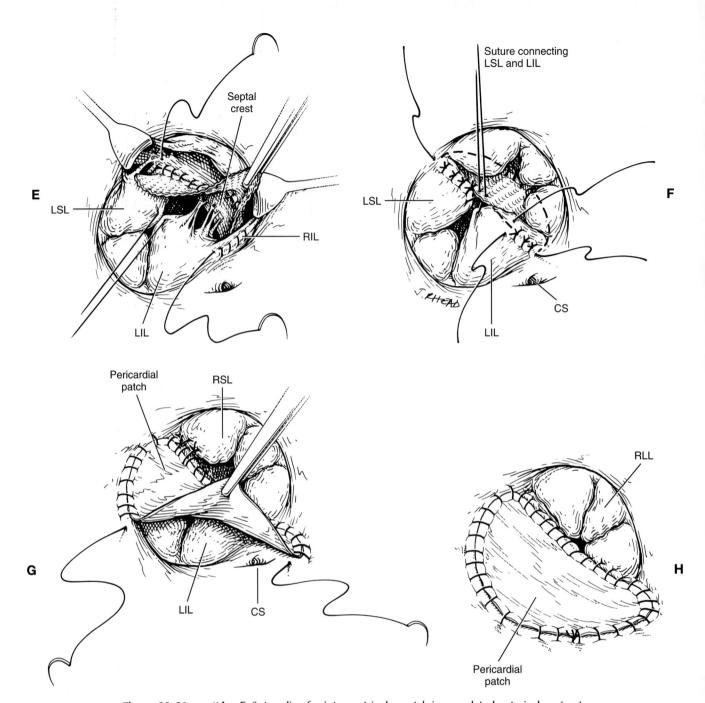

Figure 20-21, cont'd **E,** Suture line for interventricular patch is completed anteriorly, retracting the defect posteriorly and elevating the RSL to expose the aspect of the defect closest to left ventricular outflow tract. Width of the patch at the valve level will be less than its width deeper on ventricular septum level. **F,** Left superior leaflet *(LSL)* and left inferior leaflet *(LIL)* are precisely anchored to ventricular septal patch using fine interrupted simple or mattress sutures. It is here that care is taken to ensure that the left-sided valve apparatus at the patch is appropriately narrow so as not to create regurgitation and at the correct height so as not to produce left ventricular outflow tract narrowing (too low) or left AV valve regurgitation (too high). To provide accuracy, the previously placed fine stay suture joining LSL and LIL is positioned approximately at midpoint of the suture line. **G,** The pericardial patch for closure of the atrial defect is trimmed to size and a new suture line is begun with bites incorporating pericardial patch, left AV valve tissue (at its junction with the top of the polyester patch), and polyester patch, sandwiching delicate left AV valve tissue between pericardium and fabric. Initial suturing at crest of polyester patch can be done with the pericardial patch folded leftward toward left AV valve. The conduction system is avoided by extending the pericardium to the right of the coronary sinus, leaving its drainage to left atrium. Competence of the left (and right) AV valve is next tested with saline injection. If necessary, small anuloplasty sutures can be placed between LSL and left lateral leaflet (LLL) and between LIL and LLL. **H,** The remainder of the pericardial patch is sutured inferiorly and then superiorly to rim of atrial defect, often also incorporating closure of foramen ovale defect.

Key: *CS,* Coronary sinus; *LIL,* left inferior leaflet; *LSL,* left superior leaflet; *RIL,* right inferior leaflet; *RLL,* right lateral leaflet; *RSL,* right superior leaflet.

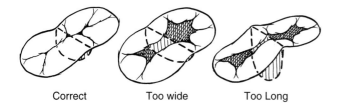

Correct   Too wide   Too Long

Figure 20-22   Depiction of ventricular septal portion of two-patch technique. If the patch is too wide, theoretically left ventricular outlet flow obstruction may be produced. If the patch is too long, with level of atrioventricular (AV) valves too high, there is a high probability of left AV valve regurgitation. (Modified from Lacour-Gayet and colleagues.[L,9])

lar papillary muscles. A few chordae may be cut for surgical exposure, because the whole anterior edge of the LSL is later attached to the patch.

The interventricular patch must have appropriate dimensions and configuration (Fig. 20-22). If the patch is excessively wide (in a superior–inferior direction), there is greater likelihood of postoperative LV outflow tract obstruction. If the patch is excessively long (deep, in a caudad–cephalad direction), there is a greater likelihood of left AV valve regurgitation.

Incising the LSL from its free edge to the anulus is rarely necessary, although in extreme cases in which a small right AV valve would otherwise result, it may be done, with both divided edges later sutured onto the interventricular polyester patch.

Repair of Complete Atrioventricular Septal Defect with Single-Patch Technique

Repair using a single patch differs from the two-patch technique in the following ways: (1) the single patch is almost always pericardium, (2) tailoring the waist of the patch (at the level of the AV valves) is critical, and (3) both the LSL and RSL and the LIL and RIL are sutured to the patch. Setup using bicaval cannulation is the same as for the two-patch technique, making sure that the IVC cannula is placed well caudad at the cavoatrial junction. CPB is established at 20° to 24°C, and antegrade cardioplegia is infused after aortic clamping. The right atrial incision is made and atrial exposure is arranged as for the two-patch technique. The most anterior point of LSL–LIL apposing edges is identified, and a No. 6-0 polypropylene suture is placed to retain that apposing relationship. Bridging leaflets superiorly and occasionally inferiorly are incised laterally to the valve anulus (Fig. 20-23, A). This maneuver allows easy later exposure for closing the intraventricular portion of the defect and accommodating the waist of the patch. The patch for the ventricular septal closure is inserted using continuous polypropylene or interrupted synthetic braided mattress sutures. Generally, the initial suture is placed at the midpoint of the ventricular defect and is continued upward anteriorly (Fig. 20-23, B). Posteriorly, the suture line stays behind the rim of the defect to avoid conduction fibers. Both left and right AV valve leaflets are then anchored to the waist of the patch using double-pledgeted horizontal mattress sutures (Fig. 20-23, C). Pledgets are generally of pericardium; often a single strip is used on the left-sided aspect. The strip is made a little shorter than the anteropos-

terior width of the anulus to somewhat narrow the anulus and contribute to AV valve competency. The level of this suture line (in a cephalad–caudad direction) must ensure that height of the AV valve anulus is such that left AV valve regurgitation is avoided (patch too high) and LV outflow obstruction is not produced (patch too low). At this point, the LV is loaded by saline injection to test valve competency and VSD closure. The left AV valve cleft is closed with fine interrupted sutures at its opposing edges to the previously placed marking suture. At this point, if necessary, anuloplasty sutures (horizontal mattress) are placed at the two lateral commissures. Repair of the remaining atrial defect proceeds as for the two-patch technique (Fig. 20-23, D), outside the rim of the coronary sinus and including the foramen ovale defect. The completed single pericardial patch has a lopsided, dumbbell-shaped configuration (Fig. 20-23, E).

Repair of Partial Atrioventricular Septal Defect with Little or No Left Atrioventricular Valve Regurgitation

Repair is similar to that just described, but no interventricular polyester patch is required. After CPB is established, intraatrial exposure is arranged, cold cardioplegic solution infused, and morphology studied. Attachments of LSL and LIL to the crest of the ventricular septum are probed to be certain there are no small interventricular communications.

The "cleft" in the AV valve is then identified and its medial and septal extremities noted (Fig. 20-24, A to C). In the past, if there was no left AV valve regurgitation, nothing was done to the valve at the cleft (commissure). More recently, most surgeons obliterate this gap (close the cleft) using several interrupted simple sutures. The margins here are characterized by slightly thickened and rolled edges, and it is at these margins that sutures are based.

An anuloplasty stitch may also be placed at the LSL–LLL commissure. The intraatrial pericardial patch is sewn into place in the same way used for repairing complete AV septal defect (Fig. 20-24, D; see also Fig. 20-21).

Small pledgeted mattress sutures of No. 6-0 polyester are passed from the right ventricular side through the base of the RIL and the bridging part of the LIL and through the pericardial patch. More cephalad, the patch is sewn to fibrous valvar tissue attached to the crest of the ventricular septum in this reinforced manner, analogous to its suturing to the top of the polyester patch (see Fig. 20-21).

Repair of Atrioventricular Septal Defect with Small Interchordal Interventricular Communications (Intermediate Form)

When two AV valve orifices are present but small interventricular communications exist between thick, short chordae attaching the LSL to the crest of the ventricular septum, repair is simple. The interventricular communication is simply closed by taking the anterior portion of the pericardial patch just to the right side of the septal crest, catching the base of the LSL with each stitch.

When the interventricular communications are beneath the LIL, the same maneuver may be followed. However, because of the bundle of His, care must be taken to keep the suture line well away from the crest of the septum and

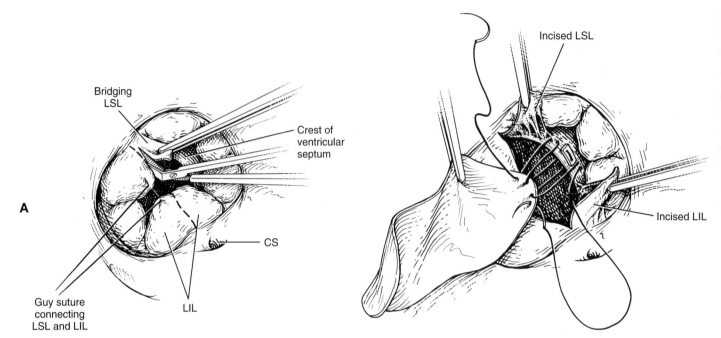

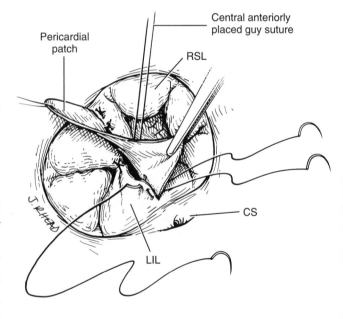

Figure 20-23   Complete atrioventricular (AV) septal defect repair, single-patch technique. **A,** Right atriotomy is made as for two-patch technique and AV valves are inspected. Saline is infused into ventricles as for two-patch technique, and apposition point of left superior leaflet *(LSL)* and left inferior leaflet *(LIL)* is identified as the leaflets float up to their systolic position. A fine guy suture is placed for alignment and left loose. Frequently, the bridging LSL or LIL is incised to gain access to the anterior portion of interventricular defect. Later, each cut edge of the superior leaflet will be attached to pericardial patch at its waist. **B,** Fresh or glutaraldehyde-treated pericardial patch is trimmed partially after measuring height and width of interventricular communication. Generally, the ventricular portion of the patch is attached to the right side of crest of ventricular septum using a continuous suture initiated at the deepest aspect (midpoint) of the rim of the ventricular septal defect. Usual precautions are taken as in the two-patch technique to avoid the bundle of His at posterior–inferior aspect of ventricular defect. **C,** AV leaflets, both left and right, are attached to pericardial patch at appropriate level. As in the two-patch technique, the central guy suture, which approximates the gap between LSL and LIL, helps to position the AV valves at correct height and midpoint on the single pericardial patch. Interrupted horizontal mattress sutures incorporate bites of right-sided valve tissue, pass through pericardium, and end with bites of left-sided valve tissue. Small pledgets of pericardium may be used to buttress sutures on left and right AV valve tissue. Several additional sutures complete closure of gap between LSL and LIL.

Key: *CS,* Coronary sinus; *LIL,* left inferior leaflet; *LSL,* left superior leaflet; *RSL,* right superior leaflet.   *Continued*

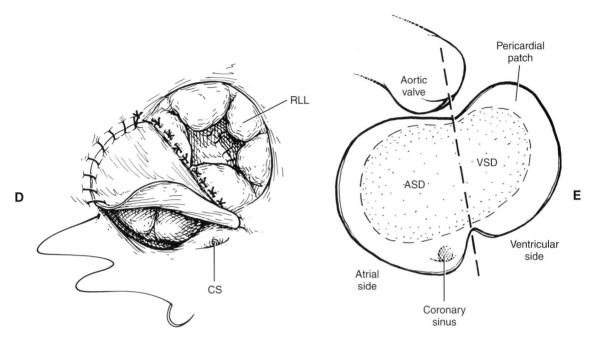

Figure 20-23, cont'd   **D,** Atrial portion of patch is completed with continuous suture extending inferiorly and medially to place coronary sinus on left atrial side, incorporating any foramen ovale defect within superior rim of patch. Before completing atrial septal patch insertion, the atrioventricular valves are tested by saline infusion and anuloplasty is done as necessary. **E,** Approximate configuration of pericardial patch for single patch technique. Height and width of waist (indicated by dashed line) are critical.

Key: *ASD,* Atrial portion of atrioventricular septal defect; *CS,* coronary sinus; *RLL,* right lateral leaflet; *VSD,* ventricular portion of atriventricular septal defect.

to attach the patch in the same manner in which the interventricular patch is attached in repair of complete AV septal defects.

Repair of Atrioventricular Septal Defect with Common Atrium

When a common atrium is present, either with or without an interventricular communication, special effort is made to ensure that there is no left superior vena cava or, if one is present, that there is not a completely unroofed coronary sinus, which would change the repair (see "Technique of Operation" in Chapter 19).

Repair is accomplished by sewing an appropriately larger pericardial patch to the atrial wall on the left atrial side of the orifice of the inferior vena cava, to the right of the right pulmonary veins, and beneath the superior vena cava (where there is usually a small septal remnant).

Repair of Complete or Partial Atrioventricular Septal Defect with Moderate or Severe Left Atrioventricular Valve Regurgitation

For repair of an AV septal defect with moderate or severe left AV valve regurgitation, results seem to vary from one institution to another, even when the same techniques have apparently been used. According to one view, relief of important regurgitation in patients with complete AV septal

defects can often be accomplished by the rather simple maneuvers discussed earlier, but this is less frequently successful in patients with partial AV septal defects. In this view, each patient with a partial or complete AV septal defect and important left AV valve regurgitation must be evaluated individually by careful study of the two-dimensional echocardiogram, cineangiogram, and valve at operation. Depending on the findings, the repair is planned. About the only tools thought to be available are (1) remodeling leaflet closure by suturing portions of LSL and LIL together in areas in which regurgitation is demonstrated ("closure of the cleft") or by plicating them, although this must be done thoughtfully to prevent narrowing the orifice or later dehiscence; and (2) narrowing of the anulus. The latter is accomplished by anuloplasty at the commissures on both sides of the LSL–LIL complex and by making the edge of the pericardial patch along it *shorter* than the combined length of the base of the leaflets. The latter maneuver can sometimes be facilitated by suturing the patch to the LSL–LIL complex 5 to 15 mm *away from* (on the orifice side of) their attachment to the crest of the septum. Thus, leaflet tissue between the crest and this suture line functionally becomes interventricular septum.

If moderate or severe left AV valve regurgitation remains, repair should be immediately reassessed. If, in the surgeon's judgment, improvement by further repair is possible, the patient is returned to CPB. If no further repair is likely, valve replacement is performed. If the patient is

Figure 20-24   Repair of partial atrioventricular (AV) septal defect. **A,** Cross-section through the defect with an atrial communication and intact ventricular septum. **B,** Right atrium is opened in a superior to inferior direction. (Inferior vena cava cannula is placed well caudal). Atrial defect (primum ASD) is seen with its inferior border comprised partially of AV valve tissue. A search is made for interventricular communications as the left-sided AV valve is tested for regurgitation by saline infusion. Extent of cleft is seen and any regurgitation through it identified.

Key: *AV,* Atrioventricular; *CS,* coronary sinus; *LIL,* left inferior leaflet; *LSL,* left superior leaflet; *RIL,* right inferior leaflet; *RSL,* right superior leaflet.

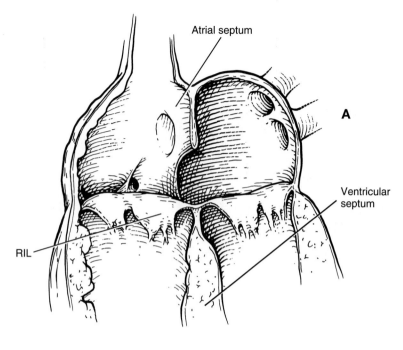

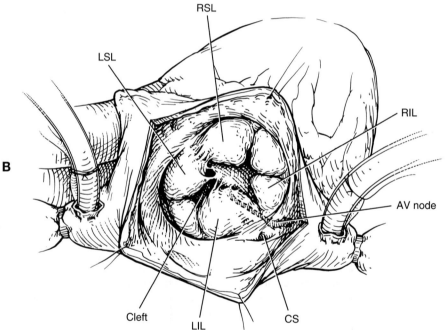

small, no further intervention is feasible and the infant is managed as well as possible postoperatively.

Right Atrioventricular Valve

In hearts with or without interventricular communications, the right AV valve usually does not require attention. Two-patch repair leaves this valve without a complete "septal leaflet," but in this and other situations, regurgitation does not result. The RSL and RIL (and the RLL) are well supported by chordae, and this, combined with their closure against the polyester patch or bare ventricular septum, generally results in adequate valve function.

Left Superior Leaflet–Right Superior Leaflet and Left Inferior Leaflet–Right Inferior Leaflet Commissures

Generally, repair of LSL–RSL and LIL–RIL commissures can be made without disturbing the commissural leaflet tissue in these areas. Occasionally, however, these commissural leaflet areas are larger than usual and handicap exposure. Then they may be incised back to the anulus, *once it is certain that this is commissural tissue!* Tissue on the LV side is incorporated into the repair along with the LSL or LIL. That on the right side should be reattached to the patch with a few sutures at the end of the repair.

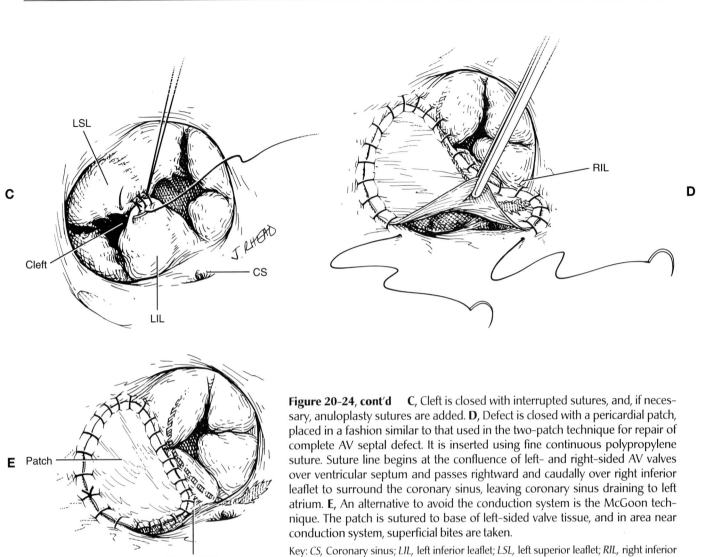

Figure 20-24, cont'd   C, Cleft is closed with interrupted sutures, and, if necessary, anuloplasty sutures are added. **D,** Defect is closed with a pericardial patch, placed in a fashion similar to that used in the two-patch technique for repair of complete AV septal defect. It is inserted using fine continuous polypropylene suture. Suture line begins at the confluence of left- and right-sided AV valves over ventricular septum and passes rightward and caudally over right inferior leaflet to surround the coronary sinus, leaving coronary sinus draining to left atrium. **E,** An alternative to avoid the conduction system is the McGoon technique. The patch is sutured to base of left-sided valve tissue, and in area near conduction system, superficial bites are taken.

Key: *CS,* Coronary sinus; *LIL,* left inferior leaflet; *LSL,* left superior leaflet; *RIL,* right inferior leaflet.

Replacement of Left Atrioventricular Valve

When severe left AV valve regurgitation cannot be repaired, or when it persists or develops postoperatively, left AV valve replacement may be necessary.[C4] Because the left AV valve nearly always encroaches on the LV outflow tract (see Figs. 20-5, *A* and 20-10), valve replacement may accentuate or produce subaortic stenosis. The prosthesis must therefore be kept away from the subaortic area. This may be accomplished by attaching a rectangular piece of polyester to the anulus of the left AV valve in the subaortic area (Fig. 20-25).[M13] (Poirier and colleagues describe outcome of 8 patients in which similar augmentation was used at reoperation to increase deficient bridging leaflet coaptation without valve replacement.[P10]) The prosthesis is then sutured to this artificial mitral–aortic anulus and to the natural anulus for the rest of its circumference. Particular care is taken anteriorly and inferiorly to sew only to the fringe of left AV valve that has been preserved to minimize the chance of damage to the AV node and His bundle. Alternatively, the prosthesis can be attached in a supraanular position using atrial wall to base the sewing ring. When possible, valve replacement should be deferred until childhood, when risk is less.[K9] This decision is particularly difficult in infants for whom no device of appropriate size is available. Then, even moderate or severe left AV valve regurgitation must be accepted.

Ebels and colleagues have suggested a somewhat different method for avoiding encroachment on the LV tract by the prosthesis.[E7,E9] Their technique involves resecting the atrial fold lying external to the area of fibrous continuity between aortic leaflets and LSL, presumably along with part of the fibrous continuity. The prosthesis then lies against the aortic valve, rather than in a subvalvar, obstructing position. Clinical evaluation of this method is limited.

Repair of Complete Atrioventricular Septal Defect with Tetralogy of Fallot

In complete AV septal defect associated with tetralogy of Fallot, the large VSD is also juxtaaortic. The LSL bridges moderately (grade 3) or markedly (grades 4 or 5) and is not

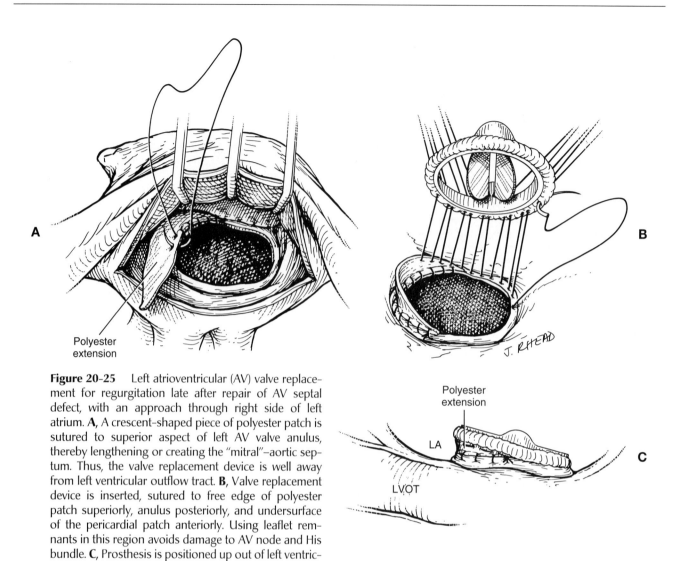

Figure 20-25   Left atrioventricular (AV) valve replacement for regurgitation late after repair of AV septal defect, with an approach through right side of left atrium. **A,** A crescent-shaped piece of polyester patch is sutured to superior aspect of left AV valve anulus, thereby lengthening or creating the "mitral"–aortic septum. Thus, the valve replacement device is well away from left ventricular outflow tract. **B,** Valve replacement device is inserted, sutured to free edge of polyester patch superiorly, anulus posteriorly, and undersurface of the pericardial patch anteriorly. Using leaflet remnants in this region avoids damage to AV node and His bundle. **C,** Prosthesis is positioned up out of left ventricular outflow tract and into left atrium.

Key: *LA*, Left atrium; *LVOT*, left ventricular outflow tract.

attached to the crest of the ventricular septum. Any of the types of right ventricular outflow tract obstruction associated with tetralogy of Fallot may be present (see "Convenient Morphologic Categories of Right Ventricular Outflow Obstruction" under Morphology in Section 1 of Chapter 24), and anterior deviation of the infundibular septum is always present and must be considered in the repair. Preoperative cineangiographic studies are often necessary to delineate the surgically important details of right ventricular outflow obstruction and morphology of the pulmonary arteries.

Operation is begun as for repair of any complete AV septal defect. Before heparinization, however, if a right ventricular outflow patch is required, an appropriately sized patch is prepared as described in Section 1 of Chapter 24 (see "Decision and Technique for Transanular Patching" under Technique of Operation). The VSD patch is trimmed with a wide superior aspect, which is important in preventing *left* ventricular outflow obstruction.

Usually the anteriorly deviated parietal extension of the infundibular septum (band) can be seen through the AV valve, and it is cut and mobilized (see "Repair of Uncomplicated Tetralogy of Fallot with Pulmonary Stenosis via Right Atrium" under Technique of Operation in Section 1 of Chapter 24). Other muscular infundibular obstructions can be visualized and resected. The pulmonary valve can be visualized and fused commissures opened. The right ventricular outflow tract is sized with Hegar dilators. At this point the surgeon may decide on a combined right atrial–right ventricular (RA–RV) approach. If so, a small vertical incision is made in the right ventricular outflow tract, and parietal and septal extensions are mobilized and partially resected. This incision is later closed with a small patch.

The interventricular communication is closed by suturing into place a polyester or pericardial patch from this right atrial approach, sequencing the repair exactly as described for other complete AV septal defects. This can be accomplished with a one- or two-patch technique. With either, the shape of the ventricular component of the patch must be modified to account for the anterior–superior extension of the interventricular communication. Familiarity with the atrial approach for repair of isolated VSD (see

"Technique of Operation" in Section 1 of Chapter 21) and for the repair of the VSD in simple tetralogy of Fallot (see "Repair of Uncomplicated Tetralogy of Fallot with Pulmonary Stenosis via Right Atrium" under Technique of Operation in Section 1 of Chapter 24), as well as familiarity with repair of uncomplicated complete AV septal defects, are important preparations for this procedure. Stay sutures are placed as usual for transatrial repair. Repair is begun at the AV valve anulus superiorly, where the atrial septal remnant meets the anulus.

Care must be taken that repair does not begin too far rightward, in which case the right side of the surgically partitioned AV valve orifice will be too small. Because of the dextroposed aorta, attachment of the VSD patch to tissue over the aortic root (and beneath the commissural tissue and RSL) is particularly important. The patch is generally beneath (on the *left* ventricular side of) chordae attached to the right extremity of the bridging LSL and beneath this leaflet itself. Because this leaflet will be attached to the VSD patch, some of these chordae may be cut to facilitate exposure. In the one-patch technique, the entire bridging leaflet is incised. The suture line is then carried around the interventricular communication and along the base of the RIL as described earlier for the usual complete AV septal defect. When the aorta overrides the interventricular septum to a considerable degree (and when double outlet right ventricle is present), the juxtaaortic portion of the repair may be completed through a small infundibular incision. Remainder of the AV septal defect is repaired as described earlier.

The right ventricular outflow tract is again sized with Hegar dilators. If it is adequate, nothing further is done. Otherwise, the right ventricular outflow tract is enlarged by an infundibular patch, or, if necessary, a transanular patch (see "General Plan and Details of Repair Common to All Approaches" under Technique of Operation in Section 1 of Chapter 24.) Moderate or severe pulmonary regurgitation must be avoided because associated right ventricular dilatation may result in severe right AV valve regurgitation from deficiency of right-sided AV valve tissue. Therefore, the threshold for inserting a valve (monocusp or allograft) in the right ventricular outflow tract is lower than usual.

Repair of Complete Atrioventricular Septal Defect with Double Outlet Right Ventricle

When the interventricular communication is large and subaortic, configuration and insertion of the interventricular patch are similar to that just described for tetralogy of Fallot. Pulmonary stenosis, when coexisting, is also treated similarly.

When the interventricular communication is *not* subaortic and cannot be converted into one by septal excision (see "Intraventricular Tunnel Repair of Double Outlet Right Ventricle with Noncommitted Ventricular Septal Defect" under Technique of Operation in Chapter 39), a Fontan repair (see "Technique of Operation" in Section 4 of Chapter 27) is necessary if pulmonary stenosis coexists.

Repair with Transposition of the Great Arteries

When size of the LV allows it, usual repair of the AV septal defect is carried out, and an arterial switch operation is performed (see "Arterial Switch Operation" under Technique of Operation in Chapter 38).

SPECIAL FEATURES OF POSTOPERATIVE CARE

Usual care as described in Chapter 5 is accorded patients after repair of AV septal defects, but certain features require emphasis. Because of the complexity of repair and despite the generally good results now obtained, vigilance must be exercised to detect any important imperfections in the repair. Thus, transesophageal or transthoracic echocardiography (if the infant is small) is of great help in the operating room and a few hours after the patient's return to the intensive care unit to verify complete closure of the interatrial and interventricular communications and absence of important AV valve regurgitation. Left atrial pressure more than 6 mmHg higher than right atrial pressure raises the possibility of either severe left AV valve regurgitation or stenosis, although it can result simply from small size and low compliance of the LV (see Chapter 5). Height of the *v* wave is not helpful because, as in all circumstances, this correlates more with height of mean left atrial pressure than with degree of regurgitation. Usual prophylaxis is taken against pulmonary hypertensive crises. Generally, this includes introducing a pulmonary artery catheter intraoperatively. Because average age at repair has decreased, this complication is seen less frequently now (see "General Care of Neonates and Infants," Section 4 of Chapter 5).

If the patient's condition is not optimal and important residual left AV valve regurgitation is suspected—particularly if deterioration continues over several hours—repeat echocardiographic study in the intensive care unit is advisable. If results of this study are inconclusive, left ventriculographic studies (or some other reliable method of quantifying left AV valve regurgitation) should be considered. Indirect indications, both in the operating room and early postoperatively (including absence of a murmur), are not reliable. If severe regurgitation is demonstrated, reoperation is indicated. Likewise, if the patient's condition is unsatisfactory and a large residual left-to-right shunt is present, reoperation is indicated.

When the patient does not convalesce normally, echocardiographic and possibly left ventriculographic studies before hospital discharge are indicated. Because left AV valve repair failure predisposes the patient to death within the first year after operation, consideration should be given to early reoperation if severe regurgitation is found.

RESULTS
Survival
Early (Hospital) Death

Hospital mortality after repair of *partial AV septal defects* has been low for a long time, dating back to the early experience reported from the Mayo Clinic.[R2] Although in recent years overall hospital mortality after repair of this malformation has been 3% to 4% when the septal defect is an isolated one and without important AV valve regurgitation, hospital mortality generally is less than 1%.

Hospital mortality after repair of uncomplicated *complete AV septal defects* was 30% to 50% during the early years of cardiac surgery, but has become steadily lower in recent years. This has been the result of greatly improved understanding of the morphology of this complex malformation, better surgical techniques, and general improvements in cardiac surgery in infants.[G4,K12,M6,M10] These improvements are evident in the UAB experience, among others (Fig. 20-26), in which hospital mortality for repair of complete AV septal defect was 3% from 1982 to 1986. Improvement in hospital mortality has been particularly evident in infants (Table 20-12), and young age is no longer a risk factor for hospital death after repair of this malformation.[A5,B1,B12,G8,K14,M16,S2] Weintraub and colleagues, from the group directed by Mee, have reported a 3% hospital mortality (CL 1%-7%) among 62 infants whose median age at operation was 4.3 months, and when the two-patch technique described in this chapter was used, Bailey and Watson have reported hospital mortality of 6% (CL 2%-14%) in infants.[B22,W7] These reports may convey overly optimistic records of accomplishment. As is often the case, results from individual centers of excellence are superior to results from unselected institutional studies. The Pediatric Cardiac Care Consortium reported the results of 10 years' activity in 25 institutions within the United States.[M17] Overall operative mortality was 14% and did not differ between Down and non-Down cases. There was a total of 768 cases, averaging three cases per year per institution. This report should be contrasted to individual institutional reports demonstrating low mortality representing caseloads of 20 to 50 yearly (Table 20-13).

Even when complete AV septal defect coexists with other major cardiac anomalies such as tetralogy of Fallot, hospital mortality remains low (Table 20-14).[K13] However, a few uncommon combinations with both partial and complete AV septal defects impose a considerable increase in hospital mortality (Table 20-15).

Time-Related Survival

Fig. 20-27 shows time-related survival for patients undergoing repair of all types of AV septal defects at UAB between 1967 and 1982. Hazard function for death after operation had an early declining phase, which gave way at about 6 to 9 months to an appreciable constant hazard phase for as long as the patients were followed up (Fig. 20-28). It is noteworthy that the declining early phase of hazard does not give way to the constant phase until 6 to 9

months after operation, meaning that "hospital" or "30-day mortality" considerably underestimates the early risks of operation in this malformation. Weintraub and colleagues indicate that the constant hazard phase is lower in the current era, but it is still present because of problems late

■ **TABLE 20-12 Hospital Deaths According to Age at Operation, after Repair of Isolated Atrioventricular Septal Defects without Major Associated Cardiac Anomalies**

Age			Hospital Deaths		
≤ months <		*n*	No.	%	CL (%)
	1	1	0	0	0-85
1	3	0	–	–	–
3	6	13	1	8	1-24
6	12	16	0	0	0-11
12	24	4	0	0	0-38
24		24	0	0	0-8
TOTAL		58	1	2	0.2-6
$P(x^2)$				0.5	

(Data from UAB, 1984 to September 1985.)

Key: *CL*, 70% confidence limits.

■ **TABLE 20-13 Complete Atrioventricular Septal Defect: Operative Mortality According to Age, for all Patients and for those with Down Syndrome**

Age	All cases			Down Syndrome		
	n	Deaths	%	*n*	Deaths	%
≤ months <						
1	5	3	60	1	0	0
1 3	70	15	21	45	5	11
3 6	203	27	13	157	17	11
6 12	268	36	13	223	31	14
≤ years <						
1 5	183	23	13	122	18	15
5 10	26	2	7.7	20	1	5.0
10 21	12	1	8.3	8	1	12
21	1	0	0.0	1	0	0.0
TOTAL	768	107	14	577	73	13

(Data from Moller.[M17])

Figure 20-26 Observed hospital mortality after repair (1984 to September 1985) of complete and partial atrioventricular septal defects with or without major associated cardiac anomalies; mortality is shown as open circles, and vertical bars represent 70% confidence limits. Note that these mortalities lie on the nomogram lines representing an extrapolated solution of a multivariable equation. Solid lines represent 8-day mortality, and dashed lines enclose 70% confidence limits. The widely dotted depiction extends solid lines into a time period (1982 to 1986) not included in the experience used to derive equations and coefficients. (See original publication for details, coefficients, and *P* values of multivariable equation.) (From Kirklin and colleagues.[K14])

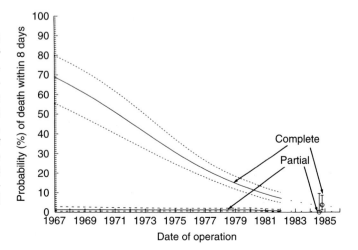

postoperatively with the left AV valve.[W7] Shapes of the separate time-related survival depictions for partial and complete AV canal defects are similar, but that for the partial defects is more favorable (Fig. 20-29).[C7]

Modes of Death

In the UAB experience, most early deaths (67%) after repair of AV septal defects were in acute cardiac failure, and at least some were caused by failure (stenosis or regurgitation) of left AV valve repair.[S2] Pulmonary dysfunction accounted for about 10% of early deaths. The few late deaths were in chronic or subacute cardiac failure, related to failure of the left AV valve repair.

■ **TABLE 20-14   Repair of Complex Complete Atrioventricular Septal Defects** [a]

Age ≤ months <		n	No.	%	CL (%)
	6	3	0	0	0-47
6	12	1	1	100	14-100
12	24	4	0	0	0-38
24	48	8	0	0	0-21
48		13	0	0	0-14
TOTAL		29	1	3.5	0.4-11
$P(\chi^2)$				<.0001	

(Data from UAB, 1982 to 1986.)

Key: *CL,* 70% confidence limits.

[a] Includes 7 patients with atrial isomerism, 10 with double outlet right ventricle, and 12 with tetralogy of Fallot.

■ **TABLE 20-15   Hospital Mortality after Repair of Atrioventricular Septal Defects and Major Associated Cardiac Anomalies**

	Without Interventricular Communication				With Interventricular Communication			
		Hospital Deaths				Hospital Deaths		
Associated Anomaly [a]	n	No.	%	CL (%)	n	No.	%	CL (%)
Tetralogy of Fallot (1982-1986)	0	–	–	–	12	0	0	0-15
DORV [b] (1982-1986)	0	–	–	–	10	1	10	1-30
Atrial isomerism [c] (1982-1986)	0	–	–	–	7	0 [d]	0	0-24
TGA	0	–	–	–	1	0	0	0-85
TAPVC	0	–	–	–	2	1	50	7-93
Pulmonary stenosis	1	0	0	0-85	0	–	–	–
LV outflow obstruction	2	1	50	7-93	0	–	–	–
Supravalvar LAVVS	0	–	–	–	1	0	0	0-85
Completely unroofed coronary sinus	5	0	0	0-32	4	1	25	3-63
Ebstein malformation	1	1	100	15-100	0	–	–	–
Additional VSDs	1	0	0	0-85	4	3	75	37-97
Patent ductus arteriosus	2	0	0	0-61	29	12	41	31-53
Coarctation	0	–	–	–	1	1	100	15-100
Dextrocardia with situs solitus	0	–	–	–	1	1	100	15-100

(Data from UAB, 1967 to 1982.)

Key: *CL,* 70% confidence limits; *DORV,* double outlet right ventricle; *LAVVS,* left atrioventricular valve stenosis; *LV,* left ventricular; *TAPVC,* total anomalous pulmonary venous connection; *TGA,* transposition of the great arteries; *VSD,* ventricular septal defect.

[a] Categories are not mutually exclusive.

[b] Two also had pulmonary stenosis.

[c] Left atrial isomerism in four, right in three; ventricular D-loop in six, L-loop in one; ventriculoarterial connection discordant in four, concordant in two, and DORV in one.

[d] Two patients died late postoperatively, one at 24 months and one at 29 months, both of cardiac failure.

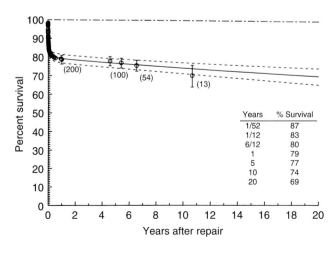

Figure 20-27   Survival after repair of atrioventricular septal defects of all types in a heterogeneous group of 310 patients operated on at UAB from 1967 to 1982. Hospital deaths are included. Individual deaths are indicated by open circles and 70% confidence limits by vertical bars. Solid line enclosed within dashed 70% confidence limits represents parametric estimates of survival. Only one patient among the 310 was untraced. Numbers in parentheses are numbers of patients at risk at that time. Dash-dot-dash line represents survival of an age-gender-ethnicity–matched general population. (From Kirklin and colleagues.[K14])

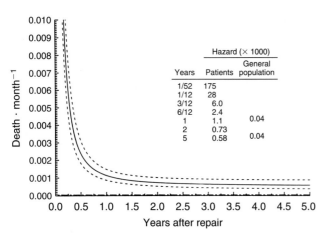

Figure 20-28 Hazard function (two phases) for death at any moment after repair of atrioventricular septal defects (1967 to 1982; *n* = 310; deaths = 70). Dashed lines enclose 70% confidence limits. Barely visible is the hazard function for an age–gender–ethnicity–matched population. (From Kirklin and colleagues.[K14])

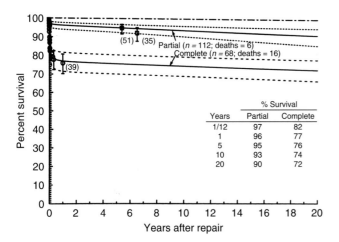

Figure 20-29 Survival after repair of atrioventricular (AV) septal defects in patients with uncomplicated partial and complete AV septal defects. Depiction is as in Fig. 20-26. To achieve the risk adjustment described, patients were excluded if they were preoperatively in New York Heart Association class IV or V, if they had preoperative AV valve regurgitation grade IV or V, or if they had major associated cardiac anomalies (UAB, 1967 to 1982).

Incremental Risk Factors for Premature Death

Earlier Date of Operation

An earlier date of operation as a risk factor in a surgical experience that covers a large number of years, such as that at UAB (Table 20-16), demonstrates that many risks of repair have been neutralized across the experience.[K14,S2] Others report similar experiences.[A5,B1,H4,M2] This effect has already been depicted for hospital mortality in the case of partial and complete AV septal defects (see Fig. 20-25). The effect of date of operation on outcome is just as evident in long-term events as it is in hospital mortality. This is

TABLE 20-16 Incremental Risk Factors (Hazard Function Domain) for Premature Death after Repair of Atrioventricular Septal Defects[a]

Risk Factor	Hazard Phase	
	Early and Decreasing	Constant
Demographic Variables		
Younger age	•	
Clinical Variables		
Higher NYHA class	•	•
Greater severity of preoperative AV valve regurgitation		•
Morphologic Variables		
Interventricular communication	•	
Accessory valve orifice		•
Major associated cardiac anomalies	•	
Surgical Variables		
Earlier date of operation	•	
Interaction with age	•	

(Data from Kirklin and colleagues[K14]; see source for *P* values.)

Key: *AV*, Atrioventricular; *NYHA*, New York Heart Association.

[a] Data are from a study of 310 patients operated on from 1967 to 1982.

dramatically evident in predicted 10-year survival after repair of partial and complete AV septal defects in patients operated on in 1967 versus 1977 and 1985 (Fig. 20-30).

Higher New York Heart Association Functional Class

As in most cardiac surgery, severe preoperative disability (higher New York Heart Association [NYHA] functional class) is a risk factor for premature death in both the early and constant hazard phases (see Table 20-16).

Important Pre-Repair Atrioventricular Valve Regurgitation

Important pre-repair regurgitation of either the left AV valve in partial AV canal defects or the common AV valve in complete AV septal defects increases risk of premature death, but only in the constant hazard phase (see Table 20-16). This suggests that postrepair regurgitation, the prevalence of which is almost surely increased by severe preoperative regurgitation in patients with partial AV septal defects but probably not in patients with complete AV septal defects, is reasonably well tolerated early postoperatively, but becomes more serious several months later.[W7]

Interventricular Communication

An interventricular communication (complete AV septal defect) has been an important risk factor, but only in the early declining hazard phase (see Table 20-16). The effect of this aspect of morphology indicates that outcomes after repair of complete AV septal defects currently approximate those of partial AV septal defects, which have been excellent for many years (see Figs. 20-29 and 20-30).[M7,R2] Residual interventricular communication after repair of complete AV septal defect may be an infrequent cause for reoperation and a risk factor for premature death. Early postoperative residual VSD should be suspected in the

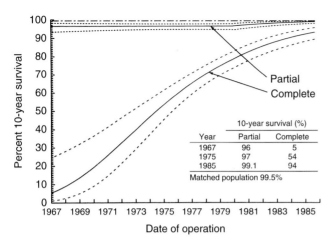

Figure 20-30 Nomogram representing predicted 10-year survival (including hospital deaths) after repair of partial and complete atrioventricular septal defects with or without major associated cardiac anomalies, according to year in which operation was performed. Solid lines are survival estimates, and dashed lines are 70% confidence limits (See original publication for details, risk factors, coefficients, and *P* values of multivariable equation.) (From Kirklin and colleagues.[K14])

presence of "pulmonary hypertensive crisis" and low cardiac output.

Accessory Valve Orifice

An accessory valve orifice is an incremental risk factor for premature death (see Table 20-16), almost surely because of its potentially adverse effect on function of the surgically created left AV valve (see description under "Morphology" earlier in this chapter).[C2,C8,L10,S2] Despite the realization that the accessory orifice should not be "tampered with," this risk factor has not been neutralized.[H4]

Major Associated Cardiac Anomalies

Included among important risk factors are major associated cardiac anomalies (see Table 20-16), but some of them, particularly tetralogy of Fallot, have been largely neutralized.

Young Age

Young age has been an incremental risk factor for death, usually hospital death, in all experiences that go back 30 years or so.[B3,M2] However, it has been virtually eliminated as a risk factor,[B23,H4,K14,P8,W7] primarily because of overall improvement in knowledge and techniques of repair, but also because of advances in intraoperative and early postoperative care of infants.

Down Syndrome

Risk-adjusted analysis does not show that Down syndrome affects risk of premature death early or late after repair, except when complete AV septal defect is associated with tetralogy of Fallot (Table 20-17).[K13,K14,N3,S2] However, in view of the considerably decreased prevalence of LV inflow and outflow obstruction in patients with AV septal defects and Down syndrome, these patients may in fact have a better early and intermediate-term survival than patients without Down syndrome. The left AV valve may also be

■ TABLE 20-17 Mortality and Reoperation Classified by Presence of Down Syndrome and Left Atrioventricular Valve Anomaly

Patients	*n*	Early Deaths		Reoperation	
		No.	%	No.	%
Down syndrome[a]	235	23	10	18	8
Non–Down syndrome[a]	128	15	12	27	21
Parachute LAVV	40	3	8	8	20
Double-orifice LAVV	21	6	29	6	29

(Data from Najm and colleagues.[N3])

Key: *LAVV*, Left atrioventricular valve.

[a] *P* = .39.

■ TABLE 20-18 Risk Factors Associated with Perioperative Deaths in Complete Atrioventricular Septal Defect According to Univariable Analysis

Risk Factor	Parameter Estimate	Risk Ratio	*P*
General Variables [a]			
Prematurity	1.39 ± 0.53	4.01	.009
Down syndrome	-0.63 ± 0.35	0.53	.08
Year of operation	-0.17 ± 0.04	0.85	.0001
Morphologic Variables [b]			
Double-orifice left AV valve	1.71 ± 0.60	5.52	.005
Single left papillary muscle	1.01 ± 0.53	2.75	.06
Procedural Variables [c]			
Circulatory arrest	0.03 ± 0.02	1.03	.05
Total CPB time	0.01 ± 0.00	1.01	.003
Postoperative Physiologic Variables [d]			
Absence of sinus rhythm	1.89 ± 0.43	6.60	.0001
Postop left AV valve regurgitation	1.00 ± 0.39	2.72	.01
Left atrial pressure	0.09 ± 0.02	1.10	.0001
Right atrial pressure	0.09 ± 0.05	0.90	.06
Pulmonary artery pressure	0.06 ± 0.03	1.07	.02
Reoperation Variables [b]			
For pacemaker	1.73 ± 0.48	5.66	.0003
For VSD	1.45 ± 0.48	4.25	.003
For left AV valve regurgitation	1.00 ± 0.37	2.72	.007

(Data from Hanley and colleagues.[H4])

Key: *AV*, Atrioventricular; *CPB*, cardiopulmonary bypass; *Postop*, postoperative; *VSD*, ventricular septal defect.

[a] *P* > .1 for age, weight, and previous palliation.

[b] *P* > .1 for multiple ventricular septal defects, patent ductus arteriosus, left-sided obstructive lesions, left superior vena cava, Rastelli type, atrioventricular valve regurgitation (severe), and ventricular dominance.

[c] *P* > .1 for cleft repair, left atrioventricular valve valvuloplasty (other than cleft closure or anuloplasty), left atrioventricular valve anuloplasty, cardioplegia, aortic clamp time, inotropic support, and single or double patch.

[d] *P* > .1 for right atrial–pulmonary artery saturation step-up, pulmonary artery saturation, and mean arterial blood pressure.

easier to repair, lessening the likelihood of late death from mitral regurgitation.[W8]

Need for Reoperation

Although reoperation within 30 days postoperatively may contribute to a good long-term outcome, need for reoperation to insert a pacemaker, close a residual interventricular communication, or deal with important left AV valve regurgitation has been associated with added risk of death (Table 20-18). These technique-related variables can be

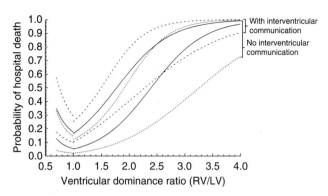

Figure 20-31   Nomogram of hospital mortality after repair of atrioventricular septal defects according to ventricular dominance. Solid lines are survival estimates, and dashed lines are 70% confidence limits. (See the original publication for details of variables examined and of the logistic regression equation for the nomogram.) (From Studer and colleagues.[S2])

Key: *LV*, Left ventricular area measured angiographically; *RV*, right ventricular area measured angiographically.

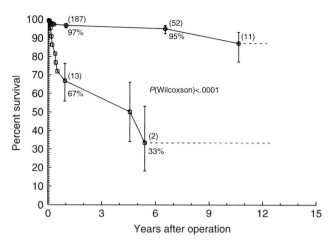

Figure 20-32   Survival after hospital discharge of 259 patients undergoing repair of atrioventricular (AV) septal defects, according to whether failure of the AV valve repair occurred. Squares represent patients with AV valve repair failure ($n = 23$) and circles those without ($n = 236$), with one untraced patient. The two deaths after 5 postoperative years in the latter group were of patients with known severe preoperative and postoperative pulmonary vascular disease. (From Studer and colleagues.[S2])

considered to apply more frequently in complex malformations. Additionally, in the experience of Hanley and colleagues, each of these three reasons for reoperation has decreased over time.[H4]

Other Risk Factors

Other incremental risk factors for premature death after repair have been reported. A single papillary muscle (see description under "Morphology" earlier in this chapter) becomes a serious problem after repair because of its tendency to result in LV inflow obstruction. It may therefore be a contraindication to typical two-ventricle repair. Severe ventricular hypoplasia is a risk factor for hospital death after a two-ventricle repair (Fig. 20-31). Severe LV hypoplasia is more common in patients with complete AV septal defects than is severe right ventricular hypoplasia. However, van Son and colleagues have suggested in a right-dominant unbalanced AV septal defect, leftward septal bowing may cause underestimation of LV volume and thus preclude operation. A preoperative LV volume of 15 mL · m^{-2} increased to greater than 30 mL · m^{-2} postoperatively in five patients, four of whom survived through use of a technique to orient the ventricular patch rightward at operation.[V11] However, most hearts with this defect are properly classified and treated as part of hypoplastic left heart syndrome.

Heart Block and Other Arrhythmias

Since Lev described the architecture of the conduction system in AV septal defects in 1958, prevalence of surgically induced permanent complete heart block has been approximately 1%.[L4] It is more frequent after repair of AV septal defect associated with tetralogy of Fallot and after AV valve replacement.[N3,S2]

First-degree AV block, present in about 30% of patients preoperatively, has been found in about 50% of patients after repair.[F5] Right bundle branch block is common after

repair of complete AV septal defects but uncommon after repair of partial AV septal defects.[F5]

In the UAB experience, when left AV valve replacement was required, heart block occurred in 4 of 20 patients (20%; CL 10%-33%).[S2] This is because sutures placed in the left AV valve anulus at about the 2-o'clock position overlie the AV node. A fringe of AV valve tissue must be left in this area so valve replacement sutures can be placed there and, more anteriorly, in the interatrial pericardial patch rather than along the ventricular septal crest. Placing the prosthesis in supraanular position is also helpful.[K2] With these precautions, complete heart block is minimized.

Functional Status

Most long-term survivors are in excellent health. In one center, 88% of surviving patients were in NYHA functional class I, and 11% were in class II.[K14,S2]

Atrioventricular Valve Function

Advent of Doppler color flow interrogation combined with two-dimensional echocardiography has increased considerably the knowledge about postrepair left AV valve function. Also, the reinforced leaflet method of repair has appeared to improve results.[B17,R8,S2,W7] Better techniques for repairing the left AV valve have played a major role in improving overall results, because patients whose repair fails are likely to have a considerably higher death rate in the intermediate and long term than are patients whose valve repair is good (Figs. 20-32 and 20-33; Table 20-19).

After repair of *partial AV septal defects,* about 10% of patients have late, severe left AV valve regurgitation, and such patients are more likely to have had severe regurgita-

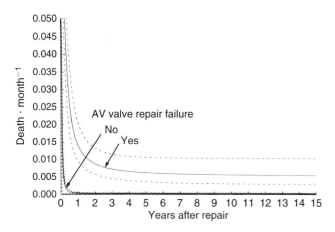

Figure 20-33   Hazard functions for death after repair of atrioventricular (AV) septal defects, one determined from analysis of those patients known to have had failure of the AV valve repair (*n* = 32; deaths = 19) and the other from analysis of those without valve repair failure (*n* = 278; deaths = 51). (From Kirklin and colleagues.[K14])

Key: *AV,* Atrioventricular.

■ **TABLE 20-19   Early Mortality Associated with Reoperation for Complete Atrioventricular Septal Defect**

	n	% of 363	Death		
			No.	%	CL (%)
LAVV repair[a]	26	7.2	3	12	5–22
LAVV replacement	8	2.2	0	0	0–21
Subaortic stenosis	5	1.4	0	0	0–32
Residual VSD	7	1.9	1	14	2–41
Permanent pacemaker	5	1.4	0	0	0–32
Other	10	2.8	2	20	7–41

(Data from Najm and colleagues.[N3])

Key: *LAVV,* Left atrioventricular valve; *VSD,* ventricular septal defect.

[a] Two patients had residual VSD.

tion prior to the repair.[A6,K15,L6,L7,M7,M15,S2] Generally, these patients have a deficiency of the LIL of the AV valve; to date, valve replacement has been the only certain method of achieving left AV valve competence in such patients.[B9,M15] Lesser degrees of regurgitation are present late postoperatively in about half of patients[M15]; 30% to 40% have essentially no left AV valve regurgitation late postoperatively.

In patients undergoing repair of *complete AV septal defects,* there appears to be little relationship between preoperative severity of AV valve regurgitation and that present late postoperatively,[W7] in contrast to the earlier findings of Studer and colleagues (before echocardiography was available).[S2] Even so, 10% to 20% of infants and older patients have important regurgitation late postoperatively, with the remainder having little or no regurgitation.[S2,W7] In many of these patients, re-repair may restore competence to the valve, but in some cases valve replacement is required.[P10]

Repair of uncomplicated partial and complete AV septal defects uncommonly results in stenosis of the left AV valve.

More often, this complication results when an accessory valve orifice or single papillary muscle coexists with the AV septal defect.

Important regurgitation or stenosis of the right AV valve is rare after repair of AV septal defects.

Left Ventricular Outflow Tract Obstruction

Uncommonly, LV outflow tract obstruction develops after repair of AV septal defects. As predicted on anatomic grounds by Ebels and colleagues, the AV septal defect has usually been the partial form.[E7] King and colleagues reported that 3 of 188 (1.6%; CL 0.7%-3.2%) hospital survivors of partial AV septal defect repair required reoperation for this condition, but with long-term follow-up, the true prevalence may be closer to 5%. [K15]

When LV outflow obstruction develops, it may be associated with worsening left AV valve regurgitation; its relief usually permits regression of the regurgitation.

Prevalence of subaortic LV outflow tract obstruction late after repair of complete AV septal defect is unknown but not negligible. Obstruction may have the appearance characteristic of discrete subaortic stenosis, with an "acquired fibromuscular ridge" (see "Resection of Localized Subvalvar Aortic Stenosis" in Section 2 of Chapter 33), or it may appear to result from the long narrow LV outflow tract itself.[S13] In either case, simple resection rarely suffices. Extensive transaortic myectomy or the modified Konno operation, without aortic valve replacement, is indicated (see "Modified Konno Operation" in Section 2 of Chapter 33).

Residual Pulmonary Hypertension

When important pulmonary hypertension is present preoperatively, it can be expected to regress postoperatively if the pulmonary blood flow is large and the patient receives a timely operation, usually when younger than age 6 months.[B1,C2,C5,L3]

INDICATIONS FOR OPERATION

Presence of an AV septal defect indicates need for operation, because an important hemodynamic derangement is nearly always present, and spontaneous closure does not occur.

Partial Atrioventricular Septal Defects

In partial AV septal defects, pulmonary hypertension is usually absent, and the optimal age for operation is 1 to 2 years, assuming a competent left AV valve. If AV valve regurgitation is present, earlier operation is indicated to prevent further damage to valve tissue. Also, when heart failure or severe growth failure is evident earlier in life, operation is indicated at that time.

Complete Atrioventricular Septal Defects

Operation is indicated early in the first year of life. When the infant's general condition is good, repair can be delayed until about age 2 to 4 months. When refractory heart failure or severe growth failure is evident at an earlier age, repair at that time is indicated. Often in patients who are older than 1 year, and occasionally in those in the last part of the first year of life, pulmonary vascular disease may already be too severe to permit repair. Criteria of inoperability are the same as described for patients with VSD (see "Indications for Operation" in Section 1 of Chapter 21). Lung biopsy is not recommended as an aid in grading severity of pulmonary vascular disease because of its associated morbidity and mortality and because of the scatter between histopathologic findings and pulmonary vascular resistance. Down syndrome is not generally considered a contraindication. However, Bull and colleagues have supported the alternative point of view, but on bases that have been disputed.[B19,K14,M14,W6]

Coexisting Cardiac Anomalies

Although certain major associated cardiac anomalies increase risk of repair of AV septal defects (see Table 20-15), their presence rarely alters the indication for operation. Thus, although a coexisting large patent ductus arteriosus has in the past increased risk of repair of complete AV septal defects, it increases the urgency of early repair rather than contraindicating it. When tetralogy of Fallot coexists, indication and timing of repair are similar to that for tetralogy of Fallot in general (see "Indications for Operation" in Section 1 of Chapter 24). When complete AV septal defect with juxtaaortic VSD is combined with double outlet right ventricle without pulmonary stenosis, life history and indications for operation are the same as for isolated complete AV septal defect; in the past, risk of repair has been high, but in the current era, early risk has been much less (see Table 20-14) and intermediate-term results good.[P3,P8]

SPECIAL SITUATIONS AND CONTROVERSIES

Pulmonary Trunk Banding

Pulmonary trunk banding has been used episodically as initial management for small infants with complete AV septal defects, and some excellent results have been reported.[E4,W5] This approach has been used only sparingly in recent years. However, Silverman and colleagues, as well as Williams and colleagues, demonstrated in the early era that some very sick, small infants can be well managed initially by banding and deferral of repair for 1 to 2 years.[S10,W5] In the absence of other contraindications to repair (unbalanced ventricles, comorbid conditions), banding is not indicated because age, left AV valve regurgitation, and many other risk factors have been neutralized and overall results of complete repair are excellent.

Septal Patches

There have been several reports of near-fatal hemolysis from the regurgitant jet of a left AV valve striking a synthetic interatrial patch after repair of AV septal defect.[H2,S1,V4] Therefore, for maximal safety, the interatrial patch material should be pericardium.

Avoiding Heart Block

For years, McGoon and colleagues successfully used a method that involved keeping the suture line on the *left* and *superior sides* of the conduction tissue, rather than on the right side and inferiorly.[M6] Starr's group has used the same general method with good results.[A5] The patch is sutured to the LSL–LIL complex on the *left* ventricular side of its attachment to the crest of the ventricular septum. Inferiorly, the suture line then goes to the *edge* of the ostium primum defect, posterior and central to the AV node and bundle of His, and posteriorly along the atrial septal edge. This method keeps the suture line to the *left* of, and away from, the AV node and bundle of His (see Fig. 20-24, *E*).

Hypoplastic Ventricle

When one ventricle is severely hypoplastic, a repair resulting in a two-ventricle system usually fails. Theoretically, a Fontan-type repair should be applicable to patients with this type of major associated cardiac anomaly. In the small number of patients treated in this manner, however, hospital mortality was extremely high.[C7,K14] This may be related to very early development of pulmonary vascular disease in patients with complete AV septal defects.

In a subset of patients characterized by small size and questionable functional status of the right ventricle, and success of classic biventricular repair in question, a "1½ ventricle repair" as suggested by Alvarado and colleagues and others may be appropriate.[A8,V12] In this repair, the usual procedure to correct the AV septal defect is accompanied by a bidirectional cavopulmonary anastomosis. Pulmonary blood flow is augmented, and the right ventricle is unloaded. A potential but unusual problem is pulmonary artery to right atrial circular flow if superior vena cava to right atrium continuity is maintained.

Late Reoperation

The only residual condition that remains an important cause of late reoperation is left AV valve regurgitation. Najm and colleagues reported that 9.4% of 363 patients operated on for complete AV septal defect underwent subsequent repair or replacement of the left AV valve; 3 of 34 (8.8%; CL 3.9%-17%) patients died (Table 20-19).[N3] Intraoperative echocardiography reduces the occurrence of residual important left AV valve regurgitation. The report of Reddy and colleagues is illustrative.[R10] Seventy-two infants (median age 3 to 9 months) underwent repair of complete AV septal defect. Cleft closure or anuloplasty was done in 70. Based on transesophageal echocardiography, 10 were returned to CPB for revision of the left AV valve. Among all 72 patients, there was one early death. There were five late reoperations with a median follow-up of 24 months: two were for AV valve regurgitation and three for subaortic obstruction. Although there may have been mild deterioration of AV valve function in patients with mild to moderate regurgitation early postoperatively, there was a 90% probability of not having severe late AV valve regurgitation at a mean follow-up of 45 months (range 3 to 169 months).[R11]

Wilcox Method of Extended Atrial Patch Repair of Complete Atrioventricular Septal Defect

Wilcox[W9] and subsequently Nicholson and colleagues[N4] used a single atrial patch extended downward to close the interventricular communication along with the interatrial defect. The common AV valve at its intersection with the ventricular septum is sutured along with the atrial patch to the right side of the crest of the ventricular septum, thereby obliterating the defect. The suture line is supported by a polyester strip shortened to 80% of the length of the exposed septal crest to serve as an anuloplasty for the medial portions of the AV valves. Thus, the bridging leaflets close the ventricular portion of the defect.

In both reports, there has been no heart block, no outflow tract obstruction, and no greater prevalence of left AV valve regurgitation than reported for the methods previously described. Frequently, there are trivial residual interventricular communications. Advocates of this approach claim shorter myocardial ischemic times.

REFERENCES

A

1. Alfieri O, Subramanian S. Successful repair of complete atrioventricular canal with undivided anterior common leaflet in a 6-month-old infant. Ann Thorac Surg 1975;19:92.
2. Abbott ME. Atlas of congenital cardiac disease. New York: The American Heart Association, 1936, pp. 34 and 50.
3. Alivizatos P, Anderson RH, Macartney FJ, Zuberbuhler JR, Stark J. Atrioventricular septal defect with balanced ventricles and malaligned atrial septum: double-outlet right atrium. Report of two cases. J Thorac Cardiovasc Surg 1985;89:295.
4. Anderson RH, Neches WH, Zuberbuhler JR, Penkoske PA. Scooping of the ventricular septum in atrioventricular septal defect. J Thorac Cardiovasc Surg 1988;95:146.
5. Abruzzese PA, Livermore J, Sunderland CO, Nunley DL, Issenberg H, Khonsari S, et al. Mitral repair in complete atrioventricular canal: ease of correction in early infancy. J Thorac Cardiovasc Surg 1983; 85:388.
6. Abbruzzese PA, Napoleone A, Bini RM, Annecchino FP, Merlo M, Parenzan L. Late left atrioventricular valve insufficiency after repair of partial atrioventricular septal defects: anatomical and surgical determinants. Ann Thorac Surg 1990;49:111.
7. Adatia I, Gittenberger-de Groot AC. Unroofed coronary sinus and coronary sinus orifice atresia. Implications for management of complex congenital heart disease. J Am Coll Cardiol 1995;25:948.
8. Alvarado O, Sreeram N, McKay R, Boyd IM. Cavopulmonary connection in repair of atrioventricular septal defect with small right ventricle. Ann Thorac Surg 1993;55:729.
9. Anderson R, Baker E, Ho S, Rigley M, Ebels T. The morphology and diagnosis of atrioventricular septal defects. Cardiol Young 1991; 1:291.

B

1. Bender HW Jr, Hammon JW Jr, Hubbard SG, Muirhead J, Graham TP. Repair of atrioventricular canal malformation in the 1st year of life. J Thorac Cardiovasc Surg 1982;84:515.
2. Bailey LL, Takeuchi Y, Williams WG, Trusler GA, Mustard WT. Surgical management of congenital cardiovascular anomalies with the use of profound hypothermia and circulatory arrest. Analysis of 180 consecutive cases. J Thorac Cardiovasc Surg 1976;71:485.
3. Berger TJ, Kirklin JW, Blackstone EH, Pacifico AD, Kouchoukos NT. Primary repair of complete atrioventricular canal in patients less than 2 years old. Am J Cardiol 1978;41:906.
4. Baron MG, Wolf BS, Steinfeld L, Van Mierop LH. Endocardial cushion defects. Specific diagnosis by angiocardiography. Am J Cardiol 1964;13:162.
5. Bharati S, Lev M. The spectrum of common atrioventricular orifice (canal). Am Heart J 1973;86:553.
6. Baron MG. Abnormalities of the mitral valve in endocardial cushion defects. Circulation 1972;45:672.
7. Bargeron LM Jr, Elliott LP, Soto B, Beam PR, Curry GC. Axial cineangiography in congenital heart disease. I. Concept, technical and anatomic considerations. Circulation 1977;56:1075.
8. Berger TJ, Blackstone EH, Kirklin JW, Bargeron LM Jr, Hazelrig JB, Turner ME Jr. Survival and probability of cure without and with operation in complete atrioventricular canal. Ann Thorac Surg 1979; 27:104.
9. Bharati S, Lev M, McAllister HA Jr, Kirklin JW. Surgical anatomy of the atrioventricular valve in the intermediate type of common atrioventricular orifice. J Thorac Cardiovasc Surg 1980;79:884.
10. Brandt PW, Clarkson PM, Neutze JM, Barratt-Boyes BG. Left ventricular cineangiocardiography in endocardial cushion defect (persistent common atrioventricular canal). Australas Radiol 1972; 16:367.

11. Barratt-Boyes BG, Calder AL. Double outlet ventricle: classification and surgical management. In Davila JC, ed. Second Henry Ford Hospital International Symposium on Cardiac Surgery. E. Norwalk, Conn.: Appleton & Lange, 1977, p. 285.

12. Barratt-Boyes BG. Correction of atrioventricular canal defects in infancy using profound hypothermia. In Barratt-Boyes BG, Neutze JM, Harris EA, eds. Heart disease in infancy: diagnosis and surgical treatment. Edinburgh: Churchill Livingstone, 1973, p. 110.

13. Bharati S, Kirklin JW, McAllister HA Jr, Lev M. The surgical anatomy of common atrioventricular orifice associated with tetralogy of Fallot, double outlet right ventricle and complete regular transposition. Circulation 1980;61:1142.

14. Ben-Shacher G, Moller JH, Castaneda-Zuniga W, Edwards JE. Signs of membranous subaortic stenosis appearing after correction of persistent common atrioventricular canal. Am J Cardiol 1981; 48:340.

15. Binet JP, Losay J, Hvass U. Tetralogy of Fallot with type C complete atrioventricular canal: surgical repair in three cases. J Thorac Cardiovasc Surg 1980;79:761.

16. Bloom KR, Freedom RM, Williams CM, Trusler GA, Rowe RD. Echocardiographic recognition of atrioventricular valve stenosis associated with endocardial cushion defect: pathologic and surgical correlates. Am J Cardiol 1979;44:1326.

17. Bove EL, Sondheimer HM, Kavey RE, Byrum CJ, Blackman MS. Results with the two-patch technique for repair of complete atrioventricular septal defect. Ann Thorac Surg 1984;38:157.

18. Bharati S, Lev M, Kirklin JW. Cardiac surgery and the conduction system, 2nd Ed. Mount Kisco, N.Y.: Futura, 1992.

19. Bull C, Rigby ML, Shinebourne EA. Should management of complete atrioventricular canal defect be influenced by coexistent Down syndrome? Lancet 1985;1:1147.

20. Bano-Rodrigo A, Van Praagh S, Trowitzsch E, Van Praagh R. Double-orifice mitral valve: a study of 27 postmortem cases with developmental, diagnostic and surgical considerations. Am J Cardiol 1988;61:152.

21. Becker AE, Anderson RH. Atrioventricular septal defects: what's in a name? J Thorac Cardiovasc Surg 1982;83:461.

22. Bailey SC, Watson DC. Atrioventricular septal defect repair in infants. Ann Thorac Surg 1991;52:33.

23. Backer CL, Mavroudis C, Alboliras ET, Zales VR. Repair of complete atrioventricular canal defects: results with the two-patch technique. Ann Thorac Surg 1995;60:530.

C

1. Cooley DA. Results of surgical treatment of atrial septal defects: particular consideration of low defects including ostium primum and atrioventricular canal. Am J Cardiol 1960;6:605.

2. Chin AJ, Keane JF, Norwood WI, Castaneda AR. Repair of complete common atrioventricular canal in infancy. J Thorac Cardiovasc Surg 1982;84:437.

3. Cooper DK, de Leval MR, Stark J. Results of surgical correction of persistent complete atrioventricular canal. Thorac Cardiovasc Surg 1979;27:111.

4. Castaneda AR, Nicholoff DM, Moller JH, Lucas RV Jr. Surgical correction of complete atrioventricular canal utilizing ball-valve replacement of the mitral valve: technical considerations and results. J Thorac Cardiovasc Surg 1971;62:926.

5. Culpepper W, Kolff J, Lin CY, Vitullo D, Lamberti J, Arcilla RA, et al. Complete common atrioventricular canal in infancy: surgical repair and postoperative hemodynamics. Circulation 1978;58:550.

6. Carpentier A. Surgical anatomy and management of the mitral component of atrioventricular canal defects. In Anderson RH, Shinebourne EA, eds. Pediatric cardiology. London: Churchill Livingstone, 1978, p. 477.

7. Clapp SK, Perry BL, Farooki ZQ, Jackson WL, Karpawich PP, Hakimi M, et al. Surgical and medical results of complete atrioventricular canal: a ten year review. Am J Cardiol 1987;59:454.

8. Corwin RD, Singh AK, Karlson KE. Double-outlet right atrium: a rare endocardial cushion defect. Am Heart J 1983;106:1156.

9. Chang CI, Becker AE. Surgical anatomy of left ventricular outflow tract obstruction in complete atrioventricular septal defect. A concept for operative repair. J Thorac Cardiovasc Surg 1987;94:897.

10. Chan KY, Redington AN, Rigby ML. Color flow mapping in atrioventricular septal defects: does it have an important role in diagnosis and management? Cardiol Young 1991;1:315.

11. Clapp S, Perry BL, Farooki ZQ, Jackson WL, Karpawich PP, Hakimi M, et al. Down's syndrome, complete atrioventricular canal, and pulmonary vascular obstructive disease. J Thorac Cardiovasc Surg 1990;100:115.

D

1. Draulans-Noë HA, Wenink AC, Quaegebeur J. Single papillary muscle ("parachute valve") and double-orifice left ventricle in atrioventricular septal defect convergence of chordal attachment: surgical anatomy and result of surgery. Pediatr Cardiol 1990;11:29.

2. Dubost C, Blondeau P. Canal atrio-ventriculaire et ostium primum. J Chir 1959;78:241.

3. DuShane JW, Weidman WH, Brandenburg RO, Kirklin JW. Differentiation of interatrial communications by clinical methods: ostium secundum, ostium primum, common atrium, and total anomalous pulmonary venous connection. Circulation 1960;21:363.

4. D'Allaines C, Colvez P, Fevre C, Levasseur P, Facquet J, Dubost C. A rare congenital cardiopathy: association of tetralogy of Fallot and complete A-V canal. Arch Mal Coeur 1969;62:996.

5. David I, Castaneda AR, Van Praagh R. Potentially parachute mitral valve in common atrioventricular canal: pathological anatomy and surgical importance. J Thorac Cardiovasc Surg 1982;84:178.

6. De Biase L, Di Ciommo V, Ballerini L, Bevilacqua M, Marcelletti C, Marino B. Prevalence of left-sided obstructive lesions in patients with atrioventricular canal without Down's syndrome. J Thorac Cardiovasc Surg 1986;91:467.

7. Draulans-Noë HA, Wenink AC. Anterolateral muscle bundle of the left ventricle in atrioventricular septal defect: left ventricular outflow tract and subaortic stenosis. Pediatr Cardiol 1991;12:83.

E

1. Ellis FH, McGoon D, Kirklin JW. Surgical management of persistent common atrioventricular canal. Am J Cardiol 1960;6:598.

2. Edwards JE. The problem of mitral insufficiency caused by accessory chordae tendineae in persistent common atrioventricular canal. Mayo Clin Proc 1960;35:299.

3. Ellis FH Jr, Kirklin JW, Swan HJ, DuShane JW, Edwards JE. Diagnosis and surgical treatment of common atrium (cor triloculare-biventriculare). Surgery 1959;45:160.

4. Epstein ML, Moller JH, Amplatz K, Nicoloff DM. Pulmonary artery banding in infants with complete atrioventricular canal. J Thorac Cardiovasc Surg 1979;78:28.

5. Emanuel R, Somerville J, Inns A, Withers R. Evidence of congenital heart disease in the offspring of parents with atrioventricular defects. Br Heart J 1983;49:144.

6. Ebels T, Meijboom EJ, Anderson RH, Schasfoort-van Leeuwen MJ, Lenstra D, Eijgelaar A, et al. Anatomic and functional "obstruction" of the outflow tract in atrioventricular septal defects with separate valve orifices ("ostium primum atrial septal defect"): an echocardiographic study. Am J Cardiol 1984;54:843.
7. Ebels T, Ho SY, Anderson RH, Meijboom EJ, Eijgelaar A. The surgical anatomy of the left ventricular outflow tract in atrioventricular septal defect. Ann Thorac Surg 1986;41:483.
8. Ebels T, Anderson RH, Devine WA, Debich DE, Penkoske PA, Zuberbuhler JR. Anomalies of the left atrioventricular valve and related ventricular septal morphology in atrioventricular septal defects. J Thorac Cardiovasc Surg 1990;99:299.
9. Ebels T. Surgery of the left atrioventricular valve and of the left ventricular outflow tract in atrioventricular septal defect. Cardiol Young 1991;1:344.

F

1. Feldt RH, ed. Atrioventricular canal defects. Philadelphia: WB Saunders, 1976.
2. Feldt RH, DuShane JW, Titus JL. The atrioventricular conduction system in persistent common atrioventricular canal defect. Circulation 1970;42:437.
3. Fisher RD, Bone DK, Rowe RD, Gott VL. Complete atrioventricular canal associated with tetralogy of Fallot: clinical experience and operative methods. J Thorac Cardiovasc Surg 1975;70:265.
4. Freedom RM, Bini M, Rowe RD. Endocardial cushion defect and significant hypoplasia of the left ventricle: a distant clinical and pathological entity. Eur J Cardiol 1978;7:263.
5. Fournier A, Young ML, Garcia OL, Tamer DF, Wolff GS. Electrophysiologic cardiac function before and after surgery in children with atrioventricular canal. Am J Cardiol 1986;57:1137.
6. Frescura C, Thiene G, Franceschini E, Talenti E, Mazzucco A. Pulmonary vascular disease in infants with complete atrioventricular septal defect. Int J Cardiol 1987;15:91.

G

1. Gerbode F, Sanchez PA, Arguero R, Kerth WJ, Hill JD, DeVries PA, et al. Endocardial cushion defects. Ann Surg 1967;166:486.
2. Gerbode F. Surgical repair of endocardial cushion defect. Ann Chir Thorac Cardiovasc 1962;1:753.
3. Goor D, Lillehei CW, Edwards JE. Further observations on the pathology of the atrioventricular canal malformation. Arch Surg 1968;97:954.
4. Gunther T, Mazzitelli D, Haehnel CJ, Holper K, Sebening F, Meisner H. Long-term results after repair of complete atrioventricular septal defects: analysis of risk factors. Ann Thorac Surg 1998;65:754.
5. Ghosh PK, Donnelly RJ, Hamilton DI, Wilkinson JL. Surgical correction of a case of common atrium with anomalous systemic and pulmonary venous drainage. J Thorac Cardiovasc Surg 1977;74:604.
6. Goor DA, Lillehei CW. Atrioventricular canal malformations. In Congenital malformations of the heart. Orlando, Fla.: Grune & Stratton, 1975, p. 132.
7. Goor DA, Lillehei CW. Atrioventricular canal malformations. In Congenital malformations of the heart. Orlando, Fla.: Grune & Stratton, 1975, p. 138.
8. Gallucci V, Mazzucco A, Stellin G, Faggian G, Bortolotti U. Repair of complete atrioventricular canal: 1975–1985. J Cardiac Surg 1986;1:261.

9. Gutgesell HP, Huhta JC. Cardiac septation in atrioventricular canal defect. J Am Coll Cardiol 1986;8:1421.

H

1. Hardesty RL, Zuberbuhler JR, Bahnson HT. Surgical treatment of atrioventricular canal defect. Arch Surg 1975;110:1391.
2. Hines GL, Finnerty TT, Doyle E, Isom OW. Near fatal hemolysis following repair of ostium primum atrial septal defect. J Cardiovasc Surg 1978;19:7.
3. Haworth SG. Pulmonary vascular bed in children with complete atrioventricular septal defect: relation between structural and hemodynamic abnormalities. Am J Cardiol 1986;57:833.
4. Hanley FL, Fenton KN, Jonas RA, Mayer JE, Cook NR, Wernovsky G, et al. Surgical repair of complete atrioventricular canal defects in infancy: twenty-year trends. J Thorac Cardiovasc Surg 1993;106:387.

I

1. Ilbawi MN, Idriss FS, DeLeon SY, Riggs TW, Muster AJ, Berry TE, et al. Unusual mitral valve abnormalities complicating surgical repair of endocardial cushion defects. J Thorac Cardiovasc Surg 1983;85:697.

K

1. Kahn DR, Levy J, France NE, Chung KJ, Dacumos GC. Recent results after repair of atrioventricular canal. J Thorac Cardiovasc Surg 1977;73:413.
2. Kadoba K, Jonas RA, Mayer JE, Castaneda AR. Mitral valve replacement in the first year of life. J Thorac Cardiovasc Surg 1990;100:762.
3. Kaiser GA, Waldo AL, Beach PM, Bowman FO Jr, Hoffman BF, Malm JR. Specialized cardiac conduction system: improved electrophysiologic identification at surgery. Arch Surg 1970;101:673.
4. Krongrad E, Malm JR, Bowman FO Jr, Hoffman BF, Kaiser GA, Waldo AL. Electrophysiological delineation of the specialized atrioventricular conduction system in patients with congenital heart disease. I. Delineation of the His bundle proximal to the membranous septum. J Thorac Cardiovasc Surg 1974;67:875.
5. Krongrad E, Malm JR, Bowman FO Jr, Hoffman BF, Waldo AL. Electrophysiological delineation of the specialized A-V conduction system in patients with congenital heart disease. II. Delineation of the distal His bundle and the right bundle branch. Circulation 1974;49:1232.
6. Kirklin JW, Daugherty GW, Burchell HB, Wood EH. Repair of the partial form of persistent common atrioventricular canal: so-called ostium primum type of atrial septal defect with interventricular communication. Ann Surg 1955;142:858.
7. Krayenbuhl CU, Lincoln JC. Total anomalous systemic venous connection, common atrium, and partial atrioventricular canal. A case report of successful surgical correction. J Thorac Cardiovasc Surg 1977;73:686.
8. Katz NM, Blackstone EH, Kirklin JW, Bradley EL, Lemons JE. Suture techniques for atrioventricular valves: experimental study. J Thorac Cardiovasc Surg 1981;81:528.
9. Kadoba K, Jonas RA. Replacement of the left atrioventricular valve after repair of atrioventricular septal defect. Cardiol Young 1991;1:383.

10. Kirklin JW, DuShane JW, Patrick RT, Donald DE, Hetzel PS, Harshbarger HG, et al. Intracardiac surgery with the aid of a mechanical pump-oxygenator system (Gibbon type): report of eight cases. Mayo Clin Proc 1955;30:201.

11. Kirklin JW, Blackstone EH, Pacifico AD, Brown RN, Bargeron LM Jr. Routine primary repair vs. two-stage repair of tetralogy of Fallot. Circulation 1979;60:373.

12. Kirklin JK, Blackstone EH, Kirklin JW, McKay R, Pacifico AD, Bargeron LM Jr. Intracardiac surgery in infants under age 3 months: incremental risk factors for hospital mortality. Am J Cardiol 1981; 48:500.

13. Kirklin JW, Blackstone EH, Jonas RA, Shimazaki Y, Kirklin JK, Mayer JE, et al. Morphologic and surgical determinants of outcome events after repair of tetralogy of Fallot and pulmonary stenosis: a two-institution study. J Thorac Cardiovasc Surg 1992; 103:706.

14. Kirklin JW, Blackstone EH, Bargeron LM Jr, Pacifico AD, Kirklin JK. The repair of atrioventricular septal defects in infancy. Int J Cardiol 1986;13:333.

15. King RM, Puga FJ, Danielson GK, Schaff HV, Julsrud PR, Feldt RH. Prognostic factors and surgical treatment of partial atrioventricular canal. Circulation 1986;74:I42.

L

1. Lillehei CW, Cohen M, Warden HE, Varco RL. The direct-vision intracardiac correction of congenital anomalies by controlled cross circulation: results in thirty-two patients with ventricular septal defects, tetralogy of Fallot, and atrioventricularis communis defects. Surgery 1955;38:11.

2. Levy MJ, Cuello L, Tuna N, Lillehei CW. Atrioventricularis communis. Clinical aspects and surgical treatment. Am J Cardiol 1964; 14:587.

3. Lillehei CW, Anderson RC, Ferlic RM, Bonnabeau RC Jr. Persistent common atrioventricular canal: recatheterization results in 37 patients following intracardiac repair. J Thorac Cardiovasc Surg 1969; 57:83.

4. Lev M. The architecture of the conduction system in congenital heart disease. I. Common atrioventricular orifice. AMA Arch Pathol 1958;65:174.

5. Lipshultz SE, Sanders SP, Mayer JE, Colan SD, Lock JE. Are routine preoperative cardiac catheterization and angiography necessary before repair of ostium primum atrial septal defect? J Am Coll Cardiol 1988;11:373.

6. Levy S, Blondeau P, Dubost C. Long-term follow-up after surgical correction of the partial form of common atrioventricular canal (ostium primum). J Thorac Cardiovasc Surg 1974;67:353.

7. Losay J, Rosenthal A, Castaneda AR, Bernhard WH, Nadas AS. Repair of atrial septal defect primum: results, course, and prognosis. J Thorac Cardiovasc Surg 1978;75:248.

8. Lev M, Agustsson MH, Arcilla R. The pathologic anatomy of common atrioventricular orifice associated with tetralogy of Fallot. Am J Clin Pathol 1961;36:408.

9. Lacour-Gayet F, Comas J, Bruniaux J, Serraf A, Losay J, Petit J, et al. Management of the left atrioventricular valve in 95 patients with atrioventricular septal defects and a common atrioventricular orifice—a ten year review. Cardiol Young 1991;1:367.

10. Lee CN, Danielson GK, Schaff HV, Puga FJ, Mair DD. Surgical treatment of double-orifice mitral valve in atrioventricular canal defect. J Thorac Cardiovasc Surg 1985;90:700.

11. Laks H, Capouya ER, Pearl JM, Elami A, Drinkwater DC Jr. Technique of management of the left atrioventricular valve in the repair of atrioventricular septal defect with a common atrioventricular orifice. Cardiol Young 1991;1:356.

M

1. Maloney JV Jr, Marable SA, Mulder DG. The surgical treatment of common atrioventricular canal. J Thorac Cardiovasc Surg 1962; 43:84.

2. McMullan MH, Wallace RB, Weidman WH, McGoon DC. Surgical treatment of complete atrioventricular canal. Surgery 1972; 72:905.

3. Mair DD, McGoon DC. Surgical correction of atrioventricular canal during the first year of life. Am J Cardiol 1977;40:66.

4. Mills NL, Ochsner JL, King TD. Correction of type C complete atrioventricular canal. Surgical considerations. J Thorac Cardiovasc Surg 1976;71:20.

5. Midgley FM, Galioto FM, Shapiro SR, Perry LW, Scott LP. Experience with repair of complete atrioventricular canal. Ann Thorac Surg 1980;30:151.

6. McGoon DC, McMullan MH, Mair DD, Danielson GK. Correction of complete atrioventricular canal in infants. Mayo Clin Proc 1973;48:769.

7. McMullan MH, McGoon DC, Wallace RB, Danielson GK, Weidman WH. Surgical treatment of partial atrioventricular canal. Arch Surg 1973;107:705.

8. Munoz-Armas S, Gorrin JR, Anselmi G, Hernandez PB, Anselmi A. Single atrium: embryologic, anatomic, electrocardiographic and other diagnostic features. Am J Cardiol 1968;21:639.

9. Mavroudis C, Weinstein G, Turley K, Ebert PA. Surgical management of complete atrioventricular canal. J Thorac Cardiovasc Surg 1982; 83:670.

10. Moreno-Cabral RJ, Shumway NE. Double-patch technique for correction of complete atrioventricular canal. Ann Thorac Surg 1982; 33:88.

11. Mitchell SC, Korones SB, Berendes HW. Congenital heart disease in 56,109 births: incidence and natural history. Circulation 1971; 43:323.

12. Macartney FJ, Rees PG, Daly K, Piccoli GP, Taylor JF, de Leval MR, et al. Angiocardiographic appearances of atrioventricular defects with particular reference to distinction of ostium primum atrial septal defects from common atrioventricular orifice. Br Heart J 1979; 42:640.

13. McGrath LB, Kirklin JW, Soto B, Bargeron LM Jr. Secondary left atrioventricular valve replacement in atrioventricular septal (AV canal) defect: a method to avoid left ventricular outflow tract obstruction. J Thorac Cardiovasc Surg 1985;89:632.

14. Menaham S, Mee RB. Complete atrioventricular canal defect in presence of Down syndrome (letter). Lancet 1985;2:834.

15. Meijboom EJ, Ebels T, Anderson RH, Schasfoort-van Leeuwen MJ, Deanfield JE, Eijgelaar A, et al. Left atrioventricular valve after surgical repair in atrioventricular septal defect with separate valve orifices ("ostium primum atrial septal defect"): an echo-Doppler study. Am J Cardiol 1986;57:433.

16. Merrill WH, Hammon JW Jr, Graham TP Jr, Bender HW Jr. Complete repair of atrioventricular septal defect. Ann Thorac Surg 1991; 52:29.

17. Moller JH. Perspectives in pediatric cardiology, Vol. 6. Surgery of congenital heart disease. Armonk, N.Y.: Futura Publishing, 1998.

N

1. Newfeld EA, Sher M, Paul MH, Nikaidoh H. Pulmonary vascular disease in complete atrioventricular canal defect. Am J Cardiol 1977;39:721.
2. Nora JJ, Nora AH. The evolution of specific genetic and environmental counseling in congenital heart diseases. Circulation 1978; 57:205.
3. Najm HK, Coles JG, Endo M, Stephens D, Rebeyka IM, Williams WG, et al. Complete atrioventricular septal defects: results of repair, risk factors, and freedom from reoperation. Circulation 1997; 96:II311.
4. Nicholson IA, Nunn GR, Sholler GF, Hawker RE, Cooper SG, Lau KC. Simplified single patch technique for the repair of atrioventricular septal defect. J Thorac Cardiovasc Surg 1999;118:642.

O

1. Ongley PA, Pongpanich B, Spangler JG, Feldt RH. The electrocardiogram in atrioventricular canal. In Feldt RH, ed. Atrioventricular canal defects. Philadelphia: WB Saunders, 1976, p. 51.

P

1. Pacifico AD, Kirklin JW. Surgical repair of complete atrioventricular canal with anterior common leaflet attached to an anomalous right ventricular papillary muscle. J Thorac Cardiovasc Surg 1973; 65:727.
2. Park JM, Ritter DG, Mair DD. Cardiac catheterization findings in persistent atrioventricular canal. In Feldt RH, ed. Atrioventricular canal defects. Philadelphia: WB Saunders, 1976, p. 76.
3. Pacifico AD, Kirklin JW, Bargeron LM Jr. Repair of complete atrioventricular canal associated with tetralogy of Fallot or double-outlet right ventricle: report of 10 patients. Ann Thorac Surg 1980; 29:351.
4. Piccoli GP, Ho SY, Wilkinson JL, Macartney FJ, Gerlis LM, Anderson RH. Left-sided obstructive lesions in atrioventricular septal defects: an anatomic study. J Thorac Cardiovasc Surg 1982;83:453.
5. Piccoli GP, Gerlis LM, Wilkinson JL, Lozsadi K, Macartney FJ, Anderson RH. Morphology and classification of atrioventricular defects. Br Heart J 1979;42:621.
6. Piccoli GP, Wilkinson JL, Macartney FJ, Gerlis LM, Anderson RH. Morphology and classification of complete atrioventricular defects. Br Heart J 1979;42:633.
7. Piccoli GP, Ho SY, Wilkinson JL, Macartney FJ, Gerlis LM, Anderson RH. Left-sided obstructive lesions in atrioventricular septal defect. J Thorac Cardiovasc Surg 1982;83:453.
8. Pacifico AD, Ricchi A, Bargeron LM Jr, Colvin EC, Kirklin JW, Kirklin JK. Corrective repair of complete atrioventricular (AV) canal defects (CAV) and major associated cardiac anomalies. Circulation 1987;76:IV72.
9. Penkoske PA, Neches WH, Anderson RH, Zuberbuhler JR. Further observations on the morphology of atrioventricular septal defects. J Thorac Cardiovasc Surg 1985;90:611.
10. Poirier NC, Williams WG, Van Arsdell GS, Coles JG, Smallhorn JF, Omran A, et al. A novel repair for patients with atrioventricular septal defect requiring reoperation for left atrioventricular valve regurgitation. Eur J Cardiothorac Surg 2000;18:54.

Q

1. Quaegebeur J, Kirklin JW, Pacifico AD, Bargeron LM Jr. Surgical experience with unroofed coronary sinus. Ann Thorac Surg 1979; 27:418.

R

1. Rastelli GC, Ongley PA, Kirklin JW, McGoon DC. Surgical repair of complete form of persistent common atrioventricular canal. J Thorac Cardiovasc Surg 1968;55:299.
2. Rastelli GC, Weidman WH, Kirklin JW. Surgical repair of the partial form of persistent common atrioventricular canal, with special reference to the problem of mitral valve incompetence. Circulation 1965;31:31.
3. Rastelli GC, Kirklin JW, Titus JL. Anatomic observations on complete form of persistent common atrioventricular canal with special reference to atrioventricular valves. Mayo Clin Proc 1966;4 1:296.
4. Rogers HM, Edwards JE. Incomplete division of the atrioventricular canal with patent interatrial foramen primum (persistent common atrioventricular ostium): report of five cases and review of the literature. Am Heart J 1948;36:28.
5. Rastelli GC, Ongley PA, McGoon DC. Surgical repair of complete atrioventricular canal with anterior common leaflet undivided and unattached to ventricular septum. Mayo Clin Proc 1969; 44:335.
6. Rastelli GC, Ongley PA, Kirklin JW. Surgical correction of common atrium with anomalously connected persistent left superior vena cava. Mayo Clin Proc 1965;40:528.
7. Rastelli GC, Rahimtoola SH, Ongley PA, McGoon DC. Common atrium: anatomy, hemodynamics, repair and surgery. J Thorac Cardiovasc Surg 1968;55:834.
8. Rizzoli G, Mazzucco A, Brumana T, Valfre C, Rubino M, Rocco F, et al. Operative risk of correction of atrioventricular septal defects. Br Heart J 1984;52:258.
9. Roberson DA, Muhiudeen IA, Silverman NH, Turley K, Haas GS, Cahalan MK. Intraoperative transesophageal echocardiography of atrioventricular septal defect. J Am Coll Cardiol 1991;18:537.
10. Reddy VM, McElhinney DB, Brook MM, Parry AJ, Hanley FL. Atrioventricular valve function after single patch repair of complete atrioventricular septal defect in infancy: how early should repair be attempted? J Thorac Cardiovasc Surg 1998;115:1032.
11. Rhodes J, Warner KG, Fulton DR, Romero BA, Schmid CH, Marx GR. Fate of mitral regurgitation following repair of atrioventricular septal defect. Am J Cardiol 1997;80:1194.

S

1. Sayed HM, Dacie JV, Handley DA, Lewis SM, Cleland WP. Haemolytic anaemia of mechanical origin after open heart surgery. Thorax 1961;16:356.
2. Studer M, Blackstone EH, Kirklin JW, Pacifico AD, Soto B, Chung GK, et al. Determinants of early and late results of repair of atrioventricular septal (canal) defects. J Thorac Cardiovasc Surg 1982;84:523.
3. Spanos PK, Fiddler GI, Mair DD, McGoon DC. Repair of atrioventricular canal associated with membranous subaortic stenosis. Mayo Clin Proc 1977;52:121.
4. Sellers RD, Lillehei CW, Edwards JE. Subaortic stenosis caused by anomalies of the atrioventricular valves. J Thorac Cardiovasc Surg 1964;48:289.
5. Stanger P, Rudolph AM, Edwards JE. Cardiac malpositions. An overview based on study of sixty-five necropsy specimens. Circulation 1977;56:159.

6. Somerville J. Ostium primum defects: factors causing deterioration in the natural history. Br Heart J 1965;27:413.

7. Sridaromont S, Feldt RH, Ritter DG, Davis GD, McGoon DC, Edwards JE. Double-outlet right ventricle associated with persistent common atrioventricular canal. Circulation 1975;52:933.

8. Soto B, Bargeron LM Jr, Pacifico AD, Vanini V, Kirklin JW. Angiography of atrioventricular canal defects. Am J Cardiol 1981; 48:492.

9. Smallhorn JF, Tommasini G, Anderson RH, Macartney FJ. Assessment of atrioventricular septal defects by two dimensional echocardiography. Br Heart J 1982;47:109.

10. Silverman N, Levitsky S, Fisher E, DuBrow I, Hastreiter A, Scagliotti D. Efficacy of pulmonary artery banding in infants with complete atrioventricular canal. Circulation 1983;68:II148.

11. Samánek M. Prevalence at birth, "natural" risk and survival with atrioventricular septal defect. Cardiol Young 1991;1:285.

12. Smallhorn JF, Perrin D, Musewe N, Dyck J, Boutin C, Freedom RM. The role of transesophageal echocardiography in the evaluation of patients with atrioventricular septal defect. Cardiol Young 1991; 1:324.

13. Silverman NH, Gerlis LM, Ho SY, Anderson RH. Fibrous obstruction within the left ventricular outflow tract associated with ventricular septal defect: a pathologic study. J Am Coll Cardiol 1995; 25:475.

14. Suzuki K, Ho SY, Anderson RH, Becker AE, Neches WH, Devine WA, et al. Morphometric analysis of atrioventricular septal defect with common valve orifice. J Am Coll Cardiol 1998;31:217.

T

1. Toscano-Barbosa E, Brandenburg RO, Burchell HB. Electrocardiographic studies of cases with intracardiac malformations of the atrioventricular canal. Mayo Clin Proc 1956;31:513.

2. Tenckhoff L, Stamm SJ. An analysis of 35 cases of the complete form of persistent common atrioventricular canal. Circulation 1973; 48:416.

3. Tandon R, Moller JH, Edwards JE. Tetralogy of Fallot associated with persistent common atrioventricular canal (endocardial cushion defect). Br Heart J 1974;36:197.

4. Takanashi Y, Anzai N, Okada T, Sano A, Ando M, Konno S. Common atrium associated with anomalous high insertion of the inferior vena cava. J Thorac Cardiovasc Surg 1975;69:912.

5. Taylor NC, Somerville J. Fixed subaortic stenosis after repair of ostium primum defects. Br Heart J 1981;45:689.

6. Thiene G, Wenink AC, Frescura C, Wilkinson JL, Gallucci V, Ho SY, et al. Surgical anatomy and pathology of the conduction tissues in atrioventricular defects. J Thorac Cardiovasc Surg 1981;82:928.

7. Thilenius OG, Vitullo D, Bharati S, Luken J, Lamberti JJ, Tatooles C, et al. Endocardial cushion defect associated with cor triatriatum sinistrum or supravalve mitral ring. Am J Cardiol 1979;44: 1339.

8. Tandon R, Moller JH, Edwards JE. Single papillary muscle of the left ventricle associated with persistent common atrioventricular canal: variant of parachute mitral valve. Pediatr Cardiol 1986;7:111.

U

1. Ugarte M, Enriquez de Salamanca F, Quero M. Endocardial cushion defects: an anatomical study of 54 specimens. Br Heart J 1976; 38:674.

V

1. Vanetti A, Dumet. Surgical treatment of severe forms of atrioventricular canal. Arch Mal Coeur Vaiss 1975;68:719.

2. Van Praagh R, Corwin RD, Dahlquist EH Jr, Freedom RM, Mattioli L, Nebesar RA. Tetralogy of Fallot with severe left ventricular anomalous attachment of the mitral valve to the ventricular septum. Am J Cardiol 1970;26:93.

3. Van Mierop LH, Alley RD, Kausel HW, Stranahan A. The anatomy and embryology of endocardial cushion defects. J Thorac Cardiovasc Surg 1962;43:71.

4. Verdon TA Jr, Forrester RH, Crosby WH. Hemolytic anemia after open-heart repair of ostium-primum defects. N Engl J Med 1963; 269:444.

5. Van Mierop LH, Alley RD. The management of the cleft mitral valve in endocardial cushion defects. Ann Thorac Surg 1966;2:416.

6. Van Mierop LH. Pathology and pathogenesis of endocardial cushion defect. Surgical implications. In Davila JC, ed. Second Henry Ford Hospital International Symposium on Cardiac Surgery. E. Norwalk, Conn.: Appleton & Lange, 1977, p. 201.

7. Virdi IS, Keeton BR, Shore DF. Atrioventricular septal defect with a well developed primary component of the atrial septum ("septum primum"). Int J Cardiol 1985;9:243.

8. Van Praagh S, Antoniadis S, Otero-Coto E, Leidenfrost RD, Van Praagh R. Common atrioventricular canal with and without conotruncal malformations. An anatomic study of 251 postmortem cases. In Nora JJ, Ta Kao A, eds. Congenital heart disease. Causes and processes. Mount Kisco, N.Y.: Futura, 1984, p. 599.

9. Vargas FJ, Coto EO, Mayer JE Jr, Jonas RA, Castaneda AR. Complete atrioventricular canal and tetralogy of Fallot: surgical considerations. Ann Thorac Surg 1986;42:258.

10. Van Arsdell GS, Williams WG, Boutin C, Trusler GA, Coles JG, Rebeyka IM, et al. Subaortic stenosis in the spectrum of atrioventricular septal defects: solutions may be complex and palliative. J Thorac Cardiovasc Surg 1995;110:1534.

11. van Son JA, Phoon CK, Silverman NH, Haas GS. Predicting feasibility of biventricular repair of right-dominant unbalanced atrioventricular canal. Ann Thorac Surg 1997;63:1657.

12. Van Arsdell GS, Williams WG, Boutin C, Trusler GA, Coles JG, Rebeyka IM, Freedom RM. Subaortic stenosis in the spectrum of atrioventricular septal defects. Solutions may be complex and palliative. J Thorac Cardiovasc Surg 1995;110:1534.

W

1. Wakai CS, Edwards JE. Development and pathologic considerations in persistent common atrioventricular canal. Proc Mayo Clin 1956; 31:487.

2. Wakai CS, Edwards JE. Pathologic study of persistent common atrioventricular canal. Am Heart J 1958;56:779.

3. Watkins E Jr, Gross RE. Experiences with surgical repair of atrial septal defects. J Thorac Cardiovasc Surg 1955;30:469.

4. Williams RG, Rudd M. Echocardiographic features of endocardial cushion defects. Circulation 1974;49:418.

5. Williams WH, Guyton RA, Michalik RE, Plauth WH Jr, Zorn-Chelton S, Jones EL, et al. Individualized surgical management of complete atrioventricular canal. J Thorac Cardiovasc Surg 1983;86:838.

6. Wilson NJ, Gavalaki E, Newman CG. Complete atrioventricular canal defect in presence of Down syndrome (letter). Lancet 1985; 2:834.

7. Weintraub RG, Brawn WJ, Venables AW, Mee RB. Two-patch repair of complete atrioventricular septal defect in the first year of life. J Thorac Cardiovasc Surg 1990;99:320.
8. Westerman GR, Norton JB, Van Devanter SH. Double-outlet right atrium associated with tetralogy of Fallot and common atrioventricular valve. J Thorac Cardiovasc Surg 1986;91:205.
9. Wilcox BR, Jones DR, Frantz EG, Brink LW, Henry GW, Mill MR, et al. Anatomically sound, simplified approach to repair of "complete" atrioventricular septal defect. Ann Thorac Surg 1997;64:487.

Y
1. Yokoyama M. The location of the coronary sinus orifice in endocardial cushion defects. Kyobu Geka 1973;26:35.

2. Yilmaz AT, Arslan M, Kuralay E, Demrkilic U, Ozal E, Tatar H, et al. Repair of the left AV valve in atrioventricular septal defect in adults. J Card Surg 1996;11:363.
3. Yamaki S, Yasui H, Kado H, Yonenaga K, Nakamura Y, Kikuchi T, et al. Pulmonary vascular disease and operative indications in complete atrioventricular canal defect in early infancy. J Thorac Cardiovasc Surg 1993;106:398.

Z
1. Zavanella C, Matsuda H, Subramanian S. Successful correction of a complete form of atrioventricular canal associated with tetralogy of Fallot. J Thorac Cardiovasc Surg 1977;74:195.

21 Ventricular Septal Defect

SECTION 1
Primary Ventricular Septal Defect

DEFINITION

Ventricular septal defect (VSD) is a hole or multiple holes in the interventricular septum. This chapter discusses VSDs that occur as the primary lesion, recognizing that hearts with primary VSDs may have minor coexisting morphologic abnormalities.[O5]

VSD may be part of another major cardiovascular anomaly, such as tetralogy of Fallot (see Chapter 24), complete atrioventricular (AV) septal defect (see Chapter 20), anatomically corrected malposition of the great arteries (see Chapter 43), truncus arteriosus (see Chapter 29), tricuspid atresia (see Chapter 27), sinus of Valsalva aneurysm (see Chapter 22), and interrupted aortic arch (see Chapter 34). VSDs also may be acquired, as discussed in Chapters 9 and 46.

HISTORICAL NOTE

In 1954, Lillehei, Varco, and colleagues, at the University of Minnesota in Minneapolis, began to repair VSDs using normothermic, low-flow, *controlled cross-circulation* based on the so-called azygos-flow principle,[A1,C1] with an adult human as the oxygenator (see "Historical Note" in Section 2 of Chapter 2).[L1,W1] This was the beginning of the era of cardiac surgery using *cardiopulmonary bypass* (CPB), a term coined by Cooley a few years later. The paper by Lillehei and colleagues in 1955 contains some excesses of enthusiasm, such as "these observations would seem to deny the classic concept that the conduction system of the human or canine heart (atrioventricular node and bundle of His) is concentrated in a small localized discrete locus which is thereby very vulnerable to mechanical injury."[L1] However, their feat was remarkable. Five of the first eight patients were in their first year of life, and only two (40%; CL 14%-71%) of the five died, a tribute to surgical skill, lack of cardiac ischemia (the aorta was not clamped), and

perfectness of their human oxygenator. The dramatic weight gain of the surgically cured infants with large VSDs was documented. Three other patients, aged 4, 5, and 5 years, also survived, one with multiple VSDs.

In 1956, DuShane and colleagues reported 20 patients who had undergone intracardiac repair of large VSDs with a *mechanical pump-oxygenator* at the Mayo Clinic beginning in March 1955.[D1] Normothermic flow of 70 mL · kg^{-1} · min^{-1} (about 2.1 L · min^{-1} · m^{-2}) were used, along with a pump-sucker system to return intracardiac blood to the machine. Duration of CPB varied from 10 to 45 minutes. Four (20%; CL 10%-33%) of the 20 patients died in hospital, a mortality that was considered low in that era.

Truex described the location of the specialized conduction tissue in hearts with VSD.[T8] In a more detailed study, Lev expanded on this topic,[L3] and his work was the basis on which Kirklin and DuShane developed a surgical technique that avoided producing heart block during VSD repair.[K3]

Lillehei showed the feasibility of an atrial approach to VSD in 1957.[S6] The technique of hypothermic circulatory arrest, with rewarming by a pump-oxygenator, was applied successfully to infants with VSD by Okamoto.[O2] Kirklin and DuShane (1961) and Sloan's group (1967) reported the feasibility of primary repair of VSD in infants.[K12,S2]

Routine primary repair of VSD in sick, small infants was found to be superior to pulmonary artery banding by Barratt-Boyes and colleagues (1969–1971).[B7]

MORPHOLOGY

Although this chapter considers VSD that occurs as the primary lesion, the method of morphologic description is applied in other chapters to VSDs that are part of other major cardiac malformations. The morphologic classification described in this edition represents an attempt to simplify VSD classification by encompassing all variations of the lesion while conforming to other systems of classification (Box 21-1). The classification used here conforms generally with the consensus of the Congenital Heart Surgery Nomenclature and Database Project[J6] and includes many of the concepts of Anderson and Wilcox.[A12,A13]

BOX 21-1   Morphologic Classification of Ventricular Septal Defect

Classification	% of VSDs	Location/Borders
Perimembranous	80	Borders tricuspid valve Conduction system in posterior rim
Muscular	5	Borders all muscle Frequently multiple Conduction system remote
Doubly committed subarterial	5-10	Borders both semilunar valves Conduction system remote
Inlet septal	<5	Atrioventricular septal type Posterior position Conduction system in posterior rim

Key: *VSD*, Ventricular septal defect.

Size

VSDs are highly variable in size, and their division into size groups is arbitrary but useful.

Large VSDs are approximately the size of the aortic orifice or larger. They offer little resistance to flow, and thus their VSD resistance index[1] is less than 20 units · m^2 in situations in which the calculation of the index is valid.[H6,S1] Right ventricular (RV) systolic pressure approximates left ventricular (LV) pressure, and the pulmonary to systemic blood flow ratio ($\dot{Q}p/\dot{Q}s$) is increased to a degree dependent on the level of pulmonary vascular resistance.

Moderate-sized VSDs, although still restrictive, are of sufficient size to raise RV systolic pressure to approximately half LV pressure and $\dot{Q}p/\dot{Q}s$ to 2.0 or greater.

Small VSDs are of insufficient size to raise RV systolic pressure, and $\dot{Q}p/\dot{Q}s$ is not increased above 1.75. Small VSDs have a VSD resistance index greater than 20 units · m^2.[H6] Multiple small defects behave in aggregate as a large defect.

Location in Septum and Relationship to Conduction System

VSDs can occur in all portions of the ventricular septum (Fig. 21-1).[2] VSDs with entirely muscular borders (muscular VSDs) may occupy several areas of the ventricular septum; other VSDs have one or several nonmuscular borders, consisting of spaces or structures against which they are juxtaposed (Box 21-2). These nonmuscular borders may be a semilunar valve, an AV valve, or the crux cordis. Some VSDs in the periphery of the ventricular septum are bordered by the ventricular free wall, but such VSDs are conventionally considered to be muscular. VSDs in the category of subarterial may be (1) *juxta-aortic,* (2) *juxta-pulmonary,* (3) *juxta-arterial* (bordered by both pulmonary and aortic valves), or (4) *juxtatruncal* (bordered by the valve of a common arterial trunk). Subarterial VSDs are typically associated with some degree of overriding of the related arterial trunk, and the margin of the VSD is actually a space over which is a semilunar valve(s).[A8]

Many VSDs are associated with *malalignment* of portions of the ventricular septum or of the atrial septum relative to the interventricular septum, in which case an AV valve usually overrides the VSD. *Malalignment VSD* terminology results from two-dimensional echocardiographic examination of the heart regarding the alignment of the trabecular and the outlet (conal) septum. In some cardiac anomalies the aorta seems displaced relative to the VSD. The malalignment is referred to as *anterior* when the outlet septum appears anterior to the trabecular septum with the VSD interposed. Tetralogy of Fallot type of defects are considered to be anterior malalignment types, with the aorta "overriding" the VSD (see Fig. 21-19, *C*). Malalignment is

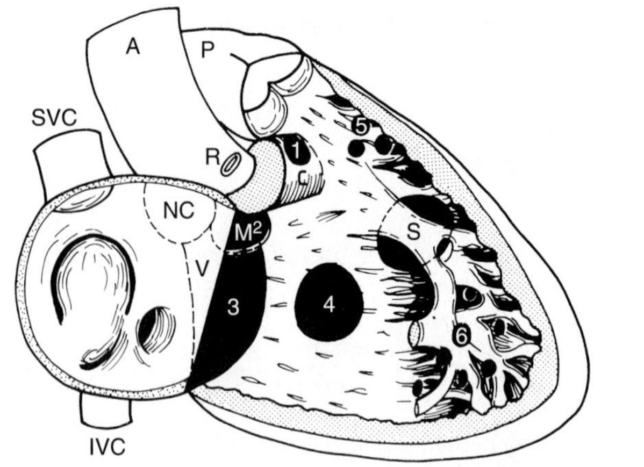

Figure 21-1   Schematic representation of position of ventricular septal defect (VSD) as seen from right ventricular side of septum. Front of right ventricle and right atrium and tricuspid valve have been removed. Shown are *(1)* doubly committed subarterial (juxta-arterial) VSD; *(2)* a perimembranous (conoventricular) VSD, which is juxta-aortic and juxtatricuspid; *(3)* an inlet septal VSD, which is juxtatricuspid and juxtamitral and, in this instance, juxtacrucial, a defect generally associated with atrial and ventricular septal malalignment and overriding tricuspid valve; and *(4, 5, 6)* trabecular VSDs. In positions 5 and 6, VSDs tend to be small and multiple, and when most of this trabeculated area and midmuscular septum are peppered with holes, the term *Swiss cheese defect* is used. Position 5 would be classified *muscular, outlet type;* position 6 is *muscular, apical.*

Key: *A,* Aorta; *c,* conal (outlet, infundibular) septum; *IVC,* inferior vena cava; *M,* membranous septum with ventricular and atrioventricular portions; *NC,* noncoronary aortic cusp; *P,* pulmonary trunk and valve; *R,* right coronary artery cut off at its origin; *SVC,* superior vena cava; *V,* muscular portion of atrioventricular septum: *S,* septal band, or trabecula septomarginalis.

BOX 21-2   Expanded Morphologic Classification of Ventricular Septal Defect

Classification	Extension
Perimembranous	Inlet
	Anterior
	Outlet
Muscular	Outlet (conal)
	Trabecula
	Inlet
	Anterior
	Apical
Doubly committed subarterial	—
Inlet septal	Atrioventricular septal type
Malalignment	Anterior (tetralogy of Fallot)
	Posterior (interrupted arch or coarctation)
	Rotational (Taussig-Bing)

---

[1] VSD resistance index $= \dfrac{P_{Lv}(peak) - P_{Rv}(peak)}{\dot{Q}p - \dot{Q}s} \times BSA$

where *BSA* is body surface area.

[2] The location is described in words that are relevant to the right ventricular aspect of the VSD (see "Right Ventricle" under Cardiac Chambers and Major Vessels in Chapter 1), because most reparative procedures are performed from that aspect.

posterior when the outlet septum appears posterior to the trabecular septum in anomalies such as interrupted aortic arch and severe coarctation of the aorta. There may also be a *rotational* malalignment in anomalies characterized under the broad category of Taussig-Bing heart.

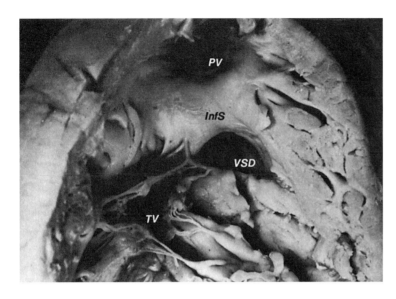

Figure 21-2 Perimembranous ventricular septal defect *(VSD)* viewed from right ventricle. VSD borders anteroseptal commissure of tricuspid valve (juxtatricuspid) and has anterior extension to VSD and midportion of muscular septum.

Key: *InfS*, Infundibular (outlet) septum; *PV*, pulmonary valve; *TV*, tricuspid valve; *VSD*, ventricular septal defect.

Anatomic location of the VSD determines its relation to the conduction system.

VSDs may also be characterized according to their *commitment* to the great arteries (Lev and colleagues[L10]): subaortic, subpulmonary, doubly committed, and noncommitted. This type of characterization, which is relational and not morphologic, preferably is restricted to hearts with double outlet ventricles, because its use in other situations has resulted in considerable confusion.

All these features of the location of VSDs should be included in descriptions of these defects.

Perimembranous Ventricular Septal Defect

Approximately 80% of patients operated on for primary VSD have a perimembranous ventricular septal defect.[S22,S23,V5] These defects could be called *junctional VSDs* because they are in the junctional area between the trabecular (sinus) and conal portions of the ventricular septum (Fig. 21-2) and usually appear to be between the posterior and anterior divisions of the septal band. Thus, these VSDs are between the outlet (conus) and inlet (ventricular) portions of the *right* ventricle, but characteristically they are in the outlet portion of the *left* ventricle.

Perimembranous VSDs are often associated with anomalies of the outlet septum[O5] and other adjacent structures, although when small, they may be truly isolated anomalies. Some perimembranous VSDs are *juxtatricuspid* (abutting the tricuspid valve), *juxtamitral*, and *juxta-aortic*.[B2] These perimembranous VSDs are also conoventricular (conotruncal) (Fig. 21-3).[S13] Such defects abut the commissural area between the noncoronary and right coronary cusps of the aortic valve. Others are only juxtatricuspid (Fig. 21-4), and in hearts with these as well as in hearts with perimembranous VSDs, the bundle of His passes along the posteroinferior border of the defect.[B2,K15,L13,S13] Some perimembranous VSDs abut none of these valvar structures and are separated from the tricuspid anulus posteriorly by a band of muscle that is part of the posterior division of the septal band (trabecula septomarginalis) joining with the ventricu-

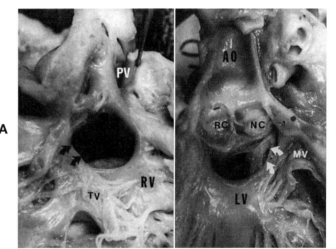

Figure 21-3 Large perimembranous ventricular septal defect, viewed from right ventricle (**A**) and left ventricle (**B**). In **A**, septal tricuspid leaflet was folded back into right atrium after its chordae were cut. Arrows indicate areas of tricuspid–mitral continuity, and defect borders the tricuspid valve; it is juxtatricuspid, juxtamitral, and juxta-aortic. This defect, viewed from the right ventricle, lies far to the right in the aortic margin of the ventricular septum and thus is beneath the commissure between noncoronary and right coronary cusps. Defect is perimembranous, and no muscle is between it and the anterior septal tricuspid commissure. Conal septum is hypoplastic but not malaligned. (From Soto and colleagues.[S23])

Key: *AO*, Aorta; *LV*, left ventricle; *MV*, mitral valve; *NC*, noncoronary cusp; *PV*, pulmonary valve; *RC*, right coronary cusp; *RV*, right ventricle; *TV*, tricuspid valve.

loinfundibular fold. The bundle of His is not in this muscular band but is in its usual position more posteriorly. Technically, although this type of defect is located in a perimembranous position, it is better classified as *muscular inlet-type VSD* because all borders are muscle.

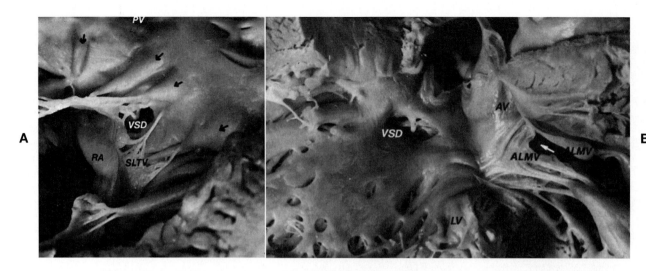

Figure 21-4   Perimembranous ventricular septal defect *(VSD)* of moderate size. **A,** VSD in region of anteroseptal commissure of tricuspid valve, viewed from right ventricle. VSD extends inferiorly beneath septal leaflet of tricuspid valve and abuts commissural area between anterior and septal tricuspid leaflets (juxtatricuspid) and remnant of membranous septum. Numerous tricuspid chordae and papillary muscles *(arrows)* are present. **B,** Same defect viewed from left ventricle. VSD lies below noncoronary cusp of aortic valve and is not juxta-aortic. Arrow indicates cleft in anterior mitral leaflet.

Key: *ALMV,* Anterior leaflet of mitral valve; *AV,* aortic valve; *LV,* left ventricle; *PV,* pulmonary valve; *RA,* right atrium; *SLTV,* septal leaflet of tricuspid valve; *VSD,* ventricular septal defect.

VSDs have also been described in the past as *typically high, infracristal, membranous,* or *perimembranous* without the original specific description.[B2,B4,S13,S22]

As already indicated, the AV node and penetrating portion of the bundle of His are in their normal position in hearts with perimembranous VSDs. As the bundle penetrates the fibrous right trigone of the central fibrous body at the base of the noncoronary cusp of the aortic valve, it lies along the posteroinferior border of perimembranous and inlet-type VSDs. As the bundle continues along the inferior border of the VSD (at times slightly to the left or right of the free edge), the left bundle branch fascicles emerge from the branching portion. Only the right bundle branch remains when the bundle reaches the level of the muscle of Lancisi.

Abnormalities of the ventricular portion of the membranous septum are often associated with perimembranous VSDs. The membranous septum may be absent or nearly so, and then the right trigone (beneath the nadir of the noncoronary aortic valve cusp) and base of the septal and anterior leaflets of the tricuspid valve are exposed and form the posteroinferior rim of the VSD (see Fig. 21-3). The bundle of His, as it penetrates the fibrous right trigone at the base of the noncoronary cusp, is intimately related to the posteroinferior angle of such a defect. This is associated with a deficiency in the posterior limb of the septal band (trabecula septomarginalis).[K14] Rarely the ventricular portion of the membranous septum may be well developed, thickened, and perforated by one or many holes, forming an *aneurysm of the membranous septum* that bulges toward the right in systole. This so-called aneurysm is simulated on

angiography by the much more common tethered anterior leaflet and the involved and usually fused chordae. Accessory fibrous tissue, not part of the tricuspid valve mechanism, may lie along the posterior or superior margin of the defect. This phenomenon is most marked in the *flap valve VSD.*

Not surprisingly, in hearts with perimembranous VSDs, still other adjacent structures may be abnormal. The medial papillary muscle characteristically joins the anteroinferior angle of the defect and receives chordae from adjacent portions of the tricuspid anterior and septal leaflets. These chordae may be increased in number and abnormally positioned around the edges of a perimembranous VSD, attached to the posterior edge, superior edge (Fig. 21-5), or most often anterior edge.[U1] A thick leash of chordae joining the center of the anterior edge of a large defect may produce an appearance on angiography or even at operation of a double defect. Chordae from the anterior leaflet may attach to all three margins, and the anterior leaflet then limits the shunt from left to right through the defect as well as hinder its repair.

Close association of some perimembranous VSDs with the commissure between anterior and septal tricuspid leaflets sometimes results in adherence of leaflet tissue to edges of the defect and shunting directly from left ventricle into right atrium (Fig. 21-6).[B8,L11] This so-called left ventricular–right atrial defect,[G4,P2,S8] which constitutes less than 5% of perimembranous VSDs in this region, rarely involves the AV septum. Adherence of tricuspid leaflet and chordal tissue is also an important mechanism of spontaneous closure of these VSDs.[C14]

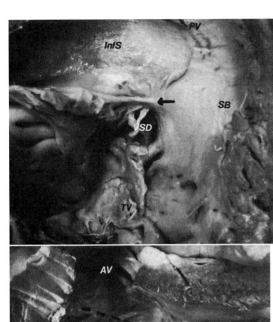

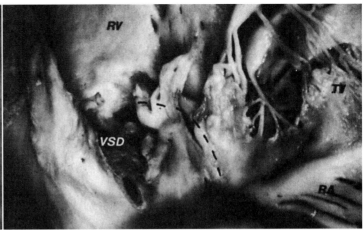

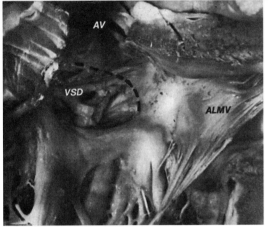

Figure 21-5   Perimembranous ventricular septal defect *(VSD)* associated with anomalous leaflet tissue. **A,** VSD viewed from right ventricle. Note chordal attachment *(arrow)* of anterior tricuspid leaflet to anterosuperior margin of defect. Normal position of infundibular (outlet) septum between two limbs of septal band is (trabecula septomarginalis) well seen. **B,** Same defect viewed from right atrium. VSD is partly obscured by tricuspid leaflet tissue, but its extent is indicated by dashed line. **C,** Same defect viewed from left ventricle. VSD is immediately beneath aortic valve (juxta-aortic), and its extent is indicated by dashed line. Abnormal tricuspid valve attachments are obvious and on an angiocardiogram are indistinguishable from an aneurysm of the membranous ventricular septum.

Key: *ALMV,* Anterior leaflet of mitral valve; *AV,* aortic valve; *InfS,* infundibular (outlet) septum; *PV,* pulmonary valve, *RA,* right atrium; *RV,* right ventricle; *SB,* septal band, or trabecula septomarginalis; *TV,* tricuspid valve; *VSD,* ventricular septal defect.

Ventricular Septal Defect in Right Ventricular Outlet (Doubly Committed Subarterial Ventricular Septal Defect)

Five percent to 10% of patients treated operatively have a single VSD, usually of moderate or large size, within the outlet portion of the *right* ventricle. VSDs in this location are also in the outlet portion of the *left* ventricle and, in contrast to perimembranous VSDs, are more beneath the right aortic cusp than the commissure between it and the noncoronary cusp. These have in the past been also termed *conal, infundibular, supracristal,* and *intracristal* defects. The complex morphology of the ventricular septum in the outlet portion of the right ventricle and many controversies concerning the term "outlet septum" support use of a simple descriptive terminology for this group of VSDs.

Important VSDs in this general location are bordered in part by a space over which lie the pulmonary and aortic valves (Fig. 21-7).[S13] As such, these VSDs are subarterial. VSDs of this type are more common in Asians than in Caucasian or African ethnicities.[T7] Subarterial VSDs may be circular, diamond shaped, or oval with the long axis lying transversely (Fig. 21-8). When viewed from the LV aspect, these defects are in the outflow portion of the ventricular septum (Fig. 21-9), beneath the right coronary cusp (or the commissure between it and the left cusp). The aortic and pulmonary valve cusps are separated by only a thin rim of fibrous tissue. The right aortic cusp and less

often noncoronary cusp may prolapse into the upper margin of the defect, with or without aortic regurgitation (see Section 2 later in this chapter).

The posteroinferior margin of RV outlet VSDs is usually well separated from the tricuspid valve anulus by a band of muscle, and consequently is well above the bundle of His. Occasionally, however, a particularly large confluent VSD may be both subarterial and perimembranous (see Fig. 21-9). The conduction system is related to such a VSD as it is to other perimembranous defects. This particular type of VSD is sometimes associated with severe overriding of the aorta, and the cardiac anomaly is then termed *double outlet right ventricle with doubly committed VSD.* The same type of VSD may also be seen in double outlet left ventricle, in which the pulmonary artery severely overrides the VSD.

Morphology of these subarterial VSDs has been particularly well elucidated in recent years by two-dimensional echocardiography and color Doppler examinations.[G9,H17,S24] Despite the potential confusion of using Lev's *relational* terminology in a morphologic sense, in the echocardiographic literature subarterial defects are usually referred to as "doubly committed ventricular septal defects." Thus, it is useful to combine morphologic and echocardiographic descriptions to characterize these VSDs occurring in the RV outlet as *doubly committed subarterial VSDs.* Echocardiography has demonstrated particularly

Figure 21-6   Type of perimembranous ventricular septal defect *(VSD)* that ejects directly into right atrium, a so-called left ventricular–right atrial defect. **A,** VSD viewed from right atrium. Posterior part of tricuspid anulus is marked by dashed line. Tricuspid septal leaflet is anomalously adherent to underlying ventricular septum and edges of VSD, which is juxta-tricuspid. Intact atrioventricular septum lies on atrial side of tricuspid anulus (beneath letters *VSD*). Bundle of His is along posterior angle of defect. **B,** Same defect viewed from left ventricle. VSD is juxta-aortic and beneath commissure between right and noncoronary aortic cusps.

Key: *ALMV,* Anterior leaflet of mitral valve; *ALTV,* anterior leaflet of tricuspid valve; *LV,* left ventricle; *NC,* noncoronary aortic cusp; *RA,* right atrium; *RV,* right ventricle; *SLTV,* septal leaflet of tricuspid valve; *VSD,* ventricular septal defect.

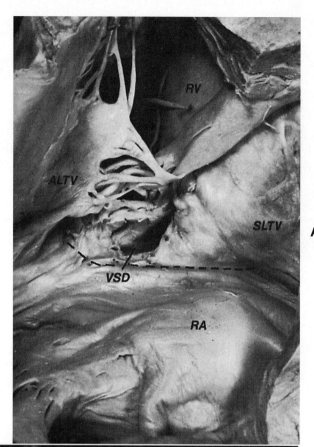

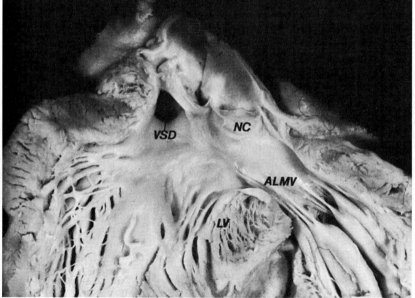

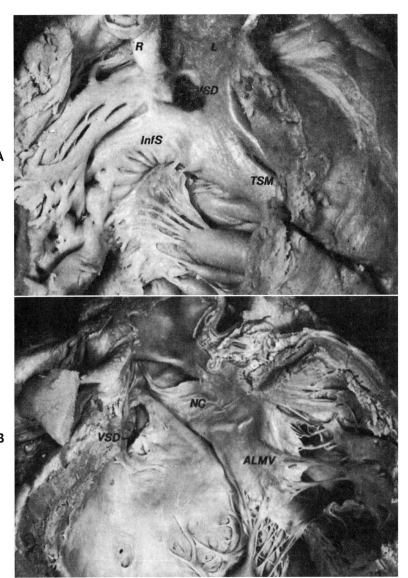

Figure 21-7   Doubly committed subarterial ventricular septal defect *(VSD)* in outlet portion of ventricular septum. **A,** VSD viewed from right ventricle. Its inferior margin is formed of thick septal tissue and its superior margin is formed by confluent right pulmonary and right aortic cusps, which are separated by a thin ridge of fibrous tissue. **B,** Same defect viewed from left ventricle. VSD is beneath right coronary cusp of aortic valve and is more anterior than is a conoventricular VSD.

Key: *ALMV,* Anterior leaflet of mitral valve; *InfS,* infundibular (outlet) septum; *L,* left pulmonary cusp; *NC,* noncoronary aortic cusp; *R,* right pulmonary cusp; *TSM,* trabecula septomarginalis; *VSD,* ventricular septal defect.

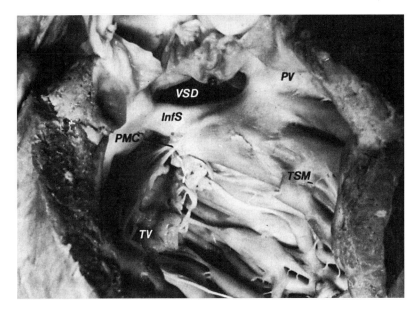

Figure 21-8   Doubly committed subarterial ventricular septal defect *(VSD)* viewed from right ventricle. VSD lies immediately beneath pulmonary valve (and, although it is unseen, the aortic valve). Inferior to defect are infundibular septum and trabecula septomarginalis. Tricuspid valve, papillary muscle of conus, and bundle of His are far from defect.

Key: *InfS,* Infundibular septum; *PMC,* papillary muscle of conus (Lancisi); *PV,* pulmonary valve; *TSM,* trabecula septomarginalis; *TV,* tricuspid valve; *VSD,* ventricular septal defect.

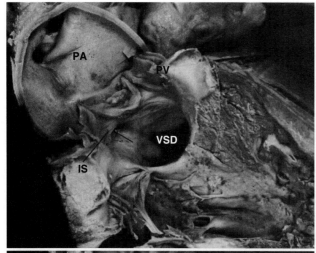

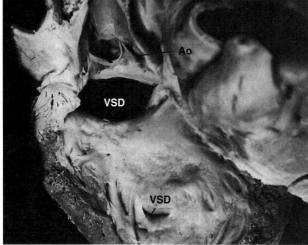

Figure 21-9   Large confluent ventricular septal defect *(VSD)* that is both subaterial and perimembranous, extending downward to reach tricuspid anulus. This type of VSD is also seen in double outlet right ventricle with doubly committed VSD and in double outlet left ventricle. **A,** VSD viewed from right ventricle. At superior margin of VSD, pulmonary and aortic cusps are in fibrous continuity. Arrow points toward aortic valve. **B,** Same defect viewed from left ventricle. Note additional small trabecular muscular defect.

Key: *Ao,* Aorta; *PA,* pulmonary artery; *PV,* pulmonary and aortic cusps; *IS,* infundibular septum.

well that the aortic and pulmonary valves are frequently at the same level in the presence of subarterial (or doubly committed) VSDs, rather than the pulmonary valve being elevated above (cephalad to) or offset relative to the aortic valve, seemingly by the RV infundibulum.[G9] This description often provides a diagnostic tool, useful in both echocardiography and angiography, along with the finding that the outlet septum appears to be absent and the subpulmonary infundibulum deficient. Echocardiography has also demonstrated well the frequently associated prolapse of an aortic cusp and aortic regurgitation present in up to half of patients with this type of VSD.[S24] Aortic cusp prolapse may nearly close the VSD during diastole. At times the fibrous

raphe between the arterial valves is displaced relative to the ventricular septum, resulting in overriding of one arterial valve and narrowing of the other.[G9]

Some VSDs in the RV outlet are only *juxta-aortic* and abut the nadir of the right coronary cusp. The cusp typically prolapses through this type of VSD, and aortic regurgitation frequently develops. This particular type of VSD and its behavior have been known for years, but its morphology has remained incompletely described until relatively recently.[S23] Rarely, VSDs in the RV outlet are only juxtapulmonary and lie far to the left.

Some defects in the outlet portion of the septum have *muscular* borders and lie in the substance of the infundibular septum (muscular VSD, outlet type), with a muscle bridge of infundibular septum superior to the defect (Fig. 21-10). The superior muscular bridge may be malaligned and displaced leftward into the aortic outflow tract (posterior malalignment type of VSD), producing muscular subaortic stenosis that lies above the VSD.[M10] This anomaly occasionally occurs in association with interrupted aortic arch and with coarctation,[A5,D8,F4,V2] although perimembranous VSDs are more common in both settings.

Inlet Septal Ventricular Septal Defect

Five percent or less of surgical patients have *inlet septal VSD* (or *AV septal type* or *AV canal type* of VSD).[N3] This defect involves the right ventricular *inlet septum* beneath the tricuspid septal leaflet and the left ventricular *outlet septum.* Its posterior margin is formed by the exposed AV valve anulus (juxtatricuspid), and its anterior margin is muscular and crescentic (Fig. 21-11). Superiorly, inlet septal defects usually extend to the membranous septum. The AV septum is intact, in contrast to the situation in hearts with AV canal septal defects (see "Morphology" in Chapter 20). The anterior (septal) mitral leaflet occasionally may be cleft, either partially or completely, with associated mitral regurgitation.

Rarely, VSDs in the inlet portion of the septum extend completely to the crux cordis and thus are also *juxtacrucial* in position. The tricuspid valve is overriding and usually straddling.

In inlet septal VSDs the AV node lies more laterally and anteriorly along the tricuspid anulus than normal and at the point at which the tricuspid anulus meets the underlying ventricular septum, because of the straddling of the tricuspid valve.[H14] The bundle of His lies along the *posteroinferior* rim of the inlet septal VSD, slightly on the left ventricular side, as in juxtatricuspid VSDs.

A *muscular VSD* can occur in the inlet portion of the ventricular septum beneath the tricuspid septal leaflet (Fig. 21-12). The posterior margin of such a defect is separated from the tricuspid ring by muscle. A muscular VSD must be distinguished from the inlet septal type of VSD because the conducting tissue runs *superior and anterior to a muscular defect.*

Muscular Ventricular Septal Defect

VSDs in other locations are generally *muscular* VSDs. Such defects are frequently multiple and may be associated with perimembranous or subarterial VSDs. Single or multiple muscular defects in the trabecular septum are more common in infants requiring operative treatment than in

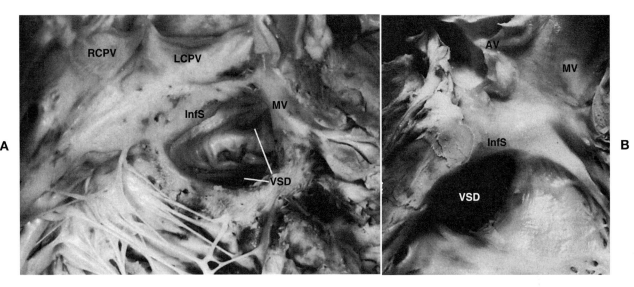

Figure 21-10   Muscular ventricular septal defect *(VSD)* in right ventricular outlet, in association with a prominent muscle bridge of infundibular septum that separates upper margin of defect from pulmonary and aortic valves. **A,** VSD viewed from right ventricle. VSD is completely surrounded by muscle, and a portion of infundibular septum is between defect and pulmonary valve. Mitral valve is seen through defect. **B,** Same defect viewed from left ventricle. Infundibular septum is malaligned and displaced leftward beneath aortic valve, producing subaortic stenosis that lies above (downstream from) VSD.

Key: *AV,* Aortic valve; *InfS,* infundibular septum; *LCPV,* left cusp of pulmonary valve; *MV,* mitral valve; *RCPV,* right cusp of pulmonary valve; *VSD,* ventricular septal defect.

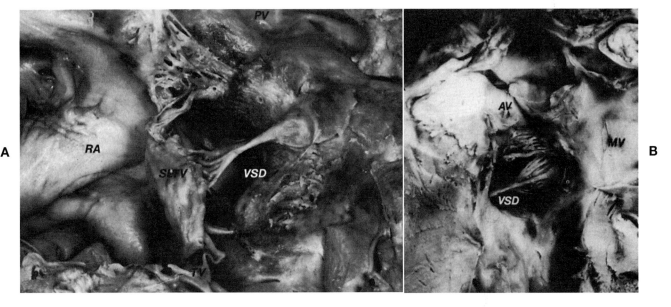

Figure 21-11   Inlet septal ventricular septal defect *(VSD)* beneath septal leaflet of tricuspid valve. Posterior margin of defect is formed by tricuspid anulus. VSD is juxtatricuspid. **A,** VSD viewed from right ventricle. Note crescentic anterior margin of defect. (A previously placed polyester patch has been removed.) **B,** Same defect viewed from left ventricle. Superiorly this defect reaches almost to the aortic valve, and posteriorly it extends to the mitral valve.

Key: *AV,* Aortic valve; *MV,* mitral valve; *PV,* pulmonary valve; *RA,* right atrium; *SLTV,* septal leaflet of tricuspid valve; *TV,* tricuspid valve; *VSD,* ventricular septal defect.

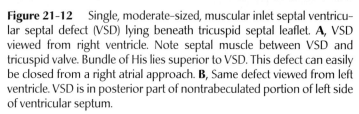
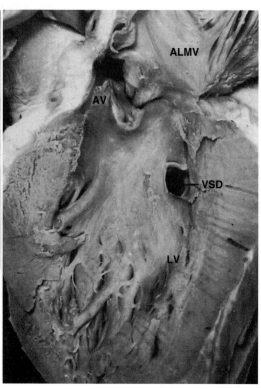

Figure 21-12   Single, moderate-sized, muscular inlet septal ventricular septal defect (VSD) lying beneath tricuspid septal leaflet. **A,** VSD viewed from right ventricle. Note septal muscle between VSD and tricuspid valve. Bundle of His lies superior to VSD. This defect can easily be closed from a right atrial approach. **B,** Same defect viewed from left ventricle. VSD is in posterior part of nontrabeculated portion of left side of ventricular septum.

Key: *ALMV,* Anterior leaflet of mitral valve; *AV,* aortic valve; *LV,* left ventricle; *PV,* pulmonary valve; *TV,* tricuspid valve; *VSD,* ventricular septal defect.

older children. For example, 16 (22%) of a group of 73 infants under 2 years of age in a surgical series at GLH had muscular defects.

Muscular defects can occur anywhere in the ventricular septum (see Fig. 21-1). Those in the middle portion of the trabecular septum are the most common (Fig. 21-13) and may be overlaid by the septal band (trabecula septomarginalis); thus, even when single on the LV side, these defects have at least two openings on the RV side. Anterior muscular defects are usually multiple and most often are in the apical and outlet (conal) portions of the septum. These defects may extend all along the anterior part of the septum, from the apex to the outlet septum. Typically, there are more openings on the RV than LV side.

A particularly important group of patients are those with many defects of variable size, not only along the anterior portion of the septum, but also throughout the midportion as well, *Swiss cheese defects* (Fig. 21-14). These defects often pass obliquely through the septum to appear on both sides of the septal band (trabecula septomarginalis) or in the anterior part of the septum. They may be associated with large or small perimembranous or subarterial defects. Major associated cardiac anomalies are common, especially severe coarctation of the aorta.

The bundle of His is not closely related to the borders of any muscular VSD.

Confluent Ventricular Septal Defect

Some unusually large, single confluent VSDs involve more than one area of the septum. Rarely a confluent VSD may involve most of the septum (Fig. 21-15), but hearts with such defects should not be classified as having a single ventricle.

Ventricular Septal Defect with Straddling or Overriding Tricuspid Valve

In rare instances, tricuspid valve chordae may *straddle* the ventricular septum in association with a large inlet septal defect resembling an inlet septal type of VSD but that extends to the crux cordis (Fig. 21-16).[L5,M7,R2] The tricuspid valve usually *overrides* both ventricles. When overriding is severe, the tricuspid anulus is usually very large, and many chordae from it are attached to the LV side of the septum (a combination of straddling and overriding).[B11] The atrial septum is malaligned relative to the ventricular septum. The right ventricle is often hypoplastic. The tricuspid valve may be regurgitant.

Associated Lesions

Nearly half of patients undergoing surgical treatment for a primary VSD have an associated cardiac anomaly (Table 21-1).[B1,B3,R5]

A moderate- or large-sized *patent ductus arteriosus* is present in about 6% of patients of all ages, but about 25% of infants in heart failure.[B3] VSD occurs in combination with moderate or severe *coarctation of the aorta* in about 5% of patients. This combination is also much more common among infants with large VSD coming to operation under age 3 months.

Congenital *aortic stenosis* occurs in about 2% of patients requiring operation for VSD. Subvalvar stenosis is more common than valvar[L8] and may also occur in association with infundibular pulmonary stenosis. The subvalvar stenosis is caused by (1) a discrete fibromuscular bar lying inferior (caudad or upstream) to the VSD; (2) a discrete fibromuscular bar located distal (downstream) to the VSD, often as noted earlier, consisting of displacement of

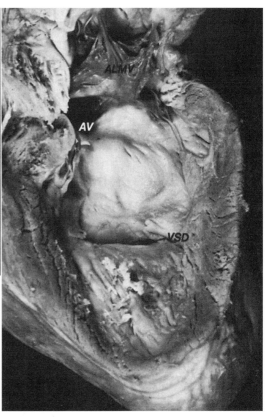

Figure 21-13 Muscular trabecular septal ventricular septal defect *(VSD)*. **A**, VSD viewed from right ventricle. VSD is actually a single one, but is covered by septal band (trabecula septomarginalis) and therefore has two openings into right ventricle (see probes). **B**, Same defect viewed from left ventricle. VSD, appearing more slitlike than it actually is, lies at junction of smooth and trabeculated portions of septum. This defect can be closed from right ventricle, provided lower end of septal band is detached.

Key: *ALMV*, Anterior leaflet of mitral valve; *AV*, aortic valve; *InfS*, infundibular septum, or crista supraventricularis; *PMC*, papillary muscle of conus (Lancisi); *PV*, pulmonary valve; *SB*, septal band, or trabecula septomarginalis; *TV*, tricuspid valve; *VSD*, ventricular septal defect.

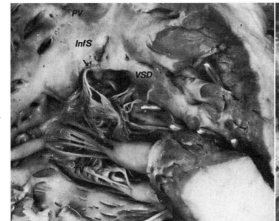

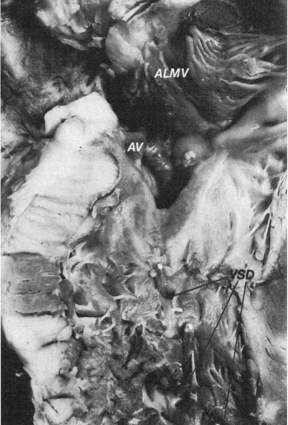

Figure 21-14 "Swiss cheese" type of multiple ventricular septal defect *(VSD)* associated with a large perimembranous VSD. **A**, VSDs viewed from right ventricle. Perimembranous defect shows anomalous chordal attachment from tricuspid valve to posterosuperior margin of defect *(arrow)*. Probes demonstrate five separate openings of small defects, one above and four below trabecula septomarginalis. **B**, Same defects viewed from left ventricle. Perimembranous defect is seen. Probes demonstrate three separate openings of Swiss cheese defects, but many more lie in grossly trabeculated lower portion of septum.

Key: *ALMV*, Anterior leaflet of mitral valve; *AV*, aortic valve; *InfS*, infundibular septum; *PV*, pulmonary valve; *TV*, tricuspid valve; *VSD*, ventricular septal defect.

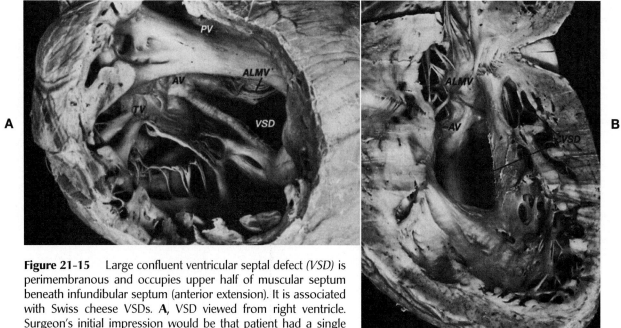

Figure 21-15 Large confluent ventricular septal defect *(VSD)* is perimembranous and occupies upper half of muscular septum beneath infundibular septum (anterior extension). It is associated with Swiss cheese VSDs. **A**, VSD viewed from right ventricle. Surgeon's initial impression would be that patient had a single ventricle. **B**, Same defect viewed from left ventricle. Malformation is clearly not a single ventricle.

Key: *ALMV*, Anterior leaflet of mitral valve; *AV*, aortic valve; *PV*, pulmonary valve; *TV*, tricuspid valve; *VSD*, ventricular septal defect.

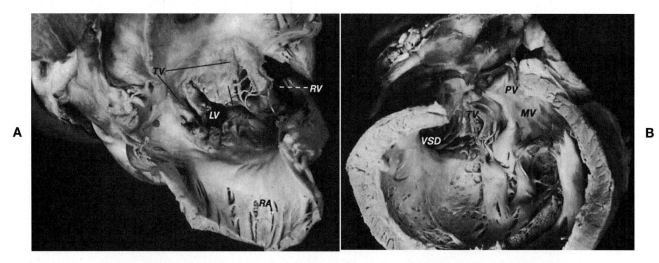

Figure 21-16 Inlet septal type of ventricular septal defect *(VSD)* with posterior extension and straddling tricuspid valve. **A**, VSD viewed from right atrium. Crest of ventricular septum forming lower boundary of defect *(black arrow)* crosses almost beneath center of large tricuspid orifice, indicating severe malalignment of atrial and ventricular septa. **B**, Same defect viewed from left ventricle. Chordal attachments of tricuspid valve cross VSD to attach to septal surface of left ventricle. This heart also exhibits transposition of the great arteries, with pulmonary artery above left ventricle.

Key: *LV*, Left ventricle; *MV*, mitral valve; *PV*, pulmonary valve; *RA*, right atrium; *RV*, right ventricle; *TV*, tricuspid valve orifice; *VSD*, ventricular septal defect.

infundibular septal muscle into the LV outflow tract (posterior malalignment) and often associated with aortic coarctation and interrupted arch[A5,D7,M6,V2,V3] (see "Morphology" in Sections 1 and 2 of Chapter 34); (3) pulmonary artery banding[F2]; and (4) excrescences of AV valvar tissue.[N4]

Congenital *mitral valve disease* occurs in about 2% of patients.[B1] One of the *pulmonary arteries* may be absent or

severely stenotic. Severe peripheral pulmonary artery stenoses occur rarely. Severe *positional cardiac anomalies,* such as isolated dextrocardia or situs inversus totalis, are uncommon in patients with VSD.

A number of minor associated cardiac anomalies may also be present in patients coming to operation for VSD (Table 21-2). Although atrial septal defects in general are

■ **TABLE 21-1   Associated Cardiac Anomalies in Surgical Patients with Primary Ventricular Septal Defect** *ᵃ*

		Hospital Deaths	
Anomaly	*n*	No.	%
None	254	16	6.3
PDA	18	4	22
Coarctation of aorta or interrupted aortic arch	11	4	36
Mitral valve disease	4	1	25
Plus straddling and cleft mitral valve	1	0	0
Plus PDA	3	1	33
Straddling tricuspid valve	4	0	0
Tricuspid regurgitation	2	0	0
Positional cardiac anomalies	4	2	50
Mesoposition of heart	1	0	0
Dextrocardia, unrepaired coarctation of aorta	1	1	100
Situs inversus totalis	1	0	0
−Plus PDA	1	1	100
Subaortic stenosis	2	0	0
Plus PDA and coarctation of aorta	1	1	100
Absence or severe stenosis of LPA or RPA	3	1	33
Absent LPA with PDA	1	0	0
Origin of RPA from ascending aorta	1	0	0
Anomalous pulmonary or systemic venous connection *ᵇ*	1	0	0
Hypoplastic RV, small tricuspid anulus	1	0	0
Unroofed coronary sinus	1	0	0

Key: *LPA*, Left pulmonary artery; *PDA*, patent ductus arteriosus; *RPA*, right pulmonary artery; *RV*, right ventricle.

ᵃ Data from UAB, 1967 to 1979; *n* = 312.

ᵇ Exclusive of persistent left superior vena cava.

■ **TABLE 21-2   Minor Associated Cardiac Anomalies in Surgical Patients with Large Primary Ventricular Septal Defect** *ᵃ*

Anomaly	*n*	% *ᵇ*
None	184	54
Atrial septal defect *ᶜ*	45	13
Mild or moderate pulmonary stenosis	50	15
Persistent left superior vena cava	28	8
Dextroposition of aorta	7	2
Aneurysm of membranous septum	5	1
Mild or moderate coarctation of aorta	8	2
Vascular ring	2	1
Right aortic arch	4	1
Tricuspid regurgitation, mild	4	1
Mitral regurgitation, mild	2	1
Pulmonary valve regurgitation	4	1
Inferior vena cava draining via azygos vein	1	0.3
Hepatic veins entering right atrium directly	1	0.3
Congenital aneurysm of anterior RV wall	2	1
Anomalous RV muscle band without pulmonary stenosis	1	0.3
Anterior descending coronary artery arising from right coronary artery	1	0.3

Key: *RV*, Right ventricle.

ᵃ Data from GLH, 1958 to 1976, and UAB, 1967 to 1976; total 343 patients.

ᵇ Sum of percentages is greater than 100% because some patients had more than one minor associated condition.

ᶜ Exclusive of simple patent foramen ovale.

BOX 21-3   Heath Edwards Classification of Pulmonary Vascular Disease Pathology

Grade 1
Medial hypertrophy without intimal proliferation

Grade 2
Medial hypertrophy with cellular intimal reaction

Grade 3
Medial hypertrophy with intimal fibrosis and possibly early generalized vascular dilatation

Grade 4
Generalized vascular dilatation areas of vascular occlusion by intimal fibrosis, and plexiform lesions

Grade 5
Other dilatation lesions such as cavernous and angiomatoid lesions

Grade 6
Necrotizing arteritis in addition to characteristics of grade 5 changes

---

not considered major associated anomalies, they may coexist with a large VSD in small infants and may be important lesions.[B3]

Pulmonary Vascular Disease

The classic description of the pathology of hypertensive pulmonary vascular disease is that of Heath and Edwards (Box 21-3).[H1]

Pulmonary vascular resistance (Rp) in patients with large VSD (and those with large patent ductus arteriosus) is positively correlated with histologic severity of the hypertensive pulmonary vascular disease by Heath and colleagues (Fig. 21-17).[H2] A close positive correlation also exists between lowest Rp at rest or with isoproterenol infusion and Heath-Edwards grade of vascular disease. Heath-Edwards grades above 3 were not found in patients with Rp index less than 7 units · m^2, whereas those with Rp greater than 8.5 units · m^2 showed changes characteristic of grade 4 or greater.[B17] Similarly, Fried and colleagues found a rather close negative correlation ($P = .001$) between magnitude of left-to-right shunt and Heath-Edwards grade in infants and children coming to VSD repair.[F6] Variability in these matters[B17] is not unexpected because Heath-Edwards classification is based on the most severe lesion seen, regardless of its frequency; as noted by Wagenvoort and colleagues[W2,W3] and by Yamaki and Tezuka,[Y1] the grading should include an assessment of the number of vessels affected. In addition, calculation of Rp is open to errors.[H11]

Hislop and colleagues provide a different view of hypertensive pulmonary vascular disease in infants with large VSD.[H7] Other investigators had noted earlier that intimal proliferation (and thus Heath-Edwards changes of grade 2 or greater) rarely develops in patients with large VSD until 1 or 2 years of age,[D6,W2] despite infants occasionally having severely elevated Rp. Hislop and colleagues found that infants dying at 3 to 6 months of age with large VSD and high (greater than 8 units · m^2) Rp with intermittent right-to-left shunting have marked medial hypertrophy affecting both large and small pulmonary arteries, including those less than 200 μm in diameter.[H7] The usual number of intraacinar vessels was present. By contrast, these investigators found that infants 3 to 10 months of age with large VSDs dying with a history of large Q̇p and heart failure and normal or slightly elevated Rp have medial hypertrophy

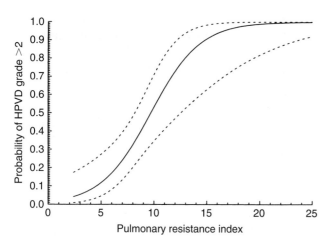

Figure 21-17 Probability of hypertensive pulmonary vascular disease greater than grade 2 in patients with ventricular septal defect, given total pulmonary resistance index (units · m²). Dotted lines enclose 70% confidence limits (P = .07). (From Heath and colleagues.[H2])

Key: *HPVD,* Hypertensive pulmonary vascular disease.

affecting mainly arteries larger than 200 mm. The intra-acinar vessels were fewer than usual, so-called lessened arterial density. These histologic features have been shown by Rabinovitch and colleagues to correlate with pulmonary hemodynamic findings after repair of VSDs.[R6] Fried and colleagues have emphasized that Heath-Edwards grade and arterial density are the best correlates of fall in pulmonary artery pressure after repair.[F6]

Histologic reversibility of pulmonary vascular disease after closure of VSD has not been documented. Favorable results in infants may be from an increase in arterial density as growth proceeds. Presumably, pulmonary vascular disease of Heath-Edwards grade 3 or greater severity is not reversible.

CLINICAL FEATURES AND DIAGNOSTIC CRITERIA

Clinical Findings

In infants, signs and symptoms of heart failure include tachypnea and liver enlargement, often associated with poor feeding and growth failure, and physical findings of a precordial pansystolic or more abbreviated systolic murmur and a hyperactive heart. These findings suggest the diagnosis of a large VSD. An apical diastolic murmur suggests large flow across the mitral valve during diastole, the result of a large $\dot{Q}p$. Cardiomegaly and evidence of large $\dot{Q}p$ are seen on the chest radiograph (Fig. 21-18). The electrocardiogram (ECG) usually shows biventricular hypertrophy. In older patients with large VSD the history is often nonspecific, but examination also shows evidence of LV and RV enlargement and a systolic murmur usually best heard in the third and fourth left interspaces. In patients with doubly committed subarterial VSDs, the systolic murmur is maximal in the second and third interspaces, and in defects shunting mainly into the right atrium, in the fourth and fifth interspaces.

A high Rp from severe pulmonary vascular disease changes the hemodynamic state and clinical findings in patients with large VSDs. A large left-to-right shunt is no longer present because the output resistances of the two pathways for LV emptying are similar, and the shunt is bidirectional and of about equal magnitude in the two directions. The heart is not enlarged and not hyperactive. A systolic murmur (which is produced by the large flow across the VSD) is soft or absent, and no apical diastolic murmur is heard. The pulmonary component of the second sound at the base is loud and sometimes palpable. Chest radiography reflects these features (see Fig. 21-18). ECG shows severe RV hypertrophy rather than combined ventricular hypertrophy and evidence of LV volume overload. When pulmonary vascular disease is even more advanced, cyanosis develops (*Eisenmenger complex*) because the shunt across the VSD becomes right-to-left as RV output resistance through the pulmonary vascular bed becomes higher than that through the VSD and aorta.

Patients with *small* VSDs have small shunts and often have no abnormal signs or symptoms other than a pansystolic murmur. Chest radiography and ECG both may be normal. When the defect is *moderate* in size, the LV is mildly or moderately enlarged, as shown by physical examination, chest radiography, and ECG, and the volume of the RV is increased.

When there is associated *pulmonary* or *aortic stenosis,* diagnostic features are changed. Thus, with important pulmonary stenosis, $\dot{Q}p$ is reduced, and the shunt may even be right to left. RV hypertrophy is increased. With important aortic stenosis, the load on the LV is increased, and if the obstruction is cephalad to the VSD, left-to-right shunt is also greater, resulting in more than the expected degree of LV hypertrophy on the ECG. Coarctation of the aorta may also produce these features in older children.

Two-Dimensional Echocardiography

High-quality two-dimensional echocardiography imaging of the VSD with color Doppler flow evaluation of shunt flow by proximal isovelocity surface area (PISA)[K21] has changed traditional views about preoperative studies. Thus, when the clinical syndrome in neonates and infants indicates a large $\dot{Q}p/\dot{Q}s$, when noninvasive imaging clearly defines the morphology, including that of the aortic arch and ductus arteriosus, and when the surgeon is experienced in the surgical identification and repair of congenital heart disease, cardiac catheterization and cineangiography are not necessary before closure of primary VSDs.[C18,M16]

For identifying a large single perimembranous VSD, combined two-dimensional echocardiography and Doppler flow interrogation is highly reliable, in combination with the clinical criteria (Fig. 21-19).[B16,O6,S18,S20] Echocardiography adds to anatomic clarification, particularly in the case of doubly committed subarterial VSDs.[G9] Particularly for small VSDs and for multiple muscular defects, two-dimensional Doppler color flow echocardiographic imaging increases the sensitivity of echocardiography (see Fig. 21-19, *A* and *B*).[H17,L12] However, and particularly in the presence of a single large VSD, multiple muscular defects can go undetected, even with refined techniques of echocardiography.[L12] Because perimembranous VSDs, infrequently (less than 3%[C17]) are accompanied by additional muscular VSDs, this does not contraindicate proceeding to repair in infants without cardiac catheterization. Malalignment VSD is diagnosed by two-dimensional echocardiography by the appearance of the alignment of the RV trabecular septum with the outlet septum. Malalignment may be *anterior* as in tetralogy of Fallot (Fig. 21-19, *C*), *posterior* as in interrupted aortic arch, or *rotational* as in Taussig-Bing heart.

Other Noninvasive Diagnostic Methods

Other noninvasive imaging modalities may come into use. At present, only magnetic resonance imaging (MRI) has shown promise to provide accurate information about the morphology of all types of VSDs.[B18] Dynamic three-dimensional echocardiographic reconstructions may refine ability to image and portray spatially VSDs.[T14]

Cardiac Catheterization

Although cardiac catheterization and cineangiography are no longer routinely used in patients with simple VSDs at many institutions, when surgical intervention is under consideration in older children, cardiac catheterization and angiography are generally indicated to assess Rp and identify precisely location, size, and number of VSDs and any associated anomalies. Furthermore, preoperative sizing of VSDs is often important in arriving at management decisions. Sizing can be especially difficult when the VSD is associated with another lesion, such as coarctation or pulmonary stenosis. The most reliable way to size the defect is to measure its diameter either by two-dimensional color flow Doppler echocardiography or cineangiography. With cineangiography the VSD must be accurately profiled and the measurement either corrected to allow for magnification or compared with aortic root diameter. In applying this method to perimembranous VSDs, the defect is smaller in a cranially tilted left anterior oblique (LAO) projection than in the conventional LAO position.

Cardiac catheterization should include both right-sided and left-sided heart studies, the latter mainly to obtain LV angiograms. Basic data obtained at cardiac catheterization should include oxygen consumption ($\dot{V}o_2$); systolic, diastolic, and mean pulmonary arterial, pulmonary artery wedge, and systemic arterial pressures; oxygen content and saturation in right atrial, pulmonary arterial, aortic, or peripheral arterial blood, and, when possible, left atrial blood. Pulmonary ($\dot{Q}p$) and systemic ($\dot{Q}s$) blood flows and $\dot{Q}p/\dot{Q}s$ are calculated[3] with Rp (Box 21-4). When left atrial (or pulmonary arterial wedge) pressure is not available, only total pulmonary resistance (TPR) can be calculated. Pulmonary vascular (arteriolar) resistance in absolute units times body surface area is of more value in predicting operability than is the ratio between resistance in the

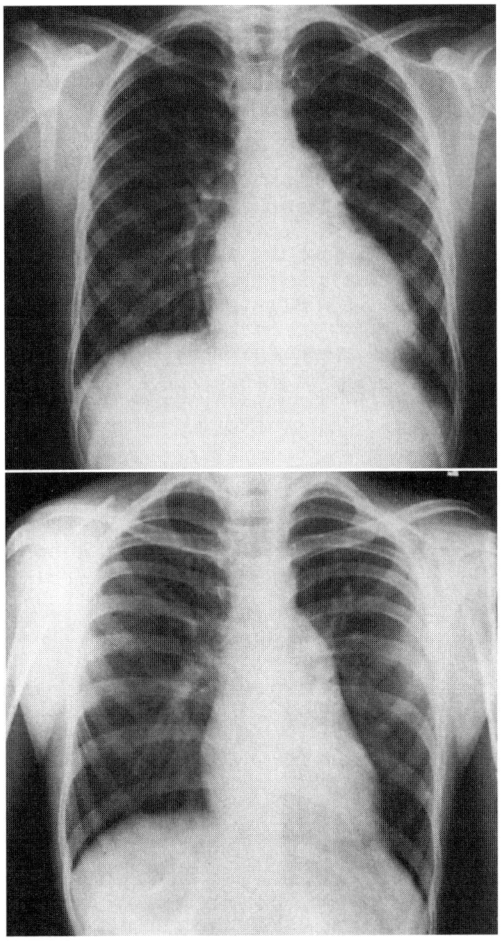

Figure 21-18   Chest radiographs of children with ventricular septal defect (VSD). **A**, Large VSD in 11-year-old girl with large left-to-right shunt, severe pulmonary hypertension, and low pulmonary vascular resistance. Cardiac enlargement and increased pulmonary vascularity are evident. Pulmonary trunk is enlarged, and aortic arch is small. Examination revealed an overactive heart with a systolic thrill and a loud (grade 4), long systolic murmur extending from lower left sternal border to apex and an apical diastolic murmur. Electrocardiogram showed evidence of left ventricular overwork. **B**, Large VSD in 10-year-old girl with severe pulmonary hypertension, pulmonary/systemic flow ratio of 1.2, and pulmonary vascular resistance of 11 units · m². Cardiac size is normal, but pulmonary trunk is enlarged. Pulmonary vascularity is not increased. Examination revealed a quiet heart, no thrill, a soft (grade 2) systolic murmur, and no apical diastolic murmur; closure of pulmonic valve was loud and palpable. Electrocardiogram demonstrated right ventricular hypertrophy without evidence of left ventricular overwork. (From Kirklin and DuShane.[K2])

---

[3] $\dot{Q}p = \dot{V}o_2/(CpvO_2 - CpaO_2)$ in $L \cdot m^{-1}$
where *pv* is pulmonary vein and *pa* is pulmonary artery. $\dot{Q}p$ may be expressed as index ($L \cdot min^{-1} \cdot m^{-2}$) by dividing by body surface area (BSA) expressed in square meters.
$\dot{Q}s = \dot{V}o_2/(CaO_2 - C\bar{v}O_2)$ in $L \cdot min^{-1}$
where *a* is aorta or arterial and $\bar{v}$ is mixed venous.
$\dot{Q}p/\dot{Q}s = (CaO_2 - C\bar{v}O_2)/(CpvO_2 - CpaO_2)$
Note that total oxygen consumption is not needed for this calculation.
$Rp = [(Ppa - Pla)/\dot{Q}p] \cdot BSA$; Rp is expressed in units · m².
$TPR = [Ppa/\dot{Q}p] \cdot BSA$; TPR is expressed in units · m².

BOX 21-4   Pulmonary Vascular Resistance

Resistance ≤ units · m² <		Description
	4	Normal
4	5	Mildly elevated
5	8	Moderately elevated
8		Severely elevated

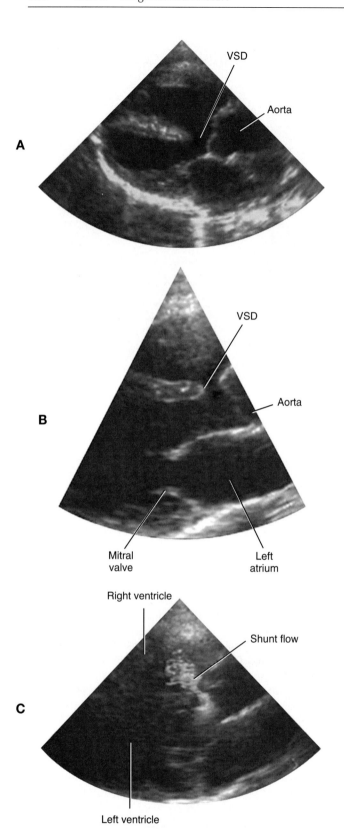

A

B

C

Figure 21-19   Two-dimensional echocardiograms with Doppler directional flow velocity in perimembranous ventricular septal defect (VSD). **A**, Four-chamber view demonstrating VSD as gap in ventricular septum between right ventricle and left ventricle. **B**, Magnified view of VSD. **C**, Turbulent blood flow through VSD is directed from left to right ventricle.

Key: *VSD*, Ventricular septal defect.

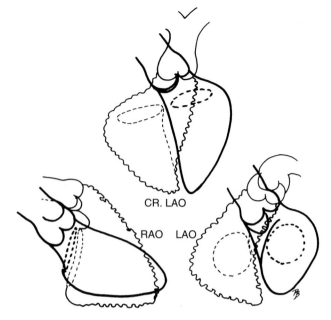

A

Figure 21-20   Line drawings of angiographic projections for assessment of ventricular septal defect (VSD). **A**, Interrelationships of left ventricle and aortic root (thick line) with right ventricle and pulmonary trunk (thin line) in 40° right anterior oblique (RAO), 50° left anterior oblique (LAO), and 40° cranially tilted (CR. LAO) projections. RAO view profiles conal (infundibular) and high anterior portions of right ventricular (RV) outlet septum below and in front of right coronary sinus and profiles atrioventricular (AV) septum beneath noncoronary sinus of aortic root. Both LAO views profile apical trabecular portion of septum. LAO view also partly profiles RV outlet septum, but superimposes it on left ventricular (LV) outflow tract and aortic root. CR. LAO projection views RV outlet septum en face and superimposes it on LV. Because orientation shows a horizontally lying heart, LAO view depicts full length (cranial to caudal) of apical and anterior trabecular portion of ventricular septum and AV valve anuli (interrupted lines), whereas CR. LAO view depicts full length of sinus portion of trabecular septum from base to apex.

Key: *CR. LAO*, Cranial left anterior oblique; *LAO*, left anterior oblique; *RAO*, right anterior oblique.   *Continued*

pulmonary and systemic circuits.[N5] When Rp is elevated, further information concerning operability should be obtained by assessing response to exercise and to isoproterenol (see "Indications for Operation" later in this chapter).

Angiography

Angiographic assessment of VSD is best performed using biplane techniques in appropriate *projections*.[B9,B12,E1] Whereas cardiologists and radiologists carry primary responsibility for these studies, appreciation of their findings and limitations is essential to the surgeon, who must also understand when the study is incomplete.[B6]

Fig. 21-20 summarizes the surgically important features of angiograms of VSD by diagram. Fig. 21-21 presents representative angiograms of the various types of VSDs.

Text continued on p. 871

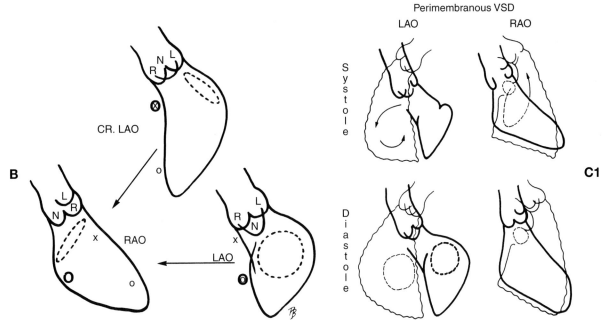

Perimembranous VSD

C1

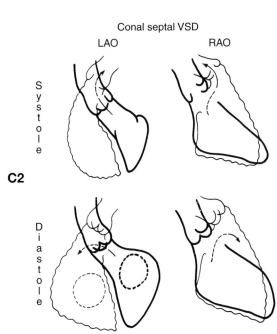

Conal septal VSD

C2

Figure 21-20, cont'd   **B**, Both cranially tilted *(CR. LAO)* and conventional left anterior oblique *(LAO)* views are required for a complete assessment of sinus septum. Basal (inlet) *(O, x)* ventricular septal defects *(VSDs)* are separated from more apical *(o)* VSDs by CR. LAO projection, whereas high *(x)* VSDs are separated from low *(O)* VSDs by LAO view. **C**, Anatomic and hemodynamic features of VSDs shown by left ventricular (LV) angiograms. LAO diagrams show a compromise between conventional and cranially tilted options. LV and aorta are shown by thick lines, right ventricle (RV) and pulmonary trunk by thin lines, and atrioventricular (AV) valves and nonprofiled VSDs by interrupted lines. **C1**, Perimembranous VSD. LAO view profiles VSD just beneath parietal band (ventriculoinfundibular fold) at upper margin of inlet septum. Flow enters base of RV above tricuspid valve, filling base before reaching infundibulum. Tricuspid valve is well seen in diastole, and lower margin of defect can be accurately related to tricuspid anulus in LAO. RAO view does not profile defect unless it extends into outlet septum. Note intact AV septum beneath noncoronary sinus of aortic root. Shunt enters RV infundibulum, crossing but not interrupting intact superior margin of LV, indicating intact conal and high anterior septal regions. **C2**, Doubly committed subarterial VSD (labeled *conal septal VSD*). LAO view shows an intact septum from aortic valve to apex. RV sinus usually fills only faintly by diastolic mixing from infundibular region, and tricuspid valve may not be seen. Defect is superimposed on aortic root.

RAO view profiles defect beneath contiguous parts of aortic and pulmonary valves. Systolic streaming through RV infundibulum to pulmonary trunk is well shown, with some mixing to more anterior part of RV in diastole, but high anterior septal region is intact.

Key: *CR. LAO,* Cranial left anterior oblique; *L,* left coronary; *LAO,* left anterior oblique; *LV,* left ventricle; *N,* noncoronary; *R,* right coronary; *RAO,* right anterior oblique; *RV,* right ventricle; *VSD,* ventricular septal defect.

Continued

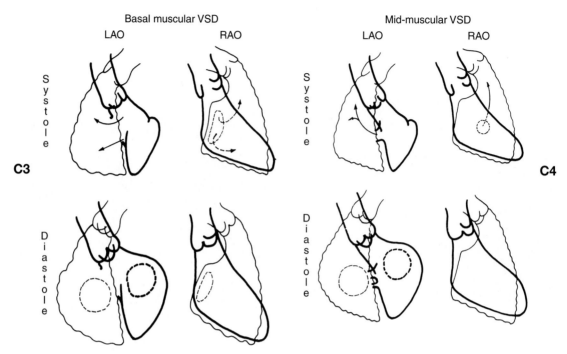

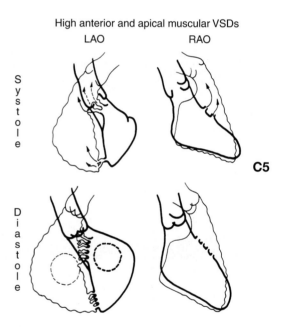

Figure 21-20, cont'd   C3, Inlet septal ventricular septal defect (VSD) (labeled *basal muscular VSD*). VSD is adjacent to tricuspid valve (atrioventricular [AV] septal type) or separated from it by a rim of muscle (muscular VSD). These two types of VSDs are not readily distinguished radiologically. In left anterior oblique *(LAO)* view, defect is profiled between AV valves, replacing full height of basal septum (conventional LAO view), perhaps extending into adjacent middle portion of ventricular septum but not into apical region (cranially tilted LAO view). Contrast medium streams directly into base of right ventricle (RV) sinus in systole, providing a good depiction of tricuspid orifice in diastole. Separate AV valves are present, in contrast to the finding in a complete AV septal defect (see Chapter 20). In right anterior oblique *(RAO)* view, VSD is not profiled. Intact AV septum distinguishes this defect from a true AV septal defect. Note intact conal and high anterior septal regions. **C4,** Muscular, trabecular VSD (labeled *mid-muscular VSD*). LAO views show an intact inlet septum and no extension into apical region, although a small additional defect is seen in diastole, closing in systole. Some of the contrast medium streams directly into RV outflow during systole. Height of defect from floor of ventricle (bottom of AV valve) is appreciated in LAO view, and separation from basal and apical regions in cranially tilted LAO view. RAO features are as in parts **C1** and **C3. C5,** Multiple muscular anterior and apical VSDs. Muscular VSDs in these regions frequently coexist and, if numerous, form a continuous series throughout trabeculated septum from high in RV infundibulum to apical sinus septum. For clarity, only highest and lowest are shown here. In LAO view, intact basal and middle septal regions are profiled. Apical defects are profiled, but high anterior defects are superimposed on LV outflow region. Contrast medium tends to stream to RV outflow tract without filling basal parts. In RAO view, high anterior defects are profiled, interrupting superior margin of LV anterior to intact outlet septum. More defects are open in diastole than in systole. (From Brandt.[B13])

Key: *LAO,* Left anterior oblique; *RAO,* right anterior oblique; *VSD,* ventricular septal defect.

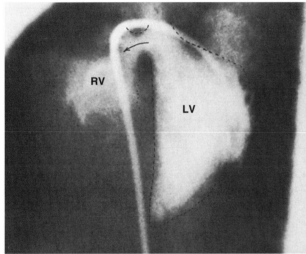

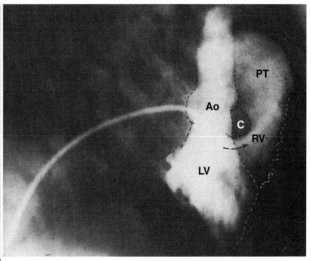

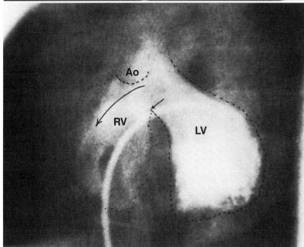

Figure 21-21   Angiograms of patients with ventricular septal defect *(VSD)*. **A,** Left ventricular *(LV)* angiograms of a perimembranous VSD. **A1,** 40° cranially tilted 60° left anterior oblique (LAO) projection, systolic frame, early in perimembranous angiographic sequence. VSD *(arrow)* lies in basal part of ventricular septum adjacent to aortic root. No additional defects are seen in middle and apical portions of septum (catheter to LV through atrial septum and mitral valve). **A2,** 30° right anterior oblique (RAO) projection, systolic frame, slightly later than *A1* in sequence. Patient was positioned to achieve cranial tilting of simultaneously exposed LAO view shown in **A1.** Note intact atrioventricular septum beneath noncoronary aortic sinus and intact outlet septum *(C)*. Contrast medium from shunt through nonprofiled VSD fills right ventricular *(RV)* outflow tract, crossing *(arrow)* but not interrupting high anterior margin of LV. **A3,** Fifty-degree LAO projection, systolic frame early in sequence (second injection). Perimembranous VSD is profiled as in **A1** beneath aortic root. Large arrow indicates flow into base of RV above tricuspid valve (identified in diastole but not illustrated). Downward extent of VSD *(small arrow)* is accurately shown, and there are no additional defects lower in septum. Perimembranous defects are frequently small, of dimensions profiled in cranially tilted LAO projection in **A1,** compared with LAO.

Key: *Ao,* Aorta; *C,* septum; *LV,* left ventricle; *PT,* pulmonary trunk; *RV,* right ventricle.   *Continued*

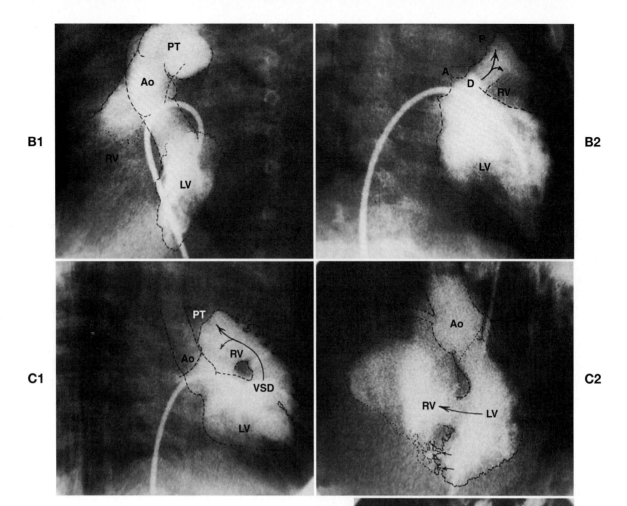

Figure 21-21, cont'd **B,** Left ventricular *(LV)* angiograms of doubly committed subarterial ventricular septal defect *(VSD).* **B1,** Sixty-degree left anterior oblique (LAO) projection, systolic frame early in sequence. Pulmonary arteries are filled by shunt through right ventricular *(RV)* outlet defect superimposed on LV outflow tract. Only slight contrast medium is seen in RV sinus, and whole of sinus septum is shown to be intact. **B2,** Thirty-degree right anterior oblique (RAO) projection, diastolic or very early systolic frame early in sequence. Doubly committed subarterial VSD is profiled immediately beneath contiguous parts of aortic and pulmonary valves, still closed. Arrows show streaming from VSD toward pulmonary valve, with some filling of remainder of RV infundibulum, but high anterior LV margin is intact. **C,** LV angiocardiograms of muscular VSDs. **C1,** Muscular anterior VSD. Thirty-degree RAO projection, diastolic or very early systolic frame early in sequence. Shunt through large, high anterior muscular VSD fills anterior part of RV infundibulum. Arrows show the main stream toward the pulmonary valve, which is still closed. There is a little mixing to RV sinus, but outlet septum is intact. **C2,** Multiple muscular VSDs (Swiss cheese septum). Forty-degree cranially tilted 60° LAO projection, systolic cine frame. A large muscular trabecular VSD *(large arrow),* accompanied by numerous small muscular apical defects *(small arrows),* is profiled, but basal part of ventricular septum beneath aortic root is intact. In diastole (not shown), more numerous apical defects were apparent. **C3,** Thirty-degree RAO projection, diastolic frame in same patient as in **C2.** Numerous muscular anterior VSDs *(arrows)* interrupt LV margin. Note intact outlet septal margin of LV near aortic valve. Earlier in sequence, intact antrioventricular septum was identified, but base of filled RV overlaps base of LV in this frame. Note that position of large muscular VSD is incompletely evaluated (trabecular); an LAO view would be necessary. Note surgically banded pulmonary trunk.

Key: *A,* Aortic valve; *Ao,* aorta; *D,* subarterial ventricular septal defect; *LV,* left ventricle; *P,* pulmonary valve; *PT,* pulmonary trunk; *R* and *RV,* right ventricle; *V,* atrioventricular septum; *VSD,* ventricular septal defect.

NATURAL HISTORY

Spontaneous Closure

VSDs tend to close spontaneously. This is relevant to decisions about operation and explains, for the most part, the infrequency with which large VSDs are encountered in adults.[C10] Spontaneous closure can be complete by 1 year of age, or the defect may have only narrowed by then, with complete closure taking considerably longer. An inverse relation exists between the probability of eventual spontaneous closure and age at which the patient is observed (Fig. 21-22).[A10,B1,H6,K5,K18] About 80% of patients with large VSDs seen at age 1 month experience eventual spontaneous closure, as do about 60% of those seen at age 3 months, about 50% of those seen at age 6 months, and about 25% of those seen at age 12 months. This decreasing tendency for spontaneous closure of a VSD as the patient becomes older has also been confirmed by Beerman and colleagues[B15] and spontaneous closure has been documented to occur in only one patient between age 21 and 31 years.[H15] Onat and colleagues studied 106 children with VSD and concluded that these patients should be followed closely through adolescence because the defects may decrease in diameter, shunt flow may diminish, and spontaneous closure may be expected in 23% of patients.[O10]

The mechanism of narrowing or closure of perimembranous VSDs is usually adherence of tricuspid leaflet or chordal tissue to the edges of the VSD.[C14,S19] Closure has erroneously been related to echocardiographic diagnosis of aneurysm of the membranous septum.[R8] Aneurysm of the membranous septum is usually considered benign, and functionally reduces the size of the VSD. It has the potential consequence of promoting tricuspid regurgitation and RV outflow tract obstruction and is a nidus for infective endocarditis.[Y4]

Perimembranous VSDs, as well as VSDs that are juxta-aortic and inlet VSDs of the AV septal type are less likely to close than are those that are juxtatricuspid or subarterial muscular.[C14]

Inferences about the tendency toward spontaneous closure seem to be in disagreement with the results of some studies. Hoffman and Rudolph's data (one of the sources for Fig. 21-22) indicate that 80% of infants age 6 weeks with large VSDs will experience spontaneous closure or reduction in size of the VSD.[H6] Rowe found that none of 11 infants (mean age 46 days) with a VSD 80% or greater in diameter than that of the aorta showed subsequent reduction in size during the period of observation.[R4] These apparent discrepancies may be explained by lack of information about location or size of VSDs.

Pulmonary Vascular Disease

A large VSD exposes the patient to risk of developing increased Rp from hypertensive pulmonary vascular disease, which tends to worsen with age.[A3,L2] Thus, the proportion of patients with large VSDs who have severely elevated Rp (see Table 20-2) is directly related to age (Fig. 21-23). The statement that some infants less than 2 years of age with large VSDs have severely elevated Rp is doubted by some, but its occurrence is well documented.[B3]

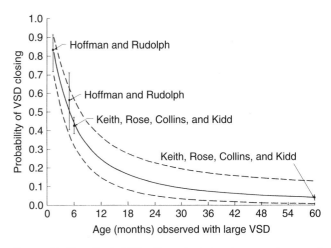

Figure 21-22   Probability of eventual spontaneous closure of a large ventricular septal defect according to age at which patient is observed. Dotted lines enclose 70% confidence limits. Specific ratios, with 70% confidence limits, reported by Hoffman and Rudolph[H6] and Keith and colleagues,[K5] are shown centered on mean or assumed ages of patients in their reports. P for age < .0001. See original sources for equations and statistics. (From Blackstone and colleagues.[B1])

Key: *VSD*, Ventricular septal defect.

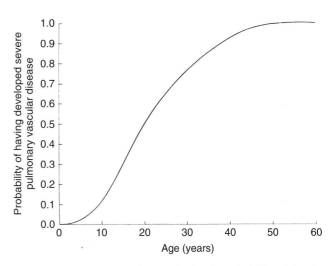

Figure 21-23   Estimated (not calculated) probability of developing severe pulmonary vascular disease (pulmonary vascular resistance 8 units · m²) in patients with large ventricular septal defects, according to age. (From Keith and colleagues.[K5])

Some infants and children with severely elevated Rp have not undergone the usual fall in Rp a few weeks to a few months after birth. Others have undergone this decrease,[J5] but later in the first 2 years of life they have developed a rapid increase in Rp.[H8]

Some infants with large VSDs and most of those with moderate-sized VSDs have normal or mildly elevated Rp and retain this through the first decade of life. Then, if their VSD is still large, more severe pulmonary vascular changes may or may not develop as they age. In infants with small VSDs, pulmonary vascular disease does not develop.[K2,K5]

Infective Endocarditis

In persons with VSD, infective endocarditis is rare, occurring at a rate of about 0.15% to 0.3% per year.[C12,C13,G7,S7] Its prevalence is greater in males and in persons over age 20 years.[G7] Infective endocarditis is more common in small and moderate VSDs than in large VSDs. Often a pulmonary process is the presenting feature, presumably developing from emboli secondary to right-sided bacterial vegetations or bacteria carried to the lungs by left-to-right–directed flow through the VSD. Prognosis with modern antibiotic treatment regimens is good.

Premature Death

Past experience and reports in the literature indicate that, without surgical treatment, about 9% of infants with *large* VSDs die from them in the first year of life.[A2,K5] Death may result from heart failure, which may develop very early, but usually occurs at about age 2 to 3 months, presumably because at that time the left-to-right shunt increases as the medial hypertrophy present in the small pulmonary arteries at birth regresses.[D6] Death may also result from recurrent pulmonary infections, often viral in origin, secondary to pulmonary edema from high pulmonary venous pressure. Death is most likely to occur in those infants with large VSDs who have associated conditions of major anatomic or functional importance, such as patent ductus arteriosus, coarctation of the aorta, or large atrial septal defect.[B3]

After the age of 1 year, few if any patients die of their VSD until the second decade of life. By then, most patients whose VSDs have remained large have pulmonary vascular disease and ultimately die with complications of Eisenmenger complex (Fig. 21-24).[C2] These include hemoptysis, polycythemia, cerebral abscess or infarction, and right-sided heart failure.

Patients with *small* VSDs die very rarely as a result of bacterial endocarditis. However, in common with patients with larger VSDs, some of these patients may develop disturbed systolic function and increased compliance in both ventricles.[O7]

Clinical Course

Patients with small VSDs rarely have symptoms related to the defect. Those with large VSDs may have symptoms of intractable heart failure in the first few months of life, with poor peripheral pulses, inability to feed, sweating, and chronic pulmonary edema. About half the patients coming to operation in the first 2 years of life do so because of intractable heart failure (Table 21-3).[B3] During early life, rapid and labored respiration and recurrent pulmonary infections may occur secondary to high pulmonary venous pressure and chronic pulmonary edema. Lobes of the lung may become chronically hyperinflated because of pressure of the large and tense pulmonary arteries on the bronchi, preventing complete escape of air during expiration.[O4] All this causes many babies with large VSDs to be small and physically underdeveloped. There is also evidence that chronic heart failure retards intellectual development. Symptomatic patients who fail to respond well to medical management are at particular risk of dying in the first year of life. Some babies who survive through the first year of

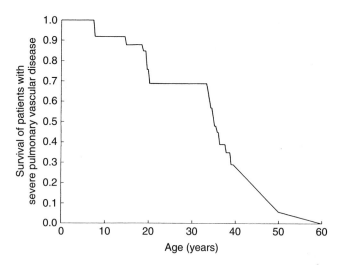

Figure 21-24   Survival after diagnosis of patients with large ventricular septal defects who had proven elevation of pulmonary vascular resistance to a level that made them inoperable (10 units · m² or greater), as demonstrated at cardiac catheterization at various ages. Note that fatalities begin to occur in the second decade of life, that about half the patients were dead by age 35, and that a few survived until 50 years of age. (Modified from Clarkson and colleagues.[C2])

■ **TABLE 21-3   Indications for Repair of Ventricular Septal Defect in Patients Undergoing Surgery in First 2 Years of Life**

Indication	n	% of Total	Average Age and Range (months)
Intractable heart failure	30	53	2.9 (1–7)
Recurrent respiratory infections	3	5	8 (6–9)
Controlled heart failure and failure to thrive	17	30	11.4 (4–21)
Increased pulmonary vascular resistance	7	12	14.6 (10–19)

(Data from Barratt-Boyes and colleagues.[B3])

life with large VSDs have controlled heart failure and failure to thrive in the second year of life as well.

Children and young adults with large VSDs are usually symptomatic and tend to be small both in height and in weight. As pulmonary vascular disease develops, symptoms may regress.

Development of Aortic Regurgitation

A small proportion of patients (about 5%) develop aortic valve regurgitation as a complication of VSD. Aortic regurgitation is more common in Asians than in Caucasians or those of African descent[T7,T14] because the VSD is frequently subarterial and may be associated with aortic valve prolapse in 36% to 79%. Regurgitation is rarely present at birth but develops during the first decade of life, then gradually worsens, so that by the end of the second decade, it is usually severe. As regurgitation increases, VSD shunt flow often decreases from occlusion of the VSD by the prolapsed aortic cusp. If the defect remains open through adolescence, about 10% of patients develop aortic valve prolapse or regurgitation.[O10]

Development of Infundibular Pulmonary Stenosis

A small proportion (5%-10%) of patients with large VSDs and large left-to-right shunt in infancy develop infundibular pulmonary stenosis.[G2,H9,K5] The mild and moderate infundibular pulmonary stenoses in patients operated on for primary VSD (see Table 21-3), as well as some of the more important pulmonary stenoses, probably develop in this way. Stenosis may become severe enough to produce shunt reversal and cyanosis, and the condition then can properly be termed *tetralogy of Fallot* (see Chapter 24).[S17] Those who undergo the transformation probably are born with a mild degree of anterior displacement of the infundibular septum and its extensions.

TECHNIQUE OF OPERATION

VSDs are repaired either through the right atrium, right ventricle, or, in special circumstances, left ventricle or pulmonary artery.[K1] Currently, RV and LV approaches are rarely used. Repair is done on conventional CPB at 20° to 24°C with direct caval cannulation and brief periods of total circulatory arrest if needed (see Sections 3 and 4 of Chapter 2).

For infants weighing less than about 3 kg, a single venous cannula is used, and the repair is performed during hypothermic circulatory arrest (see Section 4 of Chapter 2). Cold cardioplegia is used in all cases.

After the usual anesthetic and surgical preparations (see Chapter 4), a median sternotomy is made. Presence of anomalies of pulmonary or systemic venous return is determined. It should be known from preoperative study whether the ductus arteriosus is open or closed. An open ductus during open cardiotomy, particularly during hypothermic circulatory arrest, allows air to enter the aorta and later migrate to the brain; during CPB an open ductus increases intracardiac return and overdistends the pulmonary circulation. A patent ductus is ligated from the anterior approach, usually during cooling. In neonates and infants undergoing hypothermic circulatory arrest, the ductus is ligated as a routine procedure.

Repair of Perimembranous Ventricular Septal Defect

After CPB (with or without circulatory arrest) has been established, the aorta is occluded, cold cardioplegic solution injected and right atrium opened obliquely. A suction device is placed across the naturally present or surgically created foramen ovale (Fig. 21-25). Before repair is started, the defect is carefully examined to establish that all margins can be seen and reached. In the rare circumstances in which this is not possible because of chordal arrangement, an incision is made to disconnect a portion of the tricuspid valve from the anulus, and the VSD is exposed through the resulting aperture. Alternatively, the chordal group is disconnected from the anterior edge of the defect to facilitate

exposure and later is reattached. Particular attention is directed toward determining whether the VSD is juxtatricuspid, in which case it abuts the tricuspid valve in the region of the commissure between septal and anterior leaflets. If the VSD has a bar of muscle of varying width between it and the tricuspid valve, it is not juxtatricuspid. Relationship of the bundle of His to the posterior and inferior margins of the defect must be clearly understood (see "Morphology" earlier in this section) to accomplish a safe repair (Fig. 21-25, *A*).

In older infants and children the VSD is repaired with a polyester patch sewn in place with continuous polypropylene sutures (Fig. 21-25, *B*), a technique that has been confirmed to be entirely adequate in such patients. In neonates and small infants the technique may not be adequate because of the delicate nature and friability of the structures. In these patients the patch may be sewn into place using interrupted mattress sutures reinforced with small pledgets, placing all the sutures in the heart before passing them through the patch.

A ventricular approach may be used when the VSD cannot be well visualized from the right atrium. An RV approach is performed through a transverse incision. The patch is sewn into place with continuous or interrupted sutures (Fig. 21-26). Technique of repair and sequence for suturing shown in Fig. 21-26 is slightly different from that shown for the atrial approach. Suturing begins at the transition point between the septal leaflet of the tricuspid valve and the ventricular septum, 5 to 7 mm below the edge of the septal defect. This critical point is given attention by all experienced surgeons.[D5]

Usual de-airing procedures are performed, and the remainder of the operation is completed as usual.

Repair of Doubly Committed Subarterial Ventricular Septal Defect

Transverse incision in the RV infundibulum is the classic approach for repair of doubly committed subarterial VSDs (these defects were once termed subpulmonary VSDs) (Fig. 21-27).[D8] These defects should always be closed with a patch to reduce possibility of distortion of the semilunar valves. Continuous stitch technique is employed. When pledgeted sutures are used, they are placed from just above the pulmonary valve leaflets, and pledgets come to lie in the pulmonary valve sinuses. Care is taken not to damage the left main coronary artery. An approach through the pulmonary trunk is also convenient for the repair of doubly committed subarterial VSDs.

Repair of Inlet Septal Ventricular Septal Defect

Inlet septal (AV septal type) VSD is most easily repaired through the right atrium (see "Technique of Operation" in Chapter 20). Such defects are always repaired with a patch. The defect lies beneath the septal leaflet of the tricuspid valve, and care is taken to avoid damage to the leaflet or its chordae and to tailor the patch such that it is not too bulky beneath the leaflet. One method of avoiding damage to the leaflet and improving exposure is to temporarily detach the base of the septal leaflet and a portion of the anterior leaflet of the tricuspid valve and retract the leaflet anteriorly.[H12]

Text continued on p. 878

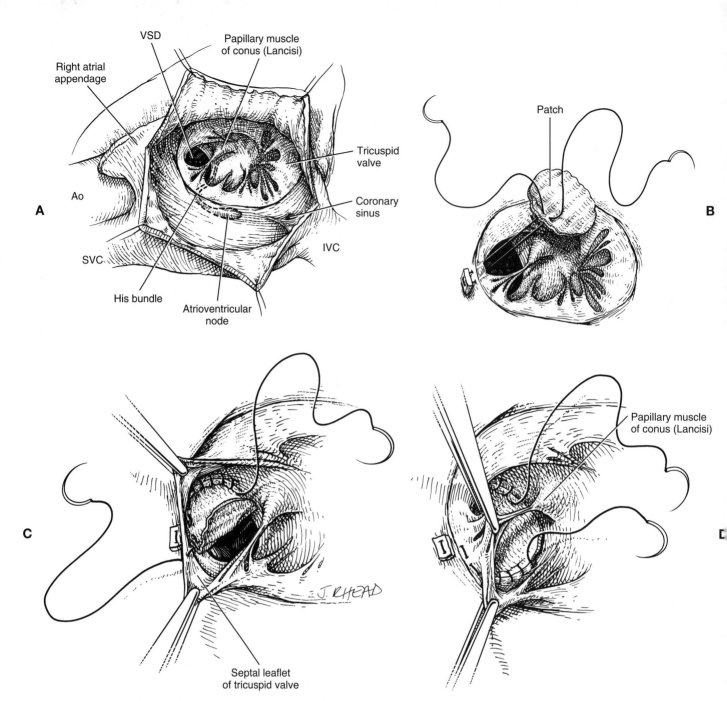

Labels in figure:

A:
- Right atrial appendage
- VSD
- Papillary muscle of conus (Lancisi)
- Tricuspid valve
- Coronary sinus
- IVC
- Atrioventricular node
- His bundle
- SVC
- Ao

B:
- Patch

C:
- Septal leaflet of tricuspid valve

D:
- Papillary muscle of conus (Lancisi)

J. RHEAD

Figure 21-25   Repair of perimembranous ventricular septal defect *(VSD)* from right atrium, continuous suture technique. **A,** Right atriotomy is parallel to atrioventricular groove from right atrial appendage toward inferior vena cava. Stay sutures are placed to expose tricuspid orifice. Superior edge of VSD is not visible because of overlying anterior leaflet of tricuspid valve. Atrioventricular node lies within triangle of Koch, with bundle of His penetrating to ventricular septum at posterior angle of VSD, where it is particularly vulnerable to injury. **B,** Repair of VSD is started at junction of septal with anterior leaflets of tricuspid valve. A pledget-reinforced No. 4-0 polypropylene suture is placed as a mattress stitch through tricuspid anulus, with pledget on atrial side of tricuspid valve. Suture is passed through a knitted double-velour polyester patch trimmed to slightly larger than size of VSD. Alternative patch material could be pericardium or polytetrafluoroethylene. **C,** Continuous stitches are placed along right side of superior rim of defect to approximate patch to ventricular septum. Simultaneous traction on suture and on patch exposes next area to be stitched and provides good visibility. Aortic valve is located to left side of septum in this area (ventriculoinfundibular fold) and must be protected from inclusion of cusp tissue in suture line. Opposite end of suture is then passed through septal leaflet of tricuspid valve as a continuous mattress stitch working inferiorly. Bundle of His crosses beneath this portion of suture line. Stitches must not penetrate tricuspid anulus or into atrial myocardium, to preserve integrity of conduction system. **D,** At a point 5 to 7 mm below inferior margin of VSD, suture line is transitioned from septal leaflet onto ventricular septum. Stitching continues along inferior rim of VSD, with stitches placed 5 to 7 mm below rim until reaching muscle of Lancisi.

Key: Ao, Aorta; IVC, inferior vena cava; SVC, superior vena cava; VSD, ventricular septal defect.

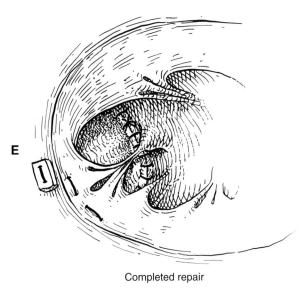

E

Completed repair

Figure 21-25, cont'd **E,** Suture line may come to edge of ventricular septal defect anterior to muscle of Lancisi and is continued until meeting previously completed superior suture line. Suture ends are joined to complete repair. Alternatively, repair may begin at point described here as end point.[D5] Initial suture line proceeds along superior edge of defect to junction of anterior and septal leaflet of tricuspid valve. Second part of suture line is carried along septum inferiorly, 5 to 7 mm below edge of defect, transitions to septal leaflet, then proceeds as a continuous mattress stitch along septal leaflet superiorly to join other end of suture to complete repair. This approach has advantages of working suture line toward surgeon and making it easier for assistant to follow suture.

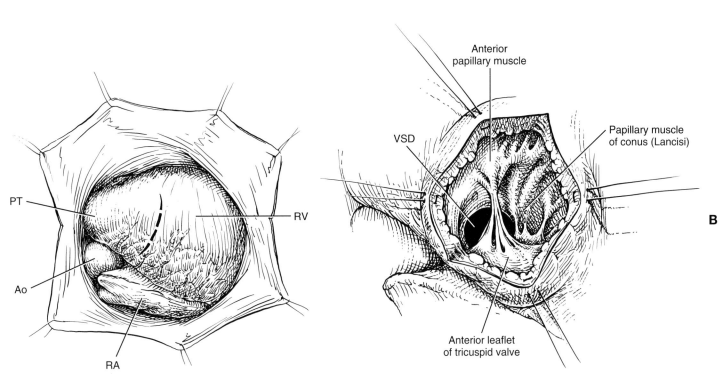

Figure 21-26 Repair of perimembranous ventricular septal defect *(VSD)* from right ventricle *(RV)*, interrupted suture technique. **A,** Transverse ventriculotomy is made low in outflow tract. A right atriotomy has been made previously to examine atrial septum for defect, with a vent device placed across patent or surgically made foramen ovale, which will be closed later. **B,** Retraction stitches are placed through myocardium superiorly and inferiorly to expose interior of RV. VSD is partially obscured by anterior leaflet of tricuspid valve, which must be retracted to expose septal leaflet.

Key: *Ao,* Aorta; *PT,* pulmonary trunk; *RA,* right atrium; *RV,* right ventricle; *VSD,* ventricular septal defect.

Continued

Figure 21-26, cont'd **C,** Septal leaflet of tricuspid valve is retracted to expose junction of tricuspid anulus with ventricular septum. A pledget-reinforced mattress stitch of No. 4-0 polypropylene suture is placed to create a transition from septal leaflet to ventricular septum. One arm of suture is placed entirely on septal leaflet, and other arm is placed into ventricular septum at hinge point of septal leaflet on ventricular septum. Stitch is at least 5 to 7 mm below rim of ventricular septal defect *(VSD)*. Suture is passed through a knitted double-velour polyester patch fashioned to be somewhat larger than VSD. Alternative patch material could be pericardium or polytetrafluoroethylene. **D,** Several pledget-reinforced mattress stitches are placed around perimeter of VSD. Stitches are placed entirely in septal leaflet tissue between transition stitch and junction of septal and anterior leaflets of tricuspid valve. Stitches are placed 5 to 7 mm below rim of defect between transition stitch and papillary muscle of conus (Lancisi), which demarcates anterior extent of specialized conduction system. Rest of stitches may be placed in rim of septal defect. All stitches are placed through ventricular septum and septal leaflet of tricuspid valve before approximating patch to ventricular septum. **E,** Patch is attached securely to ventricular septum by tying all sutures.

Key: *VSD,* Ventricular septal defect.

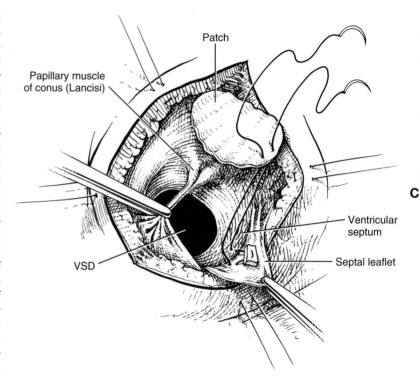

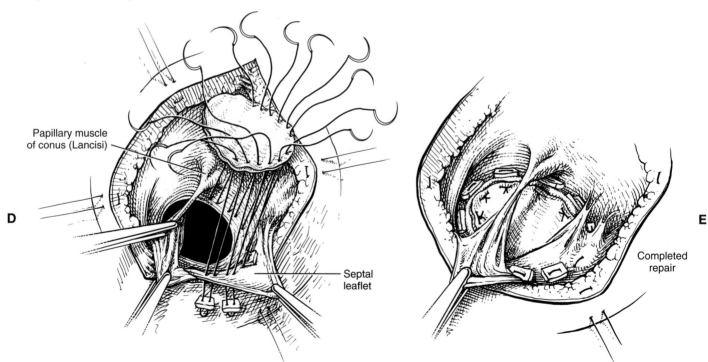

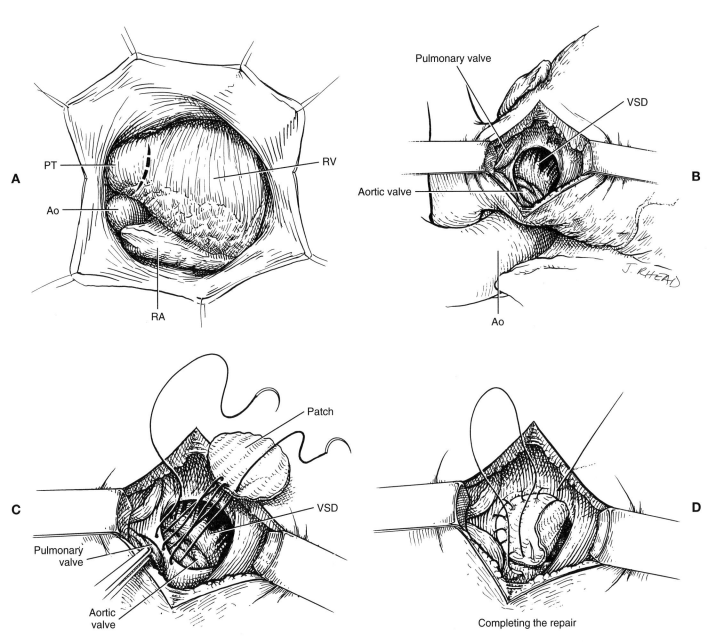

Figure 21-27   Repair of doubly committed subarterial ventricular septal defect *(VSD)*. **A,** Transverse incision is made in outflow tract of right ventricle near ventriculopulmonary arterial junction. VSD could also be approached via pulmonary trunk. **B,** VSD is subarterial, meaning that it is directly below valves of both great arteries. Superior border of VSD is pulmonary and aortic valves, and both valves are committed equally to defect. **C,** Initial stitches of No. 4-0 polypropylene suture are placed through narrow fibrous rim separating pulmonary valve anteriorly from aortic valve posteriorly. Stitches are passed through a patch (knitted double-velour polyester, polytetrafluoroethylene, or pericardium) that is slightly larger than VSD. Each stitch in this area must be placed with aortic valve in view to avoid damaging its cusps. Cardioplegic solution may be infused into aortic root or occlusion clamp removed temporarily from aorta for better visualization of aortic valve while placing stitches in this area. **D,** Remainder of defect is closed by placing stitches through rim of VSD and through patch. Bundle of His is located far posterior and is unrelated to posterior rim of VSD.

Key: *Ao,* Aorta; *PT,* pulmonary trunk; *RA,* right atrium; *RV,* right ventricle; *VSD,* ventricular septal defect.

Repair of Muscular Ventricular Septal Defect

A right-sided approach is used for repair of muscular VSDs. Left ventriculotomy provides excellent exposure,[A4,B3] and although it has been reported not to be disadvantageous in infants,[M13,S14] it can produce ventricular aneurysm and important LV dysfunction early and late postoperatively.[G8] Therefore, use of left ventriculotomy is not recommended. Defects in the lower part of the muscular septum may be obscured by trabeculations and thus difficult to visualize, resulting in incomplete closure. Wollenek and colleagues found that an apical left ventriculotomy was a useful approach in 23 patients, and in follow-up over 3 to 18 years (mean 11.3 years), echocardiography showed no residual VSD, normal LV shortening, no regional wall motion abnormality, and small LV aneurysm in only two patients.[W5]

Single or multiple muscular defects in the inlet and trabecular septum (see Figs. 21-1 and 21-13) are approached through the right atrium. When a single defect is slitlike or oval, direct suture (often in part at least with pledgeted mattress sutures) is satisfactory, but when it is large and circular, a patch is used. A cluster of defects can be closed with a single patch or individually.

Division of RV trabeculations can aid exposure of the defects, which may be difficult to close because of multiple sites of jet penetration. A heavy traction stitch passed through the defect and back through the left side of the defect may improve exposure. Use of a single patch of autologous pericardium supported by pledget-reinforced sutures covering an extensive portion of the trabecular septum is useful when there are multiple defects.[S30] Kitagawa and colleagues described resection of trabeculations to expose the defect and attaching an oversized patch to the left side of the ventricular septum by sutures passed through the septum from the left side.[K19] They also described placing pledget-supported sutures through the rim of an anterior muscular defect, passing the sutures to the outside and tying down on the epicardial surface.[4]

When a muscular VSD coexists with a perimembranous VSD, a single patch is used to avoid damage to the bundle of His.

VSDs with a single LV opening but two or more openings into the RV on both sides of the septal band are also approached through the right atrium.[S28] The defect is converted into a single LV orifice by detaching the lower end of the trabecula septomarginalis and moderator band from the septum and retracting them (see Fig. 21-13). The VSD is closed with a patch. The septal band then falls back into place.

Multiple defects in the anterior portion of the septum may be closed through a high transverse ventriculotomy. At times VSDs may be considered too numerous to close individually; these VSDs are simply compressed and often totally closed by interrupted mattress sutures between a felt strip on the anterior ventricular wall (away from the left anterior descending coronary artery) and pledgets inside the RV and inferior to the VSDs.[B5] This repair may be done from the right atrium or through a right ventriculotomy.

Apical muscular VSDs can be exposed through the right atrium and tricuspid valve or through a low vertical right ventriculotomy.[S30] This can be extended around the apex for a short distance onto the posterior wall.

The rare Swiss cheese septum, with features resembling ventricular noncompaction (spongy ventricular septum) and with defects involving all components of the ventricular septum, may not be correctable through the right side. Its repair requires an LV approach, and a patch over the entire muscular septum may be necessary. An associated perimembranous defect should be repaired through the right atrium because its repair from the LV side increases risk of heart block. Incisions into both ventricles are avoided whenever possible. Great care is used in making and closing the left ventriculotomy incision so as not to damage coronary artery branches. A continuous mattress suture over fine Teflon felt strips plus an over-and-over stitch give a secure closure. Mace and colleagues used a right atrial approach and inserted a single large patch to cover the right side of the trabecular septum, adding several intermediate fixation stitches to prevent septal bulging.[M17] Regardless of the approach employed, these patients often have poor LV function after repair and may ultimately require transplantation for heart failure.[K19] This group of patients may be better served by pulmonary trunk banding with the hope that some of these defects may close as a result of ventricular hypertrophy.[S29]

Although it is important to avoid residual shunts, multiple incisions and a prolonged search for a few small additional muscular VSDs are generally not advisable. Preoperative echocardiography should accurately delineate the size as well as position of all the defects.

Closure of Associated Patent Ductus Arteriosus

Dissection of the ductus arteriosus is done after establishing CPB to reduce the risk of hemorrhage should an error in dissection occur because of exposure, which can be difficult. After establishing CPB with the perfusate temperature at about 34°C, with caval tapes still unsnugged (so that the heart will not distend) and right atrial pressure at zero, the ductus is dissected. The heart must continue to beat; otherwise a large shunt will rapidly overdistend the right side of the heart and lungs as it steals from the systemic and cerebral circulation. If the heart does fibrillate, CPB flow rate is immediately reduced while the dissection is rapidly completed.

With downward traction on the pulmonary trunk[K4] (see "Technique of Operation" in Chapter 23), the ductus can usually be seen through its pericardial reflection and surrounding adventitial tissue. The left pulmonary artery and undersurface of the aorta both proximal and distal to the ductus are clearly identified to prevent these structures from being damaged or ligated after being mistaken for the ductus. The delicate pericardial reflection and adventitial tissue on both sides of the ductus are sharply dissected from it. The adventitia of the ductus itself and of the adjacent pulmonary artery and aorta must not be entered. The recurrent laryngeal nerve is not seen. Only when the dissection is complete, the left pulmonary artery visualized, and the ductus identified with absolute certainty is a right-angled clamp passed behind it to grasp the No. 2-0 silk ligature. One ligature, tied on the ductus while perfu-

---

[4] The pledget is a "firm" polyester mini pledget, 1/12 inch × 1/8 inch × 1/16 inch.

sion flow rate is reduced to lower intravascular pressure, is sufficient to close it. A surgical clip may be used instead. The operation then proceeds as usual.

Pulmonary Trunk Banding

Banding of the pulmonary trunk may be performed through a small left anterolateral thoracotomy. However, now that pulmonary trunk banding is reserved for special situations, often to be followed by a Fontan operation (see "Pulmonary Trunk Banding" in Section 2 of Chapter 27) or use of a valved conduit, avoiding distortion of the pulmonary trunk bifurcation by the band is crucial. To ensure this, placement of the pulmonary trunk band via median sternotomy is the best approach because it permits accurate dissection, placement, and anchoring of the band on both the left and right sides of the pulmonary trunk.

According to Trusler's rule,[A6,T2] the pulmonary trunk band is marked to a length of 20 mm, plus the number of millimeters corresponding to the child's weight in kilograms, to indicate the ultimate tightness of the band. (If the banding is done for a complex cardiac anomaly with bidirectional shunting, the length is 24 mm plus the child's weight.) A 3- to 4-mm-wide polyester tape is used. The tape may be impregnated with silicone (Silastic) for easier removal.

When a left anterolateral thoracotomy is used, a small incision is made in the pericardium, generally anterior to the phrenic nerve. When a median sternotomy is used, the pericardium is opened in the midline. The pulmonary trunk is separated from the aorta by dissecting close to the *aorta*. A right-angled clamp is passed around and behind the aorta to grasp one end of the band and pull it through. The other end of the band is retrieved by a clamp passed through the transverse sinus. Small angiocatheters are placed in the aorta and left pulmonary artery for pressure monitoring. With the band now safely around the midportion of the pulmonary trunk, the marked points on the band are joined temporarily with a hemoclip to produce the desired circumference. With proper band tightening, the systolic blood pressure rises, and in cases of complete mixing, the arterial oxygen saturation should be 80% to 85% by pulse oximetry with FIO_2 of 50%. If bradycardia or cyanosis develops, the band must be slightly loosened by placing a hemoclip more distally and removing the initial clip. If the narrowing is insufficient, as judged by the pressure difference across the band (distal pulmonary trunk pressure should be less than 50% of systemic pressure), it is tightened by adding a hemoclip more proximally. When the ideal diameter is obtained, the band is joined by sutures. It is essential that stitches be placed between the band and the pulmonary trunk adventitia to prevent migration of the band. When the banding is in preparation for a Fontan operation, the band is anchored to the commissures of the pulmonary valve, because pulmonary valve regurgitation is unimportant and distal migration highly disadvantageous. The pericardium is loosely closed to facilitate dissection at subsequent operation.

Pulmonary Trunk Debanding

When a pulmonary trunk band has been properly applied for 6 months or less, simple band removal is usually all that

is necessary. When the band must remain in place longer, reconstruction of the pulmonary trunk is usually required.

The band can almost always be cut and removed without damaging the underlying artery. The tip of the left atrial appendage actually is more likely to be damaged because it is always adherent to the banded area. Dissection is usually delayed until CPB has been established, when, if necessary, flow rate can be reduced to facilitate exposure and dissection.

The VSD is usually closed after repair of the pulmonary trunk. The pulmonary trunk is usually reconstructed. The most satisfactory technique is local excision of the short, narrowed, scarred segment of artery and reanastomosis of the divided pulmonary trunk using a continuous polypropylene suture.[D7] This technique can usually be employed even when the band lies close to the pulmonary valve by extending the incision vertically into the most anterior sinus between the valve commissures, to enlarge the diameter of the proximal end. A similar technique can be used to enlarge an orifice stenosis involving only one branch of the pulmonary trunk. When the pulmonary valve cusps have become excessively thick, their edges may require excision. If an adequate diameter is not obtainable by the technique of excision and end-to-end anastomosis, an oval-shaped patch is inserted to enlarge adequately the stenotic area (using autologous pericardium, pulmonary allograft, or thin polytetrafluoroethylene [PTFE]). An extensive reconstruction (see "Repair of Tetralogy of Fallot with Bifurcation Stenosis of Pulmonary Trunk" in Section 1 of Chapter 24) is required when the band constricts the origin of the pulmonary arteries.

SPECIAL FEATURES OF POSTOPERATIVE CARE

General measures and management of complications described in Chapter 5 are used for postoperative care of patients undergoing repair of primary VSD.

Hemodynamic state typically is good early postoperatively after closure of VSD. In the unusual situation of poor hemodynamic performance, the possibility of residual left-to-right shunting must be considered, particularly if left atrial pressure is considerably higher than right atrial pressure.[5] Also, the finding of a considerably higher oxygen

---

[5] When the two ventricles have equal stroke volumes (i.e., no shunts or valvar regurgitation is present), left and right atrial pressures are determined by the relative contractility, distensibility, and volume at zero pressure of the two ventricles.[B4] The greater each of these values is for a given ventricle, the better its performance and the lower its end-diastolic and (if the AV valves are not stenotic) atrial pressures tend to be relative to those of the other ventricle. (For a more detailed discussion of these matters, see "Cardiac Output and Its Determinants" in Section 1 of Chapter 5.) After complete repair of a large VSD through the right atrium in a patient who preoperatively had a large left-to-right shunt and a large $\dot{Q}p/\dot{Q}s$, the atrial pressures are similar, or right is slightly higher than left. When repair is through a right ventriculotomy, right atrial pressure may be 20% to 30% higher than left. Unless repair has been done through a left ventriculotomy and in the absence of other left heart lesions (e.g., aortic stenosis, coarctation), a left atrial pressure considerably greater (greater than 6 mmHg) than right suggests a residual left-to-right shunt. The high left atrial pressure under such circumstances is related to large LV stroke volume.

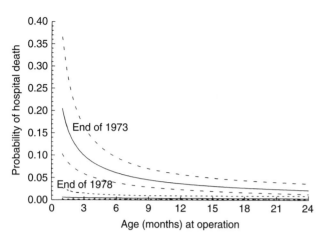

Figure 21-28   Risk-adjusted hospital mortality after repair of single large ventricular septal defects without major associated cardiac anomalies, according to age and year at operation. Nomogram represents a specific solution of logistic equation in Table 20-6. Dashed lines enclose 70% confidence limits. (From Rizzoli and colleagues.[R5])

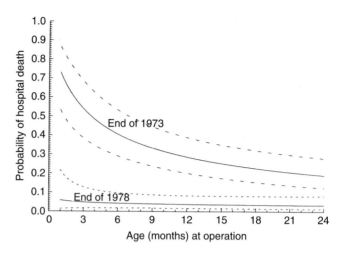

Figure 21-29   Hospital mortality after repair of multiple ventricular septal defects, according to age and year at operation (see Fig. 21-28). (From Rizzoli and colleagues.[R5])

■ **TABLE 21-4   Effect of Age on Hospital Mortality after Primary Repair of Single Large Ventricular Septal Defect**

Age at Operation			1969-1982 [a]				1974-1979 [b]			
				Hospital Deaths				Hospital Deaths		
≤	months	<	*n*	No.	%	CL (%)	*n*	No.	%	CL (%)
		3	20	3	15	7-28	11	1 [c]	9	1-28
3		6	28	0	0	0-7	10	0	0	0-17
6		12	37	1	3	0.3-9	14	0	0	0-13
12		24	28	2	7	2-16	11	0	0	0-16
24		48	71	2	2.8	0.9-6.6	15	0	0	0-12
48							33	0	0	0-6
TOTAL			184	8 [d]	4.3	2.8-6.5	94	1	1.1	0.1-3.6
$P(\chi^2)$					.10				>.9	

Key: *CL*, 70% confidence limits.

[a] Data from 184 patients with or without major associated cardiac defects operated on at GLH. Patients less than 3 months of age are presented in more detail in Table 21-8.
[b] Data from Rizzoli and colleagues.[R5]
[c] A 12-month-old baby with preoperative seizures was admitted already intubated and was ventilated; patient died on postoperative day 3 with acute cardiac failure.
[d] Six of eight deaths were of patients with major associated cardiac anomalies.

content or saturation in blood from the pulmonary artery than that from the right atrium establishes existence of a shunt.[V4] Two-dimensional Doppler color flow echocardiography can be used to settle the matter.[L12,S18] Although considerable shunting may occur for 12 to 24 hours after VSD closure with a porous patch, the usual cause of poor hemodynamic state from a left-to-right shunt is patch dehiscence. Thus, if the hemodynamic state is poor or a large left-to-right shunt is present, prompt reoperation is probably indicated. Intraoperative echocardiography at the original operation, if done, will usually have indicated residual shunting,[S27] as confirmed by postoperative echocardiography, which may be done transesophageally for greatest resolution and quality of images.

It is prudent to place temporary pacing wires on the right ventricle after VSD repair. Complete AV dissociation is often present for a short time intraoperatively. Even if this resolves promptly to normal sinus rhythm, it is advisable to leave pacing wires in place and have an external pacemaker available while the patient is hospitalized, because AV dissociation may occur temporarily.

RESULTS

Early (Hospital) Death

Hospital mortality is low for repair of single large VSDs, most of which are now repaired in early infancy (Table 21-4 and Fig. 21-28). Risk is higher when the VSDs are multiple and when major associated cardiac anomalies coexist (Fig. 21-29). As a result, overall hospital mortality after repair of primary VSDs of all types is 5% to 10% (Table 21-5). Stark and Sethia reported a hospital mortality of 12% (CL 7.8%-18%) from Great Ormond Street Hospital (1981-1985).[S21] Richardson and colleagues reported operative mortality of 3% for closure of isolated VSD in patients age 1 to 24 months.[R11]

■ **TABLE 21-5**   **Hospital Mortality after Repair of Single and Multiple Ventricular Septal Defects** [a]

| Category | Large VSD | | | | Medium VSD | | | | Small VSD | | | | Total | | | | $P(\chi^2)$ |
| | n | Hospital Deaths | | | n | Hospital Deaths | | | n | Hospital Deaths | | | n | Hospital Deaths | | | |
		No.	%	CL(%)		No.	%	CL(%)		No.	%	CL(%)		No.	%	CL(%)	
Primary	156	8	5.1	3.3-7.7	45	0	0	0-4	13	0	0	0-14	214	8	3.7	2.4-5.6	.2
Plus banded PT	24	3	12	6-24	2	0	0	0-61					26	3	12	5-22	.6
Plus AR	17	0	0	0-11	16	0	0	0-11	8	0	0	0-21	41	0	0	0-5	
Plus SVA and AR	4	0	0	0-38	2	0	0	0-61	1	0	0	0-85	7	0	0	0-24	
Total	201	11	5.5	3.8-7.7	65	0	0	0-3	22	0	0	0-8	288	11	3.8	2.7-5.4	.008
$P(\chi^2)$		.3												.11			

Key: *AR,* Aortic regurgitation; *CL,* 70% confidence limits; *PT,* pulmonary trunk; *SVA,* sinus of Valsalva aneurysm; *VSD,* ventricular septal defect.

[a] Data from 201 patients with or without major or minor associated cardiac anomalies operated on at GLH from 1965 to 1982.

■ **TABLE 21-6**   **Incremental Risk Factors for Hospital Death after Repair of Single and Multiple Ventricular Septal Defects with or without Major Associated Cardiac Anomalies** [a]

Risk Factor	Logistic Coefficient ± SD	P
Young age (months)	−2.2 ± 0.47	<.0001
Multiple VSDs		
Nontrabecular [b]	2.9 ± 1.20	.02
All others	2.2 ± 0.60	.0003
If No Major Associated Cardiac Anomaly		
Date of operation	−0.08 ± 0.020	.0001
Date of operation · age (months) interaction [c]	0.015 ± 0.0058	.008
If Major Associated Cardiac Anomaly		
Mitral lesion	3.7 ± 1.61	.02
Major associated lesions other than PDA or simultaneously repaired coarctation of aorta	1.8 ± 1.12	.10
Intercept	5.9 [d]	

(Data from Rizzoli and colleagues.[R5])

Key: *PDA,* Patent ductus arteriosus; *SD,* standard deviation; *VSDs,* ventricular septal defects.

[a] Data from an analysis of 312 surgical patients, with 30 hospital deaths.
[b] This variable applies to multiple VSDs, none of which was muscular.
[c] Interaction between age at operation and date of operation indicates that by the end of 1978, risk of young age was completely neutralized (see Figures 21-28 and 21-29).
[d] If a major associated cardiac anomaly, intercept is 1.8.

Mode of Early Death

The most common mode of death after repair of a primary VSD is acute cardiac failure.[R5] This may be related to failure of intraoperative myocardial protection in the face of myocardial dysfunction often present in sick small patients coming to operation. Occasionally, paroxysms of pulmonary arterial hypertension (see "Pulmonary Hypertensive Crises" under Pulmonary Subsystem in Section 1 of Chapter 5) precipitate acute cardiac failure.[S21] Persisting severe pulmonary dysfunction, often from viral pneumonitis present before operation, characterizes death of a few infants after repair of VSD.

■ **TABLE 21-7**   **Hospital Mortality after Repair of Large Ventricular Septal Defects in Early Era at the Mayo Clinic**

| Era | n | Hospital Deaths | | |
		No.	%	CL (%)
1955 to 1960	241	50	21	18-24
1960 to 1966	247	31	13 [a]	10-15
Total	488	81	17	15-19
$P(\chi^2)$		.02		

(Data from Cartmill and colleagues[C3] and Kirklin and DuShane.[K3])

Key: *CL,* 70% confidence limits.

[a] Between 1962 and 1966, hospital mortality in patients over age 6 months was 4.1% (CL 2.4%-6.5%).[C3]

Incremental Risk Factors for Hospital Death

Studies of experiences extending back a number of years permit identification of incremental risk factors (Table 21-6). With death after repair now less common, risk factors are now more difficult to identify.

Risk of repair has decreased, and thus *early date of operation* is an incremental risk factor (see Tables 21-5 and 21-6 and Figs. 21-28 and 21-29). Improvement from an original risk of hospital death of 20% began in the experience at the Mayo Clinic during the early 1960s (Table 21-7). This type of improvement has been demonstrated in other centers.[C6,R7]

In previous eras, *young age* increased risk of operation; identification of young age as a potential risk factor has been confirmed by Rizzoli and colleagues[R7] and Yeager and colleagues.[Y3] This risk factor has been neutralized in recent years[C5,J3,R5] (see Figs. 21-27 and 21-28). Young age may still be an incremental risk factor when major associated anomalies coexist (see Table 21-6; see also Fig. 21-28).

Multiple VSDs had increased risk of operation in the past,[F1,F5,K13] but risk has declined considerably in the current era. However, multiple VSDs complicated by additional cardiac anomalies impose a higher risk of hospital death than do uncomplicated ones.[R7] This again may not be an immutable risk and may be improved by improved myocardial management, avoidance of ventricular incisions, and device closure.[S28]

■ **TABLE 21-8** **Hospital Death after Primary Repair of Single Large Ventricular Septal Defect with or without Major Associated Cardiac Anomalies in Patients Less Than 3 Months of Age** [a]

Category	n	Hospital Deaths	
VSD alone	4	0	0/10
VSD plus large ASD	5	0	0% [b]
VSD plus partial anomalous pulmonary venous connection	1	0	CL 0%-17%
VSD plus PDA (moderate or large)	4	0	
VSD plus severe coarctation of aorta (simultaneous repair)	2	1	3/10
VSD plus moderate coarctation of aorta (not repaired)	3	1	30% [b]
			CL 14%-51%
VSD plus severe aortic stenosis (uncorrectable)	1	1	
TOTAL	20	3	15%; CL 7%-28%

Key: *ASD,* Atrial septal defect; *CL,* 70% confidence limits; *PDA,* patent ductus arteriosus; *VSD,* ventricular septal defect.

[a] Data from GLH, 1969 to 1982.

[b] *P* (Fisher) = .11.

Major associated cardiac anomalies had increased risk of hospital death in the past and continue to do so to some extent (Table 21-8), particularly when these anomalies are associated with multiple VSDs.[R7] Coexisting patent ductus arteriosus and coarctation of the aorta have not increased risk of repair of VSD to the extent that occur with more serious anomalies, such as congenital mitral valve disease. Again, better surgical techniques for managing complex anomalies and current methods of myocardial management (see Chapter 3) may neutralize much of the increased risk formerly imposed by major associated cardiac anomalies.

Neither location of the VSD (Tables 21-9 and 21-10) nor surgical approach (Table 21-11) affects risk of operation. Previous pulmonary trunk banding and associated lesions (e.g., aortic regurgitation, sinus of Valsalva aneurysm) also do not increase surgical risk.

Preoperative P_{PA} and R_p are not determinants of early mortality at present, although they affect late results.[B1] This current situation is different from earlier experiences,[C2,C3]

■ **TABLE 21-9** **Hospital Mortality According to Type of Ventricular Septal Defect (VSD) after Primary Repair of Single Large VSD** [a]

	1967-1973				1974-1979			
		Hospital Deaths				Hospital Deaths		
Type of VSD	n	No.	%	CL (%)	n	No.	%	CL (%)
Perimembranous	140	6	4.3	2.5-6.9	78	1	1.3	0.2-4.3
Subarterial	10	0	0	0-17	9	0	0	0-19
Inlet septal	7	0	0	0-24	4	0	0	0-38
Muscular	7	0	0	0-24	1	0	0	0-85
Confluent	2	0	0	0-61	2	0	0	0-61
TOTAL	166	6	3.6	2.1-5.8	94	1	1.1	0.1-3.6
$P(\chi^2)$	.9				.9			

(Data from Rizzoli and colleagues.[R5])

Key: *CL,* 70% confidence limits.

[a] Based on 260 patients without major coexisting cardiac anomalies.

■ **TABLE 21-10** **Hospital Mortality after Repair of Ventricular Septal Defects of All Types** [a]

	Perimembranous				Subarterial				Inlet Septal			
		Hospital Deaths				Hospital Deaths				Hospital Deaths		
Category	n	No.	%	CL (%)	n	No.	%	CL (%)	n	No.	%	CL (%)
Primary VSD	233 [b]	10	4.3	2.9-6.1	23	2	9	3-19	6	2	33	12-62
VSD plus banded PT	15	0	0	0-12	4	0	0	0-38	1	0	0	0-85
VSD plus AR	31	0	0	0-6	17	1	6	0.8-19				
VSD plus SVA plus AR	6	0	0	0-27	1	0	0	0-85				
TOTAL	285	10	3.5	2.4-5.0	45	3	7	3-13	7	2	29	10-55
$P(\chi^2)$	.5				.9				.5			

	Muscular				Swiss Cheese				Total				
		Hospital Deaths				Hospital Deaths				Hospital Deaths			
Category	n	No.	%	CL (%)	n	No.	%	CL (%)	n	No.	%	CL (%)	$P(\chi^2)$
Primary VSD	16	2	12	4-27					278	16	5.8	4.3-7.6	.01
VSD plus banded PT	3	2 [c]	67	24-96	3	1	33	4-76	26	3	12	5-22	.01
VSD plus AR									48	1	2	0.3-7	.17
VSD plus SVA plus AR									7	0	0	0-24	
TOTAL	19	4	21	11-35	3	1	33	4-76	359	20	5.6	4.3-7.1	.0002
$P(\chi^2)$	.03								.3				

Key: *AR,* Aortic regurgitation; *CL,* 70% confidence limits; *PT,* pulmonary trunk; *SVA,* sinus of Valsalva aneurysm; *VSD,* ventricular septal defect.

[a] Data from 359 patients with or without major coexisting cardiac anomalies operated on at GLH from 1958 to 1982.

[b] Includes 13 examples of confluent VSD.

[c] Both patients had severe recurrent coarctation of aorta at time of debanding, and one also had congenital aortic stenosis.

no doubt because the upper limit of operable Rp is better understood and perioperative management (including surgical techniques and myocardial management) has improved.

Survival

Premature late death occurs in less than 2.5% of patients when Rp is low preoperatively. Presumably, the few deaths in this setting are from arrhythmias, either ventricular fibrillation or sudden development of heart block late postoperatively.

■ **TABLE 21-11 Hospital Mortality Related to Surgical Approach after Primary Repair of Single Large Ventricular Septal Defects** [a]

| Surgical Approach | 1967-1973 | | | | 1974-1979 | | | |
| | | Hospital Deaths | | | | Hospital Deaths | | |
	n	No.	%	CL (%)	*n*	No.	%	CL (%)
Right atrium	105	2	1.9	0.6-4.5	65	1	1.5	0.2-5.1
RA → RV	4	0	0	0-38	2	0	0	0-61
Right ventricle	57	4	7	4-12	27	0	0	0-7
TOTAL	166	6	3.6	2.1-5.8	94	1	1.1	0.1-3.6
$P(\chi^2)$		.2				>.9		

(Data from Rizzoli and colleagues.[R5])

Key: *CL*, 70% confidence limits; *RA → RV*, right atrial changed to right ventricular approach.

[a] Based on 260 patients without major coexisting cardiac anomalies.

Patients with a high Rp preoperatively often die from progression of pulmonary vascular disease.

Repair of VSD during the first 1 or 2 years of life is curative for most patients, resulting in full functional activity and normal or near-normal life expectancy.

Physical Development

A prominent feature of the late postoperative course after repair of large VSDs in infants is improved physical development,[R1] and an impressive increase in weight may also be seen[B3] (Fig. 21-30, *A*), as Lillehei and colleagues first showed in 1955.[L1] There is a less impressive increase in length (Fig. 21-30, *B*) and in head circumference.[C11] This improved physical development is usually associated with complete relief of symptoms. Increase in weight postoperatively also occurs in children in whom a large VSD is repaired later in the first decade of life (Fig. 21-31).[C3]

These generalizations have been refined by Weintraub and Menahem in a definitive study.[W6] They confirmed that repair of a large VSD in the first 6 months of life results in near-normal long-term growth in most patients, so that by age 5 years, weight, length, and head circumference are normal. Low-birth-weight infants were an exception, and catch-up occurred only in their weight.

Conduction Disturbances

Conduction disturbances are frequent after repair of VSDs.

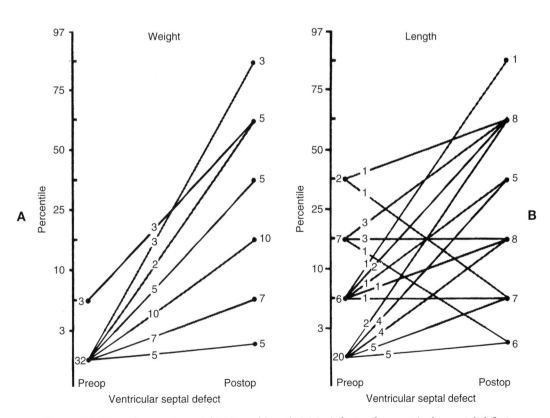

Figure 21-30 Changes in weight (**A**) and length (**B**) in infants after ventricular septal defect closure. (From Clarkson.[C11])

Key: *Preop*, Preoperative; *Postop*, postoperative.

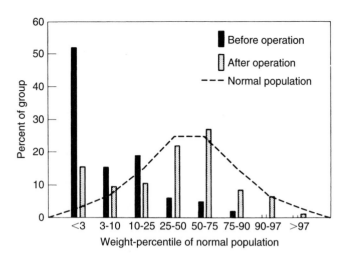

Figure 21-31   Changes in weight after repair of ventricular septal defect in 96 patients age 10 years or less with ratio of pulmonary and systemic pressures greater than 0.45 and ratio of pulmonary and systemic resistances less than 0.75 preoperatively. (From Cartmill and colleagues.[C3])

Right Bundle Branch Block

Right bundle branch block (RBBB) is present late postoperatively in many patients in whom VSDs are repaired via right ventriculotomy. In a series of infants, prevalence was 80% (CL 72%-86%).[B3] Based on their studies, Gelband and colleagues concluded that the cause is the ventriculotomy.[G3] However, Weidman and colleagues at the Mayo Clinic reported that 44% (CL 35%-54%) of 36 patients undergoing repair of perimembranous VSDs through a right atriotomy developed new RBBB.[O3] Rein and colleagues reported RBBB in 34% (CL 26%-43%) of infants undergoing repair via right atriotomy.[R1] Thus, in some patients, RBBB must result from damage to the right bundle by sutures along the inferior border of perimembranous VSDs. In any event, RBBB is less prevalent when the right atrial approach is used for VSD repair.[H18,R1,O3]

Right Bundle Branch Block and Left Anterior Hemiblock

A small proportion of patients develop the ECG pattern of RBBB and left anterior hemiblock after repair of VSD. Prevalence was 8% (CL 4%-14%) in patients repaired through right ventriculotomy[B3] and 10% (CL 6%-16%) in another group of 68 patients.[Z1] Prevalence was 17% (CL 11%-25%) in Rein and colleagues' patients repaired via right atriotomy[R1] and 12% (CL 7%-19%) in Lincoln and colleagues' patients, 72% of whom were repaired through the right atrium.[L7] Such a combination of disturbances has not yet proved to be a poor prognostic finding, but concern and some controversy have been expressed.[K10,Z1] Wolff and colleagues reported that this combination was associated with an important development of late complete heart block and sudden death after repair of tetralogy of Fallot.[W4] However, Downing and colleagues, who found this combination in 6% (CL 4%-10%) of 109 patients undergoing repair of isolated VSD, observed no late complications of any kind in patients followed 1 to 10 years.[D4] The controversy may relate in part to heterogeneity[S10]; that is, RBBB can result from damage to the main right bundle branch during repair, in which case its combination with left anterior hemiblock might be more hazardous than when RBBB results from disruption of a peripheral branch of the right bundle arborization secondary to a right ventriculotomy.[K11] Intracardiac recording techniques at cardiac catheterization may distinguish between these two groups and may be helpful prognostically.[S11]

Ventricular Arrhythmias

Serious ventricular arrhythmias and sudden death late after repair of VSDs have been rare. In a group of children ages 4 to 5 years at repair of the VSD, ventricular premature beats were identified by Holter monitoring late postoperatively in about 40%.[H18] All patients were asymptomatic, and no instances of ventricular tachycardia were observed. Prevalence was lower when an atrial rather than a ventricular approach to repair had been used and also in patients who were younger at time of repair.

Permanent Heart Block

Occurrence of permanent heart block (complete atrioventricular dissociation, with independent atrial activity not conducted to the ventricles) after repair of single VSD approaches zero with present techniques. For example, heart block was present at death or hospital dismissal in one (0.4%; CL 0.05%-1.3%) of 261 patients with single large VSDs with or without major associated cardiac anomalies in the combined GLH and UAB experience. In earlier experience at the Mayo Clinic, no heart block occurred among 146 patients with single large VSDs operated on between 1962 and 1966. Prevalence is slightly higher in patients undergoing repair of multiple VSDs, with two (4%; CL 1%-10%) of 47 such patients developing complete heart block after repair.[R5] Inlet VSDs extending posteriorly to the crux, associated with straddling tricuspid valve, also have increased prevalence of heart block after repair (4 of 6 patients; 67%; CL 8%-38%).

Cardiac Function

Late postoperative cardiac function is essentially normal when repair is done during the first 2 years of life by modern techniques through the right atrium or right ventricle. Graham's group found LV end-diastolic volume, systolic output, and ejection fraction all to be normal about 1 year after operation in a group of these patients (Fig. 21-32).[C4,J1,J2] Others have found persisting abnormalities of LV size and function after repair of large VSDs at an older age, although all patients were asymptomatic.[M1] This

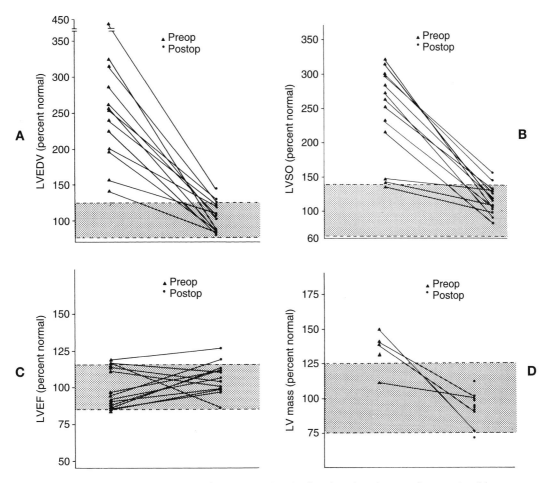

Figure 21-32   Preoperative and postoperative cardiac function 1 year after repair of large ventricular septal defect in infants. Shaded areas represent 95% confidence limits around normal value. **A,** Left ventricular end-diastolic volume, large preoperatively, returns to normal. **B,** Left ventricular systolic output returns to normal with ablation of shunt. **C,** Ejection fraction is normal preoperatively and postoperatively. **D,** Left ventricular mass returns to normal. (From Cordell and colleagues.[C4])

Key: *LVEDV,* Left ventricular end-diastolic volume; *LVEF,* left ventricular ejection fraction; *LV,* left ventricle; *LVSO,* left ventricle systolic output; *Preop,* preoperative; *Postop,* postoperative.

information suggests that in general, patients with large VSDs should be operated on before they are age 2 years, preferably during the first year of life.

Experience with LV function after left ventriculotomy for repairing VSDs in infants has been sobering because in some patients, cardiac output has been low and left atrial pressure high despite absence of a shunt. False aneurysm has occurred after closure of VSD through a left ventriculotomy.

Residual Shunting

Postoperative left-to-right shunts large enough to require reoperation are uncommon when proper techniques are used. One of 138 patients (0.7%; CL 0.1%-2%) operated on for repair of a large VSD required reoperation for an overlooked multiple muscular defect in the UAB experience.[B1] Only three (1.9%; CL 0.8%-4%) of 158 patients required reoperation in the Green Lane Hospital experience, and one patient of 48 hospital survivors (2%; CL

0%-7%) required reoperation for residual VSD in the Boston Children's Hospital study.[R1]

Small but hemodynamically unimportant residual VSDs cannot be entirely ignored because of the theoretic possibility of infective endocarditis at such sites. An accurate estimation of their incidence would require routine postoperative left ventriculography, and this has not been done. However, among 35 patients recatheterized at Green Lane Hospital for reasons other than confirmation of the presence of an important residual shunt, three (9%; CL 4%-17%) had small residual shunts detectable by oxygen saturation data. Four others (11%; CL 6%-20%) had shunts detected only by LV cineangiography, in two of whom the shunting was through small, unclosed muscular defects.

Pulmonary Hyperinflation Syndrome

When pulmonary hyperinflation syndrome is present in infants before VSD repair, it usually resolves within 1 to 2 months after repair.[O4]

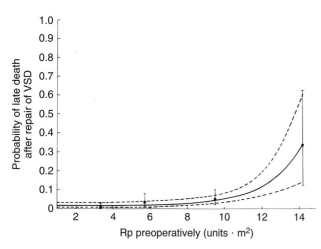

Figure 21-33   Probability of late death (within 5 years of operation) in patients who have survived early postoperative period, according to pulmonary vascular resistance *(Rp)* preoperatively. Dashed lines enclose 70% confidence limits. Actual proportions of death obtained from Cartmill and colleagues[C3] are shown with their 70% confidence limits. *P* for Rp = .0002. See Blackstone and colleagues for data, equations, and statistics.[B1]

Key: *Rp,* Pulmonary vascular resistance; *VSD,* ventricular septal defect.

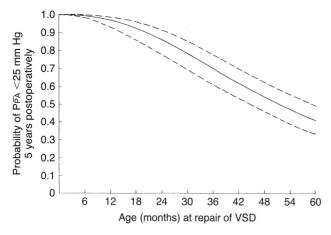

Figure 21-34   Probability of good late results (mean pulmonary artery pressure of less than 25 mmHg 5 years after repair) in patients leaving hospital alive after operation and surviving 5 years, according to age (months) at repair of a large ventricular septal defect. Dashed lines enclose 70% confidence limits (*P* for age < .0001). Equations and statistics are based on data of DuShane and Kirklin.[D2]

Key: *P$_{\overline{PA}}$,* Mean pulmonary artery pressure; *VSD,* ventricular septal defect.

Surgically Produced Aortic or Tricuspid Regurgitation

As complications of repair of primary VSD, surgically produced aortic and tricuspid regurgitation are rare.

Rarity of surgically induced tricuspid regurgitation is surprising considering how often abnormal chordae are attached around the defect. Aortic valve regurgitation occurring after patch closure of doubly committed subarterial VSD may be a special problem. Tomita and colleagues

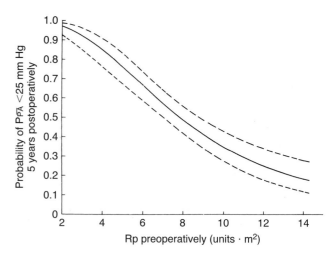

Figure 21-35   Probability of good late results (mean pulmonary artery pressure of less than 25 mmHg 5 years after repair) in patients leaving hospital alive after operation and surviving 5 years, according to preoperative pulmonary vascular resistance (Rp). Dashed lines enclose 70% confidence limits (*P* for Rp < .001). Equations and statistics are based on data of DuShane and Kirklin.[D2]

Key: *P$_{\overline{PA}}$,* Mean pulmonary artery pressure; *Rp,* pulmonary vascular resistance.

reported that aortic valve regurgitation was detected by echocardiography in 6 of 23 patients (26%; CL16%-39%) having neither aortic valve prolapse nor regurgitation before operation.[T1] Aortic valve regurgitation in these patients was silent and asymptomatic.

Pulmonary Hypertension

When severe pulmonary hypertension persists after operation, it may worsen with passage of time and may cause premature late death.[D2,F3,H3] About 25% of patients with preoperative pulmonary hypertension and high Rp (at least 10 units · m^2) die with pulmonary hypertension within 5 years of operation (Fig. 21-33).[B1] However, some patients with pulmonary hypertension and elevated Rp late postoperatively have neither progression nor regression of their disease for as long as 20 years, although they have some limitation in exercise tolerance.[D2,H10]

In general, the younger the child at time of repair, the better are the child's chances of surviving and having an essentially normal P$_{PA}$ 5 years and more later (Fig. 21-34).[B3,C8,D2,H8,L4,M2,S16,Y2] The lower the Rp at repair, the better are the chances of having normal pressure late postoperatively (Fig. 21-35). These two factors, age and preoperative Rp, interact in determining late postoperative P$_{PA}$.

A more specific correlate of survival and good outcome in patients with important preoperative pulmonary hypertension is preoperative response to infusion of a pulmonary vascular dilator, such as isoproterenol.[L14,M12,N5] Generally, outcome is good in patients of all ages when preoperative Rp is only mildly or moderately elevated (less than 8 units · m^2) (see Box 21-4). Outcome is good in patients with severely elevated Rp only when it drops

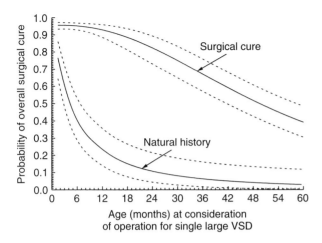

Figure 21-36   Probability of overall surgical cure (survival at least 5 years postoperatively with a mean pulmonary artery pressure of less than 25 mmHg) according to age (months) at repair for all patients with single large ventricular septal defects *(VSD).* Dashed lines enclose 70% confidence limits. Analysis is based on data of DuShane and Kirklin.[D2] Natural history is also shown, with *vertical axis* the probability of long-term survival and ultimate spontaneous closure of the defect and *horizontal axis* the age at observation of a patient with a large VSD. (From Blackstone EH, Kirklin JW: Unpublished study, 1982.)

Key: *VSD,* Ventricular septal defect.

below 7.0 units · m² with preoperative infusion of isoproterenol (Fig. 21-36).[N5] Sodium nitroprusside infusion may also be used and has the advantage of not producing tachycardia.

Surgical Cure

Combining data on P$_{PA}$ late postoperatively with the proportion of patients dying early and late postoperatively, chances of "surgical cure" (defined as surviving the early postoperative period and being alive late postoperatively with essentially normal P$_{PA}$) can be estimated for an individual patient. If repair of a large VSD is performed in a patient at 6 months of age, there is at least a 95% chance of surgical cure, unless preoperative Rp is greater than about 8 units · m² and does not fall to less than 7 units · m² with infusion of isoproterenol (which is rare at that age). This is supported by studies by Rabinovitch and colleagues, in which it was also found that surgical cure is likely to result in any infant in whom the VSD is repaired before age 6 to 9 months, irrespective of degree of pulmonary vascular disease.[R6] In a patient age 2 years, chances of cure are this good only if preoperative Rp is less than about 5 units · m². In a patient operated on for repair of large VSD at age 4 years, chances are that good only if Rp is normal preoperatively (which is unusual). This unfavorable effect of older age has been confirmed by John and colleagues.[J4] This finding supports the practice of repair of large defects at least by age 12 months and can be used to predict results of operation in individual patients.

INDICATIONS FOR OPERATION

When infants with large VSDs have severe and intractable heart failure or respiratory symptoms during the *first 3 months of life,* prompt primary repair of the VSD is indicated. Many such infants have major associated cardiac anomalies, which are repaired simultaneously when appropriate. Exceptions to this practice are made for rare infants with Swiss cheese septum, who present a special problem because of higher risk of surgery. In this setting during the first 3 months of life, pulmonary trunk banding may be indicated; when there are no complications from the band, repair of the Swiss cheese septum and debanding are postponed until age 3 to 5 years. This general plan is also followed when Swiss cheese septum coexists with coarctation of the aorta. Other exceptions to primary repair during the first 3 months of life include infants with straddling tricuspid valve.

Operation is not advised electively in the first 3 months of life in infants without serious symptoms, because the VSD may narrow or close spontaneously.

When presence of severe symptoms, important growth failure, or increasing Rp is present in infants *older than 3 months of age,* prompt primary repair is advised.

When an infant reaches *6 months of age* with a single large VSD, the infant is rarely truly thriving. Probability of cure by spontaneous VSD closure has decreased importantly (Fig. 21-37). If Rp is greater than 8 units · m², repair is advisable without undue delay because delay lessens the chances of surgical cure. If Rp is low (less than 4 units · m²) and the clinical condition reasonably good, operation can be deferred until about 12 months of age in the hope of spontaneous VSD narrowing or closure, although risks of repair are no less than at 6 months of age.

Patients with large VSDs who are first seen *after infancy* (and in some instances after 6 months of age) are considered primarily based on the extent of their pulmonary vascular disease.[K2] When Rp is truly and precisely measured at preoperative cardiac catheterization and is only mildly or moderately elevated (less than 8 units · m²), operation can be undertaken with near certainty that the early and late outcome will be good (see Fig. 21-37).[N5] Such patients usually have a large Q̇p/Q̇s. When Rp is severely elevated (greater than 8 units · m²), an isoproterenol infusion is given during cardiac catheterization (mean dose 0.14 mg · kg⁻¹ · min⁻¹), and Rp is remeasured. If Rp falls to 7 units · m² or less, the response is considered favorable and operation is advised (Fig. 21-38). Otherwise, closure of the VSD is inadvisable. In fact, VSD closure under these circumstances would prevent right-to-left shunting during exercise, resulting in a lower exercise capacity and life expectancy with the defect closed than with it open.

In older patients with a large VSD, a Q̇p/Q̇s of 1.5 to 1.8 at rest that becomes 1.0 or less during moderate exercise (from systemic peripheral vasodilatation, increased systemic blood flow, and a fixed and high Rp preventing increased Q̇p) is an indication of probable inoperability. Simple finding of an important fall in SaO₂ during exercise (from right-to-left shunting across the VSD for the reasons described) also suggests inoperability, but a more complete investigation with determination of response to infusion of isoproterenol is required for a final decision. Response of

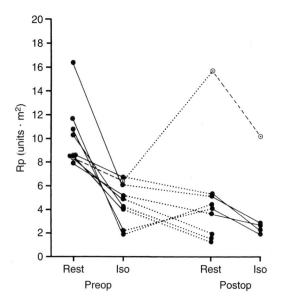

Figure 21-37 Preoperative and late postoperative pulmonary arteriolar resistance in patients with preoperatively severely elevated pulmonary vascular resistance, responsive to isoproterenol infusion. Dashed lines represent a patient whose ventricular septal defect repair dehisced postoperatively. (From Neutze and colleagues.[N5])

Key: Iso, Isoproterenol; Preop, preoperative; Postop, postoperative; Rp, pulmonary vascular resistance.

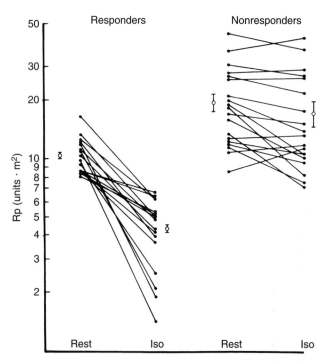

Figure 21-38 Pulmonary arteriolar resistance in patients with severe elevation of resistance (resting resistance 8 units · m² or greater) at rest and with infusion of isoproterenol. Responders experienced a fall in resistance to less than 7 units · m²; nonresponders did not. (From Neutze and colleagues.[N5])

Key: Iso, Isoproterenol; Rp, pulmonary vascular resistance.

Rp to inhalation of mixtures high in oxygen is not useful in determining operability in borderline situations.

Children with a moderate-sized VSD insufficient to raise systolic P_{PA} above 40 to 50 mmHg will not develop elevation of Rp, but it produces a $\dot{Q}p/\dot{Q}s$ of up to 3.0, moderate cardiomegaly, and pulmonary plethora, accompanied by few if any symptoms. Such patients are kept under observation for about 5 years because there may be spontaneous reduction in size or closure of the VSD. During this time, serial studies by two-dimensional echocardiography with Doppler color flow mapping are helpful in assessing change in size of the VSD.[H19] If the defect narrows appreciably or closes, surgery is no longer considered. If there is no change, closure is indicated.

Young patients with small VSDs are not advised to undergo repair. When they reach about 10 years of age, the situation is controversial. In favor of avoiding operation are (1) the possibility that the defect may still close spontaneously; (2) that its only adverse effect is possible bacterial endocarditis, which is easily treated; and (3) that operation carries a small risk. In favor of repair are (1) the possibility of infective endocarditis, with its morbidity and risk, however small; (2) the very real psychological impact of the defect on the adolescent and young adult; (3) the ventricular dysfunction that can develop even when the VSD is small; and (4) the high probability of complete cure by operation. Each patient must therefore be considered according to individual circumstances.

Doubly committed subarterial and juxtaaortic VSDs constitute a special situation.[R10] Even though apparently small, they should not be left untreated if there is any aortic cusp deformity on two-dimensional echocardiography or cineangiography, to prevent development of aortic regurgitation. These defects should be repaired promptly if an aortic diastolic murmur develops.

SPECIAL SITUATIONS AND CONTROVERSIES

Ventricular Septal Defect and Patent Ductus Arteriosus

Combination of large VSD and moderate or large patent ductus arteriosus (PDA) is particularly likely to cause severe symptoms and require operation early in infancy.[B3] During the first 6 to 8 weeks of life in patients with a very large ductus and only a moderate-sized or small VSD, the PDA alone may be repaired, because the VSD may narrow or close spontaneously. If this does not occur, the VSD is closed at an appropriate time. When the VSD is large, both it and the PDA are closed simultaneously if operation is required in early life. Risk of operation should not be higher than that for isolated VSD.

Ventricular Septal Defect and Coarctation of Aorta

Combination of VSD and aortic coarctation frequently causes severe symptoms in infancy. Both coarctation and VSD are variable in severity. Clearly, the worst combination is a large VSD and severe coarctation, but even a small VSD in association with important coarctation may produce heart failure relatively early in life.

■ **TABLE 21-12   Hospital Mortality after Initial Operation in Infants with Ventricular Septal Defect and Coarctation of Aorta** [a]

| | 1961–1969 | | | | 1969–1978 | | | |
| | | Hospital Deaths | | | | Hospital Deaths | | |
Type of Operation	*n*	No.	%	CL (%)	*n*	No.	%	CL (%)
Large VSD and Severe Coarctation								
Coarctectomy plus VSD repair					2 [b]	1	50	7–93
Coarctectomy [c]	7	4	57	32–80	5 [b]	2	40	14–71
Coarctectomy plus PT banding	4	2	50	18–82	8 [b,d]	0	0	0–21
Large VSD and Moderate Coarctation								
VSD repair	1	0	0	0–85	6	1	17	2–46
Small VSD and Coarctation								
Coarctectomy	2	0	0	0–61	7	0	0	0–24
Total	14	6	43	27–60	28	4	14	7–24

Key: *CL*, 70% confidence limits; *PT*, pulmonary trunk; *VSD*, ventricular septal defect.

[a] Data are from 42 patients operated on at GLH from 1961 to 1978.
[b] All were under age 3 months at initial operation.
[c] From 1961 to 1971, 6 (50%; CL 32%–68%) of 12 infants so treated died.
[d] Seven had a subsequent second-stage VSD repair, with 1 death (Swiss cheese septum).

■ **TABLE 21-13   Hospital Mortality in Patients with Ventricular Septal Defect and Coarctation of Aorta According to Method of Management** [a]

| | Overall Group | | Resection and End-to-End Anastomosis | | Subclavian Flap | |
Method	*n*	Hospital Deaths	*n*	Hospital Deaths	*n*	Hospital Deaths
Coarctation repair						
Without PT banding	8	1	1	1	7	0
With PT banding	8	2	4	1	3	0
One-stage primary repair	3	1 [b]	3	1		
Two-stage repair done during same hospitalization	1	0			1	0
Total	20	4	8	3	11	0
		20		38		0
CL (%)		10–33		17–62		0–16

Key: *CL*, 70% confidence limits; *PT*, pulmonary trunk.

[a] Data from 20 patients who were under age 1 year at operation at UAB, 1967 to 1981. One patient not depicted in table had patch graft repair and died of hemorrhage on postoperative day 3.
[b] Patient had multiple VSDs.

Management options for this combination of defects include simultaneous repair of both lesions,[B3] initial repair of the coarctation alone,[N2] initial coarctation repair and pulmonary trunk banding, or initial VSD closure alone.[R3] With a large VSD and severe coarctation, repair of the VSD first has certain theoretic advantages[R3] but has been practiced rarely under such circumstances. *Repair of the coarctation only* as the initial operation has the advantage of reducing afterload on the LV and, theoretically at least, reducing shunt through the defect. It also avoids a second operation if the VSD closes spontaneously.[N2] Mortality with repair of aortic coarctation in this setting has been high in the past (Table 21-12).[N2] More recent experience with this repair has been good (Table 21-13). Malm and colleagues also have had good results with this protocol, with two (11%; CL 4%-28%) hospital deaths in 17 patients so treated.[M8] Four (27%; CL 14%-43%) of the 15 survivors required repair of the VSD in early infancy, and two (13%; CL 4%-29%) required it later. Nine (60%; CL 43%-75%) hospital survivors experienced spontaneous closure or narrowing of their VSD within the follow-up period (2 to 10 years). These results have subse-

quently been corroborated.[P5] The results have also been good with *initial coarctation repair with pulmonary trunk banding* (see Table 21-12).

Simultaneous repair of both the coarctation and a large VSD in the past has carried a high risk in the first few months of life (Table 21-13).[B1,B3,N2] The only exception is the experience of Tiraboschi and colleagues, but only one of their four patients was under 3 months of age.[T10,T11] However, good results have been obtained during the current era. Simultaneous repair of both defects has been reported in five infants (ages 3 weeks to 9 months), with one death (20%; CL 3%-53%), a 3-week-old infant.[B3] A reasonable practice is as follows:

1. When the VSD is large, the coarctation severe, and the infant presents in the first few months of life with severe and intractable heart failure, which is the usual situation, the coarctation is repaired at urgent operation. The baby is closely followed. If severe heart failure persists, the VSD is repaired a few days or a few weeks later, as may be required. When Swiss cheese septum is present, the pulmonary trunk is banded, and debanding and repair

■ **TABLE 21-14   Hospital Mortality after Pulmonary Artery Banding for Ventricular Septal Defect** [a]

Type of VSD	n	Hospital Deaths			
		No.	%	CL (%)	
Swiss cheese	7	1	14	2-41	*P* = .7
Other	30	3	10	4-19	
TOTAL	37	4	11	6-19	

Key: *CL,* 70% confidence limits; *VSD,* ventricular septal defect.

[a] Data from 37 patients, including those with coexisting coarctation of aorta, operated on at GLH from 1961 to 1978.

are delayed if possible until the patient is about 5 years of age.

2. When the VSD is large, the coarctation severe, and the infant presents beyond the first few months of life, simultaneous repair of both anomalies may be performed, or occasionally the coarctation alone may be repaired and the plan outlined above followed.

3. When the coarctation is severe and VSD small, only the coarctation is repaired, and the results are those of coarctation repair in general (see Table 21-13). Subsequent repair of the VSD is rarely required.

4. When the coarctation is moderate in severity and VSD large, the VSD may be repaired initially and the coarctation repair postponed until the patient is 6 to 12 months of age. Techniques of CPB are standard, with perfusion of the lower body satisfactory in this situation. Alternatively, if both lesions seem clearly in need of repair and the infant is older than a few months of age, both lesions may be repaired simultaneously.

Pulmonary Trunk Banding

Civin and Edwards noted good prognosis and freedom from pulmonary vascular disease of patients with single ventricle and moderate pulmonary stenosis.[C7] Based on that observation, Muller and Dammann performed pulmonary trunk banding in 1952.[M3] For many years thereafter, this procedure was used by many for infants who required operation for large VSD, thereby allowing deferral of the intracardiac repair until an older age.[M4,O1,P1]

Currently, banding is seldom indicated for primary isolated large VSDs, for several reasons. Hospital mortality of patients with pulmonary trunk banding has been important, and a second operation, which carries an additional mortality, is always required.[G1,H4,H5] Hospital mortality reported in the literature for pulmonary trunk banding in the first year of life is 16%.[K6,S3-S5] Early mortality is independent of type of VSD (Table 21-14). It is difficult to adjust the tightness of the band perfectly, and reentry a few days later may be needed for modification of the tightness. Furthermore, good palliation is not always achieved by banding, and there may be an important intermediate mortality before second-stage repair. Complications result from banding in some patients, including development of infundibular and valvar pulmonary stenosis, subaortic stenosis,[F2] and migration of the band to the pulmonary trunk bifurcation (Fig. 21-39). Hospital mortality from pulmonary trunk debanding and VSD repair has been about 10% (see Table 21-10), and the debanding operation is technically more demanding than is primary repair. Furthermore, restenosis

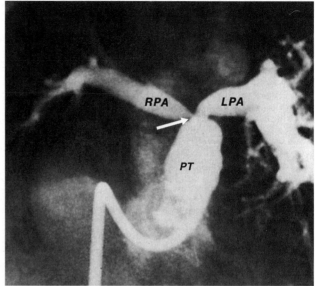

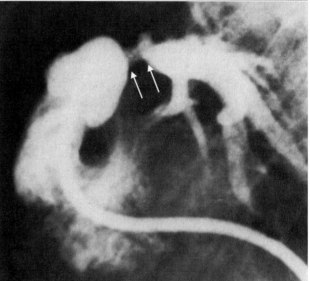

Figure 21-39   Angiograms of 4-year-old patient who had previously undergone pulmonary trunk banding. **A,** Pulmonary artery injection in frontal view of sitting-up position. Arrow indicates position of band at bifurcation of pulmonary trunk and narrowing of origin of right and left pulmonary arteries. **B,** Lateral view. Width of pulmonary band is indicated by two arrows as well as by its migration to bifurcation.

Key: *LPA,* Left pulmonary artery; *PT,* pulmonary trunk; *RPA,* right pulmonary artery.

of the pulmonary trunk may follow debanding and repair of the VSD, necessitating a third operation.[K6]

Pulmonary trunk banding as an initial palliative procedure in very young patients may still be appropriate in some centers.[S15] For a number of years, however, there have been only two indications for pulmonary trunk banding in infants with primary VSD: (1) severe heart failure from Swiss cheese septum and (2) associated severe coarctation of the aorta and severe heart failure during the first few months of life. The second is no longer an indication for banding.

Right Atrial versus Right Ventricular Approach for Perimembranous Ventricular Septal Defect

The right ventricular approach may be used for repair of perimembranous VSDs and results in a low hospital mortality even in patients with high Rp. The RV approach has the advantage that the nadir of the noncoronary cusp of the aortic valve, which is the area of the right trigone and bundle of His, can be accurately visualized, which may be helpful in choosing the suture technique that will minimize prevalence of heart block (see Fig. 21-26). The RV approach has the disadvantages of (1) leaving a scar in the RV, (2) being associated with a higher prevalence of complete RBBB than with an atrial approach, and (3) possibly resulting in more ventricular arrhythmias late postoperatively.

The right atrial approach may be used almost exclusively, a practice begun in about 1960 at the Mayo Clinic.[C3] An accurate repair can be obtained through a right atrial approach in nearly all cases. Associated infundibular pulmonary stenosis can be excised. An RV scar is avoided, and occurrence of RBBB is lower than with the transventricular approach.[H13] With the right atrial approach, however, techniques must be accurate to avoid damage to the tricuspid valve leaflets or chordae.

Percutaneous Closure of Ventricular Septal Defects

In selected cases, especially in patients with complex cardiac anomalies (e.g., multiple muscular VSDs) and those with overlooked VSDs after surgical repair of a large defect, transcatheter closure of the VSD by a percutaneously placed double umbrella can be considered.[B14,L16] This may be particularly advantageous in apical muscular defects.[K20] These devices may also be deployed intraoperatively.[A11,M18] This method in general should be considered only when surgery is contraindicated or has unusually high risks and when suitable skill and equipment are available.

A current perception is that primary multiple muscular VSDs, particularly those near the apex, are more suitably closed by a percutaneous catheter technique than by operation. This remains unproven, however, particularly in those multiple muscular VSDs that can be closed from the right atrium after taking down the septal band.[P5] The technique is a promising one, but additional experience and information are required for definitive evaluation.

Closure of Ventricular Septal Defect When Pulmonary Resistance Is High

Patients with VSD in which pulmonary hypertension is severe with P_{PA} at or above systemic blood pressure have traditionally been thought to be inoperable because of high risk of operation. Zhou and colleagues reported use of unidirectional valve patch closure of cardiac septal defects with severe pulmonary hypertension.[Z2] There was a ventricular septal defect in 22 of 24 patients in the series. All had marked elevation of P_{PA} (80 ± 12 mm Hg) and increased pulmonary to systemic pressure ratio (1.1 ± 0.11). SaO_2 was reduced to $88\% \pm 4\%$. The patch consisted of

polyester fabric with a 0.5- to 1.0-cm hole covered by a pericardial patch left open at one side to function as a one-way valve. The pericardial flap valve was placed on the systemic side of the defect. Two patients died after operation (8.3%). Pulmonary artery pressure fell to 56 ± 19 and pulmonary to systemic pressure ratio dropped to 0.7 ± 0.1 while SaO_2 rose to $96\% \pm 1\%$. Excellent improvement of functional state was also noted. These results were corroborated by Ad and colleagues while claiming earlier right of discovery of this method (see Fig. 16-27 in Chapter 16).[A14-A16]

SECTION 2

Ventricular Septal Defect and Aortic Regurgitation

DEFINITION

Ventricular septal defect and aortic regurgitation (AR) syndrome includes hearts in which AR is of congenital origin, although rarely present at birth, caused by cusp prolapse or a bicuspid aortic valve. The VSD is either doubly committed subarterial or perimembranous (with outlet extension or simply juxta-aortic). These locations are in fact a continuum, with the subarterial VSD lying farthest to the patient's left (and anteriorly), the perimembranous VSD with outlet extension lying more rightward (and slightly inferior) than the subarterial, and the perimembranous juxta-aortic VSD lying still more rightward (and inferiorly).

VSD–AR syndrome is related to congenital sinus of Valsalva aneurysm (see Chapter 22) and tetralogy of Fallot with aortic regurgitation (see Chapter 24).

HISTORICAL NOTE

Initial description of the syndrome of VSD with AR caused by aortic cusp prolapse is attributed to Laubry and Pezzi's publication in 1921.[L6] First reports of operative correction were those of Garamella and Starr and their colleagues in 1960.[G6,S12]

Experience at the Mayo Clinic began at about the same time.[K9] On review of this experience in 1963, of the 30 patients in whom the aortic valve cusps were reconstructed and repaired, 10 (33%; CL 24%-44%) still had important AR.[E2] This and other reports in which results of cusp reconstruction were equally unsatisfactory[T3] led to adoption of aortic valve replacement using either an allograft[G5] or prosthetic valve. During this period, operations were delayed beyond childhood whenever possible to avoid valve replacement in the young age group. Renewed interest in use of cusp reconstruction dates from publications of Spencer and Trusler and their colleagues in 1973, which followed the work of Frater.[F7,S9,T4]

Tatsuno and colleagues in Japan have done much to elucidate the nature of the anomaly and document the good results obtained by closure of the VSD alone when AR is mild.[T5-T7]

MORPHOLOGY

Perimembranous VSDs are the most prevalent among predominantly Caucasian patients with VSD and AR[L15,M11] (Table 21-15). Among Asians with VSD and AR, VSDs are more prevalent in the right ventricular (RV) outlet and particularly doubly committed subarterial VSDs (Table 21-16).[H16,H17,O9] AR is most often caused by prolapse of the right cusp of the aortic valve (about two thirds of patients). The remaining one third of patients have prolapse of the noncoronary cusp or of both noncoronary and right coronary cusps, with about equal prevalence in the two groups. Infrequently, no cusp is prolapsing, but the aortic valve is bicuspid and regurgitant.

Variable degrees of RV outflow obstruction are present in many patients (see Table 21-15). In the GLH experience, no gradient was present in nine (24%) of 37 patients, a gradient of less than 20 mmHg in 51% and of 20 to 40 mmHg in 24% (the gradient was unknown in four patients). The infundibular septum may be underdeveloped and displaced anteriorly and leftward[V1] (malaligned as in tetralogy of Fallot), a feature responsible for mild infundibular stenosis that may be present. Occasionally, RV trabeculae near the junction of the infundibular septum and free wall may contribute to infundibular stenosis, as may hypertrophy of the moderator band at a lower level. Thus, Keane and colleagues found that typical low-lying infundibular pulmonary stenosis (double-chambered right ventricle) accounted for the gradient in some patients.[K7]

The aortic root and valve exhibit a variety of anomalies. Cusps may prolapse not only into but at times through the VSD. Protrusion through the VSD increases during diastole and effectively plugs the defect, limiting the shunt even when the defect is large. Extensive cusp prolapse through a large VSD can also produce some obstruction to RV outflow. In advanced cases the center of the prolapsed free margin of the cusp is thickened and retracted, a feature that makes resuspension of the leaflet relatively ineffective. Some patients have additional damage produced by endocarditis.

The sinus of Valsalva adjacent to the prolapsed leaflet is enlarged, often considerably. This enlarged sinus is associated with asymmetric splaying and dilatation of the aortic "anulus," a feature aggravated by severe AR and volume changes in the LV. It is virtually impossible to distinguish the junction between the prolapsed cusp and dilated sinus at cineangiography and at times at operation. The wall of the enlarged sinus may be thinned and aneurysmal adjacent to the cusp hinge line and rarely may protrude into the RV immediately above the prolapsed cusp. Such a finding indicates the close similarity between this condition and that of ruptured congenital sinus of Valsalva aneurysm with VSD.

Mechanism of cusp prolapse and AR is uncertain. It may result from lack of support of the aortic sinus of Valsalva and "anulus" by the infundibular septum,[T6,V1] although because most large perimembranous defects are closely adjacent to the aortic "anulus" and very few have associated regurgitation, this cannot be the entire explanation. A structural defect in the base of the sinus itself may also play a role, particularly when the VSD is small.[E3] Hemodynamic influences during both systole and diastole aggravate the tendencies toward AR.[T6] Such influences are more marked

■ **TABLE 21-15**　Characteristics of Surgical Patients with Ventricular Septal Defect and Aortic Regurgitation [a]

	Prevalence	
Characteristic	**n**	**% of 48**
VSD Location		
RV outlet	17	35
Perimembranous	31	65
VSD Size		
Small	10	21
Moderate	16	33
Large	22	46
Aortic Cusp Anomaly		
Right cusp prolapse	37	77
Noncoronary cusp prolapse	5	10
Both cusps prolapsed	4	8
Bicuspid valve	2	4
Infective endocarditis	4	8
Sinus of Valsalva		
Aneurysm (unruptured)	7	15
Magnitude of AR		
Severe	25	52
Moderate	10	21
Mild	13	27
Magnitude of PS		
Mild to moderate	9	19
Aortic Valve Procedure [b]		
Reconstruction	26	54
Valve replacement	12	25
None	10	21

Key: *AR*, Aortic regurgitation; *PS*, pulmonary stenosis (infundibular) with gradient >15 mmHg; *RV*, right ventricle; *VSD*, ventricular septal defect.

[a] Data from 48 patients operated on at GLH from 1960 to 1982. Mean age and range (years) were 17.6 (2/12 to 44).
[b] All also had repair of VSD.

■ **TABLE 21-16**　Type of Ventricular Septal Defect and Severity of Aortic Regurgitation in 86 Japanese Patients

		RV Outlet VSD		Perimembranous VSD	
Degree/Type of AR	**n**	**No.**	**%**	**No.**	**%**
Mild	40	35	88	5	12
With cusp prolapse					
Moderate	14	12	86	2	14
Severe	10	9	90	1	10
Without cusp prolapse	22	17	77	5	23
TOTAL	86	73	85	13	15

(Data from Tatsuno and colleagues.[T7])

Key: *AR*, Aortic regurgitation; *RV*, right ventricular; *VSD*, ventricular septal defect.

once AR develops, resulting in progressive prolapse and distortion.

Yacoub and colleagues proposed that the basic abnormality is discontinuity of the aortic media from the aortic "anulus" (hinge point of the aortic cusp) and the ventricular septum in the region of the right coronary sinus.[Y5] This results in weakness of the area with progressive dilatation of the sinus and downward and outward displacement of the aortic "anulus." Progressive changes are the result of hemodynamic factors operating during the cardiac cycle.

The fast jet produced by the left-to-right shunt through the slitlike VSD during early systole results in a Venturi effect, tending to displace the unsupported "anulus" outward and downward into the RV. Later in systole the aortic cusp prolapses into the VSD and is acted on by direct pressure from the cavity of the LV, displacing both "anulus" and cusp into the RV. During diastole the high pressure in the aortic root distends the dilated sinus, with further displacement of the aortic "anulus" toward the RV. As the sinus dilates, the distending force becomes greater due to increase in wall tension.

CLINICAL FEATURES AND DIAGNOSTIC CRITERIA

Potential for development of AR can be assessed by noting the possible presence of aortic cusp prolapse at cineangiography. Thus, Tatsuno and colleagues found prolapse of the right aortic cusp in 10 (42%; CL 30%-54%) of 24 patients with a subarterial defect in whom AR had not yet occurred.[T7] Exact prevalence of leaflet prolapse with or without AR in perimembranous VSDs is unknown, but it is clearly much less.

In patients with mild regurgitation, such as younger patients, signs of the VSD dominate the clinical picture, but as AR increases, the shunt decreases. Such patients characteristically have a to-and-fro murmur, which may simulate the continuous murmur of PDA but occasionally may be mistaken for that of isolated AR or combined AR and stenosis.

Studies in such patients should include two-dimensional echocardiography with Doppler flow velocity evaluation. Anatomic relationships of the aortic valve and VSD should be easily demonstrated. AR is estimated qualitatively. Aortic root dimensions are measured accurately. Usually, echocardiography provides sufficient information on which to base clinical decisions.

In some patients it is desirable to have cardiac catheterization, which should include (1) right-sided heart catheterization (for calculating shunt and measuring pressures in the pulmonary artery and RV), (2) right ventriculography (for studying possible infundibular pulmonary stenosis), (3) left ventriculography (for identifying location and size of VSD), and (4) aortography (for estimating the magnitude of AR and morphology of the aortic root). Finding a normal aortic root diameter without cusp prolapse suggests that regurgitation is caused by a bicuspid valve and may not be amenable to repair. Anatomic size of the VSD cannot be demonstrated angiographically when, as often occurs, it is occluded throughout the cardiac cycle by the prolapsed aortic cusp.

NATURAL HISTORY

Prevalence of AR among patients with VSD is uncertain; in the combined UAB–GLH surgical series the prevalence was 11%. In a review of 756 young patients with VSD studied at Boston Children's Hospital between 1948 and 1962, Nadas and colleagues reported a prevalence of 4.5%.[N1] Prevalence is related in part to age at which the population is studied, because this complication is rare before age 2 years. Prevalence is also related to the

frequency with which subarterial VSDs occur in the population studied, because AR is more common with this type of defect.[D4,P3] The latter relationship explains the relatively high prevalence of VSD and AR reported from Japan[K8,T7,T15] and China.[L9]

Aortic valve regurgitation does not usually appear until age 2 to 5 years.[C9,D3] However, three patients operated on at ages 2, 3, and 7 months had associated mild AR, and one operated on at age 22 months had moderate AR. Once AR appears, it gradually increases and within 10 years is usually severe. This rate of progression is similar whether the VSD is subarterial or perimembranous. At repair the AR is mild to moderate in about half of patients and severe in about half (see Table 21-15).

Secondary effects of AR on the LV are at least as marked as those of rheumatic AR and may be more severe because of additional volume load from the VSD. Rp is seldom if ever elevated, presumably because functionally the VSD is usually not large. Risk of infective endocarditis is high.[R10]

Aneurysms of the sinuses of Valsalva also may develop as part of the natural history of patients with doubly committed subarterial VSD or perimembranous VSD with outlet extension. This is a slower process than is development of AR, and Momma and colleagues did not observe sinus of Valsalva aneurysms before age 10 years in patients with perimembranous VSDs.[M9] Most often the aneurysm is observed during the third decade, when it may be present in 10% of patients whose VSDs of these types are still open.[M9]

TECHNIQUE OF OPERATION

In patients in whom AR is trivial or absent, only the VSD is repaired. When AR is important (moderate or severe) and often when it is mild, the aortic valve is repaired.[M5] The aortic valve is usually replaced in adults, and this is done only when the AR is moderate or severe.

Transesophageal echocardiography (TEE) is performed after induction of anesthesia and before incision for a final analysis of the aortic valve and VSD. Operation is performed on CPB, with cold cardioplegia for myocardial protection. A transverse aortotomy is made. Dimensions of the aortic root are measured at the ventriculoaortic junction ("anulus") and sinotubular junction. These dimensions are compared with normal valves adjusted for size of the patient (see "Dimensions of Normal Cardiac and Great Artery Pathways" in Chapter 1). The aortic valve is examined to assess feasibility of repair rather than replacement. If the cusp edge is retracted and thickened or the valve bicuspid, repair is usually not possible.

One or more leaflets may be repaired by the Trusler method of plication (Fig. 21-40).[T4] This procedure is carried out at the commissure adjacent to the prolapsed cusp (usually the right or noncoronary cusp). A No. 5-0 or 6-0 polypropylene suture is placed through the fibrous lacunae at the midpoint of each leaflet. Leaflets can then be assessed for elongation and attenuation. A leaflet plication is performed at the elongated free edges of the aortic valve leaflets. A No. 5-0 or 6-0 PTFE suture is woven between the right and noncoronary cusps to adjust the excessive length of the prolapsed cusp to the adjacent aortic wall. Repair may be reinforced by pledgets (pericardial or felt).

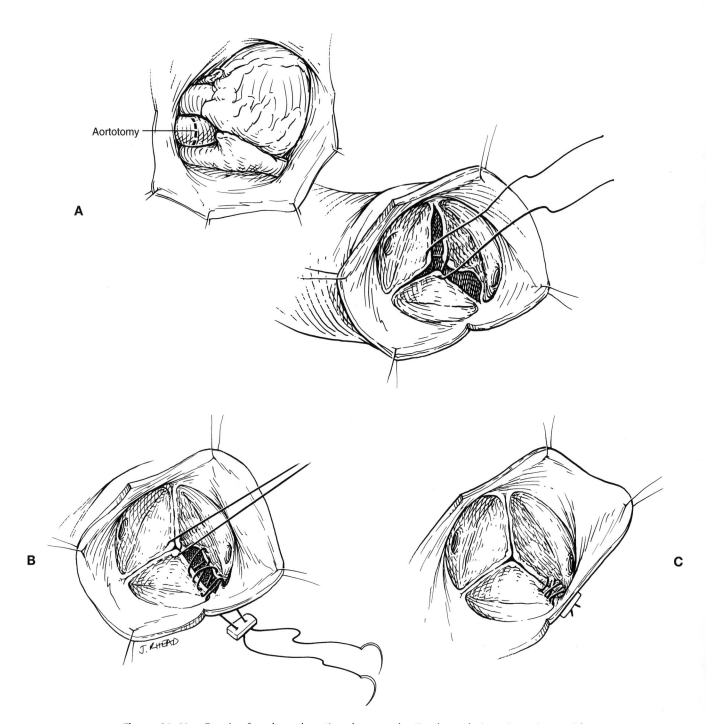

Figure 21-40   Repair of prolapsed aortic valve cusp by Trusler technique in patients with ventricular septal defect and aortic valve regurgitation. **A,** Transverse aortotomy is made at a level just downstream from commissural attachments of aortic valve. **B,** Stitch of No. 5-0 or 6-0 polypropylene is placed through midpoint of each cusp. Traction on this stitch allows identification of redundant or elongated free edges of a cusp, as shown here in the case of right coronary cusp near its commissure with noncoronary cusp. **C,** A No. 5-0 or 6-0 polytetrafluoroethylene suture is used to "reef up" redundant and attenuated portions of aortic valve. A double row of reefing stitches is used to bring ends of suture to outside of aorta at commissures. A pledget is added to strengthen repair.

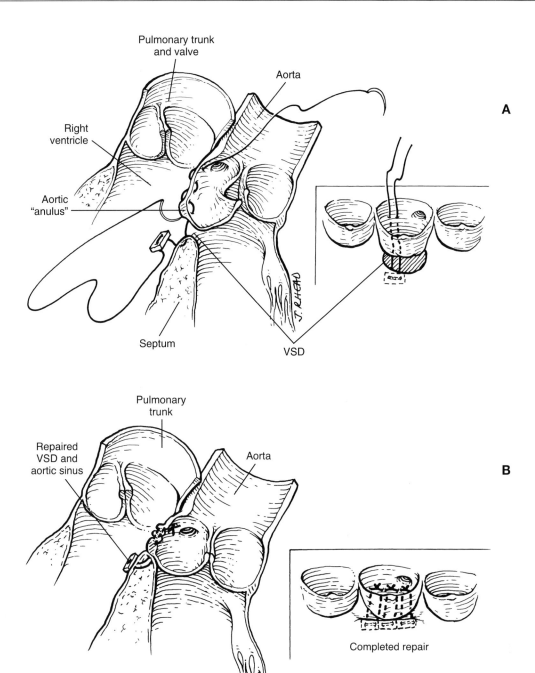

Figure 21-41   Repair of aortic valve in syndrome of ventricular septal defect *(VSD)* and aortic valve regurgitation by Yacoub technique. **A,** Aortic valve and VSD are approached through a transverse aortotomy. Morphologic defect causing lack of coaptation of aortic cusps is considered to be discontinuity between aortic media and "anulus" of aortic valve, resulting in lack of support to "anulus" and sinus of Valsalva, with downward and outward displacement of "anulus" into right ventricle. VSD is closed by plication suture, which elevates crest of septum to aortic media and plicates unsupported sinus of Valsalva. A series of interrupted mattress stitches using No. 4-0 braided polyester suture with pericardial pledgets are placed from crest of ventricular septum slightly toward its right ventricular aspect. Stitches are passed through "anulus" of aortic valve and reefed through unsupported sinus of Valsalva to strong tissue of aortic media. **B,** Stitches are tied down (knots inside aortic sinus), elevating ventricular crest to aortic valve "anulus" to close VSD as well as displacing "anulus" and aortic valve leaflet centrally to achieve greater aortic leaflet coaptation, restoring valve competence. (Modified from Yacoub and colleagues.[Y5])

Key: *VSD,* Ventricular septal defect.

Hisatomi and colleagues proposed pledget stitch aorto-plasty to make the aortic cusps protrude for even greater aortic valve coaptation.[H20,H21] The stitch at the center of the valve is removed after VSD repair.

Approach to the VSD is appropriate to the location of the defect and may be transaortic if the defect is accessible. Any infundibular stenosis is relieved by excising trabecular muscle bands between infundibular septum and free wall of the RV and, when necessary, by mobilizing and excising parietal and septal extensions of the infundibular septum and portions of the moderator bands.

An entirely different technique has been successfully used by Carpentier, Chauvaud and colleagues.[C15,C16] Its basic feature is triangular excision and reconstruction of the prolapsing cusp. Combined with this is an anuloplasty of the left ventriculoaortic junction. They also recommend that the VSD be repaired through the aortic root, using a glutaraldehyde-treated pericardial patch.

Yacoub and colleagues have proposed another alternative method of repair (Fig. 21-41) that addresses the basic morphologic defect more completely.[Y5] All anatomic components of the defect are corrected by a simple transaortic repair. A transverse aortotomy is made (Fig. 21-41, A). Extent of dilatation of the right coronary sinus and exact definition of the thin area of sinus resulting from discontinuity between aortic valve "anulus" and media of aorta are accurately defined. A series of pledget-reinforced mattress sutures are placed through the crest of the ventricular septum slightly on the RV side to avoid injuring the conduction system. The sutures are passed through the "anulus" of the aortic valve and then used to plicate the thin portion of the sinus of Valsalva and continued until strong aortic tissue supported by aortic media is reached. Tying of sutures results in closing the VSD, elevating the right coronary anulus and cusp, and reducing the size of the right coronary sinus and RV outflow tract bulge (Fig. 21-41, B). Repair of the defect is possible in all cases regardless of size of the VSD, which is usually slitlike, because there are always redundant tissues in the septum and aortic sinus in the vertical plane. Plication of redundant tissues toward the media of the aortic sinus elevates the aortic valve cusp and anulus, displacing them centrally toward the lumen of the aorta. This results in increased aortic valve coaptation and restored aortic valve competence. This operation can be applied to patients with doubly committed subarterial ventricular septal defects with AR and thus may apply to the Asian population, in whom these types of defects are common.

If the valve requires replacement, the RV (or pulmonary trunk) should be opened before valve insertion, the VSD repaired, the RV closed, and then the aortic valve replaced. This sequence is advised because occasionally it may be necessary to place sutures from the prosthetic valve ring across the upper margin of the VSD patch, where it extends between the base of the right and noncoronary cusps (in the region normally occupied by the membranous septum). Sutures in this area should be securely buttressed with pledgets of PTFE felt. Although a freehand allograft has been used successfully for valve replacement under such circumstances,[G5] degree of distortion of the aortic sinuses often makes its precise placement difficult.[B10] Allograft aortic root replacement or aortic valve replacement with a pulmonary autograft (Ross procedure) is probably a better choice (see "Autograft Pulmonary Valve" under Technique of Operation in Chapter 12).

When there is also a true thin-walled aneurysm of the sinus of Valsalva at the base of the right aortic cusp and a VSD, repair is more difficult because the sinus must also be repaired. If the aortic valve requires excision and replacement, excision should include the base of the cusp and the thinned area of the sinus wall, which becomes continuous with the VSD and is incorporated into its closure. Again, under such circumstances, the prosthetic valve suture line will cross the polyester patch. Aortic root replacement may be a simpler solution. When the valve is suitable for plication, the base of the cusp is preserved and sutured back to the patch.

RESULTS

No reliable comparison of outcomes after the various techniques of operation is currently available.

Survival

Only one of 76 patients operated on by the UAB and GLH groups died in hospital (1.3%; CL 0.2%-4.4%), and at last follow-up, no late deaths had occurred, an experience similar to that of Okita and colleagues over an 18-year follow-up and Yacoub and colleagues over 24 years with a mean follow-up of 8.4 years.[O9,Y5]

Heart Block

Heart block occurs rarely even though operation is in the region of the conduction system. In Yacoub and colleagues' series of 38 patients, there were no cases of conduction abnormality, and ECG remained normal.[Y5]

Relief of Aortic Regurgitation

When AR is mild, closure of the VSD alone usually prevents progression of regurgitation. When AR is moderate before repair, about two thirds of patients have no or trivial AR after repair using the Trusler technique (Table 21-17).[E4,H5,H16,O11,T4,T13] Infrequently, AR is severe preoperatively, and chances of a good result are decreased in this setting.

When the Carpentier method has been used, results are also reported to be good.[C15] Yacoub and colleagues reported that 38 patients were operated on using their technique over 24 years.[Y5] Aortic valve competence was restored in 25 patients (65%). In the remainder of the patients, additional plication or resection of the aortic valve was required.

Okita and colleagues have determined perimembranous VSD (rather than VSDs in the RV outlet) to be a risk factor for important residual AR, possibly because factors other than cusp prolapse are partly responsible for preoperative AR when the VSD is perimembranous.[O9] Bicuspid aortic valves are less satisfactorily repaired than are tricuspid ones.

Older age at operation also contributes to presence of important AR after repair.

■ **TABLE 21-17   Grade of Aortic Regurgitation (AR) Late after Repair of Ventricular Septal Defect and AR, According to Preoperative AR Grade** [a]

| | | Postoperative AR Grade | | | | | | | | | | |
| | | None | | Mild | | Mild to Moderate | | Moderate | | Moderate to Severe | | Severe | |
Preoperative AR Grade	n	No.	%	No.	%	No.	%	No.	%	No.	%	No.	%
Mild	10	2	20	1	10	6	60	1	10	0	0	0	0
Mild to moderate	4	0	0	1	25	1	25	1	25	0	0	1 [b]	25
Moderate	12	4	33	4	33	2	17	0	0	1	8	1 [b]	8
Moderate to severe	9	3	33	4	44	1	11	1	11	0	0	0	0
Severe	1	0	0	0	0	0	0	1	100	0	0	0	0
TOTAL	36	9	25	10	28	10	28	4	11	1	3	2	6

(Data from Maehera and colleagues.[M11])

Key: *AR,* Aortic regurgitation.

[a] Data from 36 patients operated on from 1967 to 1987. Three patients who had aortic valve replacement at the original operation after failure of Trusler repair and two other patients who had missing values for postoperative aortic regurgitation are not included.

[b] These two patients received late postoperative aortic valve replacement.

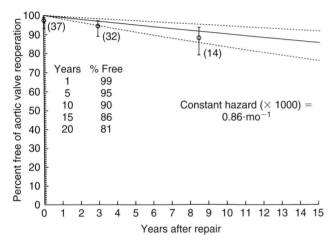

Figure 21-42   Nonparametric *(open circles)* and parametric estimates of freedom from aortic valve reoperation (one second repair, two valve replacements) after repair of ventricular septal defect and aortic regurgitation in 38 patients. (From Maehara and colleagues.[M11])

Freedom from Aortic Valve Replacement

Some patients will probably require aortic valve replacement in later life, although freedom from aortic valve reoperation was 89% at 8 years in the UAB group's series; parametrically predicted freedom at 20 years was 81% (Fig. 21-42).[M11] Elgamal and colleagues confirmed these data, reporting 15-year freedom from reoperation of 81% ± 19% after Trusler repair of the aortic valve.[E4] Adequacy of repair at operation was the most important determinant of long-term results. Yacoub and colleagues report 5 valve replacements among 38 patients 8 to 11 years after operation.[Y5]

INDICATIONS FOR OPERATION

When a child with a VSD first shows development of the murmur of AR, repair of the VSD should be promptly accomplished while the AR is still mild.[T6,T7] If cusp prolapse without AR is demonstrated on the aortogram or by two-dimensional echocardiography, in association with any perimembranous VSD, early repair is also indicated. Even if cusp prolapse has not occurred, doubly committed subarterial and moderate or large perimembranous VSDs with outlet extension should be closed before the patient is about 5 years of age to prevent cusp prolapse.[R10] Patients having doubly committed subarterial VSD should have immediate operation regardless of age, if any aortic valve deformity or regurgitation is detected, because anatomic and hemodynamic features of the VSD have great impact on development of aortic valve cusp deformity and subsequent AR.[K3,K22,O11,S31] When AR is moderate or severe and cusp prolapse is noted on the two-dimensional echocardiogram or aortogram, operation should be undertaken promptly. Operation certainly should be done before the patient is age 10 years, because reconstruction of the valve is usually possible when operation is done during the first decade of life; thus, valve replacement is prevented or at least postponed. This fact is confirmed by the UAB experience, in which the average age of patients requiring replacement was 19.5 years, compared with 12.1 years for the remainder of the group.[M11]

When two-dimensional echocardiography shows bicuspid aortic valve or when the aortogram shows minimal enlargement of the sinuses and no cusp prolapse in the presence of severe AR, a bicuspid valve is probably present, and valve replacement may be required. Operation should therefore be postponed until symptoms develop or LV enlargement indicates need for operation.

When operation is delayed until adult life, aortic valve replacement is usually required.[O8]

SPECIAL SITUATIONS AND CONTROVERSIES

Many surgeons prefer to visualize and repair VSDs through an aortotomy.[C19,L21] This practice can produce good results. However, if the VSD is perimembranous rather than in the RV outflow tract, possibility of permanent damage to the bundle of His may be increased by this essentially LV approach to repair. Because precise location of the VSD may be uncertain preoperatively, repair through the pulmonary trunk or RV is considered prudent.

Smaller incisions (minimally invasive approaches) have been used for closure of VSDs.[B19,L20] Although it is technically feasible to close a VSD successfully through a variety of minimally invasive techniques, no advantages have been demonstrated other than the smaller incision.

SECTION 3

Straddling and Overriding Tricuspid (or Mitral) Valve

A straddling and overriding tricuspid valve sometimes coexists with an otherwise isolated VSD, usually one that extends posteriorly to the crux. Straddling and overriding of an AV valve may also coexist with a VSD that is simply part of a congenital cardiac anomaly, such as transposition of the great arteries, congenitally corrected transposition of the great arteries, and univentricular AV connection. The subject is considered in its entirety in this chapter, with reference to other chapters.

Straddling and overriding of an AV valve always occur in relation to a VSD close to the valve.[K17] When straddling or overriding of an AV valve is mild, surgical considerations are usually related primarily to the associated anomalies. When straddling or overriding is severe, or when there is associated hypoplasia of the ventricle to which the AV valve is appropriately connected, surgical considerations are usually based primarily on straddling and overriding and severity of any coexisting ventricular hypoplasia.

Hypoplasia of the ventricle guarded by the straddling or overriding valve (termed the *appropriate* ventricle) usually coexists. Generally, the more severe the overriding, the greater is the ventricular hypoplasia. Occasionally, a straddling or overriding AV valve has leaflets that differ from normal in number and morphology. Overriding and straddling AV valves may occasionally produce subpulmonary or subaortic obstruction.

DEFINITION

An AV valve is considered to be *straddling* when a part of the tension apparatus of the valve crosses the VSD and the crest of the interventricular septum to attach to the septum or a papillary muscle in the opposite (inappropriate) ventricle. The tension apparatus is thus attached within both ventricles, and blood passing through the valve is directed into both ventricles. An AV valve is considered to be *overriding* when the AV junction to which the AV valve leaflets attach is connected to both ventricles. AV valve straddling and overriding usually occur in combination, and occasionally both AV valves are involved with these anomalies in the same heart.

HISTORICAL NOTE

Lambert in 1951 and Van Praagh and colleagues in 1964 appeared to be aware of AV valve straddling and overriding, although they were not explicit about it.[L17,V6] In 1966, Mehrizi and colleagues referred to overriding and straddling of the right AV valve onto the RV in hearts with double inlet LV and the LV lying posteriorly and to the left.[M14] Subsequently, de la Cruz and Miller in 1968 and Lev and colleagues in 1969 referred to this occurrence in hearts with various types of "single ventricle" (generally double inlet ventricles).[D9,L18]

Rastelli and colleagues reported "straddling right atrioventricular valves" in hearts with a large VSD, but the right AV valve in their cases appears to have been both overriding and straddling.[R2] These investigators identified malalignment of atrial and ventricular septa as the characteristic of hearts with overriding AV valves, along with cleft leaflets often present, and juxtacrucial position of the VSD. Liberthson, one of whose co-authors was Lev, clearly distinguished between overriding and straddling AV valves in hearts with double inlet ventricles in 1971, although those terms were not used or defined.[L5] Again, in the context of double inlet ventricles, Tandon and colleagues discussed "straddling AV valves."[T12] Thereafter, ease of diagnosis provided by two-dimensional echocardiography rapidly led to broader recognition and improved understanding of these abnormalities of the AV valves.[L19,S25]

Surgical management of straddling and overriding AV valves was first reported in 1979, independently by Pacifico and by Tabry and their colleagues.[D10,P4,T9] Surgical possibilities, rapidly expanding knowledge of morphology of congenital heart disease, and increased use of two-dimensional echocardiography resulted in clear perception of the morphology and implications of these AV valve anomalies.

Clarifying terminology used in this section was evolved by Milo and Ho and their colleagues in studies of straddling and overriding AV valves.[H14,M7] Milo and colleagues described disposition of the conduction system in hearts with overriding AV valves,[M7] and Anderson and colleagues formulated the basis for categorizing these hearts as well as those with univentricular AV connections ("single ventricle").[A9]

MORPHOLOGY

Morphologic Syndromes

When atria are in usual (solitus) situs, ventricular topology is right handed, and AV and ventriculoarterial (VA) connections are concordant (see "Terminology and Classification of Heart Disease" in Chapter 1), the right AV valve sometimes overrides or straddles. This anomaly is associated with a posteriorly placed (juxtacrucial) VSD in the inlet portion of the ventricular septum when viewed from the RV aspect. The interventricular septum does not attach to the crux cordis in this situation. The overriding tricuspid valve is associated with malalignment of the atrial and interventricular septa. The right ventricle is usually somewhat hypoplastic.

When there is atrial situs solitus, ventricular right-handedness (D-loop), AV concordant connection, and discordant VA connection (complete transposition of the great arteries), the left AV valve may be overriding, then over a VSD in the anterior portion of the ventricular septum.

When there is atrial situs solitus, ventricular right-handedness, AV concordant connection, and double outlet RV (one of the most common situations in which overriding and straddling of an AV valve occur[R9]), the right AV valve may be overriding and usually straddling in hearts with a VSD that is juxta-aortic and usually also perimembranous and juxtacrucial. When the VSD is juxtapulmonary and somewhat anterior (Taussig-Bing heart), the left AV valve may be straddling and overriding a VSD that does not extend to the crux cordis.[K16]

When there is atrial situs solitus, left-handed ventricular topology (L-loop), AV discordant connection, and VA discordant connection (congenitally corrected transposition of the great arteries), the right AV valve (which generally in this setting has two leaflets) may override an anteriorly situated VSD. The interventricular septum does reach the crux cordis. When overriding of the right AV valve in this setting is more than 50%, there is double-inlet RV with the RV lying to the left and more or less posterior, and an anterior, right-sided, and often hypoplastic and rudimentary (incomplete) LV.

In hearts with congenitally corrected transposition of the great arteries, the left-sided AV valve may override a posteriorly placed VSD; in these hearts, the interventricular septum does not reach the crux cordis. When overriding is more than 50%, the condition is double inlet LV with left-sided and anteriorly placed hypoplastic and rudimentary (incomplete) RV, the most common type of double inlet ventricle. A special group of cases with AV discordant connection, usually with double outlet RV, involves a VSD that is juxtacrucial and in which one or both AV valves are overriding and straddling. Ventricles in this setting are usually in an over-and-under position, and circulations appear to crisscross within the heart.

Similar patterns may occur with atrial situs inversus and with atrial situs ambiguus.

Conduction System

Knowledge of location of the AV node and bundle of His is required for satisfactory surgical treatment of cardiac malformations. When the AV valve is overriding or straddling a VSD that does not reach the crux cordis, the conduction system is usually unaffected by the overriding valve.[A7] Thus, the AV node is in its usual location in the AV septum when the ventricular topology is right handed and the AV connection concordant. When the ventricular topology is left handed and the AV connection discordant, the conduction system generally arises from an anomalous anterolateral node, and this is unaffected by the overriding valve.

When in hearts with AV concordant connection the AV valve (in this case the tricuspid valve) overrides a VSD that is juxtacrucial (such defects may be perimembranous as well), the AV node is situated anomalously.[A7] It lies at the point inferiorly at which the ventricular septum attaches to the anulus (or circumference) of the right AV valve.[M7]

When the VSD is juxtacrucial and the AV connection discordant, the left AV valve overrides and the AV node occupies an anterolateral position near the right AV valve anulus, as is usual in hearts with AV discordant connection.

CLINICAL FEATURES AND DIAGNOSTIC CRITERIA

Straddling and overriding of an AV valve are uncommon, occurring as an added anomaly in about 3% of patients with congenital heart disease. They seem to be more prevalent in hearts with AV discordant connection than in those with AV concordant connections (Table 21-18). Among hearts with

■ **TABLE 21-18   Cardiac Morphology and Mortality after Operation in Patients with Overriding and Straddling Atrioventricular Valves** [a]

Cardiac Morphology	n	Hospital Deaths	Total Deaths
AV Concordant Connection			
VSD (RAVV)	6	0	0
VSD (LAVV)	1 [b]	0	0
VSD and valvar PS (RAVV)	1	0	0
TF (RAVV)	3	0	0
TGA and PS (LAVV)	2	1	1
DORV			
Subaortic VSD and PS (RAVV)	3	2	2
Subpulmonary VSD and PS (LAVV)	4	0	2
Taussig-Bing heart (LAVV)	1	1	1
AV Discordant Connection			
CTGA (LAVV)			
PS	4	0	1
Without PS	3	0	2
TGA (RAVV) and PS	2	0	0
DORV with PS			
LAVV	2 [c]	0	0
RAVV	2	1	1
AV Ambiguous Connection			
DORV, PS (RAVV)	1	0	0
TOTAL	35	5	10

Key: *AV*, Atrioventricular; *CTGA*, Corrected transposition of the great arteries; *DORV*, double outlet right ventricle; *LAVV*, left atrioventricular valve; *PS*, pulmonary stenosis; *RAVV*, right atrioventricular valve; *TF*, tetralogy of Fallot; *TGA*, transposition of the great arteries; *VSD*, ventricular septal defect.

[a] Data from 35 patients operated on at UAB from 1967 to 1985. Total deaths include hospital deaths and those in follow-up period.

[b] Several cords from mitral valve straddled to insert on right ventricular side of septum near ventricular septal defect.

[c] One patient also had right atrioventricular valve atresia.

AV concordant connections, straddling and overriding of an AV valve occur most often in hearts with double outlet RV and in those with complete transposition of the great arteries.

Coexisting cardiac anomalies, not straddling and overriding of the AV valve, generally determine the clinical syndrome, natural history, and diagnostic features in patients with straddling or overriding of the AV valves.

Straddling and overriding AV valves are usually competent and have no features that permit their identification by history, physical examination, chest radiograph, or ECG. Echocardiography is the technique by which they are generally diagnosed, although overriding can often be diagnosed or inferred from the angiogram.[B14,S26]

TECHNIQUE OF OPERATION

When an AV valve is only overriding, repair of the associated VSD or of other cardiac anomalies can usually be done in essentially the normal manner, except for some deviation of the patch to accommodate the overriding. Straddling presents a more severe surgical challenge, particularly when the straddling is moderate or severe in degree and when the inappropriate ventricle into which the straddling cords enter is not the one in which the surgeon is working.[M15] For these reasons, the Fontan operation (see Section 4 of Chapter 27) often is the most appropriate option when severe straddling or overriding is present.

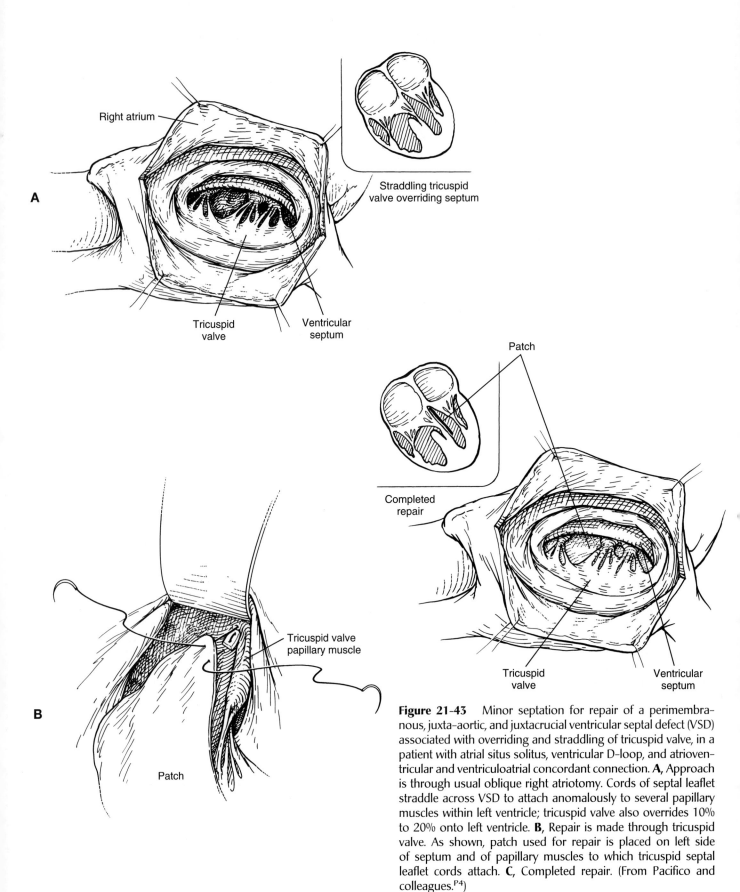

Figure 21-43   Minor septation for repair of a perimembranous, juxta–aortic, and juxtacrucial ventricular septal defect (VSD) associated with overriding and straddling of tricuspid valve, in a patient with atrial situs solitus, ventricular D-loop, and atrioventricular and ventriculoatrial concordant connection. **A,** Approach is through usual oblique right atriotomy. Cords of septal leaflet straddle across VSD to attach anomalously to several papillary muscles within left ventricle; tricuspid valve also overrides 10% to 20% onto left ventricle. **B,** Repair is made through tricuspid valve. As shown, patch used for repair is placed on left side of septum and of papillary muscles to which tricuspid septal leaflet cords attach. **C,** Completed repair. (From Pacifico and colleagues.[P4])

Section of Straddling Cords

Rarely a single straddling cord can be sectioned to permit repair of a VSD or an intraventricular tunnel repair, without rendering the AV valve regurgitant. This technique can probably be used only when straddling is mild.

Slotting of Repair Patch

Rarely, straddling cords can fit into a slot or cut made in the patch used to close the VSD or to make an intraventricular tunnel. The slot is then closed by sutures. This technique is applicable only to mild or possibly moderate straddling involving just a few cords, and it probably results in loss of free motion of the cords.

Reattachment of Sectioned Tensor Apparatus

When straddling is mild or moderate, and when the straddling tensor apparatus attaches to only one papillary muscle or area of the muscular interventricular septum in the inappropriate ventricle, and when that muscle has no other cord attachments, the muscle may be sectioned at its base. Then, along with its straddling cords, the muscle is brought back into the appropriate ventricle. The VSD is closed with a patch, or if indicated, an intraventricular tunnel repair is performed. Finally, the muscle to which the straddling cords connect is reattached to the patch or tunnel.

This technique is used infrequently and is applicable only when surgery is being performed from within the appropriate ventricle, approached either through its atrium or a ventriculotomy. Probability of dehiscence of a reattached papillary muscle or tendinous cord has not been determined.

Minor Septation

The patch used to close a VSD or create an intraventricular tunnel may be deviated around the papillary muscle and septal attachments of a straddling AV valve so that, after repair, they lie within the appropriate ventricle (Figs. 21-43 and 21-44). This approach is most easily performed when straddling is *into* the ventricle in which the surgeon is working, through its atrium or a ventriculotomy. This is usually the ventricle ejecting into the pulmonary trunk: the right-sided RV in double outlet RV with concordant AV connection, or the right-sided LV in hearts with discordant AV connection. In some cases, however, the technique of minor septation can be applied when straddling is into the ventricle ejecting into the aorta (Fig. 21-43).

Replacement of Straddling Atrioventricular Valve

When the straddling AV valve is regurgitant (a relatively unusual situation), operation usually includes valve replacement. This approach may be used as well in some cases simply because of complexity and severity of the straddling. The valve replacement device may face onto the patch used for repair of the VSD or creation of an intraventricular tunnel, because of the malalignment of the atrial and ventricular septa. This possibility emphasizes the value of a low-profile device in this setting, and even with such a device, some functional impairment may result.

Particular care and thoughtfulness are required when straddling or overriding occurs in the setting of ventricular L-loop, when valve replacement appears to be indicated. This situation, along with the sometimes associated complete heart block, may compromise long-term outlook sufficiently that a Fontan operation is preferable to a two-ventricle repair (see Chapter 27).

Fontan Operation

The Fontan operation is also the only method that can be used when moderate or severe hypoplasia of a ventricle is associated with straddling and overriding AV valves. Current information concerning early and intermediate-term results of this operation encourages its wider use when AV valve straddling or overriding is moderate or severe (see Chapter 27).

Cardiac Transplantation

Cardiac transplantation is reserved for patients with straddling and overriding AV valves in whom a severe secondary cardiomyopathy has developed.

RESULTS

Early and intermediate-term (5 to 15 years) survival after surgery in patients with straddling and overriding AV valves is determined primarily by the cardiac defect with which the AV valve anomaly is associated. However, this survival is somewhat less satisfactory than survival in general after repair of the primary cardiac defect. Exceptions are patients in whom the Fontan operation or cardiac transplantation is performed, because survival after these operations is unrelated to the cardiac anomaly for which the operation was done and is not lessened by presence of a straddling or overriding AV valve.

Heart block has occurred more frequently than usual after repair of hearts with concordant AV connection and overriding AV valves associated with a VSD extending to the crux cordis and in patients with discordant AV connection. Because position of the AV node and conduction system in such hearts is now known, heart block should now occur less frequently.

INDICATIONS FOR OPERATION

Indications for operation in patients with overriding and straddling AV valves lie with the coexisting anomalies rather than with the AV valve anomaly.

Strategy of operation is greatly influenced by the AV valve anomaly, and whenever possible that strategy should be decided in early life. If straddling is mild, the strategy can probably be that for the coexisting anomaly in general, and the AV valve anomaly can be managed by the technique of minor septation or an even lesser procedure.

When straddling is severe, these techniques seem likely to be associated with a relatively high early risk. Valve replacement in this setting carries more than the usual early and intermediate risks and imponderables. A Fontan operation probably is associated with better early and late results

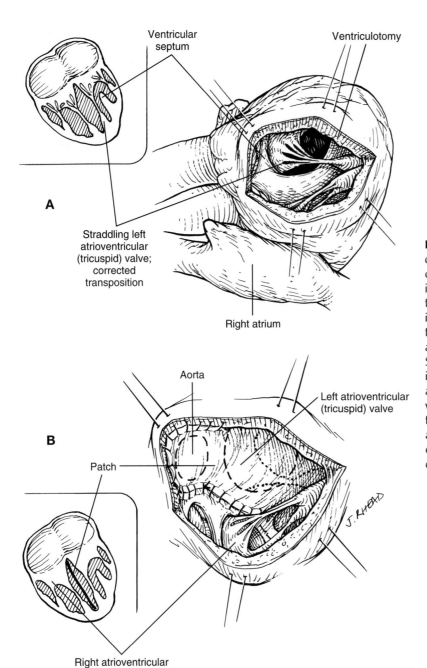

A

Ventricular septum

Ventriculotomy

Straddling left atrioventricular (tricuspid) valve; corrected transposition

Right atrium

B

Aorta

Left atrioventricular (tricuspid) valve

Patch

Right atrioventricular (mitral) valve

Figure 21-44 Intraventricular tunnel repair incorporating a minor septation for straddling and overriding left atrioventricular (AV) tricuspid valve in a patient with congenitally corrected transposition of the great arteries and about 40% overriding of aorta onto right-sided left ventricle. **A,** Vertical left (right-sided) ventriculotomy is shown, but an approach through right atrium is preferred. Straddling and overriding left AV (tricuspid) valve is shown as well as ventricular septal defect and aortic overriding. **B,** Repair patch creates an intraventricular tunnel repair conducting systemic arterial blood flow from left-sided right ventricle to aorta and keeping entire left AV valve apparatus on appropriate side of patch. (From Pacifico and colleagues.[P4])

than these procedures and is the only type of procedure that can be considered when the patient has important ventricular hypoplasia. Therefore, diagnosis of AV valve straddling or overriding should be made in early infancy. If the patient has cyanosis from reduced pulmonary blood flow, a PTFE interposition pulmonary-systemic arterial shunt or a bidirectional cavopulmonary anastomosis should be performed. If there is a large left-to-right shunt, pulmonary trunk banding should be performed in early life. In either case the Fontan operation is then performed in patients ages 1 to 2 years, before ventricular hypertrophy becomes marked (see Chapter 27).

REFERENCES

A

1. Andreasen AT, Watson F. Experimental cardiovascular surgery: "The azygos factor." Br J Surg 1952;39:548.
2. Ash R. Natural history of ventricular septal defects in childhood lesions with predominant arteriovenous shunts. J Pediatr 1964;64:45.
3. Auld PA, Johnson AL, Gibbons JE, McGregor M. Changes in pulmonary vascular resistance in infants and children with left-to-right intracardiac shunts. Circulation 1963;27:257.
4. Aaron BL, Lower BR. Muscular ventricular septal defect repair made easy. Ann Thorac Surg 1975;19:568.
5. Anderson RH, Lenox CC, Zuberbuhler JR. Morphology of ventricular septal defect associated with coarctation of aorta. Br Heart J 1983; 50:176.
6. Albus RA, Trusler GA, Izukawa T, Williams WG. Pulmonary artery banding. J Thorac Cardiovasc Surg 1984;88:645.
7. Anderson RH, Milo S, Ho SY, Wilkinson JL, Becker AE. The anatomy of straddling atrioventricular valves. In Becker AE, Loosekoot G, Marcelletti C, Anderson RH, eds. Paediatric cardiology, Vol. 3. New York: Churchill Livingstone, 1981, p. 411.
8. Anderson RH, Becker AE, Tynan M. Description of ventricular septal defects—or how long is a piece of string? Int J Cardiol 1986;13:267.
9. Anderson RH, Macartney FJ, Tynan M, Becker AE, Freedom RM, Godman MJ, et al. Univentricular atrioventricular connection: single ventricle trap unsprung. Pediatr Cardiol 1983;4:273.
10. Alpert BS, Cook DH, Varghese PJ, Rowe RD. Spontaneous closure of small ventricular septal defects: ten-year follow-up. Pediatrics 1979; 63:204.
11. Amin Z, Berry JM, Foker JE, Rocchini AP, Bass JL. Intraoperative closure of muscular ventricular septal defect in a canine model and application of the technique in a baby. J Thorac Cardiovasc Surg 1998;115:1374.
12. Anderson RH, Wilcox BR. The surgical anatomy of ventricular septal defect. J Card Surg 1992;7:17.
13. Anderson RH, Wilcox BR. The surgical anatomy of ventricular septal defects associated with overriding valvar orifices. J Card Surg 1993;8:130.
14. Ad N, Barak J, Birk E, Snir E, Vidne BA. Unidirectional valve patch (letter). Ann Thorac Surg 1996;62:626.
15. Ad N, Barak J, Birk E, Diamant S, Vidne BA. A one-way, valved, atrial septal patch in the management of postoperative right heart failure. An animal study. J Thorac Cardiovasc Surg 1994;108:134.
16. Ad N, Birk E, Barak J, Diamant S, Snir E, Vidne BA. A one-way valved atrial septal patch: a new surgical technique and its clinical application. J Thorac Cardiovasc Surg 1996;111:84.

B

1. Blackstone EH, Kirklin JW, Bradley EL, DuShane JW, Appelbaum A. Optimal age and results in repair of large ventricular septal defects. J Thorac Cardiovasc Surg 1976;72:661.
2. Becu LM, Fontana RS, DuShane JW, Kirklin JW, Burchell HB, Edwards JE. Anatomic and pathologic studies in ventricular septal defect. Circulation 1956;14:349.
3. Barratt-Boyes BG, Neutze JM, Clarkson PM, Shardey GC, Brandt PW. Repair of ventricular septal defect in the first two years of life using profound hypothermia-circulatory arrest techniques. Ann Surg 1976;184:376.
4. Berglund E. Ventricular function. VI. Balance of left and right ventricular output: relation between left and right atrial pressures. Am J Physiol 1954;178:381.
5. Breckenridge IM, Stark J, Waterston DJ, Bonham-Carter RE. Multiple ventricular septal defects. Ann Thorac Surg 1972;13:128.
6. Brandt PW, Calder AL. Cardiac connections: the segmental approach to radiologic diagnosis in congenital heart disease. Curr Probl Diagn Radiol 1977;7:1.

7. Barratt-Boyes BG, Simpson M, Neutze JM. Intracardiac surgery in neonates and infants using deep hypothermia with surface cooling and limited cardiopulmonary bypass. Circulation 1971;43:I25.
8. Braunwald E, Morrow AG. Left-ventriculo-right atrial communication: diagnosis by clinical, hemodynamic, and angiographic methods. Am J Med 1960;28:913.
9. Bargeron LM Jr, Elliott LP, Soto B, Bream PR, Curry GC. Axial cineangiography in congenital heart disease: section I. Circulation 1977;56:1075.
10. Barratt-Boyes BG, Roche AH, Whitlock RM. Six year review of the results of freehand aortic valve replacement using an antibiotic sterilized homograft valve. Circulation 1977;55:353.
11. Bharati S, McAllister HA Jr, Lev M. Straddling and displaced atrioventricular orifices and valves. Circulation 1979;60:673.
12. Bergdahl LA, Blackstone EH, Kirklin JW, Pacifico AD, Bargeron LM Jr. Determinants of early success in repair of aortic coarctation in infants. J Thorac Cardiovasc Surg 1982;83:736.
13. Brandt PW. Cineangiography of atrioventricular and ventriculoarterial connections. In Godman MJ, ed. Paediatric cardiology, Vol. 4. Edinburgh: Churchill Livingstone, 1980, p. 191.
14. Bridges ND, Perry SB, Keane JF, Goldstein SA, Mandell V, Mayer JE Jr, et al. Preoperative transcatheter closure of congenital muscular ventricular septal defects. N Eng J Med 1991;324:1312.
15. Beerman LB, Park SC, Fischer DR, Fricker FJ, Mathews RA, Neches WH, et al. Ventricular septal defect associated with aneurysm of the membranous septum. J Am Coll Cardiol 1985;5:118.
16. Bierman FZ, Fellows K, Williams RG. Prospective identification of ventricular septal defects in infancy using subxiphoid two-dimensional echocardiography. Circulation 1980;62:807.
17. Bush A, Busst CM, Haworth SG, Hislop AA, Knight WB, Corrin B, et al. Correlations of lung morphology, pulmonary vascular resistance, and outcome in children with congenital heart disease. Br Heart J 1988;59:480.
18. Baker EJ, Ayton V, Smith MA, Parsons JM, Ladusans EJ, Anderson RH, et al. Magnetic resonance imaging at a high field strength of ventricular septal defects in infants. Br Heart J 1989;62:305.
19. Burke RP. Minimally invasive techniques for congenital heart surgery. Semin Thorac Cardiovasc Surg 1997;9:337.

C

1. Cohen M, Lillehei CW. A quantitative study of the 'azygos factor' during vena caval occlusion in the dog. Surg Gynecol Obstet 1954;98:225.
2. Clarkson PM, Frye RL, DuShane JW, Burchell HB, Wood EH, Weidman WH. Prognosis for patients with ventricular septal defect and severe pulmonary vascular obstructive disease. Circulation 1968;38:129.
3. Cartmill TB, DuShane JW, McGoon DC, Kirklin JW. Results of repair of ventricular septal defect. J Thorac Cardiovasc Surg 1966;52:486.
4. Cordell D, Graham TP Jr, Atwood GF, Boerth RC, Boucek RJ, Bender HW. Left heart volume characteristics following ventricular septal defect closure in infancy. Circulation 1976;54:294.
5. Ching E, DuShane JW, McGoon DC, Danielson GK. Total correction of ventricular septal defect in infancy using extracorporeal circulation: surgical considerations and results of operation. Ann Thorac Surg 1971;12:1.
6. Cooley DA, Garrett HE, Howard HS. The surgical treatment of ventricular septal defect: An analysis of 300 consecutive surgical cases. Prog Cardiovasc Dis 1962;4:312.
7. Civin WH, Edwards JE. Pathology of the pulmonary vascular tree. I. A comparison of the intrapulmonary arteries in Eisenmenger's complex and in stenosis of ostium infundibuli associated with biventricular origin of the aorta. Circulation 1950;2:545.

8. Castaneda AR, Zamora R, Nicoloff DM, Moller JH, Hunt CE, Lucas RV. High-pressure, high-resistance ventricular septal defect: surgical results of closure through right atrium. Ann Thorac Surg 1971;12:29.

9. Chung KJ, Manning JA. Ventricular septal defect associated with aortic insufficiency: medical and surgical management. Am Heart J 1974;87:435.

10. Collins G, Calder L, Rose V, Kidd L, Keith J. Ventricular septal defect: clinical and hemodynamic changes in the first five years of life. Am Heart J 1972;84:695.

11. Clarkson PM. Growth following corrective cardiac operation in early infancy. In Barratt-Boyes BG, Neutze JM, Harris EA, eds. Heart disease in infancy: diagnosis and surgical treatment. London: Churchill Livingstone, 1973, p. 75.

12. Corone P, Doyon F, Gaudeau S, Guerin F, Vernant P, Ducam H, et al. Natural history of ventricular septal defect: a study involving 790 cases. Circulation 1977;55:908.

13. Campbell M. Natural history of ventricular septal defect. Br Heart J 1971;33:246.

14. Capelli H, Marantz P, Micheli D, Coronel AR, Kreutzer G, Becu L, et al. Type of ventricular septal defect present in patients who survived heart failure in the first year. A two-dimensional echocardiographic study. Rev Lat Cardiac Inf 1985;1:292.

15. Chauvaud S, Serraf A, Mihaileanu S, Soyer R, Blondeau P, Dubost C, et al. Ventricular septal defect associated with aortic valve incompetence: results of two surgical managements. Ann Thorac Surg 1990; 49:875.

16. Carpentier A. Cardiac valve surgery—The "French correction." J Thorac Cardiovasc Surg 1983;86:323.

17. Chin AJ, Alboliras ET, Barber G, Murphy JD, Helton JG, Pigott JD, et al. Prospective detection by Doppler color flow imaging of additional defects in infants with a large ventricular septal defect. J Am Coll Cardiol 1990;15:1637.

18. Carotti A, Marino B, Bevilacqua M, Marcelletti C, Rossi E, Santoro G, et al. Primary repair of isolated ventricular septal defect in infancy guided by echocardiography. Am J Cardiol 1997;79:1498.

19. Cooley DA, Hallman GL, Wukasch DC, Sandiford FM. Transaortic repair of ventricular septal defect. Ann Thorac Surg 1973;16:99.

D

1. DuShane JW, Kirklin JW, Patrick RT, Donald DE, Terry HR Jr, Burchell HB, et al. Ventricular septal defects with pulmonary hypertension: surgical treatment by means of a mechanical pump oxygenator. JAMA 1956;160:950.

2. DuShane JW, Kirklin JW. Late results of the repair of ventricular septal defect in pulmonary vascular disease. In Kirklin JW, ed. Advances in cardiovascular surgery. Orlando, Fla: Grune & Stratton, 1973, p. 9.

3. Dimich I, Steinfeld L, Litwak RS, Park S, Silvers N. Subpulmonic ventricular septal defect associated with aortic insufficiency. Am J Cardiol 1973;32:325.

4. Downing JW Jr, Kaplan S, Bove KE. Postsurgical left anterior hemiblock and right bundle branch block. Br Heart J 1972;34:263.

5. Doty DB, McGoon DC. Closure of perimembranous ventricular septal defect. J Thorac Cardiovasc Surg 1983;85:781.

6. Davis Z, McGoon DC, Danielson GK, Wallace RB. Removal of pulmonary artery band. Isr J Med Sci 1975;11:110.

7. Dirksen T, Moulaert AJ, Buis-Liem TN, Brom AG. Ventricular septal defect associated with left ventricular outflow tract obstruction below the defect. J Thorac Cardiovasc Surg 1978;75:688.

8. de Leval MR, Pozzi M, Starnes V, Sullivan ID, Stark J, Somerville J, et al. Surgical management of doubly committed subarterial ventricular septal defects. Circulation 1988;78:III40.

9. de la Cruz MV, Miller BL. Double-inlet left ventricle: two pathological specimens with comments on the embryology and on its relation to single ventricle. Circulation 1968;37:249.

10. Danielson GK, Tabry IF, Fulton FE, Hagler DJ, Ritter DG. Successful repair of straddling atrioventricular valve by technique used for septation of univentricular heart. Ann Thorac Surg 1979;28:554.

E

1. Elliott LP, Bargeron LM Jr, Bream PR, Soto B, Curry GC. Axial cineangiography in congenital heart disease. II. Specific lesions. Circulation 1977;56:1048.

2. Ellis H Jr, Ongley PA, Kirklin JW. Ventricular septal defect with aortic valvular incompetence. Surgical considerations. Circulation 1963; 27:789.

3. Edwards JE, Burchell HB. The pathologic anatomy of deficiencies between the aortic root and the heart including aortic sinus aneurysm. Thorax 1957;12:125.

4. Elgamal MA, Hakimi M, Lyons JM, Walters HL 3rd. Risk factors for failure of aortic valvuloplasty in aortic insufficiency with ventricular septal defect. Ann Thorac Surg 1999;68:1350.

F

1. Friedman WF, Mehrizi A, Pusch AL. Multiple muscular ventricular septal defects. Circulation 1965;32:35.

2. Freed MD, Rosenthal A, Plauth WH Jr, Nadas AS. Development of subaortic stenosis after pulmonary artery banding. Circulation 1973; 48:III7.

3. Friedli B, Kidd BS, Mustard WT, Keith JD. Ventricular septal defect with increased pulmonary vascular resistance: late results of surgical closure. Am J Cardiol 1974;33:403.

4. Freedom RM, Dische MR, Rowe RD. Pathologic anatomy of subaortic stenosis and atresia in the first year of life. Am J Cardiol 1977;39:1035.

5. Fox KM, Patel RG, Graham GR, Taylor JF, Stark J, De Leval MR, et al. Multiple and single ventricular septal defect. A clinical and haemodynamic comparison. Br Heart J 1978;40:141.

6. Fried R, Falkovsky G, Newburger J, Gorchakova AI, Rabinovitch M, Gordonova MI, et al. Pulmonary arterial changes in patients with ventricular septal defects and severe pulmonary hypertension. Pediatr Cardiol 1986;7:147.

7. Frater RW. The prolapsing aortic cusp: experimental and clinical observations. Ann Thorac Surg 1967;3:63.

G

1. Girod DA, Hurwitz RA, King H, Jolly W. Recent results of two-stage surgical treatment of large ventricular septal defect. Circulation 1974;50:II9.

2. Gasul BM, Dillon RF, Vrla V, Hait G. Ventricular septal defects: their natural transformation into those with infundibular stenosis or into the cyanotic or non-cyanotic type of tetralogy of Fallot. JAMA 1957; 164:847.

3. Gelband H, Waldo AL, Kaiser GA, Bowman FO Jr, Malm JR, Hoffman BF. Etiology of right bundle-branch block in patients undergoing total correction of tetralogy of Fallot. Circulation 1971; 44:1022.

4. Gerbode F, Hultgren H, Melrose D, Osborn J. Syndrome of left ventricular-right atrial shunt: successful surgical repair of defect in five cases, with observation of bradycardia on closure. Ann Surg 1958;148:433.

5. Gonzalez-Lavin L, Barratt-Boyes BG. Surgical considerations in the treatment of ventricular septal defect associated with aortic valvular incompetence. J Thorac Cardiovasc Surg 1969;57:422.

6. Garamella JJ, Cruz AB Jr, Heupel WH, Dahl JC, Jensen NK, Berman R. Ventricular septal defect with aortic insufficiency: successful surgical correction of both defects by the transaortic approach. Am J Cardiol 1960;5:266.

7. Gersony WM, Hayes CJ. Bacterial endocarditis in patients with pulmonary stenosis, aortic stenosis, or ventricular septal defect. Circulation 1977;56:I84.

8. Griffiths SP, Turi GK, Ellis K, Krongrad E, Swift LH, Gersony WM, et al. Muscular ventricular septal defects repaired with left ventriculotomy. Am J Cardiol 1981;48:877.
9. Griffin ML, Sullivan ID, Anderson RH, Macartney FJ. Doubly committed subarterial ventricular septal defect: new morphological criteria with echocardiographic and angiocardiographic correlation. Br Heart J 1988;59:474.

H

1. Heath D, Edwards JE. The pathology of hypertensive pulmonary vascular disease: a description of six grades of structural changes in the pulmonary arteries with special reference to congenital cardiac septal defects. Circulation 1958;18:533.
2. Heath D, Helmholz HF Jr, Burchell HB, DuShane JW, Edwards JE. Graded pulmonary vascular changes and hemodynamic findings in cases of atrial and ventricular septal defect and patent ductus arteriosus. Circulation 1958;18:1155.
3. Hallidie-Smith KA, Hollman A, Cleland WP, Bentall HH, Goodwin JF. Effects of surgical closure of ventricular septal defects upon pulmonary vascular disease. Br Heart J 1969;31:246.
4. Hunt CE, Formanek G, Levine MA, Castaneda A, Moller JH. Banding of the pulmonary artery: results in 111 children. Circulation 1971;43:395.
5. Henry J, Kaplan S, Helmsworth JA, Schreiber JT. Management of infants with large ventricular septal defects: results with two-stage surgical treatment. Ann Thorac Surg 1973;15:109.
6. Hoffman JI, Rudolph AM. The natural history of ventricular septal defects in infancy. Am J Cardiol 1965;16:634.
7. Hislop A, Haworth SG, Shinebourne EA, Reid L. Quantitative structural analysis of pulmonary vessels in isolated ventricular septal defect in infancy. Br Heart J 1975;37:1014.
8. Hoffman JI, Rudolph AM. Increasing pulmonary vascular resistance during infancy in association with ventricular septal defect. Pediatrics 1966;38:220.
9. Hoffman JI, Rudolph AM. The natural history of isolated ventricular septal defect with special reference to selection of patients for surgery. Adv Pediatr 1970,17:57.
10. Hallidie-Smith KA, Edwards RE, Wilson R, Zeidifard E. Long-term cardiorespiratory assessment after surgical closure of ventricular septal defect in childhood (abstract). Br Heart J 1975;37:553.
11. Hoffman JI. Diagnosis and treatment of pulmonary vascular disease. Birth Defects 1972;8:9.
12. Hudspeth AS, Cordell AR, Meredith JH, Johnston FR. An improved transatrial approach to the closure of ventricular septal defects. J Thorac Cardiovasc Surg 1962;43:157.
13. Hobbins SM, Izukawa T, Radford DJ, Williams WG, Trusler GA. Conduction disturbances after surgical correction of ventricular septal defect by the atrial approach. Br Heart J 1979;41:289.
14. Ho SY, Milo S, Anderson RH, Macartney FJ, Goodwin A, Becker AE, et al. Straddling atrioventricular valve with absent atrioventricular connection. Br Heart J 1982;47:344.
15. Hu DC, Giuliani ER, Downing TP, Danielson GK. Spontaneous closure of congenital ventricular septal defect in an adult. Clin Cardiol 1986;9:587.
16. Hisatomi K, Kosuga K, Isomura T, Akagawa H, Ohishi K, Koga M. Ventricular septal defect associated with aortic regurgitation. Ann Thorac Surg 1987;43:363.
17. Helmcke F, de Souza A, Nanda NC, Villacosta I, Gatewood R Jr, Colvin E, et al. Two-dimensional and color doppler assessment of ventricular septal defect of congenital origin. Am J Cardiol 1989;63:1112.
18. Houyel L, Vaksmann G, Fournier A, Davignon A. Ventricular arrhythmias after correction of ventricular septal defects: importance of surgical approach. J Am Coll Cardiol 1990;16:1224.
19. Hornberger LK, Sahn DJ, Krabill KA, Sherman FS, Swensson RE, Pesonen E, et al. Elucidation of the natural history of ventricular septal defects by serial Doppler color flow mapping studies. J Am Coll Cardiol 1989;13:1111.
20. Hisatomi K, Isomura T, Sato T, Kawara T, Kosuga K, Ohishi K, et al. Aortoplasty for aortic regurgitation with ventricular septal defect. J Thorac Cardiovasc Surg 1994;108:396.
21. Hisatomi K, Taira A, Oku S, Moriyama Y. New valid technique for ventricular septal defect associated with aortic regurgitation. J Thorac Cardiovasc Surg 1998;115:733.

J

1. Jarmakani JM, Graham TP Jr, Canent RV Jr, Capp MP. The effect of corrective surgery on left heart volume and mass in children with ventricular septal defect. Am J Cardiol 1971;27:254.
2. Jarmakani JM, Graham TP Jr, Canent RV Jr. Left ventricular contractile state in children with successfully corrected ventricular septal defect. Circulation 1972;45:I102.
3. Johnson DC, Cartmill TB, Celermajer JM, Hawker RE, Stuckey DS, Bowdler JD, et al. Intracardiac repair of large ventricular septal defect in the first year of life. Med J Aust 1974;2:193.
4. John S, Korula R, Jairaj PS, Muralidharan S, Ravikumar E, Babuthaman C, et al. Results of surgical treatment of ventricular septal defects with pulmonary hypertension. Thorax 1983;38:279.
5. Juaneda E, Gittenberger de Groot A, Oppenheimer-Dekker A, Haworth SG. Pulmonary arterial development in infants with large perimembranous ventricular septal defects associated with overriding of the aortic valve. Int J Cardiol 1985;7:223.
6. Jacobs JP, Burke RP, Quintessenza JA, Mavroudis C. Congenital Heart Surgery Nomenclature Database Project: ventricular septal defect. Ann Thorac Surg 2000;69:S25.

K

1. Kirklin JW, Harshbarger HG, Donald DE, Edwards JE. Surgical correction of ventricular septal defect: anatomic and technical considerations. J Thorac Surg 1957;33:45.
2. Kirklin JW, DuShane JW. Indications for repair of ventricular septal defects. Am J Cardiol 1963;12:79.
3. Kobayashi J, Koike K, Senzaki H, Kobayashi T, Tsunemoto M, Ishizawa A, et al. Correlation of anatomic and hemodynamic features with aortic valve leaflet deformity in doubly committed subarterial ventricular septal defect. Heart Vessels 1999;14:240.
4. Kirklin JW, Silver AW. Technique of exposing the ductus arteriosus prior to establishing extracorporeal circulation. Proc Mayo Clin 1958;33:423.
5. Keith JD, Rose V, Collins G, Kidd BS. Ventricular septal defect: incidence, morbidity, and mortality in various age groups. Br Heart J 1971;33:81.
6. Kirklin JW, Appelbaum A, Bargeron LM Jr. Primary repair versus banding for ventricular septal defects in infants. In Kidd BS, Rowe RD, eds. The child with congenital heart disease after surgery. Mount Kisco, NY: Futura, 1976, p. 3.
7. Keane JF, Fellows KE, Buckley L, Castaneda AR, Nadas AS. Ventricular septal defect with aortic regurgitation: a 33 year experience (abstract). In Godman MJ, ed. World Congress of Paediatric Cardiology. Edinburgh: Churchill Livingstone, 1981, p. 292.
8. Kawashima Y, Danno M, Shimizu Y, Matsuda H, Miyamoto T, Fujita T, et al. Ventricular septal defect associated with aortic insufficiency: anatomic classification and method of operation. Circulation 1973;47:1057.
9. Keck EW, Ongley PA, Kincaid OW, Swan HJ. Ventricular septal defect with aortic insufficiency: a clinical and hemodynamic study of 18 proved cases. Circulation 1963;27:203.
10. Kulbertus HE, Coyne JJ, Hallidie-Smith KA. Conduction disturbances before and after surgical closure of ventricular septal defect. Am Heart J 1969;77:123.
11. Krongrad E, Hefler SE, Bowman FO Jr, Malm JR, Hoffman BF. Further observations on the etiology of the right bundle branch block pattern following right ventriculotomy. Circulation 1974;50:1105.
12. Kirklin JW, DuShane JW. Repair of ventricular septal defect in infancy. Pediatrics 1961;27:961.

13. Kirklin JK, Castaneda AR, Keane JF, Fellows KE, Norwood WI. Surgical management of multiple ventricular septal defects. J Thorac Cardiovasc Surg 1980;80:485.

14. Kurosawa H, Becker AE. Modification of the precise relationship of the atrioventricular conduction bundle to the margins of the ventricular septal defects by the trabecula septomarginalis. J Thorac Cardiovasc Surg 1984;87:605.

15. Kirklin JW, McGoon DC, DuShane JW. Surgical treatment of ventricular septal defect. J Thorac Cardiovasc Surg 1960;40:763.

16. Kitamura N, Takao A, Ando M, Imai Y, Konno S. Taussig-Bing heart with mitral valve straddling: case reports and postmortem study. Circulation 1974;49:761.

17. Kirklin JW, Anderson RH, Pacifico AD, Kirklin JK, Bargeron LM Jr. Surgery for hearts with straddling and overriding atrioventricular valves. In Baue AE, Geha AS, Hammond GL, Laks H, Naunheim KS, eds. Glenn's thoracic and cardiovascular surgery, 5th Ed. East Norwalk, Conn: Appleton & Lange, 1991, p. 1069.

18. Krovetz LJ. Spontaneous closure of ventricular septal defect. Am J Cardiol 1998;81:100.

19. Kitagawa T, Durham LA 3rd, Mosca RS, Bove EL. Techniques and results in the management of multiple ventricular septal defects. J Thorac Cardiovasc Surg 1998;115:848.

20. Kumar K, Lock JE, Geva T. Apical muscular ventricular septal defects between the left ventricle and the right ventricular infundibulum: diagnostic and interventional considerations. Circulation 1997; 95:1207.

21. Kurotobi S, Sano T, Matsushita T, Takeuchi M, Kogaki S, Miwatani T, et al. Quantitative, non-invasive assessment of ventricular septal defect shunt flow by measuring proximal isovelocity surface area on colour Doppler mapping. Heart 1997;78:305.

22. Komai H, Naito Y, Fujiwara K, Noguchi Y, Nishimura Y, Uemura S. Surgical strategy for doubly committed subarterial ventricular septal defect with aortic cusp prolapse. Ann Thorac Surg 1997;64:1146.

L

1. Lillehei CW, Cohen M, Warden HE, Ziegler NR, Varco RL. The results of direct vision closure of ventricular septal defects in eight patients by means of controlled cross circulation. Surg Gynecol Obstet 1955;101:446.

2. Lucas RV Jr, Adams P Jr, Anderson RC, Meyne NG, Lillehei CW, Varco RL. The natural history of isolated ventricular septal defect: a serial physiologic study. Circulation 1961;24:1372.

3. Lev M. The architecture of the conduction system in congenital heart disease. III. Ventricular septal defect. Arch Pathol 1960;70:529.

4. Lillehei CW, Anderson RC, Eliot RS, Wang Y, Ferlic RM. Pre- and postoperative cardiac catheterization in 200 patients undergoing closure of ventricular septal defects. Surgery 1968;63:69.

5. Liberthson RR, Paul MH, Muster AJ, Arcilla RA, Eckner FA, Lev M. Straddling and displaced atrioventricular orifices and valves with primitive ventricles. Circulation 1971;43:213.

6. Laubry C, Pezzi C. Traitédes maladies carpentales du coeur. In Laubry C, Routier D, Soulie P: Les soufflés de (a maladie de Roger). Rev Med Paris 1933;50:439.

7. Lincoln C, Jamieson S, Joseph M, Shinebourne E, Anderson RH. Transatrial repair of ventricular septal defects with reference to their anatomic classification. J Thorac Cardiovasc Surg 1977;74:183.

8. Lauer RM, DuShane JW, Edwards JE. Obstruction of left ventricular outlet in association with ventricular septal defect. Circulation 1960;22:110.

9. Lue HC, Shen CT, Wang NK, Wu JR, Chu SH, Hung CR. Ventricular septal defect and coronary cusp prolapse: an assessment of some special features in Chinese (abstract). In Godman MJ, ed. World Congress of Paediatric Cardiology. Edinburgh: Churchill Livingstone, 1981, p. 291.

10. Lev M, Bharati S, Meng CC, Liberthson RR, Paul MH, Idriss F. A concept of double-outlet right ventricle. J Thorac Cardiovasc Surg 1972;64:271.

11. Leung MP, Mok CK, Lo RN, Lau KC. An echocardiographic study of perimembranous ventricular septal defect with left ventricular to right atrial shunting. Br Heart J 1986;55:45.

12. Ludomirsky A, Huhta JC, Vick GW 3rd, Murphy DJ Jr, Danford DA, Morrow WR. Color Doppler detection of multiple ventricular septal defects. Circulation 1986;74:1317.

13. Lauer RM, Ongley PA, DuShane JW, Kirklin JW. Heart block after repair of ventricular septal defect in children. Circulation 1960; 22:526.

14. Lupi-Herrera E, Sandoval J, Seoane M, Bialostozky D, Attie F. The role of isoproterenol in the preoperative evaluation of high pressure high resistance ventricular septal defect. Chest 1982;81:42.

15. Leung MP, Beerman LB, Siewers RD, Bahnson HT, Zuberbuhler JR. Long-term follow-up after aortic valvuloplasty and defect closure in ventricular septal defect with aortic regurgitation. Am J Cardiol 1987;60:890.

16. Lock JE, Block PC, McKay RG, Baim DS, Keane JF. Transcatheter closure of ventricular septal defects. Circulation 1988;78:361.

17. Lambert EC. Single ventricle with a rudimentary outlet chamber. Case report. Bull Johns Hopkins Hosp 1951;88:231.

18. Lev M, Liberthson RR, Kirkpatrick JR, Eckner FA, Arcilla RA. Single (primitive) ventricle. Circulation 1969;39:577.

19. LaCorte MA, Fellows KE, Williams RG. Overriding tricuspid valve. Echocardiographic and angiocardiographic features. Am J Cardiol 1976;37:911.

20. Lin PJ, Chang CH, Chu JJ, Liu HP, Tsai FC, Su WJ, et al. Minimally invasive cardiac surgical techniques in closure of ventricular septal defect: an alternative approach. Ann Thorac Surg 1998;65:165.

21. Leao LE, Buffolo E, Coto AE, Maluf MA, Andrade JC. Transaortic approach has a role in the surgical treatment of ventricular septal defects. Cardiovasc Surg 1996;4:250.

M

1. Mason DT, Spann JF Jr, Zelis R, Amsterdam EA. Comparison of the contractile state of the normal, hypertrophied, and failing heart in man. In Alpert N, ed. Cardiac hypertrophy. New York: Academic, 1971, p. 433.

2. Maron BJ, Redwood DR, Hirschfeld JW Jr, Goldstein RE, Morrow AG, Epstein SE. Postoperative assessment of patients with ventricular septal defect and pulmonary hypertension: response to intense upright exercise. Circulation 1973;48:864.

3. Muller WH Jr, Dammann JF Jr. The treatment of certain congenital malformations of the heart by the creation of pulmonic stenosis to reduce pulmonary hypertension and excessive pulmonary blood flow: a preliminary report. Surg Gynecol Obstet 1952;95:213.

4. Menahem S, Venables AW. Pulmonary artery banding in isolated or complicated ventricular septal defects: results and effects on growth. Br Heart J 1972;34:87.

5. Moreno-Cabral RJ, Mamiya RT, Nakamura FF, Brainard SC, McNamara JJ. Ventricular septal defect and aortic insufficiency: surgical treatment. J Thorac Cardiovasc Surg 1977;73:358.

6. Moulaert AJ, Bruins CG, Oppenheimer-Dekker A. Anomalies of the aortic arch and ventricular septal defects. Circulation 1976;53:1011.

7. Milo S, Ho SY, Macartney FJ, Wilkinson JL, Becker AE, Wenink AC, et al. Straddling and overriding atrioventricular valves: morphology and classification. Am J Cardiol 1979;44:1122.

8. Malm JR: Personal communication; 1989.

9. Momma K, Toyama K, Takao A, Ando M, Nakazawa M, Hirosawa K, et al. Natural history of subarterial infundibular ventricular septal defect. Am Heart J 1984;108:1312.

10. Moene RJ, Gittenberger-de Groot AC, Oppenheimer-Dekker A, Bartelings MM. Anatomic characteristics of ventricular septal defect associated with coarctation of the aorta. Am J Cardiol 1987;59:952.

11. Maehara T, Blackstone EH, Kirklin JW, Kirklin JK, Pacifico AD, Colvin EC. The results of the Trusler operation for ventricular septal defect and aortic valvar incompetence. In Crupi G, Parenzan L, Anderson RH, eds. Perspectives in pediatric cardiology, Vol. 2: Pediatric cardiac surgery, Part 1. Mount Kisco, NY: Futura, 1989, p. 61.

12. Momma K, Takao A, Ando M, Nakazawa M, Takamizawa K. Natural and post-operative history of pulmonary vascular obstruction associated with ventricular septal defect. Jpn Circ J 1981;45:230.

13. McDaniel N, Gutgesell HP, Nolan SP, Kron IL. Repair of large muscular ventricular septal defects in infants employing left ventriculotomy. Ann Thorac Surg 1989;47:593.

14. Mehrizi A, McMurphy DM, Ottesen OE, Rowe RD. Syndrome of double inlet left ventricle. Angiocardiographic differentiation from single ventricle with rudimentary outlet chamber. Bull Johns Hopkins Hosp 1966;119:255.

15. McGoon DC, Danielson GK, Wallace RB, Puga FJ. Surgical implications of straddling atrioventricular valves. In Becker AE, Loosekoot G, Marcelletti C, Anderson RH, eds. Paediatric cardiology, Vol. 3. New York: Churchill Livingstone, 1981, p. 431.

16. Magee AG, Boutin C, McCrindle BW, Smallhorn JF. Echocardiography and cardiac catheterization in the preoperative assessment of ventricular septal defect in infancy. Am Heart J 1998;135:907.

17. Mace L, Dervanian P, Le Bret E, Folliguet TA, Lambert V, Losay J, et al. "Swiss cheese" septal defects: surgical closure using a single patch with intermediate fixings. Ann Thorac Surg 1999;67:1754.

18. Murzi B, Bonanomi GL, Giusti S, Luisi VS, Bernabei M, Carminati M, et al. Surgical closure of muscular ventricular septal defects using double umbrella devices (intraoperative VSD device closure). Eur J Cardiothorac Surg 1997;12:450.

N

1. Nadas AS, Thilenius OG, LaFarge CG, Hauck AJ. Ventricular septal defect with aortic regurgitation: medical and pathologic aspects. Circulation 1964;29:862.

2. Neches WH, Park SC, Lenox CC, Zuberbuhler JR, Siewers RD, Hardesty RL. Coarctation of the aorta with ventricular septal defect. Circulation 1977;55:189.

3. Neufeld HN, Titus JL, DuShane JW, Burchell HB, Edwards JE. Isolated ventricular septal defect of the persistent common atrioventricular canal type. Circulation 1961;23:685.

4. Nanton MA, Belcourt CL, Gillis DA, Krause VW, Roy DL. Left ventricular outflow tract obstruction owing to accessory endocardial cushion tissue. J Thorac Cardiovasc Surg 1979;78:537.

5. Neutze JM, Ishikawa T, Clarkson PM, Calder AL, Barratt-Boyes BG, Kerr AR. Assessment and follow-up of patients with ventricular septal defect and elevated pulmonary vascular resistance. Am J Cardiol 1989;63:327.

O

1. Oldham HN Jr, Kakos GS, Jarmakani MM, Sabiston DC Jr. Pulmonary artery banding in infants with complex congenital heart defects. Ann Thorac Surg 1972;13:342.

2. Okamoto Y. Clinical studies for open heart surgery in infants with profound hypothermia. Nippon Geka Hokan 1969;38:188.

3. Okoroma EO, Guller B, Maloney JD, Weidman WH. Etiology of right bundle-branch block pattern after surgical closure of ventricular septal defects. Am Heart J 1975;90:14.

4. Oh KS, Park SC, Galvis AG, Young LW, Neches WH, Zuberbuhler JR. Pulmonary hyperinflation in ventricular septal defect. J Thorac Cardiovasc Surg 1978;76:706.

5. Oppenheimer-Dekker A, Gittenberger-de Groot AC, Bartelings MM, Wenink AC, Moene RJ, van der Harten JJ. Abnormal architecture of the ventricles in hearts with an overriding aortic valve and a perimembranous ventricular septal defect. Int J Cardiol 1985;9:341.

6. Ortiz E, Robinson PJ, Deanfield JE, Franklin R, Macartney FJ, Wyse RK. Localisation of ventricular septal defects by simultaneous display of superimposed colour Doppler and cross sectional echocardiographic images. Br Heart J 1985;54:53.

7. Otterstad JE, Simonsen S, Erikssen J. Hemodynamic findings at rest and during mild supine exercise in adults with isolated, uncomplicated ventricular septal defects. Circulation 1985;71:650.

8. Ohkita Y, Miki S, Kusuhara K, Ueda Y, Tahata T, Komeda M, et al. Reoperation after aortic valvuloplasty for aortic regurgitation associated with ventricular septal defect. Ann Thorac Surg 1986;41:489.

9. Okita Y, Miki S, Kusuhara K, Ueda Y, Tahata T, Yamanaka K, et al. Long-term results of aortic valvuloplasty for aortic regurgitation associated with ventricular septal defect. J Thorac Cardiovasc Surg 1988;96:769.

10. Onat T, Ahunbay G, Batmaz G, Celebi A. The natural course of isolated ventricular septal defect during adolescence. Pediatr Cardiol 1998;19:230.

11. Ogino H, Miki S, Ueda Y, Tahata T, Morioka K, Sakai T, et al. Surgical management of aortic regurgitation associated with ventricular septal defect. J Heart Valve Dis 1997;6:174.

P

1. Patel RG, Ihenacho HN, Abrams LD, Astley R, Parsons CG, Roberts KD, et al. Pulmonary artery banding and subsequent repair in ventricular septal defect. Br Heart J 1973;35:651.

2. Perry EL, Burchell HB, Edwards JE. Congenital communication between the left ventricle and the right atrium: co-existing ventricular septal defect and double tricuspid orifice. Mayo Clin Proc 1949;24:198.

3. Plauth WH Jr, Braunwald E, Rockoff SD, Mason DT, Morrow AG. Ventricular septal defect and aortic regurgitation: clinical, hemodynamic and surgical considerations. Am J Med 1965;39:552.

4. Pacifico AD, Soto B, Bargeron LM Jr. Surgical treatment of straddling tricuspid valves. Circulation 1979;60:655.

5. Park JK, Dell RB, Ellis K, Gersony WM. Surgical management of the infant with coarctation of the aorta and ventricular septal defect. J Am Coll Cardiol 1992;20:176.

R

1. Rein JG, Freed MD, Norwood WI, Castaneda AR. Early and late results of closure of ventricular septal defect in infancy. Ann Thorac Surg 1977;24:19.

2. Rastelli GC, Ongley PA, Titus JL. Ventricular septal defect of atrioventricular canal type with straddling right atrioventricular valve and mitral valve deformity. Circulation 1968;37:816.

3. Rowe RD, Vlad P. Diagnostic problems in the newborn: origins of mortality in congenital cardiac malformations. In Barratt-Boyes BG, Neutze JM, Harris EA, eds. Heart disease in infancy: diagnosis and surgical treatment. London: Churchill Livingstone, 1973, p. 3.

4. Rowe RD. Angiocardiography in the prognosis for young infants in congestive failure with ventricular septal defect: the value of defect/ascending aorta diameter ratio. In Barratt-Boyes BG, Neutze JM, Harris EA, eds. Heart disease in infancy: diagnosis and surgical treatment. London: Churchill Livingstone, 1973, p. 119.

5. Rizzoli G, Blackstone EH, Kirklin JW, Pacifico AD, Bargeron LM Jr. Incremental risk factors in hospital mortality rate after repair of ventricular septal defect. J Thorac Cardiovasc Surg 1980;80:494.

6. Rabinovitch M, Keane JF, Norwood WI, Castaneda AR, Reid L. Vascular structure in lung tissue obtained at biopsy correlated with pulmonary hemodynamic findings after repair of congenital heart defects. Circulation 1984;69:655.

7. Rizzoli G, Rubino M, Mazzucco A, Rocco F, Bellini P, Brumana T, et al. Progress in the surgical treatment of ventricular septal defect: an analysis of a twelve years' experience. Thorac Cardiovasc Surg 1983;31:382.

8. Ramaciotti C, Keren A, Silverman NH. Importance of (perimembranous) ventricular septal aneurysm in the natural history of isolated perimembranous ventricular septal defect. Am J Cardiol 1986;57:268.

9. Rice MJ, Seward JB, Edwards WD, Hagler DJ, Danielson GK, Puga FJ, et al. Straddling atrioventricular valve: two-dimensional echocardiographic diagnosis, classification and surgical implications. Am J Cardiol 1985;55:505.

10. Rhodes LA, Keane JF, Keane JP, Fellows KE, Jonas RA, Castaneda AR, et al. Long follow-up (to 43 years) of ventricular septal defect with audible aortic regurgitation. Am J Cardiol 1990;66:340.

11. Richardson JV, Schieken RM, Lauer RM, Stewart P, Doty DB. Repair of large ventricular septal defects in infants and small children. Ann Surgery 1982;195:318.

S

1. Savard M, Swan JHC, Kirklin JW, Wood EH. Hemodynamic alterations associated with ventricular septal defects. In Congenital heart disease. Washington, DC: American Association for the Advancement of Science, 1960, p. 141.

2. Sigmann JM, Stern AM, Sloan HE. Early surgical correction of large ventricular septal defects. Pediatrics 1967;39:4.

3. Stark J, Tynan M, Aberdeen E, Waterston DJ, Bonham-Carter RE, Graham GR, et al. Repair of intracardiac defects after previous constriction (banding) of the pulmonary artery. Surgery 1970;67:536.

4. Subramanian S, Wagner HR. Pulmonary artery banding and debanding in patients with ventricular septal defect. In Barratt-Boyes BG, Neutze JM, Harris EA, eds. Heart disease in infancy: diagnosis and surgical treatment. London: Churchill Livingstone, 1973, p. 141.

5. Stark J, Hucin B, Aberdeen E, Waterston DJ. Cardiac surgery in the first year of life: experience with 1,049 operations. Surgery 1971;69:483.

6. Stirling GR, Stanley PH, Lillehei CW. Effect of cardiac bypass and ventriculotomy upon right ventricular function. Surgical Forum 1957;8:433.

7. Shah P, Singh WS, Rose V, Keith JD. Incidence of bacterial endocarditis in ventricular septal defects. Circulation 1966;34:127.

8. Stahlman M, Kaplan S, Helmsworth JA, Clark LC, Scott HW Jr. Syndrome of left ventricular—right atrial shunt resulting from high interventricular septal defect associated with defective leaflet of the tricuspid valve. Circulation 1955;12:813.

9. Spencer FC, Doyle EF, Danilowicz DA, Bahnson HT, Weldon CS. Long-term evaluation of aortic valvuloplasty for aortic insufficiency and ventricular septal defect. J Thorac Cardiovasc Surg 1973;65:15.

10. Steeg CN, Krongrad E, Davachi F, Bowman FO Jr, Malm JR, Gersony WM. Postoperative left anterior hemiblock and right bundle branch block following repair of tetralogy of Fallot: clinical and etiologic considerations. Circulation 1975;51:1026.

11. Sung RJ, Tamer DM, Garcia OL, Castellanos A, Myerburg RJ, Gelband H. Analysis of surgically induced right bundle branch block pattern using intracardiac recording techniques. Circulation 1976;54:442.

12. Starr A, Menasche V, Dotter C. Surgical correction of aortic insufficiency associated with ventricular septal defect. Surg Gynecol Obstet 1960;111:71.

13. Soto B, Becker AE, Moulaert AJ, Lie JT, Anderson RH. Classification of ventricular septal defects. Br Heart J 1980;43:332.

14. Singh AK, de Leval MR, Stark J. Left ventriculotomy for closure of muscular ventricular septal defects. Ann Surg 1977;186:577.

15. Sandrasagra FA, Hamilton DI, Wilkinson JL. Surgery of VSD in infancy (abstract). In Godman MJ, ed. World Congress of Paediatric Cardiology. Edinburgh: Churchill Livingstone, 1981, p. 289.

16. Sigmann JM, Perry BL, Gehrendt DM, Stern AM, Kirsh MM, Sloan HE. Ventricular septal defect: results after repair in infancy. Am J Cardiol 1977;39:66.

17. Somerville J. (1980) Unpublished study.

18. Stevenson JG, Kawabori I, Stamm SJ, Bailey WW, Hall DG, Mansfield PB, et al. Pulsed Doppler echocardiographic evaluation of ventricular septal defect patches. Circulation 1984;70:I38.

19. Sutherland GR, Godman MJ, Keeton BR, Shore DF, Bain HH, Hunter S. Natural history of perimembranous ventricular septal defects: a prospective echocardiographic haemodynamic correlative study. Br Heart J 1984;51:682.

20. Sutherland GR, Godman MJ, Smallhorn JF, Guiterras P, Anderson RH, Hunter S. Ventricular septal defects: two-dimensional echocardiography and morphological correlations. Br Heart J 1982;47:316.

21. Stark J, Sethia B. Closure of ventricular septal defect in infancy. J Cardiac Surg 1986;1:135.

22. Smolinsky A, Castaneda AR, Van Praagh R. Infundibular septal resection: surgical anatomy of the superior approach. J Thorac Cardiovasc Surg 1988;95:486.

23. Soto B, Ceballos R, Kirklin JW. Ventricular septal defects: a surgical viewpoint. J Am Coll Cardiol 1989;14:1291.

24. Schmidt KG, Cassidy SC, Silverman NH, Stanger P. Doubly committed subarterial ventricular septal defects: echocardiographic features and surgical implications. J Am Coll Cardiol 1988;12:1538.

25. Seward JB, Tajik AJ, Ritter DG. Echocardiographic features of straddling tricuspid valve. Mayo Clin Proc 1975;50:427.

26. Soto B, Ceballos R, Nath PH, Bini RM, Pacifico AD, Bargeron LM Jr. Overriding atrioventricular valves. An angiographic-anatomical correlate. Int J Cardiol 1985;9:323.

27. Stümper O, Fraser AG, Elzenga N, Van Daele M, Frohn-Mulder I, Van Herwerden LA, et al. Assessment of ventricular septal defect closure by intraoperative epicardial ultrasound. J Am Coll Cardiol 1990;16:1672.

28. Serraf A, Lacour-Gayet F, Bruniaux J, Ouaknine R, Losay J, Petit J, et al. Surgical management of isolated multiple ventricular septal defects. Logical approach in 130 cases. J Thorac Cardiovasc Surg 1992;103:437.

29. Seddio F, Reddy VM, McElhinney DB, Tworetzky W, Silverman NH, Hanley FL. Multiple ventricular septal defects: how and when should they be repaired? J Thorac Cardiovasc Surg 1999;117:134.

30. Stellin G, Padalino M, Milanesi O, Rubino M, Casarotto D, Van Praagh R, et al. Surgical closure of apical ventricular septal defects through a right ventricular apical infundibulotomy. Ann Thorac Surg 2000;69:597.

31. Sim EK, Grignani RT, Wong ML, Quek SC, Wong JC, Yip WC, et al. Influence of surgery on aortic valve prolapse and aortic regurgitation in doubly committed subarterial ventricular septal defect. Am J Cardiol 1999;84:1445.

T

1. Tomita H, Arakaki Y, Ono Y, Yamada O, Tsukano S, Yagihara T, et al. Evolution of aortic regurgitation following simple patch closure of doubly committed subarterial ventricular septal defect. Am J Cardiol 2000;86:540.

2. Trusler GA, Mustard WT. A method of banding the pulmonary artery for large isolated ventricular septal defect with and without transposition of the great arteries. Ann Thorac Surg 1972;13:351.

3. Tatooles CJ, Miller RA. Palliative surgery in infants with congenital heart disease. Prog Cardiovasc Dis 1973;15:331.

4. Trusler GA, Moes CA, Kidd BS. Repair of ventricular septal defect with aortic insufficiency. J Thorac Cardiovasc Surg 1973;66:394.

5. Tatsuno K, Konno S, Sakakibara S. Ventricular septal defect with aortic insufficiency: angiocardiographic aspects and a new classification. Am Heart J 1973;85:13.

6. Tatsuno K, Konno S, Ando M, Sakakibara S. Pathogenetic mechanisms of prolapsing aortic valve and aortic regurgitation associated with ventricular septal defect. Circulation 1973;48:1028.

7. Tatsuno K, Ando M, Takao A, Hatsune K, Konno S. Diagnostic importance of aortography in conal ventricular septal defect. Am Heart J 1975;89:171.

8. Truex RC. The sinoatrial node and its connections with the atrial tissues. In Wellens HJ, Lie KI, Janse MJ, eds. The conduction system of the heart. Philadelphia: Lea & Febiger, 1976, p. 209.

9. Tabry IF, McGoon DC, Danielson GK, Wallace RB, Tajik AJ, Seward JB. Surgical management of straddling atrioventricular valve. J Thorac Cardiovasc Surg 1979;77:191.

10. Tiraboschi R, Villani M, Bianchi T, Locatelli G, Vanini V, Crupi G, et al. Surgical management of ventricular septal defect and coarctation of the aorta. Observations on 40 cases, with particular references to infancy. G Ital Cardiol 1978;8:811.

11. Tiraboschi R, Alfieri O, Carpentier A, Parenzan L. One stage correction of coarctation of the aorta associated with intracardiac defects in infancy. J Cardiovasc Surg 1978;19:11.

12. Tandon R, Becker AE, Moller JH, Edwards JE. Double inlet left ventricle. Straddling tricuspid valve. Br Heart J 1974;36:747.

13. Trusler GA, Williams WG, Smallhorn JF, Freedom RM. Late results after repair of aortic insufficiency associated with ventricular septal defect. J Thorac Cardiovasc Surg 1992;103:276.

14. Tantengco MV, Bates JR, Ryan T, Caldwell R, Darragh R, Ensing GJ. Dynamic three-dimensional echocardiographic reconstruction of congenital cardiac septation defects. Pediatr Cardiol 1997;18:184.

15. Tohyama K, Satomi G, Momma K. Aortic valve prolapse and aortic regurgitation associated with subpulmonic ventricular septal defect. Am J Cardiol 1997;79:1285.

U

1. Ueda M, Becker AE. Morphological characteristics of perimembranous ventricular septal defects and their surgical significance. Int J Cardiol 1985;8:149.

V

1. Van Praagh R, McNamara JJ. Anatomic types of ventricular septal defect with aortic insufficiency: diagnostic and surgical considerations. Am Heart J 1968;75:604.

2. Van Praagh R, Bernhard WF, Rosenthal A, Parisi LF, Fyler DC. Interrupted aortic arch: surgical treatment. Am J Cardiol 1971;27:200.

3. Vogel M, Freedom RM, Brand A, Trusler GA, Williams WG, Rowe R. Ventricular septal defect and subaortic stenosis: an analysis of 41 patients. Am J Cardiol 1983;52:1258.

4. Vincent RN, Lang P, Chipman CW, Castaneda AR. Assessment of hemodynamic status in the intensive care unit immediately after closure of ventricular septal defect. Am J Cardiol 1985;55:526.

5. Van Praagh R, Weinberg PM, Calder AL, Buckley LF, Van Praagh S. The transposition complexes: How many are there? In Davila JC, ed. Second Henry Ford Hospital International Symposium on Cardiac Surgery. East Norwalk, Conn: Appleton & Lange, 1977, p. 207.

6. Van Praagh R, Ongley PA, Swan HJ. Anatomic types of single or common ventricle in man: morphologic and geometric aspects of 60 necropsied cases. Am J Cardiol 1964;13:367.

W

1. Warden HE, Cohen M, Read RC, Lillehei CW. Controlled cross circulation for open intracardiac surgery. J Thorac Surg 1954;28:331.

2. Wagenvoort CA, Neufeld HN, DuShane JW, Edwards JE. The pulmonary arterial tree in ventricular septal defect: a quantitative study of anatomic features in fetuses, infants, and children. Circulation 1961;23:740.

3. Wagenvoort CA, Wagenvoort N. Primary pulmonary hypertension: a pathological study of the lung vessels in 156 clinically diagnosed cases. Circulation 1970;42:1163.

4. Wolff GS, Rowland TW, Ellison RC. Surgically induced right bundle branch block with left anterior hemiblock: an ominous sign in postoperative tetralogy of Fallot. Circulation 1972;46:587.

5. Wollenek G, Wyse R, Sullivan I, Elliott M, de Leval M, Stark J. Closure of muscular ventricular septal defects through a left ventriculotomy. Eur J Cardiothorac Surg 1996;10:595.

6. Weintraub RG, Menahem S. Early surgical closure of a large ventricular septal defect: influence on long-term growth. J Am Coll Cardiol 1991;18:552.

Y

1. Yamaki S, Tezuka F. Quantitative analysis of pulmonary vascular disease in complete transposition of the great arteries. Circulation 1976;54:805.

2. Yacoub MH, Radley-Smith R, de Gasperis C. Primary repair of large ventricular septal defects in the first year of life. G Ital Cardiol 1978;8:827.

3. Yeager SB, Freed MD, Keane JF, Norwood WI, Castaneda AR. Primary surgical closure of ventricular septal defect in the first year of life: results in 128 infants. J Am Coll Cardiol 1984;3:1269.

4. Yilmaz AT, Ozal E, Arslan M, Tatar H, Ozturk OY. Aneurysm of the membranous septum in adult patients with perimembranous ventricular septal defect. Eur J Cardiothorac Surg 1997;11:307.

5. Yacoub MH, Khan H, Stavri G, Shinebourne E, Radley-Smith R. Anatomic correction of the syndrome of prolapsing right coronary aortic cusp, dilatation of the sinus of Valsalva, and ventricular septal defect. J Thorac Cardiovasc Surg 1997;113:253.

Z

1. Ziady GM, Hallidie-Smith KA, Goodwin JF. Conduction disturbances after surgical closure of ventricular septal defect. Br Heart J 1972;34:1199.

2. Zhou Q, Lai Y, Wei H, Song R, Wu Y, Zhang H. Unidirectional valve patch for repair of cardiac septal defects with pulmonary hypertension. Ann Thorac Surg 1995;60:1245.

22 Congenital Sinus of Valsalva Aneurysm and Aortico–Left Ventricular Tunnel

SECTION 1

Unruptured and Ruptured Sinus of Valsalva Aneurysms

DEFINITION

Congenital sinus of Valsalva aneurysms are thin-walled saccular or tubular outpouchings usually located in the right sinus or adjacent half of the noncoronary sinus. They generally have an intracardiac course, but may protrude into the pericardial space. They may rupture into the right (or rarely the left) heart chambers to form an aortocardiac fistula, or into the pericardial cavity. Associated congenital cardiac anomalies are common.

HISTORICAL NOTE

The syndrome of acute rupture of a congenital sinus of Valsalva aneurysm was apparently first described by Hope in 1839.[H3] A year later, Thurman published the first important paper on the subject.[T2] He discussed Hope's case and added five of his own, none of which had ruptured. Eighty years later, Abbott reviewed the clinical features of acute rupture from eight previous cases and reported another case.[A2] At that time,[S4] and even as late as 1937,[S5] most ruptured and unruptured sinus of Valsalva aneurysms were considered syphilitic. Smith stated in 1914 that "the lesion, which is usually syphilitic, is not so rare as to be altogether devoid of clinical interest, but the diagnosis, perforating or otherwise, presents almost insurmountable difficulties."[S13] Jones and Langley reviewed congenital and acquired aneurysms in 1949.[J1] They accepted 25 cases as being of congenital origin and elucidated most of the important features of the condition. In 1951, Venning may have been the first to diagnose acute rupture during life,[V1] although Oram and East claimed this distinction in 1955,[O2] as did Brown and colleagues.[B4] In Oram and East's patients, cardiac catheterization confirmed the presence of a left-to-right shunt, although angiography was not performed. The earliest report of using aortography to diagnose an unruptured aneurysm was that of Falholt and Thomsen in 1953.[F1]

The first successful surgical repairs of sinus of Valsalva aneurysms were performed in 1956 at the Mayo Clinic and the University of Minnesota, using cardiopulmonary bypass (CPB).[B1,L1,M7] Spencer, Blake, and Bahnson[S10] and Morris and colleagues[M2] also reported early successful cases. In 1957, both Morrow and colleagues and Bigelow and Barnes successfully closed a ruptured congenital sinus of Valsalva aneurysm using mild hypothermia with inflow stasis,[B3,M1] but this technique was not subsequently employed. Numerous reports followed of one or two patients treated successfully using CPB. Dubost and colleagues reported eight cases in 1962,[D2] and Besterman and colleagues reported six cases in 1963.[B2] In a 1960 collective review, Kieffer and Winchell reported 78 surgical and nonsurgical patients, 59 of whom had rupture of the aneurysm into a cardiac chamber.[K2] Sakakibara and Konno noted the prevalence of this lesion in Japan and its association with ventricular septal defect (VSD) and aortic regurgitation, and were among the first to provide a comprehensive classification.[S1-S3] Their first patient underwent aneurysm repair in 1960.[S14]

MORPHOLOGY

The essential lesion of *congenital* sinus of Valsalva aneurysms is separation of the aortic media of the sinus from the media adjacent to the hinge line of the aortic valve cusp, as emphasized by Edwards and Burchell in 1957[E1] (Fig. 22-1). This defect may result from absence of normal aortic elastic tissue and media in this region.[E3,V1] The congenitally weak area gradually enlarges under aortic pressure to form an aneurysm, although the age at which this occurs is uncertain. Viewed from the aorta, the aneurysm appears as an excavation of the sinus of Valsalva that protrudes into the underlying cardiac chamber (Fig. 22-2, *A* and *B*).

Precise location of this basic congenital abnormality, which may be accompanied by an adjacent separation of the ventricular septum from the aorta to form a VSD, tends to be different in Asians and non-Asians. In Asians, the basic abnormality is located leftward and toward the commissural area between the right and left coronary cusps; thus, compared with non-Asians, rupture occurs more often into the right ventricle than the right atrium (94% versus 77%, $P[\chi^2] = .0001$).[C3] Also in Asians, the coexisting VSD is usually leftward and juxta-arterial, whereas in non-Asians it is usually rightward and only juxta-aortic (see Chapter 21 for definitions). The leftward tendency in Asians is also manifested by fewer aneurysms of the more rightward noncoronary sinus than in non-Asians (11% versus 32%, $P < .0001$). Left sinus of Valsalva aneurysms are uncommon in both Asians (2%) and non-Asians (5%) ($P[\chi^2]$ for difference = .11).[C3]

Acquired sinus of Valsalva aneurysms caused by medionecrosis,[D3] syphilis,[S13] atherosclerosis,[D1] endocarditis,[S7] Behçet's disease,[K5,W4] or penetrating injuries[M2] are usually readily distinguishable from congenital forms. They are more diffuse, involving more of the sinus or multiple sinuses and often the ascending aorta, and therefore project into the pericardium outside the heart. A congenital aneurysm is frequently diagnosed by exclusion of other etiologies as well as by presence of associated

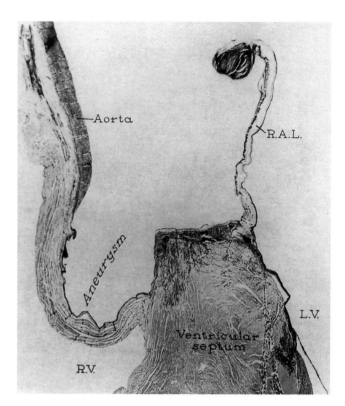

Figure 22-1 Unruptured right sinus of Valsalva aneurysm in a non-Asian patient. Low-power photomicrograph of a longitudinal section through the central portion of right aortic sinus shows separation of aortic media of the sinus from the media adjacent to the hinge line of right aortic cusp. Aneurysm is walled by atrophic muscular tissue of right ventricular outflow tract. (From Edwards and Burchell.[E1])

Key: *L.V.,* Left ventricle; *R.A.L.,* right aortic leaflet (cusp); *R.V.,* right ventricle.

congenital cardiac defects. Difficulties arise with mycotic aneurysms[J1,V1] because endocarditis complicates about 5% to 10% of congenital aneurysms,[N1] and with medionecrosis because it and Marfan syndrome and medionecrosis both occur in some patients with congenital sinus of Valsalva aneurysms.[A1,M3]

Rupture

In some patients the aneurysm gradually develops a localized windsock, which ultimately ruptures into an adjacent low-pressure cardiac chamber in an unknown percentage of patients (Fig. 22-3). The thin-walled, ruptured aneurysm characteristically has an intracardiac fistulous portion and a nipplelike projection into the cardiac chamber, with one or more points of rupture at its apex (Fig. 22-4). Rarely it projects outside the aortic root or heart. When the aneurysm coexists with a VSD, the windsock usually projects into the right ventricle through a thinned area of myocardium just downstream from the VSD; the aneurysm is separated from the VSD by the hinge line of the aortic valve cusp, at the septal portion of the left ventriculoaortic junction (Fig. 22-5; see also Fig. 22-2, *C*).

About one fourth of patients have no windsock or other suggestion of aneurysm formation, but rather have a direct

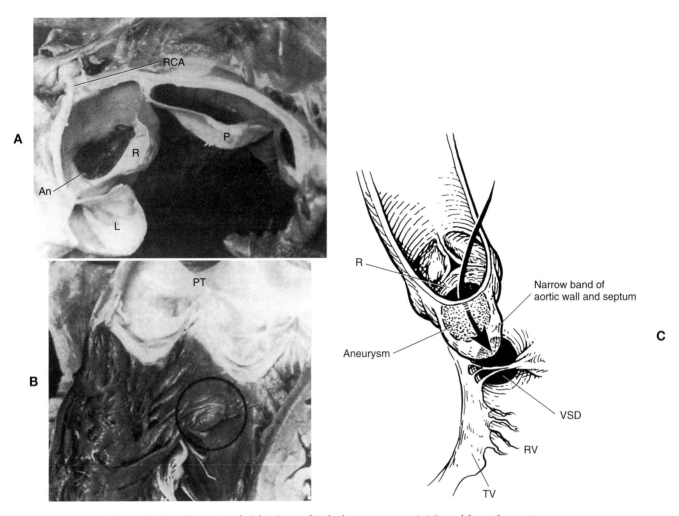

Figure 22-2   Unruptured right sinus of Valsalva aneurysm. **A,** Viewed from the aorta, aneurysm has a well-defined origin, or neck, presenting as an almost circular ostium in the base of the sinus of Valsalva just above the hinge line of the aortic cusp. **B,** Viewed from right ventricle, aneurysm protrudes into right ventricular outflow tract just below pulmonary valve. **C,** Anatomic depiction of a specimen with coexisting juxta–aortic ventricular septal defect *(VSD)* in the right ventricular outlet portion of the ventricular septum. The narrow band of aortic wall and septum separating aneurysm from VSD is located behind the aneurysm. (From Edwards and Burchell.[E1])

Key: *An,* Aneurysm of right aortic sinus of Valsalva; *L,* left aortic valve cusp; *P,* posterior (noncoronary) aortic valve cusp; *PT,* pulmonary trunk; *R,* right aortic valve cusp; *RCA,* right coronary artery; *RV,* right ventricle; *TV,* tricuspid valve; *VSD,* ventricular septal defect.

fistulous communication between the aortic sinus and the heart.[N1,R3] This defect has been recognized in a few patients at or soon after birth.[D2,K2,P1,R3] Windsock deformity is typical in lesions originating from the right sinus and communicating with the right ventricle; a direct fistula is typical in those from the noncoronary sinus to the right atrium[B1,R3]; and an extracardiac aneurysm is typical[B10,K1,K2,N1,S10] in the rare cases of left sinus origin.[E4]

Although the prevalence of aneurysms of the sinus of Valsalva in various locations is different among Asians and non-Asians, in both groups the *sinus of origin* is the main determinant of the direction of protrusion and rupture of the aneurysm, and thus of the chamber into which it ruptures (Fig. 22-6). Also in both populations, but with differing prevalence, aneurysms of the right aortic sinus of Valsalva

are most common.[C3,G2,J1,K2,N1,O2,S8] The aneurysm may arise from the leftward portion of this sinus, with the windsock projecting into the adjacent right ventricular outflow tract just below the pulmonary valve, termed *type I* by Sakakibara and Konno.[S3] It may also originate more centrally and project through the substance of the outlet portion of the right ventricular aspect of the ventricular septum (Fig. 22-7), or from the rightward portion of the sinus, entering the right ventricle beneath the parietal band (parietal extension of the infundibular septum) in the region of the membranous septum. Rarely the aneurysm may project into the pulmonary trunk.[S17]

Aneurysms from the noncoronary sinus usually originate from its anterior portion and project into the right atrium (Fig. 22-8), but in rare cases they project and rupture into

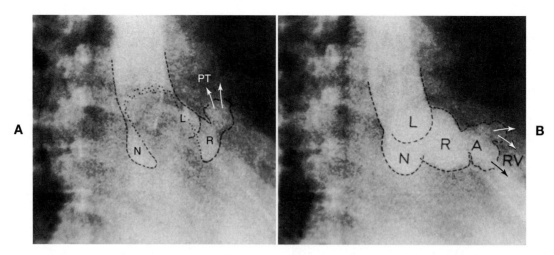

Figure 22-3   Cineangiograms in right anterior oblique projection of a right sinus of Valsalva aneurysm ruptured into right ventricle in systole (**A**) and in diastole (**B**). Noncoronary and left coronary sinuses and cusps are normal. Right coronary sinus is enlarged, and there is an aneurysm (windsock) protruding into right ventricular infundibulum. Arrows indicate contrast medium shunting through holes in aneurysm and filling right ventricular infundibulum in diastole and pulmonary trunk in systole (when the aneurysm almost prolapses through the pulmonary valve). There is no aortic regurgitation, but the ruptured aneurysm is associated with a large conoventricular juxta–aortic ventricular septal defect.

Key: *A*, Aneurysm; *L*, left coronary sinus; *N*, noncoronary sinus; *PT*, pulmonary trunk; *R*, right coronary sinus; *RV*, right ventricular infundibulum.

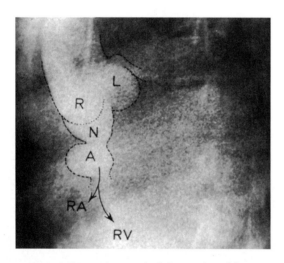

Figure 22-4   Cineangiogram in left anterior oblique projection of an aneurysm and fistula arising from the noncoronary sinus of Valsalva and rupturing into the right atrium. Aneurysm fills from nadir of noncoronary sinus. There is shunting of contrast medium to the right atrium, through the tricuspid valve, and to the right ventricle. Right and left coronary sinuses appear normal. There is no aortic regurgitation and no ventricular septal defect.

Key: *A*, Aneurysm; *L*, left coronary sinus; *N*, noncoronary sinus; *R*, right coronary sinus; *RA*, right atrium; *RV*, right ventricle.

the right ventricle. Rarely, rupture can occur simultaneously into the right ventricle and right atrium or into the muscular ventricular septum.[G1] Aneurysms arising from the posterior portion of the noncoronary sinus may rupture into the pericardium.[B11,M10] Another rare occurrence is a right sinus or noncoronary sinus aneurysm that ruptures into the left ventricle (LV).[H4,S12,W2] Rarity of rupture into the LV may be related to the relatively thick wall and high pressure in that chamber. Aneurysms arising from the left coronary sinus may rupture into the left atrium, LV, or rarely the pulmonary trunk or pericardium.[H5,K6]

Sinus of Valsalva aneurysms rupturing into areas adjacent to the tricuspid valve are also adjacent to the atrioventricular (AV) node and His bundle and may be a cause of heart block, bundle branch block, and ventricular fibrillation.[C4,H9,T1,W5]

Table 22-1 shows the overall distribution of the various sites of rupture, based on analysis by Chu and colleagues of 361 cases in the literature, including 57 from their own institution.[C3]

Associated Cardiac Anomalies
Ventricular Septal Defect

A VSD is the most common coexisting cardiac anomaly and may arise from the same congenital anomaly that produced the aneurysm. VSDs occur in 30% to 50% of patients,[A4,C3,C5,N1,O1,S2,S3,V3] but prevalence is higher when the aneurysm arises from the right sinus.[C3,C5] When the aneurysm arises from the left third of the right aortic sinus, the VSD is *juxta-arterial*, with its upper margin formed by the confluent aortic and pulmonary valves. When the aneurysm arises from the central third of the right sinus, the VSD may be *juxta-aortic* or may lie within the muscle of the septum's outlet portion. When the aneurysm arises from the right third of the right sinus (or rarely, the anterior portion of the noncoronary sinus),[E1,S2] the VSD is usually *conoventricular* and may be *perimembranous* as

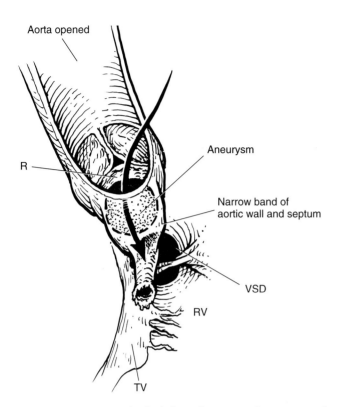

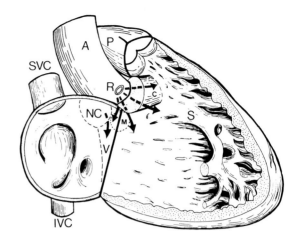

Figure 22-6   Diagrammatic representation of structures depicted in right anterior oblique view of heart. Arrows indicate common sites of rupture of sinus of Valsalva aneurysms.

Key: *A,* Aorta; *C,* conal (infundibular) septum; *IVC,* inferior vena cava; *M,* membranous septum; *NC,* noncoronary sinus; *P,* pulmonary trunk; *R,* right coronary sinus; *S,* septal band; *SVC,* superior vena cava; *V,* atrioventricular septum.

Figure 22-5   Anatomic depiction of a ruptured aneurysm of the rightward portion of the right sinus of Valsalva associated with a conoventricular, juxta-aortic ventricular septal defect *(VSD).* Rupture has occurred at apex of the windsock. Narrow band of aortic wall and septum separates aneurysm from VSD.

Key: *R,* Right coronary cusp; *RV,* right ventricle; *TV,* tricuspid valve; *VSD,* ventricular septal defect.

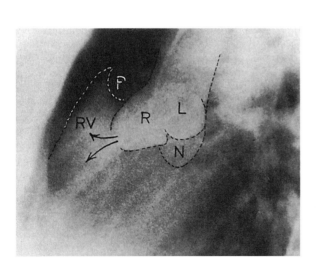

Figure 22-7   Cineangiogram in diastole (lateral projection) of an aneurysm of right coronary sinus that protrudes into right ventricular infundibulum, filled by contrast medium shunting through ruptured aneurysm. Pulmonary valve is still closed. Left coronary and noncoronary sinuses appear normal. There is no aortic regurgitation. At operation, aneurysm arose from center of right sinus, with a prominent windsock in the infundibular septum; immediately beneath it was a moderate-sized ventricular septal defect.

Key: *L,* Left coronary sinus; *N,* noncoronary sinus; *P,* pulmonary valve; *R,* right coronary sinus; *RV,* right ventricular infundibulum.

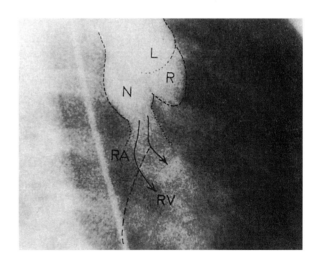

Figure 22-8   Cineangiogram in right anterior oblique projection (diastole) of a large aneurysmal connection of noncoronary sinus to right atrium. Contrast flow *(arrows)* was observed to enter right atrium close to tricuspid ring *(dashed line)* before passing through tricuspid valve to right ventricle. Right and left coronary sinuses appear normal. There is no aortic regurgitation and no ventricular septal defect. At operation a 15-mm-long windsock aneurysm was projecting into the right atrium adjacent to anteroseptal commissure of tricuspid valve.

Key: *L,* Left coronary sinus; *N,* noncoronary sinus; *R,* right coronary sinus; *RA,* right atrium; *RV,* right ventricle.

■ **TABLE 22-1   Prevalence of Sites of Rupture for Sinus of Valsalva Aneurysms**

Site of Rupture	Asian (% of 195)	Non-Asian (% of 166)	Total (% of 361)
Right atrium	13	35	23
Right ventricle	84	57	72
Right ventricle + right atrium	<1	1	<1
Left atrium	<1	1	<1
Left ventricle	<1	2	1
Right atrium + left atrium + left ventricle	<1	<1	1
Ventricular septum	1	1	<1
Pulmonary trunk	<1	<1	<1
Right ventricle + pulmonary trunk	<1	<1	<1
Pericardium	<1	2	<1

(Data from Chu and colleagues.[C3])

well (see Chapter 21 for definitions). Rarely a conoventricular VSD occurs in association with an aneurysm arising from the central or leftward third of the right sinus. Sakakibara and Konno considered this a coincidental association between two independent malformations rather than a combined developmental anomaly.[S2]

Aortic Valve Abnormalities and Aortic Regurgitation

Aortic valve abnormalities and aortic regurgitation (AR) are common in patients with sinus of Valsalva aneurysms.[A4,C3,C5,V3] When a VSD is present, AR usually results from a prolapsed aortic cusp, similar to the finding in the syndrome of VSD and AR (see Section 2 of Chapter 21). When a VSD is not present, AR usually arises from other aortic valve abnormalities, including a bicuspid valve.

As in VSD and AR, when prolapse of the aortic cusp into a VSD is the cause, severity of AR progressively worsens.[S2] If the fibrous hinge line remains intact at the base of a prolapsed cusp, a sinus of Valsalva aneurysm projects toward the ventricle superior to the hinge line, and the cusp projects through the VSD inferior to it. When the hinge line does not retain its integrity, however, as in long-standing cases, both structures form a single sac.[S1-S3] Taguchi and colleagues noted that prolonged AR produces a fixed fibrous deformity of the prolapsed cusp.[T1]

The frequency of aortic cusp prolapse in sinus of Valsalva aneurysms was undoubtedly underestimated in earlier reports, particularly when no aortograms or echocardiograms were obtained and the aorta was not opened at operation. Aortic cusp prolapse is also less common if only ruptured sinus aneurysm is considered. Thus, in the series of Taguchi and colleagues, which included unruptured cases, AR (although usually mild) was present in 75% of patients,[T1] whereas in the series of Okada and colleagues from Japan, which included only ruptured cases, the prevalence was 17%.[O1]

A complicating problem is the difficulty of determining what constitutes a true (unruptured) sinus aneurysm with combined VSD and AR. Aneurysmal enlargement of the aortic sinus is common in this setting, and the distinction from unruptured sinus aneurysm is difficult to delineate by aortography and even at operation or autopsy. However, seven (15%) of 48 surgical patients with VSD and AR had a distinct but unruptured sinus of Valsalva aneurysm (see Table 21-18).

Pulmonary Stenosis

Important pulmonary stenosis is uncommon in patients with congenital sinus of Valsalva aneurysms, but small gradients are common.[O1] The stenosis may be valvar, but is usually caused by either a projection of the windsock in front of the infundibular septum[B1] or a developmental anomaly of the right ventricular outflow tract similar to that present in tetralogy of Fallot and VSD–AR syndrome.

Other Anomalies

Infrequently, other congenital cardiac anomalies may coexist with sinus of Valsalva aneurysms, including aortic coarctation, patent ductus arteriosus, atrial septal defect, subaortic stenosis, and tetralogy of Fallot.[A4,C3,C5,V3]

CLINICAL FEATURES AND DIAGNOSTIC CRITERIA

Unruptured congenital sinus of Valsalva aneurysms are usually silent lesions; their diagnosis depends on echocardiograms or aortograms usually obtained to demonstrate associated symptomatic lesions such as VSD or AR. Diagnosis can be made incidentally during coronary angiography. Rarely, unruptured aneurysms produce tricuspid valve dysfunction or right ventricular outflow obstruction, bringing the patient to medical care.[G4,K4] These aneurysms may also produce severe myocardial ischemia by compressing the right or left main coronary artery.[B10,B12,G5,G6,T7] Embolization from unruptured sinus of Valsalva aneurysms has also been reported.[S18,W6] The presence of this anomaly should be considered in men, who represent 80% of patients with sinus of Valsalva aneurysms.[J1,S8]

Acute symptoms occur in about 35% of patients with rupture of the aneurysm.[M6,N1,T1] In 45% of patients, surprisingly, rupture is associated only with gradual onset of effort dyspnea, and in 20%, no symptoms develop. Acute symptoms consist of sudden breathlessness and pain. The pain is usually precordial and may also be epigastric, probably because of acute hepatic congestion. Precordial pain may mimic myocardial infarction, although radiation of the pain beyond the substernal area is unusual.[O2] In a few patients, death occurs within days of rupture from right-sided heart failure, but most patients improve during the *latent period,*[O2] which may last for weeks, months, or years. This improvement may occur without specific medical therapy. The latent period is usually followed by recurrence of dyspnea and signs of right-sided heart failure. Characteristic features at this final stage are aortic and tricuspid regurgitation, an unusual combination.[O2,S8]

The infrequency of severe symptoms at rupture may be due to the initially small size of the rupture in many patients. Studies by Sawyers and colleagues in dogs indicate that symptoms are severe when the fistula is greater than 5 mm in diameter.[S8] However, in humans, Taguchi and colleagues found little correlation between size of the fistulous opening at operation and a history of acute symptoms.[T1] Acute symptoms at rupture may occur less often with a VSD[S2,T1] and more often with severe AR.

Acute symptomatic ruptures may be precipitated by heavy exertion, but they also occur after serious automobile accidents and at cardiac catheterization.[B1] Rarely, an episode of infective endocarditis may be the precipitating factor. Marfan syndrome may also predispose the aneurysm to rupture.[S6]

Rupture is heralded not only by pain and dyspnea but also by a characteristic murmur that is loud, harsh, superficial, and accompanied by a coarse thrill.[S9] The murmur is usually continuous with either systolic or diastolic accentuation, but it may be to and fro, similar to that present in the VSD–AR syndrome. In the past, this murmur has been mistaken for that of patent ductus arteriosus, but it is maximal at a lower site, usually the left second, third, or fourth intercostal space. With rupture into the sinus portion of the right ventricle or right atrium, the murmur tends to be maximal at a low level over the sternum or to the right of the lower sternum.[E2,M4,M5,S1] Rarely the murmur is systolic only,[B1] possibly because the communication is small.[H2] Alternatively, the murmur may be confined to diastole in those few cases when rupture occurs into the high-pressure LV[N1,W2] or when right ventricular pressure is at systemic level, as in the neonate.[A1] When the murmur is continuous, its timing and accentuation are a function of several factors, including degree of associated AR, degree of aortic systolic murmur, functional size of the VSD, and size of the fistula.[T1] Morch and Greenwood assessed the various causes of murmurs that were believed to be continuous and associated with signs of rapid aortic runoff in their adult patients.[M6] They found that ruptured sinus aneurysm (8 cases) was the second most common cause, after patent ductus arteriosus (33 cases), VSD and AR (3 cases), aortopulmonary window (3 cases), coronary arteriovenous fistula (1 case), and pulmonary arteriovenous fistula (1 case).

Other physical signs of ruptured aneurysm include widened aortic pulse pressure, suggesting mild to severe AR. An elevated jugular venous pressure with a prominent *v* wave, suggesting tricuspid regurgitation, may be caused by direct entrance of a fistula into the right atrium, but in most cases this sign is absent until onset of right-sided heart failure, when liver enlargement and pulsation also occur.[B2]

The chest radiograph does not show enlargement of the aortic root. Plethora may be present, although the left-to-right shunt through both the fistula and any associated VSD is usually small. The electrocardiogram shows either LV or biventricular hypertrophy. Right bundle branch block may

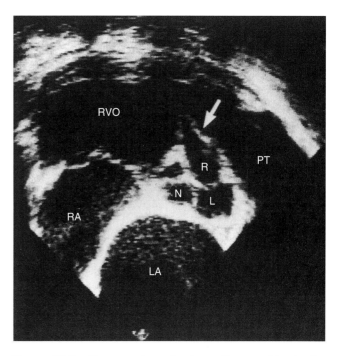

Figure 22-9   Transesophageal echocardiogram (short-axis view) of sinus of Valsalva aneurysm *(arrow)* that has ruptured into right ventricular outflow tract. (From van Son and colleagues.[V3])

Key: *L*, Left aortic sinus; *LA*, left atrium; *N*, noncoronary aortic sinus; *PT*, pulmonary trunk; *R*, right coronary sinus; *RA*, right atrium; *RVO*, right ventricular outflow tract.

occur and may be more common in aneurysms with an intracardiac course close to the AV node and bundle of His. Complete heart block can also occur.[M8,W5]

Although the diagnosis is virtually certain on clinical grounds in patients with acute symptoms and sudden appearance of a continuous murmur, two-dimensional Doppler color flow echocardiography is used for verification (Fig. 22-9).[C2,T5,V2,W1] Cardiac catheterization and angiography are generally (Figs. 22-3, 22-4, 22-7, 22-8) performed to study the site of origin and termination of the fistula and the presence of associated anomalies, particularly VSD, AR, and pulmonary stenosis. The true size of the VSD cannot be estimated angiographically when the right aortic cusp is prolapsed into the VSD. Degree of left-to-right shunting through the fistulous communication with the VSD is calculated, as is pulmonary vascular resistance (see "Cardiac Catheterization" under Clinical Features and Diagnostic Criteria in Section 1 of Chapter 21). Magnetic resonance imaging may establish the diagnosis of aneurysm in certain circumstances.[K7]

NATURAL HISTORY

In an era in which unruptured sinus of Valsalva aneurysms are being diagnosed with greater frequency (42% of those diagnosed by Chiang and colleagues were unruptured[C2]), it is unfortunate that the time-related probability of aneurysmal rupture is unknown. Such information would be useful not only in advising patients for or against operation, but also in managing an unruptured aneurysm at the time of surgical treatment of a coexisting cardiac anomaly. Occasionally, unruptured aneurysms of the sinuses of Valsalva cause important symptoms by protruding into either the right atrium, which causes tricuspid stenosis and regurgitation,[G4] or the right ventricle, which causes right ventricular outflow obstruction.[B9,K3,K4] Complete heart block and ventricular tachycardia may result from the sheer mass of a large and strategically located aneurysm of a sinus of Valsalva.[H9,M8,R2,W5]

When it ruptures, the aneurysm usually does so in the third or fourth decade of life. An exception is when there is already a small fistulous communication present at birth. This is well tolerated and is not a cause of early death.[A1,D2,S1] As already noted, in about 20% of patients, the time of rupture cannot be determined by history. Once symptoms develop, heart failure worsens, and without surgical treatment, most patients die within 1 year of rupture.[S8]

Although death after intracardiac rupture of a sinus of Valsalva aneurysm is usually from heart failure, infective endocarditis complicates heart failure in about 10% of patients[N1] and may itself be a cause of death.

When a VSD coexists with the aneurysm, the aortic valve is usually at least mildly regurgitant. The natural history then becomes similar to that of VSD and AR (see section 2 of Chapter 21).[S2] The AR becomes progressively more severe, as does prolapse of the right aortic cusp and aneurysmal sac. This process gradually reduces the size of the VSD until even an anatomically large defect becomes functionally small. Pulmonary arterial hypertension and increased pulmonary vascular resistance therefore are rare.[N1] By the time most patients with this combination of anomalies reach age 15 to 20 years, a fixed fibrous deformity of the prolapsed cusp has developed.

TECHNIQUE OF OPERATION

The many types and variations of ruptured and unruptured sinus of Valsalva aneurysms, as well as the rarity of some, make detailed description of repair of each impractical. Instead, this section details repair of three of the most common varieties, and from these the techniques of repair for most other aneurysms can be deduced. For example, an aneurysm of the right sinus of Valsalva, without VSD, that has ruptured into the right ventricle is repaired much the same as described for this type of aneurysm that has ruptured into the right atrium, but substituting "ventricle" for "atrium." Some rare and difficult types may be most simply repaired through an aortic approach, closing the origin of the aneurysm from the sinus with a patch.

Unruptured sinus of Valsalva aneurysms are probably best repaired by excision or, occasionally, by exclusion of the aneurysm and reconstruction by the identical method used for a similar but ruptured aneurysm.

Ruptured Right Sinus of Valsalva Aneurysm, with Ventricular Septal Defect

Repair of a ruptured aneurysm at the midportion of the right sinus of Valsalva with coexisting juxta-aortic VSD is described first, because the surgical principles are more easily appreciated in this setting. If the aneurysm is in the rightward portion of the right sinus, the VSD is probably conoventricular (perimembranous) and would be approached through the right atrium, often with detachment of the anterior and septal leaflets of the tricuspid valve. If the aneurysm is in the leftward portion of the right sinus of Valsalva, the associated VSD in the outlet portion of the ventricular septum would be juxta-arterial, and the approach would be through the right ventricle or pulmonary trunk. In either case, operation is usually facilitated by a combined aortic and right ventricular, pulmonary arterial, or right atrial approach.[C3,M5,S11,S14,V3]

Initial preparations follow the usual routine (see Section 3 of Chapter 2). After median sternotomy the pericardium is opened and complete external evaluation of the heart is made. The protruding nipple of the ruptured aneurysm may be palpated through the free wall of the right ventricle. It is important to note that no external evidence of the aneurysm itself is usually seen, and the aortic root appears to be normal on inspection. Intraoperative transesophageal echocardiography (TEE) is useful for defining the location of the aneurysm and the cardiac chamber into which it has ruptured (see Fig. 22-9), and for assessing completeness of the fistula and VSD repair and severity of AR before and after repair.

CPB is established after cannulation of the ascending aorta and direct caval cannulation, and body temperature is reduced. The aorta is clamped promptly, the right atrium is opened through a short oblique incision, and a sump suction catheter is placed across the foramen ovale. In most cases the aortic valve is at least mildly regurgitant. The aortic root is opened transversely (Fig. 22-10, A), and cold cardioplegic solution is infused directly into the left and right coronary ostia or retrogradely through the coronary sinus (see Chapter 3).

Exposure is obtained by placing stay sutures on the edges of the aortotomy. The orifice of the aneurysm is visualized, and elevating the right aortic cusp reveals the underlying VSD. No attempt is made to determine the feasibility of repairing the VSD through the aortic root; it may be difficult through the aortotomy to distinguish between a conoventricular VSD adjacent to the His bundle and a juxta-aortic VSD in the right ventricular outflow tract that does not border the His bundle. Any redundancy or tendency of the right coronary cusp to prolapse is noted, but its repair is deferred.

The right ventricle is opened through a transverse or vertical incision, depending on distribution of the branches of the right coronary artery. Alternatively, an approach is made through the pulmonary trunk. The anatomy is visualized (Fig. 22-10, B). The thinned-out windsock, often containing one or more perforations, is resected, creating a large defect in the right sinus of Valsalva. This defect is downstream (cephalad) from the VSD and separated from it by the hinge line of the right aortic cusp (Fig. 22-10, C). Most of the excised windsock is devoid of aortic media (see Fig. 22-1). A single polyester or pericardial patch is sewn into place to close the VSD and defect in the sinus of Valsalva, and the area of the hinge line of the right aortic cusp, which has been isolated by the resection, is sutured to the patch at an appropriate level (Fig. 22-10, D to F).

After closing the ventriculotomy (or pulmonary trunk) with polypropylene suture placed as a continuous stitch, the

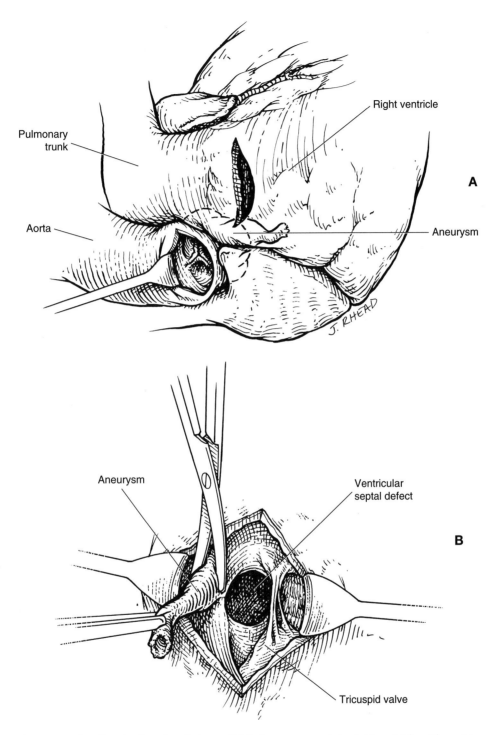

Figure 22-10   Repair of ruptured sinus of Valsalva aneurysm into right ventricle, with ventricular septal defect (VSD). **A,** Initial incision is a transverse aortotomy. The orifice of the aneurysm in the right sinus is visualized. The right ventricle is opened through a transverse incision. Care must be taken to ensure that the aortic incision does not extend into right coronary artery. **B,** Windsock of ruptured aneurysm is seen overlying VSD. The thinned-out portion of the windsock containing the perforation is excised, taking care not to damage the hinge line of the right aortic valve cusp.

Continued

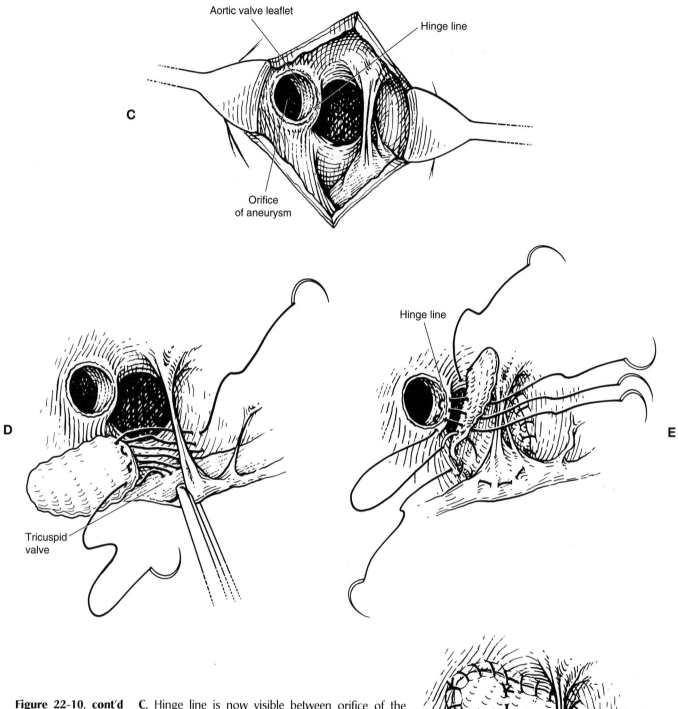

Figure 22-10, cont'd   C, Hinge line is now visible between orifice of the aneurysm and ventricular septal defect (VSD). **D,** Repair is performed using one patch and inserting it through right ventriculotomy. The patch is first sutured to inferior rim of VSD, incorporating septal leaflet of tricuspid valve and avoiding conduction system, using a continuous polypropylene suture. **E,** Midportion of patch is sutured to hinge line of right aortic leaflet using interrupted polypropylene mattress sutures. This step is accomplished before remainder of patch is sewn into place. **F,** Superior aspect of patch is sewn into place over orifice of the aneurysm in the aortic sinus, completing the repair.

interior of the aortic root is again exposed through the aortotomy. When AR coexists and the patient is young with pathology limited to prolapse, all or part of a Trusler repair of the aortic valve is then performed (see Figs. 21-40 and 21-41).[T3] In older patients with AR or when the aortic valve defect is more extensive, valve replacement is necessary (see "Cold Cardioplegia, Controlled Aortic Root Reperfusion, and [When Needed] Warm Cardioplegic Induction" in Chapter 12). Either before or after closing the aortic root, the controlled, initially hyperkalemic reperfusion is begun if indicated (see Chapter 3), the sump suction catheter is removed, and the foramen ovale and then the right atrium are closed. The remainder of the operation is completed in the usual manner (see Section 3 of Chapter 2).

Alternatively, when it is certain that the VSD is *not* conoventricular, the entire repair can be performed through the aortic root. Attachment of the base of the right coronary cusp to the patch is more conveniently accomplished from this exposure than from the right ventricular approach.

Ruptured Sinus of Valsalva Aneurysm into Right Atrium, without Ventricular Septal Defect

When the sinus of Valsalva aneurysm, usually from the noncoronary sinus but occasionally from the right coronary sinus, ruptures into the right atrium, the approach may be through both the aorta and right atrium. If AR and VSD can be securely excluded, the approach may be from the right atrium or the aorta alone. Intraoperative TEE facilitates this assessment.

In either situation, CPB is established using direct caval cannulation, an aortic root cannula is inserted, and the aorta is clamped (see Section 3 of Chapter 2). The right atrium is opened obliquely, and a sump suction catheter is inserted across the foramen ovale. A clamp can be placed across the windsock, or it can be occluded with a finger. Infusion of cardioplegic solution into the aortic root is begun. If the aortic valve is not completely competent, the root infusion is stopped, a transverse aortotomy is made, and cardioplegic solution is infused directly into the coronary ostia (see "Perfusion of Individual Coronary Arteries" in Chapter 3). Alternatively, cardioplegic solution is administered retrogradely through the coronary sinus (see "Technique of Retrograde Infusion" in Chapter 3).

A coexisting VSD is always sought, because it may be overlooked during preoperative evaluation if it is plugged by a prolapsing aneurysm or valve cusp. The windsock is then excised, remembering the precise location of the hinge line of the valve cusp. When the windsock is narrow and the bordering edges of the sinus are of good quality, direct transverse closure of the defect is safe. Usually, however, closure is made with a polyester or pericardial patch.

The remainder of the operation is completed in the usual manner (see Section 3 of Chapter 2).

Unruptured Sinus of Valsalva Aneurysm

Most unruptured sinus of Valsalva aneurysms can be repaired through the ascending aorta. CPB is established using a single cannula in the right atrium (see Section 3 of

Chapter 2). A venting catheter is placed into the left atrium through the right superior pulmonary vein. A catheter is placed into the ascending aorta for delivery of cardioplegic solution. Alternatively, a cannula can be placed into the coronary sinus for delivery of cardioplegic solution retrogradely. The ascending aorta is occluded and the cardioplegic solution administered. The aorta is opened transversely and the site of origin of the aneurysm identified (Fig. 22-11, A and B). The orifice of the aneurysm is closed with a polyester or pericardial patch, avoiding injury to the aortic cusp and ostium of the coronary artery (Fig. 22-11, C). If the aneurysm is large with associated AR, valve replacement, aortic root replacement with a composite valve-graft or aortic allograft, or a valve-sparing procedure may be necessary.[G6,T7]

SPECIAL FEATURES OF POSTOPERATIVE CARE

The usual care is given to patients after repair of sinus of Valsalva aneurysm (see Chapter 5).

RESULTS

Survival

Most patients survive the early period after operation. Hospital mortality has not exceeded 4% in the largest reported series.[A4,C3,C5,H10,O1,V3]

Long-term results are excellent, particularly when aortic valve replacement is not required. Abe and Komatsu reported 86% survival at 25 years in 31 surgical patients.[A3] All patients who died late after operation had undergone aortic valve replacement. In the report by van Son and colleagues of the entire Mayo Clinic experience, survival of 31 patients was 95% at 20 years.[V3] The single late death resulted from endocarditis 9 years after a subsequent aortic valve replacement.

Risk Factors for Premature Late Death

Severe AR accompanied by marked LV enlargement is a risk factor for premature death in the late postoperative period. Aortic valve replacement appears to be a risk factor for late death,[A3] as does dehiscence of an aortic valve prosthesis.[A4]

Functional Status

Most surviving patients are asymptomatic.[T1] Abe and Komatsu found that 22 (86%) of 26 surviving patients were in New York Heart Association (NYHA) functional class I, and the other four were in class II.[A3] Similar results were observed in the Mayo Clinic series; 25 of 28 known surviving patients were in NYHA class I (89%), and the other three were in class II.[V3] Persistent or worsening AR accounted for most of the functional disability after operation.

Complications

Direct closure of the ruptured aneurysm, with or without repair of a coexisting VSD, has resulted in a 20% to 30%

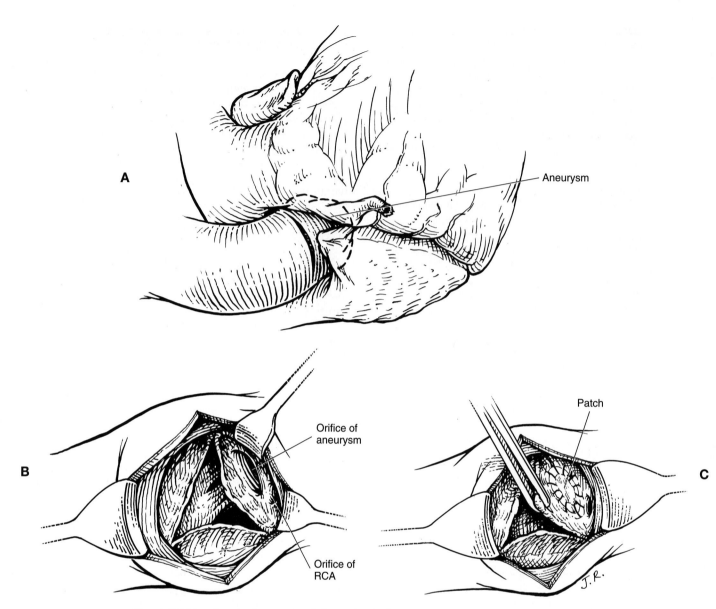

Figure 22-11   Repair of unruptured sinus of Valsalva aneurysm. **A,** Aneurysm is approached through a transverse aortotomy. **B,** Orifice of aneurysm in right coronary sinus is identified, noting its proximity to the right coronary artery and hinge point of the aortic cusp. **C,** Orifice is closed with a polyester or pericardial patch using a continuous No. 5-0 or 6-0 polypropylene suture.

Key: *RCA,* Right coronary artery.

prevalence of reoperation for recurrence of the fistula.[A3,B8] Other groups have experienced a lower prevalence of reoperations.[B1,H1,V3] When the defect left by excision of the ruptured aneurysm is repaired with a patch, reoperation is rare.

Heart block occurs in 2% to 3% of patients postoperatively,[A4,C5,V3] occasionally in the late postoperative period.[B8,C5] This complication is not surprising given the proximity of the His bundle and its branches to the area of repair.

INDICATIONS FOR OPERATION

When congenital sinus of Valsalva aneurysm ruptures or is associated with VSD or with VSD and AR, prompt operation is advisable.

Unruptured sinus of Valsalva aneurysms that are producing hemodynamic derangements, and those that are enlarging, should be repaired. Small and moderate-sized unruptured aneurysms probably should not be repaired surgically, at least with the present state of knowledge about the natural history of these lesions, although this issue is controversial.[M3]

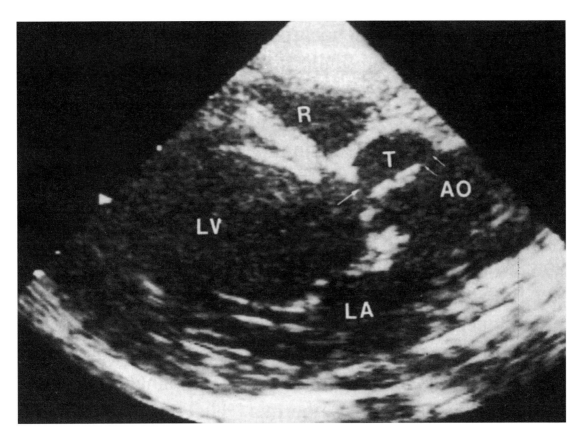

Figure 22-12 Two-dimensional echocardiogram in the parasternal long-axis view, demonstrating the entire aortico–left ventricular tunnel and dilated aortic root. Aortic and ventricular ends of the tunnel are defined by arrows. (From Sreeram and colleagues.[S19])

Key: *AO,* Aorta; *LA,* left atrium; *LV,* left ventricle; *R,* right ventricle; *T,* tunnel.

SECTION 2
Aortico–Left Ventricular Tunnel

DEFINITION

Aortico–left ventricular (LV) tunnel, or communication, is a short, abnormal pathway that begins in an aneurysmal dilatation of the aortic root and upper portion of the right sinus of Valsalva (rarely the left), just to the left of the orifice of the right coronary artery. The defect then passes through the upper end of the ventricular septum to open into the LV cavity.

HISTORICAL NOTE

Aortico–LV tunnel, a rare congenital cardiac anomaly, was first described by Levy and colleagues in 1963.[L2]

MORPHOLOGY

In its most characteristic form, the aortic orifice of the aortico–LV tunnel is anterior and just downstream from the commissural level of the aortic valve and separated from the right sinus of Valsalva by a prominent transverse supravalvar ridge.[B6,C1,G3,L2,P2] The anomaly is visible externally, and the extracardiac bulge can often be seen on the chest radiograph. The tunnel passes directly downward, alongside the aortic valve and through the junction between the aorta and ventricular septum, to communicate with the LV. The tunnel may displace the outlet portion of the ventricular septum into the right ventricle and produce important subpulmonary stenosis.[K8,T4] A VSD may coexist.[B7] Rarely the tunnel may communicate with the infundibulum of the right ventricle rather than the LV.

In one patient the orifice of the right coronary artery was shown to arise from the extracardiac portion of the tunnel.[B5] This finding, coupled with demonstration of elastic fibers in the extracardiac portion of some tunnels, suggests that some may actually be examples of coronary artery fistulae. However, most observers believe this anomaly is related to a congenital weakness in the region of the right sinus of Valsalva. In several patients the ostium and proximal portion of the right coronary artery were absent.[S15]

CLINICAL FEATURES AND DIAGNOSTIC CRITERIA

Patients with an aortico–LV tunnel usually have severe aortic regurgitation (AR) into the LV. They present with heart failure and marked cardiomegaly as well as symptoms and signs of severe AR.[L3,O3]

Diagnosis can usually be made with two-dimensional echocardiography and Doppler color flow imaging (Fig. 22-12).[B7,F2,H7,S19] Cardiac catheterization and angiography are usually performed to exclude uncommon associated cardiac anomalies.

NATURAL HISTORY

In view of the rarity of the condition, the natural history of patients with aortico–LV tunnel can be outlined only in general terms. Age at presentation and severity of symptoms are related to cross-sectional area of the tunnel and severity of AR. Some patients present as neonates with cardiomegaly and severe heart failure; others who have a smaller tunnel present in childhood without symptoms.[H6,H8] Patients rarely present beyond the second decade of life. When symptoms are present, marked LV enlargement has already occurred, and the natural history thereafter is that of severe AR (see Chapter 12). When symptoms are present in infancy and surgical repair is not accomplished, death usually occurs within a few months.

TECHNIQUE OF OPERATION

Repair is performed using CPB, and a single venous cannula may be used in most cases. In neonates and small infants, hypothermic circulatory arrest may be advantageous. The aorta must be clamped soon after cooling the patient with CPB to prevent LV distention from rapid aortic runoff. Cardioplegic solution must be infused directly into the coronary ostia or retrogradely via the coronary sinus (see "Perfusion of Individual Coronary Arteries" and "Technique of Retrograde Infusion" in Chapter 3).

A transverse aortotomy is made just downstream from the external bulge in the region of the right sinus of Valsalva. The ostium of the right coronary artery is identified and protected. Care is taken to avoid damaging the aortic cusps while visualizing the opening of the tunnel into the LV cavity through the aortic valve. If possible, both ends of the tunnel should be closed. The ventricular end is closed by sutures, usually pledgeted, or with a polyester or pericardial patch.[H8,K8,W3] The aortic end of the tunnel is closed by suturing into place a pericardial patch; direct suture closure distorts the sinus and may aggravate the tendency to develop AR postoperatively.[W3] If necessary the ostium of the right coronary artery is excised before placing the patch and is reimplanted.[H8]

The aortotomy is closed, and the remainder of the operation is completed in the usual manner. Particular care is taken to avoid LV distention from residual AR because the heart is recovering from the period of global myocardial ischemia.

SPECIAL FEATURES OF POSTOPERATIVE CARE

The usual care is given to patients after the repair (see Chapter 5).

RESULTS

The risk of hospital death has been 5% to 20%.[F2,H6,H8,T4] Most patients have at least mild AR after the operation,[M9,S16] and in about half of these the regurgitation becomes severe enough to require later aortic valve replacement.[M9,R1,S15,S16] The reason for postoperative AR is poorly understood,[T6] although in some patients it appears to be due to anuloaortic ectasia. Patients who do not require aortic valve replacement have excellent functional status.[H8,S19]

INDICATIONS FOR OPERATION

Diagnosis of aortico–LV tunnel is an indication for operation. Surgery should be performed as early in life as possible to minimize damage to the LV from chronic volume overload imposed by AR.

REFERENCES

A

1. Ainger LE, Pate JW. Rupture of a sinus of Valsalva aneurysm in an infant: surgical correction. Am J Cardiol 1963;11:547.
2. Abbott ME. Clinical and developmental study of a case of ruptured aneurysm of the right anterior aortic sinus of Valsalva: contributions to medical and biological research, Vol. 2. New York: Hoeber, 1919, p. 899.
3. Abe T, Komatsu S. Surgical repair and long-term results in ruptured sinus of Valsalva aneurysm. Ann Thorac Surg 1988;46:520.
4. Au WK, Chiu SW, Mok CK, Lee WT, Cheung D, He GW. Repair of ruptured sinus of Valsalva aneurysm: determinants of long-term survival. Ann Thorac Surg 1998;66:1604.

B

1. Bontils-Roberts EA, DuShane JW, McGoon DC, Danielson GK. Aortic sinus fistula: surgical considerations and results of operation. Ann Thorac Surg 1971;12:492.
2. Besterman EM, Goldberg MJ, Sellors TH. Surgical repair of ruptured sinus of Valsalva. Br Med J 1963;2:410.

3. Bigelow WG, Barnes WT. Ruptured aneurysm of aortic sinus. Ann Surg 1959;150:117.
4. Brown JW, Heath D, Whitaker W. Cardioaortic fistula: a case diagnosed in life and treated surgically. Circulation 1955;12:819.
5. Bharati S, Lev M, Cassels DE. Aortico–right ventricular tunnel. Chest 1973;63:198.
6. Bove KE, Schwartz DC. Aortico–left ventricular tunnel: a new concept. Am J Cardiol 1967;19:696.
7. Bash SE, Huhta JC, Nihill MR, Vargo TA, Hallman GL. Aortico–left ventricular tunnel with ventricular septal defect: two-dimensional/Doppler echocardiographic diagnosis. J Am Coll Cardiol 1985;5:757.
8. Barragry TP, Ring WS, Moller JH, Lillehei CW. Fifteen- to 30-year follow-up of patients undergoing repair of ruptured congenital aneurysms of the sinus of Valsalva. Ann Thorac Surg 1988;46:515.
9. Bulkley B, Hutchins GM, Ross RS. Aortic sinus of Valsalva aneurysms simulating primary right-sided valvular heart disease. Circulation 1975;52:696.
10. Bashour TT, Chen F, Yap A, Mason DT, Baladi N. Fatal myocardial ischemia caused by compression of the left coronary system by a large left sinus of Valsalva aneurysm. Am Heart J 1996;132:1050.

11. Brabham KR, Roberts WC. Fatal intrapericardial rupture of sinus of Valsalva aneurysm. Am Heart J 1990;120:1455.

12. Brandt J, Jogi P, Luhrs C. Sinus of Valsalva aneurysm obstructing coronary arterial flow: case report and collective review of the literature. Eur Heart J 1985;12:1069.

C

1. Cooley RN, Harris LC, Rodin AE. Abnormal communication between the aorta and left ventricle: aortico–left ventricular tunnel. Circulation 1965;31:564.

2. Chiang CW, Lin FC, Fang BR, Kuo CT, Lee YS, Chang CH. Doppler and two dimensional echocardiographic features of sinus of Valsalva aneurysm. Am Heart J 1988;116:1283.

3. Chu SH, Hung CR, How SS, Chang H, Wang SS, Tsai CH, et al. Ruptured aneurysms of the sinus of Valsalva in Oriental patients. J Thorac Cardiovasc Surg 1990;99:288.

4. Choudhary SK, Bhan A, Reddy SC, Sharma R, Murari V, Airan B, et al. Aneurysm of sinus of Valsalva dissecting into interventricular septum. Ann Thorac Surg 1998;65:735.

5. Choudhary SK, Bhan A, Sharma R, Airan B, Kumar AS, Venugopal P. Sinus of Valsalva aneurysms: 20 years' experience. J Card Surg 1997;12:300.

D

1. DeBakey ME, Lawrie GM. Aneurysm of sinus of Valsalva with coronary atherosclerosis: successful surgical correction. Ann Surg 1979;189:303.

2. Dubost C, Blondeau P, Piwnica A. Right aorta-atrial fistulas resulting from a rupture of the sinus of Valsalva: a report on 6 cases. J Thorac Cardiovasc Surg 1962;43:421.

3. DeBakey ME, Diethrich EB, Liddocoat JE, Kinard SA, Garrett HE. Abnormalities of the sinuses of Valsalva. Experience with 35 patients. J Thorac Cardiovasc Surg 1967;54:312.

E

1. Edwards JE, Burchell HB. The pathological anatomy of deficiencies between the aortic root and the heart, including aortic sinus aneurysms. Thorax 1957;12:125.

2. Evans JW, Harris TR, Brody DA. Ruptured aortic sinus aneurysm: case report, with review of clinical features. Am Heart J 1961;61:408.

3. Edwards JE, Burchell HB. Specimen exhibiting the essential lesion in aneurysm of the aortic sinus. Mayo Clin Proc 1956;31:407.

4. Eliott RS, Wolbrink A, Edwards JE. Congenital aneurysm of the left aortic sinus: a rare lesion and a rare cause of coronary insufficiency. Circulation 1963;28:951.

F

1. Falholt W, Thomsen G. Congenital aneurysm of the right sinus of Valsalva, diagnosed by aortography. Circulation 1953;8:549.

2. Fripp RR, Werner JC, Whitman V, Nordenberg A, Waldhausen JA. Pulsed Doppler and two-dimensional echocardiographic findings in aortico–left ventricular tunnel. J Am Coll Cardiol 1984;4:1012.

G

1. Gibbs NM, Harris EL. Aortic sinus aneurysms. Br Heart J 1961; 23:131.

2. Gerbode F, Osborne JJ, Johnston JB, Kerth WJ. Ruptured aneurysm of the aortic sinuses of Valsalva. Am J Surg 1961;102:268.

3. Goor DA, Lillehei CW. Congenital malformations of the heart. Orlando, Fla: Grune & Stratton, 1975, p. 301.

4. Gibbs KL, Reardon MJ, Strickman NE, de Castro CM, Gerard JA, Rycyna JL, et al. Hemodynamic compromise (tricuspid stenosis and insufficiency) caused by an unruptured aneurysm of the sinus of Valsalva. J Am Coll Cardiol 1986;7:1177.

5. Gallet B, Combe E, Saudemont JP, Tetard C, Barret F, Gandjbakhch I, et al. Aneurysm of the left aortic sinus causing coronary compression and unstable angina: successful repair by isolated closure of the aneurysm. Am Heart J 1988;115:1308.

6. Garcia-Rinaldi R, Von Koch L, Howell JF. Aneurysm of the sinus of Valsalva producing obstruction of the left main coronary artery. J Thorac Cardiovasc Surg 1976;72:123.

H

1. Howard RJ, Moller J, Castaneda AR, Varco RL, Nicoloff DM. Surgical correction of sinus of Valsalva aneurysm. J Thorac Cardiovasc Surg 1973;66:420.

2. Hong PW, Lee SS, Kim SW, Cha HD. Unusual manifestations of aneurysm of the aortic sinus: a report of 2 cases. J Thorac Cardiovasc Surg 1966;51:507.

3. Hope J. A treatise of disease of the heart and great vessels, 3rd Ed. London: Churchill, 1839.

4. Heydorn WH, Nelson WP, Fitter JD, Floyd GD, Strevey TE. Congenital aneurysm of the sinus of Valsalva protruding into the left ventricle. J Thorac Cardiovasc Surg 1976;71:839.

5. Heilman KJ, Groves BM, Campbell D, Blount SG. Rupture of left sinus of Valsalva aneurysm into the pulmonary artery. J Am Coll Cardiol 1985;5:1105.

6. Hovaguimian H, Cobanoglu A, Starr A. Aortico–left ventricular tunnel: a clinical review and new surgical classification. Ann Thorac Surg 1988;45:106.

7. Humes RA, Hagler DJ, Julsrud PR, Levy JM, Feldt RH, Schaff HV. Aortico–left ventricular tunnel: diagnosis based on two-dimensional echocardiography, color flow Doppler imaging, and magnetic resonance imaging. Mayo Clin Proc 1986;61:901.

8. Horvath P, Balaji S, Skovranek S, Hucin B, de Leval MR, Stark J. Surgical treatment of aortico–left ventricular tunnel. Eur J Cardiothorac Surg 1991;5:113.

9. Hoshino J, Naganuma F, Nagai R. Ventricular fibrillation triggered by a ruptured sinus of Valsalva aneurysm. Heart 1998;80:203.

10. Hamid IA, Jothi M, Rajan S, Monro JL, Cherian KM. Transaortic repair of ruptured aneurysm of sinus of Valsalva: fifteen-year experience. J Thorac Cardiovasc Surg 1994;107:1464.

J

1. Jones AM, Langley FA. Aortic sinus aneurysms. Br Heart J 1949; 11:325.

K

1. Kay JH, Anderson RM, Lewis RR, Reinberg M. Successful repair of sinus of Valsalva–left atrial fistula. Circulation 1959;20:427.

2. Kieffer SA, Winchell P. Congenital aneurysms of the aortic sinuses with cardioaortic fistula. Dis Chest 1960;38:79.

3. Kerber RE, Ridges JD, Driss JP, Silverman JF, Anderson ET, Harrison DC. Unruptured aneurysm of the sinus of Valsalva producing right ventricular outflow obstruction. Am J Med 1972;53:775.

4. Kiefaber RW, Tabakin BS, Coffin LH, Gibson RW. Unruptured sinus of Valsalva aneurysm with right ventricular outflow obstruction diagnosed by two-dimensional and Doppler echocardiography. J Am Coll Cardiol 1986;7:438.

5. Koh KK, Lee KH, Kim SS, Lee SC, Jin SH, Cho SW. Ruptured aneurysm of the sinus of Valsalva in a patient with Behçet's disease. Int J Cardiol 1994;47:177.

6. Killen DA, Wathanacharoen S, Pogson GW Jr. Repair of intrapericardial rupture of left sinus of Valsalva aneurysm. Ann Thorac Surg 1987;44:310.

7. Karaaslan T, Gudinchet F, Payot M, Sekarski N. Congenital aneurysm of sinus of Valsalva ruptured into right ventricle diagnosed by magnetic resonance imaging. Pediatr Cardiol 1999;20:212.

8. Knott-Craig CJ, van der Merwe PL, Kalis NN, Hunter J. Repair of aortico–left ventricular tunnel associated with subpulmonary obstruction. Ann Thorac Surg 1992;54:557.

L

1. Lillehei CW, Stanley P, Varco RL. Surgical treatment of ruptured aneurysms of the sinus of Valsalva. Ann Surg 1957;146:460.

2. Levy MJ, Lillehei CW, Anderson RC, Arnplatz K, Edwards JE. Aortico–left ventricular tunnel. Circulation 1963;27:841.

3. Levy MJ, Schachner A, Blieden LC. Aortico–left ventricular tunnel: collective review. J Thorac Cardiovasc Surg 1982;84:102.

M

1. Morrow AG, Baker RR, Hanson HE, Mattingly TW. Successful surgical repair of a ruptured aneurysm of the sinus of Valsalva. Circulation 1957;16:533.

2. Morris GC Jr, Foster RP, Dunn RJ, Cooley DA. Traumatic aortico-ventricular fistula: report of two cases successfully repaired. Am Surg 1958;24:883.

3. Mayer J, Wukasch DC, Hallman GL, Cooley DA. Aneurysm and fistula of the sinus of Valsalva. Ann Thorac Surg 1975;19:170.

4. Magidson O, Kay JH. Ruptured aortic sinus aneurysms: clinical and surgical aspects of seven cases. Am Heart J 1963;65:597.

5. Morgan JR, Rogers AK, Fosburg RG. Ruptured aneurysms of the sinus of Valsalva. Chest 1972;61:640.

6. Morch JE, Greenwood WF. Rupture of the sinus of Valsalva: a study of eight cases with discussion on the differential diagnosis of continuous murmurs. Am J Cardiol 1966;18:827.

7. McGoon DC, Edwards JE, Kirklin JW. Surgical treatment of ruptured aneurysm of aortic sinus. Ann Surg 1958;147:387.

8. Metras D, Coulibalty AO, Outtra K. Calcified unruptured aneurysm of sinus of Valsalva with complete heart block and aortic regurgitation. Br Heart J 1982;48:507.

9. Meldrum-Hanna W, Schroff R, Ross DN. Aortico–left ventricular tunnel: late follow-up. Ann Thorac Surg 1986;42:3904.

10. Munk MD, Gatzoulis MA, King DE, Webb GD. Cardiac tamponade and death from intrapericardial rupture (corrected) of sinus of Valsalva aneurysm. Eur J Cardiothorac Surg 1999;15:100.

N

1. Nowicki ER, Aberdeen E, Friedman S, Rashkind WJ. Congenital left aortic sinus–left ventricle fistula and review of aortocardiac fistulas. Ann Thorac Surg 1977;23:378.

O

1. Okada M, Muranaka S, Mukubo M, Asada S. Surgical correction of the ruptured aneurysm of the sinus of Valsalva. J Cardiovasc Surg (Torino) 1977;18:171.

2. Oram S, East T. Rupture of aneurysm of aortic sinus (of Valsalva) into the right side of the heart. Br Heart J 1955;17:541.

3. Okoroma EO, Perry LW, Scott LP 3rd, McClenathan JE. Aortico–left ventricular tunnel: clinical profile, diagnostic features, and surgical consideration. J Thorac Cardiovasc Surg 1976;71:238.

P

1. Perloff JK. Sinus of Valsalva–right heart communications due to congenital aortic sinus defects. Am Heart J 1960;59:318.

2. Perez-Martinez V, Quero M, Castro C, Moreno F, Brito JM, Merino G. Aortico–left ventricular tunnel: a clinical and pathologic review of this uncommon entity. Am Heart J 1973;85:237.

R

1. Ruschewski W, de Vivie ER, Kirchhoff PG. Aortico–left ventricular tunnel. J Thorac Cardiovasc Surg 1981;29:282.

2. Raizes GS, Smith HC, Vlietstra RE, Puga FG. Ventricular tachycardia secondary to aneurysm of sinus of Valsalva. J Thorac Cardiovasc Surg 1979;78:110.

3. Rosenberg H, Williams WG, Trusler GA, Smallhorn J, Rowe RD, Moes CA, et al. Congenital aortico–right atrial communications: the dilemma of differentiation from coronary-cameral fistula. J Thorac Cardiovasc Surg 1986;91:841.

S

1. Sakakibara S, Konno W. Congenital aneurysms of sinus of Valsalva: a clinical study. Am Heart J 1962;63:708.

2. Sakakibara S, Konno S. Congenital aneurysm of the sinus of Valsalva associated with ventricular septal defect: anatomical aspects. Am Heart J 1968;75:595.

3. Sakakibara S, Konno S. Congenital aneurysm of the sinus of Valsalva: anatomy and classification. Am Heart J 1962;63:405.

4. Scott RW. Aortic aneurysm rupturing into the pulmonary artery: report of two cases. JAMA 1924;82:1417.

5. Schuster NH. Aneurysm of the sinus of Valsalva involving the coronary orifice. Lancet 1937;1:507.

6. Szweda JA, Drake EH. Ruptured congenital aneurysms of the sinuses of Valsalva: a report of 2 cases treated surgically. Circulation 1962;25:559.

7. Shumacker HB Jr. Aneurysms of the aortic sinuses of Valsalva due to bacterial endocarditis, with special reference to their operative management. J Thorac Cardiovasc Surg 1972;63:896.

8. Sawyers JL, Adams JE, Scott HW Jr. Surgical treatment for aneurysms of the aortic sinuses with aortico atrial fistula: experimental and clinical study. Surgery 1957;41:26.

9. Segal BL, Likoff W, Novack P. Rupture of a sinus of Valsalva aneurysm. Am J Cardiol 1963;12:544.

10. Spencer FC, Blake HA, Bahnson HT. Surgical repair of ruptured aneurysm of sinus of Valsalva in two patients. Ann Surg 1960;152:963.

11. Shumacker HB Jr, King H, Waldhausen JA. Transaortic approach for the repair of ruptured aneurysms of the sinuses of Valsalva. Ann Surg 1965;161:946.

12. Shumacker HB Jr, Judson WE. Rupture of aneurysm of sinus of Valsalva into left ventricle and its operative repair. J Thorac Cardiovasc Surg 1963;45:650.

13. Smith WA. Aneurysm of the sinus of Valsalva with report of two cases. JAMA 1914;62:1878.

14. Sakakibara S, Konno S. Congenital aneurysm of the sinus of Valsalva: criteria for recommending surgery. Am J Cardiol 1963;12:100.

15. Somerville J, English T, Ross DN. Aorto–left ventricular tunnel: clinical features and surgical management. Br Heart J 1974;36:321.

16. Serino W, Andrade JL, Ross D, de Leval M, Somerville J. Aorto–left ventricular communication after closure: late postoperative problems. Br Heart J 1983;49:501.

17. Shiraishi S, Watarida S, Katsuyama K, Nakajima Y, Imura M, Nishi T, et al. Unruptured aneurysm of the sinus of Valsalva into the pulmonary artery. Ann Thorac Surg 1998;65:1458.

18. Stollberger C, Seitelberger R, Fenninger C, Prainer C, Slany J. Aneurysm of the left sinus of Valsalva. An unusual source of cerebral embolism. Stroke 1996;27:1424.

19. Sreeram N, Franks R, Arnold R, Walsh K. Aortico–left ventricular tunnel: long-term outcome after surgical repair. J Am Coll Cardiol 1991;17:950.

T

1. Taguchi K, Sasaki N, Matasuura Y, Mura R. Surgical correction of aneurysm of the sinus of Valsalva: a report of 45 consecutive patients, including 8 with total replacement of the aortic valve. Am J Cardiol 1969;23:180.

2. Thurman J. On aneurysms and especially spontaneous varicose aneurysms of the ascending aorta and sinuses of Valsalva, with cases. Med Chir Tr Lond 1840;23:323.

3. Trusler GA, Moes CA, Kidd BS. Repair of ventricular septal defect with aortic insufficiency. J Thorac Cardiovasc Surg 1973;66:394.

4. Turley K, Silverman NH, Teitel D, Mavroudis C, Snider R, Rudolph A. Repair of aortico–left ventricular tunnel in the neonate: surgical, anatomic and echocardiographic considerations. Circulation 1982;65:1015.

5. Terdjman M, Bourdarias JP, Farcot JC, Gueret P, Dubourg O, Ferrier A, et al. Aneurysms of sinus of Valsalva: two-dimensional echocardiographic diagnosis and recognition of rupture into the right heart cavities. J Am Coll Cardiol 1984;3:1227.

6. Tuna IC, Edwards JE. Aortico–left ventricular tunnel and aortic insufficiency. Ann Thorac Surg 1988;45:5.

7. Takahara Y, Sudo Y, Sunazawa T, Nakajima N. Aneurysm of the left sinus of Valsalva producing aortic valve regurgitation and myocardial ischemia. Ann Thorac Surg 1998;65:535.

V

1. Venning GR. Aneurysms of the sinuses of Valsalva. Am Heart J 1951;42:57.
2. Vered Z, Rath S, Benjamin P, Motro M, Neufeld HN. Ruptured sinus of Valsalva: demonstration by contrast echocardiography during cardiac catheterization. Am Heart J 1985;109:365.
3. Van Son JA, Danielson GK, Schaff HV, Orszulak TA, Edwards WD, Seward JB. Long-term outcome of surgical repair of ruptured sinus of Valsalva aneurysm. Circulation 1994;90:II20.

W

1. Weyman AE, Dillon JC, Feigenbaum H, Chang S. Premature pulmonic valve opening following sinus of Valsalva aneurysm rupture into the right atrium. Circulation 1975;52:556.

2. Warthen RO. Congenital aneurysm of the right anterior sinus of Valsalva (interventricular aneurysm) with spontaneous rupture into the left ventricle. Am Heart J 1949;37:975.
3. Warnke H, Bartel J, Blumenthal-Barby C. Aortico-ventricular tunnel. Thorac Cardiovasc Surg 1988;36:86.
4. Wakabayashi Y, Tawarahara K, Kurata C. Aneurysms of all sinuses of Valsalva and aortic valve prolapse secondary to Behçet's disease. Eur Heart J 1996;17:1766.
5. Walters MI, Ettles D, Guvendik L, Kaye GC. Interventricular septal expansion of a sinus of Valsalva aneurysm: a rare cause of complete heart block. Heart 1998;80:202.
6. Wortham DC, Gorman PD, Hull RW, Vernalis MN, Gaither NS. Unruptured sinus of Valsalva aneurysm presenting with embolization. Am Heart J 1993;125:896.

23 Patent Ductus Arteriosus

DEFINITION

Patent ductus arteriosus (PDA) is an abnormal persistence of a patent lumen in the fetal ductus arteriosus that usually connects the upper descending thoracic aorta with the proximal portion of the left pulmonary artery (LPA). When the aortic arch is right-sided, the ductus usually connects to the proximal right pulmonary artery. The ductus may at times connect to the adjacent subclavian or innominate artery, rather than to the upper descending thoracic aorta.

This chapter is primarily concerned with isolated PDA. Patent ductus associated with other anomalies is discussed briefly here and in more detail in other chapters (coarctation of the aorta, Chapter 34; ventricular septal defect, Chapter 21; and tetralogy of Fallot with pulmonary stenosis or pulmonary atresia, Chapter 24).

HISTORICAL NOTE

The ductus arteriosus apparently was first described by Galen (born AD 129). It was rediscovered by Botallo in the sixteenth century, although some attribute the description of its postnatal closure to Arenzio[A4,F6] and Harvey.[F7,H10] In 1888, Munro demonstrated in an infant cadaver the feasibility of dissecting and ligating a PDA.[M1] In 1900, Gibson described the characteristic continuous murmur of this anomaly.[G1] However, it was not until 1937 that Strieder, in Boston, attempted to close a PDA surgically in a patient with fulminating infective endocarditis (or endarteritis); the patient died on the fourth postoperative day with gastric distention and aspiration of vomitus.[G2]

Cardiac surgery received a great impetus on August 26, 1938, when Gross successfully ligated the PDA of a 7-year-old girl at Boston Children's Hospital.[G3] Subsequently, he developed division rather than ligation as the surgical technique of choice.[G7,G8] The first successful repair of an infected PDA was reported in 1940 by Touroff and Vesell, who later reported successful division of an infected PDA.[T3,T4] Portsmann and colleagues reported catheter closure of this anomaly in 1971.[P5] The first successful catheter closure of a PDA in a neonate or infant was performed by Rashkind and Cuaso in 1977.[R7,R8] Thus, PDA is the anomaly that initiated not only the *surgical* treatment of congenital heart disease, but also the *percutaneous* treatment of congenital heart disease.

MORPHOLOGY
Morphology of Normal Ductal Closure

At birth, the fetal ductus arteriosus is patent, resembling, according to Gittenberger-de Groot and colleagues,[G11] "a muscular artery with an intact, wavy internal elastic lamina, interrupted only underneath the intimal cushions. At those sites the elastic lamina is fragmented and is sometimes split up into several layers. The media is mainly composed of circularly arranged smooth muscle cells, with only minimal elastin fibers in between. The medial components may be widely separated, predominantly along the line of junction with intimal cushions, thereby creating large pools filled with a mucoid, slightly eosinophilic substance, the so-called mucoid lakes. In more advanced stages of anatomic closure, necrosis of cellular components of the media and a diffuse fibrous proliferation of the intima begin to appear."

Postnatal closure occurs in two stages.[C6] The first stage is complete within 10 to 15 hours after birth in full-term infants and is due to contraction of the smooth muscle in the media of the ductal wall, which produces shortening and an increase in wall thickness. This functional closure is assisted by approximation of the intimal cushions. The intimal cushions (or mounds or pillows) are swellings composed of longitudinally oriented smooth muscle cells that protrude into the lumen and lie between the endothelium and internal elastic lamina and thus within the intima.[J4] They thicken as the duct matures and are most prominent at the pulmonary end. Muscle contraction occurs both circumferentially from the circularly arranged smooth muscle cells that fill almost the entire media, and longitudinally from one or more bands of muscle in the inner media.[S4]

The second stage of closure is usually completed by 2 to 3 weeks. It is the result of diffuse fibrous proliferation of the intima, sometimes associated with necrosis of the inner layer of the media, and hemorrhage into the wall. The latter may be due to intimal tears producing a limited dissection of the ductus wall; there may also be small thrombi within the lumen, but gross luminal thrombus is rare.[C7] These changes result in permanent sealing of the lumen and produce the fibrous ligamentum arteriosum.

Closure usually begins at the pulmonary end and may remain incomplete at the aortic end, leaving an aortic ampulla from which the ligamentum arteriosum arises. Less commonly, there may be a ductus diverticulum arising from the proximal LPA.

The ductus arteriosus is completely closed by 8 weeks of age in 88% of infants with a normal cardiovascular system.[C3] When the process is delayed, the term *prolonged patency* of the ductus arteriosus is appropriate; when the process ultimately fails, *persistent patency* of the ductus arteriosus is the appropriate term. Ductus closure is mediated by release of vasoactive substances (acetylcholine, bradykinin, endogenous catecholamines, and probably others), by variations in pH, but chiefly by oxygen tension[M4] and prostaglandins (PGE_1, PGE_2, and prostacyclin PGI_2).[C8] Oxygen tension and prostaglandins act in opposite directions, with an increasing Po_2 constricting the ductus and prostaglandins relaxing it; the potency of each varies at different gestational ages.[H6] Thus, the ductus is considerably more sensitive to Po_2 in the mature fetus and to prostaglandins (specifically, PGE_1) in the immature fetus. The complex interplay of these factors is the reason that prolonged patency of the ductus is more common in premature than term infants, particularly when there is associated respiratory distress syndrome (see "Special Situations and Controversies" later in this chapter). *Intermittent patency* of the ductus arteriosus has been documented, particularly when the ductus is long and narrow.[D3]

Position and Absence

At birth, usually in subjects with other cardiac anomalies, the ductus may be unilateral, bilateral, or, rarely, completely absent. It is absent in 35% of autopsy specimens with tetralogy of Fallot with pulmonary stenosis, in 40% of those with tetralogy of Fallot with pulmonary atresia, in almost all patients with tetralogy of Fallot and absent pulmonary valve (see Chapter 24), and in truncus arteriosus (see Chapter 29). It is rarely absent in patients with pulmonary atresia and an intact ventricular septum (4%) (see Chapter 26) and in those with pulmonary atresia and other complex anomalies (15%).

Anatomic Details
Isolated Patent Ductus Arteriosus

The usual isolated PDA connects to the upper descending thoracic aorta 2 to 10 mm beyond the aortic origin of the left subclavian artery (Fig. 23-1). From the aorta, it passes centrally toward the origin of the LPA from the pulmonary trunk, either directly or angling superiorly and hugging the undersurface of the distal aortic arch.

The PDA is generally 5 to 10 mm in length, with a wide aortic orifice and a pulmonary orifice that is considerably narrower, and it is restrictive to flow. The PDA may be longer or shorter than this and may have a wide pulmonary as well as aortic orifice.

Patent Ductus Arteriosus as a Coexisting Anomaly

When other cardiac anomalies are present, orientation of the ductus to the aortic arch varies, as does the flow pattern in fetal life.[C7] When, as in the normally developing heart, the ductus delivers approximately 55% of the combined ventricular output into the descending aorta, the ductus meets the aorta at a proximal acute angle (less than 40°)

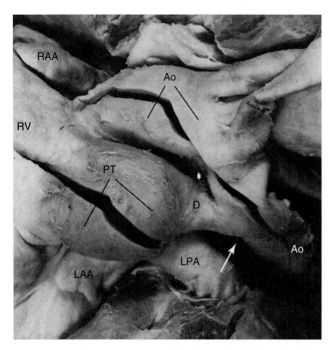

Figure 23-1 Specimen of isolated patent ductus arteriosus in an infant. Ductus passes from junction of pulmonary trunk and left pulmonary artery in an inferior and lateral direction to join the descending aorta. Angle between the superior border of the ductus *(asterisk)* and aorta (proximal angle) is acute, and that between the lower border and aorta *(arrow)* (distal angle) is obtuse. (From Calder and colleagues.[C7])

Key: *Ao,* Aorta; *D,* patent ductus arteriosus; *LAA,* left atrial appendage; *LPA,* left pulmonary artery; *PT,* pulmonary trunk; *RAA,* right atrial appendage; *RV,* right ventricle.

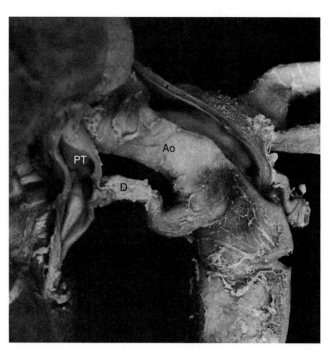

Figure 23-2 Specimen of patent ductus arteriosus in an infant with pulmonary atresia. Compared with the ductus in Fig. 23-1, it is long and relatively narrow and joins the aorta at a completely different angle. The proximal angle is obtuse and distal angle acute. (From Calder and colleagues.[C7])

Key: *Ao,* Aorta; *D,* patent ductus arteriosus; *PT,* pulmonary trunk.

■ TABLE 23-1 **Morphologic Features of Ductus Arteriosus in Fixed Autopsy Specimens**

		Age		Ductal Status		Average Length (mm)	Average Width (mm)	Average Prox Angle [a] (°)	Average Distal Angle [a] (°)
Cardiac Diagnosis	n	Range	Median	Open	Closed				
Normal [b]	13	SB–5 mo	2 d	10	3	8	5.9	29	134
Pulmonary atresia	32	SB–11 mo	8 d	13	19	9.7	3.7	83 [c]	90 [c]
Aortic atresia	13	2 d–11 wk	4 d	12	1	7.9	7.2	70 [c]	127
Coarctation	14	3 d–6 mo	14 d	8	6	5.6	6.0	70 [c]	139
Miscellaneous CHD	37	1 d–8 mo	23 d	18	19	7.1	4.6	52	124

(Data from Calder and colleagues.[C7])

Key: *CHD,* Congenital heart disease; *d,* days; *mo,* months; *prox,* proximal; *SB,* stillborn; *wk,* weeks.

[a] Angle between ductus and descending aorta.
[b] Normal hearts except for open ductus arteriosus.
[c] Difference from normal: $P < .001$.

and a distal obtuse angle (110° to 160°, mean 134°) (Table 23-1; see also Fig. 23-1).[C7,H5,M5] In striking contrast, when there is pulmonary atresia and the pulmonary circulation is ductus dependent, ductal flow in utero is from the aorta to the pulmonary artery; then the ductus becomes a downwardly directed branch of the distal aortic arch so that the proximal angle is much less acute and often obtuse, and the distal angle is often acute[C7,R5] (Fig. 23-2; see also Table 23-1) (see "Aortic Arch and Ductus Arteriosus" under Morphology in Section 1 of Chapter 24). When this is not the case, pulmonary atresia likely developed late in pregnancy.[S5] In aortic atresia and coarctation of the aorta, the distal angle is normal, but the proximal angle in these shorter, broader examples of PDA is much less acute, probably because ductal flow enters both the ascending and descending aorta.[C7]

Both the diameter and length of a PDA vary widely. In fixed autopsy specimens, diameter in otherwise normal hearts varied from 4 to 12 mm and length from 2.5 to 8 mm. In pulmonary atresia, the ductus is usually longer and narrower[C7] (see Fig. 23-2). The lumen is usually narrower at the pulmonary end and wider at the aortic end.

Uncommonly, in the presence of a left aortic arch, the ductus may arise from an aortic diverticulum (thought to represent persistence of the most distal portion of the right fourth branchial arch), which projects from the medial aspect of the left arch just distal to the origin of the left subclavian artery.[G12] In rare cases in which the ductus is bilateral, the right-sided PDA connects the right pulmonary artery to the innominate artery.

In the presence of a right aortic arch, a left-sided ductus is even more common. When there is mirror-image branching of the right arch, the left PDA arises from the distal innominate (or proximal left subclavian) artery (see Chapter 24). Much less commonly, the right PDA persists in mirror image to the normal, passing from the right arch beyond the right subclavian artery to the right pulmonary artery origin. A PDA (or ligamentum arteriosum) arising from an aortic diverticulum or from an aberrant left subclavian artery is one form of vascular ring (see Chapter 37).

Histology

Histology of a persistent PDA is different from that of simple prolonged patency of the ductus.[G6] It is also different from that of the adjoining great arteries. A persistent PDA has a relatively thick intima with an unfragmented elastic lamina separating it from the media, an additional and pronounced wavy unfragmented subendothelial elastic lamina, and variable mucoid material in the media where there is an intricate helicoid spiral muscular arrangement.[G6] The media contains variable amounts of elastic material that may form conspicuous lamellae, making the ductus wall resemble the wall of the aorta (aortification).

Aneurysms of Ductus Arteriosus

Aneurysms of the ductus arteriosus, which are rare lesions, appear to be of two types. One is the spontaneous infantile ductal aneurysm, which is present at birth or develops shortly thereafter.[H4] The other develops in childhood or adult life.

Presence of the first type may not be detected until autopsy after death from other causes.[D2] The aneurysm involves the entire length of the ductus arteriosus and is usually associated with occlusion of the pulmonary artery end and a relatively narrow but patent aortic end.[F4] It generally contains thrombus and is occasionally a site of infection and embolism. Rarely, it may be a true dissecting aneurysm of the ductal wall.[F2] This rare lesion manifests most often in newborns with a history of respiratory difficulties.[D4,H4] It produces a tumorlike shadow of variable size that projects beyond the mediastinum adjacent to the aortic knob in the posteroanterior chest radiograph. The aneurysm usually regresses spontaneously within weeks or months, presumably as a result of complete thrombosis and organization, but progressive enlargement or onset of hoarseness from recurrent laryngeal nerve involvement is an indication for surgical exploration and excision.[H4] Less marked dilatation of the ductus can be seen on the plain chest radiograph as a fusiform shadow between 6 and 18 hours after birth, disappearing by 24 to 48 hours of age.[B7] It has been called the *ductus bump.*

The second type of ductal aneurysm is thought to be unrelated to the infantile form. The ductus may be patent at both ends, but usually the pulmonary artery end is closed.[G5,T6] There is a tendency for progressive enlargement, and death may occur from rupture.[C4]

CLINICAL FEATURES AND DIAGNOSTIC CRITERIA

Symptoms and signs of a PDA are the consequence of left-to-right shunting, with the magnitude of the shunt depending on size of the communication and relationship between the systemic and pulmonary vascular resistances. In this regard, it is similar to other types of high-pressure shunts, which include those across the ventricular septum and others from the aorta.

Large Patent Ductus Arteriosus

Aortic and pulmonary artery pressures are essentially equal when the PDA is large, and the magnitude and direction of shunting are dependent on changes in pulmonary vascular resistance, because systemic vascular resistance remains fairly constant after birth.[R6] As neonatal pulmonary vascular resistance decreases, left-to-right shunting increases and severe heart failure develops within a month or so of birth. There is tachypnea, tachycardia, sweating and irritability, poor feeding, and slow weight gain.[K1] Pulmonary edema and pneumonia or less severe and recurrent respiratory infection may occur.

On examination, there is an overactive precordium, sometimes with a systolic thrill, and evidence of cardiac enlargement with a thrusting left ventricular apical impulse.[A2] The pulse is jerky or frankly collapsing, and the pulse pressure is correspondingly wide; these features become more obvious when heart failure is medically controlled. On auscultation, there is a systolic murmur maximal in the pulmonary area, with late systolic accentuation and minimal spillover into diastole.[R1] Occasionally the murmur is continuous, but sometimes with severe heart failure, no murmur is heard.[M2] The first and second heart sounds are accentuated, and there is a third sound at the apex or a prominent mid-diastolic mitral flow murmur.[R2] The liver enlarges and jugular venous pressure rises; frequently, rales are heard in the lung bases.

The electrocardiogram shows left ventricular enlargement with deep Q and tall R waves in the left ventricular leads. There may be evidence of right ventricular hypertrophy with upright T waves in the right precordial leads and evidence of left atrial enlargement with widened P waves. The chest radiograph shows marked cardiomegaly and plethora with or without interstitial or alveolar pulmonary edema. The pulmonary trunk is enlarged, as is the ascending aorta. The echocardiogram shows left atrial enlargement, and the ductus itself may be visualized with two-dimensional echocardiography.

In some infants with a large PDA, heart failure may be less marked, presumably because pulmonary vascular resistance does not fall to the usual level. Histologic changes of pulmonary vascular disease may develop within the first few months of life. The same may occur in those in whom heart failure is controlled medically and the ductus is not closed by intervention. These patients become asymptomatic and the left-to-right shunt diminishes. The murmur becomes purely systolic, the pulmonary component of the second heart sound is markedly accentuated, the apical mid-diastolic murmur disappears, and the pulse loses its jerky quality. Right ventricular hypertrophy becomes dominant in the electrocardiogram, the heart becomes smaller on the chest radiograph, and pulmonary plethora disappears. Cyanosis develops as pulmonary vascular resistance increases above systemic vascular resistance (Eisenmenger syndrome), typically earlier than with ventricular septal defect (see Chapter 21).[E4] Differential cyanosis may be noted, with blueness of the feet and sometimes the left hand, but not of the face or right hand.

Moderate-Sized Patent Ductus Arteriosus

Left-to-right shunt in moderate-sized PDA is regulated by size of the ductus arteriosus. In this setting, pulmonary artery pressure is only moderately elevated. As neonatal pulmonary vascular resistance declines, the shunt increases and heart failure may occur; by the second or third month of life, however, compensatory left ventricular hypertrophy is usually associated with clinical improvement and stabilization of symptoms. Physical development may be somewhat retarded, and breathlessness and fatigue may occur, but many individuals with moderate-sized PDA remain essentially asymptomatic until the second decade of life or later.

On examination, the pulse is jerky, the precordium is mildly overactive, and the left ventricle is palpable at the apex in association with some cardiac enlargement. The classic continuous murmur is usually heard by age 2 to 3 months, although it varies in intensity.[L1] The murmur is generally loud and often masks the heart sounds. It is maximal over the pulmonary artery and radiates upward beneath the mid-third of the clavicle. As described by Gibson in 1900, "it begins after the commencement of the first sound—it persists through the second sound and dies away gradually during the long pause. The murmur is rough and thrilling. It begins softly and increases in intensity so as to reach its acme at or immediately after the occurrence of the second sound, and from that point gradually wanes until its termination."[G1] Substandard physical growth is common; Krovetz and Warden found body weight below the third percentile in 26% of 515 surgically proven cases.[K1] The electrocardiogram may be relatively normal during infancy, but some degree of left ventricular hypertrophy develops in older children. The chest radiograph shows moderate cardiac enlargement and plethora and a prominent ascending aorta (in contrast to findings in patients with a large ventricular or atrial septal defect). In adults, the PDA may be calcified. It is rare for pulmonary vascular resistance to increase, and Eisenmenger syndrome does not develop.

Small Patent Ductus Arteriosus

Left-to-right shunt is small in early life, and pulmonary vascular resistance decreases rapidly to normal after birth.

Left ventricular failure does not occur, and symptoms are absent in infancy and childhood. They may appear much later in life, but usually attention is drawn to the condition by a murmur detected on routine physical examination.

Physical development is normal unless there is maternal rubella. The pulse is normal and the precordium not overactive. By age 2 to 3 months, a short systolic murmur is usually replaced by one that spills over into diastole, or it may be continuous in the second left intercostal space but less intense and with less radiation than when the ductus is moderate in size. The continuous murmur varies greatly in intensity between patients and sometimes is detectable only when the patient is sitting or standing upright. The electrocardiogram and chest radiograph are normal or nearly so.

Special Investigations

Most children and young adults with a PDA and continuous murmur maximal in the second left intercostal space do not need preoperative invasive studies unless other defects are suspected. Two-dimensional echocardiography can image the ductus arteriosus and may be necessary for diagnosis in atypical cases. It has identified so-called silent ductus (a PDA without auscultatory findings).[H9] Managing patients with isolated silent ductus remains controversial, although endocarditis has been reported and may be an indication for closure.[B10] Cardiac catheterization and angiography are indicated if the echocardiogram suggests elevated pulmonary vascular resistance or associated cardiac anomalies.

NATURAL HISTORY

Isolated PDA in term infants occurs in approximately 1 in 2000 live births and accounts for 5% to 10% of all types of congenital heart disease.[M6] It is twice as common in girls[C2] and may occur in siblings, suggesting a genetic factor. It is particularly common when the mother contracts rubella during the first trimester of pregnancy and may then be associated with multiple peripheral pulmonary artery stenoses and renal artery stenosis.

Because of the early introduction of surgical treatment of PDA, which antedated methods for establishing the diagnosis, its natural history is not completely documented.

Spontaneous Closure

Campbell's study concluded that spontaneous closure of isolated PDA occurs in 0.6% of patients per year and that this rate is fairly constant through the first four decades of life.[C2] If this is accepted, it means that in approximately 20% of patients, the PDA will have closed by age 40. His study involved only patients diagnosed beyond age 12 months and was based entirely on clinical findings, closure being assumed to have occurred when a typical murmur was no longer audible, regardless of size of the ductus or initial right-to-left shunt. Other experience suggests that the closure rate is much lower, and it is generally agreed that spontaneous closure is uncommon beyond age 3 to 5 months in full-term infants. Delayed closure of the ductus arteriosus in preterm infants is, however, common (see "Special Situations and Controversies" later in this chapter).

Pulmonary Vascular Disease

Prevalence and type of pulmonary vascular disease in patients with large PDA are similar to those in patients with large ventricular septal defect (see "Pulmonary Vascular Disease" under Morphology in Section 1 of Chapter 21).

Death

Mortality with untreated PDA in infancy is high, and it has been estimated that 30% of patients born with an isolated PDA die within the first year.[C2,H2] Risk of death is highest in the first few months of life (see "Patent Ductus Arteriosus in Preterm Infants" under Special Situations and Controversies later in this chapter).

After infancy, the annual death rate of patients with untreated PDA decreases dramatically to approximately 0.5% per year.[C2] By the third decade, the death rate has increased to about 1% per year; by the fourth decade, 1.8% per year; and in subsequent decades, as high as 4% per year.[C2] As a result, approximately 60% of patients with PDA die by age 45. Most of the deaths in older patients are related to development of intractable left ventricular failure secondary to long-standing volume overload.

Modes of Death

In infants with a large PDA, mode of death is usually heart failure. Recurrent respiratory infection terminating in pneumonia is a less common mode. In those with a large PDA who survive infancy, death is usually due to acute or chronic right heart failure secondary to development of severe pulmonary vascular disease by the second or third decade of life.

In patients with a moderate-sized PDA, mode of death from the third and fourth decades onward is heart failure. Excluding infants and deaths from pulmonary vascular disease, Campbell estimated that heart failure was the cause of death in 30% of patients.[C2]

Infective endocarditis occurs mainly as a complication of small PDA and less often with a moderate-sized ductus. It rarely occurs when the ductus is large. In the preantibiotic era, endocarditis was responsible for approximately 45% of deaths in patients with surgically untreated PDA.[A1,C2,K2] After the advent of antibiotics, few patients died from this cause, although they remained subject to another episode.

TECHNIQUE OF OPERATION
Closure of Patent Ductus Arteriosus

Unless the patient is an infant in severe heart failure, an intraarterial monitoring catheter is unnecessary. After the usual induction of anesthesia and preparations for operation (see Chapter 4), the patient is positioned on the right side (Fig. 23-3, *A*). A small roll or pillow may be placed under the mid-chest. The patient is positioned near the surgeon's side of the table but not so much so that the first assistant,

across the table from the surgeon, cannot see into the field well and work comfortably.

Posterolateral Thoracotomy

A curving skin incision is made, centered about 1 to 2 cm below the tip of the scapula. In infants and young children, the incision is really a lateral one, because only the latissimus dorsi and posterior part of the serratus anterior are divided. In older children, the incision is posterolateral, extending posterosuperiorly to overlie the lower 1 or 2 cm of the trapezius, which is also incised. In patients who are in the second decade of life or older, the incision extends from the anterior axillary line around the scapula and up midway between the spine and posterior scapular border over the lower 3 to 4 cm of the trapezius.

After incising the latissimus dorsi (and trapezius if indicated), the scapula is elevated with a retractor and the ribs are counted from the top down to the fifth rib. Identification of the appropriate rib or intercostal space requires an accurate point of reference. There are three possible points of reference (the second and third are more reliable than the first):

- First rib: The surgeon passes his left hand under the serratus and identifies the first rib by palpation.
- Second rib: The serratus anterior attaches superiorly to the second rib. The surgeon identifies this attachment using upward traction on the scapular retractor, which makes the prominent posterior border of this muscle taut.
- Second intercostal space: This is usually appreciably wider than the third intercostal space.

Counting down from the reference point, the fifth rib is identified and scored. Only then are the posterior and midportions of the serratus anterior divided so that the muscle incision may be directly over the fifth rib. The fourth interspace may be opened with a knife or cautery or the chest may be entered through the superior part of the bed of the nonresected fifth rib. With the latter method, the periosteum over the rib is incised, and its superior portion is elevated from the front and back with a periosteal elevator.

After extending the incision in the rib cage anteriorly and posteriorly, the rib retractor is placed with the ratcheted portion anteriorly (Fig. 23-3, *B*). The retractor is opened only partially at first, but as the operation proceeds, it is gradually opened further to obtain adequate exposure.

A retractor is gently placed on the lung, and a vertical incision is made in the mediastinal pleura over the proximal descending thoracic aorta (see Fig. 23-3, *B*).[1] Traction sutures are placed on the anterior and posterior pleural flaps. The lung retractor is removed, moist gauze is placed over the lung, and the anterior pleural traction sutures are pulled taut and anchored to the retractor or drapes. The vein that traverses the aorta obliquely on its anterior surface is divided. The PDA is completely dissected from

---

[1] Gross made an anterolateral thoracotomy incision, placed the pleural incision midway between the phrenic and vagus nerves, and retracted the vagus nerve posteriorly.[G3,G7-G9] Exposure is probably less optimal with this approach, although it may be appropriate in small patients and those with variations of situs, such as mesocardia and dextrocardia.

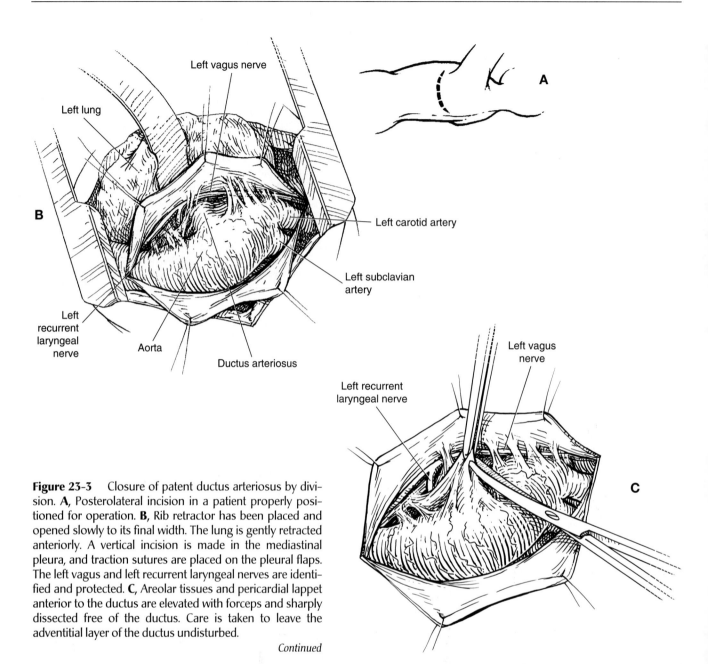

Figure 23-3   Closure of patent ductus arteriosus by division. **A,** Posterolateral incision in a patient properly positioned for operation. **B,** Rib retractor has been placed and opened slowly to its final width. The lung is gently retracted anteriorly. A vertical incision is made in the mediastinal pleura, and traction sutures are placed on the pleural flaps. The left vagus and left recurrent laryngeal nerves are identified and protected. **C,** Areolar tissues and pericardial lappet anterior to the ductus are elevated with forceps and sharply dissected free of the ductus. Care is taken to leave the adventitial layer of the ductus undisturbed.

Continued

the surrounding tissue (Fig. 23-3, *C* to *E*). In small infants, particular care is taken to be certain that the structure identified as the PDA connects the aorta and pulmonary artery and that it is not the LPA or distal aortic arch. As dissection proceeds, the left recurrent laryngeal nerve is not isolated, although it should be clearly visualized behind the areolar tissue over the LPA, just inferior and posterior to the PDA (see Fig. 23-3, *C*).

When the PDA is an uncomplicated one, either division or ligation may be performed. Both techniques, when done properly, ensure complete closure with low risk.

Division.   When division is elected and the patient is an infant or young child, one straight and two angled fine-toothed Potts ductus clamps are selected. In teenagers and adults, longer-handled vascular clamps are used. At this time, and particularly in older children and adults, the anesthesiologist reduces arterial blood pressure (see

Chapter 4) and maintains it below baseline level until the clamps are removed.

The straight clamp is placed completely across the aortic end of the PDA, making sure that its tip does not grasp the recurrent laryngeal nerve or other soft tissue deep to the ductus. The clamp is placed in the surgeon's left hand and is gently pulled anteriorly. One angled ductus clamp is placed on the aortic side of the straight clamp and usually on the aorta contiguous with the PDA rather than on the ductus itself. The straight clamp is removed. With the clamp on the aortic origin of the PDA, which is held in the surgeon's right hand, the other angled clamp is placed with the left hand on the pulmonary end of the ductus. The clamp must grasp only the ductus, and not any of the lappet of pericardium or other tissue, to avoid dislodgment from the clamp and retraction into the pericardial cavity. This clamp, like the one on the aortic end, is "squeezed" onto the

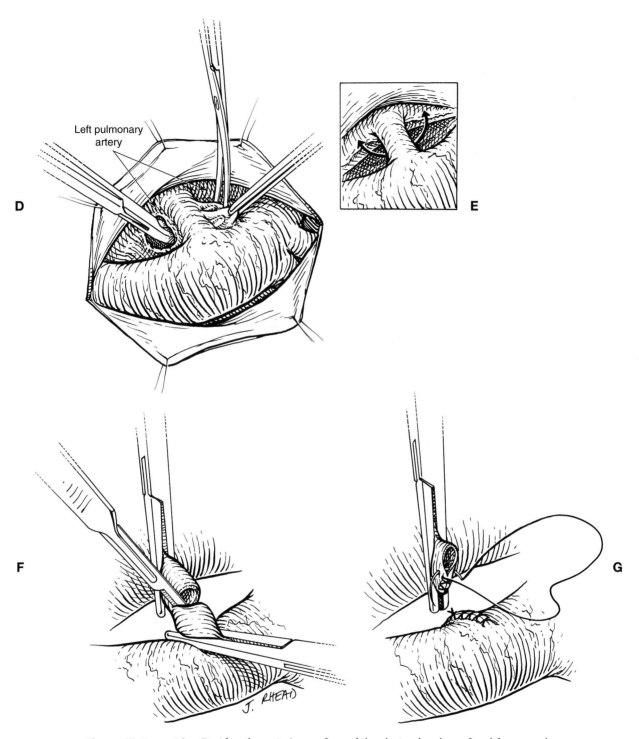

Figure 23-3, cont'd   D, After the anterior surface of the ductus has been freed far enough medially so that the junction of the patent ductus arteriosus with the left pulmonary artery is visible, the superior and inferior surfaces are similarly dissected. A right-angled clamp is passed behind the ductus. The clamp stretches the areolar tissue behind the ductus, which is then grasped with forceps and cut away. **E,** This maneuver is repeated several times and creates a space behind the ductus. **F,** Clamps are placed at the aortic and pulmonary ends of the ductus (see text), and it is divided midway between them. **G,** The aortic end of the ductus is oversewn with two rows of No. 5-0 or 6-0 polypropylene suture. The clamp on the aortic end of the ductus is generally kept in place following closure and provides traction to expose the pulmonary end, which is then oversewn in a similar fashion. The clamps are then released.

pulmonary artery as much as possible when it is being placed, to give added length to the ductus. The ductus is divided midway between these clamps by Potts scissors or a scalpel (Fig. 23-3, *F*).

The aortic end of the PDA is oversewn with two rows of No. 5-0 or 6-0 polypropylene suture placed as a whip stitch (Fig. 23-3, *G*). The pulmonary end is similarly closed. Although accurate suturing is of obvious importance, the key to a safe repair is separating the clamps widely enough so that a substantial cuff of ductus remains beyond them after the ductus is divided. This permits placement of additional sutures for hemostasis.

The clamp on the pulmonary end of the divided ductus generally is removed first. The clamp on the aortic end is then removed, and a sponge is placed between the divided ends and held in place with pressure for several minutes. Unless the original placement of the clamps has been faulty or the suture closure is inadequate, the bleeding that occurs when the clamps are released usually stops within this period. If not, and if there is no major bleeding that would require replacement of one or both clamps, a No. 5-0 polypropylene suture approximating the adventitia from both sides of the suture line usually controls the bleeding. A pledget of absorbable porcine gelatin sponge (Gelfoam) is left between the divided ends of the ductus to prevent the suture lines from rubbing against each other.

Ligation. If the situation is uncomplicated and the PDA is pliable, it may be ligated rather than divided. The technique is basically that described by Blalock in 1946.[B6] The operation proceeds exactly as described for ductal division until the PDA is completely dissected. Using a double-armed No. 5-0 or 6-0 polypropylene suture, adventitial stitches are placed into the accessible superior, inferior, and anterior aspects of the aortic wall contiguous with the PDA (Fig. 23-4, *A*). One end of the suture is passed beneath the ductus, and the ends are held. A similar stitch is placed on the pulmonary end of the ductus (Fig. 23-4, *B*). The aortic stitch is pulled up and snugly tied, and then the suture at the pulmonary end is tied. This leaves a long length of ductus between the tied sutures. Finally, a transfixion ligature of No. 5-0 or 6-0 polypropylene is placed at the middle of the ductus, and the ends are passed in the opposite direction around the ductus and tied to complete the repair (Figs. 23-4, *C* to *F*).

The mediastinal pleura is closed with interrupted sutures, leaving a small opening at each end. In the unlikely event that there is substantial bleeding from the suture lines after operation, this closure will contain it and may be lifesaving.

The rib retractor is removed, a small catheter is inserted into the posterior part of the pleural space through a stab wound in the sixth or seventh intercostal space at the midaxillary line, and suction of 15 to 25 cm water is placed on it. The ribs on either side of the incision are approximated with interrupted sutures. The muscles are individually sutured with a slowly absorbable synthetic material (polyglycolic acid), and the skin edges are approximated with a subcutaneous stitch. In infants, the chest tube may be removed in the operating room.

Transaxillary Muscle-Sparing Lateral Thoracotomy

A 3- to 4-cm incision is made over the third intercostal space in the axilla. The serratus anterior is reflected inferiorly and laterally, and the pectoralis major is reflected anteriorly. The third intercostal space is entered and a rib retractor inserted. The lung is retracted anteriorly, and the pleura overlying the descending thoracic aorta is incised. The PDA is identified at its junction with the aorta, and the recurrent laryngeal nerve is identified and protected. The PDA is dissected circumferentially and is divided or ligated using the techniques just described. Alternatively, it may be occluded with a medium-sized surgical clip.[C12] The lung is inflated as the chest is closed.

Fluid and air can be aspirated as the chest wall is closed with interrupted pericostal sutures, making a chest tube unnecessary. The muscle and soft tissue layers are approximated with a slowly absorbable synthetic suture (polyglycolic acid), and the skin edges are approximated with a subcutaneous stitch. This technique is applicable to premature infants, neonates, older children, and adults.[G10,K4,M9,T2,T7]

Closure of Patent Ductus Arteriosus in Association with Repair of Intracardiac Lesions

Closure of a PDA may be required during operations to correct intracardiac anomalies that require the use of cardiopulmonary bypass (CPB). This occurs in two distinct clinical situations. When the PDA is an incidental finding and relatively small and restrictive, such as with a large ventricular septal defect, dissection of the ductus is usually performed after CPB has been established, because exposure of the adjacent aorta and pulmonary artery is facilitated when the heart is decompressed, and injury to the ductus or surrounding structures can be avoided. The technique for closure of the PDA under these circumstances is described in "Technique of Operation" in Chapter 21. In the second situation, as in the neonate with transposition of the great arteries with intact ventricular septum, the ductus is large. It must be exposed and controlled before initiating CPB, so that it can be ligated immediately after bypass is established.

Closure of Patent Ductus Arteriosus in Older Adults

When a PDA requires closure in the fifth to seventh decades of life, the aortic end is often calcified and the ductus very short. A technique using CPB, described by Goncalves-Estella and colleagues[G4] and later by O'Donovan and Beck,[O1] is appropriate in this circumstance.

With the usual preparations (see Chapter 2), a median sternotomy is performed and the usual stay sutures and purse-string sutures placed. The aorta and pulmonary trunk are dissected apart. CPB is established with a single venous cannula, and cooling of the patient by the perfusate is begun. The head of the table is lowered to place the patient in a moderate Trendelenburg position. As the heart begins to slow from the cold perfusion, the ductus is obliterated

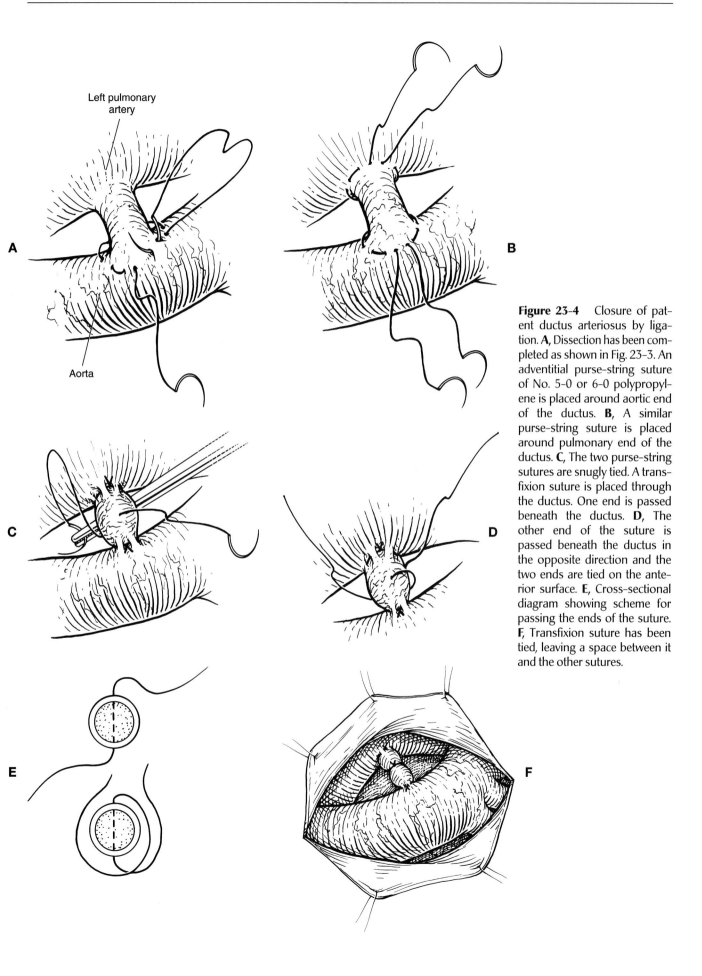

Figure 23-4 Closure of patent ductus arteriosus by ligation. **A,** Dissection has been completed as shown in Fig. 23-3. An adventitial purse-string suture of No. 5-0 or 6-0 polypropylene is placed around aortic end of the ductus. **B,** A similar purse-string suture is placed around pulmonary end of the ductus. **C,** The two purse-string sutures are snugly tied. A transfixion suture is placed through the ductus. One end is passed beneath the ductus. **D,** The other end of the suture is passed beneath the ductus in the opposite direction and the two ends are tied on the anterior surface. **E,** Cross-sectional diagram showing scheme for passing the ends of the suture. **F,** Transfixion suture has been tied, leaving a space between it and the other sutures.

Left pulmonary artery

Aorta

A

B

C

D

E

F

by compressing the front wall of the LPA against it with the index finger. This is essential, because otherwise ductal flow into the pulmonary artery will overdistend the pulmonary vascular bed and the right ventricle (this does not occur when the heart is ejecting adequately). When the nasopharyngeal temperature reaches 20° to 22°C, the aorta is clamped and cold cardioplegic solution is infused into the aortic root or retrogradely into the coronary sinus (see "Technique of Retrograde Infusion" in Chapter 3). The perfusion temperature is stabilized at 20° to 22°C, and flow is reduced to $0.5 \text{ L} \cdot \text{min}^{-1} \cdot \text{m}^{-2}$. The finger is removed, the distal pulmonary trunk is opened anteriorly and longitudinally, and the incision is continued into the LPA opposite the ductus. If external pressure on the LPA does not control ductal flow during CPB cooling, perfusion is temporarily reduced to a low level and the pulmonary artery incision is made so that the finger can be placed directly over the ostium of the ductus to control the flow from it into the LPA. CPB flow rate is then increased until cooling is completed.

The intracardiac sucker is positioned within the LPA beyond the ductus to aspirate blood entering it. The ductal orifice is closed by placing and tying one or more pledgeted mattress sutures of No. 3-0 or 4-0 polypropylene. This is readily accomplished, because the pulmonary artery end of the ductus is rarely calcified, and the pulmonary artery tissues are strong enough to hold sutures well. If the orifice of the pulmonary artery end of the PDA is too large or immobile for this technique, an impervious patch of bovine pericardium, woven polyester, or polytetrafluorethylene can be used to close it, sewing the patch in place with continuous No. 4-0 or 5-0 polypropylene suture. Flows are then restored, the table leveled, and rewarming of the patient with the perfusate begun. Any leak from the ductus closure site is secured with additional sutures. The pulmonary arteriotomy is closed with a running stitch of fine polypropylene.

With strong suction on the aortic root catheter, the aortic clamp is released. The remainder of the operation is completed in the usual fashion (see "Completing Cardiopulmonary Bypass" in Section 3 of Chapter 2).

Closure of Patent Ductus Arteriosus in Premature Infants

Perioperative management and technique of operation are different when surgical closure of the ductus is indicated in the premature infant, most of whom weigh approximately 1000 g and some as little as 400 g. Precise management of ventilation, fluid administration, and body temperature, as well as a precise surgical technique, are essential for success.[S1]

Operation is usually performed in the neonatal intensive care unit. This simplifies the logistics and, when properly organized, can provide outcomes as good as those obtained in a conventional operating room.[C11,E7]

If the procedure is to be performed in the operating room, the infant is intubated in the neonatal nursery, and proper position of the tube is verified by a chest radiograph. The patient, covered by a plastic wrap blanket and cloth cap, is transported to the operating room in a prewarmed (37°C) transport isolette.

The room is prewarmed to approximately 30°C, and the patient is placed on the right side on an infant operating table with overhead servocontrolled radiant warmers set at 37°C.

After preparation and draping, a short left lateral incision approximately 2.5 cm in length is made, cutting or reflecting the latissimus dorsi and posterior aspect of the serratus anterior. The chest is entered through the third or fourth interspace, and a small rib retractor is put into place. With a narrow malleable retractor, the lung is held forward by the first assistant. The ductus is usually large, but is variable in position. It may course superiorly as well as anteriorly from the aorta and be immediately adjacent to the distal aortic arch. In this location it can be easily mistaken for the arch. It may course directly anteriorly and be well inferior to the arch.

The friable vascular tissue makes the usual complete dissection of the ductus inadvisable.[G10,K3,M3,T2] The mediastinal pleura is incised with fine scissors just superior to the aortic end of the ductus and then just inferior to it. The tissue plane is developed by gently spreading fine scissors. As the inferior tissue plane is developed, the back wall (or right side) of the ductus is seen; no attempt is made to pass an instrument around it. The ductus is temporarily and lightly occluded with a fine forceps, and a pulse oximeter on the foot confirms that it is the ductus, not aorta, and that the aortic arch is intact without interruption or coarctation. A medium-sized hemoclip on a holder is positioned well across the ductus at its aortic end; the tip of the clip must be *beyond* the ductus posteriorly. The adventitia of the aorta may be grasped and gently retracted toward the surgeon as the clip is placed. By closing the holder the ductus is closed.

A No. 12 catheter is brought out through a stab wound in the chest wall and placed on suction. Placement of a chest tube is usually not necessary. The chest wall is closed with two pericostal sutures. The muscles are closed with a continuous fine absorbable suture (polyglycolic acid), and the closure is completed with a subcuticular stitch of fine absorbable sutures. When the procedure is performed in the operating room, the infant is transferred back to the neonatal intensive care unit in the same prewarmed transfer isolette.

SPECIAL FEATURES OF POSTOPERATIVE CARE

Care after division or ligation of PDA is simple and follows the principles described in Chapter 5. The patient is usually extubated and the drainage catheter removed in the operating room or within a few hours of leaving it. When the transaxillary muscle-sparing technique is used, most patients can be discharged from the hospital within 24 hours.[C12,H7]

When the operation is done with CPB, care is also simple and usual (see Chapter 5).

RESULTS

Early (Hospital) Death

Within 10 years of Gross and Hubbard's first successful case, hospital mortality for surgical closure of uncomplicated PDA had become very low. Gross and Longino, in 1951, reported eight deaths (1.9%; CL 1%-3%) among their

■ **TABLE 23–2   Associated Anomalies in a Surgical Series of Essentially Isolated Patent Ductus Arteriosus**

Associated Anomalies	No. of Cases [a]
Mild congenital aortic stenosis and/or regurgitation	5
Mild congenital mitral valve disease	5
Small VSD	8
Right or left pulmonary artery stenosis	3
Congenital complete heart block	1
Preterm infant	14 [b]
Rubella syndrome	16 [c]
Somatic congenital anomalies	9 [c]
Congenital lobar emphysema	1
Laryngeal web	1

(Data from GLH group, 1966 to 1984.)

Key: *VSD*, Ventricular septal defect.

[a] Categories shown are not mutually exclusive.

[b] Operation done in 4 patients age 2 to 5 months and in 10 patients age 1 to 13 years.

[c] Includes one example of Larsen syndrome and one of Cornelia de Lang syndrome.

■ **TABLE 23–3   Distribution of Pulmonary Artery Pressure in 50 Patients Undergoing Surgical Closure of Patent Ductus Arteriosus**

$P\bar{P}A$ [a]			
≤ mmHg <		*n*	% of 50
20	30	13	26
30	40	7	14
40	50	15	30
50	60	12	24
60	70	1	2
Uncertain		2	4
Total		50	100

(Data from GLH group, 1966 to 1984.)

Key: *P$\bar{P}A$*, Mean pulmonary artery pressure.

[a] Only patients whose preoperative mean pulmonary artery pressure was 20 mmHg or greater are included. Cardiac catheterization was done in these 50 patients because there was a clinical suggestion that pulmonary vascular resistance was elevated.

■ **TABLE 23–4   Distribution of Preoperative Pulmonary Vascular Resistance Among Patients Undergoing Surgical Closure of Patent Ductus Arteriosus**

Rpl			
≤ units · m² —	<	*n*	% of 50
	2	8	16
2	5	25	50
5	7	10	20
7		0	0
NA		7	14
Total		50	100

(Database is as in Table 23–3.)

Key: *NA*, Not available because oxygen consumption was not measured; *Rpl*, pulmonary vascular resistance index.

first 412 surgically treated cases.[G9] In 1955, Ash and Fischer reported no deaths (0%; CL 0%-6%) among 116 consecutive children (ages 4 months to 14 years) undergoing surgical closure.[A2] Other similar experiences reinforce the idea that the operation is safe and that hospital mortality approaches zero.[M10]

Incremental Risk Factors for Early Death

No risk factors for early death can currently be identified. Operation in infancy or childhood, associated congenital anomalies (Table 23-2), pulmonary hypertension (Table 23-3), and mild or moderate increase of pulmonary vascular resistance (Table 23-4) do not increase the risk of hospital death, nor does the surgical technique used. However, by considering the entire span of time since Gross first successfully closed a PDA in 1938, certain situations can be presumed to increase risk.

When pulmonary vascular disease is severe and the shunt is bidirectional or dominantly right to left, risk is high; 5 of 14 such patients (36%; CL 21%-53%) died in the hospital in the early Mayo Clinic experience.[E4] Death was due to hemorrhage during operation (from the pulmonary artery suture line, because pulmonary artery pressure after closure was *higher* than systemic arterial pressure and the pulmonary artery was large and thin walled), or it occurred suddenly some days later without any demonstrable cause.[E4] However, no distinction with regard to reactivity of the pulmonary vascular bed was made in these patients. Thus, it is likely that with preoperative provocative testing, a subgroup of patients could be identified that would have lower operative risk.

When pulmonary vascular disease is mild or moderate, and thus when a large left-to-right shunt is present, there is no increased risk. Even in the early era, 16 among 271 patients undergoing repair of PDA at the Mayo Clinic had severe pulmonary hypertension but only mild or moderate pulmonary vascular disease and a large left-to-right shunt, and there were no (0%; CL 0%-11%) early or late deaths.[E4]

Older age mildly increases risk of surgical closure even in the absence of severe pulmonary vascular disease. This increase is from the technical problems posed by the friable and often calcified ductal wall in older patients and the tendency of the long-standing volume overload of the left ventricle to predispose them to fatal arrhythmias. The mildly increased risk in the older age group is illustrated by the report of Black and Goldman in 1972, which described one death (2%; CL 0.2%-6%) in 53 adults (age 14 to 55 years) undergoing surgical closure of a PDA. Death occurred at early reoperation for postoperative bleeding from a tear in the aorta.[B3] In recent years, the technical problems in older patients have been eased by the use of an open technique (see "Technique of Operation" earlier in this chapter).

Time-Related Survival

Life expectancy is normal after surgical closure of an uncomplicated PDA in infancy or childhood. When moderate or severe pulmonary vascular disease has developed preoperatively, late deaths may result from its progression, as is the case in children with ventricular septal defect (see "Pulmonary Hypertension" under Results in Section 1 of Chapter 21).

When the operation is performed in adults with advanced chronic heart failure, premature late death is at times unavoidable. This is because the cardiomyopathy secondary to long-standing left ventricular volume overload is irreversible in some patients, in a way entirely analogous to the situation in patients with long-standing aortic valve regurgitation (see "Left Ventricular Structure and Function" under Results in Chapter 12).

Symptomatic and Functional Status

Disappearance of the signs and symptoms of heart failure is dramatic after surgical closure of a large PDA. Ash and Fischer recount that the marked hepatomegaly and splenomegaly in a 3-year-old girl with cardiac cachexia and advanced heart failure were no longer detectable 3 hours after surgical closure of the ductus, and cardiac size on chest radiography had returned to near normal within 4 months.[A2]

Physical Development

It has been presumed that when a large isolated PDA is closed in infancy, growth pattern becomes normal. However, growth retardation, particularly in regard to height, tends to persist, particularly when the operation is delayed beyond infancy or if the child has a rubella syndrome.[E6] The same may occur after repair of ventricular septal defect (see "Physical Development" under Results in Section 1 of Chapter 21).

Recurrence of Ductal Patency

Currently, prevalence of recurrent or persistent ductal patency approaches zero when division or appropriate ligation techniques are used.[E2,L2,M10] In an earlier era, it did occur. In 1965, Jones reported 12 patients (20%; CL 14%-26%) with recurrent or persistent ductal patency out of 61 patients who had ductal ligation with heavy tape.[J1] Later, it became less common; Panagopoulos and colleagues reported only four cases (0.4%; CL 0.2%-0.8%) among 936 patients undergoing ductal closure, mostly by ligation.[P1] Trippestad and Efskind reported 20 among 639 traced cases (3.1%; CL 2.4%-4.0%).[T5]

False Aneurysm

False aneurysm is a rare complication of surgical ductal closure that usually occurs after ligation rather than division.[P3,P4,R3] Only rare cases of false aneurysm have been reported after ductal division, and these probably resulted from technical errors or infection.[C1,E8,H1,R4]

Development of a false aneurysm is an indication for urgent reoperation.

Left Vocal Cord Paralysis

Transient and occasionally permanent left vocal cord paralysis resulting from manipulation or injury of the left recurrent laryngeal nerve occurs in 1% to 4% of patients following division or ligation of a PDA.[F3,M10]

Prevalence is higher among infants with low birth weight.[D5,F3,Z1]

Phrenic Nerve Paralysis

Phrenic nerve paralysis with elevation of the hemidiaphragm is an uncommon complication of PDA closure, occurring in approximately 4% of patients.[F3] It usually occurs on the left side, usually in infants, and most frequently in preterm babies.[F3] It is not necessarily due to surgical damage to the phrenic nerve, because it may develop on the right side. It often regresses spontaneously, but may persist for many months or indefinitely.

Chylothorax

Chylothorax is a rare complication of surgical ductal closure. Its management is discussed in Section 2 of Chapter 5.

INDICATIONS FOR OPERATION

Persistent PDA is an indication for closure, and the optimal age for operating is during the first year of life.[A2] Patients, either term or preterm, with *prolonged* PDA require closure in early life only when a large left-to-right shunt results in heart failure. In practice, this means that in term infants in the first month of life, PDA closure is indicated only when symptoms of heart failure are present. (For a discussion of the special situation in preterm infants, see "Patent Ductus Arteriosus in Preterm Infants" under Special Situations and Controversies later in this chapter).

Beyond the first month of life, prophylactic closure of the PDA is indicated. In the absence of symptoms, operation may be delayed until about age 6 months. However, closure is indicated at any time before this when symptoms of heart failure or failure to thrive persist despite intense medical treatment.

Older age is not a contraindication to closure of an isolated PDA in the absence of severe pulmonary vascular disease.

Severe pulmonary vascular disease is a contraindication to closure. The criteria of inoperability in this setting are the same as described for patients with ventricular septal defect (see "Indications for Operation" in Section 1 of Chapter 21). In the case of patients with PDA, the ductus may be temporarily occluded at operation; if pulmonary artery pressure does not decrease but remains severely elevated with no increase in aortic pressure, the shunt is *not* dominantly left to right. Closure of the ductus, therefore, will not reduce pulmonary artery pressure or left atrial pressure and therefore cannot trigger a favorable change in pulmonary vascular resistance. Repair is contraindicated in this situation. With preoperative provocative testing, abandoning closure in the operating room should be uncommon.

Until recently, indications for "closure" of PDA were indications for *operative* closure. This is probably still true in many institutions, but percutaneous closure must be considered (see "Percutaneous [Catheter] Closure of Patent Ductus Arteriosus" under Special Situations and Controversies later in this chapter).

SPECIAL SITUATIONS AND CONTROVERSIES

Patent Ductus Arteriosus in Preterm Infants

Historical Note

In 1963, both Powell and De Cancq, independently, were apparently the first to close a PDA in a preterm infant by operation.[D1,P2] Subsequently, improvement in the cardiovascular status of preterm infants after surgical closure of a PDA has been clearly demonstrated.[B2,J2]

Clinical Features and Diagnostic Criteria

The preterm infant with a PDA may have a continuous murmur, and under these circumstances diagnosis is made with confidence.[C9,E5] The shunt is considered large enough to be important if there is pulmonary plethora and cardiomegaly on the chest radiograph, if peripheral pulses are bounding, or, if by echocardiography, the left atrial–aortic ratio is greater than or equal to 1.5 and Doppler color flow interrogation demonstrates a large left-to-right shunt.[J3]

A systolic murmur is less specific for PDA, but the diagnosis is made clinically if the murmur is associated with a hyperactive precordium, increased pulse pressure, or positive chest radiograph or echocardiogram. A few preterm infants have these positive clinical and laboratory findings of PDA without a murmur.[M2,T1]

Natural History

A high proportion of preterm infants have prolonged patency of the ductus arteriosus after birth. The frequency increases with decreasing gestational age and decreasing birth weight.[H5] Siassi and colleagues reported the presence of a PDA (based on presence of a long systolic murmur) in 77% of premature infants with a gestational age of 28 to 30 weeks, 44% with a gestational age of 31 to 33 weeks, and 21% with a gestational age of 34 to 36 weeks.[S3] Birth weights of less than 1000 g, 1000 to 1500 g, and 1500 to 2000 g were associated with a PDA prevalence of 83%, 47%, and 27%, respectively. Frequency of hemodynamically important PDA is less, however: approximately 40% when the birth weight is less than 1000 g and 10% when it is less than 1750 g.[E5,V1]

A PDA has the same hemodynamic effects in preterm infants as in term infants, as evidenced by collapsing pulses and radiographic evidence of increased pulmonary blood flow, left atrial enlargement, and cardiomegaly. Furthermore, experimental studies in preterm lambs have shown that the left-to-right shunt through the open ductus is associated with reduced effective systemic blood flow and organ hypoperfusion.[B1] This has led to the hypothesis that necrotizing enterocolitis in preterm infants may be associated with a large PDA, which is supported by results of a randomized trial of ductal closure in preterm babies and by other studies.[C10,V1]

A strong correlation exists between patency of the ductus arteriosus and idiopathic respiratory distress syndrome, although these may not be causally related.[E1,E3,T1] There is also an association between fluid administration and ductal patency; thus, PDA is less frequent in neonatal units that restrict fluids in preterm infants.[B5]

Technique of Operation

See "Technique of Operation" earlier in this chapter.

Special Features of Postoperative Care

Because surgical closure of a PDA is only one facet of care of a preterm infant, the patient is returned to the care of the neonatologist in the neonatal intensive care unit.[S1] The drainage catheter may be left until mechanical ventilation is no longer necessary, because pneumothorax occasionally develops in preterm infants maintained on a ventilator.

Early Results

Hospital mortality is approximately 10% to 20%.[P7,P8,T8] It is not related to the interval between birth and operation, but, as in other circumstances in preterm infants, it is probably related to birth weight and gestational age. Death may be from continuing respiratory distress, intracranial hemorrhage, necrotizing enterocolitis, or a diffuse coagulopathy,[B4,P8] but it rarely occurs during the immediate perioperative period. There is no evidence that prevalence of intracranial hemorrhage is increased by surgical closure of the ductus.[S2]

Cardiac status usually improves immediately, and left atrial size is promptly reduced.[B4] At least one randomized study indicates overall benefit of early surgical closure of a PDA in preterm infants weighing less than 1500 g and requiring mechanical ventilation.[C5] Another randomized study of infants weighing 1000 g or less and requiring supplemental oxygen demonstrated reduction ($P = .001$) in necrotizing enterocolitis among those treated by early ligation.[C10]

Late Results

Among preterm infants requiring PDA closure, only half the hospital survivors are well 1 to 5 years later.[B4] Approximately one third have bronchopulmonary dysplasia on chest radiograph, with variable clinical findings. About one sixth have more severe complications, such as retrolental fibroplasia, blindness, and cerebral palsy.[B4]

Indications for Operation

Indications for operative closure of a PDA include respiratory distress (ventilator dependency and need for high F_{IO_2} in the absence of important shunt) and demonstration of a large PDA (collapsing pulses, left atrial enlargement by echocardiography, and a large $\dot{Q}p/\dot{Q}s$ by radionucleotide scanning). In many centers, closure is reserved for infants who do not respond to medical management, including a course of indomethacin therapy.[F1,H3,P6] Failure of indomethacin treatment approaches 40% to 50%, particularly in low-birth-weight infants (<800 g).[P7,P8,T8] Surgical ligation should be considered the primary form of treatment in small preterm infants who have either a lower probability of PDA closure with indomethacin or an increased risk for development of complications from this therapy.[C10,G13,P8]

Percutaneous (Catheter) Closure of Patent Ductus Arteriosus

Technical improvements and operator experience have made percutaneous closure of PDA an intervention of proven efficacy. In earlier years, approximately 65% of patients had complete ablation of the shunt with this technique.[A3,R8] Currently, closure can be achieved in a high percentage of patients with umbrella or button coils or plugs.[B8,L4,L5,M12,R9,S6,S7,T9] Effective occlusion (no or trivial residual shunt) can be accomplished in approximately 85% to 90% of patients.[M11,R10,U1] The procedures are performed under local anesthesia and on an outpatient basis in many centers.[F5,M7,M8,P9,W1] (In patients with a PDA of large diameter or short length, surgical closure is advisable.)

The ultimate role of outpatient closure of a PDA will be determined by its costs compared with those of operative closure, reproducibility of the results obtained, prevalence of complete and permanent closure, and occurrence of late complications resulting from a device residing in the ductus arteriosus.[F5,G14,G15,P7]

Thoracoscopic Closure of Patent Ductus Arteriosus

An alternative to percutaneous catheter closure of a PDA is thoracoscopic closure without thoracotomy. It is performed under general anesthesia using three or four incisions 3 to 7 mm in length in the left hemithorax.[L3,L6] The surgical field is viewed on a video screen. Once the ductus is dissected from the surrounding tissue, one or more clips are applied to close it. The technique has been used in neonates, children of all ages, and adults.[B9,C13,H8,L6] In the experience of Laborde and colleagues with 332 consecutive pediatric patients, mortality was zero and morbidity minimal.[L6] Three patients with persistent ductal patency required surgical closure.

REFERENCES

A

1. Abbott M. Atlas of congenital heart disease. New York: American Heart Association, 1936.
2. Ash R, Fischer D. Manifestations and results of treatment of patent ductus arteriosus in infancy and childhood. An analysis of 138 cases. Pediatrics 1955;16:695.
3. Ali Khan MA, Mullins CE, Nihill MR, Yousef SA, Oufy SA, Abdullah M, et al. Percutaneous catheter closure of the ductus arteriosus in children and young adults. Am J Cardiol 1989;64:218.
4. Acierno LJ. History of cardiology. New York: Parthenon, 1994.

B

1. Baylen BG, Ogata H, Ikegami M, Jacobs HC, Jobe AH, Emmanouilides GC. Left ventricular performance and regional blood flows before and after ductus arteriosus occlusion in premature lambs treated with surfactant. Circulation 1983;67:837.
2. Baylen BG, Emmanouilides GC. Patent ductus arteriosus in the newborn. In Gregory GA, Thibeault DW, eds. Neonatal pulmonary care. Menlo Park, Calif: Addison-Wesley, 1979, p. 318.
3. Black LL, Goldman BS. Surgical treatment of the patent ductus arteriosus in the adult. Ann Surg 1972;175:290.
4. Brandt B, Marvin WJ, Ehrenhaft JL, Heintz S, Doty DB. Ligation of patent ductus arteriosus in premature infants. Ann Thorac Surg 1981;32:167.
5. Bell EF, Warburton D, Stonestreet BS, Oh W. Effect of fluid administration on the development of symptomatic patent ductus arteriosus and congestive heart failure in premature infants. N Engl J Med 1980;302:598.
6. Blalock A. Operative closure of the patent ductus arteriosus. Surg Gynecol Obstet 1946;82:113.
7. Baden M, Kirks DR. Transient dilatation of the ductus arteriosus—the "ductus bump." J Pediatr 1974;84:858.
8. Bridges ND, Perry SB, Parness I, Keane JF, Lock JE. Transcatheter closure of a large patent ductus arteriosus with the clamshell septal umbrella. J Am Coll Cardiol 1991;18:1297.
9. Burke RP, Wernovsky G, van der Velde M, Hansen D, Castaneda AR. Video-assisted thoracoscopic surgery for congenital heart disease. J Thorac Cardiovasc Surg 1995;109:499.
10. Balzer DT, Spray TL, McMullin D, Cottingham W, Canter CE. Endarteritis associated with a clinically silent patent ductus arteriosus. Am Heart J 1993;125:1192.

C

1. Crafoord G. Discussion of paper by Gross RE. Complete division for the patent ductus arteriosus. J Thorac Surg 1947;16:314.
2. Campbell M. Natural history of persistent ductus arteriosus. Br Heart J 1968;30:4.
3. Christie A. Normal closing time of the foramen ovale and the ductus arteriosus. Am J Dis Child 1930;40:323.
4. Cruickshank B, Marquis RM. Spontaneous aneurysms of the ductus arteriosus. Am J Med 1958;25:140.
5. Cotton RB, Stahlman MT, Bender HW, Graham TP, Catterton WZ, Kovar I. Randomized trial of early closure of symptomatic patent ductus arteriosus in small preterm infants. J Pediatr 1978;93:647.
6. Cassels DE. The ductus arteriosus. Springfield, Ill: Charles C Thomas, 1973, p. 75.
7. Calder AL, Kirker JA, Neutze JM, Starling MB. Pathology of the ductus arteriosus treated with prostaglandins: comparisons with untreated cases. Pediatr Cardiol 1984;5:85.
8. Clyman RI, Heymann MA. Pharmacology of the ductus arteriosus. Pediatr Clin North Am 1981;28:77.
9. Clarkson PM, Orgill AA. Continuous murmurs in infants of low birth weight. J Pediatr 1974;84:208.
10. Cassady G, Crouse DR, Kirklin JW, Strange MJ, Joiner CH, Godoy G, et al. A randomized controlled trial of very early prophylactic ligation of the ductus arteriosus in babies who weighed 1000 g or less at birth. N Engl J Med 1989;320:1511.
11. Coster DD, Gorton ME, Grooters RK, Thieman KC, Schneider RF, Soltanzadeh H. Surgical closure of the patent ductus arteriosus in the neonatal intensive care unit. Ann Thorac Surg 1989;48:386.
12. Cetta F, Deleon SY, Roughneen PT, Graham LC, Lichtenberg RC, Bell TJ, et al. Cost-effectiveness of transaxillary muscle-sparing same-day operative closure of patent ductus arteriosus. Am J Cardiol 1997;79:1281.
13. Chu JJ, Chang CH, Lin PJ, Liu HP, Tsai FC, Wu D, et al. Video-assisted thoracoscopic operation for interruption of patent ductus arteriosus in adults. Ann Thorac Surg 1997;63:175.

D

1. De Cancq HE Jr. Repair of patent ductus arteriosus in a 1417 g infant. Am J Dis Child 1963;106:402.
2. Das JB, Chesterman JT. Aneurysms of the patent ductus arteriosus. Thorax 1956;11:295.

3. DuBrow IW, Fisher E, Hastreiter A. Intermittent functional closure of patent ductus arteriosus in a ten-month old infant: hemodynamic documentation. Chest 1975;68:110.

4. d'Udekem Y, Rubay JE, Sluysmans T. A case of neonatal ductus arteriosus aneurysm. Cardiovasc Surg 1997;5:338.

5. Davis JT, Baciewicz FA, Suriyapa S, Vauthy P, Polamreddy R, Barnett B. Vocal cord paralysis in premature infants undergoing ductal closure. Ann Thorac Surg 1988;46:214.

E

1. Edmunds LH Jr. Operation or indomethacin for the premature ductus. Ann Thorac Surg 1978;26:586.

2. Emmanouilides GC. Persistent patency of the ductus arteriosus in premature infants. In Seventy-fifth Ross Conference on Pediatric Research, Palm Beach, Fla, Dec 4-7, 1977.

3. Edmunds LH Jr, Gregory GA, Heymann MA, Kitterman JA, Rudolph AM, Tooley WH. Surgical closure of the ductus arteriosus in premature infants. Circulation 1973;48:856.

4. Ellis FH Jr, Kirklin JW, Callahan JA, Wood EH. Patent ductus arteriosus with pulmonary hypertension. J Thorac Surg 1956;31:268.

5. Ellison RC, Peckham GJ, Lang P, Talner NS, Lerer TJ, Lin L, et al. Evaluation of the preterm infant for patent ductus arteriosus. Pediatrics 1983;71:364.

6. Engle MA, Holswade GR, Goldbert HP, Glenn F. Present problems pertaining to patency of the ductus arteriosus. I. Persistence of growth retardation after successful surgery. Pediatrics 1958;21:70.

7. Eggert LD, Jung AL, McGough EC, Ruttenberg HD. Surgical treatment of patent ductus arteriosus in preterm infants. Four-year experience with ligation in the newborn intensive care unit. Pediatr Cardiol 1982;2:15.

8. Egami J, Tada Y, Takagi A, Sato O, Idezuki Y. False aneurysm as a late complication of division of a patent ductus arteriosus. Ann Thorac Surg 1992;53:901.

F

1. Friedman WF, Hirschlau MJ, Printz MP, Pitlick PT, Kirkpatrick SE. Pharmacologic closure of patent ductus arteriosus in the premature infant. N Engl J Med 1976;295:526.

2. Falcone MW, Perloff JK, Roberts WC. Aneurysm of the nonpatent ductus arteriosus. Am J Cardiol 1972;29:422.

3. Fan LL, Campbell DN, Clarke DR, Washington RL, Fix EJ, White CW. Paralyzed left vocal cord associated with ligation of patent ductus arteriosus. J Thorac Cardiovasc Surg 1989;98:611.

4. Fripp RR, Whitman V, Waldhausen JA, Boal DK. Ductus arteriosus aneurysm presenting as pulmonary artery obstruction: diagnosis and management. J Am Coll Cardiol 1985;6:234.

5. Fedderly RT, Beekman RH 3rd, Mosca RS, Bove EL, Lloyd TR. Comparison of hospital charges for closure of patent ductus arteriosus by surgery and by transcatheter coil occlusion. Am J Cardiol 1996;77:776.

6. French RK. The thorax in history. V. Discovery of the pulmonary transit. Thorax 1978;33:555.

7. Franklin KJ. Ductus venosus (Arantii) and ductus arteriosus (Botalli). Bull Hist Med 1941;9:580.

G

1. Gibson GA. Persistence of the arterial duct and its diagnosis. Edinb Med J 1900;8:1.

2. Graybial A, Strieder JW, Boyer NH. An attempt to obliterate the patent ductus arteriosus in a patient with subacute bacterial endocarditis. Am Heart J 1938;15:621.

3. Gross RE, Hubbard JP. Surgical ligation of a patent ductus arteriosus. Report of first successful case. JAMA 1939;112:729.

4. Goncalves-Estella A, Perez-Villoria J, Gonzalez-Reoyo F, Gimenez-Mendez JP, Castro-Cels A, Castro-Llorens M. Closure of a complicated ductus arteriosus through the transpulmonary route using hypothermia. J Thorac Cardiovasc Surg 1975;69:698.

5. Graham EA. Aneurysm of the ductus arteriosus, with a consideration of its importance to the thoracic surgeon. Arch Surg 1940;41:324.

6. Gittenberger-de Groot AC. Persistent ductus arteriosus: most probably a primary congenital malformation. Br Heart J 1977;39:610.

7. Gross RE. Complete surgical division of the patent ductus arteriosus. Surg Gynecol Obstet 1944;78:36.

8. Gross RE. Complete division of the patent ductus arteriosus. J Thorac Surg 1947;16:314.

9. Gross RE, Longino LA. The patent ductus arteriosus. Observations from 412 surgically treated cases. Circulation 1951;3:125.

10. Gunning AJ. A simple, safe, surgical technique for closing the persistent ductus arteriosus in the preterm neonate. Ann R Coll Surg Engl 1983;65:214.

11. Gittenberger-de Groot AC, Moulaert AJ, Harinck ME, Becker AE. Histopathology of the ductus arteriosus after prostaglandin E$_1$ administration in ductus dependent cardiac anomalies. Br Heart J 1978; 40:215.

12. Grollman JH Jr, Harris CH, Hamilton LC. Congenital diverticula of the aortic arch. N Engl J Med 1967;276:1178.

13. Grosfeld JL, Chaet M, Molinari F, Engle W, Engum SA, West KW, et al. Increased risk of necrotizing enterocolitis in premature infants with patent ductus arteriosus treated with indomethacin. Ann Surg 1996;224:350.

14. Gray DT, Fyler DC, Walker AM, Weinstein MC, Chalmers TC. Clinical outcomes and costs of transcatheter as compared with surgical closure of patent ductus arteriosus. The Patent Ductus Arteriosus Closure Comparative Study Group. N Engl J Med 1993; 329:1517.

15. Gray DT, Weinstein MC. Decision and cost-utility analyses of surgical versus transcatheter closure of patent ductus arteriosus: should you let a smile be your umbrella? Med Decis Making 1998;18:187.

H

1. Hallman AL, Cooley DA. False aortic aneurysm following division and suture of a patent ductus arteriosus. Successful excision with hypothermia. J Cardiovasc Surg 1964;5:23.

2. Hay JD. Population and clinic studies of congenital heart disease in Liverpool. Br Med J 1966;2:661.

3. Heymann MA, Rudolph AM, Silverman NH. Closure of the ductus arteriosus in premature infants by inhibition of prostaglandin synthesis. N Engl J Med 1976;295:530.

4. Heikkinen ES, Simila S, Laitinen J, Larmi T. Infantile aneurysm of the ductus arteriosus. Diagnosis, incidence, pathogenesis, and prognosis. Acta Paediatr Scand 1974;63:241.

5. Heymann MA. Patent ductus arteriosus. In Adams FH, Emmanouilides GC, eds. Heart disease in infants, children, and adolescents, 3rd ed. Baltimore: Williams & Wilkins, 1983.

6. Heymann MA, Rudolph AM. Control of the ductus arteriosus. Physiol Rev 1975;55:62.

7. Hawkins JA, Minich LL, Tani LY, Sturtevant JE, Orsmond GS, McGough EC. Cost and efficacy of surgical ligation versus transcatheter coil occlusion of patent ductus arteriosus. J Thorac Cardiovasc Surg 1996;112:1634.

8. Hines MH, Bensky AS, Hammon JW Jr, Pennington G. Video-assisted thoracoscopic ligation of patent ductus arteriosus: safe and outpatient. Ann Thorac Surg 1998;66:853.

9. Houston AB, Gnanapragasam JP, Lim MK, Doig WB, Coleman EN. Doppler ultrasound and the silent ductus. Br Heart J 1991;65:97.

10. Harvey W. The circulation of the blood. Franklin KJ, translator. Springfield, Ill: Charles C Thomas, 1958.

J

1. Jones JC. Twenty-five years' experience with the surgery of patent ductus arteriosus. J Thorac Cardiovasc Surg 1965;50:149.

2. Jacob J, Gluck L, DiSessa T, Edwards D, Kulovich M, Kurlinski J, et al. The contribution of PDA in the neonate with severe RDS. J Pediatr 1980;96:79.

3. Johnson GL, Breart GL, Gewitz MH, Brenner JI, Lang P, Dooley KJ, et al. Echocardiographic characteristics of premature infants with patent ductus arteriosus. Pediatrics 1983;72:846.

4. Jager BV, Wollenman OF Jr. An anatomical study of the closure of the ductus arteriosus. Am J Pathol 1942;18:595.

K

1. Krovetz LJ, Warden HE. Patent ductus arteriosus. An analysis of 515 surgically proved cases. Dis Chest 1962;42:241.

2. Keys A, Shapiro MJ. Patency of the ductus arteriosus in adults. Am Heart J 1943;25:158.

3. Kron IL, Mentzer RM Jr, Rheuban KS, Nolan SP. A simple, rapid technique for operative closure of patent ductus arteriosus in the premature infant. Ann Thorac Surg 1984;37:422.

4. Karwande SV, Rowles JR. Simplified muscle-sparing thoracotomy for patent ductus arteriosus ligation in neonates. Ann Thorac Surg 1992;54:164.

L

1. Levine SA, Geremia AE. Clinical features of patent ductus arteriosus with special reference to cardiac murmurs. Am J Med Sci 1947;213:385.

2. Lucht U, Sondergaard T. Late results of operation for patent ductus arteriosus. Scand J Thorac Cardiovasc Surg 1971;5:223.

3. Laborde F, Noirhomme P, Karam J, Batisse A, Bourel P, Saint Maurice O. A new video-assisted thoracoscopic surgical technique for interruption of patent ductus arteriosus in infants and children. J Thorac Cardiovasc Surg 1993;105:278.

4. Lloyd TR, Fedderly R, Mendelsohn AM, Sandhu SK, Beekman RH 3rd. Transcatheter occlusion of patent ductus arteriosus with Gianturco coils. Circulation 1993;88:1412.

5. Lloyd TR, Rao PS, Beekman RH 3rd, Mendelsohn AM, Sideris EB. Atrial septal defect occlusion with the buttoned device (a multi-institutional U.S. trial). Am J Cardiol 1994;73:286.

6. Laborde F, Folliguet TA, Etienne PY, Carbognani D, Batisse A, Petrie J. Video-thoracoscopic surgical interruption of patent ductus arteriosus. Routine experience in 332 pediatric cases. Eur J Cardiothorac Surg 1997;11:1052.

M

1. Munro JC. Surgery of the vascular system. Ligation of patent ductus arteriosus. Ann Surg 1907;46:335.

2. McGrath RL, McGuinness GA, Way GL, Wolfe RR, Nora JJ, Simmons MA. The silent ductus arteriosus. J Pediatr 1978;93:110.

3. Mavroudis C, Cook LN, Fleischaker JW, Nagaraj HS, Shott RJ, Howe WR, et al. Management of patent ductus arteriosus in the premature infant: indomethacin versus ligation. Ann Thorac Surg 1983;36:561.

4. McMurphy DM, Heymann MA, Rudolph AM, Melmon KL. Developmental change in constriction of the ductus arteriosus: response to oxygen and vasoactive substances in the isolated ductus arteriosus of the fetal lamb. Pediatr Res 1972;6:231.

5. Mancini AJ. A study of the angle formed by the ductus arteriosus with the descending thoracic aorta. Anat Rec 1951;109:535.

6. Mitchell SC, Korones SB, Berendes HW. Congenital heart disease in 56,109 births. Incidence and natural history. Circulation 1971;43:323.

7. Mullins CE. Pediatric and congenital therapeutic cardiac catheterization. Circulation 1989;79:1153.

8. Musewe NN, Benson LN, Smallhorn JF, Freedom RM. Two-dimensional echocardiographic and color flow Doppler evaluation of ductal occlusion with the Rashkind prosthesis. Circulation 1989;80:1706.

9. Majid AA. Closure of the patent ductus arteriosus with a Ligaclip through a minithoracotomy. Chest 1993;103:1512.

10. Mavroudis C, Backer CL, Gevitz M. Forty-six years of patent ductus arteriosus division at Children's Memorial Hospital of Chicago. Ann Surg 1994;220:402.

11. Magee AG, Stumper O, Burns JE, Godman MJ. Medium-term follow up of residual shunting and potential complications after transcatheter occlusion of the ductus arteriosus. Br Heart J 1994;71:63.

12. Masura J, Walsh KP, Thanopoulous B, Chan C, Bass J, Goussous Y, et al. Catheter closure of moderate- to large-sized patent ductus arteriosus using the new Amplatzer duct occluder: immediate and short-term results. J Am Coll Cardiol 1998;31:878.

O

1. O'Donovan TG, Beck W. Closure of the complicated patent ductus arteriosus. Ann Thorac Surg 1978;25:463.

P

1. Panagopoulos PH, Tatooles CJ, Aberdeen E, Waterston DJ, Bonham-Carter RE. Patent ductus arteriosus in infants and children: a review of 936 operations (1946-69). Thorax 1971;26:1937.

2. Powell ML. Patent ductus arteriosus in premature infants. Med J Aust 1963;2:56.

3. Payne RF, Jordan SC. Postoperative aneurysms following ligation of the patent ductus arteriosus. Br J Radiol 1968;42:858.

4. Punsar S, Scheinin T, Tala P, Telivuo L. Postoperative aneurysm of the patent ductus arteriosus. Ann Chir Gynaecol (Fenn) 1962;51:385.

5. Portsmann W, Wierny L, Warnke H, Gerstberger G, Romaniuk PA. Catheter closure of patent ductus arteriosus, 62 cases treated without thoracotomy. Radiol Clin North Am 1971;9:203.

6. Peckham GJ, Miettinen OS, Ellison RC, Kraybill EN, Gersony WM, Zierler S, et al. Clinical course to 1 year of age in premature infants with patent ductus arteriosus: results of a multicenter randomized trial of indomethacin. J Pediatr 1984;105:285.

7. Palder SB, Schwartz MZ, Tyson KR, Marr CC. Association of closure of patent ductus arteriosus and development of necrotizing enterocolitis. J Pediatr Surg 1988;23:422.

8. Perez CA, Bustorff-Silva JM, Villasenor E, Fonkalsrud EW, Atkinson JB. Surgical ligation of patent ductus arteriosus in very low birth weight infants: is it safe? Am Surg 1998;64:1007.

9. Prieto LR, DeCamillo DM, Konrad DJ, Scalet-Longworth L, Latson LA. Comparison of cost and clinical outcome between transcatheter coil occlusion and surgical closure of isolated patent ductus arteriosus. Pediatrics 1998;101:1020.

R

1. Rowe RD, Lowe JB. Auscultation in the diagnosis of persistent ductus arteriosus in infancy: a study of 50 patients. N Z Med J 1964;63:195.

2. Ravin A, Karley W. Apical diastolic murmur in patent ductus arteriosus. Ann Intern Med 1950;33:903.

3. Ross RJ, Feder FP, Spencer FC. Aneurysms of the previously ligated patent ductus arteriosus. Circulation 1961;23:350.

4. Rosenkrantz JG, Kelminson LL, Paton BC, Vogel JH. False aneurysm after ligation of a patent ductus arteriosus. Ann Thorac Surg 1967;3:353.

5. Rudolph AM, Heymann HA, Spitznas U. Hemodynamic considerations in the development of narrowing of the aorta. Am J Cardiol 1972;30:514.

6. Rudolph AM: The changes in the circulation after birth. Their importance in congenital heart disease. Circulation 1970;41:343.

7. Rashkind WJ, Cuaso CC. Transcatheter closure of patent ductus arteriosus: successful use in a 3.5 kg infant. Pediatr Cardiol 1979;1:63.

8. Rashkind WJ, Mullins CE, Hellenbrand WE, Tait MA. Nonsurgical closure of patent ductus arteriosus: clinical application of the Rashkind PDA Occluder System. Circulation 1987;75:583.

9. Rosenthal E, Qureshi SA, Reidy J, Baker EJ, Tynan M. Evolving use of embolisation coils for occlusion of the arterial duct. Heart 1996;76:525.

10. Rao PS, Kim SH, Choi JY, Rey C, Haddad J, Marcon F, et al. Follow-up results of transvenous occlusion of patent ductus arteriosus with the buttoned device. J Am Coll Cardiol 1999;33:820.

S

1. Strange M, Philips J, Kirklin JK, Lell W, Cassady G. Perioperative management of the tiny infant undergoing ligation of the patent ductus arteriosus (PDA). American Academy of Pediatrics, Spring Meeting, 1984.
2. Strange M, Myers G, Kirklin JK, Pacifico AD, Cassady G. Lack of effect of patent ductus arteriosus ligation on intraventricular hemorrhage in preterm infants. Clin Res 1983;31:913A.
3. Siassi B, Blanco C, Cabal LA, Coran AG. Incidence and clinical features of patent ductus arteriosus in low-birthweight infants: a prospective analysis of 150 consecutively born infants. Pediatrics 1976;57:347.
4. Silver MM, Freedom RM, Silver MD, Olley PM. The morphology of the human newborn ductus arteriosus: a reappraisal of its structure and function with special reference to prostaglandin E_1 therapy. Hum Pathol 1981;12:1123.
5. Santos MA, Moll JN, Drumond C, Araujo WB, Romano N, Reiss NB. Development of the ductus arteriosus in right ventricular outflow tract obstruction. Circulation 1980;62:818.
6. Sievert H, Niemoller E, Franz K, Kaltenbach M, Kober G, Rufenacht D, et al. Detachable balloon technique for transvenous closure of patent ductus arteriosus. J Interv Cardiol 1994;7:25.
7. Schrader R, Hofstetter R, Fassbender D, Berger F, Bubmann WD, Ernst JM, et al. Transvenous closure of patent ductus arteriosus with Ivalon plugs. Multicenter experience with a new technique. Invest Radiol 1999;34:65.

T

1. Thibeault DW, Emmanouilides GC, Nelson RJ, Lachman RS, Rosengart RM, Oh W. Patent ductus arteriosus complicating the respiratory distress syndrome in preterm infants. J Pediatr 1975;86:120.
2. Traugott RC, Will RJ, Schuchmann GF, Treasure RL. A simplified method of ligation of patent ductus arteriosus in premature infants. Ann Thorac Surg 1980;29:263.
3. Touroff AS, Vesell H. Experiences in the surgical treatment of subacute *Streptococcus viridans* endarteritis complicating patent ductus arteriosus. J Thorac Surg 1940;10:59.

4. Touroff AS, Vesell H. Subacute *Streptococcus viridans* endarteritis complicating patent ductus arteriosus: recovery following surgical treatment. JAMA 1940;115:1270.
5. Trippestad A, Efskind L. Patent ductus arteriosus. Surgical treatment of 686 patients. Scand J Thorac Cardiovasc Surg 1972;6:38.
6. Tutassaura H, Goldman B, Moes CA, Mustard WT. Spontaneous aneurysm of the ductus arteriosus in childhood. J Thorac Cardiovasc Surg 1969;57:180.
7. Tovar EA, Vana M Jr. VATS versus minithoracotomy for interruption of PDA in adults. Ann Thorac Surg 1997;64:1517.
8. Trus T, Winthrop AL, Pipe S, Shah J, Langer JC, Lau GY. Optimal management of patent ductus arteriosus in the neonate weighing less than 800 g. J Pediatr Surg 1993;28:1137.
9. Tometzki A, Chan K, De Giovanni J, Houston A, Martin R, Redel D, et al. Total UK multi-centre experience with a novel arterial occlusion device (Duct Occlud pfm). Heart 1996;76:520.

U

1. Uzun O, Dickinson D, Parsons J, Gibbs JL. Residual and recurrent shunts after implantation of Cook detachable duct occlusion coils. Heart 1998;79:220.

V

1. van de Bor M, Verloove-Vanhorick SP, Brand R, Ruys JH. Patent ductus arteriosus in a cohort of 1338 preterm infants: a collaborative study. Paediatr Perinat Epidemiol 1988;2:328.

W

1. Wessel DL, Keane JF, Parness I, Lock JE. Outpatient closure of the patent ductus arteriosus. Circulation 1988;77:1068.

Z

1. Zbar RI, Chen AH, Behrendt DM, Bell EF, Smith RJ. Incidence of vocal fold paralysis in infants undergoing ligation of patent ductus arteriosus. Ann Thorac Surg 1996;61:814.

SECTION 1

Tetralogy of Fallot with Pulmonary Stenosis

DEFINITION

Tetralogy of Fallot (TF) is a congenital cardiac malformation characterized by underdevelopment of the right ventricular (RV) infundibulum with anterior and leftward displacement of the infundibular (conal, outlet) septum and its parietal extension. Displacement (malalignment) of the infundibular septum is associated with RV outflow (pulmonary) stenosis (in extreme forms, atresia) and a large ventricular septal defect (VSD). Typically, the VSD is subaortic in position, but it may be beneath both the aorta and pulmonary trunk (juxta-arterial VSD). RV and left ventricle (LV) are of equal thickness, and their systolic pressures are usually the same. The atrioventricular (AV) connection is concordant, and the aorta is biventricular in origin, overriding onto the RV. The malformation may be called TF with double outlet RV if the aorta arises more than 50% from the RV (see description of aorta under "Morphology" later in this section). However, an interventricular tunnel repair (see "Intraventricular Tunnel Repair of Simple Double Outlet Right Ventricle" under Technique of Operation in Chapter 39), rather than VSD closure, is required only when more than 90% of the aorta arises from the RV.

This section considers only TF with pulmonary stenosis.

HISTORICAL NOTE

TF was first treated surgically by Blalock and Taussig in 1945, when they performed a palliative subclavian–pulmonary arterial shunt.[B4] Other types of systemic–pulmonary arterial shunts were introduced by Potts and colleagues in 1946,[P2] Waterston in 1962,[W1] Klinner in 1961,[K14,K20] Davidson in 1955,[D9] Laks and Castaneda in 1975,[L7] and de Leval and colleagues in 1981,[D6] among others. Palliation by direct relief of pulmonary stenosis with a closed technique was introduced by Sellors[S15] and Brock[B7,B27] in 1948.

TF was first successfully repaired by Lillehei and colleagues at the University of Minnesota in 1954 using "controlled cross-circulation" with another person serving as oxygenator.[L3] First successful repair of TF with a pump-oxygenator was done by Kirklin and colleagues at the Mayo Clinic in 1955.[K1] Warden and Lillehei and colleagues introduced patch enlargement of the RV infundibulum in 1957,[W4] and Kirklin and colleagues reported using transanular patching in 1959.[K2] Use of an RV–pulmonary trunk conduit for TF with pulmonary atresia was reported by Kirklin and colleagues in 1965,[R1] and Ross and Somerville first reported use of a valved extracardiac conduit for this purpose in 1966.[R19] It was recognized very early that repairing TF in infants was associated with high mortality, and two-stage repair soon evolved. In 1969 at GLH, a policy of routine one-stage repair was adopted and later shown to provide good results.[B9,B26] However, a selective and more conservative approach with routine two-stage repair continued to be used by many surgeons.[A2,R24] Subsequently, a two-institution comparative study demonstrated one-stage repair to be equal or preferable to the two-stage approach.[K19]

MORPHOLOGY

TF with pulmonary stenosis encompasses a wide spectrum of morphologic subsets that vary primarily in details of RV outflow obstruction, VSD, and aortic overriding.

Right Ventricular Outflow Tract

Infundibulum

Infundibular stenosis associated with specific alterations in position of the infundibular (conal, outlet) septum is the hallmark of TF. Specifically, the septal (leftward) end of the infundibular septum is displaced anteriorly, inserting in front of the left anterior division of the trabecula septomarginalis (septal band) (Fig. 24-1)[A13,V2] rather than between its two divisions, as in the normal heart (see Chapter 1, Fig. 1-5). In addition, the parietal (rightward) end of the conal septum is rotated anteriorly and passes anteriorly and inferiorly to reach the free wall of the RV (Fig. 24-2), so that the infundibular septum and its parietal extension may come to lie almost in a sagittal rather than the usual coronal (frontal) plane. Parietal and septal ends of the conal septum give rise to prominent muscle bands that attach to the right and left sides of the anterior RV free wall.[B21] The anterior free wall may show additional trabeculations or moderate thickening.

There is frequently a localized narrowing, the *os infundibulum*, which in 72% of cases lies in a transverse plane at the lower conal septal edge (see Fig. 24-2). This siting

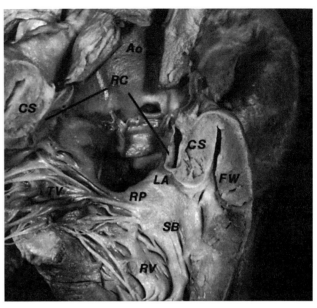

Figure 24-1 Autopsy specimen of tetralogy of Fallot with pulmonary stenosis, with right ventricle *(RV)* opened vertically and incision continued into overriding ascending aorta, dividing conal (infundibular, outlet) septum and right aortic cusp transversely. Right aortic cusp clearly originates within the RV (overrides), its belly attaching to the conal septum and almost reaching its inferior edge. Septal end of conal septum is displaced anteriorly in front of the left anterior division of the septal band (trabecula septomarginalis). Right posterior division of septal band gives origin to tricuspid chordae (papillary muscle of the conus or medial papillary muscle). The gap between these two limbs of the septal band, which in a normal heart is occupied by the septal insertion of the conal septum, now forms inferior and anterior margin of ventricular septal defect, which is clearly related to this malalignment of the conal septum relative to the septal band. (In this and subsequent photographs of autopsied specimens, orientation is the traditional anatomic one. To view morphology as the surgeon does at operation, photograph needs to be rotated 90 degrees counterclockwise.)

Key: *Ao,* Aorta; *CS,* conal (infundibular) septum; *FW,* anterior free wall; *LA,* left anterior division of septal band; *RC,* right coronary cusp; *RP,* right posterior division of septal band; *RV,* right ventricle; *SB,* septal band (trabecula septomarginalis); *TV,* tricuspid valve.

means that when the conal septum is well developed, there is a large infundibular chamber (or "third ventricle"; see Fig. 24-2), which in older patients occasionally becomes aneurysmal. In older patients, however, the os infundibulum is surrounded by fibrosis, which, when the chamber is small or absent, may extend into the RV–pulmonary trunk junction (pulmonary "anulus"). Less commonly (about 15% of cases), the major stenotic zone at the lower infundibular (conal) septal edge lies almost in a coronal plane, extending inferiorly from the lower infundibular septal edge. This occurs when hypertrophied muscle bands at the parietal end of the infundibular septum pass more inferiorly to join the free wall nearer to the RV apex, while on the septal (medial or leftward) aspect, there are not only inferiorly directed additional trabeculae, but also often an undue prominence and hypertrophy of the septal band. Under these circumstances the inferior boundary of the os

Figure 24-2   Autopsy specimen of tetralogy of Fallot with low-lying infundibular stenosis. Death occurred without surgical correction at age 3 years. **A,** Isolated infundibular stenosis viewed from below through opened right ventricle. **B,** Stenosis viewed from above after removing anterior wall of large infundibular chamber and opening front of pulmonary trunk. Stenosis is localized at lower border of conal septum (os infundibulum). Note that lateral (parietal) end of the septum is deviated anteriorly into almost a sagittal plane. Posterosuperior angle of ventricular septal defect is well seen *(arrow)*, as is its proximity to right aortic cusp. Infundibular chamber is dilated and thin walled in association with the low, transversely placed infundibular stenosis. Pulmonary valve is tricuspid and not stenotic.

Key: *Ao,* Aorta; *CS,* conal septum; *OsInf,* os infundibulum; *PT,* pulmonary trunk; *PV,* pulmonary valve; *RAA,* right atrial appendage; *RC,* right coronary cusp; *RV,* right ventricle; *TV,* tricuspid valve; *VSD,* ventricular septal detect.

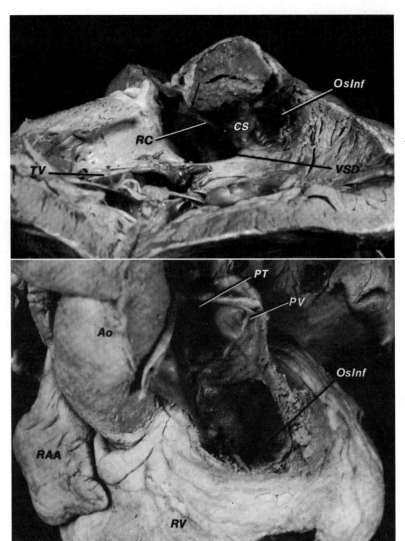

infundibulum may be formed by a prominent superiorly displaced moderator band.[A13] (When this type of low-lying infundibular stenosis is associated with a small or moderate-sized VSD, it is not termed TF; see Section 5.) Both transverse and coronal plane stenoses are occasionally present (12% of cases in the GLH experience).

When an *infundibular chamber* is present, its walls laterally and medially consist of numerous trabeculated spaces, some of which may form prominent blind recesses that do not lead directly to the valve "anulus," and occasionally an accessory opening is present. Endocardial fibrosis is not seen during the first 6 to 9 months of life and is seldom marked before age 2 years.[C13] Later, fibrosis seems to progress, which may lead to acquired infundibular atresia.

Generally, the infundibulum is somewhat longer, relative to total RV length, than it is in normal hearts.[B35,H23] When the infundibular (conal) septum is short (hypoplastic), infundibular stenosis reaches the pulmonary valve "anulus" without an intervening chamber. When the infundibular septum is absent, the VSD is juxta-arterial (doubly committed), extending superiorly to reach the pulmonary valve; infundibular stenosis is absent, and the posterior

aspect of the RV outflow tract is formed by the VSD (Fig. 24-3).[N4] The pulmonary valve and sometimes its "anulus" are the main sites of the usually moderate stenosis in these hearts. However, once a VSD patch is in position, the hypertrophied RV walls and dextroposed aorta may combine with the patch to form severe subvalvar stenosis.

The infundibulum may be diffusely narrowed and hypoplastic. This is often the situation when operation is performed in neonates. There is no localized os infundibulum (Fig. 24-4); neither is there increased trabeculations nor important muscular hypertrophy. Nevertheless, stenosis is usually severe because narrowing occurs throughout the outflow tract (Fig. 24-5). This tubular stenosis is usually short but may be of moderate length, depending on conal septal development (see Fig. 24-4).

Pulmonary Valve

The pulmonary valve is stenotic to some degree in 75% of cases of TF. Approximately two thirds of stenotic valves are bicuspid (Table 24-1);[L1,N1] three-cusp configuration occurs more commonly in nonstenotic valves. Even when nonstenotic, valve area is usually smaller than that of the aortic valve, which is the reverse of normal.

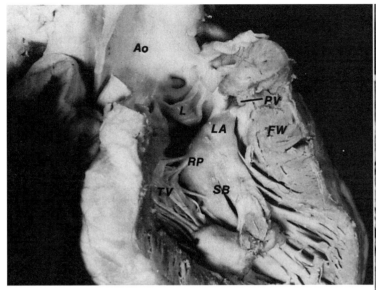

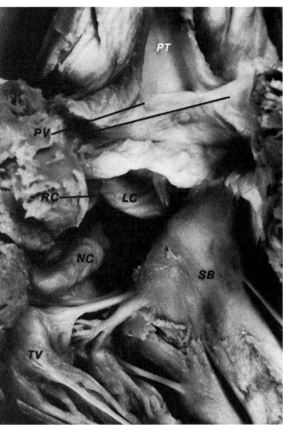

Figure 24-3   Autopsy specimen of tetralogy of Fallot with juxta-arterial ventricular septal defect (VSD). **A,** Viewed from opened right ventricle (RV) with incision carried across right cusp of aortic valve. **B,** Viewed after opening RV across pulmonary valve and trunk. Conal septum appears to be absent, and VSD is bounded superiorly by fused aortic and pulmonary valve "anuli." Septal band (trabecula septomarginalis) and RV free wall are severely hypertrophied. There is marked narrowing of pulmonary "anulus" and trunk and thickening and tethering of the valve cusps.

Key: *Ao,* Aorta; *FW,* right ventricular free wall; *L,* left coronary cusp; *LA,* left anterior division at septal band; *LC,* left coronary aortic cusp; *NC,* noncoronary aortic cusp; *PT,* pulmonary trunk; *PV,* pulmonary valve; *RC,* right coronary aortic cusp; *RP,* right posterior division of septal band; *SB,* septal band; *TV,* tricuspid valve.

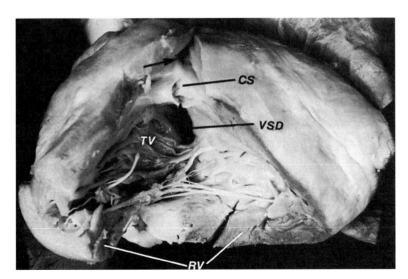

Figure 24-4   Autopsy specimen of tetralogy of Fallot with diffuse right ventricular *(RV)* outflow hypoplasia (same specimen as in Fig. 24-1). View is through opened RV. Stenotic infundibulum *(arrow)* is relatively short with a well-formed anteriorly displaced infundibular (conal) septum. There is no os infundibulum, but rather diffuse outflow tract narrowing without increased trabeculation or free wall thickening. Ventricular septal defect is conoventricular and perimembranous.

Key: *CS,* Conal septum; *RV,* right ventricle; *TV,* tricuspid valve; *VSD,* ventricular septal defect.

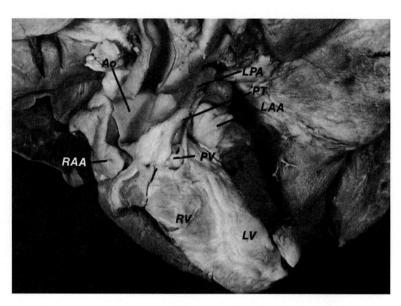

Figure 24-5   Specimen of tetralogy of Fallot with infundibular, valvar, and supravalvar pulmonary stenosis viewed from front. Aorta and pulmonary trunk have been opened. Pulmonary trunk is also diffusely narrowed and continues directly into a left pulmonary artery of satisfactory size without any stenosis at its origin. Right pulmonary artery origin is not visible, passing at right angles directly beneath aorta.

Key: *Ao*, Aorta; *LAA*, left atrial appendage; *LPA*, left pulmonary artery; *LV*, left ventricle; *PT*, pulmonary trunk; *PV*, pulmonary valve; *RAA*, right atrial appendage; *RV*, right ventricle.

■ **TABLE 24-1**   **Pulmonary Valve Morphology in Tetralogy of Fallot** *ᵃ*

Morphology	n	%
Valve Configuration		
Bicuspid	93	66
Three-cusp	21	15
Vestigial	14	10
Not recorded	13	9
TOTAL	141	100
Valve Lesion		
Tethering alone	89	63
Commissural fusion alone	20	14
Tethering + fusion	8	6
Vestigial valve	14	10
Atretic valve (acquired)	2	1
Not recorded	8	6
TOTAL	141	100

ᵃ Based on 141 patients undergoing repair (GLH experience, 1968 to 1978) of tetralogy of Fallot with pulmonary stenosis (excluding patients with subarterial ventricular septal defect, absent pulmonary valve, or congenital pulmonary atresia).

Stenotic valve cusps are usually thickened, frequently severely so, a feature that increases the amount of obstruction at valve level (Fig. 24-6). In approximately 10% of cases, cusps are replaced by sessile nubbins of fibromyxomatous tissue that offer little obstruction. Such vestigial valves are usually associated with a stenotic pulmonary "anulus." When the "anulus" is not narrowed and the valve is vestigial, pulmonary regurgitation results, a condition called *TF with absent pulmonary valve* (see Section 3).

Pulmonary valve stenosis is usually caused by cusp tethering rather than commissural fusion (see Table 24-1). The free edge of tethered cusps is considerably shorter than the diameter of the pulmonary trunk, so that the valve cannot open adequately, and the pulmonary trunk is pulled inward at the point of commissural attachment. This produces a localized narrowing or corseting of the trunk at distal valve level. Thus, both the valve and trunk are tethered (see Fig. 24-6). In this situation the sinuses of

Valsalva are frequently well formed, but entry into them between the cusp edge and pulmonary trunk wall is often also stenotic, resulting in slow filling of the sinuses with contrast medium on cineangiography. Uncommonly, cusps of a tethered valve may be fused for a short distance. Tethering is more common in a bicuspid valve, but can occur in a three-cusp valve.

Less commonly, thickened cusps are associated with congenital commissural fusion, resulting in a concentric or eccentric stenotic orifice. An eccentric orifice can also result from a unicuspid configuration.

A fused stenotic pulmonary valve orifice may be beaded with tiny "vegetations" of fibrin. Progressive deposition of fibrin is presumably the mechanism of *acquired valvar atresia*.

Right Ventricular–Pulmonary Trunk Junction

The RV–pulmonary trunk junction is normally a muscular structure and, like the infundibulum, varies in diameter during the cardiac cycle. In TF, it is almost always smaller in diameter than the aortic "anulus" (the reverse of normal), but may not be obstructive. It is rarely stenotic when infundibular stenosis is low lying. The pulmonary "anulus" may become thick from fibrosis, which is usually an extension of endocardial thickening surrounding an intermediate- or high-level infundibular stenosis; in such cases, it is variably obstructive. It is small and obstructive when there is diffuse infundibular hypoplasia, resulting in diffuse RV outflow hypoplasia.

Pulmonary Trunk

Like the pulmonary valve and "anulus," the pulmonary trunk is nearly always smaller than the aorta. Reduction is most marked when there is diffuse RV outflow hypoplasia. Then, the pulmonary trunk is less than half the aortic diameter and is short (see Fig. 24-6), directed sharply posterior to its bifurcation. It is thus largely hidden from view at operation by the prominent aorta, which also displaces the origin of the trunk leftward and posteriorly.

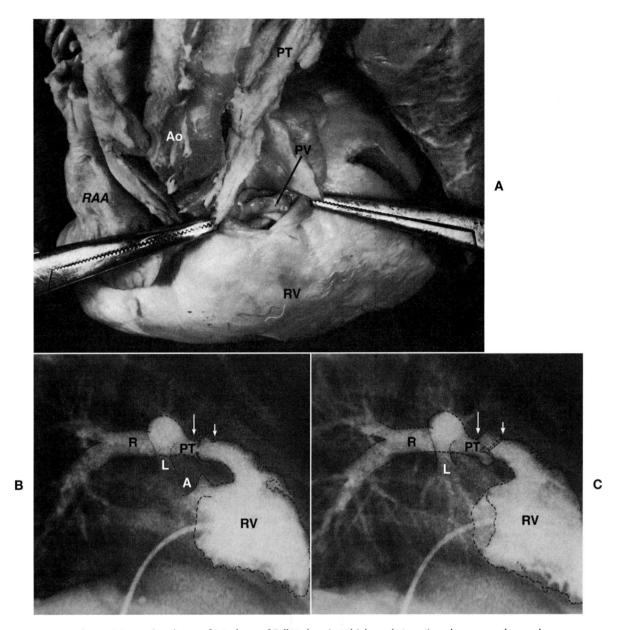

Figure 24-6   Specimen of tetralogy of Fallot showing thickened stenotic pulmonary valve, and right ventricular cineangiograms in the right anterior oblique projection showing same feature. **A**, Specimen showing stenotic pulmonary valve viewed through opened pulmonary trunk. There are two thickened cusps that are not fused, but pulmonary trunk wall is drawn inward where commissures attach (tethering). **B**, Early systolic frame. Pulmonary valve stenosis is due to valve tethering. Cusps are thickened and form a dome in systole from their attachments to pulmonary "anulus" *(small arrow)*. Supravalvar pulmonary trunk narrowing *(large arrow)* is localized to region between pulmonary sinuses and pulmonary trunk. **C**, Diastolic frame. Distal edges of thickened cusps remain approximated to narrowed pulmonary trunk wall, and the prominent sinuses may be slow to fill with contrast. Note shortness of pulmonary trunk. (From Calder and colleagues.[C17])

Key: *A*, Aortic valve; *Ao*, aorta; *L*, left pulmonary artery; *PT*, pulmonary trunk; *PV*, pulmonary valve; *R*, right pulmonary artery; *RAA*, right atrial appendage; *RV*, right ventricle.

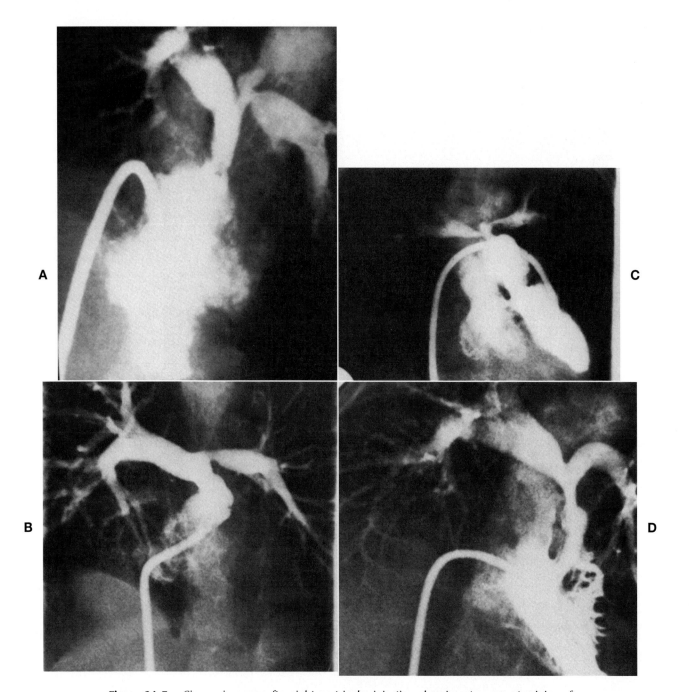

Figure 24-7   Cineangiograms after right ventricular injection showing stenoses at origins of pulmonary arteries in tetralogy of Fallot with pulmonary stenosis. **A**, Stenosis at origin of left pulmonary artery (LPA) in region of ductus arteriosus, which is closed at its aortic end. **B**, Stenosis at origin of LPA. This arrangement is unusual in that the LPA comes off at right angles. **C**, Bifurcation stenosis. Note that, as usual, the right pulmonary artery comes off at right angles to the pulmonary trunk. **D**, Severe narrowing of distal pulmonary trunk. Note that first portion of LPA appears to be a continuation of pulmonary trunk.

When the pulmonary valve is markedly tethered, the pulmonary trunk is also tethered or corseted at its commissural attachments (see Fig. 24-6), and it may be very angulated or kinked at this point. This is the usual mechanism of supravalvar narrowing, and it is not associated with wall thickening. Rarely, however, there may be a discrete supravalvar narrowing beyond commissural level with diffuse wall thickening.

Pulmonary Trunk Bifurcation

The left pulmonary artery (LPA) is usually a direct continuation of the pulmonary trunk, with the right pulmonary artery (RPA) arising almost at right angles and close to it, but this pattern varies (Fig. 24-7). Uncommonly, the distal pulmonary trunk and origin of RPA and LPA are moderately or severely narrowed *(bifurcation stenosis),* and in this situation the bifurcation may have a Y shape.

■ **TABLE 24-2   Abnormalities of Pulmonary Trunk Bifurcation and Right or Left Pulmonary Artery Origin in Tetralogy of Fallot** [a]

PA Branch Lesion	Degree of Narrowing		Total	
	Severe	Moderate	n	% of 365
Congenital				
Left + right origin stenosis [b]	11	8	19	5.2
Left origin stenosis	6	4	10	2.7
Right origin stenosis	0	1	1	0.3
Left origin atretic or absent	0	0	5	1.4
Right origin absent [c]	0	0	1	0.3
Diffuse narrowing left + right or left alone	5	0	5	1.4
Iatrogenic				
Right stenosis or occlusion	3	0	3	0.8
TOTAL	25	13	44	12.1

Key: *PA*, Pulmonary artery.

[a] Based on 365 patients undergoing repair (GLH experience, 1960 to 1978) of tetralogy of Fallot with pulmonary stenosis (including those with juxta-arterial ventricular septal defect and absent pulmonary valve syndrome). Categories are mutually exclusive.

[b] Bifurcation stenosis.

[c] Origin of right pulmonary artery from ascending aorta.

Right and Left Pulmonary Arteries

Anomalies of the RPA and LPA are common in TF with pulmonary atresia (see Section 2) but uncommon in TF with pulmonary stenosis, although any of the anomalies present in pulmonary atresia may occur in patients with pulmonary stenosis (Table 24-2). Fellows and colleagues found pulmonary artery anomalies in 30% of infants having TF with pulmonary stenosis presenting in the first year of life.[F4]

Distal Pulmonary Arteries and Veins

Pulmonary arteries and veins beyond the hilar positions are about normal in size in most patients.[H6,S16] Intraacinar arteries are smaller than in normal individuals, and their media are thinner.[J5] In addition, lung volume, alveolar size, and total alveolar number tend to be reduced.[H6,J5]

Dimensions of Right Ventricular Outflow Tract and Pulmonary Arteries

Morphology, and particularly dimensions, of pathways between the RV and pulmonary arterioles in TF with pulmonary stenosis has been confusing in the past because of failure to realize that, in general, these are quite different from those of TF with pulmonary atresia. This confusion is one reason for considering TF in separate sections in this text.

Hypoplasia, or narrowness, in these pathways in patients having TF with pulmonary stenosis is most marked centrally in the RV infundibulum and pulmonary trunk (Fig. 24-8).[S16] This is true on average and also for minimum Z values, representing the most extreme hypoplasia. (Z value is defined later in this chapter and discussed in detail

under "Dimensions of Normal Cardiac and Great Artery Pathways" in Chapter 1. Nomograms for determining Z values from cineangiographic and echocardiographic measurements are in Appendix 1C of Chapter 1.) On average, the RPA and LPA and their branches are not abnormally small. This does not deny the occasional existence of severe narrowing at the origin of the LPA or RPA (see Fig. 24-7). Elzenga and colleagues found juxtaductal proximal stenoses of the LPA in 10% of patients having TF with pulmonary stenosis[E11]; about 90% are free of these severe findings (see Table 24-2). There is great variability in these dimensions, however, making their careful pre-repair study important.

Convenient Morphologic Categories of Right Ventricular Outflow Obstruction

The nearly infinitely variable spectrum of RV outflow obstruction in TF can be conveniently categorized in a way that is surgically useful because it relates to difficulty in obtaining good relief of the pulmonary stenosis and therefore to surgical techniques and mortality (Box 24-1). Their frequency of occurrence in the GLH experience is given in Table 24-3, and Figures 24-9 and 24-10 illustrate some categories. This supplements earlier discussion of patterns of the infundibular portion of the obstruction. It might be inferred that transanular patching to relieve outflow tract obstruction would be more frequently required in those with "anulus" stenosis or diffuse hypoplasia, but a blanket rule is probably inappropriate.

Iatrogenic Pulmonary Arterial Problems

Functional absence of the central portion of the pulmonary artery is produced by a classic Glenn anastomosis and by an end-to-end Blalock-Taussig (B-T) shunt. A palliative transanular patch may later produce severe stenosis at the origin of the LPA or, less commonly, of the RPA.[F8] Important stenosis or kinking of an RPA or LPA may be produced by an imprecise shunting operation, particularly of the Waterston or Potts type (see "Techniques of Shunting Operations" later in this section). The distal pulmonary artery may then become relatively hypoplastic because of poor pulmonary blood flow ($\dot{Q}p$).

Collateral Pulmonary Arterial Blood Flow

Patients virtually always have increased collateral pulmonary arterial blood flow, primarily from true bronchial arteries. Occasionally (less than 5% of patients), large aortopulmonary (AP) collateral arteries are present (see detailed discussion in "Alternative Sources of Pulmonary Blood Flow" in Section 2).

Ventricular Septal Defect

In classic TF, the VSD is juxta-aortic and usually lies adjacent to or involves the membranous septum (conoventricular and perimembranous). It differs from the usual isolated VSD, however, in that it is associated with malalignment of the conal (infundibular) septum (see Fig. 24-2) and is virtually always large. It is presumed anterior displacement and hypoplasia of the conal septum leaves a

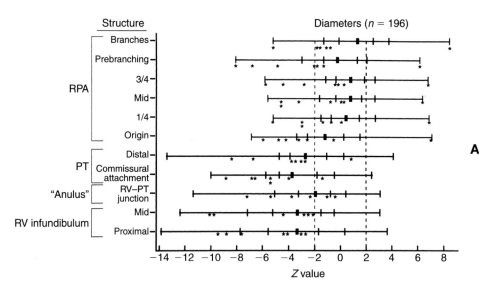

Figure 24-8 Distribution of dimensions (expressed as *Z* values) of right ventricular (RV) and pulmonary arterial pathways in tetralogy of Fallot with pulmonary stenosis. Median values, represented by solid upright rectangles along horizontal lines, are abnormally small (*Z* value less than -2) in RV infundibulum and pulmonary trunk, and minimum *Z* values (represented by most leftward short vertical bar) are also smallest in this part of the pathway. (Vertical bars just left of the median represent the 25th percentile, and next most leftward the 10th percentile. Vertical bars just right of the median represent the 75th percentile, next most rightward the 90th, and most rightward the maximum.) Median *Z* values at all levels in the right and left pulmonary arteries (RPA and LPA) are within normal range (-2 to +2). Asterisks (*) represent *Z* values for each patient (*n* = 7) who had large aortopulmonary collateral arteries. This study indicates the tendency of such patients to have unusually severe pulmonary artery hypoplasia. **A**, Depiction includes RPA. **B**, Depiction includes LPA. (From Shimazaki and colleagues.[S16])

Key: *LPA*, Left pulmonary artery; *PT*, pulmonary trunk; *RPA*, right pulmonary artery; *RV*, right ventricle.

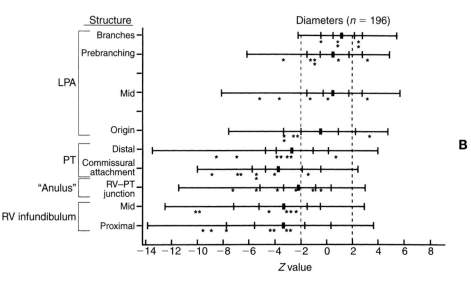

BOX 24-1 Convenient Morphologic Categories of Right Ventricular Outflow Obstruction in Tetralogy of Fallot with Pulmonary Stenosis

The following patterns of right ventricular infundibular obstruction are surgically useful, although they arbitrarily categorize what is in reality a continuous spectrum (see Table 24-3).

■ **Isolated Infundibular Stenosis**
This obstruction is encountered in a minority of cases (26% in the GLH experience). An infundibular chamber is usual when the level of stenosis is intermediate or low, but it may be absent when stenosis is high. When stenosis is at a low level, it is usually transversely oriented but may be in the coronal plane, and the infundibular chamber is usually large. Isolated infundibular stenosis may be at an intermediate level and transversely oriented. In this case the infundibular septum is shorter than in the preceding type, and a moderate-sized or small chamber separates the stenotic zone from the pulmonary valve.

■ **Infundibular Plus Valvar Stenosis**
A combination of infundibular and valvar stenosis occurs in most cases (74% in the GLH experience). In 26% of cases the infundibulum and pulmonary valve are stenotic to a variable degree, but the pulmonary "anulus" is of good size. Low-level infundibular stenosis is less common than in isolated infundibular stenosis, but, again, when present it may be in either a transverse or coronal plane, or both. The pulmonary trunk may be diffusely small or tethered, but bifurcation stenosis is rare.

■ **Infundibular Plus Valvar Plus "Anular" Stenosis**
This combination is present less frequently (16% in the GLH

experience). The os infundibulum lies either close to the valve without an intervening chamber (high infundibular stenosis) or at mid-infundibular level. The infundibular stenosis is rarely at a low level. Diffuse narrowing or tethering of the pulmonary trunk is common.

■ **Diffuse Right Ventricular Outflow Hypoplasia**
This morphologic subset is commonly seen in infants presenting with severe cyanosis. There is rarely (4% in the GLH experience) an additional proximal conal stenosis. The pulmonary valve is usually bicuspid with thickened, tethered, stenotic cusps; the pulmonary "anulus" is small and obstructive; and the pulmonary artery trunk is half or less that of the aorta, often with associated tethering. The more severe the hypoplasia of the infundibulum and pulmonary trunk, the more severe is the narrowing of the first part of the right and left pulmonary arteries (see Fig. 24-9), although the *Z* values of these structures are usually larger than those of the pulmonary trunk (see Fig. 24-10).

■ **Dominant Valvar Stenosis**
This obstruction is rare. The pulmonary "anulus" is frequently also stenotic, and when valve stenosis is produced by cusp tethering, the pulmonary trunk is also tethered. Infundibular stenosis is mild, but the conal (infundibular) septal deviation characteristic of TF is present. Examples of important valvar stenosis and a large VSD without developmental anomalies of TF type in the infundibulum are uncommon (see Section 5).

■ **TABLE 24-3   Morphology and Sites of Right Ventricular Outflow Obstruction in Patients Undergoing Repair of Tetralogy of Fallot** [a]

Morphology of RV Outflow Obstruction	Site of Infundibular Stenosis									
	High		Intermediate		Low		Diffuse		Total	
	No.	%	No.	%	No.	%	No.	%	No.	%
Isolated infundibular	6	3	18 (1)	9	25	13	0	0	49 (1)	26
Infundibular + valvar	9	5	31 (1)	16	9	5	0	0	49 (1)	26
Infundibular + valvar + anular	11	6	20 (1)	11	0	0	0	0	31 (1)	16
Diffuse hypoplasia	0	0	0	0	0	0	52 (17)	27	52 (17)	27
Valvar [b]	0	0	0	0	0	0	0	0	9 (1)	5
TOTAL	26	14	69 (3)	36	34	18	52 (17)	27	190 (21)	100

Key: *RV*, Right ventricular.

[a] Based on 190 patients undergoing repair (GLH experience, 1968 to 1978) of tetralogy of Fallot with pulmonary stenosis, excluding cases with juxta-arterial ventricular septal defect, absent pulmonary valve, or congenital pulmonary atresia. Figures in parentheses indicate number of patients who had diffuse pulmonary arterial narrowing, pulmonary artery branch origin stenosis or bifurcation stenosis of pulmonary trunk, or absence of central portion of right or left pulmonary artery (11% of the total). Percentages indicate percentage of the total group of 190. "High" refers to superior-level stenoses and "low" to inferior-level stenoses.

[b] With or without "anular" stenosis.

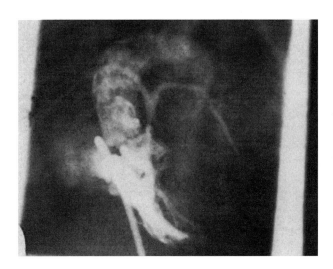

Figure 24-9   Cineangiogram following right ventricular (RV) injection in infant with tetralogy of Fallot with and pulmonary stenosis without major associated cardiac anomalies. The striking feature is diffuse hypoplasia of right and left pulmonary arteries. Pulmonary trunk, pulmonary "anulus," and RV infundibulum are also very narrow.

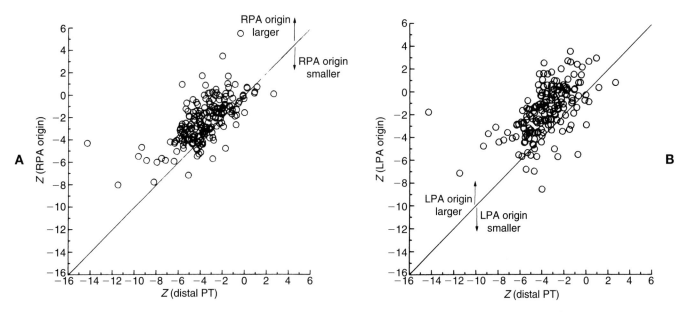

Figure 24-10   Scattergrams illustrating relationship between diameters (expressed as *Z* value) of the origins of right (**A**) and left (**B**) pulmonary arteries and diameter of distal pulmonary trunk. (From Shimazaki and colleagues.[S16])

Key: *LPA*, Left pulmonary artery; *PT*, pulmonary trunk; *RPA*, right pulmonary artery.

Figure 24-11   Specimen of tetralogy of Fallot demonstrating ventricular septal defect (VSD) and position of bundle of His. A narrow muscular bridge separates VSD from anterior tricuspid leaflet and tricuspid anulus. Right ventricle (RV) has been opened and the incision carried across conal septum and right coronary cusp out into the ascending aorta, as shown in Fig. 24-1. Narrow muscular bridge separating VSD from tricuspid valve is the continuity between right posterior division of septal band (trabecula septomarginalis) and ventriculoinfundibular fold. Ventriculoinfundibular fold joins the undersurface of the parietal end of infundibular (conal) septum. Sutures can be passed safely into this ridge along dashed line (or, alternatively, in base of tricuspid leaflet), but the margin for error is small because the course of the bundle of His (*dotted line*) is not far removed. Note marked RV overriding of right aortic cusp.

Key: *CS,* Conal (infundibular) septum; *NC,* noncoronary cusp; *RC,* right coronary cusp; *RP,* right posterior division of septal band (trabecula septomarginalis); *T,* tricuspid anterior leaflet; *VI,* ventriculoinfundibular fold.

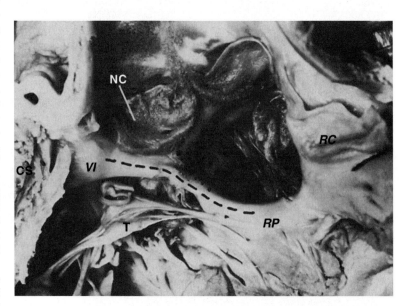

defect (VSD) at the junction of the base of the ventricular septum with the aorta.

The "junctional" defect is more U shaped than circular and is bounded superiorly and anteriorly by the conal (infundibular) septum (see Fig. 24-4). The septum may support part or most of the right aortic cusp, depending on the degree of aorta overriding the RV (see Fig. 24-1). Because of the anterior and leftward deviation of the parietal end (parietal extension) of the conal septum, the *posterosuperior* angle of the defect extends higher than that of the usual, isolated conoventricular VSD (see Fig. 24-2, *A*) and can be more difficult to expose surgically, particularly if the parietal band is not fully mobilized (transected). When the conal septum is hypoplastic, the defect is larger and extends closer to the pulmonary valve; when the conal septum is absent, the VSD becomes juxta-pulmonary (and juxta-arterial).

Posterosuperiorly, the VSD is bounded by muscle (the ventriculoinfundibular fold) adjacent to the rightward edge of the noncoronary aortic cusp (Fig. 24-11). This cusp may override considerably onto the RV (Fig. 24-12); then, the aortic "anulus" (LV–aortic junction) adjacent to the noncoronary cusp forms this boundary.

The *posterior* margin is variable. It is related to the base of the tricuspid anteroseptal leaflet commissure and to the right fibrous trigone (central fibrous body) at the nadir of the noncoronary aortic cusp. In most instances, there is tricuspid–aortic–mitral fibrous continuity at this margin, and the membranous septum is absent—characteristics of a true perimembranous VSD. In some hearts the VSD extends inferiorly beneath the tricuspid septal leaflet more than usual. When there is marked clockwise rotation of the overriding aortic root, the right trigone may form the posteroinferior angle of the defect, and the bundle of His (which perforates at this point) is exposed along the edge of the defect (Fig. 24-13). Occasionally the posterior margin may be formed by a remnant of fibrous tissue (membranous septum) projecting upward from the right trigone region.

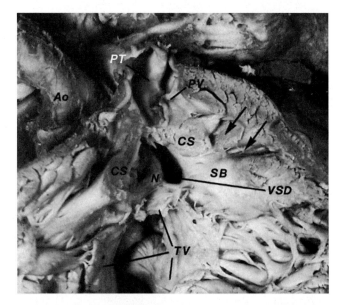

Figure 24-12   Specimen of tetralogy of Fallot with right ventricle and pulmonary trunk opened with an anterior incision and conal septum divided to expose ventricular septal defect. Accessory prominent muscular trabeculations are present in front of septal attachment of conal septum (*arrows*), contributing to stenosis. Pulmonary valve is bicuspid and tethered, with mild cusp thickening. Marked overriding of aorta is visible, involving rightward margin of noncoronary cusp.

Key: *Ao,* Aorta; *CS,* conal septum; *N,* noncoronary cusp; *PT,* pulmonary trunk; *PV,* pulmonary valve; *SB,* septal band; *TV,* tricuspid valve; *VSD,* ventricular septal defect.

This tissue, also called the *membranous flap,* does not contain conduction tissue, and theoretically it can receive some of the sutures used to secure the VSD patch.[K43] Suzuki and colleagues found such a flap in about half of 158 TF hearts.[S29] Kurosawa and Imai[K40] found at least a

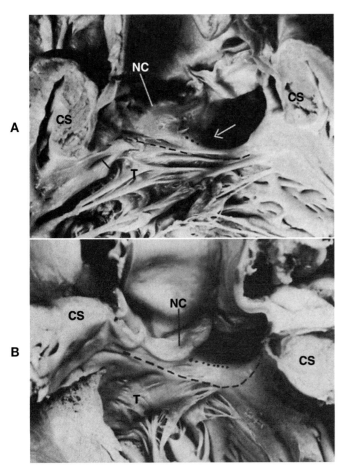

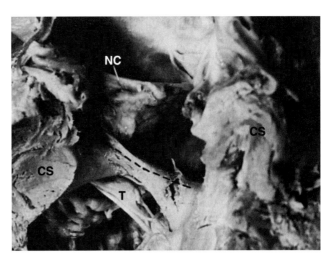

Figure 24-14 In this heart with tetralogy of Fallot the posterior muscular bridge is bulky and entirely hides the right trigone that lies several millimeters caudal and leftward of the margin of the ventricular septal defect. The His bundle will not be damaged by sutures passed into the ridge along dashed line.

Key: *CS,* Conal septum; *NC,* noncoronary cusp; *T,* tricuspid valve.

Figure 24-13 Two specimens of tetralogy of Fallot with perimembranous ventricular septal defect (VSD), opened as in Fig. 24-11. There is tricuspid–aortic–mitral fibrous continuity at the posterior margin (leftward in the photograph) of the VSD. **A,** Right fibrous trigone at nadir of noncoronary aortic cusp has been perforated by a pin passed from right atrial side at point of penetration of bundle of His; bundle extends from this point forward and slightly leftward along margin of VSD *(dotted line)*. White arrow points to this area. VSD patch suture line must pass into base of septal tricuspid leaflet *(dashed line)* and not along lower VSD margin. **B,** Position of right fibrous trigone when there is important clockwise rotation of aortic root and right ventricular overriding of noncoronary and right aortic cusps. Bundle position is shown by dotted line and position of VSD suture line (passing into base of anterior tricuspid leaflet) by dashed line.

Key: *CS,* Conal septum; *NC,* noncoronary cusp; *T,* tricuspid valve.

remnant in all 68 of their surgical cases. In at least 20% of hearts, the posterior margin is formed by a muscular ridge of variable size that separates the right trigone from the base of the anterior tricuspid leaflet.[A16,B13,R9,S9] This ridge is formed by the right posterior division of the septal band as it becomes continuous with the ventriculoinfundibular fold (Fig. 24-14; see also Fig. 24-11). It displaces the right trigone and therefore the bundle of His away from the defect edge.

The *inferior* margin of the VSD is formed by the septal band as it cradles the VSD between its limbs. The papillary

muscle of the conus (or corresponding chordae only) arises from the right posterior division of the septal band at the *anteroinferior* angle of the defect. Anomalous tricuspid chordal attachments to other margins of the defect are rare, in contrast to the situation in isolated perimembranous VSD.

The *anterior* margin of the VSD is formed by the leftward anterior division of the septal band as it becomes continuous with the inferior margin of the conal septum. When the septal band is poorly developed, the defect extends further anteriorly.

When the infundibular (conal) septum is absent, the VSD is juxta-arterial.[N4] Posteriorly, this type of VSD is commonly separated from the tricuspid anulus by a 2- to 5-mm strip of muscle, but it may extend to the anulus. Aortic and pulmonary valve "anuli" are contiguous over about one third of their circumferences, being separated at this point by only a thin fibrous ridge (see Fig. 24-3). The two valves are often side by side, with the aorta more than usually dextroposed.[S9] TF with this type of VSD is morphologically similar to double outlet RV with a doubly committed (juxta-arterial) VSD (see Chapter 39).

In 3% to 15% of patients (Table 24-4), one or more additional VSDs coexist with the typical juxta-aortic one (Fig. 24-15).[F4] Usually the additional VSD is muscular, and multiple muscular defects sometimes occur. It may also be in the inlet septum, either as an inlet septal VSD or a muscular defect (see "Inlet Septal Ventricular Septal Defect" under Morphology in Section 1 of Chapter 21).

Conduction System

The *sinus and AV nodes* are in their normal locations (see "Conduction System" in Chapter 1), and the bundle of His follows the same general course as in patients with isolated perimembranous and juxta-tricuspid VSDs (see "Location in Septum and Relationship to Conduction System" under

■ TABLE 24-4   Major Associated Cardiac Anomalies in Patients Undergoing Repair of Tetralogy of Fallot [a]

Anomaly	UAB, 1967 to 1982 (n = 713)		GLH, 1968 to 1978 (n = 205)		Total (n = 918)	
	n	%	n	%	n	%
Multiple VSDs	20	2.8	2	1.0	22	2.4
Complete atrioventricular septal defect	20	2.8	0	0	20	2.2
Patent ductus arteriosus	29	4.1	8	3.9	37	4.0
Anomalous origin of LCA from PA	1	0.1	0	0	1	0.1
AP window	2	0.3	0	0	2	0.2
Subaortic stenosis	3	0.4	1	0.5	4	0.4
Moderate or severe aortic regurgitation	0	0	1	0.5	1	0.1
PAPVC	7	1.0	2	1.0	9	1.0
TAPVC	1	0.1	0	0	1	0.1
Unroofed coronary sinus	2	0.3	4	2.0	6	0.6
Straddling tricuspid valve	3	0.4	0	0	3	0.3
Small tricuspid valve anulus	2	0.3	0	0	2	0.2
Severe tricuspid regurgitation	2	0.3	1	0.5	3	0.3
Mitral stenosis	1	0.1	0	0	1	0.1
Dextrocardia	6	0.8	3	1.5	9	1.0
Situs ambiguous	2	0.3	0	0	2	0.2
Situs inversus totalis	2	0.3	3	1.5	5	0.5
Ebstein malformation	1	0.1	0	0	1	0.1
Underdeveloped RV	–	NT	3	1.5	3	0.3
RPA origin from ascending aorta	0	0	1	0.5	1	0.1
Pulmonary vascular disease	0	0	2	1.0	2	0.2
Endocarditis, RV outflow	0	0	2	1.0	3	0.2
TOTAL PATIENTS	87	12.2	26	13	113	12.3

Key: *AP*, Aortopulmonary; *LCA*, left coronary artery; *NT*, not tabulated; *PA*, pulmonary artery; *PAPVC*, partial anomalous pulmonary venous connection; *RV*, right ventricle; *RPA*, right pulmonary artery; *TAPVC*, total anomalous pulmonary venous connection; *VSD*, ventricular septal defect.

[a] Categories are not mutually exclusive.

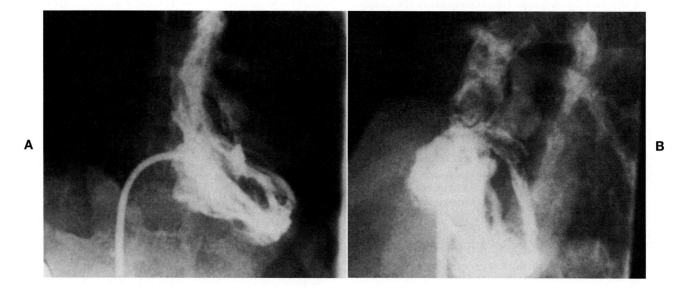

Figure 24-15   Cineangiograms of tetralogy of Fallot, pulmonary stenosis, and multiple ventricular septal defects (VSD). Note large trabecular VSD near apex as well as usual conoventricular VSD. **A,** Systolic frame. **B,** Diastolic frame.

Morphology in Section 1 of Chapter 21). Thus, the His bundle emerges through the right fibrous trigone at the base of the noncoronary cusp of the aortic valve and courses forward toward the papillary muscle of the conus along the inferior VSD margin or slightly to the left side of the defect edge.[F12,L12] In hearts showing marked clockwise rotation of the aortic root with RV overriding, the right trigone (and along with it the penetrating portion of the His bundle) is carried more rightward and superiorly and directly onto VSD margins (see Fig. 24-13).

By contrast, the bundle of His does not lie on the VSD margin when a muscle ridge is present (see Figs. 24-11 and

24-14),[D11] because the ridge projects superiorly above the right fibrous trigone; when the ridge is bulky, sutures can be safely placed into it.[B12]

Aorta

The aorta is biventricular in origin and more anteriorly placed than normal, often almost obscuring the smaller pulmonary trunk from view at operation. These changes are due to RV overriding, rotation, and enlargement of the aortic root. The proportion of aorta lying above the RV varies between 30% and 90%.[A13] Generally, about 50% of the aortic orifice is over the RV.

Aortic overriding is associated with a variable degree of clockwise rotation of the aortic root (as viewed from below). This rotation moves the base of the noncoronary cusp rightward and superiorly onto the posterosuperior margin of the VSD and away from the base of the anterior mitral leaflet so that in extreme cases, it may no longer be continuous with this structure. This cusp may then lie in part just beneath the extension of the infundibular (conal) septum. Rightward rotation of the left aortic cusp results in more of it becoming continuous with the anterior mitral leaflet. Simultaneously, the superiorly positioned right cusp moves to the left, and in extreme examples it may be just beneath the uppermost extension of the left anterior division of the trabecula septomarginalis at the anterosuperior VSD margin.

Degree of overriding and clockwise rotation of the aortic root relates to degree of underdevelopment of the RV outflow tract and to deviation (malalignment) of the infundibular septum. When these are minimal, as seen with isolated low-lying infundibular stenosis, the aorta is minimally affected; when there is diffuse RV outflow tract hypoplasia in association with a small, markedly deviated infundibular septum and posterior and leftward movement of the pulmonary trunk origin, the aorta is markedly rotated and dextroposed. Degree of overriding or dextroposition may be so extreme that it may be called double outlet RV with pulmonary stenosis, rather than TF. The overriding is well assessed cineangiographically in both left anterior oblique and right anterior oblique views (Fig. 24-16).

In patients with severe TF, the aortic root is larger than normal, even in infants. Occasionally in adults, it is greatly dilated. This may result in aortic valve regurgitation.

Aortic Arch and Ductus Arteriosus

The *ductus arteriosus* (or ligamentum arteriosum) is absent in about 30% of patients with TF (GLH experience autopsy series of 120 cases). Absence of ductus or ligamentum is about twice as common when there is a right rather than left aortic arch. Patent ductus arteriosus is more common in TF with pulmonary atresia than with pulmonary stenosis. Ductus closure and ductal tissue involution may contribute to bifurcation abnormalities and origin stenosis of the LPA often seen in TF.

A *left aortic arch* is present in about 75% of patients. In these, arch branching pattern is usually normal (Fig. 24-17). If a patent ductus arteriosus is present, its orientation and position on the left side are normal and flow in utero is from pulmonary artery through ductus arteriosus to aorta. The ductus may give origin to the LPA (Fig. 24-18).

A *right aortic arch* is present in about 25% of patients having TF with pulmonary stenosis. In 90% of them, there is mirror-image branching of the arch. Should a patent ductus arteriosus be present, it usually arises from the innominate or proximal left subclavian artery and joins the LPA.[S14] Rarely, there may be a right-sided ductus arteriosus to the RPA, usually arising from the upper descending thoracic aorta. In about 10% of instances, there is an aberrant left subclavian artery, analogous to the aberrant right subclavian artery of dysphagia lusoria in left aortic arch (see "Right Aortic Arch with Aberrant Left Subclavian Artery" in Section 1 of Chapter 37). In right aortic arch with aberrant left subclavian artery, the subclavian artery may arise directly from the descending aorta or from an aortic diverticulum. Thus, a ductus arteriosus may arise from the aortic diverticulum and pass to the left behind the esophagus to join the LPA.

Rarely, the left subclavian artery is sequestered or isolated from its aortic arch origin, but remains connected to the LPA by a patent ductus arteriosus (see Fig. 24-17). Often in these circumstances, there is vertebral steal, and on angiography the subclavian artery fills with contrast from the vertebral artery.

Right Ventricle

External dimensions of the sinus (inflow) portion of the RV are larger than normal due to hypertrophy, so that the interventricular groove is displaced leftward and the LV lies more posteriorly than usual (clockwise rotation of ventricles). The RV sinus may be clearly separated from the infundibulum during systole by a transverse depression that represents the site of maximal infundibular stenosis inferior to an infundibular chamber. RV wall thickness equals that of the LV and is therefore never excessive unless the large VSD is made restrictive by a fibrous flap valve on its right side (see Section 4). Normal trabeculations are, however, bulky and prominent. RV end-diastolic volume may be reduced and ejection fraction mildly depressed,[G1] possibly the result of chronic hypoxia. Rarely (1.5% of cases), the sinus portion of the RV and tricuspid valve are underdeveloped (see Table 24-4).

Left Ventricle

The LV is usually normal in wall thickness[M3] but variable in volume. In patients with severe forms of TF with severe cyanosis, LV end-diastolic volume is normal or somewhat small,[J1,L1,L2,M3,N1] but wall thickness remains normal. Uncommonly, the LV and mitral valve are truly hypoplastic,[G7] and rarely this may be so severe (end-diastolic volume less than $30 \text{ mL} \cdot \text{m}^{-2}$) as to contraindicate primary repair.[G7,N13]

The physiologic contributors to LV size are complex. The small pulmonary and thus left atrial blood flow tend to result in a small left atrium[M3,N1] and LV. However, the RV ejects blood into the LV as well as the aorta,[M3] and this tends to increase LV size. Mild or moderate degrees of LV hypoplasia may result from these physiologic factors, but true hypoplasia is of morphologic rather than functional origin.

LV systolic function as estimated by ejection fraction is also mildly reduced, particularly in severely cyanotic patients,[G8,J1,M3] presumably because of chronic hypoxia.

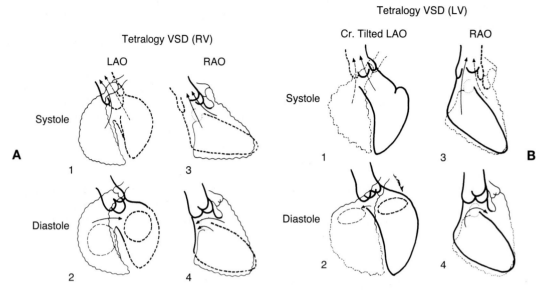

Figure 24-16 Diagrammatic cineangiocardiographic assessment of intracardiac anatomy in tetralogy of Fallot. Right ventricle *(RV)* and pulmonary trunk are indicated by thin line, left ventricle *(LV)* and aorta by thick line. Continuous line is for structures primarily demonstrated; interrupted line is for those faintly or variably demonstrated. **A,** RV injection in steep (75° to 80°) left anterior oblique *(LAO)* *(1, 2)* and 30° to 40° right anterior oblique *(RAO)* projections *(3, 4)* in systole *(1, 3)* and diastole *(2, 4).* In steep LAO projection, VSD is profiled beneath right coronary sinus at aortic root, adjacent to upper margin of tricuspid valve seen in diastole. Any inferior extension of VSD into basal sinus septum between the AV valves is accurately shown. In systole, contrast medium from RV streams up into aortic root with relatively non-opaque blood from LV. In diastole, contrast medium mixes in LV, showing left side of basal septum. This projection shows little aortic valve overriding in the region of the noncoronary sinus and adjacent commissure with the right coronary sinus. The RV infundibulum, pulmonary valve, and proximal pulmonary trunk are usually superimposed on the aortic root, but distal pulmonary trunk and proximal left pulmonary artery are well seen (although not illustrated in these diagrams).

In RAO projection, conal septum is well profiled and anatomy of RV infundibulum, pulmonary valve, pulmonary trunk, and proximal right pulmonary artery (not diagramed) are well displayed. Contrast medium streaming into anterior part of aorta through VSD delineates its margin in relationship to tricuspid anulus. Contrast medium passing beneath conal septum enters aortic root directly, because this part overrides. Degree of overriding of aorta in region of right coronary sinus relates to degree of conal septal displacement into RV from its proper connection to superior margin of LV. Degree of this displacement and extent of override, however, are not shown, because LV margin is obscured by RV contrast. In diastole, aortic valve closes and contrast medium passing beneath conal septum and through VSD into LV outlines the atrioventricular septum, usually projected behind the tricuspid valve anulus, confirming LV origin of posterior part of noncoronary sinus. **B,** LV injection is 50° to 60° LAO projection with 30° to 40° cranial tilting *(1, 2)* and 30° to 40° RAO *(3, 4)* projection. In cranially tilted LAO projection, the VSD is again profiled beneath right coronary aortic sinus, although it often looks smaller than in LAO projection. Aortic override can be assessed in relation to noncoronary sinus (not diagrammed) as in LAO projection. Extent of VSD inferiorly is less well seen and tricuspid orifice is foreshortened. Middle and apical parts of sinus septum are better separated than in LAO projection, and additional sinus septal defects are therefore more accurately excluded.

In RAO projection, contrast medium outlines atrioventricular septum and superior LV margin and streams into noncoronary and left coronary portions of aortic root. Initially, the anterior right coronary sinus portion of the aortic root may not outline owing to non-opaque RV streaming. In diastole, however, contrast medium passing through the VSD shows the right coronary aortic cusp and conal septum in RV. Degree of displacement of conal septum from superior LV margin at edge of VSD is accurately shown, indicating extent of anterior aortic override at midportion of right coronary sinus. Additional high anterior muscular VSDs, if present, are profiled in RAO projection.

Key: *Cr.,* Cranial; *LAO,* left anterior oblique; *LV,* left ventricle; *RAO,* right anterior oblique; *RV,* right ventricle; *VSD,* ventricular septal defect.

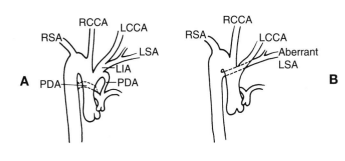

Right aortic arch

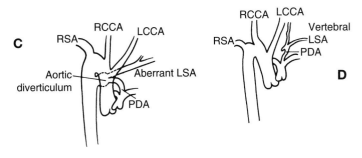

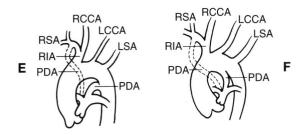

Left aortic arch

Figure 24-17 Aortic branching pattern and ductus origin in tetralogy of Fallot (TF). A *right aortic arch* is present in about 25% of hearts with pulmonary stenosis and 30% with pulmonary atresia. A patent ductus arteriosus is uncommon when there is pulmonary stenosis and common when there is pulmonary atresia. **A,** Usual branching pattern in TF with right aortic arch, present in almost 90% of cases, is the mirror image of normal. The first branch is the left innominate, second the right common carotid, and last the right subclavian artery. A left ductus, when present, arises from the innominate artery. Rarely, there may be a right ductus to the right pulmonary artery, usually from the upper descending aorta *(dashed lines)*. **B,** Less commonly (about 10% of hearts with TF and right aortic arch), there is an aberrant left subclavian artery. A ductus, if present, may arise near the origin of the left common carotid artery or from the aberrant left subclavian artery. **C,** Rarely (about 2% of hearts with TF and right aortic arch), an aberrant left subclavian artery may arise from an aortic diverticulum, which also gives origin to a left ductus arteriosus. The ductus then passes behind the esophagus. (This is the usual pattern in situs solitus with right aortic arch without TF.) **D,** Least often (in TF and right aortic arch), there is an isolated (sequestered) left subclavian artery. This vessel fills by retrograde flow in the vertebral artery and is connected to the left pulmonary artery (LPA) by a ductus arteriosus that may or may not be patent. **E,** When a left aortic arch is present in TF with pulmonary stenosis, the arch branching pattern is usually normal, and if a patent ductus is present, its orientation and position are the normal ones. A right patent ductus is rare and would come off either the right subclavian or innominate artery *(dashed lines)*; if arising in conjunction with an aberrant right subclavian via an aortic diverticulum (not shown in diagram), it passes behind the esophagus. **F,** When a left aortic arch is present in TF with pulmonary atresia, the frequently left patent ductus is long and has a downward orientation from the undersurface of the aortic arch, indicating flow in utero from aorta to LPA. A right ductus may also be present as in (**E**), and rarely, both left and right ductus may be patent.

Key: *LCCA*, Left common carotid artery; *LIA*, left innominate artery; *LSA*, left subclavian artery; *PDA*, patent ductus arteriosus; *RCCA*, right common carotid artery; *RIA*, right innominate artery; *RSA*, right subclavian artery.

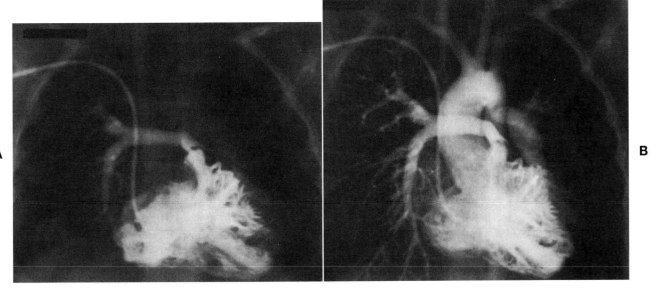

Figure 24-18 Cineangiogram of tetralogy of Fallot and absence of central portion of left pulmonary artery (LPA). **A,** Right ventricular injection shows lack of connection between pulmonary trunk and LPA. **B,** Later phase shows that hilar portion of LPA originates from ductus arteriosus.

Coronary Arteries

As in other cyanotic conditions, the coronary arteries become dilated and tortuous in children and adults. A large conal branch of the right coronary artery (RCA) usually courses obliquely across the free wall of the RV. A vertical or transverse ventriculotomy can usually be made downstream from this.

The left anterior descending coronary artery (LAD) arises anomalously from the RCA in about 5% of patients (Table 24-5).[D5,F4,F5] The entire LAD may originate from the RCA and cross the anterior wall of the infundibulum a variable distance from the pulmonary valve, or only the distal part of the LAD may arise anomalously, in this case usually from the large conal branch of the RCA.

Rarely, the RCA originates from the left coronary artery, and equally uncommonly, there is anomalous origin of the left coronary artery from the pulmonary artery (see Section 2 of Chapter 32).[A10]

Major Associated Cardiac Anomalies

Major associated cardiac anomalies are relatively uncommon (see Table 24-4). *Patent ductus arteriosus, multiple VSDs,* and *complete AV septal defect*[Z1] are most often seen.

Rarely, the RPA[K15] or LPA[M6] arises anomalously from the ascending aorta[K7] (see Chapter 31). This complicates the pathophysiology and repair, because the lung supplied by the pulmonary artery arising from the aorta usually has overcirculation, and the other usually has restricted of flow due to the intracardiac anatomy of TF.

Infrequently, *aortic valve regurgitation* coexists. This may be from typical cusp prolapse in TF with subarterial VSD (see Section 2 in Chapter 21).[M8] A bicuspid aortic valve occurs rarely in TF and may result in aortic regurgitation.[G10,V1] Occasionally, ill patients with TF in the second decade of life or older develop aortic regurgitation from endocarditis.[B11,C12] Massive dilatation of the aortic root from anuloaortic ectasia may result in aortic valve regurgitation,[C12] particularly in patients with large natural or surgically created systemic–pulmonary arterial shunts (see "Anastomotic" under Morphology in Chapter 53).

Minor Associated Cardiac Anomalies

Most infants undergoing repair of TF have a patent foramen ovale; when all ages are considered, a true atrial septal defect is found at operation in about 10%. Other minor associated cardiac anomalies are listed in Table 24-5.

CLINICAL FEATURES AND DIAGNOSTIC CRITERIA

Clinical Presentation

The usual clinical presentation is with cyanosis, which varies with severity of the pulmonary stenosis. Infants with diffuse RV outflow hypoplasia, severe infundibular plus valvar plus anular stenosis, or severe infundibular plus valvar stenosis (see Box 24-1) are deeply cyanotic from birth and do not develop heart failure. They are breathless on feeding or other exertion. Hypoxic spells are rare, the cyanosis being constant and gradually worsening. It is seldom lessened by propranolol.

This situation contrasts with that in infants having dominant infundibular stenosis, where onset of cyanosis is delayed and hypoxic (cyanotic) spells due to infundibular spasm may occur. These spells are often prevented or lessened in frequency by propranolol. Characteristically, they become less frequent with age, presumably because stenosis becomes fixed as a result of acquired endocardial fibrosis and thickening.

In up to 10% of patients who require surgical relief in infancy, presentation is initially as a large VSD with pulmonary plethora and sometimes heart failure at age 2 to 3 months, followed by gradually increasing cyanosis, frequently with cyanotic spells, at about age 6 months. In this group, stenosis is purely infundibular.

A minority of patients are acyanotic at rest and only mildly cyanotic during exercise because pulmonary stenosis is mild and right-to-left shunting minimal. In some the shunt is predominantly left to right. These individuals may remain acyanotic without spells and present at any age within the first or second decades of life with gradually increasing cyanosis and breathlessness as stenosis slowly increases in severity.

In patients with severe cyanosis and polycythemia, cerebral thrombosis may precipitate hemiplegia at any age (particularly in association with dehydration), or hemiplegia may follow paradoxical embolism or a brain abscess. The latter is heralded by fever, headache, and sometimes seizures. Massive hemoptysis may occur in older patients who are severely cyanotic, presumably from rupture of bronchial collateral vessels.

Cyanosis is always accompanied by effort dyspnea that is sometimes the dominant symptom, and as the child begins to walk (frequently much later than for a healthy child), cyanosis is often accompanied by squatting, which lessens its severity.[K16] There may be increased occurrence of respiratory infection, but not to the same extent as in patients with large isolated VSD. Failure to thrive is also less striking than in patients with large isolated VSD.

■ TABLE 24–5   **Minor Associated Cardiac Anomalies in Patients Undergoing Repair of Tetralogy of Fallot with Pulmonary Stenosis or Atresia (n = 836)** [a]

Anomaly	n	% of 836
Atrial septal defect	75	9
Persistent left superior vena cava	68	8
Anomalous origin of LAD from RCA	34	4
Aberrant origin of right subclavian artery	2	0.3
Absent right superior vena cava	1	0.2
Azygos extension of inferior vena cava	1	0.2
Congenital heart block	1	0.2
Juxtaposition of atrial appendages	1	0.2
Vascular ring	1	0.2

Key: *LAD,* Left anterior descending coronary artery; *RCA,* right coronary artery.

[a] UAB experience (1967 to July 1982).

Physical Examination

Cyanosis of variable degree is generally evident. Deeply cyanotic infants are often obese (in contrast to infants with isolated VSD). Severe symmetric clubbing of the fingers and toes is often present in children and adults, but not in infants. Older patients may also have marked acne of the face and anterior chest. Jugular venous pressure is normal, and pulse is of low volume with low blood pressure (relative hypotension may persist into the early postoperative period). The heart is not enlarged and is relatively quiet with an unimpressive RV lift. In those few patients with increased $\dot{Q}p$, the lift may be more marked than usual.

A precordial systolic thrill is rare. There is a moderate-intensity midsystolic pulmonary (ejection) murmur maximal in the second and third left intercostal spaces that becomes less prominent or even disappears when the stenosis is severe. When there is still a reasonable blood flow in the presence of moderate pulmonary stenoses, the systolic murmur is well heard posteriorly and in the axilla. In the presence of important cyanosis and low $\dot{Q}p$, the second heart sound is single, but in acyanotic patients it may be finely split with a low-intensity pulmonary component. Splitting is also present in moderately cyanotic patients with only a mildly reduced $\dot{Q}p$ when there are important pulmonary artery origin stenoses.

Signs of heart failure with venous pressure elevation and liver enlargement occur in patients with too large a systemic–pulmonary arterial shunt (usually Waterston or Potts). Heart failure may also appear in untreated severely cyanotic adults in the fourth or fifth decade of life, presumably secondary to myocardial fibrosis or in association with systemic hypertension or aortic regurgitation.

Laboratory Studies

Neonates or young infants who have severe TF with pulmonary stenosis usually present with marked reduction of arterial oxygen pressure (PaO_2) and saturation (SaO_2) and sometimes with metabolic acidosis. Polycythemia is rarely present, and, in fact, such infants are often anemic.

In older infants and children, red blood cell count and hematocrit are usually elevated, and degree of elevation is correlated with degree of arterial desaturation and thus with severity of the pulmonary stenosis. In older patients, hematocrit may reach 90%.

Most cyanotic patients have depressed platelet count and prolongation of most coagulation tests.

Chest Radiography

Chest radiographs in children usually show the typical boot-shaped heart of TF. In neonates and young infants the heart may be strikingly small, with an absent pulmonary artery segment along the left upper cardiac border and oligemic lung fields. In older patients, there may be a prominence of the left upper cardiac border caused by a large infundibular chamber. Large AP collaterals may alter the pulmonary blood flow pattern in one or both lungs. Plethora of one lung and oligemia of the other suggest anomalous origin of one pulmonary artery from the ascending aorta (see Chapter 31).

If there is a right aortic arch, posterior indentation of the shadow of the barium-filled esophagus results from an aberrant left or right subclavian artery.

Rib notching of the upper ipsilateral ribs may develop in the presence of a long-standing B-T shunt, secondary to development of a rich collateral blood flow to the arm. Rarely, collaterals from the pleura to the lung may be sufficiently large, especially after poudrage or pleural stripping procedures, to result in bilateral rib notching in the lower half of the thorax. Patients in the second or third decade of life may show progressive kyphoscoliosis.

Electrocardiography

Electrocardiography (ECG) shows moderate RV hypertrophy consistent with RV pressure that is equal to but not greater than systematic pressure (in contrast to flap valve VSD; see Section 4). Occasionally, there is minimal RV hypertrophy, and in these circumstances RV underdevelopment should be suspected, although it may not be present. Left precordial leads are characterized by absent Q waves and low-voltage R waves. Occasionally the frontal plane vectorcardiographic pattern characteristic of AV septal defect is found in patients with typical TF.

Echocardiography

The VSD, aortic overriding, and narrowing of the RV infundibulum can usually be seen with echocardiography (Fig. 24-19). Also, in experienced hands, two-dimensional echocardiography with Doppler color-flow interrogation has the same sensitivity and specificity for multiple VSDs in TF as does cineangiography. Morphologic details of the pulmonary trunk and central portions of the LPA may not be reliably visualized. However, because cardiac catheterization and cineangiography impose risks, particularly in patients with recent onset of hypoxic spells, echocardiography is considered the definitive diagnostic procedure in many small patients.

Cardiac Catheterization and Angiography

Preoperative cardiac catheterization and angiography, although not routinely required when expertly interpreted echocardiography is available, precisely portray the hemodynamic state and morphology. Peak pressure in the RV cavity (PRV) is similar to that in the left (PLV), and pulmonary artery pressure (PPA) is below normal. A systolic pressure gradient can often be demonstrated at infundibular and valvar levels when both zones are stenotic, but rarely at a more peripheral site, even when severe stenosis is present. When proximal stenoses are severe, however, it may be impossible to enter the pulmonary trunk with a catheter.

There is right-to-left shunting at ventricular level and low $\dot{Q}p$, the severity of which reflect severity of stenosis. In acyanotic patients, there is minimal right-to-left shunting at rest or even a slight increase in $\dot{Q}p$, but in most patients, right-to-left shunting occurs on exercise. In severely cyanotic patients, PPA and resistance (Rp) are not elevated preoperatively, even in the presence of important peripheral pulmonary artery stenosis or thrombosis, because of low $\dot{Q}p$. PPA may be elevated when there is a large $\dot{Q}p$ and an increase in Rp.

Biplane cineangiography demonstrates all the morphologic features of the malformation, as well as morphology

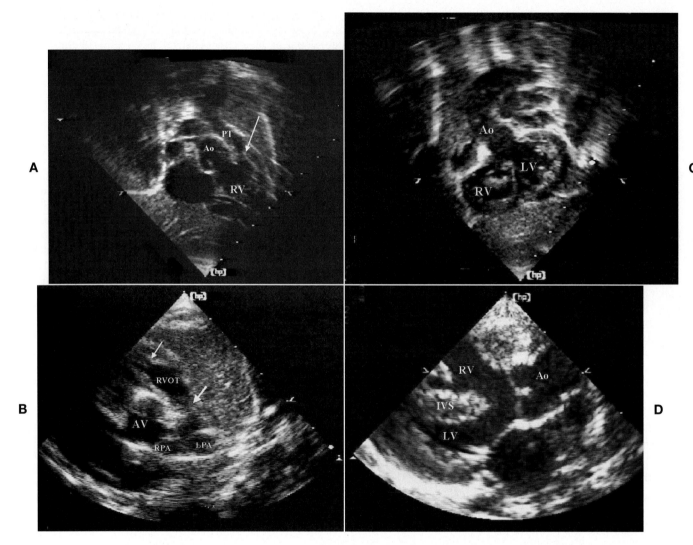

Figure 24-19   Echocardiograms of tetralogy of Fallot. **A,** Subxiphoid view. Narrowed right ventricular *(RV)* outflow tract due to infundibular hypertrophy *(arrow)* and anterior malalignment of conus. **B,** Parasternal short axis view. Narrowed RV outflow tract due to infundibular hypertrophy *(thin arrow).* Pulmonary "anulus" and area distal to it are narrowed as well *(thick arrow).* **C,** Sagittal view from subxiphoid position. Overriding aorta is demonstrated. **D,** Parasternal long axis view. Aorta is overriding interventricular septum and junctional ventricular septal defect is imaged.

Key: *Ao,* Aorta; *AV,* aortic valve; *C,* conus; *IVS,* interventricular septum; *LPA,* left pulmonary artery; *LV,* left ventricle; *PT,* pulmonary trunk; *RA,* right atrium; *RPA,* right pulmonary artery; *RV,* right ventricle; *RVOT,* right ventricular outflow tract.

and dimensions of the RV–pulmonary trunk junction, pulmonary trunk, and RPA and LPA and their branches. Oblique[C17] and angled views[B5,S10] are used. Configuration of the RV sinus and infundibulum and degree and morphology of the RV outflow obstruction are studied. Morphology of the pulmonary valve and any tethering or narrowing of the pulmonary trunk at the level of the commissural attachment of the valve or beyond are noted. Bifurcation of the pulmonary trunk and origins of the LPA and RPA are studied with particular care because the surgeon cannot accurately assess presence or severity of stenoses in this area at the time of operation. The sitting-up position (cranially tilted frontal view) generally offers the best view, although oblique views also usually demonstrate

origins of both pulmonary arteries. Presence, size, and morphology of various portions of the RPA and LPA are studied with care.

With proper profiling of the ventricular septum, the typical large VSD and overlying dextroposed aorta are identified (see Fig. 24-16). Additional VSDs, if present, are identified as well.

Coronary arterial anatomy can usually be seen following LV injection. Particular search is made for anomalous origin of the LAD from the RCA and for the rare but surgically important associated origin of the left coronary artery from the pulmonary artery.

Follow-through frames are examined for evidence of large AP collateral arteries, and injection is made into

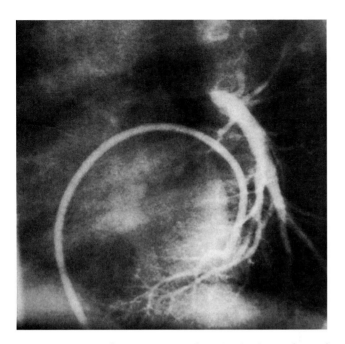

Figure 24-20 Pulmonary vein wedge injection in tetralogy of Fallot and absent central portion of left pulmonary artery demonstrating a left hilar pulmonary artery and its normal continuation. The artery was not visualized by right ventricular or aortic injection.

the thoracic aorta[R4] and/or selectively into the collateral arteries[P10] if these are present. When the true LPA or RPA is not visualized following these injections, which must include late filming and sometimes also digital subtraction techniques, a *pulmonary vein wedge injection* is made to fill, retrogradely, the pulmonary arterial tree (Fig. 24-20).[F13,N9,S10,T5] When all techniques, including this one, fail to outline a central or hilar portion of a pulmonary artery, it can be safely assumed to be absent.

Any major associated cardiac anomalies are identified by the study. Previous palliative shunts or transanular patches are visualized, the former by selective injections if necessary. Any iatrogenic pulmonary arterial problems are defined in detail. Particular care is taken to visualize these to help the surgeon avoid misidentifying structures at the time of repair.

NATURAL HISTORY

The natural history of patients having TF with pulmonary stenosis without major associated cardiac anomalies is variable[M5] and is determined primarily by severity of RV and pulmonary arterial outflow obstruction.[R13]

Symptoms and Survival

Twenty-five percent of surgically untreated infants die in the first year of life, but uncommonly in the first month (Fig. 24-21). These are the patients with the most severe obstruction to pulmonary blood flow. Forty percent are dead by age 3, 70% by age 10, and 95% by age 40. Instantaneous risk of death (hazard function) is greatest in the first year of life (see Fig. 24-21, *C*). Risk then stays

constant until about age 25, when it begins again to increase.

Hypoxic spells in the first few years of life are related to hyperactivity of the infundibulum. This and contraction of the infundibular septum and its parietal extension earlier in systole than in normal subjects[G3] produce variable and sometimes severe episodes of RV outflow tract obstruction and symptoms. Any sudden reduction of systemic vascular resistance also may precipitate a hypoxic spell.

About 25% of patients are acyanotic at birth and become cyanotic in the ensuing weeks, months, or years as pulmonary stenosis increases.[B2,B3,G2,G3] Progression of arterial desaturation, cyanosis, and polycythemia is variable and is furthered not only by increasing pulmonary stenosis but also by widespread tendency to thrombosis of the smaller pulmonary arteries, with progressive reduction in $\dot{Q}p$.[F1,M4,R2] As part of this same tendency, death may result from cerebral thromboses or abscesses.

In those few patients surviving into the fourth and fifth decades of life, death is commonly from chronic heart failure due to secondary cardiomyopathy that results from RV pressure overload and chronic hypoxia and polycythemia.

Pulmonary Artery Thromboses

In severely cyanotic and polycythemic patients, diffuse pulmonary arterial thrombosis can occur. This is initially visible only microscopically,[F1] but rarely it progresses to occlusion of a lobar pulmonary artery or even an entire RPA or LPA. Usually, Rp is not importantly increased by this process, but rarely the thrombosis is so widespread and severe as to be a cause of immediate and sometimes fatal pulmonary hypertension and RV failure following repair.

Pulmonary Vascular Disease

Pulmonary vascular disease rarely develops in surgically untreated patients. It may develop following too large a systemic–pulmonary arterial shunt (see "Interim Results after Classic Shunting Operations" later in this section). When a surgical shunt appears to be the cause, it is possible that preexistent pulmonary arterial thrombosis has compounded the problem.

Genetic History

Offspring of a parent who has TF are more likely to have the anomaly than offspring of parents without congenital heart disease. It is estimated that about 0.1% of live births have TF under the latter circumstances and about 1.5% under the former.[S3]

TECHNIQUE OF OPERATION

General Plan and Details of Repair Common to All Approaches
Surgical Evaluation

Outcome of repair of TF depends mainly on relief of pulmonary stenosis, whether infundibular, valvar, pulmonary arterial, or, as is usual, a combination of these. Therefore, the surgeon must come to the operating room with a clear mental image of the morphology as it has been

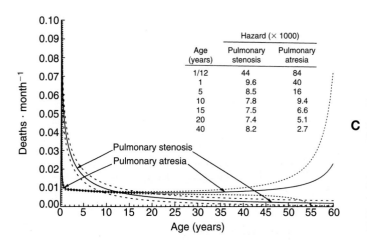

Figure 24-21 Natural history of surgically untreated patients having tetralogy of Fallot with pulmonary stenosis or pulmonary atresia. **A**, Survival to age 60 years. Smooth lines represent survival of each group, and dashed lines enclose 70% confidence limits. **B**, Survival to age 10 years (expanded time scale). **C**, Hazard function according to age. (From Bertranou and colleagues.[B13])

displayed in the echocardiogram or cineangiogram, particularly as it relates to the RV and pulmonary arterial outflow obstruction. Degree of narrowing can be expressed quantitatively by a Z value, that is, the number of standard deviations (usually smaller) from normal. When the Z value of the pulmonary valve "anulus" has been determined from echocardiography or from corrected and transformed cineangiographic measurements to be larger than −3, the surgeon's bias should be that a transanular patch is probably unnecessary (Fig. 24-22); when it is −3 or smaller, a patch is probably required. The surgeon's bias should also

be that, even with a transanular patch, when the Z value of the "anulus" is less than −7 (less than 10% of cases), postrepair $P_{RV/LV}$ (ratio of peak pressure in the RV to that in the LV) may be 1 or higher, even with a properly placed transanular patch (Fig. 24-23).

After median sternotomy, external anatomy of the heart is studied, with particular attention to RV and pulmonary artery anatomy and configuration of coronary arteries crossing the RV. The cineangiogram and echocardiogram are mentally reviewed; these and observation of the heart determine the incision and details of repair.

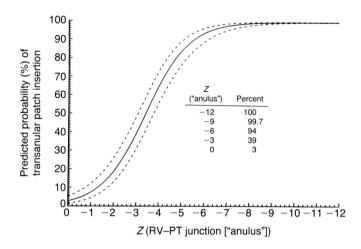

Figure 24-22 Probability of transanular patch insertion during repair of tetralogy of Fallot with pulmonary stenosis (solid curve), according to dimension (Z value) of right ventricular–pulmonary trunk junction (pulmonary valve "anulus"). (See original paper for data and equation.) Dashed lines are 70% CLs. (From Kirklin and colleagues.[K19])

Key: *PT,* Pulmonary trunk; *RV,* right ventricular.

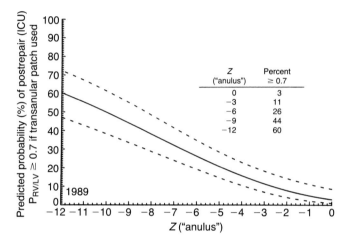

Figure 24-23 Probability of postrepair (ICU) $P_{RV/LV}$ being greater than 0.7 after a repair that includes insertion of a transanular patch, according to dimension (Z value) of pulmonary "anulus" as determined on preoperative cineangiogram. (See original paper for data and equation.) Depiction as in Fig. 24-22. (From Kirklin and colleagues.[K19])

Key: $P_{RV/LV}$, Ratio of peak pressure in right ventricle to that in left ventricle.

Surgical Approach

Approach to the repair must:

- Provide excellent exposure
- Avoid damaging major coronary artery branches
- Avoid excessive division of muscular bands in the RV

First, the procedure must relieve RV hypertension by mobilizing, transecting, and, infrequently, resecting parietal and septal extensions (bands) of the crista supraventricularis. Second, the VSD must be closed completely while avoiding the conduction system. When the first criterion (excellent exposure) is met by a right atrial approach, it is considered the method of choice.[B10,E2,E3,H2] A small vertical incision primarily in the infundibulum also meets the requirements for repair; it is particularly advised in cases in which a transanular patch is likely to be required. A transverse right ventriculotomy has been preferred by some, but care must be taken not to extend it into the RCA by strong retraction. Initial approach through the pulmonary artery and right atrium is preferred in all situations by some.[K10,K15,K42,P16]

Preparations for Cardiopulmonary Bypass

Before establishing cardiopulmonary bypass (CPB), the ascending aorta is dissected free from the pulmonary trunk so that when the aortic clamp is in position, the pulmonary trunk and RPA are undistorted. Unless it is clear from the cineangiogram that the pulmonary trunk bifurcation and central and hilar portions of the LPA and RPA are free of stenoses or diffuse hypoplasia, these too are mobilized. On the left side, this is aided by cutting the pericardium down to the LPA, dissecting away and preserving the left phrenic nerve. The ligamentum (or ductus) arteriosum is seen and dissected also, and in neonates and infants it is ligated. On the right side, the aorta is retracted anterior and to the left, and the RPA is dissected completely away from it out to the superior vena cava and beneath it if necessary.

Any surgically created shunts are at least partially dissected before establishing CPB (see later sections on repair after various shunts).

Repair

Immediately after CPB is established, all surgically created shunts and the ductus (if patent) are controlled and ligated or divided. Thereafter, the right ventriculotomy or right atriotomy is made and the internal anatomy further visualized and conceptualized. The plan is to:

- Dissect and resect the infundibular stenosis (recalling that this may be at several levels)
- Visualize the pulmonary valve and open it if necessary
- If possible, estimate dimensions of the outflow tract, valve, and anulus with a Hegar dilator[D2]
- Repair the VSD

Figure 24-24 Anatomic substrate of repair of tetralogy of Fallot with pulmonary stenosis from right ventricular (RV) approach, shown as if RV free wall were in part translucent. Separation of pulmonary valve from aortic valve by infundibular septum is evident. Parietal extension arches to the right and over the RV outflow tract, blending in its termination with RV free wall. Posteriorly, the ventricular septal defect (VSD) abuts the tricuspid anulus. Ventriculoinfundibular fold borders VSD posterosuperiorly, but is unseen because it is overhung by the parietal extension. VSD comes into relationship anterosuperiorly and anteriorly with the anteriorly displaced infundibular septum. This partially borders the aorta as well in many patients, with an aortic cusp on its inferior surface. Anteroinferiorly, a valley-like area may be seen where the infundibular septum merges with the trabecula septomarginalis (septal band) that forms the inferior border of the VSD.

Key: *AV*, Atrioventricular; *RAA*, right atrial appendage; *VSD*, ventricular septal defect.

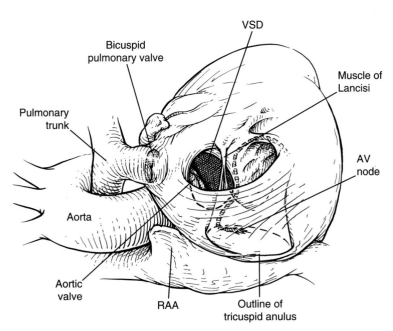

Pulmonary valvotomy, if needed, may be done through a vertical pulmonary arteriotomy or from below via the right ventriculotomy or right atriotomy. When a vertical right ventriculotomy limited to the infundibulum is used, it is closed with a patch of woven polyester or other material (see "Decision and Technique for Transanular Patching" later in this section); this particular incision is chosen in large part because of a narrow infundibulum and because, in any event, direct closure could narrow the outflow tract. When a transanular patch is needed, a woven polyester or glutaraldehyde-treated or untreated pericardial[H7] one is inserted after extending the infundibular incision across the pulmonary "anulus" (see footnote 2, "Pericardial Patch Preparation," under Technique of Operation in Chapter 16).

Repair is basically the same whether an RV (through a vertical or transverse incision) or right atrial approach is chosen and is represented in Figs. 24-24 through 24-27, which should be studied in parallel to obtain the most complete understanding of the pathologic anatomy and its repair.

Typically, in the *infundibular dissection,* the parietal extension of the infundibular (conal) septum is dissected away from the RV free wall and from the ventriculoinfundibular fold and is divided transversely 5 mm or so to the right of the attachment of the right coronary cusp of the aortic valve to the undersurface of the conal (infundibular) septum. This increases diameter of the infundibulum at its rightward end and improves exposure of the VSD from an RV approach. Any obstructive trabeculae along the left side of the outflow tract are also incised and partially removed. The aim is to increase the circumference of the infundibulum by enlarging each lateral recess in front of the conal (infundibular) septum. An obstruction at a low level (coronal plane) is relieved by dividing anomalous trabeculae above the moderator band while protecting adjacent papillary muscles; the moderator band is divided only when this is necessary to relieve the obstruction. When an os infundibulum is present at the level of the inferior edge of the infundibular septum, the *fibrous thickening* all around the

ostial orifice is excised, as is any fibrous obstruction extending upstream toward the pulmonary valve.

This type of anatomic dissection is not possible in the presence of diffuse RV outflow hypoplasia and is often not possible when there is combined infundibular, valvar, and anular stenosis. The structures are all hypoplastic, a situation frequently encountered in patients who have become importantly symptomatic as neonates or infants, and patch graft enlargement is often all that can be accomplished. In any event, particularly in infants, resection or even transection of RV muscle bundles that are not obstructive must be avoided,[C19] because this unnecessarily impairs RV function.

If *pulmonary valvotomy* is needed, a vertical incision is made in the pulmonary trunk, taking care to avoid damaging the valve commissures (Fig. 24-28), or the valve is examined from below through the RV or right atrial incision. The pulmonary arteriotomy is not made through a commissure between the leaflets, because placing a patch in such an incision renders the valve regurgitant. Rarely can an adequate valvotomy be performed by simply dividing one or more sites of commissural fusion, because fusion is present in only 20% of stenotic valves and is almost always associated with important cusp thickening, particularly at the cusp free edge (see "Morphology" earlier in this section). After valvotomy, therefore, the surgeon may elect to excise the thickened cusp edge to relieve the stenosis, although some pulmonary valve regurgitation results. When there is cusp tethering only, the most common situation, the cusp edge may be cut from its attachment to the pulmonary artery wall over about 3 mm. This is done to one cusp at each commissure. Here, too, excising thickened cusp tissue may be required. Regurgitation from minor detachment of a cusp may be less than that from a transanular patch.[R16] If considerable cusp incision and detachment are required, regurgitation results; if there is also important residual narrowing, it is preferable to excise the cusps and place a transanular patch after completing the intraventricular part

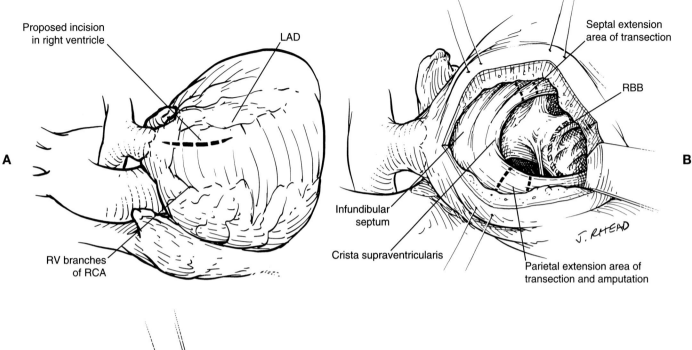

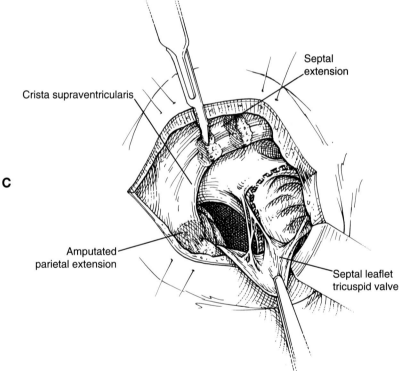

Figure 24-25   Repair of tetralogy of Fallot via right ventricular *(RV)* approach using a vertical incision. **A,** Superiorly the incision stops short of the pulmonary valve "anulus" and may vary according to presence and direction of a large conal branch of right coronary artery. **B,** RV incision is spread widely by retraction sutures. Parietal extension of infundibular septum is transected where it begins to fuse with RV free wall, dissected away from ventriculoinfundibular fold, and then amputated from the infundibular septum. This uncovers the ventricular septal defect (VSD) and tricuspid valve. Ventriculoinfundibular fold remains unseen because it is overhung by the tricuspid valve anterior leaflet. **C,** Parietal extension has been mobilized (divided and partially amputated). Septal extension is likewise mobilized to maximize circumference of infundibular outflow tract.

Key: *LAD,* Left anterior descending coronary artery; *RBB,* right bundle branch; *RCA,* right coronary artery; *RV,* right ventricular.   *Continued*

of the repair. If a transanular patch is not needed (see "Decision and Technique for Transanular Patching" later in this section), the pulmonary arteriotomy is closed, usually with a pericardial patch.

In children and adults the *VSD is closed* with a filamentous polyester or polytetrafluoroethylene (PTFE) patch; in infants, glutaraldehyde-treated pericardium works well. The patch is trimmed to be slightly larger than the VSD, but not so large as to preclude pulling the infundibular septum down onto the patch during repair. Exposure may be obtained entirely with stay sutures; alternatively, the VSD is exposed through the right ventriculotomy by the assistant using two small curved retractors, one beneath both ends of the conal (infundibular) septum, which are pulled upward and apart. A third retractor is positioned in the lower margin of the ventriculotomy for gentle inferior traction. Sequencing of the suturing depends on whether the repair is from the right atrium or RV and is similar to that used for isolated VSD (see Figs. 24-24 through 24-27; see also Chapter 21 and Figs. 21-25 and 21-26). For example,

Text continued on p. 975

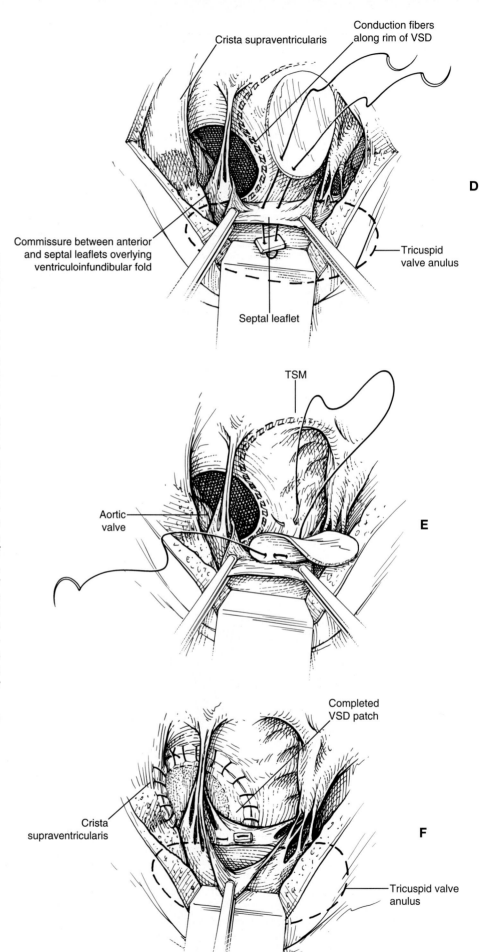

Figure 24-25, cont'd   D, Pledgeted mattress suture is placed from right atrial side through base of commissural tissue between septal and posterior tricuspid leaflets and through patch. A few more stitches are taken, working posteriorly between base of septal leaflet and patch, followed by stitches through ventriculoinfundibular fold and patch. **E,** Suturing is continued onto parietal extension and infundibular septum, visualizing and staying close to aortic valve leaflets to avoid leaving a hole between muscular bands. The suture is then held. With the other arm of the suture, a few stitches are taken, working anteriorly between septal tricuspid leaflet and patch, weaving beneath any chordae crossing the VSD. When this has taken the suture line about 5 mm inferior to edge of the VSD, stitches are taken in septum, well back from VSD edge. **F,** Repair of VSD is completed. Note that suture line is away from bundle of His and its branches, except where it crosses the right bundle branch anteroinferiorly. The crista supraventricularis is pulled downward by the patch, which helps increase the infundibular outflow circumference.

Key: *TSM,* Trabecula septomarginalis; *VSD,* ventricular septal defect.

Crista supraventricularis

Conduction fibers along rim of VSD

Commissure between anterior and septal leaflets overlying ventriculoinfundibular fold

Septal leaflet

Tricuspid valve anulus

TSM

Aortic valve

Completed VSD patch

Crista supraventricularis

Tricuspid valve anulus

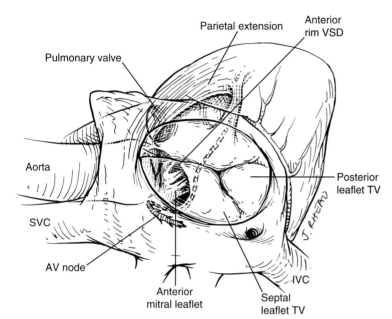

Figure 24-26   Anatomy of tetralogy of Fallot from perspective of right atrial approach, shown as if right atrial free wall and tricuspid valve were translucent. The striking difference from the right ventricular (RV) perspective (see Fig. 24-25) is apparent position of parietal extension. From right atrial perspective, the surgeon is looking beneath this, as parietal extension arches over the RV outflow tract. Ventriculoinfundibular fold is easily seen through tricuspid valve.

Key: *AV*, Atrioventricular; *IVC*, inferior vena cava; *SVC*, superior vena cava; *TV*, tricuspid valve; *VSD*, ventricular septal defect.

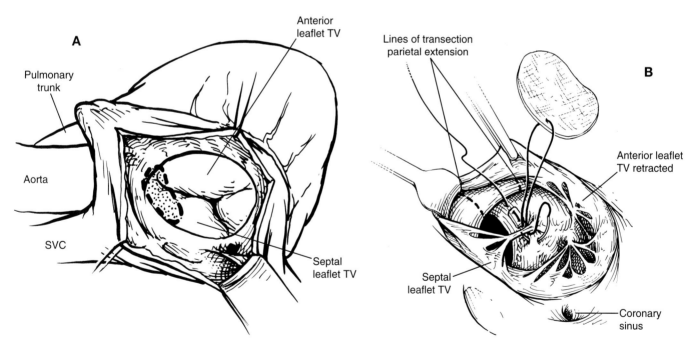

Figure 24-27   Repair of tetralogy of Fallot, right atrial approach. **A**, A high right atrial incision made close to the atrioventricular groove aids exposure. Ventricular septal defect (VSD) is located beneath anteroseptal commissure, indicated by dashed line. **B**, VSD is closed before amputating parietal extension. A pledgeted double-armed suture is begun at the anteroinferior aspect of VSD about 5 mm away from rim to avoid conduction fibers.

Key: *SVC*, Superior vena cava; *TV*, tricuspid valve.   *Continued*

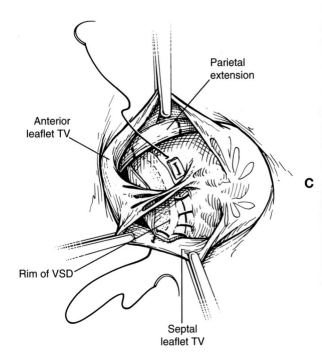

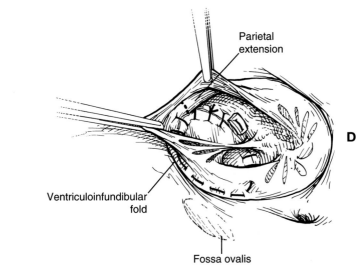

Figure 24-27, cont'd **C,** Suture line securing ventricular septal defect *(VSD)* patch is carried posteriorly to base of septal leaflet and then upward toward ventriculoinfundibular fold. **D,** Patch suture is completed, carrying second end of continuous suture anteriorly and superiorly at rim of VSD near base of aorta. This suture line thus marks the limit of infundibular resection at parietal extension. **E,** Parietal extension is transected at its origin from infundibular septum (staying outside VSD patch suture line). Remaining parietal muscle band is dissected up toward free wall and amputated. Exposure for accurate dissection is not as good as when using the RV approach.

Key: *TV,* Tricuspid valve; *VSD,* ventricular septal defect.

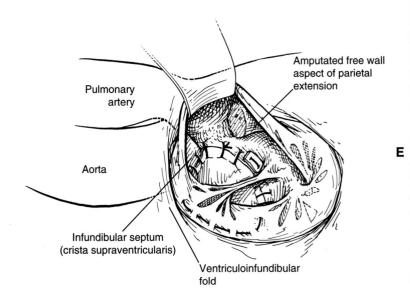

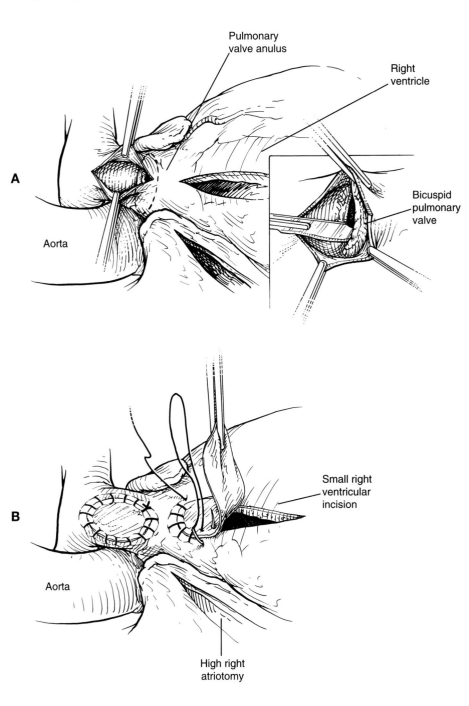

Figure 24-28   Repair of tetralogy of Fallot with separate infundibular and pulmonary arterial patches. **A,** Pulmonary trunk incision is shown extending to but not into pulmonary valve "anulus" *(dashed line).* Vertical ventriculotomy is also shown. *Inset,* Stenotic pulmonary valve seen through pulmonary arteriotomy. Fused commissures are incised with a knife to the pulmonary trunk wall. Fine tissue forceps steady the cusps on each side of commissure and provide even tension as incision is made. **B,** Unless pulmonary trunk is of normal width, which is uncommon, incision is closed with an oval pericardial or polytetrafluoroethylene patch. Patch is cut in the form shown, and its dimensions ensure that it is convex rather than flat.

through the RV it is usual to begin the continuous suture at the base of the tricuspid septal leaflet at the posterior–inferior aspect of the VSD. Via the right atrial approach, the suture is often begun anterior to the insertion of the medial papillary muscle (muscle of Lancisi).

Decision and Technique for Transanular Patching

The surgeon's bias regarding transanular patching is that it generally should not be necessary when the pulmonary "anulus" has a Z value larger than -3 as measured on the preoperative echocardiogram or cineangiogram. This is based on the high probability under these circumstances that the postrepair ratio between the peak pressure in the sinus portion of the RV and that in the LV (postrepair $P_{RV/LV}$) will be less than about 0.7,[K19] and on the anticipated increased need for insertion of a pulmonary valve very late postoperatively when a transanular patch has been placed.[K29] When the patient has TF with *subarterial* VSD, the "Asian" variant of TF, the surgeon's bias is that there is a 3 in 4 chance that a transanular patch is necessary.[V6]

Reassessment after closing the VSD is accomplished by estimating the diameter of the "anulus" with a Hegar dilator that passes snugly but not tightly through it. This diameter is transformed to the Z value as described in Chapter 1, Appendix Fig. 1D-1; generally this finding is similar to that obtained from the cineangiogram (but slightly smaller when the body surface area of the patient is less than 0.7 m^2 and slightly larger in patients with a body

Figure 24-29 Use of transanular patch in repair of tetralogy of Fallot with pulmonary stenosis. **A,** Entire incision is made initially when a transanular patch is clearly indicated; otherwise, only a partial incision is made *(inset)*. Note that the incision extends beyond the narrowest portion of the pulmonary trunk, but only a short distance onto right ventricle. Pulmonary valve is excised completely and ventricular septal defect repaired. **B,** A double-velour woven polyester (or polytetrafluoroethylene or pericardium) patch is trimmed to appropriate size and shape. When a polyester tube is used, it is elongated slightly by traction and cut to the correct length. It is then cut in half longitudinally and the ends trimmed. Note that the distal end remains essentially square, with only the corners trimmed off. When inserted, it forms a roof that is convex in all directions (inset).

Key: *VSD,* Ventricular septal defect.

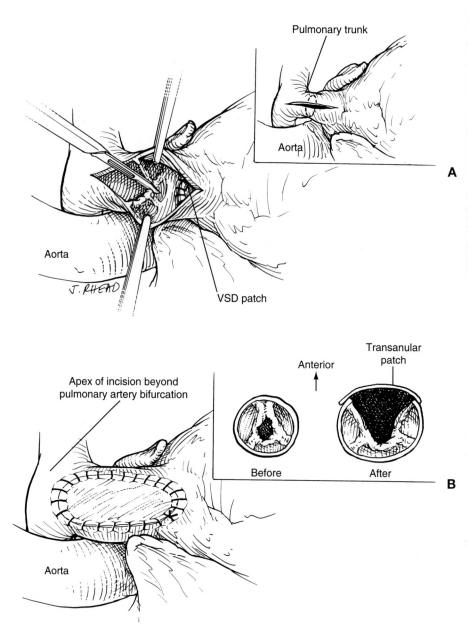

surface area greater than about 0.7 m²).[B1] Generally, a transanular patch should not be placed when the Z value is larger than −3. Otherwise, the incision is carried across the "anulus," the pulmonary valve excised, and the patch inserted. If the situation is borderline, the lesser risk lies with inserting a transanular patch.

When a transanular patch is used, a major consideration is the distal extent of the incision in the pulmonary trunk, because this must be into an area of *distinctly greater diameter* than that of the "anulus," which is usually the narrowest area (Fig. 24-29). Otherwise, a transanular patch relieves only the small component of the high resistance produced by the length of the narrowing, and the gradient will persist essentially unchanged and be at the junction of the patch and distal pulmonary trunk. In some patients the distal pulmonary trunk is narrower than the anulus (Fig. 24-30); in these cases the incision is extended into the LPA, which usually continues in the same general

direction as the pulmonary trunk and is usually proportionally larger than the distal pulmonary trunk. If the origin of the LPA is proportionally *no* larger than the distal pulmonary trunk, then the incision and patch reconstruction should be carried into the midportion of the LPA, which is nearly always wider than the origin.[S16] Care must be taken not to damage the left phrenic nerve or left superior pulmonary vein.

The transanular patch may be of glutaraldehyde-treated or untreated pericardium, or cut from a cylinder of preclotted double-velour woven polyester, collagen-impregnated knitted polyester or PTFE. Pericardium may be used routinely or only in very small patients. Collagen-impregnated polyester is preferred otherwise, because it facilitates precise sizing of the patch (an important consideration[F6,I5]), and when properly trimmed, its convexity is ensured, as is a relatively "square cut" of its distal end (see Fig. 24-29). Glutaraldehyde-treated pericardium has similar advantages.

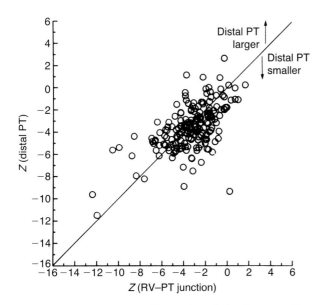

Figure 24-30   Scattergram illustrating relation between diameters of right ventricular–pulmonary trunk junction and those of distal portion of pulmonary trunk in patients having tetralogy of Fallot with pulmonary stenosis. In some patients with an anular Z value of −4 or smaller, the distal pulmonary trunk is narrower than the "anulus." (From Shimazaki and colleagues.[516])

Key: *PT,* Pulmonary trunk; *RV,* right ventricle.

When a polyester tube is used, one is selected whose diameter corresponds to a Z value of 0 to +2. Too large a transanular patch increases postoperative pulmonary regurgitation.[F7,I5,K41,O4,O5]

When the time comes for inserting the patch and the distal end of the incision is on the pulmonary trunk, the polyester tube is stretched *slightly* and cut to the length of the incision, cutting both ends squarely (see Fig. 24-29). The corrugated (crimped) nature of the tube provides sufficient length that it is convex longitudinally; the curve makes it a convex "roof" transversely. The tube is then cut longitudinally so that about three fifths of the circumference remains as the roof. Only the corners are trimmed at the distal end, leaving it very broad, while the proximal (RV) end is tapered. It is then sewn into place with a continuous No. 5-0 polypropylene suture (see Fig. 24-29).

When the incision has been carried onto the LPA, a slightly different technique is used, in the belief that the result is more apt to be geometrically correct. For this, a rectangular piece of pericardium is cut about 1½ times wider than the apparent diameter of the LPA and about 1½ times longer than the incision in the LPA. It is sewn into place with continuous No. 6-0 polypropylene sutures placed slightly farther apart in the patch than in the wall of the LPA. A polyester tube is used for the remainder of the reconstruction (Fig. 24-31). Alternatively, glutaraldehyde-treated pericardium can be used for both the transanular patch and the extension onto the LPA. Its length can be determined by measuring length of the incision from the RV to the pulmonary artery and its maximum width is determined visually by holding the edges of the incision open at valve level and judging the size of the roof required

to create a new pulmonary "anulus" whose diameter is no larger than three fourths the diameter of the ascending aorta. Alternatively, in infants, an 8-, 9-, or 10-mm Hegar dilator can be placed through the divided "anulus" and the width of the patch required to complete the roof over it measured. Usually, the patch is about 50 mm long and 15 mm wide at its center. Both ends are cut almost transversely to create a blunt patch, particularly distally, and the patch is positioned using continuous No. 5-0 polypropylene sutures, commencing at the distal end of the incision. The suture is mattressed at the end and over and over elsewhere, placing the first two or three throws along each side before pulling the pericardial patch into position as the suture is tightened. Suturing is continued down each side to anulus level; then the remainder of the right ventriculotomy is closed by incorporating the pericardial patch into it with continuous sutures. Deep bites of muscle are taken down each side and at the angle.

A monocusp may be attached to the pericardial roofing patch. The cusp diameter is fashioned somewhat larger than the planned roofed RV outflow. It is cut more or less circular and sutured to the patch when the latter suturing from distally reaches the valve "anulus."

Measuring Postrepair (OR) $P_{RV/LV}$

After repair, and preferably with the cannulae for CPB still in place, postrepair (OR) $P_{RV/LV}$ is obtained (OR meaning "operating room"). For this, a long, thin needle attached to a strain gauge manometer is passed into the RV and across the septum into LV. P_{LV} is recorded; the needle is withdrawn into the RV, and P_{RV} recorded.

If a transanular patch has not been placed and postrepair (OR) $P_{RV/LV}$ is greater than 0.7, CPB should be reestablished and a transanular patch placed.

When a transanular patch has been placed and the ratio is greater than about 0.8, localizing the site of the gradient is vigorously pursued by pressure manometry or transesophageal echocardiography. If pressure gradient or localized obstruction is identified *between* the sinus portion of the RV *and* distal end of the patch, CPB is reestablished and the situation corrected. If the operation has been properly performed (in which case the gradient is located at the distal end of the patch) and if the patch has been extended into a widened portion of the pulmonary trunk or artery, little more can be done to relieve the obstruction.

If no correctable cause of the elevation of postrepair (OR) $P_{RV/LV}$ is found, and if the elevation is not extreme and the patient's condition is good, the patient should be sent to the intensive care unit (ICU) with continuous monitoring of RV pressure. There, over a few hours, postrepair (ICU) $P_{RV/LV}$ may fall to reasonable levels (see "Special Features of Postoperative Care" later in this section). If the patient's condition in the operating room is not good or if right atrial pressure is considerably elevated above left, then the situation is precarious, although uncommon, and requires action. CPB is reestablished, and a large hole is cut in the VSD patch, usually during a brief period of aortic clamping and through a right atriotomy.

Closure of Foramen Ovale

During repair a patent foramen ovale (present in about two thirds of patients[L1,R3]) should generally be closed in older

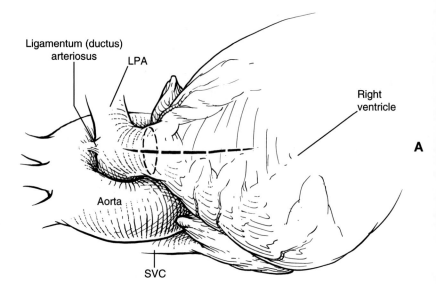

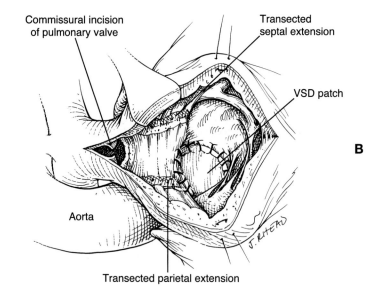

Figure 24-31   Repair of tetralogy of Fallot in neonates. **A,** A transanular right ventricular–pulmonary trunk incision is almost always used, keeping ventricular portion as cephalad as practicable. **B,** Pulmonary valve is incised fully to arterial wall and, if grossly distorted, resected fully. Parietal and septal extensions are incised at their origins from the infundibular septum, but resection of muscle is kept to a minimum. Ventricular septal defect *(VSD)* is closed as for the right ventricular approach (see Fig. 24-25). Often pericardium is used for VSD patch. **C,** Transanular incision is closed with a polyester, polytetrafluoroethylene, or pericardial patch large enough to attain a mildly convex contour in all directions.

Key: *LPA,* Left pulmonary artery; *SVC,* superior vena cava; *VSD,* ventricular septal defect.

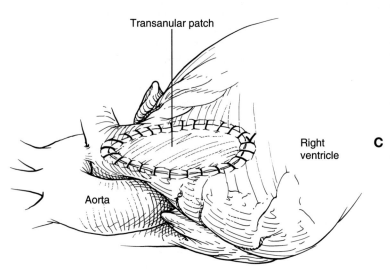

infants and children. Rarely, a persistent atrial communication can be the source of paradoxical cerebral emboli late postoperatively[L4] if a true atrial septal defect is not closed, there may be left-to-right shunting at atrial level. In neonates and infants, a patent foramen ovale is left unclosed to allow decompression of any right atrial hypertension caused by acute RV failure.[C19,D16] Some arterial desaturation may be present in the first few postoperative days, but it then disappears. A foramen ovale atrial septal defect should be narrowed to a diameter of 3 to 4 mm.

Repair of Uncomplicated Tetralogy of Fallot with Pulmonary Stenosis via Right Ventricle

After usual intraoperative preparations (see "Preparation for Cardiopulmonary Bypass" in Section 3 of Chapter 2), a median sternotomy is performed. Prompt control of major bleeding from collaterals is accomplished with diathermy. The usual dissections are made (see "General Plan and Details of Repair Common to All Approaches" earlier in this section) and purse-string sutures and tapes placed. A polyester tube (see "Decision and Technique for Transanular Patching" earlier in this section) may be selected and pericardium may be removed and treated with glutaraldehyde (see footnote 2, "Pericardial Patch Preparation" under Technique of Operation in Chapter 16).

CPB is established at 24° to 30°C using direct or indirect vena caval cannulation (see "Preparation for Cardiopulmonary Bypass in Section 3 of Chapter 2). In very small patients, hypothermic circulatory arrest may be used for most of the procedure. Two venous cannulae may be used as described or a single venous cannula may be preferred[C19] (see "One Versus Two Venous Cannulae" under Special Situations and Controversies in Section 3 of Chapter 2). The cardioplegic catheter (or needle) is secured into the ascending aorta. An efficient system for venting the left heart is essential for precise repair of TF, because 20% or more of the total flow from the pump-oxygenator to the patient passes through collaterals into the pulmonary circulation and then into the left heart.[M1,M2] For this, a short right atriotomy may be made after snugging down the caval tapes, and a pump-oxygenator sump sucker placed partially across the natural or surgically created foramen ovale. Alternatively, the left atrial suction line may be inserted through the base of the right superior pulmonary vein through a purse-string suture. The aorta is clamped and cold cardioplegic solution injected (see "Cold Cardioplegia, Controlled Aortic Root Reperfusion, and [When Needed] Warm Cardioplegic Induction" in Chapter 3). Efflux from the coronary sinus is aspirated and discarded or allowed to escape from the right atrium. The perfusate is made as cold as possible and is kept there until the patient's body temperature is 18° to 25°C; 18°C is selected in small patients and in those in whom repair may be unusually difficult to allow periods of low flow (0.5 L · min^{-1} · m^{-2}) or circulatory arrest with reasonable safety; 25°C is selected in other circumstances.

The RV is opened through a vertical (longitudinal) or transverse incision (see "General Plan and Details of Repair Common to All Approaches" earlier in this section for indications for each), and large conal and anterior branches of the RCA that cross the RV are spared. The

vertical incision is made in the midportion of the RV infundibulum and extended nearly to, but not into, the pulmonary valve superiorly and just into the sinus portion of the RV (see Fig. 27-25, A).[K8] Two pledgeted stay sutures placed through each side of the incision are placed on traction for exposure (see Fig. 27-25, B).

A transverse incision in the RV is used only when the infundibulum has adequate lateral width. Site of the os infundibulum is often indicated by a transverse indentation of the RV free wall over it. Ideally, the transverse incision is made at this level, but a large marginal RCA branch may overlie this. The incision is then made just downstream from this level (if the infundibular chamber is large) or just upstream to it (if there is inadequate infundibular width).

Infundibular dissection is performed (see "General Plan and Details of Repair Common to All Approaches" earlier in this section and Fig. 24-24, C). The pulmonary valve is examined, and if it is stenotic, a valvotomy is performed, perhaps through a pulmonary arteriotomy (see Fig. 24-28, A). Diameter of the valve anulus is estimated with Hegar dilators. If a transanular patch is considered necessary (see "Decision and Technique for Transanular Patching" earlier in this section), the ventriculotomy is carried across the "anulus" (see Fig. 24-29), because this aids exposure of the VSD. Otherwise, stay sutures are inserted and the VSD repaired (see Fig. 27-25, D to F). If the decision earlier in the operation has been not to use a transanular patch, measurements with Hegar dilators are repeated from the RV. If no further narrowing has resulted from VSD repair, the pulmonary arteriotomy (if one has been made) is closed with a pericardial patch, and the vertical infundibular incision, if made, is closed with polyester, PTFE, or a glutaraldehyde-treated pericardial patch (see Fig. 24-28, B). When a transverse incision has been used, it is closed directly. Rewarming of the patient is begun, controlled aortic root reperfusion (see "Cold Cardioplegia, Controlled Aortic Root Reperfusion, and [When Needed] Warm Cardioplegic Induction" in Chapter 3) is commenced or the aortic clamp released, the sump sucker is removed and the foramen ovale is usually closed, the right atrium is closed, and the usual de-airing procedures are accomplished (see "Completing Cardiopulmonary Bypass" in Section 3 of Chapter 2).

Repair of Uncomplicated Tetralogy of Fallot with Pulmonary Stenosis via Right Atrium

This procedure is identical to repair through the RV until CPB has been established. After commencing CPB, caval tapes are snugged and a long right atriotomy is carried well inferiorly a little anterior to the inferior vena cava cannula site (see Fig. 24-27, A). The incision lies quite anteriorly near the AV groove. The pump-oxygenator sump sucker is placed partially across the natural or surgically created foramen ovale to keep the left and right atria and pulmonary arterial tree free of blood. The aorta is clamped, cold cardioplegic solution is injected, and perfusate temperature is stabilized as described in the previous text. Stay sutures are applied to the right atrial wall for exposure, and the interior of the RV and its outflow tract are studied through the tricuspid valve (see Fig. 24-27, A).

With properly placed No. 6-0 polypropylene traction sutures on the septal and anterior leaflets of the tricuspid valve, edges of the VSD can usually be visualized,[1] although with more difficulty in TF than an isolated VSD because of the leftward and anterior displacement of the infundibular septum and its parietal extension.[K12] The pathway from sinus to outflow portion of the RV is examined. The obstructive nature of the prominent parietal extension of the infundibular septum (see Figs. 24-26 and 24-27, *B*) is particularly well appreciated from this approach, and the infundibular chamber, if present, is easily visualized. The pulmonary valve can usually also be well seen.

The parietal extension is deeply incised 2 to 4 mm beyond its origin (toward the free wall) from the infundibular septum and 4 to 5 mm above the aortic cusps, which are visualized as the cut is made (see Fig. 24-27, *E*). The parietal extension is then dissected away from the ventriculoinfundibular fold (inner curvature of the RV) and from the anterior free wall of the RV and excised. The free wall of the RV is palpated occasionally from outside during this dissection to avoid perforating it. Any hypertrophied and obstructive trabeculae along the left side of the outflow tract are incised and removed together with the fibrous margins of the infundibulum. The infundibular chamber and areas just upstream to the pulmonary valve are examined to determine (in concert with the preoperative imaging studies) whether they need widening by an infundibular patch. The pulmonary valve is examined to determine whether a valvotomy should be done through the pulmonary artery. Diameter of the narrowest part of the pulmonary arterial outflow tract is estimated by passage of a Hegar dilator. The VSD is repaired by sewing into place a polyester velour patch with continuous No. 4-0 or 5-0 polypropylene (Fig. 24-27, *B* to *D*). Alternatively, it may be closed before mobilizing and resecting the parietal band (as illustrated in Fig. 24-27). Often this allows better visualization of the borders of the VSD and, importantly, defines the area of parietal extension to be resected (Fig. 24-27, *B*). The VSD patch protects the aortic valve and crista during subsequent relief of outflow stenosis. It is probably better to use an interrupted suture technique with this method, because there is potential to cut the continuous patch suture anteriorly when resecting the parietal band.

If a pulmonary valvotomy is needed, it is usually done through a vertical incision in the pulmonary trunk (see Fig. 24-28). After valvotomy, RV outflow diameter is estimated by sizing the pulmonary valve orifice with Hegar dilators, which is usually best done through the right atrium. If a transanular patch is not to be used, the pulmonary arteriotomy is closed, usually with a pericardial patch. (It is

recommended [see "General Plan and Details of Repair Common to All Approaches" earlier in this section] that the right atrial approach be restricted to patients thought not to need infundibular or transanular patches. If unexpectedly one or the other is necessary, they can be placed through appropriate incisions.)

Next, the sump sucker is withdrawn from the foramen ovale and positioned in the right atrium, and controlled aortic root reperfusion is begun (see "Cold Cardioplegia, Controlled Aortic Root Reperfusion, and [When Needed] Warm Cardioplegic Induction" in Chapter 3) or the aortic clamp is released. The foramen ovale is closed in older infants and children, the right atriotomy is closed, and the caval tapes are loosened. Remainder of the operation proceeds as described for repair through the RV.

Repair of Tetralogy of Fallot in Infancy Using Hypothermic Circulatory Arrest

This technique combines some elements of surface cooling and hypothermia using short periods of circulatory arrest and low-flow CPB (0.5-1.0 L $\cdot$ min^{-1} $\cdot$ m^2) (see "Technique in Neonates, Infants, and Children" in Section 4 of Chapter 2). A median sternotomy is performed and the heart exposed. If the echocardiogram or cineangiogram indicates that a transanular patch is required, and in borderline cases, the front of the pericardium is removed from where it joins the diaphragm to its most superior reflection from the aorta. This secures a piece of pericardium at least 6 cm long and 3 cm wide, tapering at both ends. The pericardium is stretched with its epicardial surface downward onto moist gauze or cardboard (see footnote 2, "Pericardial Patch Preparation," under Technique of Operation in Chapter 16) and is set aside for later use. Dissection of the pulmonary trunk, RPA and LPA is easily and rapidly achieved.

CPB is established, cooling to a nasopharyngeal temperature of 18°C (14°C rectal) accomplished, and circulatory arrest established. When imaging studies indicate that a transanular patch is not required and when dissection of the pulmonary trunk confirms that it is of adequate diameter, a vertical incision is made into the RV (see Fig. 24-25). The infundibular stenosis is completely relieved. This often involves simple transection of the parietal and septal extensions of the crista, rather than resection. The pulmonary valve is examined from below and any stenosis relieved in the manner already described. The VSD is closed.

The tricuspid valve is retracted and the atrial septum exposed. If a patent foramen ovale is present, it is often possible to close it from this approach; if not, or if there is a more extensive atrial septal defect, the right atrium is opened and the defect closed through this approach with continuous polypropylene suture. The right atrium is closed. The ventriculotomy is then closed with a small patch.

When a transanular patch is indicated, the incision is carried across the "anulus" and out along the pulmonary trunk almost to the origin of the LPA, and a transanular pericardial patch is placed (see Fig. 24-31, *A*). Should there be LPA origin stenosis, the incision passes beyond this to reach the normal diameter LPA (Fig. 24-32). When a transanular patch is needed, VSD repair may be performed after the patch has been inserted onto the pulmonary artery.

---

[1] In about 5% of patients, aortic dextroposition is sufficiently severe that the cephalad (superior) borders of the VSD cannot be seen except with extreme traction on the tricuspid valve. In these cases, rather than using such strong traction, either the right atrial approach is aborted or a circumferential incision is made in the anterior and septal tricuspid leaflets, about 2 mm from the anulus, beginning in the anterior leaflet about 15 to 20 mm anterior to the commissural leaflet tissue between it and the septal leaflet. Stay sutures of No. 6-0 polypropylene are placed (see Chapter 41, Fig. 41-11).

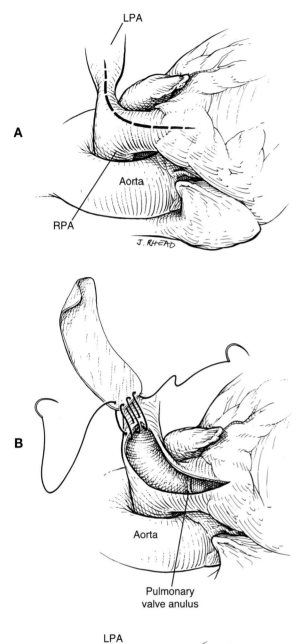

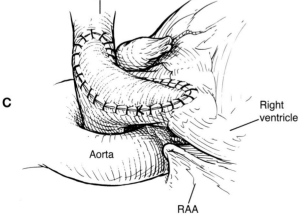

Figure 24-32   Repair when incision for transanular patch has been carried onto left pulmonary artery *(LPA)*. **A,** Dashed line indicates extent of incision. **B,** Pericardial patch is sewn into place to enlarge LPA. Note that it is cut in rectangular shape to permit maximum convexity after insertion. At first, distal suturing of patch is done "at a distance." **C,** Completed patch attains a rounded convex contour.

Key: *LPA,* Left pulmonary artery; *RAA,* right atrial appendage; *RPA,* right pulmonary artery.

If the duration of circulatory arrest approaches 45 minutes before repair is completed (which is uncommon when the procedure is done accurately and efficiently), CPB is recommended by reinserting the single cannula into the right atrial appendage if only the RV pericardial patch suture line requires completion or, otherwise, by inserting two small caval cannulae via the opened right atrium.

Repair of Tetralogy of Fallot with Stenosis at Origin of Left Pulmonary Artery

In this situation, there is usually sufficient hypoplasia of the pulmonary anulus and trunk that a transanular patch is also required (see "Morphology" earlier in this section). Repair is usually accomplished in exactly the manner described for situations in which the incision for placement of a transanular patch must be extended onto the LPA (see "Decision and Technique for Transanular Patching" earlier in this section; see Fig. 24-32). In those uncommon instances in which a transanular patch is not needed, an incision is made across the stenosis in the origin of the LPA. A rectangular patch of pericardium is trimmed and sewn into place as described.

When there is virtual or total occlusion of the LPA origin, patch graft enlargement is not satisfactory. Instead, after locating the patent portion of the LPA beyond the zone of occlusion by dissecting along the chord of tissue that still connects it to the pulmonary artery bifurcation, the patent LPA is opened longitudinally on its anterior surface (or aspect) for a short distance. The opened end is then sutured to the adjacent leftward edge of the pulmonary trunk with a running fine polypropylene suture to create a new posterior wall. The anterior wall is next created by a pericardial patch positioned as for reconstruction of a zone of stenosis (see earlier text). When the LPA is totally disconnected from the pulmonary trunk or is too small for the previously described reconstruction, repair entails locating the LPA in or adjacent to the lung hilum (usually by intrapleural dissection) and disconnecting it from any vessel that supplies it. It is then usually possible to anastomose the LPA end to side to the leftward edge of the distal pulmonary trunk (mobilizing the trunk completely so that it will swing more easily to the left). If the LPA is narrowed proximally, however, a technique similar to that described earlier is employed.

Repair of Tetralogy of Fallot with Stenosis at Origin of Right Pulmonary Artery

This situation occurs uncommonly without associated LPA stenosis. In contrast to the LPA, the RPA is usually *not* an extension of the pulmonary trunk but comes off its side at a right angle. This makes the simple type of repair used for origin stenosis of the LPA less satisfactory, although it can be used when stenosis is not too severe.

Operation proceeds as usual until the VSD has been repaired. Then a small longitudinal incision is made in the pulmonary trunk so that the orifice of the RPA can be visualized (Fig. 24-33, *A*). The origin of the RPA is excised from the pulmonary trunk. Lateral incisions are made to enlarge the orifice in the side of the pulmonary trunk

(Fig. 24-33, *B*). The RPA is incised from its narrow orifice back into its wide portion. A rectangular piece of pericardium is trimmed and sewn to the RPA to make a markedly enlarged proximal RPA (Fig. 24-33, *C*). The proximal end of the reconstructed RPA is then sutured to the enlarged orifice in the side of the RPA using No. 6-0 polypropylene sutures and closely placed sutures, while taking care to avoid any purse-string effect (Fig. 24-33, *D*). Alternatively, the posterior edge of the opened RPA is sutured to the back wall of the opened pulmonary trunk; the rectangular piece of pericardium is then sewn to the remaining opening to widen it further.

Transection of the ascending aorta improves exposure, but generally is not necessary.

Repair of Tetralogy of Fallot with Bifurcation Stenosis of Pulmonary Trunk

This condition requires appropriate reconstruction based on proper understanding of the morphology, although few papers discuss details of this repair.[L9] Both the LPA and RPA ostia are usually stenosed to a similar degree and over a short distance (less than 15 mm), and the distal pulmonary trunk is often similarly narrowed. The pulmonary trunk may be short and the carina between the two branches prominent and unusually proximal, making the bifurcation more Y shaped than usual.

In patients age 5 years or older, the optimal procedure may be to replace the pulmonary valve, trunk, bifurcation, and proximal RPA and LPA with a pulmonary allograft (Fig. 24-34).[B30,C21] It is a less desirable operation in infants, however, because the allograft will almost certainly be outgrown and require earlier replacement than when used in older children. However, this procedure has the greatest probability of providing a good hemodynamic result in this complex situation.

Otherwise, and surely in infants, repair rather than replacement is indicated. Complete mobilization of aorta, pulmonary trunk, RPA, and LPA is required, preferably before CPB. Before or after repairing the VSD, the vertical ventriculotomy is carried across the anulus, into the pulmonary trunk and extended across the narrow LPA origin and into the dilated portion. Repair is made after fashioning a similar anterior incision across the RPA origin stenosis. Superior edges of both opened arteries are sutured together with No. 5-0 polypropylene over a distance of about 10 mm (tissue at the original carina may need to be trimmed away to make this area less bulky). This suture line is intended to create a single widely open distal ostium, and a rectangular-shaped pericardial patch of appropriate size is sutured onto its edges to create a new front wall, carrying the patch proximally into the pulmonary trunk and right ventriculotomy.

Alternatively, the identical repair described earlier is used for the RPA (see Fig. 24-33), and the usual steps are taken to enlarge the first part of the LPA (see Fig. 24-32). The transanular patch is then made from a polyester tube.

In view of the complexity of both the geometry and the repair, these procedures are indicated only when *bifurcation* stenosis is severe. Otherwise, only the origin of the LPA is enlarged.

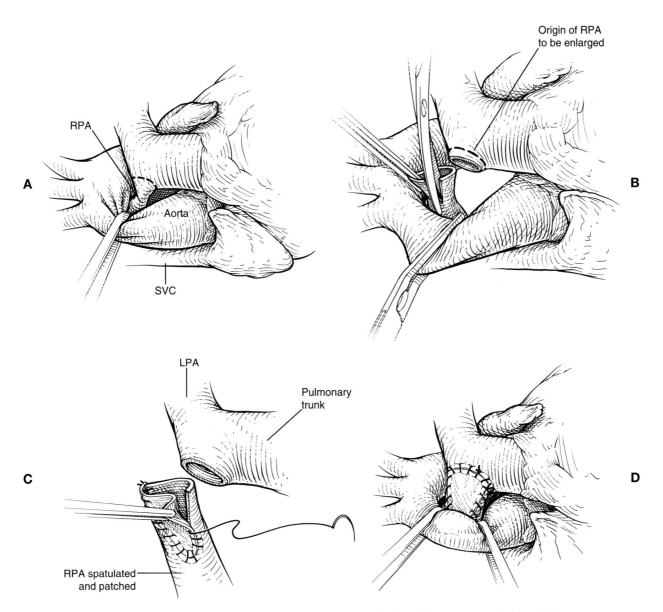

Figure 24-33   One type of repair of stenosis at origin of right pulmonary artery *(RPA)*. Initially, a small incision is made in pulmonary trunk through which stenotic orifice of RPA can be viewed from within. **A,** Ascending aorta has been mobilized to expose origin of RPA. Proposed incision for disconnecting RPA from pulmonary trunk is shown. **B,** RPA has been disconnected from pulmonary trunk. Resulting orifice in RPA is enlarged as shown, but enlargement by *incision* is preferable. An incision is made down anterior aspect of RPA. **C,** RPA is enlarged with a pericardial patch. **D,** Enlarged RPA is reattached to enlarged aperture in pulmonary trunk. (At times, it may be easier to suture posterior wall of RPA to posterior aspect of pulmonary trunk orifice before making pericardial enlargement of RPA.)

Key: *LPA,* Left pulmonary artery; *RPA,* right pulmonary artery; *SVC,* superior vena cava.

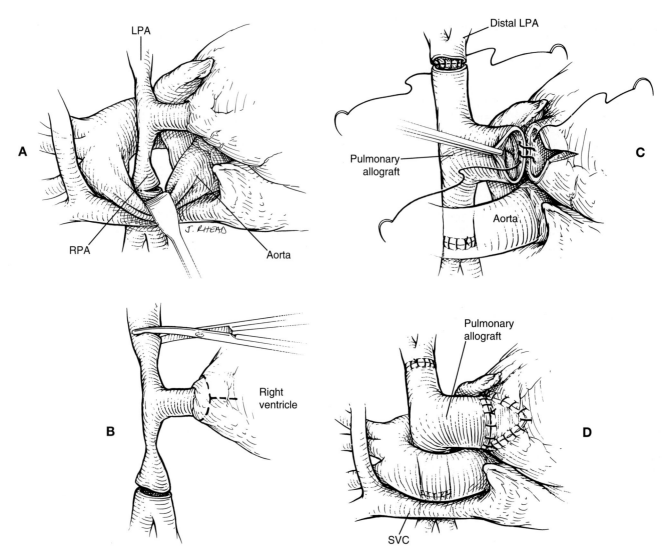

Figure 24-34 Repair of severe pulmonary trunk and bifurcation stenosis using a pulmonary valve allograft and its bifurcation. **A,** Dissection must be complete. For this, entire ascending aorta is completely freed from its posterior connections and from pulmonary trunk and its bifurcation. **B,** Superior vena cava is completely mobilized, and right and left pulmonary arteries (*RPA* and *LPA*) are dissected at least to the point where the first branch is visualized, that is, beyond the immediately prebranching level. **C,** Ascending aorta may be divided, but often the procedure can be performed without this step. Distal anastomoses are made first, taking care to transect LPA and RPA beyond the narrow areas and to leave some redundancy in allograft bifurcation. **D,** Completion of the proximal anastomosis, often with a polyester (or pericardial) hood as shown. If transected, aorta is brought together end to end. Importantly, however, if aorta is enlarged and compresses the underlying allograft bifurcation or RPA, then a short segment of polyester or polytetrafluoroethylene tube should be interposed between the two ends of the aorta.

Key: *LPA,* Left pulmonary artery; *RPA,* right pulmonary artery; *SVC,* superior vena cava.

Repair of Tetralogy of Fallot with Anomalous Origin of Left Anterior Descending Coronary Artery from Right Coronary Artery

In hearts in which there is a large coronary artery crossing the RV outflow tract close to the pulmonary "anulus" (usually an anomalously arising LAD from the RCA, but sometimes the entire left coronary artery coming from the RCA), relief of pulmonary stenosis must neither divide nor compromise flow through this vessel. Because such a vessel is occasionally buried in muscle or fat and is not apparent on surface inspection at operation, preoperative cineangiographic or two-dimensional echocardiographic study must be of sufficient quality to exclude this anomaly. When there is uncertainty, site of the usual course of the first part of the

LAD is investigated, and if the LAD is not there, it arises anomalously. When anomalous origin is present, technique of repair depends on morphology of the RV outflow obstruction, as usual. When the pulmonary "anulus" is of adequate diameter, a transverse right ventriculotomy is made low in the outflow tract and the infundibular stenosis relieved from below. Alternatively, repair is accomplished via the right atrium. Any valvar stenosis is relieved either from below or via the pulmonary trunk.

When there is a small pulmonary "anulus" and proximal pulmonary trunk, a vertical ventriculotomy may be made after dissecting up the anomalous artery from its bed in the RV wall over almost its entire length from its origin to near the interventricular groove. The incision is then carried beneath it and across the "anulus" into the pulmonary trunk. Infundibular stenosis is relieved in the usual fashion and a patch sufficiently large to relieve the stenosis positioned beneath the artery across the "anulus." If this is done, care is taken to avoid making the native pulmonary valve regurgitant by injudicious valvotomy. Alternatively, the surgeon may consider this approach dangerous and use an allograft valved conduit between the RV and pulmonary artery to bypass the area.

If the left coronary artery is damaged by the right ventriculotomy, the left internal thoracic artery can be taken down (see "Internal Thoracic Artery" under Technique of Operation in Chapter 7) and anastomosed to the distal left coronary artery. This procedure can be life saving.

Repair of Tetralogy of Fallot after Blalock–Taussig or Polytetrafluoroethylene Interposition Shunt

Median sternotomy in an older patient with TF and a *classic B-T shunt* is usually accompanied by profuse bleeding from arteries in front of and behind the sternum that have developed as part of the collateralization that follows ligation of the subclavian artery. While this bleeding is being controlled, rapid volume replacement should not be made with banked blood. This blood passes directly across the VSD into the aorta and coronary arteries. If unmodified banked blood is infused rapidly, because it is cold and has low calcium content and low pH, the heart may slow and even develop asystole (warmed calcium-enriched blood may be used).

Commonly, when a systemic–pulmonary arterial shunt was made in neonates or small infants having a left aortic arch, a left PTFE tube graft was placed between the left subclavian artery and LPA. In part this was motivated by the ease with which it can be closed during repair. After sternotomy is performed, hemostasis secured, and rib spreader inserted, when the patient's condition is good, initial dissection is made. Because the graft lies deeply in the left chest, the approach is not beneath the thymus gland but over it, directly into the left pleural space. The few adhesions between the mediastinal pleura and lung are divided with the electrocautery. The PTFE tube graft is somewhat rigid and easily palpated. A small incision is made directly over it and is carried down to it. At times a plane of dissection between the graft wall and surrounding tissue is easily established; if so, this dissection is carried out. Otherwise, the pericardium is opened and CPB is established at about 32°C. The lungs are collapsed, and a plane of dissection is easily established around the graft. CPB flow is reduced to about $1 \, L \cdot min^{-1} \cdot m^{-2}$, and an appropriate-sized hemostasis clip[2] is placed accurately and securely across the tube graft. It is not divided, because as the child grows, the LPA is not pulled up and distorted but rather the left subclavian artery is pulled down (and infrequently occluded), although not dividing the graft is controversial (see "Technique of Operation" in Chapter 41). Remainder of the operation is carried out as usual.

When a classic right B-T shunt is present in a patient with a left aortic arch, the pericardium is opened and a piece removed if needed, pericardial stay sutures and purse-string sutures are placed as usual, tubing to the pump-oxygenator is divided and positioned, and, as the assistant elevates and retracts the ascending aorta to the left, the RPA is visualized coming from beneath the aorta, and the superior vena cava is dissected off from it and gently retracted rightward.[K3] (In a few cases, exposure of the subclavian artery may be easier with the superior vena cava retracted to the left.) Possible distortions of the RPA by the shunt are known from the preoperative cineangiogram, and these are kept in mind as dissection proceeds. Course of the right subclavian artery coming down to the RPA usually can be suspected from observation and palpation of a continuous thrill. The entire circumference of the subclavian artery may be freed along a short length by sharp dissection well superior to the anastomosis, and two heavy ligatures are placed loosely around it. The artery is then temporarily occluded, and if vessel identification has been correct, the continuous thrill disappears, systolic and diastolic systemic arterial pressures increase, and pulse pressure narrows. If these things do not occur, then the RPA has been misidentified as the subclavian artery, or the shunt is small. The heart is cannulated and CPB begun. Ligatures around the subclavian artery are tied, and the operation proceeds as usual. An alternative, preferred method is closure with a sturdy clip (see footnote 2), in which case the back wall of the subclavian artery is not dissected and temporary ligatures are not placed.

When a classic *left* B-T shunt is present in a patient with a left or right aortic arch, the subclavian artery is approached from outside the pericardium. For this, the upper left pericardial stay sutures are placed on strong traction to the patient's right. Level of the LPA is noted before this maneuver; just cephalad (superior) to this level, the thymus gland and left phrenic nerve are dissected up from the pericardium, sharply and over a limited area, because excessive dissection in this region can result in major bleeding that is difficult to control. A narrow Deaver retractor is slipped under the thymus, and the region of the subclavian artery is located by gentle palpation and sharp dissection beneath the thymus gland. The subclavian artery is dissected out as described for the right side, and the same tests are made for accuracy of identification. Operation then proceeds as described earlier.

If the left subclavian artery cannot be located by going over the thymus gland and phrenic nerve, an alternative

---

[2] The Weck medium-large (10) or large (15) hemoclip or the Ethicon medium large (LC300) or large (LC400) Ligaclip serves well for this.

method is used in patients with a right aortic arch. The innominate artery is identified beneath the innominate vein and traced distally to the point at which it bifurcates into left subclavian and left common carotid arteries. After identifying the left subclavian artery positively by the maneuvers described and by the fact that the anesthesiologist can feel the left common carotid (or left superficial temporal) pulse when the vessel is temporarily occluded, the operation proceeds as described.

In many centers, median sternotomy has replaced lateral thoracotomy for primary systemic–pulmonary arterial shunts in neonates. Generally a PTFE tube graft is used. At complete repair, access is appreciably better because the conduit lies on the right, medial to the superior vena cava and apposed to the lateral aspect of the ascending aorta, and on the left, just leftward of the descending aorta. Interruption is as discussed earlier, generally using a hemostasis clip with or without graft disconnection.

Repair of Tetralogy of Fallot after Waterston Shunt

Initially, preparation for TF repair proceeds as usual, and pericardial stay sutures are placed. The superior vena cava is carefully dissected off the RPA and retracted laterally, while the right atrial appendage is retracted inferiorly and the ascending aorta is retracted to the patient's left. Medial to the superior vena cava, the RPA is dissected back to its point of anastomosis with the aorta. Then the ascending aorta is retracted to the right, the pulmonary trunk and RPA origin are dissected away from the left side of the ascending aorta, and tapes are placed around the aorta—one proximal to the Waterston anastomosis and another distal to it. Purse-string sutures and left atrial catheter are placed, positioning the aortic purse strings well distally so that there is ample room for the aortic clamp between them and the Waterston anastomosis.[A1]

When CPB is begun, a soft vascular clamp is placed across the Waterston anastomosis. Caval tapes are snugged and left atrial suction system positioned. The aorta is clamped between the arterial cannula and Waterston anastomosis, cold cardioplegic solution is infused, perfusate temperature is made as cold as possible until the patient's temperature is about 25°C and is then stabilized at that temperature, and the clamp is removed from the anastomosis when the cardioplegic infusion has been completed (see "Cold Cardioplegia, Controlled Aortic Root Reperfusion, and [When Needed] Warm Cardioplegic Induction" in Chapter 3). The aorta is rolled to the patient's right by the tapes, and medially the RPA is freed further from the leftward posterior wall of the aorta. The aorta is next retracted to the patient's left and an incision made through the most accessible part of the suture line between aorta and RPA. This allows a view of the anastomosis from within the aorta; working first from above and then below, the incision through the suture line is extended until the two vessels are completely separated.

A two-row transverse closure of the aorta is made. The first row is placed as a continuous whipstitch of No. 4-0 polypropylene, brought back to the starting point as an over-and-over adventitial stitch that covers the first row. Occasionally the RPA is small and the opening cannot be closed transversely without narrowing it. In such cases a generous square of pericardium, at least 1½ times larger than the diameter of the RPA, is sewn into the opening with continuous No. 5-0 or 6-0 polypropylene.

Alternative methods of managing this situation have been described and used in the past, but are no longer recommended. Closure of the anastomosis from within the aorta is a simple method that works well in the uncommon patient with *no* distortion of a large RPA. The more radical method of transecting the ascending aorta at the level of the anastomosis[E4,Y1] gives superb exposure of the entire central portion of the RPA and pulmonary trunk bifurcation and facilitates extensive reconstruction in this area. The proximal and distal aortic segments must be well mobilized, or else when reconstructed the ascending aorta will compress the RPA. This method is necessary only when simple complete mobilization of all structures fails to give good exposure.

Remainder of the repair is accomplished as usual.

Repair of Tetralogy of Fallot after Potts Shunt

Usual preparations for TF repair are made, but a femoral (or external iliac) artery is exposed through a small vertical groin incision (or a transverse iliac fossa incision for retroperitoneal exposure of the iliac artery) before median sternotomy. After sternotomy the usual stay and purse-string sutures are applied, and the anterior aspect of the LPA is freed where it exits through the pericardium (see "General Plan and Details of Repair Common to All Approaches" earlier in this section). This dissection is carried as far distally as possible, usually to a point at which the left superior pulmonary vein crosses the artery. Origins of the innominate and left common carotid arteries from the transverse aortic arch are dissected and a single tape placed around them so that an angled arterial clamp can later be placed across their aortic origins.

The heart is usually grossly enlarged and distorted in the presence of a long-standing Potts anastomosis. The aorta may be very large, and aortic regurgitation may be present from anular dilatation. Acquired infundibular or pulmonary valvar atresia is sometimes present.

After placing the arterial cannula in the femoral or iliac artery and cannulating the cavae as usual, CPB is established (see "Cardiopulmonary Bypass Established by Peripheral Cannulation" in Section 3 of Chapter 2). A large-bore cold cardioplegia catheter is secured in the ascending aorta. The perfusate is made as cold as possible, caval tapes are left open, head of the operating table is lowered,[G9] flow is momentarily reduced to about $1.0 \text{ L} \cdot \text{min}^{-1} \cdot \text{m}^{-2}$, and a longitudinal incision is made in the LPA. The Potts stoma is identified by blood exiting from it and is digitally occluded.[K6] Full perfusion rate can then be reestablished. When the patient's nasopharyngeal temperature reaches about 20°C, perfusion flow is reduced to about $0.5 \text{ L} \cdot \text{min}^{-1} \cdot \text{m}^{-2}$, and the surgeon can relinquish digital occlusion of the Potts stoma. A small intracardiac sucker placed in the pulmonary artery returns blood escaping from it to the circuit. An angled vascular clamp is placed across the superior aspect of the aortic arch so that origins of the innominate and carotid arteries are completely excluded. An aortic clamp is placed *between* the cardioplegic catheter and heart.

If the stoma is small, repair can be made during low-flow perfusion. However, the exposure usually is inadequate even then, and circulatory arrest must be established. The Potts stoma must be accurately identified to avoid closing the orifice of a branch of the LPA because of misidentification. Accurate identification is aided by giving a 1- or 2-second burst of perfusion through the arterial cannula, identifying the Potts stoma as the one from which blood escapes. Usually the stoma has tough edges and can be closed by a two-row whipstitch of polypropylene and one or two previously placed pledgeted mattress sutures. Occasionally a pericardial patch is needed for closure.

Often the LPA incision can be closed directly. However, it may be narrow in the region of the Potts stoma. If so, incision is made across the stenosis and it is reconstructed with a rectangular piece of pericardium that is 1½ times as long as the incision and 1½ times as wide as the diameter of the LPA before the stricture.[3] Usually all this can be accomplished in about 20 minutes of circulatory arrest.

Low-flow CPB is reestablished at 28°C. Strong suction is placed on the cardioplegic catheter, as in the de-airing process (see "De-airing Heart" in Section 3 of Chapter 2), and full flow is reestablished. Air in the aorta is driven superiorly into the arch by blood coming up from the femoral cannula and is removed via the aortic root catheter. After determining that all air has been removed, the clamp excluding the innominate and left common carotid arteries is removed, as is the aortic clamp. The table is leveled. If the heart fibrillates, it is defibrillated. About 5 minutes of a beating heart is allowed. The perfusate is then made very cold, left atrial suction system positioned, aorta clamped, cold cardioplegic solution given, perfusate temperature stabilized at 25°C, and repair performed.

Technique of Shunting Operations

Fig. 24-35 is a composite illustration of various positions used for systemic–pulmonary arterial shunts for augmenting pulmonary blood flow. Details of each follow.

Classic Right Blalock-Taussig Shunt

Occasionally an intraarterial needle is not placed for classic right B-T shunt operation, but a pulse oximeter is useful. However, in critically ill infants, a needle is placed in the left radial artery, primarily so that any metabolic acidosis can be identified and treated.

With the patient in left lateral decubitus position, a right lateral thoracic incision is made (Fig. 24-36, *A*, insert). The thorax is entered through either the top of the bed of the nonresected fourth rib or the third interspace. A rib spreader is positioned and gradually opened (see Fig. 24-36, *A*).

The first step in dissection is to securely identify the right superior pulmonary vein as it courses obliquely downward (medially and inferiorly) toward the heart to pierce the pericardium posterior to the phrenic nerve. The right superior pulmonary vein partially overlies the RPA;

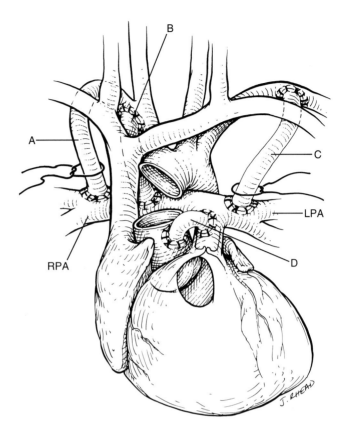

Figure 24-35   Composite diagram illustrating various positions of the usual systemic–pulmonary arterial shunts for augmenting pulmonary blood flow. *A,* Classic right Blalock-Taussig subclavian–pulmonary artery shunt with left (normal) aortic arch. *B,* Usual polytetrafluoroethylene (PTFE) interposition tube graft, shown between right pulmonary artery and innominate artery bifurcation. *C,* Left-sided PTFE interposition tube graft, shown between left pulmonary artery and left subclavian artery. *D,* Central shunt utilizing short PTFE tube between ascending aorta and pulmonary trunk.

Key: *LPA,* Left pulmonary artery; *RPA,* right pulmonary artery.

however, the artery, in contrast to the vein, follows a straight course medially. With the lung retracted toward the surgeon, often best done in the initial stages of dissection by the surgical nurse standing on the surgeon's right using his or her left hand, the periarterial sheath over the RPA is incised. Usually the superior branch of the artery is first freed, in the process of which the main RPA (lying in a slightly different plane of dissection) can be easily overlooked. To find it, the superior surface of the right superior pulmonary vein is cleared, and it and the superior vena cava are elevated (Fig. 24-36, *A*). Dissection is carried centrally until the proximal RPA is identified as a single vessel, proximal to its first branch. With lateral traction on a loop of heavy suture placed around the artery, the RPA is dissected in the periarterial tissue plane as far centrally as possible. The loop is then removed so that the artery does not inadvertently become obstructed during the next phase of the operation.

The lung is packed off and retracted inferiorly. An incision is made in the mediastinal pleura over the azygos vein and carried superiorly to the top of the chest, parallel

---

[3] This latter assumes that the pericardium will form the entire anterior half of the circumference of the enlarged LPA. The circumference is roughly three times the diameter and half of this is 1½ times the diameter.

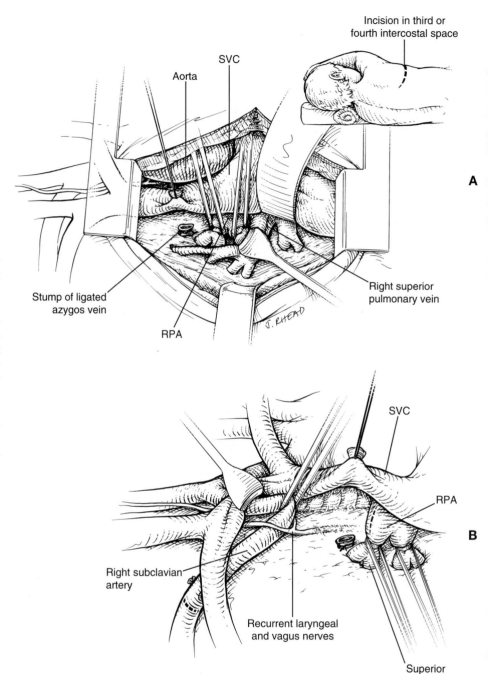

Figure 24-36   Classic right Blalock-Taussig shunt (left aortic arch). **A,** Right lateral thoracotomy is made in third or fourth intercostal space *(inset).* Right pulmonary artery *(RPA)* and its branches are mobilized and azygos vein ligated and transected. **B,** Right subclavian artery is completely dissected, mobilized, and ligated just proximal or distal to its first branch. It is then divided as shown by dashed line and brought out from beneath the vagus nerve.

Key: *RPA,* Right pulmonary artery; *SVC,* superior vena cava.

and posterior to the phrenic nerve. The azygos vein is divided between ligatures, and the soft tissue and right paratracheal lymph nodes are divided to provide a free pathway for the turned-down right subclavian artery. Any small veins overlying it are ligated and divided. Vagus and recurrent laryngeal nerves are identified, and the periarterial plane over the right subclavian artery is incised. By grasping only the adventitia of the often delicate subclavian artery, dissection is carried distally in the periarterial plane until the origins of internal thoracic and vertebral arteries are identified. These vessels are divided between ligatures, taking care that the proximal ligature is placed 1 to 2 mm away from the subclavian artery (Fig. 24-36, *B*). Anomalies

in the branching of the subclavian artery are frequent. The vagus nerve is gently retracted laterally, and the periarterial plane over the subclavian artery medially is opened and dissected. The subclavian artery is divided between ligatures placed beyond the first two large branches, and a right-angled clamp is passed beneath the vagus nerve from its medial aspect superior to the recurrent laryngeal nerve (Fig. 24-36, *C*). The subclavian artery beyond the ligature is grasped with the clamp and pulled out from under the vagus nerve. Holding the artery *beyond* the ligature, dissection is carried centrally in the periarterial plane until the distal portion of the innominate artery and nearly the entire right common carotid artery are liberated. As dissection

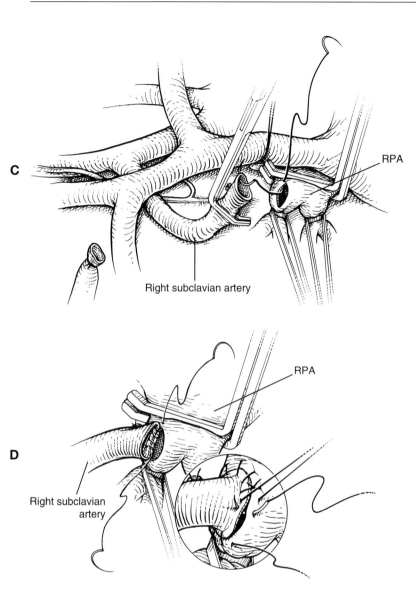

C

RPA

Right subclavian artery

D

RPA

Right subclavian
artery

Figure 24-36, cont'd **C,** Subclavian artery has been divided and appropriate occluding devices placed on right pulmonary artery *(RPA).* Incision in RPA is made on its very superior aspect. **D,** Anastomosis is made using interrupted or continuous No. 7-0 polypropylene sutures, starting posteriorly from within vessels. Inset shows completion of anastomosis.

Key: *RPA,* Right pulmonary artery.

proceeds, a small artery is occasionally found arising from the origin of the subclavian from the innominate artery, and this must be ligated and divided. The only thing limiting the turned-down length of the subclavian artery is the common carotid artery. Any obstructing bands in the paratracheal soft tissue are divided so that there is nothing in the pathway of the relocated right subclavian artery.

A light, straight arterial clamp with a handle long enough to allow easy holding by the first assistant is placed across the subclavian artery about 8 mm proximal to the point of final transection. The artery is cut squarely across just proximal to its first branch. (Rarely the first branch comes off very proximally and the subclavian artery is unusually large beyond it. In such instances, the artery can be transected beyond this branch.) Double-looped elastic ligatures are placed around the upper branch and distal main RPA, snugged, and weighted laterally with heavy Kocher clamps. An appropriate-sized Baumgartner clamp is placed across the very proximal RPA, with the surgeon passing a right-angled clamp beneath the artery for lateral retraction as the first assistant tightens the clamp. A longitu-

dinal incision is made *in the very superior surface* of the RPA (so that when the occluding devices are removed there will be no torsion of the RPA).

Anastomosis is made with continuous or interrupted double-armed No. 7-0 polypropylene or polyester sutures, the continuous suture placed from within the respective arteries posteriorly (Fig. 24-36, *D*). The first assistant holds the two clamps so that the vessels are in perfect apposition and without tension during the anastomosis. Before placing the last few sutures, the lumina are examined and any tiny thrombi or debris irrigated away. After completing the anastomosis, in rather rapid succession the two doubly looped elastic ligatures are cut and removed, the clamp on the subclavian artery removed, and the proximal RPA clamp removed. Packing is placed lightly around the anastomosis, any unusual bleeding is controlled digitally, the lung is partially reexpanded, and 5 minutes are allowed to pass. During this time a palpable continuous thrill should be present in the RPA. When the packs are removed, the field is usually dry. Rarely, an additional adventitial suture is needed.

A small chest catheter is brought out from the posterior gutter through about the seventh intercostal space and attached to gentle suction. The chest wall is closed and the lungs are well inflated before the ribs are brought together with absorbable suture. The wound is closed in layers with continuous fine polyglycolic acid sutures, and the skin approximated with a continuous subcuticular suture. With moderate positive pressure on the lung, the chest tube can be removed and small stab wound closed, generally with a subcuticular suture. Otherwise, it is removed the next day.

Interposition Shunt between Left Subclavian and Left Pulmonary Artery

Monitoring and thoracotomy are as described for the classic B-T shunt. If necessary, an arterial needle is placed in the right radial artery. The LPA is identified and dissected out. The mediastinal pleura is opened over the left subclavian artery and contiguous portion of the aortic arch, and the periarterial sheath over these structures is opened. The subclavian artery is not mobilized.

Ideally, a 5-mm PTFE tube graft is selected. In neonates or in the case of a very small LPA, a 3.5- or 4-mm PTFE tube graft is used, despite a possible small reduction in patency (see "Size" under Systemic–Pulmonary Arterial Shunt in Section 2 of Chapter 27 for discussion of criteria for selecting size of PTFE tube graft).[M11] *Before* any occluding devices are placed, the proper length of the tube graft is determined. For this, the lung is partially inflated to bring the LPA into its usual position. When the anastomosis is completed, the graft should lie without tension and without redundancy (and thus potential kinking) between the proximal half of the subclavian artery and the superior surface of the LPA. The end of the graft that will be anastomosed to the subclavian artery is beveled (Fig. 24-37), the graft is placed in a temporary position, and the other end is cut square at the point that will make the length to the LPA correct.

A delicate side-biting clamp (such as a Castaneda clamp) is placed deeply on the subclavian artery so that the handle lies inferiorly and the clamp occludes the artery both proximally and distally. A longitudinal incision is made in the excluded portion of the delicate subclavian artery, and an adventitial stay suture is placed on the anterior lip. The proximal anastomosis is made with a continuous No. 6-0 or 7-0 polypropylene suture. The clamp on the subclavian artery is not loosened or removed at this time (see variation in the detail under "Systemic-Pulmonary Arterial Shunt" under Technique of Operation in Section 2 of Chapter 27). Elastic ligatures are looped twice around the upper branch and main LPA and snugged, and heavy Kocher clamps are placed on each for lateral traction. A Baumgartner or 35-35 clamp is placed very proximally on the LPA, taking care not to compromise the ductus arteriosus. A longitudinal incision is made in the *superior* surface of the LPA, making this a little shorter than half the circumference of the PTFE tube graft. The distal anastomosis is made with continuous No. 6-0 or 7-0 polypropylene suture.

In quick succession, the doubly looped ligatures are cut and removed, the clamp on the subclavian artery is opened and carefully removed from the field, and the LPA clamp is

opened and removed. A light pack is placed about each anastomosis, with light digital pressure if needed. A continuous thrill should be present in the LPA. Other evidences of patency include registration of an immediate increase in oxygen saturation (pulse oximeter) and an immediate increase in systolic and diastolic blood pressure when the shunt is briefly occluded with forceps. Five minutes are allowed to pass. Nearly always, when the packs are removed the field is dry.

Remainder of the procedure is completed as described for the classic B-T shunt.

The interposition operation as an isolated procedure in patients with *left aortic arch* can be performed through a right thoracotomy. The PTFE tube graft is anastomosed proximally to the junction of right subclavian and innominate arteries, which is in the top of the chest. This operation is more difficult than that on the left side, but as opposed to the classic B-T anastomosis, the shunt is easier to close later.

Right-Sided Interposition Shunt through Median Sternotomy

The preferred systemic–pulmonary arterial shunt in neonates is a right PTFE interposition shunt performed through a median sternotomy (Fig. 24-38, *A*). After sternotomy, most of the thymus gland is removed. The pericardium is opened in its superior portion and stay sutures applied. The posterior pericardium is opened over the RPA between the ascending aorta and superior vena cava. A small, fine side-biting clamp is used to exteriorize the junction between the innominate and right subclavian arteries. A longitudinal incision is made, and the end of a beveled 3.5- or 4-mm PTFE tube is anastomosed to the incision (Fig. 24-38, *B*). A small, fine side-biting (C) clamp is placed on the RPA as it is elevated with fine forceps; the clamp exteriorizes essentially the full width of the RPA. The other end of the PTFE tube graft is anastomosed to this opening (Fig. 24-38, *C*). Continuous No. 6-0 or 7-0 polypropylene on a cutting needle is used for both anastomoses. The clamps are removed sequentially, removing the RPA clamp first. After hemostasis is secured, the pericardium is loosely closed. The remainder of the sternotomy is closed in the usual manner. Although this technique has been used primarily in neonates, it is likewise applicable to infants.

Classic Left Blalock-Taussig Shunt (in Patients with Right Aortic Arch)

Monitoring, left thoracotomy incision, and dissection of the LPA are as described in the preceding text. The left subclavian artery is dissected in the cupola of the chest, and maneuvers for freeing it, bringing it beneath the vagus nerve, and preparing it for anastomosis are those described for the right side (see Fig. 24-36). Occluding devices are placed, the anastomosis performed in the manner already described, and the operation completed as described.

Right-Sided Interposition Shunt (in Patients with Right Aortic Arch)

This procedure in patients with right aortic arch proceeds exactly as the procedure on the left side in patients with left aortic arch (see Fig. 24-37).

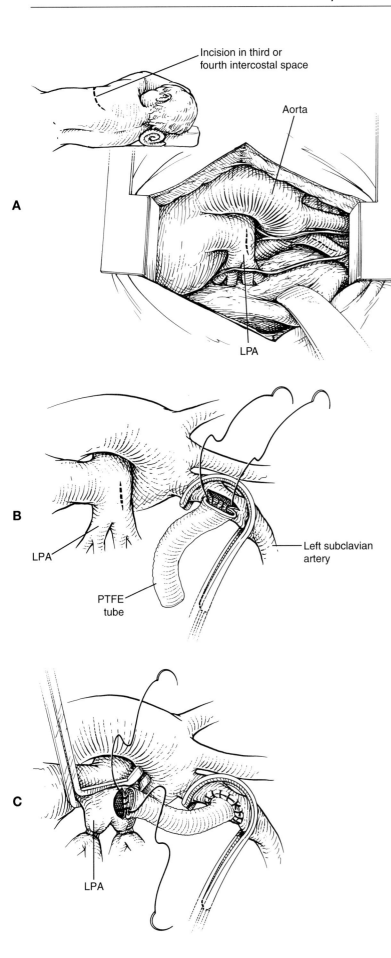

Figure 24-37   Left polytetrafluoroethylene *(PTFE)* interposition shunt (left aortic arch). **A,** Exposure and sites of incision *(dashed lines)* in pulmonary and subclavian arteries. **B,** PTFE graft has been trimmed for insertion. End-to-side anastomosis is made between graft and left subclavian artery. First portion of suture line is made by sewing from within, as shown. **C,** Distal anastomosis is made in a similar fashion. Direction of suturing (from medial to lateral) at both anastomoses minimizes possibility of tearing delicate subclavian or pulmonary artery. Note that clamp remains on subclavian artery until anastomosis is completed.

Key: *LPA,* Left pulmonary artery; *PTFE,* polytetrafluoroethylene.

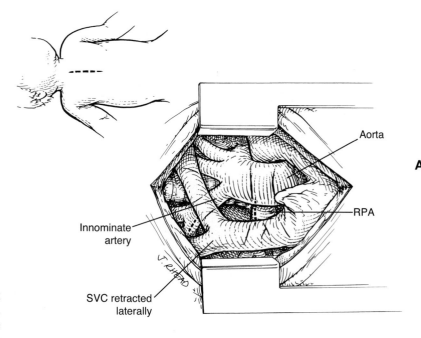

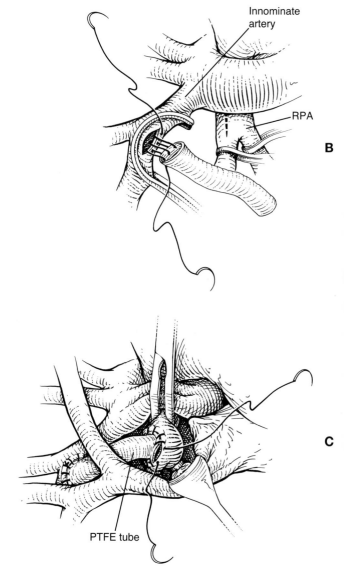

Figure 24-38 Modified Blalock-Taussig shunt performed via median sternotomy using a 3.5-, 4-, or 5-mm thin-walled polytetrafluoroethylene *(PTFE)* tube graft. **A,** Aorta and superior vena cava are mobilized enough to expose right pulmonary artery *(RPA)*. Innominate vein is elevated and right subclavian, right carotid, and innominate arteries are mobilized. Proposed incisions (indicated by dashed lines) are at cephalad aspect of RPA and junction of innominate and subclavian arteries. **B,** PTFE tube graft is cut on a bias and sutured to innominate–subclavian artery junction using continuous No. 6-0 or 7-0 polypropylene suture, beginning the anastomotic suture from within PTFE tube graft and systemic arteries. **C,** Shunt is completed after transecting PTFE tube graft squarely and using a suture technique similar to that for the systemic arterial anastomosis. Although not shown, subclavian artery clamp remains in place until RPA anastomosis is completed.

Key: *PTFE,* Polytetrafluoroethylene; *RPA,* right pulmonary artery; *SVC,* superior vena cava.

SPECIAL FEATURES OF POSTOPERATIVE CARE

Repair

Management is by the general measures described in Chapter 5. Patients with TF have a particular tendency to increase their interstitial, pleural, and peritoneal fluids early postoperatively. Like other deeply cyanotic individuals, they probably have abnormal systemic and pulmonary capillary membranes, and this may make them particularly sensitive to the damaging effects of CPB (see "Response Variables" in Section 2 of Chapter 2). Therefore, particular care is taken lest loss of intravascular plasma to extravascular spaces produces undesirable hemoconcentration early postoperatively, and attention is given to the possible development of pleural and peritoneal fluid collections. If these develop, they should be aspirated.

Evaluation is complicated by the fact that in patients convalescing normally after repair of TF, with warm feet and good pedal pulses, arterial blood pressure tends to be as much as 10% lower than that in patients who are acyanotic preoperatively. Cardiac index is usually normal for this stage of convalescence, and tendency to hypotension is related to relatively low systemic vascular resistance.[T1] In the presence of other signs of normal convalescence, treatment of arterial blood pressure is not indicated.

The hemodynamic state is assessed continuously and management constantly reviewed to be certain of its appropriateness. Measurement of cardiac output is helpful, along with other determinants of adequacy of cardiovascular subsystem function (see "Cardiovascular Subsystem" in Section 1 of Chapter 5). An important right-to-left or left-to-right shunt must be identified, either by the indicator-dilution method (see "Risk Factors for Low Cardiac Output" under Cardiovascular Subsystem in Section 1 of Chapter 5) or by two-dimensional echocardiography with Doppler color flow interrogation. This is particularly important in neonates and infants, in whom the foramen ovale may have been left open for early postoperative decompression of the right atrium. Arterial desaturation is then the rule in the early hours after operation, and demonstrating right-to-left shunting at atrial level by echocardiography using saline bubble injection reassures that desaturation is not from pulmonary dysfunction (Fig. 24-39). Desaturation from right-to-left shunting usually decreases within 48 hours as RV function improves.

In the absence of shunting, values of left (P_{LA}) and right (P_{RA}) atrial pressures provide considerable insight into the relative function of the two ventricles. After repair of TF, these are usually similar, but one may be 2 to 4 mmHg higher than the other. Rarely, P_{LA} is 5 to 10 mmHg higher than P_{RA}. When this occurs, a residual left-to-right shunt at ventricular or great artery level must be sought and, if found, promptly closed by reoperation. If no shunt is found, elevated P_{LA} indicates LV hypoplasia or severe impairment of LV systolic or diastolic function, and an inotropic agent and afterload reduction are indicated.

Rarely, P_{RA} is 5 to 10 mmHg higher than P_{LA}, indicating important volume or pressure overload of the RV or severe impairment of RV function. This situation is precarious and requires intense treatment, especially when postrepair $P_{RV/LV}$ is greater than about 0.7 (Fig. 24-40). If a transanu-

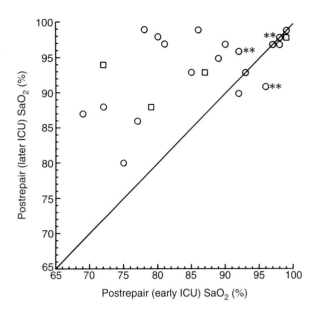

Figure 24-39   Relation of arterial oxygen saturation (SaO_2) on first arrival at intensive care unit after repair of tetralogy of Fallot (horizontal axis) to that present about 48 hours later (vertical axis), emphasizing arterial desaturation present early postoperatively when foramen ovale has been left open. Line of identity is shown. Squares represent patients who died early or late postoperatively, and circles represent survivors. Patients identified by two asterisks had the foramen ovale closed. (From Di Donato and colleagues.[D16])

Key: *ICU*, Intensive care unit; *SaO₂*, systemic arterial oxygen saturation.

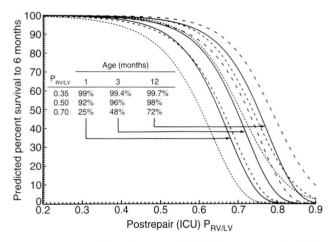

Figure 24-40   Effect of postrepair (ICU) $P_{RV/LV}$ on probability of early (6-month) survival after repair of tetralogy of Fallot. Additional effect of age at operation on this relation is also indicated. (See original paper for data and equations.) (From Kirklin and colleagues.[K19])

Key: *ICU*, Intensive care unit; $P_{RV/LV}$, ratio of peak pressure in right ventricle to that in left ventricle.

lar patch was not used, generally the patient should promptly be returned to the operating room and a patch placed. If a transanular patch is in place, as complete a repair as possible was obtained, and the patient's condition is reasonably good on only modest catecholamine support (e.g., 5 µg · kg⁻¹ · min⁻¹ of dopamine or dobutamine), then delay for a few hours is reasonable. If no improvement occurs, and particularly if postrepair $P_{RV/LV}$ is 0.8 or greater (or 0.7 or greater in a young infant), risk of death approaches 50% and intervention is indicated. A right ventriculogram and determination of site of the gradient by cardiac catheterization are indicated. If an appreciable gradient is found in the RV or at the pulmonary "anulus," or a localized important uncorrected LPA or RPA origin or bifurcation stenosis is found, correction of these areas of residual stenosis at prompt reoperation is indicated.

However, if the original repair was complete, it is likely that none of these will be found. Instead, the gradient will be located at the distal transanular patch suture line. This circumstance is uncommon (1% to 2% of patients), limited almost entirely to patients with severe hypoplasia of the "anulus" and pulmonary trunk. In that setting, and particularly without a distal widening (in the distal pulmonary trunk or LPA) into which the transanular patch can be extended, it may be impossible to make a geometrically proper patch.[K19,S16] Such a patient should be returned to the operating room and a large perforation made in the VSD patch. Optimally, this is performed through the right atrium. Outlook for survival is good, probably because systemic flow can be maintained when necessary by right-to-left shunting across the VSD. Such a situation may well be correctable by replacement of the pulmonary valve, trunk, and bifurcation with a pulmonary allograft at age 5 to 8 years (see Fig. 24-34).

Particular attention is paid to the possible need for reoperation for bleeding. Preoperative polycythemia and depletion of many clotting factors, extensive collateral circulation, and damaging effects of CPB often combine to produce a considerable bleeding tendency. Intense treatment, particularly with platelet-rich plasma, is indicated. The usual criteria for reoperation are followed (see "Bleeding" in Section 2 of Chapter 5), and prompt reoperation is advised as soon as they are violated. This practice was one factor contributing to the considerable reduction in risk of operation in the early 1960s. Currently, with careful intraoperative hemostasis and definitive repair at a young age, reoperation for bleeding is rarely necessary.

After the patient leaves the ICU, body weight is followed closely because transient fluid retention is common, particularly when a transanular patch has been used. Digoxin is particularly useful in this situation of a volume-overloaded RV and, if started, should be continued for about 6 weeks. Diuretics are used as indicated.

Systemic–Pulmonary Arterial Shunting

Although one-stage repair is advocated for TF with pulmonary stenosis, there are circumstances when systemic–pulmonary arterial shunting may be used. Except for neonates and occasionally very young infants, care after creating a systemic–pulmonary arterial shunt is simple. The patient is nursed in the ICU in a humidified oxygen-enriched atmosphere, usually provided by a head box. Oral intake is resumed 4 to 6 hours after operation.

In neonates and young infants, careful intraoperative and postoperative monitoring and control of PaO_2, pH, and buffer base are required (see "Neonates and Infants" in Section 2 of Chapter 5). An intraarterial needle may have

been placed preoperatively, and the baby is returned to the ICU still intubated. The usual intense postoperative care and protocols are applied (see Chapter 5). Support of arterial perfusion pressure is often necessary using dopamine or epinephrine to establish arterial blood pressure that is 10% to 20% greater than normal to ensure good flow through the shunt. Some centers recommend a heparin drip for 24 hours.

A chest radiograph is obtained as soon as the child reaches the ICU and is repeated about 4 hours later. Infrequently, dense opacification of the ipsilateral lung becomes apparent at this time, and nearly inevitably this localized hemorrhagic pulmonary edema produces hypoxia and clinical deterioration. It is an indication for immediately returning the patient to the operating room and narrowing the anastomosis in some way. This complication seems to be a direct effect of sudden increase in $\dot{Q}p$ on the abnormal lung of the cyanotic patient and *not* a reflection of elevated pulmonary venous pressure. This was reinforced by Ferencz,[F2] who found extravasation of red cells and localized but extensive areas of hemorrhage and edema in the lungs of many patients dying a few days after shunting operations for TF.

Infrequently, mild renal failure and rarely acute renal failure and anuria develop after a simple shunting procedure. This is related to the renal pathology sometimes present in cyanotic patients with TF and to renal damage by radiopaque dye that may have been used for the cineangiogram a few hours or days before operation. Therefore, urine flow is carefully observed postoperatively.

A surgically created shunt *must* function. Therefore, auscultation is used to assess its patency during the entire postoperative hospitalization. If doubt develops concerning shunt function, immediate two-dimensional echocardiography or cineangiographic study is indicated. If it is poorly functioning, prompt reoperation is indicated. In patients with large AP collateral arteries, a continuous murmur is present preoperatively, and therefore simple auscultation is not as useful early postoperatively. In this setting, if cyanosis has *not* improved, echocardiography or aortography is indicated.

RESULTS

Survival

Early (Hospital) Death

Although hospital mortality in a few series of heterogeneous groups of patients has been 1% or less,[A5,G26,P14,P15,S30,S31] in most series it varies between 2% and 5% (Fig. 24-41).[B8,C3,C19,G22,K19,K44,N2,R33,T8] With up to 40 centers in the United States participating from 1983 through 1993, the Pediatric Cardiac Care Consortium reported 12% mortality in all infants undergoing repair. Young age and low weight were associated with poorer survival (Fig. 24-42 and Table 24-6).[M28] In large part, deaths occurred in patients with severe or complex morphology.[K45] Better myocardial management that allows time for complete repair and provides a more robust hemodynamic state in the ICU may be required for mortality to approach zero.

Because the early rapidly declining phase of hazard does not flatten out until 3 to 6 months after operation

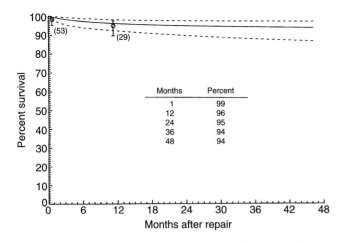

Figure 24-41   Survival after repair of tetralogy of Fallot in infancy. Circles represent two individual deaths. Vertical bars represent 70% confidence limits (CL). Solid line represents separately determined parametric estimates, and dashed lines enclose 70% CLs. (From Groh and colleagues.[G22])

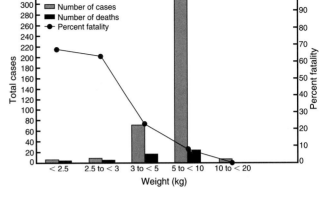

Figure 24-42   Mortality according to weight following repair of tetralogy of Fallot in infants. (From Moller.[M28])

■ **TABLE 24-6   Mortality in Infants Following Repair or Shunting Procedures for Tetralogy of Fallot**

Interval		Infundibulectomy/ VSD Closure			Central Shunt			Blalock–Taussig Shunt			Prosthetic Shunt			Absent Pulmonary Valve Syndrome		
≤ months <		n	No.	%	n	No.	%	n	No.	%	n	No.	%	n	No.	%
	0.25	6	4	67	21	3	14	12	0	0	32	2	6.3	12	6	50
0.25	1	10	4	40	14	1	7.1	17	2	12	48	2	4.2	5	4	80
1	3	58	16	28	12	1	8.3	23	1	4.3	65	4	6.2	14	10	71
3	6	93	7	7.5	8	2	25	15	0	0	50	3	6.0	6	0	0
6	12	243	17	7.0	7	0	0	19	0	0	48	0	0	4	0	0
TOTAL		410	480	12	62	7	11	86	3	3.5	243	11	4.6	41	20	49

Data from centers participating in the United States Cardiac Care Consortium 1983 to 1993.

Key: *VSD,* Ventricular septal defect.

(Fig. 24-43), hospital or 30-day mortality underestimates the risk of death early after repair.

Time-Related Survival and the Question of "Cure"

In considering survival, it must be recalled that deaths occurring *before* repair are not represented. Thus, an institution that delays repair until some specified age may have a few patients who, whether shunted or not, die before repair, whereas an institution that has a policy of one-stage repair in all symptomatic patients, no matter how young, may have an apparently higher mortality while actually saving more lives. Vobecky of Toronto Children's Hospital examined this issue in 270 TF patients younger than age 18 months.[V8] A few deaths occurred before palliation, between palliation and repair, and after repair (Table 24-7). Major noncardiac anomalies may preclude repair, and major associated malformations may increase operative risk at any age. At present, the data show nearly equal time-related survival for one-stage repair performed at any age and staged operation.

Time-related survival after repair in heterogeneous groups of patients at 1 month and at 1, 5, 10, and 20 years is about 94%, 92%, 91%, 90%, and 87%, respectively (Fig. 24-44). Patient-specific survivals and those of homogeneous groups of patients vary, with 10- and 20-year values as high as 97% in some circumstances (Fig. 24-45).

"Is the patient cured of TF?" This is a critical question that must be examined not only for the entire heterogeneous population of patients undergoing repair but also for specific patients, taking into account the strength and time-relatedness (shape) of their various risk factors.

For operation to be curative, the hazard function for death after the early postoperative period (3 to 6 months) must be no greater than that for an age-, gender-, ethnicity-matched general population and have no late increase until that imposed by older age on the general population. Hazard function for death after repair in a heterogeneous group of 814 patients (UAB, 1967 to May 1986), with follow-up out to 20 years in some patients, has a constant hazard phase (as opposed to a rising phase) late postoperatively. The same has been found in a follow-up (out to 30 years in the case of some patients) of the early Mayo Clinic patients included in the study of Fuster and colleagues[F3] and subsequently reported by Murphy and colleagues.[M29]

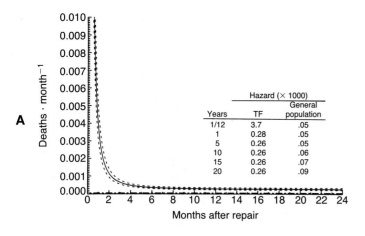

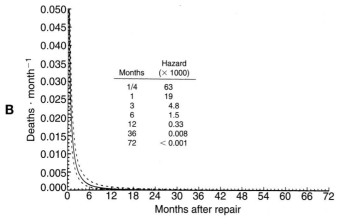

Figure 24-43 Hazard function for death after repair of tetralogy of Fallot with pulmonary stenosis from two different studies. In both, the rapidly declining early phase of hazard does not flatten appreciably until 3 to 6 months after repair. **A,** Hazard function from UAB study (1967 to May 1986; *n* = 814) with follow-up over 15 years. There is a constant phase of hazard extending for as long as patients were followed. **B,** Hazard function from combined Boston Children's Hospital–UAB study (September 1984 to 1989; *n* = 176), which has no late constant phase.[K19] Thus, the hazard function at 5 years, and presumably for a considerable period beyond, is the same as that of a matched general population (barely visible at dash-dot-dash line). (From Kirklin and colleagues.[K19])

Key: *TF,* Tetralogy of Fallot.

At 30 years, survival for patients who left the hospital alive was 86% compared with 96% in the general population (*P* <.01).

The 35-year follow-up of patients operated on by Lillehei and colleagues and the 30-year follow-up of patients operated on at Johns Hopkins Hospital are also consistent with presence of a low constant phase of hazard without a late rising phase.[H21,L18,L19]

Value of the constant hazard phase in the heterogeneous group of 814 patients is about three times higher than that of a matched general population, but many patients had numerous risk factors. The hazard function for younger patients in the combined Boston Children's Hospital–UAB data set, most of whom underwent primary (one-stage)

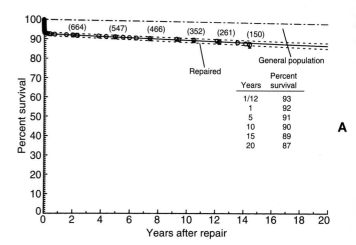

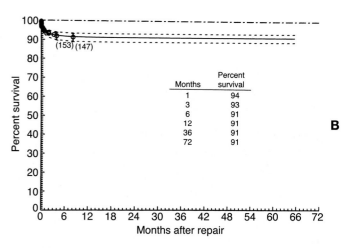

Figure 24-44 Survival after repair of tetralogy of Fallot with pulmonary stenosis in the two heterogeneous groups of patients whose hazard functions are depicted in Fig. 24-43. Each circle represents a death estimated by the Kaplan–Meier method. Vertical bars represent 70% confidence limits (CL) of these estimates. Solid line represents parametric estimate of survival, and dashed lines enclose its 70% CLs. Dash-dot-dash line represents survival of an age-gender-ethnicity–matched general population. **A,** Survival after repair in UAB study (1967 to May 1986; *n* = 814). **B,** Survival after repair in combined Boston Children's Hospital–UAB study (September 1984 to 1989; *n* = 176). (From Kirklin and colleagues.[K19])

■ **TABLE 24-7** Time of Death of Infants with Isolated Tetralogy of Fallot (*n* = 237)

Timing of Death	No.	%
None	218	92
Before palliation	3	1.3
At palliation	2	0.8
Secondary palliation	1	0.4
After palliation/before repair	8	3.4
At repair	7	3.0
After repair	1	0.4
TOTAL DEATHS	22[a]	9.3

(Data from Vobecky and colleagues.[V8])

[a] Fourteen deaths occurred before repair (5.9%; CL 4.3%–7.9%).

repair, is behaving as if the constant hazard phase will be closer to that of a matched general population when they have been followed long enough for this to be identified (see Fig. 24-43).[C1,K19] Predictions for a patient having TF with pulmonary stenosis, operated on at 6 to 18 months of age, are that (1) the value for the constant phase of hazard will be somewhere between that of a matched general population and twice that value, and (2) a late rise in the hazard function will not occur within the first 20 to 30 postoperative years (see Appendix Figs. 24F-1, *B*, 24F-2, *B*, 24F-3, *B*, and 24F-4, *B*).

Thus, the inference is that time-related survival of most patients after repair of TF with pulmonary stenosis under proper circumstances is excellent, approaching that of the general population, but that the risk of death throughout life is slightly greater than that of the general population.

Modes of Death

Most patients who died in hospital in a somewhat earlier era died in acute or chronic cardiac failure (Table 24-8); currently, this mode of death is not the most common. Considering death with multiple subsystem failure to be basically death in subacute heart failure, only half the patients who died in hospital after repair in the combined Boston Children's Hospital–UAB study died this way (see Table 24-8). Pulmonary failure, hypermetabolic state, and catastrophic surgical or early postoperative events account for more deaths than after most kinds of cardiac surgery in adults. Pathologic basis of the pulmonary insufficiency has been described by Harms and colleagues,[H1] who found in their autopsy studies that extensive alveolar and interstitial edema and hemorrhage are characteristic of the lungs of patients dying early after repair of TF. This process is probably caused by the damaging effects of CPB (see Chapter 2),[H1,K5] to which severely cyanotic and polycythemic patients seem particularly sensitive. Thus, further improvement in results of repair may demand not only improved myocardial management but also lessening of the damaging effects of CPB and improved technical proficiency in the operating room and ICU when repair is being done in very small patients.

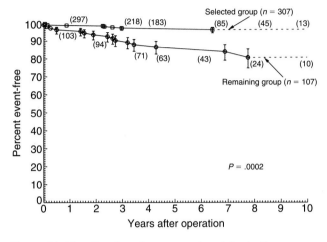

Figure 24-45 Freedom from premature late death, reoperation, arrhythmic symptoms, and heart failure among patients discharged from hospital alive after repair of tetralogy of Fallot with pulmonary stenosis. "Selected group" consisted of patients younger than age 20 years at repair, with no previous procedure or only a single Blalock-Taussig shunt, and a postrepair (OR) P$_{RV/LV}$ of 0.85 or less. (From Katz and colleagues.[K10])

■ TABLE 24-8   Modes of Death after Repair of Tetralogy of Fallot with Pulmonary Stenosis

	In Hospital				After Discharge			
	UAB [a]		BCH–UAB [b]		UAB		BCH–UAB	
Mode	No.	% of 57	No.	% of 12	No.	% of 24	No.	% of 1
Cardiac failure								
Acute	32	56	2	17	0	–	0	–
Subacute	12	21	1	8	0	–	0	–
Chronic	0	–	0	–	6	25	0	–
Multiple subsystem failure	0	–	3	25	0	–	0	–
Pulmonary failure								
Acute	2	4	1	8	0	–	1	100
Subacute	5	9	0	–	0	–	0	–
Chronic	0	–	0	–	1	4	0	–
Hypermetabolic state	1	2	1	8	0	–	0	–
Catastrophic postoperative event	0	–	3	25	0	–	0	–
Hemorrhage	2	4	0	–	0	–	0	–
Sudden	1	2	1	8	7	29	0	–
Arrhythmic	1	2	0	–	0	–	0	–
Hypoxia	0	–	0	–	1	4	0	–
Neurologic	1	2	0	–	0	–	0	–
Trauma	0	–	0	–	9	38	0	–
Subtotal	57	100	12	100	24	100	1	100
Unknown	0		0		0		2	
Total	57		12		24		3	

(Data from UAB are based on Kirklin and colleagues[K29]; data from BCH–UAB are based on Kirklin and colleagues.[K19])

Key: *BCH*, Boston Children's Hospital.

[a] 1967 to May 1986.

[b] September 1984 to 1989.

■ **TABLE 24-9   Incremental Risk Factors for Death at Any Time after Repair of Tetralogy of Fallot with Pulmonary Stenosis (analysis of patient variables only)** *a*

	Risk Factor *b*	Single Hazard Phase *P*
(Younger)	Age at repair	.003
	Down syndrome	.007
	Multiple VSDs	.0002
(Smaller)	Dimension (Z value) of RV–PT junction ("anulus")	.07
	Large AP collateral arteries	.009

(Data and analysis from Kirklin and colleagues.[K19])

Key: *AP*, Aortopulmonary; *PT*, pulmonary trunk; *RV*, right ventricle; *VSD*, ventricular septal defect.

a Details of multivariable analysis are in original paper.

b Dimensions of left and right pulmonary arteries were not risk factors.

Incremental Risk Factors for Death

Incremental risk factors for death early and late after repair have been identified from a number of different studies. The difficulties are that some variables were available for one analysis and not for another, that the risk factors may be different if procedural as well as patient characteristics are considered, and that some simultaneously determined "independent" risk factors are highly correlated and thus may be surrogates for one other (see "Variable Selection" in Section 4 of Chapter 6). However, using medical knowledge plus statistical analysis, a clear understanding is obtained of the risk factors for death after the repair of TF with pulmonary stenosis. Tables 24-9 through 24-11 present a sequential analysis of risk factors that begins with patient variables, adds details of repair, and then adds ICU factors. However, Tables 24-9 and 24-11 represent a different set of patients (the Boston Children's Hospital–UAB experience) with shorter follow-up than the larger UAB experience (see Table 24-10).

Young Age at Repair

Young age at repair[4] is a risk factor for death early after repair.[C9,C10,H13,P7,V4] This does not mean it is necessarily an immutable risk factor, because the age at which risk increases appreciably has been progressively reduced as experience and knowledge have grown. This improvement is illustrated by the UAB experience, in which risk of hospital death and predicted 20-year survival after repair in a 6-month-old infant improved considerably between 1967 and 1986 (Fig. 24-46). The incremental risk of young age, in general, is currently not apparent until age is less than 3 months and in some circumstances less than 1 month (Fig. 24-47). These trends are evident in the experience at GLH with one-stage repair of TF with pulmonary stenosis in the very young (Fig. 24-48 and Table 24-12). The incremental risk of young age may be related to inability of the very young RV to adjust to the volume overload of a transanular patch.

---

[4] Body surface area is a more statistically significant risk factor than young age in the majority of multivariable analyses, but most groups prefer to think in terms of age. Therefore, a regression analysis has been made of the relation of age to body surface area so that one can be used to estimate the other (see Appendix Fig. 24G-1).

■ **TABLE 24-10   Incremental Risk Factors for Death at Any Time after Repair of Tetralogy of Fallot with Pulmonary Stenosis (analysis of both patient and surgical variables)** *a*

	Risk Factor	Early	Constant
	Demographic		
(Smaller)	Body surface area	●	
(Older)	Age	●	●
	Clinical		
(Higher)	Hematocrit	●	
	Previous Potts anastomosis		●
	More than 1 previous palliative operation	●	
	Previous palliative direct approach to RV outflow tract obstruction		●
	Morphologic		
	Absence of unbranched hilar portion of one PA	●	
	Multiple VSDs	●	
	Dextrocardia	●	
	Surgical		
(Earlier)	Date of operation	●	
	Transanular patch	●	
(Higher)	Postrepair (OR) $P_{RV/LV}$	●	●

(Data from Kirklin and colleagues.[K29])

Key: *LV*, Left ventricle; *OR*, operating room; *PA*, pulmonary artery; $P_{RV/LV}$, ratio of peak pressure in right ventricle to that in left ventricle; *RV*, right ventricle; *VSD*, ventricular septal defect.

a Details of multivariable analysis are in original paper.[K29]

■ **TABLE 24-11   Incremental Risk Factors for Death at Any Time after Repair of Tetralogy of Fallot with Pulmonary Stenosis (analysis of patient surgical, and early postoperative variables)** *a*

	Risk Factor *b*	Hazard Single Phase *P*
(Younger)	Age at repair	.001
	Multiple VSDs	.002
(Higher)	Postrepair (ICU) $P_{RV/LV}$	<.0001

(Data from Kirklin and colleagues.[K19])

Key: *ICU*, Intensive care unit; $P_{RV/LV}$, ratio of peak pressure in right ventricle to that in left ventricle; *VSD*, ventricular septal defect.

a Patient, surgical, and institutional variables as well as postrepair $P_{RV/LV}$ were entered into the analysis.

b Institution, surgical approach, use of transanular patch, and postrepair (OR) $P_{RV/LV}$ were not risk factors in the final equation.

Reduction of the age at which risk is increased is due, in part, to increasing technical expertise in intracardiac surgery and early postoperative care in the very young.[T8] Further improvements in these areas may completely neutralize the increased risk of young age. Control of the damaging effects of CPB (see Chapter 2) and improvement in the function of the heart early postoperatively, brought about by more effective intraoperative myocardial management, will assist in this effort (Table 24-13).

Older Age at Repair

Older age is a risk factor for death early and late after repair (see Tables 24-10 and 24-14). Its effect on survival late after repair is probably truly immutable (Fig. 24-49). This is because the bases of the incremental risk of older age lie in the adverse, and to a considerable extent irreversible, effect of long-standing RV hypertension, cyanosis, and

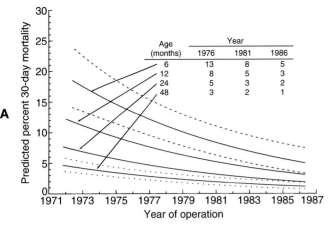

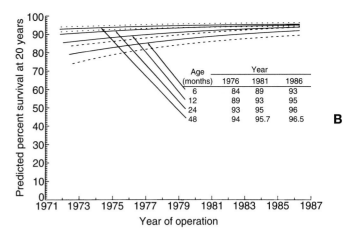

Figure 24-46 Nomograms illustrating decreasing strength across year of operation of the incremental risk of young age on early and late survival after repair of tetralogy of Fallot with pulmonary stenosis. (Nomogram is specific solution of multivariable risk factor equation represented by Table 24-10. Values entered for other variables in equation are in Appendix 24H.) **A,** Predicted 30-day mortality. **B,** Predicted 20-year survival, including early deaths. (From Kirklin and colleagues.[K29])

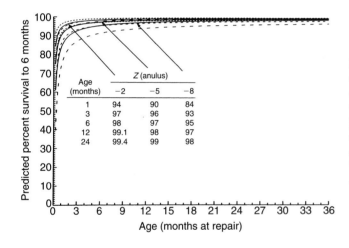

Figure 24-47 Nomogram illustrating incremental risk of young age and of dimension of pulmonary "anulus" on early survival after repair of tetralogy of Fallot with pulmonary stenosis in recent era. Note that effect of young age is stronger and more evident in patients with a very small "anulus" (Z value of -8) than in the others, reflecting the usual incremental effect of one risk factor on another. (Nomogram is specific solution of multivariable risk factor equation represented by Table 24-9. Values for other variables are in original publication.) (From Kirklin and colleagues.[K19])

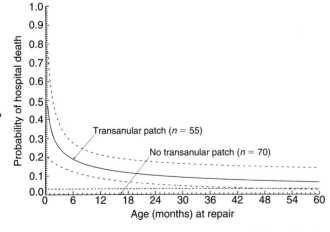

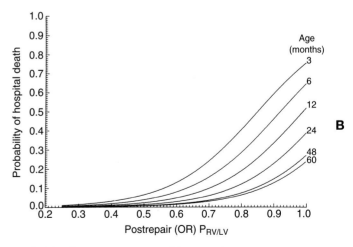

Figure 24-48 Nomograms illustrating incremental risk of young age, use of transanular patching and postrepair (OR) $P_{RV/LV}$ on hospital mortality after repair of tetralogy of Fallot with pulmonary stenosis (GLH experience, 1970 to 1978; $n = 125$) (Nomogram is specific solution of multivariable logistic regression analysis of patients without major coexisting cardiac anomalies undergoing one-stage repair. **A,** Effect of age $(P = .06)$ at operation and use of a transanular patch $(P = .001)$ on hospital mortality. **B,** Effect of postrepair (OR) $P_{RV/LV}$ $(P = .003)$ and of age at repair $(P = .001)$ on hospital mortality.

■ **TABLE 24-12   Hospital Mortality after Repair of Tetralogy of Fallot during First 2 Years of Life**

			Transanular Patch														
			No						**Yes**						**Total**		
Age				**Hospital Deaths**						**Hospital Deaths**						**Hospital Deaths**	
≤	**months**	<	*n*	**No.**	**%**	**CL (%)**		*n*	**No.**	**%**	**CL (%)**		*n*	**No.**	**%**	**CL (%)**
		1	2	1	50	7-93	⎫	1	0	0	0-85	⎫	3	1	33	4-76
1		3	2	0	0	0-61	⎬ 1/8 (12%)	7	2	29	10-55		9	2	22	8-45
3		6	4	0	0	0-38	⎬ CL 2%-36%	11	1	9	1-28	⎬ 6/34 (18%)	15	1	7	0.9-21
6		12	21	0	0	0-9		15	2	13	4-29	⎬ CL 11%-27%	36	2	6	2-13
12		24	13	1	8	1-24	⎭	13	0	0	0-14	⎭	26	1	4	0.5-12
TOTAL			42	2	5	2-11		47	5	11	6-17		89	7	8	5-12

(Data from GLH experience, 1970 to 1980.)

Key: *CL*, 70% confidence limits.

■ **TABLE 24-13   Modes of Death Following Repair of Tetralogy of Fallot during First 2 Years of Life** [a]

Age (months)	Mode of Death
0.4	Low cardiac output
1.2	Pulmonary dysfunction
1.3	Pulmonary dysfunction
3	Low cardiac output ($P_{RV/LV}$ = 1.1)
6	Low cardiac output ($P_{RV/LV}$ = 1.2)
11	Hemorrhage
22	Pulmonary dysfunction

[a] Based on same patients (GLH experience, 1970 to 1980) as in Table 24-12. In the patient 0.4 months of age, toxic serum propranolol levels were present immediately preoperatively on a dose of 10 μg^{-1} · kg^{-1} · day $^{-1}$ in the patient 1.3 months of age; patent foramen ovale was not closed; in the patient 11 months of age, ruptured polypropylene sutures were found at pulmonary artery bifurcation suture line. Preoperative pulmonary arterial problems were present in the patients 0.4 and 11 months of age.

Key: $P_{RV/LV}$, Ratio of peak pressure in right ventricle to that in left ventricle.

■ **TABLE 24-14   Risk Factors for Time-Related Survival among Hospital Survivors of Repair of Tetralogy of Fallot (*n* = 160)** [a]

	Rick Factor [b]	Hazard Ratio (95% CL)	P
(Older)	Age at operation [c]	1.6 (1.1-2.2)	.02
(Higher)	Post-repair $P_{RV/LV}$ [d]	1.4 (1.1-1.8)	.008
	History of heart failure	4.5 (0.9-22.8)	.068

(Data from Murphy and colleagues.[M25])

Key: *CL*, Confidence limits; $P_{RV/LV}$, ratio of peak pressure in right ventricle to that in left ventricle.

[a] Cox proportional hazards analysis.

[b] Variables not predictive of survival in patients surviving repair were presence and type of previous palliative shunt, surgical patch repair of pulmonary outflow tract, cardiopulmonary bypass or clamp time, degree of hypothermia during surgery, pulmonary blood flow, size of ventricular septal defect, history of palpitations or syncope, and temporary perioperative heart block.

[c] Per 10-year increment.

[d] For increments of 0.10 in the ratio.

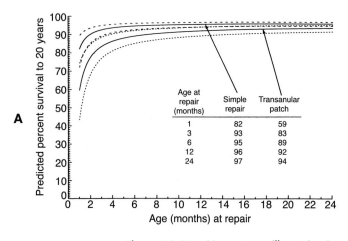

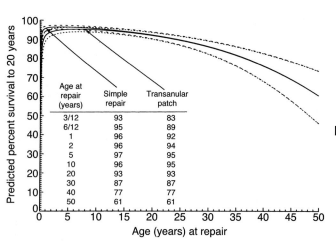

Figure 24-49   Nomograms illustrating incremental risk of older age at repair of tetralogy of Fallot with pulmonary stenosis in patients with and without a transanular patch. Note that adverse effects of older age on predicted, risk-adjusted survival begin at about age 5 to 7 years, but remain rather weak until after about age 20. Also noteworthy is lack of any adverse effect of transanular patching in older patients. (Nomograms are specific solutions of multivariable risk factor equation represented by Table 24-10. Values entered for other variables in equation are in Appendix 24H.) **A,** Effect of young age (expanded horizontal axis). **B,** Effect of older age. (From Kirklin and colleagues.[29])

polycythemia on cardiac structure and function,[B19] of cyanosis and polycythemia on renal function, and of volume overload on the LV of surgically created palliative shunts. For example, RV hypertrophy begins shortly after birth, continues as the child grows, and begins to be irreversible by age 4 years.[M26] It is in part to prevent these irreversible changes that repair is advisable early in life. A contraindication to early repair may be presence of an anomalous LAD from the RCA.[S31] Relative contraindications include complex pulmonary artery anatomy or very small pulmonary arteries. However, independent reports from Reddy, Stellin, Sousa-Uva, Starnes, and Groh and their colleagues[G22,R33,S30-S32] document excellent results when early one-stage repair is applied routinely in neonates and infants.

Severity of Right Ventricle–Pulmonary Trunk Junction Hypoplasia

Severe hypoplasia of the RV–pulmonary trunk junction ("anulus") is a risk factor for death, at least early after repair (see Fig. 23-47 and Appendix Fig. 23D-1). This may be related in part to the need for a *transanular patch* when the hypoplasia is severe, and to the correlation between severity of anular hypoplasia and *postrepair* $P_{RV/LV}$, even when a transanular patch is used and particularly when there is coexisting hypoplasia of the distal pulmonary trunk (see "Decision and Technique for Transanular Patching" earlier in this section). Thus, severity of anular hypoplasia, use of a transanular patch, and postrepair $P_{RV/LV}$ are all surrogates for one another in a complex manner that is difficult to quantify (Fig. 24-50).[K28]

Small Size of Right and Left Pulmonary Arteries

Important localized or diffuse hypoplasia of the RPA and LPA is uncommon in patients having TF with pulmonary stenosis.[S16] It is not surprising, then, that the diameters of these arteries are not correlates of postrepair $P_{RV/LV}$ and are not risk factors for premature death after repair.[G22,K19]

Transanular Patch

It remains arguable whether presence of a transanular patch is, per se, an incremental risk factor for premature death after repair of TF with pulmonary stenosis, although most studies find a higher mortality by univariable analysis among patients in whom a patch was used (see Table 24-12; see also Fig. 24-50).[K26]

In one analysis, transanular patching was a risk factor for early death (see Table 24-10), but in other analyses it was not (see Tables 24-9 and 24-11). Even so, in the latter analyses survival through the early postoperative period (up to 6 months) was lower in patients receiving a transanular patch than in those in whom simple repair of TF had been performed (Fig. 24-50; see also Figs. 24-48, 24-49, and Appendix Figs. 24D-2 and 24D-3). The question is whether the difference is due to presence of a transanular patch or to differing characteristics of patients in the two studies. Appendix Figs. 24D-2 and 24D-3 strongly suggest transanular patching is not an independent risk factor for death in the early phase. (These analyses were performed before the advent of sophisticated methods for analysis of nonrandomized clinical experiences as described under "Clinical Studies with Nonrandomly Assigned Treatment" in Section 1 of Chapter 6).

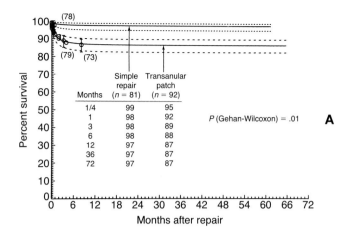

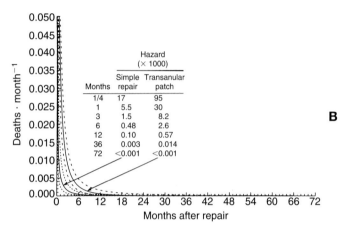

Figure 24-50   Survival after repair of tetralogy of Fallot with pulmonary stenosis with and without use of transanular patch. **A,** Survival. Depiction is as in Fig. 24-44. **B,** Hazard function. Note that the adverse effect of transanular patching on rate of death was no longer evident about 18 months after repair. (From Kirklin and colleagues.[K19])

Although multivariable analysis (see Table 24-10) does not indicate that transanular patching is a risk factor later postoperatively (in the constant hazard phase), nor does the late postrepair study of earlier Mayo Clinic patients,[F3,M29] the increased chance of needing later reoperation and its attendant risk suggest that in a sufficiently large and well-matched comparison, use of a transanular patch will have a late increased risk (see "Reoperation and Other Reinterventions for Right Ventricular Outflow Problems" later in this section). Strength of the effect of transanular patching is weak when postrepair $P_{RV/LV}$ is low and more important when it is elevated. Apparently, the pulmonary regurgitation allowed by a transanular patch, and the increase in RV volume, are usually (unless postrepair $P_{RV/LV}$ is high) well tolerated acutely, chronically, and late postoperatively out to about 20 years by the previously hypertrophied RV.[M30] However, the natural history of patients with isolated congenital pulmonary valvar regurgitation[S19] suggests that by about 40 years after repair, RV dysfunction will have developed in some and could lead to premature death.

Postrepair $P_{RV/LV}$

Important residual pulmonary stenosis after repair, expressed as postrepair $P_{RV/LV}$, is a risk factor for premature

■ **TABLE 24-15   Hospital Mortality after One-stage Repair of Tetralogy of Fallot with Pulmonary Stenosis, According to Postrepair (OR) $P_{RV/LV}$**

Postrepair (OR) $P_{RV/LV}$				Hospital Deaths		
≤ ratio <			n	No.	%	CL (%)
	0.40		35	0	0	0-6
0.40	0.65		47	4	9	4-15
0.65	0.75		18	0	0	0-10
0.75	0.85		11	1	9	1-28
0.85	1.0		6	2	33	12-62
1.0			1	1	100	14-100
TOTAL			118	8	6.8	4.4-10.1
P (logistic)					.002	

(Based on 118 patients undergoing repair at GLH [1970 to 1978]).

Key: *CL*, 70% confidence limits; *OR*, operating room; $P_{RV/LV}$ ratio of peak pressure in right ventricle to that in left ventricle.

■ **TABLE 24-16   Incremental Risk Factors for Death after Repair of Tetralogy of Fallot with Pulmonary Stenosis, Determined after Entering into the Analysis Only Patient Variables and Including Patients in Whom the Patch Was Perforated after Repair (Intent-to-Treat Analysis) [a]**

Risk Factor [b]		Single Hazard Phase P
(Younger)	Age at repair	.003
	Down syndrome	.007
	Multiple VSD	.0002
(Smaller)	Dimension (Z value) of RV–PT junction ("anulus")	.07
	Large AP collateral arteries	.009

(Data from Kirklin and colleagues.[K46])

Key: *AP*, Aortopulmonary; *PT*, pulmonary trunk; *RV*, right ventricle; *VSD*, ventricular septal defect.

[a] Data from combined Boston Children's Hospital–UAB experience, September 1984 to 1989; n = 196, repairs = 176.

[b] Dimensions of left and right pulmonary arteries were not risk factors.

■ **TABLE 24-17   Incremental Risk Factors for Death after Repair of Tetralogy of Fallot with Pulmonary Stenosis, Determined after Entering into the Analysis Patient Institution, Operation, and Postrepair $P_{RV/LV}$ (Intent-to-Treat Analysis) Variables [a]**

Risk Factor [b]		Single Hazard Phase P
(Younger)	Age at repair	.001
	Multiple VSDs	.002
(Higher)	Postrepair (ICU) $P_{RV/LV}$	<.0001

(Data from Kirklin and colleagues.[K28])

Key: *ICU*, Intensive care unit; $P_{RV/LV}$ ratio of peak pressure in right ventricle to that in left ventricle; *VSD*, ventricular septal defect.

[a] Data from combined Boston Children's Hospital–UAB experience, September 1984 to 1986; n = 196.

[b] Institution, surgical approach, use of transanular patch, and postrepair (OR) $P_{RV/LV}$ were not identified as risk factors.

death early and late after operation (Table 24-15; see also Table 24-10, Table 24-11, Fig. 24-14, Fig. 24-48, and Appendix Fig. 24D-8). The effect of a high postrepair $P_{RV/LV}$ was also observed in the early Mayo Clinic experience[K2,K4,K7] and has been reported by others.[H14,L11,R7,R35] This is true of postrepair (OR) $P_{RV/LV}$, but the ratio as measured in the ICU about 24 hours after operation is a more powerful and precise predictor (see Fig. 24-40, Appendix Figs. 24C-5 and 24D-8, and Appendix Table 24C-4). The interaction of young age (or small patient size), small anulus, transanular patching, and postrepair $P_{RV/LV}$ is apparent when Tables 24-11, 24-16, and 24-17 and Fig. 24-50 are compared. Here among patient-related variables, smaller Z value of the pulmonary "anulus" is a moderately strong risk factor for death after repair (Table 24-16). After adding operative variables (Table 24-17), the level of $P_{RV/LV}$ has a clear association with risk of death. In the same group of patients, transanular patching (see Fig. 24-50) was also associated with a higher risk of death early after repair.[K28] Although identified as a risk factor, postrepair $P_{RV/LV}$ is inversely correlated with size of the pulmonary valve "anulus" and of the distal pulmonary trunk.

Previous Palliative Operations

A single previously performed classic shunting operation is not a risk factor for death after repair (see Table 23-7), but more than one palliative operation is. When a pulmonary artery has been importantly distorted by a shunting operation, an unusual occurrence under proper circumstances, risks of repair are increased.

Multiple Ventricular Septal Defects

Multiple VSDs are present in only 1% to 3% of patients having TF with pulmonary stenosis, but they are a strong risk factor for death in the early hazard phase (see Tables 24-10, 24-11, 24-16, and 24-17), as evident in Fig. 24-51.[K28]

Coexisting, Related Cardiac Anomalies

Although a coexisting *complete AV septal defect* complicates repair of TF with pulmonary stenosis, it is *Down syndrome* that appears to be the incremental risk factor

(Tables 24-16 and 24-18).[K19,K28] Complete AV septal defect itself adds only a small increment to risk in institutions properly prepared to care for this combination of anomalies. Thus, between July 1, 1982, and December 31, 1986, no hospital deaths (CL 0%-15%) occurred at UAB among 12 such patients undergoing repair.[P19] Likewise, Ilbawi and colleagues reported one death (11%; CL 1%-33%) among nine similar patients undergoing repair.[I6]

Large AP collateral arteries are risk factors for death early after repair of TF with pulmonary stenosis but this may be due to the greater frequency of important RPA and LPA hypoplasia in such patients, and of discontinuity between the pulmonary trunk and RPA or LPA.[K28]

Other Risk Factors

Other uncommonly encountered risk factors are included in Tables 24-10, 24-14, and 24-16. Although *high hematocrit* was frequently observed in an earlier era of delayed surgery, it is uncommon today; when seen, it is a strong risk factor.[K11,R5]

Graham and colleagues proposed that small LV *end-diastolic volume* (less than 55% of normal for age) is an important risk factor for early death after repair.[G7] Nomoto

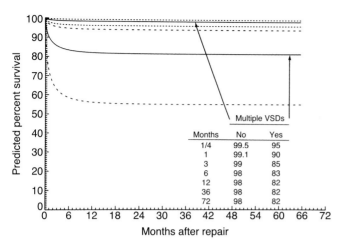

Figure 24-51   Nomogram illustrating adverse effect of multiple ventricular septal defects on survival early after repair of tetralogy of Fallot with pulmonary stenosis. Analysis is based on 176 patients undergoing repair at Boston Children's Hospital and UAB, 1985 to 1989. (Nomogram is specific solution of multivariable risk factor equation represented by Table 24-9. Values entered for other variables in equation are in Appendix 24H.) (From Kirklin and colleagues.[K19])

Key: *VSD*, Ventricular septal defect.

■ **TABLE 24-18   Confounding Effects of Down Syndrome and Coexisting Complete Atrioventricular Septal Defects on Non–Risk-Adjusted Survival in Patients with Tetralogy of Fallot**

Category	n	Total Deaths after Entry		
		No.	%	CL (%)
No Down syndrome	177	13	7	5-10
No AV septal defect	173	13	8	5-10
AV septal defect	4	0	0	0-38
P (Fisher)			.7	
Down syndrome	19	9	47	34-62
No AV septal defect	10	2	20	7-41
AV septal defect	9	4	44	24-66
P (Fisher)			.3	
P (Normal vs. Down syndrome, χ^2)			.001	

(Data from Kirklin and colleagues.[K19])

Key: *AV*, Atrioventricular; *CL*, 70% confidence limits.

and colleagues also reported that small LV volume is a risk factor, with a demonstrable increase in risk when preoperative LV end-diastolic volume is less than about 65% of normal.[N7] Oberhansli and Friedli reported similar findings.[O8]

Heart Block

Complete heart block is uncommon after repair. It occurred in 1.3% of patients from 1963 to 1978 at GLH, in 7 of 814 patients (0.9%; CL 0.5%-1.3%) from 1967 to May 1986 at UAB, and in 0.6% (CL 0.1%-1.9%) of patients from September 1984 to 1989 in the Boston Children's Hospital–UAB study.[K19] Right bundle branch block and left anterior hemiblock[B18,R29,W6] occur in about the same frequency as after repair of isolated VSD (see "Conduction Disturbances" under Results in Chapter 21), and the combination is usually associated with a favorable course late postoperatively.[C11]

Junctional Ectopic Tachycardia

Junctional ectopic tachycardia occurs infrequently after repair of TF. Survival depends on aggressive treatment in

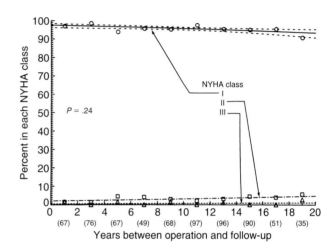

Figure 24-52   New York Heart Association (NYHA) functional class after repair of tetralogy of Fallot with pulmonary stenosis, according to interval between operation and last follow-up. Numbers in parentheses along horizontal axis represent number of patients available for functional class categorization at the odd-numbered interval below which number is positioned. Squares represent proportion of patients in functional class I at each interval, circles those in class II, and triangles those in class III. Solid line represents slope of solution of ordinal logistic (longitudinal) regression analysis, although the P value of .24 for the difference from zero slope indicates that change across time in the distribution of patients according to their NYHA functional class could be due to chance alone. (From Kirklin and colleagues.[K29])

the ICU with moderate core cooling and amiodarone (see "Atrial Arrhythmias" in Section 1 of Chapter 5).[W10] Thereafter, there is probably little risk of complete heart block.

Functional Status

About 98% of patients are considered by themselves or their parents to be in New York Heart Association (NYHA) functional class I after repair.[K10,K19,P1,R23] Most importantly, this proportion has not declined over time, at least out to 20 years (Fig. 24-52).

■ **TABLE 24-19** **Exercise Performance under Standardized Conditions 1 or More Years after Repair of Tetralogy of Fallot** [a]

Characteristic	10 Highest Performers [b]	10 Lowest Performers [c]	P (for Difference)
CT ratio	0.49	0.58	.001
Prv (mmHg)	39	76	.001
Age at repair (years)	5.83	10.7	.001
Pulmonary valve regurgitation (patients)	0/10	8/10	.0004
Previous Potts anastomosis (patients)	0/10	4/10	.04

(Data from Wessel and colleagues.[W2])

Key: *CT*, Cardiothoracic; *Prv*, right ventricular pressure.

[a] Mean values are given for continuous variables.

[b] Duration of exercise greater than 100% of normal for age.

[c] Duration of exercise 43% of normal for age.

■ **TABLE 24-20** **Exercise Performance under Standardized Conditions 1 or More Years after Repair of Tetralogy of Fallot, according to Right Ventricular Pressure and Presence of Pulmonary Regurgitation** [a]

Right Ventricular Pressure Range and Regurgitation	Duration of Exercise (% of Normal Controls) Mean ± SD	P (for Difference)
Prv <50 mmHg		
Pulmonary regurgitation: No	98 ± 20	
Pulmonary regurgitation: Yes	75 ± 8.9	<.05
Prv > 50 mmHg		
Pulmonary regurgitation: No	88 ± 16	
Pulmonary regurgitation: Yes	51 ± 30	<.02

(Data from Wessel and colleagues.[W2])

Key: *Prv*, Right ventricular pressure; *SD*, standard deviation.

[a] Exclusive of patients with residual ventricular septal defects.

Some asymptomatic patients have reduced exercise capacity,[D8,W2] some have normal functioning capacity as judged by quantitative testing (Table 24-19), and some have the capacity of a trained athlete.[W2] Some patients with normal response exercise to testing have other abnormalities, such as limitation in chronotropic response to exercise.[P17]

Risk factors for impaired exercise tolerance have been identified, and these include *age at repair.* Repair in the first 5 years of life results in a normal response to objective exercise testing.[J3,M15,P17] Patients averaging 12 years of age at operation have subnormal exercise capacity late postoperatively.[J3] *Residual RV hypertension,* expressed as Prv, $P_{RV/LV}$, or RV to pulmonary artery gradient, adversely affects functional status late after complete repair.[O3,P8,W2] Wessel and colleagues suggest that in the absence of other problems, Prv greater than 50 mmHg (corresponding roughly to $P_{RV/LV}$ greater than 0.7) is likely to exert this effect (Table 24-20) although Prv greater than 70 mmHg may be a more realistic number (indeed, the relation is likely continuous, but nonlinear).[W2] *Pulmonary valve regurgitation* after repair results in reduced exercise capacity regardless of RV systolic pressure.[D8,D19,M27,P8,R32,V7,W2] Consistent with this is the tendency of patients with transanular patches to have larger cardiothoracic ratios and RV volumes[E5] late postoperatively.

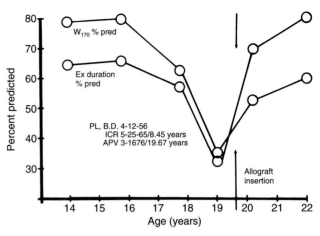

Figure 24-53 Results of serial exercise testing (work capacity above, exercise duration below, expressed as percentage of predicted value for age) after repair of tetralogy of Fallot with absent pulmonary valve. Intracardiac repair was performed without a valve in a patient age 8.45 years, and exercise and work capacity steadily decreased. An allograft pulmonary valve was inserted when the patient was 19 years old, with subsequent improvement in performance. (From Ilbawi and colleagues.[I1])

Key: *APV*, Allograft pulmonary valve; *B.D.*, birth date; *Ex*, Exercise; *ICR*, intracardiac repair; *PL*, patient identifier; *Pred*, predicted; *W*, work.

In patients who have undergone repair without insertion of a valve for TF with absent pulmonary valve (Section 3), subsequent insertion of a valve improves exercise capacity (Fig. 24-53).[I1] *Residual or recurrent VSDs* decrease exercise capacity.[W2,Z2] Furthermore, large residual or recurrent VSDs (Q̇p/Q̇s greater than 2) strongly predispose the patient to chronic heart failure late postoperatively.[R17]

Maximal oxygen uptake during exercise is only 30% to 40% of normal in patients corrected at an average age of 19.5 years.[B20] When repair is made at a still older age, the functional result is clearly worse than when it is performed in infancy or early childhood.[S5]

Right Ventricular Function

RV systolic and diastolic functions are variable late postoperatively and depend on preoperative status of the ventricle, extensiveness of the right ventriculotomy (if any) and muscular resection within the ventricle, care with which RV coronary arteries have been preserved, amount (if any) of postoperative RV systolic hypertension, and amount of pulmonary regurgitation. Relation of these to late RV systolic and diastolic function has not been well quantified, but general relations are evident.

Pulmonary regurgitation has its most evident effect on RV function. When a transanular patch has not been used and the pulmonary valve is competent, RV systolic function (ejection fraction) and end-diastolic volume may be normal late postoperatively.[B6,G1] However, even in this circumstance, RV ejection fraction may not increase normally with exercise (Fig. 24-54).[M31,R9] Global RV function (RV ejection fraction estimated by ventriculography) and contractile response to isoproterenol are better preserved after trans-

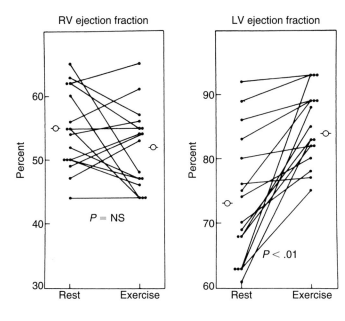

Figure 24-54 Right ventricular and left ventricular systolic function at rest and during exercise after repair of tetralogy of Fallot. Mean value for each set of data is indicated by open circle. (From Reduto and colleagues.[R9])

Key: *LV*, Left ventricular; *NS*, not significant; *RV*, right ventricular.

atrial repair than after transventricular repair when measured in the early postoperative period. Later clinical performance in the two groups is unknown.[M31] Also, in some patients with little or no pulmonary regurgitation, RV ejection fraction is depressed,[R27] no doubt related to other variables that affect it. When the pulmonary valve is regurgitant, RV systolic function and end-diastolic volume are less likely to be normal, and their decrement correlates with amount of regurgitation.[R27] When a transanular patch has been used in the repair, ejection fraction is more likely to be low, and RV end-diastolic volume is increased, often severely so (Fig. 24-55).[B15,F7,G1] However, it has been suggested that increased RV wall thickness and consequently decreased ventricular compliance may limit volume expansion and RV enlargement. Reduced compliance may also protect against detrimental effects of pulmonary valve regurgitation.[G27] Decrease in ejection fraction is correlated with the increase in end-diastolic volume.

Postrepair RV systolic and diastolic function and a resting systolic pressure up to 60 to 70 mmHg have little adverse effect. Higher systolic pressures produce dysfunction, but this is not well quantified.

Other potential determinants of postrepair RV function have not been correlated with it in a quantitative fashion.

Right Ventricular Aneurysms

RV aneurysms adversely affect RV function, but they are uncommon. Only 0.9% of patients having TF with pulmonary stenosis underwent reoperation for RV aneurysms in the UAB experience, and in all (three patients, two of whom had transanular patches), postrepair (OR) $P_{RV/LV}$ was greater than 0.79.

The aneurysm may be a false one, but it is usually a true aneurysm, presumably related to excessive thinning or devascularization of the RV free wall or thinning and bulging of pericardium if it has been used as an infundibular or transanular patch.[S6] The latter is rare; aneurysm of a pericardial transanular patch requiring reoperation developed in only one patient in the GLH experience in associa-

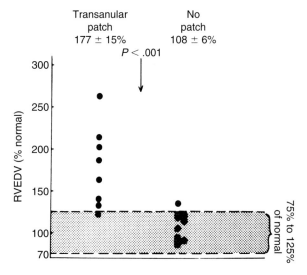

Figure 24-55 Right ventricular end-diastolic volume late after repair of tetralogy of Fallot. Patients are separated into those with and without a transanular patch. Stippled area represents normal values. (From Graham and colleagues.[G1])

Key: *RVEDV*, Right ventricular end-diastolic volume.

tion with a residual high P_{RV} caused by unrelieved bifurcation stenosis. Most RV aneurysms develop within 6 months of operation, and true aneurysms stabilize and rarely progress, whereas false ones may progress rapidly and rupture.[R11]

Residual Right Ventricular Outflow Obstruction

Residual narrowing in the infundibulum, at the RV–pulmonary trunk junction (with or without a transanular patch) or more distally, can result in at least some residual RV outflow obstruction. Magnitude of obstruction is not

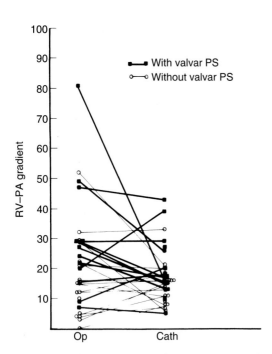

Figure 24-56 Right ventricular–pulmonary artery peak pressure gradient after repair of tetralogy of Fallot without a transanular patch. Thirty-three patients were operated on at age 2 to 8 years and restudied an average of 26 months later. All had low or midlevel infundibular stenosis. (From patients operated on at GLH.)

Key: *Cath,* Catheterization; *Op,* operation; *PA,* pulmonary artery; *PS,* pulmonary stenosis; *RV,* right ventricle.

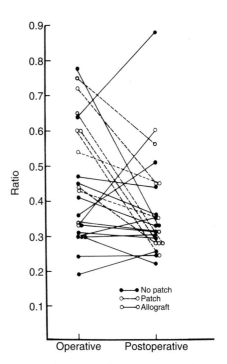

Figure 24-57 Right ventricular to aortic systolic pressure ratios (analogous to postrepair $P_{RV/LV}$) in the operating room after repair and at postoperative catheterization an average of 30 months later in 23 infants age 0.7 to 21 months at the time at operation. The child whose ratio increased to 0.87 had an inadequately relieved high-level infundibular and pulmonary "anulus" stenosis. (From Calder and colleagues.[C17])

Key: *Ratio,* Right ventricular to aortic peak pressure ratio.

evident at the end of operation, because both the gradient between the RV and distal pulmonary trunk and the postrepair $P_{RV/LV}$ are usually somewhat less late postoperatively than when measured in the operating room (Figs. 24-56 and 24-57).[B16] Dimensions of the RV–pulmonary junction grow, but proportionally to the growth of the child after repair, whether or not a transanular patch was used (Fig. 24-58). However, disproportionate growth of the "anulus" does not occur without a transanular patch, and it cannot be expected that an "anulus" that is relatively small preoperatively and intraoperatively will become normal sized late postoperatively (Table 24-21).

Progression of originally unimportant residual RV outflow obstruction to important obstruction occurs uncommonly. Stiffening, thickening, and eventually even calcification of pulmonary valve cusps may occur and produce increasing RV hypertension, whether they are left in an intact "anulus" or beneath a transanular patch.[H3]

Important residual or recurrent RV outflow obstruction is an indication for reintervention if the obstruction is considered treatable. This is because of its adverse effect on RV function, particularly when considerable pulmonary regurgitation coexists.[I5]

Reoperation and Other Reinterventions for Right Ventricular Outflow Problems

Reoperations and other reinterventions (percutaneous technique) are uncommonly required after repair of TF with pulmonary stenosis (Table 24-22).[K29]

Reoperations for pulmonary valvar regurgitation (insertion of a pulmonary valve) are of particular interest, because they relate to indications for transanular patching. They occur most frequently in patients in whom a transanular patch has been used, and rate of reoperation increases as time passes (Fig. 24-59).[K45] However, few patients in whom a transanular patch has been inserted have required reoperation, unless their postrepair (OR) $P_{RV/LV}$ was greater than about 0.7 (Fig. 24-60). Onset of symptoms including fatigue and dyspnea, ventricular arrhythmias, or tricuspid regurgitation in patients with pulmonary valve regurgitation should prompt consideration for reoperation. In the Toronto experience,[Y3] 85 patients (1.2% of total number repaired) underwent reoperation a mean of 12 years (range 0.4 to 36 years) following initial correction. A transanular patch had been used in 66%. In many of these patients (66%), pulmonary valve regurgitation was associated with another structural problem, and the latter might have been the primary reason for reoperation. Operative mortality was low (one patient, 1.2%; CL 0.2%-4.0%) and functional class improved.[Y3] Insertion of an allograft aortic or pulmonary valve may be indicated in this setting because it increases RV ejection fraction, decreases RV end-diastolic dimensions, and improves symptomatic status.[B33,F19]

Reoperation for residual pulmonary stenosis has been more common, but is still relatively rare, with 95% of patients being free from it for at least 20 years (see Fig. 24-61). Although rate of reoperation is highest early after

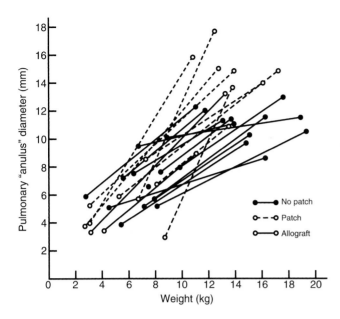

Figure 24-58   Diameter of right ventricular–pulmonary trunk junction ("anulus"), measured cineangiographically and corrected for magnification, in 23 infants age 0.7 to 21 months at repair. Leftward circle is immediately preoperative value, and rightward one is value obtained an average of 30 months later. (From Calder and colleagues.[C17])

■ **TABLE 24-21   Change in Size of the Right Ventricular–Pulmonary Trunk Junction ("Anulus") after Repair of Tetralogy of Fallot** [a]

	Pulmonary "Anulus"		
Type of Repair	**Z (Preop) Mean ± SD**	**Z (Late Postop) Mean ± SD**	**P (for Difference)**
No transanular patch or allograft (n = 12)	-2.2 ± 1.54	-2.0 ± 1.25	.7
Transanular patch (n = 11)	-2.4 ± 1.78	1.1 ± 1.77	.004

(Data from Calder and colleagues.[C17])

Key: *Postop,* Postoperative; *Preop,* preoperative; *SD,* standard deviation.

[a] Change over a 30-month period in 23 infants aged 0.7 to 21 months.

■ **TABLE 24-22   Reasons for Reintervention after Repair of Tetralogy of Fallot with Pulmonary Stenosis** [a]

Cause of Reintervention [b]	**No.**	**% of 757**
Persistent or recurrent RV outflow obstruction [c]	17	2
Pulmonary regurgitation	5	1
Residual or recurrent VSD	3	0.3
Large left-to-right shunt [d]	1	0.1
Valved conduit obstruction	2	0.2
Miscellaneous (four different categories)	4	1
TOTAL	32	4

Key: *RV,* Right ventricular; *VSD,* ventricular septal defect.

[a] Based on follow-up and analysis of 757 hospital survivors (UAB experience, 1967 to May 1986).

[b] Reoperation: n = 31; balloon dilatation, n = 1.

[c] Obstruction was isolated and in the infundibulum in 4, at anulus in 1, at bifurcation of pulmonary trunk in 2, at origin of one or both pulmonary arteries in 2, and at multiple sites in 4. In one person each, it was associated with a small ventricular septal defect (VSD), a right ventricular aneurysm, a small VSD and a right ventricular aneurysm, and severe tricuspid regurgitation.

[d] Through a recanalized classic Blalock-Taussig shunt and residual VSD.

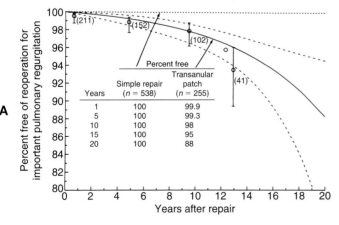

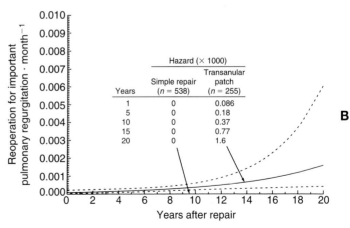

Figure 24-59   Reoperation (insertion of a xenograft or allograft pulmonary valve) for important pulmonary valvar regurgitation after repair of tetralogy of Fallot with pulmonary stenosis. **A,** Freedom from reoperation according to whether a transanular patch was used. Note greatly expanded vertical axis. Depiction is as in Fig. 24-44. **B,** Hazard function. (From Kirklin and colleagues.[K29])

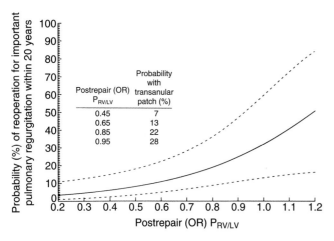

Figure 24-60 Nomogram illustrating effect of postrepair (OR) $P_{RV/LV}$ on probability of reoperation for pulmonary regurgitation within 20 years after repair of tetralogy of Fallot with pulmonary stenosis using a transanular patch. (Nomogram is specific solution of multivariable risk factor equation in original publication.) (From Kirklin and colleagues.[K29])

Key: *OR*, Operating room; $P_{RV/LV}$, ratio of peak pressure in right ventricle to that in left ventricle.

repair, there is a constant phase of hazard as well, lasting as long as patients have been followed (see Fig. 24-61). The higher the postrepair (OR) $P_{RV/LV}$, the greater the probability of this type of reintervention, and the prevalence increases particularly steeply when the value is greater than about 0.7 (Fig. 24-62).

Left Ventricular Function

LV systolic and diastolic function are variable late after operation. Risk factors for poor LV function include older age at repair, pre-repair status of LV (affected as it is by previous palliative operations), and residual or recurrent defects.

Patients undergoing repair during the first few years of life have normal or near-normal LV function not only at rest but also during stress.[B19,S8] Patients who are older at the time of repair[J1,O8] often have depressed LV ejection fraction at rest that intensifies during stress.[B19,J1] Less satisfactory function in patients undergoing repair at an older age may be due to myocardial damage from chronic preoperative hypoxia and to long-standing LV overload from systemic–pulmonary arterial shunts in most patients who are older at repair.[L13,R26]

The age range at repair within which late postoperative LV function at rest and during exercise can be expected to be normal is not clearly defined. Some studies indicate that it extends to only age 2 to 3 years,[B19,S8] while others suggest that it extends to as late as age 10 if shunting operations have not been necessary.[R9,R10]

Pulmonary Function

Patients with an optimal hemodynamic result from repair of TF in infancy or early childhood (closed VSD, P_{RV} less than 50 mmHg, and no pulmonary valve regurgitation)

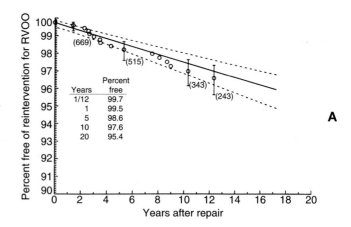

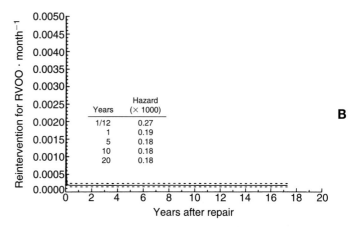

Figure 24-61 Reintervention for residual or recurrent right ventricular outflow obstruction after repair of tetralogy of Fallot with pulmonary stenosis (*n* = 793). (Based on the study used for Table 24-10, exclusive of those patients in whom a valved conduit was used in the repair [*n* = 21].) **A**, Time-related freedom from reintervention. Note greatly expanded vertical axis. Depiction is as in Fig. 24-44. **B**, Hazard function, which has a steeply declining early phase and a constant phase.

Key: *RVOO*, Right ventricular outflow obstruction.

have normal lung volumes and capacities late postoperatively.[G25,W7] Conversely, patients with a less than optimal hemodynamic result and those operated on later in life have distinctly subnormal lung function. Postoperative pulmonary valve regurgitation has a particularly adverse effect on late postoperative lung volume and function.[W7]

Recurrent (Residual) Ventricular Septal Defects

Important recurrent or residual VSDs are uncommon, with reoperation being necessary in less than 1% of cases in the UAB experience.[K11] Even small and hemodynamically unimportant leakage is infrequent.[B17] Routine left ventriculography done an average of 23 months postoperatively in 23 infants showed a tiny residual VSD in one (4%; CL 0.6%-14%).[C17] Others have reported small leakage in up to 10% of patients.[A3]

When important shunts are present, they are usually from inaccurate repair or dehiscence at the posteroinferior angle of the VSD.[C5]

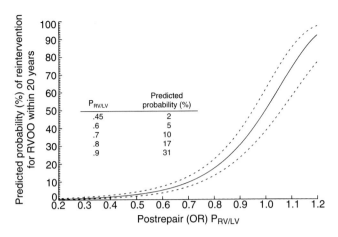

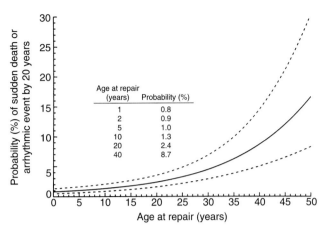

Figure 24-62 Nomogram illustrating relationship between postrepair (OR) $P_{RV/LV}$ and probability of reintervention for right ventricular outflow obstruction within 20 years. Analysis is based on 814 patients undergoing repair of tetralogy of Fallot and pulmonary stenosis at UAB from 1967 to May 1986. (Nomogram is specific solution of multivariable risk factor equation represented by Appendix Table 24C-5.) (From Kirklin and colleagues.[K29])

Key: *OR,* Operating room; *$P_{RV/LV}$,* ratio of peak pressure in right ventricle to that in left ventricle; *RVOO,* right ventricular outflow obstruction.

Figure 24-63 Nomogram illustrating relationship between age at repair and probability of sudden death or an important arrhythmic event within 20 years of repair of tetralogy of Fallot with pulmonary stenosis. (Multivariable equation is a specific solution of multivariable risk factor equation in original publication, as are values entered for other variables equation.) (From Kirklin and colleagues.[K30])

Sudden Death and Important Arrhythmic Events

There has been much discussion about the possibility of sudden or arrhythmic death late after repair of TF with pulmonary stenosis,[G18,H5,Q1] but there is a lack of information about the circumstances under which this is likely to occur.

These events are more likely to occur in patients *not operated on in early life* and are unlikely when patients are repaired in the first few years of life.[D12,S26,T8] Thus, probability of sudden death or an important arrhythmic event (defined as a clearly arrhythmic death, intractable ventricular tachycardia, or insertion of a pacemaker for bradycardia developing late postoperatively) within 20 years of repair has occurred in less than 1% of patients who were younger than age 5 years at operation (Fig. 24-63).[K30] When the patient underwent repair in adult life, probability was 5% to 10%. Castaneda and colleagues have found no sudden deaths and no important ventricular electrical instability in long-term follow-up of patients undergoing repair in infancy.[C19,C20,W9] Others have reported similar experiences with the relation between age and prevalence of sudden death late postoperatively.[K23,K27]

When *repairs are incomplete,* and particularly when this results in postoperative cardiomegaly, prevalence of ventricular arrhythmias and sudden death is higher.[W5] During long-term follow-up of the early Mayo Clinic patients, only 2% experienced sudden death; most had important cardiomegaly.[F3] Similar findings have been reported by others.[K25,W2]

When there is *important residual pulmonary stenosis,* prevalence of late postoperative arrhythmic events may be somewhat higher,[G5,G6] but the correlation is weak. Strong correlation has been demonstrated between *pulmonary re-*

gurgitation and important ventricular arrhythmias late postoperatively.[Z6]

Rarely, the *right ventriculotomy scar* may be arrhythmogenic. This should be considered as a possibility in patients with life-threatening ventricular arrhythmias only when cardiomegaly is absent and there is neither important pressure nor volume overload of the RV. Under these circumstances, electrophysiologic mapping is indicated; when the source of the arrhythmia can be localized to the right ventriculotomy scar, excising the scar and inserting a patch graft have been reported to be beneficial.

Infective Endocarditis

Infective endocarditis is rare after repair. No instances were observed in the 10-year follow-up of 414 patients by Katz and colleagues[K10] nor in the combined Boston Children's Hospital–UAB study.[K19]

Interim Results after Classic Shunting Operations

Survival

Classic B-T and PTFE interposition shunts have a hospital mortality approaching zero when done for palliation of TF with pulmonary stenosis (Table 24-23).[K9] Even in the first month of life, hospital mortality was 0.6% (CL 0.1%-2.3%) in the UAB experience. Similarly low risks have been reported by other groups.[A4,A8,B32,G11,I3,K28,L17,S2,T3]

Other types of shunting operations have a higher hospital mortality, in part because the shunt rather easily becomes too large or too small. Arciniegas and colleagues found hospital mortality after the Waterston shunt to be more than twice that after the B-T shunt.[A4]

■ **TABLE 24-23   Hospital Mortality after First-stage Palliative Operations for Tetralogy of Fallot** [a]

| | Pulmonary Stenosis | | | | Pulmonary Atresia | | | | Total | | | |
| | | Hospital Deaths | | | | Hospital Deaths | | | | Hospital Deaths | | |
Shunt	n	No.	%	CL (%)	n	No.	%	CL (%)	n	No.	%	CL (%)
Classic B-T	44	0	0	0-4	40 [b]	4	10	5-17	84	4	5	2-9
PTFE interposition	9	0	0	0-19	11	2 [c]	18	6-38	20	2	10	3-22
TOTAL	53	0	0	0-4	51	6	12	7-18	104	6	6	3-9
Waterston	17	4	24	12-39	6	2	33	12-62	23	6	26	16-39
Palliative RV–PT connection												
Transanular patch	2	1	50	7-93	6	2	33	12-62	8	3	38	17-62
Valved conduit	0	–	–		1	0	0	0-85	1	0	0	0-85
Miscellaneous	1	0	0	0-85	4	0	0	0-38	5	0	0	0-32
TOTAL	73 [d]	5	7	4-11	68 [d]	10	15	10-21	141	15	11	8-14

Key: *B-T*, Blalock-Taussig; *CL*, 70% confidence limits; *PT*, pulmonary trunk; *PTFE*, polytetrafluoroethylene; *RV*, right ventricle.

[a] Based on 141 patients undergoing palliative operations (UAB experience, 1967 to July 1982).

[b] Ages 1, 3 days, 1.7, 3 months.

[c] Ages 2, 3 days.

[d] In addition, 1 patient with pulmonary stenosis survived both inadvertent left subclavian artery anastomosis to left pulmonary vein and later complete repair; 1 patient with pulmonary atresia had polytetrafluoroethylene interposition graft inadvertently to AP collateral artery and died after central shunt 1 day later.

Probably the most important risk factor for early death after classic shunting procedures is *pulmonary arterial problems.*[K22]

Young age adds an increment of risk to shunting operations, but a relatively small one (Fig. 24-64).

Interim Events

Early (less than 30 days) *nonfatal shunt closure* or narrowing occurs uncommonly (7%) in patients undergoing classic B-T or PTFE interposition shunt operations.

Intermediate-term shunt closure or narrowing requiring reoperation occurs in 3% to 20% of heterogeneous groups of infants and children (Table 24-24).[B32,D4,D10,K22,M11] Closure or important narrowing is considerably more common in neonates and young infants than in older patients (74% versus 90% freedom at 2 years).[K22] However, closure may be less common in neonates and young infants when a PTFE interposition graft is used.[U1] Overall, shunt closure or narrowing results in unsatisfactory palliation within 3 years of shunting in about 40% of patients.[C22] This prevalence does not seem to differ among patients receiving a classic B-T shunt and those receiving a PTFE interposition graft.[C22] Use of aspirin seemingly does not increase long-term patency or reduce occurrence of localized shunt stenosis.[C23]

One manifestation of *reduced blood flow* in the arm on the side of a classic B-T shunt is that it becomes slightly shorter and smaller during the intermediate term after operation.[H9] Likewise, strength of the arm on the side of the shunt has been demonstrated to be less than normal, even though the patient is unaware of this.[Z5] When blood flow reduction is more severe than usual, gangrene of the hand can occur, although rarely (see Table 24-24).

Sudden death, without explanation or autopsy, is uncommon after classic shunting procedures. It occurred 4 months after operation in one patient in the UAB experience. Nonfatal brain abscess is also uncommon, occurring in one patient in that experience. These two events represent a prevalence of 1.9% (CL 0.6%-4.5%) of patients undergoing classic shunting operations for TF.[K9] A similar low preva-

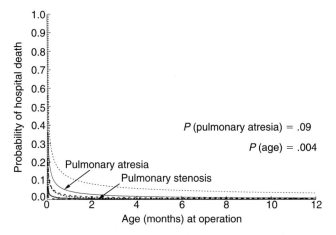

Figure 24-64   Nomogram of illustrating effect of age on hospital mortality after repair of tetralogy of Fallot with pulmonary atresia versus pulmonary stenosis in patients with previous classic shunts. (Nomogram is specific solution of multivariable risk factor equation in original publication. Values entered for other variables are also given in original publication.) (From Kirklin and colleagues.[K9])

lence of unfavorable interim events has been reported by others.[A2,S2] Improperly performed shunts of any kind result in a higher prevalence of unsatisfactory interim results primarily because of iatrogenic pulmonary arterial problems.

Iatrogenic pulmonary arterial problems are probably uncommon after classic shunting or PTFE interposition shunting operations. For example, none was identified in the UAB experience or by Bove and colleagues.[B32] However in the present era, because shunts are done more frequently in patients with small pulmonary arteries, especially neonates, angiographic evidence of pulmonary artery distortion is fairly common late postoperatively and must be dealt with at the time of repair.[G28] Problems occur

■ **TABLE 24-24   Events Other than Hospital Death after One-Stage Classic Shunting Operation for Tetralogy of Fallot** [a]

Event	Pulmonary Stenosis (n = 53)			Pulmonary Atresia (n = 51)			Total (n = 104)		
	No.	%	CL (%)	No.	%	CL (%)	No.	%	CL (%)
Early (<30 days) shunt closure, with successful reoperation	4	8	4-13	3	6	3-11	7 [b]	7	4-10
Premature repair because of shunt closure	2	4	1-9	1	2.0	0.3-6.5	3	2.9	1.3-5.7
Later shunting operations	0	0	0-4	7 [c]	14	9-21	7	7	4-10
Sudden death	1 [d]	1.9	0.2-6.3	0	0	0-4	1	1.0	0.1-3.2
Brain abscess	1 [e]	1.9	0.2-6.3	0	0	0-4	1	1.0	0.1-3.2
Gangrene of hand	1	1.9	0.2-6.3	0	0	0-4	1	1.0	0.1-3.2

Key: CL, 70% confidence limits.

[a] Based on 104 hospital survivors (UAB experience, 1967 to July 1982).

[b] None occurred after 1979; none had initial polytetrafluoroethylene interposition shunts; three were younger than 30 days old.

[c] None for shunt closure.

[d] Four months postoperatively, cause unknown; date of operation 1980.

[e] Nonfatal; age 28 months at shunt in 1971; occurred 15 months postoperatively.

after Waterston shunts, and their prevalence varies from 16%[G13,P6,R14,T2] to 64%[N5] of cases.

The key *beneficial interim results* of shunting procedures are increased $\dot{Q}p$, with consequent reduction in cyanosis and polycythemia, and improved functional capacity. NYHA functional class is usually I or II after shunting. SaO_2 at rest is usually 80% to 90%, but it always decreases with exercise, at times to as low as 50%.[H9,J2] These benefits are obtained at the expense of increased LV stroke volume, a stimulus to gradual development of LV dysfunction.

Another benefit of classic shunting procedures is diffuse increase in size of the RPA and LPA.[G12,K17] and to some extent of the pulmonary "anulus" and pulmonary trunk.[R24] These enlargements may occasionally be enough to allow subsequent repair to be done without a transanular patch.[V4] (Enlargement of the "anulus" and pulmonary trunk is even greater after a Waterston anastomosis,[A11] but the higher prevalence of iatrogenic pulmonary arterial problems offsets this advantage.)

Occasionally, severe infundibular or valvar stenoses becomes complete atresia after a palliative shunting operation.[F10,M12,R12] This, however, does not complicate later repair.

Important pulmonary vascular disease may develop after a classic B-T shunt but rarely before 7 years have passed.[H10] Beyond this time, the proportion of patients developing hypertensive pulmonary vascular disease increases with increasing shunt duration[D3,H11,R12] and is still greater after a Potts anastomosis[C8,V3]; again, however, the prevalence is time related, and important pulmonary vascular disease is uncommon before 5 years.[N8]

INDICATIONS FOR OPERATION

Diagnosis of TF is generally an indication for repair. When diagnosis is made in the first 3 months of life and the infant is importantly symptomatic, prompt one-stage repair may be indicated. Early repair is advisable because of the unfavorable natural history of the disease, particularly in the first year of life (see Fig. 24-21), advantages of repair before irreversible secondary myocardial and pulmonary changes occur, and low risks of repair in

the current era. When severe symptoms develop in the first 1 or 2 months of life, an initial shunting operation followed within 12 months by repair is a reasonable alternative.

When diagnosis is made early in life and the patient is essentially asymptomatic or only mildly symptomatic, and the morphology of the TF is uncomplicated, one-stage repair is deferred until age 3 to 24 months.

Overall results with a two-stage protocol with an initial shunting operation for patients younger than about age 6 months and repair between age 6 and 24 months appear to be similar to those of one-stage repair, although such a protocol is not ideal.[K19] However, two-stage repair is probably prudent for institutions not well prepared for the intraoperative and early postoperative care required by neonates and small children undergoing intracardiac operations. It is also reasonable for surgeons who are not yet certain of their ability to achieve comparable results with one-stage repair in neonates and infants younger than about age 6 months.

When the LAD arises from the RCA, repair can be accomplished with usual techniques unless a transanular patch is required. Thus, its presence in a neonate or infant need not affect indications for operation unless study demonstrates possible need for a transanular patch. Then, a systemic–pulmonary arterial shunt is indicated in small symptomatic patients, with the hope of deferring repair and probable insertion of an allograft valved conduit until age 3 to 5 years, when a reasonable-sized one can be used. This deferral may not be necessary if techniques for conduit growth prove to be clinically effective.[S18] In the unusual circumstance of severe stenosis of the distal pulmonary trunk and origins of the RPA and LPA, deferral might be considered for similar reasons, although a one-stage non-conduit repair is often successful.

Multiplicity of VSDs in very young patients increases the risk of repair. Closure of apical muscular defects can often be accomplished percutaneously (see "Percutaneous Closure of Ventricular Septal Defects" under Special Situations and Controversies in Chapter 21). Thus, an initial shunting operation may be prudent, with subsequent percutaneous closure of muscular VSDs, followed by repair.

SPECIAL SITUATIONS AND CONTROVERSIES

Rationale for Use of Postrepair P$_{RV/LV}$

P$_{RV/LV}$ is easily measured in the operating room after repair, and therefore, when pulmonary artery pressure is known to be low, it is a convenient way of assessing adequacy of relief of pulmonary stenosis. It has the disadvantage of being difficult to measure late postoperatively, so in its place the ratio of peak P$_{RV}$ to peak radial, femoral, or aortic pressure is generally used. P$_{RV/LV}$ is neither better nor worse for assessing relief of pulmonary stenosis than is the theoretically more useful gradient between RV and pulmonary artery. This, too, has disadvantages: (1) measuring pulmonary artery pressure distal to the last stenotic lesion (which may be in the hilar portion of the RPA or LPA) can be difficult in the operating room or early postoperatively[L8] and (2) interpreting the gradient requires measuring flow through the area, which is not easily accessible in the operating room. The scanty data available concerning the relationship both of the postrepair (OR) RV–pulmonary artery gradient to that of the next day or late postoperatively[G17,L8,S1] and of the gradient to late results are compatible with information and conclusions drawn from postrepair P$_{RV/LV}$. P$_{RV}$ alone is perhaps the least useful measurement, because by itself it conveys no information about the possible effect of the patient's hemodynamic state on the measurement.

Postrepair P$_{RV/LV}$ is related to pulmonary arteriolar resistance, size of the RPA and LPA,[M14] presence and severity of localized or segmental stenoses or incomplete distributions of the pulmonary arteries, and residual pulmonary trunk or RV outflow obstructions. It is also related to flow through the RV outflow tract, which is increased postoperatively by residual left-to-right shunting across the VSD and by pulmonary valve regurgitation.

Initial Palliative Operations

The classic B-T shunt, performed using the subclavian artery arising from the innominate artery on the side opposite that of the aortic arch, is used by some as the initial palliative procedure except in infants younger than 2 to 3 months of age. However, in most institutions a PTFE interposition shunt between innominate or subclavian artery and pulmonary artery via a median sternotomy is preferred in all age groups. This operation, using older PTFE (Teflon) or polyester rather than PTFE (Gore-Tex), was reported by Klinner in 1961[K14,K18] and later by de Leval and colleagues.[D6] The PTFE shunt, introduced by Gazzaniga and colleagues in 1976,[G15,G16] is reliable even in very young infants, with few late occlusions (see "Interim Results after Classic Shunting Operations" earlier in this section).

Although at one time the Waterston ascending aorta–RPA shunt was popular, most groups find it has higher mortality in infants,[A4,D1] a considerably higher proportion of iatrogenic RPA problems, and a relatively high prevalence of late pulmonary hypertension because of excessive Q̇p.[G13] The same disadvantages pertain for the Potts descending aorta–LPA anastomosis[D3] in addition, it is more difficult to perform than other shunts and more difficult to close later.

A central shunt between ascending aorta and pulmonary trunk has, in most instances, no advantage over a properly performed laterally placed PTFE interposition shunt.

Initial Palliation by Beta-Adrenergic Blockade

The possible advantage of beta-adrenergic blockade with, for example, propranolol therapy for severe cyanosis and hypoxic spells in early infancy is that surgery may be deferred. Disadvantages are that propranolol does not always provide good palliation, and risk of repair may be higher in patients who are taking it.

Honey and colleagues showed in 1964 that beta-adrenergic-blockade usually alleviates paroxysmal hypoxic spells,[H4] and this has been confirmed by many others.[C7,K13,P4] When doses of about 2.5 mg · kg^{-1} · day^{-1} of propranolol are used, relief of the hypoxic spells for at least 3 months occurs in 80% of patients.[G4] However, Garson and colleagues found this regimen to be more effective in patients older than 1 year, when it could be considered unnecessary, and less successful in infants age 6 months or less.[G4] However, their conclusion was that the drug was effective in very young patients if the dose was adequate (2 to 6 mg · kg^{-1} · day^{-1} and serum propranolol levels about 100 ng · mL^{-1}).

Initial Palliation by Balloon Valvotomy

Percutaneous balloon dilatation of the infundibulum and pulmonary valve, and percutaneous infundibular myectomy, have been reported to provide good relief of cyanosis and symptoms, with little risk, in some small patients.[B28,Q2,Q3,S19] However, the reports are anecdotal, and risks and effectiveness of the procedure in safely deferring repair remain to be clearly defined.

Monocusp Valves beneath Transanular Patches

Many informal reports suggest that constructing monocusp valves, usually made of pericardium, beneath a transanular patch is of value.[A15,F7,I2,M13,S11,Z1] These usually support the idea that these valves are competent in the early postrepair period but that they usually become regurgitant later, but over the long term they do not appear to result in less pulmonary regurgitation than does a simple transanular patch.[G29,R15] Subsequent calcification of the cusp is potentially obstructive. Some enthusiastic formal reports have appeared,[P17] but evidence favoring their use is not persuasive.

SECTION 2 ▮▮▮▮▮▮▮▮

Tetralogy of Fallot with Pulmonary Atresia

DEFINITION

The definition of TF with pulmonary stenosis applies to TF with pulmonary atresia, except that in the latter there is no luminal continuity between the RV and pulmonary trunk (or both RPA and LPA). Atresia is usually congenital but may be acquired.

HISTORICAL NOTE

As noted in Section 1, Lillehei and colleagues first successfully repaired TF, and their original paper included a patient with pulmonary atresia.[L3] Rastelli and Kirklin reported the first use of an RV–pulmonary trunk extracardiac conduit to repair this anomaly in 1965.[R1] Ross and Somerville first reported use of a valved conduit for this purpose in 1966,[R19] as did Weldon and colleagues soon thereafter.[W3] Enlarging very hypoplastic pulmonary arteries by increasing pulmonary artery pressure and flow using a conduit connecting the RV to pulmonary arteries or by a systemic–pulmonary arterial shunt was reported by McGoon and colleagues and Kirklin and colleagues in 1977.[G14,K17]

The important role of large AP collateral arteries in many patients having TF with pulmonary atresia appears to have been first addressed in a constructive manner by Macartney and colleagues.[M16] These investigators reported on the hemodynamic characteristics of these arteries in 1973[M16] and again in 1974.[M17] They introduced the concept of a multifocal blood supply to the pulmonary circulation through both the central pulmonary arteries and large AP collateral arteries.[M17] In 1980, Haworth and Macartney described in detail the large AP collateral arteries supplying blood to some pulmonary arterial segments by end-to-end anastomosis, and to others by end-to-side anastomosis.[H12] By then, the UAB group had described, in 1978, the adverse effect of incomplete distribution (arborization) of the pulmonary arteries on survival after repair of TF with pulmonary atresia.[A7] In 1981, Haworth, Macartney, and colleagues introduced the concept of unifocalization of pulmonary arterial supply as a first step to repair in patients with multifocal supply and large AP collateral arteries.[H14] Subsequently the surgical results of these procedures have accumulated (see "Results after Staged Palliative Operations for Unifocalization" later in this section). The systematic approach of one-stage complete repair in infancy involving bilateral unifocalization and intracardiac repair via median sternotomy was introduced by Reddy and Hanley in 1992 and reported in 1995.[R34] Percutaneous catheter dilatation of localized stenoses in the RPA and LPA was reported by Lock and colleagues in 1983,[L11] and closure of large AP collateral arteries using this technique was reported by Yamamoto and colleagues in 1979.[Y2]

MORPHOLOGY

Tetralogy of Fallot with Congenital Pulmonary Atresia

General morphology of the heart in TF with pulmonary atresia is similar to that in TF with pulmonary stenosis. The most important differences are that in TF with pulmonary atresia,

- No blood passes from RV to lungs; consequently, all pulmonary blood flow arises from the ductus arteriosus, collateral vessels, or fistulae
- Pulmonary arterial anomalies are common
- Large AP collateral arteries are common

Right Ventricular Outflow Tract

The atresia, when congenital, may be in the infundibular area or at the RV–pulmonary trunk junction ("anulus").

Infundibular atresia is the most severe manifestation of RV outflow atresia in TF, occurring in about 70% of hearts with TF and pulmonary atresia.[A12] The RV infundibulum seems to be totally absent in such cases (and these may be analogous to cases of TF with pulmonary stenosis and subarterial VSD), or the conal septal elements may be present but nearly fused with the anterior RV free wall (Fig. 24-65). The VSD is usually large and extends nearly to the free wall of the RV anteriorly, as does the aortic valve. The RV in such hearts is usually massively hypertrophied.

When the *atresia is at the RV–pulmonary trunk junction,* the infundibulum is usually present, but the pathway is narrowed by marked hypertrophy of the infundibular structures (Fig. 24-66). Obstruction consists of a thick fibrous membrane (analog of the pulmonary valve) above the infundibulum. Length and width of the infundibulum is variable.

Pulmonary Trunk

The pulmonary trunk may be present and of reasonable size, but more commonly it is importantly hypoplastic (Fig. 24-67). Occasionally, it is represented by only a fibrous cord without a lumen. In about 5% of patients, it appears to be completely absent.[A17]

No clear correlation has been developed between location and type of atresia and morphology of the pulmonary trunk.

An unusual variation of pulmonary trunk morphology has been recognized with increasing frequency recently, especially in patients with arborization abnormalities of the pulmonary artery branches. In this variant, the pulmonary trunk arises from the proximal coronary artery system. Origins from the left main, right, and circumflex coronaries have all been identified.[A18] The true prevalence of this variant is not known, because most cases have been reported in isolation or in small groups[B36,K39,M32,W12,Y4]; however, when systematically sought in a population of patients with arborization abnormalities of the pulmonary artery branches, it has been found to occur in up to 10%.[A18]

Right and Left Pulmonary Arteries

Confluence of right and left pulmonary arteries. About 20% to 30% of patients have nonconfluent RPAs and LPAs (discontinuity).[E1] This usually results from absence of the central portion of one or both of these arteries.[S20] Rarely, it is caused by atresia of at least the distal pulmonary trunk and origins of both pulmonary arteries. (Patients having TF with pulmonary stenosis rarely have discontinuity of the RPA and LPA.)

Confluent RPA and LPA may be associated with either a patent or atretic pulmonary trunk.

Stenoses of origins of pulmonary arteries. Among patients with confluence of RPA and LPA, about 10% have stenosis of the origin (central portion) of the RPA and about 20% have stenosis of the LPA.[S20] The latter anomaly seems clearly related to the extension onto the LPA of the process of ductal closure.[E9]

Distribution (arborization) of pulmonary arteries. An important feature of the morphology of TF with pulmonary atresia is the frequent failure of the pulmonary arteries to distribute to all 20 pulmonary vascular segments.[A7,H12,S20] In this regard, patients with relatively

Figure 24-65   Specimen of tetralogy of Fallot with congenital infundibular atresia. Conal (infundibular) septum is small and divisions of the septal band (trabecula septomarginalis) prominent. The ventricular septal defect is perimembranous but extends anteriorly and superiorly almost to anterior free wall of ventricle. The danger of inadvertently cutting into the aortic root when making the right ventriculotomy is evident. There is marked overriding of noncoronary aortic cusp.

Key: *FW,* Anterior free wall; *L,* left coronary cusp of aortic valve; *LA,* left anterior division of septal band; *N,* noncoronary cusp of aortic valve; *R,* right coronary cusp of aortic valve; *RP,* right posterior division of septal band; *SB,* septal band (trabecula septomarginalis); *TV,* tricuspid valve.

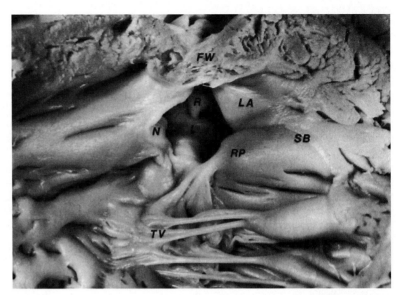

Figure 24-66   Autopsy specimen of tetralogy of Fallot with pulmonary atresia from a newborn. Anterior and leftward displacement of septal end of an unusually bulky conal (infundibular) septum is shown, inserting in front of left anterior division of septal band rather than between the two septal band divisions. Anterior and leftward deviation of parietal end of conal septum is also obvious, with the septum lying partway between a coronal and sagittal plane. There is a diminutive blind right ventricular outflow tract *(arrow)* in front of the conal septum.

Key: *CS,* Conal (infundibular) septum; *FW,* anterior free wall; *LA,* left anterior division of septal band; *LC,* left coronary cusp of aortic valve; *P,* parietal end of conal (infundibular) septum; *RP,* right posterior division of septal band; *SB,* septal band (trabecula septomarginalis); *TV,* tricuspid valve.

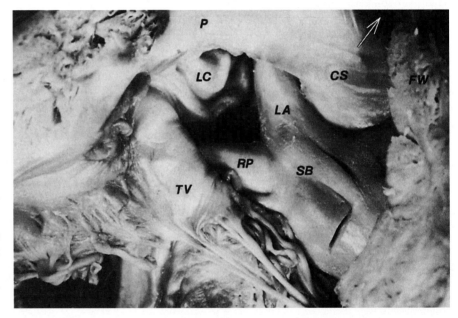

normal caliber confluent central portions of the RPA and LPA are very different from those with either hypoplastic confluent branches or nonconfluent ones. In fact, patients who have a pulmonary trunk and normal caliber confluent RPA and LPA and valvar pulmonary atresia usually receive pulmonary blood flow from the ductus arteriosus, rarely have incomplete distribution of the RPA or LPA, and rarely have large AP collateral arteries.[H12]

Distribution of the pulmonary arteries is complete to all 20 pulmonary arterial segments in slightly more than half (53%; CL 48%-58%)[S20] the patients with confluent RPA and LPA, and normal distribution is associated with relatively normal caliber of the confluent LPA and RPA (Table 24-25). In contrast, more than 80% of those with nonconfluent RPA and LPA or confluent but hypoplastic pulmo-

nary arteries have incomplete distribution of one or both arteries, and in slightly more than one third of this group less than 10 pulmonary vascular segments are in continuity with a central or proximal extrapericardial portion of an ipsilateral pulmonary artery[S20] (see Table 24-25). Pulmonary arterial segments that are not connected to a central pulmonary artery usually receive large AP collateral arteries. In contrast, most patients having TF with pulmonary stenosis have all 20 pulmonary arterial segments in continuity with a central or proximal extrapericardial portion of an ipsilateral pulmonary artery.

Stenoses of pulmonary arteries.   Stenoses of the pulmonary arteries beyond their origins are identified in only a small percentage of cases. However, when these small pulmonary arteries are subjected to increased pressure and

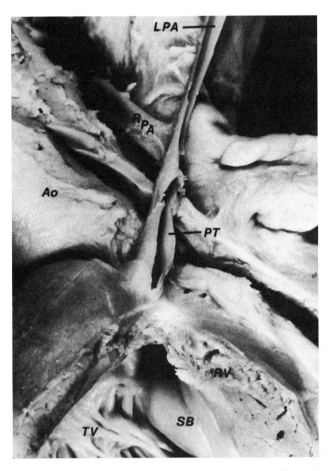

Figure 24-67 Autopsy specimen of tetralogy of Fallot with congenital pulmonary atresia (same specimen as Fig. 24-65). Proximally, the pulmonary trunk ends blindly; distally, it extends directly into small left pulmonary artery. By contrast, the right pulmonary artery arises almost at right angles from pulmonary trunk.

Key: *Ao*, Aorta; *LPA*, left pulmonary artery; *PT*, pulmonary trunk; *RPA*, right pulmonary artery; *RV*, opened right ventricular anterior wall; *SB*, septal band (trabecula septomarginalis); *TV*, tricuspid valve.

◨ TABLE 24-25 Confluence or Nonconfluence of Central Pulmonary Arteries and Number of Pulmonary Artery Segments Centrally Connected in Patients with Tetralogy of Fallot with Pulmonary Atresia

No. of Pulmonary Artery Segments	Confluent (n = 132)		Nonconfluent [a] (n = 28)	
	No. of Patients	%	No. of Patients	%
20	62	47	5	18
19	8	6	2	7
18	8	6	2	7
17	13	10	0	0
16	6	5	0	0
15	8	6	0	0
14	6	5	1	4
13	6	5	0	0
12	5	4	0	0
11	4	3	0	0
10	2	2	8	29
9	2	4	1	4
8	0	0	0	0
7	0	0	2	7
6	1	1	0	0
5	0	0 *(4 (3%))*	1	4 *(10 (36%))*
4	1	1	0	0
3	0	0	0	0
2	0	0	0	0
1	0	0	0	0
0	0	0	6	21
TOTAL	132	100	28	100

(Data from Shimazaki and colleagues.[S20])

[a] Absence of one or both central pulmonary arteries.

flow after a palliative or corrective operation, they may enlarge in some areas and not in others.[F8,H14,K18] Thus, localized areas of noncompliance in the pulmonary arterial walls may not present as stenoses until after a procedure that increases pulmonary blood flow.

Overall, stenoses are most common at the origin of the pulmonary artery on the side of the ductus arteriosus. Such juxtaductal stenoses (pulmonary artery coarctations) were found in 65% of patients studied by Elzenga and colleagues.[E11]

Size of pulmonary arteries. The immediately prebranching portion of the RPA and LPA varies widely, from normal caliber in some patients to extremely small in others, with McGoon ratios[P3] of about 0.5 (Table 24-26), which corresponds to a Nakata index[N12] of about 20 and a Z value of about −10. These dimensions are particularly small in the subset with discontinuity (nonconfluence) of the RPA and LPA (see Table 24-26).[S20] In a subset of

patients, intrapericardial pulmonary arteries are completely absent. In general, patients with TF with pulmonary atresia have considerably smaller RPA and LPA than do those with TF with pulmonary stenosis; in the latter group, these dimensions are not very different from those in normal individuals.[B1,S16,S20]

Abnormal hilar branching patterns. Even when the pulmonary arteries distribute to all parts of the right and left lung, hilar branching patterns may be abnormal, particularly in patients with large AP collateral arteries.

Alternative Sources of Pulmonary Blood Flow

Large aortopulmonary collateral arteries. The most dramatic route of collateral flow is through large AP collateral arteries, which are present in about two thirds of patients with TF having pulmonary atresia (Fig. 24-68).[S20] In this context, "large" implies embryologic rather than acquired origin of the collaterals, the latter typically resulting in smaller, more numerous collateral vessels. Large collaterals occur rarely in TF with pulmonary stenosis. AP collateral arteries are large, discrete arteries, typically from one to six in number but sometimes more, originating from the upper or mid-descending thoracic aorta.[R4] They generally pursue a somewhat serpiginous course, occasionally passing through the esophageal wall, and most commonly terminate by joining an interlobar or intralobar pulmonary artery that arborizes normally within a pulmonary lobe or segment.[H12,M16] Occasionally a collateral originates from the intraabdominal aorta.

■ **TABLE 24-26** McGoon Ratio in Patients with Tetralogy of Fallot vs. Normal Subjects

$\frac{D_{RPA} + D_{LPA}}{D_{DescAo}}$ (McGoon Ratio)		TF with Pulmonary Atresia				TF with Pulmonary Stenosis (n = 85)		Normal (n = 21)	
		Confluent Central Pulmonary Arteries (n = 117)		Nonconfluent Central Pulmonary Arteries [a] (n = 15)					
≤ ratio <		No.	%	No.	%	No.	%	No.	%
	0.50	6	5	4	27	0	0	0	0
0.50	0.75	20	17	2	13	0	0	0	0
0.75	1.00	22	19	4	27	1	1	0	0
1.00	1.25	23	20	2	13	1	1	0	0
1.25	1.50	16	14	0	0	3	4	0	0
1.50	2.0	22	19	2	13	24	28	6	29
2.0	2.5	4	3	0	0	39	46	14	67
2.5		4	3	1	7	17	20	1	5
Subtotal		117	100	15	100	85	100	21	100
Missing Data		15		13		0		0	
TOTAL		132		28		85		21	

(Data from Shimazaki and colleagues.[S20])

Key: *D*, Diameter; *DescAo*, descending aorta; *LPA*, left pulmonary artery; *RPA*, right pulmonary artery; *TF*, tetralogy of Fallot.

[a] Absence of one or both.

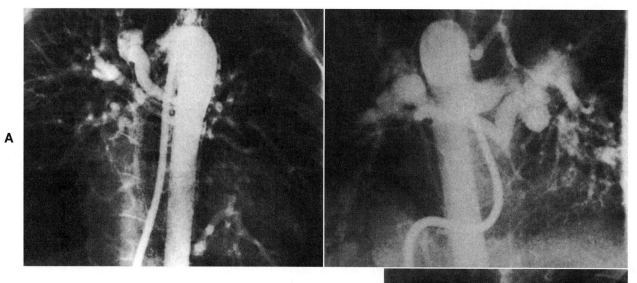

Figure 24-68 Large aortopulmonary (AP) collateral arteries in tetralogy of Fallot with pulmonary atresia. **A,** Two large AP collateral arteries come off right and anterior aspects of upper descending thoracic aorta and connect end to end with hilar arteries of right upper lobe. A smaller collateral artery supplies part of the lingula of left lower lobe. **B,** Large AP collateral artery passes to the left and joins end to side to hilar portion of left pulmonary artery (LPA) in a manifold. The Y-shaped distal pulmonary trunk and central LPA and right pulmonary artery (RPA) fill from this manifold. Another large AP collateral passes to the right above RPA. **C,** Branches of large AP collateral artery join end to end with hilar branches to left upper lobe, left lower lobe, and right lower lobe.

AP collateral arteries arise from the aorta either as elastic vessels with a wide lumen or as muscular arteries with stenotic areas.[H15] In either event, beyond their origins they resemble muscular systemic arteries. Areas of intimal proliferation (intimal pads) are frequent and result in stenoses. Extensive areas of these are prominent at branching points and at the junction of AP collateral arteries with pulmonary arteries. This process eventually results in stenoses in about 60% of collateral arteries.[H12,M18,M19] In most patients, stenoses are sufficient in number to prevent pulmonary overcirculation; when this is not the case, pulmonary overcirculation is present early in life, and pulmonary vascular disease develops in patients surviving past infancy.[H15,H16,T4] Even in the absence of clinical overcirculation, however, an unobstructed collateral may cause pulmonary vascular disease in the area of the lung it supplies.

Although stenoses are undoubtedly primarily related to structural abnormalities in the collateral vessel wall in some cases, in others they are clearly acquired, the result of abnormal postnatal flow patterns. Severe stenoses have been documented angiographically in patients as young as age 3 to 4 months in vessels that showed normal caliber at neonatal angiography.[R35] Stenoses can evolve quite variably and unpredictably.

An AP collateral artery that joins end to end with an intrapulmonary artery changes in histologic appearance as it becomes a pulmonary artery and changes its positional relation to the bronchi. Thus, peripherally, its histologic appearance and position become typical for "true" pulmonary arteries.[H12] In this situation the distal pulmonary arterial branches may be abnormally small[H12] and fewer in number than in normal individuals.

In about 50% of patients with large AP collateral arteries, the collateral enters end to side into a complex manifold in the hilum of the lung. This manifold usually includes the hilar portion of the pulmonary artery, and from this manifold interlobar and intralobar pulmonary arteries distribute distally, and central pulmonary arteries may fill retrogradely.[F11] In other cases the collateral distribution distally into the lung does not communicate with the central pulmonary artery system.

Less commonly, an AP collateral artery may connect end to side to a central pulmonary artery. Rarely, a single AP collateral artery on each side connects end to end with the hilar portion of the ipsilateral pulmonary artery.[J4,M17] It is this last form that gave origin to the appellation "truncus type IV."

AP collateral arteries are usually associated with abnormal branching patterns and incomplete distribution of the hilar portion of the pulmonary arteries. There may be associated single or multiple, localized or segmental pulmonary arterial stenoses, or diffuse hypoplasia.[H12,O1]

Paramediastinal collateral arteries. A large right or left paramediastinal collateral artery occasionally arises from the right or left subclavian artery, most often on the side opposite that of the aortic arch, and cineangiographically closely resembles a surgically created B-T shunt. It usually connects end to side to the right or left central or hilar pulmonary artery, but it may distribute end to end to the intrapulmonary arteries of the upper lobe. It may be difficult to distinguish such a collateral from an unusually positioned and tortuous patent ductus

arteriosus if the collateral is the sole vascular supply to one lung.

These collateral arteries usually occur in patients who have TF with pulmonary atresia, but they are found, uncommonly, in those with pulmonary stenosis.

Bronchial collateral arteries. Most patients with TF with pulmonary atresia (as well as some with pulmonary stenosis) have a diffusely enlarged network of bronchial collateral arteries. These provide a nondiscrete source of pulmonary blood flow; in some patients, particularly older and deeply cyanotic individuals, the collateral blood flow through them is large.

Increased use of various collateral arteries in surgical reconstruction has stimulated their careful pathologic evaluation. This seems to suggest that distinction between bronchial collaterals and other AP collaterals, and between intraparenchymal and extraparenchymal vessels, is simplistic; rather, the course and structure of those vessels is highly variable and unpredictable. This observation corresponds to recent embryologic evidence that AP collateral artery formation can occur over relatively extended periods during development.[D17]

Intercostal collateral arteries. When pleural adhesions develop spontaneously or because of a previous thoracotomy or poudrage treatment, a large amount of flow may pass to the lungs through acquired collaterals originating from the intercostal arteries, and extensive rib notching then develops. This collateral circulation may be so well developed as to make even the most careful mobilization of the lung hazardous and, on rare occasions, impossible without exsanguinating hemorrhage. Such situations are not encountered in infants who have not undergone previous surgical procedures.

Other collaterals. Small collateral channels may pass from coronary arteries to the bronchial arteries.[D5] Relatively large communications between the proximal right or left coronary artery and the central pulmonary artery confluence occur in up to 10% of cases.[A18] In rare cases a *fistula* between RCA and pulmonary trunk may be the sole large collateral source of pulmonary blood flow in TF with pulmonary atresia.[K21] Even more rarely, an aortopulmonary window may serve this function (see Chapter 30).[C2]

Iatrogenically aggravated collaterals. After a classic B-T shunt a large collateral arterial supply develops to the arm on the side of the shunt and parts of it eventually become collateral pulmonary blood flow. Large collateral arteries may develop between the two internal thoracic arteries as part of this, and these may produce massive bleeding at sternotomy.

Ductus Arteriosus

In patients having TF with pulmonary atresia in the absence of AP collaterals, pulmonary circulation at birth is dependent on ductal flow to the site of pulmonary artery confluence. Ductus orientation and position are usually abnormal—a downwardly directed branch coming from beneath the left aortic arch.[C18] It is also longer and more tortuous than is otherwise the case (Fig. 24-69) and is often narrowed at its pulmonary end. In the setting of left aortic arch, a right-sided patent ductus arteriosus is rare. When present, it comes off the right subclavian or innominate artery, or, if associated with an aberrant right subclavian

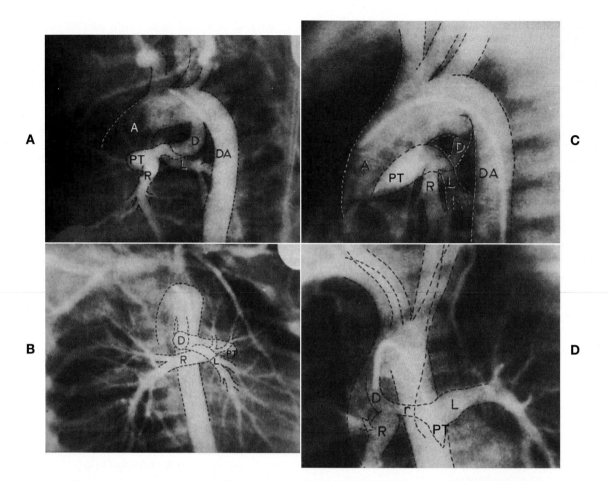

Figure 24-69 Arch aortography in tetralogy of Fallot (TF) with pulmonary atresia. Cineangiograms in (**A**) left anterior oblique (LAO) and (**B**) right anterior oblique projections show typical orientation of a left patent ductus arteriosus with left aortic arch. Ductus joins origin of left pulmonary artery (LPA). Contrast medium fills pulmonary trunk and right pulmonary artery (RPA) as well. LAO view shows normal (usual) brachiocephalic artery origins. Cineangiograms in lateral (**C**) and frontal (**D**) projections show typical orientation of patent ductus arteriosus when aortic arch is right sided. Here the right-sided ductus arises from distal arch to join the RPA. Contrast medium also fills the pulmonary trunk and LPA through narrowed proximal RPA.

Key: A, Ascending aorta; D, patent ductus arteriosus; DA, descending aorta; L, left pulmonary artery; PT, pulmonary trunk; R, right pulmonary artery; r, proximal right pulmonary artery.

artery, it may come from an aortic diverticulum and pass to the right behind the esophagus (see Fig. 24-17).

When the pulmonary arteries are confluent, presence of large (embryologic rather than acquired) AP collaterals essentially always means that there will not be a ductus arteriosus. When the pulmonary arteries are not confluent, a ductus arteriosus may or may not be present. When present, it provides flow to one entire lung (usually the left), while the other receives flow through AP collaterals. In this situation the ductus connects to a normally arborizing branch pulmonary artery, and no other AP collateral vessels supply the ipsilateral lung.

Tetralogy of Fallot with Acquired Pulmonary Atresia

Pulmonary atresia may develop spontaneously after birth in patients born with TF with pulmonary stenosis, or its development may be stimulated by a palliative operation.[F10,N6] Ac-

quired atresia is usually valvar, but it may develop in the immediately subvalvar region or in the os infundibulum. TF with this type of pulmonary atresia has the morphologic characteristics of TF with pulmonary stenosis.

CLINICAL FEATURES AND DIAGNOSTIC CRITERIA

When the patient has TF with congenital pulmonary atresia and no AP or other large collateral arteries, cyanosis is usually evident during the first few days of life, becoming extreme as the ductus narrows and closes. This rapid progression is modified when there are large collaterals supplying the pulmonary bed, when the ductus stays open, or when an operation is performed. Infants with pulmonary atresia and large AP collateral arteries have only mild cyanosis at birth. In a few, presentation is with heart failure, which usually develops at age 4 to 6 weeks as neonatal Rp decreases and Q̇p becomes large.

Primary and secondary airway problems have been recognized with increasing frequency. The reasons are many, including upper airway extrinsic compression from a large aorta or collateral vessel[M33] to small airway hyper-responsiveness.[A12]

Another feature that distinguishes patients having TF with pulmonary atresia from those having TF with pulmonary stenosis is the association of pulmonary atresia with chromosome 22q11 deletion. The association is particularly high in those with pulmonary artery arborization abnormalities and large AP collaterals.[A14,C24,D18,H25,M34] This deletion is associated with clinical evidence of DiGeorge syndrome, or velocardiofacial syndrome, in approximately 90% of cases. In those cases, careful consideration must be given to the typical immunologic, calcium metabolism, and neurodevelopmental abnormalities that may be part of this syndrome.

Children who first present at an older age are usually symptomatic, cyanotic, and polycythemic no matter what the source of collateral blood flow, because it has become inadequate by that time.

Physical examination discloses findings similar to those of patients who have TF with pulmonary stenosis. In pulmonary atresia, however, a systolic murmur is usually absent. There is frequently a continuous murmur from large AP collateral arteries, a patent ductus arteriosus, or rarely a coronary–pulmonary artery fistula.[O2] This murmur is maximal over the site of the collateral at its point of stenosis and may therefore be heard to the left or right of the sternum or posteriorly.

Clinical presentation, examination, and special studies are similar to those described for TF with pulmonary stenosis, with some important distinctions.

Echocardiography

Echocardiography is diagnostic for all cases of TF with pulmonary atresia, but it is definitive only if confluent normal caliber branch pulmonary arteries connected to a patent ductus arteriosis can be identified.

Angiography

Angiography should be performed at birth in all patients with an echocardiographic diagnosis of TF with pulmonary atresia and non–duct-dependent pulmonary blood flow as just defined. The origin, course, and distribution of every collateral should be clearly identified. Characterization of the collateral blood supply to a given lung segment should be further assessed to determine whether the collateral vessel provides the sole blood supply or is part of dual or multiple sources of blood flow coming from other collaterals or from the central or "true" pulmonary arteries. Further assessment is performed to identify whether any of the sources of blood supply come from a ductus arteriosus or the coronary artery system. Central and peripheral stenoses are identified both external to and within the lung parenchyma. Finally, specific effort should be made to fully characterize the central true pulmonary arteries using specific collateral and pulmonary wedge injections. Only after this level of definition is achieved can an appropriate surgical management plan be formulated.

Although clinical status of the patient and specifics of the management plan may influence the need for repeat study at any time, in almost all cases repeat cardiac catheterization and detailed angiography are required in a matter of months. The reason may be to reevaluate an infant at age 3 to 4 months, immediately before a one-stage unifocalization and intracardiac repair, because collaterals may change dramatically in the first few months of life, or it may be to assess the results of a previous palliative procedure performed in the neonatal period. Clinical stability (i.e., a thriving infant with SaO$_2$ of 80% ± 5%) is not an indication to postpone cardiac catheterization. Such infants are likely to have important maldistribution of pulmonary blood flow despite their clinical stability, putting some lung segments at risk of developing pulmonary vascular disease due to overcirculation and other segments at risk of being lost due to collateral occlusion.

In patients with ductus-dependent pulmonary blood flow with normally developed confluent pulmonary arteries, early repeat catheterization is typically not necessary, whether the initial neonatal procedure was one-stage repair or shunt placement. Although cardiac catheterization and standard angiography are absolute necessities in the workup of TF with pulmonary atresia and complex pulmonary arteries, newer imaging modalities, such as angiography combined with three-dimensional computed tomography or magnetic resonance imaging, currently provide an adjunctive role and may eventually take on increasing diagnostic importance in defining the complex morphology of abnormal pulmonary arteries and AP collaterals.[L20] Echocardiography is important in defining the intracardiac morphology, but has a subordinate role in the arterial assessment.[S33]

NATURAL HISTORY

The natural history of patients with TF and congenital pulmonary atresia cannot be described simply, in part because of the great variability of morphology.[M20] This is reflected in the more complex hazard function for death compared with that for TF and pulmonary stenosis (see Fig. 23-20, *C*).[B13] It consists of a short-lasting early hazard phase considerably more acute than for TF with pulmonary stenosis, that merges with a constant hazard phase (exponentially decreasing survival) that lasts to about age 50, followed by an increasing late hazard (with wide confidence limits). Unfortunately, morphologic characteristics of the anomaly corresponding to early death were not available to Bertranou and colleagues for their study of natural history, nor is it certain that reported groups of patients were a reasonably unselected sample of all patients born with this condition. This is particularly unfortunate in this condition, because treatment for some subsets of patients is not optimal and noninterventional therapy may be a reasonable option.

Nevertheless, knowledge of the pathophysiology of the anomaly suggests that the shape of the natural history hazard function (see Fig. 24-21, *C*) may result from a mixture of different morphologic and physiologic subgroups that have been conveniently formed because of their surgical significance.

- *Confluent and normally distributing RPA and patent ductus arteriosus.* In this group the only source of pulmonary blood flow is a patent ductus arteriosus, and the RPA and LPA are confluent, usually minimally hypoplastic, and distribute to all 20 pulmonary arterial segments.

- *Confluent RPA and LPA distributing to the majority of pulmonary arterial segments.* In this group the pulmonary arteries are confluent, often moderately or severely hypoplastic, and distribute to the majority of the pulmonary arterial segments, but not all; some large AP collateral arteries are present.
- *Confluent or nonconfluent RPA and LPA distributing to a minority of pulmonary arterial segments.* In this group, in which the RPA and LPA may or may not be confluent, the majority (and at times all) of pulmonary arterial segments are not connected to the central pulmonary arteries, but are supplied by large AP collateral arteries.[D15]

Although there is a discrete separation between the first and second groups defined by the normal pulmonary artery distribution and complete absence of collaterals in group one, the second and third groups blend together imperceptibly.

Natural History of Pathophysiologic Subgroups

Confluent and Normally Distributing Right and Left Pulmonary Arteries and Patent Ductus Arteriosus

At least 50% of patients are in this category. The ductus arteriosus appears to have its usual tendency to close, albeit probably more slowly than normal; without treatment, half of this group is probably dead of hypoxia by age 6 months and 90% by age 1 year.

Confluent Right and Left Pulmonary Arteries Distributing to the Majority of Pulmonary Arterial Segments

About 25% of patients are in this category. The distribution, or arborization, abnormality of the confluent central pulmonary arteries almost always indicates an absent ductus arteriosus. Cyanosis and symptoms may develop, depending on the number, size, and behavior of collateral vessels, but not as quickly or as severely as in the first group. Without interventional therapy, 10% of this group may die within the first few years of life, half by age 3 to 5 years, and 90% by age 10.

Confluent or Nonconfluent Right and Left Pulmonary Arteries Distributing to Minority of Pulmonary Arterial Segments

About 25% of patients are in this category, with AP collateral arteries supplying the majority (and occasionally all) of the pulmonary arterial segments. These patients often have a large Q̇p early after birth, but only rarely large enough to produce severe symptoms and signs of heart failure. Often they are mildly cyanotic and essentially asymptomatic in the early years of life, and the majority probably survive in reasonably good health until the age of about 15 years. Cyanosis often then begins to worsen, and without interventional therapy, probably most are dead by about age 30 years. The similarity of their course to that of patients with Eisenmenger syndrome is apparent.

Occasionally in the setting of nonconfluent RPA and LPA, a ductus arteriosus gives rise to a normally arborizing, typically left, pulmonary artery. The ductus closes rapidly following birth, and the natural history depends on adequacy of collateral supply to the right lung; ductal closure may be silent clinically if right-sided collateral flow is generous.

Pulmonary Arterial Disease

Patients with pulmonary atresia and AP collateral arteries probably differ from other patients with TF in the matter of pulmonary arterial disease. The phrase *pulmonary arterial disease,* rather than "pulmonary vascular disease," is used because of uncertainty regarding how much of their increased pulmonary vascular resistance is due to hypoplasia and stenoses of the distal pulmonary arteries themselves and of the distal portions of the AP collateral arteries, and how much is due to hypertensive pulmonary vascular disease.[R18] In any event, evidence suggests that pulmonary arterial disease tends to develop in those pulmonary arterial segments that are centrally connected and that it progresses at a considerably accelerated rate, and perhaps even in fetal life or in the first few months after birth, in segments whose only, or major, source of pulmonary blood flow is large AP collateral arteries.[S21] Patients who survive without correction into the second and third decades of life often develop massive and sometimes fatal hemoptysis related to the large AP collaterals.[K38]

In previous editions of this book, the phrase pulmonary *vasculature* resistance, as opposed to pulmonary *vascular* resistance, was used to denote this same concept.

TECHNIQUE OF OPERATION

Repair of Tetralogy of Fallot with Acquired Pulmonary Atresia

Occasionally, and particularly in patients with pulmonary atresia that has developed after a shunting procedure, atresia is at the level of the infundibulum. The operation described for TF with pulmonary stenosis can then be done (see "Technique of Operation" in Section 1), often without a transanular patch. When acquired atresia is at the pulmonary "anulus" and the pulmonary trunk is present (which it usually is), a transanular patch repair can be used, as described below under "Repair of Tetralogy of Fallot with Pulmonary Atresia and Confluent and Normally Distributing Right and Left Pulmonary Arteries and Patent Ductus Arteriosus." In about 90% of patients with TF and *acquired* pulmonary atresia, these straightforward repairs are feasible.

Repair of Tetralogy of Fallot with Pulmonary Atresia and Confluent and Normally Distributing Right and Left Pulmonary Arteries and Patent Ductus Arteriosus

This operation is usually performed in neonates and young infants in whom atresia is usually at the pulmonary "anulus," and the pulmonary trunk and confluence of the RPA and LPA are usually patent and of reasonable size. Occasionally, it is performed in older infants and in children who have been palliated by a shunting operation early in life.

Operation proceeds much as described in Section 1 (see "Decision and Technique for Transanular Patching" and "Repair of Uncomplicated Tetralogy of Fallot with Pulmonary Stenosis via the Right Ventricle" under Technique of Operation). A difference is that the patent ductus arteriosus must be controlled and that the transanular patch, if used, is contoured differently. Commonly a valved conduit is used instead.

Aortic cannulation is accomplished in the usual fashion using a single venous cannula or two venous cannulae inserted directly into the cavae (see "Venous Cannulation" under Preparation for Cardiopulmonary Bypass in Section 3 of Chapter 2). CPB is established at about 34°C so that cardiac action remains good and the large pulmonary venous blood flow (because of the ductus) is well handled by the beating LV. With the heart decompressed by CPB, the ductus arteriosus is expeditiously dissected and closed with two ligatures (see "Closure of Associated Patent Ductus Arteriosus" in Technique of Operation in Section 1 of Chapter 21). Alternatively, the ductus is carefully dissected and suture ligatures positioned prior to beginning CPB. The ligations are tied as CPB is begun. The aortic root catheter is inserted, cold cardioplegia is established (see "Cold Cardioplegia, Controlled Aortic Root Reperfusion, and [When Needed] Warm Cardioplegic Induction" in Chapter 3), the perfusate is made cold, and the procedure described in Section 1 begins.

Preferably, a valved conduit is used to connect RV to pulmonary trunk as described under "Establishing Right Ventricle to Pulmonary Artery Continuity" later in this section.

Although the lumens of the RV and pulmonary trunk are separated by an atretic area, it may be possible in some cases to make a single vertical incision in the RV infundibulum and extend it through the atresia and to an appropriate point distally on the pulmonary trunk. Sufficient tissue is present posteriorly at the site of the atresia that growth of the area should proceed satisfactorily. The transanular patch must be appropriately contoured at the atretic area to accomplish satisfactory widening. Great care is taken to avoid damage to the LAD and RCA by the patch suture line. Severe pulmonary regurgitation will be present immediately when this technique is used. Remainder of operation, including closure of the VSD, is completed as described in Section 1.

Repair of Tetralogy of Fallot with Pulmonary Atresia and Large Aortopulmonary Collaterals

Vascular supply of blood to the lungs in this condition represents, arguably, the most variable and complex "lesion," both morphologically and physiologically, in congenital heart disease. As such, no single operative approach is applicable to all patients. That having been said, recent techniques have been developed, supported by mid-term follow-up data, demonstrating that a majority of patients with TF with pulmonary atresia and large AP collaterals can be managed with one-stage repair in early infancy, involving left and right lung unifocalization, VSD closure, and RV outflow tract reconstruction.[L21,M35-M38,R34,R35,T9]

This approach can be applied to patients having relatively large confluent true pulmonary arteries, minor or moderate arborization abnormalities, severely hypoplastic confluent true pulmonary arteries with major arborization abnormalities and dominant collaterals, or completely absent intrapericardial true pulmonary arteries and collaterals only.

There are specific subpopulations, both morphologic and physiologic, in which the one-stage approach is contraindicated; these are discussed under "Alternatives to One-Stage Unifocalization and Intracardiac Repair" under Special Situations and Controversies later in this section. It should also be emphasized that individual surgeons selectively use one-stage repair based on morphologic details and their own experience.[C25,I7,M37,P18,P21,R36,R37,S27,W13]

One-Stage Unifocalization and Intracardiac Repair

In the text that follows, various components of the operation are described, including preliminary procedures leading up to it. These components include:

■ Assessing intrapericardial true pulmonary artery system
■ Identifying and assessing collateral system
■ Managing sources of pulmonary blood flow on CPB
■ Completing unifocalization
■ Assessing adequacy of unifocalization
■ Performing intracardiac repair
■ Establishing RV to pulmonary arterial continuity
■ Assessing complete repair

This procedure is typically performed in infants at approximately 3 to 4 months of age. Occasionally, it is performed in neonates or younger infants whose condition is unstable because of either profound cyanosis or severe pulmonary overcirculation, or in whom there is a ductus arteriosus providing blood flow to one of the lungs with collateral supply to the contralateral lung.[R34]

Exposure is through median sternotomy. The skin incision is extended from the suprasternal notch to well below the xiphoid to provide adequate exposure for the extensive dissection that is necessary. If a thymus gland is present, it is subtotally removed, leaving a small remnant of thymic lobes above the innominate vein. The pericardium is opened anteriorly with a longitudinal incision; a piece of anterior pericardium may be removed and treated in glutaraldehyde for later use in the operation (see footnote 2, "Pericardial Patch Preparation," under Technique of Operation in Chapter 16).

Assessing true pulmonary artery system. The first task is to assess the intrapericardial true pulmonary artery system. Commonly there are confluent and very hypoplastic central pulmonary arteries with a small pulmonary trunk segment that ends blindly at the level of an atretic pulmonary valve (Fig. 24-70). The pulmonary trunk and branch pulmonary arteries are dissected over their entire course beginning centrally and moving to the periphery, clearly identifying major branches of the RPA and LPA as they enter the lung parenchyma.

Identifying and assessing collateral system. The next task is to identify and assess the collateral system. This requires a clear mental image of it based on careful study of the preoperative angiograms. This part of the procedure is variable and depends on the number and positions of large collateral arteries. Each large collateral artery is identified at its systemic source and dissected over its entire length to

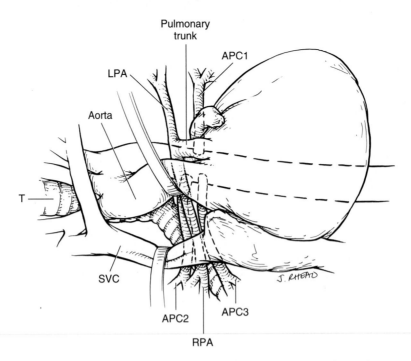

Figure 24-70 Anatomy of tetralogy of Fallot with pulmonary atresia, hypoplastic confluent central pulmonary arteries, and large aortopulmonary collateral arteries. This illustration provides a single example; however, it should be emphasized that extreme variability in number, origin, course, and size of large collateral arteries and true pulmonary arteries is found.

Small pulmonary trunk extends to atretic pulmonary valve and is physically connected to the infundibulum. True pulmonary arteries are confluent and severely hypoplastic, and these central pulmonary arteries have limited distribution to the lungs. True left pulmonary artery *(LPA)* bifurcates to upper lobe and lingula only, and true right pulmonary artery *(RPA)* distributes to upper and middle lobes only. Three collateral vessels are present: one distributes to the left lower lobe (APC1) and two distribute to the right lung, one to the right upper lobe (APC2) and one to right lower lobe (APC3). Note that APC2 communicates with upper branch of true RPA, whereas APC1 and 3 have no proximal communication to true RPA and LPA. Thus, the right upper lung field is said to have "dual-supply" blood flow from both the collateral system (APC2) and the true RPA, while the left upper lung field has isolated blood supply from the true LPA, and the right lower lobe and left lower lobe have isolated blood supply, each from one collateral.

Prior to beginning cardiopulmonary bypass *(CPB)*, true pulmonary arteries and all major collaterals are identified at their origin and dissected throughout their course until the vessels enter lung parenchyma. This often requires extensive dissection. Although collateral arteries may arise from many systemic arterial sites (see text for detailed description), the most common site of origin is the upper descending thoracic aorta, as illustrated. These collaterals are best identified, dissected, and rerouted for unifocalization by working through the central mediastinum as shown. Based on evaluation of preoperative angiograms, it may be beneficial to dissect and identify all major communications between collateral vessels and true pulmonary arteries.

As illustrated, ascending aorta is retracted anteriorly and to the left, either with a rigid retractor or a heavy stay suture placed into the adventitia. The superior vena cava *(SVC)* is mobilized completely, and commonly the azygos vein is ligated and divided. The SVC is then retracted laterally to the right. This exposes the central mediastinum in the midline. If true central pulmonary arteries are present, these are fully dissected first so they can be mobilized, allowing direct dissection into the central mediastinum. To accomplish this, pericardial reflection in transverse sinus is opened in the midline, and the space below tracheal bifurcation and above dome of left atrium is entered. Dissection transitions from central to posterior mediastinum, and upper thoracic descending aorta and esophagus are completely exposed. Collateral arteries are encountered in this dissection, and their origins from the upper thoracic aorta are easily identified. These collaterals are then dissected along their entire course until they enter lung parenchyma. It should be noted that collateral arteries commonly pass superficially through esophageal musculature; this must be recognized during the process of collateral dissection to avoid injuring the esophagus. Collaterals are commonly intertwined with secondary vagal nerve fibers, and it may be necessary to divide these to fully mobilize the collateral arteries. Once the true pulmonary arteries and all the collateral vessels have been fully identified and mobilized, preparation is made for CPB.

Key: Ao, Aorta; *APC,* aortopulmonary collateral artery; *LPA,* left pulmonary artery; *PT,* pulmonary trunk; *RPA,* right true pulmonary artery; *SVC,* superior vena cava; *T,* trachea.

the point where it enters the lung parenchyma. The specific approach to each collateral depends on its point of origin. The most common site of origin is the upper descending aorta with the collaterals coursing anteriorly through the posterior mediastinum into the middle mediastinum and then into the lung hilum (see Fig. 24-70). It is best to approach these collaterals through direct mediastinal dissection rather than by entering the pleural space. With the ascending aorta retracted anteriorly and to the left and the superior vena cava retracted to the right (see Fig. 24-70), the posterior pericardial reflection is opened in the midline within the space bordered above by the tracheal bifurcation and below by the dome of the left atrium. If confluent central pulmonary arteries are present, it may be necessary to work around them as the posterior dissection proceeds. Once the posterior pericardium is opened and the soft tissue of the posterior mediastinum is entered, collateral vessels are easily identified. Further posterior dissection exposes the esophagus and descending aorta, allowing access to the origin of collaterals that arise from this aortic position (see Fig. 24-70).

Occasionally, large collateral arteries arise lower on the descending aorta or from the major head and neck vessels. Those arising from head and neck arteries can be accessed directly by dissecting the artery of origin and then exposing the collateral along its length until it enters lung parenchyma. Collaterals originating from the lower thoracic and occasionally intraabdominally are best exposed by opening the appropriate pleural space anterior to the phrenic nerve and gently retracting the lung out of the pleural space to expose the descending aorta and collateral origin. These lower collaterals may enter the hilum of the lung directly or travel in the inferior pulmonary ligament before entering the lung parenchyma. It is not uncommon for collateral vessels to pass through the muscle of the esophagus before entering the lung tissue.

Managing sources of pulmonary blood flow in cardiopulmonary bypass. Once the true pulmonary artery system and all collateral vessels have been identified and fully dissected, cannulation sutures are placed in preparation for CPB. Aortic and bicaval cannulation are standard (see Section 3 of Chapter 2). After full heparinization and aortic cannulation, but before venous cannulation, collateral vessels are rapidly ligated at their aortic or systemic vessel origin using appropriately sized permanent metal clips. Then, venous cannulation and CPB are initiated. Patients with TF generally have a large intracardiac return during repair because of large collateral flow to the pulmonary arteries; those with pulmonary atresia, and especially those with the large AP collateral arteries, may have a particularly large intracardiac return requiring special consideration. Thus, an important goal in patients who will be placed on CPB is to have control of as much pulmonary blood flow as possible. The surgeon should be aware of all sources of pulmonary flow. This is accomplished by detailed review of the preoperative cardiac catheterization and angiographic data. Possible sources include the ductus arteriosus, surgically created systemic–pulmonary arterial shunts, large AP collateral arteries, and acquired AP collaterals. Before commencing CPB, all sources should be surgically identified and dissected to the degree that instantaneous control can be achieved. This is most easily accomplished with the

ductus or with surgically created shunts. Although more difficult, it is also possible to dissect the origin of all large AP collaterals as described in the preceding text. Acquired collaterals, usually smaller in size but more numerous and diffuse, pose the greatest challenge. They usually arise from the internal thoracic artery, intercostal arteries, bronchial arteries, or other unnamed mediastinal vessels. If previous surgery has been performed, acquired collaterals may form at sites of pleural fusion. Some, and sometimes many, acquired collaterals can be coil occluded by an interventional cardiologist at preoperative catheterization. The surgeon should attempt to control remaining acquired collaterals during the operation before placing the patient on CPB (still, it is not unusual for intracardiac return to increase once CPB is established).

CPB is established with the perfusate at about 34°C and with ionized calcium at a normal level, so that ventricular fibrillation does not occur before proper preparations are made for managing intracardiac return. After aortic and bicaval cannulation is accomplished, CPB is slowly established with the heart continuing to beat vigorously. An LV vent of appropriate size (No. 10 French for patients weighing 4.0 kg or less; No. 13 French for patients weighing 4 to 10 kg; adult size for patients weighing more than 10 kg) is placed via a purse-string suture into the right upper pulmonary vein and the vent tip is passed across the mitral valve into the LV. At this point, full CPB and vigorous venting are established, and immediately all sources of pulmonary blood flow, previously identified and dissected at their systemic origin, are permanently closed using metal clips. If appropriate pre-CPB dissection has been accomplished, all major sources, including complex situations with up to eight large AP collaterals, can be controlled in 30 to 90 seconds. Commonly, especially in patients with baseline SaO_2 greater than 80%, a substantial portion of the multiple sources can be closed before initiation of CPB, with this process limited only by decrease in SaO_2. It is not unusual, particularly if the patient is in early infancy and has not undergone prior palliation, for these maneuvers to reduce intracardiac return to normal levels.

In older children who have been chronically cyanotic or palliated, acquired collateral vessels from the systemic to the pulmonary circulation have often developed. In these cases, control of the embryologic large AP collaterals may still leave substantial cardiac return through the acquired collaterals. Then, a larger LV vent and higher perfusion flow rates may be needed to account for the abnormally high runoff. Once CPB is established, perfusion temperature is gradually reduced, aiming for a core body temperature of 25°C.

In addition to these precautions against damage from large intracardiac return, cerebral perfusion can be further maintained at an adequate level by blood gas control despite rapid aortic runoff. Arterial P_{CO_2} is maintained at 45 mmHg or greater to maximize cerebral blood flow.

Completing unifocalization. The next task is to complete the unifocalization process. This again depends on number and positions of the collateral arteries and status of the central pulmonary artery system. Most collateral arteries can be connected directly to the central pulmonary artery system by working within the central mediastinal space previously dissected. Most commonly, long side-to-side anastomoses between the collaterals and true pulmonary arteries, extending from a midline position all the way to the periphery where the arteries enter the lung parenchyma, are performed using No. 7-0 absorbable monofilament suture (Fig. 24-71). Occasionally, collateral arteries arising from head and neck vessels or from much lower on the descending thoracic aorta can be connected in end-to-side fashion to the central system. Collateral arteries are usually connected to the superior–posterior, direct posterior, or inferior–posterior circumferential aspect of the central pulmonary artery system, leaving its anterior aspect untouched. Typically, collateral vessels that are candidates for unifocalization will not reach the true pulmonary artery easily if the collateral artery is rerouted over the hilum of the lung, and this technique is avoided.

Once all collateral vessels have been unifocalized, it is often beneficial to incise the remaining anterior aspect of the central true pulmonary arteries from left hilum to right hilum and then patch them with a segment of cryopreserved allograft pulmonary artery. In this fashion a completely unifocalized pulmonary artery system, with newly reconstructed branch pulmonary arteries that are of normal or even supranormal diameter, can be achieved with no areas of circumferential pulmonary artery patch throughout the system.

If there is complete absence of true pulmonary arteries within the pericardium, then collateral vessels from the right and left lungs can be easily connected to each other across the midline within the central mediastinal space. Most frequently, all ipsilateral collateral vessels are first connected to one another with long side-to-side anastomoses, with the anastomoses beginning at the transected systemic end of the collaterals and extending to the lung parenchyma. Then, the left side is connected to the right, achieving complete unifocalization and left–right confluence. Occasionally the older child or young adult will present as a good candidate for unifocalization. In this case more liberal use of circumferential synthetic material (no growth potential) is acceptable (see Fig. 24-72). This should be avoided if possible in the growing infant and child.

Assessing adequacy of unifocalization. Once unifocalization is complete, an assessment must be made regarding whether the pulmonary artery system will have adequately low resistance to allow intracardiac repair with subsequent low RV and pulmonary artery pressure. Following intracardiac repair, peak RV pressure should be less than 60% of peak systemic arterial pressure. Experienced surgeons can often predict this by size of the true pulmonary arteries and collateral arteries and adequacy of the unifocalization. In such cases, proceeding directly to intracardiac repair is indicated. In other circumstances, typically those in which neither the true pulmonary artery system nor the collateral system is sufficiently large to ensure low pulmonary arterial resistance, or in which unifocalization was difficult and a question remains regarding adequacy of anastomoses or positioning of the unifocalized vessels, it is most prudent to assess pulmonary arterial resistance objectively before deciding whether to move ahead with intracardiac repair.

Objective assessment can be made using an intraoperative blood flow study.[R36] The perfusionist primes a separate circuit, which draws blood from the venous reservoir and perfuses a cannula that is placed into the central portion of the newly unifocalized pulmonary artery system. Based on body surface area, controlled perfusion into the pulmonary artery circuit is then performed in incremental steps beginning at 20% of baseline cardiac output and increasing in increments of 20% cardiac outputs up to 100% indexed cardiac output. At each increment, after a steady state is achieved, pressure is measured using a small catheter placed into the pulmonary artery system and connected to a pressure transducer. During the assessment, careful attention is paid to the left atrial appendage. If the heart is not beating vigorously because of hypothermia or hypocalcemia, or if the heart is fibrillating, the left atrium and LV can be quickly overdistended by pulmonary venous return. To counter this, the LV vent is placed on vigorous suction and the vent pop-off valve is completely occluded. Even then, careful attention should be paid to the left atrial appendage to be sure that the vent system is not overwhelmed by pulmonary blood flow at higher incremental flows.

If mean P_{PA} remains less than 25 mmHg at full indexed cardiac output in a 3- to 4-month-old infant, then intracardiac repair can proceed. These values have been shown to predict accurately that $P_{RV/LV}$ will be less than 0.5 following intracardiac repair.[R36] In older children, a mean P_{PA} of 25 to 30 mmHg at full indexed cardiac output usually indicates ability to move ahead with intracardiac repair. If pressures increase to more than these threshold values at any incremental step in the pulmonary blood flow study, then the test is terminated and intracardiac repair is not performed. In this case, a central aorta to pulmonary artery shunt is performed from the left side of the ascending aorta to the central portion of the unifocalized system using standard techniques for creating systemic–pulmonary arterial shunts (see "Techniques of Shunting Operations" in Section 1). Size of the shunt is based on body size and on total pulmonary arterial resistance as assessed from the pulmonary blood flow study just completed. If resistance is particularly high, then a slightly larger shunt may be needed.

Intracardiac repair. If pulmonary arterial resistance is acceptable, intracardiac repair commences. The aorta is clamped and cardioplegic solution introduced into the aortic root in the usual manner (see "Cold Cardioplegia, Controlled Aortic Root Reperfusion, and [When Needed] Warm Cardioplegic Induction" in Chapter 3). After adequate cardiac arrest is achieved, superior and inferior caval tapes are tightened around the venous cannulae to isolate systemic venous return. A longitudinal incision is made in the infundibulum of the RV and the ventricular cavity is entered. Hypertrophied muscle is removed from the septal and parietal bands and infundibular free wall. This adequately exposes the VSD, which is then closed with either a glutaraldehyde-treated autologous pericardial patch or a woven polyester patch. Depending on the surgeon's preference, either a running nonabsorbable monofilament suture or interrupted pledgeted mattress sutures are used for attaching the patch to the borders of the VSD. All the same considerations are addressed in this situation as in VSD closure in more typical TF (see "Technique of Operation" in Section 1).

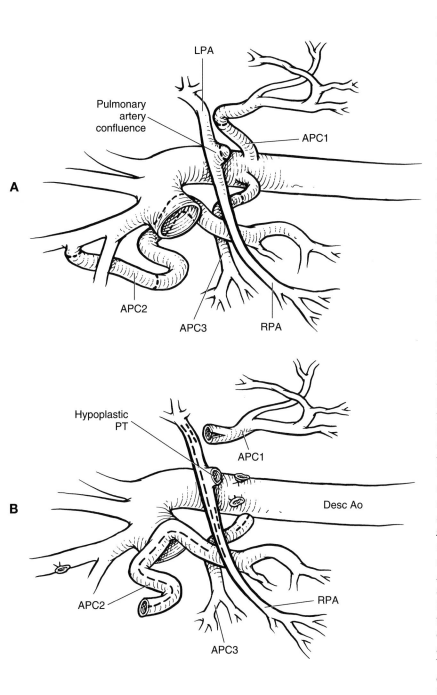

Figure 24-71   One-stage complete unifocalization and intracardiac repair via median sternotomy for tetralogy of Fallot with pulmonary atresia and large aortopulmonary collateral arteries. Median sternotomy preliminary dissection of true pulmonary arteries and collaterals, and cardiopulmonary bypass (CPB) details are described in the text, in Section 3 of Chapter 2, and in Fig. 24-70. Once CPB is established, previously dissected collateral vessels are immediately ligated at their systemic origin. This preserves entire length of each collateral so that this tissue can be utilized in the reconstruction that results in complete unifocalization. For clarity, heart, ascending aorta, and trachea have been eliminated in this figure. **A,** Hypoplastic centrally confluent true pulmonary arteries are present. Hypoplastic left pulmonary artery distributes to left upper lobe and hypoplastic right pulmonary artery *(RPA)* distributes to lateral aspect of right lower lobe. Three large collateral arteries are present. One arises from right carotid artery and takes a tortuous course *(dashed lines)* to provide blood flow to medial aspect of right lower lobe (APC2). Two other collaterals arise from typical upper descending thoracic aortic position. One courses to right upper and middle lobes (APC3) and the second to left lower lobe (APC1). The surgeon should be acutely aware, based on careful preoperative evaluation of the angiograms, of all stenotic areas within each collateral artery. Stenotic areas must be eliminated *(dashed lines on APC2)* if they are proximal within the collateral, or addressed surgically with either patching or some other form of augmentation if they are more distal. **B,** All three collateral arteries have been ligated and divided at their systemic origins. Hypoplastic pulmonary trunk has been transected just distal to atretic pulmonary valve. Unifocalization sites *(dashed lines)* have been chosen on the true pulmonary arteries in accordance with positions and lengths of collateral arteries to be unifocalized. In this case the two *short* dashed lines on the true pulmonary artery represent sites of implantation of the left and right mid-thoracic collateral vessels (APC1 and APC3). These incisions on the true pulmonary arteries are placed directly posterior. APC1 has been incised over part of its length to allow a side-to-side anastomosis within left hilum. Dashed line on APC3 identifies intended incision that will allow a side-to-side anastomosis with the true RPA. Tortuous APC2 has been mobilized, and the dashed line along its length indicates proposed incision that will allow performing an extensive side-to-side anastomosis onto the true pulmonary arteries beginning in the left hilum and extending all the way to the right hilum. The long incision on the true pulmonary artery, represented by the dashed line, is positioned on the superior–posterior aspect of the true pulmonary arteries.

Key: *APC,* Aortopulmonary collateral artery; *Desc Ao,* descending thoracic aorta; *LPA,* left pulmonary artery; *PT,* pulmonary trunk; *RPA,* right pulmonary artery.

Continued

Figure 24-71, cont'd   **C**, The three collateral vessels have been connected to the true pulmonary artery system as shown using running No. 7-0 absorbable monofilament sutures. Exquisite attention to detail and a three-dimensional vision of the result are required to avoid kinking, overstetching, and twisting of the delicate vessels. In this particular case the large tortuous collateral APC2 provides a large degree of "raw material" to augment the central pulmonary artery system adequately. In the absence of such abundant raw material, a less extensive anastomosis of the collateral to the true pulmonary artery would be performed, similar to the other two collateral anastomoses in this example, and the central pulmonary artery system would be augmented centrally from hilum to hilum with a patch of pulmonary arterial allograft tissue. At this point in the operation the decision is made whether to perform an intraoperative pulmonary blood flow study as an aid in designing the remainder of the operation. **D**, In this case operation is completed by ventricular septal defect (VSD) closure and right ventricular outflow tract conduit (see text for other options). The small opening at transected pulmonary trunk is enlarged to the left and right sides in order to perform distal anastomosis of valved allograft conduit into newly reconstructed central pulmonary artery system. This aspect of the procedure and remaining VSD closure and proximal conduit to right ventricular anastomosis is performed in standard fashion for tetralogy with pulmonary atresia without large aortopulmonary collateral arteries.

Key: *APC,* Aortopulmonary collateral artery.

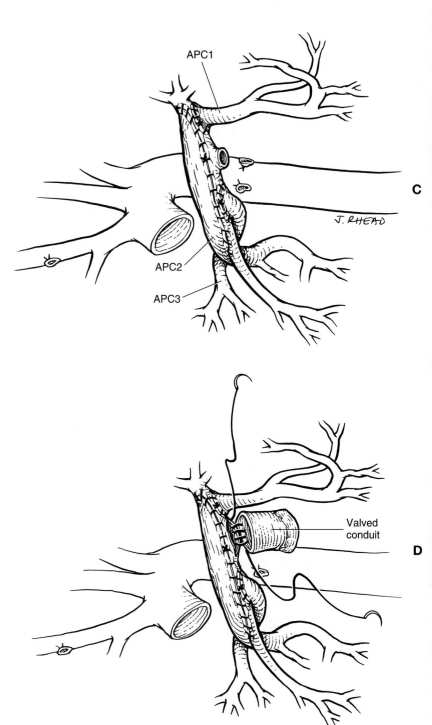

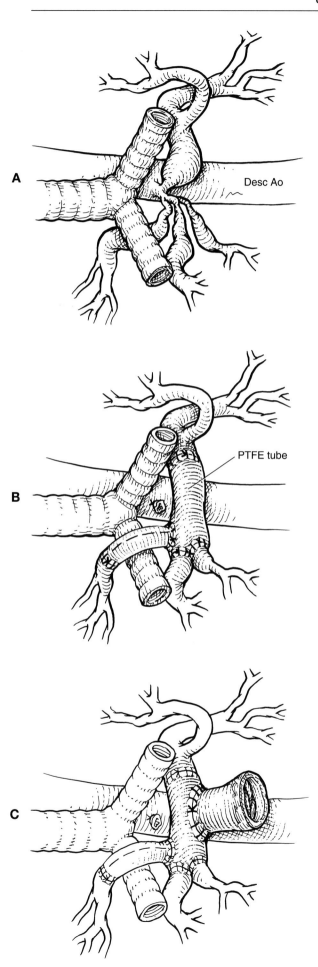

Desc Ao

PTFE tube

Figure 24-72   Alternative unifocalization repair of tetralogy of Fallot (TF) with pulmonary atresia and large aortopulmonary collateral arteries with absent true pulmonary arteries. In most cases when true pulmonary arteries are completely absent, central confluence between left- and right-sided collaterals is provided by creating direct continuity between collateral arteries from each side, working within the dissected space in central mediastinum, as described in Fig. 24-70. This is especially important in infants and young children, who require growth potential of living tissue. Occasionally a patient will present at an older age with stenotic but open collaterals with well-developed distal vasculature, as shown in this case. Under these conditions, native tissue-to-tissue anastomoses are not critical because growth potential is not required. For clarity, the heart and ascending aorta are eliminated from this figure. **A,** Four collateral vessels are shown arising from the upper mid-thoracic aorta. They have been exposed according to the dissection process described in the text and in Fig. 24-70. There is one large collateral vessel supplying the entire left lung; it is stenotic at its origin. Three separate collateral vessels, all stenotic at their origins and in their proximal segments, supply the right lung—one each to the right upper, right middle, and right lower lobes. **B,** All collaterals have been ligated and divided at their aortic origins. A polytetrafluoroethylene *(PTFE)* conduit of appropriate diameter is used to connect left and right sides. The large left-sided collateral is connected end to end to the PTFE tube graft, and the three right-sided collaterals are unifocalized either directly or with a separate smaller PTFE tube, after resecting proximal stenotic segments. **C,** Conduit placement and ventricular septal defect closure are performed as for typical TF with pulmonary atresia without large aortopulmonary collateral arteries.

Key: *Desc Ao,* Descending thoracic aorta; *PTFE,* polytetrafluoroethylene.

A small right atriotomy is made and status of the atrial septum examined. If a competent but patent foramen ovale is present, it is usually left as is. A secundum atrial septal defect is typically closed either primarily or, if needed, with a pericardial or polyester patch attached with running nonabsorbable monofilament suture. If the atrial septum is intact, it is left in this state. If appropriate decisions have been made with respect to Rp, presence of a competent RV to pulmonary artery valved conduit usually allows for adequate RV function early postoperatively, minimizing the potential benefits of an open atrial septum (as described in the text that follows). The right atrial incision is then closed in standard fashion and the aortic clamp removed, allowing reperfusion of the myocardium.

At this point, RV to pulmonary artery reconstruction is undertaken. With adequate unifocalization and central pulmonary artery augmentation as described earlier, the conduit procedure is the same as used in the more straightforward case with duct-dependent TF, pulmonary atresia, and normally arborizing confluent central pulmonary arteries.

Establishing right ventricle to pulmonary artery continuity. Valved polyester conduits were used in the early era of this type of surgery; today, allograft conduits, either aortic valve with ascending aorta or pulmonary valve with pulmonary trunk, with or without the bifurcation, is preferred. Their preparation and storage by cryopreservation and their reconstitution in the operating room are described in Appendix 12A of Chapter 12. The allograft pulmonary valved conduit with its bifurcation is often the optimal replacement device.[B30,C21] When a bifurcated graft is not required, there is no secure evidence that the pulmonary or aortic valve allograft has an advantage over the other; however, the thinner wall of the pulmonary allograft may have more tendency to become aneurysmal if pulmonary artery pressure becomes importantly elevated.

During the early stages of the procedure, the allograft valved conduit is selected, thawed, and rinsed. In neonates and infants, depending on their size, a 10- to 18-mm-diameter valve can be used; in children older than age 5, a 22- to 25-mm-diameter valve can be used. These sizes should not be flow limiting.

Two somewhat different techniques of allograft insertion are used. In one (preferable), the proximal end of the allograft is sunk into the RV outflow tract and a piece of pericardium or polyester is used as a roof over the ventriculotomy (in previous editions of the textbook, this has been termed "orthotopic" placement) (Fig. 24-73). The distal end of the allograft is attached to the pulmonary trunk or (in unifocalization cases) the newly reconstructed transverse central pulmonary artery system before making the proximal anastomosis of the allograft conduit directly onto the right ventriculotomy site. This method has the advantages of minimal use of foreign material on which a thick neointima may develop, and freedom from sternal compression. However, care must be taken that the allograft valve anulus retains its proper circular geometry and that the opening from RV into allograft is large.

In the second method, a woven polyester tube 2 to 5 mm larger than the diameter of the allograft valve anulus is sutured to the proximal end of the allograft. Before insertion, the proximal polyester end is cut in a severely beveled

fashion so that it serves primarily as a roof on the ventriculotomy incision with only a few millimeters of fully circular polyester conduit just proximal to the allograft. With care, the conduit can be kept completely away from the sternum. This technique has the advantage that the perfectly circular geometry of the allograft valve is well maintained and that with it all types of RV and pulmonary trunk morphology can be managed. It has the disadvantage of a very short 2- to 3-mm cylinder of polyester in the proximal end of the conduit.

There are situations in which one or the other method is mandated, depending on RV morphology and availability of the pulmonary trunk, but more often selection is one of preference.

Using either technique, the proximal end of the allograft is cut transversely about 5 mm below the nadir of the valve cusps, leaving the muscular remnant at least 4 mm thick (thicker than when the valve is used for aortic valve replacement). The conduit is not trimmed distally until the nature of the pulmonary artery confluence is established following either complete dissection of the native pulmonary artery or completed unifocalization and central pulmonary artery augmentation and the distance between this and the right ventriculotomy is measured.

With the first method (see Fig. 24-73, *A*), a limited longitudinal incision is made in the superior RV wall where the pulmonary trunk would normally arise. Care is taken in extending the incision distally so that the anterior margin of the VSD and right coronary cusp of the aortic valve are not damaged. The RV opening is also enlarged proximally, and any thick trabeculations arising from the free wall, particularly inferiorly, are excised. The VSD is repaired in a fashion similar to that described for TF with pulmonary stenosis (see Fig. 24-25). The distal end of the allograft conduit is cut so that it is the correct shape and the conduit is the correct length. It must not be too long or it may kink and possibly compress either branch of the pulmonary artery. The pulmonary artery confluence (or reconstruction, in the case of unifocalization) is opened with an incision extending out along the RPA and LPA. The opening is made long enough to match exactly the diameter of the allograft. Occasionally, it may need to extend further out along one branch to relieve a long zone of stenosis (usually in the LPA). The allograft conduit may be cut with an appropriately shaped flanged extension that extends into and enlarges this new opening, or the branch may be widened with a separate pericardial or allograft arterial wall patch (see "Repair of Tetralogy of Fallot with Stenosis at Origin of Left Pulmonary Artery" in Section 1). The distal anastomosis is made with continuous No. 5-0 or 6-0 polypropylene suture (Fig. 24-73, *B*). The proximal conduit anastomosis is made by commencing the suturing posteriorly where the allograft is apposed to the superior margin of the ventriculotomy and any remnant of infundibular septum. A No. 4-0 polypropylene suture is used, and often both the RV wall and superior edge of the VSD patch are picked up in the suture line to make it particularly secure posteriorly. The suture line is continued from the midline along both sides around about half the circumference of the conduit, and the sutures are held. A patch of pericardium, polyester, or allograft arterial wall is cut to an approximate semilunar shape and sutured into place to complete the

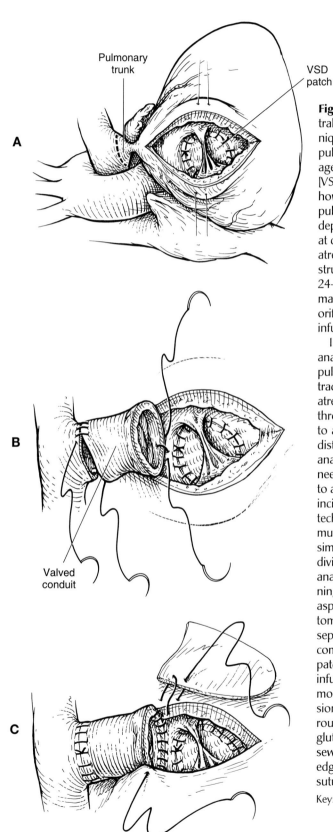

Figure 24-73   Right ventricular outflow tract conduit placement for tetralogy of Fallot (TF) with pulmonary atresia. Much of the surgical technique for repair of TF with pulmonary atresia is similar to that for TF with pulmonary stenosis (e.g., cardiopulmonary bypass [CPB], myocardial management, and intracardiac management of the ventricular septal defect [VSD] and the atrial septum). Management of these two malformations, however, deviates at several important points. Specific management of the pulmonary arteries depends on the form of pulmonary atresia. For duct-dependent atresia, ligation and division of ductus arteriosus is performed at commencement of CPB. For more complex forms of TF with pulmonary atresia and large aortopulmonary (AP) collateral arteries, complex reconstruction of the pulmonary vasculature is often required (see Figs. 24-70 to 24-72). Although in TF with pulmonary stenosis the VSD closure may be managed through a right atrial incision working through the tricuspid valve orifice, in TF with pulmonary atresia the VSD is always closed through an infundibular incision in the right ventricle (RV).

In the various parts of this figure (and in Fig. 24-74), pulmonary artery anatomy is that of normally arborizing, normal diameter, confluent branch pulmonary arteries with patent ductus arteriosus. However, RV outflow tract conduit placement is the same for more complex TF with pulmonary atresia in which the pulmonary artery system has been reconstructed through unifocalization. **A,** Ductus arteriosus has been ligated, taking care to avoid narrowing the left branch pulmonary artery. Dashed line on the distal pulmonary trunk shows site of transaction in preparation for distal anastomosis of valved conduit to it. Opening in the pulmonary trunk may need to be extended with incisions along left and right pulmonary arteries to accommodate circumference of the conduit. A longitudinal infundibular incision has been made and VSD closed with a patch and running suture technique. Note in this case that VSD has an inlet component. Hypertrophic muscle of the RV infundibulum and VSD closure are handled in a manner similar to that in TF with pulmonary stenosis. **B,** Ductus arteriosus has been divided. A pulmonary allograft valved conduit is shown with the distal anastomosis performed end to end, allograft to pulmonary trunk. A running suture technique using fine monofilament suture is used. Proximal aspect of conduit is then attached to RV. Conduit is placed into ventriculotomy with the suture line attaching its proximal end to the infundibular septum within the ventricular incision. Although not shown in this figure, commonly the proximal suture line incorporates the upper aspect of VSD patch, which is also attached to the anteriorly displaced edge of the infundibular septum. **C,** Posterior suture line of proximal conduit anastomosis is completed as it transitions onto free edge of infundibular incision. Proximal component of the reconstruction is completed using a roughly hemi-oval patch made of polyester, polytetrafluoroethylene, or glutaraldehyde-treated autologous pericardium. Straight edge of patch is sewn around remaining anterior aspect of proximal conduit, and curved edge is sewn around ventriculotomy site to complete the reconstruction. All sutures lines are running nonabsorbable monofilament suture.

Key: *VSD,* Ventricular septal defect.

anterior half of the anastomosis (Fig. 24-73, *C*). Its straight superior edge is anastomosed to the muscular portion of the graft as the first step, and its curved inferior edge is attached to the edges of the right ventriculotomy. Good bites of muscle are taken all around and care is used to avoid damaging the valve cusps of the graft or the LAD. The conduit arises from the RV in nearly the same position as a normal pulmonary artery and passes superiorly and posteriorly directly to the pulmonary artery bifurcation. It is in little danger of being compressed by the sternum.

In the second method, a longitudinal incision is made in the downstream portion of the RV (Fig. 24-74, *A*). If a rudimentary infundibular septum and parietal extension are present, these are dissected away from the RV free wall. The VSD is repaired as described for TF with pulmonary stenosis, and preparations are made for inserting the conduit. The conduit, once in position, should be directed toward the patient's left shoulder as it comes off the right ventriculotomy (it need not be oriented parallel to the ventriculotomy) and then curve gently back to the right to approach the pulmonary artery with just a little redundancy and in an undistorted fashion. This is accomplished by cutting the distal end of the allograft exactly transversely (not obliquely). The proximal end of the conduit is cut obliquely so that the tubular part of the proximal polyester extension is only a few millimeters long and the rest is merely a hood (Fig. 24-74, *B*). The distal and proximal anastomoses are made using a running polypropylene suture (Fig. 24-74, *C*).

Assessing complete repair. After completing the procedure, the surgeon must continue to pay close attention to preventing overdistention of the LV and left atrium by the potentially large pulmonary venous return secondary to the large collateral pulmonary blood flow. The remainder of the procedure is completed as described for TF with pulmonary stenosis (see "Technique of Operation" in Section 1).

Immediately after discontinuing CPB, postrepair (OR) $P_{RV/LV}$ is measured (see "Measuring Postrepair [OR] $P_{RV/LV}$" under Technique of Operation in Section 1). A polyvinyl catheter is advanced from the RV through the conduit for a withdrawal tracing to be made the next morning. The level of postrepair (OR or ICU) $P_{RV/LV}$ that is acceptable in this situation is arguable. Although disquieting in an abstract sense, it seems reasonable to accept a higher postrepair (OR or ICU) $P_{RV/LV}$ in these patients than in patients with TF with pulmonary stenosis, in part because this repair is usually their last option. Thus, repair is left if the $P_{RV/LV}$ is less than about 0.9 and the patient is clinically stable, because probability of death is low (Fig. 24-75). Otherwise, CPB is reestablished and the VSD patch is perforated, usually through a right atriotomy. This situation, however, should be encountered rarely if the intraoperative blood flow study is utilized appropriately.

SPECIAL FEATURES OF POSTOPERATIVE CARE

Postoperative care is similar to that described for TF with pulmonary stenosis (see Section 1).

When the patient has come from the operating room with a complete repair, including closure of the VSD, and

postrepair (ICU) $P_{RV/LV}$ (or some surrogate for it) is consistently less than about 0.9, further intervention is seldom needed. However, if the ratio approaches that level, there is a considerable probability of death (see Fig. 24-75), and either the cause of the residual obstruction must be removed or ameliorated or the VSD patch perforated. Emergency study by echocardiography or cineangiography is indicated. If there are pulmonary arterial stenoses that can be dilated effectively, this should be done. If there are surgically correctable causes of residual obstruction, prompt reoperation and repair are indicated. If no central gradients are detected, this implies peripheral hypoplasia or microvascular disease. In this case the patient is returned to the operating room and the VSD patch is perforated.

Occasionally, pulmonary hypertension is caused by reactivity in the microvascular bed rather than by proximal or fixed distal obstruction. This is more likely if the P_{PA} and P_{RV} had been low earlier postoperatively. Increased ventilatory support, sedation, and a trial of inhaled nitric oxide are typical maneuvers that are both diagnostic and therapeutic.

Postoperative airway difficulties are more common in TF with pulmonary atresia than in TF with pulmonary stenosis, especially if complex unifocalization was performed. *Large airway problems* caused by external compression by the aorta, unifocalized collaterals, or conduits can occur.[M33] Unmasking of subclinical, or exacerbation of clinically important, preoperative tracheobronchial malacia can also occur. Phrenic nerve injury is an important concern when extensive dissection has been performed. *Small airway reactivity* also appears to be more common than in TF with pulmonary stenosis, possibly related to an intrinsic predisposition,[M19] but also almost certainly related to direct trauma, autonomic nerve disruption, or airway blood supply disruption.[R34,S34] Careful and aggressive pulmonary toilet is an important component of treatment, both intraoperatively after CPB and in the ICU. Tracheobronchial suctioning and lavage, and even bronchoscopy may be needed to keep airways free of both clear and bloody secretions.

If the P_{LA} is considerably higher than the P_{RA} (see "Risk Factors for Low Cardiac Output" in Section 1 of Chapter 5), a left-to-right shunt may be present at some level. Unless the patient is convalescing well, an echocardiographic and cineangiographic search is made for sites of shunting that can be closed percutaneously or surgically.

RESULTS

After Repair

Early (Hospital) Death

Overall hospital mortality after repair in a heterogeneous population varies between less than 3% and up to 20%, depending on era, patient characteristics, and institution.

Most recent studies report hospital mortality of less than 5% for a heterogeneous population[H26] and less than 3% when patients undergoing extensive unifocalization procedures are excluded.[H27] When examining clinical series dealing only with complete repair involving unifocalization, hospital mortality has generally been less than 10%[L9,M37,R35,T9]; as experience with surgical management of this difficult group of patients accumulates, hospital mortality of less than 5% should be achievable.

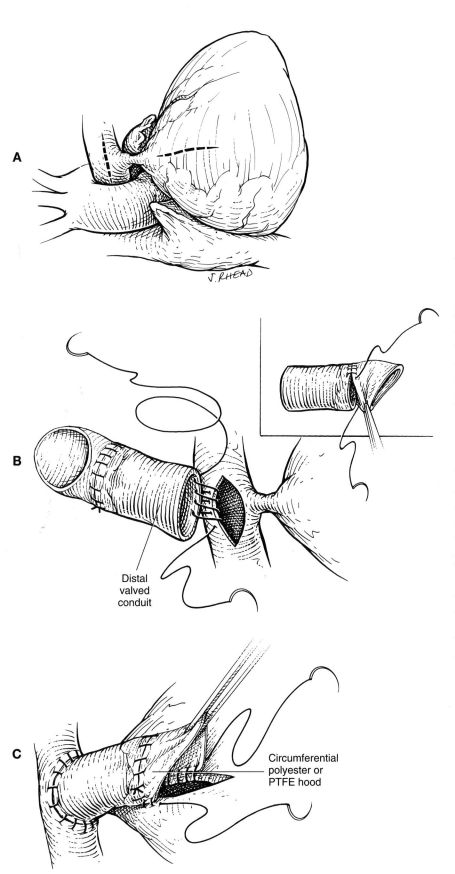

Figure 24-74   Alternative method for right ventricular (RV) outflow tract valved conduit placement in tetralogy of Fallot with pulmonary atresia. General operative management is similar to that described in Fig. 24-73. Using this method, a circumferential polyester conduit is attached to proximal end of allograft valved conduit to facilitate ventricle-to-conduit anastomosis. **A,** Dashed lines indicate incisions to be made on the central pulmonary artery and on RV infundibulum. **B,** Inset shows the polyester conduit being connected to proximal end of allograft valved conduit with a running monofilament suture. In the main figure, the distal anastomosis between the allograft conduit and incision in pulmonary trunk is performed, leaving the atretic pulmonary trunk intact. The proximal polyester extension of the allograft is tailored with a sharp bevel to accommodate its connection to the RV. **C,** Beveled free edge of polyester conduit is connected to ventriculotomy to complete operation. As seen here, there may be only several millimeters of length to the circumferential component of the polyester extension of the conduit, which mostly serves as a proximal hood, similar to the freestanding patch used for the hood in the technique shown in Fig. 24-73.

Key: *PTFE,* Polytetrafluoroethylene.

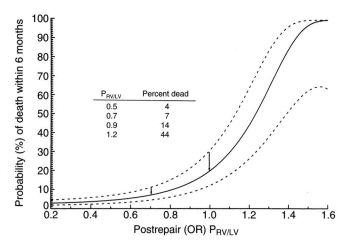

Figure 24-75 Nomogram illustrating relation between postrepair (OR) $P_{RV/LV}$ and death within 6 months of repair of tetralogy of Fallot with pulmonary atresia using a valved conduit. (Nomogram is specific solution of multivariable risk factor equation in original publication. Values entered for other variables are in original publication.) (From Kirklin and colleagues.[K30])

Key: $P_{RV/LV}$, Ratio of the peak pressure in right ventricle to that in left ventricle.

Time-Related Survival

Overall time-related survival after repair in a heterogeneous group of patients is somewhat less than that after repair of TF with pulmonary stenosis (Fig. 24-76). This is because of both a higher and more prolonged early phase of risk and a constant phase of hazard that is higher than that for TF with pulmonary stenosis (see Figs. 24-43 and 24-44).

Time-related survival has improved in recent years, with an approximately 90% 5-year survival for patients undergoing early repair without unifocalization[H22,H26] and 88% 2-year survival for patients undergoing one-stage repair with unifocalization.[R35]

Modes of Death

Most early postoperative deaths are attributable to acute cardiac failure, although some are due to acute or subacute pulmonary failure and a few to hypoxia or hemorrhage.[K31] Most late postoperative deaths are due to chronic heart failure, although an appreciable number are sudden. These latter may be arrhythmic deaths.

Incremental Risk Factors for Death

Variables relating to morphology of the pulmonary arterial circulation are the strongest risk factors for death after repair. Their presence probably accounts for most of the differences in outcome between these patients and those having TF with pulmonary stenosis. Whether they can be neutralized by an informed and aggressive surgical approach remains to be determined definitively; however, available data in patients who do not require unifocalization, as well as in those who do, suggest that these variables can and are being neutralized.[H27,R35]

Size of central and proximal extracardiac right and left pulmonary arteries. Among patients undergoing repair, in some of whom an effort has been made to enlarge the pulmonary arteries by increasing pulmonary blood flow by a palliative operation, small size of the proximal portions of the RPA and LPA is a strong risk factor for death after repair.[K31] However, in the absence of large AP collateral arteries, small pulmonary arteries have only a slight incremental risk effect (Fig. 24-77).

Pulmonary arteries that remain small locally or generally after a palliative procedure to enlarge them have abnormal wall characteristics. This is uncommon in TF with pulmo-

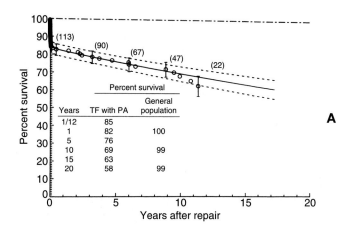

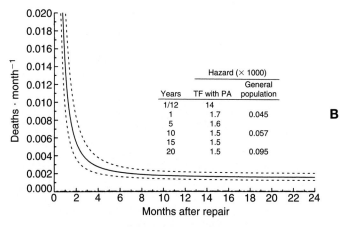

Figure 24-76 Time-related survival after repair of tetralogy of Fallot with pulmonary atresia in a heterogeneous group of patients. **A,** Survival. Presentation is as in Fig. 24-44. **B,** Hazard function for death. Note expanded horizontal axis. (From Kirklin and colleagues.[K31])

Key: *PA,* Pulmonary atresia; *TF,* tetralogy of Fallot.

nary stenosis. In TF with pulmonary atresia, current surgical techniques allow reliable relief of central and proximal branch hypoplasia.

Congenitally nonconfluent right and left pulmonary arteries. When considering only patient variables, noncon-

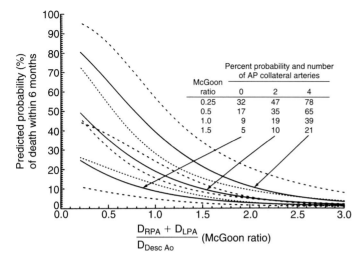

Figure 24-77   Nomogram illustrating incremental adverse effects of small proximal portions of right and left pulmonary arteries (just before repair and after palliative procedures) and of number of large aortopulmonary collateral arteries (*before* any percutaneous or surgical closures). (Nomogram is a specific solution of multivariable risk factor equation in original publication. Values entered for other variables are in original publication.) (From Kirklin and colleagues.[K30])

Key: *AP,* Aortopulmonary; *D,* diameter; *Desc Ao,* descending thoracic aorta; *LPA,* left pulmonary artery; *RPA,* right pulmonary artery.

A

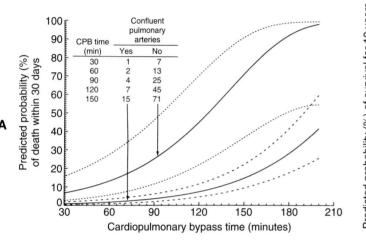

B

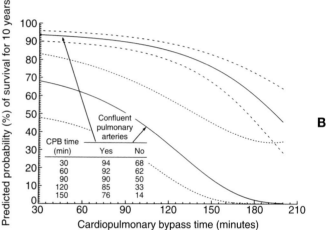

Figure 24-78   Nomograms illustrating effect of confluence (or lack thereof) of right and left pulmonary arteries and total cardiopulmonary bypass time on survival after repair of tetralogy of Fallot with pulmonary atresia. (Nomograms are specific solutions of multivariable risk factor equation in original publication, and values entered for other variables are in Appendix 24H.) **A,** Probability of death within 30 days. **B,** Probability of survival for 10 years. (From Kirklin and colleagues.[K30])

Key *CPB,* Cardiopulmonary bypass.

fluence of the LPA and RPA, either congenital or acquired, is also a strong risk factor for death after repair (Fig. 24-78).[K31] This can possibly be overcome by improved surgical methods, including bifurcated pulmonary allografts; better control of the damaging effects of CPB, especially those leading to bleeding; and improved myocardial management.[H27,P9]

Number of large aortopulmonary collateral arteries. Some studies suggest that the greater the number of large AP collateral arteries, the greater the early risks of the operation (see Fig. 24-77).[K31] This risk factor must be a surrogate for other as yet poorly defined but more fundamental ones. One of the most important of these may be pulmonary arterial and vascular resistance. Shimizaki and colleagues found that late postrepair pulmonary vasculature (arterial and vascular) resistance is inversely related to number of pulmonary arterial segments connected (by nature) to an ipsilateral central pulmonary artery.[S21] Other

studies and common experience indicate that the number of centrally connected pulmonary arterial segments is inversely related to the number of large AP collateral arteries.[S20] Thus, the incremental risk of the latter is probably a surrogate for that of increased pulmonary arterial and vascular resistance (see definition in "Pulmonary Arterial Resistance" under Natural History earlier in this section).

It seems logical that early and aggressive attempts to surgically achieve complete unifocalization of all collateral vessels and patch augment centrally hypoplastic pulmonary arteries may eliminate the association between higher pulmonary arterial resistance and pulmonary arterial arborization abnormalities, in essence by surgically correcting arborization. Recent experience seems to support his hypothesis.[M35,M38,R34-R36,T9]

Age (size). Very young age is a risk factor for death, primarily early after repair; age older than about 5 to 8 years is also a risk factor for death, primarily late after

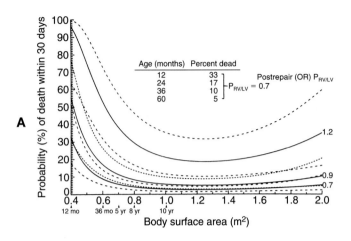

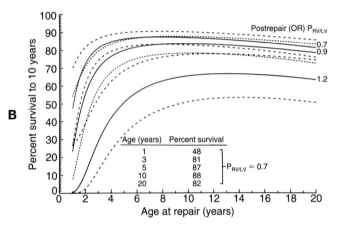

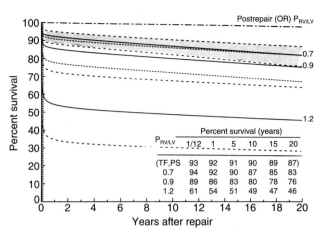

Figure 24-80 Nomogram illustrating effect of postrepair (OR) $P_{RV/LV}$ on survival after repair of tetralogy of Fallot with pulmonary atresia. Cross-hatched area represents 70% confidence interval of survival when postrepair (OR) $P_{RV/LV}$ is 0.7. For comparison, percent survival in a heterogeneous group of patients having tetralogy of Fallot with pulmonary stenosis is included in the table (top line designated TF, PS) (see Fig. 24-44). (Nomogram is specific solution of multivariable risk factor equation in original publication. Values entered for other variables are in original publication.) (From Kirklin and colleagues.[K30])

Key: $P_{RV/LV}$, Ratio of the peak pressure in right ventricle to that in left ventricle; *PS*, pulmonary stenosis; *TF*, tetralogy of Fallot.

Figure 24-79 Nomograms illustrating relation between size and age of patient, postrepair (OR) $P_{RV/LV}$, and risk of death after repair of tetralogy of Fallot with confluent right and left pulmonary arteries. (Nomograms are specific solutions of multivariable risk factor equation in original publication. Values entered for other variables are in original publication.) **A**, Probability of death within 30 days of repair. **B**, Probability of survival for at least 10 years. (From Kirklin and colleagues.[K30])

Key: *OR*, Operating room; $P_{RV/LV}$, ratio of the peak pressure in right ventricle to that in left ventricle.

repair (Fig. 24-79). The incremental risk of young age may be overcome by improved myocardial management, but those of older age are probably immutable for the same reasons as in TF with pulmonary stenosis (see "Results" in Section 1). This possibility of neutralizing the increased risk of young age is evident in more recent experiences from institutions in which one-stage repair is typically performed in neonates and young infants.[D16,L21,R34,T9]

Postrepair $P_{RV/LV}$. Postrepair $P_{RV/LV}$ is a risk factor for death after repair, probably an immutable one. Although it is a surrogate at least for size of pulmonary arteries and magnitude of pulmonary arterial and vascular resistance, and probably also accuracy of the repair within limits set by morphology, it is valuable as a synthesis of these variables. It is also the most influential on survival of any risk factor after repair of TF with pulmonary stenosis (see Appendix Figs. 24C-5 and 24D-8), and may by itself account for the

difference in time-related survival after repair between the two groups (Fig. 24-80).

Probability of a postrepair (OR) $P_{RV/LV}$ equal to or greater than 1, which is strongly suggestive that complete repair cannot be safely accomplished, is related primarily to size of the RPA and LPA and number of large AP collateral arteries (Fig. 24-81).[B29] Thorough surgical correction of arborization abnormalities and central hypoplasia within the pulmonary vasculature seems to neutralize the relationship between elevated $P_{RV/LV}$ and both number of large AP collaterals and size of RPA and LPA.[R34,R35]

Duration of cardiopulmonary bypass. Duration of CPB is a risk factor for death, particularly in the early period after repair (see Fig. 24-78). Neutralization requires eliminating or minimizing the damaging effects of CPB.

Heart Block

Heart block is rare after repair, just as it is in TF with pulmonary stenosis.

Functional Status

Most patients who survive repair have a good functional status (Table 24-27). Importantly, a tendency to declining functional status across time exists, but this may be attributable to chance alone (Fig. 24-82). Few objective studies of exercise performance have been reported.

Pulmonary Artery Pressure and Resistance

As with other postoperative outcome events, information about Ppa and Rp is limited. RV pressure can in no way substitute for Ppa and Rp, because almost all patients have

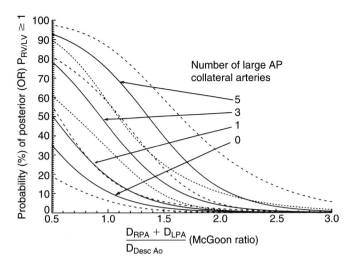

Figure 24-81 Nomogram illustrating relation between size of the prebranching point of right and left pulmonary arteries (McGoon ratio) just before repair and original number of large aortopulmonary collateral arteries, and probability of postrepair (OR) $P_{RV/LV}$ equal to or greater than 1 after repair of tetralogy of Fallot with pulmonary atresia. (Nomogram is specific solution of multivariable risk factors equation in original publications. Values entered for other variables are in original publication.) (From Blackstone and colleagues.[B29])

Key: *AP*, Aortopulmonary; *D*, diameter; *Desc Ao*, descending thoracic aorta; *LPA*, left pulmonary artery; *OR*, operating room; $P_{RV/LV}$, ratio of the peak pressure in right ventricle to that in left ventricle; *RPA*, right pulmonary artery.

■ **TABLE 24-27   New York Heart Association Functional Class after Repair of Tetralogy of Fallot with Pulmonary Atresia**

NYHA Class at Last Follow-up	n	% of 95
I	89	94
II	5	5
III	1	1
IV	0	0
Subtotal	95	100
Dead	39	
Alive, unknown class	5	
TOTAL	139	

(Data from Kirklin and colleagues.[K31])

a pressure gradient between the RV and pulmonary arteries after repair. Shimazaki and colleagues found that 75% of patients had a gradient of at least 20 mmHg late after repair, and 10% had one of 60 mmHg.[S21]

Data indicate that about 50% of a heterogeneous group of patients have an elevated PPA and Rp late after repair (Fig. 24-83).[S21] Type of repair did not correlate with late postoperative Rp, but number of centrally connected pulmonary arterial segments was highly and inversely ($P < .001$) correlated (Fig. 24-84). Surgical management plans that include early and complete correction of pulmonary artery arborization abnormalities have resulted in relatively low PPA and Rp, regardless of degree of original arborization,[R34,R35] indicating that this correlation is not immutable.

Reintervention

Reoperations other than those on valved conduits are rare. Reintervention is infrequently needed to repair a residual or recurrent VSD or to close an overlooked large AP collateral artery (both 3% of patients[K31]). Progressing dilatation of the aortic root and development of aortic valve regurgitation has required aortic valve replacement in 1% of patients.[K31] For patients undergoing early aggressive unifocalization, reoperation on the peripheral pulmonary arterial

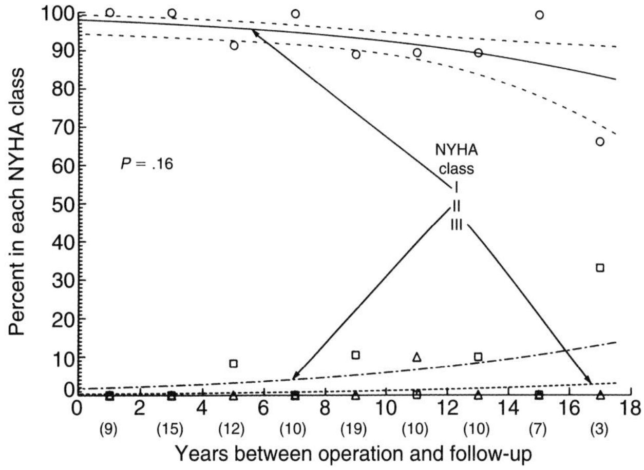

Figure 24-82 New York Heart Association (NYHA) functional class after repair of tetralogy of Fallot with pulmonary atresia, according to interval between operation and last follow-up. Details of the presentation are similar to those of Fig. 24-52. The *P* value of .16 for time trend in this ordinal logistic (longitudinal) regression analysis indicates that change across time in distribution of patients according to their NYHA functional class may be due to chance alone. (From Kirklin and colleagues.[K31])

Key: *NYHA*, New York Heart Association.

vasculature for persistent or recurrent obstruction is less than 15% at 5-year follow-up.[R35]

The most common reoperation is replacement of an obstructed xenograft or allograft valved conduit.[A6,B25,C6,I4,J6,M9,N3] Among a heterogeneous group of patients receiving these conduits for a variety of conditions, but most commonly for TF with pulmonary atresia, freedom from reoperation for conduit obstruction was 99%, 95%, 59%, and 11% at 3.5, 5, 10, and 15 years, respectively.[I5,K32,S22]

Among very young patients receiving 12-mm porcine valve xenografts in a polyester conduit, 3.5-, 5-, and 10-year freedom from replacement was 60%, 35%, and 9%,

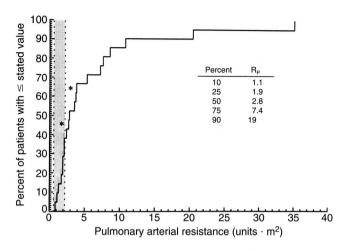

Figure 24-83   Cumulative frequency distribution of pulmonary arterial resistance late after repair among a heterogeneous group of patients undergoing repair of tetralogy of Fallot with pulmonary atresia. (From Shimazaki and colleagues.[S21])

Key: *Rp,* Pulmonary arterial resistance.

A

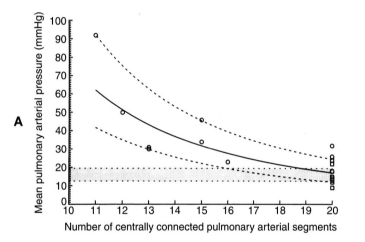

B

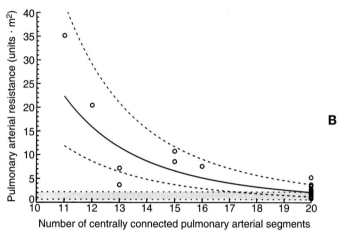

Figure 24-84   Nomograms expressing relation between (**A**) mean pulmonary arterial pressure and (**B**) pulmonary vasculature resistance (pulmonary arterial and vascular resistance), and number of originally centrally connected pulmonary arterial segments, late after repair of tetralogy of Fallot with pulmonary atresia. Parallel dotted lines indicate mean values and their 70% confidence limits in normal individuals. (Analysis and regression equation are in original publication.) (From Shimazaki and colleagues.[S21])

respectively, related in part to rapid growth of the patient.[B31] Time-related freedom from reoperation on allograft aortic and pulmonary valved conduits larger than about 21 mm is not yet known with a high degree of certainty. Currently, for properly preserved allograft aortic conduits, this appears to be about 95% at 5 years, falling to about 90% at 10 years and 60% at 20 years (Fig. 24-85, *A*).[K32,K33] The hazard function for reoperation has a steadily rising single phase (Fig. 24-85, *B*), suggesting that all such conduits may ultimately require replacement. Small patients require small allograft valved conduits, and the very small conduits required in neonates and infants clearly have a shorter reoperation-free interval than do larger conduits that can be used in children (Fig. 24-86). Young children can have a prolonged reoperation-free interval (Table 24-28).

Prevalence and rate of reoperation for conduit obstruction are considerably greater when an allograft valved conduit is extended with a polyester cylinder than when it

is not.[A16,A21] It is not known whether this applies to proximal or distal extensions, or to both. A proximal polyester gusset in the RV does not seem to have this effect.[H24] Oversizing the conduit by too great a degree results in earlier reoperation, as shown by a recent multicenter study.[A21]

After Palliative Operations for Increasing Pulmonary Blood Flow

Effect on Size of Pulmonary Arteries

Important enlargement of at least some portions of the pulmonary arteries can be obtained by increasing pulmonary blood flow and pressure.[G23,K34] This observation has influenced a number of institutions to follow management plans in patients with small pulmonary arteries that include staging procedures to achieve increased flow and pressure into both the pulmonary arteries and collateral vessels. Various ways of achieving this have been described, includ-

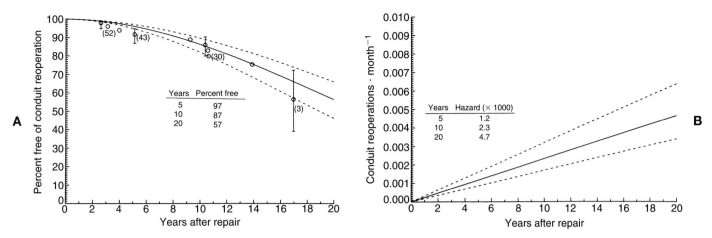

Figure 24-85 Freedom from conduit reoperation after placing of allograft valved conduit between ventricle and pulmonary trunk as part of a cardiac repair. A polyester tube was used as a distal prolongation in a few patients, and this appeared to be disadvantageous. (Analysis is based on 58 patients operated on between 1966 and 1985. Data were supplied by DN Ross and J Somerville.) **A,** Freedom from reoperation. Depiction is as in Fig. 24-44. **B,** Hazard function.

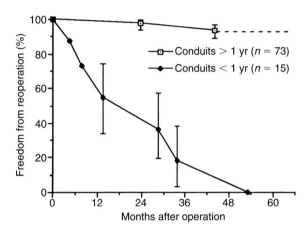

Figure 24-86 Freedom from reoperation for conduit obstruction according to age of patient (less than age 1 year and more than age 1 year) at time of insertion. Analysis includes patients in whom an allograft pulmonary or aortic valve conduit was used to construct right ventricular–pulmonary trunk continuity. (There was no difference in freedom between allograft pulmonary and allograft aortic valve conduits.) In patients younger than 1 year, the most common operation was repair of truncus arteriosus; in older patients, it was repair of tetralogy of Fallot with pulmonary atresia. (From Hawkins and colleagues.[H24])

Key: *yr,* Year.

■ **TABLE 24-28** Results of Follow-up Cardiac Catheterization after Repair Using an Allograft Aortic Valve Conduit in First 2 Years of Life [a]

Age at Repair (mo)	Interval [b] (years)	Pressure (mmHg)					NYHA Class	Interval [c] (years)
		AO	RV	PT	LPA	RPA		
Tetralogy of Fallot with Pulmonary Atresia								
1	3	95	36	33	–	25	I	10
16	5	130	80	56	–	33	I	5
17	3	130	44	26	15	13	I	9
Complex Tetralogy of Fallot								
3	3	90	48	35	21	33	I	10
14	2	110	37	33	–	25	I	8
Truncus Arteriosus								
1	3	–	50	31	14	29	I	9
2	3	115	42	32	16	–	II	9
3	3	110	60	29	–	–	I	4
Double Outlet Left Ventricle								
18	2	120	30	26	26	26	I	9
24	3	95	36	28	–	20	I	9
TGA + VSD + PS								
13	2	105	40	26	24	24	I	8
20	10	100	80	18	–	–	II	10

Key: *Ao,* Aorta; *LPA,* left pulmonary artery; *mo,* months; *NYHA,* New York Heart Association; *PS,* pulmonary stenosis; *PT,* pulmonary trunk; *RPA,* right pulmonary artery; *RV,* right ventricle; *TGA,* transposition of the great arteries; *VSD,* ventricular septal defect.

[a] Based on GLH experience, 1970 to 1976.

[b] Internal from repair to cardiac catheterization.

[c] Internal from repair to follow-up inquiry of functional status.

ing placing PTFE systemic–pulmonary arterial shunts, directly connecting central pulmonary arteries to the ascending aorta, placing RV–pulmonary trunk conduits or patches, and constructing shunts into individual or partially unifocalized collateral vessels.[M39,M40,P18,R37,S27,S35,W13] Although vessel growth clearly results from these procedures, it is difficult to document how frequently they lead to intracardiac repair with acceptable RV and pulmonary artery pressure. Reports suggest that approximately 20% of anastomoses performed in the palliative setting will occlude, and about half the patients undergoing staged palliative procedures will eventually undergo intracardiac repair. A substantial portion of these patients will have unacceptably high pulmonary artery pressure.[I7,I9,M39,Y5]

Also well established is the fact that enlargement is not always diffuse, and there may remain areas of stenosis, presumably because pulmonary arterial walls are not uniformly compliant. Reasons for the noncompliance are not completely clear. Intrinsic abnormalities within the vessel wall and persistently abnormal blood flow patterns related to the palliative procedure may both play a role. These areas can be approached by percutaneous balloon dilatation or stenting. An immediate favorable response can be achieved in more than 80% of cases; however, later stenosis and occlusion are common.[B22,E12,R6,R37,V9,Z7]

Likewise, the degree of enlargement that can be obtained in individual patients cannot be accurately predicted. However, it is correlated with the magnitude of increase in the $\dot{Q}p$ and P_{PA} that can be brought about by the palliative procedure.[A14,G24] When the central pulmonary arteries are small, palliative RV–pulmonary trunk and systemic–pulmonary arterial shunts can provide maximal stimulus for pulmonary arterial enlargement. There is no reason to believe that this growth is any greater than that occurring in the pulmonary arteries and unifocalized collaterals following reparative surgery. Although there is no definitive data, there is a suggestion that focal areas of stenosis may be reduced in the setting of the normal pulmonary blood flow patterns that attend reparative, as opposed to palliative, operations.

Survival

Hospital mortality has been 12% (see Table 24-23),[K9] with most of the deaths in very small (young) infants with severe hypoplasia of the pulmonary arteries or other kinds of pulmonary arterial anomalies. Survival for at least 12 years has been good (75%) in patients receiving a systemic–pulmonary arterial shunt and no further procedures (Fig. 24-87). These patients were deemed unsuitable for repair in the era of 1967 to 1983. There is no way, it seems, to compare in a risk-adjusted manner this survival with that had these same patients undergone one-stage repair after repair or received no treatment. Most of the deaths occurred within the first 3 postoperative months.

Modes of Death

Death early after operation was usually due to acute cardiac failure, whereas late postoperatively it was usually from hypoxia.

Functional Status

Of the 38 patients in the UAB subset who were known to be alive at last follow-up, 54% considered themselves to be

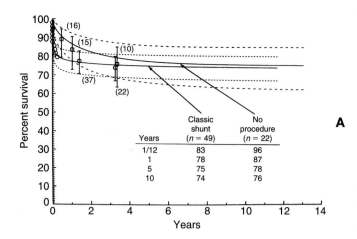

A

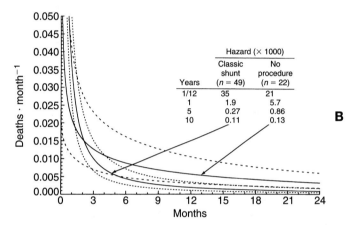

B

Figure 24-87 Time-related survival in patients having tetralogy of Fallot (TF) with pulmonary atresia who underwent no interventional therapy (*n* = 22) and who underwent only a systemic–pulmonary arterial shunt with no further intervention (*n* = 49). (Analysis is based on cross-sectional follow-up of 244 patients having TF with pulmonary atresia seen at UAB between 1967 and July 1983; follow-up was in mid-1986.) **A**, Survival. Depiction is as in Fig. 24-44. **B**, Hazard function for death.

without limitations (NYHA class I), 16% in NYHA class II, and 3% (one patient) in class NYHA III.

Results of No Interventional Therapy
Historical Perspective

Because there has been increasing recognition over the past 20 years that surgical or other interventional therapy is beneficial to patients with all forms of TF with pulmonary atresia, unselected patient cohorts receiving no intervention no longer exist.

Survival

Survival for at least 12 years in 22 patients receiving no interventional treatment was 75% (see Fig. 24-87). These were patients considered unsuitable for complete repair and too well oxygenated to require a systemic–pulmonary arterial shunt when they presented between 1967 and 1983. Most were older children who had fewer than 10 pulmonary arterial segments in continuity with central or hilar RPA or LPA. Again, there is no way to know the proportion of patients with TF and pulmonary atresia who are born with this condition nor to make a risk-adjusted comparison of their survival with that of patients who received interventional therapy. It is, however, almost a certainty that this patient group is highly selected and does not represent the newborn population with this malformation. Most of the deaths occurred within a year of presentation (see Fig. 24-87).

Modes of Death

Among the four patients who died within the follow-up period, one died of hypoxia and one of massive pulmonary hemorrhage. Mode of death was unknown in the other two.

Functional Status

Functional status of living patients was unknown, except in four. Two of these considered themselves to be fully active (NYHA class I), whereas one each was in NYHA classes II and III.

After Staged Palliative Operations for Unifocalization

Results of unifocalization operations, performed as a preliminary step before complete repair in patients who have TF with pulmonary atresia and considerably incomplete distribution of the RPA and LPA, are not yet clear (see "Special Situations and Controversies" later in this section). Some reports refer only to a few patients; others contain information that is insufficient for assessing results. The best estimate based on available reports is that as many as half, but often less, actually undergo repair. Of those who do, a substantial percentage, even a majority, will have $P_{RV/LV}$ greater than 0.67.[17,M39,P18,S27,W13,Y5]

One exemplary report from the Hospital for Sick Children at Great Ormond Street, London,[S25] states that among 26 infants and children undergoing staged unifocalization operations of various types through a lateral thoracotomy, most commonly with interposition of prosthetic tubes, 4 (15%; CL 8%-26%) died in hospital postoperatively. Eleven of 20 patients restudied had 10 or fewer pulmonary artery segments connected to central pulmonary arteries before the unifocalization procedure, whereas at restudy 9 were in this state (Fig. 24-88). Patency of the unifocalizing anastomoses varied between 5% and 100%, depending on the type of procedure. Seven (27%; CL 17%-39%) of the original group of 26 patients either underwent complete repair or were suitable for it.

A large experience has also been reported from the Mayo Clinic.[P18] Among 38 patients undergoing unifocalization, hospital mortality was 5% (CL 2%-12%), similar to that at Great Ormond Street. Sixty-one percent (CL 51%-70%) underwent complete repair, a higher prevalence than at Great Ormond Street; however, there is insufficient information to determine whether patient groups were comparable. Among the 23 patients undergoing complete repair, 21 (91%; CL 81%-97%) survived; these represent 55% (CL 46%-65%) of the original group, a higher prevalence than at Great Ormond Street. Of the 23 patients undergoing repair, 13% had postrepair (OR) $P_{RV/LV}$ greater than 0.85, and the mean value was 0.63.

Fifty-eight patients with TF and pulmonary atresia were reported from the Royal Children's Hospital in Melbourne,

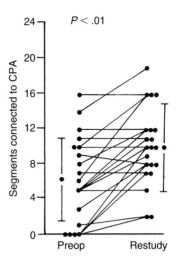

Figure 24-88   Number of pulmonary arterial segments connected centrally before and after unifocalization in 20 patients. $P < .01$ for difference in means (vertical bar represents one standard deviation). (From Sullivan and colleagues.[S25])

Key: *CPA,* Central pulmonary arteries; *Preop,* preoperative.

Australia, 34 of whom had unifocalization procedures. It is difficult to determine the outcome in these 34 separately from that of the entire group. However, among the 58 patients, 27 (47%; CL 39%-54%) either died after preliminary procedures or were ultimately considered unsuitable for repair. Results were good among the 30 patients who underwent repair, with one early death and three late deaths. In 2 of the 30 patients, late VSD patch fenestration was required because of $P_{RV/LV}$ greater than 1. Among 27 survivors who have undergone postoperative hemodynamic study, 5 (29%; CL 17%-45%) had postrepair $P_{RV/LV}$ of 0.7 to 0.9.[17]

Thirty-four similar patients were reported from the Heart Institute of Japan at the Tokyo Women's Medical Colleges.[S27] Twenty-two had incomplete distribution of one or both pulmonary arteries. Among 16 of the 34 patients who underwent the final repair, postrepair $P_{RV/LV}$ ranged between 0.36 and 1.00, with a mean of 0.71. In four other patients, a perforated VSD patch was used because severe elevation of postrepair $P_{RV/LV}$ was predicted if complete repair was done.

Clearly, some patients are correctable after a staged unifocalization operation and successfully undergo complete repair. For those whose repair is not successful, many factors may come into play, including natural attrition of healthy lung segments that occurs over time due to either vessel occlusion or pulmonary vascular obstructive disease, iatrogenic loss of lung segments directly related to palliative surgery, inability to create vascular continuity between lung segments due to scarring from prior palliative operations, and general cardiovascular complications related to chronic mixed circulation. Risk-adjusted, time-related probabilities of death and of importantly elevated postrepair $P_{RV/LV}$ are not yet available.

INDICATIONS FOR OPERATION

Proper indications for operation, and their sequencing in the various subsets of patients who have TF with congenital pulmonary atresia, cannot be identified with certainty. This is not surprising, because the necessary patient-specific (risk-adjusted) comparisons of outcomes after no interventional treatment versus the various types and combinations of procedures are not yet available. Therefore, indications can only be discussed in general terms for the major groups.

Confluent and Normally Distributing Right and Left Pulmonary Arteries and Patent Ductus Arteriosus

The highly unfavorable natural history of newborns in this subset, coupled with the fact that at least 80% survive complete repair in early life and 75% of those undergoing repair are alive and in good health for at least 10 years, indicates that complete repair as early in life as possible should be undertaken, often meaning repair in neonates. It must be emphasized, however, that equal outcomes appear to be achievable with neonatal shunting followed by later repair.

In those patients first seen after the neonatal period and usually living because of an AP anastomosis of some type, repair as soon as possible is likewise advisable.

Pulmonary Arteries with Arborization Abnormalities

Although the natural history is much more variable in this morphologic group, rarely do patients reach adult life in a healthy state if left untreated. Based on early surgical outcomes before 1990, it has been argued by some that surgical intervention is not indicated unless the individual is very symptomatic. More recent surgical results following both staged unifocalization and one-stage unifocalization and intracardiac repair demonstrate that repair with low P_{RV} and P_{PA} can be achieved in a high percentage of patients whether symptomatic or not. Although long-term outcome using these newer techniques is not yet known, the combination of low operative mortality and resultant low P_{RV} suggests that outcomes over the long term are likely, in many cases, to be comparable to those achieved in the more favorable morphologic subset of patients with TF with pulmonary atresia and ductus-dependent, confluent, normally distributing pulmonary arteries. The most important principles in achieving results comparable to this more favorable group are incorporating blood supply from all lung segments into the central pulmonary artery system and achieving this in a timely manner such that the microvasculature in each lung segment remains undamaged.

SPECIAL SITUATIONS AND CONTROVERSIES

Alternatives to One-Stage Unifocalization and Intracardiac Repair

Situations may arise in the setting of large AP collaterals and true pulmonary artery arborization abnormalities in which one-stage unifocalization and intracardiac repair are not indicated. One of these is described earlier in which one-stage unifocalization through a midline sternotomy is accomplished, but pulmonary arterial resistance is proven to be elevated, intracardiac repair is aborted, and unifocalized pulmonary arteries are connected to the systemic circulation by a shunt. It has been demonstrated that approximately 80% to 90% of patients with large AP collaterals can achieve complete bilateral unifocalization through a midline sternotomy in one procedure in early infancy, and of these, approximately two thirds can undergo intracardiac repair at the same time. Of the one third of patients who undergo complete unifocalization, but in whom pulmonary arterial resistance is too high to permit immediate intracardiac repair, most achieve repair within 2 years.[R35]

There are various reasons why midline complete unifocalization is contraindicated in approximately 10% to 20% of patients with major AP collaterals. The most important is a lack of pulmonary vascular "raw materials." Raw materials are defined as the combination of true pulmonary arteries and major AP collaterals taken together. If both the true pulmonary artery system and AP collateral system are severely underdeveloped, an alternative approach should be considered. In the setting of poorly developed collaterals and absent true pulmonary arteries, a lateral thoracotomy with single lung unifocalization connected to an AP shunt may be the procedure of choice. This would be followed by a similar procedure on the contralateral lung at a future time. At a third procedure, a median sternotomy approach would be used to achieve vascular confluence between the left and right lungs, with later intracardiac repair and takedown of the previously placed shunts. Many techniques, using native tissue as well as prosthetic material, have been described to accomplish this type of reconstruction.[C25,I9,M39,P18,P21,R37,S27,Y5] In other situations the true central pulmonary arteries are present, confluent, but extremely hypoplastic in the mediastinum; however, they communicate to the collateral system extensively within the lung parenchyma. In this situation, there are few, if any, isolated segments of lung that are supplied by only collateral flow. In this setting, creation in the neonatal or early infancy period of a central native tissue anastomosis between ascending aorta and blind end of the pulmonary trunk can be performed to promote growth of the central system with communication to most lung segments. Following an interim period of central pulmonary artery growth, a second procedure with ligation of the dual-supply collateral sources at their systemic origin, and subsequent intracardiac repair and placement of an RV to pulmonary artery conduit, can be accomplished.[I7,R29,W13]

It should be emphasized that there is wide variability among experienced surgeons in the approach to TF with pulmonary atresia and large AP collaterals. Experienced surgical teams may prefer one of the alternative surgical approaches described earlier as their procedure of choice.[P18,P21,R37,W13] One common approach is to perform an initial procedure that provides increased blood flow and pressure into the confluent hypoplastic central artery system whenever there exists confluent central pulmonary arteries. This can be accomplished through many techniques, for example, by creating the central systemic–pulmonary tissue-to-tissue connection described earlier.[R29,W13] Another approach is to create an RV to pulmonary trunk conduit using various tissue or synthetic prostheses, leaving the VSD open.[R37] A third approach is to create a prosthetic systemic–pulmonary arterial shunt to the pulmonary trunk or one of its branches. A major concern about all of these approaches when they are used unselectively as first-line management, especially when the central pulmonary arteries have limited arborization, is that they leave collateral flow untouched, allowing time for detrimental changes to occur in the lung vasculature, either in the form of overcirculation with development of pulmonary vascular obstructive changes or in the form of stenosis and occlusion leading to loss of lung segments. These negative effects inevitably lead to reduction in healthy lung cross-sectional area, increasing pulmonary arterial resistance. Another concern is that any surgical procedure is followed by scarring and adhesions, markedly reducing the ability of the surgeon to manipulate, reroute, and unifocalize collaterals at subsequent operations.

Percutaneous Balloon Dilatation of Stenoses of Right and Left Pulmonary Arteries

Lock and colleagues first demonstrated the feasibility of this procedure.[L10,L11,R28] Intimal disruption with tearing of the media is one mechanism of dilatation, with the tears being subsequently filled in by scar tissue.[E10] In a multi-institutional study of a heterogeneous group of 156 patients, the largest subset of which had some form of pulmonary atresia, systolic pressure gradient across the stenosis was reduced only 10 to 14 mmHg, on average.[K35] A single-institution analysis of results in 135 patients indicated that about 60% of the procedures were satisfactory, defining this as a decrease of 20% or more of the peak pressure ratio between RV and aorta.[R25] Risk of death or other major complication was 1% to 3%. Patient age had no correlation with outcome. Effectiveness may be increased in the future by use of expandable stents.[M28,O9]

Effectiveness of balloon dilatation can also be assessed by its effect on normalizing the flow distribution in the lungs as measured by nuclear lung perfusion scan, even if P_{RV} is not reduced. Following complete repair, normalization of homogeneous flow to the lungs can be promoted by balloon dilatation of lobar and segmental stenoses within the unifocalized pulmonary artery system.[R35]

Percutaneous Closure of Large Aortopulmonary Collateral Arteries

Yamamoto first demonstrated the feasibility of this procedure in 1979,[Y2] and Szarnicki and colleagues accomplished it by embolizing a Gianturco wire coil device in 1981.[S23] Subsequently, a number of studies have demonstrated the effectiveness and safety of percutaneous closure of large AP collateral arteries as long as proper precautions are taken. When wire coil uniformly coated with thrombogenic polyester strands is used, occlusion by thrombosis usually occurs within about 10 minutes.[F17] Other devices for promoting thrombosis have been used, including bucrylate adhesive[Z4] and detachable silicone balloons.[G19,T7] With wire coil and proper techniques, complete occlusion is achieved in about 70% of instances and subtotal occlusion in another 25%.[P16]

A large AP collateral artery should never be closed surgically or percutaneously when it connects end to end to distal pulmonary arteries and thus is the sole, or major, source of blood flow to one or more pulmonary segments. Even when blood supply to a pulmonary segment occurs from dual sources, occlusion of the collateral source may not be indicated; for example, if upon review of detailed angiograms it is determined that the collateral tissue can be used productively in surgical unifocalization, then it should not be occluded prematurely. In this case the collateral should be left open at catheterization and then ligated and divided, with its tissue used in the unifocalization and pulmonary artery augmentation process. When it is determined that tissue from a dual-supply collateral is not needed in surgical reconstruction and coil occlusion is being considered, it is prudent to occlude the vessel temporarily to be certain that its presence is not necessary for maintaining reasonable SaO_2.

SECTION 3 ▦
Tetralogy of Fallot with Absent Pulmonary Valve

DEFINITION

TF with absent pulmonary valve is a subset of TF in which the pathologic and clinical states are determined largely by the vestigial, severely hypoplastic, nonfunctioning pulmonary valve cusps at the RV–pulmonary trunk junction.

HISTORICAL NOTE

Apparently the first description was by Royer and Wilson in 1908.[R31] A second example was not reported until Kurtz and colleagues described their case in 1927.[K43]

MORPHOLOGY

The pulmonary valve cusps are myxomatous nubbins of valvar tissue at the RV–pulmonary trunk junction.[Z3] They are so severely hypoplastic that they are both nonfunctioning and only minimally stenotic. The pulmonary "anulus" is moderately narrow.[L6]

The VSD is large and similar to that in TF with pulmonary stenosis. The typical associated malalignment of the outlet septum contributes to infundibular narrowing. In addition, and perhaps related to the large flow, the RV outflow tract is often dilated and elongated.[Z2] The sinus portion of the RV is hypertrophied and its volume large.

The pulmonary trunk and central portions of the RPA and LPA are often aneurysmally dilated at birth.[S4] This dilatation may extend into hilar portions of these arteries, particularly the right, which then produces tracheobronchial compression. This often results in either hyperexpansion from air trapping or collapse of lobes or even an entire lung.[L6]

Beyond their hilar portions, pulmonary arteries are usually of normal size. Rarely are distal branches hypoplastic or hilar branching pattern abnormal.[R11] However, segmental distribution of the RPA and LPA is abnormal. Instead of single segmental arteries, tufts of arteries entwine and compress the interpulmonary bronchi in some patients. This pathology, when present, may in part account for symptoms of severe pulmonary dysfunction seen in some neonates and young infants.[R8]

There is controversy regarding the histopathology of the dilated pulmonary arteries in this syndrome. Arensman and colleagues report a normal pulmonary arterial wall in five of six children, with one child having a reduction in the amount of elastic tissue.[A9] Osman and colleagues have reported similar findings,[O6] but histopathologic abnormalities have been reported by others.[M7,M10,O7,R7,R8] Whatever the histology, physiologic studies indicate a marked decrease in RPA compliance in sick small babies.[H8]

Cause of massive dilatation of the pulmonary arteries in utero is unclear, but when there are severe pulmonary regurgitation and a large VSD, absence of ductal flow between the pulmonary trunk and aorta seems to be essential to intrauterine survival.[Z2] Thus, a ductus arteriosus (or ligamentum) is almost always absent at autopsy[E8] (unless the ductus connects to a pulmonary artery isolated from the pulmonary trunk).

There may be origin of the RPA or LPA from the ascending aorta,[C4] or a pulmonary artery may originate from a patent ductus arteriosus.[Z2]

CLINICAL FEATURES AND DIAGNOSTIC CRITERIA

TF with absent pulmonary valve generally results in both severe pulmonary regurgitation and a somewhat increased $\dot{Q}p$. Narrowing at the pulmonary "anulus," in combination with the large VSD, results in low P_{PA} and similar peak pressures in both ventricles.[L6] Part of the pressure gradient between RV and pulmonary trunk is related to large $\dot{Q}p$ (the $\dot{Q}p/\dot{Q}s$ is generally 1.5 to 2.0). Part is related to mild "anular" and infundibular narrowing.

When pulmonary regurgitation is severe, $\dot{Q}p$ increased, and pulmonary arteries dilated and compressing the tracheobronchial tree, presentation is in early infancy, often in the first weeks of life, with heart failure and severe intractable tracheobronchitis and respiratory distress responding poorly to routine medical measures. Cyanosis is absent unless hypoxia develops from pulmonary complications. There is marked failure to thrive, and there may be low cardiac output, acidemia, and death.

When pulmonary regurgitation is less severe (in association with slightly more pulmonary stenosis, a near normal $\dot{Q}p$, and less marked aneurysmal dilatation of the pulmonary arteries), presentation is later in life and less severe, usually confined to recurrent respiratory infections or mild heart failure.

Physical Examination

Severely affected infants are in considerable respiratory distress with tachypnea, subcostal retraction, and wheeze with rales and rhonchi audible throughout both lung fields. The heart is overactive and its rate rapid, pulse is of low volume, and there is obvious cardiomegaly, hepatomegaly, and raised venous pressure. There may be a precordial bulge. The infant is frail, cachectic, and febrile. On auscultation a to-and-fro murmur is audible along the left sternal

edge, with the diastolic component often the more prominent. The second heart sound is single, and there may be an apical gallop.

Chest Radiography

Chest radiography is distinctive, showing from birth marked supracardiac mediastinal widening caused by aneurysmal dilatation of central and hilar pulmonary arteries, usually equal on both sides although sometimes asymmetric, with relatively oligemic lung fields. Segmental or lobar atelectasis is common, and sometimes an entire lung is collapsed. Aerated portions of the lung may be overinflated. Atelectasis is associated with mediastinal shift, and in cases with partial or complete lung collapse, with acquired dextrocardia.[M7] In severe cases, there is considerable cardiomegaly. The left atrium may be pushed downward[M10] and the carina splayed with compression of lower trachea and both main bronchi.

Other Studies

The ECG is typical for patients with TF. Two-dimensional echocardiography and cardiac catheterization, including angiography, are required for definitive diagnosis and demonstrate the pulmonary artery dilatation and the tetralogy-type VSD.

NATURAL HISTORY

TF with absent pulmonary valve is present in about 5% of patients born with a large VSD and pulmonary stenosis. A high percentage (perhaps 50%) die in the first year of life if untreated, and most in the first few months of life, from respiratory distress caused by the massively dilated RPA and LPA compressing the tracheobronchial tree.[A9,C4,D7,L6] Such critically ill infants also have heart failure associated with a left-to-right shunt, and the RV is markedly enlarged and systolic function reduced.[H8]

Patients who survive infancy, however, generally do well for 5 to 20 years, because RV outflow obstruction is only moderate and cyanosis mild or absent.[S17] They tend to become symptomatic ultimately and die of intractable RV failure as a result of its chronic pressure and volume overload.

TECHNIQUE OF OPERATION

When operation is delayed to age 3 to 5 years or older, the usual procedure is repair of the VSD and orthotopic insertion of an allograft aortic or pulmonary valve cylinder (see "Establishing Right Ventricle to Pulmonary Artery Continuity" under Technique of Operation in Section 2; see also Fig. 24-73). An end-to-end anastomosis is usually made between the distal end of the conduit and the divided pulmonary trunk. Usually no "roofing" of the right ventriculotomy is required, because the large infundibulum permits direct approximation.

In critically ill neonates and infants, a number of palliative operations have been used, but the corrective repair just described is preferred. In addition, however, an ellipse of arterial wall is removed from the anterior aspect of the RPA, LPA, and pulmonary trunk bifurcation; the resultant defect is closed with a continuous suture before inserting the allograft valve cylinder.[G30,K37,S24,S28] This takes pressure off the underlying tracheobronchial tree. Watterson[W11] and Godart and colleagues[G30] report good results in infants using extensive pulmonary arterioplasty, closure of the VSD, infundibular resection, and placement of a transanular patch; a valved conduit is not used. Often the large pulmonary trunk can be transected, shortened, and moved ventrally and caudally to roof the infundibulum and relieve pressure from the tracheal bifurcation.

SPECIAL FEATURES OF POSTOPERATIVE CARE

When operation is performed electively in a patient age 3 to 5 years or older, care is the same as that usually given to patients after intracardiac surgery.

When operation has been performed urgently in neonates, infants, or young children, severe respiratory distress has usually been present and the patient receiving intensive treatment. This treatment (see "Indications for Operation" later in this section) is intensified in the postoperative period and then slowly withdrawn as the patient's condition improves.

RESULTS

Survival

Early (Hospital) Death

Absent pulmonary valve syndrome has been associated with a high probability of hospital death after repair in young infants.[A9,I1,M24,P5] In the current era, emphasizing pulmonary arterioplasty, Watterson and colleagues[W11] report 16% mortality (CL 7%-29%) in infants, and Godart and colleagues[G30] 20% mortality (CL 6%-41%) in infants and 3.7% (CL 0.5%-12%) in children older than 1 year. Mortality in infants is related in part to their poor preoperative condition and severe respiratory problems. When operation is undertaken beyond the first year of life, respiratory problems have usually resolved or not been present, and hospital mortality is low.

Time-Related Survival

This, and the incremental risk factors for premature death, as well as other outcome events, are similar to those in other patients with TF whose repair includes insertion of an allograft valved conduit.

INDICATIONS FOR OPERATION

Help is urgently needed for small babies with this morphologic variant who present with severe respiratory distress. Some have unrelated congenital hypertrophic lobar emphysema, and a few have severe hypoplasia of the RPA LPA; in either event, salvage may be impossible. In the others an intense medical program is begun as soon as the condition is recognized. It includes nursing the baby continuously in a prone position on a hinged board placed in head-up position.[A9] This allows the pulmonary arteries to fall forward and away from the bronchi, particularly the RPA.[A9]

If the infant responds well, operation is deferred. At times infants improve sufficiently to allow treatment to be

gradually diminished so that operation can be performed electively at age 3 to 5 years. More often, babies with this condition remain seriously ill and operation is required.

In patients with this morphology who require no special care in early life, repair is advised electively at 3 to 5 years of age.

Although various procedures have been recommended from time to time, that described under Technique of Operation is considered indicated. This is because alternative palliative procedures[B14,L5,O7] have not resulted in improved long-term outcomes.

Tetralogy of Fallot with Flap Valve Ventricular Septal Defect

DEFINITION

TF with flap valve VSD is a subset of TF characterized by a thick, fibrous flap hinged on the right side of a large VSD that narrows the interventricular communication and thereby limits right-to-left shunting.

MORPHOLOGY

The VSD is typical for TF. Its inferior margin either reaches the tricuspid anulus or is separated from it by a ridge of muscle (see "Ventricular Septal Defect" under Morphology in Section 1). A fibrous flap is attached posteriorly to the aortic margin of the VSD, and its inferior margin may or may not be fused with the base and superior margin of the anterior tricuspid leaflet. Elsewhere, the flap is unattached, and it rarely plays any part in tricuspid valve function (Fig. 24-89). It can hinge freely toward the right, but its thickness and bulk prevent movement through the VSD into the LV. Therefore, in the presence of severe pulmonary stenosis and raised RV pressure, it virtually occludes the defect.[N11]

Pulmonary stenosis is typical of TF, but the infundibular component is made more evident by the severe degree of RV hypertrophy that involves chiefly the sinus portion of the ventricle, because of high ventricular pressure. Thus, there may be a localized high-, intermediate-, or low-level infundibular stenosis or the narrowing may be diffuse, and the valve may or may not be stenotic. Congenital pulmonary atresia is occasionally present and pulmonary artery branch origin stenosis may occur.

This subset of TF is one of the group of conditions in which there is an *accessory fibrous flap* or *pouch* or *excrescence* arising in the region of the AV valve apparatus and sometimes from the leaflets themselves.[C16,F16,I8] They have sometimes been called, usually erroneously, "aneurysms of the membranous septum."[P13] Such anomalies associated with the tricuspid valve may prolapse into the RV outflow tract and pulmonary valve and cause severe pulmonary stenosis,[C15,F15,P12] a phenomenon that may occur in the absence of a VSD.[E7] A mobile mass of fibrous tissue related to the tricuspid valve may prolapse through a VSD and produce LV outflow tract obstruction.[M22,N10,S13] This type of subaortic stenosis is easily corrected by opera-

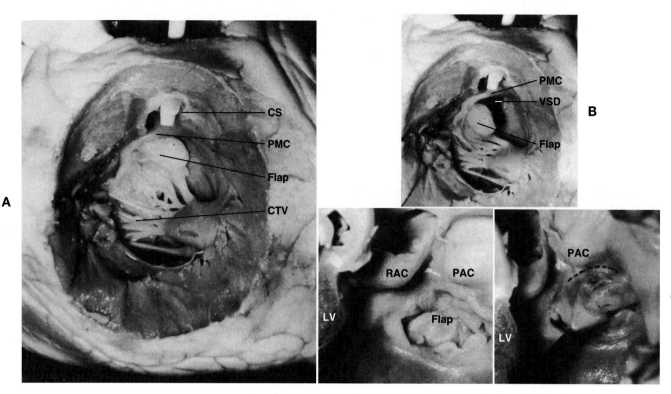

Figure 24-89 Tetralogy of Fallot with flap valve ventricular septal defect *(VSD)* and severe infundibular pulmonary stenosis. In this heart the pulmonary valve was normal and pulmonary trunk of near-normal size. **A** and **B,** Viewed from right ventricle (RV). Note extreme degree of RV hypertrophy and tight infundibular stenosis (probe). In this specimen the flap is continuous with anterior tricuspid leaflet. **B,** Flap has been moved rightward to expose large VSD. **C** and **D,** Viewed from left ventricle. Flap is hinged posteriorly *(dashed line)* beneath noncoronary aortic cusp and adjacent right cusp, where it becomes continuous with membranous septum.

Key: *CS,* Conal (infundibular) septum; *CTV,* chordae of tricuspid valve; *LV,* left ventricle; *PAC,* posterior (noncoronary) aortic cusp; *PMC,* papillary muscle of conus (muscle of Lancisi); *RAC,* right aortic cusp; *VSD,* ventricular septal defect.

tion.[M25] When transposition of the great arteries and VSD coexist, prolapse of accessory tricuspid valve tissue through the VSD results again in LV outflow tract obstruction, which is then subpulmonary (see Chapter 38).[H20,R22] In cases with congenitally corrected transposition of the great arteries (see Chapter 41), accessory valvar tissues of the right-sided, morphologically left AV valve may coexist. In this situation the tendency is for the accessory tissue to prolapse in ball-valve fashion into the morphologically LV outflow tract, producing subpulmonary stenosis.[L16] This may occur with or without an associated VSD. Such prolapsing accessory tissue is uncommon, but appears to be more often associated with the systemic venous rather than the pulmonary venous (systemic) AV valve. Maclean and colleagues[M23] and Levy and colleagues[L16] each report such a case in which subaortic obstruction resulted. Such a phenomenon may rarely coexist with TF.[V5]

CLINICAL FEATURES AND DIAGNOSTIC CRITERIA

Right-to-left shunting through the restricted VSD may be large enough to produce important cyanosis; usually it is not, so that when the atrial septum is also intact, the patient is acyanotic or only mildly cyanotic despite severe pulmonary stenosis, and presentation in the first year of life is uncommon. When pulmonary stenosis is severe, the virtually intact ventricular septum results in severe RV hypertrophy on ECG (in contrast to the moderate RV hypertrophy typical of TF), near normal splitting of the second heart sound (because $\dot{Q}p$ and P_{PA} are maintained at a near normal level), and a prominent *a* wave in the jugular venous pulse. These features and the larger cardiac silhouette on chest radiograph than in classic TF make the diagnosis likely. On cardiac catheterization, P_{RV} is nearly always suprasystemic. The flap can frequently be visualized on cineangiography and echocardiography.[F1]

TECHNIQUE OF OPERATION

Intracardiac repair is similar to that for TF with pulmonary stenosis. However, severe RV hypertrophy makes relief of pulmonary stenosis more difficult and may also limit exposure of the VSD. Usually, wide excision of muscle is required. The fibrous flap is identified and excised unless it is atypical and part of the AV valve mechanism, which is rare. Then, its herniation into the VSD is simply reduced and the VSD repaired in the usual way. It may be necessary

■ **TABLE 24-29   Hospital Mortality after Repair of Tetralogy with Flap Valve Ventricular Septal Defect (VSD) and of Other Types of Pulmonary Stenosis and VSD**

| | UAB (1967 to July 1983) | | | | GLH (1959 to 1983) | | | |
| | Hospital Deaths | | | | Hospital Deaths | | | |
Category	*n*	No.	%	CL (%)	*n*	No.	%	CL (%)
Tetralogy of Fallot with flap valve VSD	5	2	40	14-71	12	2	17	6-35
Low-lying infundibular PS[a]	48	1	2	0.3-7	45	2[b]	4	1-10
With VSD	41	1[c]	2	0.3-8	32	2	6	2-14
Without VSD	7	0	0	0-24	13	0	0	0-14
Other forms of infundibular PS[a]	22	0	0	0-8	—			
With VSD	17	0	0	0-11				
Without VSD	5	0	0	0-32				
Valvar PS with VSD	8	0	0	0-21	6	0	0	0-27
Valvar and infundibular PS (or atresia) with VSD	11	2	18	6-38	NA			

Key: *CL*, 70% confidence limits; *NA*, not available; *PS*, pulmonary stenosis; *VSD*, ventricular septal defect.

[a] In the GLH material, these two subsets are combined.

[b] Both deaths occurred in 1960, one in association with underdeveloped right ventricle.

[c] Operation in 1971; death with low cardiac output.

to attach the herniated portion to the tricuspid valve to prevent it from obstructing the RV outflow tract.

RESULTS

Hospital mortality after repair has, in the past, been relatively high.[F16] Four (24%; CL 12%-39%) of 17 patients in the GLH and UAB experiences died in hospital after repair (Table 24-29). One UAB death occurred in association with anomalous origin of the left main coronary artery from the pulmonary trunk and one GLH death in association with pulmonary atresia and a large fistulous communication between the left coronary artery and RV. Severe RV hypertrophy appears to be the primary incremental risk factor, and improved myocardial management may neutralize it. Late results in hospital survivors have been good.

INDICATIONS FOR OPERATION

Palliative shunting operations are inappropriate because they do not relieve the progressive RV pressure overload. Similarly, blind (or open) pulmonary valvotomy could result in excessive shunting from left to right through the VSD. One-stage repair is the proper treatment and is advisable when diagnosis is made.

SECTION 5
Low-Lying Infundibular Pulmonary Stenosis and Ventricular Septal Defect

DEFINITION

Low-lying infundibular pulmonary stenosis, so-called double-chamber RV, is a type of intraventricular stenosis that clearly separates the sinus (inflow) portion of the RV from a large and thin-walled infundibulum.[H17,L14] It is usually, but not always, associated with a small or moderate-sized and occasionally large VSD, which is usually juxtatricuspid in position, but it may have a narrow bar of muscle between it and the valve anulus. Also included in

this section are similar cases with an intact ventricular septum, because they may be considered part of this overall spectrum.

Low-lying infundibular pulmonary stenosis may coexist with otherwise typical TF (see Section 1).[L14] Low-lying infundibular pulmonary stenosis may also coexist with double outlet RV (see Chapter 39).[G20]

HISTORICAL NOTE

Like many cardiac anomalies, low-lying infundibular pulmonary stenosis was encountered by cardiac surgeons during the mid- and late 1950s, before the malformation was well recognized by morphologists as a discrete entity.[K24,S12,W8] However, case 1 in the 1933 report by Eakin and Abbott[E6] and cases 1 and 3 in the 1959 report by Blount and colleagues[B24] were examples of the entity, and Grant and colleagues clearly discussed this malformation in their 1961 publication.[G21] However, credit for the first description of the entity is generally given to Tsifutis and colleagues, who published their paper in the same year.[T6]

MORPHOLOGY

The most striking morphologic finding is the large thin-walled infundibular chamber, which gives rise to the appellation "two-chambered RV."[H17] The pulmonary valve and "anulus" are normal sized or large, as is the pulmonary trunk, and the RPA and LPA are virtually always large and free of stenoses or distributional anomalies.

The stenosis is formed by accessory bulky muscle bundles concentrated at the junction of the sinus portion of the RV and infundibulum. In the most florid form, there is a bulky, trabeculated muscular shelf lying almost in a coronal plane that separates a large, thin-walled infundibular chamber from a hypertrophied, thick-walled sinus portion containing the tricuspid valve apparatus and VSD. The shelf is often formed by medial and lateral anomalous muscle bundles that join the anterior free wall about halfway between ventricular apex and base.[B24] However, the shelf may be, in part, hypertrophied septoparietal bands.[R30] The stenotic ostium is usually centrally located, and in older patients it is surrounded by a bulky fibrous collar that

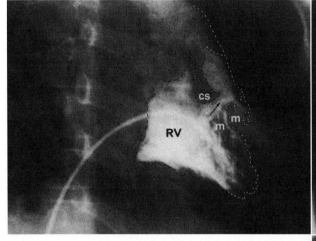
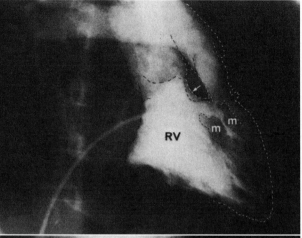
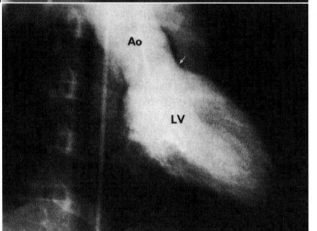

Figure 24-90 Right anterior oblique cineangiograms of low-lying infundibular pulmonary stenosis and a large ventricular septal defect (VSD) that has characteristics tending to distinguish it from tetralogy of Fallot (TF). **A,** Early frame after right ventricular *(RV)* injection. Anomalous muscle bundles form an extensive coronal plane stenosis between RV sinus and infundibulum, with an ostium *(arrow)* lying immediately below normally positioned conal septum. **B,** In this later frame, right-to-left shunting through VSD (not profiled in this view) outlines not only the aorta but also superior margin of left ventricle *(LV)* *(arrow).* **C,** LV injection, confirming a normally aligned connection *(arrow)* between superior margin of LV (formed by the conal or infundibular septum) and aorta. In TF, this view shows overriding of aorta onto RV secondary to conal (infundibular) septal displacement (see Fig. 24-16, *A*).

Key: *Ao,* Aorta; *cs,* conal septum; *LV,* left ventricle; *m,* muscle bundles; *RV,* right ventricle.

further increases stenosis. There may be more than one ostium. This obstructing muscular diaphragm inserts so far inferiorly on the free wall that it lies nearly in a coronal plane, which predisposes the ventricular incision to be in the infundibular chamber. The muscular band on the right side usually seems to be the parietal extension of the infundibular septum.

The VSD is usually small or moderate in size, although it may be large or it may have closed to only by a dimple. It is usually perimembranous and juxta-tricuspid and is overhung by thick tricuspid chordae, but it may have a bar of muscle at its posterior margin rather than abutting the tricuspid anulus.

In about 5% of cases, important and otherwise typical subaortic stenosis (see Section 2 of Chapter 33) coexists with low-lying infundibular pulmonary stenosis.[R21] Why this relatively large proportion exists is unknown.[B23]

CLINICAL FEATURES AND DIAGNOSTIC CRITERIA

Patients usually present with mild cyanosis in the midpart of the first decade of life, but they may present in the second decade or even in adult life. On examination the most striking feature is the loud systolic murmur, often grade 6 (heard with the stethoscope off the chest wall).

Chest radiography is not specific, but the pulmonary trunk shadow along the upper left cardiac border is usually prominent.

Diagnosis can be made by two-dimensional echocardiography, but cardiac catheterization and cineangiography are often performed, particularly to confirm presence and location of the VSD and the amount of displacement of the infundibular septum and overriding of the aorta (Fig. 24-90).

NATURAL HISTORY

Natural history can only be surmised. Because in some cases only a dimple remains in the perimembranous area at operation, the VSD presumably has a tendency to close spontaneously. Because few patients with this entity present in infancy, it is not surprising that the stenosis has been demonstrated to increase gradually in severity as the child grows.[C14,D14,F14,H18,H19] The progression can lead to complete infundibular atresia.[P11]

TECHNIQUE OF OPERATION

Preparations for CPB median sternotomy, and placement of stay sutures and purse-string sutures are as usual (see "Preparation for Cardiopulmonary Bypass" in Section 3 of

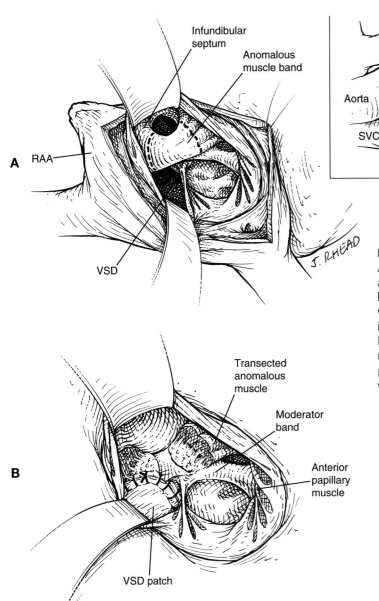

Figure 24-91   Low-lying infundibular pulmonary stenosis. **A**, Inset: Usual high right atriotomy is made as for right atrial approach to repair tetralogy of Fallot (TF). Anomalous muscle band arises from moderator band and is downstream from ventricular septal defect *(VSD)*. Proposed incisions for resecting obstructing anomalous bands are shown *(dashed lines)*. **B**, After relief of the obstruction, VSD is closed in the same manner as for TF.

Key: *RAA*, Right atrial appendage; *SVC*, superior vena cava; *VSD*, ventricular septal defect.

Chapter 2). Examination of the heart may confirm presence of a characteristically large, thin-walled infundibular chamber, but this is not always evident externally. Usually a marginal branch of the RCA courses over the underlying infundibular stenosis and should be preserved by making the ventriculotomy just downstream (cephalad) from it.

CPB is established at 32° to 35°C, employing direct caval cannulation or caval cannulation via the right atrium (see Fig. 2-21 in Chapter 2). The aortic root infusion catheter is inserted, the aorta clamped, and cold cardioplegia is given (see "Cold Cardioplegia, Controlled Aortic Root Reperfusion, and [When Needed] Warm Cardioplegic Induction" in Chapter 3). Temperature is then stabilized at 25°C. If the RV approach is chosen, a preliminary small right atriotomy is made and a pump-oxygenator sump sucker is passed into the left atrium across a natural or surgically created foramen ovale. A transverse low infundibular incision or right atrial incision (see later text) is made, [F20] and stay sutures are inserted.[P20]

The view is interesting and unique from the RV approach, because the interior of the smooth thin-walled infundibulum is exposed, and in its depth inferiorly is seen the ostium of the low-lying infundibular stenosis. A moment of carelessness could lead to misidentifying it as the VSD,[C13,L15] but further examination confirms it as the infundibulum because the tricuspid valve apparatus, lying entirely in the sinus portion of the RV, cannot be visualized.

Incision is made in the obstructing muscle mass anteriorly and to the left, which allows visualization of the interior of the sinus portion (proximal chamber) of the RV, tricuspid apparatus, and VSD. The part of the obstructing muscle mass that arches up and to the right from the infundibular septum (probably the parietal extension of the infundibular septum) is dissected and largely resected. Before resecting the left side of the obstructive muscular collar, which is usually in part moderator band, location of the tricuspid papillary muscles is visualized, and they are protected as the left-sided heavy muscular band is dissected and largely amputated. There is then a wide exposure of the sinus portion of the RV and VSD. Although the VSD is small, it is repaired with a patch, just as for other VSDs in this area. If the VSD is small and overhung by thick chordae, a completely interrupted suture technique is preferable.

From the right atrial approach (Fig. 24-91, *A*), the obstructing muscle is located at its insertion anteriorly at the region of the moderator band. The anterior papillary muscle of the tricuspid valve is retracted. Relief of the muscular narrowing is accomplished much as for the atrial approach to classic TF, but exposure is easier because the obstruction is less anteriorly placed and more proximal in the RV. After muscle resection, the VSD is closed with a patch in a fashion similar to patch closure for isolated VSD by way of the right atrium (Fig. 24-91, *B*) (see "Technique of Operation" in Section 1 of Chapter 21). The right ventriculotomy or right atriotomy is closed directly, and remainder of the procedure is completed as usual.

The morphology is so well suited to repair that usually no gradient is present after repair, nor are murmurs present postoperatively.

SPECIAL FEATURES OF POSTOPERATIVE CARE

Postoperative care is as usual (see Chapter 5).

RESULTS

Early (Hospital) Death

Hospital mortality after repair should approach zero, but the UAB experience (Table 24-30) is marred by an unexplained death in 1971, with low cardiac output and high left atrial

■ **TABLE 24-30 Hospital Mortality after Repair of Low-Lying Infundibular Pulmonary Stenosis** [a]

VSD	Age at Operation		Hospital Deaths		
	≤ years <		*n*	No.	%
Yes		1	1	0	
	1	5	9 [b]	0	
	5	10	9 [c]	1	
	10	20	11 [b]	0	
	20	40	6	0	
	40		5 [d]	0	
TOTAL			41	1	2.4 (CL 0.3-8.1)
No		1	0	–	
	1	5	1	0	
	5	10	2	0	
	10	20	4	0	
	20		0	–	
TOTAL			7	0	0 (CL 0-24)
ALL CASES			48	1	2.1 (CL 0.3-7)

Key: *CL*, 70% confidence limits; *VSD*, ventricular septal defect.

[a] Based on repair in 48 patients (UAB experience, 1967 to July 1983). Thirty-three of 41 patients had a small or moderate-sized VSD, and among the 33 the infundibular stenosis was severe in 31 and moderate in 2; 8 had a large VSD and moderate stenosis. Among the 7 who had no VSD, 6 had severe and 1 moderate pulmonary stenosis.

[b] One patient had associated subaortic stenosis requiring resection.

[c] One patient (surviving) had associated severe tricuspid regurgitation.

[d] One patient had concomitant coronary artery bypass grafting.

pressure. Neither heart block nor other complications have occurred.

Time-Related Survival

Long-term results are excellent, with no late deaths and all patients asymptomatic.[H19] In the University of Michigan experience, among 20 patients followed up for at least 20 years, 85% were in NYHA functional class I and only one (5%) had hemodynamically important impairment of cardiac function.[K42]

INDICATIONS FOR OPERATION

Diagnosis of the malformation is an indication for elective repair.

SECTION 6 ■

Other Forms of Infundibular Pulmonary Stenosis and Ventricular Septal Defect

A few patients with infundibular pulmonary stenosis, with or without a VSD, do not meet the criteria for diagnosis of TF or for low-lying infundibular stenosis. These are included in this section.

Some of these malformations may be similar in origin to low-lying infundibular pulmonary stenosis, except that there is infundibular hypoplasia and the anomalous muscle bundles arise from the infundibular septum a little more distally (downstream). Other examples in this subset probably represent instances in which the only discernible malformation at birth is a large VSD. With time, the parietal extension of the infundibular septum hypertrophies out of proportion to the rest of the RV, and in some cases the VSD narrows or closes.[C14] In view of this, cases with only mild infundibular pulmonary stenosis associated with an important VSD are included in Chapter 21, while those with more severe stenosis are included here.[5]

Age distribution at operation of the 22 patients in this subset is similar to that of patients with low-lying infundibular pulmonary stenosis and, not surprisingly, consists mostly of children and young adults, not infants. In all cases the surgeon believed the stenosis was severe enough to require resection. Among the 17 patients with associated VSD, stenosis was severe in five and moderate in 12. Eight of the VSDs were conoventricular and large, and eight were small; one was subarterial in position. Among the five patients without VSD, stenosis was severe in three and moderate in two.

Diagnosis, natural history, and techniques of repair are similar to those for low-lying infundibular pulmonary stenosis, except that a vertical ventriculotomy and infundibular patching should probably be used routinely. It is important to recognize the infundibular stenosis at time of repair

---

[5] Five of the cases included in this section were by error included in the 312 cases of VSD published by Rizzoli and colleagues.[R20]

of the VSD, because otherwise it can persist or worsen and reoperation may be required for relief.[D13,M21] Results of complete repair are excellent (see Table 24-30).

Indications for operation are the same as for low-lying infundibular pulmonary stenosis.

SECTION 7
Valvar Pulmonary Stenosis and Ventricular Septal Defect

Surprisingly, isolated valvar pulmonary stenosis rarely co-exists with VSD. Only eight patients with this combination were encountered in the UAB experience from 1967 to July 1983 (see Table 24-29), and their age distribution was similar to that of patients described in Sections 5 and 6. Valvar pulmonary stenosis was anatomic and not "functional" and was severe in five of the eight patients and moderately severe in three. The VSD was conoventricular and large in four patients and small in two; two patients had small muscular VSDs.

This combination may merely represent chance coexistence of these two malformations. The combination is an indication for elective operation by the techniques described earlier.

SECTION 8
Combined Valvar and Infundibular Pulmonary Stenosis or Atresia and Ventricular Septal Defect

Ten patients encountered during the 1967 to July 1983 UAB experience had combined valvar and infundibular pulmonary stenosis (or atresia, one additional case) and VSD but were morphologically *not* TF (see Table 24-29). In one, situs solitus of the atria, ventricular D-loop, and dextrocardia, as well as an LV diverticulum, coexisted. In one, mesocardia coexisted. In 4 of the 11, VSDs were muscular and multiple. In one of these four, a 10-month-old who died after repair, there was also severe stenosis at the origin of the LPA. In the other patient who died, there was also severe mitral regurgitation and prolapse of tricuspid valve tissue through a perimembranous VSD, causing subaortic stenosis (see Section 4). These seem to be unique cases whose management must be individualized.

APPENDIXES

APPENDIX 24A

Tetralogy of Fallot with Pulmonary Stenosis: Early Mayo Clinic Experience (1955 to 1967)

■ **TABLE 24A-1   Effect of Previous Operation on Hospital Mortality after Intracardiac Repair of Tetralogy of Fallot** [a]

	Hospital Deaths									
	1960		**1961**		**1962**		**1963**		**1964**	
	No.	**%**	**No.**	**%**	**No.**	**%**	**No.**	**%**	**No.**	**%**
None (one-stage repair) [b]	40	13	26	12	30	10	25	8	22	5
Repair after functioning Blalock-Taussig anastomosis [c]	18	33	14	7	15	7	20	5	23	0
Repair after functioning Potts anastomosis	7	14	11	18	4	25	3	67	10	10
Repair after nonfunctioning shunt	8	13	2	50	3	33	3	33	1	0
TOTAL	73	18	53	13	52	12	51	12	56	4

(Data from Kirklin and colleagues.[K7])

[a] Based on 285 patients with moderate or severe forms of tetralogy of Fallot with pulmonary stenosis undergoing operation at the Mayo Clinic from 1960 to 1965.

[b] A few patients had a previous closed Brock operation.

[c] Some patients had a previous bilateral Blalock-Taussig anastomosis.

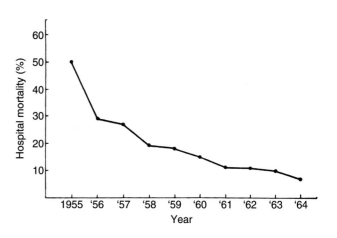

Figure 24A-1 Hospital mortality after repair of tetralogy of Fallot with pulmonary stenosis in a heterogeneous group of patients. (Figure based on 509 patients operated on at the Mayo Clinic from 1955 to 1965.) (From Kirklin and colleagues.[K7])

Figure 24A-2 Percentage of cases in which a transanular patch was used *(dashed line between open circles)* in repair of tetralogy of Fallot with pulmonary stenosis in a heterogeneous group of patients, according to year of operation. Also shown are (1) percentage of patients classified as having severe form of the disease *(dashed line between x's)*, (2) postrepair (OR) $P_{RV/LV}$ in patients in whom a transanular patch was used *(solid line between open circles)*, (3) this ratio in patients in whom a transanular patch was not used *(solid line between solid circles)*. $P_{RV/LV}$ was higher in patients with a transanular patch than in those without one, paradoxically, and this was again found in another study 20 years later.[K19] (Figure based on 285 patients operated on at the Mayo Clinic from 1960 to 1965.) (From Kirklin and colleagues.[K7])

Key: $P_{RV/LV}$, Ratio of the peak pressure in right ventricle to that in left ventricle.

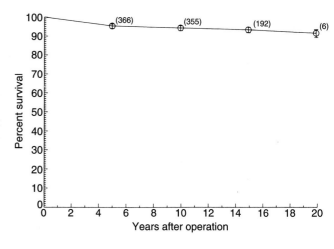

Figure 24A-3 Survival (actuarial method) of hospital survivors of repair of tetralogy of Fallot and pulmonary stenosis. Depiction is as in Fig. 24-44. (Figure based on 396 patients operated on at the Mayo Clinic from 1955 to 1965). (From Fuster and colleagues.[F3])

APPENDIX 24B

Tetralogy of Fallot with Pulmonary Stenosis: Early Green Lane Hospital Experience (1959 to 1978)

■ **TABLE 24B-1   Hospital Mortality after Repair of Tetralogy of Fallot without Major Associated Cardiac Anomalies** [a]

		Hospital Deaths		
Category	n	No.	%	CL (%)
Tetralogy of Fallot with pulmonary stenosis	341	24	7.0	5.6–8.8
Tetralogy of Fallot with pulmonary atresia	31 [b]	14	45	35–56
Tetralogy of Fallot with sub-arterial VSD	15	2	13	4–29
Tetralogy of Fallot with pulmonary regurgitation	6	2	33	12–62
Tetralogy of Fallot with flap-valve VSD	10	1	10	1–30
TOTAL	403	43	10.7	9.1–12.5

Key: *CL,* 70% confidence limits; *VSD,* ventricular septal defect.

[a] Based on 403 patients operated on at GLH from 1959 to 1978.

[b] One patient had flap-valve ventricular septal defect.

■ **TABLE 24B-2   Hospital Mortality after Repair of Tetralogy of Fallot with Pulmonary Stenosis and without Major Associated Cardiac Anomalies** [a]

		Hospital Deaths		
Treatment of Pulmonary Stenosis	n	No.	%	CL (%)
Without transanular patch	70	0	0	0–3
Transanular patch	55	8	15	10–21
Orthotopic valve insertion	2	0	0	0–61
TOTAL	127	8	6.3	4.1–9.4

[a] Based on patients operated on at GLH from 1970 to 1978.

■ **TABLE 24B-3   Prevalence of Transanular Patching in Repair of Tetralogy of Fallot with Pulmonary Stenosis, According to Age at Repair** [a]

Age			Transanular Patch			
≤ months <		n	No.	%	CL (%)	
	6	19	13	68	54–80	
6	12	28	9	32	22–44	30/65 = 46%
12	24	18	8	44	30–59	(39%–53%)
24	48	22	10	45	33–59	
48		38	15	39	30–49	

Key: *CL,* 70% confidence limits.

[a] Based on 125 patients undergoing repair at GLH from 1970 to 1978. Two additional patients received an orthotopic allograft valve insertion.

■ **TABLE 24B-4   Hospital Mortality after Repair of Tetralogy of Fallot with Pulmonary Stenosis, According to Age at Repair** [a]

Age			Hospital Deaths		
≤ months <		n	No.	%	CL (%)
	3	12	4	33	18–52
3	6	8	0	0	0–21
6	12	29	1	3	0.4–11
12	24	23	1	4	0.6–14
24	48	45	5	11	6–18
48	60	37	6	16	10–25
≤ years <					
5	10	98	3	3.1	1.3–6.1
10	20	49	2	4.1	1–9
20	30	22	0	0	0–8
30		18	2	11	4–24
TOTAL		341	24	7.0	5.6–8.8

Key: *CL,* 70% confidence limits.

[a] Based on 341 patients operated on at GLH from 1959 to 1978.

APPENDIX 24C

Tetralogy of Fallot with Pulmonary Stenosis: UAB Experience (1967 to May 1986)

■ **TABLE 24C-1   Hospital and Total Deaths (Hospital and Late) after Repair of Tetralogy of Fallot with Pulmonary Stenosis** [a]

Previous Palliative Operations	n	Hospital Deaths			Total Deaths	
		No.	%	CL (%)	No.	%
None (one-stage repair)	483	29	6.0	4.9-7.3	37	7.7
After a single classic shunt	204	10	4.9	3.4-7.0	17	8.3
After a single Waterston shunt	47	5	11	6-17	6	13
After a single Potts shunt	23	1	4	0.6-14	5	22
After a single central shunt	4	1	25	3-63	1	25
After other shunts [b]	4	2	50	18-82	2	50
After two or more shunts	29	4	14	7-24	4	14
After RV outflow tract procedure	16	3	19	8-34	7	44
After other procedures [c]	4	2	50	18-82	2	50
TOTAL	814	57	7.0	6.1-8.1	81	10.0

Key: *CL,* 70% confidence limits; *RV,* right ventricular.

[a] Based on 814 patients undergoing repair at UAB from 1967 to May 1986. A multivariable analysis has been made of time-related survival after repair (see Fig. 24-44).

[b] Three end-to-end left Blalock-Taussig (2 hospital deaths, 2 total deaths); 1 internal thoracic to left pulmonary artery (survivor).

[c] One Blalock-Hanlon operation, followed by left Blalock-Taussig shunt (hospital death); 1 left Blalock-Taussig shunt followed by classic Glenn shunt (hospital death).

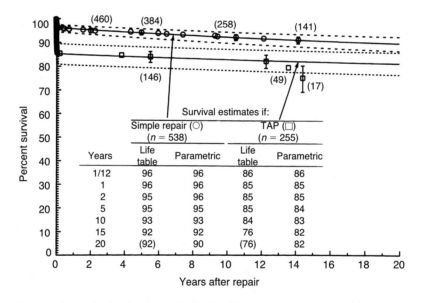

Figure 24C-1 Survival of patients stratified according to type of repair, and the parametrically predicted survivorship of each group using the multivariable risk factor equation (see Table 24-9). This and the subsequent appendix figures concerning survival after repair of tetralogy of Fallot with pulmonary stenosis (UAB; 1967 to May 1986; *n* = 814) represent (1) a validation of the parametric method[B34] and (2) the strength and time-relatedness of the effect of the risk factors. In each instance, the life-table method (Kaplan–Meier) was used to depict survivorship of the subset (represented by symbols; vertical bars represent 70% confidence limits; and numbers in parentheses patients at risk),[K36] and the parametric survivorship in each of the stratified subsets was obtained by determining, from the multivariable equation (Table 24-10), the probability of survival of each individual patient in the subset and averaging these using the method described by Ferrazzi and colleagues.[F18] In the figures, the 20-year values from the life-table analyses are assumed to be the same as the 15-year value and are therefore in parentheses. The multivariable equation is described in detail in the paper by Kirklin and colleagues.[K29]

Key: *TAP,* Transanular patch.

■ TABLE 24C-2   Hospital Mortality after Repair of Tetralogy of Fallot with Pulmonary Stenosis, According to Whether Repair Was Simple or with a Transanular Patch[a]

| Repair | 1967 to 1972 | | | | 1972 to 1977 | | | | 1977 to 1982 | | | | 1982 to 1986 | | | | Total | | | |
| | | Hospital Deaths | | | | Hospital Deaths | | | | Hospital Deaths | | | | Hospital Deaths | | | | Hospital Deaths | | |
	n	No.	%	CL (%)	n	No.	%	CL (%)	n	No.	%	CL (%)	n	No.	%	CL (%)	n	No.	%	CL (%)
Simple	119	6	5.0	3.0–8.0	159	8	5.0	3.3–7.5	101	2	2.0	0.7–4.6	90	1	1.1	0.1–3.7	469	17	3.6	2.7–4.7
Transanular patch	20	2	10	3–22	93	9	9.7	6–14	53	6	11	7–18	46	2	4.3	1–10	212	19	9.0	6.9–11.5
Subtotal	139	8	5.8	3.7–8.6	252	17	6.7	5.1–8.8	154	8	5.2	3.4–7.8	136	3	2.2	1.0–4.4	681	36	5.3	4.4–6.3
P(χ²)		.4				.16				.01				.22				.004		
Valved conduit	2	0	0	0–61	4	0	0	0–38	3	0	0	0–47	2	0	0	0–61	11	0	0	0–16
Total	141	8	5.7	3.7–8.5	256	17	6.6	5.0–8.7	157	8	5.1	3.3–7.6	138	3	2.2	1.0–4.3	692	36	5.2	4.3–6.2

Key: *CL,* 70% confidence limits.

[a] Based on 814 patients undergoing repair of tetralogy of Fallot with pulmonary stenosis at UAB from 1967 to May 1986, but excluding patients with multiple ventricular septal defects, dextrocardia, and nonconfluent right and left pulmonary arteries, and those with previous palliative procedures other than a single classic shunt.

■ TABLE 24C-3 Hospital Mortality after Repair of Tetralogy of Fallot with Pulmonary Stenosis, According to Age of Repair[a]

Age at Repair (months)		1967 to 1972 Hospital Deaths				1972 to 1977 Hospital Deaths				1977 to 1982 Hospital Deaths				1982 to 1986 Hospital Deaths				Total Hospital (30-Day) Deaths			
≤	<	n	No.	%	CL (%)	n	No.	%	CL (%)	n	No.	%	CL (%)	n	No.	%	CL (%)	n	No.	%	CL (%)
	6	—				10	3	30	14-51	7	2	29	10-55	4	0	0	0-38	21	5	24	14-37
6	12	—				26	4	15	8-26	12	1	8.3	1-26	13	0	0	0-14	51	5	10	6-16
12	24	1	0	0	0-85	39	2	6.9	2-16	24	1	4.2	0.5-13	37	0	0	0-5	91	3	3.3	1.4-6.5
24	48	4	0	0	0-38	38	4	11	5-18	44	3	6.8	3-13	46	3	6.5	3-13	132	10	7.6	5.2-10.7
48		136	8	5.9	3.8-8.8	153	4	2.6	1.3-4.7	70	1	1.4	0.2-4.8	38	0	0	0-5	397	13	3.3	2.4-4.5
TOTAL		141	8	5.7	3.7-8.5	256	17	6.6	5.0-8.7	157	8	5.1	3.3-7.6	138	3	2.2	1.0-4.3	692	36	5.2	4.3-6.2
P(χ²)								.002				.03				.19					

Key: CL, 70% confidence intervals.

[a] Based on the data set described in Table 24C-2.

■ TABLE 24C-4   **Hospital Mortality after Repair of Tetralogy of Fallot with Pulmonary Stenosis, According to the Postrepair (OR) $P_{RV/LV}$[a]**

Postrepair $P_{RV/LV}$ ratio	1967 to 1972				1972 to 1977				1977 to 1982				1982 to 1986				Total			
		Hospital Deaths				Hospital Deaths				Hospital Deaths				Hospital Deaths				Hospital Deaths		
	n	No.	%	CL (%)	n	No.	%	CL (%)	n	No.	%	CL (%)	n	No.	%	CL (%)	n	No.	%	CL (%)
≤ 0.35	18	0	0	0-10	83	4	4.8	2-9	28	0	0	0-7	18	0	0	0-10	147	4	2.7	1.4-4.9
0.35 <...≤ 0.55	79	4	5.1	3-9	116	8	6.9	4-10	72	8	11	7-16	76	0	0	0-3	343	20	5.8	4.5-7.4
0.55 <...≤ 0.75	55	3	5.5	2-11	66	7	11	7-16	52	3	5.8	3-11	41	3	7.3	3-14	214	16	7.5	5.6-9.8
0.75 <...≤ 0.95	19	4	21	11-35	11	2	18	6-38	19	1	5.3	0.7-17	12	1	8.3	1-26	61	8	13	9-19
0.95 <	4	0	0	0-38	10	2	20	7-41	6	2	33	12-62	3	2	67	24-96	23	6	26	16-39
SUBTOTAL	175	11	6.3	4.4-8.8	286	23	8.0	6.4-10.1	177	14	7.9	5.8-10.6	150	6	4.0	2.4-6.4	788	54	6.9	5.9-7.9
P (logistic)			.11				.02				.21				.0001				<.0001	
Unknown	6	1	17	2-46	4	1	25	3-63	6	1	17	2-46	10	0	0	0-17	26	3	12	5-22
TOTAL	181	12	6.6	4.7-9.1	290	24	8.3	6.6-10.3	183	15	8.2	6.1-10.9	160	6	3.8	2.2-6.0	814	57	7.0	6.1-8.1

Key: *CL*, 70% confidence limits.

[a] Based on 814 patients undergoing repair at UAB from 1967 to May 1986.

■ **TABLE 24C-5** **Incremental Risk Factors for Continuing or Recurring Right Ventricular Outflow Tract Obstruction after Repair of Tetralogy of Fallot with Pulmonary Stenosis** [a]

		Hazard Phase	
	Risk Factor	Early	Constant
(Smaller)	Demographic		•
	BSA		
(Higher)	Surgical	•	•
	Postrepair (OR) $P_{RV/LV}$		

(Data from Kirklin and colleagues.[K29])

Key: *BSA*, Body surface area; $P_{RV/LV}$, ratio of peak pressure in right ventricle to that in left ventricle.

[a] Based on 814 patients undergoing repair of tetralogy of Fallot with pulmonary stenosis at UAB from 1967 to May 1986.

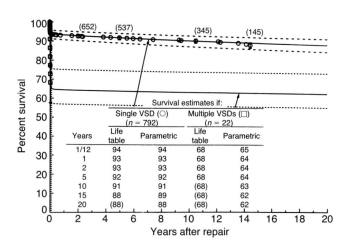

Figure 24C-2 Survival of patients stratified according to whether ventricular septal defect was single or multiple, and their parametrically predicted survivorship.

Key: *VSD*, Ventricular septal defect.

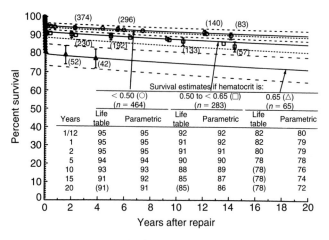

Figure 24C-3 Survival of patients stratified according to the value for hematocrit, and their parametrically predicted survivorship.

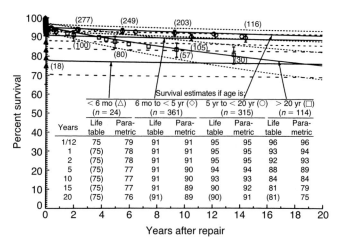

Figure 24C-4 Survival of patients stratified according to age, and their parametrically predicted survivorship.

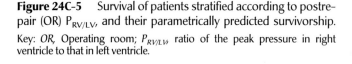

Figure 24C-5 Survival of patients stratified according to postrepair (OR) $P_{RV/LV}$, and their parametrically predicted survivorship.

Key: *OR*, Operating room; $P_{RV/LV}$, ratio of the peak pressure in right ventricle to that in left ventricle.

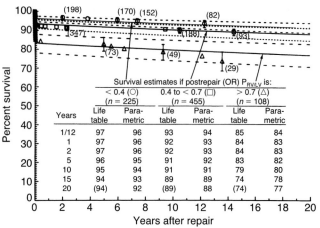

APPENDIX 24D

Tetralogy of Fallot with Pulmonary Stenosis: Combined Boston Children's Hospital–UAB Experience (September 1984 to 1989)

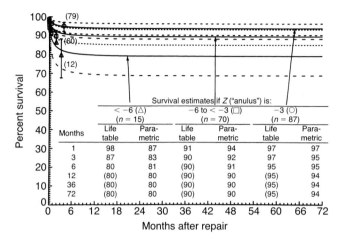

Figure 24D-1   Survival of patients stratified according to pre-repair diameter (expressed as Z value) of right ventricular–pulmonary trunk junction ("anulus") as determined from pre-repair cineangiograms, and their parametrically predicted survivorship. Note: This and subsequent appendix figures concerning survival after repair of tetralogy of Fallot with pulmonary stenosis are based on 196 patients undergoing 176 repairs at Boston Children's Hospital and UAB from September 1984 to 1989. The multivariable equation used is depicted in Table 24-9, which includes patient variables only; it and the data set are described in detail in the publication by Kirklin and colleagues.[K22] The method for parametric depiction is as described for Figure 24C-1.

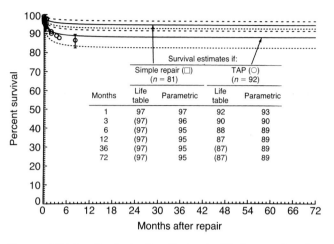

Figure 24D-2   Survival of patients stratified according to whether repair was a simple one or included a transanular patch, and their parametrically predicted survivorship.

Key: *TAP*, Transanular patch.

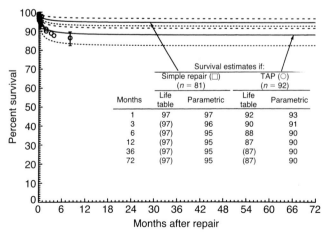

Figure 24D-3   Survival of patients stratified according to whether repair was a simple one or included a transanular patch, and their parametrically predicted survivorship. Multivariable equation (see Table 24-11) included patient and procedural variables.

Key: *TAP*, Transanular patch.

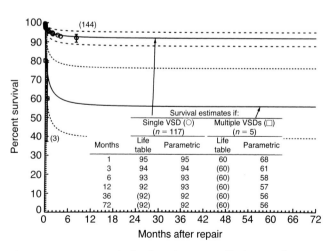

Figure 24D-4   Survival of patients stratified according to whether the ventricular septal defect was single or multiple, and their parametrically predicted survivorship. Multivariable equation used is depicted in Table 24-9.

Key: *VSD*, Ventricular septal defect.

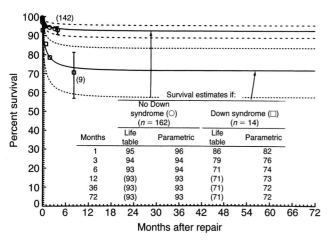

Figure 24D-5 Survival of patients stratified according to whether Down syndrome was or was not present, and their parametrically predicted survivorship. Multivariable equation used is depicted in Table 24-9.

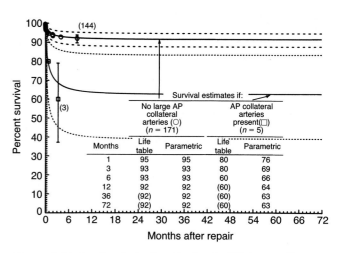

Figure 24D-6 Survival of patients stratified according to whether there were or were not large aortopulmonary collateral arteries, and their parametrically predicted survivorship. The equation used is depicted in Table 24-9.

Key: *AP*, Aortopulmonary.

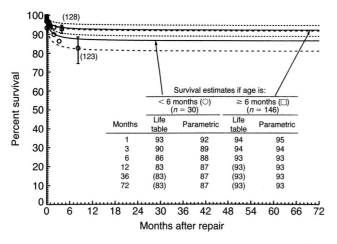

Figure 24D-7 Survival of patients stratified according to whether patients were younger than age 6 months or older, and their parametrically predicted survivorship. The equation used is depicted in Table 24-9.

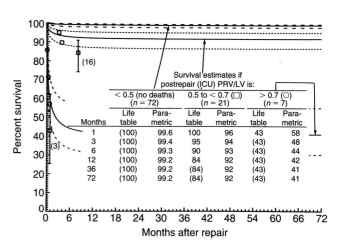

Figure 24D-8 Survival of patients stratified according to three ranges of values of postrepair (ICU) $P_{RV/LV}$, and their parametrically predicted survivorship. The equation used is depicted in Table 24-11.

Key: *ICU*, Intensive care unit; $P_{RV/LV}$, ratio of the peak pressure in right ventricle to that in left ventricle.

APPENDIX 24E

Tetralogy of Fallot with Pulmonary Atresia: UAB Experience (1967 to May 1986)

■ TABLE 24E-1   **Validation of Multivariable Logistic Regression Equation for Probability that Postrepair (OR) $P_{RV/LV}$ Will Be Equal to or Greater than 1**

No. of Large AP Collaterals	n	No. of Patients with $P_{RV/LV} \geq 1$		
		Actual	Predicted	P
0	40	4	4.7	.7
1	20	5	3.6	.4
2	8	2	1.9	.96
3	17	5	5.7	.7
4	8	4	4.1	.9
5	1	0	0.2	.6
6	2	1	0.7	.6

(McGoon Ratio) of RPA and LPA			n	No. of Patients with $P_{RV/LV} \geq 1$		
≤	ratio	<		Actual	Predicted	P
		0.5	2	2	1.2	.2
0.5		1	25	7	8.8	.4
1		1.5	28	6	5.1	.7
1.5		2	17	1	0.8	.8
2			8	0	0.1	.7

(Data from Blackstone and colleagues.[29])

Key: *AP*, Aortopulmonary; *LPA*, left pulmonary artery; *P_{RV/LV}*, ratio of peak pressure in right ventricle to that in left ventricle, *RPA*, right pulmonary artery.

APPENDIX 24F

Patient-Specific Predictions and Comparisons of Outcome in Patients with Tetralogy of Fallot with Pulmonary Stenosis

Distillation of the GLH, UAB, and BCH experiences (Appendixes 24A through 24E), indicates that the large volume of available information on outcomes after repair of TF with pulmonary stenosis is internally consistent. Unfortunately, it cannot all be put into a single analysis to permit development of a multiinstitutionally based multivariable risk factor equation for predicting and comparing outcome events (results) in a time-related manner. However, available analyses can be focused on an individual patient to provide therapeutically and inferentially useful predictions and comparisons (for a more detailed discussion, see "Decision-Making for Individual Patients" in Section 5 of Chapter 6). A hypothetical patient is presented to illustrate this.

Case 1

A 6-month-old moderately cyanotic but otherwise normal-appearing infant (no Down syndrome) has TF with a single typical VSD. RPA and LPA are confluent and distribute to all pulmonary arterial segments. They appear to be somewhat small. No large AP collateral arteries are present. There is infundibular and valvar pulmonary stenosis, and the Z value for diameter of the pulmonary "anulus" (calculated from measurements on the cineangiogram corrected for magnification) is −3.9. A transanular patch is judged likely to be needed at repair, and postrepair (ICU) $P_{RV/LV}$ is speculated to be about 0.6. If an equation from the era 1967 to 1986 is used (see Table 24-10) predicted probability of hospital (30-day) survival after one-stage repair of the TF with a transanular patch is 89% (CL 85%-94%) and 10-year survival is 88% (CL 84%-92%) (Fig. 24F-1, *A*). If the equation from the era of 1984 to 1989 is used, predicted hospital and 10-year survivals with a transanular patch and a postrepair (ICU) $P_{RV/LV}$ of 0.6 are similar: 93% (CL 86%-97%) and 87% (CL

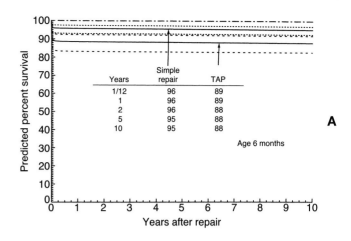

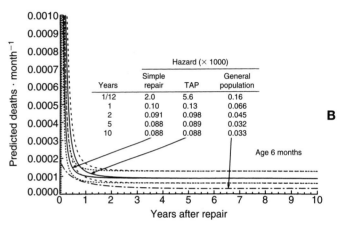

Figure 24F-1   Nomogram of patient-specific solutions of the multivariable risk factor equation (UAB, 1967 to May 1986; n = 814; see Table 24-10) illustrating patient-specific predicted percent survival (**A**) if simple repair is done or a transanular patch is used at 6 months of age. In this and subsequent depictions, solid line represents the continuous point estimate, and the dashed lines enclose its 70% confidence limits. Dash-dot-dash line represents the survival of an age–gender–ethnicity–matched general population. **A**, Survival. **B**, Hazard function for death.

Key: *TAP*, Transanular patch.

79%-94%), respectively (Fig. 24F-2, *A*). (In this series of figures, each depiction of survival is followed by a figure depicting the time-related hazard function for death.)

Predicted probability of the child's survival to age 18 months without operation is 91% to 96% (see Fig. 24-21); predicted probability of hospital survival after repair with a transanular patch at that age is 95% (CL 92%-97%) and that 10-year survival is 93% (CL 91%-96%) (Fig. 24F-3, *A*). Using the equations from the more recent era, predicted postrepair hospital and 10-year survivals for this 18-month-old are, respectively, 96% (CL 94%-98%) and 93% (CL 88%-96%) (Fig. 24F-4, *A*).

Thus, *overall* probability of survival for at least 10 years if repair is deferred from age 6 months to age 18 months, which is a combination of survival to age 18 months and survival after repair, would be about 84% to 91% using the equation from an earlier era. The deferral would have no predicted advantage over primary repair at 6 months of age, after which the 10-year predicted survival was 83% to 92%. With the equation from the more recent era, overall predicted probability of survival for at least 10 years, with deferral of repair to 18 months, would be 81% to 91%; the inference of no advantage from deferral remains.

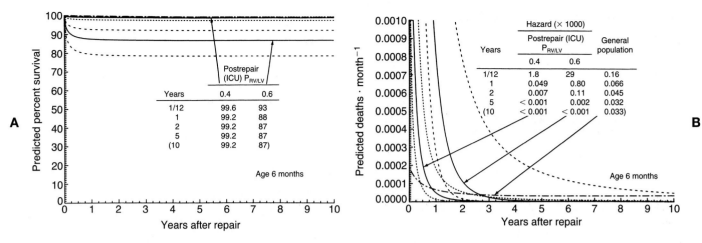

Figure 24F-2 Nomograms of patient-specific solutions of the multivariable risk factor equation (Boston Children's Hospital–UAB, September 1984 to 1989; see Table 24-11) illustrating patient-specific (for same patient described in Fig. 24F-1) predicted survival (A), according to postrepair (ICU) $P_{RV/LV}$. **A**, Survival. **B**, Hazard function for death.

Key: *ICU*, Intensive care unit; $P_{RV/LV}$, ratio of the peak pressure in right ventricle to that in left ventricle.

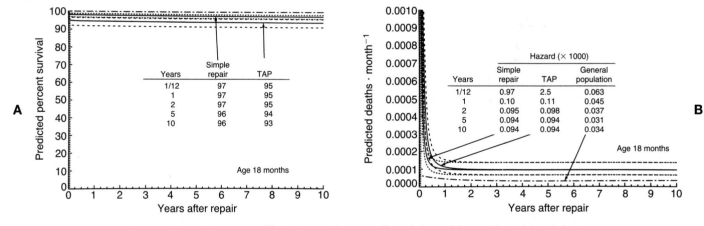

Figure 24F-3 Nomogram illustrating patient-specific solution of the multivariable risk factor equation (UAB, 1967 to May 1986; $n = 814$) for patient described in the previous figures, with the repair deferred until 18 months of age and with or without (simple) a transanular patch. **A**, Survival. **B**, Hazard function for death.

Key: *TAP*, Transanular patch.

Another possibility is to perform a systemic–pulmonary arterial shunt at age 6 months, and repair at age 18 months. No single equation summarizes survival after repair in this situation. However, the combination of the probabilities of (1) death occurring within 1 year of creating the shunt, (2) important distortion of a pulmonary artery produced by the shunt, and (3) the patient not returning for repair until the shunt has virtually closed with resultant increase in hematocrit, make it unlikely that this protocol will yield long-term survival as good or better than primary repair at age 6 months.

The therapeutic possibilities can be similarly analyzed for a patient presenting at age *3 months*. It again indicates that probabilities of long-term survival are similar after primary repair and delayed repair.

Comment
Patient-specific predictions and comparisons must be supplemented by the physician's general knowledge and judgment, as well as his or her assessment of institutional capabilities.

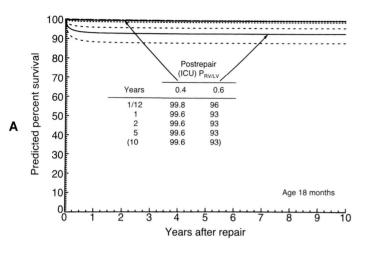

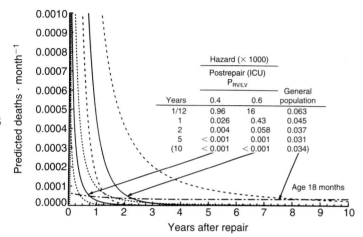

Figure 24F-4   Nomogram illustrating patient-specific solution of the multivariable risk factor equation (Boston Children's Hospital–UAB, September 1984 to 1989) for the patient described in the previous figures, with the repair deferred until 18 months of age, stratified according to post repair (ICU) $P_{RV/LV}$. **A**, Survival. **B**, Hazard function for death.

Key: *ICU*, Intensive care unit; $P_{RV/LV}$, ratio of the peak pressure in right ventricle to that in left ventricle.

APPENDIX 24G

Relation of Body Surface Area to Age

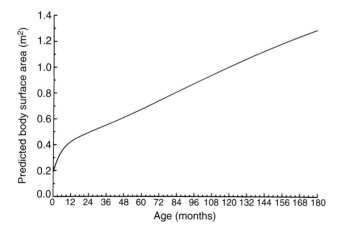

Figure 24G-1   Nomogram of equation relating body surface area to age in patients with tetralogy of Fallot. Equation is based on data from 1533 patients with tetralogy of Fallot and pulmonary stenosis or atresia (UAB experience). They ranged in age from 1 day to 57 years and in body surface area from 0.12 to 2.3 m². The equation is as follows:

$$Ln\ (BSA) = -4.504 + 27.82 \cdot a^3 - 45.51 \cdot a^4 + 26.39 \cdot a^5 - 5.238 \cdot a^6$$

where a = Ln [Ln(age + 9)], age is in months, and Ln is the natural logarithm double logarithmic transformation, and Ln [BSA(m²)] = natural logarithm of body surface area.

APPENDIX 24H
Values of Variables Used in Nomograms

Values in Fig. 24-46: Specific values entered into the multivariable equation were hematocrit 50%, no more than one previous palliative operation, no Potts anastomosis, no previous direct approach to RV outlet obstruction, no multiple VSDs, no dextrocardia, no absence of unbranched hilar portion of one pulmonary artery, average prevalence of transanular patch placement (31%), and postrepair (OR) $P_{RV/LV}$ of 0.55. For age 6 months, 12 months, 24 months, and 48 months, body surface area was entered as 0.345 m², 0.4125 m², 0.5025 m², and 0.630 m², respectively.

Values in Fig. 24-49: Specific values entered into the multivariable equation were hematocrit 50%, no more than one previous palliative operation, no Potts anastomosis, no previous direct approach to RV outlet obstruction, no multiple VSDs, no dextrocardia, no absence of unbranched hilar portion of one pulmonary artery, date of operation 1988, and postrepair (OR) $P_{RV/LV}$ of 0.6.

Values in Fig. 24-51: Specific values entered into the multivariable equation were age 6 months at repair and postrepair (ICU) $P_{RV/LV}$ of 0.45.

Values in Fig. 24-78: Specific values entered into the multivariable equation were age 5 years at repair, body surface area 0.695 m², no more than one previous palliative operation, extracardiac valved conduit used, and postrepair (OR) $P_{RV/LV}$ of 0.7.

REFERENCES

A

1. Alfieri O, Locatelli G, Bianchi T, Vanini V, Parenzan L. Repair of tetralogy of Fallot after Waterston anastomosis. J Thorac Cardiovasc Surg 1979;77:826.

2. Arciniegas E, Farooki ZQ, Hakimi M, Green EW. Results of two-stage surgical treatment of tetralogy of Fallot. J Thorac Cardiovasc Surg 1980;79:876.

3. Albertal G, Swan HJ, Kirklin JW. Hemodynamic studies two weeks to six years after repair of tetralogy of Fallot. Circulation 1964;29:583.

4. Arciniegas E, Farooki ZQ, Hakimi M, Perry BL, Green EW. Classic shunting operations for congenital cyanotic heart defects. J Thorac Cardiovasc Surg 1982;84:88.

5. Arciniegas E, Farooki ZQ, Hakimi M, Perry BL, Green EW. Early and late results of total correction of tetralogy of Fallot. J Thorac Cardiovasc Surg 1980;80:770.

6. Agarwal KC, Edwards WD, Feldt RH, Danielson GK, Puga FJ, McGoon DC. Pathogenesis of nonobstructive fibrous peels in right-sided porcine-valved extracardiac conduits. J Thorac Cardiovasc Surg 1982;83:584.

7. Alfieri O, Blackstone EH, Kirklin JW, Pacifico AD, Bargeron LM Jr. Surgical treatment of tetralogy of Fallot with pulmonary atresia. J Thorac Cardiovasc Surg 1978;76:321.

8. Arciniegas E, Blackstone EH, Pacifico AD, Kirklin JW. Classic shunting operations as part of two-stage repair of tetralogy of Fallot. Ann Thorac Surg 1979;27:514.

9. Arensman FW, Francis PD, Helmsworth JA, Benzing G 3rd, Schreiber JT, Schwartz DC, et al. Early medical and surgical intervention for tetralogy of Fallot with absence of pulmonic valve. J Thorac Cardiovasc Surg 1982;84:430.

10. Akasaka T, Itoh K, Ohkawa Y, Nakayama S, Miyamoto H, Nishi T, et al. Surgical treatment of anomalous origin of the left coronary artery from the pulmonary artery associated with tetralogy of Fallot. Ann Thorac Surg 1981;31:469.

11. Alfieri O, Blackstone EH, Parenzan L. Growth of the pulmonary anulus and pulmonary arteries after the Waterston anastomosis. J Thorac Cardiovasc Surg 1979;78:440.

12. Ackerman MJ, Wylam ME, Feldt RH, Porter CJ, Dewald G, Scanlon PD, et al. Pulmonary atresia with ventricular septal defect and persistent airway hyperresponsiveness. J Thorac Cardiovasc Surg 2001;122:169.

13. Anderson RH, Allwork SP, Ho SY, Lenox CC, Zuberbuhler JR. Surgical anatomy of tetralogy of Fallot. J Thorac Cardiovasc Surg 1981;81:887.

14. Anaclerio S, Marino B, Carotti A, Digilio MC, Toscano A, Gitto P, et al. Pulmonary atresia with ventricular septal defect: prevalence of deletion 22q11 in the different anatomic patterns. Ital Heart J 2001;2:384.

15. Abdulali SA, Silverton NP, Yakirevich VS, Ionescu MI. Right ventricular outflow tract reconstruction with a bovine pericardial monocusp patch. J Thorac Cardiovasc Surg 1985;89:764.

16. Almeida RS, Wyse RK, de Leval MR, Elliott MJ, Stark J. Long-term results of homograft valves in extracardiac conduits. Eur J Cardiothorac Surg 1989;3:488.

17. Anderson RH, Devine WA, Del Nido P. The surgical anatomy of tetralogy of Fallot with pulmonary atresia rather than pulmonary stenosis. J Card Surg 1991;6:41.

18. Amin Z, McElhinney DB, Reddy VM, Moore P, Hanley FL, Teitel DF. Coronary to pulmonary artery collaterals in patients with pulmonary atresia and ventricular septal defect. Ann Thorac Surg 2000;70:119.

B

1. Blackstone EH, Kirklin JW, Bertranou EG, Labrosse CJ, Soto B, Bargeron LM Jr. Preoperative prediction from cineangiograms of postrepair right ventricular pressure in tetralogy of Fallot. J Thorac Cardiovasc Surg 1979;78:542.

2. Bonchek LI, Starr A, Sunderland CO, Menashe VD. Natural history of tetralogy of Fallot in infancy. Circulation 1973;48:392.

3. Becu L, Ikkos D, Ljungqvist A, Rudhe U. Evolution of ventricular septal defect and pulmonary stenosis with left to right shunt into classic tetralogy of Fallot. Am J Cardiol 1961;7:598.

4. Blalock A, Taussig HB. The surgical treatment of malformations of the heart in which there is pulmonary stenosis or pulmonary atresia. JAMA 1945;128:189.

5. Bargeron LM Jr, Elliott LP, Soto B, Bream PR, Curry GC. Axial cineangiography in congenital heart disease. Section I. Concept, Technical and Anatomic Considerations. Circulation 1977;56:1075.

6. Barnard CN, Schrire V. The surgical treatment of the tetralogy of Fallot. Thorax 1961;16:346.

7. Brock RC, Campbell M. Infundibular resection or dilatation for infundibular stenosis. Br Heart J 1950;12:403.

8. Bender HW Jr, Fisher RD, Conkle DM, Martin CE, Graham TP. Selective operative treatment for tetralogy of Fallot. Ann Surg 1976;183:685.

9. Barratt-Boyes BG, Simpson M, Neutze JM. Intracardiac surgery in neonates and infants using deep hypothermia with surface cooling and limited cardiopulmonary bypass. Circulation 1971;43:I25.

10. Binet JP, Hvass U, Bruniaux J, Langlois J, Planche C, Dreyfus G, et al. Complete correction of tetralogy of Fallot without opening the right ventricle. Arch Mal Coeur Vaiss 1980;73:1185.

11. Beach PM Jr, Bowman FO Jr, Kaiser GA, Malm JR. Total correction of tetralogy of Fallot in adolescents and adults. Circulation 1971;43:I37.

12. Bharati S, Lev M, Kirklin JW. Cardiac surgery and the conduction system, 2nd Ed. Mount Kisco, NY: Futura, 1992.

13. Bertranou EG, Blackstone EH, Hazelrig JB, Turner ME, Kirklin JW. Life expectancy without surgery in tetralogy of Fallot. Am J Cardiol 1978;42:458.

14. Byrne JP, Hawkins JA, Battiste CE, Khoury GH. Palliative procedures in tetralogy of Fallot with absent pulmonary valve: a new approach. Ann Thorac Surg 1982;33:499.

15. Bove EL, Byrum CJ, Thomas FD, Kavey RE, Sondheimer HM, Blackman MS, et al. The influence of pulmonary insufficiency on ventricular function following repair of tetralogy of Fallot. Evaluation using radionuclide ventriculography. J Thorac Cardiovasc Surg 1983; 85:691.

16. Barratt-Boyes BG. The surgery of tetralogy of Fallot, pulmonary atresia with ventricular septal defect and transposition of the great vessels. Aust Radiol 1968;12:311.

17. Blondeau PH, Nottin R, d'Allaines C, Carpentier A, Soyer R, Bouchard F, et al. Communications interventriculaires residuelles aprés reparation compléte de la tetralogie de Fallot. Coeur 1977;3:31.

18. Bocala RR, Guller B, Danielson GK, Feldt RH. Left anterior hemiblock and complete repair of tetralogy of Fallot (abstract). Pediatr Res 1974;8:347.

19. Borow KM, Green LH, Castaneda AR, Keane JF. Left ventricular function after repair of tetralogy of Fallot and its relationship to age at surgery. Circulation 1980;61:1150.

20. Bjarke B. Oxygen uptake and cardiac output during submaximal and maximal exercise in adult subjects with totally corrected tetralogy of Fallot. Acta Med Scand 1975;197:177.

21. Bharati S, Paul MH, Idriss FS, Potkin RT, Lev M. The surgical anatomy of pulmonary atresia with ventricular septal defect: pseudotruncus. J Thorac Cardiovasc Surg 1975;69:713.

22. Brown SC, Eyskens B, Mertens L, Dumoulin M, Gewillig M. Percutaneous treatment of stenosed major aortopulmonary collaterals with balloon dilation and stenting: what can be achieved? Heart 1998;79:24.

23. Baumstark A, Fellows KE, Rosenthal A. Combined double chambered right ventricle and discrete subaortic stenosis. Circulation 1978; 57:299.

24. Blount SG Jr, Vigoda PS, Swan H. Isolated infundibular stenosis. Am Heart J 1959;57:684.

25. Bailey WW, Kirklin JW, Bargeron LM Jr, Pacifico AD, Kouchoukos NT. Late results with synthetic valved external conduits from venous ventricle to pulmonary arteries. Circulation 1977;56:II73.

26. Barratt-Boyes BG, Neutze JM. Primary repair of tetralogy of Fallot in infancy using profound hypothermia with circulatory arrest and limited cardiopulmonary bypass: a comparison with conventional two-stage management. Ann Surg 1973;178:406.

27. Brock RC. Pulmonary valvulotomy for relief of congenital pulmonary stenosis. Report of 3 cases. Br Med J 1948;1:1121.

28. Boucek MM, Webster HE, Orsmond GS, Ruttenberg HD. Balloon pulmonary valvotomy: palliation for cyanotic heart disease. Am Heart J 1988;115:318.

29. Blackstone EH, Shimazaki Y, Maehara T, Kirklin JW, Bargeron LM Jr. Prediction of severe obstruction to right ventricular outflow after repair of tetralogy of Fallot and pulmonary atresia. J Thorac Cardiovasc Surg 1988;96:288.

30. Burczynski PL, McKay R, Arnold R, Mitchell DR, Sabino GP. Homograft replacement of the pulmonary artery bifurcation. J Thorac Cardiovasc Surg 1989;98:623.

31. Boyce SW, Turley K, Yee ES, Verrier ED, Ebert PA. The fate of the 12 mm porcine valved conduit from the right ventricle to the pulmonary artery. A ten-year experience. J Thorac Cardiovasc Surg 1988;95:201.

32. Bove EL, Kavey RE, Byrum CJ, Sondheimer HM, Blackman MS, Thomas FD. Improved right ventricular function following late pulmonary valve replacement for residual pulmonary insufficiency or stenosis. J Thorac Cardiovasc Surg 1985;90:50.

34. Blackstone EH, Naftel DC, Turner ME Jr. The decomposition of time-varying hazard into phases, each incorporating a separate stream of concomitant information. J Am Stat Assoc 1986;81:615.

35. Becker AE, Connor M, Anderson RH. Tetralogy of Fallot: a morphometric and geometric study. Am J Cardiol 1975;35:402.

36. Bogers AJ, Rohmer J, Wolsky SA, Quaegebeur JM, Huysmans HA. Coronary artery fistula as source of pulmonary circulation in pulmonary atresia with ventricular septal defect. Thorac Cardiovasc Surg 1990;38:30.

C

1. Castaneda AR, Freed MD, Williams RG, Norwood WI. Repair of tetralogy of Fallot in infancy. Early and late results. J Thorac Cardiovasc Surg 1977;74:372.

2. Castaneda AR, Kirklin JW. Tetralogy of Fallot with aorticopulmonary window. Report of two surgical cases. J Thorac Cardiovasc Surg 1977;74:467.

3. Castaneda AR, Norwood WI. Fallot's tetralogy. In Stark J, de Leval M, eds. Surgery for congenital heart defects. Orlando, Fla.: Grune & Stratton, 1983.

4. Calder AL, Brandt PW, Barratt-Boyes BG, Neutze JM. Variant of tetralogy of Fallot with absent pulmonary valve leaflets and origin of one pulmonary artery from the ascending aorta. Am J Cardiol 1980;46:106.

5. Castaneda AR, Sade RM, Lamberti J, Nicoloff DM. Reoperation for residual defects after repair of tetralogy of Fallot. Surgery 1974; 76:1010.

6. Ciaravella JM Jr, McGoon DC, Danielson GK, Wallace RB, Mair DD, Ilstrup DM. Experience with the extracardiac conduit. J Thorac Cardiovasc Surg 1979;78:920.

7. Cumming GR, Carr W. Relief of dyspneic attacks in Fallot's tetralogy with propranolol. Lancet 1966;l:519.

8. Cole RB, Muster AJ, Fixler DE, Paul MH. Long-term results of aortopulmonary anastomosis for tetralogy of Fallot. Circulation 1971;43:263.

9. Chiariello L, Meyer J, Wukasch DC, Hallman GL, Cooley DA. Intracardiac repair of tetralogy of Fallot. Five-year review of 403 patients. J Thorac Cardiovasc Surg 1975;70:529.

10. Clayman JA, Ankeney JL, Liebman J. Results of complete repair of tetralogy of Fallot in 156 consecutive patients. Am J Surg 1975; 130:601.

11. Cairns JA, Dobell AR, Gibbons JE, Tessler I. Prognosis of right bundle branch block and left anterior hemiblock after intracardiac repair of tetralogy of Fallot. Am Heart J 1975;90:549.

12. Capelli H, Ross D, Somerville J. Aortic regurgitation in tetrad of Fallot and pulmonary atresia. Am J Cardiol 1982;49:1979.

13. Coates JR, McClenathan JE, Scott LW 3rd. The double-chambered right ventricle. A diagnostic and operative pitfall. Am J Cardiol 1964;14:561.

14. Corone P, Doyon F, Gaudeau S, Guerin F, Vernant P, Ducam H, et al. Natural history of ventricular septal defect. A study involving 790 cases. Circulation 1977;55:908.

15. Cosio FG, Wang Y, Nicoloff DM. Membranous right ventricular outflow obstruction. Am J Cardiol 1973;32:1000.

16. Chesler E, Korns ME, Edwards JE. Anomalies of the tricuspid valve, including pouches, resembling aneurysms of the membranous ventricular septum. Am J Cardiol 1968;21:661.

17. Calder AL, Barratt-Boyes BG, Brandt PW, Neutze JM. Postoperative evaluation of patients with tetralogy of Fallot repaired in infancy. J Thorac Cardiovasc Surg 1979;77:704.

18. Calder AL, Kirker JA, Neutze JM, Starling MB. Pathology of the ductus arteriosus treated with prostaglandins. Comparison with untreated cases. Pediatr Cardiol l984;5:85.

19. Castaneda AR. Classical repair of tetralogy of Fallot: timing, technique, and results. Semin Thorac Cardiovasc Surg 1990;2:70.

20. Castaneda AR, Mayer J, Jonas R, Walsh EP, Lang P. Tetralogy of Fallot: Repair in infancy. In Crupi G, Parenzan L, Anderson RH, eds. Perspectives in pediatric cardiology, Vol. 2. Pediatric cardiac surgery, Part 1. New York: Futura Publishing, 1989.

21. Clarke DR, Campbell DN, Pappas G. Pulmonary allograft conduit repair of tetralogy of Fallot. An alternative to transanular patch repair. J Thorac Cardiovasc Surg 1989;98:730.

22. Calder AL, Chan NS, Clarkson PM, Kerr AR, Neutze JM. Progress of patients with pulmonary atresia after systemic to pulmonary arterial shunts. Ann Thorac Surg 1991;51:40l.

23. Centazzo S, Montigny M, Davignon A, Chartrand C, Fournier A, Marchand T. Use of acetylsalicylic acid to improve patency of subclavian to pulmonary artery Gore-Tex shunts. Can J Cardiol 1993;9:243.

24. Chessa M, Butera G, Bonhoeffer P, Iserin L, Kachaner J, Lyonnet S, et al. Relation of genotype 22q11 deletion to phenotype of pulmonary vessels in tetralogy of Fallot and pulmonary atresia-ventricular septal defect. Heart 1998;79:186.

25. Carotti A, Di Donato RM, Squitieri C, Guccione P, Catena G. Total repair of pulmonary atresia with ventricular septal defect and major aortopulmonary collaterals: an integrated approach. J Thorac Cardiovasc Surg 1998;116:914.

D

1. Daily PO, Stinson EB, Griepp RB, Shumway NE. Tetralogy of Fallot. Choice of surgical procedure. J Thorac Cardiovasc Surg 1978;75:338.

2. Dobell AR, Charrette EP, Chughtai MS. Correction of tetralogy of Fallot in the young child. J Thorac Cardiovasc Surg 1968;55:70.

3. Daoud G, Kaplan S, Helmsworth JA. Tetralogy of Fallot and pulmonary hypertension. Am J Dis Child 1966;111:166.

4. Donahoo JS, Gardner TJ, Zahka K, Kidd BS. Systemic-pulmonary shunts in neonates and infants using microporous expanded polytetrafluoroethylene: immediate and late results. Ann Thorac Surg 1980;30:146.

5. Dabizzi RP, Caprioli G, Aiazzi L, Castelli C, Baldrighi G, Parenzan L, et al. Distribution and anomalies of coronary arteries in tetralogy of Fallot. Circulation 1980;61:95.

6. de Leval MR, McKay R, Jones M, Stark J, Macartney FJ. Modified Blalock-Taussig shunt. Use of subclavian artery orifice as flow regulator in prosthetic systemic-pulmonary artery shunts. J Thorac Cardiovasc Surg 1981;81:112.

7. D'Cruz I, Lendrum BL, Novak G. Congenital absence of the pulmonary valve. Am Heart J 1964;68:728.

8. Delisle G, Olley PM. Submaximal effort test in children with Fallot's tetralogy before and after surgical correction. Union Med Can 1974;103:886.

9. Davidson JS. Anastomosis between the ascending aorta and the main pulmonary artery in the tetralogy of Fallot. Thorax 1955;10:348.

10. Di Benedetto G, Tiraboschi R, Vanini V, Annecchino P, Aiazzi L, Caprioli C, et al. Systemic-pulmonary artery shunt using PTFE prosthesis (Gore-Tex). Early results and long-term follow-up on 105 consecutive cases. Thorac Cardiovasc Surg 1981;29:143.

11. Dickinson DF, Wilkinson JL, Smith A, Hamilton DI, Anderson RH. Variations in the morphology of the ventricular septal defect and disposition of the atrioventricular conduction tissues in tetralogy of Fallot. Thorac Cardiovasc Surg 1982;30:243.

12. Deanfield JE, Ho SY, Anderson RH, McKenna WJ, Allwork SP, Hallidie-Smith KA. Late sudden death after repair of tetralogy Fallot: a clinicopathologic study. Circulation 1983;67:626.

13. Dolara A, Dellocchio T, Diligenti LM, Manetti A, Vergassola R. Pulmonary infundibular stenosis developing after closure of ventricular septal defect. Acta Cardiol 1975;30:221.

14. Danilowicz D, Hoffman JI, Rudolph AM. Serial studies of pulmonary stenosis in infancy and childhood. Br Heart J 1975;37:808.

15. Doty DB, Kouchoukos NT, Kirklin JW, Barcia A, Bargeron LM Jr. Surgery for pseudotruncus arteriosus with pulmonary blood flow originating from upper descending thoracic aorta. Circulation 1972;45:I121.

16. Di Donato RM, Jonas RA, Lang P, Rome JJ, Mayer JE Jr, Castaneda AR. Neonatal repair of tetralogy of Fallot with and without pulmonary atresia. J Thorac Cardiovasc Surg 1991;101:126.

17. DeRuiter MC, Gittenberger-de Groot AC, Bogers AJ, Elzenga NJ. The restricted surgical relevance of morphologic criteria to classify systemic-pulmonary collateral arteries in pulmonary atresia with ventricular septal defect. J Thorac Cardiovasc Surg 1994;108:692.

18. Digilio MC, Marino B, Grazioli S, Agostino D, Giannotti A, Dallapiccola B. Comparison of occurrence of genetic syndromes in ventricular septal defect with pulmonic stenosis (classic tetralogy of Fallot) versus ventricular septal defect with pulmonic atresia. Am J Cardiol 1996;77:1375.

19. D'Allaines C, Sover R, Rioux C, Blondeau P, Cachera JP, Dubost C. Tetralogies de Fallot: Resultats à distance de la correction compléte. Nouv Presse Med 1973;2:961.

E

1. Edwards JE, McGoon DC. Absence of anatomic origin from heart of pulmonary arterial supply. Circulation 1973;47:393.

2. Edmunds LH Jr, Saxena NC, Friedman S, Rashkind WJ, Dodd PF. Transatrial resection of the obstructed right ventricular infundibulum. Circulation 1976;54:117.

3. Edmunds LH Jr, Saxena NC, Friedman S, Rashkind WJ, Dodd PF. Transatrial repair of tetralogy of Fallot. Surgery 1976;80:681.

4. Ergin MA, Griepp RB. Total correction of tetralogy of Fallot. How to deal with complicated ascending aorta-right pulmonary artery anastomosis. J Thorac Cardiovasc Surg 1979;77:469.

5. Ebert PA. Second operations for pulmonary stenosis or insufficiency after repair of tetralogy of Fallot. Am J Cardiol 1982;50:637.

6. Eakin WW, Abbott ME. Stenosis of the pulmonary conus at the lower bulbar orifice (conus a separate chamber) and closed interventricular septum with two illustrative cases. Presented at the Meeting of the American Association of Pathologists and Bacteriologists, Washington, DC, May 9, 1933.

7. Ehrenhaft JL, Theilen EO, Fisher J. Ectopic tricuspid leaflet producing symptoms of infundibular pulmonic stenosis. Ann Surg 1959;150:937.

8. Emmanoulides GC, Thanopoulos B, Siassi B, Fishbein M. "Agenesis" of ductus arteriosus associated with the syndrome of tetralogy of Fallot and absent pulmonary valve. Am J Cardiol 1976;37:403.

9. Elzenga NJ, Gittenberger-de Groot AC. The ductus arteriosus and stenoses of the pulmonary arteries in pulmonary atresia. Int J Cardiol 1986;11:195.

10. Edwards BS, Lucas RV Jr, Lock JE, Edwards JE. Morphologic changes in the pulmonary arteries after percutaneous balloon angioplasty for pulmonary arterial stenosis. Circulation 1985;71:195.

11. Elzenga NJ, von Suylen RJ, Frohn-Mulder I, Essed CE, Bos E, Quaegebeur JM. Juxtaductal pulmonary artery coarctation. An underestimated cause of branch pulmonary artery stenosis in patients with pulmonary atresia or stenosis and a ventricular septal defect. J Thorac Cardiovasc Surg 1990;100:416.

12. El-Said HG, Clapp S, Fagan TE, Conwell J, Nihill MR. Stenting of stenosed aortopulmonary collaterals and shunts for palliation of pulmonary atresia/ventricular septal defect. Catheter Cardiovasc Interv 2000;49:430.

F

1. Ferencz C. The pulmonary vascular bed in tetralogy of Fallot. I. Changes associated with pulmonary stenosis. Bull Johns Hopkins Hosp 1960;106:81.

2. Ferencz C. The pulmonary vascular bed in tetralogy of Fallot. II. Changes following a systemic-pulmonary arterial anastomosis. Bull Johns Hopkins Hosp 1960;106:100.

3. Fuster V, McGoon DC, Kennedy MA, Ritter DG, Kirklin JW. Long-term evaluation (12 to 22 years) of open heart surgery for tetralogy of Fallot. Am J Cardiol 1980;46:635.

4. Fellows KE, Smith J, Keane JF. Preoperative angiocardiography in infants with tetrad of Fallot. Review of 36 cases. Am J Cardiol 1981;47:1279.

5. Fellows KE, Freed MK, Keane JF, Praagh R, Bernhard WF, Castaneda AC. Results of routine preoperative coronary angiography in tetralogy of Fallot. Circulation 1975;51:561.

6. Furuse A, Mizuno A, Shindo G, Yamaguchi T, Saigusa M. Optimal size of outflow patch in total correction of tetralogy of Fallot. Jpn Heart J 1977;18:629.

7. Furuse A, Mizuno A, Shindo G, Yamaguchi T, Saigusa M. Pulmonary regurgitation following total correction of tetralogy of Fallot. Jpn Heart J 1977;18:621.

8. Freedom RM, Pongiglione G, Williams WG, Trusler GA, Rowe RD. Palliative right ventricular outflow tract construction for patients with pulmonary atresia, ventricular septal defect, and hypoplastic pulmonary arteries. J Thorac Cardiovasc Surg 1983;86:24.

9. Finnegan P, Haider R, Patel RG, Abrams LS, Singh SP. Results of total correction of the tetralogy of Fallot. Long-term haemodynamic evaluation at rest and during exercise. Br Heart J 1976;38:934.

10. Fabricius J, Hansen PF, Lindeneg O. Pulmonary atresia developing after a shunt operation for Fallot's tetralogy. Br Heart J 1961;23:556.

11. Faller K, Haworth SG, Taylor JF, Macartney FJ. Duplicate sources of pulmonary blood supply in pulmonary atresia with ventricular septal defect. Br Heart J 1981;46:263.

12. Feldt RH, DuShane JW, Titus JL. The anatomy of the atrioventricular conduction system in ventricular septal defect and tetralogy of Fallot: correlations with the electrocardiogram and vectorcardiogram. Circulation 1966;34:774.

13. Freedom RM, Pongiglione G, Williams WG, Trusler GA, Moes CA, Rowe RD. Pulmonary vein wedge angiography: indications, results, and surgical correlates in 25 patients. Am J Cardiol 1983;51:936.

14. Forster JW, Humphries JO. Right ventricular anomalous muscle bundle. Clinical and laboratory presentation and natural history. Circulation 1971;43:115.

15. Flege JB Jr, Vlad P, Ehrenhaft JL. Aneurysm of the triscuspid valve causing infundibular obstruction. Ann Thorac Surg 1967;3:446.

16. Flanagan MF, Foran RB, Van Praagh R, Jonas R, Sanders SP. Tetralogy of Fallot with obstruction of the ventricular septal defect: spectrum of echocardiographic findings. J Am Coll Cardiol 1988; 11:386.

17. Fuhrman BP, Bass JL, Castaneda-Zuniga W, Amplatz K, Lock JE. Coil embolization of congenital thoracic vascular anomalies in infants and children. Circulation 1984;70:285.

18. Ferrazzi P, McGiffin DC, Kirklin JW, Blackstone EH, Bourge RC. Have the results of mitral valve replacement improved? J Thorac Cardiovasc Surg 1986;92:186.

19. Finck SJ, Puga FJ, Danielson GK. Pulmonary valve insertion during reoperation for tetralogy of Fallot. Ann Thorac Surg 1988;45:610.

20. Ford DK, Bullaboy CA, Derkac WM, Hopkins RA, Jennings RB Jr, Johnson DH. Transatrial repair of double-chambered right ventricle. Ann Thorac Surg 1988;46:412.

G

1. Graham TP Jr, Cordell D, Atwood GF, Boucek RJ Jr, Boerth RC, Bender HW, et al. Right ventricular volume characteristics before and after palliative and reparative operation in tetralogy of Fallot. Circulation 1976;54:417.

2. Gasul BM, Dillon RF, Urla V. The natural transformation of ventricular septal defects into ventricular septal defects with pulmonary stenosis and/or into tetralogy of Fallot. Am J Dis Child 1957;94:424.

3. Gotsman MS. Increasing obstruction to the outflow tract in Fallot's tetralogy. Br Heart J 1966;28:615.

4. Garson A Jr, Gillette PC, McNamara DG. Propranolol: the preferred palliation for tetralogy of Fallot. Am J Cardiol 1981;47:1098.

5. Garson A Jr, Nihill MR, McNamara DG, Cooley DA. Status of the adult and adolescent after repair of tetralogy of Fallot. Circulation 1979;59:1232.

6. Garson A Jr, Gillette PC, Gutgesell HP, McNamara DG. Stress-induced ventricular arrhythmia after repair of tetralogy of Fallot. Am J Cardiol 1980;46:1006.

7. Graham TP Jr, Faulkner S, Bender H Jr, Wender CM. Hypoplasia of the left ventricle: rare cause of postoperative mortality in tetralogy of Fallot. Am J Cardiol 1977;40:454.

8. Graham TP Jr, Erath HG Jr, Boucek RJ Jr, Boerth RC. Left ventricular function in cyanotic congenital heart disease. Am J Cardiol 1980; 45:1231.

9. Gross RE, Bernhard WF, Litwin SB. Closure of Potts anastomoses in the total repair of tetralogy of Fallot. J Thorac Cardiovasc Surg 1969;57:72.

10. Glancy DL, Morrow AG, Roberts W. Malformations of the aortic valve in patients with the tetralogy of Fallot. Am Heart J 1968;76:755.

11. Guyton RA, Owens JE, Waumett JD, Dooley KJ, Hatcher CR Jr, Williams WH. The Blalock-Taussig shunt: low risk, effective palliation, and pulmonary artery growth. J Thorac Cardiovasc Surg 1983;85:917.

12. Gale AW, Arciniegas E, Green EW, Blackstone EH, Kirklin JW. Growth of the pulmonary anulus and pulmonary arteries after the Blalock-Taussig shunt. J Thorac Cardiovasc Surg 1979;77:459.

13. Gay WA Jr, Ebert PA. Aorta-to-right pulmonary artery anastomosis causing obstruction of the right pulmonary artery. Ann Thorac Surg 1973;16:402.

14. Gill CC, Moodie DS, McGoon DC. Staged surgical management of pulmonary atresia with diminutive pulmonary arteries. J Thorac Cardiovasc Surg 1977;73:436.

15. Gazzaniga AB, Elliott MP, Sperling DR, Dietrick WR, Eiseman JT, McRae DM, et al. Microporous expanded polytetrafluoroethylene arterial prosthesis for construction of aortopulmonary shunts. Experimental and clinical results. Ann Thorac Surg 1976;21:322.

16. Gazzaniga AB, Lamberti JJ, Siewers RD, Sperling DR, Dietrick WR, Arcilla RA, et al. Arterial prosthesis of microporous expanded polytetrafluoroethylene for construction of aorto-pulmonary shunts. J Thorac Cardiovasc Surg 1976;72:357.

17. Goor DA, Smolinsky A, Mohr R, Caspi J, Shem-Tov A. The drop of residual right ventricular pressure 24 hours after conservative infundibulectomy in repair of tetralogy of Fallot. J Thorac Cardiovasc Surg 1981;81:897.

18. Gillette PC, Yeoman MA, Mullins CE, McNamara DG. Sudden death after repair of tetralogy of Fallot. Electrocardiographic and electrophysiologic abnormalities. Circulation 1977;56:566.

19. Grinnell VS, Mehringer CM, Hieshima GB, Stanley P, Lurie PR. Transaortic occlusion of collateral arteries to the lung by detachable valved balloons in a patient with tetralogy of Fallot. Circulation 1982;65:1276.

20. Gallucci V, Scalia D, Thiene G, Mazzucco A, Valfre C. Double-chambered right ventricle: surgical experience and anatomical considerations. Thorac Cardiovasc Surg 1980;28:13.

21. Grant RP, Downey FM, MacMahon H. The architecture of the right ventricular outflow tract in the normal human heart and in the presence of ventricular septal defects. Circulation 1961;24:223.

22. Groh MA, Meliones JN, Bove EL, Kirklin JW, Blackstone EH, Lupinetti FM, et al. Repair of tetralogy of Fallot in infancy: effect of pulmonary artery size on outcome. Circulation 1991;84:III206.

23. Gill CC, Moodie DS, McGoon DC. Staged surgical management of pulmonary atresia with diminutive pulmonary arteries. J Thorac Cardiovasc Surg 1977;73:436.

24. Gale AW, Arciniegas E, Green EW, Blackstone EH, Kirklin JW. Growth of the pulmonary anulus and pulmonary arteries after the Blalock-Taussig shunt. J Thorac Cardiovasc Surg 1979;77:459.

25. Gaultier C, Boule M, Thibert M, Leca F. Resting lung function in children after repair of tetralogy of Fallot. Chest 1986;89:561.

26. Gustafson RA, Murray GF, Warden HE, Hill RC, Rozar GE Jr. Early primary repair of tetralogy of Fallot. Ann Thorac Surg 1988;45:235.

27. Gatzoulis MA, Clark AL, Cullen S, Newman CG, Redington AN. Right ventricular diastolic function 15 to 35 years after repair of tetralogy of Fallot. Circulation 1995;91:1775.

28. Gladman G, McCrindle BW, Williams WG, Freedom RM, Benson LN. The modified Blalock-Taussig shunt: clinical impact and morbidity in Fallot's tetralogy in the current era. J Thorac Cardiovasc Surg 1997;114:25.

29. Gundry SR, Razzouk AJ, Boskind JF, Bansal R, Bailey LL. Fate of the pericardial monocusp pulmonary valve for right ventricular outflow tract reconstruction: early function, late failure without obstruction. J Thorac Cardiovasc Surg 1994;107:908.

30. Godart F, Houyel L, Lacour-Gayet F, Serraf A, Sousa Uva M, Bruniaux J, et al. Absent pulmonary valve syndrome: surgical treatment and considerations. Ann Thorac Surg 1996;62:136.

H

1. Harms D, Hansen P, Fischer K, Bernhard A. Pathology of the "Fallot Lung." Virchows Arch Abt A Path Anat 1973;361:77.

2. Hudapeth AS, Cordell AR, Johnston FR. Transatrial approach to total correction of tetralogy of Fallot. Circulation 1963;27:796.

3. Hawe A, McGoon DC, Kincaid OW, Ritter DG. Fate of outflow tract in tetralogy of Fallot. Ann Thorac Surg 1972;13:137.

4. Honey M, Chamberlain DA, Howard J. The effect of beta sympathetic blockade on arterial oxygen saturation in Fallot's tetralogy. Circulation 1964;30:501.

5. Harken AH, Horowitz LN, Josephson ME. Surgical correction of recurrent sustained ventricular tachycardia following complete repair of tetralogy of Fallot. J Thorac Cardiovasc Surg 1980;80:779.

6. Hislop A, Reid L. Structural changes in the pulmonary arteries and veins in tetralogy of Fallot. Br Heart J 1973;35:1178.

7. Hjelms E, Pohlner P, Barratt-Boyes BG, Gavin JB. Study of autologous pericardial patch-grafts in the right ventricular outflow tracts in growing and adult dogs. J Thorac Cardiovasc Surg 1981;81:120.

8. Hiraishi S, Bargeron LM, Isabel-Jones JB, Emmanouilides GC, Friedman WF, Jarmakani JM. Ventricular and pulmonary artery volumes in patients with absent pulmonary valve. Factors affecting the natural course. Circulation 1983;67:183.

9. Harris AM, Segel N, Bishop JM. Blalock-Taussig anastomosis for tetralogy of Fallot. A ten-to-fifteen year follow-up. Br Heart J 1964; 26:266.

10. Hofschire PJ, Rosenquist GC, Ruckerman RN, Moller JH, Edwards JE. Pulmonary vascular disease complicating the Blalock-Taussig anastomosis. Circulation 1977;56:124.

11. Hancock EW, Hultgren HN, March HW. Pulmonary hypertension after Blalock-Taussig anastomosis. Am Heart J 1964;67:817.

12. Haworth SG, Macartney FJ. Growth and development of pulmonary circulation in pulmonary atresia with ventricular septal defect and major aortopulmonary collateral arteries. Br Heart J 1980;44:14.

13. Hamilton DI, Di Eusanio G, Piccoli GP, Dickinson DF. Eight years experience with intracardiac repair of tetralogy of Fallot. Early and late results in 175 consecutive patients. Br Heart J 1981;46:144.

14. Haworth SG, Rees PG, Taylor JF, Macartney FJ, de Leval M, Stark J. Pulmonary atresia with ventricular septal defect and major aortopulmonary collateral arteries: effect of systemic-pulmonary anastomosis. Br Heart J 1981;45:133.

15. Haworth SG. Collateral arteries in pulmonary atresia with ventricular septal defect. A precarious blood supply. Br Heart J 1980;44:5.

16. Haworth SG, Reid L. Quantitative structural study of pulmonary circulation in the newborn with pulmonary atresia. Thorax 1977; 32:129.

17. Hartmann AF Jr, Tsifutis AA, Arvidsson H, Goldring D. The two-chambered right ventricle. Report of nine cases. Circulation 1962;26:279.

18. Hartmann AF Jr, Goldring D, Carlsson E. Development of right ventricular obstruction by aberrant muscular bands. Circulation 1964;30:679.

19. Hartmann AF Jr, Goldring D, Ferguson TB, Burford WH, Smith CH, Kissane JM, et al. The course of children with two chambered RV. J Thorac Cardiovasc Surg 1970;60:72.

20. Hu DC, Seward JB, Puga FJ, Fuster V, Tajik AJ. Total correction of tetralogy of Fallot at age 40 years and older: long-term follow-up. J Am Coll Cardiol 1985;5:40.

21. Horneffer PJ, Zahka KG, Rowe SA, Manolio TA, Gott VL, Reitz BA, et al. Long-term results of total repair of tetralogy of Fallot in childhood. Ann Thorac Surg 1990;50:179.

22. Hofbeck M, Sunnegardh JT, Burrows PE, Moes CA, Lightfoot N, Williams WG, et al. Analysis of survival in patients with pulmonic valve atresia and ventricular septal defect. Am J Cardiol 1991;67:737.

23. Howell CE, Ho SY, Anderson RH, Elliott MJ. Variations within the fibrous skeleton and ventricular outflow tracts in tetralogy of Fallot. Ann Thorac Surg 1990;50:450.

24. Hawkins JA, Bailey WW, Dillon T, Schwartz DC. Mid-term results with cryopreserved allograft valved conduits from the right ventricle to the pulmonary arteries. J Thorac Cardiovasc Surg 1992;104:910.

25. Hofbeck M, Leipold G, Rauch A, Buheitel G, Singer H. Clinical relevance of monosomy 22q11.2 in children with pulmonary atresia and ventricular septal defect. Eur J Pediatr 1999;158:302.

26. Hadjo A, Jimenez M, Baudet E, Roques X, Laborde N, Srour S, et al. Review of the long-term course of 52 patients with pulmonary atresia and ventricular septal defect. Anatomical and surgical considerations. Eur Heart J 1995;16:1668.

27. Hirsch JC, Mosca RS, Bove EL. Complete repair of tetralogy of Fallot in the neonate: results in the modern era. Ann Surg 2000;232:508.

I

1. Ilbawi MN, Idriss FS, Muster AJ, Wessel HU, Paul MH, DeLeon SY. Tetralogy of Fallot with absent pulmonary valve. Should valve insertion be part of the intracardiac repair? J Thorac Cardiovasc Surg 1981;81:906.

2. Ionescu MI, Tandon AP, Macartney FJ. Long-term sequential hemodynamic evaluation of right ventricular outflow tract reconstruction using a valve mechanism. Ann Thorac Surg 1979;27:426.

3. Ilbawi MN, Grieco J, DeLeon SY, Idriss FS, Muster AJ, Berry TE, et al. Modified Blalock-Taussig shunt in newborn infants. J Thorac Cardiovasc Surg 1984;88:770.

4. Ilbawi MN, Idriss FS, DeLeon SY, Muster AJ, Berry TE, Paul MH. Long-term results of porcine valve insertion for pulmonary regurgitation following repair of tetralogy of Fallot. Ann Thorac Surg 1986;41:478.

5. Ilbawi MN, Idriss FS, DeLeon SY, Muster AJ, Gidding SS, Berry TE, et al. Factors that exaggerate the deleterious effects of pulmonary insufficiency on the right ventricle after tetralogy repair. Surgical implications. J Thorac Cardiovasc Surg 1987;93:36.

6. Ilbawi M, Cua C, DeLeon S, Muster A, Paul M, Cutilletta A, et al. Repair of complete atrioventricular septal defect with tetralogy of Fallot. Ann Thorac Surg 1990;50:407.

7. Iyer KS, Mee RB. Staged repair of pulmonary atresia with ventricular septal defect and major systemic to pulmonary artery collaterals. Ann Thorac Surg 1991;51:65.

8. Idriss FS, Muster AJ, Paul MH, Backer CL, Mavroudis C. Ventricular septal defect with tricuspid pouch with and without transposition: anatomic and surgical considerations. J Thorac Cardiovasc Surg 1992;103:52.

9. Ishizaka T, Yagihara T, Yamamoto F, Nichigaki K, Matsuki O, Uemura H, et al. Results and unifocalization for pulmonary atresia, ventricular septal defect and major aortopulmonary collateral arteries: patency of pulmonary vascular segments. Eur J Cardiothorac Surg 1996;10:331.

J

1. Jarmakani JM, Graham TP Jr, Canent RV Jr, Jewett PH. Left heart function in children with tetralogy of Fallot before and after palliative or corrective surgery. Circulation 1972;46:478.

2. Jarmakani JM, Nakazawa M, Isabel-Jones J, Marks RA. Right ventricular function in children with tetralogy of Fallot before and after aortic to pulmonary shunt. Circulation 1976;53:555.

3. James FW, Kaplan S, Schwartz DC, Chou TC, Sandker MJ, Naylor V. Response to exercise in patients after total surgical correction of tetralogy of Fallot. Circulation 1976;54:671.

4. Jefferson K, Rees S, Somerville J. Systemic arterial supply to the lungs in pulmonary atresia and its relation to pulmonary artery development. Br Heart J 1972;34:418.

5. Johnson RJ, Haworth SG. Pulmonary vascular and alveolar development in tetralogy of Fallot: a recommendation for early correction. Thorax 1982;37:893.

6. Jonas RA, Freed MD, Mayer JE Jr, Castaneda AR. Long-term follow-up of synthetic right heart conduits. Circulation 1985;72:II77.

K

1. Kirklin JW, DuShane JW, Patrick RT, Donald DE, Hetzel PS, Harshbarger HC, et al. Intracardiac surgery with the aid of a mechanical pump-oxygenator system (Gibbon type): Report of eight cases. Mayo Clin Proc 1955;30:201.

2. Kirklin JW, Ellis FH Jr, McGoon DC, DuShane JW, Swan HF. Surgical treatment for the tetralogy of Fallot by open intracardiac repair. J Thorac Surg 1959;37:22.

3. Kirklin JW, Payne WS. Surgical treatment for tetralogy of Fallot after previous anastomosis of systemic to pulmonary artery. Surg Gynecol Obstet 1960;110:707.

4. Kirklin JW, Payne WS, Theye RA, DuShuane JW. Factors affecting survival after open operation for tetralogy of Fallot. Ann Surg 1960;152:485.

5. Kirklin JK, Westaby S, Chenoweth D, Blackstone EH. Kirklin JW, Pacifico AD. Complement and the damaging effects of cardiopulmonary bypass. J Thorac Cardiovasc Surg 1983;86:845.

6. Kirklin JW, Devloo RA. Hypothermic perfusion and circulatory arrest for surgical correction of tetralogy of Fallot with previously constructed Potts' anastomosis. Dis Chest 1961;39:87.

7. Kirklin JW, Wallace RB, McGoon DC, DuShane JW. Early and late results after intracardiac repair of tetralogy of Fallot: 5-year review of 337 patients. Ann Surg 1965;162:578.

8. Kawashima Y, Kitamura S, Nakano S, Yagihara T. Corrective surgery for tetralogy of Fallot without or with minimal right ventriculotomy and with repair of the pulmonary valve. Circulation 1981;64:II147.

9. Kirklin JW, Blackstone EH, Kirklin JK, Pacifico AD, Aramendi J, Bargeron LM Jr. Surgical results and protocols in the spectrum of tetralogy of Fallot. Ann Surg 1983;198:251.

10. Katz NM, Blackstone EH, Kirklin JW, Pacifico AD, Bargeron LM Jr. Late survival and symptoms after repair of tetralogy of Fallot. Circulation 1982;65:403.

11. Kahn DR. Discussion of paper by Dobell et al.[D2] J Thorac Cardiovasc Surg 1968;55:78.

12. Kawashima Y, Mori T, Kitamura S, Hirose H, Nakano S, Yagihara T. Trans-pulmonary arterial, trans-right atrial repair of tetralogy of Fallot. J Jpn Surg Soc 1979;80:1259.

13. Keck EW, Brode P. Beta-receptor blockade in Fallot's tetralogy. Dtsch Med Wochenschr 1970;95:766.

14. Klinner W. Klinische und experimentelle untersuchungen zur operativen korrektur der Fallotschen tetralogie. Aus der Chirurgischen Klinik der Universitat Munchen, 1961.

15. Kuers PF, McGoon DC. Tetralogy of Fallot with aortic origin of right pulmonary artery. J Thorac Cardiovasc Surg 1973;65:327.

16. Kirklin JW, Karp RB. The tetralogy of Fallot. Philadelphia: WB Saunders, 1970.

17. Kirklin JW, Bargeron LM Jr, Pacifico AD. The enlargement of small pulmonary arteries by preliminary palliative operations. Circulation 1977;56:612.

18. Kirklin JW. Reviewer's comment of paper by Freedom et al.[F8] J Thorac Cardiovasc Surg 1983;86:24.

19. Kirklin JW, Blackstone EH, Jonas RA, Shimazaki Y, Kirklin JK, Mayer JE Jr, et al. Morphologic and surgical determinants of outcome events after repair of tetralogy of Fallot and pulmonary stenosis: a two-institution study. J Thorac Cardiovasc Surg 1992;103:706.

20. Klinner VW, Pasini M, Schaudig A. Anastomose zwischen system- und lungenarterie mit hilfe von kunststoffprothesen bei cyanotischen herzvitien. Thoraxchirurgie 1962;10:68.

21. Krongrad E, Ritter DG, Hawe A, Kincaid OW, McGoon DC. Pulmonary atresia or severe stenosis and coronary artery-to-pulmonary artery fistula. Circulation 1972;46:1005.

22. Kay PH, Capuani A, Franks R, Lincoln C. Experience with the modified Blalock-Taussig operation using polytetrafluoroethylene (Impra) grafts. Br Heart J 1983;49:359.

23. Kavey RE, Blackman MS, Sondheimer HM. Incidence and severity of chronic ventricular dysrhythmias after repair of tetralogy of Fallot. Am Heart J 1982;103:342

24. Kirklin JW, Openshaw CR, Tompkins RG. Surgical treatment of infundibular stenosis with intact ventricular septum. Ann Surg 1953;137:228.

25. Kavey RE, Thomas FD, Byrum CJ, Blackman MS, Sondheimer HM, Bove EL. Ventricular arrhythmias and biventricular dysfunction after repair of tetralogy of Fallot. J Am Coll Cardiol 1984;4:126.

26. Klinner W, Reichart B, Pfaller M, Hatz R. Late results after correction of tetralogy of Fallot necessitating outflow tract reconstruction. Comparison with results after correction without outflow tract patch. Thorac Cardiovasc Surg 1984;32:244.

27. Kobayashi J, Hirose H, Nakano S, Matsuda H, Shirakura R, Kawashima Y. Ambulatory electrocardiographic study of the frequency and cause of ventricular arrhythmia after correction of tetralogy of Fallot. Am J Cardiol 1984;54:1310.

28. Kirklin JW, Blackstone EH, Jonas RA, Shimazaki Y, Kirklin JK, Mayer JE Jr, et al. Morphologic and surgical determinants of outcome events after repair of tetralogy of Fallot and pulmonary stenosis. J Thorac Cardiovasc Surg 1992;103:706.

29. Kirklin JK, Kirklin JW, Blackstone EH, Milano A, Pacifico AD. Effect of transanular patching on outcome after repair of tetralogy of Fallot. Ann Thorac Surg 1989;48:783.

30. Kirklin JK, Kirklin JW, Blackstone EH, Pacifico AD, McConnell ME, Colvin EV, et al. Sudden death and arrhythmic events after repair of tetralogy of Fallot. In Crupi G, Parenzan L, Anderson RH, eds. Perspectives in pediatric cardiology, Vol. 2. Pediatric cardiac surgery, Part 1. Mount Kisco, N.Y.: Futura, 1989, p. 204.

31. Kirklin JW, Blackstone EH, Shimazaki Y, Maehara T, Pacifico AD, Kirklin JK, et al. Survival, functional status, and reoperations after repair of tetralogy of Fallot with pulmonary atresia. J Thorac Cardiovasc Surg 1988;96:102.

32. Kirklin JW, Blackstone EH, Maehara T, Pacifico AD, Kirklin JK, Pollock S, et al. Intermediate-term fate of cryopreserved allograft and xenograft valved conduits. Ann Thorac Surg 1987;44:598.

33. Kay PH, Ross DN. Fifteen years' experience with the aortic homograft: The conduit of choice for right ventricular outflow tract reconstruction. Ann Thorac Surg 1985;40:360.

34. Kirklin JW, Bargeron LM Jr, Pacifico AD. The enlargement of small pulmonary arteries by preliminary palliative operations. Circulation 1977;56:612.

35. Kan JS, Marvin WJ Jr, Bass JL, Muster AJ, Murphy J. Balloon angioplasty-branch pulmonary artery stenosis: Results from the Valvuloplasty and Angioplasty of Congenital Anomalies registry. Am J Cardiol 1990;65:798.

36. Kaplan EL, Meier P. Nonparametric estimation from incomplete observations. J Am Stat Assoc 1958;53:457.

37. Karl TR, Musumeci F, de Leval M, Pincott JR, Taylor JF, Stark J. Surgical treatment of absent pulmonary valve syndrome. J Thorac Cardiovasc Surg 1986;91:590.

38. Kaufman SL, Kan JS, Mitchell SE, Flaherty JT, White RI Jr. Embolization of systemic to pulmonary artery collaterals in the management of hemoptysis in pulmonary atresia. Am J Cardiol 1986;58:1130.

39. Kaneko Y, Okabe H, Nagata N, Kobayashi J, Murakami A, Takamoto S. Pulmonary atresia, ventricular septal defect, and coronary-pulmonary artery fistula. Ann Thorac Surg 2001;71:355.

40. Kurosawa H, Imai Y. Surgical anatomy of the atrioventricular conduction bundle in tetralogy of Fallot. New findings relevant to the position of the sutures. J Thorac Cardiovasc Surg 1988;95:586.

41. Kusuhara K, Miki S, Ueda Y, Ohkita Y, Tahata T, Komeda M, et al. Evaluation of corrective surgery for tetralogy of Fallot from late results by multivariate statistical analysis. Eur J Cardiothorac Surg 1988;2:124.

42. Kveselis D, Rosenthal A, Ferguson P, Behrendt D, Sloan H. Long-term prognosis after repair of double-chamber right ventricle with ventricular septal defect. Am J Cardiol 1984;54:1292.

43. Kurtz CM, Sprague HB, White PD. Congenital heart disease. Am Heart J 1927;3:77.

44. Karl TR, Sano S, Pornviliwan S, Mee RB. Tetralogy of Fallot: favorable outcome of nonneonatal transatrial, transpulmonary repair. Ann Thorac Surg 1992;54:903.

45. Knott-Craig CJ, Elkins RC, Lane MM, Holz J, McCue C, Ward KE. A 26-year experience with surgical management of tetralogy of Fallot: risk analysis for mortality or late reintervention. Ann Thorac Surg 1998;66:506.

L

1. Lev M, Eckner FA. The pathologic anatomy of tetralogy of Fallot and its variations. Dis Chest 1964;45:251.

2. Lev M, Rimoldi HJ, Rowlatt DF. Quantitative anatomy of cyanotic tetralogy of Fallot. Circulation 1964;30:531.

3. Lillehei CW, Cohen M, Warden HE, Read RC, Aust JB, De Wall RA, et al. Direct vision intracardiac surgical correction of the tetralogy of Fallot, pentalogy of Fallot, and pulmonary atresia defects: report of first ten cases. Ann Surg 1955;142:418.

4. Levine FH, Reis RL, Morrow AG. Incidence and significance of patent foramen ovale after correction of tetralogy of Fallot. Ann Thorac Surg 1972;13:464.

5. Litwin SB, Rosenthal A, Fellows K. Surgical management of young infants with tetralogy of Fallot, absence of the pulmonary valve, and respiratory distress. J Thorac Cardiovasc Surg 1973;65:552.

6. Lakier JB, Stanger P, Heymann MA, Hoffman JI, Rudolph AM. Tetralogy of Fallot with absent pulmonary valve. Natural history and hemodynamic considerations. Circulation 1974;50:167.

7. Laks H, Castaneda AR. Subclavian arterioplasty for the ipsilateral Blalock-Taussig shunt. Ann Thorac Surg 1975;19:319.

8. Lang P, Chipman CW, Siden H, Williams RG, Norwood WI, Castaneda AR. Early assessment of hemodynamic status after repair of tetralogy of Fallot: a comparison of 24 hour (intensive care unit) and 1 year postoperative data in 98 patients. Am J Cardiol 1982; 50:795.

9. Lecompte Y, Hazan E, Baillot F, Jarreau MM, Mathey J. La reparation chirurgicale de la voie pulmonaire dans la tetralogie de Fallot. Coeur 1977;3:739.

10. Lock JE, Niemi T, Einzig S, Amplatz K, Burke B, Bass JL. Transvenous angioplasty of experimental branch pulmonary artery stenosis in newborn lambs. Circulation 1981;64:886.

11. Lock JE, Castaneda-Zuniga WR, Fuhrman BP, Bass JL. Balloon dilation angioplasty of hypoplastic and stenotic pulmonary arteries. Circulation 1983;67:962.

12. Lev M. The architecture of the conduction system in congenital heart disease. II. Tetralogy of Fallot. AMA Arch Pathol 1958;67:572.

13. Lange PE, Onnasch DG, Bernhard A, Heintzen PH. Left and right ventricular adaptation to right ventricular overload before and after surgical repair of tetralogy of Fallot. Am J Cardiol 1982;50:786.

14. Li MD, Coles JC, McDonald AC. Anomalous muscle bundle of the right ventricle. Its recognition and surgical treatment, Br Heart J 1978;40:1040.

15. Lucas RV Jr, Varco RL, Lillehei CW, Adams P Jr, Anderson RC, Edwards JE. Anomalous muscle bundle of the right ventricle. Hemodynamic consequences and surgical considerations. Circulation 1962;25:443.

16. Levy MJ, Lillehei CW, Elliott LP, Carey LS, Adams P Jr, Edwards JE. Accessory valvular tissue causing subpulmonary stenosis in corrected transposition of great vessels. Circulation 1963;27:494.

17. Lamberti JJ, Carlisle J, Waldman JD, Lodge FA, Kirkpatrick SE, George L, et al. Systemic-pulmonary shunts in infants and children. J Thorac Cardiovasc Surg 1984;88:76.

18. Lillehei CW. Discussion of paper by Horneffer and colleagues.[H21] Ann Thorac Surg 1990;50:184.

19. Lillehei CW, Varco RL, Cohen M, Warden HE, Gott VL, DeWall RA, et al. The first open heart corrections of tetralogy of Fallot. A 26-31 year follow-up of 106 patients. Ann Surg 1986;204:490.

20. Le Bret E, Mace L, Dervanian P, Folliguet T, Bourriez A, Zoghy J, et al. Images in cardiovascular medicine. Combined angiography and three-dimensional computed tomography for assessing systemic-to-pulmonary collaterals in pulmonary atresia with ventricular septal defect. Circulation 1998;98:2930.

21. Lofland GK. The management of pulmonary atresia, ventricular septal defect, and multiple aorta pulmonary collateral arteries by definitive single stage repair in early infancy. Eur J Cardiothorac Surg 2000;18:480.

M

1. Monties JR, Goudard A, Fogliani J, Bandini A, Blanc-Gauthier T. Correction of Fallot's tetralogy before the age of 5 years. Indications and results with reference to 42 cases. Ann Chir Thorac Cardiovasc 1975;14:229.

2. Moffitt EA, Kirklin JW, Theye RA. Physiologic studies during whole-body perfusion in tetralogy of Fallot. J Thorac Cardiovasc Surg 1962;44:180.

3. Miller GA, Kirklin JW, Rahimtoola SH, Swan HJ. Volume of the left ventricle in tetralogy of Fallot. Am J Cardiol 1965;16:488.

4. De Matteis A. The vascular pathology of the lung in congenital malformations of the heart with severe pulmonary stenosis or atresia and right-to-left shunt. Respiration 1969;26:337.

5. McCord MC, van Elk J, Blount G Jr. Tetralogy of Fallot clinical and hemodynamic spectrum of combined pulmonary stenosis and ventricular septal defects. Circulation 1957;16:736.

6. Morgan JR. Left pulmonary artery from ascending aorta in tetralogy of Fallot. Circulation 1972;45:653.

7. Miller RA, Lev M, Paul MH. Congenital absence of the pulmonary valve. The clinical syndrome of tetralogy of Fallot with pulmonary regurgitation. Circulation 1962;26:266.

8. Matsuda H, Ihara K, Mori T, Kitamura S, Kawashima Y. Tetralogy of Fallot associated with aortic insufficiency. Ann Thorac Surg 1980;29:529.

9. McGoon DC, Danielson GK, Puga FJ, Ritter DG, Mair DD, Ilstrup DM. Late results after extracardiac conduit repair for congenital cardiac defects. Am J Cardiol 1982;49:1741.

10. Macartney FJ, Miller GA. Congenital absence of the pulmonary valve. Br Heart J 1970;32:483.

11. McKay R, de Leval MR, Rees P, Taylor JF, Macartney FJ, Stark J. Postoperative angiographic assessment of modified Blalock-Taussig shunts using expanded polytetrafluoroethylene (Gore-Tex). Ann Thorac Surg 1980;30:137.

12. Mizuno A, Sato F, Hasegawa T, Tsuzuki M, Furuse A. Acquired obstruction of the right ventricular outflow tract in tetralogy of Fallot after Blalock-Taussig anastomosis. Report of two cases successfully treated with total correction. Jpn Heart J 1970;11:113.

13. Marchand P. The use of a cusp-bearing homograft patch to the outflow tract and pulmonary artery in Fallot's tetralogy and pulmonary valvular stenosis. Thorax 1967;22:497.

14. McGoon DC, Baird DK, Davis GD. Surgical management of large bronchial collateral arteries with pulmonary stenosis or atresia. Circulation 1975;52:109.

15. Murphy JD, Freed MD, Keane JF, Norwood WI, Castaneda AR, Nadas AS. Hemodynamic results after intracardiac repair of tetralogy of Fallot by deep hypothermia and cardiopulmonary bypass. Circulation 1980;62:I168.

16. Macartney F, Deverall P. Scott O. Haemodynamic characteristics of systemic arterial blood supply to the lungs. Br Heart J 1973;35:28.

17. Macartney FJ, Scott O, Deverall PB. Haemodynamic and anatomical characteristics of pulmonary blood supply in pulmonary atresia with ventricular septal defect—including a case of persistent fifth aortic arch. Br Heart J 1974;36:1049.

18. McGoon MD, Fulton RE, Davis GD, Ritter DG, Neill CA, White RI Jr. Systemic collateral and pulmonary artery stenosis in patients with congenital pulmonary valve atresia and ventricular septal defect. Circulation 1977;56:473.

19. Mocellin R, Krettek M, Sauer U, Buhlmeyer K. Pulmonary atresia with ventricular septal defect. Follow up and surgical results from 1963 to 1976 and diagnostic measures with special reference to large systemic-pulmonary collaterals. Z Kardiol 1977;66:382.

20. Miller WW, Nadas AS, Bernhard WF, Gross RE. Congenital pulmonary atresia with ventricular septal defect. Review of the clinical course of fifty patients with assessment of the results of palliative surgery. Am J Cardiol 1968;21:673.

21. Maron BJ, Ferrans VJ, White RI Jr. Unusual evolution of acquired infundibular stenosis in patients with ventricular septal defect. Clinical and morphologic observations. Circulation 1973;48:1092.

22. Macedo ME, Sena Lino JA, Lima M, Salomao CS. Left ventricular outflow tract obstruction due to tricuspid valve prolapse through a high ventricular septal defect. Thorac Cardiovasc Surg 1983;31:110.

23. Maclean LD, Culligan JA, Kane DJ. Subaortic stenosis due to accessory tissue on the mitral valve. J Thorac Cardiovasc Surg 1963;45:382.

24. McCaughan BC, Danielson GK, Driscoll DJ, McGoon DC. Tetralogy of Fallot with absent pulmonary valve. J Thorac Cardiovasc Surg 1985;89:280.

25. Mullins CE, O'Laughlin MP, Vick GW III, Mayer DC, Myers TJ, Kearney DL, et al. Implantation of balloon-expandable intravascular grafts by catheterization in pulmonary arteries and systemic veins. Circulation 1988;77:188.

26. Manabe H. Recent advance in total correction of tetralogy of Fallot. Jpn Circ J 1984;48:1.

27. Marx GR, Hicks RW, Allen HD, Goldberg SJ. Noninvasive assessment of hemodynamic responses to exercise in pulmonary regurgitation after operations to correct pulmonary outflow obstruction. Am J Cardiol 1988;61:595.

28. Moller JH, ed. Perspectives in pediatric cardiology: surgery of congenital heart disease, Vol. 6. Pediatric Cardiac Care Consortium 1984-1995, New York: Futura, 1998, p. 207.

29. Murphy JG, Gersh BJ, Mair DD, Fuster V, McGoon MD, Ilstrup DM, et al. Long-term outcome in patients undergoing surgical repair of tetralogy of Fallot. N Engl J Med 1993;329:593.

30. Mulla N, Simpson P, Sullivan NM, Paridon SM. Determinants of aerobic capacity during exercise following complete repair of tetralogy of Fallot with a transanular patch. Pediatr Cardiol 1997;18:350.

31. Miura T, Nakano S, Shimazaki Y, Kobayashi J, Hirose H, Sano T, et al. Evaluation of right ventricular function by regional wall motion analysis in patients after correction of tetralogy of Fallot. J Thorac Cardiovasc Surg 1992;104:917.

32. McMahon CJ, Nihill MR. Origin of the main pulmonary artery from the left coronary artery in complex pulmonary atresia. Pediatr Cardiol 2001;22:347.

33. McElhinney DB, Reddy VM, Pian MS, Moore P, Hanley FL. Compression of the central airways by a dilated aorta in infants and children with congenital heart disease. Ann Thorac Surg 1999; 67:1130.

34. Marino B, Digilio MC, Toscano A, Anaclerio S, Giannotti A, Feltri C, et al. Anatomic patterns of conotruncal defects associated with deletion 22q11. Genet Med 2001;3:45.

35. Murthy KS, Rao SG, Naik SK, Coelho R, Krishnan US, Cherian KM. Evolving surgical management for ventricular septal defect, pulmonary atresia, and major aortopulmonary collateral arteries. Ann Thorac Surg 1999;67:760.

36. Moritz A, Marx M, Wollenek G, Domanig E, Wolner E. Complete repair of PA-VSD with diminutive or discontinuous pulmonary arteries by transverse thoracosternotomy. Ann Thorac Surg 1996;61:646.

37. Murthy KS, Krishnanaik S, Coelho R, Punnoose A, Arumugam SB, Cherian KM. Median sternotomy single stage complete unifocalization for pulmonary atresia, major aorto-pulmonary collateral arteries and VSD—early experience. Eur J Cardiothorac Surg 1999;16:21.

38. McElhinney DB, Reddy VM, Haley FL. Tetralogy of Fallot with major aortopulmonary collaterals: early total repair. Pediatr Cardiol 1998;19:289.

39. Metras D, Chetaille P, Kreitmann B, Fraisse A, Ghez O, Riberi A. Pulmonary atresia with ventricular septal defect, extremely hypoplastic pulmonary arteries, major aorto-pulmonary collaterals. Eur J Cardiothorac Surg 2001;20:590; discussion 596.

40. Marelli AJ, Perloff JK, Child JS, Laks H. Pulmonary atresia with ventricular septal defect in adults. Circulation 1994;89:243.

N

1. Nagao GI, Daoud GI, McAdams AJ, Schwartz DC, Kaplan S. Cardiovascular anomalies associated with tetralogy of Fallot. Am J Cardiol 1967;20:206.

2. Naito Y. Study on total correction of tetralogy of Fallot: factors affecting operative mortality and surgical measures to improve operative results. Jpn J Assoc Thorac Surg 1972;20:131.

3. Norwood WI, Freed MD, Rocchini AP, Bernhard WF, Castaneda AR. Experience with valved conduits for repair of congenital cardiac lesions. Ann Thorac Surg 1977;24:223.

4. Neirotti R, Galindez E, Kreutzer G, Rodriguez Coronel A, Pedrini M, et al. Tetralogy of Fallot with subpulmonary ventricular septal defect. Ann Thorac Surg 1978;25:51.

5. Norberg WJ, Tadavarthy M, Knight L, Nicoloff DM, Moller JH. Late hemodynamic and angiographic findings after ascending aorta–pulmonary artery anastomosis. J Thorac Cardiovasc Surg 1978; 76:345.

6. Norwood WI, Rosenthal A, Castaneda AR. Tetralogy of Fallot with acquired pulmonary atresia and hypoplasia of pulmonary arteries. Report of surgical management in infancy. J Thorac Cardiovasc Surg 1976;72:454.

7. Nomoto S, Muraoka R, Yokota M, Aoshima M, Kyoku I, Nakano H. Left ventricular volume as a predictor of the postoperative hemodynamics and a criterion for total correction of the tetralogy of Fallot. J Thorac Cardiovasc Surg 1984;88:389.

8. Newfeld EA, Waldman D, Paul MH, Muster AJ, Cole RB, Idriss F, et al. Pulmonary vascular disease after systemic-pulmonary arterial shunt operations. Am J Cardiol 1977;39:715.

9. Nihill MR, Mullins CE, McNamara DG. Visualization of the pulmonary arteries in pseudotruncus by pulmonary vein wedge angiography. Circulation 1978;58:140.

10. Nanton MA, Belcourt CL, Gillis DA, Krause VW, Roy DL. Left ventricular outflow tract obstruction owing to accessory endocardial cushion tissue. J Thorac Cardiovasc Surg 1979;78:537.

11. Neufeld HN, McGoon DC, DuShane JW, Edwards JE. Tetralogy of Fallot with anomalous tricuspid valve simulating pulmonary stenosis with intact septum. Circulation 1960;22:1083.

12. Nakata S, Imai Y, Takanashi Y, Kurosawa H, Tezuka K, Nakazawa M, et al. A new method for the quantitative standardization of cross sectional areas of the pulmonary arteries in congenital heart diseases with decreased pulmonary blood flow. J Thorac Cardiovasc Surg 1984;88:610.

13. Naito Y, Fujita T, Yagihara T, Isobe F, Yamamoto F, Tanaka K, et al. Usefulness of left ventricular volume in assessing tetralogy of Fallot for total correction. Am J Cardiol 1985;56:356.

O

1. Olin CL, Ritter DG, McGoon DC, Wallace RB, Danielson GK. Pulmonary atresia: surgical considerations and results in 103 patients undergoing definitive repair. Circulation 1976;54:III35.

2. Ongley PA, Rahimtoola SH, Kincaid OW, Kirklin JW. Continuous murmurs in tetralogy of Fallot and pulmonary atresia with ventricular septal defect. Am J Cardiol 1966;18:821.

3. Oku H. Operative results and postoperative hemodynamic results in total correction of tetralogy of Fallot with special reference to patient's age and enlargement of right ventricular outflow tract. Nippon Geka Hokan 1976;45:87.

4. Oku H, Shirotani H, Yokoyama T, Yokota Y, Kawai J, Makino S, et al. Right ventricular outflow tract prosthesis in total correction of tetralogy of Fallot. Circulation 1980;62:604.

5. Oku H, Shirotani H, Yokoyama T, Yokota Y, Kawai J, Mori A, et al. Postoperative size of the right ventricular outflow tract and optimal age in complete repair of tetralogy of Fallot. Ann Thorac Surg 1978;25:322.

6. Osman MZ, Meng CC, Girdany BR. Congenital absence of the pulmonary valve. Report of eight cases with review of the literature. Am J Roentgenol Radium Ther Nucl Med 1969;106:58.

7. Opie JC, Sandor GG, Ashmore PG, Patterson MW. Successful palliation by pulmonary artery banding in absent pulmonary valve syndrome with aneurysmal pulmonary arteries. J Thorac Cardiovasc Surg 1983;85:125.

8. Oberhansli I, Friedli B. Echocardiographic study of left and right ventricular dimension and left ventricular function in patients with tetralogy of Fallot, before and after surgery. Br Heart J 1979;41:40.

9. O'Laughlin MP, Perry SB, Lock JE, Mullins CE. Use of endovascular stents in congenital heart disease. Circulation 1991;83:1923.

P

1. Poirier RA, McGoon DC, Danielson GK, Wallace RB, Ritter DG, Moodie DS, et al. Late results after repair of tetralogy of Fallot. J Thorac Cardiovasc Surg 1977;73:900.

2. Potts WJ, Smiths S, Gibson S. Anastomosis of the aorta to a pulmonary artery. JAMA 1946;132:627.

3. Piehler JM, Danielson GK, McGoon DC, Wallace RB, Fulton RE, Mair DD. Management of pulmonary atresia with ventricular septal defect and hypoplastic pulmonary arteries by right ventricular outflow construction. J Thorac Cardiovasc Surg 1980;80:552.

4. Ponce FE, Williams LC, Webb HM, Riopel DA, Hohn AR. Propranolol palliation of tetralogy of Fallot: experience with long-term drug treatment in pediatric patients. Pediatrics 1973;52:100.

5. Pinsky WW, Nihill MR, Mullins CE, McNamara DG. Management of absent pulmonary valve syndrome. Am J Cardiol 1977;39:311.

6. Parenzan L, Alfieri O, Vanini V, Bianchi T, Villani M, Tiraboschi R, et al. Waterston anastomosis for initial palliation of tetralogy of Fallot. J Thorac Cardiovasc Surg 1981;82:176.

7. Puga FJ, DuShane JW, McGoon DC. Treatment of tetralogy of Fallot in children less than 4 years of age. J Thorac Cardiovasc Surg 1972;64:247.

8. Piccoli GP, Dickinson DF, Musumeci F, Hamilton DI. A changing policy for the surgical treatment of tetralogy of Fallot: early and late results in 235 consecutive patients. Ann Thorac Surg 1982;33:365.

9. Puga FJ, McGoon DC, Julsrud PR, Danielson GK, Mair DD. Complete repair of pulmonary atresia with nonconfluent pulmonary arteries. Ann Thorac Surg 1983;35:36.

10. Pacifico AD, Kirklin JW, Bargeron LM Jr, Soto B. Surgical treatment of common arterial trunk with pseudotruncus arteriosus. Circulation 1974;50:II20.

11. Perloff JK, Ronan JA Jr, de Leon AC Jr. Ventricular septal defect with the "two chambered right ventricle." Am J Cardiol 1965;16:894.

12. Pate JW, Richardson RL Jr, Giles HH. Accessory tricuspid leaflet producing right ventricular outflow obstruction. N Engl J Med 1968;279:867.

13. Perasalo O, Halonen PI, Pyorala K, Telivuo L. Aneurysm of the membranous ventricular septum causing obstruction of the right ventricular outflow tract in a case of ventricular septal defect. Acta Chir Scand 1961;283:123.

14. Pacifico AD, Sand ME, Bargeron LM Jr, Colvin EC. Transatrial-transpulmonary repair of tetralogy of Fallot. J Thorac Cardiovasc Surg 1987;93:919.

15. Pacifico AD, Kirklin JK, Colvin EV, McConnell ME, Kirklin JW. Transatrial-transpulmonary repair of tetralogy of Fallot. Semin Thorac Cardiovasc Surg 1990;2:76.

16. Perry SB, Radtke W, Fellows KE, Keane JF, Lock JE. Coil embolization to occlude aortopulmonary collateral vessels and shunts in patients with congenital heart disease. J Am Coll Cardiol 1989;13:100.

17. Perrault H, Drblik SP, Montigny M, Davignon A, Lamarre A, Chartrand C, et al. Comparison of cardiovascular adjustments to exercise in adolescents 8 to 15 years of age after correction of tetralogy of Fallot, ventricular septal defect or atrial septal defect. Am J Cardiol 1989;64:213.

18. Puga FJ, Leoni FE, Julsrud PR, Mair DD. Complete repair of pulmonary atresia, ventricular septal defect, and severe peripheral arborization abnormalities of the central pulmonary arteries. J Thorac Cardiovasc Surg 1989;98:1018.

19. Pacifico AD, Ricchi A, Bargeron LM Jr, Colvin EC, Kirklin JW, Kirklin JK. Corrective repair of complete atrioventricular canal defects and major associated cardiac anomalies. Ann Thorac Surg 1988;46:645.

20. Penkoske PA, Duncan N, Collins-Nakai RL. Surgical repair of double-chambered right ventricular with or without ventriculotomy. J Thorac Cardiovasc Surg 1987;93:385.

21. Permut LC, Laks H, Aharon A. Surgical management of pulmonary atresia with ventricular septal defect and multiple aortopulmonary collaterals. Isr J Med Sci 1994;30:215.

Q

1. Quattlebaum TG, Varghese J, Neill CA, Donahoo JS. Sudden death among postoperative patients with tetralogy of Fallot. Circulation 1976;54:289.

2. Qureshi SA, Kirk CR, Lamb RK, Arnold R, Wilkinson JL. Balloon dilatation of the pulmonary valve in the first year of life in patients with tetralogy of Fallot: a preliminary study. Br Heart J 1988;60:232.

3. Qureshi SA, Parsons JM, Tynan M. Percutaneous transcatheter myectomy of subvalvar pulmonary stenosis in tetralogy of Fallot: a new palliative technique with an atherectomy catheter. Br Heart J 1990; 64:163.

R

1. Rastelli GC, Ongley PA, Davis GD, Kirklin JW. Surgical repair for pulmonary valve atresia with coronary-pulmonary artery fistula: report of case. Mayo Clin Proc 1965;40:521.

2. Rich AR. A hitherto unrecognized tendency to the development of widespread pulmonary vascular obstruction in patients with congenital pulmonary stenosis (tetralogy of Fallot). Bull Johns Hopkins Hosp 1948;82:389.

3. Rowe RD, VIad P, Keith JD. Experiences with 180 cases of tetralogy of Fallot in infants and children. Can Med Assoc J 1955;73:23.

4. Rees S, Somerville J. Aortography in Fallot's tetralogy and variants. Br Heart J 1969;31:146.

5. Richardson JP, Clarke CP. Tetralogy of Fallot. Risk factors associated with complete repair. Br Heart J 1976;38:926.

6. Redington AN, Somerville J. Stenting of aortopulmonary collaterals in complex pulmonary atresia. Circulation 1996;94:2479.

7. Ruttenberg HD, Carey LS, Adams P, Edwards JE. Absence of the pulmonary valve in tetralogy of Fallot. Am J Roentgenol Radium Ther Nucl Med 1964;91:500.

8. Rabinovitch M, Grady S, David I, Van Praagh R, Sauer U, Buhlmeyer K, et al. Compression of intrapulmonary bronchi by abnormally branching pulmonary arteries associated with absent pulmonary valves. Am J Cardiol 1982;50:804.

9. Reduto LA, Berger HJ, Johnstone DE, Hellenbrand W, Wackers FJ, Whittemore R, et al. Radionuclide assessment of right and left ventricular exercise reserve after total correction of tetralogy of Fallot. Am J Cardiol 1980;45:1013.

10. Rosing DR, Borer JS, Kent KM, et al. Long-term hemodynamic and electrocardiographic assessment following operative repair of tetralogy of Fallot. Circulation 1978;58:I209.

11. Rosenthal A, Gross RE, Pasternac A. Aneurysms of right ventricular outflow patches. J Thorac Cardiovasc Surg 1972;63:735.

12. Roberts WC, Friesinger GC, Cohen LS, Mason DT, Ross RS. Acquired pulmonic atresia. Total obstruction to right ventricular outflow after systemic to pulmonary arterial anastomoses for cyanotic congenital cardiac disease. Am J Cardiol 1969;24:335.

13. Rygg IH, Olesen K, Boesen I. The life history of tetralogy of Fallot. Dan Med Bull 1971;18:25.

14. Reitman MJ, Galioto FM Jr, el-Said GM, Cooley DA, Hallman GL, McNamara DG. Ascending aorta to right pulmonary artery anastomosis. Immediate results in 123 patients and one month to six year follow-up in 74 patients. Circulation 1974;49:952.

15. Regensburger D, Sievers HH, Lange PE, Heintzen PH, Bernhard A. Reconstruction of the right ventricular outflow tract in tetralogy of Fallot and pulmonary stenosis with a monocusp patch. Thorac Cardiovasc Surg 1981;29:345.

16. Rohmer J, Van Der Mark F, Zijlstra WG. Pulmonary valve incompetence. II. Application of electromagnetic flow velocity catheters in children. Cardiovasc Res 1976;10:46.

17. Rocchini AP, Rosenthal A, Freed M, Castaneda AR, Nadas AS. Chronic congestive heart failure after repair of tetralogy of Fallot. Circulation 1977;56:305.

18. Rabinovitch M, Herrera-deLeon V, Castaneda AR, Reid L. Growth and development of the pulmonary vascular bed in patients with tetralogy of Fallot with or without pulmonary atresia. Circulation 1981;64:1234.

19. Ross DN, Somerville J. Correction of pulmonary atresia with a homograft aortic valve. Lancet 1966;2:1446.

20. Rizzoli G, Blackstone EH, Kirklin JW, Pacifico AD, Bargeron LM Jr. Incremental risk factors in hospital mortality rate after repair of ventricular septal defect. J Thorac Cardiovasc Surg 1980;80:494.

21. Rowland TW, Rosenthal A, Castaneda AR. Double-chamber right ventricle: experience with 17 cases. Am Heart J 1975;89:455.

22. Riemenschneider TA, Goldberg SJ, Ruttenberg HD, Gyepes MT. Subpulmonic obstruction in complete (d) transposition produced by redundant tricuspid tissue. Circulation 1969;39:603.

23. Rosenthal A, Behrendt D, Sloan H, Ferguson P, Snedecor SM, Schork A. Long-term prognosis (15 to 26 years) after repair of tetralogy of Fallot. I. Survival and symptomatic status. Ann Thorac Surg 1984; 38:151.

24. Rittenhouse EA, Mansfield PB, Hall DG, Herndon SP, Jones TK, Kawabori I, et al. Tetralogy of Fallot: selective staged management. J Thorac Cardiovasc Surg 1985;89:772.

25. Rothman A, Perry SB, Keane JF, Lock JE. Early results and follow-up of balloon angioplasty for branch pulmonary artery stenoses. J Am Coll Cardiol 1990;15:1109.

26. Rocchini AP, Keane JF, Freed MD, Castaneda AR, Nadas AS. Left ventricular function following attempted surgical repair of tetralogy of Fallot. Circulation 1978;57:798.

27. Redington AN, Oldershaw PJ, Shinebourne EA, Rigby ML. A new technique for the assessment of pulmonary regurgitation and its application to the assessment of right ventricular function before and after repair of tetralogy of Fallot. Br Heart J 1988;60:57.

28. Ring JC, Bass JL, Marvin W, Fuhrman BP, Kulik TJ, Foker JE, et al. Management of congenital stenosis of a branch pulmonary artery with balloon dilation angioplasty. Report of 52 procedures. J Thorac Cardiovasc Surg 1985;90:35.

29. Rodefeld MD, Reddy VM, Thompson LD, Suleman S, Moore PC, Teitel DF, et al. Surgical creation of aortopulmonary window in selected patients with pulmonary atresia with poorly developed aortopulmonary collaterals and hypoplastic pulmonary arteries. J Thorac Cardiovasc Surg 2002;123:1147.

30. Restivo A, Cameron AH, Anderson RH, Allwork SP. Divided right ventricle: a review of its anatomical varieties. Pediatr Cardiol 1984;5:197.

31. Royer BF, Wilson JD. Incomplete heterotaxy with unusual heart malformations: case report. Arch Pediatr 1908;25:881.

32. Rowe SA, Zahka KG, Manolio TA, Horneffer PJ, Kidd L. Lung function and pulmonary regurgitation limit exercise capacity in postoperative tetralogy of Fallot. J Am Coll Cardiol 1991;17:461.

33. Reddy VM, Liddicoat JR, McElhinney DB, Brook MM, Stanger P, Hanley FL. Routine primary repair of tetralogy of Fallot in neonates and infants less than three months of age. Ann Thorac Surg 1995;60:S592.

34. Reddy VM, Liddicoat JR, Hanley FL. Midline one-stage complete unifocalization and repair of pulmonary atresia with ventricular septal defect and major aortopulmonary collaterals. J. Thorac Cardiovasc Surg 1995;109:832.

35. Reddy VM, McElhinney DB, Amin Z, Moore P, Parry AJ, Teitel DF, et al. Early and intermediate outcomes after repair of pulmonary atresia with ventricular septal defect and major aortopulmonary collateral arteries: experience with 85 patients. Circulation 2000; 101:1826.

36. Reddy VM, Petrossian E, McElhinney DB, Moore P, Teitel DF, Hanley FL. One-stage complete unifocalization in infants: when should the ventricular septal defect be closed? J Thorac Cardiovasc Surg 1997;113:858.

37. Rome JJ, Mayer JE, Castaneda AR, Lock JE. Tetralogy of Fallot with pulmonary atresia. Rehabilitation of diminutive pulmonary arteries. Circulation 1993;88:1691.

S

1. Starr A, Bonchek LI, Sunderland CO. Total correction of tetralogy of Fallot in infancy. J Thorac Cardiovasc Surg 1973;65:45.

2. Stephenson LW, Friedman S, Edmunds LH Jr. Staged surgical management of tetralogy of Fallot in infants. Circulation 1978;58:837.

3. Sanchez Cascos A. Genetics of Fallot's tetralogy. Br Heart J 1971;33: 899.

4. Stafford EG, Mair DD, McGoon DC, Danielson GK. Tetralogy of Fallot with absent pulmonary valve. Surgical considerations and results. Circulation 1973;48:III24.

5. Strieder DJ, Aziz K, Zaver AG, Fellows KE. Exercise tolerance after repair of tetralogy of Fallot. Ann Thorac Surg 1975;19:397.

6. Seybold-Epting W, Chiariello L, Hallman GL, Cooley DA. Aneurysm of pericardial right ventricular outflow tract patches. Ann Thorac Surg 1977;24:237.

7. Steeg CN, Krongrad E, Davachi F, Bowman FO Jr, Malm JR, Gersony WM. Postoperative left anterior hemiblock and right bundle branch block following repair of tetralogy of Fallot. Circulation 1975; 51:1026.

8. Sunderland CO, Rosenberg JA, Menashe VC, Lees MH, Bonchek LI, Starr A. Total correction of tetralogy of Fallot under two years of age. Postoperative hemodynamic evaluation (abstract). Circulation 1972; 45:98.

9. Soto B, Pacifico AD, Ceballos R, Bargeron LM Jr. Tetralogy of Fallot: an angiographic-pathologic correlative study. Circulation 1981; 64:558.

10. Singh SP, Rigby ML, Astley R. Demonstration of pulmonary arteries by contrast injection into pulmonary vein. Br Heart J 1978;40:55.

11. Sievers HH, Lange PE, Regensburger D, Yankah CA, Onnasch DG, Bursch J, et al. Short-term hemodynamic results after right ventricular outflow tract reconstruction using a cusp-bearing transanular patch. J Thorac Cardiovasc Surg 1983;86:777.

12. Swan H, Hederman WP, Vigoda PS, Blount SG Jr. The surgical treatment of isolated infundibular stenosis. J Thorac Cardiovasc Surg 1959;38:319.

13. Sellers RD. Lillehei CW, Edwards JE. Subaortic stenosis caused by anomalies of the atrioventricular valves. J Thorac Cardiovasc Surg 1964;48:289.

14. Shuford WH, Sybers RG. The aortic arch and its malformations with emphasis on the angiographic features. Springfield, Ill.: Charles C Thomas, 1974.

15. Sellors H. Surgery of pulmonary stenosis. A case in which the pulmonary valve was successfully divided. Lancet 1948;1:988.

16. Shimazaki Y, Blackstone EH, Kirklin JW, Jonas RA, Mandell V, Colvin EV. The dimensions of the right ventricular outflow tract and pulmonary arteries in tetralogy of Fallot and pulmonary stenosis. J Thorac Cardiovasc Surg 1992;103:692.

17. Shimazaki Y, Blackstone EH, Kirklin JW. The natural history of isolated congenital pulmonary valve incompetence: surgical implications. Thorac Cardiovasc Surg 1984;32:257.

18. Sawatari K, Kawata H, Armiger LC, Jonas RA. Growth of composite conduits utilizing longitudinal arterial autograft. J Thorac Cardiovasc Surg 1992;103:47.

19. Sreeram N, Saleem M, Jackson M, Peart I, McKay R, Arnold R, et al. Balloon pulmonary valvuloplasty for palliation of tetralogy of Fallot (abstract). J Am Coll Cardiol 1991;17:18A.

20. Shimazaki Y, Maehara T, Blackstone EH, Kirklin JW, Bargeron LM Jr. The structure of the pulmonary circulation in tetralogy of Fallot with pulmonary atresia. J Thorac Cardiovasc Surg 1988;95:1048.

21. Shimazaki Y, Tokuan Y, Lio M, Nakano S, Matsuda H, Blackstone EH, et al. Pulmonary artery pressure and resistance late after repair of tetralogy of Fallot with pulmonary atresia. J Thorac Cardiovasc Surg 1990;100:425.

22. Schaff HV, DiDonato RM, Danielson GK, Puga FJ, Ritter DG, Edwards WD, et al. Reoperation for obstructed pulmonary ventricle-pulmonary artery conduits. J Thorac Cardiovasc Surg 1984;88:334.

23. Szarnicki R, Krebber HJ, Wack J. Wire coil embolization of systemic-pulmonary artery collaterals following surgical correction of pulmonary atresia. J Thorac Cardiovasc Surg 1981;81:124.

24. Stellin G, Jonas RA, Goh TH, Brawn WJ, Venables AW, Mee RB. Surgical treatment of absent pulmonary valve syndrome in infants: relief of bronchial obstruction. Ann Thorac Surg 1983;36:468.

25. Sullivan ID, Wren C, Stark J, de Leval MR, Macartney FJ, Deanfield JE. Surgical unifocalization in pulmonary atresia and ventricular septal defect. A realistic goal? Circulation 1988;78:III5.

26. Sullivan ID, Presbitero P, Gooch VM, Aruta E, Deanfield JE. Is ventricular arrhythmia in repaired tetralogy of Fallot an effect of operation or a consequence of the course of the disease? A prospective study. Br Heart J 1987;58:40.

27. Sawatari K, Imai Y, Kurosawa H, Isomatsu Y, Momma K. Staged operation for pulmonary atresia and ventricular septal defect with major aortopulmonary collateral arteries. New technique for complete unifocalization. J Thorac Cardiovasc Surg 1989;98:738.

28. Snir E, de Leval MR, Elliott MJ, Stark J. Current surgical technique to repair Fallot's tetralogy with absent pulmonary valve syndrome. Ann Thorac Surg 1991;51:979.

29. Suzuki A, Ho SY, Anderson RH, Deanfield JE. Further morphologic studies on tetralogy of Fallot with particular emphasis on the prevalence and structure of the membranous flap. J Thorac Cardiovasc Surg 1990;99:528.

30. Stellin G, Milanesi O, Rubino M, Michielon G, Bianco R, Moreolo GS, et al. Repair of tetralogy of Fallot in the first six months of life; transatrial versus transventricular approach. Ann Thorac Surg 1995; 60:S588.

31. Sousa-Uva M, Lacour-Gayet F, Komiya T, Serraf A, Bruniaux J, Touchot A, et al. Surgery for tetralogy of Fallot at less than six months of age. J Thorac Cardiovasc Surg 1994;107:1291.

32. Starnes VA, Luciani GB, Latter DA, Griffin ML. Current surgical management of tetralogy of Fallot. Ann Thorac Surg 1994;58:211.

33. Smyllie JH, Sutherland GR, Keeton BR. The value of Doppler color flow mapping in determining pulmonary blood supply in infants with pulmonary atresia with ventricular septal defect. J Am Coll Cardiol 1989;14:1759.

34. Schulze-Neick I, Ho SY, Bush A, Rosenthal M, Franklin RC, Redington AN, Penny DJ. Severe airflow limitation after the unifocalization procedure: clinical and morphological correlates. Circulation 2000; 102:III142.

35. Sabri MR, Sholler G, Hawker R, Nunn G. Branch pulmonary artery growth after Blalock-Taussig shunts in tetralogy of Fallot and pulmonary atresia with ventricular septal defect: a retrospective, echocardiographic study. Pediatr Cardiol 1999;20:358.

T

1. Theye RA, Kirklin JW. Physiologic studies early after repair of tetralogy of Fallot. Circulation 1963;28:42.

2. Tay DJ, Engle MA, Ehlers KH, Levin AR. Early results and late developments of the Waterston anastomosis, Circulation 1974;50:220.

3. Tyson KR, Larrieu AJ, Kirchmer JT Jr. The Blalock-Taussig shunt in the first two years of life: a safe and effective procedure. Ann Thorac Surg 1978;26:38.

4. Thiene G, Frescura C, Bini RM, Valente M, Gallucci V. Histology of pulmonary arterial supply in pulmonary atresia with ventricular septal defect. Circulation 1979;60:1066.

5. Takamiya M, Tauge I, Tadokoro M. Retrograde pulmonary arteriography: a new approach to opacification of pulmonary artery in pulmonary atresia, in Proceedings of the Thirteenth International Congress of Radiology, Madrid (abstract). International Congress Series No. 301. Amsterdam: Excerpta Medica, 1973, p. 233.

6. Tsifutis AA, Hartmann AF Jr, Arvidsson H. Two-chambered right ventricle: report on seven patients. Circulation 1961;24:1058.

7. Terry PB, White RI Jr, Barth KH, Kaufman SL, Mitchell SE. Pulmonary arteriovenous malformations: physiologic observations and results of therapeutic balloon embolization. N Engl J Med 1983;308:1197.

8. Touati GD, Vouhe PR, Amodeo A, Pouard P, Mauriat P, Leca F, et al. Primary repair of tetralogy of Fallot in infancy. J Thorac Cardiovasc Surg 1990;99:396.

9. Tchervenkov CI, Salasidis G, Cecere R, Beland MJ, Jutras L, Paquet M, et al. One-stage midline unifocalization and complete repair in infancy versus multiple-stage unifocalization followed by repair for complex heart disease with major aortopulmonary collaterals. J Thorac Cardiovasc Surg 1997;114:727.

U

1. Ullom RL, Sade RM, Crawford FA Jr, Ross BA, Spinale F. The Blalock-Taussig shunt in infants: standard versus modified. Ann Thorac Surg 1987;44:539.

V

1. Van Praagh R, McNamara JJ. Anatomic types of ventricular septal defect with aortic insufficiency: diagnostic and surgical considerations. Am Heart J 1968;75:604.

2. Van Praagh R, Van Praagh S, Nebesar RA, Muster AJ, Sinha SN, Paul MH. Tetralogy of Fallot: underdevelopment of the pulmonary infundibulum and its sequelae. Am J Cardiol 1970;26:25.

3. Von Bernuth G, Ritter DG, Frye RL, Weidman WH, Davis GD, McGoon DC. Evaluation of patients with tetralogy of Fallot and Potts anastomosis. Am J Cardiol 1971;27:259.

4. Villani M, Gamba A, Tiraboschi R, Crupi G, Parenzan L. Surgical treatment of tetralogy of Fallot. Recent experience using a prospective protocol. Thorac Cardiovasc Surg 1983;31:151.

5. Van Praagh R, Corwin RD, Dahlquist EH Jr, Freedom RM, Mattioli L, Nebesar RA. Tetralogy of Fallot with severe left ventricular anomalous attachment of the mitral valve to the ventricular septum. Am J Cardiol 1970;26:93.

6. Vargas FJ, Kreutzer GO, Pedrini M, Capelli H, Coronel AR. Tetralogy of Fallot with subarterial ventricular septal defect. Diagnostic and surgical considerations. J Thorac Cardiovasc Surg 1986;92:908.

7. Vetter HO, Reichart B, Seidel P, Kleinhans E, Bull U, Klinner W. Non-invasive assessment of right and left ventricular volumes 11 to 24 years after corrective surgery on patients with tetralogy of Fallot. Eur J Cardiothorac Surg 1990;4:24.

8. Vobecky SJ, Williams WG, Trusler GA, Coles JG, Rebeyka IM, Smallhorn J, et al. Survival analysis of infants under age 18 months presenting with tetralogy of Fallot. Ann Thorac Surg 1993;56:944.

9. Vranicar M, Teitel DF, Moore P. Use of small stents for rehabilitation of hypoplastic pulmonary arteries in pulmonary atresia with ventricular septal defect. Catheter Cardiovasc Interv 2002;55:78.

W

1. Waterston DJ. Treatment of Fallot's tetralogy in children under one year of age. Rozhl Chir 1962;41:181.

2. Wessel HU, Cunningham WJ, Paul MH, Bastanier CK, Muster AJ, Idriss FS. Exercise performance in tetralogy of Fallot after intracardiac repair. J Thorac Cardiovasc Surg 1980;80:582.

3. Weldon CS, Rowe RD, Gott VL. Clinical experience with the use of aortic valve homografts for reconstruction of the pulmonary artery, pulmonary valve, and outflow portion of the right ventricle. Circulation 1968;37:II51.

4. Warden HE, DeWall RA, Cohen M, Varco RL, Lillehei CW. A surgical-pathologic classification for isolated ventricular septal defects and for those in Fallot's tetralogy based on observations made on 120 patients during repair under direct vision. J Thorac Surg 1957;33:21.

5. Wessel HU, Bastanier CK, Paul MH, Berry TE, Cole RB, Muster AJ. Prognostic significance of arrhythmia in tetralogy of Fallot after intracardiac repair. Am J Cardiol 1980;46:843.

6. Wolff GS, Rowland TW, Ellison RC. Surgically induced right bundle branch block with left anterior hemiblock. Circulation 1972;46:587.

7. Wessel HU, Weiner MD, Paul MH, Bastanier CK. Lung function in tetralogy of Fallot after intracardiac repair. J Thorac Cardiovasc Surg 1981;82:616.

8. Williams GR, Richardson WR, Cayler GC, Campbell GC. Infundibular pulmonic stenosis with intact ventricular septum. Am Surg 1961;27:307.

9. Walsh EP, Rockenmacher S, Keane JF, Hougen TJ, Lock JE, Castaneda AR. Late results in patients with tetralogy of Fallot repaired during infancy. Circulation 1988;77:1062.

10. Walsh EP, Saul JP, Sholler GF, Triedman JK, Jonas RA, Mayer JE, et al. Evaluation of a staged treatment protocol for rapid automatic junctional tachycardia after operation for congenital heart disease. J Am Coll Cardiol 1997;29:1046.

11. Watterson KG, Malm TK, Karl TR, Mee RB. Absent pulmonary valve syndrome: operation in infants with airway obstruction. Ann Thorac Surg 1992;54:1116.

12. Wu QY, Yang XB. Anomalous origin of the pulmonary artery from the right coronary artery. Ann Thorac Surg 2001;72:1396.

13. Watterson KG, Wilkinson JL, Karl TR, Mee RB. Very small pulmonary arteries: central end-to-side shunt. Ann Thorac Surg 1991; 52:1132.

Y

1. Yamamoto N, Reul GJ, Kidd JN, Cooley DA, Hallman GL. A new approach to repair of pulmonary branch stenosis following ascending aorta-right pulmonary artery anastomosis. Ann Thorac Surg 1976; 21:237.

2. Yamamoto S, Nozawa T, Aizawa T, Honda M, Mohri M. Transcatheter embolization of bronchial collateral arteries prior to intracardiac operation for tetralogy of Fallot. J Thorac Cardiovasc Surg 1979; 78:739.

3. Yemets IM, Williams WG, Webb GD, Harrison DA, McLaughin PR, Trusler GA, et al. Pulmonary valve replacement late after repair of tetralogy of Fallot. Ann Thorac Surg 1997;64:526.

4. Yoshigi M, Momma K, Imai Y. Coronary artery–pulmonary artery fistula in pulmonary atresia with ventricular septal defect. Heart Vessels 1995;10:163.

5. Yagihara T, Yamamoto F, Nishigaki K, Matsuki O, Uemura H, Isizaka T, et al. Unifocalization for pulmonary atresia with ventricular septal defect and major aortopulmonary collateral arteries. J Thorac Cardiovasc Surg 1996;112:392.

Z

1. Zavanella C, Matsuda H, Subramanian S. Successful correction of a complete form of atrioventricular canal associated with tetralogy of Fallot. Case report. J Thorac Cardiovasc Surg 1977;74:195.

2. Zerbini EJ. The surgical treatment of the complex of Fallot: late results. J Thorac Cardiovasc Surg 1969;58:158.

3. Zach M, Beitzke A, Singer H, Hofler H, Schellmann B. The syndrome of absent pulmonary valve and ventricular septal defects—Anatomical features and embryological implications. Basic Res Cardiol 1979; 74:54.

4. Zuberbuhler JR, Dankner E, Zoltun R, Burkholder J, Bahnson HT. Tissue adhesive closure of aortic-pulmonary communications. Am Heart J !974;88:41.

5. Zahka KG, Manolio TA, Rykiel MJ, Abel DL, Neill CA, Kidd L. Handgrip strength after the Blalock-Taussig shunt: 14 to 34 year follow-up. Clin Cardiol 1988;11:627.

6. Zahka KG, Horneffer PJ, Rowe SA, Neill CA, Manolio TA, Kidd L, et al. Long-term valvular function after total repair of tetralogy of Fallot. Relation to ventricular arrhythmias. Circulation 1988; 78:III14.

7. Zahn EM, Lima VC, Benson LN, Freedom RM. Use of endovascular stents to increase pulmonary blood flow in pulmonary atresia with ventricular septal defect. Am J Cardiol 1992;70:411.

Index